KAROLYI

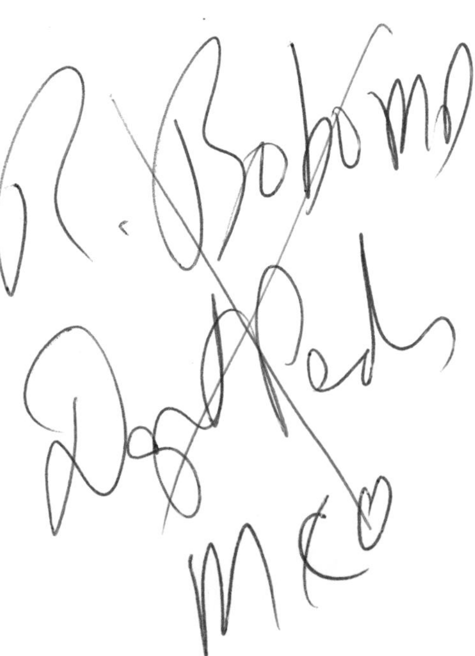

Pediatric Gastrointestinal Disease

Pathophysiology • Diagnosis • Management

W. Allan Walker, M.D.

Professor of Pediatrics, Harvard Medical School; Chief, Combined Program in Pediatric Gastroenterology and Nutrition, Children's Hospital and Massachusetts General Hospital, Boston, Massachusetts

Peter R. Durie, B.Sc., M.D., FRCPC

Associate Professor, University of Toronto Faculty of Medicine; Senior Scientist, Research Institute, and Staff Physician, Division of Gastroenterology, Department of Paediatrics, The Hospital for Sick Children, Toronto, Ontario, Canada

J. Richard Hamilton, M.D., FRCPC

Professor and Chairman, Department of Pediatrics, Faculty of Medicine, McGill University; Physician-in-Chief, Montreal Children's Hospital, Montreal, Quebec, Canada

John A. Walker-Smith, M.D. (Syd.), F.R.C.P. (Lon., Edin.), F.R.A.C.P.

Professor of Paediatric Gastroenterology, The Medical College of St. Bartholomew's Hospital; Consultant Paediatrician, Queen Elizabeth Hospital for Children, London, England

John B. Watkins, M.D.

Professor of Pediatrics, University of Pennsylvania School of Medicine; Director, Division of Gastroenterology and Nutrition, The Children's Hospital of Philadelphia, Philadelphia, Pennsylvania

VOLUME TWO

Pediatric Gastrointestinal Disease

Pathophysiology • Diagnosis • Management

B.C. Decker Inc.
Philadelphia • Toronto

Publisher

B.C. Decker Inc
3228 South Service Road
Burlington, Ontario L7N 3H8

B.C. Decker Inc
320 Walnut Street
Suite 400
Philadelphia, Pennsylvania 19106

Sales and Distribution

United States and Puerto Rico
Mosby-Year Book Inc.
11830 Westline Industrial Drive
Saint Louis, Missouri 63146

Canada
Mosby-Year Book Limited
5240 Finch Avenue E., Unit 1
Scarborough, Ontario M1S 5A2

Australia
McGraw-Hill Book Company Australia Pty. Ltd.
4 Barcoo Street
Roseville East 2069
New South Wales, Australia

Brazil
Editora McGraw-Hill do Brasil, Ltda.
rua Tabapua, 1.105, Itaim-Bibi
Sao Paulo, S.P. Brasil

Colombia
Interamericana/McGraw-Hill de Colombia, S.A.
Carrera 17, No. 33-71
(Apartado Postal, A.A., 6131)
Bogota, D.E. Colombia

Europe
McGraw-Hill Book Company GmbH
Lademannbogen 136
D-2000 Hamburg 63
West Germany

France
MEDSI/McGraw-Hill
6, avenue Daniel Lesueur
75007 Paris, France

Hong Kong and China
McGraw-Hill Book Company
Suite 618, Ocean Centre
5 Canton Road
Tsimshatsui, Kowloon
Hong Kong

India
Tata McGraw-Hill Publishing Company, Ltd.
12/4 Asaf Ali Road, 3rd Floor
New Delhi 110002, India

Indonesia
Mr. Wong Fin Fah
P.O. Box 122/JAT
Jakarta, 1300 Indonesia

Italy
McGraw-Hill Libri Italia, s.r.l.
Piazza Emilia, 5
I-20129 Milano MI
Italy

Japan
Igaku-Shoin Ltd.
Tokyo International P.O. Box 5063
1-28-36 Hongo, Bunkyo-ku,
Tokyo 113, Japan

Korea
Mr. Don-Gap Choi
C.P.O. Box 10583
Seoul, Korea

Malaysia
Mr. Lim Tao Slong
No. 8 Jalan SS 7/6B
Kelana Jaya
47301 Petaling Jaya
Selangor, Malaysia

Mexico
Interamericana/McGraw-Hill de Mexico, S.A. de C.V.
Cedro 512, Colonia Atlampa
(Apartado Postal 26370)
06450 Mexico, D.F., Mexico

New Zealand
McGraw-Hill Book Co. New Zealand Ltd.
5 Joval Place, Wiri
Manukau City, New Zealand

Portugal
Editora McGraw-Hill de Portugal, Ltda.
Rua Rosa Damasceno 11A–B
1900 Lisboa, Portugal

South Africa
Libriger Book Distributors
Warehouse Number 8
"Die Ou Looiery"
Tannery Road
Hamilton, Bloemfontein 9300

Singapore and Southeast Asia
McGraw-Hill Book Co.
21 Neythal Road
Jurong, Singapore 2262

Spain
McGraw-Hill/Interamericana de Espana, S.A.
Manuel Ferrero, 13
28020 Madrid, Spain

Taiwan
Mr. George Lim
P.O. Box 87–601
Taipei, Taiwan

Thailand
Mr. Vitit Lim
632/5 Phaholyothin Road
Sapan Kwai
Bangkok 10400
Thailand

United Kingdom, Middle East and Africa
McGraw-Hill Book Company (U.K.) Ltd.
Shoppenhangers Road
Maidenhead, Berkshire
SL6 2QL England

Venezuela
Editorial Interamericana de Venezuela C.A.
2da. calle Bello Monte
Local G-2
Caracas, Venezuela

NOTICE

The authors and publisher have made every effort to ensure that the patient care recommended herein, including choice of drugs and drug dosages, is in accord with the accepted standards and practice at the time of publication. However, since research and regulation constantly change clinical standards, the reader is urged to check the product information sheet included in the package of each drug, which includes recommended doses, warnings, and contraindications. This is particularly important with new or infrequently used drugs.

Pediatric Gastrointestinal Disease

ISBN 1–55664–261–X (set)
1–55664–122–2 (Volume 1)
1–55664–209–1 (Volume 2)

Library of Congress catalog card number: 89–50930

10 9 8 7 6 5 4 3 2 1

Contributors

MARVIN E. AMENT, M.D.
Professor of Pediatrics, and Chief, Division of Pediatric Gastroenterology and Nutrition, University of California, Los Angeles, School of Medicine, Los Angeles, California
Endoscopy: Fiberoptic Upper Intestinal Endoscopy
Nutritional Therapy: Home Total Parenteral Nutrition

JOEL M. ANDRES, M.D.
Associate Professor, University of Florida College of Medicine, Gainesville, Florida
The Liver and Biliary Tree: Congenital Infections of the Liver

MAGDALENA ARAYA, M.D.
Professor of Pediatrics, and Member, Gastroenterology Unit, Institute of Nutrition and Food Technology, University of Chile, Santiago, Chile
The Intestines: The Gut in Malnutrition

SALVATORE AURICCHIO, M.D.
Professor, Department of Pediatrics, II Faculty of Medicine, University of Naples, Naples, Italy
The Intestines: Genetically Determined Disaccharidase Deficiencies

ALBERT AYNSLEY-GREEN, M.A., D. Phil., M.B., B.S., F.R.C.P. (Lon., Edin.)
James Spence Professor of Child Health, University of Newcastle-Upon-Tyne Medical School; Senior Consultant Paediatrician, Royal Victoria Infirmary, Newcastle-Upon-Tyne, England
Endocrine Function of the Gut in Early Life

PAUL BABYN, M.D.C.M.
Assistant Professor, University of Toronto Faculty of Medicine; Staff Radiologist, The Hospital for Sick Children, Toronto, Ontario, Canada
Imaging: Radiography: Plain Film; Sonography; Computed Tomography

WILLIAM F. BALISTRERI, M.D.
Dorothy M.M. Kersten Professor of Pediatrics, and Director, Division of Pediatric Gastroenterology and Nutrition, University of Cincinnati College of Medicine; Attending Physician, Children's Hospital Medical Center, Cincinnati, Ohio
The Liver and Biliary Tree: Prolonged Neonatal Obstructive Jaundice

GRAEME L. BARNES, M.D., Ch.B., F.R.A.C.P.
Director of Gastroenterology, Royal Children's Hospital, Melbourne, Australia
The Intestines: Intestinal Viral Infections

LEWIS A. BARNESS, M.D.
Professor of Pediatrics, University of South Florida College of Medicine, Tampa, Florida; Visiting Professor of Pediatrics, University of Wisconsin School of Medicine, Madison, Wisconsin
Nutritional Therapy: Special Dietary Therapy for Specific Disease States

RONALD G. BARR, M.A., M.D.C.M., FRCPC
Associate Professor of Pediatrics, McGill University Faculty of Medicine; Director, Child Development Programme, Montreal Children's Hospital, Montreal, Quebec, Canada
Colic and Gas

GERARD T. BERRY, M.D.
Associate Professor of Pediatrics, University of Pennsylvania School of Medicine; Senior Physician, The Children's Hospital of Philadelphia, Philadelphia, Pennsylvania
The Liver and Biliary Tree: Disorders of Amino Acid Metabolism

RAVI BERRY, M.D.
Former Fellow in Pediatric Gastroenterology, Mayo Graduate School of Medicine, Rochester, Minnesota; Pediatric Gastroenterologist, Riverside Medical Clinic, Riverside, California
Gastrointestinal Bleeding

JULIE E. BINES, M.B.B.S.
Fellow, Harvard Medical School; Fellow, Combined Program in Pediatric Gastroenterology and Nutrition, The Children's Hospital and Massachusetts General Hospital, Boston, Massachusetts
Endoscopy: Lower Endoscopy

ROBERT E. BLACK, M.D., M.P.H.
Professor and Chair, Department of International Health, The Johns Hopkins University School of Medicine, Baltimore, Maryland
The Intestines: Idiopathic Prolonged Diarrhea

EDGAR C. BOEDEKER, M.D.
Associate Professor, Department of Medicine, Uniformed Services University of the Health Sciences, Bethesda, Maryland; Chief, Department of Gastroenterology, Walter Reed Army Institute of Research, Washington, D.C.
Flora of the Gut and Protective Function

JOHN T. BOYLE, M.D.
Associate Professor of Pediatrics, Case Western Reserve University School of Medicine; Chief, Division of Gastroenterology and Nutrition, Rainbow Babies and Children's Hospital, Cleveland, Ohio
Chronic Abdominal Pain

KENNETH H. BROWN, M.D.
Professor, Department of Nutrition, and Director, Program in International Nutrition, University of California, Davis, School of Medicine, Davis, California
The Intestines: Idiopathic Prolonged Diarrhea

OSCAR BRUNSER, M.D.
Professor of Pediatrics, and Chief, Gastroenterology Unit, Institute of Nutrition and Food Technology, University of Chile, Santiago, Chile
The Intestines: The Gut in Malnutrition

PATRICIA E. BURROWS, M.D., FRCPC
Assistant Professor, University of Toronto Faculty of Medicine; Staff Radiologist, The Hospital for Sick Children, Toronto, Ontario, Canada
Imaging: Angiography

GEOFFREY J. CLEGHORN, M.B.B.S., F.R.A.C.P.
Senior Lecturer, Department of Child Health, University of Queensland; Director of Paediatric Gastroenterology, Mater Misericordiae Children's Hospital; Visiting Gastroenterologist, Royal Children's Hospital, Brisbane, Australia
Drug Therapy: Pharmacologic Treatment of Exocrine Pancreatic Insufficiency

PAUL M. COATES, Ph.D.
Research Professor of Pediatrics, University of Pennsylvania School of Medicine; Director, Fellowship Research, and Director, Center for Mitochondrial Biology, Division of Gastroenterology and Nutrition, The Children's Hospital of Philadelphia, Philadelphia, Pennsylvania
The Liver and Biliary Tree: Lysosomal Acid Lipase Deficiency: Cholesteryl Ester Storage Disease and Wolman's Disease; Inherited Abnormalities in Mitochondrial Fatty Acid Oxidation

MERVYN D. COHEN, M.B., Ch.B., M.D., F.R.C.R., M.R.C.P.
Professor of Radiology, Indiana University School of Medicine; Chief of Pediatric Radiology, James Whitcomb Riley Hospital for Children, Indianapolis, Indiana
Imaging: Magnetic Resonance Imaging of the Gastrointestinal Tract

JEAN A. CORTNER, M.D.
Professor of Pediatrics, University of Pennsylvania School of Medicine; Director, Lipid-Heart Research, and Director, Nutrition Center, Division of Gastroenterology and Nutrition, The Children's Hospital of Philadelphia, Philadelphia, Pennsylvania
The Liver and Biliary Tree: Lysosomal Acid Lipase Deficiency: Cholesteryl Ester Storage Disease and Wolman's Disease

RICHARD COUPER, M.B., Ch.B., F.R.A.C.P.
Research Fellow in Gastroenterology, The Hospital for Sick Children, Toronto, Ontario, Canada
Pancreatic Function Tests

GEOFFREY P. DAVIDSON, M.D., F.R.C.P.
Clinical Senior Lecturer, Department of Paediatrics, University of Adelaide; Director, Gastroenterology Unit, Adelaide Children's Hospital, North Adelaide, South Australia, Australia
The Intestines: Idiopathic Villus Atrophy

MURRAY DAVIDSON, M.D.
Professor of Pediatrics, State University of New York at Stony Brook School of Medicine, Stony Brook, New York
The Intestines: Idiopathic Constipation

JEHAN-FRANÇOIS DESJEUX, M.D.
Director, Nutrition Research Center, Institut National de la Santé et de la Recherchie Medicali (INSERM U290); Consultant in Pediatric Gastroenterology, Hôpital Saint-Lazare, Paris, France
Transport of Water and Ions
The Intestines: Congenital Transport Defects

VIVIAN L. DILLARD, R.N., M.S.N., C.P.N.P.
Nurse Practitioner, Division of Pediatric Gastroenterology and Nutrition, University of Virginia Children's Medical Center, Charlottesville, Virginia
Nutritional Therapy: Enteral Nutrition

JOHN A. DODGE, M.D., F.R.C.P. (Lon., Edin., Ire.), D.C.H.
Professor and Head, Department of Child Health, The Queen's University of Belfast; Consultant Paediatrician, Royal Belfast Hospital for Sick Children, Belfast, North Ireland, United Kingdom
Vomiting and Regurgitation
The Stomach and Duodenum: Trauma and Foreign Substances

BRENDAN DRUMM, M.B., Ch.B. FRCPC
Assistant Professor of Paediatrics, University of Toronto Faculty of Medicine; Staff Gastroenterologist, The Hospital for Sick Children, Limerick, Ireland
The Stomach and Duodenum:Gastritis in Childhood

PETER R. DURIE, B.Sc., M.D., FRCPC
Associate Professor, University of Toronto Faculty of Medicine; Senior Scientist, Research Institute, and Staff Physician, Division of Gastroenterology, Department of Paediatrics, The Hospital for Sick Children, Toronto, Ontario, Canada
The Pancreas: Cystic Fibrosis; Pancreatitis
Pancreatic Function Tests
Book Editor

EDMUND J. EASTHAM, M.B., B.S., F.R.C.P.
Honorary Lecturer, University of Newcastle-Upon-Tyne Medical School; Consultant Paediatric Gastroenterologist, Department of Child Health, Royal Victoria Infirmary, Newcastle-Upon-Tyne, England
The Stomach and Duodenum: Peptic Ulcer

SIGMUND H. EIN, M.D.C.M., FRCSC, F.A.C.S., F.A.A.P.
Assistant Professor, Department of Surgery, University of Toronto Faculty of Medicine; Staff Surgeon, Division of General Surgery, The Hospital for Sick Children; Consultant Staff, Division of Pediatric, Women's College Hospital; Associate Staff, Department of Surgery, Mount Sinai Hospital, Toronto, Ontario
Surgical Treatment: General Principles; Pediatric Ostomy

JULIO ESPINOZA, M.D.
Professor of Pediatrics, and Member, Gastroenterology Unit, Institute of Nutrition and Food Technology, University of Chile, Santiago, Chile
The Intestines: The Gut in Malnutrition

MICHAEL J.G. FARTHING, B.Sc., M.D., F.R.C.P.
Reader in Gastroenterology, The Medical College of St. Bartholomew's Hospital; Honorary Consultant Physician, St. Bartholomew's and St. Mark's Hospitals, London, England
The Intestines: Parasitic and Fungal Infections of the Digestive Tract

MILTON J. FINEGOLD, M.D.
Professor of Pathology and Pediatrics, Baylor College of Medicine; Head, Department of Pathology, Texas Children's Hospital, Houston, Texas
The Liver and Biliary Tree: Liver Tumors

JOSEPH F. FITZGERALD, M.D.
Professor of Pediatrics, Indiana University School of Medicine; Director, Gastrointestinal Disease Section, James Whitcomb Riley Hospital for Children, Indianapolis, Indiana
The Liver and Biliary Tree: Chronic Hepatitis

GORDON FORSTNER, M.D., FRCPC
Professor, Department of Paediatrics, University of Toronto Faculty of Medicine; Chief, Division of Gastroenterology, The Hospital for Sick Children, Toronto, Ontario, Canada
The Intestines: Bacterial Overgrowth
The Pancreas: Cystic Fibrosis

MELVIN H. FREEDMAN, M.D., FRCPC
Professor, Department of Paediatrics, University of Toronto Faculty of Medicine; Head of Clinical Hematology and Senior Staff Physician, The Hospital for Sick Children, Toronto, Ontario, Canada
Laboratory Studies: Hematologic Studies

PATRICIA FYVIE, R.N., E.T.
Enterostomal Therapist, The Hospital for Sick Children, Toronto, Ontario, Canada
Surgical Treatment: Ostomy Care

MARGARET A. GAINEY, M.D.
Associate Professor of Diagnostic Imaging, Temple University School of Medicine; Clinical Associate Professor of Radiology, Medical College of Pennsylvania and Hahnemann University; Chief, Section of Nuclear Medicine, St. Christopher's Hospital for Children, Philadelphia, Pennsylvania
Imaging: Radionuclide Diagnosis

KEVIN JOHN GASKIN, M.B., B.S., F.R.A.C.P., FRCPC
Clinical Lecturer, University of Sydney Medical School; Director, James Fairfax Institute of Paediatric Clinical Nutrition; Staff Gastroenterologist, The Children's Hospital, Sydney, Australia
The Pancreas: Hereditary Disorders of the Pancreas; Acquired Disorders of the Pancreas

FAYEZ K. GHISHAN, M.D.
Vice Chairman of Pediatrics/Research, Professor of Pediatrics and Molecular Physiology and Biophysics, and Director of Pediatric Gastroenterology, Vanderbilt University School of Medicine, Nashville, Tennessee
The Intestines: Secondary Enzyme Deficiencies

JULIUS G. GOEPP, M.D.
Research Associate, The Johns Hopkins University School of Hygiene and Public Health; Fellow in Pediatric Infectious Diseases, The Johns Hopkins University School of Medicine,

Fluid Therapy of Diarrhea: Industrialized Countries

JOHN S. GOFF, M.D.
Associate Professor, University of Colorado School of Medicine: Head of Clinical Gastroenterology, University Hospital and Veterans Administration Medical Center; Director of Endoscopy, University of Colorado Health Sciences Center, Denver, Colorado
The Esophagus: Infections

RICHARD J. GRAND, M.D.
Professor of Pediatrics, Tufts University School of Medicine; Chief, Division of Gastroenterology, The Floating Hospital for Infants and Children, New England Medical Center, Boston, Massachusetts
The Intestines: Crohn's Disease; Ulcerative Colitis
The Liver and Biliary Tree: Wilson's Disease

ANNE M. GRIFFITHS, M.D., FRCPC
Assistant Professor, Department of Paediatrics, University of Toronto Faculty of Medicine; Paediatric Gastroenterologist, The Hospital for Sick Children, Toronto, Ontario, Canada
Drug Therapy: Pharmacologic Treatment of Inflammatory Bowel Disease

JOYCE D. GRYBOSKI, M.D.
Professor of Pediatrics, Yale University School of Medicine, New Haven, Connecticut
The Esophagus: Traumatic Injury of the Esophagus

SANJEEV GUPTA, M.D., M.R.C.P.
Assistant Professor of Medicine, Albert Einstein College of Medicine; Physician, Weiler Hospital of Albert Einstein College of Medicine, Montefiore Medical Center and Bronx Municipal Hospital Center, Bronx, New York
The Liver and Biliary Tree: Molecular Biology of Hepatitis B Virus

COVA GURBINDO, M.D., Ph.D.
Postdoctoral Research Fellow, Department of Pediatrics, University of Montreal Faculty of Medicine; Postdoctoral Research Fellow, Division of Gastroenterology and Nutrition, Hôpital Ste. Justine, Montreal, Quebec, Canada
The Intestines: Gastrointestinal Manifestations of Immunodeficiency States

DANIEL E. HALE, M.D.
Assistant Professor of Pediatrics, University of Pennsylvania School of Medicine; Associate Physician, Division of Endocrinology/Diabetes, The Children's Hospital of Philadelphia, Philadelphia, Pennsylvania
The Liver and Biliary Tree: Inherited Abnormalities in Mitochondrial Fatty Acid Oxidation

J. RICHARD HAMILTON, M.D., FRCPC
Professor and Chairman, Department of Pediatrics, Faculty of Medicine, McGill University; Physician-in-Chief, Montreal Children's Hospital, Montreal, Quebec, Canada
Pediatric Gastroenterology: An Emerging Specialty
Book Editor

JAMES E. HEUBI, M.D.
Professor of Pediatrics, University of Cincinnati College of Medicine; Attending Gastroenterologist, and Acting Director, Clinical Research Center, Children's Hospital Medical Center, Cincinnati, Ohio
The Liver and Biliary Tree: Reye's Syndrome

A. CRAIG HILLEMEIER, M.D.
Associate Professor of Pediatrics, and Director, Division of Pediatric Gastroenterology, University of Michigan Medical School; Director of Pediatric Gastroenterology, C.S. Mott Children's Hospital, Ann Arbor, Michigan
The Esophagus: Reflux and Esophagitis

BARRY Z. HIRSCH, M.D.
Assistant Clinical Professor, Tufts University School of Medicine; Chief of Pediatric Nutrition, Baystate Medical Center, Springfield, Massachusetts
The Intestines: Radiation Enteritis

BERT HIRSCHHORN, M.D.
Lecturer, The Johns Hopkins University School of Hygiene and Public Health, Baltimore, Maryland; Honorary Senior Lecturer, Liverpool School of Tropical Medicine, Liverpool, England; Consultant Professor, Cairo University Faculty of Medicine, Cairo, Egypt
Fluid Therapy of Diarrhea: Industrialized Countries

PAUL E. HYMAN, M.D.
Associate Professor of Pediatrics, University of California, Los Angeles, School of Medicine; Chief, Pediatric Gastroenterology, Harbor-UCLA Medical Center, Los Angeles, California
Gastric Function Tests

ESTHER J. ISRAEL, M.D.
Instructor, Harvard Medical School; Associate Pediatrician, Massachusetts General Hospital, Boston, Massachusetts
The Intestines: Necrotizing Enterocolitis

W. DANIEL JACKSON, M.D.
Assistant Professor, Department of Pediatrics, University of Utah School of Medicine; Division of Gastroenterology, Primary Children's Medical Center, Salt Lake City, Utah
The Intestines: Crohn's Disease; Ulcerative Colitis

MOHAMED A. KARMALI, M.B., Ch.B., FRCPC
Associate Professor, University of Toronto Faculty of Medicine; Microbiologist-in-Chief, The Hospital for Sick Children, Toronto, Ontario, Canada
Laboratory Studies: Microbiologic Tests

DAVID J. KELJO, M.D., Ph.D.
Clinical Assistant Professor of Pediatrics, University of Texas Southwestern Medical School; Associate Attending, Baylor University Medical Center, Dallas, Texas
The Intestines: Secretory Tumors Affecting the Gut

RICHARD I. KELLEY, M.D., Ph.D.
Assistant Professor, Department of Pediatrics, The Johns Hopkins University School of Medicine; Staff Physician, Kennedy Institute, Baltimore, Maryland
The Liver and Biliary Tree: Disorders of Peroxisomal Metabolism

JOHN A. KERNER Jr., M.D.
Associate Professor of Pediatrics, Stanford University School of Medicine; Co-Director, Pediatric Gastroenterology and Nutrition, Stanford University Medical Center and The Children's Hospital at Stanford, Stanford, California
Nutritional Therapy: Parenteral Nutrition

BARBARA S. KIRSCHNER, M.D.
Professor of Pediatrics and Medicine, University of Chicago Pritzker School of Medicine; Associate Director, Pediatric Gastroenterology, Hepatology, and Nutrition, Wyler Children's Hospital, Chicago, Illinois
The Intestines: Miscellaneous Intestinal Inflammatory Disorders; Hirschsprung's Disease

RONALD E. KLEINMAN, M.D.
Associate Professor of Medicine, Harvard Medical School, Associate Chief, Combined Program in Pediatric Gastroenterology and Nutrition, Children's Hospital and Massachusetts General Hospital, Boston, Massachusetts
The Intestines: Radiation Enteritis
The Liver and Biliary Tree: Cholestasis Associated with Parenteral Nutrition; Liver Transplantation

RAYMOND S. KOFF, M.D.
Professor of Medicine and Assistant Dean, Boston University School of Medicine, Boston; Chairman, Department of Medicine, Framingham Union Hospital, Framingham, Massachusetts
The Liver and Biliary Tree: Viral Hepatitis

HINDA KOPELMAN, M.D., FRCPC
Assistant Professor, McGill University Faculty of Medicine; Pediatric Gastroenterologist, Montreal Children's Hospital, Montreal, Quebec, Canada
The Pancreas: Congenital Anomalies; Tumors of the Pancreas

J. THOMAS LAMONT, M.D.
Professor of Medicine, Boston University School of Medicine; Chief, Section of Gastroenterology, The University Hospital, Boston, Massachusetts
The Intestines: Pseudomembranous Colitis

JOHN S. LATIMER, M.D.
Associate Professor of Clinical Pediatrics, and Chief, Division of Pediatric Gastroenterology, Uniformed Services University of the Health Sciences, Bethesda, Maryland; Chief, Division of Pediatric Gastroenterology, Walter Reed Army Medical Center, Washington, D.C.
Flora of the Gut and Protective Function

ALAN M. LEICHTNER, M.D.
Assistant Professor of Pediatrics, Harvard Medical School; Clinical Chief of Gastroenterology, The Children's Hospital, Boston, Massachusetts
The Stomach and Duodenum: Esophageal and Gastric Neoplasms
The Intestines: Intestinal Neoplasms

STEVEN LICHTMAN, M.D.
Assistant Professor of Pediatric Gastroenterology, University of North Carolina at Chapel Hill School of Medicine; Attending Physician, University of North Carolina Hospital, Chapel Hill, North Carolina
The Intestines: Bacterial Overgrowth

PETER LIU, M.D.
Assistant Professor, University of Toronto Faculty of Medicine; Staff Radiologist, The Hospital for Sick Children, Toronto, Ontario, Canada
Imaging: Radiography: Contrast Studies; Interventional Radiology

THOMAS T. MACDONALD, B.Sc.(Hon.), Ph.D., M.R.C.Path.
Wellcome Senior Lecturer, Department of Paediatric Gastroenterology, St. Bartholomew's Hospital, London, England
The Intestines: Pathogenesis of Intestinal Inflammation

DILIP MAHALANABIS, M.B.B.S., F.R.C.P.
Head, Clinical Science Division, and Associate Director, International Centre for Diarrhoeal Disease Research, Bangladesh, Dhaka, Bangladesh
Fluid Therapy of Diarrhea: Developing Countries

RUSSELL J. MERRITT, M.D., Ph.D.
Clinical Associate Professor of Pediatrics, University of Southern California; Clinical Associate Gastroenterologist, Children's Hospital of Los Angeles, Los Angeles, California
Nutritional Therapy: Nutritional Requirements

PETER J. MILLA, M.Sc., M.B.B.S., F.R.C.P.
Senior Lecturer in Child Health, Department of Child Health, Institute of Child Health, University of London; Honorary Consultant Paediatric Gastroenterologist, The Hospital for Sick Children, London, England
Feeding, Tasting, and Sucking
The Stomach and Duodenum: Motor Disorders Including Pyloric Stenosis

MARY SUSAN MOYER, M.D.
Assistant Professor of Pediatrics, Yale University School of Medicine; Attending Physician, Yale-New Haven Hospital, New Haven, Connecticut
The Liver and Biliary Tree: Prolonged Neonatal Obstructive Jaundice

M. STEPHEN MURPHY, B.Sc., M.B., B.Ch., M.R.C.P.
Clinical and Research Fellow, Harvard Medical School; Clinical and Research Fellow, Combined Program in Gastroenterology and Nutrition, Children's Hospital and Massachusetts General Hospital, Boston, Massachusetts
Constipation

SAMUEL NURKO, M.D.
Instructor in Pediatrics, Harvard Medical School; Assistant in Medicine, Children's Hospital, Boston, Massachusetts; Head of Pediatric Gastroenterology, Hospital Infantil de Mexico, Mexico
Esophageal Motility
The Esophagus: Motor Disorders

CHRISTOPHER B. O'BRIEN, M.D.
Assistant Professor of Medicine, University of Pennsylvania School of Medicine; Director of Liver Section, Hospital of the University of Pennsylvania, Philadelphia, Pennsylvania
The Liver and Biliary Tree: Systemic Conditions Affecting the Liver

JAMES A. O'NEILL Jr., M.D.
Professor of Pediatric Surgery, University of Pennsylvania School of Medicine; Surgeon-in-Chief, The Children's Hospital of Philadelphia, Philadelphia, Pennsylvania
The Liver and Biliary Tree: Vascular Disorders Involving the Liver

ANTONIO R. PEREZ-ATAYDE, M.D.
Assistant Professor, Harvard Medical School; Pathologist, The Children's Hospital, Boston, Massachusetts
Liver Biopsy Interpretation

DAVID H. PERLMUTTER, M.D.
Associate Professor of Pediatrics, Cell Biology and Physiology, Washington University School of Medicine; Associate Pediatrician, Children's Hospital, St. Louis, Missouri
The Liver and Biliary Tree: Alpha$_1$-Antitrypsin Deficiency

JAY A. PERMAN, M.D.
Associate Professor of Pediatrics, The Johns Hopkins University School of Medicine; Director, Division of Pediatric Gastroenterology and Nutrition, The Johns Hopkins Hospital and University of Maryland Medical System, Baltimore, Maryland
The Intestines: Munchausen Syndrome by Proxy
Breath Analysis

JEAN PERRAULT, M.D.
Associate Professor of Pediatrics, Mayo Medical School; Consultant in Pediatric Gastroenterology, Mayo Clinic, Rochester, Minnesota
Gastrointestinal Bleeding

MARTIN PETRIC, Ph.D.
Assistant Professor, University of Toronto Faculty of Medicine; Virologist, The Hospital for Sick Children, Toronto, Ontario, Canada
Laboratory Studies: Microbiologic Tests

MICHAEL J. PETTEI, M.D., Ph.D.
Assistant Professor of Pediatrics, State University of New York at Stony Brook School of Medicine, Stony Brook; Co-Chief, Division of Gastroenterology and Nutrition, Schneider Children's Hospital, New Hyde Park, New York
The Intestines: Idiopathic Constipation

ALAN D. PHILLIPS, B.A. (Hon.)
Principal Electron Microscopist, Queen Elizabeth Hospital for Children, London, England
Intestinal Biopsy

DAVID A. PICCOLI, M.D.
Assistant Professor of Pediatrics, University of Pennsylvania School of Medicine; Associate Physician, The Children's Hospital of Philadelphia, Philadelphia, Pennsylvania
The Liver and Biliary Tree: Neonatal Iron Storage Disease; Disorders of the Intrahepatic Bile Ducts; Disorders of the Extrahepatic Bile Ducts

C.S. PITCHUMONI, M.D., M.P.H., FRCPC, F.A.C.P.
Professor of Medicine and Professor of Community and Preventive Medicine, New York Medical College, Valhalla; Program Director, Internal Medicine, and Chief, Division of Gastroenterology, Our Lady of Mercy Medical Center, Bronx, New York
The Pancreas: Juvenile Tropical Pancreatitis

RANDI G. PLESKOW, M.D.
Assistant Professor, Tufts University School of Medicine; Pediatric Gastroenterologist, The Floating Hospital for Infants and Children, New England Medical Center, Boston, Massachusetts
The Liver and Biliary Tree: Wilson's Disease

DON W. POWELL, M.D.
Professor and Associate Chairman, Department of Medicine, Chief, Division of Digestive Diseases and Nutrition, and Director, Center for Gastrointestinal Biology and Disease, University of North Carolina at Chapel Hill School of Medicine, Chapel Hill, North Carolina
Diarrhea

ROY PROUJANSKY, M.D.
Associate Professor, Department of Pediatrics, Jefferson Medical College, Philadelphia, Pennsylvania; Chief, Division of Gastroenterology and Nutrition, Alfred I. DuPont Institute, Wilmington, Delaware
The Intestines: Protein-Losing Enteropathy

JENNIFER M. PUCK, M.D.
Assistant Professor of Pediatrics, University of Pennsylvania School of Medicine; Staff Physician, Division of Infectious Diseases, The Children's Hospital of Philadelphia, Philadelphia, Pennsylvania
The Liver and Biliary Tree: Bacterial, Parasitic, and Other Infections of the Liver

JON MARC RHOADS, M.D.
Assistant Professor of Pediatrics, University of North Carolina at Chapel Hill School of Medicine, Chapel Hill, North Carolina
Diarrhea

SUSAN E. RICHARDSON, B.Sc., M.D., C.M.
Assistant Professor, University of Toronto Faculty of Medicine; Medical Microbiologist, The Hospital for Sick Children, Toronto, Ontario, Canada
Laboratory Studies: Microbiologic Tests

PAUL I. RICHMAN, M.B.B.S., Ph.D., M.R.C.Path.
Senior Lecturer and Consultant in Histopathology, The Medical College of St. Bartholomew's Hospital, London, England
Intestinal Biopsy

CAROLINE A. RIELY, M.D.
Professor of Medicine and Pediatrics, University of Tennessee, Memphis, School of Medicine; Attending Physician, The William F. Bowld Hospital, The Regional Medical Center at Memphis, Le Bonheur Children's Medical Center, Memphis, Tennessee
The Liver and Biliary Tree: Familial Intrahepatic Cholestasis: An Overview

EVE A. ROBERTS, M.D., FRCPC
Assistant Professor of Paediatrics and Medicine, University of Toronto Faculty of Medicine; Staff Physician, Division of Gastroenterology, Department of Paediatrics, The Hospital for Sick Children, Toronto, Ontario, Canada
The Liver and Biliary Tree: Drug-induced Hepatotoxicity in Children
Drug Therapy: Treatment of Acid-Peptic Disease; Drug Therapy for Liver Disease

ARTHUR J. ROSS, III, M.D.
Assistant Professor of Pediatric Surgery, University of Pennsylvania School of Medicine; Attending Surgeon, The Children's Hospital of Philadelphia, Philadelphia, Pennsylvania
Acute Abdominal Pain
Abdominal Masses

DAVID C. RULE, B.D.S., F.D.S., D.Orth., M.C.C.D.
Honorary Senior Lecturer, Institute of Dental Surgery, University of London; Consultant, Department of Children's Dentistry, Eastman Dental Hospital, London, England
The Mouth: Disorders of the Oral Cavity

WILLIAM E. RUSSELL, M.D.
Assistant Professor of Pediatrics, Harvard Medical School; Assistant Pediatrician, Massachusetts General Hospital, Boston, Massachusetts
Growth Failure and Malnutrition

PATRICK J. ST. LOUIS, Ph.D., Dip.C.C.
Lecturer, Department of Clinical Biochemistry, University of Toronto Faculty of Medicine; Clinical Chemist, Department of Biochemistry, The Hospital for Sick Children, Toronto, Ontario, Canada
Laboratory Studies: Biochemical Studies: Liver and Intestine

RICHARD H. SANDLER, M.D.
Instructor, Harvard Medical School; Research Fellow in Gastroenterology, and Assistant in Nutrition, The Children's Hospital, Boston, Massachusetts
The Liver and Biliary Tree: Cholestasis Associated with Parenteral Nutrition

JACQUES SCHMITZ, M.D.
Professor of Pediatrics, Necker-Enfants Malades School of Medicine; Department of Pediatrics, Enfants Malades Hospital, Paris, France
Malabsorption
Digestive and Absorptive Function

BRENT SCOTT, M.D.C.M., FRCPC
Associate Professor of Paediatrics, University of Calgary Faculty of Medicine; Program Director, Division of Gastroenterology and Nutrition, Alberta Children's Hospital, Calgary, Alberta, Canada
The Intestines: Drug-Induced Bowel Injury; Motility Disorders
Motility Studies

ERNEST G. SEIDMAN, M.D.
Assistant Professor, Departments of Pediatrics and Nutrition, University of Montreal Faculty of Medicine; Director, Intestinal Immunology Lab, and Attending Physician, Division of Gastroenterology and Nutrition, Hôpital Ste. Justine, Montreal, Quebec, Canada
The Intestines: Gastrointestinal Manifestations of Immunodeficiency States

KENNETH D.R. SETCHELL, Ph.D.
Associate Professor of Pediatrics, University of Cincinnati College of Medicine; Director, Clinical Mass Spectrometry Laboratory, Children's Hospital Medical Center, Cincinnati, Ohio
The Liver and Biliary Tree: Disorders of Bile Acid Synthesis

ELDON A. SHAFFER, M.D., FRCPC, F.A.C.P., F.A.C.G.
Professor of Medicine, Head, Division of Gastroenterology, and Associate Dean (Clinical Services), University of Calgary Faculty of Medicine; Head, Division of Gastroenterology, Foothills Hospital, Calgary, Alberta, Canada
Hepatobiliary System: Structure and Function
The Liver and Biliary Tree: Gallbladder Disease

DAVID A. SHAFRITZ, M.D.
Professor of Medicine and Cell Biology, and Director, Marion Bessin Liver Research Center, Albert Einstein College of Medicine; Attending Physician, Weiler Hospital of Albert Einstein College of Medicine and Bronx Municipal Hospital Center, Bronx, New York
The Liver and Biliary Tree: Molecular Biology of Hepatitis B Virus

BARRY SHANDLING, M.B., Ch.B., F.R.C.S.(Eng.), FRCSC, F.A.C.S.
Associate Professor, Department of Surgery, University of Toronto Faculty of Medicine; Senior Staff Surgeon, The Hospital for Sick Children; Director, Bowel Clinic, The Hugh MacMillan Medical Centre; Consultant Surgeon, Sunnybrook Hospital and North York General Hospital, Toronto, Ontario, Canada
The Intestines: Peritonitis; Perianal Lesions; Appendicitis; Diverticular Disease

THOMAS A. SHAW-STIFFEL, M.D., C.M., FRCPC, F.A.C.G.
Assistant Professor of Gastroenterology and Clinical Pharmacology, University of Toronto Faculty of Medicine; Staff Physician, Sunnybrook Health Science Centre, Toronto, Ontario, Canada
Drug Therapy: Treatment of Acid-Peptic Disease

ROSS W. SHEPHERD, M.D., M.R.C.P., F.R.A.C.P.
Associate Professor of Child Health, University of Queensland; Director of Gastroenterology, Royal Children's Hospital, Brisbane, Australia
The Intestines: The Gut in Systemic Endocrinopathies

PHILIP SHERMAN, M.D., FRCPC
Associate Professor of Paediatrics and Microbiology, University of Toronto Faculty of Medicine; Staff Gastroenterologist, The Hospital for Sick Children, Toronto, Ontario, Canada
The Stomach and Duodenum: Gastritis in Childhood
The Intestines: Bacterial Overgrowth

ANA ABAD SINDEN, M.S., R.D.
Pediatric Nutrition Specialist, Department of Nutrition Services, University of Virginia Medical Center, Charlottesville, Virginia
Nutritional Therapy: Enteral Nutrition

JOHN D. SNYDER, M.D.
Assistant Professor of Pediatrics, Harvard Medical School; Associate in Gastroenterology, Children's Hospital, Boston, Massachusetts
The Intestines: Bacterial Infections

JUDITH M. SONDHEIMER, M.D.
Associate Professor of Pediatrics, and Chief of Pediatric Gastroenterology and Nutrition, University of Colorado School of Medicine; Chief of Gastroenterology, The Children's Hospital, Denver, Colorado
Esophageal pH Monitoring

STEPHEN P. SPIELBERG, M.D., Ph.D.
Professor of Paediatrics and Pharmacology, University of Toronto Faculty of Medicine; Director, Division of Clinical Pharmacology and Toxicology, The Hospital for Sick Children, Toronto, Ontario, Canada
The Liver and Biliary Tree: Drug-induced Hepatotoxicity in Children
Drug Therapy: Principles of Pediatric Therapeutics

MICHAEL SPINO, B.Sc.Phm., Pharm.D.
Associate Professor, University of Toronto Faculties of Pharmacy and Medicine; Senior Scientist, Division of Clinical Pharmacology and Toxicology, The Hospital for Sick Children, Toronto, Ontario, Canada
Drug Therapy: Pharmacologic Treatment of Gastrointestinal Motility

WILLIAM SPIVAK, M.D.
Associate Clinical Professor of Pediatrics, Albert Einstein College of Medicine, New York; Associate Attending Pediatrician, Montefiore Medical Center, Bronx, New York
The Liver and Biliary Tree: Disorders of Bilirubin Metabolism

CHARLES A. STANLEY, M.D.
Professor of Pediatrics, University of Pennsylvania School of Medicine; Associate Director, Clinical Research Committee, Endocrine/Diabetes Division, The Children's Hospital of Philadelphia, Pennsylvania
The Liver and Biliary Tree: Disorders of Carbohydrate Metabolism

MARTIN STERN, M.D.
Professor of Pediatrics, Universitaets-Kinderklinik, Tuebingen, West Germany
The Intestines: Gastrointestinal Allergy

DAVID A. STRINGER, B.Sc., M.B.B.S., F.R.C.R., FRCPC
Associate Professor, University of Toronto Faculty of Medicine; Head, Divisions of Ultrasound and Gastrointestinal Radiology, The Hospital for Sick Children, Toronto, Ontario, Canada
Imaging: Overview; Radiography: Plain Film; Radiography: Contrast Studies; Sonography; Computed Tomography; Interventional Radiology

JAMES L. SUTPHEN, M.D., Ph.D.
Associate Professor, University of Virginia School of Medicine; Chief, Division of Pediatric Gastroenterology and Nutrition, University of Virginia Children's Medical Center, Charlottesville, Virginia
Nutritional Therapy: Enteral Nutrition

LESLI A. TAYLOR, M.D.
Instructor in Pediatric Surgery, University of Pennsylvania School of Medicine; Fellow in Pediatric Surgery, The Children's Hospital of Philadelphia, Philadelphia, Pennsylvania
Abdominal Masses

M. MICHAEL THALER, M.D.
Professor of Pediatrics, University of California, San Francisco, School of Medicine; Attending Physician, University of California Medical Center, San Francisco, California
The Liver and Biliary Tree: Cirrhosis

WILLIAM R. TREEM, M.D.
Assistant Professor of Pediatrics, University of Connecticut School of Medicine; Associate Director, Division of Pediatric Gastroenterology and Nutrition, Hartford Hospital, Hartford, Connecticut
Hepatic Failure

GEORGE TRIADAFILOPOULOS, M.D., D.Sc., F.A.C.P., F.A.C.G.
Assistant Professor of Medicine, University of California, Davis, School of Medicine; Chief, Section of Gastroenterology, Martinez Veterans Administration Medical Center, Martinez, California
The Intestines: Pseudomembranous Colitis

DAVID N. TUCHMAN, M.D.
Assistant Professor of Pediatrics, The Johns Hopkins University School of Medicine, Baltimore, Maryland
The Mouth: Disorders of Deglutition

JOHN N. UDALL Jr., M.D., Ph.D.
Associate Professor of Pediatrics, University of Arizona School of Medicine; Chief, Pediatric Gastroenterology, University Medical Center, Tucson, Arizona
Development of Immune Function
Nutritional Therapy: Introduction

JAY P. VACANTI, M.D.
Assistant Professor of Surgery, Harvard Medical School; Assistant in Surgery, The Children's Hospital, Boston, Massachusetts
The Liver and Biliary Tree: Liver Transplantation

JORGE VARGAS, M.D.
Assistant Professor of Pediatrics, Division of Gastroenterology, University of California, Los Angeles, School of Medicine, Los Angeles, California
Endoscopy: Fiberoptic Upper Intestinal Endoscopy

FERNANDO E. VITERI, M.D., Sci.D.
Professor, Nutritional Sciences, University of California, Berkeley, California
Nutritional Therapy: Protein Energy Malnutrition

W. ALLAN WALKER, M.D.
Professor of Pediatrics, Harvard Medical School; Chief, Combined Program in Pediatric Gastroenterology and Nutrition, Children's Hospital and Massachusetts General Hospital, Boston, Massachusetts
Book Editor

JOHN A. WALKER-SMITH, M.D.(Syd.), F.R.C.P. (Lon., Edin.), F.R.A.C.P.
Professor of Paediatric Gastroenterology, The Medical College of St. Bartholomew's Hospital; Consultant Paediatrician, Queen Elizabeth Hospital for Children, London, England
The Intestines: Celiac Disease
Intestinal Biopsy
Book Editor

JOHN B. WATKINS, M.D.
Professor of Pediatrics, University of Pennsylvania School of Medicine; Director, Division of Gastroenterology and Nutrition, The Children's Hospital of Philadelphia, Philadelphia, Pennsylvania
The Liver and Biliary Tree: Neonatal Iron Storage Disease
Book Editor

RONALD R. WATSON, Ph.D.
Research Professor, Department of Family Community Medicine, University of Arizona School of Medicine, Tucson, Arizona
Development of Immune Function

LAWRENCE T. WEAVER, M.A., M.D., M.R.C.P., D.C.H.
Scientific Staff, MRC Dunn Nutrition Unit, University of Cambridge; Honorary Consultant Paediatrician, Department of Paediatrics, Addenbrooke's Hospital, Cambridge, England
Anatomy and Embryology

WILLIAM B. WEIL Jr., M.D.
Professor of Pediatrics and Human Development, Michigan State University College of Human Medicine, East Lansing, Michigan
Nutritional Therapy: Obesity

STEVEN L. WERLIN, M.D.
Professor of Pediatrics, Medical College of Wisconsin; Director of Gastroenterology, Children's Hospital of Wisconsin, Milwaukee, Wisconsin
Exocrine Pancreas: Structure and Function

BARRY K. WERSHIL, M.D.
Instructor, Harvard Medical School; Clinical Assistant in Gastroenterology, Combined Program in Pediatric Gastroenterology and Nutrition, Children's Hospital and Massachusetts General Hospital, Boston, Massachusetts
Gastric Function

DAVID WESSON, M.D.
Associate Professor, Department of Surgery, University of Toronto Faculty of Medicine; Staff Surgeon, The Hospital for Sick Children, Toronto, Ontario, Canada
The Intestines: Congenital Anomalies; Trauma and Foreign Bodies; Acute Intestinal Obstruction; Hernias

HARLAND S. WINTER, M.D.
Assistant Professor of Pediatrics, Harvard Medical School; Associate in Medicine, Combined Program in Pediatric Gastroenterology and Nutrition, Children's Hospital and Massachusetts General Hospital, Boston, Massachusetts
The Intestines: Intestinal Polyps
Endoscopy: Lower Endoscopy

CAMILLUS L. WITZLEBEN, M.D.
Professor of Pathology and Pediatrics, University of Pennsylvania School of Medicine; Pathologist-in-Chief, The Children's Hospital of Philadelphia, Philadelphia, Pennsylvania
The Liver and Biliary Tree: Neonatal Iron Storage Disease; Disorders of the Intrahepatic Bile Ducts; Disorders of the Extrahepatic Bile Ducts

BEATRICE WOOD, Ph.D.
Clinical Assistant Professor of Psychology in Psychiatry and Pediatrics, University of Pennsylvania; Director of Psychotherapy, Child Study Institute, Department of Human Development, Bryn Mawr College, Bryn Mawr, Pennsylvania
Biopsychosocial Care

VANESSA M. WRIGHT, M.B., B.S., F.R.C.S., F.R.A.C.S.
Consultant Paediatric Surgeon, Queen Elizabeth Hospital for Children, London University College Hospital, London, England
The Esophagus: Congenital Anomalies
The Stomach and Duodenum: Congenital Anomalies

ELI ZALZSTEIN, M.D.
Fellow in Clinical Pharmacology, The Hospital for Sick Children, Toronto, Ontario, Canada
Drug Therapy: Principles of Pediatric Therapeutics

W. ALLAN WALKER

To Ted and Isabel Sattler
who are role models for life,
for their support and encouragement.

PETER R. DURIE

To Gordon Forstner,
whose insightful approach to research medicine and life
has provided continuing encouragement and direction.

J. RICHARD HAMILTON

To Andrew Sass-Kortsak and Jack French,
who stimulated my early interest in this fascinating field.

JOHN A. WALKER-SMITH

To Liz, Louise, Laura, and James Walker-Smith,
with appreciation for their patience.

JOHN B. WATKINS

To Mary, Sarah, and Leah Watkins and The Friendship Trust,
for their love, support, and encouragement.

Preface

Over the last two decades, the field of pediatric gastroenterology has developed from an obscure subspecialty to an essential component of every major academic pediatric program throughout the world. Among the many pediatric texts available, none deals extensively with the pathophysiologic basis of gastrointestinal disease in children of all ages. Contributors to this text have been asked to undertake their writing with a plan to fill this void, extending pathophysiologic considerations to their coverage of diagnosis and management as well. In tandem with development of the subspecialty the literature of gastrointestinal and hepatic entities as they pertain to the pediatric patient has grown. Accordingly, we have prepared an approach to the subject that should provide a reference text for pediatricians, gastroenterologists, and pediatric gastroenterologists alike.

This new multivolume textbook is dedicated to establishing a comprehensive approach to pediatric gastroenterology. Each author was carefully selected to provide an authoritative, comprehensive, and complete account of his assigned topic. We have devised an approach to dealing with the families of children with gastrointestinal diseases, and a pathophysiologic section examines cardinal manifestations of gastrointestinal disease as well as the development of the gastrointestinal tract. These sections help to augment an in-depth approach to disease manifestations and management. A careful and unique approach to diagnosis of gastrointestinal diseases in children follows. Finally, the principles of therapy are explored. We hope and expect that this collective approach will be beneficial to all physicians dealing with gastrointestinal problems in children.

W. Allan Walker, M.D.
Peter R. Durie, B.Sc., M.D., FRCPC
J. Richard Hamilton, M.D., FRCPC
John A. Walker-Smith, M.D., (Syd.), F.R.C.P. (Lon., Edin.), F.R.A.C.P.
John B. Watkins, M.D.

Acknowledgments

The editors wish to acknowledge the enormous and gracious efforts of our subsection editors. They include Dr. David A. Stringer (Imaging); Dr. John N. Udall Jr. (Nutrition); and Dr. Eve Roberts (Pharmacology). We would also like to thank Stacia Langenbahn for her editorial assistance. Finally we would like to thank Mary Mansor for her strong support in synthesizing the textbook and Leslie Fenton for her excellent editorial support and project management during final production.

Contents

VOLUME ONE

VOLUME TWO

SECTION V

Diagnosis of Gastrointestinal Disease in Children

Pediatric Gastrointestinal Disease

Pathophysiology • Diagnosis • Management

SECTION IV

Clinical Manifestations and Management (Continued)

CHAPTER 28

The Liver and Biliary Tree

PART 1

Prolonged Neonatal Obstructive Jaundice

Mary Susan Moyer, M.D.
William F. Balistreri, M.D.

Cholestasis, defined physiologically as a reduction in canalicular bile flow, is manifested clinically as conjugated hyperbilirubinemia with retention of other substances, such as bile acids, which are dependent on bile flow for excretion. Immature hepatic excretory function renders infants highly susceptible to infectious or metabolic insults that result in mechanical or further functional impairment of biliary excretion. Recognized disorders associated with neonatal cholestasis are numerous, and, in many cases, the precise etiology or mechanism of injury remains undetermined. Recent advances have been made in the definition of hepatic structure and physiologic function of the liver in the neonatal period. In addition, characterization and identification of specific metabolic or structural disorders have provided insight into the pathophysiology of perinatal liver dysfunction.

Evaluation of the cholestatic infant remains a difficult task, in part owing to the diversity of cholestatic syndromes and to the obscure pathogenesis of many of these disorders. Prompt identification and diagnostic assessment of the infant with cholestasis is imperative, however, in order to (1) recognize disorders amenable either to specific medical therapy (e.g., galactosemia) or to early surgical intervention, and (2) institute effective nutritional and medical support to allow optimal growth and development.

DEVELOPMENTAL PHYSIOLOGY OF HEPATOBILIARY FUNCTION

The primary motive force in the generation of bile flow is the hepatocytic secretion of bile acids that are major synthetic and excretory products of the liver. Bile flow, which is proportional to bile acid secretion, can be divided into two components: (1) *bile acid–dependent flow,* which involves active canalicular bile acid secretion accompanied by osmotic water flow and diffusion of other solutes, and (2) *bile acid–independent flow,* which is thought to be mediated by active anion and cation transport.[1-3] Effective bile flow is therefore dependent on the efficient enterohepatic cycling of bile acids. Many of the physiologic and structural mechanisms responsible for generation of bile flow are immature at birth. These unique developmental changes during the perinatal period provide a conceptual framework for understanding the cholestatic propensity of the newborn.

Substantial evidence exists for immature or altered metabolism and transport of bile acids at birth (Table 1).[4] Serum bile acid concentrations, which reflect the net efficiency of intestinal absorption and hepatobiliary function, are maintained at low levels in the fetus by net transplacental transport to the mother.[5] Postnatally, in the normal infant, concentrations of bile acids in the serum increase progressively and attain levels that are significantly elevated compared with those found in the adult.[6-8] In studies using the suckling rat model, plasma disappearance and biliary excretion of the labeled bile acid taurocholate occur at a much slower rate compared with adults, resulting in accumulation of bile acids in the systemic circulation.[7] In human infants as well, both fasting and postprandial serum bile acid concentrations are significantly higher than those found in older children and are similar to levels attained in adults with cholestatic liver disease.[6,8] These elevated serum bile acid concentrations persist through the first 4 to 6 months of life, corresponding to a period of "physiologic cholestasis" in the infant. Watkins et al have demonstrated that the bile acid pool size and synthetic rate are decreased in premature and full-term infants,[9,10] which further contributes to the decreased hepatic bile acid secretion and low bile acid concentrations in the intestinal lumen in early life. Other factors contributing to decreased bile flow and inefficient enterohepatic cycling in the neonate include (1) inefficient intestinal and hepatic bile acid uptake, (2) qualitative and quantitative deficiencies of bile acid synthesis, (3) altered bile acid metabolism, and (4) decreased hepatocellular secretion.[11]

The rate of hepatic clearance of bile acids from the portal blood is decreased during development.[12] Lower rates of hepatic uptake have been demonstrated experimentally in both isolated hepatocytes[13] and purified basolateral (sinusoidal) membrane vesicles,[14,15] reflecting immaturity of the sodium-coupled bile acid transport mechanism localized to the

TABLE 1
Manifestations of Underdeveloped Bile Acid Transport and Metabolism in Early Life

Increased serum bile acid levels (physiologic cholestasis)
Decreased hepatic uptake of bile acids
Enhanced bile acid efflux
Absent lobular gradient
Decreased conjugation, sulfation, and glucuronidation of bile acids
Qualitative and quantitative differences in bile acid synthesis
Decreased bile acid pool size
Decreased bile acid secretion rate
Low intraluminal concentrations of bile acids
Decreased or absent ileal active transport of bile acids

Modified from Balistreri and Schubert.[57]

sinusoidal domain of the hepatocyte. In the adult rat, avid extraction of bile acids by periportal hepatocytes results in a decreasing periportal to central lobular gradient for bile acid uptake.[16,17] Using similar radioautographic techniques, no acinar gradient could be demonstrated in the 14-day-old rat liver,[18] suggesting that the entire hepatic lobule must participate in uptake, even under basal conditions, in the face of decreased membrane transport. With no reserve capacity for additional recruitment throughout the lobule, bile acids enter the systemic circulation. A similar developmental pattern for the membrane transport of bile acids can be demonstrated in the ileum where active bile acid uptake is decreased or even absent during the suckling period.[19,20] This inefficient intestinal salvage of bile acids contributes to the reduced bile acid pool noted at this age.

Quantitative and qualitative differences in bile acid synthetic pathways are also apparent during early life. Bile acid synthesis begins on day 11 of the 21-day gestation in the rat[21] and near week 12 in the human fetus.[22] A 30-fold increase in the biliary concentration of the primary bile acids, cholic and chenodeoxycholic acids, has been observed in the human fetus between 16 and 20 weeks of gestation with a decreased ratio of cholate to deoxycholate compared with that in the adult (0.85 versus 1.6), indicating immaturity of hepatic alpha-hydroxylation.[23] The immaturity of bile acid synthetic function is also reflected in the presence of "atypical" bile acids, such as the cholestatic bile acid intermediate 3 beta-hydroxy-5 delta-cholenoic acid in amniotic fluid[24] and meconium,[25,26] suggesting a fetal pathway for synthesis of this compound. Bile acids with hydroxyl groups at positions one and six of the steroid skeleton have also been detected in meconium,[25] and Strandvik and Wikstrom[27] have identified significant amounts of nonsulfated tetrahydroxylated bile acids in the urine of healthy neonates. These unusual metabolites are also excreted in the urine of older children and adults with cholestatic liver disease.[25] It is of interest that polyhydroxylation may increase bile acid solubility, providing a potential pathway for excretion at a time when transformation and biliary secretion are not fully developed.

Although the mechanisms of intracellular biotransformation and transport of bile acids are not well defined, there is evidence that both the conjugation and sulfation of these organic anions are underdeveloped in early life.[28,29] Conjugation of bile acids with the amino acids taurine and glycine, an important step in bile acid metabolism that allows efficient intestinal fat digestion and absorption and provides a potential mechanism for detoxification, may be the overall rate-limiting step in hepatic excretory function. In isolated hepatocytes obtained from fetal and suckling rats, the rate of conjugation of a radiolabeled bile acid was shown to increase with postnatal age.[29] The overall capacity of rat liver homogenate to conjugate cholate with taurine was significantly lower in suckling compared with adult rats, with a marked increase apparent at the time of weaning. This increase in overall conjugation capacity paralleled an increase in the specific activities of the individual enzymes, microsomal cholyl-CoA ligase and cytosolic bile acid CoA-amino acid *N*-acyltransferase, involved in the process.[29]

There is an apparent discrepancy between the time of onset of bile acid synthesis and the development of efficient secretory processes. This is suggested by studies of the distribution of the taurocholate pool in fetal and newborn rats.[30] In the fetus, 85 percent of the pool is localized in the liver with only 10 percent found in the intestinal lumen. By postnatal day 5, this distribution is reversed with 85 percent of the bile acid pool localized in the intestine. Reduced canalicular excretion of bile acids in the fetus may be related to an immaturity of the membrane transport system for bile acids in the canalicular membrane. Data comparing the kinetics of taurocholate transport in canalicular membrane vesicles prepared from 14-day-old and adult rats suggest that the canalicular bile acid carrier is functionally mature at 14 days of age[31]; however, transport during earlier stages of development has not been examined.

Canaliculi differentiate from simple intracellular invaginations of two adjacent cell membranes during fetal development into well-defined structural lumina filled with microvilli.[32] The pericanalicular cytoskeleton, which has been implicated in promotion of bile formation, also manifests ontogenic changes. Cultured fetal hepatocytes, compared with adult cells, have a decreased frequency and force of canalicular contractions that appear to be related to a lack of pericanalicular cytoplasmic actin.[33] Structural immaturity of both the canaliculi and the pericanalicular cytoskeleton may be significant factors in impaired bile acid secretion during development.

In this setting of impaired bile secretion or *physiologic cholestasis* the immature liver may be more susceptible to injury. Bile acid transport and metabolism, enterohepatic recycling, and hepatic secretory function are all immature during early life. Transient perturbation of any of these processes may lead to further alterations in cellular bile formation, bile flow, and ultimately to the anatomic and clinical manifestations of cholestasis.

DIFFERENTIAL DIAGNOSIS OF CHOLESTASIS

The causes of prolonged conjugated hyperbilirubinemia in the newborn period are diverse (Table 2). These include specific infections, toxic insults associated with hyperalimentation and sepsis, as well as disorders of amino acid, lipid,

TABLE 2
Classification of Disorders Associated with Cholestasis in the Newborn

I. Extrahepatic disorders
  A. Biliary atresia
  B. Biliary hypoplasia
  C. Bile duct stenosis
  D. Anomalies of choledochopancreaticoductal junction
  E. Spontaneous perforation of the bile duct
  F. Mass (neoplasia, stone)

II. Intrahepatic disorders
  A. Idiopathic
    1. "Idiopathic" neonatal hepatitis
    2. Intrahepatic cholestasis, persistent
      a. Arteriohepatic dysplasia (Alagille's syndrome)
      b. Byler's disease (severe intrahepatic cholestasis with progressive hepatocellular disease)
      c. Trihydroxycoprostanic acidemia (defective bile acid metabolism and cholestasis)
      d. Zellweger's syndrome (cerebrohepatorenal syndrome)
      e. *Nonsyndromic* paucity of intrahepatic ducts (apparent absence of bile ductules)
      f. Microfilament dysfunction[112]
    3. Intrahepatic cholestasis, recurrent (syndromic?)
      a. Familial benign recurrent cholestasis
      b. Hereditary cholestasis with lymphedema (Aagenaes)
  B. Anatomic
    1. Congenital hepatic fibrosis or infantile polycystic disease (of liver and kidney)
    2. Caroli's disease (cystic dilation of intrahepatic ducts)
  C. Metabolic disorders
    1. Disorders of amino acid metabolism
      a. Tyrosinemia
    2. Disorders of lipid metabolism
      a. Wolman's disease
      b. Niemann-Pick disease
      c. Gaucher's disease
    3. Disorders of carbohydrate metabolism
      a. Galactosemia
      b. Fructosemia
      c. Glycogenosis IV
    4. Disorders of bile acid metabolism
      a. 3β-hydroxysteroid dehydrogenase/isomerase[47]
      b. $\Delta 4$-3-oxosteroid 5β-reductase[48]
    5. Metabolic disease in which the defect is uncharacterized
      a. α-antitrypsin deficiency
      b. Cystic fibrosis
      c. Idiopathic hypopituitarism
      d. Hypothyroidism
      e. Neonatal iron storage disease
      f. Infantile copper overload
      g. Multiple acyl-CoA dehydrogenation deficiency (glutaric acid type II)
      h. Familial erythrophagocytic lymphohistiocytosis
      i. Arginase deficiency[113]
  D. Hepatitis
    1. Infectious (hepatitis in the neonate)
      a. Cytomegalovirus (CMV)
      b. Hepatitis B virus (non-A, non-B virus?)
      c. Rubella virus
      d. Reovirus type 3
      e. Herpes virus
      f. Varicella virus
      g. Coxsackie virus
      h. ECHO virus
      i. Parvovirus B19[114]
      j. Toxoplasmosis
      k. Syphilis
      l. Tuberculosis
      m. Listeriosis

Table continues

TABLE 2 (*Continued*)

    2. Toxic
      a. Cholestasis associated with parenteral nutrition
      b. Sepsis with possible endotoxemia (urinary tract infection, gastroenteritis)
  E. Genetic or chromosomal
    1. Trisomy E
    2. Down's syndrome
    3. Donahue's syndrome (leprechaunism)
  F. Miscellaneous
    1. Histiocytosis X
    2. Shock or hypoperfusion
    3. Intestinal obstruction
    4. Polysplenia syndrome
    5. Neonatal lupus

and carbohydrate metabolism. Other metabolic defects such as alpha-1-antitrypsin deficiency, which have yet to be fully characterized, may present in the newborn period as chronic cholestasis. Structural anomalies of the biliary tract may result in cholestatic liver disease. The obstruction may be intrahepatic as in arteriohepatic dysplasia and congenital hepatic fibrosis, or may involve the extrahepatic biliary duct system and be amenable to surgical correction.

Although the differential diagnosis of neonatal cholestasis is varied, the clinical presentation in many of these situations is similar, reflecting a characteristic pathophysiologic response to the underlying decrease in bile flow. Specifically, these infants present with jaundice, dark urine, acholic stools, and varying degrees of hepatomegaly. Even though the presence of decreased bile flow is universal, associated synthetic dysfunction and hepatocellular necrosis are present to varying degrees.

Early recognition of cholestasis in an infant and prompt diagnosis of the underlying disorder are imperative in order to identify disorders that will respond to a specific treatment and to institute general supportive care that may ameliorate the clinical course. The majority of infants with prolonged cholestasis fall into the diagnostic category of *idiopathic cholestasis*, which is composed of extrahepatic biliary atresia or idiopathic neonatal hepatitis (Table 3). Because of the preponderance of these disorders and the clinical importance of differentiating between these two disease entities, they will be considered in some detail. Other specific disorders associated with neonatal cholestasis are discussed in subsequent chapters.

Idiopathic Infantile Cholangiopathies

Extensive evaluation of the infant with cholestasis leads to a diagnosis of either extrahepatic biliary atresia or *idiopathic* neonatal hepatitis in approximately 70 to 80 percent of infants (Table 3). These terms are descriptive and imply a clinical condition rather than an etiology. Although discrete diagnoses, such as alpha-1-antitrypsin deficiency and inborn errors in bile acid metabolism, have allowed specific definition of cases previously described as neonatal hepatitis, the precise etiology and mechanism of injury in the majority of cases of neonatal hepatitis as well as in extrahepatic biliary

TABLE 3
Relative Frequency of Various Clinical Forms of Neonatal Cholestasis*

Clinical Form	Cumulative Percentage	Estimated Frequency†
Idiopathic neonatal hepatitis	35–40	1.25
Extrahepatic biliary atresia	25–30	0.70
α_1-antitrypsin deficiency	7–10	0.25
Intrahepatic cholestasis syndromes		
(Alagille's, Byler's, etc.)	5–6	0.14
Bacterial sepsis	2	<0.1
Hepatitis		
Cytomegalovirus	3–5	<0.1
Rubella, herpes	1	<0.1
Endocrine (hypothyroidism,		
panhypopituitarism)	1	<0.1
Galactosemia	1	<0.1

*Compilation of several published series (>500 cases).
†Per 10,000 live births.
Modified from Balistreri.[111]

atresia remain obscure. The term *idiopathic obstructive or obliterative cholangiopathy* has been used to include disorders that manifest a range of pathology from predominantly hepatocellular injury to predominantly extrahepatic biliary tract injury.

Several hypotheses exist that attempt to conceptually unify the pathogenesis of these disorders. The "ductal plate theory," set forth initially by Jorgensen[34] and subsequently expanded by Desmet,[35] suggests that altered embryogenesis is responsible for clinically apparent disorders of neonatal cholestasis. During normal embryogenesis, the earliest form of the bile duct is a cylindric ductal plate that is then remodeled through an interaction between the ingrowing mesenchyme and disappearing ductal plate. Defective remodeling or incomplete dissolution with failure of recanalization leads to malformation of the ductal plate and subsequent anatomic abnormalities such as biliary atresia or cystic diseases of the hepatobiliary system.

Landing set forth the concept of "infantile obstructive cholangiopathy,"[36] suggesting that these cholestatic disorders represent the pathophysiologic continuum of a single underlying disease process. According to this hypothesis, an initial insult leads to inflammation at various levels of the hepatobiliary tract. The clinical sequelae represent a static or a progressive inflammatory process at the specific site of injury. If the site of injury is predominantly the bile duct epithelium, the resulting cholangitis could lead to progressive sclerosis and obliteration of the bile duct, clinically manifest as extrahepatic biliary atresia. If, on the other hand, the inflammation is primarily hepatocellular, the clinical picture may be one of neonatal hepatitis. The initial injury and sustaining mechanisms proposed in the Landing hypothesis remain largely undefined; however, recent studies examining specific viral etiologies as well as the identification of metabolic errors in bile acid metabolism may represent specific insults that subsequently result in the nonspecific generalized hepatobiliary response.

Although no specific virus has been consistently identified in patients with obliterative cholangiopathies, recent interest in reovirus type 3 as a candidate pathogen arose from observations of the similarity between histologic lesions found in the porta hepatis of weanling mice with a reovirus type 3 infection and those of infants with extrahepatic biliary atresia.[37] In two large series of patients, serologic evidence of reovirus infection, using an indirect immunofluorescent antibody assay, was detected in approximately 60 percent of cases of biliary atresia or idiopathic neonatal hepatitis compared with less than 12 percent of controls or patients with other cholestatic disorders.[38,39] In addition, reovirus type 3 antigens have been detected in the tissue from the porta hepatis resected from an infant with biliary atresia.[40] Reovirus antibodies were also identified in the serum of an infant rhesus monkey who spontaneously developed biliary atresia.[41] The clinical course, unlike the histologic lesion, of reovirus 3 infection in mice[37] differs from that of infants with biliary atresia[42] in that these mice have the capacity to regenerate normal extrahepatic bile ducts in spite of extensive damage. This has raised interest in the possibility of a bile duct growth factor present in mice, and a protein that copurifies with immunoglobulin A has been identified as a potential candidate for this factor.[43,44] Although these studies support the association between infection with reovirus type 3 and the development of idiopathic obstructive cholangiopathies in infants, a recent large series using a different assay system for detection of reovirus 3 infection did not substantiate these results.[45] Further studies are therefore needed to define the role of perinatal infection with reovirus type 3 as an initiating event in the development of neonatal hepatitis or extrahepatic biliary atresia.

Defects in bile acid metabolism resulting from a structural or functional block at specific steps in the metabolic pathway may also lead to biochemical defects and cholestasis.[49] These inborn errors may be related to organelle dysfunction, such as that described in peroxisomal disorders involving impaired oxidation of the cholesterol side chain, or may involve reactions that affect alteration of the steroid nucleus itself. Using fast atom bombardment ionization-mass spectrometry, two new inborn errors in bile acid synthesis associated with the clinical picture of neonatal hepatitis have been described.[47,48] Prototypic defects in the bile acid synthetic or degradative pathways may therefore result in either the absence of choleretic compounds, specifically primary bile acids, or the accumulation of potentially cholestatic substances such as intermediate metabolites. These disorders also support the contention that the neonatal liver is uniquely susceptible to injury and that the stereotypic histologic reaction and mechanism for perpetuation of injury in infantile obstructive cholangiopathy may result from a wide variety of initiating insults at any level of the hepatobiliary system.

Idiopathic Neonatal Hepatitis

This diagnosis should be restricted to cases of prolonged neonatal cholestasis in which the classic histologic changes described by Craig and Landing[49] are present on liver biopsy and known infectious or metabolic causes of neonatal hepatocellular disease have been excluded (Table 2). Idiopathic neonatal hepatitis represents the most common diagnosis in infants with neonatal cholestasis, with an incidence ranging from 1 in 4,800 to 1 in 9,000 live births.[50-52] Since the initial description by Stokes et al,[53] further extensive investigation has led to identification of specific disorders, such as alpha$_1$-antitrypsin deficiency, presenting with a clinical picture of neonatal hepatitis; however, in a majority of cases, no consistent etiologic agent has been determined. Based on epidemiologic data, two categories of neonatal hepatitis have been identified, *sporadic* and *familial*.[54] The increased incidence within certain families suggests that, at least in these cases, hereditary or metabolic factors are operant.

Clinical Presentation. Idiopathic neonatal hepatitis appears to be more common in males, and low birth weight is a frequent finding. More than 50 percent will develop jaundice, to a varying degree, within the first week of life. A significant proportion may appear to be otherwise clinically well; however, approximately one-third will manifest failure to thrive and a more fulminant course, intimating more extensive hepatocellular damage. Acholic stools are uncommon with this disorder, but may be present if the cholestasis is severe. The liver (and occasionally the spleen) is firm and enlarged and the urine dark. A bleeding diathesis resulting from vitamin K deficiency and/or decreased synthesis of clotting factors may be present. Other signs or associated anatomic abnormalities such as microcephaly, chorioretinitis, or vascular or skeletal anomalies are unusual and should suggest alternative diagnoses.

Pathology. Although several histologic features such as giant cell transformation and extramedullary hematopoiesis are nonspecific and represent a stereotypic response of the neonatal liver to injury, the biopsy can be helpful in excluding other causes of neonatal hepatitis. In general, there is disarray of the lobular architecture with hepatocellular swelling, focal hepatic necrosis, and multinucleated giant cells representing fusion of adjacent hepatocytes (Fig. 1). Portal triads are expanded with inflammatory infiltrate of lymphocytes, neutrophils, and occasional eosinophils. There is extramedullary hematopoiesis as well as varying degrees of portal fibrosis. Although canalicular bile stasis in the lobule may be prominent, bile duct proliferation and bile plugging in portal triads are usually absent. The severity of hepatocellular injury usually correlates with the degree of cholestasis.[49,55]

Management. Owing to the fact that neonatal hepatitis represents such a heterogeneous disorder with no specifically delineated causative or perpetuating factors in many cases, management is usually directed at nutritional support, vitamin supplementation, and general medical management of the clinical complications of cholestasis, such as ascites or pruritus. There has also been recent interest in the use of the bile acid ursodeoxycholate to ameliorate symptoms in certain patients with cholestasis, although the efficacy of this therapy has not been established in controlled trials. General medical management of chronic cholestasis is discussed in detail below.

Prognosis. The overall prognosis in idiopathic neonatal hepatitis is difficult to estimate, again owing to the variability of the clinical course and generally ill-defined pathogenesis. The outcome will depend, in part, on the underlying cause and the factors related to perpetuation of the cholestatic process. No specific biochemical or histologic correlates with clinical outcome have been identified, although Chang et al[56] have reported a worse outcome in infants whose peak bilirubin was greater than 15 mg per deciliter. A composite of several large series reviewing outcome of patients with idiopathic neonatal hepatitis is presented in Table 4. From these data, it would appear that sporadic cases have a more favorable outcome than familial cases. The poor prognosis in a number of the familial cases may relate to the presence of underlying inborn metabolic errors, specifically defects in bile acid metabolism, as have recently been described in familial cases of clinically defined neonatal hepatitis. As the underlying causes and pathogenesis of neonatal hepatitis are

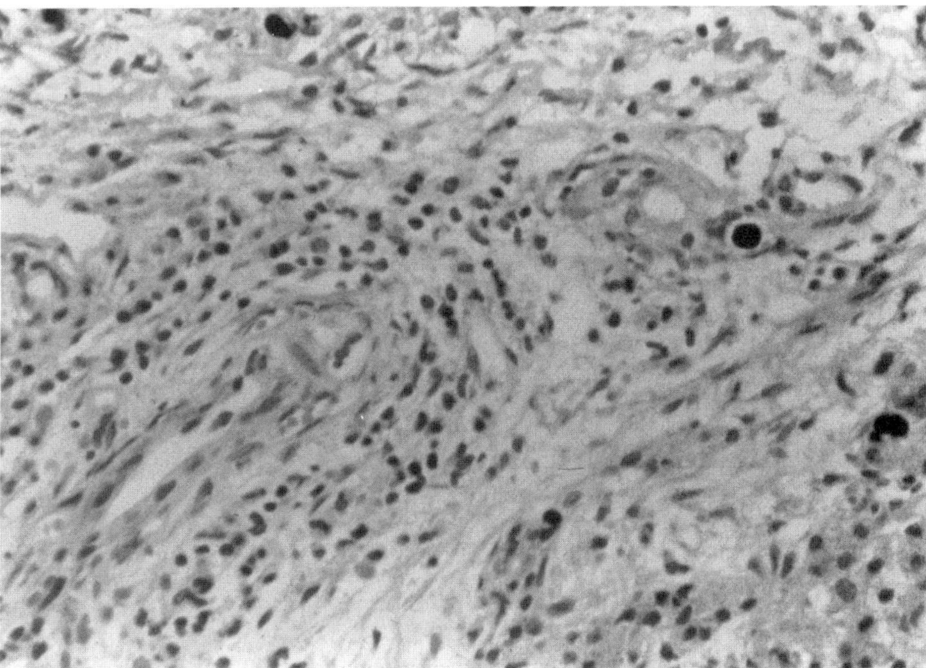

FIGURE 1 Liver histology in neonatal hepatitis. This biopsy specimen demonstrates disruption of hepatic lobular architecture with multinucleated giant cells. There are also inflammatory cells within the portal area.

TABLE 4
Outcome of Infants with Idiopathic Neonatal Hepatitis*

	Deutsch[90] n (%)	Danks[91] n (%)	Odiévre[92] n (%)	Lawson[54] n (%)	Chang[56] n (%)	Total
Sporadic Cases						
Recovered	40 (65)	31 (60)	60 (94)	11 (60)	19 (83)	161 (74)
Chronic Liver Disease	3 (5)	6 (12)	1 (2)	4 (22)	1 (4)	15 (7)
Died	19 (31)	15 (29)	3 (5)	3 (17)	3 (13)	43 (20)
Total	62	52	64	18	23	219
Familial Cases						
Recovered	2 (22)	3 (30)	2 (25)	0		7 (22)
Chronic Liver Disease	1 (11)	1 (10)	0	3 (60)		5 (16)
Died	6 (67)	6 (60)	6 (75)	2 (40)		20 (63)
Total	9	10	8	5		32

*Compilation of several published series.

further defined, more precise prognoses can be established, and newer therapeutic options, such as orthotopic liver transplant, may be considered for infants who progress to cirrhosis.

Biliary Atresia

Extrahepatic biliary atresia (EHBA) is responsible for approximately one-third of the cases of neonatal cholestasis and may also represent a spectrum of disorders. The incidence varies according to the series examined, but ranges from 1 in 8,000 to 1 in 25,000 live births.[51,57] EHBA appears to occur slightly more commonly in girls, but there is no clear racial predilection. Familial cases are not well described and studies demonstrating discordance in monozygotic and dizygotic twins do not support a genetic basis for the disease.[58,59] In some cases associated malformations, such as cardiovascular anomalies, polysplenia, malrotation, and situs inversus viscerum, are present suggesting a congenital insult.[35,60,61] There have, however, been no well-documented cases in premature infants or stillbirths, and at autopsy or re-exploration, obliteration of previously patent ducts have been found,[62,63] suggesting a failure of recanalization of the embryonic ductal system with a progressive obliterative process rather than agenesis.

Based on clinical and histopathologic findings, two types of atresia of the extrahepatic bile ducts have been recognized; (1) an *embryonic* or fetal type and (2) a *perinatal* type.[35,64] In a series compiled by Schweizer, the embryonic form of the EHBA constituted approximately 34 percent of the cases.[64] This form was characterized by the early onset of cholestasis with no decline in bilirubin noted following the usual period of physiologic elevation in the perinatal period. In these cases, no identifiable bile duct remnants were seen in the porta hepatis and associated malformations were often present. It would appear that the onset of the pathologic process in this proposed form of EHBA occurs early in fetal life with obliteration of bile ducts present at the time of birth. The perinatal type was found in approximately 66 percent of the cases and was characterized by a later onset of jaundice following a relatively jaundice-free period. Bile duct remnants were present in the porta hepatis, and there were usually no associated malformations. In these cases the fibro-obliterative process appears to have started late in gestation or in the immediate postnatal period. Therefore, the clinical presentation, histopathologic findings, and ultimately the prognosis correlate with the developmental stage at which the obliterative process begins.

Clinical Presentation. In general, the birth weight of infants with EHBA is normal and jaundice may be present from birth or be inapparent until 3 to 5 weeks of life or later. Acholic stools are common, occurring earlier and more frequently than in neonatal hepatitis. A consistent absence of stool pigment suggests biliary obstruction. The liver is usually firm and enlarged, and splenomegaly may develop rapidly, suggesting portal hypertension. As the disease progresses and biliary cirrhosis develops, the infant may manifest failure to thrive, nutritional deficiencies, and the sequelae of portal hypertension. As discussed above, anomalies of other organs may be present, such as polysplenia, malrotation, or congenital heart disease.[60,61]

Pathology. The extrahepatic anatomy in infants with EHBA is variable. In 90 percent there is inflammatory obliteration of all or portions of the extrahepatic biliary tract. Early in the disease the hepatic lobular architecture is generally intact. There are variable degrees of canalicular and cellular bile stasis, and bile duct proliferation is prominent. The finding of bile plugs in the portal ducts is relatively specific for biliary obstruction, although this feature is noted in approximately 40 percent of cases (Fig. 2).[65] There may be portal or perilobular fibrosis within large portal triads, but with little or no increase in cellularity. In a small number of cases, portal inflammation and giant cell transformation may be present, complicating the histologic differentiation from neonatal hepatitis.

From histopathologic examination of the extrahepatic biliary tree, Witzleben[66] proposed that EHBA resulted from persistent epithelial cell injury with inflammation, which eventually caused fibrosis and compromise of the ductal lumen. Subsequent studies have supported this hypothesis,[67,68] noting changes in biliary remnants in the porta hepatis that were consistent with an inflammatory, ascending "cholangitic" process accompanied by obliteration of the biliary ducts. Immunoglobulin deposits were noted along the basement membrane of these duct remnants, suggesting that perpetuation of the injury may involve an immune mechanism.[69]

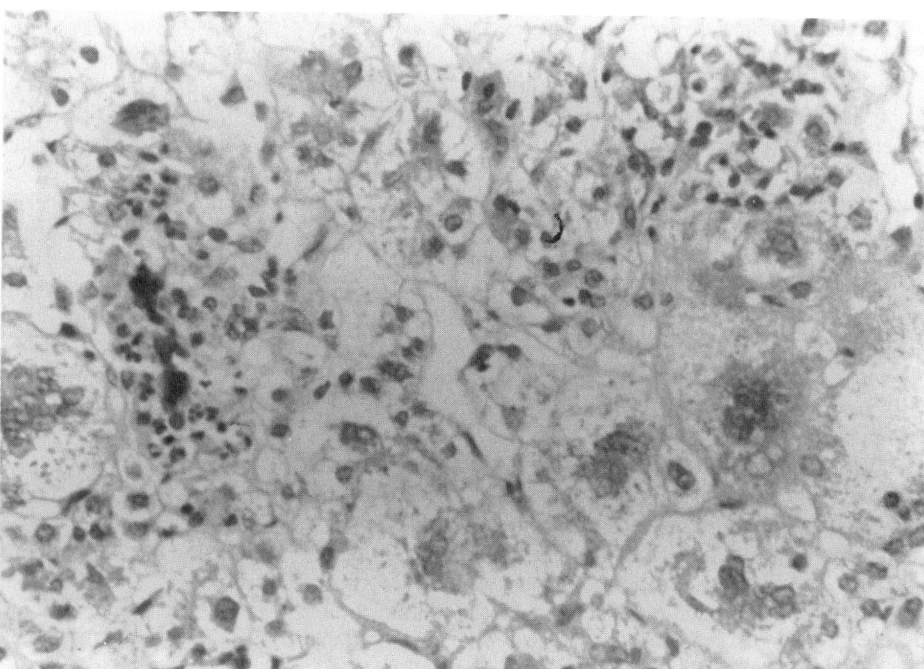

FIGURE 2 Liver histology in extrahepatic biliary atresia. This biopsy specimen demonstrates bile duct proliferation, fibrotic portal areas, and bile plugs. The lobular architecture outside of the portal areas is fairly well preserved.

Management. EHBA should be confirmed by an intraoperative cholangiogram performed prior to surgical intervention (Fig. 3). On the basis of the anatomy of the extrahepatic bile ducts the lesion is categorized as either correctable or noncorrectable.[70,71] Correctable lesions involve distal atresia along with a patent proximal portion of the extrahepatic duct to the level of the porta hepatis. This situation allows direct drainage of the biliary system. A noncorrectable lesion, involving obstruction at or above the porta hepatis, occurs in 75 to 85 percent of the cases of EHBA. The surgical success rates in these cases are highly variable despite an operable potential of 15 to 25 percent. The surgical procedure employed in cases of EHBA is the hepatoportoenterostomy with Roux-en-Y enteroanastomosis (Kasai procedure) to attempt bile drainage.[72] This procedure involves the excision of the obliterated extrahepatic ducts with apposition of the resected surface of the porta hepatis to the bowel mucosa. Although a portion of infants may derive a significant long-term benefit from this procedure, the majority will continue to manifest signs and symptoms of hepatic dysfunction with progression of their intrahepatic disease. Success in establishing biliary drainage appears to depend on the age at operation as well as on the size of the bile duct remnants. Bile flow was established in approximately 80 percent of infants who underwent the operative procedure at less than 2 months of age.[72] This success rate decreased to less than 20 percent in infants who were older than 90 days at the time of surgery. Also important in ultimately establishing effective bile flow is the size of the visualized ducts, although this tenet is not universally accepted and the reported size of the lumen necessary for successful bile drainage varies. Chandra and Altman,[73] by examining the resected intrahepatic biliary system in 65 patients who had undergone hepatoportoenterostomy, correlated a lumen size of greater than 150 μm with an excellent chance for subsequent bile flow. In the ser-

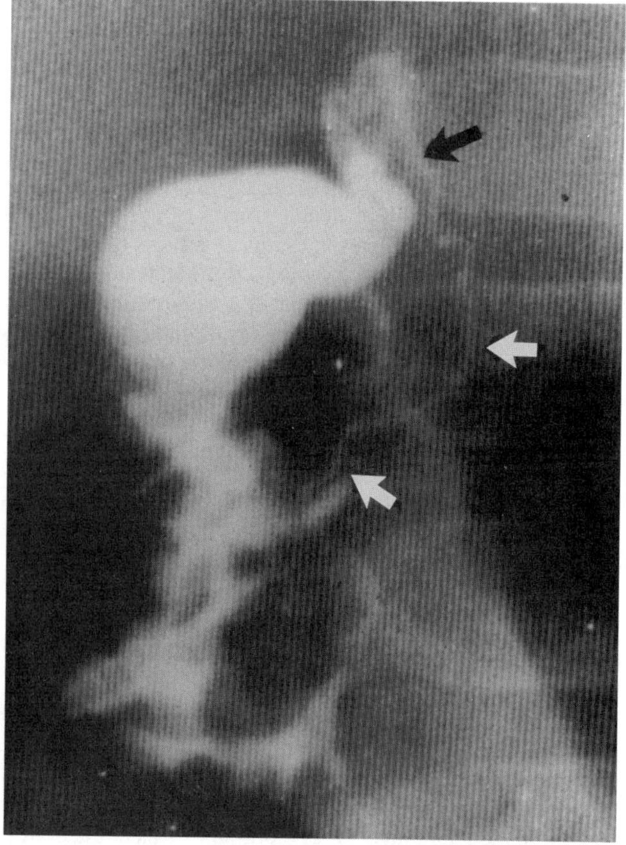

FIGURE 3 Operative cholangiogram in extrahepatic biliary atresia. The gallbladder is filled with contrast material, and no proximal duct system is visualized. A hypoplastic common duct (*arrows*) is seen distally entering the duodenum. (From Balistreri and Schubert.[57])

ies reported by Schweizer, postoperative bile flow was correlated with a lumen size of 450 μm or greater.[64]

The most significant postoperative complication appears to be ascending cholangitis,[74,75] which presents with acute onset of fever, leukocytosis, bacteremia or endotoxemia, and a concomitant decrease in bile drainage and elevation of the total and conjugated bilirubin. Bacterial cholangitis can lead to reobstruction of a previously patent biliary tract. Patients in whom effective bile flow has been established appear to be more susceptible to the development of cholangitis. In one series, 78 percent of patients with good bile flow versus 13 percent with no obvious postoperative bile flow developed cholangitis.[74] In addition, the number of episodes of cholangitis was inversely correlated with maintenance of good biliary drainage.

Prognosis. The average life expectancy for a patient with untreated biliary atresia is approximately 2 years,[76] with morbidity and mortality related to liver failure and/or the consequences of portal hypertension. The prognosis following hepatoportoenterostomy depends primarily on the outcome of the initial surgery and ultimately on the extent and activity of the biliary tract disease as well as on the development of postsurgical complications. Despite successful surgical relief of extrahepatic obstruction, the intrahepatic disease process will progress in a majority of patients, resulting in the development of cirrhosis and portal hypertension.[77] Therefore, the pathologic process that damages the extrahepatic bile ducts involves the intrahepatic biliary tree as well, with progressive destruction of ducts—even in situations of adequate surgical drainage. The overall 10-year survival rate in a series of 149 patients reported by Kasai et al was 33 percent.[78] The survival ranged from 75 percent in patients whose age at operation was less than 2 months to 10 percent in those who were greater than 3 months of age at the time of surgery, reflecting in part the surgical success rates for establishing bile flow.[72] The prognosis for infants with EHBA has been improved by the advent of orthotopic liver transplantation, which offers a viable option for patients who have progressed to end-stage liver disease. Even those who attain less than adequate biliary drainage following the initial surgery may derive short-term benefit from the procedure by achieving sufficient growth to allow transplantation.

EVALUATION OF THE INFANT WITH CHOLESTASIS

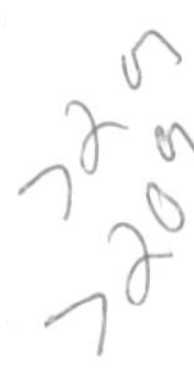

Conjugated hyperbilirubinemia in the newborn period always requires further evaluation. Fractionation of the bilirubin, which allows identification of patients with cholestatic (as opposed to physiologic) jaundice, should be obtained in any infant with prolonged hyperbilirubinemia. Cholestasis is defined as the presence of a conjugated (or direct-reacting) fraction of greater than 2 mg per deciliter or greater than 20 percent of the total bilirubin. The primary goals of the evaluation of neonatal cholestasis are to differentiate intrahepatic from extrahepatic disorders, to identify those disease entities for which specific therapy is available, and to recognize the clinical sequelae of cholestasis for which general empiric therapy may be efficacious. Extrahepatic biliary obstruction must be differentiated from intrahepatic disorders as soon as possible in order to institute and optimize appropriate surgical intervention. This remains a difficult diagnostic problem owing to overlap in the clinical presentation and laboratory profile of patients with idiopathic cholangiopathies, specifically EHBA and neonatal hepatitis. In addition, early recognition of treatable causes of cholestasis, such as sepsis, galactosemia, or endocrinopathies, will allow initiation of appropriate therapy that may prevent further damage to the liver and/or reverse the existing injury. Finally, recognizing the presence of clinical complications of cholestasis in general, including coagulopathy due to hypoprothrombinemia or vitamin K deficiency and the nutritional consequences of fat malabsorption, can direct empiric therapy and may improve the ultimate outcome and the general quality of life.

History and Physical Examination

During the evaluation of the cholestatic infant, the family history, prenatal and postnatal clinical course, and physical examination on presentation may provide important clues. Specific clinical features may aid in differentiating intrahepatic cholestasis from extrahepatic obstruction (Table 5). Irritability, poor feeding, and vomiting may indicate a metabolic disorder such as galactosemia or tyrosinemia, whereas vertebral arch anomalies, posterior embryotoxon, and the murmur of peripheral pulmonic stenosis suggest the diagnosis of arteriohepatic dysplasia or a syndromatic paucity of intrahepatic bile ducts.[79] Although characteristic facies have been described in the latter disorder, they appear to be nonspecific and may be present in infants with other forms of intrahepatic cholestasis.[80]

The general presentation of infants with EHBA is one of increasing jaundice, acholic stools, dark urine, hepatomegaly, and eventually splenomegaly. Persistently acholic stools are highly suggestive of extrahepatic obstruction; however, they may also be associated with severe intrahepatic cholestatic disease. Conversely, the presence of pigmented stools suggests patency of the extrahepatic biliary system and generally precludes the diagnosis of EHBA. Although these findings

TABLE 5
Discriminant Value ($P < 0.001$) of Various Clinical and Histologic Features in Infants with Cholestasis

Feature	Extrahepatic Cholestasis	Intrahepatic Cholestasis
Birth weight, g (mean)	3,200	2,700
Stool color within 10 days of admission, (% acholic)	79	26
Age of onset of acholic stools (days)	16	30
Abnormal size or consistency of liver (%)	87	53
Biopsy		
Portal fibrosis, (% positive)	94	47
Bile ductular proliferation (% positive)	86	30
Intraportal bile thrombi (% positive)	63	1

Modified from Alagille.[81]

are nonspecific. Alagille[81] has emphasized the importance of specific clinical information by performing discriminant analysis of several clinical signs and routine biochemical tests (Table 5). This analysis identified four clinical features that supported the correct diagnosis of intrahepatic or extrahepatic cholestasis in 82 percent of cases. These clinical parameters included stool color within 10 days of admission, birth weight, age at onset of acholic stools, and the features of hepatic involvement, specifically the presence of hepatomegaly and consistency of the liver on palpation. In this study, addition of liver histology to the evaluation increased diagnostic accuracy by only 3 percent (Table 5).

Laboratory Evaluation

No single test is consistently reliable in differentiating intrahepatic from extrahepatic forms of cholestasis; nevertheless, several tests may help identify specific causes of cholestasis and assess and monitor the degree of hepatobiliary dysfunction. The laboratory data (Table 6) must be analyzed in the context of the clinical setting. For example, urine-reducing substances may be falsely negative if the infant is not receiving a galactose-containing formula or is vomiting. In these situations, the diagnosis of galactosemia may be made by measuring the RBC galactose-1-phosphate and uridyl transferase activity, providing the infant has received no recent blood transfusions. Elevated methionine and tyrosine on a serum metabolic screen may reflect severe liver disease and not necessarily be diagnostic of an underlying metabolic defect. Evaluation for alpha-1-antitrypsin deficiency should include not only a serum level of the protein, but a phenotype as well. TORCH (*t*oxoplasmosis, *r*ubella, *c*ytomegalovirus, and *h*erpes simplex) titers and other serologies should be compared with maternal serum titers. Finally, an adequate quantity of sweat must be obtained for a sweat chloride test to accurately identify the infant with cystic fibrosis.

Duodenal intubation with analysis of fluid for bilirubin content is a highly sensitive test and is particularly helpful in situations in which skilled personnel are not available to perform and interpret liver biopsy specimens.[82,83] If the drainage is bilious, EHBA is virtually excluded. Although severe intrahepatic disease may result in the absence of bilirubin in the duodenal drainage, the majority of patients with neonatal hepatitis will have bile-stained fluid. Of 151 infants subsequently confirmed to have EHBA, none had bile pigment in the duodenal fluid.[83] Other serum tests, such as lipoprotein-X, 5′-nucleotidase and alpha-fetoprotein, initially reported to have discriminatory value, have not been found to be of consistently significant diagnostic efficacy.

Radiographic Evaluation

Ultrasonography. Real-time ultrasonography is an important adjunct to the diagnosis of neonatal cholestasis.[84] The study is most helpful in ascertaining the presence of a choledochal cyst, which can have a clinical presentation similar to that of EHBA. The absence of a gallbladder on a fasting study is suggestive, but not diagnostic, of biliary atresia. Dilated ducts are usually not present in EHBA, reflecting the fibro-obliterative or sclerotic nature of the coincident intrahepatic duct lesion.

TABLE 6
Staged Evaluation of Neonatal Cholestasis

1. Clinical evaluation (history, physical examination)
2. Fractionated bilirubin (±bile acids)
3. SGOT, SGPT
4. Stool color
5. Index of hepatic "synthetic function" (serum albumin, prothrombin time)
6. Viral and bacterial cultures (blood, urine)
7. Viral serology (HBsAg, TORCH) and VDRL titers
8. Alpha-$_1$-antitrypsin phenotype and level
9. T_4 and TSH
10. Sweat chloride
11. Metabolic screen (urine and serum amino acids, urine-reducing substances); ferritin
12. Ultrasonography
13. Imaging (hepatobiliary scintigraphy)
14. Duodenal intubation (bilirubin)
15. Liver biopsy

SGOT = serum glutamic-oxaloacetic acid; SGPT = serum glutamic-pyruvic transaminase; HBsAg = hepatitis B surface antigen; VDRL = Venereal Disease Research Laboratories; T_4 = thyroxine; TSH = thyroid-stimulating hormone.

Radionuclide Imaging. Hepatobiliary scintigraphy, using technetium-labeled iminodiacetic acid analogues, is highly useful in differentiating biliary atresia from nonobstructive causes of cholestasis. The hepatic uptake and secretion into bile of these derivatives of iminodiacetic acid occur by a carrier-mediated organic anion pathway and depend on the structure of the specific analogue, the integrity of hepatocellular function, and biliary tract patency.[85] In patients with EHBA, particularly early in the disorder, parenchymal function is not compromised; therefore uptake, or clearance, of the radioisotope is unimpaired, although subsequent excretion into the intestine is absent (Fig. 4*A*). Conversely, uptake is usually delayed in infants with neonatal hepatitis owing to hepatocellular dysfunction, but eventual excretion into the bile and intestine does occur (Fig. 4*B*). Pretreatment with oral phenobarbital (5 mg per kilogram per day for 5 days) enhances or maximizes biliary excretion of the isotope and can increase sensitivity to 94 percent.[86,87] Although the discriminating value of this test is excellent, nonexcretion may be related to severe intrahepatic cholestasis and not to extrahepatic obstruction. In addition, the 5 days required for phenobarbital administration in order to optimize diagnostic yield may ultimately affect outcome by delaying surgical intervention.

Other radiographic studies such as percutaneous transhepatic cholangiography or endoscopic retrograde cholangiopancreatography are rarely of diagnostic value in these infants.

Liver Biopsy

The liver biopsy remains the most reliable and definitive procedure in the evaluation of the neonate with persistent conjugated hyperbilirubinemia. Tissue may be obtained, in most cases, using a percutaneous technique with local anesthesia.[88] Careful interpretation by an experienced pathologist yields the correct diagnosis in 90 to 95 percent of cases.

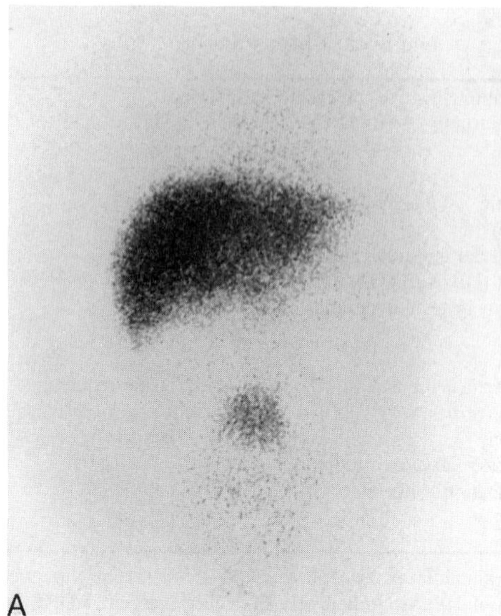

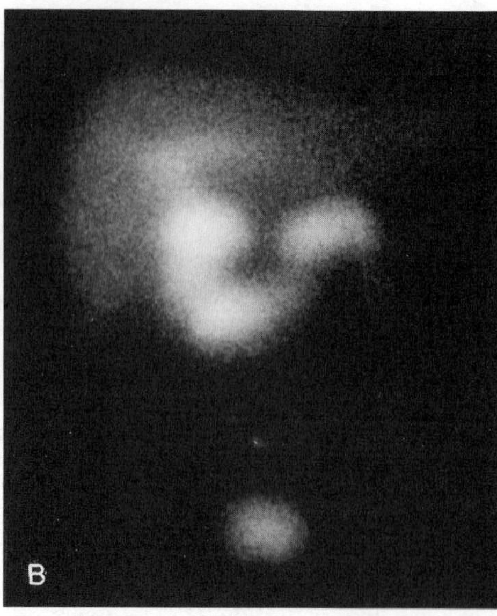

FIGURE 4 *A*, Radioisotope scan in extrahepatic biliary atresia. On a delayed scan, there is good uptake of the isotope by the liver, but no intestinal excretion is demonstrated. *B*, Radioisotope scan in neonatal hepatitis. Uptake of the isotope by the liver is delayed and decreased; however, excretion into the intestine is noted.

Prompt diagnosis may expedite surgery for EHBA and preclude unnecessary surgical exploration. The typical histologic findings in EHBA and neonatal hepatitis are summarized in Table 5.

Conclusions Regarding Evaluation

If EHBA is suggested, based on histology as well as imaging studies, an exploratory laparotomy with intraoperative cholangiogram is performed to verify the nature and site of the obstruction prior to hepatoportoenterostomy. If no specific etiology is determined, but extrahepatic obstruction is unlikely, the infant is followed and re-evaluated frequently. Empiric therapy may also be instituted to optimize growth and development and ameliorate the consequences of chronic cholestasis.

The need to correctly differentiate EHBA from intrahepatic disorders is illustrated in a report by Markowitz et al,[89] in which four patients who underwent hepatoportoenterostomies on the basis of hepatobiliary scans, and intraoperative cholangiograms were subsequently found to have arteriohepatic dysplasia on histologic and clinical criteria. None had adequate drainage postoperatively, two progressed to cirrhosis, and one died from hepatic failure, indicating that the intervening surgery had adversely altered the course of a usually benign disorder. If careful consideration is given to the history, physical examination, and these selected diagnostic tests (see Table 4), institution of appropriate surgery may be expedited, unnecessary surgery avoided, and, in many cases, the precise etiology determined.

MEDICAL MANAGEMENT OF CHRONIC CHOLESTASIS

In infants with intrahepatic cholestasis or those with EHBA in whom surgical attempts at establishing adequate biliary drainage are unsuccessful, the presence of the clinical consequences of persistent cholestasis directs medical therapy. These complications are related, either directly or indirectly, to diminished bile flow and reflect (1) retention of substances dependent on bile secretion such as bile acids, bilirubin, and cholesterol, (2) decreased bile acid delivery to the intestine with resultant fat and fat-soluble vitamin malabsorption, and (3) progressive hepatocellular damage leading to portal hypertension and eventual liver failure (Fig. 5). Currently, no specific therapy either reverses existing cholestasis or prevents ongoing liver damage; therefore, therapy is empiric and aimed at maximizing growth potential and nutritional status and minimizing discomfort.[93] The success of this therapeutic intervention is limited by the residual functional capacity of the liver and by the rate of progression of the underlying disorder.

Malabsorption and Malnutrition

One of the major and more immediate complications of chronic cholestasis is fat malabsorption related to decreased intraluminal bile acids, which leads to malnutrition and fat-soluble vitamin deficiency. Owing to decreased excretion of bile acids into the intestine, intraluminal long-chain triglyceride lipolysis and absorption are ineffective. Medium-chain triglycerides (MCT) are more readily absorbed in the face of low concentrations of bile acids and therefore are a better source of fat calories either as MCT-containing formulas or as a dietary supplement of MCT oil.

Intestinal absorption of fat soluble vitamins (D,E,A,K) that require solubilization by bile acids into mixed micelles is also compromised, and supplementation of at least two to four times the RDA is often necessary. Serum vitamin levels as well as laboratory tests such as Ca, PO_4, and prothrombin time are useful indices of adequate supplementation. Chronic vitamin E (alpha-tocopherol) deficiency has been associated recently with a progressive neuromuscular syndrome characterized by areflexia, cerebellar ataxia, posterior column dysfunction, and peripheral neuropathy.[94,95] The most reliable index of vitamin E status is the ratio of serum vitamin E to

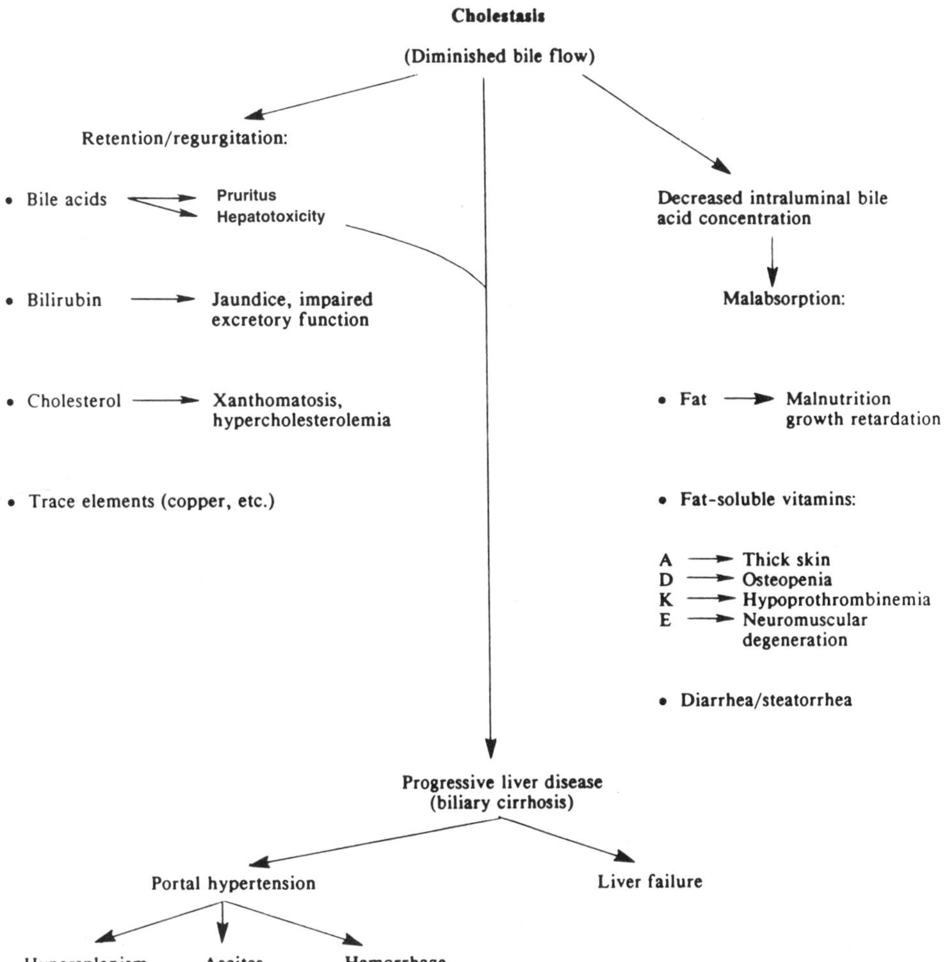

FIGURE 5 Clinical sequelae of chronic cholestasis. Numerous consequences of cholestasis become clinically manifest and result from retention of substances excreted in bile, reduction of intestinal bile acids, and progressive damage to the liver.

total serum lipids, since elevated lipids, as seen in chronic cholestasis, allow vitamin E to partition into the nonpolar phase (plasma lipoprotein fraction), artificially raising the serum vitamin E concentration. In infants and children less than 12 years of age a ratio of less than 0.6 mg per gram indicates vitamin E deficiency.[96] Large doses of vitamin E or even parenteral administration may be necessary.[95,96] Oral administration of a water-soluble form of vitamin E, *d*-alpha-tocopheryl polyethylene glycol-1000 succinate (TPGS), has recently been tested and found to correct biochemical vitamin E deficiency in doses of 15 to 25 IU per kilogram per day.[97] Further studies are under way to confirm these results.

Pruritus/Xanthomas

Significant clinical morbidity may result from pruritus. Xanthomas and itching may reflect retention and elevation of serum cholesterol and bile acids, respectively. Therapy is directed at decreasing the concentrations of these substances by enhancing conversion of cholesterol to bile acids and by stimulating the excretion and elimination of these bile acids. The efficacy of these therapeutic agents depends on generating increased bile flow and therefore requires a patent biliary tract. Cholestyramine is an anion exchange resin that enhances bile flow by interrupting the enterohepatic circulation and by increasing the pool size of cholic acid which is choleretic. Problems with the clinical use of this agent include obstruction, hyperchloremic acidosis, and exacerbation of steatorrhea, as well as poor compliance because the resin is not palatable. Phenobarbital, in therapeutic doses, stimulates bile acid independent flow and decreases the bile acid pool size.[98] The drug has been shown to be efficacious in relieving pruritus and decreasing serum bilirubin and bile acids.[99,100] The sedative side effect of phenobarbital may be a limiting factor in its clinical usefulness. Preliminary results suggest that the administration of an experimental agent (ursodeoxycholic acid), which alters bile acid composition, may be of benefit in ameliorating pruritus.[101] This observation, however, must be confirmed in controlled clinical trials.

Portal Hypertension

Progressive fibrosis and cirrhosis ultimately lead to the development of portal hypertension and its sequelae, the most clinically significant being ascites and variceal hemorrhage. The medical management of ascites should be dictated by patient comfort and by the relative risk of peritoneal bacterial infection. The judicious use of sodium restriction and diuretics may be helpful in controlling ascites accumulation. Initial steps include restricting sodium to 1 to 2 mEq per kilogram per day and introducing a diuretic such as spironolactone, which inhibits the effects of aldosterone. Refractory ascites with respiratory compromise may be managed with intravenous administration of albumin and furosemide under close observation or by therapeutic paracentesis with concomitant administration of intravenous colloid such as albumin.[102] Head-out water immersion, shown to be efficacious in some adult patients with ascites,[103] has not been systematically examined in infants.

Esophageal and gastric varices are a potentially life-threatening complication of portal hypertension. Acute variceal hemorrhage is managed in an intensive care unit with intravenous fluids and blood products, gastric lavage, and intravenous vasopressin infusion as indicated. Balloon tamponade, used for severe or prolonged hemorrhage, may be associated with significant complications such as esophageal rupture, airway obstruction, and pulmonary aspiration.[104] Endoscopic sclerotherapy is being used more extensively in infants and children for the acute and ongoing management of esophageal varices and may be superior to surgical alternatives,[105] particularly if eventual liver transplant is anticipated. There has also been continued interest in long-term administration of beta-blocking agents such as propranolol to reduce portal pressure and prevent recurrent variceal bleeding.[106]

In recent years, orthotopic liver transplantation has become a viable option for infants and children who progress to end-stage liver disease.[107] The ability to determine the optimum time in the clinical course to pursue transplantation requires careful monitoring and sequential evaluation of hepatic function.[108] Although no one specific functional measure has been shown to reliably assess hepatocellular reserve, prognostic scores have been developed for predicting outcome without transplantation,[108,109] which may then be compared with operative survival statistics for a particular patient group and thus aid in decision-making.

One of the major limiting factors for successful transplantation in infants has been the supply of appropriate-sized organs. This situation has been somewhat alleviated by introduction of the technique of segmental or volume reduction liver transplantation.[110] However, more effective means for supporting and monitoring infants with chronic liver disease are needed. Ultimately a better understanding of the pathophysiology of specific underlying disease processes may lead to more efficacious treatment of the sequelae of persistent infantile cholestasis and, one hopes, to therapeutic interventions that will prevent or reverse the development of chronic liver disease.

REFERENCES

1. Blitzer BL, Boyer JL. Cellular mechanisms of bile formation. Gastroenterology 1982; 83:346–357.
2. Javitt NB. Hepatic bile formation. N Engl J Med 1976; 295:1464–1469, 1511–1516.
3. Boyer JL, Bloomer JR. Canalicular bile secretion in man. Studies utilizing the biliary clearance of [^{14}C] mannitol. J Clin Invest 1974; 54:773–781.
4. Suchy FJ, Bucuvalas JC, Novak DA. Determinants of bile formation during development: Ontogeny of hepatic bile acid metabolism and transport. Semin Liver Dis 1987; 7:77–84.
5. Itoh S, Onishi S, Isobe K, Manabe M, Inukai K. Foetal maternal relationship of bile acid pattern estimated by high pressure liquid chromatography. Biochem J 1982; 204:141–145.
6. Suchy FJ, Balistreri WF, Heubi JE, Searcy JE, Levin RS. Physiologic cholestasis. Elevation of primary bile acid concentrations in normal infants. Gastroenterology 1981; 80:1037–1041.
7. Klaassen CD. Hepatic excretory function in the newborn rat. J Pharmacol Exp Ther 1975; 184:721–728.
8. Barbara L, Lazzari R, Roda A, Aldini R, Festi D, Sama C, Morselli AM, Collina A, Bazzoli F, Mazzella G, Roda E. Serum bile acids in newborns and children. Pediatr Res 1980; 14:1222–1225.
9. Watkins JB, Ingall D, Szczepanik P, Klein P. Bile-salt metabolism in the newborn. N Engl J Med 1973; 288:431–434.
10. Watkins JB, Szczepanik P, Gould JB, Klein P, Lester R. Bile-salt metabolism in the human premature infant. Gastroenterology 1975; 69:706–713.
11. Balistreri WF, Heubi JE, Suchy FJ. Immaturity of the enterohepatic circulation in early life: Factors predisposing to "physiologic" malabsorption and cholestasis. J Pediatr Gastroenterol Nutr 1983; 2:346–354.
12. Belknap WM, Balistreri WF, Suchy FJ, Miller PC. Physiologic cholestasis: II. Serum bile acid levels reflect the development of the enterohepatic circulation in rats. Hepatology 1981; 1:613–616.
13. Suchy FJ, Balistreri WF. Uptake of taurocholate by hepatocytes isolated from developing rats. Pediatr Res 1982; 16:282–285.
14. Suchy FJ, Bucuvalas JC, Goodrich AL, Moyer MS, Blitzer BL. Taurocholate transport and $Na^{+}K^{+}$-ATPase activity in fetal and neonatal rat liver plasma membrane vesicles. Am J Physiol 1986; 251:G655–G673.
15. Suchy FJ, Courchene SM, Blitzer BL. Taurocholate transport by basolateral membrane vesicles isolated from developing rat liver. Am J Physiol 1985; 248:G648–G654.
16. Jones AL, Hradek GT, Renston RH, Wong KY, Karlaganis G, Paumgartner G. Autoradiographic evidence for hepatic lobular concentration gradient of bile acid derivative. Am J Physiol 1980; 238:G233–G237.
17. Groothius GM, Hardonk MJ, Keulemans KP, Nieuwenhuis P, Meijer DKF. Autoradiographic and kinetic demonstration of acinar heterogeneity of taurocholate transport. Am J Physiol 1982; 243:G455–G462.
18. Suchy FJ, Balistreri WF, Breslin JS, Dumaswala R, Setchell KD, Garfield SA. Absence of an acinar gradient for bile acid uptake in developing rat liver. Pediatr Res 1987; 21:417–421.
19. deBelle RC, Vaupshas V, Vitullo BB, Haber LR, Shatter E, Mackie GG, Owen H, Little JM, Lester R. Intestinal absorption of bile salts: Immature development in the neonate. J Pediatr 1979; 94:472–476.
20. Moyer MS, Heubi JE, Goodrich AL, Balistreri WF, Suchy FJ. Ontogeny of bile acid transport in brush border membrane vesicles from rat ileum. Gastroenterology 1986; 90:1188–1196.
21. Danielsson H, Rutter WJ. The metabolism of bile acids in the developing rat liver. Biochemistry 1968; 7:346–351.
22. Subbiah TR, Hassan AS. Development of bile acid biogenesis and its significance in cholesterol homeostasis. Adv Lipid Res 1982; 19:137–161.
23. Columbo C, Zuliani G, Rochi M, Breidenstein J, Setchell KDR. Biliary bile acid composition of the human fetus in early gestation. Pediatr Res 1987; 21:197–200.
24. Deleze G, Paumgartner G, Karlaganis G, Giger W, Reinhard M, Sidiropoulos D. Bile acid pattern in human amniotic fluid. Eur J Clin Invest 1978; 8:41–45.
25. Back P, Walter K. Developmental pattern of bile acid metabolism as revealed by bile acid analysis of meconium. Gastroenterology 1980; 78:671–676.
26. St Pyrek J, Sterzycki R, Lester R, Adcock E. Constituents of human meconium II: Identification of steroidal acids with 21 and 22 carbon atoms. Lipids 1982; 17:241–249.
27. Strandvik B, Wikstrom SA. Tetrahydroxylated bile acids in healthy human newborns. Eur J Clin Invest 1982; 12:301–305.
28. Balistreri WF, Zimmer L, Suchy FJ, Bove KE. Bile salt sulfotransferase: alteration during maturation and noninducibility during substrate ingestion. J Lipid Res 1984; 25:228–235.
29. Suchy FJ, Courchene SM, Balistreri WF. Ontogeny of hepatic bile acid conjugation in the rat. Pediatr Res 1985; 19:97–101.
30. Little JM, Richey JE, VanThiel DH, Lester R. Taurocholate pool size and distribution in the fetal rat. J Clin Invest 1979; 63:1042–1048.

31. Novak DA, Suchy FJ. Postnatal expression of the canalicular bile acid transport system in rat liver. (Abstract) Hepatology 1987; 7:1037.
32. DeWolf-Peeters C, DeVos R, Desmet V, Bianchi L, Rohr HP. Electron microscopy and morphometry of canalicular differentiation in fetal and newborn rat liver. Exp Mol Pathol 1974; 21:339–350.
33. Miyairi M, Wantanabe S, Phillips MJ. Cell motility of fetal hepatocytes in short term culture. Pediatr Res 1985; 19:1225–1229.
34. Jorgensen MJ. The ductal plate malformation. Acta Pathol Microbiol Scand 1977; 257:7–88.
35. Desmet VJ. Cholangiopathies: Past, present and future. Semin Liver Dis 1987; 7:67–76.
36. Landing BH. Consideration of the pathogenesis of neonatal hepatitis, biliary atresia and choledochal cyst. The concept of infantile obstructive cholangiopathy. Prog Pediatr Surg 1974; 6:113–139.
37. Bangaru B, Morecki R, Glaser JH, Gartner LM, Horwitz MS. Comparative studies of biliary atresia in the human newborn and reovirus-induced cholangitis in weanling mice. Lab Invest 1980; 43:456–462.
38. Morecki R, Glaser JH, Cho S, Balistreri WF, Horwitz MS. Biliary atresia and reovirus 3 infection. N Engl J Med 1982; 307:481–484.
39. Glaser J, Morecki R, Balistreri WF, Collins J, Horwitz MS. Neonatal obstructive cholangiopathy and reovirus 3 infection. (Abstract) Hepatology 1982; 2:719A.
40. Morecki R, Glaser JH, Johnson AB, Kress Y. Detection of reovirus type 3 in the porta hepatis of an infant with extrahepatic biliary atresia: ultrastructural and immunocytochemical study. Hepatology 1984; 4:1137–1142.
41. Rosenberg DP, Morecki R, Lollini LO, Glaser J, Cornelius CE. Extrahepatic biliary atresia in a rhesus monkey (Macaca mulatta). Hepatology 1983; 3:577–580.
42. Gautier M, Jehan P, Odiévre M. Histologic study of biliary fibrous remnants in 48 cases of extrahepatic biliary atresia: correlation with post-operative bile flow restoration. J Pediatr 1976; 89:704–709.
43. Glaser JH, Morecki R, Fallon-Friedlander S, Horwitz MS. An extrahepatic bile duct growth factor: detection and preliminary characterization. Hepatology 1987; 7:272–276.
44. Fallon-Friedlander S, Boscamp JR, Morecki R, Lilly F, Horwitz MS, Glaser JH. IgA stimulates growth of the extrahepatic bile duct in BALB/c mice. Proc Natl Acad Sci 1987; 84:3244–3248.
45. Brown WR, Sokol RJ, Levin MJ, Silverman A, Tamaru T, Lilly JR, Hall RJ, Cheney M. Lack of correlation with reovirus 3 and extrahepatic biliary atresia or neonatal hepatitis. J Pediatr 1988; 113:670–676.
46. Setchell KDR, Street JM. Inborn errors of bile acid synthesis. Semin Liver Dis 1987; 7:85–99.
47. Clayton PT, Leonard JV, Lawson AM, Setchell KD, Andersson B, Egestad B, Sjövall J. Familial giant cell hepatitis associated with synthesis of 3β, 7α-dihydroxy- and 3β, 7α 12α-tri-hydroxy-5-cholenoic acids. J Clin Invest 1987; 79:1031–1038.
48. Setchell KDR, Suchy FJ, Welsh MB, Zimmer-Nechemias L, Heubi J, Balistreri WF. Δ^4-3 Oxosteroid 5β-reductase deficiency described in identical twins with neonatal hepatitis. A new inborn error in bile acid synthesis. J Clin Invest 1988; 2:2148–2157.
49. Craig JM, Landing BH. Form of hepatitis in the neonatal period simulating biliary atresia. Arch Pathol 1952; 54:321–333.
50. Danks DM, Campbell PE, Jack I, Rogers J, Smith AL. Studies of the aetiology of neonatal hepatitis and biliary atresia. Arch Dis Child 1977; 52:360–367.
51. Henriksen NT, Drablos PA, Aegenaes O. Cholestatic jaundice in infancy. The importance of familial and genetic factors in aetiology and prognosis. Arch Dis Child 1981; 56:62–67.
52. Balistreri WF. Neonatal cholestasis. In: Leventhal E, ed. The textbook of pediatric gastroenterology in infancy and childhood. New York: Raven Press, 1981: 1081.
53. Stokes J Jr, Wolman IJ, Blanchard MC, Farquhar JD. Viral hepatitis in the newborn; clinical features, epidemiology and pathology. Am J Dis Child 1951; 82:213–216.
54. Lawson EE, Boggs JD. Long-term follow-up of neonatal hepatitis: safety and value of surgical exploration. Pediatrics 1974; 53:650–655.
55. Montgomery CK, Ruebner BH. Neonatal hepatocellular giant cell transformation: a review. Perspect Pediatr Pathol 1976; 3:85–101.
56. Chang MH, Hsu HC, Lee CY, Wang TR, Kao CL. Neonatal hepatitis: a follow-up study. J Pediatr Gastroenterol Nutr 1987; 6:203–207.
57. Balistreri WF, Schubert WK. Liver disease in infancy and childhood. In: Schiff L, Schiff ER, eds. Diseases of the liver. Philadelphia: JB Lippincott 1987: 1337.
58. Hyams JS, Glaser JH, Leichtner AM, Morecki R. Discordance for biliary atresia in two sets of monozygotic twins. J Pediatr 1985; 107:420–422.
59. Strickland AD, Shannon K, Coln CD. Biliary atresia in two sets of twins. J Pediatr 1985; 107:418–420.
60. Miyamoto M, Kajimoto T. Associated anomalies in biliary atresia patients. In: Kasai M, ed. Biliary atresia and its related disorders. Amsterdam-Oxford-Princeton: Excerpta Medica 1983: 13.
61. Chandra RS. Biliary atresia and other structural anomalies in the congenital polysplenia syndrome. J Pediatr 1974; 85:649–655.
62. Danks DM, Campbell PE. Extrahepatic biliary atresia: comments on the frequency of potentially operable cases. J Pediatr 1966; 69:21–29.
63. Holder TM. Atresia of the extrahepatic bile duct. Am J Surg 1964; 107:458–462.
64. Schweizer P, Müller G, eds. Gallengangsatresie. Cholestase-Syndrome in Neugeborenen-und Sanglingsalter. Bibliothek für Kinderchirurgie. Stuttgart: Hippokrates, 1984.
65. Brough AJ, Bernstein J. Conjugated hyperbilirubinaemia in early infancy. A re-assessment of liver biopsy. Hum Pathol 1974; 5:507–516.
66. Witzleben CL. Bile duct paucity (intrahepatic atresia). Perspect Pediatr Pathol 1982; 9:185–201.
67. Gautier M, Eliot N. Extrahepatic biliary atresia. Morphologic study of 98 biliary remnants. Arch Pathol Lab Med 1981; 105:397–402.
68. Chandra RS. Bile duct and hepatic morphology in biliary atresia: correlation with bile flow following portoenterostomy. In: Daum F, Fisher SE, eds. Extrahepatic biliary atresia. New York: Marcel Dekker. 1983:43.
69. Hadchouel M, Hugon RN, Odiévre M. Immunoglobulin deposits in the biliary remnants of extrahepatic biliary atresia: a study by immunoperoxidase staining in 128 infants. Histopathology 1981; 5:217–221.
70. Kasai M, Kimura S, Asakura Y, Suzuki H, Taira Y, Ohashi E. Surgical treatment of biliary atresia. J Pediatr Surg 1968; 3:665–675.
71. Kasai M. Intra- and extrahepatic bile ducts in biliary atresia. In: Javitt NB, ed. Neonatal hepatitis and biliary atresia. Washington DC: United States Department of Health, Education and Welfare. Publication No. (NIH) 79-1296, 1977:351.
72. Kasai M. Treatment of biliary atresia with special reference to hepatic portoenterostomy and its modifications. Prog Pediatr Surg 1974; 6:5–52.
73. Chandra RS, Altman RP. Ductal remnants in extrahepatic biliary atresia. A histopathologic study with clinical correlation. J Pediatr 1978; 93:196–200.
74. Ecoffey C, Rothman E, Bernard O, Hadchouel M, Valayer J, Alagille D. Bacterial cholangitis after surgery for biliary atresia. J Pediatr 1987; 111:824–829.
75. Kobayashi A, Utsunomiya T, Ohbe Y, Shimizu K. Ascending cholangitis after successful surgical repair of biliary atresia. Arch Dis Child 1973; 48:697–703.
76. Hays D, Snyder W. Life-span in untreated biliary atresia. Surgery 1973; 54:373–375.
77. Ito T, Horisawa M, Ando H. Intrahepatic bile ducts in biliary atresia—a possible factor determining prognosis. J Pediatr Surg 1983; 18:124–130.
78. Kasai M, Ohi R, Chiba T. Long-term survivors after surgery for biliary atresia. In: Ohi R, ed. biliary atresia: proceedings of the 4th international symposium on biliary atresia. Tokyo: Professional Postgraduate Services, 1986: 277.
79. Alagille D, Odiévre M, Gautier M, Dommergues JP. Hepatic ductular hypoplasia associated with characteristic facies, vertebral malformations, retarded physical, mental and sexual development and cardiac murmur. J Pediatr 1975; 86:63–71.
80. Sokol RJ, Heubi JE, Balistreri WF. Intrahepatic "cholestasis facies": is it specific for Alagille's syndrome? J Pediatr 1983; 103:205–208.
81. Alagille D. Cholestasis in the first three months of life. Prog Liver Dis 1979; 6:471–485.
82. Greene HL, Helinek GL, Moran R, O'Neill J. A diagnostic approach to prolonged obstructive jaundice by 24-hour collection of duodenal fluid. J Pediatr 1979; 95:412–414.
83. Kawai S, Kobayashi A, Ohbe Y. Duodenal aspiration in the differentiation of biliary atresia and neonatal hepatitis. (Abstract) Jpn J Pediatr Surg 1978; 10:619.
84. Franken EA, Smith WL, Siddiqui A. Noninvasive evaluations of liver disease in pediatrics. Radiol Clin North Am 1980; 18:239–252.
85. Krishnamurthy S, Krishnamurthy GT. Technetium-99m iminodiacetic acid organic anions: review of biokinetics and clinical application in hepatology. Hepatology 1989; 9:139–153.
86. Miller JH, Sinatra FR, Thomas DW. Biliary excretion disorders in

infants: evaluation using ^{99m}Tc-PIPIDA. Am J Radiol 1980; 135:47–52.
87. Majd M, Reba RC, Altman RP. Hepatobiliary scintigraphy with ^{99m}Tc-PIPIDA in the evaluation of neonatal jaundice. Pediatrics 1981; 67:140–145.
88. Hong R, Schubert WK. Menghini needle biopsy of the liver. Am J Dis Child 1960; 100:42–46.
89. Markowitz J, Daum F, Kahn EL, Schneider KM, So HB, Altman RP, Aiges HW, Alperstein G, Silverberg M. Arteriohepatic dysplasia. I. Pitfalls in diagnosis and management. Hepatology 1983; 3:74–76.
90. Deutsch J, Smith AL, Danks DM, Campbell PE. Long-term prognosis for babies with neonatal liver disease. Arch Dis Child 1985; 60:447–451.
91. Danks DM, Campbell PE, Smith AL, Rogers J. Prognosis of babies with neonatal hepatitis. Arch Dis Child 1977; 52:368–372.
92. Odiévre M, Hadchouel M, Landrieus P, Alagille D, Eliot N. Long-term prognosis for infants with intrahepatic cholestasis and patent extrahepatic biliary tract. Arch Dis Child 1981; 56:373–376.
93. Sokol RJ. Medical management of the infant or child with chronic liver disease. Semin Liver Dis 1987; 7:155–167.
94. Rosenblum JL, Keating JP, Prensky AL, Nelson JS. A progressive neurologic syndrome in children with chronic liver disease. N Engl J Med 1981; 304:503–508.
95. Sokol RJ, Heubi JE, Iannaccone ST, Bove KE, Balistreri WF. Mechanism causing vitamin E deficiency during chronic childhood cholestasis. Gastroenterology 1983; 85:1172–1182.
96. Sokol RJ, Heubi JE, Iannaccone ST, Bove KE, Balistreri WF. Vitamin E deficiency with normal serum vitamin E concentrations in children with chronic cholestasis. N Engl J Med 1984; 310:1209–1212.
97. Sokol RJ, Heubi JE, Butler-Simon NA, McClung HJ. Oral *d*-alpha tocopheryl polyethylene glycol-1000 succinate (TPGS) treatment for vitamin E deficiency in chronic childhood cholestasis. (Abstract) Pediatr Res 1986; 20:249A.
98. Bloomer JR, Boyer JL. Phenobarbital effects in cholestatic liver disease. Ann Intern Med 1985; 82:310–317.
99. Sharp HL, Mirkin BL. Effect of phenobarbital on hyperbilirubinemia, bile acid metabolism and microsomal enzyme activity in chronic intrahepatic cholestasis of childhood. J Pediatr 1972; 81:116–126.
100. Stiehl A, Thaler MM, Admirand WH. The effects of phenobarbital on bile salts and bilirubin in patients with intrahepatic and extrahepatic cholestasis. N Engl J Med 1972; 286:858–861.
101. Balistreri WF, Heubi JE, Whitington P, Perrault J, Bancroft J, Setchell KDR. Ursodeoxycholic acid (UDCA) therapy in pediatric hepatobiliary disease. (Abstract) Hepatology 1989; 10:602.
102. Ginès P, Titó L, Arroyo V, Planas R, Panés J, Viver J, Torres M, Humbert P, Rimola A, Llach J, Badalamenti S, Jiménez W, Gaya J, Rodés J. Randomized comparative study of therapeutic paracentesis with and without intravenous albumin in cirrhosis. Gastroenterology 1988; 94:1493–1502.
103. Bichet DG, Groves BM, Schrier RW. Mechanisms of improvement of water and sodium excretion by immersion in decompensated cirrhotic patients. Kidney Int 1983; 24:788–794.
104. Chojkier M, Conn HO. Esophageal tamponade in the treatment of bleeding varices: a decadal progress report. Dig Dis Sci 1980; 25:267–272.
105. Howard ER, Stringer MD, Mowat AP. Assessment of injection sclerotherapy in the management of 152 children with oesophageal varices. Br J Surg 1988; 75:404–408.
106. Sheen IS, Chen TY, Liaw YF. Randomized controlled study of propranolol for prevention of recurrent esophageal varices bleeding in patients with cirrhosis. Liver 1989; 9:1–5.
107. Starzl TE, Iwatsuki S, VanThiel DH, Gartner JC, Zitelli BJ, Malatack JJ, Schade RR, Shaw BW, Hakala TR, Rosenthal JT, Porter KA. Evolution of liver transplantation. Hepatology 1982; 2:614–636.
108. Bircher J. Assessment of prognosis in advanced liver disease: to score or to measure, that's the question. Hepatology 1986; 6:1036–1037.
109. Malatack JJ, Schaid DJ, Urbach AH, Gartner JC Jr, Zitelli BJ, Rockette H, Fischer J, Starzl TE, Iwatsuki S, Shaw BW. Choosing a pediatric recipient for orthotopic liver transplantation. J Pediatr 1987; 111:479–489.
110. deHemptinne B, deVille de Goyet J, Kestens PJ, Otte JB. Volume reduction of the liver graft before orthotopic transplantation: report of a clinical experience in 11 cases. Transplant Proc 1987; 19:3317–3322.
111. Balistreri WF. Neonatal cholestasis: lessons from the past, issues for the future. Semin Liver Dis 1987; 7:61–66.
112. Weber AM, Tuchweber B, Yousef I, Brochu P, Turgeon C, Gabbiani G, Morin CL, Roy CC. Severe familial cholestasis in North American Indian children: a clinical model of microfilament dysfunction? Gastroenterology 1981; 81:653–662.
113. Grody WW, Argyle C, Kern RM, Dizikes GJ, Spector EB, Strickland AD, Klein D, Cederbaum SD. Differential expression of the two human arginase genes in hyperargininemia. Enzymatic, pathologic and molecular analysis. J Clin Invest 1989; 83:602–609.
114. Metzman R, Anand A, DeGiulio PA, Knisely AS. Hepatic insufficiency with bile duct proliferation and marked periportal fibrosis due to intrauterine parvovirus B19 infection in a premature infant. (Abstract) Lab Invest 1989; 60:5p.

PART 2

Congenital Infections of the Liver

Joel M. Andres, M.D.

ACQUIRED IMMUNODEFICIENCY SYNDROME

Acquired immunodeficiency syndrome (AIDS) was first described in 1981.[1] It is now known to be caused by an infectious agent, the human immunodeficiency virus (HIV),[2,3] and affected individuals have rapidly expanded to include infants and young children. HIV, also known as human T-cell lymphotropic virus type III (HTLV-III),[4] is a retrovirus with a glycoprotein envelope and a characteristic core protein that surrounds genomic RNA.

Pathogenesis. HIV selectively replicates in T4 lymphocytes (helper/inducer T cells).[5] In addition, a CD4 molecule on these T lymphocytes may be the HIV receptor. The envelope glycoprotein (gp120) component of the virus binds to the CD4 molecule on T4 inducer lymphocytes,[6] in addition to monocytes and macrophages.[7,8] HIV enters the T4 cells by an unknown mechanism, followed by viral replication and subsequent cell lysis. Monocytes and macrophages, with their lower surface density of CD4 molecules necessary for cell-to-cell fusion, are relatively refractory to HIV-induced cell killing.[8] Therefore, HIV infection of the above cells may cause host immunodeficiency by T4 cell lysis, defects in chemotaxis,[9] and deficiencies of macrophage-derived cytokines such as interferons, interleukins, and tumor necrosis factors.[10,11] Cytokine deficiencies then result in monocyte/macrophage dysfunction and abnormalities of T cell–specific immunity and B cell–antibody production. The consequences of these immune defects is susceptibility to opportunistic and common bacterial infections of many organs, including the liver. Furthermore, infection of relatively resistant cells such as monocytes and macrophages may lead to persistence of virus in the host.

Epidemiology. In the United States, AIDS has been recognized primarily among homosexual men, intravenous drug users, and recipients of blood or blood products. Cases of pediatric AIDS account for about 1.5 percent of the total AIDS cases reported to the Centers for Disease Control,[16] and the majority are younger than 6 years of age. For children, there are two important routes of transmission—maternal transfer of virus during pregnancy or the perinatal period and viral transfer through blood products. Approximately 80 percent of cases of AIDS in children are acquired via the perinatal route; most of these children are born to mothers who have AIDS or are at risk of developing the disease.[12,13] A large percentage of mothers of congenitally infected children are asymptomatic at the time of birth, but they have immunologic evidence of HIV infection. For these children, the risk of perinatal acquisition of HIV and subsequent development of AIDS or AIDS-related complex (ARC) is estimated to be as high as 50 percent,[14,15] although the precise rate of perinatal transmission is not known. The seroprevalence of HIV among childbearing women was recently estimated by measurement of antibodies contained in routinely collected neonatal blood specimens, i.e., screening for phenylketonuria (PKU).[17] HIV antibody by immunofluorescence assay or enzyme-linked immunosorbent assay (ELISA) was positive in 2.1 per 1,000 women (8.0 per 1,000 in inner-city hospitals). Breast milk has also been implicated in the transmission of HIV[18]; it is recommended that HIV infected mothers refrain from breast-feeding.

Clinical Manifestations. For perinatal HIV infection clinical symptoms can develop as early as 1 month of age, but the median interval from birth to symptoms is 8 months.[19] The most common early manifestations of disease in infants include the triad of poor growth, interstitial pneumonitis, and hepatosplenomegaly.[12–14,20–22] Infected alveolar macrophages may have a role in the lymphocytic interstitial pneumonitis seen in children with AIDS.[23] Similar involvement of hepatic macrophages has not been noted in the liver; however, it is likely that Kupffer cell hyperplasia occurs in infants and children with hepatomegaly and AIDS.

Clinical symptoms of pediatric AIDS are similar to those of adult AIDS, including fever, malaise, and recurrent and chronic infections.[20,22] Children also have central nervous system infections and associated progressive loss of developmental milestones. As in adult AIDS, opportunistic infections are frequent with pathogens such as *Pneumocystis carinii*, *Cryptosporidium*, *Mycobacterium avium-intracellulare* (MAI), cytomegalovirus (CMV), and *Herpes virus hominis*.

Craniofacial dysmorphism has been reported in patients with congenital AIDS; the features include prominent box-like head, hypertelorism, obliquity of eyes, long palpebral fissures, blue sclerae, depressed bridge of nose, prominent upper vermilion border, and triangular philtrum.[24,25] Others have not been able to confirm these findings of altered craniofacial morphogenesis in children exposed to perinatal HIV infection.[26]

Although multiorgan involvement is common in all patients with AIDS, a systematic description of the spectrum of liver disease and pathologic features in neonates and young infants with AIDS has not been reported. A form of chronic active hepatitis was discovered in four older infants (1.5 to 6 years of age) with clinical and immunologic characteristics of AIDS and ARC.[27] There was prominent T8 (cytotoxic and/or suppressor) lymphocytic infiltration in both the portal and lobular areas, piecemeal necrosis, and bridging fibrosis, in addition to prominent sinusoidal cell hyperplasia but no obvious intranuclear viral inclusions. Clinically evident opportunistic infection was not present in three of the four patients, although two had a positive serology for CMV, one had positive antibody titers to herpes simplex, and Epstein-Barr virus (EBV) serology was positive in all four patients. The precise etiology remained unclear, since marked sinusoidal cell hyperplasia and lymphocytic infiltration have been previously described in CMV[28]- and EBV[29]-induced hepatitis. Further, EBV infections of the liver are difficult to document in AIDS patients because antibodies to this virus are frequent in these patients. Of Interest is the report of one 10-year-old child with clinical AIDS, documented opportunistic infections with *Cryptosporidium* and MAI, and small epithelioid granulomas on liver histology.[30] Granulomatous involvement of the liver occurs in adult intravenous drug abusers with AIDS.[31] Cultures of liver tissue were positive for mycobacteria in the patients with abundant acid-fast bacilli (Ziehl-Nielsen method), usually MAI. MAI is the most commonly diagnosed hepatic infection in adult AIDS.[32] Generally, mycobacteria are not visualized and cultures are negative for the liver specimens of immunocompetent patients with hepatic tuberculosis.[33] The finding of hepatic granulomas with numerous bacilli is highly suggestive of AIDS, but biopsy specimens must be cultured for mycobacteria. Prolonged duration of illness and a high serum alkaline phosphatase level were significantly associated with the presence of hepatic granulomas.[39] Other opportunistic infections associated with hepatic granulomas in AIDS patients are *Mycobacterium tuberculosis*,[34] histoplasmosis,[35,38] cryptococcosis,[31,34] and rarely toxoplasmosis and CMV.[36] CMV has also been implicated as an etiologic factor in AIDS patients with a cholestatic syndrome caused by sclerosing cholangitis.[36a] Also, CMV may perturb bile ductular epithelium in the neonate,[36b] but a sclerosing cholangitis syndrome has not been described in pediatric AIDS.

In a large series of homosexual adults with AIDS, macrosteatosis and nonspecific portal inflammation were the most common histologic abnormalities.[37,38] Liver histology was seldom normal, and characteristic histologic features for AIDS were not identified. It was concluded that since the liver was frequently involved in opportunistic disseminated infections, biopsy may be useful as a diagnostic tool in selected patients with AIDS. This may be especially true in pediatric AIDS, since transplacental passage of antibody can delay the diagnosis of HIV and intrahepatic diseases cannot reliably be predicted on the basis of clinical (e.g., unexplained fever and hepatomegaly) and laboratory data.

Hepatitis B virus (HBV) has no etiologic or opportunistic role in AIDS; however, the modes of transmission of HBV and HIV are similar and the epidemiology of the two diseases has common features. The markers of past HBV infection, anti-HBs and anti-HBc, are found in about 90 percent of AIDS patients, not substantially different from their incidence in homosexuals and intravenous drug abusers without AIDS.[32,35,40] The prevalence of chronic HBV carriers (positive for HBsAg) among AIDS patients with evidence of past HBV infection is approximately 10 percent, which is similar to that of the general population.[32,35,40] Despite this widespread exposure to HBV and the inability to protect against many other viral agents, chronic active hepatitis and cirrhosis are uncommon in patients with AIDS. Perhaps this is not true for neonates and infants,[27] but the most likely explanation is that acquisition and clearance of HBV occurred prior to the onset of immunodeficiency.[37] Interestingly, in a recent study of concomitant HBV infections in patients with AIDS or ARC, DNA sequences of HBV were found in lymphocytes from patients with AIDS even in the absence of conventional HBV serologic markers.[41] This should prompt additional studies to re-evaluate a possible role of HBV as a co-factor in AIDS in addition to the HIV causal agent[41]—perhaps in the modulation of immunologic abnormalities.

Laboratory Findings. The most useful studies for AIDS screening are a complete blood count and differential, quantitative immunoglobulins, T-helper/T-suppressor cell ratios (looking for a reversal of the normal helper-to-suppressor ratio of 2:1), and HIV antibody. Polyclonal hypergammaglobulinemia often precedes abnormalities of T-cell immunity, and normal immunologic studies in an HIV antibody–positive child do not preclude the development of immunodeficiency. Immunologic abnormalities include decreased lymphocyte cytotoxicity against virus-infected cells, decreased cytokine production (e.g., interleukin), and decreased natural killer cell activity.[22] The presence of HIV antibody to the core and envelope regions of the virus antibody by ELISA screening must be confirmed by a Western blot assay. In infants, the diagnosis of HIV infection may be difficult because mothers with HIV produce IgG antibodies that are tranplacentally transferred to the fetus and may persist for longer than 12 months.[43] Because of this and the limited antibody response to HIV infection, these neonates make difficult-to-detect amounts of HIV-specific IgM antibody.[14,42] Recently, an early appearance and more specific pattern of response of anti-HIV antibody (IgM and later the IgG3 subclass) was demonstrated, suggesting perinatal infection.[43] Some infants remain antibody-negative when infected with HIV; culture of the virus may be necessary in this situation, but the methods are not readily available. The need for studies to identify opportunistic infections, pulmonary dysfunction, significant coagulopathy or anemia, and liver disease is determined by each clinical situation.

Treatment. No curative therapy exists for HIV infection, but antiviral agents such as AZT (3-azido-3-deoxythymidine) are now being actively investigated. Also, development of an effective vaccine may become a reality in the future. Patients with AIDS generally do not die from liver disease, although there can be significant morbidity related to the hepatic involvement with pathogens such as CMV and MAI.

Currently, there is no effective therapy for CMV infection, although recent adult studies suggest that the antiviral agent DHPG (dihydroxypropoxymethyl-guanine, ganciclovir) may be effective in some patients.[44] MAI is considered a low-grade pathogen, but it displays a high degree of resistance to most antimycobacterial agents. The experimental drugs ansamycin and clofazimine have shown some clinical promise.[45] The hepatitis associated with toxoplasmosis is usually a self-limited disease; however, treatment with pyrimethamine isethionate and sulfadiazine is needed in the treatment of AIDS patients. Fungal hepatitis should always be confirmed by isolation of the organism. Histoplasmosis is usually a disseminated infection in patients with AIDS and is treated with amphotericin B.[46] Amphotericin[22] combined with flucytosine is suggested for treating *Candida* hepatitis (the less common disseminated visceral involvement in children with AIDS) and disseminated cryptococcal infections involving the liver.

HEPATITIS B VIRUS

Since the discovery of a serologic marker for HBV,[47] viral hepatitis in infancy has been extensively studied and the virus is now recognized to be endemic throughout many parts of the world. It is a DNA virus and consists of surface and inner core antigens. The surface antigen (HBsAg) is the earliest indicator of the presence of acute infection. The other antigens are core antigen (HBcAg) in addition to e antigen (HBeAg) and DNA polymerase, which correlate with HBV replication. Corresponding antibodies are designated anti-HBs, anti-HBc, and anti-HBe. During recovery from HBV infection patients acquire anti-HBs, and anti-HBc is found during the acute phase of infection (IgM) or during recovery (IgG).[48] The immunobiology of HBV had led to important information regarding the mechanisms of disease, including oncogenesis, viral replication, and cellular damage. This agent was the first human virus to be unequivocally linked to the development of cancer in man.[49] Cytotoxicity of lymphocytes for liver cell antigens may be the mechanism of tissue injury rather than a direct cytopathic effect of HBV.

Epidemiology. Hepatitis B is seldom transmitted congenitally. In fact, it has been established that vertical transmission of HBV occurs from mother to infant during late pregnancy or during the perinatal period.[50] The modes of transmission include (1) possible transplacental passage of HBV; (2) transmission of contaminated maternal blood directly from mother to neonate during the birth process; (3) oral inoculation of the newborn infant by ingestion of maternal blood on passage through the dilated cervix and vagina at the time of delivery (caesarean section does not protect against HBV transmission); and (4) contact with the mother during early infancy, including the ingestion of contaminated breast milk.[51]

Most infants who develop HBV infection are probably exposed at the time of delivery, although a number of infants born to asymptomatic chronic carriers of the HBV are infected in utero.[50,52] This is especially true in women with active hepatitis during the last trimester of pregnancy. It has been estimated that 70 percent of infants born under these latter conditions receive HBV and become chronic carriers of the antigen.[50] Women who have acute hepatitis B in the first or second trimester rarely transmit HBV to their newborn infant.[50,55] HBeAg has been discovered to be more closely associated with actual HBV infection than is HBsAg; its presence in serum also appears to correlate more closely with development of the chronic carrier state in infants of HBsAg-positive mothers, up to 90 percent of infected infants.[54] Infants born to anti-HBe–positive mothers are less likely to become chronic carriers than those born to mothers with HBeAg. The exact mechanisms of transmission in the perinatal period are not clear, and, as noted above, the risks for the neonate are different depending on the time of maternal infection. This suggests that HBV passes the placenta poorly, the infant acquires passive immunization, or chronic carrier mothers have low antigen levels that do not readily traverse the placenta. The infants infected late in pregnancy or in the postpartum period are not protected by antibody and must rely on their own immature immunocompetence. These infants born to HbsAg-positive mothers do not usually manifest serologic or clinical evidence of HBV infection until 1 to 3 months of age; this also suggests that HBV transmission most likely occurs during birth. Susceptible infants are always at risk of HBV infection in families in which the HBsAg carrier rate is high.

From a world-wide perspective, the perinatal transmission of HBV is an extremely important public health problem. The highest rates of vertical transmission and HBV prevalence occur in the Far East, Africa, and Southeast Asia. In Taiwan, 20 percent of the general population are HBsAg carriers, an 18 percent prevalence of HBsAg occurs in pregnant women, and 30 to 70 percent of children born to these mothers are infected.[56] Prior to an extensive, controlled hepatitis B vaccine trial in Senegal, striking endemicity of HBV infection occurred with 12 percent of HBsAg-positive blood donors, and 80 percent of the population of 6- and 7-year-old children had at least one serum marker of past or present HBV infection.[57] In contrast, the HBV carrier rate in the United States and Europe is less than 0.5 percent.[58] Where HBV is endemic, the relative risk of primary hepatocellular carcinoma in carriers to that of noncarriers is over 200 to 1.[49]

Clinical Manifestations. The HBV-infected neonate is usually asymptomatic, but mild clinical hepatitis may become apparent. After perinatal acquisition of HBV, most infants develop the chronic carrier state.[59] In rare instances, fulminant hepatitis can occur[60]; this may be more common in infants of mothers who are chronic HBV carriers.[63] Some children have mild abnormalities of liver function and eventually develop chronic liver dysfunction, but no data are available about the frequency with which HBsAg-carrier infants and children develop chronic active hepatitis and cirrhosis.[58] It is known, however, that even in countries with a high frequency of perinatal HBV transmission, chronic hepatitis and cirrhosis occur most often among adults—not in infancy and childhood.[58] The long-term consequences of asymptomatic HBV in neonates are more worrisome, especially the high risk of hepatocellular carcinoma among middle-aged men.[49] Another alarming finding is that approximately 50 percent of Taiwanese male HBsAg carriers die from the consequences hepatocellular carcinoma or cirrhosis.[61] The prevention of neonatal HBV hepatitis could eventually decrease the incidence of hepatocellular carcinoma and cirrhosis in many parts of the world.[62]

Screening and Prevention. It is appropriate to screen pregnant women at high risk for the HBV carrier state. If possible, this should be done before delivery of the in utero HBV-exposed child. There are certain aspects of a mother's history that indicate a need for prenatal HBsAg and anti-HBc–IgM screening, e.g., occupational exposure (Table 1). All infants born to high-risk mothers should be tested after birth if prenatal screening was not completed. The diagnosis of HBV infection is confirmed by detection of HBsAg or anti-HBc–IgM in the newborn's serum. Treatment with hepatitis B immunoglobulin and vaccine is instituted immediately if the neonate is found to be serologically negative.

Excellent HBV vaccines (e.g., Heptavax B) have been prepared using noninfectious HBsAg particles from the blood of HBsAg-positive donors.[64] They are subjected to extensive purification and inactivation steps; no bacterial or viral agent has been known to survive this process, including HIV.[65] Recombivax-HB, a yeast recombinant (DNA) vaccine with comparable immunogenicity, was recently licensed by the Food and Drug Administration.[66] Primary vaccination for perinatal postexposure prophylaxis consists of three intramuscular 10-μg doses of HBV vaccine, with the first given within 12 hours of birth and the second and third given 1 and 6 months, respectively, after the initial dose. The anterolateral thigh muscle is used in neonates and infants, but vaccines should be given in the deltoid muscle in older children to guarantee high immunogenicity. For the neonate, 0.5 ml of hepatitis B immunoglobulin (HBIG) is given with HBV vaccine (concurrently but at a separate site) within 12 hours of birth.

TABLE 1
Aspects of a Mother's History That Make Careful Prenatal HBsAg Screening Mandatory*

1. Asian, Alaskan Eskimo, or Pacific island descent
2. Haitian, sub-Saharan African, Far Eastern, Southeast Asian birth
3. History of:
   - Acute or chronic liver disease
   - Occupational exposure (e.g., institution for mentally retarded, hospital, hemodialysis unit)
   - Rejection as a blood donor
   - Numerous blood transfusions
   - Intravenous drug abuse
   - Multiple episodes of venereal disease
   - AIDS
   - Household contact with HBV carrier

*Adapted from CDC[71] and Snydman.[62]

It has been demonstrated that no statistically significant advantage is gained from multiple doses of HBIG compared with a single dose.[67,68] Conclusive evidence from two important studies also favored the combination of active and passive immunization[67,68] for infants born to HBsAg-positive chronic carrier mothers. The overall protective efficiency rate in the HBV vaccine and HBIG groups of the Taiwan study exceeded 93 percent, which was substantial improvement over administration of either HBV or HBIG prophylaxis alone.[67] The Hong Kong study[68] used a higher dose of HBIG (1 ml versus 0.5 ml), HBV vaccine was inactivated by heat rather than formalin, and a smaller dose of HBV vaccine was given (20 μg versus 3 μg) within 1 hour of birth. Despite the above differences, the findings of both studies were similar; i.e., efficacy rates were above 90 percent (even with the smaller 3-μg dose of HBV vaccine the immunogenicity was high). It is noteworthy that administration of HBIG to infants born to mothers with acute hepatitis B during the third trimester of pregnancy was effective in preventing perinatal transmission of HBV.[69] However, with the availability of HBV vaccine, the current recommendation that ensures long-lasting immunity is use of combination therapy as previously described. Mothers who are positive for HBsAg and anti-HBe are not necessarily noninfectious; their infants should also receive combination prophylaxis. HBV vaccine offers no therapeutic benefit when given to HBV carriers.[70] The issue of booster immunizations after the third dose of HBV vaccine awaits future study.

HEPATITIS A; NON-A, NON-B; AND D VIRUSES

Hepatitis A (HAV), an RNA virus, is transmitted by the fecal-oral route (ingestion of contaminated food or water). Pregnant women with hepatitis A infection probably do not transmit HAV to their infants, and it is generally assumed that this virus does not pose a risk to the fetus.[55] However, neonates may be at a small risk of HAV infection if acute hepatitis occurs less than 2 weeks before the termination of pregnancy.[58] Under these circumstances, it would be prudent to administer a single 0.5-ml dose of intramuscular immune serum globulin (ISG) shortly after birth. A chronic carrier state for HAV has never been demonstrated. Therefore, isolation of infants from mothers convalescing from HAV hepatitis is not necessary.[58]

Until recently there have been no serologic markers for *non-A, non-B (NANB) virus*, and it has been impossible to detect a carrier state during pregnancy. However, there have been infants born to mothers with abnormal liver function; in this situation, fetal transmission of virus could potentially occur, since NANB virus appears to have epidemiologic characteristics similar to those of HBV.[55] Despite the controversy in older children and adults about efficacy of ISG for the prevention of post-transfusion hepatitis, it is reasonable to administer intramuscular ISG (0.5 ml) to the neonate acutely exposed to NANB virus soon after birth and 1 month later.[72]

Transmission of the *hepatitis D virus (delta agent)* from mother to infant has been reported.[73] This RNA virus requires HBV for replication; therefore, it is possible that the transmission of delta agent and HBV to the infant, and prevention of disease for both, are similar. The delta agent frequently is responsible for more serious liver disease such as fulminant hepatitis. No therapy is available to treat this viral infection, which is currently not common in the United States.

PERINATAL BACTERIAL INFECTIONS

Clinical Manifestations and Diagnosis. The temporal association between hyperbilirubinemia and sepsis (or bacteremia) has been well documented in neonates and infants.[74–76] The prompt diagnosis of sepsis is often difficult because jaundice may be the only clinical manifestation in an otherwise healthy-appearing neonate, and its relationship to infection should never be overlooked. Disproportionate hyperbilirubinemia is probably less common in infants with bacteremia than in older children and adults, except for neonates with hemolysis during the early phase of sepsis, when they experience elevated indirect bilirubin levels.[76] Despite this, jaundice should not divert attention from other systemic (extrahepatic) problems such as urinary tract infection.[74,77–79] In fact, the agent most commonly reported in neonates with sepsis is the gram-negative bacterium *Escherichia coli*, and the most common site of infection is the urinary tract. Jaundice is usually prominent in the second week of life after the illness becomes established. At this time, serum bilirubin levels may exceed 10 mg per deciliter and are predominantly direct-reacting with serum transaminase levels mildly elevated or normal. A variety of other clinical manifestations generally become apparent at the end of the first week of life, including anorexia, lethargy, and unsatisfactory progression of weight gain. Urinary tract symptoms are difficult to detect and fever is rare. Therefore, the routine evaluation of infants with jaundice must always include a urinalysis and urine culture in addition to blood cultures. Pyuria is often discovered, urine cultures are diagnostic, and structural anomalies of the genitourinary tract are not commonly found.[79] Liver histologic findings include Kupffer cell hyperplasia and cholestasis; liver biopsy is not required to make the correct diagnosis.

Pathogenesis. Neonates have a greater susceptibility to gram-negative bacterial infections. However, the mechanism(s) for hyperbilirubinemia associated with sepsis is not known. Bilirubin "overload" from brisk hemolysis and hepatocellular damage is more likely to occur in infancy. This may reflect immaturity of their biliary excretory mechanisms.[80] and the unique pathologic response of the neonatal liver (e.g., lobular disorganization, giant cell transformation, and active fibroblast proliferation) to a variety of insults including infection. One mechanism may be inhibition of membrane Na^+,K^+-ATPase by the lipid A moiety of endotoxin, which interferes with the excretion of direct-reacting bilirubin into the bile canaliculi.[81–83] Even though all bacteria do not produce toxin, there is little evidence that direct invasion of liver parenchyma is responsible for the hepatic abnormalities in sepsis. Bacteria are rarely isolated from the liver—even organisms that infect the liver in unique ways, e.g., gonococcal infection causing perihepatitis. This is intriguing, since the liver is exposed to bacteria from both the systemic and portal circulations. In this regard, Kupffer cells, which can interact with other cellular components of the hepatic sinusoids and with hepatocytes, are capable of clearing bacteria from the blood. An inflammatory stimulus may lead to elaboration of secretory products from hepatic parenchymal macrophages producing local hepatocyte damage. Endotoxin-exposed Kupffer cells can exert potentially harmful effects on hepatocyte function during sepsis[84] and after interaction with inflammatory macrophages are able to induce liver injury via leukotrienes.[85]

Gram-positive infections are common in neonates, but associated liver abnormalities are distinctly uncommon. Infection with *Listeria monocytogenes* is an exception in that hepatic manifestations are always present.[86] The modes of transmission include transplacental passage or inoculation of the neonate on passage through an infected cervix or vagina. These neonates are critically ill and most develop meningitis, but some have jaundice and hepatomegaly. The liver pathology is highly abnormal, and two histologic forms are described: (1) diffuse hepatitis and (2) the more common demarcated areas of necrosis or microabscesses that contain the pleomorphic gram-positive bacilli.

Less common hepatic infections include tuberculosis resulting from transplacental dissemination to the fetus.[63] MAI, the most commonly diagnosed hepatic infection in adult AIDS,[32] could be recognized in the future as a potential problem for infants born to mothers with this devastating disease.

TABLE 2
TORCH Infections: Clinical Manifestations That Suggest a Specific Diagnosis*

Agent	Clinical Findings
Toxoplasmosis	Hydrocephalus with intracranial calcifications Microcephaly Chorioretinitis AIDS
Syphilis	Rhinitis (snuffles) Rash Osteitis
Rubella	Cataracts, cloudy cornea Deafness Petechiae ("blueberry muffin") Cardiac malformations
Cytomegalovirus	Microcephaly with periventricular calcifications Deafness AIDS
Herpes	Rash (skin vesicles) Keratoconjunctivitis Acute central nervous system disease

*Adapted from Alpert and Plotkin.[88]

TORCH INFECTIONS

The acronym TORCH (*t*oxoplasmosis, *r*ubella, *c*ytomegalovirus, and *h*erpes simplex) was coined to call attention to a specific group of pathogens that share similar features in the infected fetus and neonate.[87] Infections by these agents are often clinically indistinguishable and can be inapparent in both the neonate and mother. Unfortunately, serious sequelae commonly occur even in asymptomatic infants.[88] Although additional agents are reported to produce similar congenital problems, only the original pathogens will be discussed: *Toxoplasma gondii, Treponema pallidum,* rubella virus, cytomegalovirus, and *Herpes virus hominis*. The incidence of these infections is high, occurring in 0.5 to 2.5 percent of births.[88]

Subsequent discussion will focus on the liver, which is frequently involved in congenital infections. In addition to hepatosplenomegaly and liver dysfunction, other organ systems can be affected, causing neurologic impairment (microcephaly, chorioretinitis), skin manifestations, and congenital anomalies (especially involving the heart and eye). As listed in Table 2, certain clinical features are associated with specific pathogens.

Toxoplasmosis

Epidemiology. When acute *T. gondii* infection occurs during pregnancy, it can cross the placenta and infect the fetus; the earlier the transmission, the more severe are the congenital lesions. Acquisition of maternal infection during the first two trimesters almost always leads to severe disease, whereas later acquisition usually results in subclinical or no fetal infections.[89] Also, fetuses of women with prepregnancy antibodies in their serum are not at risk of being infected by *Toxoplasma*. In addition to placental transmission, this organism can be acquired by ingestion of poorly cooked or raw infected meat and through direct exposure to *Toxoplasma* oocysts excreted in the feces of infected cats.[90] This parasite is an obligate intracellular organism that can live in most cells except non-nucleated erythrocytes.[91]

Clinical Manifestations and Diagnosis. The infant with severe congenital infection has hydrocephalus or microcephaly, chorioretinitis, and psychomotor retardation. The parasite is widely distributed in the host including in the liver, but isolation of *Toxoplasma* from the liver is rare. Hepatomegaly and jaundice are only occasionally noted. Surprisingly, the hepatic histology is not unique; there can be periportal inflammation and marked extramedullary hematopoiesis.[63] Hepatitis may be the only manifestation of the disease.[89] Microcalcifications have been noted in the liver on plain films of the abdomen.[92]

Toxoplasmosis frequently occurs in HIV-infected individuals. Serologic screening for *Toxoplasma* infection should be completed in pregnant females with AIDS to assist in early diagnosis and consideration of prenatal therapy[93] if there is a wish to continue the pregnancy. Toxoplasmic encephalitis is now the most commonly recognized cause of opportunistic infection of the central nervous system in patients with AIDS.[94]

The IgM-ELISA test is highly sensitive and specific for the diagnosis of congenital *Toxoplasma* infection.[95] It avoids the false-negative results caused by high levels of maternal IgG antibody that occur in the IgM-IFA test. In the congenitally infected infant, antibody titer may drop initially, and only after 6 to 12 months will an increase in antibody titer be detected.[88]

Treatment. If seroconversion is noted, pyrimethamine isethionate and sulfadiazine should be given.

Congenital Syphilis

Clinical Manifestations and Diagnosis. Congenital syphilis infection occurs in utero. It was a frequent cause of neonatal death before the discovery of penicillin and continues to be a major problem in developing countries. When the typical features of this infection (rash, snuffles, and bone lesions) are associated with hepatosplenomegaly, the diagnosis is easy to make at birth. Jaundice is often present, appearing in the first 24 hours after birth, or a delayed onset may be observed.[63] The liver histologic findings may be a characteristic centrilobular fibrosis with mononuclear infiltration or a more typical neonatal hepatitis pattern consisting of cellular infiltration of the parenchyma with lobular disorganization and giant cell transformation, or they may be completely normal.[96]

The diagnosis of congenital syphilis is based on serologic testing. First, a nontreponemal test such as Venereal Disease Research Laboratory (VDRL) or rapid plasma reagin (RPR) should be performed. Confirmatory tests are for specific treponemal antibodies, e.g., the fluorescent treponemal antibody absorption (FTA-ABS) test.[88] Confusion with passive transfer of maternal antibody should not be a problem after 4 months of age.

Treatment. Cases of treatment failure have been seen in infants given benzathine penicillin. Hence, the most appropriate approach to active infection is the 10-day regimen of crystalline or procaine penicillin. However, the administration of penicillin can precipitate or exacerbate liver dysfunction in patients with congenital syphilis.[115] It is speculated that the products of *Treponema* lysis cause a toxic reaction, e.g., a hepatic Herxheimer reaction.

Rubella

Epidemiology. The transplacental origin of rubella infection has been well documented.[97] Prenatal infection can occur during the first trimester and result in chronic multisystem disease. Widespread use of the rubella vaccine, however, has had a profound effect on the epidemiology of rubella in the United States; i.e., there has been a progressive decline in the number of reported cases.

Clinical Manifestations and Diagnosis. When this disease occurs the most commonly reported problems include visual impairment, congenital heart disease, microcephaly, and deafness. Also, liver involvement is frequent in congenital rubella, and hepatomegaly is a constant feature. Results of liver function tests are nonspecific. Histologically, mononuclear inflammatory infiltrates are prominent in the portal tracts and intralobular fibrosis and persistence of extramedullary hematopoiesis are present.[98] More characteristic findings of hepatitis also occur and persist well into the first year.[99]

Congenital rubella infection should be diagnosed by a culture of the virus because all infected neonates shed the rubella virus. If this is not possible, serologic tests are available. A latex agglutination test has recently become available.[88,100] If it is positive, an attempt should be made to detect specific IgM antirubella antibody.

Cytomegalovirus

Epidemiology. Neonates are infected with CMV in utero, at the time of birth, or later in the postpartum period from maternal saliva or milk.[101] It is a significant problem throughout the world and may occur in up to 2 percent of all live births.[102] Few of these infants demonstrate clinical symptoms. Maternal immunity to CMV, unlike immunity to rubella and toxoplasmosis, does not prevent virus reactivation, nor does it control the spread of virus that can produce congenital infection.[107]

Clinical Manifestations and Diagnosis. A well-described syndrome of microcephaly, cerebral calcifications, deafness, and hepatosplenomegaly occurs in congenital CMV infection. The onset of hepatomegaly and jaundice usually occurs within the first day of life. The histopathology of the liver reveals a severe inflammatory reaction. Intranuclear and intracytoplasmic inclusion bodies are rarely detected in bile duct epithelia and in hepatocytes.[103] Radiographic evidence of calcifications in the liver has been noted in congenital CMV disease.[109] Generally, there is no evidence of severe liver disease after prolonged follow-up evaluation, in contrast to the devastating effects on the central nervous system.[103,108] However, CMV has been reported to be a common associated infection in Chinese infants with neonatal hepatitis of poor outcome[106]; also, biliary cirrhosis and noncirrhotic portal fibrosis have been rarely described in children.[104,114]

As previously mentioned, a newly recognized complication of AIDS, papillary stenosis with sclerosing cholangitis, has been associated with CMV.[36a] A large percentage of adults with AIDS have CMV infection or viremia.[105] Defective cell-mediated immunity presumably predisposes to reactivation of latent CMV disease.

All CMV-infected neonates shed the virus in their urine from the time of birth. The diagnosis is confirmed by demonstrating the presence of CMV in the urine. Serology has a limited role; however, a new CMV-specific IgM-ELISA test may prove reliable in the future.[88]

Treatment. No effective drug therapy exists for CMV infection. However, therapeutic trials with DHPG[44] are being conducted in older children and adult transplant recipients.[110]

Herpes Simplex

Epidemiology. Maternal herpes (HSV) infection can result in congenital and perinatal infections in the neonate, even subsequent to a first episode of genital herpes, because of asymptomatic cervical shedding of the virus.[111] There is a 40 percent serious perinatal morbidity in affected women, especially those who acquire infection in the third trimester of pregnancy, making preventive measures, including antiviral chemotherapy, extremely important.[111] Neonates born to mothers with a recurrent HSV infection are likely to have HSV antibody at birth.

Clinical Manifestations and Diagnosis. Within the first hours of life, the neonate with HSV infection appears seriously ill with generalized acute disease, and there are usually signs of encephalitis. The associated ulcerative, vesicular, or purpuric skin lesions are diagnostic. HSV hepatitis may be part of the acute disease[112]; it is often severe, with jaundice and coagulation abnormalities. Liver histologic findings reveal multifocal necrosis of the hepatic parenchyma, in addition to characteristic intranuclear inclusions in hepatocytes.

The smear of a skin vesicle or ulceration is the most rapid way to make a diagnosis. Scrapings are examined for giant cells, which are diagnostic for HSV infection.[88] Viral cultures are needed to confirm the diagnosis.

Treatment. Acyclovir is useful in pregnant women with disseminated HSV infections. Intravenous vidarabine therapy of neonates with HSV is valuable in that mortality can be decreased in infants with disseminated and central nervous system disease.[113] Infection in the neonate may be prevented by caesarean section delivery.

REFERENCES

1. Gottlieb MS, Schroff R, Schanker HM, Weisman JD, Fan PT, Wolf RA, Saxon A. *Pneumocystis carinii* pneumonia and mucosal candidiasis in previously healthy homosexual men: evidence of a new acquired cellular immunodeficiency. N Engl J Med 1981; 305:1425–1431.
2. Barre-Sinoussi F, Chermann JC, Rey F, Nugeyre MT, Chamaret S, Gruest J, Dauguet C, Axler-Blin C, Vezinet-Brun F, Rouzioux C, Rozenbaum W, Montagnier L. Isolation of a T-lymphotropic retrovirus from a patient at risk for the acquired immune deficiency syndrome (AIDS). Science 1983; 220:868–871.
3. Gallo RC, Salahuddin SZ, Popovic M. Frequent detection and isolation of cytopathic retroviruses (HTLV-III) from patients with AIDS and at risk for AIDS. Science 1984; 224:500–503.
4. Popovic M, Sarngatharan MG, Read E, Gallo RC. Detection, isolation, and continuous production of cytopathic retroviruses (HTLV-III) from patients with AIDS and pre-AIDS. Science 1984; 224:497–500.
5. Klatzmann D, Barre-Sinoussi F, Nugeyre MT, Danguet C, Vilmer E, Griscelli C, Vezinet-Brun F, Rouzioux C, Gluckman JC, Cherman JC, Montagnier L. Selective tropism of lymphadenopathy associated virus (LAV) for helper-inducer T lymphocytes. Science 1984; 225:59–64.
6. Ho DD, Pomerance RJ, Kaplan JC. Pathogenesis of infection with human immunodeficiency virus. N Engl J Med 1987; 317:278–286.
7. Ho DD, Rota TR, Hirsch MS. Infection of monocytes/macrophages by human T lymphotropic virus type III. J Clin Invest 1986; 77:1712–1715.
8. Gartner S, Markovits P, Markovitz DM, Kaplan MH, Gallo RC, Popovic M. The role of mononuclear phagocytes in HTLV-III/LAV infection. Science 1986; 233:215–219.
9. Smith PD, Ohura K, Masur H, Lane HC, Funci AS, Wahl SM. Monocyte function in the acquired immune deficiency syndrome: defective chemotaxis. J Clin Invest 1984; 74:2121–2128
10. Ammann AJ. The immunology of pediatric AIDS. In: Report of the Surgeon General's Workshop on Children with HIV Infection and Their Families. DHHS publication No. HRS-D-MC 87-1, 1987:13–16.
11. Seligmann M, Chess L, Fahey JL, Fauci AS, Lachmann PJ, L'Age-Stehr J, Ngu J, Pinching AJ, Rosen FS, Spira TJ, Wybran J. AIDS—an immunologic re-evaluation. N Engl J Med 1984; 311:1286–1292.
12. Rogers MF, Thomas PA, Starcher ET, Noa MC, Bush TJ, Jaffe HW. Acquired immunodeficiency syndrome in children: report of the Centers for Disease Control National Surveillance, 1982-1985. Pediatrics 1987; 79:1008–1014.
13. Shannon KM, Ammann AJ. Acquired immune deficiency syndrome in childhood. J Pediatr 1985; 106:332–342.
14. Pahwa S, Kaplan M, Fifrig S, Pahwa R, Sarngadharan MG, Popovic M, Gallo RC. Spectrum of human T-cell lymphotropic virus type III infection in children: recognition of symptomatic, asymptomatic, and seronegative patients. JAMA 1986; 255:2299–2305.
15. Rubinstein A, Bernstein L: The epidemiology of pediatric acquired immunodeficiency syndrome. Clin Immunol Immunopathol 1986; 40:115–121.
16. Osterholm MT, MacDonald KL. Facing the complex issues of pediatric AIDS: a public health perspective. JAMA 1987; 258:2736–2737.
17. Hoff R, Berardi VP, Weiblen BJ, Mahoney-Trout L, Mitchell ML, Grady GF. Seroprevalence of human immunodeficiency virus among childbearing women. N Engl J Med 1988; 318:525–530.
18. Ziegler JB, Cooper DA, Johnson RO, Gold J. Postnatal transmission of AIDS associated retrovirus from mother to infant. Lancet 1985; i:896–897.
19. Rogers MF. AIDS in children: a review of the clinical epidemiologic and public health aspects. Pediatr Infect Dis 1985; 4:230–236.
20. Oleske J, Minnefor A, Cooper R, Thomas K, delaCruz A, Houman A, Guerrero I, Joshi VV, Desposito F. Immune deficiency syndrome in children. JAMA 1983; 249:2345–2349.
21. Scott GB, Buck BE, Leterman JG, Bloom FL, Parks WP. Acquired immunodeficiency syndrome in infants. N Engl J Med 1984; 310:76–81.
22. Ammann AJ, Shannon KM. Recognition of acquired immune deficiency syndrome (AIDS) in children. Pediatr Rev 1985; 7:101–107.
23. Chayt KJ, Harper ME, Marselle LM, Lewin EB, Rose RM, Oleske JM, Epstein LG, Wong-Staal F, Gallo RC. Detection of HTLV-III RNA in lungs of patients with AIDS and pulmonary involvement. JAMA 1986; 256:2356–2359.
24. Marion RW, Wizma AA, Hutcheon RG, Rubinstein A. Fetal AIDS syndrome score: correlation between severity of dysmorphism and age at diagnosis of immunodeficiency. Am J Dis Child 1987; 141:429–431.
25. Iosub S, Bamji M, Store RK, Gromisch DS, Wasserman E. More on human immunodeficiency virus embryopathy. Pediatrics 1987; 80:512–516.
26. Qazi QH, Sheikh TM, Fikrig S, Menikoff H. Lack of evidence for craniofacial dysmorphism in perinatal human immunodeficiency virus infection. J Pediatr 1988; 112:7–11.
27. Duffy LF, Daum F, Kahn E, Teichberg S, Pahwa R, Fagin J, Kenigsberg K, Kaplan M, Fisher SE, Pahwa S. Hepatitis in children with acquired immune deficiency syndrome: histopathologic and immunocytologic features. Gastroenterology 1986; 90:173–181.
28. Sack SL, Freeman HJ. Cytomegalovirus hepatitis: evidence for direct hepatic viral infection using monoclonal antibodies. Gastroenterology 1984; 86:346–350.
29. Carter RL, Penman HG. Histopathology of infectious mononucleosis. In: Carter RL, Penman HS, eds. Infectious mononucleosis. London: Blackwell Scientific, 1969: 146.
30. Patrick CC, Hawkins EP, Guerra C, Taber LH. A patient with leukemia in remission and acute abdominal pain (clinical conference). J Pediatr 1987; 111:624–628.
31. Orenstein MS, Tavitian A, Yonk B, Dincsoy HP, Zerega J, Iyer SK, Straus EW. Granulomatous involvement of the liver in patients with AIDS. Gut 1985; 26:1220–1225.
32. Lebovics E, Dworkin BM, Heier SK, Rosenthal WS. The hepatobiliary manifestations of human immunodeficiency virus infection. Am J Gastroenterol 1988; 83:1–7.
33. Korn RJ, Kellow WF, Heller P, Chomet B, Zimmerman HJ. Hepatic involvement in extrapulmonary tuberculosis: histologic and functional features. Am J Med 1959; 27:60–71.
34. Devars du Mayne JF, Marche C, Penalba C. Atteintes hépatiques au cours du syndrome d'immunodépression acquiré: étude de 20 case. Presse Med 1985; 14:1177–1180.
35. Dworkin BW, Stahl RE, Giardina MA, Wormser GP, Weiss L, Jankowski R, Rosenthal WS. The liver in acquired immune deficiency syndrome: emphasis on patients with intravenous drug abuse. Am J Gastroenterol 1987; 82:231–236.
36. Clarke J, Craig RM, Saffro R, Murphy P, Hidijiro Y. Cytomegalovirus granulomatous hepatitis. Am J Med 1979; 66:264–269.

36a. Jacobson MA, Cello JP, Sande MA. Cholestasis and disseminated cytomegalovirus disease in patients with the acquired immunodeficiency syndrome. Am J Med 1988; 84:218–224.

36b. Finegold MJ, Carpenter RJ. Obliterative cholangitis due to cytomegalovirus: a possible precursor of paucity of intrahepatic bile ducts. Hum Pathol 1982; 13:662–665.

37. Schneiderman DM, Arenson DM, Cello JP, Margaretten W, Weber TE. Hepatic disease in patients with the acquired immune deficiency syndrome (AIDS). Hepatology 1987; 7:925–930.
38. Lebovics E, Thung SN, Schnaffner F, Radensky DW. The liver in the acquired immunodeficiency syndrome: a clinical and histologic study. Hepatology 1985; 5:293–298.
39. Kahn SA, Saltzman BR, Klein RS, Mahadevia PS, Friedland GH, Brandt LJ. Hepatic disorders in the acquired immune deficiency syndrome: a clinical and pathological study. Am J Gastroenterol 1986; 81:1145–1148.
40. Rustgi VK, Hoofnagle JH, Gerin JC, Gelmann EP, Reichert CM, Cooper JN, Macher AM. Hepatitis B virus infection in the acquired immunodeficiency syndrome. Ann Intern Med 1984; 101:795–797.

41. Laure F, Zaqury D, Sannot AG, Gallo RC, Hahn BH, Brechot C. Hepatitis B virus DNA sequences in lymphoid cells from patients with AIDS and AIDS-related complex. Science 1985; 229:561–563.
42. Johnson JP, Nair P, Alexander S. Early diagnosis of HIV infection in the neonate. N Engl J Med 1987; 316:273–274.
43. Pyun KO, Ochs HD, Dufford MTW, Wedgwood RJ. Perinatal infection with human immunodeficiency virus: specific antibody responses by the neonate. N Engl J Med 1987; 317:611–613.
44. Collaborative DHPG Treatment Study Group. Treatment of serious cytomegalovirus infections with 9-(1,3 dihydroxy-2-propoxymethyl) guanine in patients with AIDS and other immunodeficiencies. N Engl J Med 1986; 314:801–805.
45. Murray JF, Felton CR, Garay SM, Gottlieb MS, Hopewell PC, Stover DE, Teirstein AS. Pulmonary complications of the acquired immunodeficiency syndrome. N Engl J Med 1984; 310:1682–1688.
46. Wheat LJ, Slama TG, Zeckel ML. Histoplasmosis in the acquired immune deficiency syndrome. Am J Med 1985; 78:203–210.
47. Blumberg BS, Alter HJ, Visnich S. A "new" antigen in leukemia sera. JAMA 1965; 191:541–546.
48. Werner BG, Dienstag JL, Kuter BJ. Immunologic responses to hepatitis B virus and their interpretations. In: Millman J, Eisenstein TK, Blumberg BS, eds. Hepatitis B: the virus, the disease, and the vaccine. New York: Plenum, 1984: 105.
49. Beasley RP, Hwang SY, Lin CC, Chien SC. Hepatocellular carcinoma and HBV: A prospective study of 22707 men in Taiwan. Lancet 1981; ii:1129–1133.
50. Schweitzer IL, Dunn AEG, Peters RL, Spears RL. Viral hepatitis B in neonates and infants. Am J Med 1973; 55:762–771.
51. Boxall EH, Flewett TH, Dane DS, Cameron CH, MacCallum FO, Lee TW. Hepatitis B surface antigen in breast milk. Lancet 1974; ii:1007–1008.
52. Wong VCW, Lee AKY, Ip Hm. Transmission of hepatitis B antigens from symptom free carrier mothers to the fetus and the infant. Br J Obstet Gynecol 1980; 87:958–965.
53. Magnius LO, Lindholm A. Lundin P, Iwarson S. A new antigen- antibody system: clinical significance of long term carriers of hepatitis B surface antigen. JAMA 1975; 231:356–359.
54. Okada K, Kamiyama I, Inomata M, Imai M, Miyakawa Y, Mayumi M. e-Antigen and anti-e in the serum of asymptomatic carrier mothers as indicators of positive and negative transmission of hepatitis B virus to their infants. N Engl J Med 1976; 294:746–749.
55. Tong MJ, Thursby M, Rakela J, McPeak C, Edwards VM, Mosley JW. Studies on the maternal-infant transmission of viruses which cause hepatitis. Gastroenterology 1981; 80:999–1004.
56. Chen DS, Hsu NH, Sung JL, Hsu TC, Hsu ST, Kuo YT, Lo KJ. A mass vaccination program in Taiwan against hepatitis B virus infection in infants of hepatitis B surface antigen-carrier mothers. JAMA 1987; 257:2597–2603.
57. Maupas P, Barin F, Chiron JP, Coursaget P, Goudeau A, Perrin J, Denis F, Diop Mar I. Efficacy of hepatitis B vaccine in prevention of early HBsAg carrier state in children: controlled trial in an endemic area (Senegal). Lancet 1981; i:289–292.
58. Stevens CE, Krugman S, Szmuness W, Beasley RP. Viral hepatitis in pregnancy: problems for the clinician dealing with the infant. Pediatr Rev 1980; 2:121–125.
59. Schweitzer IL, Dunn AEG, Peters RL, Spears RL. Viral hepatitis B in neonates and infants. Am J Med 1973; 55:762–771.
60. Delaplane D, Yoger R, Crussi F, Shulman ST. Fatal hepatitis B in early infancy: the importance of identifying HBsAg-positive pregnant women and providing immunoprophylaxis to their newborns. Pediatrics 1983; 72:176–180.
61. Beasley RP, Hwang LY. Epidemiology of hepatocellular carcinoma. In: Vyas GN, Dientag JL, Hoofnagle JH, eds. Viral hepatitis and liver disease. New York: Grune and Stratton, 1984; 209.
62. Snydman DR. Hepatitis in pregnancy. N Engl J Med 1985; 313:1398–1401.
63. Watkins JB, Sunaryo FP, Berezin SH. Hepatic manifestations of congenital and perinatal disease. Clin Perinatol 1981;8:467–480.
64. Hilleman MR, Buynak EB, McAleer WJ, McLean AA, Provost PJ, Tytell A. Hepatitis A and hepatitis B vaccines. In: Szmuness W, Alter HJ, Maynard JE, eds. Viral hepatitis 1981 International Symposium. Philadelphia: Franklin Institute Press, 1982: 385.
65. Stevens CE, Taylor PE, Rubinstein P, Ting RC, Bodner AJ, Sarhgadharan MG, Gallo RC. Safety of the hepatitis B vaccine. N Engl J Med 1985; 312:375–376.
66. Stevens CE, Taylor PE, Tong MJ, Toy PY, Vyas GN, Nair PV, Weissman JY, Krugman S. Yeast-recombinant hepatitis B vaccine: efficacy with hepatitis B immune globulin in prevention of perinatal hepatitis B virus transmission. JAMA 1987; 257:2612–2616.
67. Beasley RP, Lee GCY, Roan CH, Wang LYH, Lan CC, Huang FY, Chen CC. Prevention of perinatally transmitted hepatitis B virus infection with hepatitis B immune globulin and hepatitis B vaccine. Lancet 1983; ii:1099–1102.
68. Wong VCW, Ip HMH, Reesink HW, Nco Lelie P, Reerink-Brongers EE, Yeung CY, Ma HK. Prevention of the HBsAg carrier state in newborn infants of mothers who are chronic carriers of HBsAg and HBeAg by administration of hepatitis B vaccine and hepatitis B immunoglobulin. Lancet 1984; i:921–926.
69. Tong MJ, Nair PV, Thursby M, Schweitzer IL. Prevention of hepatitis B infection by hepatitis B immune globulin in infant born to mothers with acute hepatitis during pregnancy. Gastroenterology 1985; 89:160–164.
70. Dienstag JL, Stevens CE, Bhan AK, Szmuness W. Hepatitis B vaccine administered to chronic carriers of hepatitis B surface antigen. Ann Intern Med 1982; 96:575–579.
71. Recommendations for protection against viral hepatitis. MMWR 1985; 4:313–335.
72. Seeff LB, Hoofnagle JH. Immunoprophylaxis of viral hepatitis. Gastroenterology 1979; 77:161–182.
73. Zanetti AR, Ferroni P, Magliano EM. Perinatal transmission of the hepatitis B virus and of the HBV-associated delta agent from mothers to offspring in northern Italy. J Med Virol 1982; 9:139–148.
74. Hamilton JR, Sass-Kortsak A. Jaundice associated with severe bacterial infection in young infants. J Pediatr 1963; 63:121–132.
75. Bernstein J, Brown AK. Sepsis and jaundice in early infancy. Pediatrics 1962; 29:873–882.
76. Franson TR, Hierholzer WJ, LaBrecque DR. Frequency and characteristics of hyperbilirubinemia associated with bacteremia. Rev Infect Dis 1985; 7:1–9.
77. Seeler RA, Hahn K. Jaundice in urinary tract infection in infancy. Am J Dis Child 1969; 118:553–558.
78. Rooney JC, Hill DJ, Danks DM. Jaundice associated with bacterial infection in the newborn. Am J Dis Child 1971; 122:39–41.
79. Littlewood JM. 66 Infants with urinary tract infection in first month of life. Arch Dis Child 1972; 47:218–226.
80. Watkins JB, Ingall D, Szczepanik P, Klein PD, Lester R. Bile salt metabolism in newborn. Measurement of pool size and synthesis by stable isotope technique. N Engl J Med 1973; 288:431–434.
81. Utili R, Abernathy CO, Zimmerman HJ. Cholestatic effects of *Escherichia coli* endotoxin on the isolated perfused rat liver. Gastroenterology 1976; 70:248–253.
82. Utili R, Abernathy CO, Zimmerman HJ. Inhibition of Na, K- adenosine triphosphatase by endotoxin: a possible mechanism for endotoxin-induced cholestasis. J Infect Dis 1977; 136:583–587.
83. Nolan JP. The role of endotoxin in liver injury. Gastroenterology 1975; 69:1346–1356.
84. Keller GA, West MA, Harty JT, Wilkes LA, Cerra FB, Simmons RL. Modulation of hepatocyte protein synthesis by endotoxin activated Kupffer cells. Ann Surg 1985; 201:436–443.
85. Keppler D, Hagmann W, Rapp S, Denzlinger C, Koch HK. The relation of leukotrienes to liver injury. Hepatology 1985; 5:883–891.
86. Becroft DMO, Farmer K, Seddon RJ, Sowden R, Stewart JH, Vines A, Wattie DA. Epidemic listeriosis in the newborn. Br Med J 1971; 3:747–751.
87. Nahmias AJ. The TORCH complex. Hosp Pract 1974; (May):65–72.
88. Alpert G, Plotkin SA. A practical guide to the diagnosis of congenital infections in the newborn infant. Pediatr Clin North Am 1986; 33:465–479.
89. Desmonts GD, Couvreur J. Congenital toxoplasmosis: a prospective study of 378 pregnancies. N Engl J Med 1974; 290:1110–1115.
90. Stagno S, Dykes AC, Amas CS, Head RA, Juranek DO, Walls K. An outbreak of toxoplasmosis linked to cats. Pediatrics 1980; 65:706–712.
91. Feldman HA. Toxoplasmosis. N Engl J Med 1968; 279:1370–1375.
92. Remington JS, Desmonts G. Toxoplasmosis. In: Remington JS, Klein JO, eds. Infectious diseases of the fetus and newborn. Philadelphia: WB Saunders Co, 1976: 191.

93. Daffas F, Forestier F, Pavlovsky MC, Thulliez P, Aufrant C, Valenti D, Cox WL. Prenatal management of 746 pregnancies at risk for congenital toxoplasmosis. N Engl J Med 1988; 318:271–275.
94. Luft BJ, Remington JS. Toxoplasmic encephalitis. J Infect Dis 1988; 157:1–6.
95. Noat Y, Desmonts G, Remington JS. IgM enzyme-linked immunosorbent assay test for the diagnosis of congenital toxoplasma infection. J Pediatr 1981; 98:32–36.
96. Watkins JB, Katz AJ, Grand RJ. Neonatal hepatitis. A diagnostic approach. Adv Pediatr 1977; 24:399–454.
97. Dudgeon JA. Congenital rubella. J Pediatr 1975; 87:1078–1086.
98. Esterly JR, Slusser RJ, Ruebner BH: Hepatic lesions in the congenital rubella syndrome. J Pediatr 1967; 71:676–685.
99. Strauss L, Bernstein J. Neonatal hepatitis in congenital rubella. Arch Pathol 1968; 86:317–327.
100. Meegan JM, Evans BK, Horstmann DM. Comparison of the latex agglutination test with the hemagglutination inhibition test, enzyme-linked immunosorbent assay, and neutralization test for detection of antibodies to rubella virus. J Clin Microbiol 1982; 16:644–649.
101. Reynolds DW, Stagno S, Hosty TS, Tiller M, Alford CA. Maternal cytomegalovirus excretion and perinatal infection. N Engl J Med 1973; 289:1–5.
102. Griffiths PD. Cytomegalovirus and the liver. Semin Liver Dis 1984; 4:307–312.
103. McCracken GH, Shinefield HR, Cobb K, Rausen AR, Dische MR, Eichenwald HF. Congenital cytomegalic inclusion disease: a longitudinal study of 20 patients. Am J Dis Child 1969; 117:522–539.
104. Berenberg W, Nankervis G. Long-term follow-up of cytomegalic inclusion disease of infancy. Pediatrics 1970; 46:403–410.
105. Quinnan GV, Masur H, Rook AH. Herpes virus infections in the acquired immune deficiency syndrome. JAMA 1984; 252:72–77.
106. Chang MH, Hsu HC, Lee CY, Wang TR, Kao CL. Neonatal hepatitis: a follow-up study. J Pediatr Gastroenterol Nutr 1987; 6:203–207.
107. Stagno S, Whitley RJ. Herpes infections of pregnancy. I. Cytomegalovirus and Epstein-Barr virus infections. N Engl J Med 1985; 313:1270–1274.
108. Grishan FK, Green HL, Halter S, Barnard JA, Moran JR. Noncirrhotic portal hypertension in congenital cytomegalovirus infection. Hepatology 1984; 4:684–686.
109. Ansari BM, Davies DB, Jones MR. Calcification in liver associated with congenital cytomegalic inclusion disease. J Pediatr 1977; 90:661–662.
110. Hirsch MS, Schooley RT. Treatment of herpes virus infections. N Engl J Med 1983; 309:1032–1033.
111. Brown ZA, Vontver LA, Benedetti J, Critchlow CW, Sells CJ, Berry S, Corey L. Effects on infants of a first episode of genital herpes during pregnancy. N Engl J Med 1987; 317:1246–1251.
112. Nahmias AJ, Visintine AM, Reimer CB, Del Buono L, Shore SL, Starr SE. Herpes simplex virus infection of the fetus and newborn. Prog Clin Biol Res 1975; 3:63–65.
113. Whitley RJ, Yeager A, Kartus P, Bryson Y, Connor JD, Alford CA, Nahmias A, Soong SJ. Neonatal herpes simplex virus infection: follow-up evaluation of vidarabine therapy. Pediatrics 1983; 72:778–785.
114. Dresler S, Linder D. Noncirrhotic portal fibrosis following neonatal cytomegalic inclusion disease. J Pediatr 1978; 93:887–888.
115. Long WA, Ulshen MH, Lawson EE. Clinical manifestations of congenital syphilitic hepatitis: implications for pathogenesis. J Pediatr Gastroenterol Nutr 1984; 3:551–555.

PART 3

Viral Hepatitis

Raymond S. Koff, M.D.

Viral hepatitis is a systemic infection in which the liver is the major target organ; the principal hepatic lesions are hepatocyte necrosis and panlobular infiltration with mononuclear cells. At least six distinct viral agents are believed to be responsible. All produce clinically similar acute infections ranging from asymptomatic, inapparent infections to fulminant hepatitis leading to death. Persistent infections associated with viral hepatitis may be subclinical or may lead to overt, progressive chronic liver disease complicated by cirrhosis or the development of primary hepatocellular carcinoma.

HISTORY

Outbreaks of jaundice, presumably due to viral hepatitis, have a long and well-established recorded history among ancient civilizations. Hepatitis also occupies a prominent position in the history of warfare; it has been a regular concomitant of military conflicts in antiquity as well as in modern times, afflicting both combatants and disrupted and displaced civilians (both adults and children). The high frequency with which young children were infected during community-wide outbreaks, recognition of outbreaks among children inoculated with hepatitis-contaminated vaccines, and outbreaks and endemic cases in institutions for the mentally retarded and in day-care centers for preschool children attest to the importance of viral hepatitis in the pediatric age group. Furthermore, there is now considerable evidence that among aysmptomatic hepatitis B virus (HBV) carriers, as many as one-third become infected during the perinatal period, whereas the majority develop the infection during childhood or early adulthood.[1] The important long-term implications of viral hepatitis beginning early in life, e.g., the sequela of persistent infection, also have been recognized only recently.

It is possible to consider the history of knowledge of viral hepatitis in four overlapping stages. The first, which lasted several millennia, provided limited recognition of the clinical manifestations of hepatitis. The second stage, which began just before World War II, provided evidence for infectivity, transmissibility, and distinct etiologic agents with different incubation periods and routes of spread. The third stage began in the mid-1960s with the serendipitous discovery of the Australia antigen (the hepatitis B surface antigen) and its association with HBV. It continued with the identification of the hepatitis A virus (HAV) a decade later and shortly thereafter, when specific methods to identify both HAV and HBV infections became available, confirmation of the existence of the hepatitis D (delta agent) virus (HDV), and two blood-borne and one enterically transmitted non-A, non-B hepatitis viruses. The fourth, current stage is characterized by the use of biotechnology to prevent the transmission of infection and to develop techniques to treat established infections. Unfortunately, acquisition of information about each of the hepatitis agents has been asynchronous. As a consequence, a firm scientific basis for control of all hepatitis virus infections remains elusive.

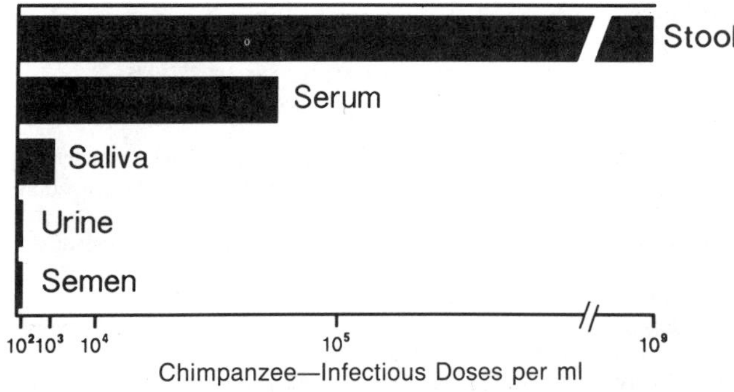

FIGURE 1 Infectivity titers of clinical specimens (body fluids and excretions) from patients with hepatitis A, tested in chimpanzees, show that the highest titers of HAV are detected in acute-phase stool samples. (Courtesy of the Clinical Teaching Project, American Gastroenterological Association.)

THE AGENTS

Hepatitis A Virus

HAV is a 27-nm RNA virus that has been classified as enterovirus type 72.[2] Only one serotype of HAV has been recognized in human beings. While it has many characteristics of a picornavirus, the amino acid sequences of HAV appear to be more heterogeneous than those of the other picornaviruses.[3] The complete sequence of the single-stranded RNA of HAV, comprising 7,478 nucleotides, has been determined, and HAV has been propagated in several primate cell lines. Four structural virion polypeptides typical of enteroviruses have been identified in the viral capsomere.[4] While replication of enteroviruses typically occurs in the gut, replication of HAV appears to occur predominantly in the liver. HAV in stool is derived from hepatic bile rather than from replication in intestinal epithelium. HAV may also infect human bone marrow in vitro, inhibiting the differentiation and proliferation of bone marrow stem cells.[5] HAV has been demonstrated in serum but in low titers compared with those in stool specimens (Fig. 1). The infectivity of saliva, urine, and semen from patients with acute HAV infection remains uncertain; the role of these body fluids in the transmission of HAV is ill defined.

Hepatitis B Virus

Human HBV, classified as hepadnavirus type 1, was the first recognized member of the hepadnavirus family. These hepatotropic DNA-containing, small, double-shelled animal viruses are morphologically similar; each virus is about 42 nm in diameter. In addition to human HBV, hepadnaviruses also have been described in the woodchuck, the ground squirrel, the tree squirrel, and the domestic duck.[6] Although geese may be infected by the duck HBV and chipmunks may be infected by the ground squirrel hepatitis virus,[7] no evidence that humans can be infected by any of the nonhuman hepadnaviruses is currently available.

Thus, HBV is the sole member of the hepadnavirus family known to infect human beings and nonhuman primates (chimpanzees). Nonetheless, a number of HBV-related variants capable of infecting human beings have been postulated.[8-10] These agents may induce human hepatitis B–like infections, in which conventional markers of HBV infection cannot be found. The responsible agents are incompletely defined; in fact, their existence requires independent confirmation of reported experimental transmission studies.[9]

HBV has been propagated in vitro by the transfection of mammalian cell lines derived from human hepatic tumors with cloned HBV DNA. The HBV produced by transfected cell lines has been shown to be the intact, complete virus capable of causing acute HBV infection in chimpanzees.[11]

The molecular biology of HBV is described in detail in Chapter 28, Part 4. The genome of HBV consists of small, circular, partially double-stranded and partially single-stranded DNA. The long strand of the DNA is about 3,200 nucleotides long; four open reading frames (genes) have been recognized. The liver appears to be the major target organ and the principal but not the only site of viral replication.

HBV is associated with three particulate forms: (1) complete 42-nm virus particles, (2) spherical particles about 22 nm in diameter, and (3) tubular particles with a width of 22 nm and a variable length of up to 200 nm. The 22-nm spherical and tubular particles are present in exceedingly large numbers in the circulation of infected individuals, far in excess of the number of complete virus particles. The 22-nm particles lack DNA but are composed chiefly of the proteins, lipid, and carbohydrate of the envelope of the HBV particle. The major protein and antigenic material is called the hepatitis B surface antigen (HBsAg). Other proteins, the pre-S proteins, are also expressed on the surface of the HBV particle, as well as on the small spherical and tubular HBsAg particles.

Multiple serotypes based on antigenic subdeterminants of HBsAg have been recognized. However, a common group "a" antigenic determinant has been found in all HBV isolates. Antibodies directed against this determinant provide protection against infection by all HBV serotypes.

The core of HBV contains its DNA, an endogenous DNA polymerase, which serves as a reverse transcriptase, and a protein kinase activity, which served to phosphorylate the proteins of the nucleocapsid core.[12] Expressed on the surface of the core is a distinct antigenic material, the hepatitis B core antigen (HBcAg). A third antigenic component of the nucleocapsid core is the hepatitis B e antigen (HBeAg), a nonparticulate, soluble antigen present on the same protein as HBcAg. HBeAg appears to be derived from HBcAg by proteolytic self-cleavage.[13] HBeAg is almost never found in HBsAg-negative sera; its presence indicates ongoing viral replication, and it serves as an indirect marker of infectivity.

Hepatitis D Virus

Hepatitis D virus (HDV), also known as the delta agent or hepatitis delta virus, is a defective RNA virus. HDV cannot replicate by itself; it requires the helper function of the hepadnaviruses (HBV in human beings). HDV appears to be related to viroids, simple infectious RNAs, and plant satellite viruses. The HDV particle is about 36 nm in diameter and comprises an outer coat of HBsAg and a core containing antigenic material—the HDV antigen—and single-stranded circular RNA with a length of about 1,700 nucleotides.[14,15] HDV isolates demonstrate genetic heterogeneity[16]; the importance of such heterogeneity remains uncertain. While in vivo replication of HDV is probably limited to the liver, the precise mechanisms of replication are poorly understood.[17]

Non-A, Non-B Hepatitis Viruses

Blood-Borne Agents. At least two distinct agents appear to be responsible for blood-borne non-A, non-B (NANB) hepatitis. Evidence of their existence is the occurrence of multiple attacks of NANB hepatitis with short or long incubation periods, cross-challenge experiments with multiple inocula in chimpanzees, and apparently distinctive physicochemical properties of the agents.[18,19] One of the agents is chloroform- and heat-sensitive and induces smooth endoplasmic reticulum tubular structures in the cytoplasm of hepatocytes in infected chimpanzees. This agent, termed the hepatitis C virus (HCV), appears to be an RNA virus with about 10,000 nucleotides.[19a] It is probably related to but distinct from the flavivirus family. Highly specific serologic assays for circulating antibodies to HCV have been developed.[19b] Limited studies with these assays suggest that HCV is the major but not the sole agent of blood-borne NANB hepatitis.

Enterically Transmitted Agent. Experimental transmission of enterically transmitted NANB viral hepatitis to nonhuman primates and serial passage of 27- to 34-nm virus-like particles in nonhuman primates have been successfully undertaken.[20] Preliminary studies suggest that the responsible agent, currently termed the hepatitis E virus (HEV), may be a RNA virus with a genome length of about 7,000 nucleotides. A serologic test is under development.

PATHOLOGY AND PATHOGENESIS

The predominant morphologic lesions in acute viral hepatitis are the presence of multiple foci of hepatocyte necrosis, dropout, and degeneration, with ballooned hepatocytes and acidophilic bodies (councilman-like bodies), the latter representing dead, mummified hepatocytes. A diffuse mononuclear cell inflammatory reaction and Kupffer cell hyperplasia are prominent features. Portal triads are expanded and contain numerous small, round, mononuclear cells. Segmental erosion of the limiting plate, i.e., the hepatocytes adjacent to the portal triad, is characteristically found. Despite these changes, the lobular architecture is intact.

The predominant inflammatory cell type identified in liver biopsies of patients with acute hepatitis is the T8 (helper) lymphocyte, which is found associated with hepatocytes.[21] Natural killer T cells also are common in acute hepatitis but are localized to the sinusoids and perisinusoidal spaces but not in close proximity to hepatocytes. Hepatocyte injury in acute hepatitis may result from the activity of cytolytic T lymphocytes against target viral antigens expressed on the surface of hepatocyte membranes; some cytolytic T cells may be activated independently of virus-associated antigens. Immunocytolysis is preceded by T lymphocyte recognition of infected hepatocytes, which is believed to require surface membrane display of viral antigen and display of HLA class I antigens.[22] Whether these mechanisms are responsible for hepatic injury in all etiologic forms of viral hepatitis remains to be determined.

CLINICAL FEATURES OF ACUTE HEPATITIS

Clinical Expression

None of the known etiologic forms of viral hepatitis are important causes of neonatal hepatitis, although maternal-neonatal transmission of HBV, HDV, and the NANB hepatitis agents, but not HAV, is reasonably well documented. Affected neonates are usually but not invariably asymptomatic.

In general, viral hepatitis is expressed in two major forms representing a broad spectrum of infection: symptomatic hepatitis and asymptomatic infection. Patients with symptomatic hepatitis may or may not be jaundiced. Symptomatic hepatitis without jaundice is termed *anicteric hepatitis*. Signs and symptoms of anicteric hepatitis are similar to those of icteric hepatitis, but the intensity of symptoms may be reduced and their duration is often abbreviated in anicteric disease. Transient and unexplained fever, upper respiratory symptoms, or gastrointestinal (GI) symptoms—either alone or in combination—may be the sole clinical manifestations of anicteric hepatitis. The characteristic malaise, weakness, and anorexia of hepatitis with jaundice (see below) may be entirely absent.

Asymptomatic infection can be further classified into two categories of infection: subclinical and inapparent infection. In subclinical infection, neither jaundice nor symptoms are present, but biochemical features of hepatitis, e.g., elevated serum aminotransferase levels, can be detected. In patients with inapparent infection, neither clinical symptoms nor biochemical abnormalities are detected; inapparent infections can be identified only by serologic studies. Since serologic markers of acute infection are available only for the identification of HAV, HBV, and HDV infections, inapparent NANB hepatitis infections are not yet an established entity. Nonetheless, based on analogy with the spectrum of disease seen with other hepatitis viruses and the occurrence of subclinical and symptomatic NANB infections, inapparent NANB hepatitis infections undoubtedly occur as well. Proof of this notion requires the development of specific serologic markers for these infections.

The relative frequency of symptomatic hepatitis and asymptomatic infection has been reasonably well identified for hepatitis A and appears to be strikingly age-dependent. About 85 percent of HAV infections in children 1 to 2 years old are asymptomatic, about 50 percent of infections in children 3 to 4 years old are asymptomatic, and only 20 percent of infections in children 5 years of age or older are asymptomatic.[23] In older children and in adults, the bulk of HAV infections are symptomatic and may be associated with jaundice. In fact, symptomatic hepatitis has been reported in 75 to 97 percent of adults with hepatitis A, and 40 to 70 percent of the cases were associated with jaundice.[24] Transmissibility is probably unrelated to whether infection is symptomatic or asymptomatic. Individuals with inapparent HAV infection have been shown to shed HAV in feces.[25]

Asymptomatic infection is the rule of thumb in neonates and extremely young children with HBV infection; the precise proportions of subclinical and inapparent infections have not been well defined. Symptomatic disease becomes increasingly prevalent in adolescents and adults with acute hepatitis B. About 25 percent of symptomatic cases are accompanied by jaundice. Although early studies of HDV-HBV co-infections or HDV superinfections of HBsAg carriers suggested that symptomatic or severe disease was highly common, increasing experience has made it apparent that many asymptomatic cases occur. The ratio of subclinical cases to inapparent ones is not certain.

In the absence of serologic markers, only limited data are available concerning the spectrum of disease induced by blood-borne NANB hepatitis in children. The few neonatal infections described have been subclinical.[26] In adults with transfusion-associated NANB hepatitis, as defined by serial measurement of serum aminotransferase levels after transfusion, symptomatic disease accompanied by jaundice is recognized in less than 25 percent of cases.

In outbreaks of enterically transmitted NANB hepatitis, clinical disease is common among adults but infrequently recognized among children. The attack rate of symptomatic hepatitis with jaundice has been highest among young adults in the 15- to 39-year age group.[27] In children under 14 years of age the attack rate of symptomatic hepatitis with jaundice is lower, but the frequency of subclinical hepatitis and inapparent infection remains uncertain. Sporadic cases of enterically transmitted NANB hepatitis may be acquired early in life, and subclinical infections may be highly common in the young in developing nations in which these NANB infections are endemic.

Incubation Period

The mean incubation period of hepatitis A, defined as the interval between exposure to HAV and elevation of the serum aminotransferase levels, is about 4 weeks. The average incubation period of hepatitis B is usually between 60 and 90 days, with a range of 30 to 180 days. The incubation period of HDV is probably several weeks long. In experimentally infected chimpanzees it varied from 24 days in an animal given an undiluted inoculum to as long as 51 days in an animal given a highly diluted inoculum.[28] Evidence for two distinct blood-borne NANB agents includes the observation that the incubation period of transfusion-associated NANB hepatitis appears to have two modes, at 4 and 8 weeks, with a range of 2 to 26 weeks (mean of 9.5 weeks).[29] The mean incubation period of enterically transmitted NANB hepatitis is about 6 weeks, with a range in some outbreaks from as short as 2 weeks to as long as 9 weeks.[27]

Features of Symptomatic Hepatitis

Symptoms of acute hepatitis are highly similar in all etiologic forms; some features are suggestive of specific etiologic agents. For example, in older children and adults with acute hepatitis A, the onset of illness appears to be so abrupt that the patient can identify a specific day during which symptoms were first experienced. In the other forms of viral hepatitis, the onset of symptoms is usually insidious and a specific first day of illness cannot be pinpointed as readily. Fever and headache are also more commonly described in hepatitis A than in the other etiologic forms. However, only serologic testing can be relied upon to distinguish among the etiologic agents.

Duration of the Prodrome

During the acute phase of infection, a number of preicteric, prodromal symptoms may be identified. In a few patients, no symptoms occur prior to the onset of jaundice. The prodromal phase may be variable in duration but tends to be shorter in hepatitis A than in the other forms. The average duration of preicteric symptoms is from a few days to about 1 week for hepatitis A. The preicteric phase may exceed 1 week in less than 10 percent of cases, but in some cases it may last as long as 2 weeks. In hepatitis B, the preicteric phase may be considerably prolonged—in some cases as long as 2 months. In fact, short preicteric phases of less than 1 week are seen in only 25 percent of hepatitis B cases. Prodromal features of HDV infection and NANB viral hepatitis may be so brief that they are not recognized before the onset of jaundice. However, a prodrome closely resembling that of hepatitis B, with a serum sickness–like syndrome, has been reported with NANB viral hepatitis.[30] In sporadic NANB viral hepatitis, a preicteric phase of more than 2 weeks' duration has been reported in 95 percent of cases.[31]

Prodromal Features

A variety of constitutional, GI, and respiratory symptoms and an extrahepatic serum sickness–like syndrome may be seen during the preicteric prodrome. Lassitude, fatigue, anorexia, nausea and vomiting, right upper quadrant abdominal discomfort, fever (usually below 39 °C), chilliness (without shaking chills), headache, flulike symptoms, nasal discharge, sore throat, and cough are the major complaints. Anorexia intensifies as the day progresses; dinner is less well tolerated than lunch, which is less well tolerated than breakfast. Abnormalities in gustatory and olfactory acuity are accompanied by loss of taste for food. Vomiting is common but is rarely severe or prolonged. Persistent vomiting, leading to dehydration and electrolyte abnormalities, suggests a more serious variant of viral hepatitis or the presence of an unrelated complicating disorder. A mild weight loss may occur during the prodrome and the acute phase of illness.

Myalgias and photophobia and, in as many as one-third of patients, diffuse arthralgias may be seen. Arthralgias may be less common in patients with hepatitis A.[32,33] Combinations of arthritis, angioedema, urticaria, and maculopapular eruptions, and, rarely, hematuria and proteinuria that are indicative of glomerular involvement are the major extrahepatic, immunologically mediated manifestations observed during the prodrome of hepatitis B. Arthritis, occurring as a component of a serum sickness–like syndrome, is most closely associated with HBV infection; 3 to 10 percent of patients with hepatitis B may have evidence of an acute, migratory polyarthritis during the prodrome. A similar syndrome is rarely found in NANB viral hepatitis[30] and has been reported in relapsing HAV infection, with vasculitis and cryoglobulinemia.[34]

The polyarthritis of hepatitis B is typically symmetric, affects the distal joints, e.g., the proximal interphalangeal joints, and, to a lesser extent, the larger axial and appendicular joints. Joint involvement usually subsides with the development of jaundice, and residual joint disease has yet to be reported. Rashes have been reported in as many as one-third of patients with viral hepatitis[36] and have been described in all etiologic forms (its occurrence in HDV infection is uncertain, since rashes in this setting may be attributable to HBV). Urticaria and angioedema may develop during the prodrome of hepatitis B in association with arthritis. A transient macular erythema is the most common rash, regardless of etiologic form. Papular eruptions are also seen and a papulovesicular eruption localized to the trunk and anterior surfaces of the upper extremities, with or without pruritus, has been described in blood-borne NANB viral hepatitis.[35] Skin biopsies in affected patients failed to reveal deposition of immunoglobulin or complement components in tissue samples. The specific mechanisms underlying these lesions remain to be determined.

An unusual skin lesion in the United States, but one not uncommonly reported in Japan and Italy, the Gianotti-Crosti syndrome or papular acrodermatitis of childhood, has been associated with HBV, HAV, and other nonhepatitis infections.[36] The syndrome is characterized by the occurrence of nonpruritic, symmetric, flat papules on the face, extremities, and buttocks, associated with lymphadenopathy predominantly in infants and children with anicteric hepatitis B. The cutaneous lesions may persist for several weeks before subsiding.

In the absence of fulminant hepatitis, neurologic involvement is a rare prodromal or acute-phase manifestation of acute viral hepatitis.[37] The Guillain-Barré syndrome has been recognized during the preicteric phase of hepatitis B[38] and following the onset of jaundice in hepatitis A.[39] Mononeuritis (cranial or peripheral nerve) has been reported in both hepatitis A and hepatitis B during the preicteric and icteric phases of illness.[40]

Physical examination of the patient in the prodrome of viral hepatitis may be unrewarding or may reveal minimal hepatomegaly or evidence of joint, skin, or other extrahepatic manifestations.

In patients with HBV infection in whom prodromal extrahepatic manifestations are recognized, tests for circulating HBsAg are invariably positive (see below), and elevated serum aminotransferase levels (see below) may be found within a few days to a week or so after the onset of these symptoms. After running its course, this immune complex–mediated disorder is followed by the development of the icteric phase of illness. In patients in whom extrahepatic manifestations are not seen, the same icteric phase may be seen.

Icteric and Convalescent Phases

Before jaundice is recognized, darkening of the urine to a brownish color and lightening of stool color may be observed. As the jaundice appears, the anorexia, malaise, and weakness seen in the preicteric phase may transiently worsen. Nausea and vomiting also become more severe before remitting. In general, as jaundice deepens, constitutional symptoms become less severe. In half of patients with icteric acute viral hepatitis, pruritus is noted concomitantly with jaundice or a few days later.

Jaundice disappears gradually, usually within 2 to 6 weeks after its onset. In children and particularly in patients with hepatitis A, jaundice tends to be relatively brief, persisting for no longer than 2 weeks in 85 percent. In hepatitis B and blood-borne NANB viral hepatitis, the duration of jaundice may be considerably longer than in typical hepatitis A.

Serum aminotransferase (ALT and AST) elevations are found during the late prodromal phase and may reach peak levels shortly after jaundice is recognized. Peak levels are 10 to 100 times the upper limits of normal. Serum bilirubin levels rise and peak 1 to 8 days after peak aminotransferase levels. Serum bilirubin levels subsequently decline fairly rapidly during the convalescent phase, reaching normal levels within 4 to 6 weeks in most patients. Although serum aminotransferase levels also decline rapidly from their peak values, the rate of fall is not maintained. As a consequence, in many patients minor elevations persist for a few months. In typical cases, only minimal alterations in hepatic synthetic function may be observed; the prothrombin time and serum albumin are either normal or mildly abnormal.

During the physical examination, direct palpation may reveal slight tenderness over the liver, which is usually mildly enlarged. Striking tenderness is rarely found; its presence suggests other diagnoses. The liver edge is usually rounded, and nodularity is not found. In 10 to 15 percent of patients the spleen tip may be palpated and posterior cervical lymphadenopathy is detected. In a variable proportion of patients, small spider angiomata are recognized. These physical findings disappear during convalescence. Ascites and peripheral edema are atypical findings that suggest the presence of a severe variant of hepatitis or another diagnosis. Impaired mentation, drowsiness, insomnia, and asterixis, reflecting the development of hepatic encephalopathy, suggest the presence of fulminant hepatitis (see below).

CLINICAL VARIANTS

Fulminant Hepatitis

In considerably less than 1 percent of patients, symptoms of hepatic encephalopathy and marked prolongation of the prothrombin time, developing within 8 weeks of the onset of illness in patients in whom prior liver disease has not been identified, signal the development of fulminant hepatitis. Pregnant women appear to be highly susceptible to the development of fatal, fulminant enterically transmitted NANB hepatitis.[41] In this group case fatality rates approach 20 percent.

In patients with the disorder, examination of liver tissue reveals massive hepatic necrosis. The surviving hepatocytes form irregular, thickened plates or pseudoductular structures. A diffuse inflammatory reaction, consisting of small round cells, plasma cells, and polymorphonuclear leukocytes may be present.

A progressive constellation of complications can be anticipated with the development of fulminant hepatitis. Among these, cerebral edema is the most important. It may herald the development of brain death or brain stem involvement leading to cardiopulmonary arrest and central hypotension. The profound coagulopathy of fulminant hepatitis may be complicated by GI bleeding, and sepsis may be prominent. Severe hypoglycemia or insulin-resistant nonketotic hyperglycemia[42] may dominate the clinical picture in some patients. Chances for survival appear to fall as, one after another, organ systems fail. Among patients who develop fulminant hepatitis, the fatality rate in those with severe encephalopathy often exceeds 75 percent.[43]

With the possible exception of orthotopic liver replacement, the mortality of fulminant hepatitis has not been diminished by modern management in the intensive care unit.[44] Controlled clinical trials have shown that corticosteroids and exchange transfusion are ineffective.[45] Total body washout and extracorporeal support systems are of uncertain value. Early recognition and appropriate treatment of complications with concentrated glucose, lactulose, fresh frozen plasma, and antibiotics may be beneficial. Intracranial pressure monitoring and mannitol treatment of patients with cerebral edema has been reported to have a favorable influence on survival in one study.[46] In contrast, prophylactic treatment with H_2-receptor antagonists reduced the risk of GI bleeding but did not increase survival.[47] Therapy designed to stimulate or expedite hepatic regeneration and restitution is not currently available.

Cholestatic Hepatitis

This highly rare syndrome is characterized by prolonged jaundice with total serum bilirubin levels that exceed 10 mg per deciliter, accompanied by pruritus, fever, diarrhea, and weight loss.[48] Most patients feel reasonably well and recover completely, although the course of cholestatic hepatitis may last more than 12 weeks. Hepatitis A appears to be responsible for most cases.

Relapsing Hepatitis

Recurrent symptoms and secondary rises in serum aminotransferase levels have been observed 2 to 8 weeks after the initial onset of symptoms in hepatitis A.[49] In general, the height of the aminotransferase elevation is lower in the secondary rise than in the initial episode. Bilirubin levels during the relapse may be either higher or lower than at the initial bout. Although relapsing hepatitis may be a prolonged illness, resolution is expected.

SEROLOGY

HAV Infection

Measurement of IgM anti-HAV is the mainstay in the serologic diagnosis of hepatitis A and the method of choice, since testing a single specimen is sufficient. IgM anti-HAV appears in the serum during the acute phase of illness, reaches a peak within a few weeks, and then declines in titer, becoming undetectable in most patients at 3 to 4 months after infection (Fig. 2).[50,51] Demonstration of a rising titer of IgG anti-HAV by commercial immunoassays also permits detection of hepatitis A but requires repeated testing over time. IgG anti-HAV, which persists indefinitely in slowly declining titers, is believed to be responsible for immunity following natural infection.

Identification of fecal HAV in patients with acute HAV infection is possible but is not a practical means of diagnosis.[52] A highly sensitive molecular hybridization assay for the detection of HAV RNA in fecal extracts also has been described, but it too seems impractical as a clinical laboratory tool and remains limited to research facilities.[53,54]

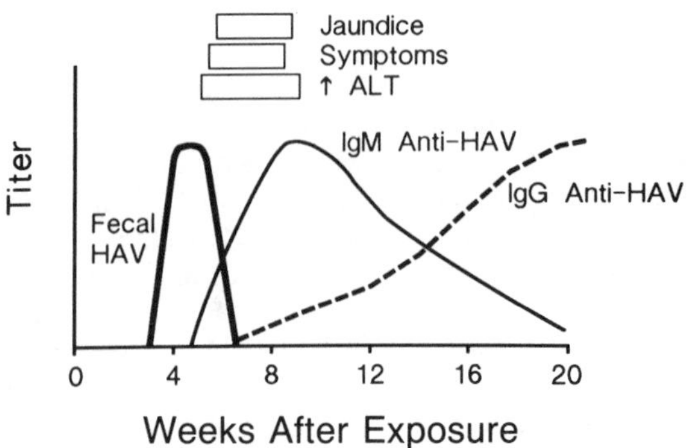

FIGURE 2 The sequence of serologic and clinical events seen during hepatitis A is shown in this schematic illustration. Fecal HAV appears during the late phase of the incubation period, peaks near the onset of symptoms, and then declines rapidly; detection of fecal HAV is not used in clinical diagnosis. Diagnosis of acute hepatitis A is usually based on detection of IgM anti-HAV. (Courtesy of the Clinical Teaching Project, American Gastroenterological Association.)

HBV Infection

The first measurable antigen to appear in acute HBV infection is the HBsAg. As shown in Figure 3, it is present before the development of elevated levels of serum alanine aminotransferase (ALT), symptoms of hepatitis, or jaundice. In most patients HBsAg becomes serologically undetectable, with conventional radioimmunoassays, either before or by the end of the fourth to sixth month following its appearance. In 5 to 15 percent HBsAg disappears by the time symptoms develop and sera are tested. It should be noted that a monoclonal radioimmunoassay detected HBsAg 1 to 9 weeks longer than the conventional polyclonal assay.[55]

The second antigen measurable in acute HBV infection, usually detected within a few days to a few weeks after the appearance of HBsAg, is the hepatitis B e antigen (HBeAg).[56] HBeAg is an imperfect marker of active HBV replication. Its presence in serum is correlated with the occurrence of complete HBV particles in the circulation. In acute HBV infection associated with recovery, HBeAg disappears before HBsAg disappears. The disappearance of HBeAg is followed by the appearance of its corresponding antibody, anti-HBe, which persists for prolonged periods.[57]

Pre-S proteins, expressed on the surface of the HBV particle, as well as on the small spherical and tubular HBsAg forms,[58] have been detected in acute-phase sera of HBV-infected patients during the period of active HBV replication. These proteins persist for a few weeks to months and then disappear as the corresponding anti–pre-S antibodies develop.[59] IgM and IgG anti–pre-S antibodies have been detected.[60] Anti–pre-S are also transient and disappear with the development of circulating anti-HBs.[61] Commercial assays for pre-S proteins and antibodies are not yet available.

The best marker of active HBV replication during the acute infection is HBV DNA. HBV DNA is detectable in sera during the early phase of acute HBV infection but 6 to 8 weeks later is generally not detectable.[62] Persistent detection of HBV DNA beyond this period indicates continuing viral replication and infectivity. HBV DNA can be identified in an extrachromosomal site within the hepatocyte of patients with active HBV replication. HBV DNA has also been detected in peripheral mononuclear cells of blood, i.e., T cells, B cells, and monocytes, as well as in bone marrow stem cells.[63]

As the titer of HBsAg declines with time, its corresponding antibody, the antibody to HBsAg (anti-HBs), is detectable and reaches peak levels within a few months. During late convalescence from hepatitis B, anti-HBs titers begin to decline slowly and continue to do so for many years to decades. In some patients, anti-HBs may eventually become undetectable.

Antibody to the hepatitis B core antigen (anti-HBc) is routinely detected prior to the appearance of anti-HBs during acute hepatitis B.[64] In fact, anti-HBc becomes measurable shortly after HBsAg is detected. The initial and predominant immunoglobulin class of anti-HBc is IgM. This IgM anti-HBc reaches peak levels within several weeks of the onset of infection and persists long after the disappearance of HBsAg. As a consequence, testing for IgM anti-HBc is the most sensitive test for the identification of acute HBV infection. Early in the development of serologic tests for HBV infection, a ''window'' period between the loss of HBsAg and the appearance of anti-HBs was recognized, during which the sole marker of acute HBV infection could be the detection of IgM anti-HBc. This ''window'' is infrequently encountered with the currently available tests for HBsAg and anti-HBs.

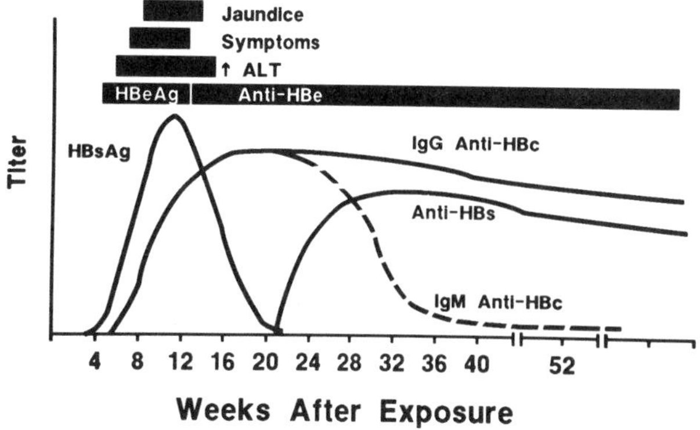

FIGURE 3 In this schematic illustration of the serologic events of acute hepatitis B, HBsAg appears before the development of increased serum alanine aminotransferase (ALT) levels, symptoms of hepatitis, or jaundice. The sequential appearance and disappearance of HBeAg and IgM anti-HBc and the late appearance of anti-HBs are depicted. (From Seeff LB, ed. Current perspectives in hepatology. New York: Plenum Press, 1989.)

After reaching an early peak, IgM anti-HBc titers fall and become undetectable in nearly all patients with acute hepatitis B 4 to 8 months after the onset of symptoms.[65] Total anti-HBc levels tend to decline at a much slower rate. The predominant immunoglobulin form of anti-HBc found during late convalescence is IgG. IgG anti-HBc persists in slowly declining titers for many years to decades after acute infection.

Although persistence of IgM anti-HBc is highly unusual on complete recovery from HBV infection, among patients who became HBV carriers after acute infection, 15 percent remained reactive for IgM anti-HBc.[66] Similarly, in patients with chronic hepatitis B, about 15 percent were found to be IgM anti-HBc positive. HBV carriers with active viral replication[67] as well as those with reactivation[68] also may express IgM anti-HBc.

Anti-HBc, without IgM anti-HBc, HBsAg, or anti-HBs, also may indicate the existence of the HBV carrier state in which HBsAg is below the level of detectability, remote infection with failure to develop anti-HBs, passive transfer of anti-HBc by transfusion (unlikely since anti-HBc screening of blood donors was initiated), or a false-positive test result. Isolated anti-HBc also may reflect waning immunity following infection.[69] During the late phase of recovery from HBV infection, the titer of anti-HBs declines with time, and in some individuals anti-HBs becomes undetectable. As a consequence, anti-HBc may be the sole marker of prior HBV infection. The conversion of individuals with low levels of anti-HBs and anti-HBc to anti-HBc alone has been reported.[70]

Acute hepatitis in an HBsAg-positive individual is not pathognomonic of acute HBV infection. The differential diagnosis includes reactivation of chronic HBV infection (see below), superinfection by other hepatitis viruses, and liver injury due to other causes such as drug-induced or alcoholic hepatitis. Accuracy in serologic diagnosis requires testing for multiple markers and sequential studies.

HDV Infection

HDV infection should be considered only in patients shown to be positive for HBsAg, since HDV has rarely, if ever, been found in persons who are HBsAg-negative. Acute HDV and acute HBV infection occur together as co-primary infections, or acute HDV infection may be a superinfection imposed on the HBsAg carrier state. When it is a superinfection, the majority of HDV infections become chronic. Because HDV infection cannot persist after recovery from infection with HBV, and because most acute HBV infections resolve, the expression of HDV is limited during acute hepatitis B. Detection of HDV antigen and HDV RNA in serum and liver tissue is available only in research laboratories, but testing for IgM and IgG antibodies to HDV (total anti-HDV) is commercially available.

During acute co-infection, HDV antigen and HDV RNA (measured by a hybridization probe) appear in serum during the late incubation period or early acute phase of illness. Both markers disappear before the clearance of HBsAg.[71] IgM anti-HDV is measurable, transiently, during the acute illness but may be detectable for no longer than a few weeks to 1 or 2 months. IgM anti-HDV is followed by IgG anti-HDV, which also may disappear by 6 months after the onset of illness. In acute HDV co-infection, one or more of these markers may be absent.[72]

During HDV superinfection, a brisk and sustained IgM and IgG anti-HDV response may be detected. HDV antigen and HDV RNA may be detected in serum; these markers and IgM anti-HDV tend to correlate with the presence of HDV in the liver.[71] Persistent HDV infection may result from superinfection. In affected patients large quantities of HDV antigen may be detected in hepatocytes, and high titers of IgM and IgG anti-HD are maintained.[73]

Non-A, Non-B Hepatitis Infections

Diagnosis of blood-borne HCV requires identification of anti-HCV and serologic exclusion of HAV and HBV infections. Initial studies of assays for anti-HCV suggest that seroconversion to anti-HCV positivity may often be delayed for many weeks after hepatitis is recognized. Immunoassays for the second agent of blood-borne NANB viral hepatitis are not yet available. Assays for serologic markers of HEV infection are presently under development.

EPIDEMIOLOGY

The relative proportions of HAV, HBV, HDV, and NANB agents responsible for clinically recognized hepatitis vary by geographic area and age group. For example, among consecutively hospitalized patients with acute viral hepatitis observed in China, HAV was identified in 51 percent, HBV in 30 percent, and NANB hepatitis in 19 percent. Hepatitis A accounted for 89 percent of the cases under 15 years of age; hepatitis B was identified in 49 percent of those above 15 years.[74]

HAV Infection

The epidemiology of HAV infection is conditioned by the fact that the highest titers of HAV are detected in acute-phase stool samples of infected patients.[75] HAV appears in the stools of infected patients during the late phase of the incubation period, reaches a peak near the onset of symptoms, and then declines rapidly over 1 to 2 weeks. Peak infectivity of HAV-infected individuals occurs in the week before and a few days after the onset of clinical illness. A similar pattern of infectivity is probable in patients with subclinical or inapparent infection; peak infectivity occurs about 4 weeks after the HAV exposure that leads to infection. Fecal-oral spread of HAV from infected individuals to their contacts is the major route of transmission. Intrahousehold and intrafamilial contacts of index cases are at greatest risk.

Poor hygienic conditions and inadequate sanitary standards lead to outbreaks in custodial institutions, e.g., institutions for the mentally retarded and day-care centers for preschool children. In the latter setting, the risk appears to be largely confined to day-care centers that accept young, non–toilet-trained children. About 10 to 15 percent of reported cases of hepatitis A in the United States are day-care center–associated. HAV-contaminated water, food, and bivalve mollusks have been incriminated as vehicles of HAV transmission in common-source outbreaks and in nonepidemic periods.[76]

Percutaneous spread is a minor mode of transmission; microepidemics have only occasionally been described among parenteral drug abusers, and HAV transmission by blood transfusion is a rare occurrence.

Maternal-neonatal transmission of HAV has yet to be recognized as an epidemiologic entity. In developing countries, in which the prevalence of HAV infection is often high, e.g., North Africa and the Middle East, or moderately high, e.g., Central and South America, southern Africa, and the Indian subcontinent, HAV infection occurs predominantly in young children. The prevalence of IgG anti-HAV may reach 100 percent at or shortly after 5 to 10 years of age.[77] As a consequence of infection early in life, symptomatic hepatitis A is infrequently reported in the adult population of these regions. Susceptible visitors to such areas of high or moderate HAV prevalence are at considerable risk of acquiring HAV infection.

In developed nations, HAV prevalence rates are low in all age groups without the abrupt rise seen in early childhood in developing areas. While HAV infection rates appear to increase slightly with increasing age, cross-sectional data strongly suggest that this phenomenon is due in large part to an aging cohort of individuals who experienced HAV infection several decades earlier, when HAV infection was endemic in the population.[78,79] Improved socioeconomic and sanitary conditions are likely to be responsible for the current declining frequency of new HAV infections. HAV acquired by susceptible adults during travel to endemic, developing areas may also be responsible for the minimal rise in HAV prevalence seen with increasing age.

HBV Infection

In highly endemic areas, HBV infections occur early in life. HBV markers are identified in most of the population by the end of the first decade; maternal-neonatal transmission and horizontal transmission between very young children are probably responsible. An example of one such high-prevalence area is found in the rural communities of Senegal, West Africa, where HBV infection is present in 25 percent of the population by 2 years of age[70]; 50 percent of the population is infected by age 7; and by age 15, 80 percent is infected. In this endemic area the incidence of HBV infection among susceptibles was estimated to be 6 percent per year at any age.

In areas of lower but still moderately high prevalence, infection rates are shifted to the right, with peak rates occurring considerably later. Nearly half of the population in such areas may be seropositive by 25 years of age. Transmission via intimate contact plays a key role in this epidemiologic pattern.

In contrast, in areas of low to very low prevalence such as the United States, parenteral drug abuse, occupationally acquired infection, and imported cases among travelers or immigrants appear to be responsible for transmission.[80] In the United States, the risk of transmission of HBV in day-care centers and nursery schools appears to be low.[81] On the other hand, in Japan, a higher-prevalence region, the transmission of HBV in nursery schools appears to be epidemiologically important, although the responsible mechanisms remain uncertain.[82]

Contact Transmission

Contact transmission of HBV from mentally retarded HBsAg-positive children to susceptible students and staff in day schools for the mentally retarded or after mainstreaming of HBsAg-positive retarded children into regular schools has been documented.[83,84] Direct classroom contact appears to be responsible.

The mechanisms of contact transmission are not entirely understood, either in children or in adults. Transfer of HBV-contaminated secretions, such as saliva and semen, may play a key role. The finding of HBV DNA in saliva and semen of HBsAg carriers[85,86] is consistent with experimental transmission studies using these secretions as inocula. Peripheral blood leukocytes were the probable source of HBV DNA in saliva; both spermatozoa and leukocytes contained HBV DNA in semen specimens.

In certain high-prevalence areas, intrafamilial spread of HBV infection among household members not engaging in sexual contact is an important route of infection.[87]

Maternal-Neonatal Transmission

HBV infection in utero may result from the transplacental leakage of HBV-contaminated maternal blood, induced by uterine contractions and disruption of placental barriers.[88,89] In utero infection accounts for no more than 10 percent of neonatal HBV infections.[90] The majority of HBV infections in the neonate appear to be a consequence of maternal-neonatal HBV transmission during labor, delivery, or shortly thereafter in the early postpartum period. Delivery by caesarean section or prohibition of breast feeding does not reduce the risk of infection. The risk of HBV transmission to the neonate is highest (Fig. 4) when the mother is an HBV carrier and is also HBeAg-positive or when the mother develops acute HBV infection during the third trimester or early postpartum period.[91]

HDV Infection

HDV infection occurs throughout the world in two epidemiologic patterns: endemic and nonendemic. The endemic pattern is found in the Mediterranean basin, in the Balkan peninsula, in European Soviet Union, in parts of Africa, in the Middle East, and in the Amazon basin of South America. In a prevalence study undertaken in the latter area, new HDV infections (superinfections of HBsAg carriers) occurred at a rate of 2.9 infections per 100 patient-years of follow-up; highest infection rates were seen in children under 10 years of age and in males.[92]

Maternal-neonatal transmission of HDV is uncommon. HDV is spread chiefly by direct contact of HBsAg carriers with HDV-HBV–infected individuals; household-family members and intimate contacts of HDV-HBV–infected persons appear to be at greatest risk.[93] The introduction of HDV into susceptible HBsAg carrier populations, resulting in devastating outbreaks,[94] may also lead to the development of an endemic epidemiologic pattern.

In areas like North America and northern Europe, a nonendemic pattern has been observed; HDV is uncommon in the general population. However, in certain populations, e.g., HBsAg-positive parenteral drug abusers, hemophiliacs, homosexual men, and hemodialysis patients, HDV infection

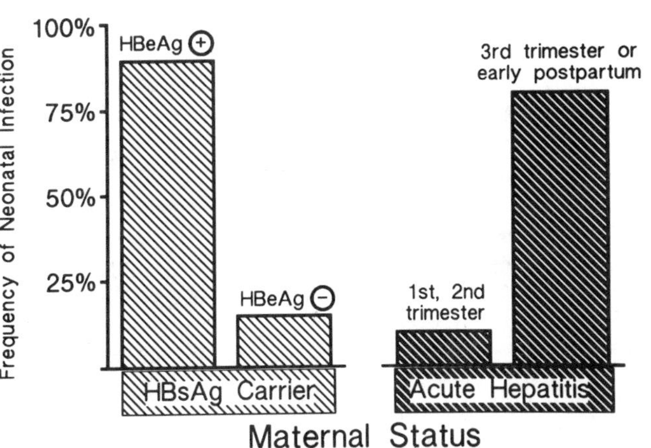

FIGURE 4 Maternal-neonatal HBV transmission. The risk of maternal-neonatal transmission of HBV is greatest when the mother is an HBeAg-positive carrier or when the mother develops acute hepatitis B in the third trimester or early postpartum period. (Courtesy of the Clinical Teaching Project, American Gastroenterological Association.)

occurs with a moderate frequency. Explosive outbreaks of HDV infection have been noted in HBsAg-positive parenteral drug abusers and their intimate contacts.[95]

Non-A, Non-B Hepatitis Infections

Blood-Borne Non-A, Non-B Hepatitis

Percutaneous spread of the blood-borne agents is believed to be one of the predominant modes of transmission in the United States. HCV has been shown to be the major complication of transfusion of blood and blood products and is commonly encountered in parenteral drug abusers who share injection equipment.[19b] Inapparent percutaneous inoculations also may be responsible for occupationally acquired HCV infections among health-care workers. Person-to-person spread of HCV and the second agent of blood-borne NANB hepatitis also appears to be responsible for transmission between sexual contacts.[96] It should be noted, however, that the route of spread of NANB hepatitis cannot be identified in nearly 40 percent of cases. Such cases, usually labeled *sporadic*, may result from contact transmission with asymptomatic carriers of HCV or the other blood-borne agent.

Enterically Transmitted Non-A, Non-B Hepatitis

Enterically transmitted NANB viral hepatitis has been responsible for large outbreaks in the Indian subcontinent, Asia, the Soviet Union, northern Africa, and Mexico.[97] In the United States, only imported cases have been recognized.[98] Water-borne transmission is the presumed enteric route of spread in most of the described outbreaks. Secondary attack rates in household members may approach 20 percent.[27]

TREATMENT

Only supportive and symptomatic therapy is available; restriction of physical activity is determined solely by the patient's sense of well-being. Similarly, no specific dietary program is offered other than a well-balanced diet. Pharmacologic antiviral therapy is not yet available but is under development. Corticosteroids should not be used. In acute hepatitis B and NANB viral hepatitis, antiviral therapy, when available, might be targeted for those individuals at risk of developing persistent infection. Similarly, antiviral therapy for HDV superinfection of HBV carriers might prevent persistent HDV infection. Early treatment of persistent HBV infection might inhibit or prevent chromosomal integration of HBV DNA and the development of certain sequelae.

SEQUELAE

Hepatitis A

HAV infections are invariably self-limited. No viremic or fecal carrier state follows infection, and chronic liver disease is not seen.

Hepatitis B

In contrast to acute HBV infection, in patients with chronic HBV infection HBsAg remains detectable for more than 6 months. In many patients HBsAg persists for decades, since the spontaneous HBsAg clearance rate is no higher than 1 to 2 percent annually. Spontaneous elimination of HBV among those individuals infected in childhood is unusual.[99] Asymptomatic persistently HBsAg-positive individuals are labeled HBsAg carriers. Other persistently HBsAg-positive individuals have clinical or laboratory evidence of chronic liver disease, i.e., chronic hepatitis B.

The prevalence of the HBsAg carrier state is variable. In the United States, as many as 0.1 to 0.9 percent of the general population are persistently HBsAg-positive. Carrier rates 5 to 10 times higher have been found in Asian-Americans, homosexual men, recipients of multiple blood transfusions or blood products, parenteral drug abusers, institutionalized individuals with Down's syndrome, and patients with immunologic defects. Among Alaskan Eskimos HBsAg carrier rates approaching 25 percent have been recognized. In parts of southeast Asia, the South Pacific, the Mediterranean littoral, and sub-Saharan Africa, HBsAg carrier rates in excess of 5 percent are commonly encountered; in a few remote and culturally isolated regions prevalence rates approaching 50 percent have been reported.

Serology of Persistent HBV Infection

Anti-HBc is present in all chronic HBV infections (Fig. 5). IgM anti-HBc is a minor fraction of total anti-HBc reactivity or is entirely absent. Persistence of IgM anti-HBc in high titer is uncommon; it reflects prolonged, active viral replication. In contrast to acute self-limited HBV infection, HBeAg may remain detectable in sera for many months to years in chronically infected individuals. Circulating HBV

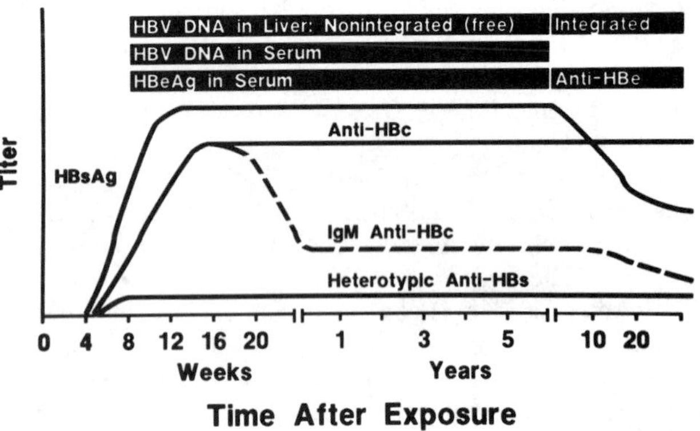

FIGURE 5 HBsAg remains detectable for prolonged periods in persistent HBV infection. Anti-HBc is present and HBeAg may remain detectable during the phase of active HBV replication, which is marked by the presence of HBV DNA in serum and liver (in a free, nonintegrated form). Subsequently, HBV replication diminishes and HBV DNA becomes integrated into the DNA of the infected hepatocyte. Low levels of heterotypic anti-HBs may be found. (From Seeff LB, ed. Current perspectives in hepatology. New York: Plenum Press, 1989.)

DNA may also be readily detected and is highly correlated with the presence of intact virions and potential infectivity. HBV DNA is also detectable in the hepatocytes of individuals with chronic HBV infection. Early after the onset of infection, this hepatic HBV DNA is present in a free, episomal, replicating form. Eventually, in some patients, replication decreases and HBV DNA becomes integrated into the genome of the host hepatocyte. This phenomenon is often signaled by the disappearance of serum HBV DNA and HBeAg and the appearance of anti-HBe in the circulation. Total anti-HBc reactivity and IgM anti-HBc level, if present, may also fall at this time. Anti-HBs is present concurrently with HBsAg in 10 to 40 percent of patients with chronic HBV infection. In contrast to typical anti-HBs seen on recovery from acute HBV infection, this anti-HBs is a low-titer, low-affinity antibody directed at a heterotypic subdeterminant of HBsAg. Its presence indicates neither reduced infectivity nor likely clearance of HBsAg.[100,101]

Determinants of Persistent HBV Infection

One risk factor for persistent HBV infection is intrinsic or iatrogenic immunosuppression. Immunosuppressed persons, whether children or adults, are at increased risk of becoming carriers after HBV infection. Gender is also a determinant of persistent infection. Women and girls are more likely than men or boys to clear HBsAg. As a consequence, among nearly all populations of HBsAg carriers, males predominate.

Age at the time of initial HBV infection is a major determinant of persistent HBV infection.[102] Available data from areas of high HBV prevalence, such as the far East, suggest that most HBsAg carriers acquire infections before 3 years of age.[103] In contrast, HBV infections after 3 years of age infrequently result in the carrier state. The development of the HBsAg carrier state occurs in an extraordinary number of infected neonates. However, as shown in Figure 6, the rate falls progressively with increasing age at time of initial infection. The crucial role of maternal-neonatal infection in the perpetuation of persistent HBV infection in certain high-prevalence areas of the world is well established (Fig. 7). Ninety percent of the neonates of HBeAg-positive carrier women are infected at or near the time of birth. Furthermore, 90 percent of the infected neonates of HBeAg-positive carrier mothers themselves become HBsAg carriers. Hence, 80 percent of the neonates born to HBeAg-positive, HBsAg carrier women become HBsAg carriers.[104] Female carriers may remain infectious at reproductive age and subsequently infect their neonates. Most carrier women are asymptomatic; in a small proportion chronic liver disease develops. In contrast, male carriers, while playing a relatively small role in the perpetuation of infection, appear to be at increased risk for the development of chronic liver disease (chronic hepatitis and cirrhosis), primary hepatocellular carcinoma (PHC), and premature death from liver disease.[105]

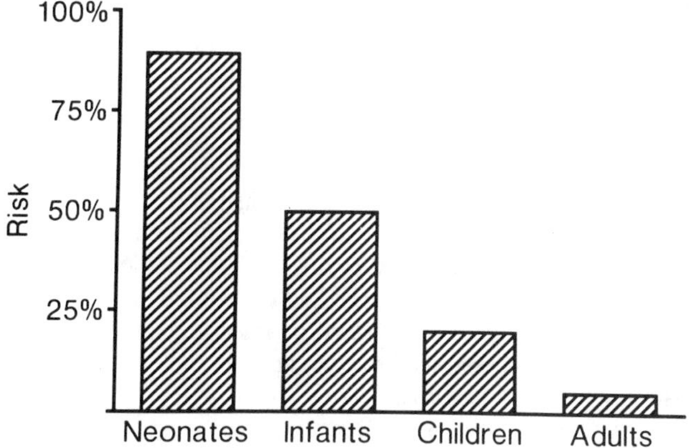

FIGURE 6 Risk of carrier state after acute HBV infection. As depicted here, there is a striking inverse relationship between age at the time of initial HBV infection and the risk of the development of the HBsAg carrier state. (Courtesy of the Clinical Teaching Project, American Gastroenterological Association.)

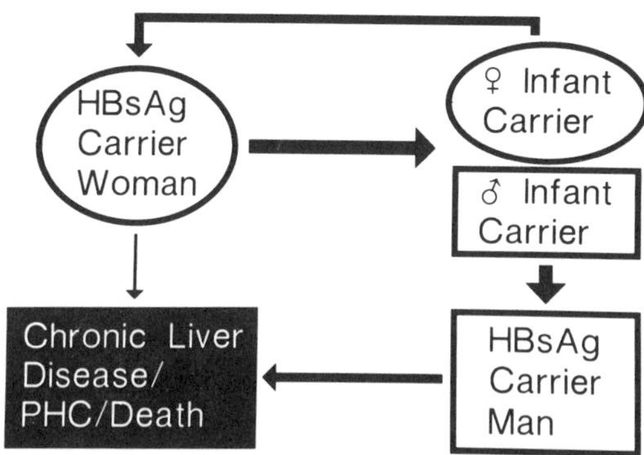

FIGURE 7 Cycle of maternal-neonatal HBV infection. Maternal-neonatal transmission plays a critical role in the perpetuation of persistent HBV infection. The infants of HBsAg carrier mothers themselves become HBsAg carriers, and their offspring may become carriers. Chronic liver disease, primary hepatocellular carcinoma (PHC), and premature death are more commonly seen in male than in female carriers. (Courtesy of the Clinical Teaching Project, American Gastroenterological Association.)

Chronic Liver Disease

Limited studies of HBsAg carrier children infected perinatally suggest that the majority are asymptomatic.[106] Serum aminotransferase levels may be mildly elevated or fluctuate in and out of the normal range. Liver biopsy reveals minimal mononuclear cell infiltration of the portal triads or evidence of chronic persistent hepatitis. Chronic active hepatitis and cirrhosis are infrequently recognized in asymptomatic HBsAg-positive children. In contrast, among symptomatic HBsAg-positive children, chronic active hepatitis and cirrhosis may be the predominant lesions found.[107]

HBV-Associated Primary Hepatocellular Carcinoma

Persistent HBV infection is an extremely important precursor in the development of PHC. In sub-Saharan Africa and in the far East PHC appears to be extraordinarily prevalent and a major cause of death from malignancies. A highly positive correlation between PHC and the prevalence of the HBV carrier state has been recognized.[108] In a classic follow-up study of asymptomatic HBsAg carriers and noncarriers in Taiwan, the relative risk of PHC in carriers compared to noncarriers was estimated to be 94 (95 percent confidence limits of 50 to 193)[109] (R.P. Beasley: personal communication). In other regions, estimates of the relative risk of PHC in HBsAg carriers are lower but still highly significant.[102]

Although PHC occurs predominantly in middle-aged to elderly male HBsAg carriers, many of whom acquired HBV infection early in life, HBsAg-positive children are also at risk of developing this malignancy.[110] As in adults with HBV-associated PHC, a male predominance has been seen in affected children. Surveillance of HBsAg-positive persons for early detection of PHC should probably begin relatively early after the carrier state is recognized, particularly in high-risk regions.

Reactivation

Occasional patients with chronic HBV infection (either chronic hepatitis B or the asymptomatic HBsAg carrier state) who have lost serologic markers of HBV replication (HBeAg or HBV DNA) may develop biochemical, clinical, and histologic exacerbations simulating acute hepatitis B.[111,112] The term "reactivation" is applied to these episodes, since HBV multiplication recurs. HBV DNA, DNA polymerase, and HBeAg usually reappear in serum concurrently with elevation of alanine aminotransferase. In some patients IgM anti-HBc also may become detectable.[113] Reactivations can be brief, asymptomatic, and self-limited or may last several months and be clinically severe.

Miscellaneous

In some areas of the world in which HBV prevalence is high, patients with membranous nephropathy, IgA nephropathy, and mesangial proliferative glomerulonephritis are HBsAg carriers in whom glomerular deposits of HBsAg or HBcAg can be detected in renal biopsy specimens.[114]

Hepatitis D

HDV superinfection of HBV carriers may lead to persistent HDV infection associated with chronic hepatitis and cirrhosis.

Non-A, Non-B Hepatitis

Among patients with transfusion-associated NANB hepatitis, chronic hepatitis, detected by persistent, if fluctuating, serum aminotransferase levels, develops in nearly half. Available data, predominantly in adults, suggest that in as many as 20 percent of those with NANB chronic hepatitis, histologic evidence of cirrhosis will appear on prolonged (5- to 10-year) follow-up. While most patients are asymptomatic, deaths due to portal hypertension and other complications of cirrhosis have been reported.[115] Primary hepatocellular carcinoma may be a sequela of NANB hepatitis associated with chronic active hepatitis with cirrhosis. The etiologic linkage requires further definition.

In a small number of patients, most of whom have NANB viral hepatitis or, less frequently, hepatitis B, clinical evidence of aplastic anemia may be recognized during the icteric or convalescent phase of illness.[116] HAV infection has rarely been implicated.[117] While the precise mechanism responsible for this devastating complication is uncertain, a direct attack of the hepatitis agents on the bone marrow has been postulated.

PREVENTION

While a variety of prevention strategies are available, immunoprophylaxis is key.

Hepatitis A

Passive Immunization

Despite the observation that HAV strains isolated in nature from nonhuman primates are distinct from HAV stains isolated from human beings,[118] human immunoglobulin appears to be highly effective in the immunoprophlaxis of HAV infection in all human populations studied. Furthermore, evidence has been presented suggesting that human HAV possesses only a single antibody-dependent immunodominant neutralization site on its capsid.[119]

The presence of IgG anti-HAV in immunoglobulin is believed to be responsible for the protective efficacy of this material. In many individuals immune globulin administration, after exposure to HAV, completely aborts HAV infection and totally suppresses clinical manifestations of hepatitis.[4,120,121] Because anti-HAV is not induced in this setting, susceptibility to infection is not altered. In perhaps 15 to 20 percent of individuals given immunoglobulin after HAV exposure, subclinical infection develops accompanied by production of anti-HAV and prolonged protection against reinfection. Immunoglobulin prophylaxis is ineffective in less than 10 percent of patients, in whom clinical illness may be seen. In these globulin failures, endogenous anti-HAV develops, leading to immunity to reinfection.

Immunoglobulin prophylaxis is recommended for household and intimate contacts of index cases with HAV infection; all children and adults within the household should be immunized. Persons exposed during the late incubation period or early acute phase of illness should be promptly immunized. Casual contacts of HAV-infected patients, e.g., co-workers, neighbors, or schoolmates, are not appropriate candidates for immunoglobulin prophylaxis.

Immunoglobulin has also been used in the control of outbreaks of HAV infections in high-risk institutions, such as day-care centers and institutions for the mentally retarded. The protective efficacy of immunoglobulin in the control of common-source outbreaks is uncertain, since such outbreaks may be identified too late to prevent infection in exposed individuals.

For pre-exposure immunoprophylaxis of HAV infection for children or adults traveling to tropical and developing countries, the United States Public Health Service Advisory Committee on Immunization Practices recommends immunoglobulin in the following dose schedules: for those spending less than 2 months abroad, 0.02 ml per kilogram of body weight, and for prolonged travel, 0.06 ml per kilogram of body weight.[122] For extended travel, additional injections of United States–made immunoglobulin at 4- to 6-month intervals should be arranged.

Active Immunization

Three approaches to the development of HAV vaccines are under study. The first approach is an attempt to produce a live, attenuated virus vaccine. Nucleotide deletions and base substitutions in the RNA of HAV result in attenuation of virulence and its adaptation to cell culture.[123] Such attenuated strains are being evaluated as prototype vaccines.[124] The second approach utilizes inactivated HAV in vaccine development.[125,126] Prototypes have been produced by chemical inactivation of HAV either isolated from the livers of nonhuman primates experimentally infected with HAV or propagated in tissue culture.[127] The third approach, the development of a recombinant vaccine containing the immunodominant neutralization site, requires considerable further research.

Hepatitis B

Anti-HBs is believed to be the protective, neutralizing antibody responsible for immunity to reinfection. However, not all anti-HBs reactivity is protective. In a small number of individuals, as well as in nonprimate animals, anti-HBs reactivity in sera may be due to the IgM antibody, which does not provide protection against HBV infection.[128,129]

The immune response to natural infection with HBV involves induction of both anti-HBc and anti-HBs, whereas the response to active immunization by vaccination is limited to anti-HBs alone.[130] Passive immunization refers to the administration of anti-HBs in the form of hepatitis B immunoglobulin (HBIG). In practice, passive immunization is rarely used alone. Active immunization and combined active-passive immunization are the preferred approaches.

The anti-HBs responses induced in human beings by equivalent doses of the plasma-derived (Heptavax-B) and recombinant (Recombivax-HB and Engerix-B) HBV vaccines, licensed for use in the United States, against a putative group "a" epitope are quantitatively and qualitatively equivalent.[131] Although data are still limited and important dose questions remain unanswered,[132, 133] it appears that the vaccines offer similar protective efficacy. Even years after initial vaccination, HBV vaccine continues to protect against clinical hepatitis B and persistent hepatitis B infection, despite the fall in titer of anti-HBs.[134]

HBsAg is the active immunogenic material of both the plasma-derived and yeast-recombinant HBV vaccines. The plasma-derived HBsAg particle is largely glycosylated, whereas that in the yeast-recombinant vaccine is nonglycosylated. Pre-S determinants might enhance the immunogenicity of HBV vaccines[135]; they are not present in the licensed preparations. Whether or not pre-S proteins should be incorporated into newly formulated HBV vaccines remains controversial.[61] Recombinant vaccines have been formulated to contain 10–20 μg of HBsAg protein per milliliter, compared with 20 μg per milliliter for the plasma-derived vaccine. Pepsin, urea, and formaldehyde are used in an inactivation phase in the production of the plasma-derived vaccine, whereas only formaldehyde is used in the preparation of one of the recombinant vaccine. The acquired immunodeficiency syndrome (AIDS) or seroconversion to anti–human immunodeficiency virus (anti-HIV) has not been identified in recipients of these vaccines.

Age appears to be a critically important factor influencing the response to vaccination. Neonates respond superbly to the HBV vaccine, with development of anti-HBs in 100 percent of vaccinees.[136,137] Children between 6 months and 10 years of age also respond far better than do adults. Immunosuppressed individuals may not respond to HBV vaccination. The role of infection by the human immunodeficiency virus (HIV) in the response to HBV vaccine remains controversial.[138,139]

Dose and Vaccine Schedule

Both the plasma-derived and yeast-recombinant vaccines have been given intramuscularly (deltoid muscle in children and adults and anterolateral muscle of the thigh in infants) in a three-dose schedule (0, 1, and 6 months). The third dose of this schedule boosts anti-HBs levels to a peak at 7 to 10 months after the first dose. The titer of anti-HBs after vaccination is generally lower and falls more rapidly than after natural infection. Protection against reinfection is therefore thought to be briefer after vaccination than after natural infection.[130]

The most cost-effective dose schedule has yet to be firmly established in children. Children receiving as little as 2 μg of hepatitis B vaccine at 0, 1, and 6 months demonstrate satisfactory anti-HBs seroconversion responses.[140] The long-term efficacy of low-dose regimens remains to be established. If the intradermal rather than the intramuscular route is utilized, revaccination at shorter intervals may be necessary,[141] since the duration of protective efficacy induced by intradermal inoculation remains uncertain.

Side Effects of HBV Vaccines

The major side effect of HBV vaccine is transient pain at the injection site. Although no definitive epidemiologic linkage between any neurologic adverse event and receipt of the plasma-derived HBV vaccine has been established, in some analyses the Guillain-Barré syndrome appeared to occur more frequently than expected.[142]

While the risk of fetal damage following administration of HBV vaccine to pregnant women is probably extremely low, it has been generally accepted that the vaccine should not be given unless clearly needed. No untoward side effects were noted in the newborn of women vaccinated during the third trimester[143]; the safety of earlier vaccination, when teratogenic effects might be more likely, remains incompletely defined.

Alternative HBV Vaccines

Glycosylated and nonglycosylated polypeptides prepared from 22-nm HBsAg particles, formulated into micelles and alum-absorbed, appear to be immunogenic in human subjects and may serve as alternative HBV vaccines.[144] Construction of recombinant vaccinia virus containing coding sequences for HBsAg[145] or construction of genetically engineered fusion proteins into which HBsAg has been inserted[146] may be used to prepare vaccines in the future. Other alternative vaccines involve the use of anti-idiotype antibodies containing the internal image of HBsAg as surrogates for HBsAg.[147]

Prevention of Maternal-Neonatal Infections

Several studies support the recommendation that prenatal HBsAg screening of all pregnant women, rather than only high-risk pregnant women, should be initiated in the United States.[148–151] Routine screening and immunoprophylaxis for the newborns of HBsAg-positive women have been estimated to be cost-effective even though the United States is usually considered a low HBV prevalence country.[152]

Inoculation, in the standard three-dose schedule, with the yeast-recombinant HBV vaccine, licensed in the United States, was shown to be as effective as inoculation with the plasma-derived HBV vaccine when given together with a single dose of hepatitis B immunoglobulin to neonates born to HBsAg- and HBeAg-positive mothers.[153] Only 5 to 10 percent of the vaccine-treated infants became HBsAg carriers. The protective efficacy rate was high (85 to 95 percent). Vaccine failures usually occurred within the first 6 months. Infants in whom venous blood samples obtained at birth were HBsAg-positive are believed to have been infected in utero. The hepatitis B immunoglobulin (0.5 ml) and vaccine (10 μg of the plasma-derived or 5 or 10 μg of the recombinant preparations) should be given at different sites in the anterolateral muscle of the thigh.

In certain high-risk areas of the developing world, mass vaccination programs designed to interrupt maternal-neonatal HBV transmission have been initiated and shown to be feasible but sufficiently costly that their adoption in the developing world will be difficult.[154] If smaller doses of the HBV vaccines can be demonstrated to have immunogenicity equivalent to that of the larger doses currently in use in neonates,[155] the economic benefits would be vast.

The duration of protective efficacy in infants given HBV vaccine in an endemic area appears to be at least 4 years, suggesting that booster inoculations may be required about 5 to 6 years after the first injection of vaccine.[156]

Immunoprophylaxis for Intimate Contacts

Sexual contacts of persons with acute hepatitis B should receive a single dose of 0.06 ml of HBIG per kilogram of body weight within 14 days of exposure; for susceptible male homosexuals HBV vaccine should be initiated at the same time.[122]

HBV vaccine has been recommended for susceptible intimate and household contacts of index cases with chronic HBV infection. Members of families in which HBsAg-positive infants or children are adopted should be vaccinated as soon as the HBsAg-positive individual is identified. Immunoprophylaxis is not recommended for the casual contacts of HBsAg-positive persons, whether acutely or chronically infected.

Hepatitis D

The only practical means of preventing HDV infection is the appropriate utilization of HBV vaccine to prevent HBV infection. For those individuals with established HBV infection (either chronic hepatitis B or the carrier state), prevention must rely on the avoidance of percutaneous exposures to HDV and the avoidance of contaminated secretions from individuals likely to be infected by HBV-HDV.

Non-A, Non-B Hepatitis

Blood-Borne Non-A, Non-B Hepatitis

Restrictions on donor eligibility and testing for HIV infection, combined with use of alanine aminotransferase and anti-HBc surrogate tests of donor blood may reduce the frequency of transfusion-associated hepatitis.[157–160] Screening of blood donors for anti-HCV should identify the majority of asymptomatic infectious HCV carriers.[160a] Data supporting a decreased risk resulting from these control measures are not yet available.[161] Until such data become available, it is reasonable to minimize the amount of blood transfused and to avoid untreated pooled blood products whenever possible, to use treated products in lieu of untreated ones, and, as much as possible, to rely on autologous transfusion.

Immunoglobulin prepared in the United States may have some efficacy in the prevention of endemic, sporadic icteric NANB hepatitis in southeast Asia.[162] In contrast, immunoglobulin, regardless of site of manufacture, is not recommended for the prophylaxis of post-transfusion hepatitis. Three clinical trials of the efficacy of immunoglobulin in this setting provided conflicting results.[163–165] There is also no evidence that HBIG would be effective.

Enterically Transmitted Non-A, Non-B Hepatitis

Immunoglobulin prophylaxis, utilizing globulin prepared from healthy donors residing in countries in which enterically transmitted NANB hepatitis occurs, may be effective in reducing the risk of disease in travelers to those countries.[166]

REFERENCES

1. Nayak NC, Panda SK, Zuckerman AJ, Bhan MK, Guha DK. Dynamics and impact of perinatal transmission of hepatitis B virus in north India. J Med Virol 1987; 21:137–145.
2. Gust ID, Coulepis AG, Feinstone SM, et al. Taxonomic classification of hepatitis A virus. Intervirology 1983; 20:1–7.

3. Cohen JI, Ticehurst JR, Purcell RH, et al. Complete nucleotide sequence of wild-type hepatitis A virus: comparison with different strains of hepatitis A virus and other picornaviruses. J Virol 1987; 61:50–59.
4. Lemon SM. Type A viral hepatitis. New developments in an old disease. N Engl J Med 1985; 313:1059–1067.
5. Busch FW, de Vos S, Flehmig B, et al. Inhibition of in vitro hematopoiesis by hepatitis A virus. Exp Hematol 1987; 15:978–982.
6. Feitelson MA, Millman I, Halbherr T, et al. A newly identified hepatitis B type virus in tree squirrels. Proc Natl Acad Sci USA 1986; 83:2233–2237.
7. Trueba D, Phelan M, Nelson J, et al. Transmission of ground squirrel hepatitis virus to homologous and heterologous hosts. Hepatology 1985; 5:435–439.
8. Fujita YK, Kamata K, Kameda H, et al. Detection of hepatitis B virus infection in hepatitis B surface antigen-negative hemodialysis patients by monoclonal radioimmunoassays. Gastroenterology 1986; 91:1357–1363.
9. Wands JR, Fujita YK, Isselbacher KJ, et al. Identification and transmission of hepatitis B virus-related variants. Proc Natl Acad Sci USA 1986; 83:6608–6612.
10. Coursaget P, Yvonnet B, Vourdil C, et al. HBsAg positive reactivity in man not due to hepatitis B virus. Lancet 1987; ii:1354–1358.
11. Acs G, Sells MA, Purcell RH, et al. Hepatitis B virus produced by transfected Hep G2 cells causes hepatitis in chimpanzees. Proc Natl Acad Sci USA 1987; 84:4641–4644.
12. Tiollais P, Pourcel C, Dejean A. The hepatitis B virus. Nature 1985; 317:489–495.
13. Miller RH. Proteolytic self-cleavage of hepatitis B virus core protein may generate serum e antigen. Science 1987; 236:722–725.
14. Wang K-S, Choo Q-L, Weiner AJ, et al. Structure, sequence and expression of the hepatitis delta (δ) viral genome. Nature 1986; 323:508–514.
15. Kos A, Dijkema R, Arnberg AC, et al. The hepatitis delta (δ) virus possesses a circular RNA. Nature 1986; 323:558–560.
16. Saldanha JA, Thomas HC, Monjardino JP. Cloning and characterization of a delta virus cDNA sequence derived from a human source. J Med Virol 1987; 22:323–331.
17. Chen P-J, Kalpana G, Goldberg J, et al. Structure and replication of the genome of the hepatitis δ virus. Proc Natl Acad Sci USA 1986; 83:3774–8778.
18. Bradley DW, Maynard JE, Popper H, et al. Postransfusion non-A, non-B hepatitis: physicochemical properties of two distinct agents. J Infect Dis 1983; 148:254–265.
19. Bradley DW, Maynard JE. Etiology and natural history of post-transfusion and enterically-transmitted non-A, non-B hepatitis. Semin Liver Dis 1986; 6:56–66.
19a. Choo Q-L, Kuo G, Weiner AJ, et al. Isolation of a cDNA clone derived from a blood-borne non-A, non-B viral hepatitis genome. Science 1989; 244:359–362.
19b. Kuo G, Choo Q-L, Alter HJ, et al. An assay for circulating antibodies to a major etiologic virus of human non-A, non-B hepatitis. Science 1989; 244:362–364.
20. Bradley DW, Krawczynski K, Cook EH Jr, et al. Enterically-transmitted non-A, non-B hepatitis: serial passage of disease in cynomolgus macaques and tamarins and recovery of disease-associated 27- to 34-nm viruslike particles. Proc Natl Acad Sci USA 1987; 84:6277–6281.
21. Dienes HP, Hutteroth T, Hess G, et al. Immunoelectron microscopic observations on the inflammatory infiltrates and HLA antigens in hepatitis B and non-A, non-B. Hepatology 1987; 7:1317–1325.
22. Pignatelli M, Waters J, Brown D, et al. HLA class I antigens on hepatocyte membrane during recovery from acute hepatitis B virus infection and during interferon therapy in chronic hepatitis B virus infection. Hepatology 1986; 6:349–353.
23. Hadler SC, Webster HM, Erben JJ, et al. Hepatitis A in day-care centers. A community-wide assessment. N Engl J Med 1980; 302:1222–1227.
24. Lednar WM, Lemon SM, Kirkpatrick JW, et al. Frequency of illness associated with epidemic hepatitis A virus infections in adults. Am J Epidemiol 1985; 122:226–233.
25. Yang N-Y, Yu PH, Mao Z-X, et al. Inapparent infection of hepatitis A virus. Am J Epidemiol 1988; 127:599–604.
26. Tong MJ, Thursby M, Rakela J, et al. Studies on the maternal-infant transmission of the viruses which cause acute hepatitis. Gastroenterology 1981; 80:999–1004.
27. Gust ID, Purcell RH. Report of a workshop: waterborne non-A, non-B hepatitis. J Infect Dis 1987; 156:630–635.
28. Ponzetto A, Hoyer BH, Popper H, et al. Titration of the infectivity of hepatitis D virus in chimpanzees. J Infect Dis 1987; 155:72–78.
29. Colombo M, Oldani S, Donato MF, et al. A multicenter, prospective study of postransfusion hepatitis in Milan. Hepatology 1987; 7:709–712.
30. Perrillo RP, Pohl DA, Roodman ST, et al. Acute non-A, non-B hepatitis with serum sickness-like syndrome and aplastic anemia. JAMA 1981; 234:494–496.
31. Shammaa MH. Acute viral hepatitis in Lebanon: Evidence for an HAV-like non-A, non-B hepatitis. Liver 1984; 4:39–44.
32. Routenberg JA, Dienstag JL, Harrison WO, et al. Foodborne outbreak of hepatitis A: clinical and laboratory features of acute and protracted illness. Am J Med Sci 1979; 278:123–137.
33. Bamber M, Thomas HC, Bannister B, et al. Acute type A, B, and non-A, non-B hepatitis in a hospital population in London: clinical and epidemiological features. Gut 1983; 24:561–564.
34. Inman RD, Hodge M, Johnston MEA, et al. Arthritis, vasculitis, and cryoglobulinemia associated with relapsing hepatitis A virus infection. Ann Intern Med 1986; 105:700–703.
35. Liehr H, Seelig R, Seelig HP. Cutaneous papulo-vesicular eruptions in non-A, non-B hepatitis. Hepatogastroenterology 1985; 32:11–14.
36. Draelos ZK, Hansen RC, James WD. Gianotti-Crosti syndrome associated with infections other than hepatitis B. JAMA 1986; 256:2386–2388.
37. Tabor E. Guillain-Barré syndrome and other neurologic syndromes in hepatitis A, B, and non-A, non-B. J Med Virol 1987; 21:207–216.
38. Ng PL, Powell LW, Campbell CB. Guillain-Barré syndrome during the pre-icteric phase of acute type B viral hepatitis. Aust N Z J Med 1975; 5:367–369.
39. Bosch VV, Dowling PC, Cook SD. Hepatitis A virus immunoglobulin M antibody in acute neurological disease. Ann Neurol 1983; 14:685–687.
40. Pelletier G, Elghozi D, Trepo C, et al. Mononeuritis in acute viral hepatitis. Digestion 1985; 32:53–56.
41. Centers for Disease Control Enterically transmitted non-A, non-B hepatitis—East Africa. MMWR 1987; 36:241–244.
42. Vilstrup H, Iversen J, Tygstrup N. Glucoregulation in acute liver failure. Eur J Clin Invest 1986; 16:193–197.
43. Gimson AES, White YS, Eddleston ALWF, et al. Clinical and prognostic differences in fulminant hepatitis type A, B and non-A, non-B. Gut 1983; 24:1194–1198.
44. Bismuth H, Samuel D, Gugenheim J, et al. Emergency liver transplantation for fulminant hepatitis. Ann Intern Med 1987; 107:337–341.
45. European Association for the Study of the Liver (EASL). Randomised trial of steroid therapy for acute liver failure. Gut 1979; 20:620–623.
46. Canalese J, Gimson AE, Davis C, et al. Controlled trial of dexamethasone and mannitol for the cerebral edema of fulminant hepatic failure. Gut 1982; 23:625–629.
47. MacDougall BRD, Williams R. H_2-receptor antagonists and antacids in the prevention of acute upper gastrointestinal haemorrhage in fulminant hepatic failure. Two controlled trials. Lancet 1977; i:617–619.
48. Gordon SC, Reddy KR, Schiff L, et al. Prolonged intrahepatic cholestasis secondary to acute hepatitis A. Ann Intern Med 1984; 101:635–637.
49. Jacobson IM, Nath BJ, Dienstag JL. Relapsing viral hepatitis type A. J Med Virol 1985; 16:163–169.
50. Decker RH, Kosakowski SM, Vanderbilt AS, et al. Diagnosis of acute hepatitis A by HAVAB-M, a direct radioimmunoassay for IgM anti-HAV. Am J Clin Pathol 1981; 76:140–147.
51. Storch GA, Bodicky C, Parker M, et al. Use of conventional and IgM-specific radioimmunoassays for anti-hepatitis A antibody in an outbreak of hepatitis A. Am J Med 1982; 73:663–668.
52. Tassopoulas NC, Roumeliotou-Karayannis A, Sakka M, et al. An epidemic of hepatitis A in an institution for young children. Am J Epidemiol 1987; 125:302–307.
53. Sjogren M, Tanno H, Fay O, et al. Hepatitis A virus in stool during clinical relapse. Ann Intern Med 1987; 106:221–226.

54. Tassopoulos NC, Papaevangelou GJ, Ticehurst JR, et al. Fecal excretion of Greek strains of hepatitis A virus in patients with hepatitis A and in experimentally infected chimpanzees. J Infect Dis 1986; 154:231–237.
55. Ben-Porath E, Wands J, Gruia M, Isselbacher K. Clinical significance of enhanced detection of HBsAg by a monoclonal radioimmunoassay. Hepatology 1984; 4:803–807.
56. Krugman S, Overby LR, Mushahwar IK, et al. Viral hepatitis, type B. Studies on natural history and prevention re-examined. N Engl J Med 1979; 300:101–106.
57. Aldershvile J, Frosner GG, Nielsen JO, et al. Hepatitis B e antigen and antibody measured by radioimmunoassay in acute hepatitis B surface antigen-positive hepatitis. J Infect Dis 1980; 141:293–298.
58. Neurath AR, Kent SBH, Strick N, et al. Hepatitis B virus contains pre-S gene-encoded domains. Nature 1985; 315:154–156.
59. Budkowska A, Riottot M-M, Dubreuil P, et al. Monoclonal antibody recognizing pre-S(2) epitope of hepatitis B virus: characterization of pre-S(2) epitope and anti-pre-S(2) antibody. J Med Virol 1986; 20:111–125.
60. Klinkert M-Q, Theilmann L, Pfaff E, Schaller H. Pre-S1 antigens and antibodies early in the course of acute hepatitis B virus infection. J Virology 1986; 58:522–525.
61. Hellstrom U, Sylvan S, Kuhns M, et al. Absence of pre-S2 antibodies in natural hepatitis B virus infection. Lancet 1986; ii:889–893.
62. Hoofnagle JH, Schafer DF. Serologic markers of hepatitis B virus infection. Semin Liver Dis 1986; 6:1–10.
63. Zeldis JB, Mugishima H, Steinberg HN, Emanuel N, Gale RP. In vitro hepatitis B virus infection of human bone marrow cells. J Clin Invest 1986; 78:411–417.
64. Mushawar IK, Dienstag JL, Polesky HF, et al. Interpretation of various serological profiles of hepatitis B virus infection. Am J Clin Pathol 1981; 76:773–777.
65. Chernesky M, Mahony J, Castriciano S, et al. Diagnostic significance of anti-HBc IgM prevalence related to symptoms in Canadian patients acutely or chronically infected with hepatitis B virus. J Med Virol 1986; 20:269–277.
66. Papavangelou G, Roumeliotou-Karayannis A, Tassopoulos N, et al. Diagnostic value of anti-HBc IgM in high HBV prevalence areas. J Med Virol 1984; 13:393–399.
67. Sjogren M, Hoofnagle JH. Immunoglobulin M antibody to hepatitis B core antigen in patients with chronic type B hepatitis. Gastroenterology 1985; 89:252–258.
68. Koike K, Iino S, Kurai K, Mitamura K, Endo Y, Oka H. IgM anti-HBc in anti-HBe positive chronic type B hepatitis with acute exacerbations. Hepatology 1987; 7:573–576.
69. Draelos M, Morgan T, Schifman RB, et al. Significance of isolated antibody to hepatitis B core antigen determined by immune response to hepatitis B vaccination. JAMA 1987; 258:1193–1195.
70. Feret E, Larouze B, Diop B, et al. Epidemiology of hepatitis B virus infection in the rural community of Tip, Senegal. Am J Epidemiol 1987; 125:140–149.
71. Rasshofer R, Buti M, Esteban R, Jardi R, Roggendorf M. Demonstration of hepatitis D virus RNA in patients with chronic hepatitis. J Infect Dis 1987; 157:191–195.
72. Aragona M, Caredda F, Lavarini C, Farci P, Macagno S, Crivelli O, Maran E, Purcell RH, Rizzetto M. Serological response to the hepatitis delta virus in hepatitis D. Lancet 1987; i:478–480.
73. Govindarajan S, De Cock KM, Redeker AG. Natural course of delta superinfection of chronic hepatitis B virus-infected patients: histological study with multiple liver biopsies. Hepatology 1986; 6:640–644.
74. Xu D-Z, Zhou W-Y, Zou H-K, et al. Etiological types and clincial and epidemiological features of acute viral hepatitis in Xi'an in China. J Med Virol 1987; 21:283–287.
75. Purcell RH, Feinstone SM, Ticehurst JR, et al. Hepatitis A virus. In: Vyas GN, Dienstag JL, Hoofnagle JH, eds. Viral hepatitis and liver disease. Orlando: Grune & Stratton, 1984: 9.
76. Koff RS, Grady GF, Chalmers TC, et al. Viral hepatitis in a group of Boston hospitals. III. Importance of exposure to shellfish in a nonepidemic period. N Engl J Med 1967; 276:703–710.
77. Szmuness W, Dienstag JL, Purcell RH, et al. The prevalence of antibody to hepatitis A antigen in various parts of the world: a pilot study. Am J Epidemiol 1977; 106:392–398.
78. Ikematsu H, Kashiwagi S, Hayashi J, et al. A seroepidemiologic study of hepatitis A virus infections: statistical analysis of two independent cross-sectional surveys in Okinawa, Japan. Am J Epidemiol 1987; 126:50–54.
79. Frosner GG, Papaevangelou G, Butler R, et al. Antibody against hepatitis A in seven European countries. I. Comparison of prevalence data in different age groups. Am J Epidemiol 1979; 110:63–69.
80. Francis DP, Favero MS, Maynard JE. Transmission of hepatitis B virus. Semin Liver Dis 1981; 1:27–32.
81. Shapiro ED. Lack of transmission of hepatitis B in a day-care center. J Pediatr 1987; 110:90–92.
82. Hayashi J, Kashiwagi S, Nomura H, et al. Hepatitis B virus transmission in nursery schools. Am J Epidemiol 1987; 125:492–498.
83. Breuer B, Friedman SM, Millner ES, et al. Transmission of hepatitis B virus to classroom contacts of mentally retarded carriers. JAMA 1985; 254:3190–3195.
84. Remis RS, Rossignol MA, Kane MA. Hepatitis B infection in a day school for mentally retarded students: transmission from students to staff. Am J Publ Health 1987; 77:1183–1186.
85. Davison F, Alexander GJM, Trowbridge R, et al. Detection of hepatitis B virus DNA in spermatozoa, urine, saliva, and leucocytes of chronic HBsAg carriers. J Hepatol 1987; 4:37–44.
86. Jenison SA, Lemon SM, Baker LN, et al. Quantitative analysis of hepatitis B virus DNA in saliva and semen of chronically infected homosexual men. J Infect Dis 1987; 156:299–307.
87. Lok A S-F, Lai C-L, Wu P-C, et al. Hepatitis B virus infection in Chinese families in Hong Kong. Am J Epidemiol 1987; 126:492–499.
88. Lin H-H, Lee T-Y, Chen D-S, et al. Transplacental leakage of HBeAg-positive maternal blood as the most likely route in causing intrauterine infection with hepatitis B virus. J Pediatr 1987; 111:877–881.
89. Ohto H, Lin H-H, Kawana T, et al. Intrauterine transmission of hepatitis B virus is closely related to placental leakage. J Med Virol 1987; 21:1–6.
90. Stevens CE, Toy PT, Tong MJ, et al. Perinatal hepatitis B virus transmission in the United States. Prevention by passive-active immunization. JAMA 1985; 253:1740–1745.
91. Stevens CE, Neurath AR, Beasley RP, et al. HBeAg and anti-HBe detection by radioimmunoassay: correlation with vertical transmission of hepatitis B virus in Taiwan. J Med Virol 1979; 3:237–241.
92. Bensabath G, Hadler SC, Soares MCP, et al. Hepatitis delta virus infection and Labrea hepatitis. Prevalence and role in fulminant hepatitis in the Amazon basin. JAMA 1987; 258:479–483.
93. Bonino F, Smedile A. Delta agent (type D) hepatitis. Semin Liver Dis 1986; 6:28–33.
94. Hadler SC, de Monzon M, Ponzetto A, et al. Delta virus infection and severe hepatitis. An epidemic in the Yucpa Indians of Venezuela. Ann Intern Med 1984; 100:339–344.
95. Lettau LA, McCarthy JG, Smith MH, et al. Outbreak of severe hepatitis due to delta and hepatitis B viruses in parenteral drug abusers and their contacts. N Engl J Med 1987; 317:1256–1262.
96. Dienstag JL. Non-A, non-B hepatitis. I. Recognition, epidemiology, and clinical features. Gastroenterology 1983; 85:439–462.
97. Centers for Disease Control. Enterically transmitted non-A, non-B hepatitis—Mexico. MMWR 1987; 36:597–602.
98. De Cock KM, Bradley DW, Sandford NL, et al. Epidemic non-A, non-B hepatitis in patients from Pakistan. Ann Intern Med 1987; 106:227–230.
99. Coursaget P, Yvonnet B, Chotard J, et al. Age- and sex-related study of hepatitis B virus chronic carrier state in infants from an endemic area (Senegal). J Med Virol 1987; 22:1–5.
100. Tsang T-K, Blei AT, O'Reilly DJ, et al. Clinical significance of concurrent hepatitis B surface antigen and antibody positivity. Dig Dis Sci 1986; 31:620–624.
101. Shiels MT, Taswell HF, Czaja AJ, et al. Frequency and significance of concurrent hepatitis B surface antigen and antibody in acute and chronic hepatitis B. Gastroenterology 1987; 93:675–680.
102. Seeff LB, Koff RS. Evolving concepts of the clinical and serologic consequences of hepatitis B virus infection. Semin Liver Dis 1986; 6:11–22.
103. Hsu H-Y, Chang M-H, Chen D-S, et al. Baseline seroepidemiology of hepatitis B virus infection in children in Taipei, 1984: a study just before mass hepatitis B vaccination program in Taiwan. J Med Virol 1986; 18:301–307.
104. Stevens CE, Beasley RP, Tsui J, et al. Vertical transmission of hepatitis B antigen in Taiwan. N Engl J Med 1975; 292:771–774.

105. Beasley RP. Hepatitis B virus as the etiologic agent in hepatocellular carcinoma—epidemiologic considerations. Hepatology 1982; 2:21S-26S.
106. Chang MH, Hwang LY, Hsu HC, et al. Prospective study of asymptomatic HBsAg carrier children infected in the perinatal period: clinical and liver histologic studies. Hepatology 1988; 8:374-377.
107. Hsu HC, Lin YH, Chang MH, et al. Pathology of chronic hepatitis B virus infection in children: with special reference to the intrahepatic expression of hepatitis B virus antigens. Hepatology 1988; 8:378-382.
108. Kew M. The hepatitis-B virus and hepatocellular carcinoma. Semin Liver Dis 1981; 1:59-67.
109. Beasley RP, Hwang L-Y. Epidemiology of hepatocellular carcinoma. In: Vyas GN, Dienstag JL, Hoofnagle JH, eds. Viral hepatitis and liver disease. Orlando: Grune & Stratton, 1984.
110. Hsu HC, Wu MZ, Chang MH, et al. Childhood hepatocellular carcinoma develops exclusively in hepatitis B surface antigen carriers in three decades in Taiwan: report of 51 cases strongly associated with rapid development of liver cirrhosis. J Hepatol 1987; 5:260-267.
111. Tong MJ, Sampliner RE, Govindarajan S, et al. Spontaneous reactivation of hepatitis B in Chinese patients with HBsAg-positive chronic active hepatitis. Hepatology 1987; 7:713-718.
112. Davis GL, Hoofnagle JH. Reactivation of chronic hepatitis B virus infection. Gastroenterology 1987; 92:2028-2031.
113. Koike K, Iino S, Kurai K, et al. IgM anti-HBc in anti-HBe positive chronic type B hepatitis with acute exacerbations. Hepatology 1987; 7:573-576.
114. Lai KN, Lai F M-M, Chan KW, et al. The clinico-pathologic features of hepatitis B virus-associated glomerulonephritis. Q J Med 1987; 63:323-333.
115. Dienstag JL, Alter HJ. Non-A, non-B hepatitis: evolving epidemiologic and clinical perspective. Semin Liver Dis 1986; 6:67-81.
116. Zeldis JB, Dienstag JL, Gale RP. Aplastic anemia and non-A, non-B hepatitis. Am J Med 1983; 74:64-68.
117. Domencech P, Palomeque A, Martinez-Gutierrex A, et al. Severe aplastic anemia following hepatitis A. Acta Haematol 1986; 76:227-229.
118. Lemon SM, Chao S-F, Jansen RW, et al. Genomic heterogeneity among human and nonhuman strains of hepatitis A virus. J Virol 1987; 61:735-742.
119. Stapleton JT, Lemon SM. Neutralization escape mutants define a dominant immunogenic neutralization site on hepatitis A virus. J Virol 1987; 61:491-498.
120. Drake ME, Ming C. Gamma globulin in epidemic hepatitis: comparative value of two dosage levels, apparently near the minimal effective level. JAMA 1954; 155:1302-1305.
121. Krugman S. Effect of human immune serum globulin on infectivity of hepatitis A virus. J Infect Dis 1976; 134:70-74.
122. Centers for Disease Control. Recommendations for protection against viral hepatitis. MMWR 1985; 34:313-324, 329-335.
123. Cohen JI, Rosenblum B, Ticehurst JR, et al. Complete nucleotide sequence of an attenuated hepatitis A virus: Comparison of wild-type virus. Proc Natl Acad Sci USA 1987; 84:2497-2501.
124. Karron RA, Daemer R, Ticehurst J, et al. Studies of prototype live hepatitis A virus vaccines in primate models. J Infect Dis 1988; 157:338-345.
125. Flehmig B, Haage A, Pfisterer M. Immunogenicity of a hepatitis A virus vaccine. J Med Virol 1987; 22:7-16.
126. Provost PJ, Hughes JV, Miller WJ, et al. An inactivated hepatitis A viral vaccine of cell culture origin. J Med Virol 1986; 19:23-31.
127. Heinricy U, Stierhof YD, Pfisterer M, et al. Properties of a hepatitis-A virus candidate vaccine strain. J Gen Virol 1987; 68:2487-2494.
128. Hoofnagle JH, Schafer DF, Ferenci P, et al. Antibody to hepatitis B surface antigen in nonprimate animal species. Gastroenterology 1983; 84:1478-1482.
129. Brotman B, Prince AM. Occurrence of AUSAB test positivity unrelated to prior exposure to hepatitis B virus. J Infect Dis 1984; 150:714-720.
130. Stevens CE, Taylor PE. Hepatitis B vaccine: issues, recommendations, and new developments. Semin Liver Dis 1986; 6:23-27.
131. Waters JA, O'Rourke SM, Richardson SC, et al. Qualitative analysis of the humoral immune response to the "a" determinant of HBs antigen after innoculation with plasma-derived or recombinant vaccine. J Med Virol 1987; 21:155-160.
132. Hollinger FB, Troisi CL, Pepe PE. Anti-HB_s responses to vaccination with a human hepatitis B vaccine made by recombinant DNA technology in yeast. J Infect Dis 1986; 153:156-159.
133. Hollinger FB. Hepatitis B vaccines—to switch or not to switch. JAMA 1987; 257:2634-2636.
134. Hadler SC, Francis DP, Maynard JE, et al. Long-term immunogenicity and efficacy of hepatitis B vaccine in homosexual men. N Engl J Med 1986; 315:209-214.
135. Milich DR, Thornton GB, Neurath AR, et al. Enhanced immunogenicity of the pre-S region of hepatitis B surface antigen. Science 1985; 228:1195-1199.
136. McClean AA, Hilleman MR, McAleer WJ, et al. Summary of worldwide experience with H-B-vax (B, MSD). J Infect 1983; 7:95-104.
137. Deinhardt F. Aspects of vaccination against hepatitis B, passive-active immunization schedules and vaccination responses in different age groups. Scand J Infect Dis 1983; 38(suppl):17-23.
138. Carne CA, Weller IVD, Waite J, et al. Impaired responsiveness of homosexual men with HIV antibodies to plasma derived hepatitis B vaccine. Br Med J 1987; 294:866-868.
139. Ostrow DG, Goldsmith J, Kalish SB, et al. Nonresponse to hepatitis B vaccine in homosexual men. Sex Transm Dis 1987; 14:92-97.
140. Milne A, Dimitrakakis M, Allwood G, et al. Immunogenicity of low doses of hepatitis B vaccine in children: a study in 650 New Zealand children. J Med Virol 1987; 23:401-405.
141. Frazer IH, Jones B, Dimitrakakis M, et al. Intramuscular versus low-dose intradermal hepatitis B vaccine. Assessment by humoral and cellular immune response to hepatitis B surface antigen. Med J Aust 1987; 146:242-245.
142. Shaw FE, Graham DJ, Guess HA, et al. Postmarketing surveillance for neurologic adverse events reported after hepatitis B vaccination. Experience of the first three years. Am J Epidemiol 1988; 127:337-352.
143. Ayoola EA, Johnson AOK. Hepatitis B vaccine in pregnancy: immunogenicity, safety and transfer of antibodies to infants. Int J Gynecol Obstet 1987; 25:297-301.
144. Hollinger FB, Troisi C, Heiberg D, et al. Response to a hepatitis B polypeptide vaccine in micelle form in a young adult population. J Med Virol 1986; 19:229-240.
145. Cheng K-C, Smith GL, Moss B. Hepatitis B virus large surface protein is not secreted but is immunogenic when selectively expressed by recombinant vaccinia virus. J Virol 1986; 60:337-344.
146. Phalipon A, Kaczorek M. Genetically engineered diptheria toxin fusion proteins carrying the hepatitis B surface antigen. Gene 1987; 232:220-223.
147. Kennedy RC, Eichberg JW, Lanford RE, et al. Anti-idiotype antibody vaccine for type B viral hepatitis in chimpanzees. Science 1986; 232:220-223.
148. Summers PR, Biswas MK, Pastorek JG, et al. The pregnant hepatitis B carrier: evidence favoring comprehensive antepartum screening. Obstet Gynecol 1987; 69:701-704.
149. McQuillan GM, Townsend TR, Johannes CB, et al. Prevention of perinatal transmission of hepatitis B virus: the sensitivity, specificity, and predictive value of the recommended screening questions to detect high-risk women in an obstetric population. Am J Epidemiol 1987; 126:484-491.
150. Kumar ML, Dawson NV, McCullough AJ, et al. Should all pregnant women be screened for hepatitis B? Ann Intern Med 1987; 107:272-277.
151. Jonas MM, Schiff ER, O'Sullivan MJ, et al. Failure of Centers of Disease Control criteria to identify hepatitis B infection in a large municipal obstetrical population. Ann Intern Med 1987; 107:335-337.
152. Arevalo JA, Washington AE. Cost-effectiveness of prenatal screening and immunization for hepatitis B virus. JAMA 1988; 259:365-369.
153. Stevens CE, Taylor PE, Tong MJ, et al. Yeast-recombinant hepatitis B vaccine. Efficacy with hepatitis B immune globulin in prevention of perinatal hepatitis B virus transmission. JAMA 1987; 257:2612-2616.
154. Chen D-S, Hsu N H-M, Sung J-L, et al. A mass vaccination program in Taiwan against hepatitis B virus infection in infants of hepatitis B surface antigen-carrier mothers. JAMA 1987; 257:2597-2603.
155. Moyes CD, Milne A, Dimitrakakis M, et al. Very-low-dose hepatitis B vaccine in newborn infants: an economic option for control in endemic areas. Lancet 1987; i:29-31.
156. Coursaget P, Yvonnet B, Chotard J, et al. Seven-year study of hepatitis B vaccine efficacy in infants from an endemic area (Senegal). Lancet 1986; ii:1143-1145.
157. Aach RD, Szmuness W, Mosley JW, et al. Serum alanine aminotransferase of donors in relation to the risk of non-A, non-B hepatitis

in recipients: the Transfusion-Transmitted Viruses study. N Engl J Med 1981; 304:989–994.
in recipients: the Transfusion-Transmitted Viruses study. N Engl J Med 1981; 304:989–994.
158. Alter HJ, Purcell RH, Holland PV, et al. Donor transaminase and recipient hepatitis. JAMA 1981; 246:630–634.
159. Stevens CE, Aach RD, Hollinger FB, et al. Hepatitis B virus antibody in blood donors and the occurrence of non-A, non-B hepatitis in transfusion recipients: an analysis of the Transfusion-Transmitted Viruses study. Ann Intern Med 1984; 101:733–738.
160. Koziol DE, Holland PV, Alling DW, et al. Antibody to hepatitis B core antigen as a paradoxical marker for non-A, non-B hepatitis agents in donated blood. Ann Intern Med 1986; 104:488–494.
160a. Alter HJ, Purcell RH, Shih JW, et al. Detection of antibody to hepatitis C virus in prospectively followed transfusion recipients with acute and chronic non-A, non-B hepatitis. N Engl J Med 1989; 321:1494–1500.
161. Bove JR. Transfusion-associated hepatitis and AIDS. N Engl J Med 1987; 317:242–245.
162. Conrad ME, Lemon SM. Prevention of endemic icteric viral hepatitis by administration of immune serum gamma globulin. J Infect Dis 1987; 156:56–63.
163. Kuhns WJ, Prince AM, Brotman B, et al. A clinical and laboratory evaluation of immune serum globulin from donors with a history of hepatitis: attempted prevention of post-transfusion hepatitis. Am J Med Sci 1976; 272:255–261.
164. Knodell RG, Conrad ME, Ginsberg AL, et al. Efficacy of prophylactic gamma-globulin in preventing non-A, non-B post-transfusion hepatitis. Lancet 1976; i:557–561.
165. Seeff LB, Zimmerman HJ, Wright EC, et al. A randomized double-blinded controlled trial of the efficacy of immune serum globulin for the prevention of post-transfusion hepatitis: a Veterans Administration cooperative study. Gastroenterology 1977; 72:111–121.
166. Joshi YK, Babu S, Sarin S, et al. Immunoprophylaxis of epidemic non-A, non-B hepatitis. Indian J Med Res 1985; 81:18–19.

PART 4

Molecular Biology of Hepatitis B Virus

Sanjeev Gupta, M.D., M.R.C.P.
David A. Shafritz, M.D.

Hepatitis B virus (HBV) was physically demonstrated by electron microscopy almost 20 years ago and identified as the agent responsible for "serum hepatitis."[1,2] However, because of the narrow host range of HBV, which is limited to humans and higher primates, and the earlier inability to effectively propagate HBV in cultured cells, progress in elucidating its biology has been limited. Nonetheless, within the past decade advances in molecular biology, development of animal models of HBV infection, and most recently successful infection with HBV of certain differentiated liver-derived cells in culture, have offered means for significant progress. Our current knowledge of the biology of HBV indicates a remarkably complex life cycle.[3,4] Unusual and unique strategies are employed for virus replication utilizing reverse transcription of an RNA intermediate in similarity to retroviruses, and expression of several gene products from overlapping viral transcripts. Despite insights into viral pathogenesis and potential targets of antiviral therapy, however, much remains unknown regarding host factors regulating HBV gene expression and the specific pathophysiologic contribution of individual viral components. Recognition of an epidemiologic association between HBV and hepatocellular carcinoma (HCC)[5-7] has generated great interest in elucidating possible roles that HBV might play in oncogenesis. This discussion focuses on the genomic organization and replication of HBV, as well as the viral transcripts and proteins. Additionally, information is presented regarding HBV and hepatocarcinogenesis. Epidemiology and clinical features of HBV are discussed in Chapter 28, Part 3.

VIRION STRUCTURE

Human HBV[3] is the most important of the five currently recognized members of the hepadna (*hep*atitis-*a*ssociated *DNA*) virus family. Other related hepadna viruses exist in the woodchuck HV (WHV),[8,9] the ground squirrel HV (GSHV),[8,10] the tree squirrel HV (TSHV),[11] and the Pekin duck HV (DHBV).[8,12] All share similar virion structures, genome organizations, and mechanisms of virus replication as well as species specificity and hepatotropism.[3,4] Recent evidence indicates that, besides hepatocytes, hepadna viruses may exist and replicate in a wide variety of other cell types,[13-24] predominantly in cells of hematopoietic origin,[13-20] and also elsewhere, including bile-duct epithelial cells, pancreas, kidney, and spermatozoa.[21-24]

HBV is found primarily in liver and serum. Purified preparations of HBV from human serum demonstrate three different types of viral particles (Fig. 1).[1,2] The infectious virion is represented by the "Dane particle," which has a diameter of 42 nM and consists of an outer envelope of protein and membrane lipids, surrounding an inner core structure or nucleocapsid (27 nM diameter), which contains the viral nucleic acid (illustrated schematically in Fig. 1*A* and demonstrated by electron microscopy of material purified from human serum in Fig. 1*B*). Found in far greater amounts (usually 10^3- to 10^6-fold excess) are 16- to 25-nM spherical particles and filaments of 22 nM diameter and variable length up to 1,000 nM that contain host-derived lipids but no viral nucleic acids and therefore are noninfectious. All three types

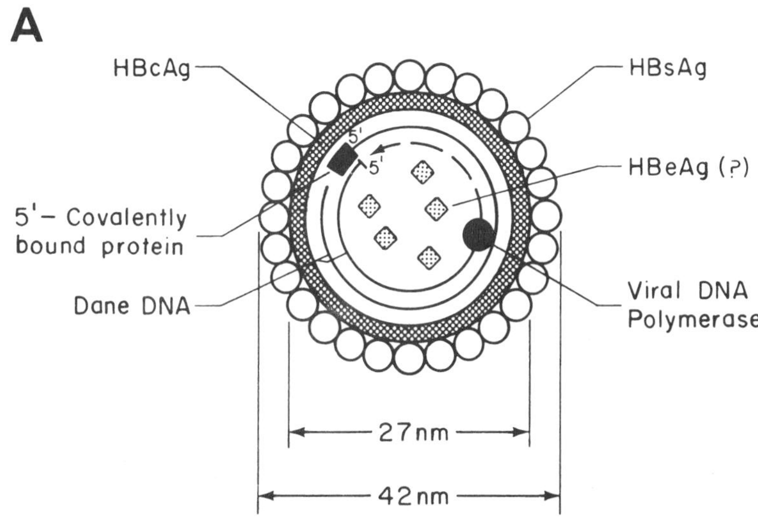

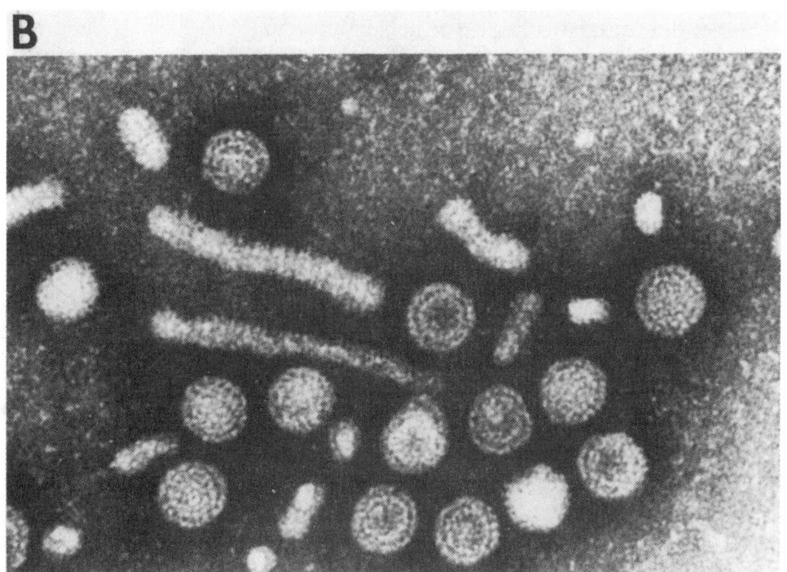

FIGURE 1 HBV particles as found in human serum. *A*, Schematic diagram of the virion (Dane particle). *B*, Electron micrograph of virion particles (42 nm) and both spherical and filamentous aggregates of HBsAg (22-nm diameter).

of particles display an externally located 24 Kd glycoprotein termed the hepatitis B surface antigen (HBsAg). The infectious nature of Dane particles was originally demonstrated by Robinson and colleagues.[2,25,26]

Treatment of Dane particles with the nonionic detergent Triton X-100, releases an inner nucleocapsid core[27] composed of a 21-Kd basic phosphoprotein termed hepatitis B core antigen (HBcAg). Such nucleocapsid cores also possess a DNA polymerase activity that is capable of filling in missing nucleotides in the unique partially double-stranded and circular viral genome.[28,29] Significant amounts of another protein called hepatitis B e antigen (HBeAg) may also be found in the serum of patients with HBV. This protein was initially distinguished from HBcAg by serologic means.[30] Treatment with proteases or certain detergents can convert HBcAg[31] into HBeAg following the removal of a C-terminal sequence.[32,33] However, HBeAg is produced independently of HBcAg from the same gene by a unique expression mechanism using an optional signal sequence (see below) and does not simply represent a HBcAg degradation product.[34–36] Nucleocapsid cores are identified within the nuclei of infected hepatocytes and are associated with HBV replication.[37] Recent evidence suggests, however, that presence of HBeAg in serum may not correlate with HBV replication.[38–40]

Virion size varies in non–human hepadna viruses from 40 nM in DHBV to 47 nM in GSHV. Both WHV and GSHV produce surface antigen in spheres and filaments similar to those of HBV with partial cross-reactivity to anti-HBs.[10,41,42] Only minor antigenic determinants are shared between WHsAg and HBsAg,[41] whereas one-third of the peptides generated by tryptic digestion of GSHsAg and HBsAg are identical. Immunodiffusion demonstrates antigenic similarity of WHcAg and HBcAg, and sequence analysis shows a 73 percent amino acid homology and 66 percent nucleic acid homology between these two antigens.[43] In DHBV infections, serum contains larger, 40 to 60 nM, spherical convoluted particles.[8] Although these particles do not cross-react with anti-HBs, they are presumed to be homologous to the other surface antigen-containing particles. Cross-reactivity with anti-HBc is demonstrated for WHV and GSHV but not with DHBV core antigens.

GENOME ORGANIZATION

The genome of HBV is a small circular DNA of 3,200 to 3,300 base pairs (for recent reviews, see Tiollais et al[3] and Ganem and Varmus.[4]) Its unique asymmetric structure was determined following isolation from Dane particles.[25,26,44–48] The genome (Fig. 2) is arranged in two strands; one DNA strand is of unit length while the other is shorter. The full-length DNA strand (L) is complementary to the viral mRNAs and is designated as minus (−) strand. This strand is complete, except for a nick of one or a few nucleotides at a fixed point (1,800 nucleotides from the EcoRl site). The short DNA strand (S), which is designated as plus (+) strand, lacks from 15 to 50 percent of its potential sequence complement.[49] The 5′ end of the S strand is located at nucleotide 1,560, but its length and consequently the position of its 3′ end varies considerably. The circular configuration of the genome is maintained by base pairing of the 5′ termini of both DNA strands, which overlap by about 250 to 300 nucleotides and form the "cohesive end" region.[50] As indicated earlier, endogenous DNA polymerase activity associated with the nucleocapsid repairs this single-stranded region of the plus (S) strand DNA by addition of nucleotides to the 3′ end. This DNA polymerase is distinct from bacterial or other serum polymerases because its activity is retained or enhanced at high salt concentrations. In vitro, the DNA polymerase reaction does not join the 3′ and 5′ ends of the S strand so that, although a complete circle is formed, it is not covalently closed. Nonetheless, particles containing covalently closed, circular double-stranded DNA (so-called superhelical forms), have been identified in liver persistently infected with HBV[51] or other members of the hepadna virus family.[52–54] The DNA molecule exhibits other asymmetries at the 5′ termini with a covalently linked protein at the (−) strand and an oligoribonucleotide attached to the (+) strand DNA.[55,56] Within the cohesive end region, there are also two 11-base-pair direct repeats, called DR1 and DR2, which may serve important functions in the virus life cycle or replication mechanism (for further details, see Tiollais et al[3] and Ganem and Varmus.[4]) Another conserved sequence is the element TATAAA within the 5′ end of the core antigen coding sequence, which serves as part of the cleavage/polyadenylation signal specifying the common 3′ termini of viral mRNAs.

Studies of cloned HBV DNA have shown significant heterogeneity in nucleotide sequence. Particles isolated from a single patient are homogeneous with respect to DNA sequences, as determined by restriction enzyme mapping,[57] and within a single HBV subtype only occasional differences are noted.[58] However, different serologic subtypes show considerable variation in restriction endonuclease maps. Nucleotide sequences of cloned HBV DNA may differ by up to 10 percent with small additions or deletions scattered throughout the genome.[59]

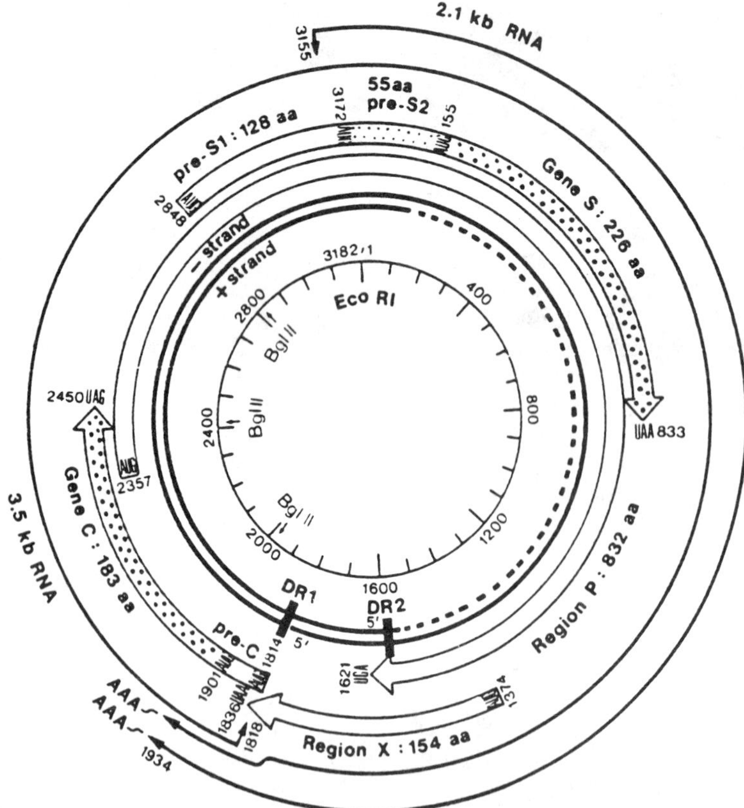

FIGURE 2 Structural and genetic organization of the HBV genome. The four transcriptional open reading frames S, C, P, and X and the position and orientation of the two major known HBV RNA transcripts are shown. (From Tiollais et al.[3])

STRUCTURAL GENES

Four translational open reading frames (ORFs) located on the minus (L) DNA strand of HBV code for polypeptides of substantial length.[3,4] The coding region for HBsAg (ORF S) extends from map positions 833 to 2,848 and in fact constitutes the 3′ portion of a larger coding region. An upstream reading frame (ORF pre-S) with two conserved in-phase ATG codons directs the synthesis of additional HBsAg-related proteins termed pre-S1 and pre-S2, which are also present in the virion envelope.[60] The coding region for HBcAg (ORF C), map positions 1,836 to 2,450, is also preceded by an upstream in-phase ORF (pre-C), which could encode a larger HBcAg-related polypeptide. The presumptive viral polymerase is encoded by ORF P, map positions 1,621 to 2,357. Another coding region that similarly overlaps ORFs S and C constitutes ORF X, map positions 1,374 to 1,818. Studies suggest that the ORF X gene product may be a transactivating protein that effects expression of homologous and heterologous genetic regulatory elements (see below).

All ORFs are well conserved among members of the hepadna virus family. One exception is that the ORF X is not present in DHBV. There is also considerable nucleotide sequence homology between the human and animal viruses (≃70, 55 and 40 percent with WHV, GSHV, and DHBV, respectively) and a greater than 80 percent homology between WHV and GSHV.[3] The plus (S) DNA strand contains only very short ORFs that could encode polypeptides smaller than 10 Kd. The positions of these ORFs on the (+) DNA strand are not well conserved in different HBV clones, suggesting that this strand may not be involved in transcription of specific viral gene products.[3]

GENOME REPLICATION

The mechanism for hepadna virus replication (Fig. 3), originally elucidated by Summers and Mason for DHBV[61] and subsequently confirmed for HBV,[62-65] is uniquely distinct from that of other DNA viruses (see Ganem and Varmus[4] for a full discussion). The asymmetric virion DNA is first converted to covalently closed circular DNA (ccc DNA) within the nucleus of infected hepatocytes.[61] Although several observations indicate this to be the initial event in genome replication, other events or enzymatic activities that lead to conversion of HBV DNA to ccc DNA are currently uniden-

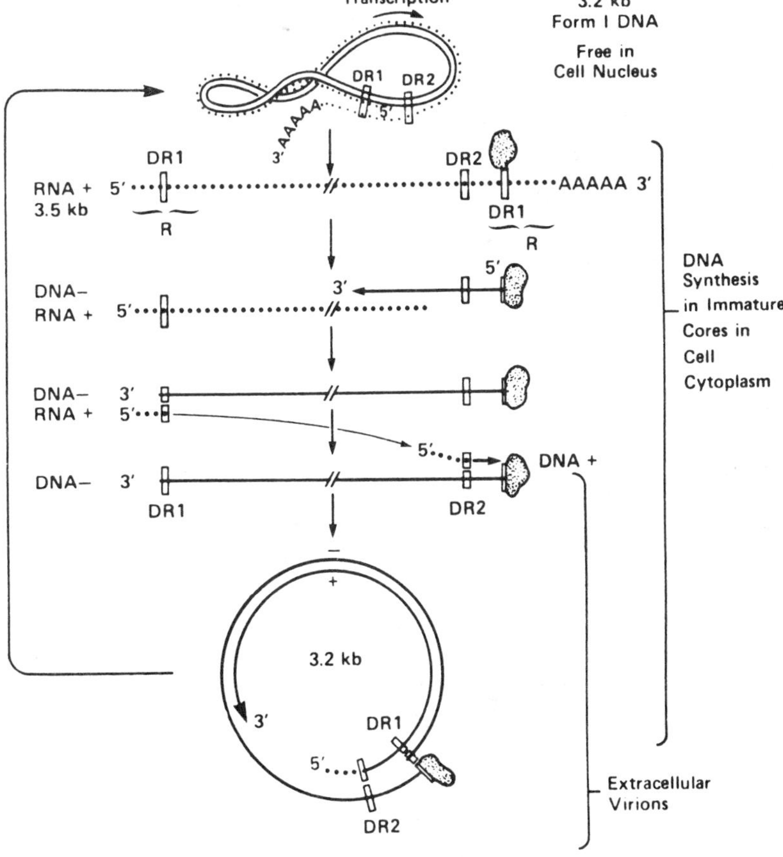

FIGURE 3 Replication scheme for various members of the hepadna virus family.

tified. The 3.5 Kb full-length copy of the (−) strand of ccc DNA is then transcribed by host RNA polymerase that generates an RNA template termed the *pregenome*. Reverse transcription of the pregenome ensues within a nuclear core particle, which is then transported to the cytoplasm. The precise timing of synthesis of the (+) DNA strand is not known. Within the cytoplasm the core particle becomes enveloped by viral surface antigen proteins to form a virion particle.

The 3.5 Kb "genomic" RNAs are heterogeneous with several choices for 5′ ends over a 31 base pair region, which includes the first ATG in the ORF C.[66] Since transcription of genomic RNA is initiated near the start of ORF pre-C upstream of the only polyadenylation site that exists in the viral genome, the signals for cleavage and polyadenylation are read only during the second cycle around the genome, leading to a terminal redundancy in the molecule ranging from 130 to 270 base pairs.[66–68] Only the shortest of several 3.5 Kb RNA species serves as a template for reverse transcription.

Synthesis of the (−) strand DNA is initiated within the short DR1 sequence probably near the 3′ end, although initiation near the 5′ end is also possible.[4] It is postulated that a protein primer participates in (−) strand synthesis similar to primers associated with other viral DNAs, although this protein has not yet been identified. However, 5′ ends of growing (−) strands are linked to a protein within the virus cores and it has been suggested that a single polypeptide encoded by ORFs P, C, or X may generate both the polymerase and the primer protein within the viral core.[4] An RNAse H function of the polymerase probably degrades RNA sequences progressively as the (−) strand elongates.

The plus (S) strand is transcribed from an initiation site at the 3′ end of DR2. However, the priming mechanism utilizes an RNA oligomer containing DR1 from either the 5′ or 3′ end of the terminal redundancy mentioned above, which is then transposed to the DR2 site of the (−) strand.[69] Extension of the growing (+) strand across the "nick" occurs by an unknown mechanism for which transfer of the primer may be facilitated by the redundancy in the pregenome sequence. As a result of unknown constraints upon the reverse transcriptase, (+) strands remain incomplete, rather than form long terminal repeats (LTRs) similar to retroviruses.[70] Serum-derived HBV particles may also contain RNA-DNA hybrids, indicating that on occasion the replication strategy is not fully completed.[65]

SIMILARITIES BETWEEN HEPADNA VIRUS AND RETROVIRUS GENOME ORGANIZATION AND REPLICATION

Analogies have been made between hepadna viruses and other viruses, particularly retroviruses and cauliflower mosaic viruses (CaMV), since they all replicate by reverse transcription.[4,71] If the nicked but repaired viral DNA were linearized and the overlapping ends filled, HBV would resemble a retrovirus proviral DNA with a long terminal repeat at both ends (Fig. 4). Organization of the structural genes of HBV is reminiscent of retroviruses in as much as all are coded from the (−) strand. Comparison of HBV and retroviral sequences reveals considerable homology between the terminal portion of the ORF C, middle portion of ORF P, and a large segment of ORF X.[72] In HBV, however, the ORF P overlaps the other ORFs. Evidence has been presented recently for ORF C and P fusion products of 35, 38, and 69 Kd.[73] Such polypeptides would have features similar to the *gag-pol* fusion gene products of retroviruses. In the linearized form of HBV, since ORF X is at the 3′ end of the genome, its location would be similar to the *tat* gene of retroviruses that encodes a transactivating protein.[74] As discussed below, recent evidence suggests that the X protein possesses a transactivating function.

Despite the apparent similarities between hepadna viruses and retroviruses, fundamental differences also exist.[4,71] In contrast to hepadna viruses, retroviruses package a single-stranded RNA, use a host tRNA as primer for (−) strand DNA synthesis, and initiate the first DNA strand outside the terminal redundancy in the RNA template. In addition, an oligomer of genomic RNA is used as primer for the (+) DNA strand; the retroviral polymerase fully extends both (+) and (−) DNA strands leading to LTRs; ccc DNA is formed from a linear rather than open circular precursor containing LTRs; viral DNA integrates into the host chromosome as a part of the virus life cycle; synthesis of viral RNA takes place from an integrated proviral template with little or no transcription of ccc DNA; and cytoplasmic cores of retroviral particles are released from the cell membrane before reverse transcription, with DNA synthesis commencing after entry of RNA containing virus particles into a new cell. The life cycle of CaMV incorporates features of both retroviruses and hepadna viruses.[4] Nonetheless, it is undisputed that hepadna

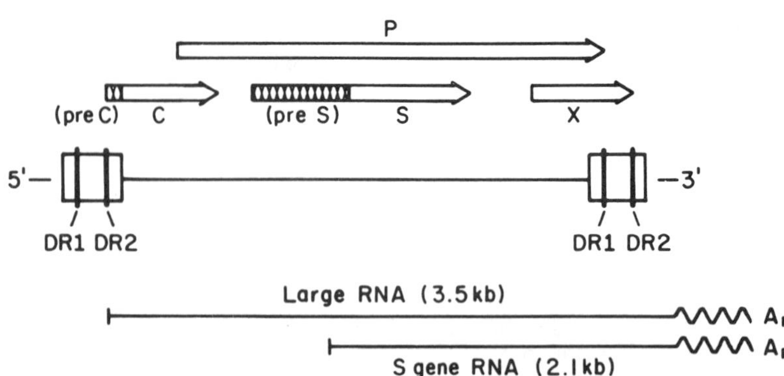

FIGURE 4 Linearized version of the HBV genome showing the orientation and overlapping nature of the known ORFs and the similarity between the genetic organization of HBV and that of retroviruses.

viruses are unique because of their unlikely DNA structure and also because of shared features with both DNA and RNA viruses.

HBV TRANSCRIPTS

Two classes of RNAs, 3.5 Kb (genomic) and 2.4 or 2.1 Kb (subgenomic), serve the replicative and transcriptive functions of hepadna viruses (see Fig. 2).[75,76] All HBV RNA transcripts reported to date are polyadenylated and derived from the (+) strand. The 5′ end of the 3.5 Kb genomic RNA has been mapped to the pre-C region and the 3′-end to the beginning of the C gene, where a specific polyadenylation signal is located.[77] The genomic RNA covers the complete genome plus an additional ~100 nucleotides. This implies that the 3.5 Kb RNA is produced from covalently closed double-stranded DNA and that the polyadenylation signal is skipped over during the initial phase of transcription (i.e., during the first cycle around the genome).

The 2.4 and 2.1 Kb subgenomic RNA species display heterogeneous 5′ ends similar to genomic RNAs. The 2.4 Kb RNA is believed to encode the pre-S1 protein, although it includes the genes for the pre-S2, S, and X proteins.[4] The 5′ end of the 2.1 Kb RNA has been mapped to ~20 bp upstream of the pre-S2 region, and these mRNA species code for the pre-S2 and S proteins.[75,76] Although minor RNA species of larger and smaller sizes are recognized, RNAs for ORF X or P have not yet been identified. Whether this is because of their low abundance or unknown mechanisms is not clear. Cell transfection experiments with cloned HBV DNA fragments and oligomers of HBV DNA have confirmed that the 2.1 Kb RNA is the mRNA for the major protein of the envelope and the 3.5 Kb RNA the mRNA for the core protein and possibly for the DNA polymerase.[78,79] Presence of other candidate RNAs has also been suspected in these in vitro systems. Indirect evidence has suggested the involvement of host RNA polymerases in transcription of hepadna viral genomes. For example, nonpermissive cells that express only HBsAg are capable of accurate transcription of subgenomic HBV RNAs. While subgenomic RNA species may be produced in a variety of nonhepatocyte cell types, occasionally including those in transgenic mice, the production of genomic RNA species is dependent upon host factors found in only hepatocytes or well-differentiated liver-derived cell lines.[4]

Transcripts of HBV in liver tissue from patients who are chronic HBV carriers demonstrate the two major classes of mRNA when both HBc and HBs proteins are expressed.[80] However, novel species of HBV transcripts may be found in liver or liver-derived cell lines bearing HBV DNA integrants that may represent fusion transcripts of viral DNA and flanking cellular sequences.[81]

CIS- AND TRANSACTING ELEMENTS REGULATING HBV GENE EXPRESSION

Several putative HBV promoters have been identified: pre-S1 (map position 2,786–2,791) with a TATAA element,[78] pre-S2 (map position 3,122–3,130) with an SV40 promoter-like sequence,[75] core (map position, 1,653–1,660), which does not contain a TATAA element,[82,83] and a promoter for X (map position 1,374–1,818).[84] Additionally, an enhancer element has been located at map position 1,080–1,234.[85] The HBV enhancer functions with both homologous (HBV) and heterologous (SV40) promoters. Another genomic region that is a glucocorticoid-responsive element is also present in HBV.[86] this glucocorticoid-responsive element, located at map position 355–366, contains all but the first nucleotide of the core consensus sequence ACAA—TGT$^{T}_{C}$CT found in the 5′-regulatory region of other glucocorticoid responsive genes, e.g., the mouse mammary tumor virus LTR, human metallothionein IIA, and human growth hormone.[86] The TGT$^{T}_{C}$CT segment is also present in multiple tandem copies, as also observed for the mouse mammary tumor virus LTR. Termination of viral transcription may be regulated by a conserved TATAAA element within the ORF C.[4] This element represents the functional homologue of the consensus AATAAA element similarly located in other *pol II* transcripts (and DHBV) and is known to be critical for RNA cleavage and polyadenylation. Downstream nucleotides also play a role in correct polyadenylation of HBV transcripts.

Evidence exists that the HBV enhancer may function in a tissue-specific manner,[87-89] although broader specificity of the enhancer has also been found.[90,91] Recent studies suggest that both viral and cellular transacting factors are involved in HBV gene expression.[92,93] By means of DNAse footprinting, regions within and adjacent to the HBV enhancer have been identified that serve as protein binding sites for factors that may be involved in tissue-specific HBV gene expression.[92] Studies in other systems suggest that tissue specificity for eukaryotic gene transcription may also partly reside in sequences of the promoter.[94]

The ORF X of HBV occupies a position similar to the trans-activating *tat* gene, which is necessary for the replication of HIV.[95] By using a combination of plasmid expression vectors containing specific promoters, enhancers, and/or other regulatory elements, it is now possible to explore the interaction of different viral and host gene products in regulating both virus and host cell functions. Such factors could play a major role in determining the hepatotropism of HBV and/or persistence of infection by modulating specific viral gene expression. Similar mechanisms could also interfere with HBV gene expression as observed during intercurrent viral infection, such as with delta agent. In vitro experiments utilizing transfection of cloned HBV DNA have shown that the X protein may transactivate a variety of viral enhancer and promoter elements.[96-98] It has been suggested that following binding of the X protein to cellular cytoplasmic protein, such complexes may be transported to the nucleus and function as a transcriptional transactivator.[99]

Studies on the in vivo role of X protein as a transactivator are not yet available, although expression of the X gene is thought to be well controlled at the cellular level.[4] Using competition experiments, preliminary evidence has recently been obtained for a possible role of cellular transacting factors in activating the HBV enhancer.[97] For some time, it has been known that the adenovirus early gene product E1A initiates transcription of other adenovirus genes and modifies cellular gene expression.[100,101] Examples of other viruses that exhibit similar regulatory phenomena include SV40, EBV,

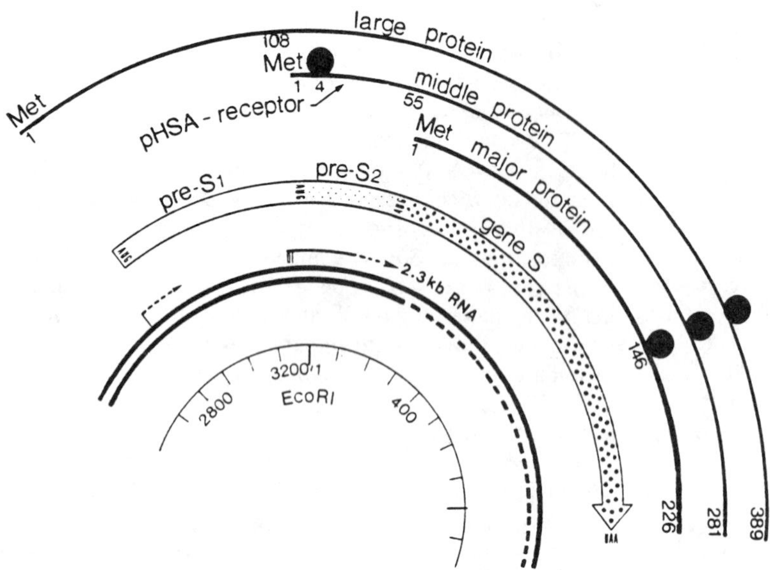

FIGURE 5 Detailed representation of the HBV surface antigen gene. The relationship of the large, middle, and small polypeptides coded by this gene is shown in detail. (From Tiollais et al.[3])

papilloma virus, and HIV. In the HIV system, several mechanisms for viral transactivation have recently been proposed. In HIV-1 and HIV-2 viruses, the viral *tat* genes produce a protein that transactivates the HIV LTR enhancer-promoter to increase transcription.[74] In contrast, the HIV-3 *tat* gene product increases translation rather than transcription of HIV-3 mRNAs, perhaps by increased mRNA binding to ribosomes (W. Haseltine: personal communication). Recent in vitro studies have clearly demonstrated that the X gene product transactivates several heterologous viral promoters or enhancers, including the LTR of human retroviruses.[97,98] A synergistic effect of X-transactivator and the HIV-1 *tat* gene may be governed by specific cellular factors.[97] Since the HBV enhancer influences the surface and core promoters, stimulation of the HBV enhancer influences the surface and core promoters, stimulation of the HBV enhancer by X protein may have widespread effects upon viral gene expression. In view of the obvious importance of these regulatory elements and factors, much current research on control of HBV gene expression is now focused on regulatory sequences in the HBV genome and how these sequences might function.

HBV GENE PRODUCTS

As indicated above, the four ORFs of hepadna viruses could encode at least four polypeptides of substantial length. However, multiple gene products result from these ORFs: six polypeptides from ORF S, two from ORF C, and three from ORF P (for details see references 3, 4, and 60).

Surface Proteins

The ORF S encodes three coterminal proteins of different sizes by the use of three functional initiation codons for protein translation and only one stop codon (Fig. 5).[60] Initially, only the smallest protein, S or small (226 amino acids), was recognized in HBsAg particles obtained from chronic HBV carriers. Two further proteins were subsequently detected: pre-S2 plus S or middle (281 amino acids) and pre-Sl plus pre-S2 plus S or large (389 to 400 amino acids, dependent upon viral subtype) (see Fig. 3). Each polypeptide can be glycosylated, and the native proteins found in virions are dimers linked through disulfide bridges. The 24-Kd small HBs protein exists in both unglycosylated ($P24^s$) and glycosylated ($GP\ 27^s$) forms, as does the large protein (unglycosylated $P39^s$ and glycosylated, $GP\ 42^s$), whereas the middle protein is found in two glycosylated forms ($GP\ 33^s$ and $GP\ 36^s$). The only difference between these latter glycosylated forms of middle HBs is that $GP\ 36^s$ has a complex glycan linked at the same site as $GP\ 27^s$.[102] The 3′ or S portion of these proteins is constant, whereas the 5′ portion varies, depending either on which S gene promoter-initiation site is used (pre-Sl or pre-S2) or on whether hitherto undescribed polypeptide processing events occurred.

The HBs polypeptides are principally found in 22-nM particles that contain about 24 percent lipid derived from the host cytoplasm. The lipids are phospholipids, free and esterified cholesterol, and small amounts of triglycerides.[60] The morphology and lipid content of GSHV and WHV surface antigen particles is similar to HBsAg, whereas the DHBV particles are larger, more heterogeneous, and have a higher lipid content.[4] Small HBs protein particles are resistant to proteases, heat, and chaotropic substances but highly sensitive to ionic detergents and reduction. Resistance to proteases is less marked in middle and large HBs proteins. The precise mechanism regulating the synthesis or level of these various ORF S products has not been elucidated. However, development of specific antibodies to the pre-Sl, pre-S2, and S regions has permitted additional analysis of the function of various S gene polypeptide regions.[60] From these studies, it is clear that 80 to 90 percent of the total S gene product on the virion surfaces is small HBs protein. The filamentous form of HBs aggregates in serum have a similar composition but the 20 nm spherical particles contain little large HBs protein. In the absence of viral replication, spherical particles contain less than 1 percent middle HBs protein and no large HBs protein. In highly viremic HBV carriers, the proportion of middle HBs molecules may be higher, approaching 5 to 10 percent. Presence of the pre-S2 moiety in middle HBs and of the pre-S1 moiety in large HBs protein has been confirmed by specific antibodies. Although the pre-S2 domain covers the external sites of the S domain in middle HBs, it is not clear whether folding in large HBs protein allows pre-S2 and S domains to be covered by pre-S1.[60]

The HBs protein contains a major antigenic group specific determinant called "a" and subtype determinants d, y, w, and r, producing four main serotypes adw, ayw, adr, and ayr. Each of these viral subtypes has a separate worldwide distribution. A hydrophilic region between amino acids 120 and 148 of small HBs protein is exposed and confers the group and subtype antigenic specificity.[102] Major B-cell epitopes of this region are conformational and dependent upon disulfide bonds. However, induction of protective antibodies, for example, in the development of HBV vaccines has required consideration of other complexities in antigen presentation, including intramolecular assembly, particle size, and denaturation of the molecule.[60]

Secretion of various HBs proteins following synthesis occurs by different mechanisms. Small HbsAg protein is extruded into the endoplasmic reticulum with an amino-terminal signal peptide. Middle HBs protein utilizes the first signal sequence within the S domain for this translocation. Although the S polypeptide is rapidly secreted from cells as compared with pre-S1 protein, secretion of the viral particles may require 24 hours.[103] In cells producing excess amounts of large HBs protein, presence of pre-S1 may prevent secretion.[104] Similar findings have been observed in reconstructed systems using frog oocytes or other eukaryotic cells into which plasmids containing expressible HBV sequences were introduced, as well as in long-term hepatitis B virus carriers (S.J. Hadziyannis, D.A. Shafritz, and J. Sninsky: unpublished observations). Cells retaining large HBs comprise the so-called ground-glass hepatocytes observed in long-term HBV carriers[105] and contain filamentous forms of HBsAg. Identical phenomena have been described in hepatocytes of transgenic mice that overproduce large HBS protein.[104] Although expression of large HBs protein is not fully understood, it is possible that the ratio of large to smaller HBs proteins may be regulated by the differentiated nature of the infected cell and its growth condition. Cells with integration of functionally active large HBs DNA sequences may overexpress this protein. Under certain conditions, a negative transcriptional factor that binds to pre-S1 sequences may inhibit expression of large HBs. While a small proportion (less than 3 percent) of large HBs protein has no influence upon the morphology of spherical HBsAg particles, a moderate proportion (10 to 20 percent) generates filamentous structures. Particles containing greater than 20 percent pre-S1 protein are probably not secreted.[60]

The pre-S2 region encodes a species-specific receptor for polymerized serum albumin.[60] The biologic significance of this binding to serum albumin is uncertain, although it has been postulated that this receptor may mediate virion attachment to hepatocyte membrane. The roles of the pre-S2 domain in eliciting a protective immune response against HBV or an immunosuppressive effect are unclear. Early appearance of pre-S2 antibodies after acute hepatitis B and its absence in chronic HBV carriers has been reported.[106] The large pre-S1 polypeptide also binds to hepatocyte membranes and may be involved in attachment of HBV particles to hepatocytes.[107,108]

Core Proteins

The ORF C contains two functional initiation codons and codes for the major polypeptides, HBc protein of 22 Kd and HBe protein of 15 to 16 Kd. As a result of post-translational modification, HBc proteins may exist in several different sizes between 16 and 25 Kd. Nucleocapsids that enclose viral DNA are composed primarily of HBc protein and are called core particles. The C-terminus of core antigen is rich in arginine, serine, and proline residues and contains a tandem repeat of an octapeptide, which is very similar to protein sequences of protamine and other DNA binding proteins.[59] During viral replication, HBc protein packages the pregenomic RNA and viral polymerase. An endogenous protein kinase activity is also present in hepadna viral core particles. This leads to phosphorylation of the HBc protein on multiple serine and threonine residues. Low-density core particles that do not contain endogenous DNA polymerase possess greater endogenous protein kinase activity. The functional significance of core phosphorylation is presently unknown.[4]

The 5′ end of ORF C (pre-C region) contains a short, in-phase sequence with an ATG codon ~80 nucleotides upstream to the core ATG that serves as the initiation site for HBe protein.[60] The mRNA for the HBeAg is longer than that for HBcAg because it contains the additional pre-C signal sequence. Expression of the pre-C gene generates a 25 Kd HBe protein, which enters the secretory pathway and undergoes removal of 19 aminoterminal amino acids to form a 23 Kd protein (P23). The processed P23 has a transmembranous location and may either be modified in the cytoplasm to P24 or is cleaved at the carboxy-terminal domain to be secreted as P16 to P20 dependent upon HBV subtype. The HBeAg does not contain a glycosylation site, whereas HBcAg is glycosylated. Therefore, production of HBeAg relies upon a unique strategy of gene expression utilizing a signal sequence to generate different proteins from the same gene.

Although the presence of HBeAg in sera of HBV carriers was recognized over 15 years ago, its function continues to be ill understood.[30] Whether HBe proteins participate in viral replication or development and maintenance of viremia is not known.

X Protein

In comparison to other hepadna viral proteins, much less is known about the expression of the ORF X (map positions 1,374 to 1,818) and its protein product. The ORF X could encode a polypeptide of 154 residues (~15 Kd). Several types of evidence suggest that this region has specific gene function, including the presence of a transcriptional promoter at map position ~1,300 and synthesis of a specific 16 Kd polypeptide when an expression vector containing this sequence is transfected into in vitro expression systems.[109] Both genomic and subgenomic mRNAs contain X sequences; however, the initial ATG codon of the X region is believed to be in a poor sequence context for translation.[4] Evidence for X gene expression in natural HBV infections is limited to the finding of antibodies to synthetic X polypeptides in the sera of patients.[110,111] Additionally, antibodies directed against X synthetic peptides recognize a 17 Kd protein in Western blots of infected liver extracts.[110] This suggests that X protein may be expressed as a fusion gene product, perhaps with a portion of the core or pol gene.[110] An X transcript of appropriate length (~750 nucleotides) has been found in liver tissue from both acute and chronic WHV infection.[112] Attempts to demonstrate either a nuclear or cytoplasmic subcellular location for the putative X gene product in either natural HBV infection or HBV transfected eukaryotic cells have produced conflicting results. Recent evidence for possible role of the X protein as a transactivator has been discussed above.

Viral Polymerase

The ORF P protein product has recently been identified as a putative 70 Kd protein with reverse transcriptase activity. Virion particles secreted by cultured cells were analyzed by activity gel analysis and found to contain polymerase activities that migrate as 90 and 70 Kd proteins.[113,114] The latter peptide contains the major polymerase activity and reacts with antisera against the carboxy terminus of the *pol* gene product. Evidence has been obtained that indicates that the ORF P product results from direct translation initiation at an internal initiation (AUG) codon.[115] Unlike retroviruses, in which the *pol* gene product is processed from a *gag-pol* fusion protein, examination of the DHBV reverse transcriptase by mutational analysis has excluded *gag-pol* fusion intermediates.[116] Presence of antibodies against ORF P domains in human sera indicate that this ORF is expressed.[117]

Other Virion Products

Other viral proteins include a protein covalently bound to the 5′ end of the minus (L) DNA strand that serves as a primer for viral replication.[55] This protein has not been further characterized at present. Another protein is produced possessing serine or threonine kinase activity that can phosphorylate HBc protein.[4] It is not known whether these two proteins are derived from the viral genome or host cellular sequences. At least three other viral polypeptides containing sequence regions derived from both the ORFs C and P have been identified.[73] For example, core-*pol* fusion polypeptides of 35 Kd, 38 Kd, and 69 Kd are found in HBV infected tumors or peritumor tissue.

SIGNIFICANCE OF SERUM HBV DNA

Sera from HBV carriers has been found to contain HBV DNA mostly as partially double-stranded DNA, although full-length genomes and DNA-RNA hybrids have been found.[51,65] Serum HBV DNA is thought to represent virion DNA, and its presence correlates with replicating and infectious HBV.[118] During acute viral hepatitis, HBV DNA is detected in the serum at the end of symptoms and is cleared rapidly during resolution of infection.[119] In immunosuppressed patients where viremia is marked, serum HBV DNA levels may be high, although a relationship between necroinflammatory activity, cellular immune function, and circulating HBV DNA is lacking.[120] In chronic HBV carriers in whom viral replication occurs, initial studies suggested that serum HBeAg correlates with HBV DNA and hepatic HBcAg.[37,121] However, several recent studies have indicated discordance between the HBeAg–anti-HBe system and serum HBV DNA for assessing viral replication.[38-40] Furthermore, in chronic HBV carriers, HBV DNA may be cleared far in advance of HBeAg[39,40]; therefore, in general, serum HBV DNA is a better indicator of HBV infectivity than HBeAg. Patients with chronic HBV infection who are HBsAg and anti-HBe positive and have no circulating HBV DNA demonstrate normal hepatic histologic findings. On the other hand, presence of serum HBV DNA in HBsAg and anti-HBe positive HBV carriers is associated with chronic liver disease.[38,121-124] The latter serologic combination is more common than previously suspected. Such patients remain potentially infectious, despite being anti-HBe positive, and demonstrate a virulent form of chronic active hepatitis that rapidly progresses to cirrhosis.[121] Recently, analysis of HBV DNA purified and amplified by PCR from sera of HBsAg positive, HBeAg negative–anti-HBe positive patients has revealed mutations in two codons of the pre-core region of ORF C, one of which leads to generation of a TAG translational stop signal. These patients continue to replicate HBV without producing HBeAg, which is initiated at the pre-core ATG, thus providing an explanation for the discordance between serum HBV DNA and HBeAg in some patients.[125] Serum HBV DNA is also frequently detected in HBV carrier mothers and their offspring at birth. Recent studies suggest that measurement of maternal serum HBV DNA has a predictive value for the efficacy of HBV immunization in preventing perinatal HBV transmission.[126,127]

HBV DNA is frequently absent from the serum of patients with hepatocellular carcinoma (HCC).[128] When present, it is generally in a low concentration. Additionally, HBV DNA may be detected in the sera of some patients who are anti-HBs positive, as well as in patients who have anti-HBc as the only markers of HBV infection. Furthermore, integrated HBV DNA sequences have been detected in HCC from some patients who are HBsAg negative and anti-HBs positive, as well as in others with no serologic marker of current or remote HBV infection.[129] Therefore, measurement of immunologic markers of HBV has certain limitations, particularly if viral antigens and their specific antibodies exist in serum simultaneously. The formation of immune complexes may interfere with competitive binding assays (radioimmunoassay or enzyme-linked immunosorbent assay) used for detection of viral antigens. In some instances, these immune complexes may be detected by using monoclonal antibodies to HBsAg.[129] With advances and simplification of molecular hybridization technology, however, it is likely that HBV DNA determinations will be used clinically as an adjunct to or replacement for some of these immunologic assays. Amplification of serum HBV DNA by the polymerase chain reaction (PCR) technique may provide greatly increased sensitivity (e.g., ~10^4 fold over slot-blot hybridization).[130] Rapid performance of such assays will be advantageous for detecting HBV and yield further information regarding its biology and pathogenetic role in liver disease.

REPLICATING AND NONREPLICATING STATES OF PERSISTENT HBV INFECTION

Various histologic, cellular, and molecular studies have indicated two states of persistent HBV infection: permissive and nonpermissive.[121,131] Features of the replicating or permissive state include active inflammatory liver disease (chronic persistent or active hepatitis), randomly distributed intracellular HBsAg and HBcAg in the hepatic parenchyma, and free virions as well as lower-molecular-weight replicating forms of HBV. The features of nonpermissive infection include the absence of active inflammatory liver disease (the liver may show no histologic evidence of HBV other than ground-glass hepatocytes or inactive cirrhosis due to remote viral infection), continued HBsAg (but not HBcAg) production, and integrated HBV DNA molecules.

In permissive infection, the bulk of HBV DNA in hepatocytes is in free virion or replicating forms, and integration into host genome is not observed by Southern blot analysis. As various studies have shown, however, viral DNA integration may be occurring randomly throughout the host genome during the infectious process.[132-135] Replication of HBV may continue long term in chronic HBV carriers or may resume following a period of interruption. While immunosuppression facilitates viral replication and reactivation of infection, other host factors regulating HBV replication are at present unknown.[136] In nonpermissive infection, it is often possible to observe these random integrations as a smear of hybridization in the high-molecular-weight region on Southern blot analysis. In these cases, free virion DNA is not found in the liver and HBV is not secreted into the circulation. In some nonpermissive infections, Southern blot analysis has demonstrated similar HBV DNA integrations, suggesting that the cells from which the DNA was derived are of a common clonal origin.[121,137] In several of these cases, clusters of HBsAg producing cells having the appearance of a focal clonal growth have been noted.[121,137] A mixed type of persistent infection may also occur in which features of replicating and nonreplicating infection are found in different cells or regions of the same liver.

During viral reactivation in chronic HBV carriers, expression of HBcAg and presence of free replicating viral forms has been demonstrated in several patients.[138] Substantial quantities of viral replicative intermediates and other extrachromosomal forms of HBV DNA were also identified in several tissue specimens (liver or tumor) from patients in whom HBV was not being secreted into the serum.[139] In the latter individuals, it may be that the virus replication, assembly, or secretion pathway is defective or blocked. Under these circumstances, there is intracellular accumulation of HBV DNA replicative forms, which may augment the viral DNA integration process.[138]

HBV AND DEVELOPMENT OF HCC

Epidemiologic and other studies have clearly established a relationship between the HBV carrier state and development of HCC.[5-7] The most striking observations were made in 22,707 Taiwanese government employees in whom HBV carriers were found to have a 217-fold greater relative risk for HCC (113 cases) compared to HBsAg negative controls (3 cases).[6] Similar conclusions were reached from a study of Japanese railroad workers.[7] In nearly all ethnic populations around the world, an increased HBsAg carrier rate is associated with an increased incidence of HCC.[140] The converse, that among patients with HCC the HBV carrier state is highly prevalent, has also been demonstrated.[1] Association between HCC and other hepadna viruses has been found particularly in woodchucks, but also in Pekin ducks and ground squirrels.[9] HCC appears to develop in HBV carriers only after long-term carriage of the virus. On the average, HCC is detected 20 or more years after persistent infection, although the onset of infection is usually unknown. However, the shortest recorded period in an HBV carrier for development of HCC is in a 4-year-old oriental boy who probably acquired HBV at birth.[141]

A causal relationship between HBV and HCC has not yet been proven. Integration of HBV DNA into one or a discrete number of sites has been reported in HCC, as well as into regions adjacent to the tumor. Nevertheless, despite enormous efforts in exploring a molecular basis for the association between HBV and HCC, as summarized below, the precise basis for the association continues to be obscure.

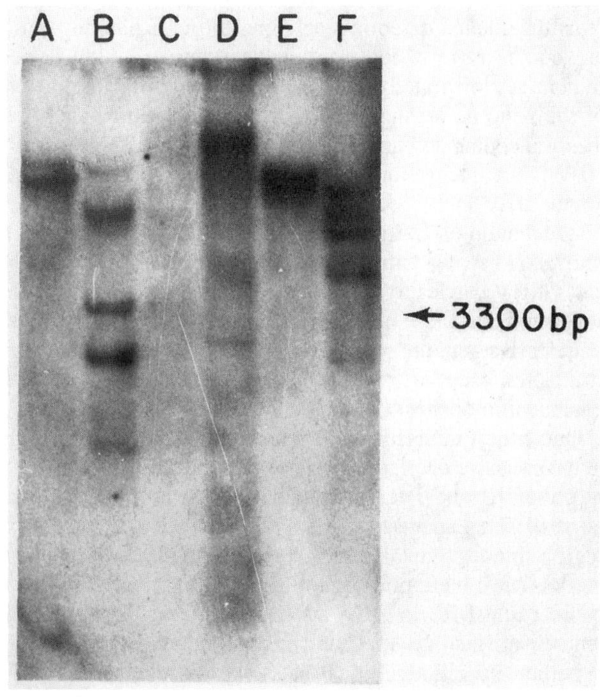

FIGURE 6 Southern blot analysis with Hind III restriction endonuclease depicting integration of HBV DNA sequences into unique sites in HCC from HBV carriers. Arrow indicates the expected position of full-length double-stranded free HBV DNA.

HBV DNA INTEGRATION IN HCC

Integration of HBV DNA was initially described in an HCC-derived cell line termed PLC/PRF/5[142–145] and all of the viral integrations in this cell line have been cloned and characterized.[146,147] Several investigators have subsequently analyzed HBV DNA integrations in HCC from HBV carriers and others negative for serum HBsAg.[132–134,137] Most of the tumors from HBsAg-positive patients have shown HBV DNA integrated in unique banding patterns varying with individual tumors and in several instances, free HBV DNA is also noted (Fig. 6). The presence of free HBV DNA indicates either continued viral replication or mingling of HBV containing hepatocytes into the tumor tissue. Although the presence of integrated HBV DNA was noted in HCC from patients with alcoholic cirrhosis lacking markers of current or remote HBV infection,[148] subsequent studies failed to confirm these observations.[149,150]

Viral DNA integration may occur during the replicative or nonreplicative phase of persistent infection and is evidenced by the presence of HBV DNA sequences spread throughout the cellular genome (a smear pattern on Southern blot analysis). In other cases, the presence of one or more unique bands of HBV DNA (Fig. 6) indicates that a clone of cells containing HBV molecules integrated into identical sites has become expanded.[137] The majority of HCC occurring in HBV carriers demonstrate the latter pattern of HBV DNA integration.

Detailed analysis of integrated HBV DNA from tumor-derived cell lines, hepatic tumors, and chronically infected woodchuck liver tissue has provided broadly similar information.[151–154] The structure of integrated HBV DNA sequences may vary from relatively simple to multiple rearrangements, deletions including those of flanking cellular sequences, inversions, or direct and inverted duplications. In general, integrated HBV DNA is oligomeric with portions of the genome arranged in inverted orientations, such that the viral coding domains are often interrupted. However, some HBV DNA integrations in HCC contain a greater-than-unit-length HBV DNA sequence with an apparently intact copy of the genome. Extrachromosomal high-molecular-weight "novel" forms of viral DNA have also been found in WHV and GSHV carrier liver but not yet in humans.[152] It has been suggested that these novel forms may represent a by-product of defective genome replication during viral persistence and could represent a precursor of integrations involved in hepatocarcinogenesis.[152]

One end of the HBV DNA integration is commonly within the cohesive overlap region between the 11 base pair direct repeats DR1 and DR2, although wide variations have been noted.[155] This suggests that a specific sequence within this region might be involved in a recombination event. Several models have been proposed to account for the involvement of DR1 and DR2 in HBV DNA integration, but no consistently satisfactory mechanism has been identified.[156,157] Whether specific cellular sites exist where HBV DNA preferentially integrates, such as in certain repetitive DNA sequences or specific histone-rich regions of cellular DNA, is also not clear.

The HBV X gene encodes a polypeptide for which antibodies have been identified in the sera from patients with chronic liver disease and HCC.[110,111] In view of extensive interruptions and disorganization of X gene sequences, it is unlikely that the X polypeptide could be produced within cells bearing integrated HBV DNA. However, it is possible that transactivating fusion proteins may result from X and flanking cellular sequences and play a role in hepatocarcinogenesis.

HBV-DIRECTED MUTAGENESIS

The ability of HBV to integrate into cellular DNA during chronic infection is consistent with its potential function as a hepatocarcinogen. For other viruses, this has been shown to occur either by direct transfer of viral oncogenes or by activation of proto-oncogenes by insertion of viral promoters or enhancers into the cellular genome. Recently, one HBV integration was found in the exon of a coding gene bearing partial sequence homology to the erb A proto-oncogene, which is structurally related to the steroid receptor.[158] This integration is located on chromosome 3. Nevertheless, augmented expression of this gene as a result of HBV DNA integration has not been demonstrated. Other HBV integrations in HCC have been found to be located on a number of chromosomes including 2, 3, 7, 9, 11, 12, 15, and 18, with also a translocation between chromosomes 17q and 18q.[153,159] However, hepadna viruses have not been shown to contain an oncogene and transfection experiments utilizing HBV DNA have failed to yield cell transformation, indicating that a direct mutagenic effect of HBV is probably limited.

An alternative explanation has begun to emerge with the recognition of recessive oncogenes, loss of both alleles of which may lead to tumorigenesis.[159] This hypothesis has gained substantiation with the study of Wilms' tumor and retinoblastoma, which may develop following loss of a recessive oncogene (also termed *tumor suppressor gene*). An HBV integration has been found that is located on chromosome site 11p13, which is in the same region that contains the Wilms' tumor locus. It is also near the locus for Beckwith-Wiedmann syndrome, which is associated with multisystem organomegaly, hepatoblastoma, and HCC. Recent studies show that in some HCCs and adjacent tissue in WHV carriers, expression of a gene located on chromosome 11p, insulin-like growth factor II, which is expressed in fetal liver and is a mitogen for cultured cells, is enhanced.[159] Whether this represents a direct cause and effect relationship between WHV and HCC is, however, not known.

HBV, PROTO-ONCOGENES, AND HCC

A number of proto-oncogenes have now been identified that produce proteins serving critical functions in growth control and cell transformation.[160] Augmented expression of proto-oncogenes occurs in spontaneous rodent HCC, WHV carriers with HCC, experimental hepatocarcinogenesis, HCC-derived cell lines, and in human HCC.[161–171] Among the commonly expressed proto-oncogenes in HCC, genes of the *ras* and *myc* families are prevalent; several other genes have also been identified. Spontaneous rodent hepatomas express the constitutive c-Ha-*ras* gene, as well as a mutated c-Ha-*ras* gene, which produces abnormal *ras* p21 proteins. Chemically induced HCC may also express a mutated c-*ras*. That activated *ras* genes may be transforming for liver tissue has been shown by transfection of an activated c-Ha- or N-*ras* gene into stable liver cell lines of parenchymal or nonparenchymal epithelial cell origin.[172,173]

Expression of c-Ha-*ras*, N-*ras*, and c-*myc* has been found in human HCC, as well as in HCC- derived cell lines.[168-171] In several instances, rearrangements and amplification of *ras* genes were found by DNA restriction fragment length polymorphism analysis. Increased c-*myc* expression has been demonstrated in chemically induced rodent tumors and WHV induced HCC in woodchucks.[166,167] Another transforming gene, *hst*, has been isolated from human HCC.[174] The *hst* gene product is a putative growth factor. Although expression of this gene was enhanced in cells transformed by purified DNA from HCC, *hst* DNA rearrangements or amplification were not present. Besides known oncogenes, which might be involved in hepatocarcinogenesis, a presumptive liver-derived oncogene, termed *lca* has been isolated from human HCC tissue by utilizing the NIH 3T3 transformation assay.[175] The transforming activity of *lca* is considerably less than that of other oncogenes. Whether this unique gene is involved in the pathogenesis of HCC remains to be demonstrated. Another liver-derived oncogene, termed *htf-1*, has also recently been isolated from the FOCUS cell line (J. Wands et al: unpublished observations).

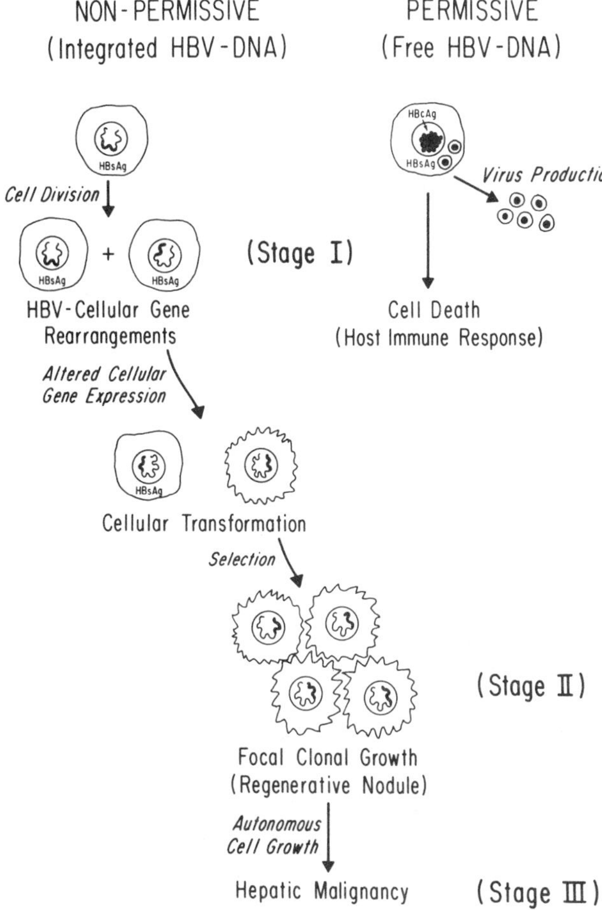

FIGURE 7 Schematic diagram illustrating various stages in persistent HBV infection and their potential relationship to the development of hepatocellular carcinoma. (From Shafritz and Rogler.[181])

Except for an HBV DNA integration next to v-*erb A* sequences, as mentioned above, HBV DNA sequences have not been found to enhance proto-oncogene expression. In fact, expression of c-Ha-*ras* and c-*myc* genes in HCC is similar irrespective of the presence of integrated HBV DNA.[166,171,176] This indicates that the probable mechanism by which HBV leads to hepatocarcinogenesis does not involve an effect of the virus upon these proto-oncogenes. In other instances, integrated WHV DNA sequences have been sited distant from regions of proto-oncogene (c-*myc*) rearrangements.[166] The prolonged latency between HBV infection and appearance of HCC is also an argument that these viruses do not carry an oncogene.

Insights into the association between HBV and HCC have also been provided by recently developed transgenic mouse systems.[177-180] The transgenic lineages that produce HBsAg particles, particularly large HBs protein, have been found to cause striking hepatocellular changes, including hepatocyte degeneration, hepatocellular necrosis, and ground-glass cells.[180] These changes are independent of host immunoresponse, because HBV antigens are recognized as "self" in the transgenic mice.[177] Overproduction of large HBs protein in transgenic mice is associated over a long term with marked hepatomegaly and nodular regenerative hyperplasia,[180] which may be a premalignant lesion. On the other hand, lineages that do not overproduce the large HBs protein have histologically normal livers throughout their life span.[180] Therefore, it appears that the mechanisms of hepatocellular injury following HBV infection are a consequence of HBV gene expression.

UNIFYING HYPOTHESIS RELATING VIRAL AND NONVIRAL FACTORS IN HEPATOCARCINOGENESIS

Although evidence from molecular studies indicates that HBV DNA integrates into host genome, this phenomenon by itself does not prove that HBV is a complete carcinogen. Were neoplasia to occur frequently in HBV infected livers and if HBV DNA integration were equally frequent, then HCC would often contain integrated HBV DNA by chance alone. This, of course, does not absolve HBV of a role in hepatocarcinogenesis but merely implies that neoplasia may result from an epigenetic mechanism.

From the currently available information, it is possible to develop a unifying hypothesis (Fig. 7). At some stage during the progression of the HBV carrier state, or perhaps as early as the initial acute infection, HBV DNA integration occurs (stage I). Hepatocytes expressing all, or at least some, specific viral proteins are efficiently removed by host defense mechanisms. However, integration of HBV DNA may alter expression of viral antigens and lead to preferential retention of such cells compared with hepatocytes with actively replicating HBV. At this stage, HBV DNA would become integrated into multiple sites within the host genome and would appear as a diffuse smear on Southern blot hybridization analysis. Hepatocyte necrosis and subsequent cell turnover may result in a selective growth advantage to cells bearing HBV DNA integrants. Repeated cycles of cell proliferation may potentiate these early selection events. Factors that stimulate cycles of hepatocyte necrosis and regeneration, such as ethanol, hepatotoxins, chemical carcinogens, infection with other viruses including non-A, non-B, and delta agent, may facilitate this process.

Subsequently, a clone or multiple clones of hepatocytes containing integrated HBV DNA might become selected for preferential survival and/or multiplication by factors unknown at present. These cells are not yet neoplastic, although presence of integrated HBV DNA, by definition, classifies them as transformed (stage II). On Southern blot analysis, these cells would show discrete, integrated HBV DNA bands. Under the influence of still further factors, environmental, genetic (such as the loss of tumor suppressor genes), or cellular (such as activation of proto-oncogenes or effects of specific growth factors), one or more of these clones may eventually give rise to a malignant clone (stage III).

The above hypothesis implies that HBV does not act alone in hepatocarcinogenesis but rather that this is a multistep process involving host, viral, and possibly other factors. In the future, the use of cell and molecular biology techniques will in great measure contribute to our eventual understanding of this complex process.

NEW MODEL SYSTEMS FOR HBV

Progress in issues related to HBV life cycle, host-virus interactions, viral pathogenesis, and antiviral therapy would be greatly facilitated by development of models of the disease in common laboratory animals and ability to infect cultured hepatocytes that support replication of HBV. Although considerable advances have been made with the use of some available natural animal models[9]—WHV for hepatocarcinogenesis, GSHV for viral replication and DHBV for in vitro viral studies—their use has inherent limitations. However, other systems have recently become available that offer powerful means of addressing a whole host of previously unanswered questions. One of these systems is the generation of transgenic mice containing integrated copies of cloned HBV genome.[177-180] This system in particular allows the in vivo analysis of the regulation of individual viral gene expression and immune response to HBV. Another recent development is the ability to support viral replication and produce complete and infectious HBV particles following transfection of cloned HBV DNA into certain differentiated liver-derived cell lines.[182-184] Means have been discovered to allow primary hepatocytes in culture to be successfully infected with HBV.[185,186] A model in nude mice has also been developed, in which a chronic HBV carrier state occurs following injection of cloned HBV DNA.[187] The morphology, kinetics, and distribution of infectious HBV particles can now be examined with these systems. Viral replication can also be studied and the influence of antiviral agents upon viral replication rapidly determined.

REFERENCES

1. Dane DS, Cameron CM, Briggs M. Virus-like particles in serum of patients with Australia-antigen-associated hepatitis. Lancet 1970; i:695–698.
2. Robinson WS, Lutwick LI. The virus of hepatitis, type B. N Engl J Med 1976; 295:1168–1175, 1232–1236.
3. Tiollais P, Pourcel C, Dejean A. The hepatitis B virus. Nature 1985; 317:489–495.
4. Ganem D, Varmus HE. The molecular biology of the hepatitis B viruses. Ann Rev Biochem 1987; 56:651–693.
5. Smuzness W. Hepatocellular carcinoma and hepatitis B virus: evidence for a causal association. Prog Med Virol 1978; 24:40–69.
6. Beasley RP, Hwang LY. Epidemiology of hepatocellular carcinoma. In: Vyas GN, Dienstag JL, Hoofnagle JH, eds. Viral hepatitis and liver disease. New York: Grune & Stratton, 1984: 209.
7. Obata H, Hatashi N, Motoike Y. A prospective study in the development of hepatocellular carcinoma in liver cirrhosis with persistent B virus infection. Int J Cancer 1979; 25:741–747.
8. Summers J, Smolec JM, Snyder R. A virus similar to hepatitis B virus associated with hepatitis and hepatomas in woodchucks. Proc Natl Acad Sci (USA) 1978; 75:4533–4537.
9. Summers J. Three recently described animal virus models for human hepatitis B virus. Hepatology 1981; 1:179–183.
10. Marion PL, Oshiro LS, Regnery DC. A virus in Beechey ground squirrels that is related to hepatitis B virus of humans. Proc Natl Acad Sci (USA) 1980; 77:2941–2945.
11. Fietelson MA, Millman I, Blumberg BS. Tree squirrel hepatitis B virus: antigenic and structural characterization. Proc Natl Acad Sci (USA) 1986; 83:2994–2997.
12. Mason WS, Seal G, Summers J. Virus of Pekin ducks with structural and biological relatedness to human hepatitis B virus. J Virol 1980; 36:829–836.
13. Blum HE, Walter E, Teubner K, Offensperger WB, Offensperger SS, Gerok W. Hepatitis B virus in non-hepatocytes. In: Bannash P, Keppler D, Weber G, eds. Liver cell carcinoma. Dordrecht: Kluwer Academic Publishers. 1989: 169.
14. Lie-Injo LE, Balasegaram M, Lopez CG, Herrera AR. Hepatitis B virus DNA in liver and white blood cells of patients with hepatoma. DNA 1983; 2:301–308.
15. Elfassi E, Romet-Lemone JL, Essex M, Frances-McLane M, Haseltine WA. Evidence of extrachromosomal forms of hepatitis B viral DNA in a bone marrow culture obtained from a patient recently infected with hepatitis B virus. Proc Natl Acad Sci (USA) 1984; 81:3526–3568.
16. Pontisso P, Poon MC, Tiollais P, Brechot C. Detection of hepatitis B virus DNA in mononuclear blood cells. Br J Med 1987; 288:1563–1566.
17. Gu JR, Chen YC, Jiang HR, et al. State of hepatitis B virus DNA in leucocytes of hepatitis B patients. J Med Virol 1985; 17:73–81.
18. Korba BE, Wells F, Tennant BC, Yoakum GH, Purcell RM, Gerin JL. Hepadnavirus infection of peripheral blood lymphocytes *in vivo*: Woodchuck and chimpanzee models of viral hepatitis. J Virol 1986; 58:1–8.
19. Yoffe B, Noonan CA, Melnick JL, Hollinger FB. Hepatitis B virus DNA in mononuclear cells and analysis of cell subsets for the presence of replicative intermediates of viral DNA. J Infect Dis 1986; 153:471–477.
20. Lieberman HM, Tung WW, Shafritz DA. Splenic replication of HBV in the chimpanzee chronic carrier. J Med Virol 1987; 21:347–360.
21. Blum HE, Stowring L, Figus A, Montgomery CK, Haase AT, Vyas GN. Detection of hepatitis B virus DNA in hepatocytes, bile duct epithelium, and vascular elements by *in situ* hybridization. Proc Natl Acad Sci (USA) 1983; 80:6685–6688.
22. Shimoda T, Shikata T, Karaasawa T, Tsukagoshi S, Yoshimura M, Sakurai I. Light microscopic localization of hepatitis B virus antigens in the human pancreas. Possibility of multiplication of hepatitis B virus in the human pancreas. Gastroenterology 1981; 81:998–1005.
23. Dejean A, Lugassy C, Zafrani S, Tiollais P, Brechot C. Detection of hepatitis B virus DNA in pancreas, kidney and skin of two human carriers of the virus. J Gen Virol 1984; 65:651–655.

24. Davison F, Alexander GJM, Trowbridge R, Fagan EA, Williams R. Detection of hepatitis B virus DNA in spermatozoa, urine, saliva and leucocytes of chronic HBsAg carriers. J Hepatol 1987; 4:37–44.
25. Hruska JE, Clayton DA, Rubenstein JLR, Robinson WS. Structure of hepatitis B Dane particle DNA before and after the Dane particle DNA polymerase reaction. J Virol 1977; 21:666–672.
26. Landers TA, Greenberg HB, Robinson WS. Structure of hepatitis B Dane particle DNA and nature of the endogenous DNA polymerase reaction. J Virol 1977; 23:368–376.
27. Almeida JD, Rubenstein D, Stott ED. New antigen-antibody system in Australia-antigen positive hepatitis. Lancet 1971; 2:1225–1227.
28. Gerlich WH, Goldmann U, Muller R, Stibbe W, Wolff W. Specificity and localization of the hepatitis B virus associated protein kinase. J Virol 1982; 42:761–766.
29. Hantz O, Fourel I, Buendia B, Baginski I, Trepo C. Specificity of the woodchuck hepatitis virus-associated protein kinase. In: Zuckerman AJ, ed. Viral hepatitis and liver disease. New York: Alan R. Liss, 1988: 471.
30. Magnius LO, Epsmark JA. New specificities in Australia antigen positive sera distinct from the Le Bouviert determinants. J Immunol 1972; 109:1017–1021.
31. Stahl S, Mackay P, Magazin M, Bruce SA, Murray K. Hepatitis B virus core antigen: Synthesis in *Escherichia coli* and application in diagnosis. Proc Natl Acad Sci (USA) 1982; 79:1606–1610.
32. MacKay P, Lees J, Murray K. The conversion of hepatitis B core antigen synthesized in *E. coli* into e antigen. J Med Virol 1981; 8:237–243.
33. Takahashi K, Machida A, Funatsu G, et al. Immunochemical structure of hepatitis B e-antigen in the serum. J Immunol 1983; 130:2903–2907.
34. Ou J, Laub O, Rutter W. Hepatitis B virus gene function: The precore region targets the core antigen to cellular membranes and causes the secretion of the e antigen. Proc Natl Acad Sci (USA) 1986; 83:1578–1582.
35. Junker M, Galle P, Schaller H. Expression and replication of the hepatitis B virus genome under foreign promoter control. Nucl Acids Res 1987; 15:10117–10132.
36. Schlict MJ, Salfeld J, Schaller H. The pre-C region of the duck hepatitis B virus is essential for synthesis and secretion of processed core proteins but not for virus formation. J Virol 1987; 61:3701–3709.
37. Govindarajan S, Fong TL, Valinluck B, Edwards V, Redeker AG. Markers of viral replication in patients with chronic hepatitis B virus infection. Am J Clin Pathol 1988; 89:233–237.
38. Matsuyama Y, Omata M, Yokosuka O, Imazeki F, Ito Y, Okuda K. Discordance of hepatitis B e antigen/antibody and hepatitis B virus deoxyribonucleic acid in serum. Gastroenterology 1985; 89:1104–1108.
39. Alberti A, Pontisso P, Fattovich G, et al. Changes in serum hepatitis B virus (HBV) DNA positivity in chronic HBV infection: results of a long-term follow-up study of 138 patients. J Infect Dis 1986; 154:562–569.
40. Tassopoulos NC, Papevangelou GJ, Roumeliotou-Karayannis A, Ticehurst JR, Feinstone SM, Purcell RH. Detection of hepatitis B virus DNA in asymptomatic hepatitis B surface antigen carriers: relation to sexual transmission. Am J Epidemiol 1987; 126:587–591.
41. Werner BG, Smolec JM, Snyder R, Summers J. Serological relationship of woodchuck hepatitis virus to human hepatitis B virus. J Virol 1979; 314–322.
42. Gerlich WM, Feitelson MA, Marion PL, Robinson WS. Structural relationships between the surface antigens of ground squirrel hepatitis virus and human hepatitis B virus. J Virol 1980; 36:787–795.
43. Galibert F, Chen TN, Mandart El. Nucleotide sequence of a cloned woodchuck hepatitis virus genome: comparison with the hepatitis B virus sequence. J Virol 1982; 41:51–65.
44. Kaplan PM, Greenman RL, Gerin JL, Purcell RH, Robinson WS. DNA Polymerase associated with human hepatitis B antigen. J Virol 1973; 12:995–1005.
45. Robinson WS, Greenman RL. DNA polymerase in the core of the human hepatitis B virus candidate. J Virol 1974; 13:1231–1236.
46. Robinson WS, Clayton DA, Greenman RL. DNA of a human hepatitis B virus candidate. J Virol 1974; 14:384–391.
47. Robinson WS. The genome of hepatitis B virus. Ann Rev Microbiol 1977; 31:357–377.
48. Summers J, O'Connell A, Millman I. Genome of hepatitis B virus: restriction enzyme cleavage and structure of DNA extracted from Dane particles. Proc Natl Acad Sci (USA) 1975; 72:4597–4601.
49. Delius H, Gough NM, Cameron CH, Murray K. Structure of the hepatitis B virus genome. J Virol 1983; 47:337–343.
50. Sattler F, Robinson WS. Hepatitis B viral DNA molecules have cohesive ends. J Virol 1979; 32:226–233.
51. Ruiz-Opazo N, Chakraborty PR, Shafritz DA. Evidence for supercoiled hepatitis B virus DNA in chimpanzee liver and serum Dane particles: possible implications in persistent HBV infection. Cell 1982; 29:129–138.
52. Mason WS, Aldrich C, Summers J, Taylor JM. Asymmetric replication of duck hepatitis B virus DNA in liver cells: free minus-strand DNA. Proc Natl Acad Sci (USA) 1982; 79:3997–4001.
53. Rogler CE, Summers J. Novel forms of woodchuck hepatitis B virus DNA isolated from chronically infected woodchuck liver nuclei. J Virol 1982; 44:852–863.
54. Weiser B, Ganem D, Seeger C, Varmus HE. Closed circular viral DNA and asymmetrical heterogeneous forms in livers from animals infected with ground squirrel hepatitis virus. J Virol 1983; 48:1–9.
55. Gerlich W, Robinson WS. Hepatitis B virus contains protein covalently attached to the 5'-terminus of its complete DNA strand. Cell 1980; 21:801–809.
56. Will H, Reiser W, Weimer T. Replication strategy of human hepatitis B virus. J Virol 1987; 61:904–911.
57. Sninsky JJ, Siddiqui A, Robinson WS, Cohen SN. Cloning and endonuclease mapping of the hepatitis B viral genome. Nature 1979; 279:346–348.
58. Siddiqui A, Sattler F, Robinson WS. Restriction endonuclease cleavage map and location of unique features of the DNA of hepatitis B virus, subtype adw2. Proc Natl Acad Sci (USA) 1979; 76:4664–4668.
59. Tiollais P, Charnay P, Vyas GN. Biology of hepatitis B virus. Science 1981; 213:406–411.
60. Gerlich WH, Heermann KH, Bruss V, et al. Structure, expression, and potential oncogenicity of hepatitis B virus proteins. In: Bannasch P, Keppler D, Weber G, eds. Liver cell carcinoma. Dordrecht: Kluwer Academic Publishers, 1989: 139.
61. Summers J, Mason WS. Replication of the genome of a hepatitis B-like virus by reverse transcription of an RNA intermediate. Cell 1982; 29:403–415.
62. Miller RH, Tran CT, Robinson WS. Hepatitis B virus particles of plasma and liver contain viral DNA-RNA hybrid molecules. Virology 1984; 139:53–63.
63. Miller RH, Marion PL, Robinson WS. Hepatitis B virus DNA-RNA hybrid molecules in particles from infected liver are converted to viral DNA molecules during an endogenous DNA polymerase reaction. Virology 1984; 139:64–72.
64. Blum HE, Haase AT, Harris JD, Walker D, Vyas GN. Asymmetric replication of hepatitis B virus DNA in human liver: demonstration of cytoplasmic minus—strand DNA by blot analyses and in situ hybridization. Virology 1984; 139:87–96.
65. Fowler MJ, Monjardino J, Tsiquaye KN, Zuckerman AJ, Thomas MC. The mechanism of replication of hepatitis B virus: evidence of asymmetric replication of the two DNA strands. J Med Virol 1984; 13:83–91.
66. Enders GH, Ganem D, Varmus H. Mapping the major transcripts of ground squirrel hepatitis virus: the presumptive template for reverse transcriptase is terminally redundant. Cell 1985; 42:297–308.
67. Buscher M, Reiser W, Will H, Schaller H. Transcripts and the putative RNA pregenome of duck hepatitis B virus: implications for reverse transcription. Cell 1985; 40:717–724.
68. Moroy T, Etreimble J, Trepo C, Tiollais P, Buendia MA. Transcription of woodchuck hepatitis virus in the chronically infected liver. EMBO J 1985; 4:1507–1514.
69. Lien JM, Aldrich EC, Mason WS. Evidence that a capped RNA is the primer for duck hepatitis B virus plus-strand DNA synthesis. J Virol 1986; 57:229–236.
70. Seeger C, Ganem D, Varmus HE. Biochemical and genetic evidence for the hepatitis B virus replication strategy. Science 1986; 232:477–483.
71. Varmus HE, Swanstrom R. Replication of retroviruses. In: Weiss R, Teich N, Varmus H, Coffin J, eds. RNA tumor viruses. 2nd ed. Cold Spring Harbor: Cold Spring Harbor Laboratory, 1985: 75.

72. Miller RH, Robinson WS. Common evolutionary origin of hepatitis B virus and retroviruses. Proc Natl Acad Sci (USA) 1986; 83:2531–2535.
73. Will H, Salfeld J, Pfaff E, Manso C, Thielman L, Schaller H. Putative reverse transcriptase intermediates of human hepatitis B virus in primary liver carcinomas. Science 1986; 231:594–596.
74. Rosen CA, Sodroski JG, Haseltine WA. Location of *cis*-acting regulatory sequences in the human T-cell leukemia virus type I long terminal repeat. Proc Natl Acad Sci (USA) 1985; 82:6502–6507.
75. Cattaneo R, Will H, Hernandez N, Schaller H. Signals regulating hepatitis B surface antigen transcription. Nature 1983; 305:336–338.
76. Cattaneo R, Will H, Schaller H. Hepatitis B virus transcription in the infected liver. EMBO J 1984; 3:2191–2196.
77. Enders G, Ganem D, Varmus H. 5'-terminal sequences influence the segregation of ground squirrel hepatitis virus RNAs into polyribosomes and viral core particles. J Virol 1987; 61:35–41.
78. Pourcel C, Louise A, Gervais M, Chenciner N, Dubois MF, Tiollais P. Transcription of the hepatitis B surface antigen gene in mouse cells transformed with cloned viral DNA. J Virol 1982; 42:100–105.
79. Gough NM. Core and E antigen synthesis in rodent cells transformed with hepatitis B virus DNA is associated with greater than genome length viral messenger RNAs. J Mol Biol 1983; 165:683–699.
80. Yokosuka O, Omata M, Imazeki F, Ito Y, Okuda K. Hepatitis B virus RNA transcripts and DNA in chronic liver disease. N Engl J Med 1986; 315:1187–1192.
81. Imazeki F, Yaginuma K, Omata M, Okuda K, Kobayashi M, Koike K. RNA transcripts of hepatitis B virus in hepatocellular carcinoma. Hepatology 1987; 7:753–757.
82. Chakraborty PR, Ruiz-Opazo N, Shafritz DA. Transcription of human hepatitis B virus core antigen gene sequences in an in vitro HeLa cellular extract. Virology 1981; 111:647–652.
83. Rall LB, Standring DN, Laub O, Rutter WJ. Transcription of hepatitis B virus by RNA polymerase II. Mol Cell Biol 1983; 3:1766–1773.
84. Treinin M, Laub O. Identification of a promoter element located upstream from the hepatitis B virus X gene. Mol Cell Biol 1987; 7:545–548.
85. Shaul Y, Rutter WJ, Laub O. A human hepatitis B viral enhancer element. EMBO J 1985; 4:427–430.
86. Tur-Kaspa R, Burk RD, Shaul Y, Shafritz DA. Hepatitis B virus DNA contains a glucocorticoid responsive element. Proc Natl Acad Sci (USA) 1986; 83:1627–1631.
87. Karpen S, Banerjee R, Zelent A, Price P, Acs G. Identification of protein-binding sites in the hepatitis B virus enhancer and core promoter domains. Mol Cell Biol 1988; 8:5159–5165.
88. Honigwachs J, Faktor O, Dikstein R, Shaul Y, Laub O. Liver-specific expression of hepatitis B virus is determined by the combined action of the core gene promoter and the enhancer. J Virol 1989; 63:919–924.
89. Antonucci TK, Rutter WJ. Hepatitis B virus (HBV) promoters are regulated by the HBV enhancer in a tissue-specific manner. J Virol 1989; 63:579–583.
90. Elfassi E. Broad specificity of the hepatitis B enhancer function. Virology 1987; 160:259–262.
91. Vannice JL, Levinson AD. Properties of the human hepatitis B enhancer: position effects and cell-type nonspecificity. J Virol 1988; 62:1305–1313.
92. Shaul Y, Ben-Levy R. Multiple nuclear proteins in liver cells are bound to hepatitis B virus enhancer element and its upstream sequences. EMBO J 1987; 6:1913–1920.
93. Chon HW, Harrell D, Forough R, Watabe K. Binding of tissue-specific factors to the enhancer sequence of hepatitis B virus. FEBS Lett 1988; 229:349–354.
94. Bulla GA, Siddiqui A. The hepatitis B virus enhancer modulates transcription of the hepatitis B virus surface antigen gene from an internal location. J Virol 1988; 62:1437–1441.
95. Wong-Staal F, Gallo RC. Human T-lymphotropic retroviruses. Nature 1985; 317–403.
96. Spandau DF, Lee CH. Trans-activation of viral enhancers by the hepatitis B virus X protein. J Virol 1988; 62:427–434.
97. Twu JS, Robinson WS. Hepatitis B virus X gene can transactivate heterologous viral sequences. Proc Natl Acad Sci (USA) 1989; 86:2046–2050.
98. Siddiqui A, Gaynor R, Srinivasan A, Mapoles J, Farr RW. Transactivation of viral enhancers including long terminal repeat of the human immunodeficiency virus by the hepatitis B virus X protein. Virology 1989; 169:479–484.
99. Siddiqui A, Jameel S, Mapoles J. Expression of hepatitis B virus X gene in mammalian cells. Proc Natl Acad Sci (USA) 1987; 84: 2513–2517.
100. Nevins JR. Induction of the synthesis of a 70,000 dalton mammalian heat shock protein by the adenovirus E1A gene product. Cell 1982; 29:913–919.
101. Treisman R, Green R, Maniatis R. *Cis* and *trans*-activation of globin gene transcription in transcription assays. Proc Natl Acad Sci (USA) 1983; 80:7428–7432.
102. Peterson DL, Noth N, Gavilanes F. Structure of hepatitis B surface antigen. J Biol Chem 1982; 257:10414–10420.
103. Patzer EJ, Nakamura GR, Simonsen CC, Levinson AD, Brands R. Intracellular assembly and packaging of hepatitis B surface antigen particles occur in the endoplasmic reticulum. J Virol 1986; 58:884–892.
104. Chisari FV, Filippi P, Buras J. Structural and pathological effects of synthesis of hepatitis B virus large envelope polypeptide in transgenic mice. Proc Natl Acad Sci (USA) 1987; 84:6909–6913.
105. Hadziyannis SJ. Use of a monoclonal antibody in the detection of HBsAg in the liver by immunofluorescence. Devel Biol Standard 1983; 55:517–521.
106. Budkowska A, Dubreuil P, Capel F, Pillot J. Hepatitis B virus pre-S gene-encoded antigenic specificity and anti-pre S antibody: Relationship between anti-pre-S response and recovery. Hepatology 1986; 6:360–368.
107. Neurath AR, Kent SBH, Strick N, Parker K. Identification and chemical synthesis of a host cell receptor binding site on hepatitis B virus. Cell 1986; 46:429–436.
108. Pontisso P, Petit MA, Bankowski MJ, Peeples ME. Human liver plasma membranes contain receptors for the hepatitis B virus pre-S1 region and, via polymerized serum human albumin, for the pre-S2 region. J Virol 1989; 63:1981–1988.
109. Koshy R, Zahm P, Wollersheim M, Hofschneider PH. Transactivation by HBV X gene product. In: Bannasch P, Keppler D, Weber G, eds. Liver cell carcinoma. Dordrecht: Kluwer Academic Publishers, 1989: 117.
110. Moriarty AM, Alexander H, Leuner RA. Antibodies to peptides detect new hepatitis B antigen: Serological correlation with hepatocellular carcinoma. Science 1985; 227:429–433.
111. Meyers ML, Trepo LV, Nath N, Sninsky JJ. Hepatitis B virus polypeptide X: Expression in *Eschericia coli* and identification of specific antibodies in sera from hepatitis B virus—infected humans. J Virol 1986; 57:101–109.
112. Kaneko S, Miller RH. X-region–specific transcript in mammalian hepatitis B virus–infected liver. J Virol 1988; 62:3979–3984.
113. Bevand MR, Laub O. Two proteins with reverse transcriptase activities associated with hepatitis B virus-like particles. J Virol 1988; 62:626–628.
114. Bevand M, Feitelson M, Laub O. The hepatitis B virus–associated reverse transcriptase is encoded by the virol *pol* gene. J. Virol 1989; 63:1019–1021.
115. Chang LJ, Pryciak P, Ganem D, Varmus HE. Biosynthesis of the reverse transcriptase of hepatitis B viruses involves de novo translational initiation not ribosomal frameshifting. Nature 1989; 337:364–368.
116. Schlicht HJ, Radziwill G, Schaller H. Synthesis and encapsidation of duck hepatitis B virus reverse transcriptase do not require formation of core-polymerase fusion proteins. Cell 1989; 56:85–92.
117. Stemler M, Hess J, Braun R, Will H, Schroder CH. Serological evidence for expression of the polymerase gene of human hepatitis B virus in vivo. J Gen Virol 1988; 69:689–693.
118. Bonino F, Hoyer B, Nelson J, Engle R, Verme G, Gerin J. Hepatitis B virus DNA in the sera of HB_sAg carriers: a marker of active hepatitis B virus replication in the liver. Hepatology 1981; 1:386–391.
119. Wood JR, Taswell MF, Czaja AJ, Rabe D. Pattern and duration of MBV DNA seropositivity in acute hepatitis B. Dig Dis Sci 1988; 33:477–480.
120. Rector WG Jr, Govindarajan S, Horsburgh CR Jr, Penley KA, Cohn DL, Judson FN. Hepatic inflammation, hepatitis B replication, and cellular immune function in homosexual males with chronic hepatitis B and antibody to human immunodeficiency virus. Am J Gastroenterol 1988; 83:262–266.
121. Hadziyannis SJ, Lieberman HM, Karvountzis GG, Shafritz DA. Analysis of liver disease, nuclear HBcAg, viral replication, and hepatitis B virus DNA in liver and serum of HBeAg vs. anti-HBc positive carriers of hepatitis B virus. Hepatology 1983; 3:656–662.
122. Negro F, Chiaberge E, Oliviero S, et al. Hepatitis B virus DNA (HBV-DNA) in anti-HBe positive sera. Liver 1984; 4:177–183.

123. Bonino F, Rosina F, Rizzetto M, et al. Chronic hepatitis in HBsAg carriers with serum HBV-DNA and anti-HBe. Gastroenterology 1986; 90:1268–1273.
124. Karayiannis P, Fowler MJF, Lok ASF, Greenfield C, Monjardino J, Thomas HC. Detection of serum HBV-DNA by molecular hybridization. Correlation with HBeAG/Anti-HBe status, racial origin, liver histology and hepatocellular carcinoma. J Hepatol 1985; 1:99–106.
125. Carman WF, Jacyna MR, Hadziyannis S, et al. Mutation preventing formation of hepatitis B e antigen in patients with chronic hepatitis B infection. Lancet 1989; ii:588–591.
126. Lee SD, Lo KJ, Wu JC, et al. Prevention of maternal-infant hepatitis B virus transmission by immunization: the role of serum hepatitis B virus DNA. Hepatology 1986; 6:369–373.
127. Ip HM, Lelie PN, Wong VC, Kuhns MC, Reesink HW. Prevention of hepatitis B virus carrier state in infants according to maternal serum levels of HBV DNA. Lancet 1989; i:406–410.
128. Lieberman HM, LaBrecque DR, Kew ML, Hadziyannis SJ, Shafritz DA. Detection of hepatitis B virus DNA directly in human serum by a simplified molecular hybridization test: comparison to HBeAg/Anti-HBC status in HBeAG carriers. Hepatology 1983; 3:285–291.
129. Shafritz DA, Lieberman HM, Isselbacher KJ, Wands JR. Monoclonal radioimmunoassays for hepatitis B surface antigen: demonstration of hepatitis B virus DNA or related sequences in serum and viral epitopes in immune complexes. Proc Natl Acad Sci (USA) 1982; 79:5675–5679.
130. Kaneko S, Miller RH, Feinstone SM, et al. Detection of serum hepatitis B virus DNA in patients with chronic hepatitis using the polymerase chain reaction assay. Proc Natl Acad Sci (USA) 1989; 86:312–316.
131. Popper H, Shafritz DA, Hoofnagle JH. Relation of the hepatitis B virus carrier state to hepatocellular carcinoma. Hepatology 1987; 7:764–772.
132. Brechot C, Hadchouel M, Scotto J, et al. State of hepatitis B virus DNA in hepatocytes of patients with hepatitis B surface antigen positive and negative liver disease. Proc Natl Acad Sci (USA) 1981; 78:3906–3910.
133. Kam A, Rall LB, Smuckler EA, Schmid R, Rutter WJ. Hepatitis B viral DNA in liver and serum of symptomatic carriers. Proc Natl Acad Sci (USA) 1982; 79:7522–7526.
134. Shafritz DA, Shouval D, Sherman HI, et al. Integration of hepatitis B virus DNA into the genome of liver cells in chronic liver disease and hepatocellular carcinoma. N Engl J Med 1981; 305:1067–1073.
135. Koshy R, Maupas P, Muller R, Hofschneider PH. Detection of hepatitis B virus—specific DNA in the genomes of human hepatocellular carcinoma and liver cirrhosis tissues. J Gen Virol 1981; 57:95–102.
136. Davis GL, Hoofnagle JH. Reactivation of chronic hepatitis B virus infection. Gastroenterology 1987; 92:2028–2031.
137. Shafritz DA, Hadziyannis SJ. Hepatitis B virus DNA in liver and serum, viral antigens and antibodies, virus replication and liver disease activity in patients with persistent hepatitis B virus infection. In: Chisari FV, ed. Advances in hepatitis research. New York: Masson Press, 1984: 80.
138. Lai MY, Chen DS, Lee SC, et al. Reactivation of hepatitis B virus in anti-HBc positive chronic active type B hepatitis: molecular and immunohistochemical studies. Hepato Gastroenterol 1988; 35:17–21.
139. Raimondo G, Burk RD, Lieberman HM, et al. Interrupted replication of hepatitis B virus in liver tissue of HBsAg carriers with hepatocellular carcinoma. Virology 1988; 166:103–111.
140. Beasley RP, Hwang LY. Epidemiology of hepatocellular carcinoma. In: Vyas GN, Dienstag JL, Hoofnagle JH, eds. Viral hepatitis and liver disease. New York: Grune & Stratton, 1984: 209.
141. Tanaka T, Miyamoto H, Hino O, et al. Primary hepatocellular carcinoma with hepatitis B virus—DNA integration in a 4 year old boy. Hum Pathol 1986; 17:202–204.
142. Marion PL, Salazan FH, Alexander JJ, Robinson WS. State of hepatitis B viral DNA in a human hepatoma cell line. J Virol 1980; 33:795–806.
143. Chakraborty PR, Ruiz-Opazo N, Shouval D, Shafritz DA. Identification of integrated hepatitis B virus DNA and expression of viral RNA in an HBsAg producing human hepatocellular carcinoma cell line. Nature 1980; 286:531–533.
144. Brechot C, Pourcel C, Louise A, et al. Presence of integrated hepatitis B virus DNA sequences in cellular DNA of human hepatocellular carcinoma. Nature 1980; 286:533–535.
145. Edman JC, Gray P, Valenzuela P, et al. Integration of hepatitis B virus sequences and their expression in a human hapatoma cell. Nature 1980; 286:535–537.
146. Shaul Y, Ziemer M, Garcia PD, et al. Cloning and analysis of integrated hepatitis virus sequences from a human hepatoma cell line. J Virol 1984; 51:776–787.
147. Ziemer M, Garcia P, Shaul Y, Rutter WJ. Sequence of hepatitis B virus DNA incorporated into the ganome of a human hepatoma cell line. J Virol 1985; 53:885–892.
148. Brechot C, Nalpas B, Courouce AM, et al. Evidence that hepatitis B virus has a role in liver-cell carcinoma in alcoholic liver disease. N Engl J Med 1982; 306:1384–1387.
149. Fong TL, Govindarajan S, Valinluck B, Redeker AG. Status of hepatitis B virus DNA in alcoholic liver disease: a study of a large population in the United States. Hepatology 1988; 8:1602–1604.
150. Walter E, Blum HE, Meier P, et al. Hepatocellular carcinoma in alcoholic liver disease: no evidence for a pathogenetic role of hepatitis B virus infection. Hepatology 1988; 8:745–748.
151. Ogsten CW, Jonak GJ, Rogler CE, et al. Cloning and structural analysis of integrated woodchuck hepatitis virus sequences from hepatocellular carcinomas of woodchucks. Cell 1982; 29:385–394.
152. Rogler CE, Summers J. Cloning and structural analysis of integrated woodchuck hepatitis virus sequences from a chronically infected liver. J Virol 1984; 50:832–837.
153. Hino O, Shows TB, Rogler CE. Hepatitis B virus integration site in hepatocellular carcinoma at chromosome 17:18 translocation. Proc Natl Acad Sci (USA) 1986; 83:8338–8342.
154. Tokino T, Fukushige S, Nakamura T, et al. Chromosomal translocation and inverted duplications associated with integrated hepatitis B virus in hepatocellular carcinomas. J Virol 1987; 61:3848–3854.
155. DeJean A, Sonigo P, Wain-Holson S, Tiollais P. Specific hepatitis B virus integration in hepatocellular carcinoma DNA through a viral 11-base pair direct repeat. Proc Natl Acad Sci (USA) 1984; 81:5350–5354.
156. Yaginama K, Kobayashi M, Yoshida E, Koike K. Hepatitis B virus integration in hepatocellular carcinoma DNA. Duplication of cellular flanking sequences at the integration site. Proc Natl Acad Sci (USA) 1985; 82:4458–4462.
157. Shih C, Burke K, Shou MJ, et al. Tight clustering of human hepatitis B virus integration sites in hepatomas near a triple-stranded region. J Virol 1987; 61:3491–3498.
158. Dejean A, Bouguelert L, Grzeschik KH, Tiollais P. Hepatitis B virus DNA integration in a sequence homologous to v-*erb*-A and steroid receptor genes in a hepatocellular carcinoma. Nature 1986; 322:70–72.
159. Rogler CE, Hino O, Yang D. Shafritz DA. Viral DNA integration, chromosome aberrations and growth factor activation in hepatocellular carcinomas of hepadna virus carriers. In: Bannash P, Keppler D, Weber G, eds. Liver cell carcinoma. Dordrecht: Kluwer Academic Publishers, 1989: 93.
160. Bishop JM. The molecular genetics of cancer. Science 1957; 235:305–311.
161. Fox TR, Watanabe PG. Detection of a cellular oncogene in spontaneous liver tumors of B6C3F1 mice. Science 1985; 228:296–297.
162. Reynolds SH, Stowers SJ, Meronpot RR, Anderson MW, Aaronson SA. Detection and identification of activated oncogenes in spontaneously occurring benign and malignant hepatocellular tumors of the B6C3F1 mouse. Proc Natl Acad Sci (USA) 1986; 83:33–37.
163. Makino R, Hayashi K, Sato S, Sugimura T. Expression of C-Ha-*ras* and c-*myc* genes in rat liver tumors. Biochem Biophys Res Commun 1984; 119:1097–1102.
164. Yaswen P, Goyette M, Shank PR, Fausto N. Expression of c-Ki-*ras*, c-Ha-*ras* and c-*myc* in specific cell types during hepatocarcinogenesis. Mol Cell Biol 1985; 5:780–786.
165. Stowers SJ, Wiseman RW, Ward JM, et al. Detection of activated protooncogenes in N-nitrosodiethylamine-induced liver tumors: a comparison between B6C3F1 mice and Fischer 344 rats. Carcinogenesis 1988; 9:271–276.
166. Moroy T, Marchio A, Etiemble J, et al. Rearrangement and enhanced expression of c-*myc* in hepatocellular carcinoma of hepatitis virus infected woodchucks. Nature 1986; 324:276–279.
167. Hsu TY, Moroy T, Etiemble J, et al. Activation of c-myc by woodchuck hepatitis virus insertion in hepatocellular carcinoma. Cell 1988; 55:627–635.
168. Gupta S, Parimoo S, Valinluck B, Govindarajan S, Epstein A, Roy-

Burman P. Protooncogene expression in five human hepatocellular carcinoma (HCC) cell lines. Hepatology 1987; 7:1127.

169. Su TS, Lin LH, Lui Wy, et al. Expression of c-*myc* gene in human hepatoma. Biochem Biophys Res Commun 1985; 132:264–268.
170. Nonomura A, Ohta G, Hayashi M, et al. Immunohistochemical detection of ras oncogene p 21 product in liver cirrhosis and hepatocellular carcinoma. Am J Gastroenterol 1987; 82:512–518.
171. Gupta S, Parimoo S, Valinluck B, Govindarajan S, Roy-Burman P. Protooncogene expression in human primary hepatocellular carcinoma (HCC). Hepatology 1987; 7:1163.
172. Sinha S, Marshall CJ, Neal GE. Gamma-glutamyl transpeptidases and the *ras*-induced transformation of a rat liver cell line. Cancer Res 1986; 46:1440–1445.
173. Braun L, Goyette M, Yaswen P, Thompson NL, Fausto N. Growth in culture and tumorigenicity after transfection with the *ras* oncogene of liver epithelial cells from carcinogen-treated rats. Cancer Res 1987; 47:4116–4124.
174. Nakagama H, Ohnishi S, Imawari M, et al. Identification of transforming genes as hst in DNA samples from two human hepatocellular carcinomas. Jpn J Cancer Res 1987; 78:651–654.
175. Ochiya T, Fujiyana A, Fukushige S, et al. Molecular cloning of an oncogene from a human hepatocellular carcinoma. Proc Natl Acad Sci (USA) 1986; 83:4993–4997.
176. Lee HS, Rajgopalan MS, Vyas GN. A lack of direct role of hepatitis B virus in the activation of *ras* and c-*myc* oncogenes in human hepatocellular carcinogenesis. Hepatology 1988; 8:1116–1120.
177. Chisari FV, Pinkert CA, Milich DR, et al. A transgenic mouse model of the chronic hepatitis B surface antigen carrier state. Science 1985; 1157–1160.
178. Farza H, Hadchouel M, Scotts J, Tiollais P, Babinet C, Pourcel C. Replication and gene expression of hepatitis B virus in a transgenic mouse that contains the complete viral genome. J Virol 1988; 62:4144–4152.
179. Burke RD, DeLoia JA, ElAwady MK, Gearhart JD. Tissue preferential expression of the hepatitis B virus (HBV) surface antigen gene in two lines of HBV transgenic mice. J Virol 1988: 62:649–654.
180. Chisari FV, Filippi P, Buras J, et al. Structural and pathological effects of synthesis of hepatitis B virus large envelope polypeptide in transgenic mice. Proc Natl Acad Sci (USA) 1987; 84:6909–6913.
181. Shafritz DA, Rogler, CE. Molecular characterization of viral forms observed in persistent hepatitis infections, chronic liver disease and hepatocellular carcinoma in woodchucks and humans. In: Vyas GN, Dienstag JL, Hoofnagle JH, eds. Viral hepatitis and liver disease. Orlando, FL: Grune & Stratton, 1984: 225.
182. Chang CM, Jeng KS, Hu CP. Production of hepatitis B virus in vitro by transient expression of cloned HBV DNA in a hepatoma cell line. EMBO J 1987; 6:675–680.
183. Gerber MA, Sells MA, Chen ML. Morphologic, immunohistochemical, and ultrastructural studies of the production of hepatitis B virus in vitro. Lab Invest 1988; 59:173–180.
184. Acs G, Sells MA, Purcell CH. Hepatitis B virus produced by transfected HepG2 cells causes hepatitis in chimpanzees. Proc Natl Acad Sci (USA) 1987; 84:4641–4644.
185. Ochiya T, Tsurimoto T, Ueda K, Okuba K, Shiozawa M, Matsubara K. An in vitro system for infection with hepatitis B virus that uses primary human fetal hepotocytes. Proc Natl Acad Sci (USA) 1989; 86:1875–1879.
186. Gripon P, Diot C, Th'ez'e N, et al. Hepatitis B virus infection of adult human hepatocytes cultured in the presence of dimethyl sulfoxide. J Virol 1988; 62:4136–4143.
187. Feitelson MA, DeTolla LJ, Zhou XD. A chronic carrierlike state is established in nude mice injected with cloned hepatitis B virus DNA. J Virol 1988; 62:1408–1415.

PART 5

Bacterial, Parasitic, and Other Infections of the Liver

Jennifer M. Puck, M.D.

The etiologies and incidence of infections of the liver vary widely in different parts of the world. In the United States, most pyogenic hepatic infections are liver abscesses due to bacteria and amebae. These infections are uncommon, particularly in children, in whom the incidences have been estimated at around 0.35 percent in fatal cases coming to autopsy in St. Louis from 1917 to 1967[1] and as low as 3 per 100,000 admissions to Milwaukee Children's Hospital between 1957 and 1977.[2] Although more recent large pediatric series have not been published, a review of trends in liver abscess in adults[3] indicates that with the advent of antibiotics and improved sanitation in the first half of this century, the number of postappendicitis and amebic abscesses has decreased dramatically, whereas those relating to biliary tract disease and impaired host defenses have increased. Continuous improvement in diagnosis and treatment has greatly decreased the mortality during this time from as high as 80 percent before 1965 to 16 to 48 percent in the 1970s,[3] with much of the current mortality attributable to patients with severe underlying diseases.

In addition to liver abscess, this discussion deals with selected systemic infections and parasitic infestations in which hepatic abnormalities may be prominent, or indeed the only localizing manifestations of illness. Clinical presentation of many of these conditions is nonspecific; there may be nothing more than fatigue or low-grade fever with generalized abdominal or right upper quadrant pain and mild abnormalities of liver function tests. Fortunately, recognition of the significance of liver involvement often helps to generate an appropriate differential diagnosis in these enigmatic cases. Serologic investigations, noninvasive imaging tests, or liver biopsy may then yield the information that solves the mystery and identifies a specific, treatable illness.

PYOGENIC LIVER ABSCESS

Infectious organisms can invade the liver in any of five different ways, as listed in Table 1. Although one must consider all pathogenetic mechanisms in each patient with liver in-

TABLE 1
Pathogenesis of Liver Abscesses

Source of Infecting Organisms	Typical Clinical Settings
1. Portal system introduction	Intraperitoneal sepsis Pancreatitis Inflammatory bowel disease Umbilical vein catheter Amebiasis
2. Spread from contiguous structures	Ascending cholangitis After correction of biliary atresia Other peritoneal and retroperitoneal infections
3. Systemic bacteremia	Pyelonephritis, cystitis Endocarditis Pneumonia Endometritis Osteomyelitis Extensive burns Indwelling venous catheters Neonatal sepsis Impaired host defenses
4. Direct inoculation	Penetrating abdominal trauma Abdominal surgery Kasai procedure Liver transplant
5. Cryptogenic	Fever of unknown origin

fection, some patterns are seen most often in a particular clinical setting. Distinct classes of infecting organisms are associated with each of the sources of infection, such as in immunosuppressed patients or those who have had surgical correction of biliary atresia.

Introduction of bacteria through the portal blood stream is seen as a complication of intraperitoneal infection with portal sepsis, as occurred often in the preantibiotic era as a complication of ruptured appendix.[4,5] Other abdominal conditions with similar potential for portal sepsis include perforated viscus, pancreatitis, and diverticulitis. Liver abscess occurred in 6 of 1,277 adult patients with Crohn's disease[3] and has been reported as the first manifestation of Crohn's disease in a 24-year-old, previously healthy man.[6] In the newborn period, omphalitis and umbilical venous catheters have been associated with introduction of bacteria into the liver through the portal vein,[7,8] causing overt infection immediately or after a delay of up to several weeks after catheter removal. Largely for this reason, umbilical vein catheters are no longer widely used. In amebic liver abscess, (see later in this discussion) the portal vein is also the route by which invasive trophozoites arrive from the colon.

The second pathogenetic mechanism for development of liver abscess is spread of infection from contiguous structures. The most common source is ascending cholangitis. The gallbladder and bile ducts may become infected as a result of obstruction from gallstones or pancreatitis, but more commonly in the pediatric age group infection occurs after surgical correction of biliary atresia by direct anastomosis of small bowel to liver. Other peritoneal infections, such as postsurgical infections, subphrenic abscess,[5] or ruptured renal carbuncle,[1] can lead to liver abscess, particularly if unrecognized and untreated for several days.

Systemic bacteremia can result in infection in the liver via the hepatic artery even though the liver is relatively well protected owing to its excellent blood circulation and the fact that it is a reticuloendothelial organ whose Kupffer cells, a form of tissue macrophage, are normally involved in ingestion and destruction of invading organisms. Any organism that is associated with bacteremia can cause liver abscess. The source is often a focal infection such as pyelonephritis, cystitis, endocarditis, pneumonia, endometritis,[9] or osteomyelitis.[1,2] Patients with severe burns and those with long-term indwelling catheters for venous access or parenteral nutrition, having a higher risk of bacteremia, consequently also have a greater chance of seeding the liver as well as other organs with bacteria that can form abscesses. Moreover, neonates, diabetics, and patients with impaired host defenses are much more likely than normal individuals to develop a focus of infection from bacteremia.

Direct penetrating trauma and surgical incision of the liver can also lead to introduction of pathogenic organisms causing liver abscess. In a multicenter review of combined adult and pediatric hepatic trauma,[10] 10 percent of patients with severe liver injuries requiring laparotomy and liver packing or drainage developed abscesses in or around the liver. Infections related to hepatic surgery also fall into this category.

Finally, there are some "cryptogenic"[1] liver infections in which a source cannot be proven. Although this group accounts for a smaller and smaller percentage of patients as diagnostic technologies improve, idiopathic liver abscess has been recognized as a cause of liver enlargement without symptoms[11] and of fever of unknown origin. Kaplan[12] reported two cases in 6- and 7-year-old boys of single liver abscess caused by *Staphylococcus aureus* without any other nidus of infection or impairment of host defense mechanisms detected, despite detailed investigations. Hepatic abscess therefore becomes a consideration in the work-up of patients with prolonged fever of unknown origin.

Special Settings

Sickle Cell Hemoglobinopathies

Children with sickle cell disease have been noted to have a predilection for liver abscess, which can be the presenting illness in a previously undiagnosed child.[13] These patients have several abnormalities that may contribute to their increased risk: (1) Impairment of hepatic microcirculation due to sickling can lead to liver infarcts that serve as a nidus for infection. (2) Splenic dysfunction prevents efficient clearance of bacteremias. (3) Sickled erythrocytes in capillaries of the gut endothelium cause microinfarcts and increase permeability of the gastrointestinal tract to resident organisms including *Salmonella*. (4) The development of gallstones in a large proportion of older children with sickle cell disease results in a high incidence of cholangitis.

Congenital Defects in Host Defenses

There is a striking association of liver abscess and defects in the intracellular killing of bacteria. X-linked chronic granulomatous disease (CGD), the most common form of this disorder, is caused by defects in the gene, now cloned, encoding one chain of cytochrome *b* 245, a component of the phagocytic cell oxidase system.[14,15] In a review of 92 CGD patients by Johnston and Baehner,[16] the most common findings were adenopathy in 94 percent, pneumonitis in 87 percent, and male sex in 87 percent; but 41 out of 92, or 45 percent, had abscesses in or around the liver. This incidence is so high that any child who presents with liver abscess without a known underlying cause should have his neutrophils evaluated for CGD with a nitroblue tetrazolium dye test or bactericidal test. Liver abscesses in CGD are caused primarily by *S. aureus,* but gram-negative enteric bacteria and *Candida albicans,* which also have catalase and therefore do not accumulate H_2O_2 intracellularly, are significant pathogens in this disease. More recent reports[17] suggest that continuous antibiotic administration, usually with trimethoprim and sulfamethoxazole, decreases the number of staphylococcal infections, including liver abscesses, in these children. Successful bone marrow transplantation may cure immune defect.[18] Although CGD has the highest incidence of liver abscess, other immunodeficiencies, including congenital neutropenia,[2] complement deficiencies, agammaglobulinemia, and severe combined immunodeficiency, have been associated with liver abscess.

Acquired Immunodeficiency Syndrome (AIDS)

Children infected with HIV are at risk of primary liver injury due to the virus[19] and secondary infections with both virulent organisms and opportunistic pathogens (see Part 2 of this chapter). In addition to the usual bacterial, fungal, and viral etiologies for liver abscess, one must be alert for amebiasis,[20] toxoplasmosis, and mycobacterial disease. Liver abscess due to *Mycobacterium tuberculosis* can be the presenting infection in AIDS.[21]

Immunocompromised Patients

Patients with severely impaired host defenses due to malignancies and cytotoxic chemotherapy account for a growing proportion of liver abscesses in pediatric medical centers. Better success in curing acute leukemia with stringent drug regimens and the growing number of bone marrow and other organ transplants have meant more patients are at risk for longer periods of time. In addition to bacterial liver abscesses, fungal infections of the liver have been recognized as a particular problem in newborns and immunocompromised patients.[22,23] Focal hepatic candidiasis is characterized by macroscopic or microscopic nodular or necrotic lesions occurring throughout the liver with or without evidence of candidal infection in the blood or other organs. It occurs in patients with prolonged neutropenia, previous treatment with broad-spectrum antibiotics, and gastrointestinal (GI) colonization with *Candida* and is associated with fever, abdominal symptoms, and elevated liver enzymes. The prognosis is grave, and survival may depend at least in part on recovery of the patient's neutrophil population; prompt treatment is indicated with amphotericin and 5-glucytosine. Unfortunately, in many institutions the proportion of *Candida* species resistant to amphotericin is rising, and fungal sensitivity testing is not routinely available.

Post-Kasai Operation and Post-Liver Transplantation

The abnormal anatomy of the GI tract of patients who have undergone as Kasai operation for biliary atresia predisposes them to the development of ascending cholangitis and infection of the liver, particularly in the first year of life. These infections are difficult to diagnose because of the nonspecific nature of the presentation, typically with fever, irritability, and increased abdominal distention. Because the variety of pathogenic organisms is wide and resistant GI flora common in these infants who receive many courses of antibiotics, specific diagnosis is critical. Liver biopsy has been found superior to blood culture in recovering pathogenic organisms; in a series of 32 episodes of cholangitis at Children's Hospital of Philadelphia,[24] liver biopsy culture was positive in 68 percent, whereas blood culture was positive in only 31 percent. Organisms include the gram-negative *Klebsiella, Escherichia coli, Pseudomonas,* and *Enterobacter,* as well as gram-positive enterococcus. All patients in this study had been on antibiotics prior to the development of cholangitis and liver infection, and their liver biopsy isolates were frequently resistant to multiple antibiotics, including those most recently administered, calling into question the use of prophylactic antibiotics in post-Kasai patients. Identification and sensitivity testing of liver pathogens in this setting are critical for optimal antibiotic treatment, and surgical drainage or revision of the portal enterostomy may be required in patients with multiple or persistent episodes of cholangitis after Kasai operation.

Infections are also one of the major complications of liver transplantation. Risk factors include presurgical debilitation, the surgical procedure itself, the anatomy of biliary reconstruction, and the condition of the transplanted organ, as well as postsurgical immunosuppressive treatment to combat rejection. Series from the University of California at Los Angeles,[25] the Mayo Clinic,[26] and the University of Pittsburgh[27] found serious bacterial and fungal infections in 26 to 88 percent of their transplanted patients, most of which were bacteremias or abdominal infections. Viral infections, especially with cytomegalovirus, which may be introduced by the donor liver or by transfusion, and *Pneumocystis,* were also important problems. As this procedure becomes more widely used in pediatric patients, better approaches to the prevention of infectious complications may be developed. Currently the best guidelines are to use the minimal immunosuppressive treatment necessary and to maintain vigilant surveillance, prompt specific diagnosis, and appropriate antimicrobial and surgical treatment for infections that develop.

Microbiology

The variety of pathogenic organisms found in liver abscesses is wide (Table 2), and some specific organisms associated with particular clinical settings have already been addressed. Determination of the route by which organisms have invaded the liver leads the clinician to suspect a particular group of pathogens. When infection is introduced through the portal system or from infections arising in the GI tract, the organisms are most likely to be the anaerobic and aerobic

TABLE 2
Organisms Cultured from Liver Abscesses (Often Polymicrobial)

Aerobes
Escherichia coli
Klebsiella-Enterobacter
Pseudomonas
Proteus
Serratia
Salmonella
Staphylococcus aureus
Streptococci, hemolytic and nonhemolytic
Enterococcus
Anaerobes[13]
Bacteroides fragilis and other *Bacteroides* species
Microaerophilic and anaerobic streptococci
Fusobacterium
Clostridium
Actinomyces
Mycobacteria (typical and atypical, seen with HIV infection)
Fungi (especially in immunocompromised hosts)
Entamoeba histolytica

bacteria that constitute normal GI flora. *E. coli, Klebsiella, Pseudomonas, Proteus,* and other gram-negative enteric organisms are commonly found, over half the time in mixed infection. With improved anaerobic culturing techniques, modern studies have emphasized the importance of anaerobic organisms[13] and the possibility of synergistic action between aerobic and anaerobic bacteria together in liver abscesses.[29] Frequently isolated anaerobes include *Bacteroides* species, anaerobic and microaerophilic streptococci, *Fusobacterium, Clostridium,* and *Actinomyces.* Because the use of antibiotics is associated with derangements of GI flora and acquisition of antibiotic-resistant strains, patients with previous antibiotic administration may have liver abscesses involving unusual or resistant organisms, including *Pseudomonas,* enterococcus, *Staphylococcus epidermidis,* and fungi. In this setting a microbiologic diagnosis is critical in order to ensure effective therapy. *Salmonella* liver abscess occurs in patients with sickle cell disease, but also in immunosuppressed and apparently normal individuals. *Entamoeba histolytica* must also always be considered a possible etiologic agent.

Liver abscess following bacteremia is much more common in children than in adults, and *S. aureus* and *Streptococci* accounted for more than 40 percent of liver abscesses in the St. Louis series.[1] If organisms from the source of bacteremia have been identified, such as with a *S. aureus* osteomyelitis in an otherwise normal host, the cause of the liver abscess can be inferred to be the same; but because of the wide range of microorganisms that can be associated with liver abscess in patients with underlying disease or immunodeficiency, culture of aspirated material may be very helpful. Streptococcal abscesses occur as a complication of endocarditis, but also in association with GI tract disease with *Streptococcus milleri.*[30] Patients with chronic granulomatous disease have a very high frequency of *S. aureus* abscesses but also infections with gram-negative enteric organisms, which produce catalase. These patients and other immunosuppressed individuals, particularly those with HIV disease, are at increased risk of mycobacterial liver abscesses due to *M. tuberculosis* and *Mycobacterium avium-intracellulare,* and abscesses caused by fungi, such as *Candida* species and *Nocardia.*

Clinical Features

Because the clinical presentation of liver abscess is nonspecific, the diagnosis has in the past often been overlooked until late in the course. There can be an acute septic picture or insidious onset over weeks to months. It is extremely important to be aware of any history of previous abdominal surgery or trauma, underlying immune deficiency disease, or other risk factors. Presenting symptoms may be minimal but frequently include fever, nausea, vomiting, weakness, fatigue, weight loss, and abdominal pain, with or without localization to the right upper quadrant. In the 50 percent of cases occurring in the first year of life, symptoms are difficult to evaluate. In adult series, single abscesses, usually in the right lobe of the liver, are generally chronic and indolent and have a more favorable course, whereas multiple abscesses present more acutely, are correlated with underlying disease, and have a poorer outcome.[3] However, in pediatrics these generalizations do not hold.[2]

Physical signs may include elevated temperature, hepatomegaly in 40 to 80 percent of patients,[31] and right upper quadrant tenderness. Jaundice, abdominal distention, splenomegaly, dullness to percussion, and decreased breath sounds in the right lower lung field may also be noted.[31,32]

Laboratory Diagnosis

Routine laboratory studies, like clinical presentation, are not specific for liver abscess and generally reflect any underlying disease of the patient. White blood counts are generally elevated, except in neutropenic patients, such as those receiving chemotherapy for malignancy. Although there are no comparable pediatric figures available, anemia is found in 50 percent and elevated sedimentation rate in 90 percent of adult patients.[31] Liver function tests reveal elevated bilirubin and alkaline phosphatase in the presence of biliary obstruction. Transaminases are usually mildly elevated rather than extremely high and may be in the normal range.[31,32] Chest radiographs were found to be abnormal in more than 50 percent of adults with liver abscess, with findings including right-sided atelectasis, infiltrates, pleural effusion, and elevated hemidiaphragm.

The importance of blood cultures, both aerobic and anaerobic, cannot be overemphasized. Although positive only approximately half the time, they document that bacteremia is occurring and aid in the choice of antibiotics for treatment. Pediatric patients with multiple abscesses are even more likely to have positive blood cultures than those with single abscesses.[32]

New noninvasive techniques for visualization of the liver have revolutionized the diagnosis of these infections. Radioactive technetium liver-spleen scans, used primarily before 1978, can detect abscesses of 4 cm but are less sensitive for smaller and multiple abscesses. Since that time ultrasonography has become a valuable, rapid, and inexpensive first step in evaluation of liver abscesses. This technique, which can detect cavities as small as 2 cm in diameter, diagnosed 86 percent of abscesses in a recent adult study[33]; however, microabscesses can be missed,[31,34] and abscesses in which protein and lipid content are high can be echogenic.[35] Computed tomography (CT) and magnetic resonance (MRI) scanning are considerably more sensitive although more costly approaches to diagnosing liver abscess. With both techniques abscesses as small as 1 cm can be visualized. MRI is still in its developmental stages but promises to be the most sensitive way to detect multiple small abscesses. The clinician should remember that these imaging tests are complementary; one may pick up an abnormality that another has missed, and repeating the tests over time can be very helpful when liver abscess is suspected.

Finally, biopsy of the liver, with ultrasound guidance in cases with a well-delineated abscess cavity, but even blind biopsy in post-Kasai and post–liver transplant patients, has proved very useful in cases in which a bacteriologic diagnosis is critical. Infection can be documented and the specific etiologic agent or agents determined early in the course, often before an actual walled-off abscess has formed. Furthermore, tissue can be used for histologic examination and mycobacterial, fungal, and viral cultures.

Treatment and Outcome

Improvements in three areas of management of liver abscess have made a dramatic difference in survival rates in the past 15 years. The most important is that the diagnosis is being made earlier in the course, still requiring a high index of suspicion but greatly facilitated by new advances in imaging techniques. In one retrospective report of adults, the mean delay from onset to diagnosis prior to 1977 was 90 days, with a 46 percent mortality rate; from 1978 to 1986 the mean delay was reduced to 28 days, and there were no deaths.[33] Clearly, there is still room for further improvement in shortening the time to diagnosis.

Second, new approaches to surgical drainage, always a mainstay of treatment, have been made available by the better delineation and localization of abscess cavities. There are now several alternative methods for drainage. In addition to transperitoneal open drainage and extraserous drainage, which avoid exposing the peritoneal cavity to possible contamination with infected material, it is now possible to perform percutaneous aspiration and placement of drains under ultrasonic or CT guidance in patients who might not tolerate abdominal surgery.[34,36]

Antibiotic therapy, without which almost all patients with liver abscess would die,[33,34] has also made important advances. While penicillinase-resistant penicillins, such as oxacillin, nafcillin, and methicillin, are the mainstay for liver abscesses due to *S. aureus,* rifampicin, a drug with excellent intracellular bactericidal function, has been found to be an effective addition in patients with chronic granulomatous disease.[17] While gram-negative enteric organisms are often successfully treated with aminoglycosides, such as gentamicin, recently developed third-generation cephalosporins achieve high tissue levels and may work better in the acidic environment produced by bacteria and necrotic debris in abscess cavities. Because *Bacteroides* and other anaerobic organisms are now frequently resistant to penicillin, for anaerobic coverage one should use clindamycin, chloramphenicol, cefoxitin, or metronidazole as effective adjuncts for treatment of liver abscesses related to the GI tract. Fungal abscesses are generally treated with amphotericin B, in some cases with the addition of 5-fluorocytosine. The increasing frequency of fungi resistant to amphotericin appearing as etiologic agents of infections in immunosuppressed individuals has stimulated the development of new antifungal agents such as fluconazole, which may have an important role in the future as the number of liver transplants increases.

Although drainage by surgery or aspiration is desirable, multiple abscesses and those not amenable to complete surgical drainage have been successfully cured with prolonged antibiotic therapy alone.[37] Controlled studies addressing the optimal management of pediatric liver abscesses have not been published, but treatment of underlying risk factors is of paramount importance. Duration of treatment with parenteral antibiotics should be a minimum of 2 to 4 weeks and up to several weeks to months in immunosuppressed patients, depending on their underlying condition.[31,32,34] Serial imaging studies may be required to document appropriate response and shrinking of abscess cavities.

SYSTEMIC ILLNESSES AFFECTING THE LIVER

The liver, a major organ of the reticuloendothelial system, is a window through which clues to the presence of many systemic diseases, including infections, may be viewed. Some infections which may be nonspecific in their presentation but in which liver abnormalities may be seen are listed in Table 3. Any child presenting with significant but nonlocalizing symptoms and signs, including fever of unknown origin, should be carefully evaluated for signs of liver involvement. A careful physical examination for liver enlargement and tenderness should be emphasized for all patients, and liver function tests and imaging studies should be considered in individual cases depending on the patient's history and the acuity of the illness. Liver biopsy and/or bone marrow aspiration for histologic examination and bacterial, viral,

TABLE 3
Other Systemic Infectious Diseases That Can Present with Abnormalities Primarily or Solely Localizing to the Liver

Tuberculosis
Brucellosis
Syphilis
Leptospirosis
Bacterial (gram-negative) sepsis in infants
Typhoid, enteric fever
Sexually acquired perihepatitis (gonoccocal, chlamydial, anaerobic bacterial)
Fungal disseminated histoplasmosis, paracoccidioidomycosis (S. Am), candidiasis
Viral diseases (HIV, CMV, EBV)

mycobacterial, and fungal cultures may yield a specific diagnosis. More extensive reviews of the diseases mentioned below can be found in Feigin and Cherry's *Textbook of Pediatric Infectious Diseases.*[38]

Disseminated tuberculosis is one of the most common causes of fever of unknown origin. The tuberculin skin test, while generally positive in pulmonary disease, may be negative on presentation with systemic involvement owing to anergy,[39] and the chest radiograph may be normal or show diffuse miliary infiltration. In critically ill children it may be advisable to start antituberculosis therapy while awaiting the results of diagnostic studies.

Brucellosis is acquired through contact with infected livestock, but in children in the United States it is seen primarily after ingestion of unpasteurized dairy products. *Brucella* organisms are ingested by the macrophages of the reticuloendothelial system, so that hepatosplenomegaly is common. Although most infections in children are mild and self-limited, severe disease and fatalities occur, especially in conjunction with endocarditis. Successful isolation of the organism from blood, liver, and other tissues requires special notification to the microbiology laboratory so that appropriate media and prolonged incubation times will be used. Serologic tests, generally by the standard tube agglutination (STA) method, can be used to document infection and follow response to treatment. Recovery is faster and relapses and complications are less frequent when patients are treated with tetracycline, which can be given in combination with rifampin or an aminoglycoside. Children under age 9 years are given trimethoprim sulfamethoxazole rather than tetracycline.[40]

Syphilis, Lyme disease, and leptospirosis are all caused by spirochetes. The involvement of the liver with syphilis in pediatrics is covered elsewhere in Chapter 28. In the acute stage, 5 percent of patients with Lyme disease had hepatomegaly and 19 percent had elevated SGOT values, but isolated hepatitis due to Lyme disease is not generally seen.[41] Leptospirosis[42] is acquired through direct or indirect contact with animal urine. It is usually a biphasic illness, with an initial septicemic phase of constitutional symptoms and generalized illness followed by a vasculitic immune phase, in which jaundice as well as rash, renal failure, and other complications can occur. Diagnosis is made by serology or culture of organisms from urine using special media. Although late recognition of the diagnosis often precludes institution of penicillin therapy in time to modify the course, it is used in treatment along with meticulous supportive management of complications.

Jaundice appearing in infants in the first 6 weeks of life can be the first sign of sepsis or urinary tract infection (discussed in detail elsewhere in Chapter 28).

Enteric fever caused by *Salmonella typhi*,[43] but also by other *Salmonella* strains,[44] is unusual in the United States. A septic picture with fever, rash (often undetected, especially in black patients), and abdominal pain with hepatosplenomegaly is the presenting finding; diarrhea, if it occurs, develops later in the course. Blood cultures are usually positive. As opposed to *Salmonella* gastroenteritis, in which treatment is not generally indicated, enteric fever should be treated with antibiotics such as ampicillin plus chloramphenicol until the sensitivity pattern of the patient's organism is known.

Perihepatitis is a complication of pelvic inflammatory disease in sexually active females. Ascent of sexually acquired infection from the vagina, endocervics, and endometrium and through the fallopian tubes can lead to pelvic inflammatory disease, and in advanced cases, perihepatic infection, also known as Fitz-Hugh-Curtis syndrome, which presents with right upper quadrant pain.[45] Although classically caused by *Neisseria gonorrhoeae,* there has been a large increase in the 1980s in chlamydial disease, which may accompany gonococcal infection or independently cause the same clinical syndrome.[46] In addition, anaerobic bacteria, gram-negative enteric bacteria, and ureaplasmal and mycoplasmal organisms have been increasingly implicated in pelvic inflammatory disease and its complications.[40] Patient evaluation should include pelvic examination with endocervical cultures for gonococcal, aerobic, and anaerobic bacteria, and rapid chlamydia antigen detection; abdominal and pelvic ultrasonography may reveal abscesses. Initial therapy should be chosen to cover increasingly frequent ampicillin-resistant *N. gonorrhoeae,* anaerobes, and *Chlamydia trachomatis.* Regimens include cefoxitin plus doxycycline; or a third-generation cepohalosporin, plus clindamycin or metronidazole, plus doxycycline. Further treatment should be tailored according to culture results and clinical response. Identification and treatment of sexual contacts of the patient are part of the management of this disease.

Fungal disease involving the liver has already been discussed in the context of immunocompromised patients. Most systemic fungal infections of individuals with no known defects in host defenses involve other organs, such as lung, sinuses, bones, eyes, central nervous system, or lymph nodes in addition to the liver, but occasionally liver infiltration may be the first or only clinical manifestation, particularly in the case of *Candida species, Histoplasma capsulatum,* and *Paracoccidioides brasiliensis.*[33,47] Liver biopsy for histologic examination and culture can be invaluable in making the diagnosis.

Of the rickettsial diseases, generally characterized by fever, headache, and rash, an exception is Q fever, caused by *Coxiella burnetii*. This organism, acquired by humans through animal contact rather than from ticks as with other rickettsiae, does not cause rashes and is more associated with pulmonary infiltrates. Liver enlargement is common, and histologic examination of liver biopsies reveals a distinctive granulomatous hepatitis.[48,49] Specific serologic tests are available. Although most patients recover uneventfully even without treatment, complications including gastroenteritis, hemolytic anemia, and carditis occur. The treatment of choice is tetracycline.

Hepatitis viruses are covered in detail in another part of Chapter 28, but it should be re-emphasized that systemic viral diseases, including HIV, cytomegalovirus (CMV), and Epstein-Barr virus (EBV) can also be manifest most significantly in the liver. HIV hepatitis in congenitally infected children may not always be accompanied by a positive antibody response, so that a high index of suspicion and determination of maternal HIV antibody are critical.[19] CMV and EBV are usually associated with either inapparent infection or the mononucleosis syndrome, characterized by fatigue, fever, exudative pharyngitis, lymphadenopathy, and hepatosplenomegaly, accompanied by atypical lymphocytes in the blood.

However, there is great variability in symptoms; liver tenderness and enlargement with elevated liver function tests may be the major abnormalities, and rapidly fatal hepatic necrosis is a well-recognized complication of EBV disease.[50,51] Rapid mononucleosis tests based on the presence of heterophil antibodies are not positive in CMV disease and are frequently negative in children with EBV infections who are under 5 years of age.[52] Specific serology for EBV[53] and serology and urine culture for CMV aid in establishing the diagnosis, and liver biopsy may also be indicated.

PARASITIC DISEASES

Parasites are an important world-wide cause of infection of the liver and are acquired by pediatric patients in both foreign countries and the United States. The most important aid in diagnosis of these diseases is a high index of suspicion prompting the physician to obtain a complete history of diet and travel, exposure to pets or other animals, and pica. Several parasitic diseases are primarily associated with liver involvement, including amebiasis, toxocariasis, echinococcosis, schistosomiasis, and infections with liver flukes.[38,54–56] More detailed discussions of parasitic infections of the liver can be found in the references.

Entamoeba histolytica has a world-wide distribution and is spread by the fecal-oral route through ingestion of cysts. The large majority of human infestations are asymptomatic and confined to the lumen of the gut, but occasionally invasion of the mucosa by activated trophozoites occurs, resulting in amebic dysentery or liver invasion through the portal blood stream. Most commonly liver abscesses are single and in the right lobe; clinical presentation is the same as for bacterial liver abscess. Diagnosis is suggested if stool examination is positive for trophozoites or cysts, but the recently developed ELISA test for antibody to *E. histolytica* is more sensitive. Because of the risk of peritoneal contamination, surgical drainage is avoided unless spontaneous rupture of a very large abscess is a concern. Treatment with metronidazole for 10 days is recommended,[40] after which cavitary lesions on serial ultrasonography or CT scans should resolve and ELISA titer should progressively decrease.

Toxocariasis is an abortive infection with roundworms *Toxocara canis* and *Toxocara cati*, whose natural hosts are dogs and cats, respectively. It is easily acquired in the United States by children, especially in the 1- to 4-year-old age group, through ingestion of larvae found in soil or sandbox sand contaminated with animal feces. Although most infections are asymptomatic, a heavy innoculum or a vigorous allergic response can lead to fever, cough or wheezing, weight loss, and hepatomegaly. Laboratory investigation reveals leukocytosis with hypereosinophilia, elevated isohemagglutinin titers to the A and B blood group antigens, high serum levels of IgE, and occasionally pulmonary infiltrates associated with the migration of larvae from the portal system of the liver to the lungs. The diagnosis can be confirmed by demonstration of *Toxocara* antibodies using an ELISA test. Visceral larva migrans can rarely be associated with serious complications due to invasion of the eye, brain, myocardium, or other organs. These may require steroid treatment in addition to use of an antiparasitic agent such as thiabendazole or diethylcarbamazine (still considered investigational for this use in the United States),[40] but most infections are self-limited if the patient is removed from the source of infection.

Echinococcosis is also caused by abortive infection in humans with a natural parasite of dogs and other carnivorous animals, the tapeworm *Echinococcus granulosis.* Acquired in warm climates, this disease causes hepatomegaly secondary to the formation of large single or multiple hepatic cysts, usually in the right lobe. Eosinophilia and lung involvement are common. The cysts can be demonstrated by ultrasonography, radionuclide scanning, or CT scan; diagnosis is confirmed by specific serology or histology after surgical removal, which is the treatment of choice.[57]

Acquisition of schistosomiasis occurs when infective cercaria maturing from snails penetrate the skin of humans exposed to infected water. Two species of schistosomes, or blood flukes, mature and persist in the mesenteric venous system, from which large numbers of eggs can be introduced into the liver, resulting in an intense local inflammatory reaction. These are *Schistosoma mansoni*, found in Africa, Asia, South America, and the Caribbean, and *Schistosoma japonicum,* found in the far East. The exuberant immune response to the eggs can produce fever, eosinophilia, and serum sickness; liver enlargement, cirrhosis, portal hypertension, and liver failure may eventually occur. The diagnosis is made by detection of ova in stool or rectal biopsy. Praziquantel is the drug of choice for treatment.[40,58]

Liver flukes, primarily *Opisthorchis sinensis* and *Opisthorchis viverrini*, are a major cause of hepatic injury in the far East, where they are acquired by ingestion of uncooked fresh water fish. The worms migrate through the intestinal wall and liver capsule to the biliary tree, where a large innoculum can cause inflammation and eventually blockage of the bile ducts with jaundice, hepatomegaly, and cirrhosis. Eosinophilia is generally present, but specific diagnosis is made by examination of stools for eggs. Again, praziquantel is considered the best therapeutic agent, although it is considered investigational for this use in the United States.

REFERENCES

1. Dehner LP, Kissane JM. Pyogenic hepatic abscesses in infancy and childhood. Pediatrics 1969; 75:763–773.
2. Chusid MJ. Pyogenic hepatic abscesses in infancy and childhood. Pediatrics 1978; 62:554–559.
3. Greenstein AJ, Sachar DB. Pyogenic and amebic abscesses of the liver. Semin Liver Dis 1988; 8:210–217.
4. de la Maza LM, Naeim F, Berman LD. The changing etiology of liver abscess. JAMA 1974; 227:161–163.
5. Greenstein AJ, Lowenthal D, Hammer GS, Schaffner F, Aufses AH Jr. Continuing changing patterns of disease in pyogenic liver abscess: a study of 38 patients. Am J Gastroenterol 1984; 79:217–226.
6. Teague M, Baddour LM, Wruble LD. Liver abscess: a harbinger of Crohn's disease. Am J Gastroenterol 1988; 83:1412–1414.
7. Brans YW, Ceballos R, Cassaday G. Umbilical catheters and hepatic abscesses. Pediatrics 1974; 53:264–266.
8. Williams JW, Rittenberry A, Dillard R, Allen RG. Liver abscess in a newborn: complications of umbilical vein catheterization. Am J Dis Child 1972; 125:111–113.
9. Ezzell JH Jr, Wickliffe JM Jr. *Gardnerella vaginalis*: an unusual case of pyogenic liver abscess. Am J Gastroenterol 1988; 83:1409–1411.
10. Cogbill TH, Moore EE, Jurkovich GJ, Feliciano DV, Morris JA, Mucha P. Severe hepatic trauma: a multi-center experience with 1,335 liver injuries. J Trauma 1988; 28:1433–1438.

11. Palmer ED. The changing manifestations of pyogenic liver abscess. JAMA 1975; 231:192–194.
12. Kaplan SL, Feigin RD. Pyogenic liver abscess in normal children with fever of unknown origin. Pediatrics 1976; 58:614–616.
13. Shulman ST, Beem MO. A unique presentation of sickle cell disease: pyogenic hepatic abscess. Pediatrics 1971; 47:1019–1022.
14. Royer-Pokora B, Kunkel LM, Monaco AP, Goff SB, Newburger PE, Baehner RL, Cole FS, Curnutte JT, Orkin SH. Cloning the gene for an inherited human disorder—chronic granulomatous disease—on the basis of its chromosomal location. Nature 1986; 322:32–38.
15. Segal AW. Absence of both cytochrome b-245 subunits from neutrophils in X-linked chronic granulomatous disease. Nature 1987; 326:88–91.
16. Johnston RB Jr, Baehner RL. Chronic granulomatous disease: correlation between pathogenesis and clinical findings. Pediatrics 1971; 48:730–739.
17. Forrest CB, Forehand JR, Axtell RA, Roberts RL, Johnston RB Jr. Clinical features and current management of chronic granulomatous disease. Hematol Oncol Clin North Am 1988; 2:253–266.
18. Kamani N, August CS, Douglas SD, et al. Bone marrow transplantation in chronic granulomatous disease. J Pediatr 1984; 105:42.
19. Witzleben CL, Marshall GS, Wenner W, Piccoli DA, Barbour SD. HIV as a cause of giant cell hepatitis. Hum Pathol 1988; 19:603–605.
20. Stanley PJ. Amoebic liver abscess in a bisexual man. J Infection 1988; 17:163–165.
21. Weinberg JJ, Cohen P, Malhotra R. Primary tuberculous liver abscess associated with the human immunodeficiency virus. Tubercle 1988; 69:145–147.
22. Tashjian LS, Abramson JS, Peacock JE Jr. Focal hepatic candidiasis: a distinct clinical variant of candidiasis in immunocompromised patients. Rev Infect Dis 1984; 6:689–703.
23. Haron E, Feld R. Hepatic candidiasis: an increasing problem in immunocompromised patients. Am J Med 1987; 83:17–26.
24. Piccoli DA, Mohan P, McConnie RM. Cholangitis post-Kasai: diagnostic value of blood cultures and liver biopsy. Pediatr Res 1986; 20:247A.
25. Colonna JO, Winston DJ, Brill JE, Goldstein LI, Hoff MP, Hiatt JR, Quinones-Baldrich W, Ramming KP, Busuttil RW. Infectious complications in liver transplantation. Arch Surg 1988; 123:360–364.
26. Krom RA, Wiesner RH, Rettke SR, Ludwig J, Southorn PA, Hermans PE, Taswell HF. The first 100 liver transplantations at the Mayo Clinic. Mayo Clin Proc 1989; 64:84–94.
27. Kusne S, Dummer JS, Singh N, Iwatsuki S, Makowka L, Esquivel C, Tzakis AG, Starzl TE, Ho M. Infection after liver transplantation: an analysis of 101 consecutive cases. Medicine 1988; 67:132–143.
28. Sabbaj J. Anaerobes in liver abscess. Rev Inf Dis 1984; 6(Suppl):S152–S156.
29. Nielsen ML, Asnaes S, Justesen T. Susceptibility of the liver and biliary tract to anaerobic infection in extrahepatic biliary tract obstruction. III. Possible synergistic effect between anaerobic and aerobic bacteria. An experimental study in rabbits. Scand J Gastroenterol 1976; 11:263–272.
30. Chua D, Reinhart HH, Sobel JD. Liver abscess caused by *Streptococcus milleri*. Rev Infect Dis 1989; 11:197–202.
31. Kandel G, Marcon NE. Pyogenic liver abscess: new concepts of an old disease. Am J Gastroenterol 1984; 79:65–71.
32. Kaplan SL. Pyogenic liver abscess. In: Feigin RD, Cherry JD, eds. Textbook of pediatric infectious diseases. 2nd ed. Philadelphia: WB Saunders, 1987: 746.
33. Farges O, Leese T, Bismuth H. Pyogenic liver abscess: an improvement in prognosis. Br J Surg 1988; 75:862–865.
34. Miedema BW, Dineen P. The diagnosis and treatment of pyogenic liver abscesses. Ann Surg 1984; 200:328–335.
35. Bunney RG. Pyogenic liver abscess with two normal ultrasound scans. Postgraduate Med J 1988; 64:373–374.
36. Stenson WF, Eckert T, Avioli LA. Pyogenic liver abscess. Arch Intern Med 1983; 143:126–128.
37. Reynolds TB. Medical treatment of pyogenic liver abscess. Ann Intern Med 1982; 96:373–374.
38. Feigin Rd, Cherry JD, eds. Textbook of pediatric infectious diseases 2nd ed. Philadelphia: WB Saunders, 1987.
39. Steiner P, Rao R, Victoria MS, Jahbar H, Steiner M. Persistently negative tuberculin reactions: their presence among children with culture positive for *M. tuberculosis*. Am J Dis Child 1982; 134:747–750.
40. Committee on Infectious Diseases, American Academy of Pediatrics. 1988 Red Book: Report of the committee on infectious diseases. 21st ed. Elk Grove Village, IL: American Academy of Pediatrics, 1988: 140.
41. Steere AC, Bartenhagen NH, Craft JE, et al. The early clinical manifestations of Lyme disease. Ann Intern Med 1983; 99:22–26.
42. Peter G. Leptospirosis: a zoonosis of protean manifestations. Pediatr Infect Dis 1982; 1:282–288.
43. Hormick RB, Greisman SE. On the pathogenesis of typhoid fever. Arch Intern Med 1979; 138:357–359.
44. Meadow WL, Schneider H, Beem M. *Salmonella enteritidis* bacteremia in childhood. J Infect Dis 1985; 152:185–189.
45. Litt IF, Cohen M. Perihepatitis associated with salpingitis in adolescents. JAMA 1978; 240:1253.
46. Center for Disease Control, 1985 STD Treatment Guidelines. MMWR 1985; 34(suppl):1–35.
47. Strickland GT, ed. Tropical medicine. 6th ed. Philadelphia: WB Saunders, 1984: 451.
48. Pellegrin M, Delsol G, Anvergnat JC, et al. Granulomatous hepatitis in Q fever. Hum Pathol 1980; 11:51–57.
49. Hoffman CE, Heaton JW Jr. Q fever hepatitis: clinical manifestations and pathological findings. Gastroenterology 1982; 83:474–479.
50. Andiman WA. Epstein-Barr virus-associated syndromes: a critical reexamination., Pediatr Infect Dis 1984; 3:198–203.
51. White NJ, Jeal-Jense BE. Infectious mononucleosis hepatitis. Semin Liver Dis 1984; 4:301–306.
52. Fleisher G. Incidence of heterophil antibody responses in children with infectious mononucleosis. J Pediatr 1979; 94:723–728.
53. Heule W, Heule G. Serodiagnosis of infectious mononucleosis. Resident Staff Physician 1981; 1:37–43.
54. Marks M. Pediatric infectious diseases for the practitioner. New York: Springer-Verlag, 1985; 441.
55. Najarian H. Patterns in medical parisitology. 2nd ed. Malabar, FL: RE Krieger, 1982.
56. Dunn MA, Sodeman WA Jr. Liver diseases. In: Strickland GT, ed. Hunter's tropical medicine. 6th ed. Philadelphia: WB Saunders, 1984; 27.
57. Haddad CG, Agrawal N, Litwin MS. Diagnosis and treatment of echinococcal cyst of the liver. South Med J 1983; 76L:300–303.
58. Laughlin LW. Schistosomiasis. In: Strickland GT, ed. Hunter's tropical medicine. 6th ed. Philadelphia: WB Saunders, 1984: 708.

PART 6

Drug-induced Hepatotoxicity in Children

Eve A. Roberts, M.D., FRCPC
Stephen P. Spielberg, M.D., Ph.D.

The liver plays a central role in drug action. It chemically transforms many drugs to their active form, and it acts upon most drugs to expedite their excretion from the body. These functions put the liver at risk for toxicity from these chemicals and their metabolites. Because of its anatomic and physiologic complexity, drug-induced liver disease represents a broad spectrum of biochemical, histologic, and clinical abnormalities. This can make it difficult to diagnose drug-induced liver disease or determine its pathogenesis. The problem of drug-induced liver disease in children is further complicated by a widely held notion that drug hepatotoxicity does not happen often in children. Children may indeed be protected in some way from drug hepatotoxicity. Whether or not this is true, because the child's liver is in the process of metabolic maturation, the manifestations of drug-induced liver disease may differ from those in adults. Since drug hepatotoxicity often imitates other more common diseases, arriving at a diagnosis of drug hepatotoxicity in a child can be especially difficult.

The purpose of this discussion is to address special features of drug hepatotoxicity in children. Mechanistic information gained from studying such processes in children is important for understanding the pathogenesis of drug hepatotoxicity. However, much more is known about the diversity of hepatic drug reactions in adults than in children. For encyclopedic reviews of what hepatotoxicities a given drug has ever caused in anyone, the reader should consult broader references[1-3] or computerized adverse drug reaction indices.

ROLE OF THE LIVER IN DRUG METABOLISM

Hepatic drug metabolism, or biotransformation, contributes to drug hepatotoxicity and to some hepatic neoplasia. Biotransformation in the liver is divided into two broad aspects: activation (phase I) and detoxification (phase II) (Fig. 1). For hepatotoxicity, the *balance* between these two processes is critical. Factors that influence this balance include age or stage of development, fasting or undernutrition, coadministered drugs, and immunomodulators resulting from viral infection. Inducing chemicals may affect phase I and phase II processes differently. The pharmacokinetics of the toxic drug also affect subsequent hepatic biotransformation. Whether the drug is taken as a single dose or many doses chronically may also change its hepatic metabolism. Finally, polymorphisms of cytochromes P–450 and various phase II enzymes also influence this balance.

The cytochromes P-450 are hemoproteins that are found throughout body tissues but are particularly important in the liver. They carry out most phase I reactions. These reactions are diverse and include various types of hydroxylation, dealkylation, and dehalogenation. The common feature in all reactions is that one atom of molecular oxygen is inserted into the substrate while the other combines with protons to form water. Hence, these enzymes are *mono-oxygenases*. Cytochromes P-450 themselves are diverse, and they have overlapping substrate specificity. An important characteristic of many cytochromes P-450 is inducibility.

The cytochromes P-450 were initially classified on the basis of the predominant inducing chemical: basically either *phenobarbital* or the polycyclic aromatic hydrocarbon *3-methylcholanthrene*.[4] Thirteen families of cytochromes P-450 have recently been distinguished on the basis of similarities in primary amino acid sequence. The cytochrome P450I family includes those cytochromes induced by polycyclic aromatic hydrocarbons. (Some authors refer to these as "cytochrome P-448.") Two major forms within the cytochrome P450IA subfamily have been found in the rat, mouse, rabbit, and human. Apart from various carcinogens, other chemicals such as caffeine and theophylline are metabolized by these cytochromes to a varying extent. Induction of the cytochrome P450IA subfamily is regulated through a cytoplas-

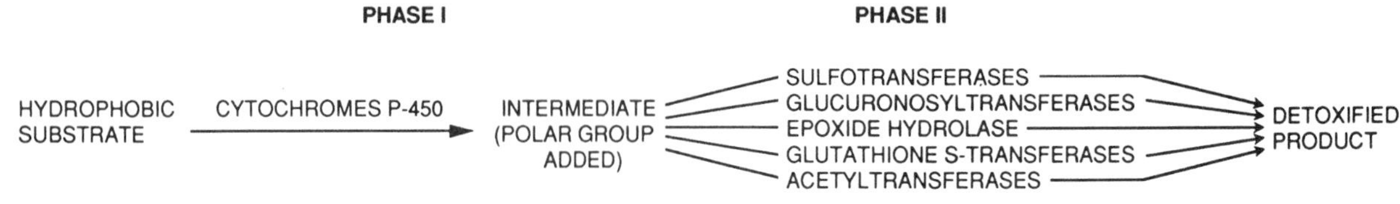

FIGURE 1 Phase I and phase II metabolism. Although the main objective is to convert a hydrophobic substance to a detoxified, water-soluble product so that it can be excreted from the body, phase I metabolism is also capable of converting some drugs to their active form or transforming other chemicals to toxic intermediates.

mic receptor protein, which has been detected and characterized in humans.[5,6] This is the only cytochrome P-450 subfamily whose regulation is understood in detail. The cytochrome P450IIB subfamily includes cytochromes induced by phenobarbital. Cytochrome P450IIE represents ethanol-inducible cytochrome P-450. The cytochrome P450III family includes cytochromes induced by pregnenolone and by glucocorticoids. Drugs that cause proliferation of peroxisomes appear to induce yet another cytochrome P-450 family, P450IV. As the hepatic metabolism of common drugs is studied more extensively, these cytochrome families are found to be involved. This has important implications for hepatotoxicity.

Polymorphisms for certain cytochromes P-450 have also been identified in human populations and in laboratory animals. In general these polymorphisms relate to differences in the rate of enzyme action. An important polymorphism is that for debrisoquine 4-hydroxylation, for which individuals may be "extensive metabolizers" (EM) or "poor metabolizers" (PM).[7] Other drugs whose metabolism shows the same pattern include sparteine, metoprolol, and dextromethorphan.[8] The difference in metabolism appears to be due to changes in the catalytic site of the cytochrome in PM[9]; enzyme induction does not affect the rate of metabolism in PM.[10] It has been speculated that this phenotype also relates to potential for developing certain cancers.[11] A clear relationship to any specific hepatotoxicity has been sought but not proven. Polymorphisms have also been found for antipyrine and theophylline metabolism.[12]

For many drugs the effect of phase I biotransformation reactions is to create a more polar chemical with a substituent poised for substitution via a phase II reaction. Phase II detoxifying reactions are performed by a variety of different types of enzymes, including glutathione S-transferases, glucuronosyl transferases, epoxide hydrolase, sulfotransferases, and *N*-acetyltransferases. In general these reactions complete the transformation of a hydrophobic chemical to a hydrophilic one that can be excreted easily in urine or bile. Certain phase II enzymes, such as some glucuronosyl transferases, are subject to induction. Some are polymorphic, notably *N*-acetyltransferase (either rapid or slow acetylators). In some metabolic diseases the activity of phase II enzymes may be abnormal; for example, in 5-oxoprolinuria, conjugation to glutathione is reduced because of deficiency of glutathione due to decreased levels of glutathione synthetase.[13] In hereditary tyrosinemia, glutathione S-transferase activity is depressed because intermediates in the abnormal tyrosine pathway consume glutathione.[14]

Hepatic drug metabolism shows developmental changes. Caffeine, which is metabolized in part by cytochromes P450IA, exemplifies these changes. The elimination half-life is very long in the newborn period[15] and drops to approximately 3 to 4 hours around 6 months of age.[16] For the balance of childhood—that is, until puberty—caffeine metabolism remains somewhat more rapid than in adults.[17] Clearance of many drugs is more rapid in children than in adults. Prominent examples include theophylline, phenobarbital, and phenytoin. Among phase II processes, a well-known example of late maturation of a detoxifying enzyme is the glucuronosyl transferase for bilirubin conjugation, which is frequently deficient for a short time after birth.

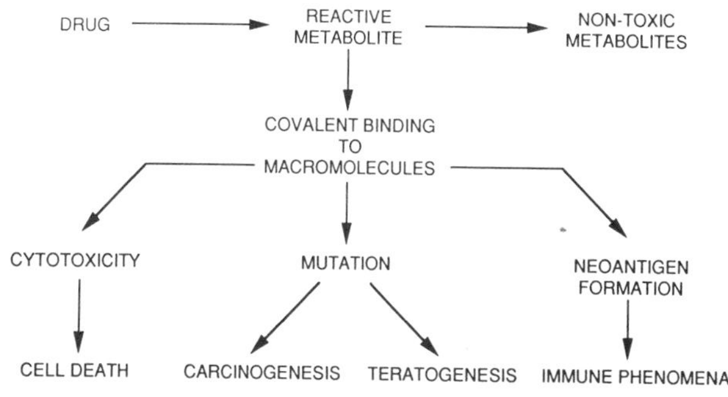

FIGURE 2 The potential fates of a toxic intermediate.

Hepatic bile acid metabolism also shows maturational changes in the first months of life. These variations may influence the occurrence and character of hepatotoxicity in children.

The product of a phase I reaction, especially when cytochromes of the P450IA subfamily are involved, may be an unstable or reactive metabolite. Phase II reactions may inactivate such chemicals before they do much harm. However, it is possible, as in the case of benzo(*a*)pyrene, for the product of phase I to recycle through the same cytochrome a second time and thence be metabolized to a proximate carcinogen.[18] Apart from the adequacy of the detoxification systems, whether reactive metabolites actually damage the cell also depends on how much reactive metabolite actually binds to cellular components, whether these components are critical to cellular function, and whether they can be repaired.[19] If the reactive metabolite binds to intracellular proteins or membranes that are vital to cellular integrity, the hepatocyte may die. If it binds to genetic apparatus, mutagenesis, carcinogenesis, or teratogenesis may ensue (Fig. 2).

Toxic metabolites are electrochemically unstable, and thus highly reactive, species derived from drugs, xenobiotics, or endogenous chemicals. Electrophilic intermediates (or *electrophiles*) are formed when electrons are lost from the original chemical; they carry a net positive charge. Examples include hydroxylamines, quinoneimines, and arene oxides. Tissue nucleophiles, such as glutathione, preferentially combine with these species. Not all nucleophiles are necessarily protective. Reactions that involve activation of oxygen produce negatively charged species, which are nucleophiles. They tend to bind to intracellular lipids, leading to lipid peroxidation. Examples include halocarbon and nitroso radicals. Besides lipid peroxidation, membranes can be altered by *alkylation* (addition of an aliphatic radical such as methyl or ethyl groups), *arylation* (addition of an aromatic group such as a phenyl group), or *acylation* (adding a radical derived from a carboxy acid). Glutathione, which is found in most mammalian cells in high concentrations, can react with electrophiles via conjugation reactions catalyzed by glutathione S-transferases. It can also interact with hydrogen peroxide and activated oxygen species via a different enzyme, glutathione peroxidase.[20] In general, when toxic metabolites are the important cause of cell damage, high tissue concentrations of the parent drug are not found. Metabolite(s) covalently bound to cellular constituents may be detected.

The cellular specialization of hepatocytes accounts in part for the diversity of patterns of hepatotoxicity. Binding to certain subcellular elements may interfere with specific metabolic functions such as protein or lipid synthesis or energy production. The parent compound or its reactive metabolites may interfere with uptake of other chemicals destined ordinarily for biliary excretion or perturb the apparatus for biliary excretion. Binding to DNA may lead to carcinogenesis. Drug-induced injury may occur to other cells in the liver besides hepatocytes. Cytotoxic damage to bile duct cells, Ito cells, or endothelial cells accounts for some of the clinical diversity of drug-induced liver disease.

CLASSIFICATION OF DRUG HEPATOTOXICITY

The clinical spectrum of drug hepatotoxicity in adults is wide. The classification presented in Table 1 forms the basis for considering hepatotoxicity in children. It encompasses a combination of clinical presentations, histologic findings, and other factors. Nonspecific elevation of serum aminotransferases is omitted. This form of hepatotoxicity is probably the most common of all, but its causes are heterogeneous and the least understood.

Most drug-induced disease is cytotoxic. Clinically, aminotransferases are elevated and hepatic insufficiency may develop. The exact mechanism of cell death is not known and is probably different for different drugs and toxins. Hepatocyte damage may be zonal, reflecting metabolic specialization in various parts of the hepatic lobule. Specifically, hepatocytes in zone 3 of the Rappaport acinus have the highest concentration of drug-metabolizing enzymes and thus the greatest potential for producing toxic intermediates.[21] Zonal hepatocellular necrosis suggests that metabolic activation of toxic metabolites has an important role in the pathogenesis of the toxicity, but spotty necrosis scattered throughout the lobule does not necessarily exclude a mechanism involving toxic metabolites. The same drugs that can cause this spotty hepatocyte damage can, on occasion, cause damage affecting most hepatocytes, leading to massive hepatocellular necrosis. Whenever hepatocellular damage is sufficiently severe, some degree of cholestasis develops.

TABLE 1
The Spectrum of Drug-Induced Liver Disease

Type	Examples
Acute hepatitis	Methyldopa, isoniazid, halothane, phenytoin
Hepatitis-cholestasis	Erythromycin, chlorpromazine, azathioprine, nitrofurantoin, cimetidine
Zonal liver cell necrosis	Acetaminophen
Bland cholestasis	Estrogens, cyclosporine
Steatonecrosis (like alcoholic hepatitis)	Perhexiline, amiodarone
Phospholipidosis	Amiodarone
Microvesicular steatosis	Valproic acid, tetracycline
Granulomatosis	Sulfonamides, phenylbutazone, carbamazepine
Biliary cirrhosis	Practolol, chlorpropamide
Sclerosing cholangitis	Floxuridine via hepatic artery
Hepatic vascular changes	
Peliosis	Estrogens, androgens
Hepatic vein thrombosis	Estrogens (oral contraceptives)
Veno-occlusive disease	Thioguanine, busulfan, pyrrolizidine (*Senecio*) alkaloids
Noncirrhotic portal hypertension	Vinyl chloride, arsenic
Liver cell adenoma	Estrogens (oral contraceptives), anabolic steroids
Malignant tumors	Estrogens, anabolic steroids, vinyl chloride
Porphyria	2,3,7,8-Tetrachlorodibenzo-*p*-dioxin, chloroquine

Some drug-induced liver disease, however, is predominantly cholestatic. Clinically, this type of reaction is characterized by jaundice, pruritus, prominent elevation of alkaline phosphatase, and mild elevations of aminotransferases. Classically these cholestatic injuries have been classified on the basis of histologic inflammation. In "hepatocanalicular jaundice," with agents such as chlorpromazine or erythromycin, liver cell injury and inflammation are relatively prominent. In "bland cholestasis," with agents such as contraceptive steroids, these histologic features are minimal.[2]

It is sometimes useful to think about drug hepatotoxicity in terms of the duration of the hepatotoxic process. Acute hepatotoxic injuries develop over a relatively short time and cause a lesion without any features of chronicity. Subacute hepatotoxicity refers to lesions that have developed over a period of weeks to months, as indicated by areas of fibrosis and possibly regeneration. Chronic hepatotoxic lesions include those with fibrosis or cirrhosis, vascular changes, and neoplasia. Some drugs can cause clinical liver disease indistinguishable from autoimmune chronic active hepatitis: These include oxyphenisatin, methyldopa, isoniazid, and nitrofurantoin.[2]

Our knowledge of mechanisms of hepatotoxicity is evolving. For many years, hepatotoxicity has been categorized on the basis of predictability. Intrinsic hepatotoxins are differentiated from idiosyncratic hepatotoxins. The intrinsic hepatotoxin causes predictable hepatic damage in almost any individual. The toxicity is dose-related in that higher doses cause more severe damage, and animal models can be developed that exhibit the same type of hepatotoxicity. However, most instances of hepatotoxicity, mainly those associated with medications, are unpredictable, infrequent, and apparently sporadic. If such a reaction is accompanied by systemic features such as fever, rash, eosinophilia, atypical lymphocytosis, and possibly other major organ involvement, then classically it has been regarded as an idiosyncratic hypersensitivity reaction, in which "hypersensitivity" with its connotation of allergy is left undefined.

An alternate explanation is that idiosyncratic hepatotoxicity has a biochemical basis and is due to *metabolic* idiosyncrasy. It occurs in individuals who have specific abnormalities in drug metabolism. If this abnormal metabolism is expressed in liver cells, then these rare individuals develop hepatotoxicity if exposed to the appropriate drug. In most instances a metabolite, not the drug itself, is responsible for hepatotoxicity (Fig. 2). Frequently, the problem seems to be a defect in detoxification of the reactive metabolite because the detoxification system is itself focally defective and cannot meet the normal demands of metabolite production. Sometimes these individuals show systemic features interpreted as hypersensitivity; it is likely that interaction of the reactive metabolite with cellular components, such as the cell membrane, elicits an immune response. Thus, in such cases, hypersensitivity is itself the consequence of metabolic idiosyncrasy, not a separate mechanism of drug hepatotoxicity. There may be strictly allergic drug hepatotoxicity, but investigations of the mechanism of drug-induced hepatotoxicity suggest that metabolic idiosyncrasy is much more common than formerly supposed. It seems likely to account for hepatotoxicity with drugs that show two main patterns: mild reversible toxicity in a comparatively large segment of patients and severe hepatotoxicity in a few individuals. Toxic metabolites are probably involved in both. The severe reactions occur in rare persons with abnormalities in toxification or detoxification, irrespective of the appearance of drug allergy.

A major implication of the metabolic idiosyncrasy thesis is that most drug hepatotoxicity is predictable if one understands the pathways of hepatic biotransformation and detoxification for each drug. Given the plethora of drugs and hepatic biotransformation pathways, it is no wonder that most clinically important drug hepatotoxicity appears sporadic and fortuitous. However, there are enough experimental data available now to warrant rethinking the intrinsic–idiosyncratic-allergic classification of drug hepatotoxicity. These definable metabolic defects in hepatic drug metabolism are particularly common in the types of drug hepatotoxicity that occur in children.

INCIDENCE OF DRUG-INDUCED LIVER DISEASE IN CHILDREN

Drug-induced liver disease is generally regarded as rare in children. In a recent survey of 10,297 pediatric hospital admissions to teaching and community hospitals in Boston, Mitchell et al[22] found that only 2 percent of hospital admissions were due to any sort of adverse drug reaction. In a subset of 725 patients with cancer, however, 22 percent of admissions were related to adverse drug reactions. Adverse drug reactions in the entire population were somewhat more common in the 0- to 5-year-old age group than in older children. The most commonly implicated drugs included phenobarbital, aspirin, phenytoin, ampicillin or amoxicillin, and sulfa. Only phenytoin-associated hepatitis was specifically mentioned in this large survey as drug hepatotoxicity. An outpatient study of 1,590 children in Britain also failed to detect drug hepatotoxicity as a problem in children.[23]

The reason for the uncommonness of childhood drug hepatotoxicity is not certain. Underdiagnosis along with under-reporting remains a possibility. Another simple reason is that most children take relatively few medications, and in particular they rarely take the cardiovascular, antihypertensive, and anxiolytic medications associated with hepatotoxicity in adults. They do not use ethanol chronically or smoke cigarettes; most have a lean body mass. Thus they are free of many factors predisposing one to drug hepatotoxicity. Finally, there is evidence that the aging liver metabolizes some drugs more slowly.[24,25] Advanced age is a risk factor for severe hepatotoxic reactions. In view of the increased risk attached to some drug hepatotoxicities in women, one can speculate that changes in drug metabolism possibly associated with puberty may influence the differing incidence of drug hepatotoxicity in childhood and adulthood. However, there is no question that some children are vulnerable to drug hepatotoxicity.

SPECIFIC DRUG HEPATOTOXICITIES IN CHILDREN

Hepatotoxicity due to all of the following drugs except isoniazid, halothane, and erythromycin has been diagnosed in children at the Hospital for Sick Children in Toronto during the past 5 years.

Acetaminophen

Acetaminophen is an effective antipyretic and analgesic. It is commonly used in most children because its metabolism is rapid enough that it does not accumulate and is not influenced by dehydration. Taken in a single large dose, however, it is a potent hepatotoxin. The mechanism for this toxicity involves the formation of a toxic metabolite.[26-29] The important role of drug metabolism in this hepatotoxicity is reflected in the predominance of hepatocellular injury in zone 3 (Fig. 3). Acetaminophen is usually metabolized via sulfation and glucuronidation (Fig. 4). If a sufficiently large amount is taken, these pathways are saturated, and an otherwise relatively minor pathway through cytochromes P-450 becomes quantitatively more important. The product of this pathway is a highly reactive species *N*-acetyl-*p*-benzoquinone-imine (NAPQI),[30,31] a potent electrophile. It is conjugated by glutathione, as long as sufficient glutathione is available. Otherwise NAPQI reacts with cellular proteins, causing cell damage and cell death. The exact details of the mechanism of cell damage in fact remain unclear. NAPQI can act directly as an oxidizing agent,[32] but the role of oxygen-mediated injury in this cytotoxicity is disputed.[33,34] Orrenius and colleagues have shown that the characteristic morphologic changes of acetaminophen toxicity in isolated hepatocytes in vitro are associated with changes in cellular calcium metabolism.[35] *N*-Acetylcysteine acts by providing substrate for making more glutathione[36] and thus can minimize hepatotoxicity if given early enough. It does not reverse the toxic effects of the toxic intermediate once they have occurred.[37] Other factors may influence the metabolism of acetaminophen. Cimetidine, which blocks cytochrome P-450, interferes with acetaminophen toxicity in laboratory animals if given early.[38] Unfortunately, the comparable dose for humans is likely to be toxic in itself. Fasting decreases the amount of glutathione in cells and thus may increase acetaminophen toxicity.

The clinical course of acetaminophen toxicity is distinctive. Immediately after taking the drug there is nausea and vomiting. These symptoms clear and there is an interval before hepatic toxicity becomes clinically apparent. At that point, jaundice, abnormal aminotransferases, and coagulopathy develop. Aminotransferases may be extremely high in this

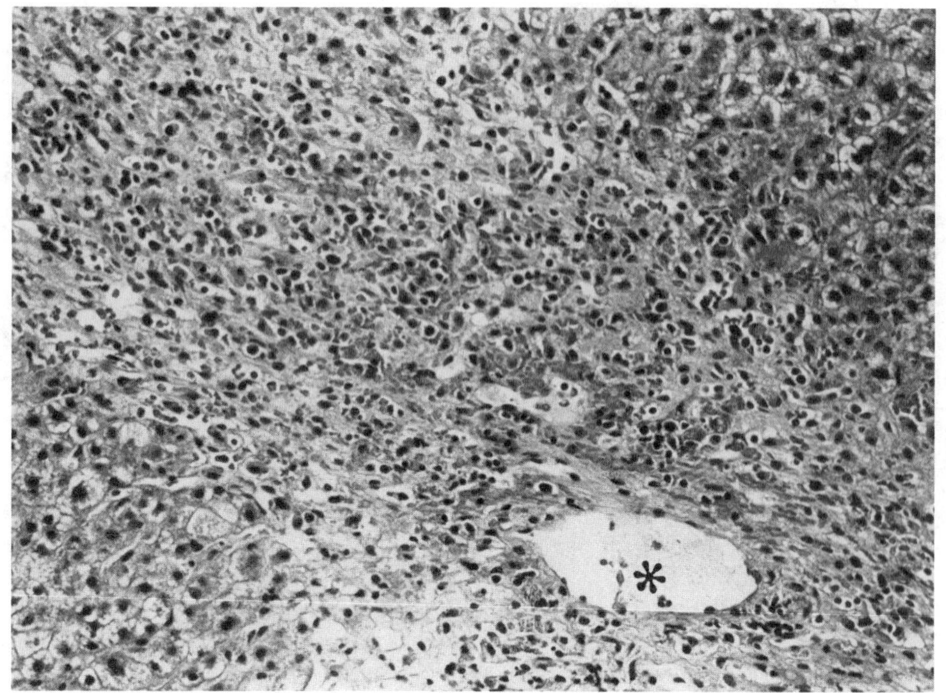

FIGURE 3 Liver biopsy in acetaminophen hepatotoxicity. There is a wide zone of necrosis occupying zone 3 of the liver, to which there is only a modest inflammatory cell response. The transition between the necrotic cells and the surrounding hepatocytes, which are swollen, vacuolated, and contain fat, is abrupt. In zone 1 (not shown) the liver parenchyma is normal. This zonal distribution of necrosis surrounded by swollen fatty hepatocytes is characteristic of acetaminophen hepatotoxicity. Terminal hepatic venule (*asterisk*) (hematoxylin and eosin, ×250). (Courtesy of Dr. M.J. Phillips.)

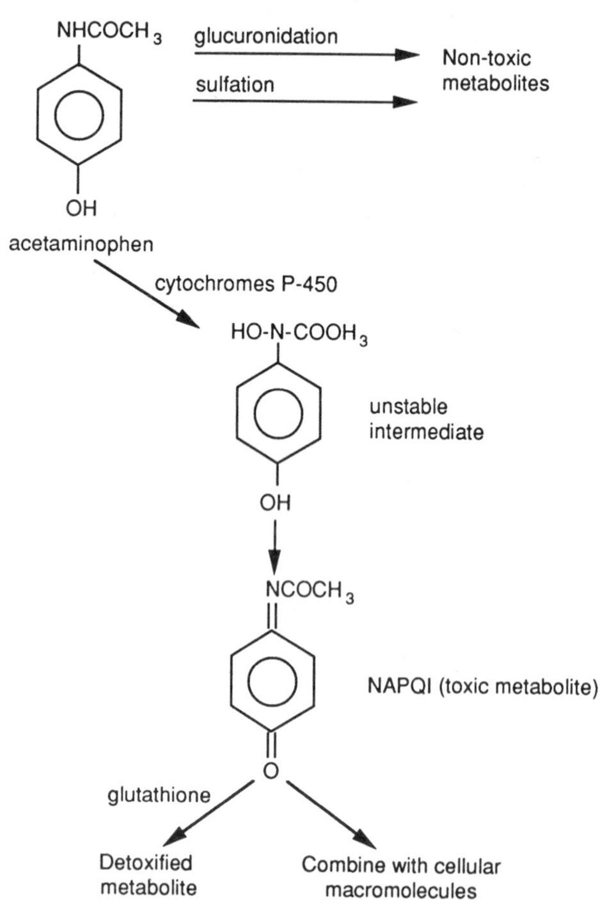

FIGURE 4 Metabolism of acetaminophen.

condition, and the degree of abnormality is not necessarily predictive of outcome. Finally, hepatic failure may supervene with progressive coma.

Whether or not to use *N*-acetylcysteine can be decided on the basis of plotting on a semilogarithmic graph the patient's plasma acetaminophen concentration against time[39]; if it falls in the zone for probable hepatic toxicity, *N*-acetylcysteine should be given. *N*-Acetylcysteine is most effective if given within 10 hours of acetaminophen ingestion, and it is usually of no benefit more than 24 hours after ingestion of the acetaminophen. However, if there is any doubt as to its usefulness, it can be given anyway. A 72-hour regimen of oral *N*-acetylcysteine appears to be as effective as the 20-hour intravenous regimen; the oral regimen may be more effective if treatment is delayed.[40] Other measures, such as inducing vomiting and using charcoal, may also be effective early, although acetaminophen ingestion itself typically causes vomiting. Hemodialysis, if it is to be effective at all, must be used early when acetaminophen plasma concentrations are high.

Extensive reviews of acetaminophen poisoning in children substantiate the impression that children tend to be resistant to this hepatotoxicity.[41–43] Various studies of acetaminophen pharmacokinetics, metabolism, and toxicity in children suggest a biochemical basis for this observation. The elimination half-life is essentially the same in children and adults, although with interindividual variation it ranges from 1 to 3.5 hours.[44] The elimination half-life is somewhat longer (2.2 to 5 hours) in neonates. The profile of metabolites differs greatly in early childhood from that in adolescence and adulthood: sulfation predominates over glucuronidation.[45] The switch to the adult pattern seems to occur around 12 years of age. However, even in newborns,[46,47] urinary metabolites reflecting cytochrome P-450–generated intermediates can be found; thus, the capacity for producing toxic metabolites seems to be present from an early age. In vitro studies with fetal human hepatocytes have shown that the cytochrome P-450–generated intermediates can be formed and conjugated to glutathione as early as 18 weeks of gestation, but the rate of formation is approximately 10 percent of that in adult human hepatocytes; sulfation, but not glucuronidation, of acetaminophen also can be detected in the human fetal liver cells.[48] An early study of neonatal mouse hepatocytes showed resistance to acetaminophen hepatotoxicity despite reduced concentrations of glutathione; this is due to even more reduced levels of cytochromes P-450.[49] Subsequent studies of susceptibility to acetaminophen hepatotoxicity in young mice disputed these findings and showed susceptibility equal to that in the adult.[50] Meanwhile, studies in young rats showed less susceptibility to hepatotoxicity in the 11-day-old rat than in the adult rat.[51] In other studies hepatocytes from young rats were shown to have a higher capacity for synthesizing glutathione than those from older rats and to be able also to increase synthesis when glutathione is depleted.[52] Perhaps human infants also have a greater capacity for synthesis of glutathione than do adults and thus can detoxify acetaminophen toxic metabolites more effectively.

Despite the relative resistance to this type of hepatotoxicity, it is also clear that young children can develop severe hepatotoxicity from acetaminophen.[53–58] Acetaminophen hepatotoxicity has also occurred in infants less than 2 months old.[59] The threshold dose for severe toxicity in children has not been determined. Some children can develop hepatotoxicity after taking repeated doses of relatively small amounts of acetaminophen (three to four times the recommended dose),[60] but most reports involve predictably toxic amounts of drug. Hepatotoxicity and extreme prolongation of the elimination half-life of acetaminophen have been found in infants born after maternal self-poisoning with acetaminophen.[46,47] Nevertheless, in aggregate, reports suggest that young children are generally resistant to acetaminophen hepatotoxicity and tend to recover when it does occur. The incidence of hepatotoxicity was 5.5 percent in a study of 417 children 5 years old or less, compared with 29 percent in adolescents and adults at comparable toxic blood levels.[41] In these young children acetaminophen ingestion occurs as part of the spectrum of household poison ingestions, whereas in young adolescents the trend to self-destruction appears.[43] As the metabolism of acetaminophen in adolescents is similar to that in adults, treatment should be appropriately aggressive. Younger children also require the benefit of antidote and supportive treatment: it may be that they respond to it better than older individuals.

Initial studies on the mechanism of acetaminophen toxicity showed that toxicity was worse when animals were pretreated with the polycyclic aromatic hydrocarbon 3-methylcholanthrene, a potent inducer of cytochrome P450IA1. Subsequently it has become evident that chronic alcoholics are more sensitive to acetaminophen than nonalcoholics in that they can develop subacute acetaminophen hepatotoxicity after taking ordinary therapeutic doses over time.[61] Cytochrome P450IIE, which is induced by ethanol, has been shown to be capable of metabolizing acetaminophen[62] and thus may enhance its toxicity. Some adolescents may be at risk for this type of acetaminophen hepatotoxicity. Whether exposure to environmental chemicals such as polychlorinated biphenyls or aromatic hydrocarbons increases susceptibility to acetaminophen hepatotoxicity remains unproven.

Phenytoin

Phenytoin is a commonly used anticonvulsant medication that has been associated with a broad range of adverse effects. Phenytoin-induced hepatitis often causes liver failure with severe hepatic necrosis. The perception that it occurs infrequently in children is misleading. Phenytoin-associated hepatitis was the only hepatitis mentioned specifically among adverse drug reactions in a large prospective study of adverse drug reactions in children.[22] The literature contains 17 cases[63] and an additional 18 cases of hepatic dysfunction in patients (nine of whom were children) whose adverse reaction to phenytoin was dominated by other organ system involvement.[64]

Phenytoin hepatotoxicity typically presents as part of a systemic disease with fever, rash (including morbilliform rash, Stevens-Johnson syndrome, and toxic epidermal necrolysis), lymphadenopathy, leukocytosis, eosinophilia, and atypical lymphocytosis. Aminotransferases are elevated, and the patient may be moderately jaundiced. In severe cases, clinical features of hepatic failure (coagulopathy, ascites, altered level of consciousness) are also present. Histopathologic examination of the liver shows spotty necrosis of hepatocytes, along with features reminiscent of mononucleosis in some cases and of viral hepatitis in others. Cholestasis may complicate more severe hepatocellular injury, and granulomas are sometimes found.[65] Reports of phenytoin-induced cholestatic hepatitis are unconvincing; although treatment with high-dose corticosteroids has not been tested in a controlled trial and anecdotal reports do not show a clear benefit, their use has appeared effective in some patients.

The typical clinical presentation of phenytoin hepatotoxicity is termed a "drug hypersensitivity reaction." There is reason to believe that this clinical syndrome develops as a result of abnormal handling of a toxic metabolite of phenytoin. Phenytoin is metabolized via an arene oxide intermediate that is ordinarily metabolized and thus detoxified by epoxide hydrolase.[66] When lymphocytes, which are easily isolated cells complete with most phase II biotransformation pathways, are incubated in vitro with phenytoin and a murine microsomal system which can generate the intermediate metabolites of phenytoin, lymphocytes from persons who have developed the drug hypersensitivity syndrome to phenytoin are killed in excess of control lymphocytes.[66] If lymphocytes from normal individuals are pretreated with chemicals that inhibit cellular epoxide hydrolase, these lymphocytes behave like those from affected individuals.[67] Studies of parents indicate an intermediate sensitivity to the toxic metabolite(s), consistent with an inherited defect in drug detoxification. Instead of causing cell death, binding of the toxic metabolite may create haptens for initiating an immune response. This may account for the clinical appearance of hypersensitivity and for the positive immune challenges noted by others.[68,69]

Three of four children reported with fatal phenytoin hepatotoxicity were taking phenobarbital at the same time. As in vitro studies indicate that some patients who cannot detoxify toxic intermediates of phenytoin are similarly sensitive to phenobarbital, this dual treatment may have made the hepatotoxicity worse. One other patient was switched from phenytoin to phenobarbital and then relapsed; he improved when high-dose corticosteroids were given along with the phenobarbital.[63]

Carbamazepine

Carbamazepine is a dibenzazepine derivative, similar structurally to imipramine in that it has fundamentally a tricyclic chemical structure. Hepatotoxicity is relatively uncommon. In adults the predominant hepatotoxicity has been granulomatous hepatitis presenting with fever and right upper quadrant pain, suggestive of cholangitis.[70,71] In children the clinical picture has been more similar to hepatitis, sometimes dominating a drug hypersensitivity syndrome like that of phenytoin. One child died of progressive liver failure when carbamazepine was not stopped in time.[72] Two other children presented with a mononucleosis-like illness with rash, lymphadenopathy, hepatosplenomegaly, and eventually neutropenia.[73,74] This description is similar to that of a child treated at the Hospital for Sick Children in Toronto (Fig. 5), who presented with fever, rash, incipient liver failure, lymphopenia, and eosinophilia. In vitro rechallenge of her lymphocytes with metabolites of carbamazepine provided evidence of defective detoxification mechanisms. An infant boy also presented here with only hepatotoxicity, and three other children with drug hypersensitivity to carbamazepine in whom hepatitis was not the dominant feature have been described.[64] Carbamazepine may also be metabolized via arene oxides. Persons with the metabolic idiosyncrasy that renders them susceptible to carbamazepine hepatotoxicity may also be susceptible to phenytoin and phenobarbital hepatotoxicity.

An alternate explanation for some types of carbamazepine hepatotoxicity rests on its chemical similarity to imipramine, which can cause cholestasis.

Phenobarbital

Hepatitis is a rare complication of phenobarbital use. When it occurs, it too is usually part of a multisystem drug hypersensitivity reaction, but it may dominate the clinical picture.[75-77] Six of 12 patients reported in the world literature were children. Three additional children, a girl aged 3 years and boys aged 10 and 18 months, have been treated at the Hospital for Sick Children, Toronto; all had severe hepatic dysfunction with coagulopathy or ascites but ultimately survived. Two further cases in children have been treated at the Hospital for Sick Children, Toronto, but hepatitis was not the dominant clinical feature.[64] In most cases of major hepatotoxicity, jaundice began 1 to 8 weeks after starting phenobarbital, along with generalized rash and fever. Usually the liver disease was moderately severe but self-limited; however, a few patients developed severe hepatitis with coagulopathy and ascites, and one died fulminantly. One child developed chronic liver disease.

The mechanism of this hepatotoxicity remains unclear. Results from in vitro rechallenge indicate an inherited defect in detoxification of active metabolite. Phenobarbital may also be metabolized via arene oxide intermediates, which are typically detoxified via epoxide hydrolase. In in vitro rechallenge,

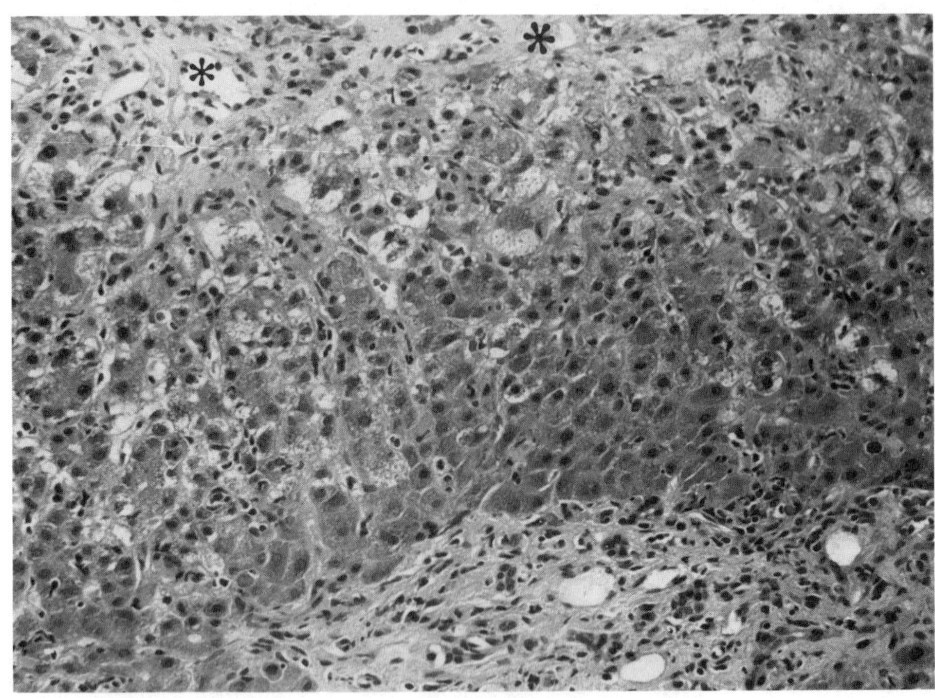

FIGURE 5 Liver biopsy in carbamazepine hepatotoxicity. The portal area shows widening with fibrosis, ductular proliferation, and mild chronic inflammatory changes. The lobular parenchyma shows variability in the size of the hepatocytes, with many swollen ballooned hepatocytes in zones 2 and 3 and occasional inflammatory cells. In zone 3 there is central bridging necrosis (*asterisks*). The pathologic diagnosis is drug-induced acute hepatitis with bridging necrosis; these findings are fully representative of the hepatic lesion with carbamazepine (hematoxylin and eosin, ×250). (Courtesy of Dr. M.J. Phillips.)

if lymphocyte epoxide hydrolase is inhibited, the extent of cytotoxicity of metabolites generated from phenobarbital, as from phenytoin, increases.[67]

Persons who develop hepatotoxicity from phenobarbital also cannot detoxify other barbiturates and their condition may become worse if they are so treated. Sedation for a diagnostic procedure in a child is an important opportunity for such a drug exposure. It is also important to bear in mind that persons who cannot detoxify the toxic metabolite(s) of phenobarbital often cannot detoxify those of carbamazepine or phenytoin.[64] Thus, substituting either may worsen the hepatitis.

Valproic Acid

Valproic acid is chemically very different from the other three anticonvulsants above: It is an eight-carbon, branched fatty acid. Hepatotoxicity takes two main forms. A certain proportion of patients, estimated at 11 percent overall,[78] develop abnormal aminotransferase levels, typically within a short time of starting treatment. This biochemical abnormality returns to normal when the dose of valproic acid is decreased. Much more rarely, patients develop progressive liver failure, which in some cases looks similar clinically to Reye's syndrome. This severe hepatotoxicity does not always regress when the drug is withdrawn. Its occurrence cannot be predicted by regular monitoring of serum aminotransferases and other liver function tests.[79] The time from initiating treatment with valproic acid and onset of liver disease is usually less than 4 months, but longer duration of treatment does not preclude hepatotoxicity. A salient feature of severe valproic acid hepatotoxicity is that it is more common in children than in adults.[80] Special identifiable risk factors include age less than 2 years, multiple anticonvulsant treatment along with valproic acid, co-existent medical problems such as mental retardation, developmental delay, or congenital abnormalities.[81] Hyperammonemia, not associated with liver failure, is another metabolic adverse effect of valproic acid.[82]

Severe hepatotoxicity was first described only relatively recently,[83,84] probably with rising use of valproic acid, and the total experience has been reviewed in detail.[78,80,81,85] The severe hepatotoxicity typically presents with a hepatitis-like prodrome, mainly malaise, anorexia, nausea, and vomiting. Seizure control may also deteriorate over the same time period. Coagulopathy is often present early; clinical jaundice tends to develop later, along with other signs of progressive hepatic insufficiency such as ascites and hypoglycemia. Death due to liver failure, complicated by renal failure or infection, is the frequently reported outcome. Liver histology reviewed in one large series[85] shows evidence of hepatocellular necrosis, which may be zonal, with outright loss of hepatocytes, and moribund hepatocytes remaining. Acidophilic bodies, ballooned hepatocytes, and cholangiolar proliferation maybe present. Microvesicular steatosis is the most common finding overall and is often present in addition to the features of cell necrosis. Hepatocellular mitochondria may be prominent on light microscopy so that the hepatocytes have a granular, highly eosinophilic appearance (Fig. 6). In cases clinically resembling Reye's syndrome, fever, coagulopathy, progressive loss of consciousness, severe acidosis, and variably abnormal aminotransferases are present, although the patient is not jaundiced.[84] Hepatocellular necrosis, as well as microvesicular fat, is found on histologic examination of the liver, unlike the histologic findings of Reye's syndrome. Electron microscopically, the mitochondrial changes associated with valproic acid toxicity differ from those of Reye's syndrome.[86]

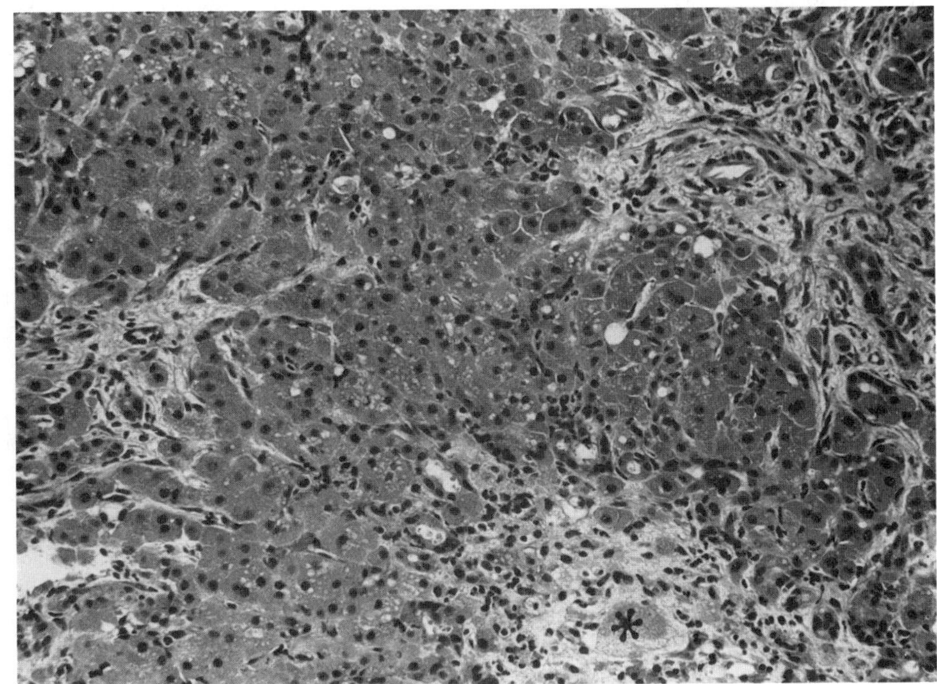

FIGURE 6 Liver biopsy in valproic acid hepatotoxicity. The liver lobule shows great reduction in the number of hepatocytes. There is portal tract widening with increased numbers of bile ducts. Hepatocytes are swollen, and most contain multiple microvesicular fat droplets. In zone 3 there is an area of necrosis (*asterisk*) with tubular transformation of hepatocytes surrounding the necrotic zone (hematoxylin and eosin, ×250). (Courtesy of Dr. M.J. Phillips.)

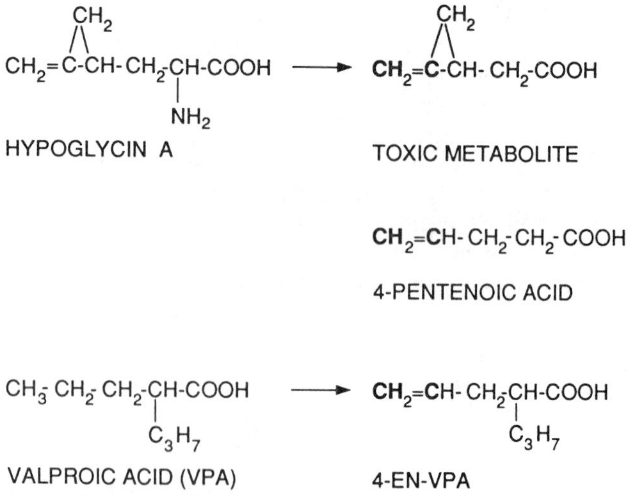

The mechanism of this severe hepatotoxicity is thought to involve generation of toxic metabolite(s) plus some type of metabolic idiosyncrasy rendering the individual susceptible. Metabolic idiosyncrasy is probable not only because severe hepatotoxicity is rare but because toxic ingestions do not necessarily lead to liver necrosis.[87] Valproic acid is related structurally to two known hepatotoxins: *hypoglycin*, which causes Jamaican vomiting sickness, characterized by microvesicular steatosis; and *4-pentenoic acid*, which causes microvesicular steatosis in rat liver and inhibits beta-oxidation (Fig. 7). The partly unsaturated metabolite 4-en-valproic acid (4-en-VPA), produced by omega oxidation, which is a minor pathway of valproic acid metabolism, is chemically similar to these toxins. Formation of 4-en-VPA has been demonstrated in a primate model[88] and in patients with liver failure developing on valproic acid treatment.[89] Several metabolites of valproic acid, including 4-en-VPA, have been shown to be toxic to isolated rat hepatocytes.[90] Administration of 4-en-VPA to rats caused accumulation of microvesicular fat in hepatocytes along with changes in hepatocyte organelles, including mitochondrial abnormalities and elaboration of myeloid bodies.[91] In the same model 4-en-VPA caused inhibition of beta-oxidation, although not to the same extent as hypoglycin.[92] Valproic acid has also been shown to inhibit ketogenesis (that is, beta-oxidation of endogenous fats such as oleic acid) in periportal rat hepatocytes, although pericentral hepatocytes are also affected; peroxisomal beta-oxidation is also decreased generally.[93] Both VPA and 4-en-VPA inhibit beta-oxidative metabolism of decanoic acid, a fatty acid of medium length; by contrast, 4-pentenoic acid is only a weak inhibitor in this system.[94] In preliminary studies 4-en-VPA has been shown to be toxic to human cells in in vitro testing. Thus valproic acid and its metabolite(s) are capable of causing adverse changes in liver cell metabolism which may lead to observed features of this hepatotoxicity. Similarities and differences in these metabolic toxicities compared with hypoglycin and 4-pentenoic acid merely reflect the complexity of this metabolic system.

In valproic acid hepatotoxicity the target organelle appears to be the mitochondrion. An individual who develops severe valproic acid hepatotoxicity may not be able to detoxify these metabolites or subsequent toxic intermediates before significant mitochondrial damage occurs. The defective detoxification pathway is not yet known. The metabolic idiosyncrasy may be a functional defect in the mitochondrion itself. Experimental data in the ornithine transcarbamylase–deficient mouse support the hypothesis of an intrinsic metabolic defect in the mitochondrion. The ornithine transcarbamylase–deficient mouse develops hepatocellular necrosis and microvesicular steatosis at doses of valproic acid which do not affect the normal control adversely.[95] The data may provide a clue to one possible metabolic abnormality in humans. Individuals who develop severe valproic acid hepatotoxicity may have mitochondria biochemically predisposed to this injury. Ornithine transcarbamylase deficiency may be one such definable abnormality and has been suspected in one instance.[96]

Serum carnitine has been found to be abnormally low in persons with Reye's syndrome. Decreased serum carnitine has also been found in valproic acid hepatotoxicity.[97,98] Serum carnitine is also low in patients treated chronically, without evidence clinically of hepatotoxicity.[98,99] One metabolic pathway for valproic acid appears to be conjugation to carnitine.[100] It is the only drug yet identified as conjugated to carnitine. Whether this pathway is important for the development of hepatotoxicity is not known. Equally, the value of carnitine repletion as treatment for severe hepatotoxicity remains unproven.

CH_2 CH_2
$CH_2=C-CH-CH_2-CH-COOH$ → $CH_2=C-CH-CH_2-COOH$
NH_2
HYPOGLYCIN A TOXIC METABOLITE

$CH_2=CH-CH_2-CH_2-COOH$
4-PENTENOIC ACID

$CH_3-CH_2-CH_2-CH-COOH$ → $CH_2=CH-CH_2-CH-COOH$
C_3H_7 C_3H_7
VALPROIC ACID (VPA) 4-EN-VPA

FIGURE 7 Chemical structural similarity of the toxic metabolite of hypoglycin A, 4-pentenoic acid, and the metabolite of valproic acid, 4-en-valproic acid.

Sulfonamides

Hepatotoxicity may be caused by any sulfonamide antibiotic. In children this problem arises most commonly in connection with treatment for otitis media and upper respiratory infections or for inflammatory bowel disease. Sulfanilamide, trimethoprim-sulfamethoxazole, and pryimethamine-sulfadoxine have all been associated with major hepatic injury.[101–104] Sulfasalazine has been associated with severe liver disease in adolescents and young adults.[105–107] Although the liver abnormality may be manifested only by elevated aminotransferases or may be a granulomatous hepatitis, the hepatic dysfunction may be severe enough to cause acute hepatic failure, in some cases fatal. In general, hepatotoxicity is part of a clinical drug hypersensitivity reaction. Fever, significant rash, periorbital edema, atypical lymphocytosis, lymphadenopathy, and renal dysfunction with proteinuria have all been described.

Sulfonamide hepatotoxicity is due to elaboration of an electrophilic toxic metabolite in the liver. The intermediate appears to be the hydroxylamine derived from the particular sulfonamide, or more likely the nitroso species derived from the hydroxylamine.[108] Patients who develop severe adverse reactions, including significant hepatotoxicity, have been shown to be slow acetylators (in the rapid/slow polymorphism for *N*-acetyltransferase) and also unable to detoxify this reactive metabolite. Upon in vitro rechallenge of their lymphocytes with sulfonamide and a metabolite-generating system, the patient's lymphocytes show significantly more cytotoxicity than controls.[103] Glutathione S-transferases may be important for detoxifying the toxic intermediate.[109] How this reactive intermediate causes hepatocellular damage is not yet known. The multisystemic hypersensitivity features of this adverse drug reaction appear to be subsequent to metabolic events, in that the reactive metabolite probably acts as a hapten to initiate the immune response. Thus, sulfa hepatotoxicity fundamentally represents metabolic idiosyncrasy, not simply allergy.

Erythromycin

Erythromycin estolate and other salts are used frequently in children. Although the estolate was originally associated with a cholestatic hepatitic lesion, it is now clear that the ethylsuccinate and other salts are also potentially hepatotoxic.[110-114] The clinical presentations are similar no matter which salt is administered: anorexia, nausea, predominantly right upper quadrant abdominal pain, and jaundice. Pruritus due to cholestasis has been reported in some adults. Hepatomegaly, sometimes accompanied by splenomegaly, appears to be frequent in children.[113] Erythromycin ethylsuccinate hepatotoxicity in a child was a relatively mild, self-limited disease.[112]

Histologic findings include prominent cholestasis which is particularly severe in zone 3, focal necrosis of hepatocytes also tending to predominate in zone 3, and eosinophils in the portal infiltrates and in the sinusoids.[110] These histologic findings are different from those of extrahepatic biliary tract obstruction, although the clinical presentation may suggest biliary tract obstruction.

The mechanism of this hepatotoxicity remains obscure. Erythromycin itself may be the cause of the hepatotoxicity because cross-reactivity between different erythromycin salts casts doubt on the hypothesis that features of certain salts themselves account for the toxicity.[111] However, in the perfused rat liver model erythromycin estolate led to decreased bile secretion, altered canalicular permeability, and decreased activities of Na^+, K^+-ATPase and Mg^{2+}-ATPase unlike erythromycin base.[115] Earlier studies in Chang liver cells suggested that erythromycin derivatives cause intrinsic hepatocellular damage. In various types of primary rat hepatocyte culture systems, erythromycin estolate leads to cytotoxicity.[116,117] Erythromycin and other macrolide antibiotics are metabolized in liver by the cytochrome P450IIIA subfamily. Hepatocellular damage may be due to a toxic metabolite, but this is by no means proven. Cholestasis may also reflect damage to the cellular biliary apparatus. The association of eosinophilia with erythromycin hepatotoxicity in some patients probably represents a forme fruste of a drug hypersensitivity syndrome.

Propylthiouracil

Hepatitis is a rare complication of propylthiouracil (PTU) treatment for hyperthyroidism. Five cases in children have been reported, and two additional cases have been treated at the Hospital for Sick Children in Toronto; all were girls.[118-121] The clinical picture typically was a nonspecific hepatitic presentation with anorexia, nausea, vomiting, and jaundice. Aminotransferases were moderately elevated. Symptoms began typically within 2 to 3 months of starting treatment, but in one child liver disease began at least 9 months after treatment began. A more cholestatic picture has been reported in some adults. Liver histology shows mild to severe hepatocellular necrosis, characterized as submassive in three patients.

Several cases of PTU-associated liver disease have been called chronic active hepatitis.[122,123] All have occurred in adults. Liver biopsy was interpreted as showing piecemeal necrosis, a histologic hallmark of chronic active hepatitis. However, no patient had had the hepatitis for more than 6 months, and thus none met the usual chronologic definition of chronic active hepatitis. In addition, the IgG and complement C′3 and C′4 concentrations were not reported, although some patients had nonspecific autoantibodies. Thyroiditis may be an accompanying feature of autoimmune chronic active hepatitis. Given the available data, it is difficult to confirm these as true cases of drug-induced chronic active hepatitis, and the association of PTU hepatotoxicity with chronic active hepatitis is dubious.

Aspirin

Hepatotoxicity has been associated with high-dose aspirin treatment. Approximately 60 percent of the 300 reported cases have been in patients with juvenile rheumatoid arthritis (not necessarily all children), and a further 10 percent have occurred in children with acute rheumatic fever.[124] Girls may tend to develop aspirin hepatotoxicity more than boys.[125] The hepatotoxicity appears to be dose-dependent, and patients without rheumatoid disease can develop hepatotoxicity. The preponderance of cases in patients with rheumatologic diseases, however, raises the possibility that these patients have a predisposition to this toxicity. One theory is that chronic inflammation increases the generation of oxygen radicals.[126]

In most cases salicylate hepatotoxicity presents with anorexia, nausea, vomiting, and abdominal pain, along with elevated aminotransferases.[127-132] Hepatomegaly is usually present, and the liver may be tender. Progressive signs of liver damage such as jaundice and coagulopathy are rare, occurring in approximately 4 percent of all reported cases.[124] However, even in uncomplicated cases aminotransferase levels may be high, greater than 1,000 IU.[130] In some cases encephalopathy (not related to Reye's syndrome) has been present.[133,134] Clinical and laboratory abnormalities resolve when aspirin is stopped. Rechallenge with aspirin may precipitate the hepatotoxicity again.[128] Liver histology frequently shows a rather nonspecific picture with acute, focal hepatocellular necrosis.[127]

A different clinical syndrome with hepatotoxicity has been reported in seven children with juvenile rheumatoid arthritis, of whom all but one received aspirin.[135] Clinical features included high fever, drowsiness, vomiting, hepatosplenomegaly, and bleeding due to disseminated intravascular coagulation and suboptimal clotting factor synthesis. Liver histology showed steatosis (predominantly large-droplet) and prominence of reticuloendothelial cells in the liver. Rechallenge with aspirin did not reproduce this syndrome, and it may have been related to other drug treatment or to intercurrent infection. Two children died of coma, but there was neither cerebral edema nor severe hyperammonemia noted, and other features were not typical of Reye's syndrome. However, Reye's syndrome can occur in children with rheumatologic diseases who receive aspirin chronically,[136] and its clinical presentation may be atypical.

Methotrexate

Methotrexate hepatotoxicity in children appears to be similar to that in adults. Chronic low-dose treatment for psoriasis or connective tissue disease can cause hepatic fibrosis with steatosis.[137,138] The appearance may be similar to alcoholic hepatitis with fibrosis. Cirrhosis can develop. Aminotransferases may not indicate ongoing liver damage, and liver biopsy prior to treatment and at regular, preferably yearly, intervals during prolonged treatment is advisable. Measurement of procollagen peptide III, proposed as a marker of liver fibrosis in adults, is probably not adequate for this sort of surveillance in children because its serum concentration is also influenced by growth.[139]

High-dose methotrexate treatment used in some oncology regimens may cause acute hepatitis.[140,141] After more protracted treatment, hepatic damage may be relatively slight, apart form ultrastructural changes including steatosis, fibrosis, and damage to some hepatocellular organelles.[142] Others have also found steatosis, portal inflammation, or portal fibrosis on light microscopic examination of liver biopsies from children with acute lymphoblastic leukemia, treated with various drugs including methotrexate.[143] Aminotransferase abnormalities did not predict histologic findings, which were, in general, mild after 2 years of treatment.[143,144]

The mechanism of this hepatotoxicity is not known. The dosage schedule may be important. Chronic intermittent administration of methotrexate may lead to recurrent hepatocellular damage superimposed on partial repair and regeneration, not unlike experimental models of carbon tetrachloride-induced hepatic fibrosis.

Antineoplastic Drugs

Besides methotrexate, many drugs used to treat neoplasia in childhood can cause hepatotoxicity.[145-147] A common and perplexing problem is elevation in aminotransferases without other evidence of severe liver toxicity. Antineoplastic drugs that commonly produce this reaction include nitrosoureas, 6-mercaptopurine, cytosine arabinoside, *cis*-platinum, and DTIC. Adriamycin, cyclophosphamide, dactinomycin, and vinca alkaloids are infrequently associated with hepatotoxicity. Adriamycin given together with 6-mercaptopurine may increase the hepatotoxic potential of 6-mercaptopurine.[148] Irradiation may increase the hepatotoxicity of dactinomycin.[149] The difficulty in assessing the hepatotoxic potential of all these drugs is that they are rarely used separately, and patients receiving them usually are at risk for multiple types of liver injury.

In children and adults L-asparaginase has been associated with more severe damage characterized by severe steatosis, hepatocellular necrosis, and fibrosis. This is usually reversible after L-asparaginase is stopped.[150] The most likely mechanism for this hepatotoxicity is a profound interference with hepatocellular protein metabolism.

Thioguanine may lead to veno-occlusive disease, and its toxicity may be enhanced by drug interactions with other antineoplastic drugs.[151] Veno-occlusive disease presents acutely with an enlarged tender liver, ascites or unexplained weight gain, and jaundice; aminotransferases may be elevated. In several reported patients the liver disease has progressed to cirrhosis with hepatic venular sclerosis and sinusoidal fibrosis.[152] Direct toxicity to zone 3 hepatocytes may occur. Several antineoplastic agents, including cytosine arabinoside, busulfan, DTIC, and carmustine (BCNU), have been associated with veno-occlusive disease at conventional or high doses.[153] Currently, veno-occlusive disease most frequently develops after allogenic bone marrow transplantation. It is difficult to say whether it is a consequence of chemotherapeutic conditioning regimens or part of the spectrum of liver injury due to graft-versus-host disease.[154,155] Irradiation can itself lead to veno-occlusive disease.[156] The combination of irradiation and chemotherapy in conditioning regimens may lead to earlier development of veno-occlusive disease than after single-agent (irradiation or chemical) injury.[157] Clinical predictors of likelihood for development of veno-occlusive disease in children have not yet been identified.

It may be difficult to distinguish between hepatic damage due to the neoplastic process and hepatoxicity. Since many antineoplastic drugs undergo biotransformation in the liver, drug regimens sometimes have to be modified to compensate for changes in hepatic reserve and hepatic drug metabolism.

Cyclosporine

Cyclosporine is a potent immunosuppressive with a novel cyclic structure composed of 11 amino acids. It is extremely lipophilic. It is metabolized in humans by cytochrome P450IIIA3.[158] Although at high dosage jaundice with abnormal aminotransferases may develop, the more common hepatic abnormality is mainly cholestasis: direct hyperbilirubinemia without other evidence of hepatocellular damage.[159,160] Cholestasis without biochemical or histologic evidence of hepatotoxicity after cyclosporine administration has been demonstrated in a rat model.[161] Cyclosporine has also been shown to inhibit taurocholate transport competitively and reversibly in an in vitro model with rat hepatocytes.[162]

As cyclosporine is metabolized by cytochromes P-450, its metabolism is subject to predictable changes due to drug interactions affecting cytochromes P-450. Phenobarbital, phenytoin, and rifampicin all increase clearance of cyclosporine because they are capable of inducing cytochrome P450IIIA3. Cimetidine and ketoconazole, nonspecific inhibitors of cytochromes P-450, decrease the clearance of cyclosporine. Erythromycin, which also is metabolized by the cytochrome P450IIIA subfamily, also inhibits cyclosporine metabolism, probably on a competitive basis.[163] At high dosages various glucocorticoids alter cyclosporine metabolism.

Isoniazid

In adults isoniazid (INH) is capable of causing a wide spectrum of toxic liver disease.[164,165] Clinically, the common finding is an asymptomatic patient with elevated aminotransferases. The development of a hepatitis-like illness with fatigue, anorexia, nausea, and vomiting is ominous. On histologic examination, INH hepatotoxicity frequently looks exactly like acute viral hepatitis. Submassive hepatic necrosis can occur, and occasionally the hepatocellular damage looks zonal.

There have been scattered reports of INH hepatotoxicity, including fatal hepatic necrosis, occurring both in children being treated for tuberculosis and in those receiving prophylaxis.[166-171] Large studies of INH hepatotoxicity as evidenced by abnormal aminotransferases in children receiving INH alone as prophylaxis showed a 7 percent incidence in a series of 369 children[172] and a 17.1 percent incidence in 239 patients aged 9 to 14 years.[173] The discrepancy in these two studies is partly methodologic. However, these findings are nearly the same as in adults, in whom the incidence of transiently elevated aminotransferases is estimated at 10 to 20 percent.[165] Several studies of children being treated with INH and rifampicin for tuberculosis also show a high incidence of hepatic dysfunction. Thirty-six of 44 patients receiving INH and rifampicin had some elevation of aminotransferases, and 15 patients (42 percent) had elevated AST and were jaundiced.[174] These children received comparatively high doses of INH and rifampicin, and many had severe infection. In another study, 37 percent had hepatotoxicity, including 4 of 7 under 17 months old.[175] These children received conventional, lower doses of INH and rifampicin and brief sequential courses of streptomycin and ethambutal. As in adults, hepatotoxicity typically developed in the first 8 to 10 weeks of treatment; in most children it resolved with either no change in dose or else a modest dose reduction. Children with more severe tuberculosis seemed to be at greater risk for hepatotoxicity. One study that showed a much lower incidence of hepatotoxicity in children on INH and rifampicin (3.3 percent of 430 via questionnaire) also found the trend to more severe hepatotoxicity in children with severe tuberculosis, notably tuberculous meningitis.[176]

Isoniazid hepatotoxicity appears to be due to a toxic metabolite, although the mechanism remains obscure. Acetylisoniazid or its derivatives have been thought to be the toxic intermediates. Susceptibility to hepatotoxicity has been linked to the polymorphism for *N*-acetylation, rapid acetylators being at greater risk.[165] Clinical studies in children have not shown a universal trend implicating rapid acetylators as more susceptible.[175] Metabolism by cytochromes P-450 may also be implicated, as pretreatment with phenobarbital appears to increase toxicity in laboratory animal models. Rifampicin may enhance INH toxicity by inducing certain cytochromes P-450.[171]

It is probably inaccurate to regard INH hepatotoxicity as uncommon in children. Some of the hepatotoxicity appears to be dose-related, and recent downward revisions of dosage recommendations may eliminate some instances of hepatoxicity. Children who have more severe tuberculosis or who receive simultaneous treatment with rifampicin, phenytoin, or phenobarbital may be at increased risk. The genetic predisposing factors remain unclear. Monitoring with frequent measurement of aminotransferases and direct inquiry for hepatitic symptoms is important in the first 10 to 12 weeks of treatment.

Halothane

Halothane hepatotoxicity shows two major clinical patterns. One is hepatitis indicated by abnormal aminotransferases in the first or second week after the anesthetic exposure. The other pattern is severe hepatitis with extensive hepatocyte necrosis and liver failure.[177] It is remarkably infrequent in children. Large retrospective studies in children estimate that the incidence is approximately 1 in 80,000 to 200,000,[178,179] in contrast to an incidence of 1 in 7,000 to 30,000 in adults.[180] The infrequency of this hepatotoxicity is not due to lack of exposure to the drug, because halothane is a mainstay of pediatric anesthetic practice. However, despite its rarity, it is now clear that halothane hepatitis *can* occur in children. Seven cases have been documented in detail in children aged 11 months to 15 years, all of whom had multiple exposures to halothane; one died of fulminant liver failure, but all others recovered.[181] In addition, there are three cases of halothane hepatitis found retrospectively[178,179] and three further children who succumbed to fulminant hepatic failure after halothane.[182-184] Other reports of hepatitis or hepatic failure in children after halothane anesthesia have been difficult to evaluate owing to inadequate data or presence of complicated, and thus confounding, systemic disease; these may amount to an additional eight cases. Clearly this problem cannot be discounted in children. There has been some speculation that children with alpha$_1$-antitrypsin deficiency may tolerate halothane poorly.[185]

Halothane is metabolized by various cytochromes P-450, and toxic metabolites are generated.[186-188] Depending on the prevailing tissue oxygen tension, oxidative or reductive metabolic pathways predominate (Fig. 8). The reductive pathway generates a toxic intermediate identified as a chlorotrifluoroethyl radical that leads to lipid peroxidation,[186] and the oxidative pathway generates a trifluoroacetyl intermediate that can acetylate cellular membranes. The contribution of these complex metabolic systems to human hepatotoxicity remains a matter of some dispute. Changes in calcium homeostasis may be the more proximate cause of liver cell necrosis.[189]

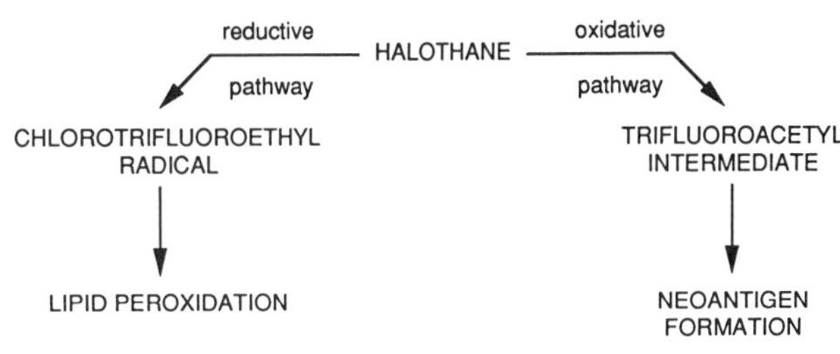

FIGURE 8 Metabolic fates of halothane. Whether the reductive or oxidative pathway predominates depends on the prevailing tissue oxygen tension.

Recent studies of the mechanism of halothane hepatotoxicity are beginning to show the connection between cytotoxic damage from reactive intermediates and immunologic phenomena often associated with this hepatotoxicity. Patients surviving halothane hepatotoxicity have been found to have an antibody to altered hepatocyte membrane constituents.[190,191] In rabbits, only oxidative metabolism of halothane has been associated with production of this altered hepatocyte membrane antigen, and the effect is greater after pretreatment with the polycyclic aromatic hydrocarbon beta-naphthaflavone.[192] Other investigators have shown that trifluoroacetyl adducts can be identified with fluorescent-tagged antibodies, mainly in zone 3 hepatocytes in the rat after phenobarbital pretreatment and also on the hepatocyte plasma membrane.[193] Antibodies to these neoantigens have now been identified in sera from patients with halothane hepatitis.[194] Further studies have shown that neoantigens, analogous to these neoantigens derived from halothane-treated animals, are expressed in human liver in individuals exposed to halothane.[195] Thus far, only one of these neoantigens has been purified and identified; this particular trifluoroactylated protein is a microsomal carboxylesterase.[196] Thus the oxidative pathway appears to be associated with hepatocellular membrane damage and immune phenomena typical of the clinical hepatotoxic syndrome.

In summary, severe halothane hepatotoxicity involves several factors whose interdependence can be partly defined. Formation of toxic metabolites depends on tissue oxygenation and possibly on which cytochromes P-450 are involved. There may be an element of idiosyncratic susceptibility with inadequate detoxification of an electrophilic intermediate.[180] The extent of immune phenomena may further depend on the immunogenicity of adducts formed and the innate immune responsiveness of the host.[193] Halothane hepatotoxicity provides the best example currently available for demonstrating a link between drug metabolism and an immune reaction in hepatotoxicity.

PRINCIPLES OF TREATMENT

Most drug-induced liver disease resolves spontaneously when the offending drug is withdrawn. Severe chronic changes should not be expected to regress. However, the histologic finding of bridging necrosis on liver biopsy does not tend to presage aggressive chronic liver damage in drug-induced liver disease.[197] Certain hepatotoxins require timely treatment with specific antidotes, such as *N*-acetylcysteine in acetaminophen hepatotoxicity. Steroid treatment has been beneficial when severe acute hepatitis dominates multisystemic hypersensitivity reaction, as with phenytoin or phenobarbital. However, the use of steroids in drug-induced liver disease remains controversial. The treatment of fulminant hepatic failure due to drug hepatotoxicity is otherwise essentially the same as in viral hepatitis. Liver transplantation may be life-saving in these circumstances.

When the major intervention is to stop a drug treatment, arriving at the diagnosis of drug-induced liver disease becomes all-important. A meticulous history of the illness with detailed attention to all drugs taken, including over-the-counter preparations, and the potential for exposure to environmental or industrial toxins is of utmost importance. In children it is important to ensure that the appropriate dosage was actually given. Liver biopsy, with electron microscopic examination if possible, is often highly informative and sometimes definitive.[198] Algorithms for determining the likelihood of an adverse drug reaction[199,200] may be helpful. In vitro rechallenge of the patient's lymphocytes with generated toxic metabolites usually provides important corroborative evidence.[201] In vitro rechallenge assays using immunologic end points have proved less informative.

SUMMARY

Drug-induced hepatotoxicity is more common in children than is generally appreciated. As in adults, the spectrum of disease is wide. Although cytotoxic processes, presenting as hepatitis, predominate, virtually every major type of hepatic pathology can occur. Hepatic drug metabolism has an important role in most of the drugs that most frequently cause hepatotoxicity in children: An imbalance between generation of toxic metabolite and detoxification processes can be identified. Focal defects in detoxification, often responsible for this imbalance, may be inherited. Developmental changes in drug disposition and metabolism further complicate the clinical spectrum of drug hepatotoxicity in children. The possibility of drug hepatotoxicity should be considered in every instance of childhood liver disease.

REFERENCES

1. Zimmerman HJ. Hepatotoxicity: the adverse effects of drugs and other chemicals on the liver. New York: Appleton-Century-Crofts, 1978.
2. Maddrey WC, Zimmerman HJ. Toxic and drug-induced hepatitis. In: Schiff L, Schiff ER, eds. Diseases of the liver. 6th ed. Philadelphia: JB Lippincott, 1987: 591.
3. Stricker BHC, Spoelstra P. Drug-induced liver injury. Amsterdam: Elsevier, 1985.
4. Okey AB, Roberts EA, Harper PA, Denison MS. Induction of drug-metabolizing enzymes: mechanisms and consequences. Clin Biochem 1986; 19:132–141.
5. Roberts EA, Golas CL, Okey AB. *Ah* receptor mediating induction of aryl hydrocarbon hydroxylase: detection in human lung by binding of 2,3,7,8-[^{3}H]tetrachlorodibenzo-*p*-dioxin. Cancer Res 1986; 47:3739–3743.
6. Manchester DK, Gordon JK, Golas CL, Roberts EA, Okey AB. *Ah* receptor in human placenta: stabilization by molybdate and characterization of binding of 2,3,7,8-tetrachlorodibenzo-*p*-dioxin, 3-methylcholanthrene, and benzo(*a*) pyrene. Cancer Res 1987; 47:4861–4868.
7. Eichelbaum M. Polymorphic drug oxidation in humans. Fed Proc 1984; 43:2298–2302.
8. Küpfer A, Schmid B, Preisig R, Pfaff G. Dextromethorphan as a safe probe for debrisoquine hydroxylation polymorphism. Lancet 1984; ii:517–518.
9. Osikowska-Evers B, Dayer P, Meyer UA, Robertz GM, Eichelbaum M. Evidence for altered catalytic properties of the cytochrome P-450 involved in sparteine oxidation in poor metabolizers. Clin Pharmacol Ther 1987; 41:320–325.
10. Eichelbaum M, Mineshita S, Ohnhaus EE, Zekorn C. The influence of enzyme induction in polymorphic sparteine oxidation. J Clin Pharmacol 1986; 22:49–53.
11. Ayesh R, Idle JR, Ritchie JC, Crothers MJ, Hetzel MR. Metabolic oxidation phenotypes as markers for susceptibility to lung cancer. Nature 1984; 312:169–170.

12. Jacqz E, Hall SD, Branch RA. Genetically determined polymorphisms in drug oxidation. Hepatology 1986; 6:1020–1032.
13. Spielberg SP, Gordon GB. Glutathione synthetase-deficient lymphocytes and acetaminophen toxicity. Clin Pharmacol Ther 1981; 29:51–55.
14. Stoner E, Starkman H, Wellner D, Wellner VP, Sassa S, Rifkind MB, Grenier A, Steinherz PG, Meister A, New MI, Levine LS. Biochemical studies of a patient with hereditary hepatorenal tyrosinemia: evidence of a glutathione deficiency. Pediatr Res 1984; 18:1332–1336.
15. Aranda JV, Cook CE, Gorman W, Collinge JM, Loughnan PM, Outerbridge EW, Aldridge A, Neims AH. Pharmacokinetic profile of caffeine in the premature newborn with apnea. J Pediatr 1979; 94:663–668.
16. Aranda JV, Collinge JM, Zinman R, Watters G. Maturation of caffeine elimination in infancy. Arch Dis Child 1979; 54:946–949.
17. Lambert GH, Schoeller DA, Kotake AN, Flores C, Hay D. The effect of age, gender and sexual maturation on the caffeine breath test. Dev Pharmacol Ther 1986; 9:375–388.
18. Oesch F. Significance of various enzymes in the control of reactive metabolites. Arch Toxicol 1987; 60:174–178.
19. Mitchell JR, Nelson SD, Thorgeirsson SS, McMurtry RJ, Dybing E. Metabolic activation: biochemical basis for many drug-induced liver injuries. Prog Liver Dis 1976; 5:259–279.
20. Moldeus P, Quanguan J. Importance of the glutathione cycle in drug metabolism. Pharmacol Ther 1987; 33:37–40.
21. Gumucio JJ, Miller DL. Functional implications of liver cell heterogenicity. Gastroenterology 1981; 80:393–403.
22. Mitchell AA, Lacouture PG, Sheehan JE, Kauffman RE, Shapiro S. Adverse drug reactions in children leading to hospital admission. Pediatrics 1988; 82:24–29.
23. Woods CG, Rylance ME, Cullen RE, Rylance GW. Adverse reactions to drugs in children. Br Med J 1987; 294:689–690.
24. Schmucker DL, Wang RK. Age-related changes in liver drug metabolism: structure as function. Proc Soc Exp Biol Med 1980; 165:178–187.
25. Vestal RE. Aging and determinants of hepatic drug clearance. Hepatology 1989; 9:331–334.
26. Mitchell JR, Jollow DJ, Potter WZ, Davis DC, Gillette JR, Brodie BB. Acetaminophen-induced hepatic necrosis. I. Role of drug metabolism. J Pharmacol Exp Ther 1973; 187:185–194.
27. Jollow DJ, Mitchell JR, Potter WZ, Davis DC, Gillette JR, Brodie BB. Acetaminophen-induced hepatic necrosis. II. Role of covalent binding *in vivo*. J Pharmacol Exp Ther 1973; 187:195–202.
28. Potter WZ, Davis DC, Mitchell JR, Jollow DJ, Gillette JR, Brodie BB. Acetaminophen-induced hepatic necrosis. III. Cytochrome P-450–mediated covalent binding *in vitro*. J Pharmacol Exp Ther 1973; 187:203–210.
29. Mitchell JR, Jollow DJ, Potter WZ, Gillette JR, Brodie BB. Acetaminophen-induced hepatic necrosis. IV. Protective role of glutathione. J Pharmacol Exp Ther 1973; 187:211–217.
30. Miner DJ, Kissinger PT. Evidence for the involvement of *N*-acetyl-*p*-quinoneimine in acetaminophen metabolism. Biochem Pharmacol 1979; 28:3285–3290.
31. Dahlin DC, Miwa GT, Lu AYH, Nelson SD. *N*-acetyl-*p*-benzoquinone imine: a cytochrome P450-mediated oxidation product of acetaminophen. Proc Natl Acad Sci USA 1984; 81:1327–1331.
32. Blair IA, Boots AR, Davies DS. Paracetamol oxidation: synthesis and reactivity of *N*-acetyl-*p*-benzoquinoneimine. Tetrahedron Lett 1980; 21:4947–4950.
33. Gerson RJ, Casini A, Gilfor D, Serroni A, Farber JL. Oxygen-mediated cell injury in the killing of cultured hepatocytes by acetaminophen. Biochem Biophys Res Commun 1985; 126:1129–1137.
34. Smith CV, Mitchell JR. Acetaminophen hepatotoxicity in vivo is not accompanied by oxidant stress. Biochem Biophys Res Commun 1985; 133:329–336.
35. Moore M, Thor H, Moore G, Nelson S, Moldeus R, Orrenius S. The toxicity of acetaminophen and *N*-acetyl-*p*-benzoquinone imine in isolated hepatocytes is associated with thiol depletion and increased cytosolic Ca2+. J Biol Chem 1985; 260:13035–13040.
36. Corcoran CB, Todd EL, Racz WJ, Hughes H, Smith CV, Mitchell JR. Effects of *N*-acetylcysteine in the disposition and metabolism of acetaminophen in mice. J Pharmacol Exp Ther 1985; 232:857–863.
37. Corcoran GB, Racz WJ, Smith CV, Mitchell JR. Effects of *N*-acetylcysteine on acetaminophen covalent binding and hepatic necrosis in mice. J Pharmacol Exp Ther 1985; 232:864–872.
38. Mitchell MC, Shenker S, Arant GR, Speeg KV. Cimetidine protects against acetaminophen heptatotoxicity in rats. Gastroenterology 1981; 81:1052–1060.
39. Rumack BH, Matthew H. Acetaminophen poisoning and toxicity. Pediatrics 1975; 55:871–876.
40. Smilkstein MJ, Knapp GL, Kulig KW, Rumack BH. Efficacy of oral *N*-acetylcysteine in the treatment of acetaminophen overdose. Analysis of the National Multicenter Study (1976 to 1985). N Engl J Med 1988; 319:1557–1562.
41. Rumack BH. Acetaminophen overdose in young children. Treatment and effects of alcohol and other additional ingestants in 417 cases. Am J Dis Child 1984; 138:428–433.
42. Peterson RG, Rumack BH. Age as a variable in acetaminophen overdose. Arch Intern Med 1981; 141:390–393.
43. Meredith TJ, Newman B, Goulding R. Paracetamol poisoning in children. Br Med J 1978; 2:478–479.
44. Peterson RG, Rumack BH. Pharmacokinetics of acetaminophen in children. Pediatrics 1978; 62:877–879.
45. Miller RP, Roberts RJ, Fischer LF. Acetaminophen elimination kinetics in neonates, children and adults. Clin Pharmacol Ther 1976; 19:284–294.
46. Lederman S, Fysh WJ, Tredger M, Gamsu HR. Neonatal paracetamol poisoning: treatment by exchange transfusion. Arch Dis Child 1983; 58:631–633.
47. Roberts I, Robinson MJ, Mughal MZ, Rutcliffe JG, Prescott LF. Paracetamol metabolites in the neonate following maternal overdose. Br J Clin Pharmacol 1984; 18:201–206.
48. Rollins DE, Von Bahr C, Glaumann H, Moldeus P, Rane A. Acetaminophen: potentially toxic metabolites formed by human fetal and adult liver microsomes and isolated fetal liver cells. Science 1979; 205:1414–1416.
49. Hart JG, Timbrell JA. The effects of age on paracetamol hepatotoxicity in mice. Biochem Pharmacol 1979; 28:3015–3017.
50. Harman AW, McCamish LE. Age-related toxicity of paracetamol in mouse hepatocytes. Biochem Pharmacol 1986; 35:1731–1735.
51. Green MD, Shires TK, Fischer LJ. Hepatotoxicity of acetaminophen in neonatal and young rats. I. Age-related changes in susceptibility. Toxicol Appl Pharmacol 1984; 74:116–124.
52. Lauterburg BH, Vaishnav Y, Stillwell WG, Mitchell JR. The effect of age and glutathione depletion on hepatic glutathione turnover in vivo determined by acetaminophen probe analysis. J Pharmacol Exp Ther 1980; 213:54–58.
53. Nogen AG, Brenner JE. Fatal acetaminophen overdosage in a growing child. J Pediatr 1978; 92:832–833.
54. Weber JL, Cutz E. Liver failure in an infant. Can Med Assoc J 1980; 123:112–117.
55. Agran PF, Zenk KE, Romansky SG. Acute liver failure and encephalopathy in a 15-month-old infant. Am J Dis Child 1983; 137:1107–1114.
56. Swetnam SM, Florman AL. Probable acetaminophen toxicity in an 18-month-old infant due to repeated overdosing. Clin Pediatr 1984; 23:104–105.
57. Lieh-Lai MW, Sarnaik AP, Newton JF, Miceli JN, Fleischman LE, Hook JB, Kauffman RE. Metabolism and pharmacokinetics of acetaminophen in a severely poisoned young child. J Pediatr 1984; 105:125–128.
58. Blake KV, Bailey D, Zientek GM, Hendeles L. Death of a child associated with multiple overdoses of acetaminophen. Clin Pharm 1988; 7:391–397.
59. Greene JW, Graft L, Gishan FK. Acetaminophen poisoning in infancy. Am J Dis Child 1983; 137:386–387.
60. Smith DW, Isakson G, Frankel LR, Kerner JA Jr. Hepatic failure following ingestion of multiple doses of acetaminophen in a young child. J Pediatr Gastroenterol Nutr 1986; 5:822–825.
61. Seeff LB, Cuccherini BA, Zimmerman HJ, Alder E, Benjamin SB. Acetaminophen hepatotoxicity in alcoholics. A therapeutic misadventure. Ann Intern Med 1986; 104:399–404.
62. Coon MJ, Koop DR. Alcohol-inducible cytochrome P-450 (P-450_{ALC}). Arch Toxicol 1987; 60:16–21.
63. Powers NG, Carson SH. Idiosyncratic reactions to phenytoin. Clin Pediatr 1987; 26:120–124.
64. Shear NH, Spielberg SP. Anticonvulsant hypersensitivity syndrome. In vitro assessment of risk. J Clin Invest 1988; 82:1826–1832.

65. Mullick FG, Ishak KG. Hepatic injury associated with diphenylhydantoin therapy. Am J Clin Pathol 1980; 74:442–452.
66. Spielberg SP, Gordon GB, Blake DA, Goldstein DA, Herlong HF. Predisposition to phenytoin hepatotoxicity assessed in vitro. N Engl J Med 1981; 305:722–727.
67. Spielberg SP, Gordon GB, Blake DA, Mellits ED, Bross DS. Anticonvulsant toxicity in vitro: possible role of arene oxides. J Pharmacol Exp Ther 1981; 217:386–389.
68. Kahn HD, Faguet GB, Agee JF, Middleton HM. Drug-induced liver injury. In vitro demonstration of hypersensitivity to both phenytoin and phenobarbitol. Arch Intern Med 1984; 144:1677–1679.
69. Kleckner HB, Yakulis V, Heller P. Severe hypersensitivity to diphenylhydantoin with circulating antibodies to the drug. Ann Intern Med 1975; 83:522–523.
70. Mitchell MC, Boitnott JK, Arregui A, Maddrey WC. Granulomatous hepatitis associated with carbamazepine therapy. Am J Med 1981; 71:733–735.
71. Williams SJ, Ruppin DC, Grierson JM, Farrell GC. Carbamazepine hepatitis: the clinicopathological spectrum. J Gastroenterol Hepatol 1986; 1:159–168.
72. Zucker P, Daum F, Cohen MI. Fatal carbamazepine hepatitis. J Pediatr 1977; 91:667–668.
73. Lewis IJ, Rosenbloom L. Glandular fever-like syndrome, pulmonary eosinophilia and asthma associated with carbamazepine. Postgrad Med J 1982; 58:100–101.
74. Brain C, MacArdle B, Levin S. Idiosyncratic reactions to carbamazepine mimicking viral infection in children. Br Med J 1984; 289–354.
75. McGeachy TE, Bloomer WE. The phenobarbital sensitivity syndrome. Am J Med 1953; 14:600–604.
76. Evans WE, Self TH, Weisburst MR. Phenobarbital-induced hepatic dysfunction. Drug Intell Clin Pharmacol 1976; 10:439–443.
77. Shapiro PA, Antonioli DA, Peppercorn MA. Barbiturate-induced submassive hepatic necrosis. Am J Gastroenterol 1980; 74:270–273.
78. Powell-Jackson PR, Tredger JM, Williams R. Hepatotoxicity to sodium valproate: a review. Gut 1984; 25:673–681.
79. Green SH. Sodium valproate and routine liver function tests. Arch Dis Child 1984; 59:813–814.
80. Zafrani ES, Berthelot P. Sodium valproate in the induction of unusual hepatotoxicity. Hepatology 1982; 2:648–649.
81. Dreifuss FE, Santilli N, Langer DH, Sweeney KP, Moline KA, Menander KB. Valproic acid hepatic fatalities. Neurology 1987; 37:379–385.
82. Coulter DR, Allen RJ. Hyperammonemia with valproic acid therapy. J Pediatr 1981; 99:317–319.
83. Suchy FJ, Balistreri WF, Buchino JJ, Sondheimer JM, Bates SR, Kearns GL, Still JD, Bove KE. Acute hepatic failure associated with the use of sodium valproate. Report of two fatal cases. N Engl J Med 1979; 300:962–966.
84. Gerber N, Dickinson RG, Harland RC, Lynn RK, Houghton D, Antonias JI. Reye-like syndrome associated with valproic acid therapy. J Pediatr 1979; 95:142–144.
85. Zimmerman HJ, Ishak KG. Valproate-induced hepatic injury: analysis of 23 fatal cases. Hepatology 1982; 2:591–597.
86. Partin JS, Suchy FJ, Bates SR. An ultrastructural analysis of sodium valproate associated hepatopathy. Gastroenterology 1983; 84:1389.
87. Schnabel R, Rambeck B, Janssen F. Fatal intoxication with sodium valproate. Lancet 1984; i:221–222.
88. Rettenmeier AW, Gordon WP, Prickett KS, Levy RH, Lockard JS, Thummel KE, Baillie TA. Metabolic fate of valproic acid in the rhesus monkey. Formation of a toxic metabolite, 2-*n*-propyl-4-pentenoic acid. Drug Metab Dispos 1986; 14:443–453.
89. Kochen W, Schneider A, Ritz A. Abnormal metabolism of valproic acid in fatal hepatic failure. Eur J Pediatr 1983; 14:30–35.
90. Kingsley E, Gray P, Tolman KG, Tweedale R. The toxicity of metabolites of sodium valproate in cultured hepatocytes. J Clin Pharmacol 1983; 23:178–185.
91. Kesterson JW, Granneman GR, Machinist JM. The hepatotoxicity of valproate in rats. I. Toxicologic, biochemical and histopathologic studies. Hepatology 1984; 4:1143–1152.
92. Granneman GR, Wang SI, Kesterson JW, Machinist JM. The hepatoxicity of valproic acid and its metabolites in rats. II. Intermediary and valproic acid metabolism. Hepatology 1984; 4:1153–1158.
93. Olson MJ, Handler JA, Thurman RG. Mechanism of zone-specific hepatic steatosis caused by valproate: inhibition of ketogenesis in periportal regions of the liver lobule. Mol Pharmacol 1986; 30:520–525.
94. Bjorge SM, Baillie TA. Inhibition of medium-chain fatty acid beta-oxidation *in vitro* by valproic acid and its unsaturated metabolite, 2-*n*-propyl-4-pentenoic acid. Biochem Biophys Res Commun 1985; 132:245–252.
95. Qureshi IA, Letarte J, Tuchweber B, Yousef I, Qureshi SR. Hepatotoxicology of sodium valproate in ornithine transcarbamylase-deficient mice. Toxicol Lett 1985; 25:297–306.
96. Hjelm M, De Silva LVK, Seakins IWT, Oberholzer VG, Rolles CJ. Evidence of inherited urea cycle defect in a case of fatal valproate toxicity. Br Med J 1986; 292:23–24.
97. Böhles H, Richter K, Wagner-Thiessen E, Schäfer H. Decreased serum carnitine in valproate induced Reye syndrome. Eur J Pediatr 1982; 139:185–186.
98. Murphy JV, Maquardt KM, Shug AL. Valproic acid associated abnormalities of carnitine of metabolism. Lancet 1985; i:820–821.
99. Matsuda I, Ohtani Y, Ninoniya N. Renal handling of carnitine in children with carnitine deficiency and hyperammonemia associated with valproate therapy. J Pediatr 1986; 109:131–134.
100. Millington DS, Bohan TP, Roe CR, Yergey AL, Liberato DJ. Valproylcarnitine: a novel drug metabolite identified by fast atom bombardment and thermospray liquid chromatography-mass spectroscopy. Clin Chim Acta 1985; 145:69–76.
101. Dujovne CA, Chan CH, Zimmerman HJ. Sulfonamide hepatic injury. Review of the literature and report of a case due to sulfamethoxazole. N Engl J Med 1967; 277:785–788.
102. Poland GA, Love KR. Marked atypical lymphocytosis, hepatitis and skin rash in sulfasalazine drug allergy. Am J Med 1986; 81:707–708.
103. Shear NH, Spielberg SP, Grant DM, Tang BK, Kalow W. Differences in metabolism of sulfonamides predisposing to idiosyncratic toxicity. Ann Intern Med 1986; 105:179–184.
104. Zitelli BJ, Alexander J, Taylor S, Miller KD, Howrie DL, Kuritsky JN, Perez TH, Van Thiel DH. Fatal hepatic necrosis due to pyrimethamine-sulfadoxine (Fansidar). Ann Intern Med 1987; 106:393–395.
105. Sotolongo RP, Neefe LI, Rudzki C, Ishak KG. Hypersensitivity reaction to sulfasalazine with severe hepatotoxicity. Gastroenterology 1978; 75:95–99.
106. Losek JH, Werlin SL. Sulfazalazine hepatotoxicity. Am J Dis Child 1981; 135:1070–1072.
107. Ribe J, Benkov KJ, Thung SN, Shen SC, Leleiko NS. Fatal massive hepatic necrosis: a probable hypersensitivity reaction to sulfasalazine. Am J Gastroenterol 1986; 81:205–208.
108. Rieder MJ, Uetrecht J, Shear NH, Cannon M, Miller M, Spielberg SP. Diagnosis of sulfonamide hypersensitivity reactions by in-vitro "rechallenge" with hydroxylamine metabolites. Ann Intern Med 1989; 110:286–289.
109. Shear NH, Spielberg SP. In vitro evaluation of a toxic metabolite of sulfadiazine. Can J Physiol Pharmacol 1985; 63:1370–1372.
110. Zafrani ES, Ishak KG, Rudzki C. Cholestatic and hepatocellular injury associated with erythromycin esters. Report of nine cases. Dig Dis Sci 1979; 24:385–396.
111. Keeffe EB, Reis TC, Berland JE. Hepatotoxicity to both erythromycin estolate and erythromycin ethylsuccinate. Dig Dis Sci 1982; 27:701–704.
112. Phillips KG. Hepatotoxicity of erythromycin ethylsuccinate in a child. Can Med Ass J 1983; 129:411–412.
113. Funck-Brentano C, Pessayre D, Benhamou JP. Hepatites dues á divers derives de l'erythromycine. Gastroenterol Clin Biol (Paris) 1983; 7:362–369.
114. Diehl AM, Latham P, Boitnott JK, Mann J, Maddrey WC. Cholestatic hepatitis from erythromycin ethylsuccinate. Am J Med 1984; 76:931–934.
115. Gaeta GB, Utili R, Adinolfi LE, Abernathy CO, Giusti G. Characterization of the effects of erythromycin estolate and erythromycin base on the excretory function of the isolated rat liver. Toxicol Appl Pharmacol 1985; 80:185–192.
116. Villa P, Begue JM, Guillouzo A. Erythromycin toxicity in primary cultures of rat hepatocytes. Xenobiotica 1985; 15:767–773.
117. Sorensen EMB, Acosta D. Erythromycin estolate-induced toxicity in cultured rat hepatocytes. Toxicol Lett 1985; 27:73–82.
118. Parker LN. Hepatitis and propylthiouracil. Ann Intern Med 1975; 82:228–229.
119. Reddy CM. Propylthiouracil and hepatitis: a case report. J Natl Med Assoc 1979; 72:1185–1186.
120. Garty BZ, Kauli R, Ben-Ari J, Lubin E, Nitzam M, Laron Z. Hepati-

tis associated with propylthiouracil treatment. Drug Intell Clin Pharm 1985; 19:740–742.
121. Jonas MM, Edison MS. Propylthiouracil hepatotoxicity: two pediatric cases and review of the literature. J Pediatr Gastroenterol Nutr 1988; 7:776–779.
122. Safani MM, Tatro DS, Rudd P. Fatal propylthiouracil-induced hepatitis. Arch Intern Med 1982; 142:838–839.
123. Fedotin MS, Leger LG. Liver disease caused by propylthiouracil. Arch Intern Med 1975; 135:319–321.
124. Benson GD. Hepatotoxicity following the therapeutic use of antipyretic analgesics. Am J Med 1983; 75:85–93.
125. Athreya BH, Moser G, Cecil HS, Myers AR. Aspirin-induced hepatotoxicity in juvenile rheumatoid arthritis. Arthritis Rheum 1975; 18:347–352.
126. Parke DV. Activation mechanisms to chemical toxicity. Arch Toxicol 1987; 60:5–15.
127. Seaman WE, Ishak KG, Plotz PH. Aspirin-induced hepatotoxicity in patients with systemic lupus erythematosus. Ann Intern Med 1974; 80:1–8.
128. Wolfe JD, Metzger AL, Goldstein RC. Aspirin hepatitis. Ann Intern Med 1974; 80:74–76.
129. Zucker P, Daum F, Cohen MI. Aspirin hepatitis. Am J Dis Child 1975; 129:1433–1434.
130. Doughty R, Giesecke L, Athreya B. Salicylate therapy in juvenile rheumatoid arthritis. Am J Dis Child 1980; 134:461–463.
131. Barron KS, Person DA, Brewer EJ. The toxicity of non-steroidal anti-inflammatory drugs in juvenile rheumatoid arthritis. J Rheumatol 1982; 9:149–155.
132. Hamdan JA, Manasra K, Ahmed M. Salicylate-induced hepatitis in rheumatic fever. Am J Dis Child 1985; 139:453–455.
133. Ulshen MH, Grand RJ, Crain JD, Gelfand EW. Hepatotoxicity with encephalopathy associated with aspirin therapy in rheumatoid arthritis. J Pediatr 1978; 93:1034–1037.
134. Petty BG, Zahka KG, Bernstein MT. Aspirin hepatitis associated with encephalopathy. J Pediatr 1978; 93:881–882.
135. Hadchouel M, Prieur AM, Griscelli C. Acute hemorrhagic, hepatic, and neurologic manifestations in juvenile rheumatoid arthritis: possible relationship to drugs or infection. J Pediatr 1985; 106:561–566.
136. Hanson JR, McCray PB, Bole JF Jr, Corbett AJ, Flanders DJ. Reye syndrome associated with aspirin therapy for systemic lupus erythematosus. Pediatrics 1985; 76:202–205.
137. Tolman KG, Clegg DO, Lee RG, Ward JR. Methotrexate and the liver. J Rheumatol 1985; 12(suppl 12):29–34.
138. Van de Kerkhof PCM, Hoefnagels WHL, Van Haelst UJGM, Mali JWH. Methotrexate maintenance therapy and liver damage in psoriasis. Clin Exp Dermatol 1985; 10:194–200.
139. Trivedi P, Cheeseman P, Portmann B, Mowat AP. Serum type III procollagen peptide as a non-invasive marker of liver damage during infancy and childhood in extrahepatic biliary atresia, idiopathic hepatitis of infancy and $alpha_1$ antitrypsin deficiency. Clin Chim Acta 1986; 161:137–146.
140. Taft LI. Methotrexate induced hepatitis in childhood leukemia. Isr J Med Sci 1965; 1:823–827.
141. Jolivet J, Cowan KH, Curt GA, Clendeninn NJ, Crabner BA. The pharmacology and clinical use of methotrexate. N Engl J Med 1983; 309:1094–1104.
142. Harb JM, Werlin SL, Camitta BM, Oechler H, Kamen BA, Blank EL. Hepatic ultrastructure in leukemic children treated with methotrexate and 6-mercaptopurine. Am J Pediatr Hematol Oncol 1983; 5:323–331.
143. Topley J, Benson J, Squier MV, Chessells JM. Hepatotoxicity in the treatment of acute lymphoblastic leukemia. Med Pediatr Oncol 1979; 7:393–399.
144. McIntosh S, Davidson DL, O'Brien RT, Pearson HA. Methotrexate hepatotoxicity in children with leukemia. J Pediatr 1977; 90:1019–1021.
145. Menard DB, Gisselbrecht C, Marty H, Reyes F, Dhumeaux D. Antineoplastic agents and the liver. Gastroenterology 1980; 78:142–164.
146. Perry MC. Hepatotoxicity of chemotherapeutic agents. Semin Oncol 1982; 9:65–74.
147. Sznol M, Ohnuma T, Holland JF. Hepatic toxicity of drugs used for hematologic neoplasia. Sem Liver Dis 1987; 7:237–256.
148. Minow RA, Stern MH, Casey JH, Rodriguez V, Luna MA. Clinicopathologic correlation of liver damage in patients treated with 6-mercaptopurine and Adriamycin. Cancer 1976; 38:1524–1528.
149. McVeagh P, Ekert H. Hepatotoxicity of chemotherapy following nephrectomy and radiation therapy for right-sided Wilms' tumor. J Pediatr 1975; 87:627–628.
150. Pratt CB, Johnson WW. Duration and severity of fatty metamorphosis of the liver following L-asparaginase therapy. Cancer 1971; 28:361–364.
151. Penta JS, Von Hoff DD, Muggia FM, Hepatotoxicity of combination chemotherapy for acute myelocytic leukemia. Ann Intern Med 1977; 87:247–248.
152. D'Cruz CA, Wimmer RS, Harcke HT, Huff DS, Naiman JL. Veno-occlusive disease of the liver in children following chemotherapy for acute myelocytic leukemia. Cancer 1983; 52:1802–1807.
153. Rollins BJ. Hepatic veno-occlusive disease. Am J Med 1986; 81:297–306.
154. Berk PD, Popper H, Krueger GF, Decter J, Herzig G, Graw RG Jr. Veno-occlusive disease of the liver after allogeneic bone marrow transplantation. Possible association with graft-versus-host disease. Ann Intern Med 1979; 90:158–164.
155. Beschorner WE, Pino J, Boitnott JK, Tutschka PJ, Santos GW. Pathology of the liver with bone marrow transplantation. Effects of busulfan, carmustine, acute graft-versus-host disease, and cytomegalovirus infection. Am J Pathol 1980; 99:369–386.
156. Fajardo LF, Colby TV. Pathogenesis of veno-occlusive disease after radiation. Arch Pathol Lab Med 1980; 104:584–588.
157. McDonald GB, Sharma P, Mathews DE, Shulman HM, Thomas ED. The clinical course of 53 patients with veno-occlusive disease of the liver after marrow transplantation. Transplantation 1985; 39:603–608.
158. Kronbach T, Fischer V, Meyer UA. Cyclosporine metabolism in human liver: identification of a cytochrome P-450 III gene family as the major cyclosporine-metabolizing enzyme explains interaction of cyclosporine with other drugs. Clin Pharmacol Ther 1988; 43:630–635.
159. Klintmalm GBG, Iwatsuki S, Starzl TE. Cyclosporine A hepatotoxicity in 66 renal allograft recipients. Transplanatation 1981; 32:488–489.
160. Schade RR, Gugliemi A, Van Thiel DH. Cholestasis in heart transplant recipients treated with cyclosporin. Transplant Proc 1983; 15:2757–2760.
161. Stone BG, Udani M, Sanghvi A, Warty V, Plocki K, Beditti CD, Van Thiel DH. Cyclosporin A–induced cholestasis. The mechanism in a rat model. Gastroenterology 1987; 93:344–351.
162. Kuhongviriyapan V, Stacey NH. Inhibition of taurocholate transport by cyclosporin A in cultured rat hepatocytes. J Pharmacol Exp Ther 1988; 247:685–689.
163. Freeman DJ, Martele R, Carruthers SG, Heinrichs D, Keown PA, Stiller CR. Cyclosporine-erythromycin interaction in normal subjects. Br J Clin Pharmacol 1987; 23:776–778.
164. Maddrey WC, Boitnott JK. Isoniazid hepatitis. Ann Intern Med 1973; 79:1–12.
165. Mitchell J, Zimmerman H, Ishak K, Thorgeirsson UP, Timbrell JA, Snodgrass WR, Nelson SD. Isoniazid liver injury: clinical spectrum, pathology and probable pathogenesis. Ann Intern Med 1976; 84:181–196.
166. Rudoy R, Stuemky J, Poley R. Isoniazid administration and liver injury. Am J Dis Child 1973; 125:733–736.
167. Casteels-Van Daele M, Igodt-Ameye L, Corbeel L, Eeckels R. Hepatotoxicity of rifampicin and isoniazid in children. J Pediatr 1975; 86:739–741.
168. Vanderhoof JA, Ament ME. Fatal hepatic necrosis due to isoniazid chemoprophylaxis in a 15-year-old girl. J Pediatr 1976; 88:867–868.
169. Litt IF, Cohen MI, McNamara H. Isoniazid hepatitis in adolescents. J Pediatr 1976; 89:133–135.
170. Walker A, Park-Hah J. Possible isoniazid-induced hepatotoxicity in a two-year-old child. J Pediatr 1977; 91:344–345.
171. Pessayre D, Bentata M, Degott C. Nouel O, Miguet JP, Rueff B, Benhamou JP. Isoniazid-rifampin fulminant hepatitis. A possible consequence of the enhancement of isoniazid hepatotoxicity by enzyme induction. Gastroenterology 1977; 72:284–289.
172. Beaudry P, Brickman H, Wise M, MacDougall D. Liver enzyme disturbances during isoniazid chemoprophylaxis in children. Am Rev Resp Dis 1974; 110:581–584.
173. Spyridis P, Sinantios C, Papadea I, Oreopoulos L, Hadjiyannis S, Papadotos C. Isoniazid liver injury during chemoprophylaxis in children. Arch Dis Child 1979; 54:65–67.
174. Tsagaropoulou-Stinga H, Mataki-Emmanouilidou T, Karadi-Kavalioti S, Manios S. Hepatotoxic reactions in children with severe tuberculosis treated with isoniazid-rifampin. Pediatr Infect Dis 1985; 4:270–273.
175. Martinez-Roig A, Cami J, Llorens-Terol J, De La Torre R, Perich F. Acetylation phenotype and hepatotoxicity in the treatment of tubercu-

losis of children. Pediatrics 1986; 77:912–915.
176. O'Brien RJ, Long MW, Cross FS, Lyle MA, Snider DE. Hepatotoxicity from isoniazid and rifampin among children treated for tuberculosis. Pediatrics 1983; 72:491–499.
177. Moult PJ, Sherlock S. Halothane-related hepatitis. A clinical study of twenty-six cases. Q J Med 1975; 44:99–114.
178. Wark HJ. Postoperative jaundice in children. Anaesthesia 1983; 38:237–242.
179. Warner LO, Beach TP, Gariss JP, Warner EJ. Halothane and children: the first quarter century. Anesth Analg 1984; 63:838–840.
180. Farrell G, Prendergast D, Murray M. Halothane hepatitis: detection of a constitutional susceptibility factor. N Engl J Med 1985; 313:1310–1314.
181. Kenna JG, Newberger J, Mieli-Vergani G, Mowat AP, Williams R. Halothane hepatitis in children. Br Med J 1987; 294:1209–1211.
182. Psacharopoulos HJ, Mowat AP, Davies M, Portmann B, Silk DBA, Williams R. Fulminant hepatic failure in childhood: an analysis of 31 cases. Arch Dis Child 1980; 55:252–258.
183. Inman WHW, Mushin WW. Jaundice after repeated exposure to halothane: a further analysis of reports to the Committee of Safety of Medicines. Br Med J 1978; 2:1455–1456.
184. Campbell RL, Small EW, Lesesne HR, Levin KJ, Moore WH. Fatal hepatic necrosis after halothane anesthesia in a boy with juvenile rheumatoid arthritis: a case report. Anesth Analg Curr Res 1977; 56:589–593.
185. Yoss BS, Lipsitz PJ. Hepatic decompensation following general anesthesia in alpha-l-antitrypsin deficiency. Am J Dis Child 1976; 130:1376.
186. DeGroot H, Noll T. Halothane hepatotoxicity: relation between metabolic activation, pyrexia, covalent binding, lipid peroxidation and liver cell damage. Hepatology 1983; 3:601–606.
187. Neuberger J, Williams R. Halothane anaesthesia and liver damage. Br Med J 1984; 289:1136–1139.
188. Farrell GC. Mechanism of halothane-induced liver injury: is it immune or metabolic idiosyncrasy? J Gastroenterol Hepatol 1988; 3:465–482.
189. Farrell GC, Mahoney J, Bilous M, Frost L. Altered hepatic calcium homeostasis in guinea pigs with halothane-induced hepatotoxicity. J Pharmacol Exp Ther 1988; 247:751–756.
190. Vergani D, Mieli-Vergani G, Alberti A, Neuberger J, Eddleston A, Davis M, Williams R. Antibodies to the surface of halothane-altered rabbit hepatocytes in patients with severe halothane-associated hepatitis. N Engl J Med 1980; 303:66–71.
191. Mieli-Vergani G, Vergani D, Tredger JM, Eddleston ALWF, Davis M, Williams R. Lymphocyte cytotoxicity to halothane altered hepatocytes in patients with severe hepatic necrosis following halothane anaesthesia. J Clin Lab Immunol 1980; 4:49–51.
192. Neuberger J, Mieli-Vergani G, Tredger JM, Davis M, Williams R. Oxidative metabolism of halothane in the production of altered hepatocyte membrane antigens in acute halothane-induced hepatic necrosis. Gut 1981; 22:669–672.
193. Satoh H, Fukuda Y, Anderson DK, Ferrans VJ, Gillette JR, Pohl LR. Immunological studies on the mechanism of halothane-induced hepatotoxicity: immunohistochemical evidence of trifluoroacetylated hepatocytes. J Pharmacol Exp Ther 1985; 233:857–862.
194. Kenna JG, Satoh H, Christ DD, Pohl LR. Metabolic basis for a drug hypersensitivity: antibodies in sera from patients with halothane hepatitis recognized liver neoantigens that contain the trifluoroacetyl group derived from halothane. J Pharmacol Exp Ther 1988; 245:1103–1109.
195. Kenna JG, Neuberger J, Williams R. Evidence for expression in human liver of halothane-induced neoantigens recognized by antibodies in sera from patients with halothane hepatitis. Hepatology 1988; 8:1635–1641.
196. Satoh H, Martin BM, Schulick AH, Christ DD, Kenna JG, Pohl LR. Human anti-endoplasmic reticulum antibodies in sera of patients with halothane-induced hepatitis are directed against a trifluoroacetylated carboxylesterase. Proc Natl Acad Sci (USA) 1989; 86:322–326.
197. Spitz RD, Keren DF, Boitnott JR, Maddrey WC. Bridging hepatic necrosis: etiology and prognosis. Am J Dig Dis 1978; 23:1076–1078.
198. Phillips MJ, Poucell S, Patterson J, Valencia P. The liver. An atlas and text of ultrastructural pathology. New York: Raven Press, 1987.
199. Naranjo CA, Busto U, Sellers EM, Sandor P, Ruiz I, Roberts EA, Janacek E, Domecq C, Greenblatt DJ. A method for estimating the probability of adverse drug reactions. Clin Pharmacol Ther 1981; 30:239–245.
200. Bégaud B, Evreux JC, Jouglard W, Lagier G. Imputabilité des effets inattendus ou toxiques des médicaments. Actualisation de la méthode utilisée en France. Thérapie 1985; 40:111–118.
201. Spielberg SP. In vitro assessment of pharmacogenetic susceptibility to toxic drug metabolites in human. Fed Proc 1984; 43:2308–2313.

PART 7

Liver Tumors

Milton J. Finegold, M.D.

Understanding and treating liver tumors of children continues to be a formidable task. Their very rarity contributes to the difficulty, as few individuals or centers compile sufficient experience to provide definitive direction. Additionally, the remarkable diversity of conditions that fall under the auspices of the term *tumor* makes it difficult to design a unifying formula to approach the subject or individual patient. Another problem is the extraordinary capacity of the liver to ignore the intruding mass, so clues to its presence often are few and so late as to make simple removal impossible. Finally, the anatomy of the liver encourages internal dissemination of neoplasms and taxes the skills of the most experienced surgeon. Nevertheless, recent advances in the molecular biology of gene expression and cellular differentiation, experimental carcinogenesis, monoclonal antibodies for diagnosis and perhaps even treatment, in imaging techniques and anesthesia, and in transplantation immunology make this a time for optimism. Of all the scientific advances, the single most important has already been achieved and merely awaits implementation: vaccination against hepatitis B virus (HBV). In regions where hepatitis B is endemic like Taiwan, hepatocellular carcinoma may account for 13 percent of all cancers in patients less than 15 years old. By interrupting the cycle of mother-to-newborn transmission, vaccination promises to eliminate the single most important cause of hepatic malignancy.

TABLE 1
Primary Liver Tumors in Children
(Eighteen Series Worldwide)

	Number	Percentage
Hepatoblastoma	539	43
Hepatocarcinoma	287	23
Adenoma	23	2
Hemangioma, hemangioendothelioma	171	13
Mesenchymal hamartoma	76	6
Sarcoma	80	6
Focal nodular hyperplasia	22	2
Other	58	5
TOTAL	1,257	100

Adapted from Weinberg and Finegold.[1]

Estimates of the incidence of primary hepatic tumors suggest that they account for about 0.04 to 0.16 per 1,000 United States hospital admissions and 0.5 to 2.0 percent of all pediatric cancers. About three-quarters of the collected tumors in large series worldwide (Table 1) are malignant, and 85 percent of those are of hepatocellular origin.[1] Hepatoblastomas comprise about 43 percent of all primary hepatic tumors. They occur in about one child per million under age 15 years (about 100 cases per year) in the United States. The Japanese Registry of childhood liver tumors recorded an average of 22 hepatoblastomas and four hepatocarcinomas per year throughout the 1970s. There is a strong possibility that all series and reports are biased toward malignancy, unusual cases, and unusual circumstances. The relative contribution of referral centers to surgical surveys and national statistics is uncertain, and the use of death certificates without autopsy verification is unreliable.

ETIOLOGY

HBV is responsible for more malignancy worldwide than any other environmental agent. Among adults there is a definite relationship to chronic hepatitis and macronodular cirrhosis, and at least 20 years of infection seem to be required for neoplastic transformation. The occurrence of hepatocarcinoma in children as young as 3 years following perinatal exposure to carrier mothers is surely an important clue to the carcinogenic process.[2] Among 173 South African blacks with hepatocarcinoma less than 30 years old only two had no serologic evidence of HBV infection, and 100 percent of affected Taiwanese children are HBV carriers. The younger the child, the less often is there evidence of active hepatitis and cirrhosis.[3-5] Hepatitis B functions like a retrovirus, with reverse transcriptase activity providing the means toward DNA replication. As with other carcinogenic retroviruses, the DNA may become integrated into the host genome,[6] and there may be associated deletions of portions of the cellular genome. In one case, the deleted material was on chromosome 11p,[7] possibly involving the same region found by Koufos et al[8] to be lost in two hepatoblastomas and in the Beckwith-Wiedemann syndrome, with which embryonal carcinomas of several organs are associated. Perhaps the reason why children exposed to hepatitis B as infants develop hepatocarcinomas so quickly is that the integration of viral

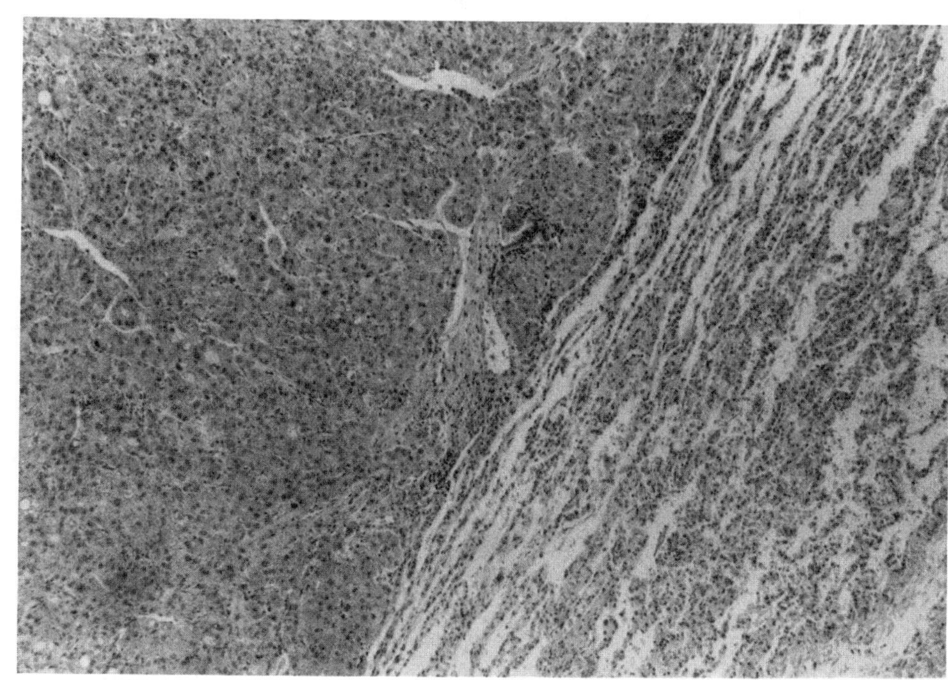

FIGURE 1 Hepatocarcinoma metastatic to the lung. A well-differentiated malignancy from a 17-year-old boy who had glucose-6-phosphatase deficiency managed successfully by frequent and nocturnal feedings. Adenomas were recognized in this liver 3 years earlier. If the illustrated tumor were in the liver, it would be impossible to predict its behavior (hematoxylin and eosin, ×63).

DNA is facilitated by the rapid rate of cell division in the developing liver. Perhaps the effects of early viral DNA integration on hepatocyte differentiation explain why three of the five hepatocarcinomas in children with HBV infection described by Ohaki et al[9] contained primitive hepatoblastic foci. The relationship of hepatitis B to oncogene expression in the genesis of hepatic malignancy remains unexplored. Baffet et al[10] found expression of N-*ras* messenger RNA in 11 of 11 hepatocarcinomas. c-Ki-*ras* and c-Ha-*ras* were detected in 7 of 11, and c-*myc* and *fos* were present in 2 of 11 tumors. The HBV status of the patients was not mentioned.

At least three-fourths of the mothers of children with HBV infection and hepatocarcinoma in Africa, China, and Japan display HB surface antigenemia. Curiously, only a minority of the fathers have antigenemia.[5] Even more perplexing is the observation by Larouze et al[11] that 27 of 28 fathers of children with hepatocarcinoma in Senegal had *no* antibody in HBs antigen, compared to 48 percent of control males of the same age in the population. Eighteen percent of those fathers had HBs antigenemia, compared with 71 percent of the mothers. The role of gender in the development of liver tumors is indeed noteworthy. Among adults the ratio of male to female for hepatocarcinomas is said to be between 8 and 10 to 1, with most of the difference attributed to chronic HBV hepatitis and cirrhosis, industrial or occupational exposure, and alcoholism. Only one of 15 antigen-positive mothers of Taiwanese children with hepatocarcinoma had a carcinoma herself, and no malignancy developed in any of the nine HBs antigen–positive sisters, but 5 of 13 HBV-carrying brothers had hepatocarcinoma.[5] Even with underlying metabolic errors having an autosomal recessive (sex neutral) basis, like type 1 glycogen storage disease or familial cholestatic cirrhosis, the incidence of carcinoma in boys is at least double that of girls.[12–14] Coire et al[15] found liver adenomas in 24 males and 12 females with von Gierke's disease. All four patients who developed carcinomas were males (Fig. 1).

It is stimulating to consider these clinical observations in the light of studies on steroid hormone receptors in normal and neoplastic liver tissue. Iqbal et al[16] found androgen receptors in fetal liver and hepatocarcinomas but not in normal adult liver, whereas estrogen receptors were detected in both tumor and adjacent liver. Nagasue et al[17] were able to detect androgen receptors in normal male liver, and 18 of 23 carcinomas had a significantly higher concentration. The cirrhotic liver of one woman also had androgen receptors, but they could be demonstrated in only one of two hepatocarcinomas in that same liver. Both Nagasue et al[17] and Ohnishi et al[18] found a loss of estrogen receptor activity in hepatocarcinomas versus the surrounding liver tissue. When aplastic or Fanconi's anemia patients of either sex are treated with C 17-alkylated anabolic steroids, tumors develop with significant frequency, and they have also been observed when testosterone was given to correct sexual immaturity in boys.[1] Of the 34 androgen-associated liver tumors in patients less than age 20 reviewed by Chandra et al,[19] 25 were in boys, half were discovered at autopsy, and two were judged to be carcinomas. Some of the tumors have regressed on withdrawal of the steroids.

Estrogens in oral contraceptives are definitely associated with the development of hepatic adenomas. After 8 years of use, the incidence of carcinoma in women is 4 to 20 times that of age-matched controls, when alcoholism, hepatitis, and cirrhosis are excluded.[20,21] Focal nodular hyperplasia is a non-neoplastic process that has to be distinguished from adenomas and carcinomas.[22] For a short time it appeared that women were more often affected, but it now seems that the lesion is more often symptomatic because oral contraceptives make the lesion more vascular and more likely to bleed. Case reports of angiosarcomas and cholangiocarcinoma in association with oral contraceptives have been limited to adults, but one 19-year-old girl was found to have a hepatoblastoma after 15 months of contraceptive pill use.[23] Prenatal exposure to synthetic estrogens and gonadotropins has been reported in two infants with hepatoblastoma.[1]

Many metabolic defects and congenital malformations are associated with and possibly contribute to hepatocellular malignancy. They are listed in Table 2 and discussed in detail by Weinberg and Finegold.[1] Of great interest is the observation by Kingston et al[24] that hepatoblastoma occurred in five families with intestinal polyposis. Garber et al[25] have expanded the number of affected families to 25. With an incidence of adenomatous polyposis of 1 per 8,300 and of hepatoblastoma of one per million children under age 15, this cannot be coincidental. There were 18 boys and seven girls. Eleven of the 25 patients have survived, including all but one of the girls, but only four of the boys. Six of the seven survivors examined developed colonic polyps as early as age 7 years. It is now possible to screen young children in families with polyposis (Gardner's syndrome) for the presence of the gene by examining the retina, where congenital hyperplasia of the pigment epithelium is readily visible. For the 50 percent who are affected, this finding should lead to periodic examinations for the presence of hepatoblastoma. How the observations by Bodmer and co-workers[26] on the localization

TABLE 2
Precursors of Hepatic Neoplasia

I. Prenatal Exposure
- Oral contraceptives
- Phenytoin
- Ethyl alcohol

II. Metabolic Disease
- Tyrosinemia
- von Gierke's disease, glycogenosis type 1

III. Malformations
- Hemihypertrophy, Beckwith-Wiedemann syndrome
- Von Recklinghausen's neurofibromatosis
- Soto's syndrome
- Multiple hemangiomatosis
- Ataxia-telangiectasia
- Fanconi's syndrome
- Budd-Chiari syndrome

IV. Biliary Tract Disease
- Extrahepatic atresia
- Familial cholestatic cirrhosis
- Alagille's syndrome
- Parenteral alimentation

V. Drugs
- Oral contraceptives
- Anabolic steroids

of the gene for familial polyposis to chromosome 5q and those of Koufos et al[8] on the 11p deletion in hepatoblastomas will be reconciled remains to be seen. When Koufos and colleagues studied the DNA from peripheral blood leukocytes of the patient we reported[1] and her parents, they were unable to detect an abnormality in chromosome 11 (personal communication).

Also noteworthy are recent case reports of hepatocarcinoma in relation to chronic biliary tract disease, adding to the few previous examples.[1] A 6-month-old boy received parenteral alimentation all his life and was found at autopsy to have a microscopic focus of carcinoma.[27] He is the second child with that background and promises not to be the last. Arteriohepatic dysplasia was previously not regarded as a preneoplastic condition, as 85 to 90 percent of affected individuals survive without serious hepatic complications of their childhood-onset cholestasis and bile duct paucity. But two patients with the syndrome have been described recently with hepatocarcinoma in the absence of biliary cirrhosis; one was a 3.5-year-old girl,[28] the other a 36-year-old man.[29]

CLINICAL MANIFESTATIONS

Regardless of cell type, the great majority of hepatic tumors are first detected as a mass or abdominal swelling. Upper abdominal pain is the next most frequent presenting complaint, followed by anorexia and weight loss, vomiting, and diarrhea. Infants with vascular hamartomas may display the signs of congestive heart failure, as have rare patients with mesenchymal hamartomas. Pruritus and frank jaundice are observed when tumors obstruct bile flow. In children, obstruction suggests rhabdomyosarcoma at any level of the biliary tract. Minor blunt trauma or apparently spontaneous hemorrhage of a liver tumor can be the earliest sign of its presence, especially among adolescent girls and young women taking estrogens for oral contraception, when tumors are especially vascular.

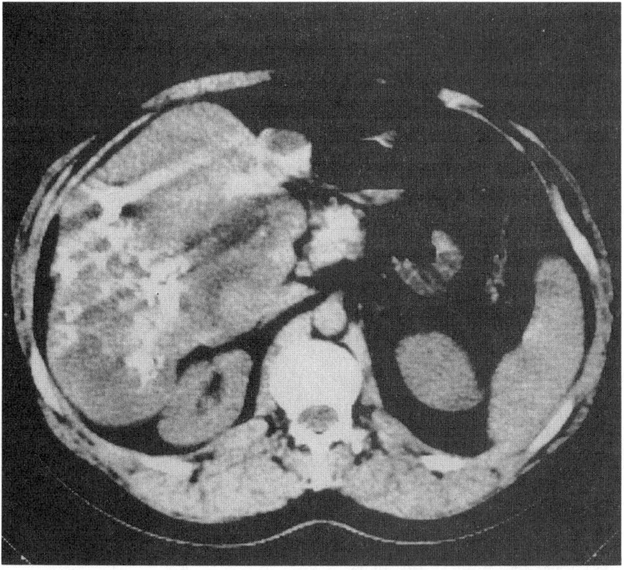

FIGURE 2 Computed tomography of the hepatoblastoma shown in Figure 4. The large inner zones of calcification are visualized as stellate radiopaque zones, whereas the epithelial portions of the mass are difficult to distinguish from host liver.

Several metabolic effects or paraneoplastic syndromes occur with a variety of hepatic tumors. Hypercalcemia with marked osteopenia can be very severe in children with either hepatoblastoma, carcinoma, or sarcoma. The mechanism, as in other malignancy-related hypercalcemias, is not fully understood, except that ectopic parathormone production is not the reason.[30] Hyperlipidemia has been associated with epithelial malignancies; particularly in infants, it has been associated with early fatality.[14,31,32] Both hyperlipidemia and hypoglycemia are thought to be secondary to injury to the remaining liver or dysfunction of the neoplastic epithelial cells, rather than a sign of underlying enzymatic error, such as glucose-6-phosphatase deficiency. The rare carcinomas in von Gierke's disease do not appear until the midteens or early twenties.[15] Thrombocytosis and polycythemia have also been observed in some hepatocarcinoma patients. Precocious puberty in males has been observed with hepatoblastomas and carcinomas. In most cases, ectopic gonadotropin production is responsible, but a few instances of testosterone synthesis have been reported.[33,34] Feminizing hepatocarcinomas are very uncommon.

IMAGING TECHNIQUES

Real-time ultrasonography is the hepatologist's stethoscope, says Okuda.[35] In Japan, where the incidence of hepatic malignancy is high and the tools and funds for screening are readily available, he and others have compared the various imaging modalities in adults and find that none of them is sufficiently sensitive to detect all hepatocarcinomas smaller than 2 cm or to completely discriminate between adenomatous and regenerating nodules of cirrhotic livers versus hepatocarcinomas or between adenomas and carcinomas. Repeat ultrasonography has shown the doubling time for carcinomas to be very variable, with growth from 1 to 2 cm taking an average of 3 months. The most rapidly growing tumors went from 1 to 3 cm in 4.6 months. By combining ultrasonography with serum alpha-fetoprotein measurements, early lesions susceptible to resection have been detected in the presence of cirrhosis.[35] Ultrasonically guided fine-needle aspirates proved to be 100 percent sensitive and 97.5 percent specific for hepatocarcinoma in 41 adult cases.[36] There has been no comparable study in children.

Arterial injections of enhancing compounds during computed tomography (CT) or magnetic resonance imaging (MRI) provide more expensive and complex means of detecting small intrahepatic lesions with questionably greater sensitivity than ultrasonography. The application of MRI is still at an early stage, but it is especially useful for distinguishing small and common hemangiomas from solid tumors.[37] MRI also shows spread of tumor into large abdominal veins very clearly. By including Lipiodol in the arterial infusate and taking delayed CT images, cancers as small as 3 mm have been observed, as the oily material is retained only by the tumor. CT is useful for scanning the abdomen for other sites of involvement when a liver mass is present. Enhanced CT and MRI have superseded angiography in delineating the extent of disease prior to partial hepatectomy (Fig. 2).[37,38] Scintigraphy with radiolabeled sulfur colloids has been used to distinguish lesions containing Kupffer cells (focal nodular hyperplasia) from those without (adenomas and carcinomas).[39] However, some hepatoblastomas have produced scintigraphic images indistinguishable from benign masses.

LABORATORY TESTS

Serum alpha-fetoprotein measurement is the most useful marker of malignant liver tumors. Eighty to 90 percent of hepatoblastomas and 60 to 90 percent of carcinomas are positive at the time of diagnosis. Except for a very few mesenchymal hamartomas in infancy and germ cell and yolk sac tumors, there are no false positives when serum alpha-fetoprotein levels exceed 500 ng per milliliter. Serum alpha-fetoprotein is elevated, although not to such high levels, in the absence of demonstrable carcinomas in both hereditary tyrosinemia and ataxia-telangiectasia. Both conditions are associated with a high frequency of hepatic malignancy, so the secretion of the fetal protein is strongly suggestive of an intrinsic defect of cell maturation in the hepatocyte. The measurement is much less sensitive than specific because poorly differentiated hepatoblastomas and fibrolamellar carcinomas and cholangiocarcinomas do not produce such high levels. Alpha-fetoprotein levels may not be elevated until ordinary hepatocarcinomas exceed 4 to 5 cm in diameter, which can take several years.[35] Regretably, intrahepatic portal vein dissemination of carcinoma has been observed with primary carcinomas less than 3 cm in diameter. Measuring serum alpha-fetoprotein to follow recurrences of resected liver tumors can be helpful. However, a fall from elevated to normal levels has been observed in some patients even though their tumors continued to grow.

Urinary cystathionine and pseudouridine are increased in the presence of hepatocarcinoma.[40,41] Pseudouridine is a catabolic product of transfer RNA. Nine of 13 patients with hepatocarcinoma whose serum alpha-fetoprotein concentration was normal had increased urinary pseudouridine.[41] Elevated serum copper in the absence of Wilson's disease has been used to detect hepatocarcinomas in adult patients with cirrhosis.[42] Plasma transcobalamin I (vitamin B_{12}-binding protein) and neurotensin have been elevated in patients with fibrolamellar carcinoma, which is potentially very useful because only 10 percent of those tumors have increased alpha-fetoprotein.[39,43,44] An abnormal form of prothrombin, des-gamma-carboxyprothrombin, was present in the serum of 74 percent of 70 adult patients with hepatocarcinoma.[45] Three children with hepatoblastoma also had detectable quantities in the blood as well as in the tumor cells. Coagulation tests were unaffected.[46]

Screening of children for hepatocarcinoma in the United States or other populations with a low incidence of disease would be unrewarding, but application of some of these sensitive tools to the small group of patients with precursor or associated conditions, such as glycogenosis type 1 and familial cholestatic cirrhosis, could be lifesaving.

PATHOLOGY

The subject has been reviewed in detail recently.[1] New data and controversial aspects will be discussed.

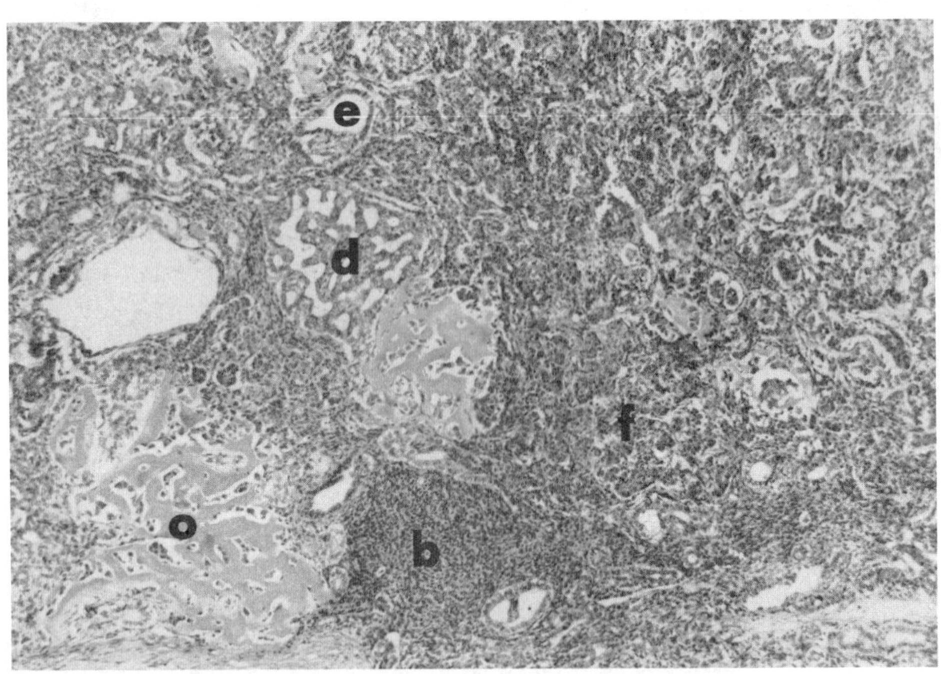

FIGURE 3 Hepatoblastoma. The diversity of cell types and varying degrees of maturation are demonstrated in this classic embryonal neoplasm. f = Fetal epithelium; e = embryonal epithelium; b = undifferentiated blastemal cells; o = osteoid; d = ductular epithelium (hematoxylin and eosin, ×63).

Hepatoblastoma

This is an embryonal tumor in the classic sense of incomplete differentiation. Ninety percent of the cases are manifest by the fourth birthday, and several have been present at birth. The usual composition reflects the complex origin of the organ, with endodermal derivatives from the original midgut outgrowth and mesodermally derived offspring of the septum transversum. Thus, parenchymal elements include hepatocytes of varying maturity, more or less closely resembling the early embryonal or later fetal liver, in association with hematopoietic cells. Primitive ducts are characteristic of the embryonal pattern, but well-differentiated ductal elements are highly unusual except in relation to diffusely infiltrating mesenchymal or blastemal cells. In that situation, they may represent residual and sometimes proliferating cholangioles of the host liver, as they are not found in metastases. However, when the ducts in the middle of a mass are in continuity with tumor cells on ultrastructural examination, it is difficult to regard them as normal remnants. It is not unusual to find portions of the epithelial component to be indistinguishable from hepatocarcinoma, even in the youngest patients.[1] Undifferentiated mesodermal or blastemal cells and stromal derivatives are present in 60 to 70 percent of cases. Usually the stroma includes osteoid and less often skeletal muscle or cartilage (Fig. 3). The osteoid is sometimes clearly related to epithelial rather than mesenchymal cells. Not infrequently, keratinizing squamous nests are found among the embryonal cells. Very rarely, the presence of ducts resembling primitive intestine, neural rosettes, and melanocytes suggests the possibility of a true teratoma.[47]

Depending on the proportions and degree of maturation of the elements, the gross appearance ranges from yellowish brown (well-differentiated epithelium) to pinkish grey (undifferentiated mesenchyme), with foci of necrosis and hemorrhage in rapidly growing tumors and firm areas when osteoid is abundant. Generally large multinodular expansile masses, hepatoblastomas appear well demarcated from the normal host liver but are not encapsulated (Fig. 4). They may invade hepatic veins and disseminate to the lungs by the time of discovery or penetrate the capsule to reach contiguous tissues and the peritoneum. Hilar lymph nodes are an early target. Staging of hepatoblastomas is done at surgery. I indicates complete resection, II microscopic residual tumor (A in liver, B outside the liver), III gross residual tumor (A spillage during surgery or gross nodal involvement, B incomplete resection with or without spillage or node involvement), and IV metastatic disease (A primary completely resected, B primary not completely resected). Among the several histologic classifications of hepatoblastoma, those of Ishak and Glunz[48] and Kasai and Watanabe[49] provide the basis for current practice. With additional suggestions from Gonzalez-Crussi et al[13] and Abenoza and colleagues,[50] we have been evaluating referrals from the Pediatric Oncology Group according to the scheme shown in Table 3.

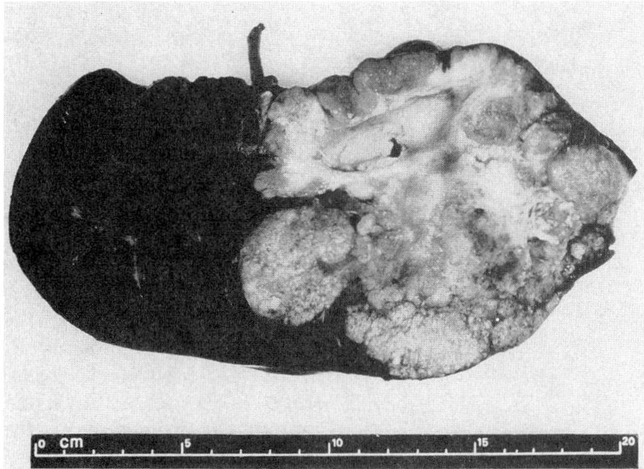

FIGURE 4 Hepatoblastoma. A multilobular expansile yellowish tan mass of mixed epithelial and mesenchymal tissues has foci of cystic degeneration and bone. It appears clearly demarcated from the host liver, which is normal, but there is no encapsulation.

TABLE 3
Classification of Hepatoblastoma

Major Categories
Epithelial
Fetal, well-differentiated
Crowded fetal
Embryonal
Macrotrabecular
Small cell undifferentiated
Mixed
Undifferentiated mesenchymal-blastemal
Minor Components
Osteoid
Keratinizing squamous epithelium
Intestinal glandular epithelium
Neuroid-melanocytic (teratoid)
Rhabdomyoblastic
Chondroid
Exceptions
Rhabdoid
Ductal (cholangioblastic)

Unresolved questions about the histologic schema are related to the following: (1) The prognostic import of the degree of differentiation of the fetal epithelial component, which often displays gradual but sometimes abrupt transition from a uniformly well-differentiated pattern with few mitoses to a more crowded but still cord- or plate-like architecture in which nuclei are more pleomorphic and mitoses more numerous (Fig. 5). Whether either or both of these types should be regarded as "favorable," as in the Wilms' tumor protocols, and subjected to less toxic adjuvant chemotherapy is uncertain. (2) The influence of the stromal derivatives on prognosis. Muraji et al[32] and Haas et al[51] suggest that mixed tumors, particularly in stage II and III cases, may respond better to chemotherapy than do pure epithelial lesions. However, the impossibility of ascertaining all the constituents or proportions of components from biopsies of unresectable tumors must be acknowledged. (3) The histogenesis of the

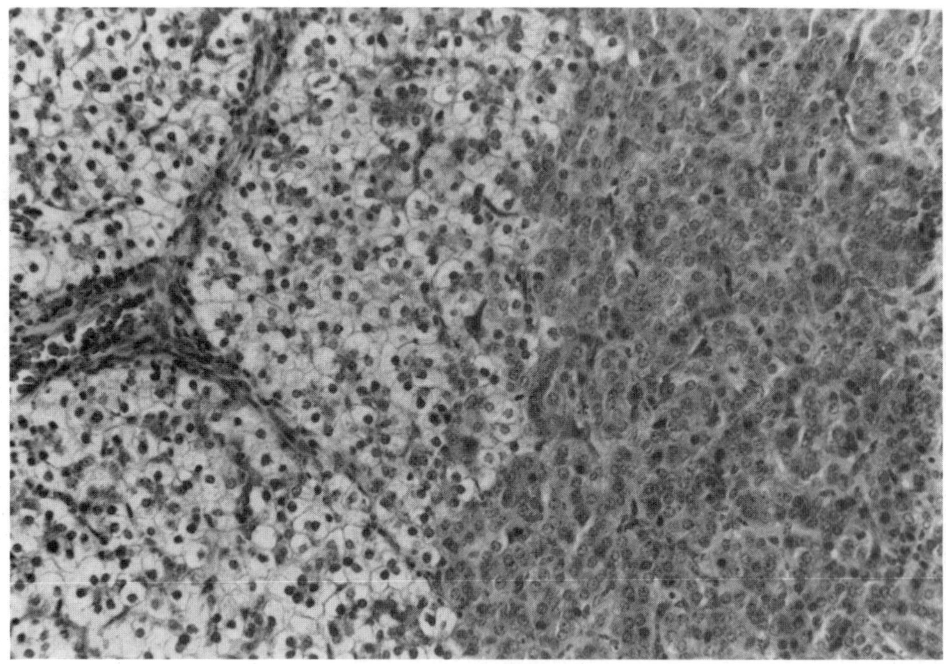

FIGURE 5 Hepatoblastoma. The well-differentiated fetal pattern is on the left. Regular cords or plates, one to three cells thick, contain hepatocytes having glycogen-rich clear cytoplasm and regular, uniform nuclei and rare mitoses (none in this picture). Immediately adjacent, on the right, the regular cordlike pattern is maintained but the cells are more numerous and crowded without being macrotrabecular (five to six cells in thickness) or primitive, as in embryonal tumors. The growth rate is increased, as reflected by the presence of two mitoses. A well-differentiated fetal pattern has been associated with an excellent rate of resection and cure. The "crowded" pattern is of uncertain prognostic significance (hematoxylin and eosin, ×160).

"rhabdoid" cell type. These are usually monomorphic malignancies of diffusely infiltrating noncohesive cells having large quantities of intermediate filaments that have been observed in several tissues. They tend to occur in young infants, to disseminate widely, and to resist chemotherapy. Immunohistochemical and ultrastructural studies indicate that the cells have both epithelial and mesenchymal characteristics.[52,53] In the liver this cell may represent a stage in the maturation of the undifferentiated mesoderm to the hepatocyte. Except for the presence of epithelial membrane antigen,[52] the immunohistochemical reactions resemble the small undifferentiated or "blastemal" cells of the hepatoblastoma exactly.[50] We have observed transition to "rhabdoid" morphology in otherwise typical hepatoblastomas (Fig. 6).

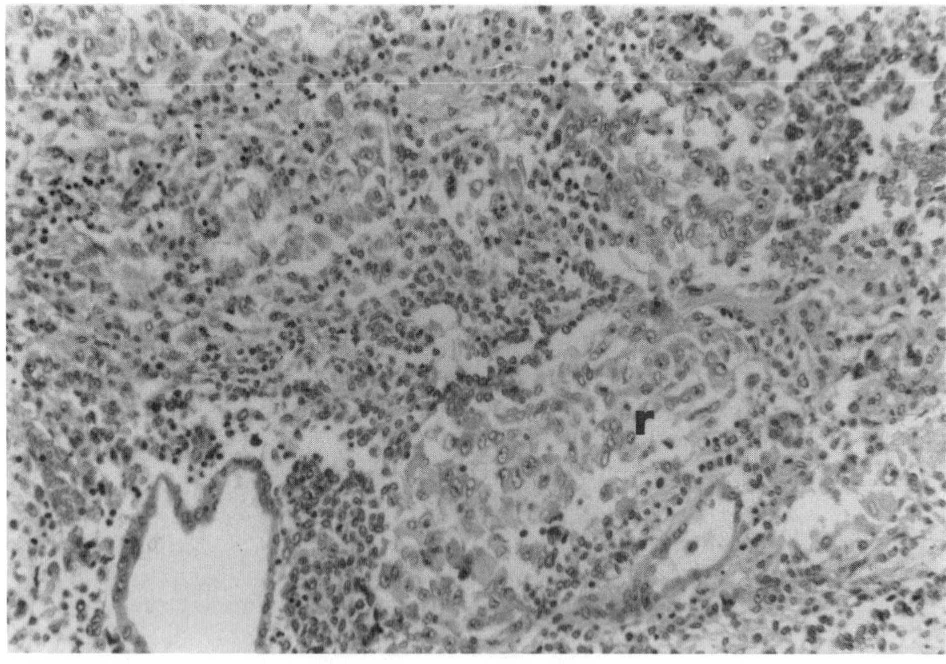

FIGURE 6 Hepatoblastoma with focal "rhabdoid" transformation. On the left, fetal-type epithelial components of the neoplasm abut what is probably a residual (non-neoplastic) bile duct. A transition to noncohesive cells of uncertain differentiation is seen in the center right (r). Those cells have larger, vesicular nuclei with prominent nucleoli and perinuclear cytoplasm that is rich in intermediate filaments, producing eosinophilic inclusions in some cells. When tumors are homogeneous for such cells, they are called "rhabdoid." In the liver they tend to occur in infants less than 1 year old and they behave badly (hematoxylin and eosin, ×160).

Hepatocarcinoma

The frequency of cirrhosis in pediatric patients with hepatocarcinoma is much less than in adults (20 to 25 percent versus 60 to 70 percent), but its presence compounds the therapeutic problem. The appearance and behavior of the tumor are the same in children as in adults, with a higher frequency of multiple nodules than with hepatoblastoma. Intrahepatic portal vein and lymphatic dissemination are often present by the time of diagnosis. There is a wide range of histologic differentiation that appears to have little or no influence on resectability or responsiveness to therapy, with only one exception, the fibrolamellar or polygonal cell tumor with fibrous stroma.

The *fibrolamellar carcinoma* is rarely associated with cirrhosis, rarely produces alpha-fetoprotein, and tends to affect young persons. Thirty-nine percent of patients are less than 20 years old and 90 percent are less than 25.[54,55] Forty-five of 80 cases were in girls and Malt[39] has called attention to the high incidence of reproductive dysfunction among the group. Fifty to 75 percent of tumors are resectable, providing a 5-year survival of 60 to 65 percent. The lesions tend to be single, large bulky masses of light tan to yellow-orange color with distinct borders. Histologically, large polygonal cells are clustered in small groups separated by bands of well-organized collagen (Fig. 7). In three teenagers, Goodman et al[56] found mucus-producing pseudoglands associated with otherwise typical fibrolamellar histology. The epidemiologic and morphologic differences between the tumor and ordinary hepatocarcinoma are also reflected in the secretion of neurotensin by this lesion and by histochemical and ultrastructural evidence of neurosecretory granules.[57] None of the cases has been associated with clinically evident hormonal effects, and the tumors do not resemble morphologically any of the several cases of primary hepatic carcinoid tumors that we have examined.[1] Thus, the exact histogenesis of this epithelial neoplasm is unresolved.

Adenoma and Focal Nodular Hyperplasia

Each condition contributed 2 percent of the collected series. They have both been observed in patients with glycogen storage disease[15] and women using oral contraceptives, but only the adenoma seems to be causally related to the pill.[19,22] Both are usually solitary and expansile, but the adenoma is more often multiple than nodular hyperplasia and is generally encapsulated. Both consist primarily of well-differentiated hepatocytes arranged in cords or plates but without the normal lobular pattern. However, the cells of adenomas may be slightly larger than normal hepatocytes and their nuclei can be slightly pleomorphic. There are no bile ducts or portal tracts in adenomas, but focal nodular hyperplasia has septa radiating from a central region of scarring in which ducts can be numerous. In a needle biopsy, these distinguishing features may be unavailable.

Vascular Tumors

Hemangioendotheliomas of infancy are the most common benign tumors of the liver and are generally regarded as hamartomas rather than neoplasms. Nevertheless, they may be symptomatic as mass lesions, because of high-output congestive heart failure due to arteriovenous shunting, or due to rupture with intraperitoneal hemorrhage. Occasionally, thrombocytopenia and intravascular coagulation have been observed.[38] Classification depends on the degree of endothelial

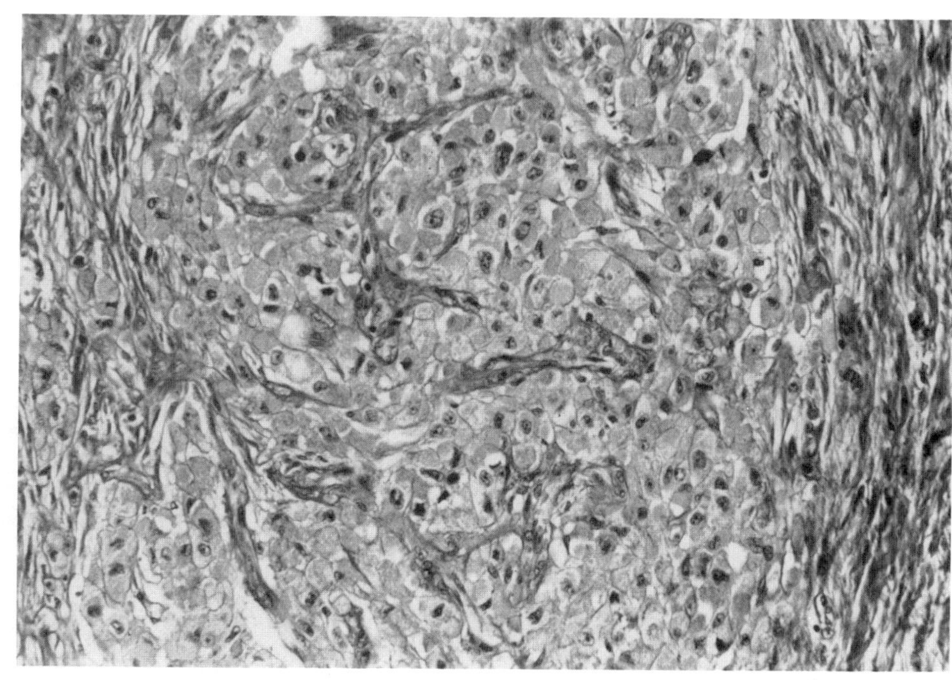

FIGURE 7 Fibrolamellar carcinoma. Nests of large polygonal cells with abundant eosinophilic cytoplasm and slightly pleomorphic nuclei are separated by distinct bundles of collagen. Ordinary hepatocarcinomas have little fibrous tissue unless there is a ductal (cholangiolar) component. This was from a 19-year-old girl with a normal serum alpha-fetoprotein. Resection was curative (trichrome, ×160).

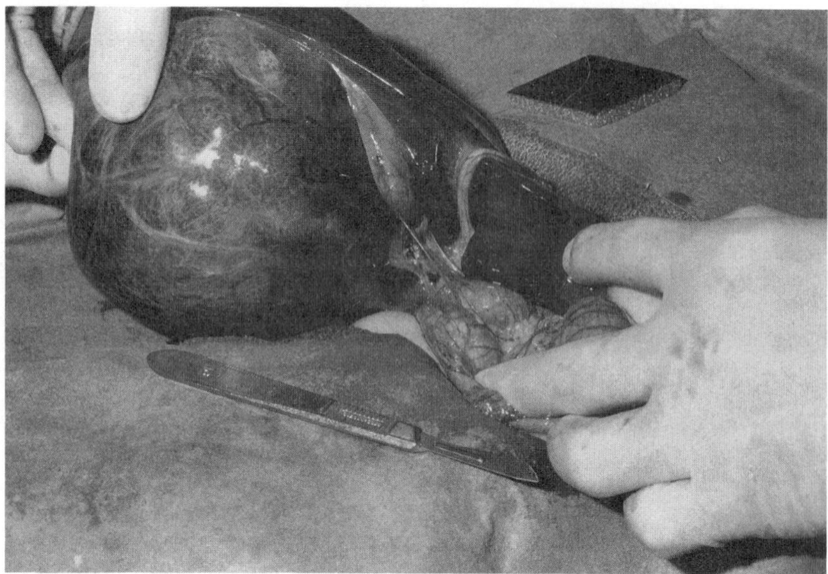

FIGURE 8 Mesenchymal hamartoma at surgery. An 11-month-old boy presented with a distended abdomen. Ultrasonography revealed a multilocular cystic mass. It protruded from the right lobe inferiorly and was completely resectable.

cell proliferation and the size of the channels. When actively dividing vasoformative cells are plentiful and not quite organized into channels, the lesions are called type II hemangioendotheliomas and occasionally have been disseminated.[58] Type I lesions are more bland, often calcified, with few mitoses. Most cases of both types regress spontaneously or respond well to corticosteroid therapy. However, perfectly bland type I lesions have been followed, on at least two occasions, by angiosarcomas of the liver 4 to 5 years later. At that point the atypical, rapidly dividing neoplastic cells were widely dispersed through the sinusoids as well as filling vascular lumina and replacing parenchymal tissues. Twenty-two angiosarcomas have been reported in children.[59] Cutaneous hemangiomas were often present, and sometimes the spleen and other organs have been involved. One infant had documented exposure to arsenicals. No other predisposing conditions were noted in children, whereas two young adults with neurofibromatosis have had hepatic angiosarcomas.[60]

Mesenchymal Tumors

The mesenchymal hamartoma of infancy can be present at birth, grown to an enormous size, and cause heart failure because of arteriovenous shunting. It may bulge from the liver and even become pedunculated, but it has no capsule (Figs.

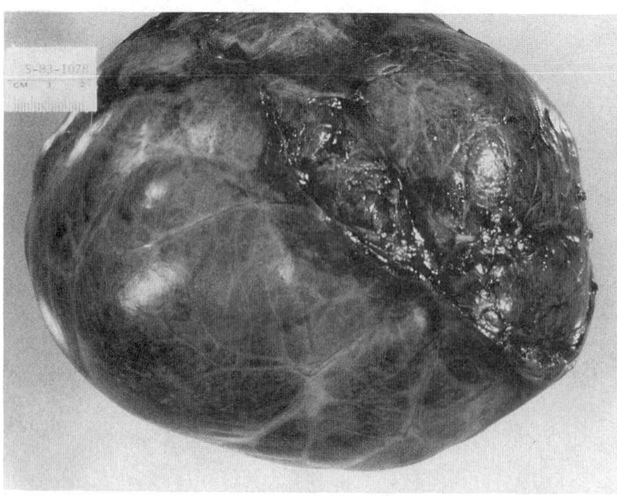

FIGURE 9 Mesenchymal hamartoma after resection. The huge bulging mass weighed 1,250 grams and consisted mainly of tense cysts. The patient had about 35 percent of the liver left and recovered uneventfully.

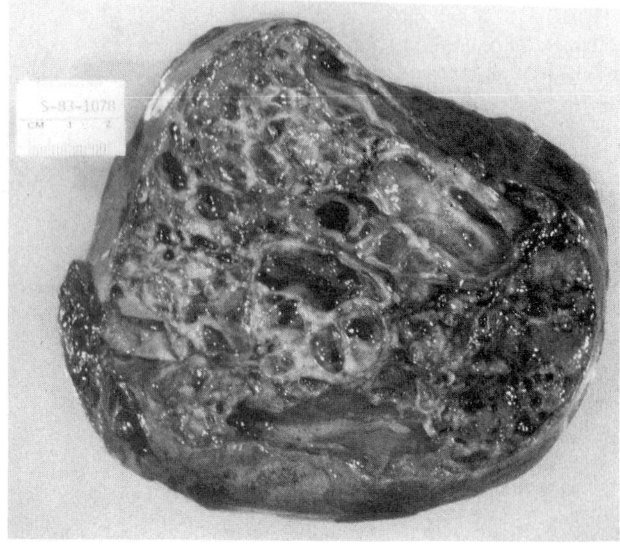

FIGURE 10 Mesenchymal hamartoma after sectioning. Multiple cysts filled with serous fluid are separated by myxomatous stroma.

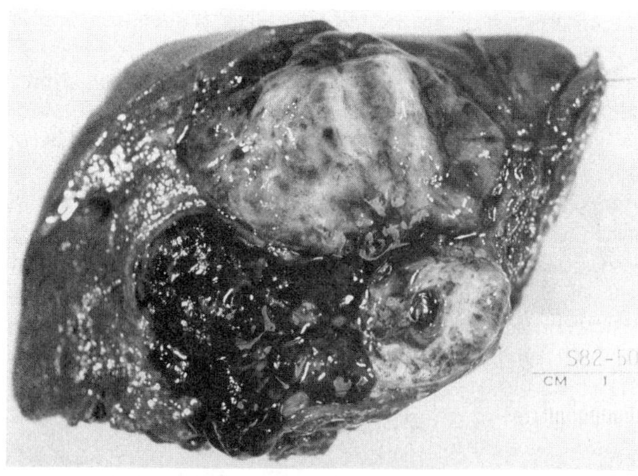

FIGURE 11 Undifferentiated sarcoma replaces most of the right lobe in a 6-year-old boy. A multinodular fleshy mass with large areas of hemorrhage and cystic degeneration, it gives the impression of encapsulation but in fact insinuates into surrounding host liver.

8 and 9). Typically, there are multiple large cystic spaces having a flat lining and serous fluid content (Fig. 10). The stroma is myxomatous and bland. At the interface with the remaining parenchyma, bile ducts proliferate actively. There is no malignant potential, so unresectable cystic lesions can be treated by drainage and marsupialization.[1]

Malignant mesenchymomas are so named because of the multiple derivatives of stromal cells they contain, including myxoid, chondroid, muscular, bony, and fibrous tissues. Since the report of Stocker and Ishak,[61] most authors have referred to the lesion as an undifferentiated sarcoma, even though many of the tumors have indeed developed regions of fibrous histiocytoma, liposarcoma, and even benign pericytoma.[1] Half the cases have presented in children at between 6 and 10 years. They tend to be huge and unresectable at discovery, when the liver is found to be replaced by a variegated, hemorrhagic, and cystic mass of greyish white soft tissue (Fig. 11). Microscopically, the undifferentiated aspect is characterized by huge, bizarre cells having prominent glycoprotein inclusions associated with small nondescript cells and abundant myxoid stroma (Fig. 12). Keating and Taylor[62] found by immunochemistry suggestions of a histiocytic origin, but histogenesis remains uncertain.

Rhabdomyosarcomas of the biliary tract tend to form polypoid masses of soft, gelatinous pinkish grey tissue that tend to obstruct bile flow. The cells are generally primitive embryonal forms with rare, ill-defined muscle filaments. Any of the ducts, including ampulla and gallbladder, can be affected. Patients have ranged in age from infancy to the teens. Two of the eight cases reported by Geoffray et al[63] were resectable, but both recurred. In the series of Mihara et al,[64] six of nine patients responded well to vigorous chemotherapy and radiotherapy.

Leiomyosarcomas have been observed in three young girls, one of whom survived after resection. Granular cell myoblastomas, which actually arise from Schwann cells, are benign tumors that can arise in the bile ducts. Eighty-seven percent of the cases in the United States have been in blacks. Two have been described in teenagers.

Bile Duct Epithelial Tumors

Biliary cystadenomas with mesenchymal stroma are benign tumors in young women but have malignant potential in middle age. Carcinomas have been observed in the remnants of choledochal cysts, so surgeons have learned to excise the affected region.[65] Two cases of biliary carcinoma have been reported in young women with chronic ulcerative colitis and sclerosing cholangitis. One patient was 17 years old.[66]

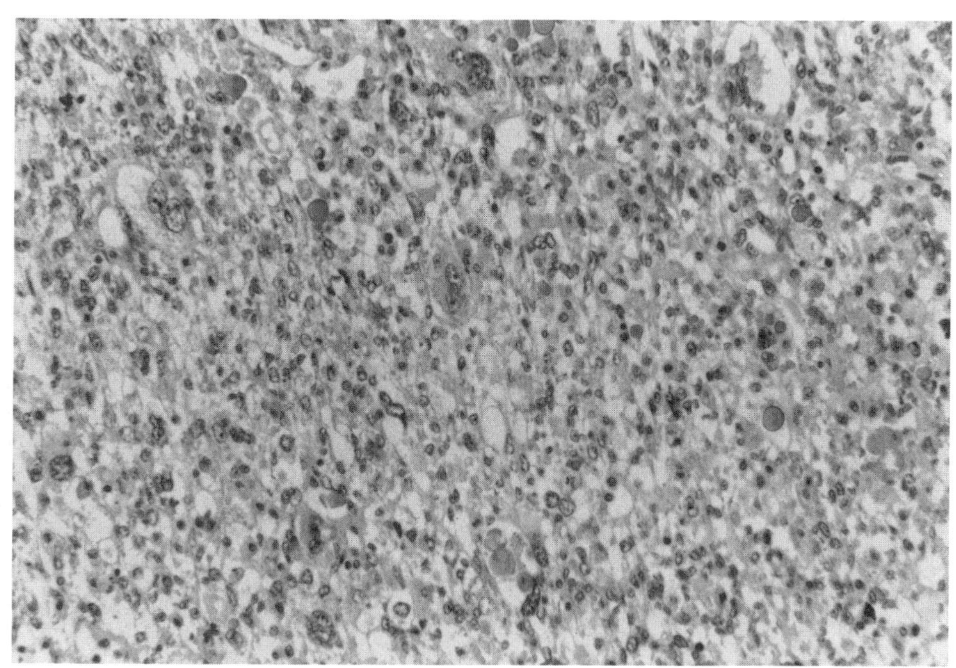

FIGURE 12 Undifferentiated sarcoma. Scattered among numerous small and nondescript cells are several giant cells with multilobate vesicular nuclei having prominent nucleoli. Large globular inclusions of glycoprotein are regularly present in the cytoplasm of such cells and sometimes spill out into the adjacent loose ground substance. Portions of such tumors have differentiated into fibroblasts and fibrohistiocytic, lipoblastic, and chondroid cells (hematoxylin and eosin, ×160).

Teratomas

Primary teratomas are rare and usually affect females, and half contain undifferentiated elements. When yolk sac tissue is present or the tumor is entirely yolk sac in type, alpha fetoprotein levels can be strikingly increased. Ninety percent of the patients are infants. Treatment is surgical.[67]

Inflammatory Pseudotumor versus Lymphoma

Inflammatory pseudotumor of the liver has been described by Anthony and Telesinghe[68] in 17 cases. Six patients were less than 12 years old. They presented with fever, abdominal pain, and/or vomiting. Jaundice was evident in four. Weight loss and diarrhea were also noted. There were solitary masses in eight patients, multiple nodules in four. The clinical impression and initial pathologic diagnosis may be confused with malignancy. But the histologic features of dense plasma cell infiltrates associated with active fibroplasia are indications of a chronic inflammatory process. The etiology is unknown, but some tumors have regressed with steroid therapy. Primary *lymphomas* of the liver of children are very rare. They are monomorphous infiltrates without fibrosis.[69] *Malignant histiocytosis* frequently involves the liver, with portal and sinusoidal infiltrates of erythrophagocytic macrophages and anaplastic precursors. Patients are often jaundiced, and needle biopsy of the liver is recommended for diagnosis in a patient with fever, weight loss, hepatosplenomegaly, and a nondiagnostic bone marrow examination.[70] It must be distinguished by surface marker studies from peripheral T-cell lymphoma.[71] Involvement of the liver in various forms of leukemia is common but only rarely of clinical significance.

Non-neoplastic Hepatic Masses

Other non-neoplastic tumors include parasitic cysts, biliary and simple cysts, and nodular regenerative hyperplasia. All but the latter tend to present as masses and rarely because of jaundice. Most are diagnosed readily by a combination of imaging techniques, particularly ultrasonography. Nodular regeneration may present with signs of portal hypertension and is sometimes associated with collagen-vascular disease. The diagnosis is difficult even on biopsy, but neoplasia can be excluded.

Secondary Neoplasia of the Liver

Secondary involvement of the liver by neuroblastoma is the most common type of metastasis in children. The primitive cells infiltrating sinusoids may be mistaken for hepatoblastoma in routine microscopic studies of small biopsies. Other malignancies spreading to the liver include Wilms' tumor, rhabdomyosarcoma, Ewing's sarcoma, and ovarian germ cell tumors.[72]

TREATMENT

The primary goal in treating liver neoplasms is complete surgical removal. The tendency of tumors to reach very large size before discovery and an anatomy that allows interlobar spread are handicaps. For benign tumors, such as vascular and mesenchymal hamartomas, focal nodular hyperplasia, and adenomas, extensive surgery may be unnecessary. Many of the lesions have responded to medical management or simple procedures, and many are stable indefinitely.[38] Therefore, vigorous efforts are made to reach a diagnosis preoperatively. When that is not possible or malignancy is suspected, surgical resection is attempted. Newer imaging modalities have been helpful in delineating the extent of involvement preoperatively.[37] When surgery for a malignancy is deemed to be too risky, preoperative chemotherapy has proved to be effective in shrinking some hepatoblastomas and some sarcomas to the point of resectability.[14,73,74] Various combinations of drugs have been tried. Doxorubicin (Adriamycin) seemed to be the most important ingredient in the study of Andrassy et al,[75] but three of six predominantly epithelial hepatoblastomas failed to respond. Since 1981, Gauthier et al[76] have routinely used Adriamycin in combination with vincristine, cyclophosphamide, 5-fluorouracil, or cisplatin, and they were successful in achieving resectability in 9 of 11 cases.

The same or similar combinations of drugs are then employed postoperatively. Nine patients with hepatoblastoma so treated by Gauthier et al[76] were cured, and there have been case reports of pulmonary metastases being eliminated by such intense regiments.[75,77] However, the incidence of severe hematologic toxicity in the Children's Cancer Study Group (CCSG)—Southwest Oncology Group (SWOG) study of 57 patients with hepatic malignancies given combination chemotherapy was 50 percent, and three children died of the complication.[78]

It seems advisable, therefore, particularly for hepatoblastomas, to re-evaluate the histologic features with the goal of defining a "favorable" histologic pattern for which chemotherapy might be reduced, as in the case of Wilms' tumor. When completely resected lesions (Stage I), which comprise 30 to 60 percent of different series, have been reviewed according to histologic subtype, the "pure" or "predominantly" fetal tumors were found in several series to have a good prognosis even without adjuvant therapy.[1,13,49,79] The most recent analysis of the 168 hepatoblastomas collected by CCSG-SWOG found 28 of 90 fetal cases to be resectable, and 87 percent of them survived 48 months.[51] Embryonal tumors performed exceptionally well in that series too, with 20 of 50 cases being resectable and 63 percent of those surviving 48 months. All received combination chemotherapy. Tumors having a macrotrabecular growth pattern were uniformly unresectable, but 9 of 18 survived 48 months, which also is much more favorable than in all other reports to date. None of the small cell undifferentiated tumors was resectable, and all 10 children died within 24 months. CCSG and the Pediatric Oncology Group are undertaking a study to treat Stage I well-differentiated hepatoblastoma with doxorubicin for 4 months, while more advanced disease and unfavorable histologic patterns will be treated with cisplatin, vincristine and 5-fluorouracil, or cisplatin and doxorubicin.

Hepatocarcinomas are resectable only 10 to 20 percent of the time. After surgery, cures are obtained with adjuvant chemotherapy in only 25 to 30 percent of cases. Ogita et al[80] were able to deliver chemotherapeutic agents suspended in Lipiodol directly into the hepatic artery of adults, with lower toxicity and longer retention of the agents by the hepatocarcinomas. This has yet to be used for children. Starzl and others have been performing liver transplants in selected cases with modest success. Many of the failures were in the precyclosporine era, so early death due to graft rejection or other complications limited evaluation. More recently, Starzl et al[81] reported success in three of six patients with unresectable fibrolamellar carcinomas. On the other hand, they also concluded that aggressive resection was preferable, as only one of eight patients having subtotal hepatectomy suffered a recurrence.

REFERENCES

1. Weinberg AG, Finegold MJ. Primary hepatic tumors in childhood. In: Finegold MJ, ed. Pathology of neoplasia in children and adolescents. Philadelphia: WB Saunders, 1986: 333.
2. DePotter CR, Robberecht E, Laureys G, Cuvelier C. Hepatitis B related childhood hepatocellular carcinoma. Cancer 1987; 60:414.
3. Kew MC, Macerollo P. Effect of age on the etiologic role of the hepatitis B virus in hepatocellular carcinoma in blacks. Gastroenterology 1988; 94:439.
4. Wu TC, Tong MJ, Hwang B, et al. Primary hepatocellular carcinoma and hepatitis B infection during childhood. Hepatology 1987; 7:46.
5. Chen WJ, Lee JC, Hung WT. Primary malignant tumor of liver in infants and children in Taiwan. J Pediatr Surg 1988; 23:457.
6. Shafritz DA, Shouval D, Sherman HI, et al. Integration of hepatitis B virus DNA into the genome of liver cells in chronic liver disease and hepatocellular carcinoma. N Engl J Med 1981; 305:1067.
7. Rogler CE, Sherman M, Su CY, et al. Deletion in chromosome llp associated with a hepatitis B integration site in hepatocellular carcinoma. Science 1985; 230:319.
8. Koufos A, Hansen MF, Copeland NG, et al. Loss of heterozygosity in three embryonal tumours suggests a common pathogenetic mechanism. Nature 1985; 316:330.
9. Ohaki Y, Misugi K, Sasaki Y, et al. Hepatitis B surface antigen positive hepatocellular carcinoma in children. Report of a case and review of the literature. Cancer 1983; 51:822.
10. Baffet G, Deugnier Y, Lehry D, et al. A study of oncogene activation in human hepatocellular carcinoma. Hepatology 1986; 6:1212.
11. Larouze B, Salmot G, Lustbader ED, et al. Host responses to hepatitis B infection in patients with primary hepatic carcinoma in their families. Lancet 1976; ii:534.
12. Dahms BB. Hepatoma in familial cholestatic cirrhosis in childhood—its occurrence in twin brothers. Arch Pathol Lab Med 1979; 103:30.
13. Gonzalez-Crussi F, Upton MP, Maurer HS. Hepatoblastoma: attempt at characterization of histologic subtypes. Am J Surg Pathol 1982; 6:599.
14. Mahour GH, Wogu GU, Siegel SE, et al. Improved survival in infants and children with primary malignant liver tumors. Am J Surg 1983; 146:236.
15. Coire CI, Qizilbash AH, Castelli MF. Hepatic adenomata in Type la glycogen storage disease. Arch Pathol Lab Med 1987; 111:166.
16. Iqbal MJ, Wilkinson ML, Johnson PJ, Williams R. Sex steroid receptor proteins in foetal, adult and malignant human liver tissue. Br J Cancer 1983; 48:791.
17. Nagasue N, Yukaya H, Chang Y-C, et al. Active uptake of testosterone by androgen receptors of hepatocellular carcinoma in humans. Cancer 1986; 57:2162.
18. Ohnishi S, Murakami T, Moriyama T, et al. Androgen and estrogen receptors in hepatocellular carcinoma and in the surrounding noncancerous liver tissue. Hepatology 1986; 6:440.
19. Chandra RS, Kapur SP, Kelleher J Jr, et al. Benign hepatocellular tumors in the young. Arch Pathol Lab Med 1984; 108:168.
20. Forman D, Vincent TJ, Doll R. Cancer of the liver and use of oral contraceptives. Br Med J 1986; 292:1357.
21. Neuberger J, Forman D, Doll R, Williams R. Oral contraceptives and hepatocellular carcinoma. Br Med J 1986; 292:1355.
22. Stocker JT, Ishak KG. Focal nodular hyperplasia of the liver: a study of 21 pediatric cases. Cancer 1981; 48:336.
23. Meyer P, LiVolsi V, Cornog J. Hepatoblastoma associated with an oral contraceptive. Lancet 1974; ii:1387.
24. Kingston JE, Herbert A, Draper GJ, et al. Association between hepatoblastoma and polyposis coli. Arch Dis Child 1983; 58:959.
25. Garber JE, Li FP, Krush AJ, et al. Familial adenomatous polyposis in hepatoblastoma survivors. J Natl Cancer Inst 1988; 80:1626.
26. Bodmer WF, Bailey CL, Bodmer J, et al. Localization of the gene for familial adenomatous polyposis on chromosome 5. Nature 1987; 328:614.
27. Patterson K, Kupur SP, Chandra RS. Hepatocellular carcinoma in a noncirrhotic infant after prolonged parenteral nutrition. J Pediatr 1985; 106:797.
28. Kaufman SS, Wood P, Shaw BW Jr, et al. Hepatocarcinoma in a child with the Alagille syndrome. Am J Dis Child 1987; 141:698.
29. Adams PC. Hepatocellular carcinoma associated with arteriohepatic dysplasia. Digest Dis Sci 1986; 31:438.
30. Mundy GR. Hypercalcemia of malignancy revisited. J Clin Invest 1988; 82:1.
31. Hanawa Y, Ise T, Hasegawa H, Sano R. Serum cholesterol in children with hepatoma. Clin Oncol 1971; 12:129.
32. Muraji T, Woolley MM, Sinatra F, et al. The prognostic implication of hypercholesterolemia in infants and children with hepatoblastoma. J Pediatr Surg 1985; 20:228.
33. Galifer RB, Sultan C, Margueritte G, Barneon G. Testosterone-producing hepatoblastoma in a 3-year old boy with precocious puberty. J Pediatr Surg 1985; 20:713.
34. Navarro C, Corretger JM, Sancho A, et al. Paraneoplastic precocious puberty. Cancer 1985; 56:1725.
35. Okuda K. Early recognition of hepatocellular carcinoma. Hepatology 1986; 6:729.
36. Tatsuta M, Yamamoto R, Kasugai H, et al. Cytohistologic diagnosis of neoplasms of the liver by ultrasonically guided fine-needle aspiration biopsy. Cancer 1984; 54:1682.
37. Stark DD. Liver. In: Stark DD, Bradley WG Jr, eds. Magnetic Resonance Imaging. St. Louis: CV Mosby, 1988: 934.
38. Holcomb GW III, O'Neill JA Jr, Mahboubi S, Bishop HC. Experience with hepatic hemangioendothelioma in infancy and childhood. J Pediatr Surg 1988; 23:661.
39. Malt RA. Fibrolamellar hepatocellular carcinoma (CPC). N Engl J Med 1987; 317:556.
40. Geiser CF, Shih VE. Cystathioninuria and its origin in children with hepatoblastoma. J Pediatr 1980; 96:72.
41. Tamura S, Amuro Y, Nakano T, et al. Urinary excretion of pseudouridine in patients with hepatocellular carcinoma. Cancer 1986; 57:1571.
42. Miatto O, Casaril M, Gabrielli GB, et al. Diagnostic and prognostic value of serum copper and plasma fibrinogen in hepatic carcinoma. Cancer 1985; 55:774.
43. Collier NA, Bloom SR, Hodgson HJF, et al. Neurotensin secretion by fibrolamellar carcinoma of the liver. Lancet 1984; i:538.
44. Wheeler K, Pritchard J, Luck W, Rossiter M. Transcobalamin 1 as a "marker" for fibrolamellar hepatoma. Med Pediatr Oncol 1986; 14:227.
45. Soulier J-P, Gozin D, Lefrere J-J. A new method to assay des-gamma-carboxy prothrombin. Gastroenterology 1986; 91:1258.
46. Motohara K, Endo F, Matsuda I, Iwamasa T. Acarboxy prothrombin (PIVKA-II) as a marker of hepatoblastoma in infants. J Pediatr Gastroenterol Nutr 1987; 6:42.
47. Manivel C, Wick MR, Abenoza P, Dehner LP. Teratoid hepatoblastoma. Cancer 1986; 57:2168.
48. Ishak KG, Glunz PR. Hepatoblastoma and hepatocarcinoma in infancy and childhood. Report of 47 cases. Cancer 1967; 20:396.
49. Kasai M, Watanabe I. Histologic classification of liver-cell carcinoma in infancy and childhood and its clinical evaluation. A study of 70 cases collected in Japan. Cancer 1970; 25:551.
50. Abenoza P, Manivel JC, Wick M, et al. Hepatoblastoma: an immunohistochemical and ultrastructural study. Hum Pathol 1987; 18:1025.
51. Haas J, Musczynski K, Krailo M, et al. Relationship of cytohistopathology to outcome in malignant epithelial hepatic tumors of childhood. Lab Invest 1988; 58:4P.
52. Parham DM, Peiper SC, Robicheaux G, et al. Malignant rhabdoid tumor of the liver. Arch Pathol Lab Med 1988; 112:61.
53. Uri A, Perilongo G, Evans A. A new subtype of hepatocellular malignancy in children distinguished from hepatoblastoma and hepatocellular carcinoma by clinical, light, electron microscopic and immunohistochemical studies. Lab Invest 1988; 58:97A.
54. Berman MM, Libbey NP, Foster JH. Hepatocellular carcinoma. Polygonal cell type and fibrous stroma—an atypical variant with a favorable prognosis. Cancer 1980; 46:1448.

55. Berman MA, Burnham JA, Sheahan DG. Fibrolamellar carcinoma of the liver: an immunohistochemical study of nineteen cases and a review of the literature. Human Pathol 1988; 19:784.
56. Goodman ZD, Ishak KG, Langloss JM, et al. Combined hepatocellular-cholangiocarcinoma. Cancer 1985; 55:124.
57. Payne CM, Nagle RB, Paplanus SH, et al. Fibrolamellar carcinoma of liver: a primary malignant oncocytic carcinoid? Ultrastruct Pathol 1986; 10:539.
58. Dehner LP, Ishak KG. Vascular tumors of the liver in infants and children. Arch Pathol 1971; 92:101.
59. Alt B, Hafez GR, Trigg M, et al. Angiosarcoma of the liver and spleen in an infant. Pediatr Pathol 1985; 4:331.
60. Lederman SM, Martin EC, Laffey KT, Lefkowitch JH. Hepatic neurofibromatosis, malignant Schwannoma, and angiosarcoma in von Recklinghausen's disease. Gastroenterology 1987; 92:234.
61. Stocker JT, Ishak KG. Undifferentiated (embryonal) sarcoma of the liver. Cancer 1978; 42:336.
62. Keating S, Taylor GP. Undifferentiated (embryonal) sarcoma of the liver: ultrastructural and immunohistochemical similarities with malignant fibrous histiocytoma. Hum Pathol 1985; 16:693.
63. Geoffray A, Couanet D, Montagne JP, et al. Ultrasonography and computed tomography for diagnosis and follow-up of biliary duct rhabdomyosarcomas in children. Pediatr Radiol 1987; 17:127.
64. Mihara S, Matsumoto H, Tokunaga F, et al. Botryoid rhabdomyosarcoma of the gallbladder in a child. Cancer 1982; 49:812.
65. Bloustein PA. Association of carcinoma with congenital cystic conditions of the liver and bile ducts. Am J Gastroenterol 1977; 67:40.
66. Ham JM, MacKenzie DC. Primary carcinoma of the extrahepatic bile ducts. Surg Gynecol Obstet 1964; 118:977.
67. Todani T, Tabuchi K, Watanabe Y, et al. True hepatic teratoma with high alpha-fetoprotein in serum. J Pediatr Surg 1977; 12:591.
68. Anthony PP, Telesinghe PU. Inflammatory pseudotumor of the liver. J Clin Pathol 1986; 39:761.
69. Miller ST, Wollner N, Meyers PA, et al. Primary hepatic or hepatosplenic non Hodgkins' lymphoma in children. Cancer 1983; 52:2285.
70. Jurco S III, Starling K, Hawkins EP. Malignant histiocytosis in childhood: morphologic considerations. Human Pathol 1983; 14:1059.
71. Kadin ME, Kamoun M, Lamberg J. Erythrophagocytic T γ lymphoma: a clinical pathologic entity resembling malignant histiocytosis. N Engl J Med 1981; 304:648.
72. Dehner LP. Pediatric surgical pathology. 2nd edition, Baltimore: Williams & Wilkins, 1987: 500.
73. Harris MB, Shen S, Weiner MA, et al. Treatment of primary undifferentiated sarcoma of the liver with surgery and chemotherapy. Cancer 1984; 54:2859.
74. Horowitz ME, Etcubanas E, Webber BL, et al. Hepatic undifferentiated (embryonal) sarcoma and rhabdomyosarcoma in children. Cancer 1987; 59:396.
75. Andrassy RJ, Brennan LP, Siegel MM, et al. Preoperative chemotherapy for hepatoblastoma in children: report of six cases. J Pediatr Surg 1970; 15:517.
76. Gauthier F, Valayer J, Thai BL, et al. Hepatoblastoma and hepatocarcinoma in children: analysis of a series of 29 cases. J Pediatr Surg 1986; 21:424.
77. Pritchard J, da Cunha A, Cornbleet NA, et al. Alpha fetoprotein (AFP) monitoring of response to adriamycin in hepatoblastoma. J Pediatr Surg 1982; 17:429.
78. Evans AE, Land VJ, Newton WA, et al. Combination chemotherapy (vincristine, adriamycin, cyclophosphamide, and 5-fluorouracil) in the treatment of children with malignant hepatoma. Cancer 1982; 50:821.
79. Lack EE, Neave C, Vawter GF. Hepatoblastoma, a clinical and pathological study of 54 cases. Am J Surg Pathol 1982; 6:693.
80. Ogita S, Tokiwa K, Taniguchi H, Takahashi T. Intra-arterial injection of anti-tumor drugs dispersed in lipid contrast medium: a choice for initially unresectable hepatoblastoma in infants. J Pediatr Surg 1987; 22:412.
81. Starzl TE, Iwatsuki S, Shaw BW Jr, et al. Treatment of fibrolamellar hepatoma with partial or total hepatectomy and transplantation of the liver. Surg Gynecol Obstet 1986; 162:145.

PART 8

Disorders of Bilirubin Metabolism

William Spivak, M.D.

Bilirubin IXα, the naturally occurring form of bilirubin in humans that is routinely called bilirubin, is the end-product of heme catabolism. It serves no physiologic function except perhaps as a biologic antioxidant.[1] In the unconjugated (or more correctly termed "unesterifed") form, it is potentially toxic to the neonatal central nervous system because of the lipophilicity it shares with the lipids of the brain and the permeability of the blood-brain barrier in the neonatal period. It is this potential toxicity that has made the study of bilirubin metabolism so important.

As part of the process of removing this toxic, nonpolar bilirubin from the serum, bilirubin is taken up by the liver and conjugated to a polar monosaccharide prior to its excretion in the aqueous milieu of bile. A small amount of conjugated bilirubin may normally reflux back into the blood. Thus, two types of bilirubin are found in the serum. Unconjugated bilirubin (indirect-reacting) is associated with noncholestatic jaundice, whereas conjugated (direct-reacting) bilirubin is most commonly associated with obstructive or cholestatic jaundice, although it does exist in trace amounts even in normal serum.[2] The diagnosis of unconjugated hyperbilirubinemia is usually established on the basis of an indirect-reacting bilirubin exceeding 85 percent of the total bilirubin. However, since measurement of bilirubin values varies considerably from laboratory to laboratory,[3] and measurement of direct-reacting bilirubin values is notoriously inaccurate at total bilirubin levels of less than 5 mg per deciliter,[3,4] it is necessary for each clinician to be familiar with the limitations of the local laboratory before establishing a diagnosis of cholestatic versus noncholestatic hyperbilirubinemia. One should also be aware of the possibility that a patient with indirect-reacting hyperbilirubinemia can occasionally develop direct-reacting hyperbilirubinemia. Thus, an infant with hemolytic disease with an initial indirect-

TABLE 1
Types of Bilirubin

I. Unconjugated Bilirubin
- A. "Free" bilirubin
  1. In Z,Z conformation: insoluble
  2. Diffuses across blood-brain barrier
  3. In Z,E; E,E; or E,Z conformation (photobilirubin): water soluble and excreted without conjugation
- B. Albumin or "bound" bilirubin
  1. Noncovalently bound
  2. Not cleared by the kidney
  3. Does not readily cross the blood-brain barrier

II. Conjugated Bilirubin (free)
- A. Predominantly conjugated with glucuronic acid
- B. Increased monoconjugates in Gilbert disease, Crigler-Najjar syndrome type II, and newborns
- C. Diconjugates are more soluble than monoconjugates
- D. Diconjugates predominate in human bile
- E. Cleared by the kidney in cholestasis

III. Protein-Bilirubin Conjugates
- A. Form in plasma by nonenzymatic covalent linkage to albumin in patients with cholestasis
- B. Not excreted in urine
- C. Remain in serum for several weeks after cause of cholestasis is resolved

reacting hyperbilirubinemia may develop conjugated hyperbilirubinemia as a result of a common bile duct gallstone or the inspissated bile syndrome. Alternatively, direct-reacting hyperbilirubinemia may persist for several weeks after the resolution of bile duct obstruction or hepatitis. This persistent direct hyperbilirubinemia occurs because of covalent linkage of conjugated bilirubin to albumin (Table 1).[5] These bile-protein conjugates are not excreted in urine as are normal bilirubin conjugates and therefore remain in serum until albumin, which has a half-life of 17 to 20 days, is degraded.

TABLE 2
Mechanisms of Unconjugated Hyperbilirubinemia in the Newborn

I. Increased "Load" of Bilirubin
- A. Increased RBC volume, especially with delayed clamping of the umbilical cord
- B. Increased RBC turnover
  1. Normal—decreased half-life of RBC
  2. Abnormal—increased intravascular erythrocyte destruction
     - a. Isoimmunization—Rh or ABO incompatibility
     - b. Erythrocyte biochemical defects—G6PD, pyruvate kinase, or hexokinase deficiency
     - c. Structural abnormalities of erythrocytes: spherocytosis, elliptocytosis, pyknocytosis
- C. Sequestered blood
  1. Subdural hematoma/cephalohematoma
  2. Ecchymoses
  3. Hemangiomas
- D. Increased enterohepatic circulation of bilirubin

II. Activity of Glucuronyl Transferase (GT)
- A. Transiently decreased in every newborn
- B. Markedly diminished GT activity in Crigler-Najjar syndrome
  1. Type I—no response to phenobarbital
  2. Type II—bilirubin decreases with phenobarbital
- C. Mild decrease with Gilbert syndrome
- D. Decreased activity in hypopituitarism or hypothyroidism

III. Decreased hepatic ligandin

IV. Multifactorial
- A. Sepsis—increased hemolysis, decreased uptake, decreased excretion
- B. Prematurity—decreased GT level, acidosis, sepsis, total parenteral nutrition, drugs, patent ductus venosus, transfusions

PHYSIOLOGIC JAUNDICE AND NEONATAL BILIRUBIN METABOLISM

Normal adult serum bilirubin levels do not exceed 2 mg per deciliter, whereas every newborn infant has serum bilirubin levels that exceed this value. In the absence of hemolytic anemia, cholestatic disease, or hereditary forms of unconjugated hyperbilirubinemia, neonatal hyperbilirubinemia is known as physiologic jaundice. Table 2 summarizes both physiologic and nonphysiologic reasons for unconjugated hyperbilirubinemia in the newborn.

Physiologic jaundice results from the interplay of a series of hematologic, hepatic, and intestinal events that are unique to the newborn. Degradation of 1 g of hemoglobin through the heme catabolic pathway (Fig. 1) results in the production of 34 mg of bilirubin. Destruction of circulating erythrocytes in the neonate accounts for approximately 75 percent of the daily bilirubin production,[6] with the remaining 25 percent occurring from heme proteins such as the cytochrome, catalase, and peroxidase and from the destruction of red cell precursors in the bone marrow.[7] The normal newborn produces an average of 8.5 ± 2.3 mg per kilogram of bilirubin per day, which is more than twice the production of the adult. This difference is due to the neonate's larger red blood cell mass per kilogram of body weight, a red cell life span that is only two-thirds that of red cells from adults, and an increased production of bilirubin from nonerythrocytic sources.

Once bilirubin is produced in the reticuloendothelial system, it must be rendered polar prior to its excretion in bile. Uptake by the hepatocyte, conjugation with polar sugars, and excretion into bile are necessary for its eventual elimination. Defects in each phase may contribute to neonatal hyperbilirubinemia.

At physiologic pH and in the crystalline form, the two carboxylic acid groups of bilirubin are internally hydrogen-bonded (Fig. 2) and therefore are not available for ionization in aqueous media. Consequently, bilirubin is lipophylic and in the free state (unbound to proteins) has no water solubility unless the pH approaches 10.[8] Consequently, it is transported in serum noncovalently linked to a hydrophobic portion of albumin. Binding to albumin occurs at at least two sites. The primary, pH-independent site has a high affinity and reversibly binds bilirubin in the dianionic state. Because the secondary site binds bilirubin in the diacid form, its binding occurs more favorably at lower pH.[9] The binding constant for the secondary site is only 10 percent of the primary. Two other potential binding sites are recognized, but their physiologic importance is uncertain. By acting as a serum reservoir of tightly bound bilirubin, albumin usually prevents mass transfer of bilirubin to the brain, where it may induce neurologic damage by adversely affecting a host of cellular activities.

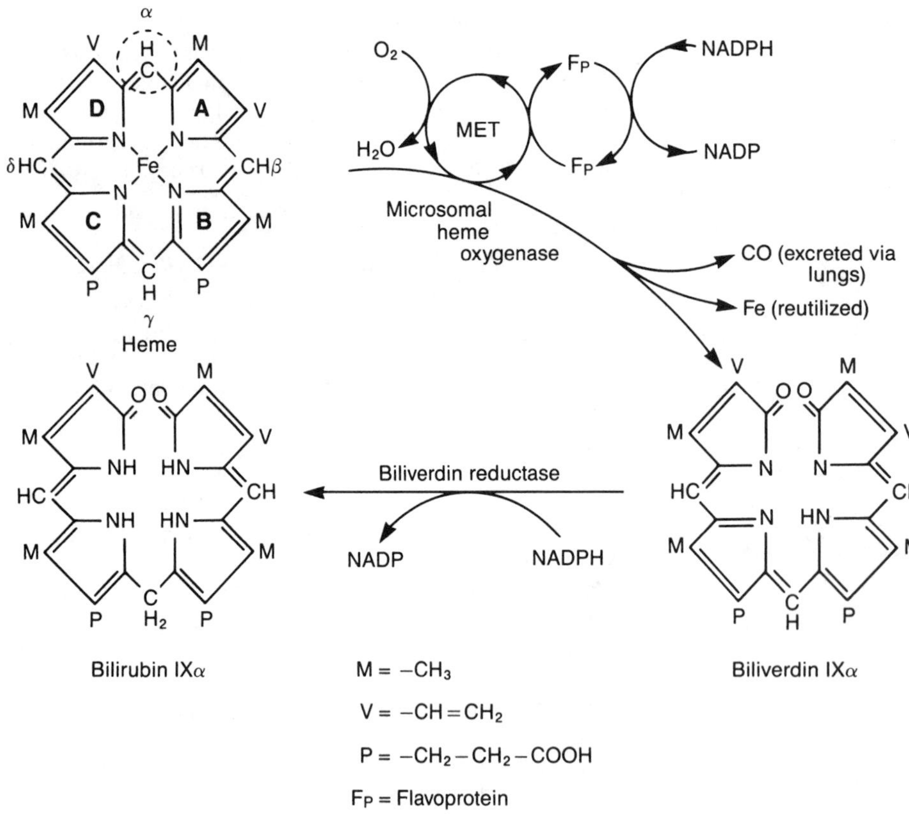

Heme

Microsomal heme oxygenase

CO (excreted via lungs)

Fe (reutilized)

Biliverdin reductase

Bilirubin IXα

Biliverdin IXα

M = $-CH_3$

V = $-CH=CH_2$

P = $-CH_2-CH_2-COOH$

Fp = Flavoprotein

FIGURE 1 Metabolic pathway for conversion of heme to bilirubin IXα by heme oxygenase and biliverdin reductase. MET = microsomal electron transport system. (Redrawn from Berlin NI, Berk PD: Blood 1981; 57:983.)

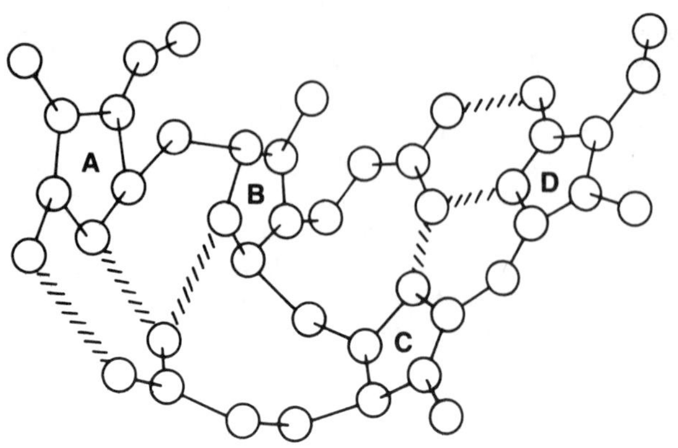

FIGURE 2 Structure of bilirubin Xα: Planar structure (*top*) and three-dimensional hydrogen-bonded structure (*bottom*). Note that intramolecular hydrogen bonding between proprionic acid groups and pyrrole C=O and N–H accounts for the insoluble nature of bilirubin at physiologic pH.

Uptake of bilirubin occurs from this bilirubin-albumin complex by an albumin receptor on the liver.[10] Bilirubin, but not albumin, is then transferred across the hepatocyte membrane[11] and is bound in the cytoplasm primarily by ligandin (also known as glutathione S-transferase B, or Y protein) but also to other glutathione S-transferases and to Z protein. Hepatic uptake of bilirubin has been shown to be impaired in the neonatal rhesus monkey, an animal model of human physiologic jaundice.[12] This impairment of uptake seems to correlate with the maturation of hepatic ligandin.

Intracellular bilirubin is then transported to the smooth endoplasmic reticulum for conjugation by the enzyme glucuronyl transferase. This enzyme is responsible for the conjugation of both propionic acid moieties of bilirubin.[13] In the presence of adequate enzyme, most of the bilirubin is conjugated with glucuronic acid (with small amounts of glucose and xylose conjugates also synthesized) (Fig. 3) at both propionic acid groups, and bilirubin diglucuronide predominates. The diglucuronide is the major bile pigment in adults.[14] However, in the presence of relative enzyme deficiency of bilirubin excess, the monoconjugated form predominates. Thus, the neonate excretes bilirubin almost exclusively in the form of the monoglucuronide during the first 2 days of life when glucuronyl transferase levels are low, with proportionally more diglucuronide being formed over the next several days. If hemolytic disease is present, then a state of excess substrate of bilirubin is present, with proportionally more bilirubin excreted in the form of the monoglucuronide, even in the older neonate.

The excretion of monoglucuronide has potential clinical importance. It may undergo hydrolysis back to unconjugated bilirubin,[15] which can then precipitate in the bile ductule in

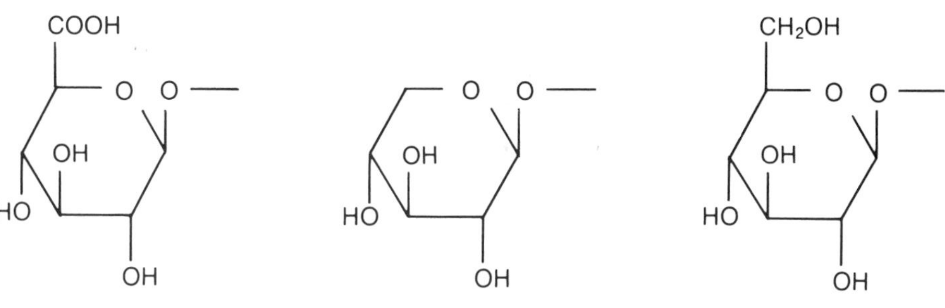

FIGURE 3 Chemical structure of bilirubin conjugates. Note that positions R_1 and R_2 are not identical, since the molecule is asymmetric with respect to the two terminal pyrrole methyl and vinyl groups. As a result, monoconjugates exist as C=8 (R_1) and C=12 (R_2) isomers.

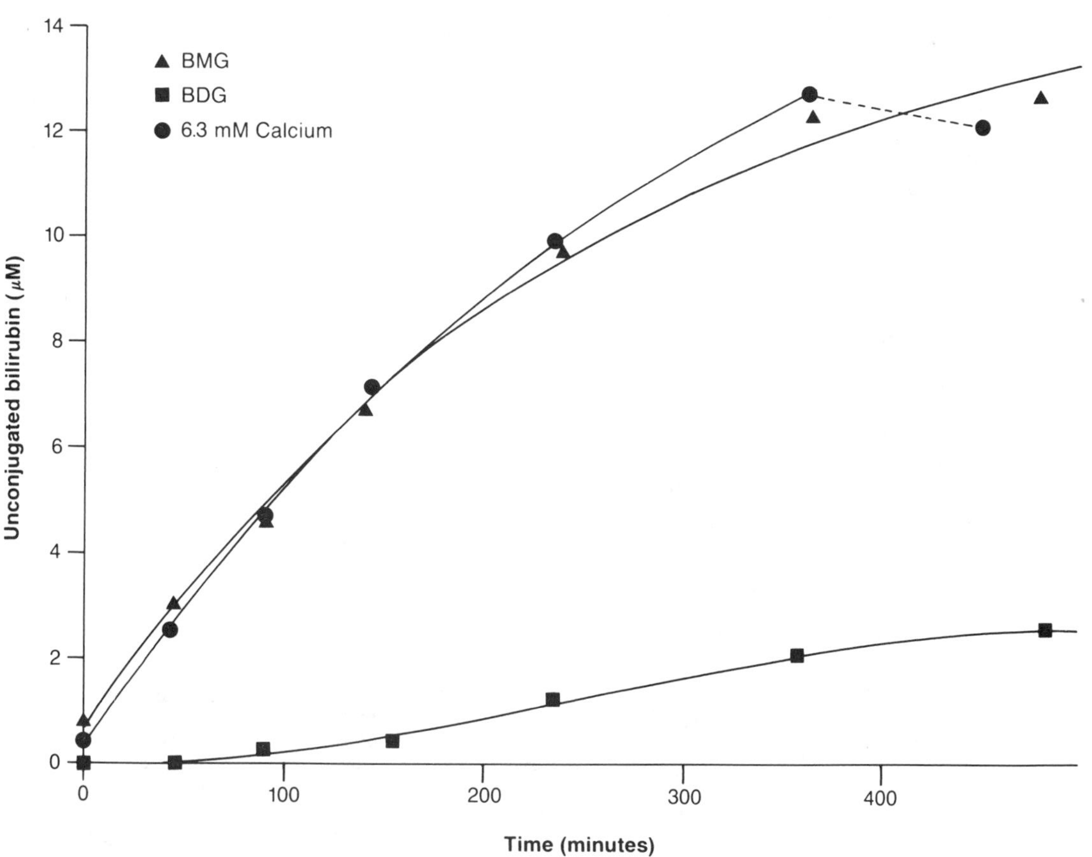

FIGURE 4 Nonenzymatic hydrolysis of bile pigments in vitro. 50 μM of bile pigment in 25 mM sodium taurocholate with imidazole-ascorbate buffer at pH 7.4. Note that hydrolysis to unconjugated bilirubin (UCB) from bilirubin monoglucuronide (BMG) is six times more rapid than from bilirubin diglucuronide (BDG). In the presence of 6.3 mM CaCl, precipitation occurs (*dashed line*). (Adapted from Spivak et al.[15])

the presence of biliary calcium to form insoluble calcium bilirubinate. In vitro experiments have shown that hydrolysis to unconjugated bilirubin occurs at rates four to six times faster for the monoglucuronide than for the diglucuronide (Fig. 4).[15] Precipitation of calcium bilirubinate in the presence of biliary proteins may be the cause of the inspissated bile syndrome in babies with rapid hemolysis and may explain the canalicular cholestasis that is seen microscopically in most forms of cholestatic jaundice. In fact, the plugging of bile ducts with bile pigment precipitates may be one of the reasons that cholestasis is prolonged, even when the original hepatocellular problem has resolved.

Enterohepatic Circulation of Bilirubin

The gut also has an important role in increasing bilirubin levels in the neonate through the enterohepatic circulation of bilirubin.[16,17] In the normal adult, bilirubin is broken down by the gut bacterial flora to polar, nonabsorbable compounds (stercobilin and urobilinogen) that are excreted in feces and urine. However, since the newborn lacks the normal bacterial flora, bilirubin conjugates are presumably hydrolyzed by intestinal beta-glucuronidase to lipophilic unconjugated bilirubin, which can diffuse across the lipophilic enterocyte membrane and be absorbed into portal blood. This absorbed bilirubin is then picked up the liver, conjugated, and re-excreted. This process of excretion, absorption, and re-excretion represents and enterohepatic circulation of bilirubin, similar to the familiar cycling of bile salts through the gastrointestinal (GI) tract and liver. Thus, in neonatal intestinal obstruction, bilirubin levels are notoriously higher because of a prolonged time for reabsorption of bilirubin. Oral charcoal[16] and agar,[17] which interfere with bilirubin absorption in the neonate, may reduce serum bilirubin levels by preventing the enterohepatic circulation of bilirubin.

Clinical Aspects of Physiologic Jaundice

Physiologic jaundice can be divided into two functionally different phases. During the first 5 days of life in the term infant (phase I), a relatively rapid rise in serum unconjugated bilirubin occurs. Mean values increase from a cord blood value of 1.5 to a mean peak value of 6 to 7 mg per deciliter by the third day of life. In the premature infant, mean peak values of 10 to 12 do not occur until the fifth to seventh day of life. In the term neonate, after the third day of life bilirubin begins to decline rapidly until the fifth day of life, during which phase II begins. It is characterized by a relatively stable serum indirect bilirubin of approximately 2 mg per deciliter that persists until the end of the second week of life. At the end of this period, serum bilirubin levels decline to values noted in normal adults. The duration of phase II in the premature infant may be 1 month or more, depending on the infant's gestational age at birth.

The National Collaborative Perinatal Project prospectively followed the serum bilirubin levels of more then 35,000 infants.[18] Bilirubin concentration was measured at 48 hours of age and then repeated daily if the initial value exceeded 10 mg per deciliter. No attempt was made to exclude infants with hemolytic disease. Of infants with birth weights of greater than 2,500 g, 4.51 percent of the black infants and 6.19 percent of the white infants had serum bilirubin levels greater than 12.9 mg per deciliter. As a result, bilirubin values of greater than 12 mg per deciliter require diagnostic evaluation,[19] although some suggest further investigation for bilirubin levels greater than 10 mg per deciliter.[20] However, 55 percent of babies with bilirubin exceeding 12 mg per deciliter have no specific etiology identified by diagnostic evaluation.[21] Since breast feeding is significantly associated with bilirubin values greater than 12 mg per deciliter, even in the first three days of life,[21] investigation of breast-fed babies for hemolytic disease with bilirubin levels above 12 mg per deciliter may not be warranted.[21] Some infants with indirect hyperbilirubinemia of greater than 12 mg per deciliter without hemolysis may have Gilbert's syndrome.

BREAST MILK JAUNDICE

Breast milk jaundice (Table 3) is a well-recognized form of unconjugated hyperbilirubinemia in which serum bilirubin concentrations rise rapidly after the fourth day of life and peak at the end of the second week. Recently, breast-feeding has been implicated as a cause of jaundice during the first 3 days of life, although the mechanism of this early form of jaundice may be related more to the poor hydrational and caloric status of some breast-fed infants than to the milk itself.[22] Therefore, it is useful to separate early onset of jaundice with breast-feeding from late onset. The estimated incidence of late onset of breast milk jaundice is 0.5 to 2 percent of otherwise healthy breast-fed infants with recurrence rates in subsequent siblings of up to 70 percent. Pooled analysis of 12 different studies, *without discriminating between late and early onset*, indicates that 12.8 percent of breast-fed infants have serum bilirubin levels that exceed 12 mg per deciliter, whereas only 4 percent of non–breast-fed infants fall into this category.[23] Severe jaundice (serum bilirubin greater than 15 mg per deciliter) occurred in 2 percent of breast-fed babies and 0.3 percent of formula-fed babies. Although bilirubin

TABLE 3
Breast Milk Jaundice

Early Onset
- Very common—12 percent of breast-fed babies affected.
- Onset during the first three days of life.
- May be related to caloric deprivation and dehydration.

Late Onset
- Occurs in approximately 0.5 to 3 percent of healthy newborns.
- Serum bilirubin rises rapidly after the fourth day of life.
- Serum bilirubin peaks at the end of the second week of life.
- Severe jaundice (bilirubin 15 mg per deciliter) occurs in 2 percent of breast-fed babies and 0.3 percent of formula-fed babies.
- Not associated with kernicterus.
- Cessation of breast-feeding for 24 to 48 hours results in a significant drop in serum bilirubin.
- "Abnormal breast milk" is associated with an increased concentration of free fatty acids.
- "Abnormal breast milk" may increase the enterohepatic circulation of bilirubin.

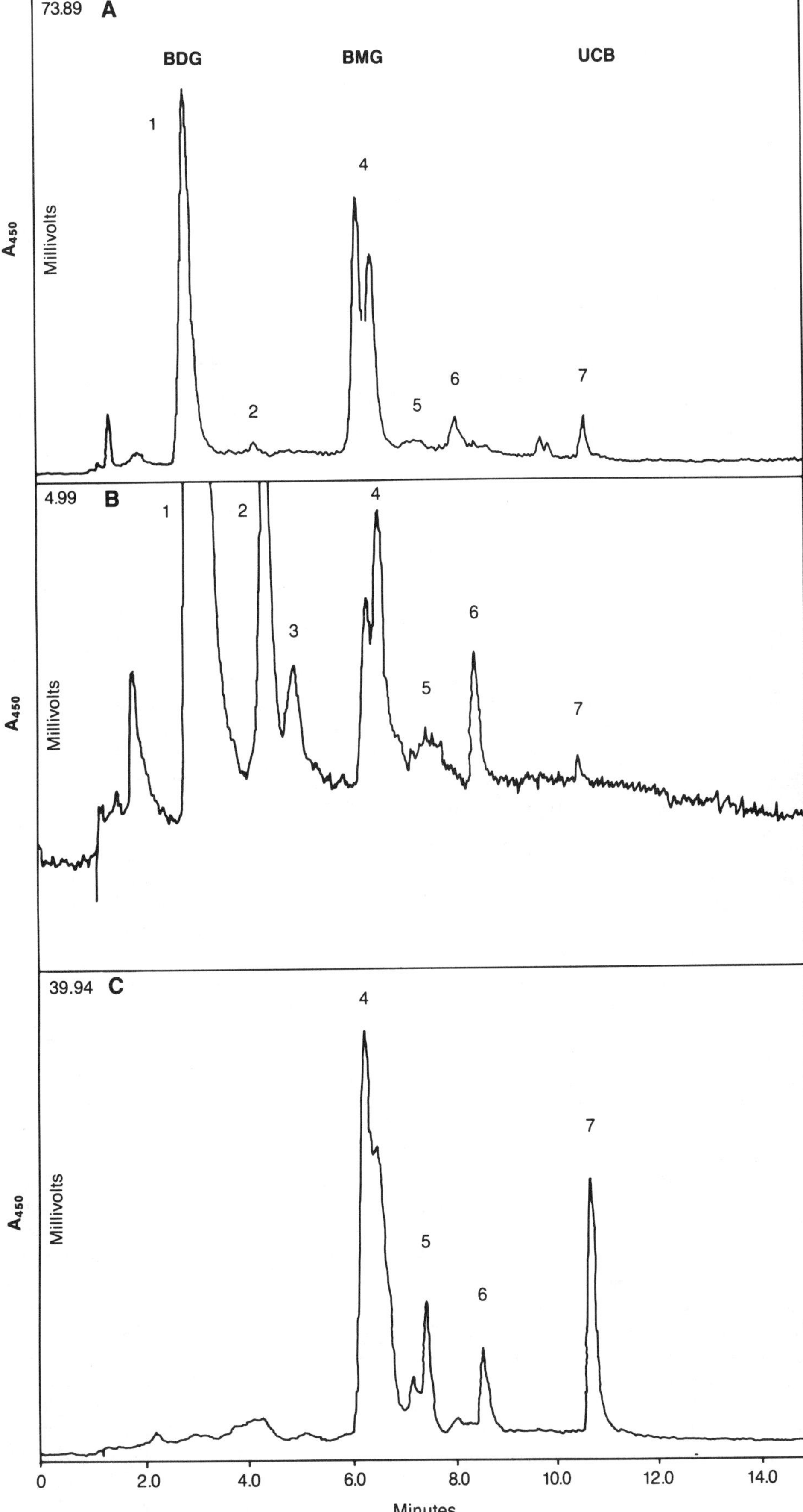

FIGURE 5 High-pressure liquid chromatography elution profiles of bilirubin. *A*, Rat bile. *B*, Normal human bile. *C*, From a child with Crigler-Najjar syndrome. Bile pigments: (1) BDG-bilirubin diglucuronide, (2) bilirubin glucuronide-glucoside, (3) bilirubin diglucoside, (4) BMG-bilirubin monoglucuronide, (5) bilirubin monoglucoside, (6) bilirubin monoxyloside, (7) unconjugated bilirubin. Note the multiplicity of conjugates in normal human bile and the absence of diconjugates in Crigler-Najjar syndrome.

levels may increase to levels that require phototherapy, kernicterus has not been reported with this form of hyperbilirubinemia in full-term infants, but long-term prospective studies have not been conducted. In the preterm infant population, which is at high risk for evolution of neurodevelopmental disabilities, infants fed on maternal or banked breast milk were four times more likely to achieve plasma bilirubin levels over 11.7 mg per deciliter than babies fed artificial preterm formula.[24] Higher bilirubin levels are also noted in preterm infants fed a combination of premature breast milk and formula than in preterm newborns fed formula alone. Seventy-six percent of preterm infants fed the combined diet met the criteria for phototherapy, whereas only 45 percent of infants fed formula alone required phototherapy. If the need for phototherapy seems likely in this disorder, it is prudent to discontinue breast feeding; a 24- to 48-hour cessation of breast-feeding usually results in a significant reduction in bilirubin levels—a test that is both diagnostic and therapeutic. Reductions of serum bilirubin with cessation of breast-feeding alone are comparable to levels achieved using phototherapy.[25] Resumption of breast-feeding is associated with either a cessation of the previous decline in serum bilirubin or a rise of only 2 to 3 mg per deciliter.

The mechanism of breast milk jaundice is not entirely clear. Older studies ascribed this form of jaundice to the inhibition of hepatic glucuronyl transferase activity by the pregnane-3 alpha, 20 beta-diol component in human milk.[26] More recent studies have not confirmed this hypothesis. Normal cow's milk and normal human milk inhibit the absorption of bilirubin from the gastrointestinal (GI) tract in rats. However, breast milk from mothers of babies with breast milk jaundice not only failed to inhibit the absorption of bilirubin but actually enhanced the absorption of bilirubin from the GI tract.[27] The mechanism for this enhanced absorption has not been defined but may be a result of an increased concentration of free fatty acids found in these abnormal breast milks.[27] Analogous to the way free fatty acids displace bilirubin from serum albumin, free fatty acids in the intestine could potentially displace bilirubin from the surface of undigested proteins and in the process increase the concentration of free bilirubin available for diffusion across the enterocytic membrane.

Mean total serum bile acids are increased in breast-fed infants with jaundice as compared with breast-fed or formula-fed infants without jaundice; however, the difference is not statistically significant.[28] The glycine-to-taurine conjugated bile acid ratio is significantly lower in breast-fed jaundiced infants than in nonjaundiced bottle- or breast-fed infants. The glycine-to-taurine ratio was always less than one in breast-fed infants, regardless of jaundice. This reflects the fact that neonates are known to conjugate bile acids predominantly as the taurine conjugate. In contrast, formula-fed infants without jaundice had a bile acid pattern with a glycine-to-taurine ratio greater than one.[29] The proportion of taurine-conjugated bile acids also increased with increasing serum bilirubin levels in breast-fed infants.[29]

The increase in mean total serum bile acids in breast-fed jaundiced infants is understandable from a pathophysiologic point of view. Just as breast milk may increase the enterohepatic circulation of bilirubin or interfere with conjugation of bilirubin, breast milk may also increase the enterohepatic circulation of bile salts or interfere with bile salt uptake and excretion. Since the immature liver of the neonate already has problems excreting bile salts (serum bile acids remain above normal adult levels in the infant for the first 6 months of life[30]), breast-feeding raises bile acid levels even further. It is not clear why there should be a difference in the bile acid pattern in breast milk jaundice.

CRIGLER-NAJJAR SYNDROME

Crigler-Najjar syndrome comprises two rare genetic disorders associated with unconjugated hyperbilirubinemia severe enough to cause kernicterus. Type I disease is associated with severe hyperbilirubinemia that is not decreased by the administration of phenobarbital. Type II Crigler-Najjar syndrome is associated with a somewhat milder form of hyperbilirubinemia that is responsive to phenobarbital.

Type I Crigler-Najjar Syndrome

In 1952 Crigler and Najjar described seven children in two related families who had extreme nonhemolytic hyperbilirubinemia with bilirubin concentration ranging from 13 to 48 mg per deciliter.[31] Six died during infancy or childhood with kernicterus. The concentrations of bilirubin are commonly between 20 and 25 mg per deciliter, although values as high as 50 mg per deciliter have been reported. Bile color has been described as very pale with this disorder, although conjugated bilirubin is present in bile in the monoconjugated form (Fig. 5).[32]

Glucuronyl transferase activity is absent in liver biopsy specimens; undoubtedly some activity is present as evidenced by the presence of monoglucuronides in bile, but the assay must be insensitive to the small amounts of transferase present. Histologically, the liver is normal by light and electron microscopy. Excretion of DISIDA, an hepatobiliary scintigraphic agent, occurs in this syndrome even with a serum bilirubin exceeding 30 mg per deciliter,[33] indicating that organic anion transport is not affected and that unconjugated bilirubin and DISIDA do not compete for the same transport sites. Occasionally, cholestasis may occur because of high levels of bilirubin found in the bile of these patients. This elevated level of bilirubin in bile is a result of direct excretion of higher than normal levels of unconjugated bilirubin, reconversion of soluble photobilirubin to insoluble unconjugated bilirubin in the bile ducts, and possible nonenzymatic hydrolysis of monoconjugated bilirubin to unconjugated bilirubin. As bile proceeds along the biliary tree, ductular pH decreases, the metastable solubility of bilirubin is exceeded, and bilirubin precipitates, leading to cholestasis.

Gunn rats are a mutant form of Wistar rats that lack glucuronyl transferase activity. Homozygous Gunn rats have been an ideal model for Crigler-Najjar syndrome. They have unconjugated hyperbilirubinemia (3 to 20 mg per deciliter) and may develop encephalopathy. As in Crigler-Najjar syndrome, there is no bilirubinuria and the bile contains only small amounts of unconjugated bilirubin. Gunn rats may also excrete bilirubin in an hydroxylated form, thereby rendering it somewhat polar.

Type II Crigler-Najjar Syndrome

The original designation of type I versus type II disease was based on three factors. First, type I Crigler-Najjar syndrome was believed to be associated with the total absence of hepatic glucuronyl transferase; hence, bilirubin conjugates were believed to be virtually absent from bile, whereas type II patients were thought to have considerable amounts of monoconjugates present in addition to unconjugated bilirubin. Second, type I patients were thought to have serum bilirubin levels that were considerably higher than those of type II patients. Third, type I patients almost always developed kernicterus if not aggressively treated for hyperbilirubinemia, whereas type II patients rarely developed this complication. More recent evidence indicates that distinctions based on the absence of conjugates, serum bilirubins, and incidence of kernicterus may not be warranted, since considerable overlap in these parameters occurs among both categories of patients. With this in mind, the distinction between the two forms should be made on a biochemical basis only—patients with type I disease have no response to phenobarbital, whereas patients with type II disease respond to this drug with a significant drop in serum bilirubin.

Diagnosis and Treatment of Crigler-Najjar Syndrome

Any child with moderate to severe nonhemolytic unconjugated hyperbilirubinemia that persists longer than physiologic jaundice should be suspected of having Crigler-Najjar syndrome. Confirmation of the diagnosis can be made by the absence of bilirubin diglucuronide in bile using reverse-phase high-pressure liquid chromatography (HPLC).[32] HPLC of serum samples may also be helpful in the diagnosis.[34] The sera of patients with this syndrome do not contain bilirubin diglucuronide, whereas sera from normals and patients with other hepatobiliary diseases contain bilirubin diglucuronide. However, since the concentration of conjugates in normal serum is at least a thousandfold less than in normal bile, some HPLC methods have difficulty in detecting conjugates in the serum of noncholestatic subjects.[35] Therefore, measurement of bile glucuronides appears less likely to lead to possible error. In addition, an elevated concentration of unconjugated bilirubin is present in bile when compared with controls.

Treatment in the neonatal period should include phototherapy and a trial of phenobarbital. Phototherapy in this syndrome and in any form of neonatal unconjugated hyperbilirubinemia works by converting the Z,Z intramolecular hydrogen-bonded bilirubin to one of three unstable, nonintramolecular hydrogen-bonded bilirubins (Fig. 6). These "E" photoisomers, along with an intramolecular cyclized form of bilirubin (lumirubin), are water soluble and thus are excreted without the need for conjugation. Beyond the age of three to four years, phototherapy becomes less effective because of thickening of the skin, increase in body mass relative to surface area, and the fact that phototherapy is practical only during sleeping hours, which decrease as the child ages. Exchange transfusion should be reserved for infants who have bilirubin levels high enough that kernicterus is feared. Agar or activated charcoal may prevent intestinal reabsorption of bilirubin. Plasmapheresis is effective in lowering bilirubin in the acute phase; however, venous access is difficult in pediatric patients, and therefore this does not appear to present a long-term solution in pediatrics, although it may be useful in older adolescents and adults, especially if plasmapheresis

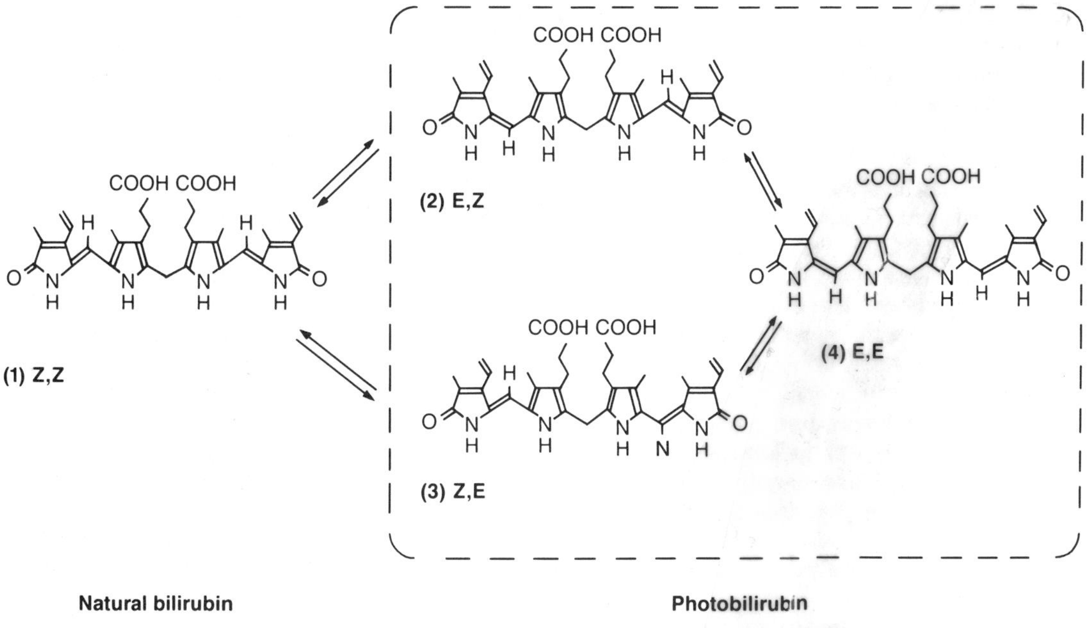

(1) Z,Z
(2) E,Z
(3) Z,E
(4) E,E

Natural bilirubin
Photobilirubin

FIGURE 6 Formation of photobilirubin (isomers) from naturally occurring Z,Z bilirubin. These photoisomers are polar because they are unable to undergo intramolecular hydrogen bonding; hence, they can be excreted in bile without prior conjugation.

becomes readily available as treatment for hyperlipidemias. Hepatic transplantation has been successful in rapidly lowering bilirubin levels[36] but should be performed when all other methods of controlling severe hyperbilirubinemia have failed and the possibility of the development of kernicterus is high. Beyond the neonatal period, kernicterus has a secondary peak of occurrence during puberty, although with very elevated bilirubin levels, it can occur at any age.

Tin Protoporphyrin

Tin (IV)-protoporphyrin-IXα (tin-heme) (a drug that is not yet approved by the FDA) is a selective inhibitor of heme oxygenase. When administered to rats, this compound reduces the endogenous production of bilirubin but does not impair hepatic uptake or excretion.[37] Excess free heme is excreted in bile. In a limited study involving 53 treated infants, tin-heme has been shown to be safe and effective in decreasing serum bilirubin levels in neonates with hemolytic anemia.[38] Similarly, since this drug is also effective in Gunn rats[39] (the animal model of type I Crigler-Najjar syndrome), it may offer in the future a long-term medical therapy for this disorder. Clinical trials of this drug in children with Crigler-Najjar syndrome should be underway shortly.

GILBERT'S SYNDROME

Gilbert's syndrome is a common form of mild unconjugated hyperbilirubinemia. Serum bilirubin levels are usually less than 3 mg per deciliter but occasionally may increase to levels as high as 8 mg per deciliter. Patients are usually noted to be jaundiced during periods of illness or stress, but fasting, hyperthyroidism, and menstrual periods may also exacerbate jaundice. Although liver biopsy is not necessary for the diagnosis, histology of the liver is normal except for nonspecific accumulation of lipofuchsin. The diagnosis is based on the presence of mild fluctuating hyperbilirubinemia (in the presence of otherwise normal liver function tests) and absence of significant hemolysis.

Hepatic glucuronyl transferase activity is diminished and is associated with an increased output of monoglucuronides in bile.[40] This increase in monoglucuronide with diminished glucuronyl transferase activity is present in the neonate during the fist few days of life, in patients with Gilbert's syndrome, and in Crigler-Najjar syndrome. However, patients with Gilbert's syndrome, unlike those with Crigler-Najjar syndrome, have bilirubin diglucuronide present in bile. Presumably because of an increase of bilirubin monoglucuronide present in bile, patients with Gilbert's syndrome may be at increased risk for the formation of pigment gallstones.

Serum bilirubin levels decrease in Gilbert's syndrome in response to phenobarbital.[41] Delayed hepatic clearance of orally administered ursodeoxycholic acid is also noted in this syndrome[41]; serum levels of this bile salt also decrease after phenobarbital administration.[41]

The Bolivian squirrel monkey is an excellent animal model for Gilbert's syndrome. This monkey has higher fasting and postcibal levels of unconjugated bilirubin than its closely related Brazilian counterpart.[42] The Bolivian monkey also has lower hepatic bilirubin glucuronyl transferase activity, a higher ratio of bilirubin mono- to diglucuronides in its bile, and a more sluggish plasma clearance of intravenously administered bilirubin than its Brazilian "cousin." Fasting hyperbilirubinemia is rapidly reversed by administration of carbohydrates but not lipids in this animal model of Gilbert's syndrome.

High-Pressure Liquid Chromatography of Bile Pigments

HPLC analysis of bile pigments (see also section on Crigler-Najjar Syndrome) allows differentiation of jaundice on the basis of serum bile pigment patterns. Normal controls have more than 96 percent of total serum bilirubin in the unconjugated form.[2] Patients with Gilbert's syndrome have levels of total conjugates comparable to normals but have mildly elevated levels of unconjugated bilirubin. In patients with hemolytic disease, the concentrations of both monoconjugated and diconjugated bilirubin were enhanced in parallel with the increase of unconjugated pigment.[34] Crigler-Najjar syndrome patients have higher unconjugated bilirubin levels and no diconjugates in serum.[34]

DUBIN-JOHNSON SYNDROME

Dubin-Johnson syndrome (Table 4) is characterized by conjugated hyperbilirubinemia and a grossly black appearance to the liver. The syndrome occurs most frequently in Persian Jews (prevalence 1:1,300), who also have an associated Factor VII deficiency. Serum bilirubin levels usually vary between 2 and 5 mg per deciliter but may be as high as 25 mg per deciliter. Unlike most hepatobiliary disorders, the serum of patients with Dubin-Johnson contains conjugated bilirubin predominantly in the diconjugated form. More than half of the serum bilirubin is present as the direct-reacting form. The direct-reacting bilirubin in this disorder may be considerably higher than with more specific methods for measuring bilirubin conjugates such as thin-layer chromatography or HPLC. This is a result of the fact that most of the latter methods have difficulty measuring covalently linked albumin-bound bilirubin, which may make up as much as 60 percent of the total conjugated bilirubin in patients with longstanding direct hyperbilirubinemia of any nature.

Serum aminotransferases, alkaline phosphatase, albumin, cholesterol, and the complete blood counts are normal in this disorder. However, oral cholecystography usually results in nonvisualization of the gallbladder. Liver biopsy, which is usually unnecessary for diagnosis reveals a grossly black liver due to the accumulation of melanin-like pigment contained in lysosomes. On electron microscopy, pericanalicular web width and area are significantly greater in Rotor's syndrome and in Dubin-Johnson syndrome than in Gilbert's syndrome, suggesting that disturbances in bile flow in Rotor's and Dubin-Johnson syndrome are related to dysfunction in pericanalicular microfilaments.[43]

Hepatic transport of organic anions conjugated in the liver (e.g., bilirubin, Bromsulphalein (BSP), indocyanine green, and iopanoic acid) is decreased; however, the transport of

TABLE 4
Principal Differences between Dubin-Johnson and Rotor's Syndromes

Characteristic	Dubin-Johnson Syndrome	Rotor's Syndrome
Appearance of liver	Grossly black	Normal
Histology of liver	Dark pigment predominantly in centrilobular areas	Normal
Serum bilirubin	Elevated levels usually between 2 and 5 mg/dl, occasionally as high as 20 mg/dl; predominantly direct bilirubin	(Same as in Dubin-Johnson syndrome)
Routine liver function tests (except bilirubin)	Normal	Normal
45-minute plasma BSP retention	Normal or elevated; secondary rise at 90 minutes	Elevated; no secondary rise
Oral cholecystogram	Gallbladder usually not seen	Gallbladder visualizes
Urinary coproporphyrin	Normal total with greater than 80 percent as isomer I	Elevated total, isomer I less than 80 percent
Mode of inheritance	Autosomal dominant	Autosomal dominant
Prognosis	Benign	Benign

organic anions that are not conjugated by the liver is not affected. BSP clearance from plasma after intravenous injection follows a characteristic biphasic pattern. BSP concentration falls initially as it does in normal patients, but after 45 minutes there is typically a secondary rise. This secondary rise is also found with other hepatobiliary disorders, but these disorders can be distinguished from Dubin-Johnson syndrome on the basis of a pathognomonic excretion of urinary coproporphyrin that occurs with the latter. Body fluids contain two forms of coproporphyrins—isomer I and isomer III. Isomer I is a byproduct of heme catabolism, whereas isomer III is a heme precursor. *Dubin-Johnson syndrome is the only form of conjugated hyperbilirubinemia in which total urinary coproporphyrin excretion is normal, and isomer I makes up more than 80 percent of urinary coproporphyrin excretion.*[44] In other disorders of conjugated hyperbilirubinemia, total urinary coproporphyrin excretion is usually elevated, and isomer I excretion accounts for less than 65 percent of the total.

Both mutant Corriedale sheep and a mutant strain of rats have some of the biochemical defects found in Dubin-Johnson syndrome.[45] The sheep have hepatic pigmentation that is probably related to melanin and also have a defective organic anion excretion. The mutant rat strain has serum bilirubin levels of 5 to 10 mg per deciliter with over 90 percent in the form of bilirubin glucuronides. Other liver function tests are normal, except the serum bile acids, which are elevated fivefold. Unlike Dubin-Johnson patients, these rats have normal liver histology, no secondary rise in the plasma BSP clearance, and a urinary coproporphyrin I level that is only 20 percent of the total isomeric excretion.

Rotor's Syndrome

Rotor's syndrome is an extremely rare and benign disorder of conjugated hyperbilirubinemia that can be distinguished from Dubin-Johnson syndrome by the fact that Rotor's syndrome patients have normal liver histology, a different pattern of BSP clearance, and a different coproporphyrin excretion. Clearance of BSP is highly delayed, and there is no secondary increase in plasma BSP.[46] Total urinary coproporphyrin in excretion is two and one-half to five times normal.

REFERENCES

1. Socker R, Yamamoto Y, McDonagh AF, Glazer AN, Ames BN. Bilirubin is an antioxidant of possible physiologic importance. Science 1987; 235:1043–1045.
2. Muraca M, Blanckaert N. Liquid-chromatographic assay and identification of mono and diesterconjugates of bilirubin in normal serum. Clin Chem 1983; 29:1767–1771.
3. Scriener RL, Glick MR. Interlaboratory bilirubin variability. Pediatrics 1982; 69:277–281.
4. Killenberg PG, Stevens RD, Wilderman RF, et al. The laboratory method as a variable in the interpretation of serum bilirubin fractionation. Gastroenterology 1980; 78:1011–1015.
5. Weiss JS, Gautman A, Lauff JJ, et al. The clinical importance of a protein bound fraction of serum bilirubin in patients with hyperbilirubinemia. N Engl J Med 1984; 309:147–150.
6. Vest M, Strebel L, Hauenstein D. The extent of "shunt" bilirubin and erythrocyte survival in the newborn infant measured by the administration of (^{15}N) glycine. Biochem J 1965; 95:11c.
7. Berk PJ, Howe RB, Bloomer JR, Berlin NI. Studies of bilirubin kinetics in normal adults. J Clin Invest 1969; 48:2176.
8. Broderson R. Bilirubin solubility and interaction with albumin and phospholipid. J Biol Chem 1979; 254:2364–2369.
9. Broderson F, Funding L, Pedersen AO, Rojgaard-Petersen H. Binding of bilirubin to low-affinity sites of human serum albumin in vitro followed by co-crystallization. Scand J Clin Lab Invest 1972; 29:433.
10. Stremmel W, Gerber MA, Glezerov V, et al. Physicochemical and immunohistological studies of a sulfobromophthalein and bilirubin binding protein from rat liver plasma membranes. J Clin Invest 1983; 71:1796–1805.
11. Bloomer JR, Berk PD, Vergalla J, Berlin NI. Influence of albumin on the extravascular distribution of unconjugated bilirubin. Clin Sci Mol Med 1973; 45:517.
12. Gartner LM, Lee KS, Vaisman S, et al. Development of bilirubin transport and metabolism in the newborn rhesus monkey. J Pediatr 1977; 90:513–531.
13. Blanckaert N, Gollan J, Schmid R. Bilirubin diglucuronide synthesis by a UDP glucuronic acid dependent enzyme system in rat liver microsomes. Proc Natl Acad Sci USA 1979; 76:2037.
14. Spivak W, Carey MC. Reverse-phase h.p.l.c. separation and preparation of bilirubin and its conjugates from native bile. Quantitative analysis of the intact tetrapyrroles based on h.p.l.c. of their ethyl anthranilate azo derivatives. Biochem J 1985; 225:787–805.
15. Spivak W, DiVenuto D, Yuey W. Non-enzymic hydrolysis of bilirubin mono-and diglucuronide to unconjugated bilirubin in model and native bile systems. Biochem J 1987; 242:323–329.
16. Ulstrom RA, Eisenklam E. The enterohepatic shunting of bilirubin in the newborn infant. J Pediatr 1964; 65:27–37.
17. Poland RL, Odell GB. Physiologic jaundice: the enterohepatic circulation of bilirubin. N Engl J Med 1964; 284:1–6.
18. Hardy JB, Drage JS, Jackson EC. The first year of life. The Collaborative Perinatal Project of the National Institutes of Neurological and Communicative Disorders and Stroke. Baltimore: The Johns Hopkins University Press, 1979: 104.
19. Behrman RE, Kliegman RM. Jaundice and hyperbilirubinemia in the newborn. In: Behrman RE, Vaughn VC III, eds. Nelson textbook of pediatrics 3rd ed. Philadelphia, WB Saunders, 1983:373.
20. Gartner LM. Hyperbilirubinemia. In: Rudolph AM, ed. Pediatrics. 17th ed. Norwalk, CT: Appleton-Century-Crofts, 1982: 1007.
21. Maisels MJ, Gifford K, Antle CE, Leib GR. Jaundice in the healthy newborn infant: a new approach to an old problem. Pediatrics 1988; 81:505–511.
22. Maisels MJ, Gifford K. Breastfeeding, weight loss and jaundice. J Pediatr 1983; 102:117–118.

23. Schneider AP II. Breast milk jaundice in the newborn. A real entity. JAMA 1986; 255:3270–3274.
24. Lucas A, Baker BA. Breast milk jaundice in premature infants. Arch Dis Child 1986; 61:1063–1067.
25. Amato M, Howald H, von-Muralt G. Interruption of breast-feeding versus phototherapy as treatment of hyperbilirubinemia in full-term infants. Helv Paediatr Acta 1985; 40:127–131.
26. Arias IM, Gartner LM, Seifter S, Furman M. Prolonged neonatal unconjugated hyperbilirubinemia associated with breast feeding and a steroid, pregnane-3(alpha), 20(beta)diol, in maternal milk that inhibits glucuronide formation in vitro. J Clin Invest 1964; 43:2037.
27. Gartner LM, Lee KS, Moscioni AD. Effect of milk feeding on intestinal bilirubin absorption in the rat. J Pediatr 1983; 103:464–471.
28. Tazawa Y, Yamada M, Nakagawa M, Konno T, Tada K. Serum bile acids and their conjugates in breast-fed infants with prolonged jaundice. Eur J Pediatr 1985; 144:37–40.
29. Yamada M, Tazawa Y, Nakagawa M, Konno T, Tada K, Goto J, Nambara T. Alterations of serum bile acid profile in breast-fed infants with prolonged jaundice. J Pediatr Gastroenterol Nutr 1985; 4:741–745.
30. Suchy FJ, Balisteri WF, Heubi JE, et al. Physiologic cholestasis: elevations of the primary serum bile acid concentrations in normal infants. Gastroenterology 1981; 80:1037–1041.
31. Crigler JF, Najjar VA. Congenital familial non-hemolytic jaundice with kernicterus. Pediatrics 1952; 10:169.
32. Spivak W, Yuey W. Application of a rapid and efficient h.p.l.c. method to measure bilirubin and its conjugates from native bile and in model bile systems. Potential use as a tool for kinetic reactions and as an aid in the diagnosis of hepatobiliary disease. Biochem J 1986; 234:101–109.
33. Ascher SA, Sarkar SD, Spivak W. Hepatic uptake of technetium-99m labeled iminodiacetic acid (DISISA) is not impaired by very high serum bilirubin levels. Clin Nucl Med 1988: 13:1–3.
34. Muraca M, Fevery J, Blanckaert N. Relationship between serum bilirubins and production and conjugation of bilirubin. Studies in Gilbert's syndrome, Crigler-Najjar disease, hemolytic disorders and rat models. Gastroenterology 1987; 92:309–317.
35. Rosenthal P, Henton D, Felber S, Sinatra FR. Distribution of serum bilirubin conjugates in pediatric hepatobiliary diseases. J Pediatr 1987; 110:201–205.
36. Kaufman SS, Wood RP, Shaw BW Jr, Markin RS, Rosenthal P, Gridelli B, Vanderhoof JA. Orthotopic liver transplantation for type I Crigler-Najjar syndrome. Hepatology 1986; 6:1259–1262.
37. Whittington PF, Moscioni AD, Gartner LM. The effect of Tin(IV)-protoporphyrin-IX on bilirubin production in the rat. Pediatr Res 1987; 21:487–491.
38. Kappas A, Drummond GS, Manola T, Petmazaki S, Valaes T. Sn-protoporphyrin use in the management of hyperbilirubinemia in term newborns with direct Coombs-positive ABO incompatibility. Pediatrics 1988; 81:485–497.
39. Sisson TR, Drummond GS, Samonte D, Calabio R, Kappas A. Sn-protoprophyrin blocks the increase in serum bilirubin levels that develops postnatally in homozygous Gunn rats. J Exp Med 1988; 167:1247–1252.
40. Berthelot P, Dhumeaux D. New insights into the classification and mechanism of hereditary, chronic, non-haemolytic hyperbilirubinaemias. Gut 1978; 19:474–480.
41. Ohkubo H, Okuda K, Shinji I, Makino I. Ursodeoxycholic acid oral tolerance test in patients with constitutional hyperbilirubinemias and effect of phenobarbital. Gastroenterology 1981; 81:126–135.
42. Portman OW, Alexander M, Chowdhurry R, Chowdhurry RN, Alexander M, Cornelius CE, Arias IM. A non-human primate model for Gilbert's syndrome. Hepatology 1984; 3:454–460.
43. Tajima J, Kuroda H. Pericanalicular microfilaments of hepatocytes in patients with familial non-hemolytic hyperbilirubinemia. Gastroenterol Jpn 1988; 23:273–278.
44. Wolkoff AW, Cohen LE, Arias IM. Inheritance of the Dubin-Johnson syndrome. N Engl J Med 1979; 288:133.
45. Jansen PLM, Peters WH, Lamers WH. Hereditary chronic conjugated hyperbilirubinemia in mutant rats caused by defective hepatic anion transport. Hepatology 1985; 5:573.
46. Wolpert E, Pascasio FM, Wolkoff AW, Arias IM. Abnormal sulfobromophthalein metabolism in Rotor's syndrome and obligate heterozygotes. N Engl J Med 1977; 296:1091.

PART 9

Disorders of Carbohydrate Metabolism

Charles A. Stanley, M.D.

The unique role of the liver in carbohydrate metabolism is most easily appreciated by considering how it functions to maintain essentially constant circulating levels of glucose in two highly different states; feeding and fasting. In the fed state, the liver must take up surplus glucose provided from dietary carbohydrate to replenish glycogen stores and must also convert the nonglucose dietary monosaccarides, fructose and galactose, to glucose. In the fasted state, the liver must switch from an organ of glucose consumption to one of glucose production, releasing glucose at rates equal to ongoing glucose oxidation by other organs of the body, particularly the brain. In the first 4 to 8 hours after a meal, the liver releases glucose from stores of glycogen; beyond 8 to 12 hours after a meal, when liver glycogen stores have been depleted, the liver must produce glucose by gluconeogenesis, utilizing chiefly the amino acids released by muscle protein degradation.

NORMAL PHYSIOLOGY

Figure 1 outlines the major metabolic pathways of carbohydrate metabolism in the liver. In the fed state, 25 to 50 percent of the glucose absorbed from the small intestine is taken up by the liver and used to replenish glycogen stores. Recent studies[1] indicate that the majority of this glucose does not enter the liver directly via the glucokinase step. Instead, glucose appears to enter the liver indirectly via lac-

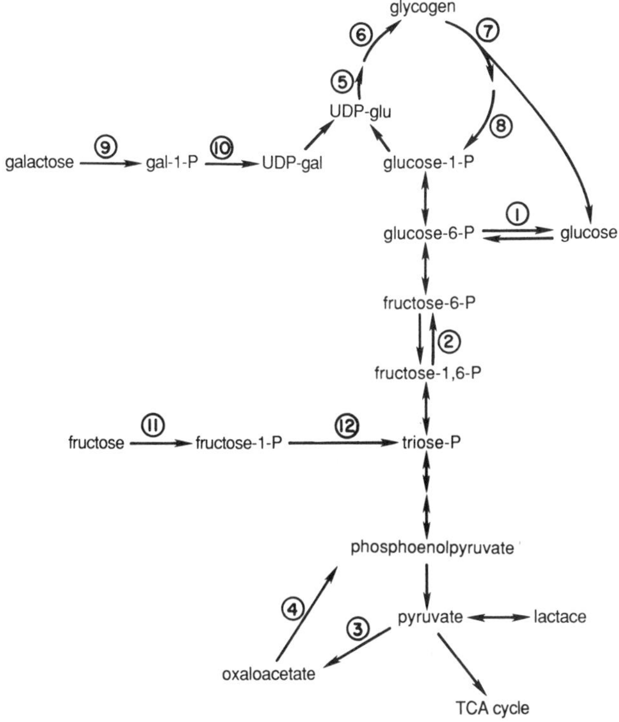

FIGURE 1 Pathways of carbohydrate metabolism in liver. Numbers identify known genetic enzyme defects: (1) glucose-6-phosphatase, (2) fructose-1,6-diphosphatase, (3) pyruvate carboxylase, (4) phosphoenolpyruvate carboxykinase, (5) glycogen synthetase, (6) brancher, (7) debrancher, (8) phosphorylase, (9) galactokinase, (10) galactose-1-phosphate uridyl transferase, (11) fructokinase, (12) fructose-1-phosphate aldolase.

tate, after first being degraded to lactate, perhaps by glycolysis in the intestine. Glycogen synthesis proceeds from glucose-6-phosphate through glucose-1-phosphate and uridine diphosphoglucose (UDP-glucose). *Glycogen synthetase* adds glucose moieties to glycogen in 1,4 linkages. The highly branched structure of glycogen is formed by *glycogen brancher enzyme*, which transfers terminal segments of 1,4-linked glucose chains to inner segments of the glycogen chain with 1,6 bonds at each branch point. Maximal glycogen levels in liver are normally about 5 to 6 g per 100 grams wet weight. Glucose taken up in excess of needs for glycogen repletion may be diverted to hepatic triglyceride synthesis.

The liver also converts other dietary monosaccharides to glucose. Galactose, derived from intestinal hydrolysis of lactose (glucose-galactose disaccharide), is converted to glucose via galactose-1-P, UDP-galactose, and UDP-glucose. Fructose, derived from intestinal hydrolysis of sucrose (glucose-fructose disaccharide), is converted to glucose via fructose-1-phosphate and the triose phosphates.

During fasting, glycogen is degraded by the combined actions of *glycogen phosphorylase* and *debrancher enzymes*. Phosphorylase releases glucose-1-phosphate, which must be converted to glucose-6-phosphate before being released as free glucose through the action of *glucose-6-phosphatase*. The action of debrancher releases one free glucose molecule from each glycogen 1,6-branch point. Glucose formation from amino acids and lactate is not a simple reversal of glycolysis. To bypass the irreversible steps between glucose and pyruvate, four gluconeogenic enzymes are required: *pyruvate carboxylase, phosphoenolpyruvate carboxykinase, fructose-1,6-diphosphatase,* and *glucose-6-phosphatase.*

The regulation of hepatic glucose uptake and production is accomplished at many of the enzyme steps shown in Figure 1 by the action of several hormones, most importantly insulin and glucagon. In the fed state, high levels of insulin and low levels of glucagon stimulate glycogen synthesis and suppress glycogenolysis and gluconeogenesis by increasing the activity of glycogen synthetase and suppressing the activities of glycogen phosphorylase, glucose-6-phosphatase, fructose-1,6-diphosphatase, and phosphoenolpyruvate-carboxykinase. In the fasted state, low levels of insulin and high levels of glucagon suppress glycogen synthesis and activate glycogenolysis and gluconeogenesis through these same enzymes. For example, insulin and glucagon exert an opposing reciprocal control of glycogen synthetase and glycogen phosphorylase activities by a cascade of protein phosphorylations and dephosphorylations.[2] Glucagon acts via adenylcyclase to increase cyclic AMP levels, which in turn activate a cascade of protein kinases that result in phosphorylation of glycogen phosphorylase to its active form and of glycogen synthetase to its inactive form. Insulin opposes this activation cascade by activating the dephosphorylation of glycogen phosphorylase to its inactive form and of glycogen synthetase to its active form. The fine-tuning of hepatic glucose uptake and release that is accomplished by these hormonal signals makes it possible for the liver to maintain plasma glucose levels within a narrow range of 80 to 120 mg per deciliter in spite of the wide swings in glucose delivery that accompany the normal cycle of feeding and fasting.

GENETIC DISORDERS OF HEPATIC CARBOHYDRATE METABOLISM

In the following description of the hepatic disorders of carbohydrate metabolism, the disorders have been divided into those that cause hypoglycemia and those that cause hepatocellular dysfunction. Table 1 outlines the major features of these disorders. Some authors have used an alternative system,[3] placing these and some additional disorders in a Roman numeral classification of glycogen storage diseases. A major disadvantage of this classification system is that it gives the misleading impression that the disorders are clinically similar. For reference, the identifiers for the numerical classification system are provided in Table 1.

Although the list of possible genetic defects in liver carbohydrate metabolism appears daunting, the most important ones are fairly easily identified by their major clinical features. The disorders that disturb the function of the liver in glucose homeostasis during fasting are usually distinguished by striking hepatomegaly and/or hypoglycemia. The two cytopathic disorders of glycogen metabolism present with either progressive cirrhosis or cardiomyopathy and skeletal muscle weakness. The two important defects in nonglucose monosaccharide assimilation present with evidence of hepatocellular damage and nephrotoxicity.

TABLE 1
Genetic Disorders of Hepatic Carbohydrate Metabolism

	Numerical Classification	Other Names	Major Features
A. Disorders of Fasting Glucose Homeostasis			
1. Glycogen pathway defects			
Debrancher deficiency	III	Cori's disease, limit dextrinosis	Hepatomegaly, hypoglycemia, growth failure
Phosphorylase deficiency	VI		Hepatomegaly, no hypoglycemia, growth failure
Phosphorylase kinase deficiency	IX		Hepatomegaly, no hypoglycemia, growth failure
Synthetase deficiency	O		No hepatomegaly, hypoglycemia, growth failure
(Enzyme defect unknown)	XI	Fanconi-Bickel syndrome	Hepatomegaly, renal Fanconi's syndrome, galactose intolerance
2. Gluconeogenesis defects			
Glucose-6-phosphatase deficiency a and b	Ia, Ib	von Gierke's disease	Hepatomegaly, hypoglycemia, growth failure
Fructose-diphosphatase deficiency			Hepatomegaly, hypoglycemia, normal growth
Phosphoenolpyruvate carboxykinase deficiency			Hepatomegaly, hypoglycemia, liver failure, early death
Pyruvate carboxylase deficiency			Severe retardation, encephalomyelopathy
B. Disorders Causing Cellular Damage			
1. Cytopathic glycogen pathway defects			
Brancher deficiency	IV	Amylopectinosis	Progressive cirrhosis
Acid maltase deficiency	II	Pompe's disease	Cardiomyopathy, skeletal muscle weakness
2. Defects in nonglucose sugar metabolism			
a. Fructose defects			
Fructokinase deficiency		Essential fructosuria	Benign
Fructose-1-phosphate aldolase deficiency		Hereditary fructose intolerance	Failure to thrive, liver failure, distress on eating sucrose
b. Galactose defects			
Galactokinase deficiency			Cataracts
Galactose-1-phosphate uridyl transferase deficiency		Galactosemia	Failure to thrive, liver failure, renal Fanconi syndrome

Disorders of Fasting Homeostasis

The distinguishing clinical features of the disorders that interfere with fasting homeostasis are outlined in Table 2. It is usually preferable to make a presumptive identification of the underlying disorder based on clinical tests prior to considering biopsies of liver or other tissues for specific biochemical assays of glycogen content or enzyme activity. For example, patients with glucose-6-phosphatase deficiency, the most common of these disorders of liver metabolism, are easily recognized by the combination of massive liver enlargement, rapid onset of hypoglycemia 3 to 4 hours after meals, elevated lactic acid levels, and marked hypertriglyceridemia. In this situation, needle liver biopsy may not be useful, since the histologic features are not specific and many laboratories require more tissue for assay of enzyme activity than can be obtained from a single needle biopsy specimen.

Defects in Glycogen Pathways

Debrancher Deficiency (Type III Glycogen Storage Disease, Limit Dextrinosis, Cori's Disease).[4–9] The function of the debrancher enzyme in glycogenolysis is outlined in Figure 2. Patients with this autosomal recessively inherited enzyme defect usually present in early infancy with massively enlarged livers and hypoglycemia occurring 4 to 6 hours after meals. The hypoglycemia may provoke seizures, but the brain is often remarkably spared, perhaps through the utilization of ketones as an alternative fuel to glucose. Levels of transaminases are often increased to 200 to 400 U per liter, but other aspects of liver function are normal. Moderate hypertriglyceridemia is common. The defect is particularly common in Israel in a group of non-Ashkenazi Jews from North Africa. In infancy, the major problems are hypoglycemia and growth retardation. With increasing age, difficulty with hypoglycemia improves; however, hepatic fibrosis cardiomyopathy and muscle weakness frequently develop during the second and third decade of life. These manifestations presumably reflect cytopathic effects of the nondegradable glycogen in these tissues. Milder forms of debrancher deficiency may present solely with myopathy later in adult life.

Several clinical findings, in addition to the hepatomegaly and hypoglycemia, are helpful in diagnosing debrancher deficiency. The rise in plasma glucose following administration of glucagon is usually normal 2 to 3 hours after a meal, when the terminal branches of glycogen are full; however, 6 to 12 hours after a meal there is no response to glucagon, since glycogen has already been degraded to its branch points. Blood lactate levels are normal or low during fasting, since there is no defect in gluconeogenesis. Lactate increases abnormally to 4 to 6 mEq per liter following an oral glucose tolerance test, as if glycogen stores are already so filled that extra glucose must be disposed of via glycolysis to pyruvate and lactate. Liver biopsy may show increased glycogen and fat and varying degrees of fibrosis. Liver glycogen is marked-

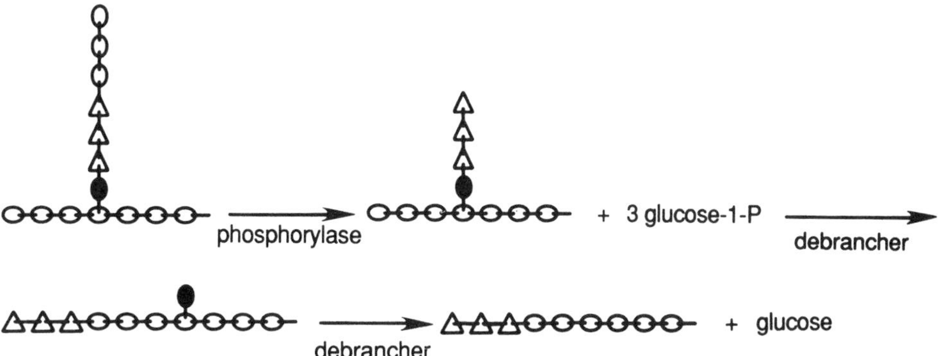

FIGURE 2 Degradation of a terminal segment of glycogen. Phosphorylase releases 1,4-linked glucose residues as glucose-1-phosphate. Debrancher combines two functions: the transfer of three glucose residues from the branch to the main glycogen chain and the release of the 1,6-linked residue at the branch point as free glucose.

ly elevated to 10 to 15 g per 100 g of tissue. Liver tissue has usually been used to demonstrate deficient enzyme activity.

Treatment in early infancy and childhood is aimed at preventing hypoglycemia and growth failure. Frequent feedings of a high-protein, low-carbohydrate diet, together with continuous overnight intragastric infusions of glucose plus protein, are commonly employed. The diet is different from that used in glucose-6-phosphatase deficiency, because gluconeogenesis is not compromised. The use of high-protein rather than high-carbohydrate, feedings blunts the tendency toward postprandial hypoglycemia. No specific therapy has been developed to alleviate or prevent the late development of cardiac and skeletal muscle disease in this disorder.

Liver Phosphorylase/Phosphorylase Kinase Deficiency (Types VI and IX Glycogen Storage Disease).[4,5,8] These two disorders are considered together, since their clinical manifestations are similar and specific assays to distinguish them are not readily available. The disorders resemble a mild form of debrancher deficiency, but with fewer problems with hypoglycemia and growth failure and without the late development of cirrhosis and myopathy. Patients with these disorders usually present with marked hepatomegaly. Hypoglycemia is rare; however, fasting adaptation may be accelerated as reflected by hyperketonemia after an overnight fast. This mild abnormality in fasting may be responsible for the mild growth failure in early infancy in these children. Liver transaminases may be mildly elevated to 100 to 200 U per liter, and triglyceride levels may be mildly increased. Phosphorylase kinase deficiency has been most clearly demonstrated in a large kindred in the Netherlands and appeared to be inherited in an X-linked manner. Liver phosphorylase deficiency is assumed to be an autosomal recessive disorder and is distinct from muscle glycogen phosphorylase deficiency (McArdle's disease).

Like debrancher deficiency, patients with these two disorders show normal levels of lactate during fasting but an abnormal rise in lactate after an oral glucose load. Surprisingly, glucagon may provoke a normal rise in glucose in either the fed or the fasted state in these patients. The enzyme defects in both disorders behave as if they were only partial.

In most cases these disorders are fairly benign, and little or no treatment is required. Catch-up growth has been described after the age of four to five years in some children who had growth failure in early infancy. If growth failure is a problem, a regimen like that used in patients with debrancher deficiency, with frequent feedings during the day and one or two nocturnal feedings or the use of nocturnal intragastric infusions, may be considered.

Glycogen Synthetase Deficiency.[10,11] This defect presents with recurrent episodes of fasting hypoglycemia without hepatomegaly. The defect has been described in only two families and appears to be either very rare or so mild that it is not easily recognized. The reported patients presented with recurrent episodes of fasting hypoglycemia beginning after nighttime feedings were stopped. In one family, the disorder presented during the first few months of life; however, in the other, the hypoglycemia was relatively asymptomatic and not recognized until 7 years of age. Hypoglycemia appears to occur 6 to 10 hours after meals and is accompanied by markedly elevated plasma ketones. Blood lactate levels rise abnormally after meals or oral glucose loading. Surprisingly, glucagon injection induces a small rise in plasma glucose in the fed but not the fasted state. Except for the absence of hepatomegaly, these features closely mimic those seen in patients with debrancher deficiency. Liver biopsy may show little besides a relatively low glycogen content. The enzyme defect appears to be limited to liver tissue. The disorder may be easily misdiagnosed as idiopathic ketotic hypoglycemia. Treatment with diet to avoid prolonged periods of fasting is the same as in the other mild glycogenoses.

Glycogenosis, Galactose Intolerance, Renal Fanconi Syndrome (Type XI Glycogen Storage Disease, Fanconi-Bickel Syndrome).[12] This is a rare disorder in which a severe renal Fanconi syndrome is associated with galactose intolerance and increased glycogen stores in liver. The underlying defect is not known. Patients present during the second 6 months of life with hepatomegaly. They have failure to grow and rickets because of renal tubular acidosis and hypophosphatemia. Hypoglycemia after 6 to 8 hours of fasting may occur but is usually not a severe problem. Galactose disposal is severely delayed. Responses to glucagon have been variable. These children have severe renal glycosuria, aminoaciduria, hypercalciuria, hyperphosphaturia, and bicarbonate wasting. Liver glycogen levels may reach 15 g per 100 g of tissue. Treatment is directed at correcting the renal tubular disturbances with phosphate and alkali supplements. The renal disease is apparently not progressive, but most patients suffer severe rachitic deformities of the bones and short stature.

Defects in Gluconeogenesis

Glucose-6-Phosphatase Deficiency a and b (Types Ia and Ib Glycogen Storage Disease, von Gierke's Disease).[4,5,8,9,13-20] Glucose-6-phosphatase deficiency is both the most common and most severe of the defects in hepatic carbohydrate metabolism which impair fasting homeostasis. While it is often grouped with the glycogen storage disorders, glucose-6-phosphatase deficiency is more appropriately considered a defect in gluconeogenesis, because the enzyme defect blocks the formation of glucose not only from glycogen stores but also from glucose precursors such as lactate and amino acids (see Fig. 1). As shown in Figure 3, glucose production from glucose-6-phosphate is a two-step process in which the sugar phosphate is first transported from the cytosol into microsomes by a specific transporter and then hydrolyzed by membrane-bound glucose-6-phosphatase. The most common form of the disorder is a defect in glucose-6-phosphatase activity itself, also termed type Ia glycogen storage disease. A less common form of the disorder results from a defect in microsomal transport of glucose-6-phosphate, also termed type Ib glycogen storage disease. In the type Ib form, glucose-6-phosphatase activity is "latent"; enzyme activity is absent in fresh tissue homogenates but is normal when microsomes are disrupted by detergents or by freezing. The two forms of the disorder have a similar presentation, but type Ib patients have additional problems with neutropenia and impaired neutrophil function.

Patients with glucose-6-phosphatase deficiency usually present in early infancy with massive hepatomegaly and growth failure. Hypoglycemia occurs within 3 to 4 hours after meals, since plasma glucose levels cannot be maintained once intestinal absorption of glucose is completed. Hypoglycemia is often asymptomatic, except for the hyperpnea associated with acidosis. This is probably because high levels of lactate can serve as an alternative fuel for the brain.

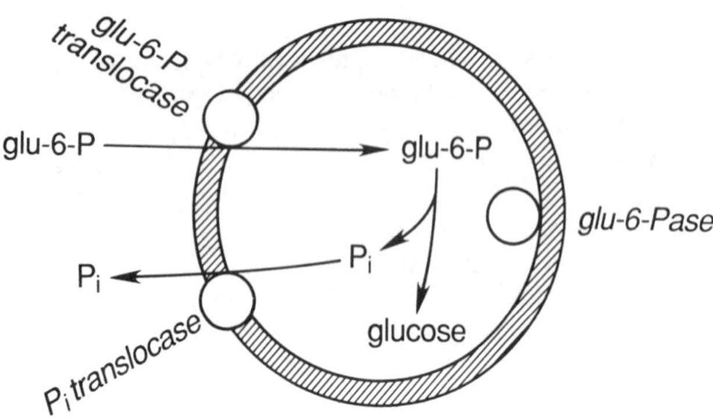

FIGURE 3 Production of free glucose from glucose-6-phosphate. Cytosolic glucose-6-phosphate is transported across the endoplasmic reticulum membrane by a specific translocase and is hydrolyzed by membrane-bound glucose-6-phosphatase to free glucose and inorganic phosphate (P_i). A second translocase carries P_i back to the cytosol. Free glucose may exit the cell via either diffusion or a third translocase.

Ketones are not likely to serve as a major fuel in this disorder, because hepatic ketogenesis is impaired. Triglyceride levels are markedly increased to as much as 2,000 to 3,000 mg per deciliter. Hyperlipidemia may impair platelet function, causing prolonged bleeding time. Apart from moderate increases in transaminases, liver function tests are normal. Hyperuricemia is common in untreated older patients as a consequence of alterations in hepatic sugar-phosphate levels, similar to those discussed under "Hereditary Fructose Intolerance," which accelerate adenosine degradation to uric acid. As shown in Table 2, the disorder is distinguished clinically by hypoglycemia early in fasting, little or no glycemic response to glucagon, and lactate levels that increase dramatically with hypoglycemia or glucagon administration and decrease following administration of glucose. Liver biopsy shows markedly increased fat and glycogen, with glycogen levels of 6 to 10 g per 100 g of tissue. Glucose-6-phosphatase is present only in liver, kidney, and intestinal mucosa. Patients with this disorder also have enlarged kidneys.

Treatment of these patients is aimed at correcting their severe growth retardation by providing exogenous glucose at rates that slightly exceed those of normal hepatic glucose production. This includes frequent carbohydrate feedings during the day and continuous overnight intragastric infusions of glucose or glucose polymers. In some patients, feedings of 1 to 2 g per kilogram of uncooked corn starch suspensions every 6 hours has been effective as a slowly absorbed form of carbohydrate. Lactose and sucrose are avoided, because galactose and fructose cannot be converted to glucose when glucose-6-phosphatase is deficient. Most patients require treatment with allopurinol to prevent hyperuricemia and renal uric acid stone formation. Portacaval shunt procedures have not been beneficial. Liver transplantation is a possible treatment, but there is little experience in these patients.

Long-term problems in these patients include the formation of large hepatic nodules that may presage development of adenomas or hepatic carcinoma. Patients with the defect in microsomal glucose-6-phosphate transport often have mild problems with bacterial infections, including poor healing of abscesses, paronychia, periodontal disease, and recurrent mouth ulcers. Recently, it has also been found that renal failure develops during the third and fourth decades in patients with both types of glucose-6-phosphatase deficiency. The cause of the renal failure is unknown, but the renal disease shares many features with diabetic nephropathy: Glomerular filtration is increased early in infancy, microalbuminuria develops in the second decade and progresses to gross proteinuria, and renal biopsies show a pattern of focal, segmental glomerulosclerosis.

Fructose-1,6-Diphosphatase Deficiency.[21,22] Patients with this rare enzyme deficiency usually present during the first year of life with life-threatening episodes of illness provoked by fasting. Features include lethargy or coma, hyperpnea, and moderate hepatomegaly. Between episodes, patients may appear quite normal. Laboratory findings at the time of acute illness include hypoglycemia and lactic acidosis as markers of the defect in gluconeogenesis. Liver biopsy may show increased fat but normal quantities of glycogen. Because of the site of the enzyme deficiency (see Fig. 1), metabolism of galactose (lactose) is normal in these patients,

TABLE 2
Distinguishing Features of the Defects in Fasting Glucose Homeostosis

	Hepatomegaly	Fasting Tolerance	Ketosis	Glucose Response to Glucagon		Lactate Response		
				Fed	Fasted	To Fasting	To Feeding	To Glucagon
Glycogen Pathway Defects								
Debrancher	3+	4–6 hr	4+	↑	–	↓	↑	↓
Phosphorylase	3+	N	4+	Varies	Varies	↓	↑	↓
Phosphorylase-kinase	3+	N	4+	Varies	Varies	↓	↑	↓
Synthetase	0	6–10 hr	4+	–/↑	–	↓	↑	
Gluconeogenesis Defects								
Glucose-6-phosphatase	4+	3–4 hr	1+	–	–	↑	↓	↑
Fructose-diphosphatase	0–2+	10–14 hr	4+	↑	–	↑	↓	
Phosphoenolpyruvate carboxykinase	+	?6–10 hr	?			N/↑	↓	
Pyruvate carboxylase	0	N	?N			N/↑	↑	

N = normal.

but the ingestion of fructose (as in sucrose) may precipitate hypoglycemia, hypophosphatemia, hyperuricemia, and lactic acidosis. The timing of the hypoglycemia in this disorder, after 12 to 16 hours of fasting, is later than in glucose-6-phosphatase deficiency, because glycogenolysis is unaffected.

The disorder is recessively inherited. Diagnosis can be made by assay of fructose-diphosphatase activity in liver. Treatment includes frequent feedings to avoid prolonged periods of fasting of more than 8 to 12 hours and the elimination of fructose (sucrose)from the diet.

Phosphoenolpyruvate-Carboxykinase Deficiency.[23] There are two distinct phosphoenolpyruvate-carboxykinase enzymes, a mitochondrial form and a cytosolic form. A very limited number of cases have been reported with deficiency of one or the other component, but the disorders remain poorly defined. Both forms can cause severe disease and have been associated with deaths in the first months of life. Hypoglycemia occurs in both forms. Ketogenesis may be suppressed. Lactic acidemia occurs in the mitochondrial but not the cytosolic enzyme defect. Moderate hepatomegaly occurs in both forms. Some patients have had chronic and progressive liver failure, with biopsies showing not only fatty infiltration but also fibrosis. One patient had renal Fanconi's syndrome. Hypotonia and developmental delay have been reported in most patients. The diagnosis has usually been made in the course of investigations of the hypoglycemia. The enzyme defect has been shown in either liver or fibroblasts. Inheritance of both forms appears to be autosomal recessive. Treatment to avoid fasting stress similar to that used in glucose-6-phosphatase or fructose-diphosphatase deficiency has been used with limited success in one case.

Pyruvate Carboxylase Deficiency.[24] A small number of cases have been reported with evidence of deficiency of the mitochondrial enzyme pyruvate carboxylase, the first step in gluconeogenesis from pyruvate. In marked contrast to the other three gluconeogenic enzyme defects, patients with pyruvate carboxylase deficiency do not present with fasting hypoglycemia but rather with a congenital lactic acidosis and progressive neurologic deterioration, including ataxia and retardation. The clinical manifestations closely resemble those of the other congenital lactic acidosis disorders, or Leigh's syndrome (subacute necrotizing encephalomyelopathy). The metabolic disturbance is primarily one of impaired pyruvate oxidation, since pyruvate carboxylase is required to produce adequate amounts of oxaloacetate to maintain the tricarboxylic acid cycle. There is no hepatomegaly or evidence of liver dysfunction. Inheritance is autosomal recessive.

Disorders Causing Cellular Damage

Cytopathic Glycogen Pathway Defects

Brancher Deficiency (Amylopectinosis, Type IV Glycogen Storage Disease).[4] Deficiency of the glycogen brancher enzyme is a rare, recessively inherited disorder characterized by progressive cirrhosis and death from liver failure within the first or second year of life. The enzyme defect causes the formation of glycogen with longer outer branches which resembles amylopectin, a form of plant starch. The abnormally structured glycogen may act as a foreign body to cause progressive cirrhosis. Patients with this disorder are normal at birth but present with failure to thrive and hepatomegaly and then splenomegaly during the first few months of life. Liver glycogen levels are not increased. The disorder affects primarily the liver, although there is some evidence of neurologic involvement. Laboratory tests show evidence of the severe liver disease; there are no specific clinical tests for the disorder. The diagnosis is based on assays of liver tissue showing abnormal structure of glycogen and deficient brancher enzyme activity. The enzyme defect has been demonstrated in cultured skin fibroblasts. Liver transplantation may be a possible mode of treatment.

Acid Maltase Deficiency (Pompe's Disease).[3,4] Acid maltase is a lysosomal enzyme that is not involved in the normal pathways of glycogen synthesis or breakdown. Deficiency of this enzyme does not cause hepatomegaly or abnormal glucose homeostasis. Instead, the acid maltase deficiency shares features with many of the other lysosomal enzyme defects, i.e., progressive multisystem disease affecting particularly cardiac and skeletal muscle. Three forms of the disease have been described. The infantile form presents with hypotonia, weakness, and massive hypertrophic cardiomyopathy. The electrocardiogram may show distinctive gigantic QRS complexes, reflecting the massive biventricular hypertrophy. Death from cardiac failure and respiratory failure usually occurs by age 1 to 2 years. The childhood form presents in later infancy or early childhood with hypotonia and progressive muscle weakness but little or no cardiomyopathy. Death usually occurs by the end of the second decade. The adult form is still milder, presenting in the second to fourth decade with gradually progressive muscle weakness.

The diagnosis is usually made on muscle biopsy, which shows both lysosomal glycogen vacuoles and a remarkable increase in cytoplasmic free glycogen by electron microscopy. Similar abnormalities may be seen in liver tissue. The enzyme deficiency can be shown in a variety of tissues, usually muscle or cultured fibroblasts. Liver size and tests of liver function and glucose homeostasis are normal. Inheritance is autosomal recessive. No specific treatment is available. Areas of research being pursued include liver transplantation, replacement enzyme infusions, and increased dietary protein to preserve muscle strength.

Defects in Metabolism of Nonglucose Sugars

Galactose Pathway Defects.[25] *Galactokinase Deficiency.* Galactokinase initiates the metabolism of galactose absorbed from the intestine following hydrolysis of lactose (see Fig. 1). In contrast to the severe disorder caused by deficiency of galactose-1-phosphate uridyl transferase, the next step in the pathway, deficiency of galactokinase, causes only cataracts. The mechanism of the cataract formation is the same as in the transferase deficiency. Through the action of aldose reductase, elevated galactose levels in the lens lead to accumulation of intracellular galactitol, a polyol that increases osmotic pressure in the lens and ultimately causes cataract formation. Following the ingestion of galactose in these patients, galactose may be detected in the urine as a nonglucose reducing sugar. Treatment is directed at elimination of galactose from the diet. The disorder is very rare. Inheritance is autosomal recessive.

Galactose-1-Phosphate Uridyl Transferase Deficiency (Galactosemia). This is a rare, life-threatening inborn error in which the ingestion of galactose has severe acute and chronic toxic effects on the liver and other organs. The disorder usually presents during the first several days of life after milk feedings containing lactose have begun. Findings include failure to thrive, vomiting, jaundice and other evidence of hepatocellular damage, and renal Fanconi's syndrome. The liver may be enlarged, and some neonates may already have evidence of early cataracts. Laboratory findings, in addition to those associated with liver dysfunction, include acidosis, proteinuria, and aminoaciduria. If lactose has been recently ingested, blood galactose levels may be elevated and galactose may be demonstrated in the urine as a nonglucose reducing sugar. Liver biopsy may show fibrosis and a characteristic acinar formation.

The disorder is due to deficiency of galactose-1-phosphate uridyl transferase, the second step in hepatic conversion of galactose to glucose (see Fig. 1). As in the defects in the fructose pathway, blocks after the formation of the sugar phosphate are many times more severe than the blocks before this point. The acute derangements of liver and kidney function are reversible with elimination of galactose in the diet. Cataracts, produced through the same mechanism as in galactokinase deficiency, may regress but not entirely disappear on a galactose-free diet. Mild to moderate mental retardation is common, probably reflecting a direct toxic effect on the developing brain. In females, the period of galactose exposure in infancy may permanently damage the ovaries, leading to hypergonadotropic hypogonadism in adulthood. Gonadal function in males is not impaired.

The enzyme deficiency can be demonstrated in a variety of tissues, including red blood cells. Galactose tolerance tests should not be used in making the diagnosis. In some states, newborn screening programs test for galactosemia. Treatment consists of the complete elimination of all sources of galactose in the diet, especially milk and milk products that contain lactose (glucose-galactose disaccharide) but also products such as breads and cakes made with milk products.

Fructose Pathway Defects.[21] *Fructokinase Deficiency (Benign Essential Fructosuria).* Genetic deficiency of fructokinase, the enzyme that initiates the metabolism of dietary fructose, causes a rare benign disorder in which the ingestion of fructose or sucrose leads to the appearance of fructose in the urine. Fructosuria may be discovered accidentally as a positive test for reducing sugars (e.g., Clinitest) but a negative test with enzyme-impregnated test strips that are specific for glucose (e.g., Diastix).

Fructose-1-Phosphate Aldolase Deficiency (Hereditary Fructose Intolerance). This is a rare, recessively inherited disorder in which the ingestion of fructose causes toxic effects on the liver, intestine, and kidney. As shown in Figure 1, the enzyme defect blocks fructose metabolism after the formation of fructose-1-phosphate. The toxic effects are largely consequences of the marked reduction in intracellular phosphate and adenosine triphosphate levels which result from the sequestration of phosphate as fructose-1-phosphate. The immediate biochemical derangements are an exaggeration of those induced by fructose infusion in normal subjects and include hyperuricemia, hypophosphatemia, lactic acidosis, and hypoglycemia. The mechanism of the hyperuricemia is the same as in glucose-6-phosphatase deficiency, i.e., overproduction of uric acid from adenosine monophosphate (AMP) as a result of deinhibition of AMP deaminase by the reduction in intracellular phosphate levels.

Infants with the disorder who are fed a diet containing fructose or sucrose may present with failure to thrive, vomiting, life-threatening hepatocellular destruction, and renal Fanconi syndrome. The liver disease may be manifest as hepatomegaly, hyperbilirubinemia, elevations of liver enzymes, and clotting factor deficiencies. Patients who are not exposed to fructose in early infancy may escape illness, because the ingestion of even small amounts of fructose causes severe distress, sweating, nausea, vomiting, and hypoglycemia. Thus, older patients frequently learn by experience to avoid fructose-containing foods.

If hereditary fructose intolerance is suspected, all sources of fructose, sucrose, and sorbitol must be immediately eliminated from the diet to prevent further liver damage. Specific diagnosis can be made with an intravenous fructose tolerance test or by assay of enzyme activity in liver biopsy.

REFERENCES

1. McGarry JD, Kuwajima M, Newgard CB, et al. From dietary glucose to liver glycogen: the full circle round. Ann Rev Nutr 1987; 7:51–73.
2. Larner J. Insulin-signaling mechanisms. Diabetes 1988; 37:262–275.
3. Hug G. Glycogen storage diseases. Birth Defects 1976; 12:145–175.
4. Howell RR, Williams JC. The glycogen storage diseases. In: Stanbury JB, et al, eds. The metabolic basis of inherited disease. 5th ed. New York: McGraw-Hill, 1983: 141.
5. Fernandes J, Leonard JV, Moses SW, et al. Glycogen storage disease; recommendations for treatment. Eur J Pediatr 1988; 147:226–228.
6. Moses SW, Gadoth N, Bashan N, et al. Neuromuscular involvement in glycogen storage disease type III. Acta Pediatr Scand 1986; 75:289–296.
7. Slonim AE, Coleman RA, Moses SW. Myopathy and growth failure in debrancher enzyme deficiency: improvement with high-protein nocturnal enteral therapy. J Pediatr 1984; 105:906–911.
8. Fernandes J, Huijing F, Van de Kamer JH. A screening method for liver glycogen diseases. Arch Dis Child 1969; 44:311.
9. Stanley CA. Intragastric feeding in glycogen storage disease and other disorders of fasting. In: Walker WA, Watkins JB, eds. Nutrition in Pediatrics Boston: Little Brown, 1985: 781.
10. Aynsley-Green A, Williamson DH, Gitzelmann R. Hepatic glycogen synthetase deficiency. Arch Dis Child 1977; 52:573–579.
11. Dykes JRW, Spencer-Peet J. Hepatic glycogen synthetase deficiency. Further studies in a family. Arch Dis Child 1972; 47:558–563.
12. Manz F, Bickel H, Brodehl J, et al. Fanconi-Bickel syndrome. Pediatr Nephrol 1987; 1:509–518.
13. Fernandes J, Berger R, Smit GPA. Lactate as a cerebral metabolic fuel for glucose-6-phosphatase–deficient children. Pediatr Res 1984; 18:335–339.
14. Binkiewicz A, Senior B. Decreased ketogenesis in von Gierke's disease (type I glycogenosis). J Pediatr 1973; 83:973.
15. Greene HL, Slonim AE, O'Neill JA, Burr IM. Continuous nocturnal intragastric feeding for management of type I glycogen storage disease. N Engl J Med 1976; 294:423–425.
16. Stanley CA, Mills JL, Baker L. Intragastric feeding in type I glycogen storage disease: factors affecting control of lactic acidemia. Pediatr Res 1981; 15:1504–1508.
17. Parker P, Burr I, Slonim A, et al. Regression of hepatic adenomas in type Ia glycogen storage disease with dietary therapy. Gastroenterology 1981; 81:534–536.
18. DiRocco M, Barrone B, Dallegri F, et al. Neutropenia and impaired neutrophil function in glycogenosis type I b. J Inher Metabol Dis 1984; 7:151–154.
19. Koven NL, Clarke MM, Cody CS, Stanley CA, Baker L, Douglas SD. Impaired chemotaxis and neutrophile (PMN) function in glycogenosis (GSD) IB. Pediatr Res 1986; 20:438–442.
20. Baker L, Dahlem S, Goldfarb S, et al. Hyperfiltration and renal disease in glycogen storage disease, type I. Kidney Int 1989; 35:1345–1350.
21. Gitzelmann R, Steinmann B, Van Den Berghe G. Essential fructosuria, hereditary fructose intolerance, and fructose-1,6-diphosphatase deficiency. In: Stanbury JB et al. eds. The metabolic basis of inherited disease. 5th ed. New York: McGraw-Hill, 1983: 118.
22. Baker L, Winegrad AL. Fasting hypoglycemia and metabolic acidosis associated with deficiency of hepatic fructose-1,6-diphosphatase activity. Lancet 1970; ii:13–16.
23. Clayton PT, Hyland K, Brand M, Leonard JV. Mitochondrial phosphoenolpyruvate carboxykinase deficiency. Eur J Pediatr 1986; 145:46–50.
24. Blass JP. Inborn errors of pyruvate metabolism. In: Stanbury JB, et al, eds. The metabolic basis of inherited disease. 5th ed. New York: McGraw-Hill, 1983; 141.
25. Segal S. Disorders of galactose metabolism. In: Stanbury JB, et al., eds. The metabolic basis of inherited disease. 5th ed. New York: McGraw-Hill, 1983: 141.

PART 10

Disorders of Amino Acid Metabolism

Gerard T. Berry, M.D.

The gastroenterologist is often confronted with the patient whose history is suggestive of a metabolic disorder and who exhibits signs of hepatic disease. The latter may take the form of isolated hepatomegaly with or without chemical evidence of hepatocellular disease. This discussion is concerned with those inborn errors that affect the metabolism of amino acids and that may be associated with hepatic abnormalities. These diseases include hereditary tyrosinemia, the various urea cycle enzyme defects (UCED), disorders of amino acid transport that affect ureagenesis, and also several disorders of organic acid metabolism that are primarily associated with defective catabolism of branched-chain amino acid metabolites.

The liver plays a major role in intermediary metabolism in man. It is the metabolic clearinghouse for many circulating metabolites, including amino acids, organic acids, and ammonia (NH_4^+). Hepatic mishandling of these compounds due to inherited enzymatic deficiencies often has widespread deleterious effects on diverse tissues or organs because levels of the affected chemicals are elevated throughout the body. Hyperammonemia as a consequence of UCED exemplifies this phenomenon. Phenylketonuria (PKU) secondary to absent hepatic phenylalanine hydroxylase activity, however, is an example of an inborn error of amino acid metabolism that results in no significant hepatic pathology but has devastating effects on the central nervous system (CNS). In some aminoacidopathies, both the liver and other organs are primarily involved because the enzyme defect not only is widespread but is associated with local pathology. Hereditary tyrosinemia is the prime example of this type of inborn error.

Because of the liver's central processing role in disposal of most amino acids and NH_4^+, hepatocellular disease, no matter what the etiology, may cause multiple secondary abnormalities in levels of circulating amino acids and NH_4^+. Relatively nonspecific metabolic screening tests performed on the body fluids of such patients may be uninformative or, worse, misleading. This may even pertain to analysis of amino acids. The ability of the clinician to arrive at the correct diagnosis is dependent on an understanding of the pathophysiology underlying the above classes of inborn errors and on ordering the appropriate metabolic tests. In this discussion, emphasis will be placed on those special metabolic tests that are essential for diagnostic ascertainment.

HEREDITARY TYROSINEMIA

Although hereditary tyrosinemia is usually classified as an aminoacidopathy, the hepatorenal form of the genetic hypertyrosinemias, termed tyrosinemia type I or tyrosinosis, is primarily a disease of organic acid metabolism.[1,2] There have been over 100 cases of this rare malady described since Baber's original report in 1956.[3] As shown in Figure 1, the defective enzyme is fumarylacetoacetic acid hydrolase (FAH) leading to impaired conversion of fumarylacetoacetate (FAA) to the Kreb's cycle intermediate, fumarate, and the ketone body, acetoacetate.[4] Oxidative metabolism of the two products will effect the complete combustion of tyrosine to carbon dioxide and water. Because of secondary inhibition of the more proximal enzyme in the tyrosine pathway, p-hydroxyphenylacetic acid oxidase (Fig. 1), probably by a metabolite of FAA,[4,5] hepatic handling of tyrosine itself is affected in this disease, resulting in accumulation of tyrosine in tissues and blood.

There are two clinical forms or phenotypes. Most patients can be readily identified as having either an acute or a chronic form. In the more common acute form, infants usually present in the first few months of life. The signs of disease are due to progressive liver destruction and the renal Fanconi syndrome. Clinical findings include failure to thrive, vomiting, jaundice, hepatomegaly, ascites, anasarca, and occasionally hyperventilatory episodes secondary to metabolic acidosis. Hemorrhages of the gastrointestinal (GI) and genitourinary (GU) tracts occur frequently and are in part evidence of a bleeding diathesis that is out of proportion to the magnitude of hepatic synthetic defects. Some patients manifest a cabbage-like odor due to a methionine metabolite. Most of these infants die by 1 year of age because of end-stage liver disease. In the chronic form, some of the above findings may be present, but vitamin D–resistant rickets due to the renal Fanconi syndrome often is the major manifestation of disease and the reason why these older infants or children usually come to clinical attention. Some infants with the acute form may also manifest rickets. Intermittent episodes of abdominal pain and neurologic abnormalities, resembling the attacks in neurovisceral porphyria, may also occur, usually in patients with the chronic form, and are secondary to accumulation of delta-aminolevulinic acid. This is due to inhibition of delta-aminolevulinic acid dehydratase by metabolites of FAA, such as succinylacetone,[6,7] which structurally is highly similar to delta-aminolevulinic acid. Hypertensive periods associated with increased catecholamine production have also been noted. Intercurrent infectious episodes may be severe.

Hepatocellular carcinoma is a frequent complication of tyrosinemia. Duration of the disease seems to be the major factor that determines the occurrence of liver cancer. In one survey, 37 percent of patients with the chronic phenotype were known to develop hepatomas.[8] However, even patients as young as 2 years of age have been noted to have microcarcinomatosis upon examination of liver tissue.[9] Patients with the "chronic" phenotype rarely survive the second decade of life because of either hepatic failure or metastatic disease. In these patients, hepatic fibrosis is often present and progressive even in the absence of overt signs of liver disease.[10]

Laboratory findings vary depending on duration of disease, organ failure, diet, and therapy. Almost all patients with the acute form are anemic. Hypoglycemia may be detected in these infants, probably because of hepatic failure. Serum bilirubin, aspartate aminotransferase (AST), alanine aminotransferase (ALT), lactate dehydrogenase, gamma glutamyltransferase, alkaline phosphatase, and alpha-fetoprotein may be increased. Even in the absence of amino acid abnormalities, levels of the latter may be increased in affected infants at birth. Depending on the extent of proximal tubular dysfunction, the renal Fanconi syndrome will variably result in glycosuria, generalized aminoaciduria, phosphaturia, hypercalciuria, hyperuricosuria, renal cation and bicarbonate wastage producing a hyperchloremic metabolic acidosis, hypophosphatemia, and hypouricemia.

The degree of tyrosine elevation in blood and urine is variable. Since tyrosine is synthesized from phenylalanine, which is an essential amino acid, tyrosine accumulation will be dependent on dietary intake or administration of hyperalimentation solutions containing phenylalanine or tyrosine. Hepatocellular disease from any cause may be associated with mishandling of methionine as well as tyrosine and phenylalanine. Hypermethioninemia, hypertyrosinemia, and hyperphenylalaninemia may be seen in patients with various disorders such as cirrhosis, acute massive hepatonecrosis, hereditary galactosemia, hereditary fructose intolerance, and Wilson's disease. These secondary biochemical abnormalities are further discussed in the chapter on liver failure. Genetic defects in tyrosine metabolism are more commonly associated with blood tyrosine levels higher than those present in liver disease per se. Nevertheless, some infants with hereditary tyrosinemia, probably due to nutritional status, have only isolated hypermethionemia with little or no elevation in blood tyrosine. Increased urinary excretion of tyrosine, phenylalanine, and methionine may be detected. Depending on blood levels and the corresponding degree of glomerular overflow, marked hypertyrosinuria, hyperphenylalaninuria, and hypermethioninuria may be superimposed on a generalized aminoaciduria. The accumulation of compounds proximal to FAA results in increased tissue (primarily liver and kidney), blood, and/or urine levels of various metabolites such as p-hydroxyphenylacetic acid, p-hydroxyphenylpyruvic acid, p-hydroxyphenyllactic acid, succinylacetoacetate, and succinylacetone. The immediate precursor, maleylacetoacetate (MAA), as well as FAA, has not been detected in liver tissue. It is generally believed that both compounds are highly reactive. Their accumulation may be the biochemical basis for liver cell death, which characterizes this progressive disease. Glutathione serves as a co-factor in the maleylacetoacetic acid isomerase reaction.[11] This peptide, which may play an important role in daily hepatic detoxification processes, becomes depleted in patients, probably secondary to adduct formation. In vitro, FAA readily forms an adduct with glutathione.[11] Laberge et al[12] reported that a mercapturic acid breakdown product of the glutathione-FAA adduct has

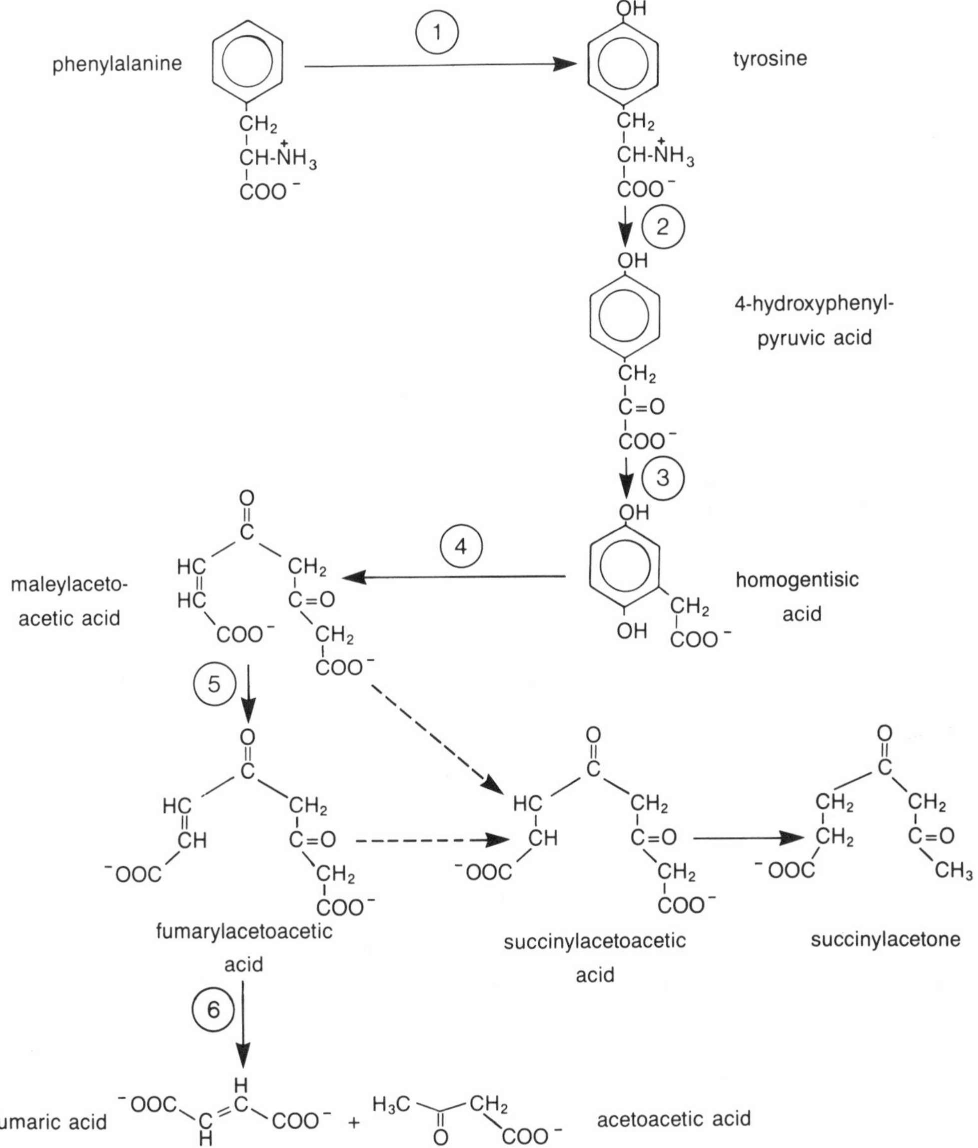

FIGURE 1 The phenylalanine-tyrosine pathway. Enzymes identified numerically include (1) phenylalanine hydroxylase, (2) tyrosine aminotransferase, (3) p-hydroxyphenylpyruvic acid oxidase, (4) homogentisate oxidase, (5) maleylacetoacetate isomerase, (6) fumarylacetoacetate hydrolase. Dotted lines indicate putative conversion of structural isomers to succinylacetoacetic acid.

been detected in urine of patients. Succinylacetone covalently linked to both glutathionine and various other amino acids has also been detected in urine.[13] Decreased activities of several hepatic enzymes such as p-hydroxyphenylacetic acid oxidase, delta-aminolevulinic acid dehydratase, S-adenosylmethionine synthetase, and the cytochrome P-450 mixed function oxidases, 7-ethoxycoumarin deethylase and aryl hydrocarbon hydroxylase, important in detoxification of potential carcinogens, have been detected, whereas others such as MAA isomerase or delta-aminolevulinic acid synthetase were unaffected or increased.[14]

Variability in patients' propensities for accumulation of toxic metabolites and development of secondary enzyme deficiencies would help to explain several perplexing features of this disease such as the variable presence of hypertyrosinemia, hypermethioninemia, isolated elevation of cord blood alpha-fetoprotein,[15] hepatoblastomas, and different phenotypes. The occurrence of an acute lethal or a chronic form in a particular patient may be related to the extent to which highly reactive molecular species can initiate hepatic damage. Environmental as well as genetic factors probably play a role in disease expression, since, while patients with the chronic phenotype usually have more residual FAA enzyme activity, both phenotypes have been detected in the same family. There are also reports of patients with infantile presentations who appeared to have "outgrown" their disease or to be relatively disease-free during the fourth decade.[8]

Pathologic findings in liver include inflammation, fatty infiltration, pseudoacinar formation, cirrhosis, and hepatocarcinoma. The pancreatic islets may be hyperplastic. The kidneys are usually enlarged with histologic evidence of renal tubular degeneration. Other lesions, such as effects on astroglial cells in the CNS, are probably secondary to hepatic failure.

Hereditary tyrosinemia should be ruled out in any infant or child with unexplained liver disease or the renal Fanconi syndrome, even if incomplete. The evaluation of renal tubular dysfunction requires quantitation of urinary amino acids. The plasma tyrosine level may be assessed by quantitation of plasma amino acids by ion exchange column chromatography. However, definitive exclusion of FAH deficiency requires analysis of urine for the organic acids succinylacetoacetate and succinylacetone by gas-liquid chromatography (GLC) in conjunction with mass spectrometry (MS). Alternatively, succinylacetone and probably other related metabolites can be detected by measuring the ability of urine to inhibit delta-aminolevulinic acid dehydratase in a radiochemical assay. The enzyme FAH may be assayed in liver tissue or cultured skin fibroblasts.[16] No enzyme protein was detected in liver of patients with the acute form using Western blotting analysis, whereas decreased amounts were present in patients with the chronic form who had measurable, residual FAH activity.[17]

As soon as the diagnosis is established, patients should be started on a low tyrosine and phenylalanine diet. A special formula devoid of tyrosine and phenylalanine may be supplemented with biologic protein to satisfy minimal daily requirements for phenylalanine while maintaining plasma at levels that are as normal as possible. With this regimen, it is highly likely that the renal Fanconi syndrome will markedly improve if not disappear. This makes management easier, because it obviates or reduces the need for oral phosphate supplementation, 1,25-dihydroxylcholecalciferol, and alkali therapy. For most patients, however, dietary therapy will not reverse the progressive liver disease. The younger infant destined to quickly develop end-stage failure will do so despite diet therapy, whereas patients with the chronic phenotype are likely to develop hepatoblastomas. Since red blood cells (RBCs) contain FAA, exchange transfusion has been tried, but for too short a period of time and in too few patients to draw conclusions about efficacy.[18] At this time, the most rational therapy is liver transplantation, particularly for infants with the acute form. Dietary therapy should be used only as a temporizing measure during the wait for the donor liver. Most of the few patients who have received transplantation have done well.[19-21] As expected, tyrosine-related liver disease was eliminated after transplantation, but several patients still showed evidence of renal tubular dysfunction or an incomplete Fanconi syndrome with persistent excretion of succinylacetone.[9,20,21] This phenomenon further serves to emphasize the local toxicity of accumulated metabolites. Depending on the severity of the renal disease, these patients may need to have phenylalanine and tyrosine intake restricted. Long-term effects on kidney function are unknown. Liver transplantation in patients with the chronic phenotype may represent a therapeutic dilemma, since during a restricted diet there may be little evidence of ongoing liver disease and no evidence of cancer. In each patient the risk of transplantation complications must be weighed against the likelihood of cancer.

There are mechanistic similarities underlying tissue destruction in hereditary tyrosemia and acute acetaminophen poisoning. In the latter, a highly reactive metabolite may lead to cell death while promoting the formation of macromolecular adducts and glutathione depletion.[22] MAA and FAA are also highly reactive compounds and may be responsible for cell injury in tyrosinemia. Laberge et al have likened them to strong alkylating agents known to be important in carcinogenesis.[12] When given appropriately in acetaminophen poisoning, pharmacologic therapy with *N*-acetylcysteine has been highly effective in minimizing the heptocellular toxicity by promoting adduct formation with the acetaminophen metabolite.[23] There have been several isolated attempts in tyrosinemic patients to enhance detoxification using glutathione, cysteine, cysteamine, and penicillamine.[10,24] Low plasma cysteine, as well as reduced RBC glutathione levels, had led to supplementation with cystine. While cystine, glutathione, and *N*-acetylcysteine have not produced dramatic clinical effects, they have not been sufficiently studied to draw any conclusions regarding long-term benefit. This form of adjunct treatment could be important in certain patients to retard the progression to cirrhosis or the development of liver cancer, particularly while awaiting liver transplantation. One patient is known to have died of metastatic liver cancer following an immediately successful liver transplantation at age 4 years.[9,21] The monitoring of serum alpha-fetoprotein levels at regular intervals may be helpful in the detection of hepatoblastoma formation.

The worldwide prevalence of this autosomal recessive disorder is approximately 1 per 100,000. The disease is most common in French Canadians, with an incidence of 0.8 per 10,000 in Quebec province. A "founder effect" is responsible for the high prevalence of the gene in the Chicoutini-Lac St. Jean region of Quebec where the carrier rate is 1 per 10 to 15 individuals. Prenatal diagnosis is feasible either by measuring FAH activity in cultured amniocytes[25] or chorionic villus samples[26] or by assaying amniotic fluid for succinylacetone by the delta-aminolevulinic acid dehydratase inhibition assay[27] or gas chromatography–mass spectrometry (GC-MS).[28,29] A false-negative result had been reported with the latter technique.[30] Negative results must be confirmed by enzyme assay. Presence of a pseudodeficiency gene within a family must be ascertained before enzyme analysis results are useful for prediction of outcome.[31] Several countries, as well as some states of the United States, have established newborn screening programs.

INHERITED DEFECTS IN UREAGENESIS

The breakdown of amino acids derived from exogenous dietary and endogenous body protein and the breakdown of urea by microorganisms in the gastrointestinal (GI) tract result in a daily load of ammonia that must be detoxified. This is accomplished by the process of ureagenesis, whereby waste nitrogen is converted into urea, which can be readily excreted in urine. The liver is the only organ that contains all of the urea cycle enzymes in sufficient quantities and is the principal site of urea formation.

The urea cycle enzymes and substrates are shown in Figure 2. Only the enzymes *N*-acetylglutamate synthetase (NAGS), carbamyl phosphate synthetase I (CPS I), and ornithine transcarbamylase (OTC) are located within the mitochondrial matrix. The rest are cytosolic. Carrier-mediated transport is

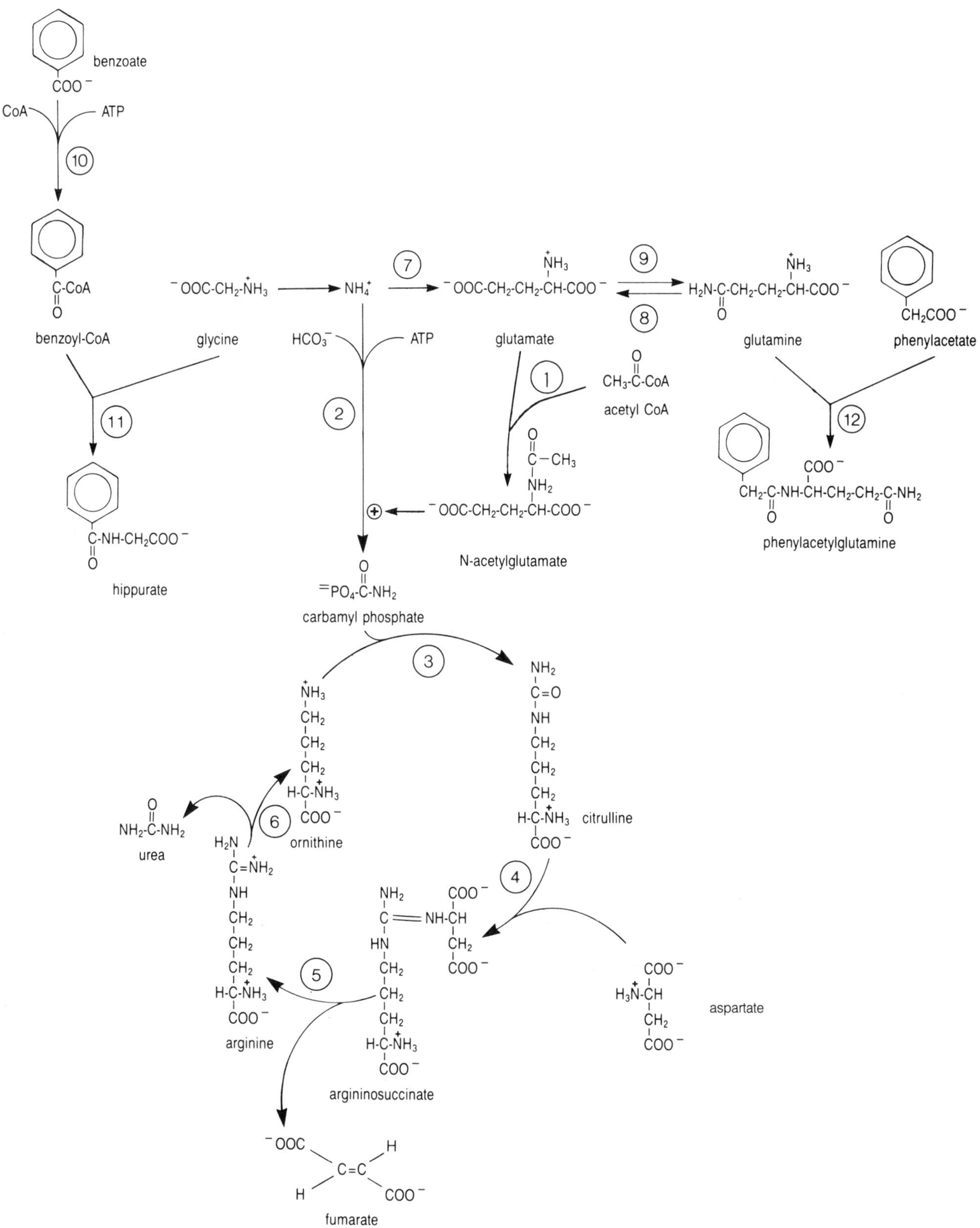

FIGURE 2 The urea cycle and other enzymatic reactions important in NH_4^+ handling. Enzymes identified numerically include (1) *N*-acetyl glutamate synthetase, (2) carbamyl phosphate synthetase I, (3) ornithine transcarbamylase, (4) argininosuccinic acid synthetase, (5) argininosuccinic acid lyase, (6) arginase, (7) glutamate dehydrogenase, (8) glutaminase, (9) glutamine synthetase, (10) thiokinase, (11) glycine *N*-acylase, (12) phenylacetylglutamine synthetase, and (13) glycine cleavage enzyme complex.

responsible for mitochondrial uptake and efflux of ornithine and citrulline, respectively. Flux through the urea cycle, i.e., conversion of ammonia to urea, is essentially governed by three factors: (1) the level of ammonia within the mitochondrial matrix; (2) adequate concentrations of the other key urea cycle substrates, adenosine triphosphate (ATP) and ornithine; and (3) sufficient quantities of urea cycle enzymes in their activated states. The mechanisms controlling intramitochondrial arginine and glutamate concentrations, both of which play a role in modulating CPS I activity and in vivo regulation of the cycle enzymes, in general, are still poorly understood. For activation, CPS I has an absolute requirement of *N*-acetylglutamate, synthesized from glutamate and acetyl-CoA by NAGS, which in turn depends on arginine as a positive effector.

Patients with inherited defects in ureagenesis have either a decrease in urea cycle enzyme activity or a defect in transport of substrate.[32] There is a marked variability in severity of a particular disease mainly related to residual total hepatic enzyme activity. The clinical findings are primarily related to the degree and duration of elevation of NH_4^+ and the age of the patient. Signs and symptoms of hyperammonemia include loss of appetite, vomiting, headache, personality changes, and psychiatric manifestations, ataxia, seizures, primary hyperventilation, lethargy, stupor, and coma. The escalation of the hyperammonemic state is reflected in the number or severity of clinical findings. Cerebral edema is an enigmatic complication of hyperammonemia. Which neurologic signs are directly attributable to ammonia or its metabolites acting as neurotoxin(s) versus those due to cerebral edema is a matter of conjecture. When a plasma specimen is collected properly, the normal range of plasma ammonia is 15 to 40 μM. In the neonate, particularly the low birth weight premature infant, the upper limit may be as high as 100 to 110 μM. Usually, when patients have a level above 500 μM, they are in stage IV coma with increased intracranial pressure and exhibit decerebrate posturing.[33]

Different phenotypes exist for almost every UCED. In general, depending on the degree of residual enzyme activity, patients present with (1) a potentially lethal neonatal-onset catastrophic disease with coma, (2) a more indolent chronic form characterized by growth failure and/or progressive psychomotor retardation, punctuated with acute episodes of severe hyperammonemia, or (3) an intermittent form in which signs and symptoms of hyperammonemia are confined to acute episodes usually precipitated by infections. Important clinical and laboratory information that pertains to the various inherited defects in ureagenesis is outlined in Table 1.

Ornithine Transcarbamylase Deficiency

OTC deficiency is the most common urea cycle enzyme deficiency,[32] with an estimated incidence in newborn infants of 1 per 50,000 while all UCED occur at a frequency of approximately 1 per 30,000. The latter figure is probably an underestimation because of failure to diagnose this rare problem. Specifically, OTC deficiency may be over-represented in this overall underestimation, as it is the only UCED inherited as a sex-linked trait, with female carriers demonstrating a spectrum of disease involvement due to variable unfavorable lyonization of the X-chromosome bearing the defective gene. When the molecular lesion is a severe one, affected males have little residual enzyme activity and exhibit catastrophic disease during the first week of life. Almost always, these male infants die unless specific therapy directed at the UCED is employed. Plasma NH_4^+ may be well over 1,000 μM by the third or fourth day of life in the presence of coma and respiratory failure. Acute hemorrhage, particularly intracranial, has been reported in these patients as well as in infants with other causes of hyperammonemia.[34] This hemizygous phenotype contrasts with the more common type of mild to moderate disease in the carrier female. Indeed, the first two patients with OTC described by Russell et al in 1962 were female first cousins whose manifestations were episodic vomiting, lethargy, mental retardation, and violent headaches with behavioral outbursts.[35] The appearance as well as the severity of signs and symptoms of illness in heterozygous females is quite variable from the first year of life to adulthood. Manifestations include feeding difficulties, episodic vomiting, protein intolerance, aversion to high-protein foodstuffs, intermittent lethargy, neuropsychiatric manifestations such as explosive behavior or even frank psychosis, headache—sometimes mimicking classic migraine, ataxia, seizures, hepatomegaly, and episodes of a Reye's syndrome–like illness. Usually, the liver is not enlarged when hyperammonemia is under control. However, during episodes even the liver function tests such as ALT and AST may become abnormal. An acute episode of hyperammonemia may lead to death in the carrier female. Attacks are usually precipitated by infections, but any state that serves to increase quickly the waste nitrogen burden via exogenous protein or amino acids or endogenous muscle proteolysis will suffice. Examples include protein ingestion, hyperalimentation, vaccinations, and surgery.

At one end of the disease spectrum in carrier females is the adult who suffers from recurrent headaches and alterations in mental alertness. However, some females with unfavorable X-chromosome inactivation have had neonatal- or infantile-onset disease. There is in addition a late-onset syndrome in males due to a less severe gene defect. Another cause of milder disease in males may be a mosaic state in which the OTC gene defect is the result of a deletion that occurred either in the oocyte prior to conception or as the result of a mitotic error in the embryo.[36] Like the carrier females, these older males may suffer from intermittent episodes of lethargy and vomiting, sometimes mimicking Reye's syndrome. However, like any patient with a significant OTC defect, they may succumb to an acute episode of hyperammonemia. Developmental delay or mental retardation is not always present in patients with a nonsevere phenotype. However, permanent brain damage, characterized by mental retardation, motor palsies, or seizures, is likely to follow an episode of prolonged hyperammonemic coma as exemplified by infants who have survived a catastrophic neonatal period. It is likely that persistent low-grade hyperammonemia during the first 2 years of critical neurodevelopment will also result in psychomotor retardation as well as failure to thrive.

Abnormal laboratory findings include plasma amino acids and urinary pyrimidine metabolites in addition to plasma NH_4^+. Several amino acids such as glutamine, glutamate, alanine, glycine, and lysine will be elevated in blood as an

TABLE 1
Inherited Defects in Ureagenesis

Disease	Genetic Defect, Inheritance	Laboratory Findings	Therapy	Notes
Ornithine transcarbamylase (OTC) deficiency	↓ OTC, X-linked	↓ Plasma cit*, arg* ↑ Urine orotate*	LPD, cit, (arg), b, p	Most common UCED X-chromosomal gene deletions and mosaic states reported Males with severe neonatal-onset disease, mild late-onset type Female carriers variably affected
Argininosuccinic aciduria	↓ ASA lyase, AR	↑ Plasma cit†, ASA† ↓ Plasma arg* ↑ Urine orotate*	LPD, arg, (b), (p)	Severe neonatal-onset disease as well as late-onset chronic type Trichorrhexis nodosa Persistent hepatomegaly
Citrullinemia	↓ ASA synthetase, AR	↑ Plasma cit† ↓ Plasma arg* ↑ Urine orotate*	LPD, arg, (b), (p)	Severe neonatal-onset disease as well as late-onset or chronic infantile, childhood, or adult types
Carbamyl phosphate synthetase (CPS) deficiency	↓ CPS, AR	↓ Plasma cit*, arg* No ↑ in urine orotate when plasma NH_4^+↑	LPD, cit, (arg), b, p	Most with severe neonatal-onset type Infantile type with ↑ residual CPS activity
N-Acetylglutamate synthetase (NAGS) deficiency	↓ NAGS, probable AR	↓ Plasma cit, arg No ↑ in urine orotate	*N*-carbamoylglutamate, (LPD), (b), (p)	Two patients with neonatal-onset disease reported *N*-Carbamoylglutamate beneficial in one patient
Argininemia	↓ Arginase, AR	↑ Plasma arg* ↑ Urine orotate†	LPD, (lysine)	Excluding NAGS, the rarest UCED Unique findings: spastic diplegia, may mimic a progressive neurodegenerative disease with leukodystrophy Plasma NH_4^+ not usually ↑
Lysinuric protein intolerance	Abnormal dibasic amino acid transport, AR	↑ Urine arg, orn, and lys	LPD, cit	Mild-moderate hyperammonemic episodes Mental retardation, poor growth, hepatosplenomegaly, diarrhea
Hyperammonemia-hyperornithinemia-homocitrullinuria syndrome	Mitochondrial ornithine transport defect, AR	↑ Plasma orn ↑ Urine homocitrulline	LPD, (orn), (arg)	Mild-moderate hyperammonemic episodes Psychomotor retardation

arg = arginine; ASA = argininosuccinic acid; AR = autosomal recessive; b= benzoate; cit = citrulline; LPD = low-protein diet; orn = ornithine; p = phenylacetate.
*Variable.
†Invariable.

indication of an increase in the total body burden of waste nitrogen, sometimes even before a substantial increase in NH_4^+ can be detected. These findings are nonspecific and can be seen in patients with any disorder of ureagenesis, even a secondary one. The degree of amino acid imbalance generally correlates with the magnitude of hyperammonemia. In OTC deficiency, plasma citrulline and arginine may be depressed. Because of the build-up of hepatic carbamyl phosphate during this state, de novo pyrimidine synthesis will be enhanced, leading to accumulation of orotic acid, uridine, and uracil. As orotic acid is readily excreted in urine, a hyperoroticaciduria will be detected, which correlates with the NH_4^+ burden. Other laboratory findings include intermittent transaminasemia and, early in the course of progressive hyperammonemia, blood gas results compatible with a primary respiratory alkalosis. Plasma urea may be in the low or normal range.

In the absence of intercurrent illness and particularly in males or females with mild to moderate disease, the liver is not enlarged. Histologic examination of liver tissue at autopsy or following biopsy has revealed fat accumulation, inflammation, portal fibrosis, and cytologic lesions. These findings are probably the consequence of NH_4^+ elevation. Brain pathology also includes abnormalities seen in any hyperammonemic disorder such as cortical atrophy with dilated ventricles and Alzheimer type II astrocytes.

The definite diagnosis of OTC deficiency can be made by assaying the enzyme in liver. Intestinal tissue is also suitable for enzyme assay. Because of the "patchy" nature of liver cells bearing the decreased OTC activity in carrier females, tissue obtained by punch biopsy may not be informative. Diagnosis can also be made by analyzing the OTC gene in any tissue such as white blood cells using a cDNA probe, provided that analysis by available restriction endonucleases is informative.[37]

Although not always positive, the heterozygous carrier state has been detected by measuring urine orotic acid after a protein load. Prenatal diagnosis has been successful following enzyme assay of biopsied fetal liver.[38] Less invasive testing, such as OTC gene analysis of amniocytes or chorionic villus tissue using a cDNA probe, is not generally useful, as most patients appear not to have gene deletions or mutations at a restriction site. However, when informative restriction fragment length polymorphisms (RFLP) in a family with an affected child have been ascertained, prenatal diagnosis is possible. Theoretically, when techniques are routinely employed to assess the most important OTC gene point mutations, prenatal diagnosis for most pregnancies will be a reality. To a large degree, prenatal counseling now centers on determination of fetal sex and its implications.

The therapy of an acute hyperammonemic crisis depends on the severity of the illness. In addition to supportive care, it is imperative to reduce NH_4^+ as quickly as possible. For the newborn infant in coma, dialysis is required. Hemodialysis is more efficacious than peritoneal dialysis, but because of technical difficulties in neonates its use is limited to a few centers. Therapy is directed toward terminating further waste nitrogen production by eliminating exogenous protein administration and reversing the catabolic state by providing calories, usually as intravenous glucose. The administration of arginine or citrulline intravenously is also beneficial in OTC-deficient patients, as it serves to replenish body arginine, necessary for protein synthesis. Intravenous administration of sodium benzoate and phenylacetate will reduce NH_4^+ levels by enhancing production and excretion of nitrogen-containing metabolic products, hippurate and phenylacetylglutamine. This is an example of the enhancement of alternate waste nitrogen excretion, first employed by Batshaw, Brusilow, and colleagues,[33,39,40] which has allowed many neonates with UCED to survive despite severe neonatal disease. Similar treatment must also be employed in the older patient during a hyperammonemic episode.[33,41] Moderate episodes may be controlled using intravenous fluids and medication alone. However, severe episodes, associated with coma, will require dialysis and potentially ICP monitoring and pressure therapy because of life-threatening cerebral edema.

Chronic management involves the use of a low-protein diet and also the UCED medications, arginine or preferably citrulline, benzoate, and phenylacetate. For the patient with severe neonatal-onset disease, even 1.5 g of protein per kilogram of body weight per day represents too great a daily load of potential waste nitrogen. To permit normal growth, this kind of infant requires a reduction in total protein intake supplemented with an essential amino acid mixture. As with other UCED patients on low-protein and relatively high-calorie diets, patients with severe OTC deficiency are likely to suffer chronic anorexia despite good metabolic control. For a carrier female or a male with a mild phenotype, a low-protein diet and benzoate alone will likely suffice to maintain health. As these patients age, many learn to modulate their own protein intake. Knowledge alone of the existence of their OTC deficiency is of tremendous benefit for the older patients with previously unexplained disease.

Argininosuccinicaciduria

Argininosuccinicaciduria, the second most common UCED, is due to a deficiency of argininosuccinic acid (ASA) lyase and is inherited as an autosomal recessive trait.[32] This block in the urea cycle impairs urea production and results in massive accumulation of ASA in tissue, blood, and urine. Depending on the degree of residual ASA lyase activity, patients present with potentially lethal neonatal-onset disease or have a chronic form characterized by failure to thrive and developmental delay with episodic vomiting, ataxia, and seizures. As with all of the UCED, the signs and symptoms referable to hyperammonemia are dependent on the degree of NH_4^+ accumulation. One of the unique findings on physical examination is trichorrhexis nodosa. This hair shaft abnormality disappears with control of hyperammonemia and improvement in nutritional status. Infants and young children with severe disease who are under good metabolic control may have massive hepatomegaly, the etiology of which is not understood.[33,42] While the liver function tests may be abnormal, particularly a sensitive one like gamma-glutamyltranspeptidase, they may be normal despite persistent enlargement. Histologic examinations have revealed steatosis, mild cellular infiltration, minimal portal fibrosis, and, in one patient on chronic arginine therapy, enlarged mitochondria with paracrystalline inclusions.[42]

Plasma and urine amino acid analysis always shows a large amount of ASA and, to a lesser degree, increased citrulline. Similar to other UCED, urine orotic acid and plasma levels of several nonessential amino acids such as glutamine, glutamate, alanine, and glycine may be increased during hyperammonemia. For enzymatic confirmation, ASA lyase may be measured in cultured skin fibroblasts as well as liver tissue. The sequence of the ASA lyase gene on chromosome 7 has been determined.[43,44] Prenatal detection is possible by enzyme assay of cultured aminocyte or measurement of ASA in amniotic fluid.

Therapy is similar to that employed in OTC deficiency. Protein restriction is the mainstay of therapy. Of all the patients with severe UCED, those with ASA lyase deficiency are most responsive to directed therapy, because ASA itself is an effective waste nitrogen vehicle. The administration of arginine increases ASA production and waste nitrogen disposal, as 100 percent of filtered ASA is excreted in urine. Essential amino acids, benzoate, and phenylacetate are usually not necessary for long-term management. In line with other UCED, while prognosis is dependent on severity of disease, any intercurrent hyperammonemic episode may prove to be lethal.

Citrullinemia

Inherited as an autosomal recessive trait, citrullinemia is due to a deficiency of ASA synthetase.[32] This enzymatic lesion impairs ureagenesis and results in a marked elevation of citrulline in blood, urine, and tissues. Phenotypes include a severe neonatal-onset form, a chronic or late-onset form in infants and children, and an adult-onset type, common among the Japanese. Clinical findings vary according to the presence and degree of hyperammonemia. Neuropsychiatric disease, including intermittent behavioral disturbances, may be more prevalent in patients with citrullinemia relative to other UCED, raising the possibility that marked hypercitrullinemia per se is toxic to the CNS. Hepatomegaly and abnormal liver function tests are usually present only during hyperammonemia.

Analogous to the plasma and urine amino acid findings in ASA lyase deficiency, citrulline is always markedly elevated, whereas glutamine, orotate, etc., are increased only during hyperammonemic episodes. Cultured skin fibroblasts are suitable for confirmatory analysis of ASA synthase. The single expressed ASA synthase gene on chromosome 9 and multiple pseudogenes have been sequenced.[45,46] Prenatal diagnosis is possible by measuring enzyme level in amniocytes or citrulline in amniotic fluid.

Therapy is similar to that for other patients with UCED. Promotion of citrulline production to further enhance waste nitrogen excretion is not as effective as with ASA because it carries only one real waste nitrogen atom and only 25 percent of filtered citrulline is excreted. In patients with severe disease, benzoate and phenylacetate, in addition to arginine and low protein diet therapy, are necessary to control hyperammonemia and enable normal growth. The prognosis is similar to that for ASA lyase deficiency and varies with the severity of the phenotype.

Carbamyl Phosphate Synthetase Deficiency

Most patients with carbamyl phosphate synthetase (CPS) deficiency have severe neonatal-onset type disease that with severe OTC deficiency in males represents the most lethal form of UCED.[32] Some patients have been reported, however, with a milder phenotype in which clinical disease does not become manifest until age 1 year and in which there is 10 to 25 percent residual enzyme activity. Both forms are inherited as autosomal recessive. The clinical findings in the severe phenotype are similar to those in OTC deficiency, and, like the latter, some newborns are unable to survive despite directed intensive therapy. Patients with the milder phenotype may be developmentally delayed, probably because moderate hyperammonemia has been persistent during infancy and/or because of acute episodes of hyperammonemia. Similar to patients with absent OTC activity, severe CPS-deficient patients may have chronic hepatomegaly and elevated severe ALT and AST levels if, despite treatment, normoammonemia cannot be maintained.

The key laboratory finding in this disease is the absence of elevated urinary orotic acid during hyperammonemia of any degree. Otherwise, plasma and urine amino acid abnormalities mimic those seen in OTC deficiency. Definite diagnosis can be made only by measuring CPS activity in liver or intestinal tissue. A CPS I gene probe is available; although no gene lesions have been defined, the presence of a restriction fragment length polymorphism may permit linkage analysis and facilitate prenatal diagnosis.[47] Fetal liver biopsy for CPS activity measurement has been successfully performed.[48]

The therapy for patients with severe or mild disease is identical to that employed in the different OTC deficiencies. For infants with the neonatal-onset form, the prognosis is guarded.

N-Acetylglutamate Synthetase Deficiency

There has been only two confirmed reports of hepatic *N*-acetylglutamate synthetase (NAGS) deficiency.[32,49] Both patients presented in the first week of life with hyperammonemia and elevated plasma glutamine but with no increase in urinary orotate levels. While CPS I activity in liver biopsy specimens was normal, NAGS was undetectable. The first patient was treated with arginine and benzoate in addition to use of a low-protein diet. However, only the use of *N*-carbamoylglutamate, a stable intermediate in the CPS reaction, was successful in controlling the hyperammonemia. Theoretically, the presence of *N*-carbamoylglutamate obviates the need for the stimulatory effect of NAG on CPS. Although two siblings had died during the neonatal period, the first patient is currently over 8 years old, has been maintained on this medication, and is mentally retarded. The second patient died in the neonatal period despite treatment. Histologic examination revealed eosinophilic inclusions in hepatocytes that may in part represent albumin accumulation within organelles such as the endoplasmic reticulum (ER).[50]

Argininemia

Prior to the reports of NAGS deficiency, argininemia within organelles such as the ER secondary to decreased arginase activity was the rarest of the UCED.[32] It is also unique among the UCED because of its peculiar clinical and biochemical findings. Almost all of the patients with this autosomal recessive disease have been Finnish and have had identical neurologic findings consisting of progressive psychomotor retardation with acquired microcephaly, spastic diplegia, and seizures. While patients may have recurrent attacks of vomiting, lethargy, headache, and behavioral changes, plasma NH_4^+ levels are usually within the normal range. When elevated, plasma NH_4^+ is rarely above 300 to 400 μM. There are no reported deaths from hyperammonemic coma. The patients do not usually demonstrate the self-imposed protein restriction so typical in other UCED patients. The liver may be enlarged. In some patients, the clinical picture is more compatible with a progressive neurodegenerative disorder that most resembles a leukodystrophy, such as metachromatic leukodystrophy. Mental retardation is the rule. The diagnosis may actually be very difficult to make. While plasma arginine is usually substantially elevated, it may approach the normal postprandial range during periods of protein restriction.

The most prominent biochemical abnormalities are the accumulation in blood, urine, and CSF of the proximal metabolite arginine and the persistent hyperoroticaciduria, which is usually present even in the absence of hyperammonemia. Ornithine levels in plasma are normal or only slightly reduced. Urinary excretion of all of the dibasic amino acids may be increased as well as several guanidine derivatives. The plasma urea may be normal or low. Hypertransaminasemia may be detected. Definitive diagnosis requires measurement of arginase in tissue such as red or white blood cells and liver but not fibroblasts or kidney, as there are two different arginase genes.[51] Prenatal diagnosis can be made by measuring enzyme in fetal erythrocytes. Histologic examination of liver tissue has revealed cytotoxic changes. Adequate treatment is difficult, since the bulk of neurotoxicity may be directly secondary to raised plasma arginine. Diets restricted in arginine have resulted in normalization of NH_4^+ levels and neurologic improvement. A low-protein diet alone is probably not sufficient for most patients; better control is dependent on the use of an essential amino acid mixture in conjunction with a low amount of biologic protein. Benzoate and phenylacetate may also be beneficial. Ornithine and lysine supplementation has also been tried to replenish the hepatic ornithine pool and stimulate brain uptake of lysine, respectively. Some of the patients treated from infancy with a suitable arginine-restricted diet have been spared the severe encephalopathy. Erythrocyte exchange transfusion, a form of enzyme replacement therapy, has been reported to be beneficial.[52]

Lysinuric Protein Intolerance

Lysinuric protein intolerance is a rare autosomal recessive disorder associated with protein intolerance and hyperammonemia and is prevalent in the Finnish.[32] Hepatic ornithine depletion, curtailing ureagenesis, is the result of a membrane transport defect involving the dibasic amino acids ornithine, arginine, and lysine and affecting intestinal and renal tubular basolateral membranes, hepatocytes, and other epithelial membranes. Hyperammonemia is the consequence of decreased urea cycle turnover due to urea cycle substrate depletion. Clinical findings include feeding problems with vomiting in infancy, poor growth, mental retardation, and episodes of mild to moderate hyperammonemia associated with lethargy or coma. In addition to liver enlargement, splenomegaly not readily attributable to portal hypertension has been a persistent finding. Diarrhea, probably secondary to the amino acid malabsorption, may also occur. Osteoporosis, myopathy, lenticular opacities, and sparse, brittle hair have also been reported.

Laboratory findings include increased urinary excretion of ornithine, arginine, and lysine and decreased levels in plasma. During hyperammonemia, plasma glutamine and alanine and urine orotic acid may be increased. It is important to note that analysis of amino acids in plasma alone is likely to cause the diagnosis to be missed. Liver function tests may be abnormal. Anemia, neutropenia, and thrombocytopenia may also occur. Plasma urea is low or normal. Hepatic pathology may include fatty infiltration and cytotoxic changes. No abnormal findings have been detected in intestinal tissue.

The goal of treatment is to replenish ornithine stores in liver to enable the cycle to turn effectively. Arginine administration is partially effective but worsens diarrhea. Probably the most suitable treatment involves protein restriction combined with citrulline supplementation. Citrulline is capable of bypassing the intestinal and hepatic transport block and can be converted to ornithine within the hepatocytes. Even on this treatment, however, some of the abnormalities, such as hepatosplenomegaly, have persisted. Acute hyperammonemic episodes are treated similarly to the UCED, although citrulline is an important addition to treatment. Most of the patients do not die from hyperammonemic coma, because episodes are usually mild. Whether prospective treatment in infancy would eliminate many of the complications is not known. Unfortunately, in this disease mental retardation is the rule.

Hyperammonemia-Hyperornithinemia-Homocitrullinuria Syndrome

This rare autosomal recessive disorder is associated with infantile-onset intermittent hyperammonemic episodes, psychomotor retardation, and occasionally hepatomegaly.[53] The basic defect is thought to reside at the level of the mitochondrial ornithine transporter leading to impaired uptake of ornithine by hepatic mitochondria and subsequent OTC substrate deficiency.

Plasma ornithine concentrations may be markedly elevated. Glutamine and alanine are increased during hyperammonemia. Increased homocitrulline production leading to increased urinary homocitrulline levels is thought to be secondary to lysine acting as a substrate for OTC, as mitochondrial lysine uptake remains unaffected in this enigmatic syndrome. Urinary orotate may be increased. Ultrastructural examination of liver tissue has revealed abnormal mitochondrial morphology with crystalline structures.

Treatment consists of protein restriction and ornithine supplementation, although chronically raised levels of plasma ornithine may not be without risk.

INHERITED DEFECTS IN BRANCHED-CHAIN ORGANIC ACID METABOLISM

Inherited defects in catabolism of the branched-chain amino acids (BCAA)—leucine, isoleucine, and valine—are responsible for most of the disorders of organic acid metabolism.[54,55] The characteristic biochemical finding in these diseases is the accumulation of branched-chain organic acids in tissues, blood, CSF, and urine. These various acids either represent the accumulated substrate from a particular enzymatic block or, more likely, are proximal metabolites in the branched-chain pathway or derivatives of the various substrates, e.g., methylmalonic acid. The branched-chain amino/organic acid pathways are outlined in Figure 3. In this section, the enzymes that are deficient in the various disorders are noted by circled numbers, which are identified in the legend of Figure 3.

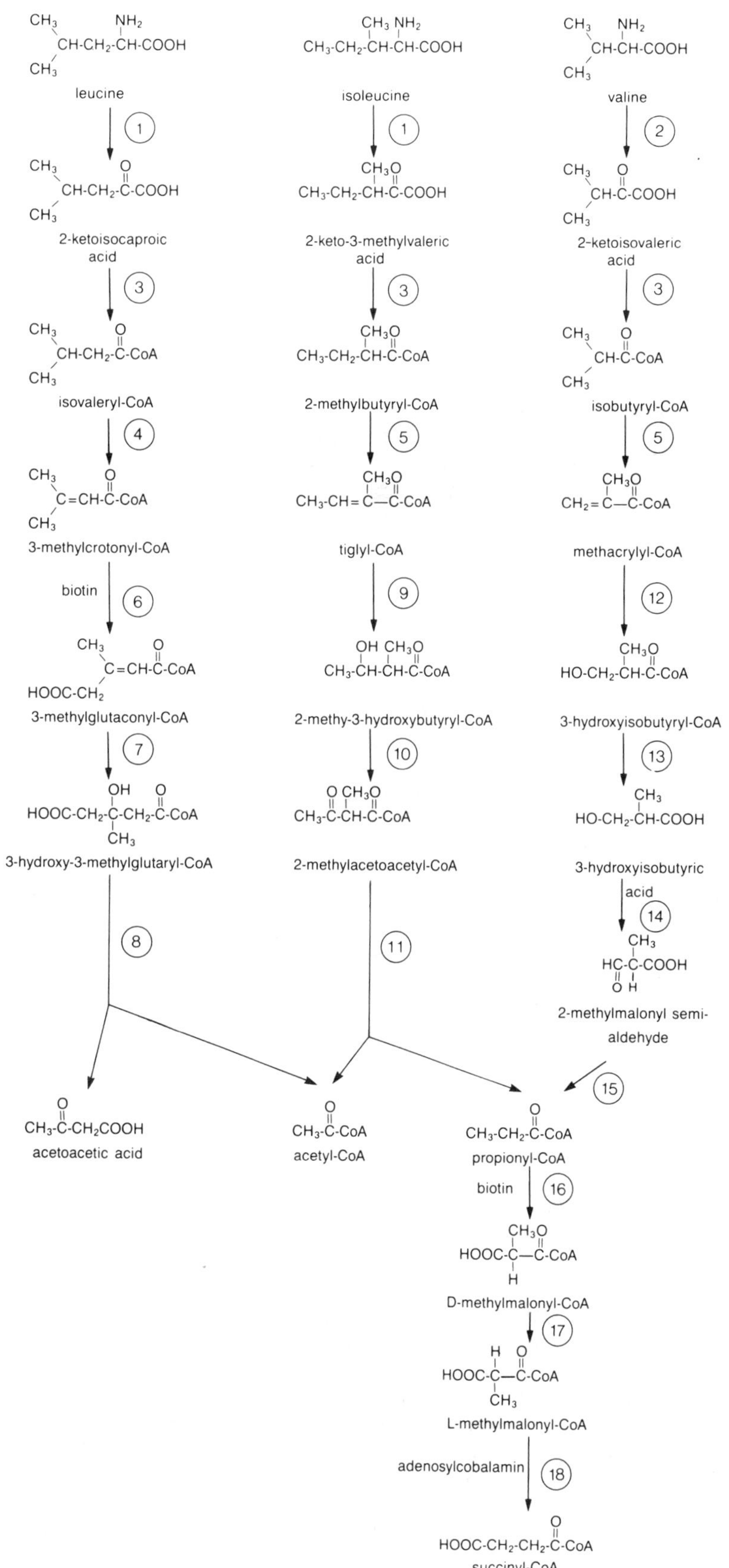

FIGURE 3 The three pathways for branched-chain amino acid catabolism. Enzymes identified numerically include (1) leucine/isoleucine transaminase, (2) valine transaminase, (3) branched-chain 2-keto acid dehydrogenase complex, (4) isovaleryl-CoA dehydrogenase, (5) isobutyryl-CoA/alpha-methylbutyryl-CoA dehydrogenase, (6) 3-methylcrotonyl-CoA carboxylase, (7) 3-methylglutaconyl-CoA hydratase, (8) 3-hydroxy-3 methylglutaryl-CoA lyase, (9) crotonase, (10) 2-methyl-3-hydroxybutyryl-CoA dehydrogenase, (11) 3-ketothiolase, (12) methylacryl-CoA hydratase, (13) 3-hydroxy-isobutyryl-CoA deacylase, (14) 3-hydroxy-isobutyrate dehydrogenase, (15) 2-methyl-malonyl semialdehyde oxidase, (16) propionyl-CoA carboxylase, (17) D-methylmalonyl-CoA racemase, and (18) L-methylmalonyl-CoA mutase.

The specialist in gastroenterology is likely to encounter an infant or child with an organicacidopathy because one of the chief clinical findings in this group of disorders is unexplained persistent or episodic vomiting. In the defects of organic acid metabolism, multiple secondary abnormalities in intermediary metabolism develop as a consequence of the accumulation of the branched-chain derivatives producing ketosis, lactic acidosis, hyperammonemia, and secondary carnitine deficiency. Poor intake and vomiting with dehydration and volume depletion may also be responsible for ketosis and lactic acidosis, respectively. High levels of some organic acids can affect the CNS, resulting in encephalopathy as well as other tissues such as bone marrow hematopoietic precursors producing diverse hematocytopenias. Laboratory findings, particularly during an acute illness, may include decreased serum HCO_3^- with an increased anion gap, increased plasma NH_4^+, increased ketone bodies in serum and urine, leukopenia, and anemia or thrombocytopenia. In some disorders, plasma and urine glycine levels may also be increased.

Similar to the UCED, phenotypic expression varies and is dependent mainly on severity of the enzyme deficiency. Major forms include severe neonatal-onset, potentially fatal disease, a chronic type with failure to thrive, developmental delay or progressive psychomotor retardation with intermittent episodes of ketoacidosis, or a completely intermittent form in which disease expression is confined to acute episodes of metabolic decompensation. Clinical features variably include feeding difficulties, vomiting, poor growth, hypotonia, developmental delay, mental retardation, seizures, ataxia, lethargy, coma, and episodes of a Reye's-like syndrome. A specific and unique odor can usually be detected in the breath, sweat, cerumen, feces, or urine of patients with maple syrup urine disease (MSUD), isovaleric acidemia, and glutaric aciduria type II. In MSUD, the odor is of maple syrup, whereas in isovaleric acidemia and glutaric aciduria type II, it resembles the odor of sweaty feet or rancid butter. A strong odor, said to resemble that of a "tom cat's urine," has been noted in some patients with deficiency of 3-methylcrotonyl-CoA carboxylase. Vomiting may be pernicious during infancy, and, unfortunately, several infants with disorders such as isovaleric acidemia and propionic acidemia have undergone surgery for presumed pyloric stenosis. This has also been true for patients with PKU.

The most common inborn error of organic acid metabolism is methylmalonic acidemia. There are several enzymatic defects that may be responsible, including L-methylmalonyl-CoA mutase deficiency,[18] D-methylmalonyl-CoA racemase deficiency,[17] and several disorders of cobalamin metabolism, all of which together account for an incidence in newborns of approximately 1 in 10,000 to 1 in 40,000. During episodes of acute metabolic decompensation associated with vomiting, dehydration, and lethargy, hepatomegaly as well as hyperammonemia may develop. These patients not uncommonly are thought to be afflicted with Reye's syndrome. With the exception of prominent ketoacidosis, this clinical picture may closely resemble that seen in the defects of fatty acid oxidation, exemplified by the medium-chain acyl-CoA dehydrogenase deficiency. The important point is that currently most patients who present with episodes that resemble Reye's syndrome have inborn errors of organic acid or fatty acid metabolism or urea cycle enzyme defects.

In addition to the BCAA, isoleucine and valine, other precursors of methylmalonic acid include methionine, threonine, thymine plus cholesterol, and odd-chain fatty acids via propionyl-CoA. Because of the effect of bowel sterilization on MMA levels, gut flora production of propionic acid from fatty acids may be an important source of MMA in some patients. Even in the absence of overt ketoacidotic decompensation, some patients with marked enzyme deficiency will demonstrate chronic anorexia, vomiting, and UGI bleeding associated with diffuse gastritis or gastric ulcers. Many patients with severe methylmalonic acidemia require gastrostomy for long-term feeding.

Other examples of organicacidopathies include MSUD due to branched-chain 2-keto acid dehydrogenase deficiency,[3] propionic acidemia,[16] and 3-methylcrotonylglycinuria[6] due to secondary deficiencies of biotin-dependent carboxylase enzymes because of impaired biotin metabolism, 3-ketothiolase deficiency,[11] isovaleric acidemia secondary to isovaleryl-CoA dehydrogenase deficiency,[4] and glutaric aciduria type II secondary to multiple acyl-CoA dehydrogenase deficiencies[4,5] involving amino acid and fatty acid, as well as branched-chain organic acid, metabolism. The 3-hydroxy-3-methyl-glutaryl-CoA lyase deficiency[8] is a unique disorder associated with nonketotic hypoglycemia which represents the most profound defect in ketogenesis as well as a defect in leucine metabolism. One patient with this potentially lethal disorder was reported to have developed acute pancreatitis and hepatomegaly with transaminasemia during an acute attack.[56] As in methylmalonic acidemia and glutaric aciduria type II, the liver enlargement is probably secondary to fatty infiltration.

The diagnosis of methylmalonic acidemia and the other rarer organicacidopathies requires directed analysis of urine for organic acids. Any patient suspected of having such a disorder must have urine analyzed by GLC and GC-MS to provide confirmatory evidence of the abnormal presence of a particular organic acid. Plasma amino acid analysis by column chromatography is also required. Quantitation of branched-chain amino acids in plasma is more informative than urinary organic acids for the patient with MSUD. Definite enzymatic analysis can usually be performed on a patient's white blood cells or cultured skin fibroblasts. Future diagnostic tests will make use of cDNA probes, which are now becoming available for many of these gene defects. The salient features of several representative inborn errors of organic acid metabolism are outlined in Table 2.

The acute management of patients suspected of an inborn error of organic acid metabolism is supportive care, intravenous fluids with glucose to eliminate hypoglycemia and suppress gluconeogenesis, correction of acid-base disturbances, and potential administration of large doses of various water-soluble vitamins such as hydroxycobalamin, biotin, and thiamine, since several disorders such as methylmalonic acidemia may be responsive to megavitamin therapy. More specific therapy of acute episodes of metabolic decompensation requires elucidation of the enzymatic lesion. Chronic management may be complicated, involving use of special diets restricted in certain amino acids and occasionally directed medications. The prognosis varies depending on the nature of the enzymatic deficiency, the delay in diagnosis, and response to dietary, vitamin cofactor, or detoxificant thera-

TABLE 2
Inherited Defects in Branched-Chain Organic Acid Metabolism

Disease	Genetic Defect Inheritance	Laboratory Findings	Therapy	Notes
Methylmalonic acidemia	↓ L-methylmalonyl-CoA mutase, AR ↓ D-methylmalonyl-CoA racemase, AR ↓ Adenosylcobalamin synthase, AR Other defects in vitamin B_{12} metabolism	↑ Urine MMA	Hydroxycobalamin Restriction of ile, val, thr, met intake Management of acute episodes* Consider bowel sterilization in some patients	Most common organicacidopathy Phenotypes range from lethal neonatal-onset disease to asymptomatic variety in adults Most severe disease due to cobalamin-unresponsive L-methylmalonyl-CoA mutase deficiency Some defects in cobalamin metabolism may also result in coexisting homocystinuria
Propionic acidemia	↓ Propionyl-CoA carboxylase, AR	↑ Urine 3-hydroxypropionate, propionylglycine, methycitrate, tiglylglycine, 2-methylglutaconate	Restriction of ile, val, thr, met intake	Usually severe phenotypes As in methylmalonic acidemia and many of the other organicacidopathies, plasma glycine and NH_4^+ may be ↑ and plasma carnitine is ↓ with ↑ in esterified carnitine fraction
Multiple carboxylase deficiency	↓ Propionyl-CoA, 3-methylcrotonyl-CoA, pyruvate and acetyl-CoA carboxylases secondary to: ↓ Holocarboxylase synthase, AR ↓ biotinidase, AR	↑ Plasma, urine, CSF lactate ↑ Urine 3-methylcrotonylglycine, 3-hydroxyisovalerate, 3-hydroxypropionate, propionylglycine, methycitrate, tiglylglycine, 2-methylglutaconate	Biotin	Adequate megatherapy with biotin allows for complete control of biotinidase deficiency Some patients with holocarboxylase synthase deficiency may not adequately respond to biotin megatherapy
Isovaleric acidemia	Isovaleryl-CoA dehydrogenase, AR	↑ Urine isovalerylglycine, 3-hydroxyisovalerate	Restriction of leu intake Glycine, L-carnitine	Acute neonatal-onset and chronic phenotype Sweaty-feet odor
Glutaric aciduria, type 2	Multiple CoA dehydrogenase deficiencies (e.g., isovaleryl-CoA, glutaryl-CoA, medium chain acyl-CoA dehydrogenase, etc.) secondary to: ↓Electron transfer flavoprotein (ETF), AR ↓ETF dehydrogenase (complex II mitochondrial electron transport chain), AR	↑ Urine isovalerylglycine, 3-hydroxyisovalerate, glutarate, adipate, suberate, sebacic, hexanoylglycine, suberylglycine, isobutyrylglycine, 2-methyl butyrylglycine, ethylmalonate	Riboflavin Restriction of leu, ile, val, lys, try intake	Several clinical types including severe riboflavin-unresponsive lethal neonatal-onset and adult-intermittent variety Occasional episodes of (non) hypoketotic hypoglycemia
HMG-CoA lyase deficiency	3-Hydroxy-3-methylglutaryl-CoA (HMG-CoA) lyase, AR	↑ Urine HMG, 3-hydroxyisovalerate	Avoid fasting IV glucose for poor intake or vomiting	Nonketotic hypoglycemia No ↑ in plasma or urine ketones during fasting/hypoglycemia
3-Ketothiolase deficiency	↓ Mitochondrial 3-ketothiolase, AR	↑ Urine ile metabolites: 2-methylacetoacetate, 2-methyl-3-hydroxybutyrate, tiglylglycine	Restriction of ile intake Avoid fasting	Different phenotypes possibly related to isozymic enzyme deficiencies May mimic ketotic hypoglycemia
Maple syrup urine disease	↓ Branched-chain 2-keto acid dehydrogenase, AR	↑ Plasma leu, ile val ↑ Urine branched-chain keto acids	Restriction of leu, ile, val intake Thiamine	Classic neonatal-onset severe disease Chronic and acute, intermittent phenotypes Maple syrup odor

AR = autosomal recessive, ile = isoleucine, leu = leucine, lys = lysine, met = methionine, MMA = methylmalonic acid, thr = threonine, try = tryptophan, val = valine.

*Management of acute episode for most organicacidopathies includes administration of intravenous fluids with glucose for rehydration, to suppress muscle protein catabolism and/or correct hypoglycemia; correction of acid-base disturbances; in some instances administration of ''nontoxic'' amino acids to promote anabolism; and occasional empirical use of megavitamins.

py, ranging from very poor for neonatal-onset cobalamin- unresponsive methylmalonic acidemia to excellent for the biotin-responsive organicacidopathies.[58-60]

REFERENCES

1. La Du BN, Gjessing LR. Tyrosinosis and tyrosinemia. In: Stanbury JB, Wyngaarden JB, Fredrickson SD, eds. The metabolic basis of inherited disease. 4th ed. New York: McGraw-Hill, 1978:256.
2. Goldsmith LA. Tyrosinemia and related disorders. In: Stanbury JB, Wyngaarden JB, Fredrickson SD, Goldstein JL, Brown MS, eds. The metabolic basis of inherited disease. 5th ed. New York: McGraw-Hill, 1983:287.
3. Baber MD. A case of congenital cirrhosis of the liver with renal tubular defects akin to those in the Fanconi syndrome. Arch Dis Child 1956; 31:335–339.
4. Lindblad B, Lindstedt S, Steen G. On the enzymic defects in hereditary tyrosinemia. Proc Natl Acad Sci USA 1977; 74:4641–4645.
5. Berger R, van Fassen H, Smith GPA. Biochemical studies on the enzymatic deficiencies in hereditary tyrosinemia. Clin Chim Acta 1983; 134:141.
6. Tschudy DP, Hess RA, Frykholm BC. Inhibition of δ-aminoleuvulinic acid dehydratase by 4,6-dioxoheptanoic acid. J Biol Chem 1981; 256:9915–9923.
7. Sassa S, Kappas A. Hereditary tyrosinemia and the heme biosynthetic pathway. J Clin Invest 1983; 71:625–634.
8. Weinberg AG, Mize CE, Worthen HG. The occurrence of hepatoma in the chronic form of hereditary tyrosinemia. J Pediatr 1976; 88:434–438.
9. Tuchman M, Freese DK, Sharp HL, Whitley CB, Ramnaraine ML, Ulstrom RA, Najarian JS, Ascher N, Buist NRM, Terry AB. Persistent succinylacetone excretion after liver transplantation in a patient with hereditary tyrosinemia type 1. J Inherited Metab Dis 1985; 8:21–24.
10. Kvittingen EA. Hereditary tyrosinemia type 1—an overview. Scand J Clin Lab Invest 1986; 46(suppl 184):24–34.
11. Edwards SW, Knox WE. Homogentisate metabolism: the isomerization of maleylacetoacetate by an enzyme which requires glutathione. J Biol Chem 1956; 220:79–91.
12. Laberge L, Lescault A, Tanguay RM. Hereditary tyrosinemias (type 1): a new vista on tyrosine toxicity and cancer. Adv Exp Med Biol 1986; 206:209–221.
13. Manabe S, Sassa S, Kappas A. Hereditary tyrosinemia. Formation of succinylacetone-amino acid adducts. J Exp Med 1985; 162:1060–1074.
14. Stoner E, Starkman H, Wellner D, Wellner VP, Sassa S, Rifkind AB, Grenier A, Steinherz PG, Meister A, New MI, Levine LS. Biochemical studies of a patient with hereditary hepatorenal tyrosinemia: evidence for a glutathione deficiency. Pediatr Res 1984; 18:1332–1336.
15. Hostetter MK, Levy HL, Winter HS, Knight GJ, Haddow JE. Evidence for liver disease preceding amino acid abnormalities in hereditary tyrosinemia. N Engl J Med 1983; 308:1265–1267.
16. Kvittingen EA, Halvorsen S, Jellum E. Deficient fumarylacetoacetate fumarylhydrolase activity in lymphocytes and fibroblasts from patients with hereditary tyrosinemia. Pediatr Res 1983; 17:541–544.
17. Tanguay RM, Laberge C, Lescault A, Valet JP, Duband JL, Quennville Y. Molecular basis of hereditary tyrosinemias: proof of the primary defect by Western blotting. In: Scott WA, Ahmand F, Black S, Schultz J, Whelan WJ, eds. Advances in gene technology: human genetic disorders. Cambridge, Cambridge University Press, 1984:250.
18. Lindblad B, Fridén J, Greter J, Holme E, Lindstedt S, Siösteen C. Treatment of hereditary tyrosinemia (fumarylacetoacetase deficiency) by enzyme substitution. J Inherited Metab Dis 1986; 9(suppl 2):257–261.
19. Staryl TE, Zitelli BJ, Shaw BW, Iwatsuki S, Gartner JC, Gordon RD, Malatack JJ, Fox IJ, Urbach AH, Van Thiel DH. Changing concepts: liver replacement for hereditary tyrosinemia and hepatoma. J Pediatr 1985; 106:604–606.
20. Kvittingen EA, Jellum E, Stokke O, Flatmark A, Bergan A, Sodal G, Halvorsen S, Schrumpf E, Gjone E. Liver transplantation in a 23-year-old tyrosinemia patient: effects on the renal tubular dysfunction. J Inherited Metab Dis 1986; 9:216–224.
21. Tuchman M, Freese DK, Sharp HL, Ramnaraine ML, Ascher N, Bloomer JR. Contribution of extrahepatic tissues to biochemical abnormalities in hereditary tyrosinemia type 1: study of three patients after liver transplantation. J Pediatr 1986; 110:399–403.
22. Mitchell JR, Jollow DJ, Potter WZ, Gillette JR, Brodie BB. Acetaminophen-induced hepatic necrosis. IV. Protective role of glutathione. J Pharmacol Exp Ther 1973; 187:211–217.
23. Smilkstein MJ, Knapp GL, Kulig KW, Rumack BH. Efficacy of oral *N*-acetylcysteine in the treatment of acetaminophen overdose: analysis of the National Multicenter Study (1976 to 1985). N Engl J Med 1988; 319:1557–1562.
24. Lindblad B. Treatment with glutathione and other sulphydryl compounds in hereditary tyrosinemia. In: Larsson A, Orrenius S, Holmgren A, Mannervik B, eds. Functions of glutathione: biochemical, physiological, toxicological and clinical aspects. New York: Raven, 1983:337.
25. Kvittingen EA, Steinman B, Gitzelmann R, Leonard JV, Andria G, Borresen AL, Mossman J, Micara G, Lindblad B. Prenatal diagnosis of hereditary tyrosinemia by determination of fumarylacetoacetase in cultured amniotic fluid cells. Pediatr Res 1985; 19:334–337.
26. Kvittingen EA, Guiband Pr P, Diury P, Mandon G, Rolland MO, Domenichini Y, Jakobs C, Christensen E. Prenatal diagnosis of hereditary tyrosinemia 1 by determination of fumarylacetoacetase in chorionic villus material. Eur J Pediatr 1986; 144:597–598.
27. Gaene R, Lescault A, Grenier A, Laberge C, Mehancon SB, Dallaire L. Prenatal diagnosis of hereditary tyrosinemia: measurement of succinylacetone in amniotic fluid. Prenatal Diagn 1982; 2:185–188.
28. Pettit BR, MacKenzie F, King GS, Leonard JV. The antenatal diagnosis and aid to the management of hereditary tyrosinemia by use of a specific and sensitive GC-MS assay for succinylacetone. J Inherited Metab Dis 1984 (suppl 2):135–136.
29. Jakobs C, Kvittingen EA, Berger R, Haagen A, Kleyer W, Niermeijer N. Prenatal diagnosis of tyrosinemia type 1 by use of stable isotope mass spectrometry. Eur J Pediatr 1985; 144:209–210.
30. Steinmann B, Gitzelmann R, Kvittingen EA, Stokke O. Prenatal diagnosis of hereditary tyrosinemia. N Engl J Med 1984; 210:855–856.
31. Kvittingen EA, Borresen AL, Stokke O, van der Hagen CB, Lie SO. Deficiency of fumarylacetoacetase without hereditary tyrosinemia. Clin Genet 1985; 27:550–554.
32. Walser M. Urea cycle disorders and other hereditary hyperammonemic syndromes. In: Stanbury JB, Wyngaarden JB, Fredrickson DS, Goldstein JL, Brown MS, eds. The metabolic basis of inherited disease. 5th ed. New York: McGraw-Hill, 1983:402.
33. Batshaw ML. Hyperammonemia. Current Probl Pediatr 1984; 14:1–69.
34. Amir J, Alpert G, Statter M, et al. Intracranial hemorrhage in siblings and ornithine transcarbamylase deficiency. Acta Paediatr Scand 1982; 71:671–673.
35. Russell A, Levin B, Oberholzer VG, Sinclair L. Hyperammonemia. A new instance of an inborn enzymatic defect of the biosynthesis of urea. Lancet 1962; ii:699.
36. Maddalena A, Sosnoski DM, Berry GT, Nussbaum RL. Mosaicism for an intragenic deletion in a boy with mild ornithine transcarbamylase deficiency. N Engl J Med 1988; 319:999–1003.
37. Rozen R, Fox JE, Hack AM, Fenton WA, Horwich AL, Rosenberg LE. DNA analysis for ornithine transcarbamylase deficiency. J Inherited Metab Dis 1986; 9(suppl 1):49–57.
38. Rodeck CH, Patrick AD, Pembrey ME, Tzannatos C, Whitfield AE. Fetal liver biopsy for prenatal diagnosis of ornithine carbamyl transferase deficiency. Lancet 1982; ii:297–299.
39. Batshaw ML, Brusilow SW. Treatment of hyperammonemic coma caused by inborn errors of urea synthesis. J Pediatr 1980; 97:893–900.
40. Batshaw ML, Brusilow S, Waber L, Blom W, Brubakk AM, Burton BK, Cann HM, Kerr D, Mamunes P, Matalon R, Myerberg D, Schafer I. Treatment of inborn errors of urea synthesis. N Engl J Med 1982; 306:1387–1392.
41. Brusilow SW, Danney M, Waber LJ, Batshaw M, Burton B, Levitsky L, Roth K, McKeethren C, Ward J. N Engl J Med 1984; 310:1630–1634.
42. Parsons HG, Scott RB, Pinto A, Carter RJ, Snyder FF. Argininosuccinic aciduria: long-term treatment with arginine. J Inherited Metab Dis 1987; 10:152–161.
43. O'Brien WE, McInnes R, Kalumuck K, Adcock M. Cloning and sequence analysis of cDNA for human argininosuccinate lyase. Proc Natl Acad Sci 1986; 83:7211–7215.
44. Matuo S, Tatsuno M, Kobayashi K, Saheki T, Miyata T, Iwanaga S, Amaya Y, Mori M. Isolation of cDNA clones of human argininosuc-

cinate lyase and corrected amino acid sequence. FEBS Lett 1988; 234:395–399.
45. Beaudet AL, Su T-S, O'Brien WE, D'Eustachio P, Barker PE, Ruddle FH. Dispersion of argininosuccinate-synthetase-like human genes to multiple autosomes and the X chromosome. Cell 1982; 30:287–293.
46. Freytag SO, Bock H-GO, Beaudet AL, O'Brien WE. Molecular structures of human argininosuccinate synthetase pseudogenes. J Biol Chem 1984; 259:3160–3166.
47. Fearon ER, Mallonee RL, Phillips JA, O'Brien WE, Brusilow SW, Adcock MW, Kirby LT. Genetic analysis of carbamyl phosphate synthetase 1 deficiency. Hum Genet 1985; 70:207–210.
48. Piceni-Sereni L, Bachmann C, Pfister U, Buscaglia M, Nicolini U. Prenatal diagnosis of carbamoyl phosphate synthetase deficiency by fetal liver biopsy. Prenat Diagn 1988; 8:307–309.
49. Bachmann C, Brandis M, Weissenbarth-Riedel E, Burghard R, Colombo JP. *N*-acetylglutamate synthetase deficiency, a second patient. J Inherited Metab Dis 1988; 11:191–193.
50. Zimmerman A, Bachmann C, Schubiger G. Liver pathology in a new congenital disorder of urea synthesis: *N*-acetylglutamate synthetase deficiency. Virchows Arch 1985; 408(2-3):259–268.
51. Dizikes GJ, Grody WW, Kern RM, Cederbaum SD. Isolation of human liver arginase cDNA and demonstration of nonhomology between the two human arginase genes. Biochem Biophys Res Comm 1986; 141:53–59.
52. Mizutani N, Hayakawa C, Maehara M, Watanabe K. Enzyme replacement therapy in a patient with hyperargininemia. Tohoku J Exp Med 1987; 151:301–307.
53. Valle D, Simell O. The hyperornithinemias. In: Stanbury JB, Wyngaarden JB, Fredrickson DS, Goldstein JL, Brown MS, eds. The metabolic basis of inherited disease. 5th ed. New York: McGraw-Hill, 1983:382.
54. Tanaka K, Rosenberg LE. Disorders of branched chain amino acid and organic acid metabolism. In: Stanbury JB, Wyngaarden JB, Fredrickson DS, Goldstein JL, Brown MS, eds. The metabolic basis of inherited disease. 5th ed. New York: McGraw-Hill, 1983:440.
55. Rosenberg LE. Disorders of propionate and methylmalonate metabolism. In: Stanbury JB, Wyngaarden JB, Fredrickson DS, Goldstein JL, Brown MS, eds. The metabolic basis of inherited disease. 5th ed. New York: McGraw-Hill, 1983:474.
56. Wilson WG, Cass MB, Sovik O, Gibson KM, Sweetman L. 3-Hydroxy-3-methylglutaryl-CoA lyase deficiency in a child with acute pancreatitis and recurrent hypoglycemia. Eur J Pediatr 1984; 142:289.
57. Matsui SM, Mahoney MJ, Rosenberg LE. The natural history of the inherited methylmalonic acidemias. N Engl J Med 1983; 308:857–861.
58. Berry GT, Yudkoff M, Segal S. Isovaleric acidemia: medical and neurodevelopmental effects of long-term therapy. J Pediatr 1988; 113:58–64.
59. Michalski AJ, Berry GT, Segal S. Holocarboxylase synthetase deficiency: nine year follow-up of a patient on chronic biotin therapy and a review of the literature. J Inherited Met Dis. In press.

PART 11

Lysosomal Acid Lipase Deficiency: Cholesteryl Ester Storage Disease and Wolman's Disease

Paul M. Coates, Ph.D.
Jean A. Cortner, M.D.

More than 100 patients have been reported to have disease associated with genetic deficiency of the lysosomal enzyme, acid lipase (E.C.3.1.1.3). There is substantial clinical heterogeneity among patients with acid lipase deficiency, ranging from the severe form of Wolman's disease (WD), in which nearly all patients have died within the first year of life, to the relatively benign form of cholesteryl ester storage disease (CESD), which has been identified in adults. In this chapter we describe the clinical, laboratory, and pathologic findings in these patients; the nature of the enzyme defect in this group of disorders and its impact on lipid and lipoprotein metabolism; and issues of management and treatment. The reader is also referred to two excellent reviews.[1,2]

Historically, the two disorders called WD and CESD were discovered independently. The first description of an infant with abdominal distention, hepatosplenomegaly, widespread lipid storage, and adrenal calcification was given in 1956 by Abramov, Schorr, and Wolman.[3] This was followed in 1961 by the report of Wolman et al that other siblings in the same family were similarly affected.[4] In the ensuing three decades, approximately 70 cases of this disease have been reported; it was first named *Wolman's disease* by Crocker et al in 1965.[5] In retrospect, it is likely that a patient described by Alexander in 1946[6] with Niemann-Pick disease and adrenal calcification actually had WD. The enzyme defect was demonstrated in 1969; Patrick and Lake described the severe deficiency of an acid ester hydrolase, or acid lipase, with activity toward both triglycerides and cholesteryl esters in liver and spleen of a patient with WD.[7] The lysosomal location of the stored lipid was confirmed by Lake and Patrick in 1970.[8]

CESD was first described briefly in 1963 by Frederickson[9] in a child with hyperlipidemia and hepatomegaly, whose liver contained significant quantities of stored cholesteryl esters. Since that time, more than 50 patients have been described under various names in addition to CESD, including hepatic cholesterol ester storage disease, polycorie cholesterolique, and Cholesterinester Speicherkrankheit. The enzyme defect in this disorder, acid lipase deficiency, was identified in 1972.[10,11]

It is now known that the same enzyme is deficient in both WD and CESD and that they most likely represent allelic variants at the same genetic locus. Furthermore, patients have been described with "intermediate" forms of disease due to this enzyme defect. Finally, a few patients with acid lipase deficiency have been reported with distinctive symptoms that do not resemble either WD or CESD.

CLINICAL MANIFESTATIONS

Wolman's Disease

A.J.[12] was the healthy first child born to unrelated parents. She was well until 8 weeks of age, when abdominal distention was noted. She was alert and otherwise appeared well. She was first admitted to hospital at 10 weeks of age, where her abdominal distention was found to be attributable to enlargement of her liver (6 cm below the right costal margin) and her spleen (4 cm below the left costal margin). There was ascites. Serum cholesterol ranged from 123 to 171 mg per deciliter and triglycerides were 148 to 232 mg per deciliter; alpha lipoproteins were markedly diminished. Initial liver function tests were normal, as was serum cortisol. Flat plate radiographs of the abdomen and intravenous pyelography revealed massive bilateral adrenal calcification. Vacuoles were observed in blood lymphocytes and in bone marrow. Her condition deteriorated over the next 2 months, during which time she developed diarrhea, forceful vomiting, severe anemia, thrombocytopenia, generalized edema, jaundice, and progressive hepatosplenomegaly. She died at 19 weeks of age in cardiorespiratory arrest. At autopsy, the liver was massively enlarged, yellow, and firm; the spleen and adrenals were also enlarged, and the latter had significant calcifications. On microscopic examination, foam cells were observed in most organ systems (pulmonary alveoli, duodenal mucosa, liver, thymus, spleen, adrenals, lymph nodes, and bone marrow). The liver showed fine fibrosis and focal canalicular bile stasis. Frozen sections stained with oil red O revealed substantial lipid accumulation, even in tissues that were not recognizably foamy (bronchial cartilage and epithelium, arterial wall). Lipid analysis revealed twice normal triglyceride content and 20 times normal cholesteryl ester content of the liver and six times normal triglyceride and cholesteryl ester content of the spleen. Acid lipase deficiency was documented in fibroblasts using triglyceride, cholesteryl ester, and 4-methylumbelliferyl ester substrates.

With few exceptions, patients with WD have had clinical and pathologic findings similar to these,[2-6,12-52,119-122] as summarized in Table 1. Onset of vomiting and diarrhea, malabsorption, hepatomegaly, splenomegaly, abdominal distention, and anemia generally begin in early infancy. Some patients have presented at birth,[6,13,119] but most have presented within the first few weeks of life. Bilateral adrenal calcification, demonstrated by flat plate radiographs of the abdomen, is a virtually universal finding[1] and has been considered pathognomonic for the disease. It should be noted, however, that not all WD patients have radiologic evidence of adrenal calcification; it may be seen only at autopsy.[17,18,22,25,27,30,42] Similarly, adrenal calcification is observed, albeit rarely and located unilaterally, in other disorders, including neuroblastoma, adrenal tumors, and tuberculosis[20,53,54]; skin eruptions have been noted, although rarely.[2] Neurologic assessment is generally within normal limits. Patients deteriorate rapidly, with increasing abdominal distention, fever, continued vomiting, diarrhea, and wasting. Of 65 reported patients, nearly 50 percent died before 3 months of age and more than 90 percent before 6 months.

Liver biopsy reveals massive accumulation of lipid, for the most part within lysosomes.[1,2] Chemical analysis of the stored lipids has revealed that these are primarily triglycerides and cholesteryl esters. Other tissues have also demonstrated significant intralysosomal lipid accumulation, including intestinal mucosa, vascular endothelium, spleen, lymph nodes, bone marrow, and circulating mononuclear leukocytes.[1,2]

TABLE 1
Clinical and Laboratory Findings in 125 Patients with Wolman's Disease, Cholesteryl Ester Storage Disease, and Their Clinical Variants

	Wolman's Disease	Intermediate Variants	Cholesteryl Ester Storage Disease
Number of patients	65	11	49
Acid lipase deficiency documented	23	8	41
Number of families	54	7	39
Consanguinity	15	1	3
Ethnic origin (% European)	65%	43%	95%
Sex (% female)	51%	46%	57%
Age at onset	Birth–5 months	Birth–7 years	3 weeks–58 years
% <1 month	62%	18%	5%
% <6 months	100%	64%	8%
Gastrointestinal symptoms	97%	82%	43%
Hepatomegaly	100%	100%	100%
Splenomegaly	95%	91%	54%
Adrenal calcification	98%	33%	0%
Hypercholesterolemia	21%	67%	93%
Hypertriglyceridemia	53%	83%	49%
Hypoalphalipoproteinemia	79%	100%	96%
Mortality	100%	55%	6%
Age at death	Birth–13 months	6 months–18 years	3 weeks–57 years
% <6 months	92%	9%	2%
% <12 months	98%	9%	2%

Notes: Information not available for all patients. From references 2–93, 119–122, and personal observations.

Cholesteryl Ester Storage Disease

Perhaps only one reason exists for separating out the group of patients with CESD from those with WD, and it is simply historical. CESD was first described in 1963 by Frederickson and since then has been noted in more than 50 patients.[1,9-11,55-83] The clinical findings in patients with CESD are, in general, dramatically different from those seen in patients with WD, as illustrated by the following previously unpublished case report (courtesy of Dr. S.V. Feinman, Toronto, Canada).

P.W. was a white male born to a 37-year-old gravida 2, para 1, Canadian woman of Irish ancestry and her 44-year-old unrelated husband. Pregnancy and delivery were uncomplicated. Hepatosplenomegaly was noted at 10 months of age during routine pediatric examination but appeared to have no clinical consequences. He was in good health until 14 years of age, when he began to complain of periodic fatigue, malaise, susceptibility to infection, and right upper quadrant pain. At 21 years, elevated plasma cholesterol and triglycerides were noted; together with his chronic hepatomegaly, this prompted the suspicion of CESD. Liver biopsy at 23 years of age revealed widespread vacuolated hepatocytes, but not Kupffer cells. Cholesteryl ester crystals were identified in hepatocytes. Acid lipase deficiency was demonstrated in liver, fibroblasts, and peripheral mononuclear leukocytes. Other members of his family were investigated, including his older brother (T.W.), mother, and maternal aunt. The brother, older by 13 years, had been noted to have an enlarged liver "in childhood" but was otherwise in excellent health. He had elevated plasma cholesterol and triglycerides and was also deficient in fibroblast and leukocyte acid lipase. Their mother and maternal aunt had heterozygote levels of acid lipase, measured in leukocytes.

The presentation of these two siblings is fairly typical of the clinical findings in CESD, summarized in Table 1. The major and often only findings are hyperlipidemia and hepatomegaly, which may or may not be symptomatic. Several patients ultimately determined to have CESD originally were evaluated for other apparently unrelated disease[78] or were evaluated as siblings of affected patients[79] and found co-incidentally to have these features.

The hepatomegaly, which may be evident very early in life, is progressive, evolving in the majority of patients into hepatic fibrosis.[55-57,61,62,64-70,72-76,79,80] Splenomegaly is found in one-half of patients, in contrast to those with fulminant WD, in whom this is a virtually constant finding. Almost invariably, CESD patients present with hyperlipidemia (see below). Given that the only signs of CESD may be hepatomegaly and hyperlipidemia, it is not surprising that patients may go undetected until relatively late in life; it is also likely that many have gone undiagnosed.

The onset of symptoms (or recognition of their disease) has ranged from 3 weeks to 58 years of age. In rare cases, the diagnosis was made only at autopsy.[70,84]

Associated findings in some patients with CESD are esophageal varices,[56,60,61] pulmonary hypertension,[85] portal hypertension,[86] abnormal liver function tests,[60] jaundice,[66] recurrent abdominal pain,[66,76] delayed onset of puberty,[56,61,67,78] and atherosclerosis.[60,70,84,85] Malabsorption and malnutrition, hallmarks of WD, have not been described in CESD. Calcified adrenals have been reported in only one case,[60] and autopsy evidence of adrenomegaly was noted in her two sisters.[86] Splenic abscess,[75] crystalline retinopathy,[78] and mesenteric lipodystrophy,[70] have each been reported in one patient.

Liver biopsy in CESD reveals many of the same abnormalities seen in WD: orange or butter-yellow color; lipid droplets in hepatic parenchymal cells; vacuoles in Kupffer cells. Although triglyceride storage is significant, it is the cholesteryl ester storage, identified as birefringent crystals, that gave the disease its name. As is the case in WD, most of the hepatic lipid is stored within lysosomes.[55,56]

Intermediate Forms

As more patients with acid lipase deficiency have been identified, it has become obvious that a spectrum of disease associated with this defect exists. The following case report describes a youngster with clinical disease intermediate between that of classic WD and that of classic CESD.

In collaboration with Dr. Y.E. Hsia, University of Hawaii, we studied a Japanese-American boy (L.H.) whose clinical findings resembled WD, with onset of gastrointestinal (GI) symptoms at 6 weeks of age and increasing abdominal distention due to hepatosplenomegaly, but in whom adrenal calcification was not demonstrable by radiologic examination. He had a lingering disease, eventually dying from hepatic failure at 18 months of age. At autopsy, his massively enlarged liver was yellow, with architecture totally destroyed, fibrotic, and heavily vacuolated, with minimal inflammation. There was prominent ascites, and fatty infiltration was noted in the enlarged spleen, the moderately calcified adrenals, lymph nodes, bone marrow, and bowel mucosa. Acid lipase deficiency was demonstrated in liver, cultured fibroblasts, and mononuclear leukocytes.

Several other patients who carried the diagnosis of WD but with prolonged survival[18,27,47] or minimal adrenal calcification,[17,18,22,25,27,30,42] as well as patients with CESD but with an insidious course,[2,10,18,60] suggest that there may be forms of acid lipase deficiency with severity intermediate between the classic forms of WD and CESD. Review of the literature suggested that 11 patients, including patient L.H. described above, could be reasonably distinguished as having an intermediate form of disease (Table 1) associated with this defect.[18,47,60,87,88,120] Two patients are worth noting in this regard. An American white male[47] had severe GI symptoms and malabsorption beginning at 4 months of age, with bilateral adrenal calcification and progressive hepatosplenomegaly, suggesting WD. Acid lipase deficiency was documented in liver and fibroblasts. Parenteral hyperalimentation was instituted[115]; the child has done moderately well and is alive at 2½ years. A Japanese male,[88] with onset of moderate GI symptoms at 5 months of age and hepatomegaly at 17 months of age, had 15 to 30 percent of control levels of acid lipase in leukocytes and liver, had no evidence of splenomegaly or adrenal calcification, and was still alive at the age of 4 years.

Triglyceride Storage Disease

Two other patients with documented acid lipase deficiency[89] have been described with clinical and pathologic findings distinctly different from any of those described in

WD, CESD, or their clinical variants. An Italian female[90,91] born to consanguineous parents presented at 8 years of age with obesity, tapetoretinal degeneration, deafness, progressive psychomotor retardation, seizures, hepatomegaly, and chronic tubulointerstitial nephropathy. She died at 10 years of age in renal failure and with uncontrollable seizures. At autopsy, she had an enlarged, yellow, fat-filled liver; fat (largely triglycerides) was found in her enlarged, atherosclerotic heart, lungs, and small intestine. Profound acid lipase deficiency was demonstrated in the liver. A Belgian female[92] presented at 2 days of age with a rapidly progressive disease involving vomiting, hypotonia, and lethargy from which she died at 6 days. She was the fourteenth child in a family in which six previous siblings had died early in life. At autopsy, she had severe fatty infiltration (largely triglycerides) of her liver and other tissues. Profound acid lipase deficiency was demonstrated in her liver. Both of these patients were considered to have "triglyceride storage disease" distinct from either WD or CESD.

Whether all of these patients represent allelic mutations at the gene locus for acid lipase remains unknown.

LABORATORY FINDINGS

Routine Laboratory Tests

Patients with WD frequently have abnormal liver function tests, severe and progressive anemia, and vacuolated lymphocytes. By contrast, patients with CESD have no consistent abnormalities in routine laboratory tests apart from the alterations in their plasma lipids and lipoproteins (see below). Hyperbilirubinemia is rarely seen, although vacuolated lymphocytes are frequently observed.

Plasma Lipids and Lipoproteins

Plasma total cholesterol and total triglyceride levels have generally been normal or low in patients with WD. However, the occasional patient has had hypercholesterolemia[17,32,38,42,51,121] or hypertriglyceridemia.[12,18,32,33,42,51,121,122] Almost invariably, WD patients have had remarkably low levels of HDL cholesterol, approaching zero in several patients in the terminal stages of their disease.[46,51]

This is in marked contrast to the almost invariable finding of hypercholesterolemia and the common finding of hypertriglyceridemia in patients with CESD. As in patients with WD, those with CESD generally have a profound reduction in plasma HDL cholesterol levels. Few detailed studies of the lipoprotein abnormalities in CESD have been reported,[1,72,76,93] but a recent study suggests that the failure of lysosomal hydrolysis to produce free cholesterol in the liver results in elevated synthesis of endogenous cholesterol and increased production of hepatic apo B–containing lipoproteins.[94]

PATHOLOGIC FINDINGS

Pathologic findings in the liver are similar in WD and CESD and hence are considered together. On gross examination, the liver is enlarged and firm, and the cut surface is yellow-orange with a greasy appearance. Normal liver architecture is rarely preserved. Hepatocytes are enlarged and vacuolated; the grossly enlarged Kupffer cells frequently are filled with vacuoles. Foamy histiocytes fill the portal and periportal areas. These areas may be fibrotic; frank cirrhosis is frequently observed. In frozen sections, hepatocytes and Kupffer cells stain intensely with oil red O. CESD liver is characterized, in addition, by the presence of massive amounts of cholesteryl ester crystals.

The enlarged adrenal glands in patients with WD are yellow and firm and sometimes contain flecks of calcified tissue, making them difficult to cut. Vascular changes include raised intimal lesions that are yellowish and resemble atheromatous lesions in some WD patients, although atherosclerosis has not been observed in WD. By contrast, significant atherosclerosis was noted at autopsy in several patients with CESD.[70,84,85] Intestinal lipid storage is prominent in WD, involving the mucosa, ganglion cells, and endothelial cells,[1] while it is less extensive in CESD.

At the ultrastructural level, liver parenchymal cells have abundant osmiophilic lipid droplets, mainly within lysosomes.[1] Similar changes have been observed by electron microscopic study of other tissues.

Chemical analysis of the stored lipid reveals significant accumulation of cholesteryl esters and triglycerides,[1] as well as several unusual storage compounds in WD tissues, including ceroid pigment,[21] oxygenated steryl esters,[35,95] and glyceryl ether lipids.[96] Triglyceride concentrations in liver may be increased 2- to 10-fold over control, and in spleen they may be increased 8- to 100-fold.[1] Free cholesterol is generally increased in liver and spleen, but cholesteryl esters may be increased 5- to 160-fold over control. Cholesteryl esters are increased in adrenal gland[97] and in aorta.[84] Fatty acid composition of these stored lipids is not consistently altered.

DIAGNOSIS

WD should be considered in the diagnosis of an infant with hepatosplenomegaly, GI signs, and failure to thrive. Flat plate radiographs of the abdomen reveal the virtually constant finding of adrenal calcification; it should be noted, however, that a few cases have been described in which adrenal calcification was absent or, at most, very slight and only demonstrable at autopsy. Bone scintigraphy[49] and computed tomography (CT)[49,98] have also been used to demonstrate the enlarged, calcified adrenals in patients with WD. Other causes of adrenal calcification (neuroblastoma, adrenal tumors, Addison's disease) can be differentiated from WD on clinical grounds and on the basis of the bilateral involvement in WD.[20,53,54] Foam cells in bone marrow and in blood films have been documented.[1] Light and electron microscopic evaluation of the liver,[1] intestinal mucosa,[99] and spleen[1] reveal significant membrane-limited lipid accumulation. The acid esterase deficiency can be detected histochemically in blood films.[100]

As noted above, CESD may be overlooked in the patient whose only signs are hepatomegaly and hyperlipidemia. Foam cells in bone marrow, vacuolated hepatocytes with membrane-limited lipid storage, and lipid analysis of tissue specimens all have been documented in CESD.

Enzymatic Diagnosis

The definitive diagnosis is made by demonstrating acid lipase deficiency. Acid lipase activity can be measured using long-chain fatty acid esters of both natural and synthetic compounds. Radiolabeled triglycerides and cholesteryl esters, esters of 4-methylumbelliferone and of *p*-nitrophenol have been used as substrates to demonstrate acid lipase deficiency in liver,[1,2,7,8,10,11] spleen,[1] aorta,[84] fibroblasts,[1,101,102] leukocytes,[12] lymphoblastoid cells,[103] and amniotic fluid cells.[12,40,50,73,104,105]

Using radiolabeled "natural" substrates (triglycerides or cholesteryl esters) and measuring activity at acid pH, tissues from patients with WD and CESD have less than 10 percent, and often as low as 1 percent, of control levels of acid lipase activity. The residual activity measured using long-chain fatty acid esters of 4-methylumbelliferone and *p*-nitrophenol is typically higher in patient tissues, most likely because these substrates are subject to hydrolysis by other intracellular esterases. Cortner et al[12] demonstrated that there are at least two enzymes that can be separated by electrophoresis that hydrolyze 4-methylumbelliferyl oleate at pH 4. The "A" enzyme is completely absent from WD and CESD tissues, whereas the "B" enzyme is unaffected. In most studies reported, there was no consistent difference in the residual activity of acid lipase between CESD and WD, using the substrates noted above. However, Fredrickson et al[84] noted that liver from a WD patient had virtually no activity toward hexadecanyl-1,2-dioleate as substrate, whereas liver from a CESD patient had normal activity.

Burton et al[106] demonstrated that both low-density lipoprotein (LDL) labeled with ^{3}H-cholesteryl linoleate and very low density lipoprotein (VLDL) labeled with ^{14}C-triolein were hydrolyzed at a slower rate in both CESD and WD fibroblasts than in controls, judged both by the appearance of radiolabeled product and by the accumulation of unhydrolyzed substrate. They also noted a significant difference between CESD and WD cells: under all conditions, WD cells hydrolyzed 10 to 20 percent of labeled lipoprotein-bound substrate, whereas CESD cells hydrolyzed 30 to 50 percent compared with controls. Burton and Reed[107] demonstrated that acid lipase activity, expressed as a function of the acid lipase cross-reacting material measured by radial immunodiffusion, was twice as high in CESD cells as in WD cells using triolein as substrate and at least 10 times as high using cholesteryl oleate as substrate. Taken together, these data suggest that (1) acid lipase protein is made in cells from both groups of patients at levels comparable to those of controls; (2) there is a higher residual activity of acid lipase in CESD than in WD under these conditions; (3) the primary defect, at least in the patients studied, is likely to be a structural mutation affecting catalytic activity; and (4) the genetic defects in WD and CESD are not the same.

Hoeg et al[47] demonstrated that liver from a patient with CESD had significantly higher residual acid lipase activity toward cholesteryl oleate than did that from a patient with WD (23 versus 4 percent of control); this might have been explained by the significantly higher neutral lipase activity (perhaps with overlapping substrate specificity) in CESD liver versus WD liver (236 versus 97 percent of control, respectively), but it is also possible, as the authors concluded, that CESD liver contains more functional acid lipase activity than does WD liver, a finding that is not reflected in cultured fibroblasts.

Hoeg et al[47] also demonstrated that culture of CESD and WD fibroblasts in medium enriched in acid lipase restored their intracellular acid lipase activity, more in CESD cells than in WD cells. These data, consistent with previous results obtained by Kyriakides et al,[108] support the now well-established pathway for the uptake of many lysosomal enzymes,[109] including acid lipase,[110] by the mannose-6-phosphate receptor. Co-culture of WD or CESD cells with normal cells[47,108,111] partially restored their enzyme activity, further suggesting that acid lipase–deficient cells can take up normal enzyme. Earlier studies by Beaudet et al[60] ruled out the possibility of a specific inhibitor of acid lipase as responsible for the enzyme deficiency in a patient with CESD. Cell fusion studies[47,124] (A. Gilbert, P.M. Coates, and J.A. Cortner: unpublished observations), in which WD × WD, CESD × CESD, and WD × CESD cell fusions were achieved with polyethylene glycol, did not lead to restoration of acid lipase activity, suggesting that the two disorders are the result of mutations in the same structural gene. Definitive molecular studies have not been reported to explain the clinical and genetic heterogeneity associated with acid lipase deficiency.

PATHOPHYSIOLOGY

Role of Acid Lipase in Cellular Metabolism

The enzyme defect, acid lipase deficiency, has been documented in many of the patients described above.[1,2,7,8,10–12,18,26,33,35,39,40,42–44,46–48,50,51,58–61,63,65,67–71,73–80,82,87–90] Acid lipase performs a critical role in the cellular disposition of triglycerides and cholesteryl esters, particularly when these are taken up as lipoprotein-bound lipids. This important function was elucidated by the work of Brown, Goldstein, and colleagues,[111,112] who demonstrated that the receptor-mediated endocytosis of plasma LDL by cultured skin fibroblasts was followed by the lysosomal degradation of cholesteryl esters (by acid lipase) and of protein components (by proteases). The cellular uptake of other lipoproteins, including triglyceride-rich particles, such as chylomicron remnants, VLDL and VLDL remnants, is also mediated by membrane receptors and also involves lysosomal degradation of their lipid and protein constituents. It is not clear that all of these lipoproteins are processed by the same receptor system, but in all cases the uptake of lipoproteins is followed by lysosomal degradation.

Acid Lipase Deficiency

The failure to hydrolyze lysosomal cholesteryl esters and triglycerides results in their accumulation in many tissues. The process of hepatic lipid accumulation evidently begins during fetal life.[40,73] Lipid infiltration of the intestinal mucosa, most marked in the proximal intestine, is undoubtedly the cause of the malabsorption syndrome in WD. It is noteworthy that, although lipid infiltration has been noted in central nervous and peripheral nervous tissue,[17] there is little clinical evidence of neurologic disease; it is likely that death from the failure of other organ systems occurs before significant degeneration of neurologic function. Adrenomegaly with fatty infiltration leading to calcification of the adrenal glands in WD is related to the normal process of fetal cortex involution, but at this time there is no obvious reason why patients with CESD are not similarly affected.

GENETIC CONSIDERATIONS

All available data point to an autosomal recessive mode of inheritance for WD, CESD, and their clinical variants. When parents have been tested, they have often[2,12,18,19,22,36,40,42,50,51,58,60,72,73,79,80,87,88] but not always[46,122] had intermediate levels of acid lipase activity. Most families with acid lipase deficiency have been of European origin, although Japanese,[14,24,31,66,88] Chinese,[34,35] Pakistani,[33] Middle Eastern,[3,4,13,15,26,29,30] Indian,[120] and American black[43,63] patients have been reported. There are no estimates of the population frequency of acid lipase deficiency. The gene for the acid lipase "A" enzyme has been assigned to human chromosome 10.[113,114] To date, no studies have been reported that examine the molecular basis of acid lipase deficiency in its various clinical forms. It is generally believed that there is more than one acid lipase–deficient allele to explain the broad clinical heterogeneity.

For the most part, affected siblings have suffered a similar disease; that is, the affected siblings of a proband with fulminant WD have had the same clinical course. There are a few notable exceptions, however, In a family described by Patrick and Lake,[2] the first child had a fulminant disease, although he died at a somewhat later age (14 months) than is typical for WD. His sister had symptoms beginning in infancy, but was still alive and in good health at 4½ years of age. Both siblings had the same degree of acid lipase deficiency and had presumably inherited the same mutant alleles from their parents, who themselves had intermediate levels of acid lipase activity. In our own experience (patient L.H., noted above), the index case had a protracted illness from which he died at 18 months of age. A younger brother, T.H., had a much more virulent disease; he demonstrated significant clinical symptoms at 4 months of age and died at 6 months, as is more commonly seen in WD. These cases of clinical heterogeneity within families are the exception rather than the rule.

Genetic counseling is possible for these disorders. Given that acid lipase activity can be measured and the "A" isozyme can be identified in chorionic villus samples and in amniotic fluid cells, prenatal diagnosis is an option. This is particularly true in families in which the proband has WD.

To our knowledge, prenatal diagnosis has been performed in 16 pregnancies in 13 families.[36,40,50,73,104,105,122,123] In 11 of these families, the indication was WD; in one, an atypical form of WD; in one, CESD. Twelve pregnancies were monitored by amniocentesis and four by chorionic villus sampling. In six pregnancies an affected fetus was predicted. Analysis of material from the aborted fetuses confirmed the prenatal diagnosis in five cases, in one case, the diagnosis was confirmed postnatally in a child who subsequently died at 6 months of age. In nine pregnancies, a normal fetus was predicted and the results confirmed postnatally. In one pregnancy the results were not conclusive; the family elected to terminate the pregnancy, which unfortunately led to the abortion of a normal fetus.

MANAGEMENT AND TREATMENT

There is no effective therapy for WD. The rapid downhill course in these patients has been unaffected by any sort of dietary management,[1] with a single exception.[115] Bile acid–binding resins, clofibrate, blood transfusions, and hormone replacement have been attempted without success. Enzyme replacement therapy is theoretically possible[116] but has not been attempted. Similarly, bone marrow and liver transplantation may offer future therapies. The recent identification of an animal model resembling WD may lead to the evaluation of therapies for this otherwise fatal disorder.[117]

Treatment of CESD is largely symptomatic, and the disease is generally benign. Iron deficiency anemia may require treatment because of intestinal involvement and esophageal varices. Bile acid–binding resins,[93] clofibrate,[118] and HMG-CoA reductase inhibitors[94] have proven effective in reducing plasma lipid levels in some CESD patients; this is particularly important in light of the fact that they are at considerably increased risk for development of premature atherosclerosis due to their hyperlipidemia.

REFERENCES

1. Schmitz G, Assmann G. Acid lipase deficiency: Wolman disease and cholesteryl ester storage disease. In: Scriver CR, Beaudet AL, Sly WS, Valle D, eds. The metabolic basis of inherited disease. 6th ed. New York: McGraw-Hill, 1989: 1623.
2. Patrick AD, Lake BD. Wolman's disease. In: Hers G, Van Hoof F, eds. Lysosomes and storage diseases. New York: Academic Press, 1973: 453.
3. Abramov A, Schorr S, Wolman M. Generalized xanthomatosis with calcified adrenals. Am J Dis Child 1956; 91:282–286.
4. Wolman M, Sterk VV, Gatt S, Frenkel M. Primary familial xanthomatosis with involvement and calcification of the adrenals: report of two more cases in siblings of a previously described infant. Pediatrics 1961; 28:742–757.
5. Crocker AC, Vawter GF, Neuhauser EBD, Rosowsky S. Wolman's disease: three new patients with a recently described lipidosis. Pediatrics 1965; 35:627–640.
6. Alexander WS. Niemann-Pick disease. Report of a case showing calcification in the adrenal glands. NZ Med J 1946; 45:43–45.
7. Patrick AD, Lake BD. Deficiency of an acid lipase in Wolman's disease. Nature 1969; 222:1067–1068.
8. Lake BD, Patrick AD. Wolman's disease: deficiency of E600-resistant acid esterase activity with storage of lipids in lysosomes. J Pediatr 1970; 76:262–266.

9. Frederickson DS. Newly recognized disorders of cholesterol metabolism. Ann Intern Med 1963; 58:718.
10. Sloan HR, Fredrickson DS. Enzyme deficiency in cholesteryl ester storage disease. J Clin Invest 1972; 51:1923–1926.
11. Burke JA, Schubert WK. Deficient activity of hepatic acid lipase in cholesterol ester storage disease. Science 1972; 176:309–310.
12. Cortner JA, Coates PM, Swoboda E, Schnatz JD. Genetic variation of lysosomal acid lipase. Pediatr Res 1976; 10:927–932.
13. Kahana D, Berant M, Wolman M. Primary familial xanthomatosis with adrenal involvement (Wolman's disease): report of a further case with nervous system involvement and pathogenetic considerations. Pediatrics 1968; 42:70–76.
14. Konno T, Fujii M, Watanuki T, Koizumi K. Wolman's disease: the first case in Japan. Tohoku J Exp Med 1966; 90:375–389.
15. Werbin BZ, Wolman M. Primary familial xanthomatosis with involvement and calcification of the adrenals. Harefuah 1968; 74:283–286.
16. Marks MI, Marcus AJ. Wolman's disease. Can Med Assoc J 1968; 99:232–235.
17. Guazzi GC, Martin JJ, Philippart M, Roels H, van der Ecken H, Vrints L, Delbeke MJ, Hooft C. Wolman's disease. Europ Neurol 1968; 1:334–362.
18. Marshall WC, Ockenden BG, Fosbrooke AS, Cumings JN. Wolman's disease: a rare lipidosis with adrenal calcification. Arch Dis Child 1968; 44:331–341.
19. Young EP, Patrick AD. Deficiency of acid esterase in Wolman's disease. Arch Dis Child 1970; 45:664–668.
20. Berdon WE, Baker DH. Radiographic findings in adrenal disease in infants and children. Adrenal hemorrhage, Wolman's familial xanthomatosis with adrenal calcifications, benign and malignant adrenal tumors. NY State J Med 1969; 69:2773–2778.
21. Lowden JA, Barson AJ, Wentworth P. Wolman's disease: a microscopic and biochemical study showing accumulation of ceroid and esterified cholesterol. Can Med Assoc J 1970; 102:402–405.
22. Kyriakides EC, Filippone N, Paul B, Grattan W, Balint JA. Lipid studies in Wolman's disease. Pediatrics 1970; 46:431–436.
23. Queloz JM, Capitanio MA, Kilpatrick JA. Wolman's disease. Roentgen observations in 3 siblings. Radiology 1972; 104:357–359.
24. Eto Y, Kitagawa J. Wolman's disease with hypolipoproteinemia and acanthocytosis: clinical and biochemical observations. J Pediatr 1970; 77:862–867.
25. Leclerc JL, Hould F, Lelievre M, Gagne F. Maladie de Wolman. Etude anatomo-clinique d'une nouvelle observation avec absence de calcifications radiologiques et macroscopiques des surrenales. Laval Med 1971; 42:461–467.
26. Wallis K, Gross M, Kohn R, Zaidman J. A case of Wolman's disease. Helv Paediatr Acta 1971; 26:98–111.
27. Nardi F, Borri P. Caratterizzazione morfologica e chimica di un caso di malattia di Wolman. Acta Neurol (Napoli) 1971; 26:270–278.
28. Sandomenico C, Tortora M, Gaetani B. La lipoidosi di Wolman. Radiol Med 1972; 58:144–148.
29. Raafat F, Hashemian MP, Abrishami MA. Wolman's disease. Report of two new cases, with a review of the literature. Am J Clin Pathol 1973; 59:490–497.
30. Kamalian N, Dudley AW, Beroukhim F. Wolman disease with jaundice and subarachnoid hemorrhage. Am J Dis Child 1973; 126:671–675.
31. Uno Y, Taniguchi A, Tanaka E. Histochemical studies in Wolman's disease. Report of an autopsy case accompanied with a large amount of milky ascites. Acta Pathol Jpn 1973; 23:779–790.
32. Lajo A, Gracia R, Navarro M, Nistal M, Rabadan B. Enfermedad de Wolman en su forma aguda infantil. An Esp Pediatr 1974; 7:438–446.
33. Ellis JE, Patrick D. Wolman's disease in a Pakistani infant. Am J Dis Child 1976; 130:545–547.
34. Ho FCS, Lin HJ, Chan WC. Wolman's disease: the first reported Chinese patient. Mod Med Asia 1978; 14:23–36.
35. Lin HJ, Ho FCS, Yu ECL, Pang S-W. Heterogeneity of tissue sterols and glycerolipids in Wolman's disease. Biochem Med 1985; 33:342–349.
36. Giambonini S, Siegrist P, Herschkowitz N, Wiesmann U, Jordan M, Hadorn B. Probleme der pranatalen und postnatalen Diagnostik bei Morbus Wolman. Helv Paediatr Acta 1977; Suppl 39:17.
37. Harrison RB, Francke P. Radiographic findings in Wolman's disease. Radiology 1977; 124:188.
38. Ozsoylu S, Gurgey A, Kocak N, Ozoran Y, Ozoran A, Kerse I, Ciliv G. Wolman's disease. A case report with lipid, chromosome and electron-microscopic studies. Turk J Pediatr 1977; 19:57–66.
39. Conde E, Fernandez P, Bureo E, Morante C, Zubizarreta A. Estudio de un caso de enfermedad de Wolman. Sangre 1978; 23:255.
40. Coates PM, Cortner JA, Mennuti MT, Wheeler JE. Prenatal diagnosis of Wolman disease. Am J Med Genet 1978; 2:397–407.
41. Young LW. Radiological case of the month. Wolman's disease. Am J Dis Child 1979; 133:959–960.
42. Schaub J, Janka GE, Christomanou H, Sandhoff K, Permanetter W, Hubner G, Meister P. Wolman's disease: clinical, biochemical and ultrastructural studies in an unusual case without striking adrenal calcification. Eur J Pediatr 1980; 135:45–53.
43. Byrd JC, Powers JM. Wolman's disease: ultrastructural evidence of lipid accumulation in central and peripheral nervous systems. Acta Neuropathol 1979; 45:37–42.
44. Bretagne MC, Rivoal-Jeanjean E, Beley G, Vidailhet M, Treheux A. La maladie de Wolman. Cause rare de calcifications surrenaliennes chez le nourrisson. Une observation. J Radiol 1981; 62:197–199.
45. Bambirra EA, Tafuri WL, Borges HHF, Carvalho C, Naves IL, Bogliolo L, Tafuri CP, Miranda D. Wolman's disease. A clinicopathologic, electron microscopic, and histochemical study. South Med J 1982; 75:595–596.
46. Fiandino G, Morgando MP, Artesani I, Iavarone A, Miniero R, Levis F. Malattia di Wolman: descrizione di un caso clinico. Riv Ital Pediatr 1983; 9:613–618.
47. Hoeg JM, Demosky SJ, Pescovitz OH, Brewer HB. Cholesteryl ester storage disease and Wolman disease: phenotypic variants of lysosomal cholesteryl ester hydrolase deficiency. Am J Hum Genet 1984; 36:1190–1203.
48. Maehira F, Nakada F, Hokama T. Characteristics of acid esterase in Wolman's disease. Biochem Med 1984; 32:322–330.
49. Dutton RV. Wolman's disease. Ultrasound and CT diagnosis. Pediatr Radiol 1985; 15:144–146.
50. Van Diggelen OP, Von Koskull H, Ammala P, Vredeveldt GTM, Janse HC, Kleijer WJ. First trimester diagnosis of Wolman's disease. Prenat Diag 1988; 8:661–663.
51. Bona G, Bracco G, Gallina MR, Iavarone A, Perona A, Zaffaroni M. Wolman's disease: clinical and biochemical findings of a new case. J Inherited Metab Dis 1988; 11:423–424.
52. Campesi G, Aragona F, Castellucci R, Vanella F. Ulteriore contributo alla conoscenza della c.d. malattia di Wolman. Arch Vecchi Anat Patol Med Clin 1977; 62:245–262.
53. Martin JF. Suprarenal calcification. Radiol Clin North Am 1965; 3:129–138.
54. Caffey J. The adrenal glands. In: Caffey J, ed. Pediatric x-ray diagnosis. Vol 2. 6th ed. Chicago: Year Book, 1972; 813.
55. Lageron A, Caroli J, Stralin H, Barbier P. Polycorie cholesterolique de l'adulte. I. Etude clinique, electronique, histochimique. Presse Med 1967; 75:2785–2790.
56. Schiff L, Schubert WK, McAdams AJ, Spiegel EL, O'Donnell JF. Hepatic cholesterol ester storage disease, a familial disorder. I. Clinical aspects. Am J Med 1968; 44:538–546.
57. Alagille D, Courtecuisse V. Surcharge hepatique a esters du cholesterol (deux observations). J Paris Pediatr 1970; 30:465–475.
58. Orme RL'E. Wolman's disease. An unusual presentation. Proc R Soc Med 1970; 63:489–490.
59. Lageron A, Lichtenstein H, Bodin F, Conte M. Polycorie cholesterolique de l'adulte. Aspects cliniques et histochimiques. Med Chir Dig 1975; 4:9–14.
60. Beaudet AL, Lipson MH, Ferry GD, Nichols B. Acid lipase in cultured fibroblasts: cholesterol ester storage disease. J Lab Clin Med 1974; 84:54–61.
61. Wolf H, Hug G, Michaelis R, Nolte K. Seltene, angeborene Erkrankung mit Cholesterinester-Speicherung in der Leber. Helv Paediatr Acta 1974; 29:105–118.
62. Keller E, Kunnert B, Braun W. Cholesterinesterspeicherkrankheit der Leber im Kindersalter. Dtsch Z Verdau Stoffwechselkr 1977; 37:231–236.
63. Arbisser A, Arbisser LB, Garcia CA, Akhtar M, Moore CM, Howell RR. Ocular findings in acid lipase deficiency. Monogr Hum Genet 1978; 9:193–197.
64. Gautier M, Lapous D, Raulin J. Maladie de surcharge a esters du cholesterol chez l'enfant. Etude biochimique comparative de cultures d'hepatocytes et de fibroblastes. Arch Fr Pediatr (Suppl) 1978; 35:38–49.
65. Lageron A. Histoenzymologie de la polycorie cholesterolique. A propos de 5 cas. Med Chir Dig 1978; 7:155–159.
66. Kawaguchi M, Hidaka S, Ikejiri N, Maeyama T, Eguchi T, Sato H,

Abe H, Tanikawa K, Nakayama T. A case of cholesterol ester storage disease. Acta Hepatol Jpn 1977; 18:786–794.
67. Pfeifer U, Jeschke R. Cholesterylester-Speicherkrankheit. Bericht uber vier Falle. Virchows Arch [B] 1980; 33:17–34.
68. Kuntz HD, May B, Schejbal V, Assmann G. Cholesterinester-Speicherkrankheit der Leber. Leber Magen Darm 1981; 11:258–263.
69. Verola O, de Roquancourt A, Chanu B, Rouffy J, Brocheriou C. Cholesterolose hepatique. Etude histologique, histochimique et ultrastructurale de deux observations. Sem Hop Paris 1983; 59:1753–1759.
70. Dincsoy HP, Rolfes DB, McGraw CA, Schubert WK. Cholesterol ester storage disease and mesenteric lipodystrophy. Am J Clin Pathol 1984; 81:263–269.
71. Besley GTN, Broadhead DM, Lawlor E, McCann SR, Dempsey JD, Drury MI, Crowe J. Cholesterol ester storage disease in an adult presenting with sea-blue histiocytosis. Clin Genet 1984; 26:195–203.
72. Kelly DR, Hoeg JM, Demosky SJ, Brewer HB. Characterization of plasma lipids and lipoproteins in cholesteryl ester storage disease. Biochem Med 1985; 33:29–37.
73. Desai PK, Astrin KH, Thung SN, Gordon RE, Short MP, Coates PM, Desnick RJ. Cholesteryl ester storage disease: pathologic changes in an affected fetus. Am J Med Genet 1987; 26:689–698.
74. Tylki-Szymanska A, Maciejko D, Wosniewicz B, Muszynska B. Two cases of cholesteryl-ester storage disease (CESD) acid lipase deficiency. Hepatogastroenterology 1987; 34:98–99.
75. Edelstein RA, Filling-Katz MR, Pentchev P, Gal A, Chandra R, Shawker T, Guzzetta P, Comly M, Kaneski C, Brady RO, Barton N. Cholesteryl ester storage disease: a patient with massive splenomegaly and splenic abscess. Am J Gastroenterol 1988; 83:687–692.
76. Longhi R, Vergani C, Valsasina R, Riva E, Galluzzo C, Agostini C, Giovaninni M. Cholesteryl ester storage disease: risk factors for atherosclerosis in a 15-year-old boy. J Inherited Metab Dis 1988; 11 (Suppl 2):143–145.
77. Van Erum S, Gnat D, Finne C, Blum D, Vanhelleput C, Vamos E, Vertongen F. Cholesteryl ester storage disease with secondary lecithin cholesterol acyl transferase deficiency. J Inherited Metab Dis 1988; 11(Suppl 2):146–148.
78. Hanak J, Elleder M. Nemoc ze stradani esteru cholesterolu (CESD). Cesk Pediatr 1984; 39:721–725.
79. D'Agostino D, Bay L, Gallo G, Chamoles N. Cholesterol ester storage disease: clinical, biochemical, and pathological studies of four new cases. J Pediatr Gastroenterol Nutr 1988; 7:446–450.
80. Giambartolomei G, Scarabicchi S, Lombardo C, Gatti R. Un caso di malattia da accumulo di esteri di colesterolo (CESD). Aspetti clinici e biochimici. Riv Ital Pediatr 1985; 11:301–303.
81. Burgin M, Neyer U, Kostner G. Lipidose mesangiale associe a une polycorie cholesterolique. Nephrologie 1982; 3:124–126.
82. Latalova E, Talas M, Prasilova J, Zupkova H. Porod u vzacne poruchy metabolismu cholesterolu (nemoc ze stradani cholesterolovych esteru). Cesk Gynekol 1987; 52:459–460.
83. Stozicky F, Liska J, Varvarovska J, Dobiasova M, Dura J, Elleder M. Odchylky v transportu a metabolismu lipoproteinu u nemoci ze stradani esteru cholesterolu. Cesk Pediatr 1985; 40:515–517.
84. Fredrickson DS, Sloan HR, Ferrans VJ, Demosky SJ. Cholesteryl ester storage disease: a most unusual manifestation of deficiency of two lysosomal enzyme activities. Trans Am Assoc Phys 1972; 85:109–120.
85. Cagle PT, Ferry GD, Beaudet AL, Hawkins EP. Clinicopathologic conference: pulmonary hypertension in an 18-year-old girl with cholesteryl ester storage disease (CESD). Am J Med Genet 1986; 24:711–722.
86. Beaudet AL, Ferry GD, Nichols BL, Rosenberg HS. Cholesterol ester storage disease: clinical, biochemical, and pathological studies. J Pediatr 1977; 90:910–914.
87. Lee JES, Chen RG, Ng WG, Koch R, Oizumi J, Davos I, Fleisher DR. Late infantile onset acid lipase deficiency. Am J Hum Genet 1981; 33:83A.
88. Suzuki Y, Kawai S, Kobayashi A, Ohbe Y, Endo H. Partial deficiency of acid lipase with storage of triglycerides and cholesterol esters in liver. Genetic variant of Wolman's disease? Clin Chim Acta 1976; 69:219–224.
89. Aubert-Tulkens G, Van Hoof F. Acid lipase deficiency: clinical and biochemical heterogeneity. Acta Paediatr Belg 1979; 32:239–245.
90. Philippart M, Durand P, Borrone C. Neutral lipid storage with acid lipase deficiency: a new variant of Wolman's disease with features of the Senior syndrome. Pediatr Res 1982; 16:954–959.
91. Durand P, Bugiani O, Palladini G, Borrone C, Della Cella G, Siliato F. Nephropathie tubulo-interstitielle chronique, degenerescence tapetoretinienne et lipidose generalisee. Analyse d'une observation anatomoclinique. Arch Fr Pediatr 1971; 28:915–927.
92. Peremans J, de Graef PJ, Strubb G, de Block G. Familial metabolic disorder with fatty metamorphosis of the viscera. J Pediatr 1966; 69:1108–1112.
93. Kostner GM, Hadorn B, Roscher A, Zechner R. Plasma lipids and lipoproteins of a patient with cholesteryl ester storage disease. J Inherited Metab Dis 1985; 8:9–12.
94. Ginsberg HN, Le N-A, Short MP, Ramakrishnan R, Desnick RJ. Suppression of apolipoprotein B production during treatment of cholesteryl ester storage disease with lovastatin. Implications for regulation of apolipoprotein B synthesis. J Clin Invest 1987; 80:1692–1697.
95. Assmann G, Fredrickson DS, Sloan HR, Fales HM, Highet RJ. Accumulation of oxygenated steryl esters in Wolman's disease. J Lipid Res 1975; 16:28–38.
96. Lin HJ, Lie Ken Hie MSF, Ho FCS. Accumulation of glyceryl ether lipids in Wolman's disease. J Lipid Res 1976; 17:53–56.
97. Lough J, Fawcett J, Wiegensberg B. Wolman's disease. An electron microscopic, histochemical, and biochemical study. Arch Pathol 1970; 89:103–110.
98. Hill SC, Hoeg JM, Dwyer AJ, Vucich JJ, Doppman JL. CT findings in acid lipase deficiency: Wolman disease and cholesteryl ester storage disease. J Comput Assist Tomogr 1983; 7:815–818.
99. Partin JC, Schubert WK. Small intestinal mucosa in cholesterol ester storage disease. A light and electron microscope study. Gastroenterology 1969; 57:542–558.
100. Lake BD. Histochemical detection of the enzyme deficiency in blood films in Wolman's disease. J Clin Pathol 1971; 24:617–620.
101. Hoeg JW, Demosky SJ, Brewer HB. Characterization of neutral and acid ester hydrolase in Wolman's disease. Biochim Biophys Acta 1982; 711:59–65.
102. Burton BK, Emery D, Mueller HW. Lysosomal acid lipase in cultivated fibroblasts: characterization of enzyme activity in normal and enzymatically deficient cell lines. Clin Chim Acta 1980; 101:25–32.
103. Negre A, Salvayre R, Maret A, Vieu C, Bes JC, Borrone C, Durand P, Douste-Blazy L. Lymphoid cell lines as a model system for the study of Wolman's disease: enzymatic, metabolic and ultrastructural observations. J Inherited Metab Dis 1986; 9:193–201.
104. Patrick AD, Willcox P, Stephens R, Kenyon VG. Prenatal diagnosis of Wolman's disease. J Med Genet 1976; 13:49–51.
105. Christomanou H, Cap C. Prenatal monitoring for Wolman's disease in a pregnancy at risk. First case in the Federal Republic of Germany. Hum Genet 1981; 47:440–441.
106. Burton BK, Remy RT, Rayman L. Cholesterol ester and triglyceride metabolism in intact fibroblasts from patients with Wolman's disease and cholesterol ester storage disease. Pediatr Res 1984; 18:1242–1245.
107. Burton BK, Reed SP. Acid lipase cross-reacting material in Wolman disease and cholesterol ester storage disease. Am J Hum Genet 1981; 33:203–208.
108. Kyriakides EC, Paul B, Balint JA. Lipid accumulation and acid lipase deficiency in fibroblasts from a family with Wolman's disease and their apparent correction in vitro. J Lab Clin Med 1972; 80:810–816.
109. Natowicz MR, Chi MM-Y, Lowry OH, Sly WR. Enzymatic identification of mannose-6-phosphate on the recognition marker for receptor-mediated pinocytosis of β-glucuronidase by human fibroblasts. Proc Natl Acad Sci USA 1979; 76:4322–4326.
110. Sando GN, Henke VL. Recognition and receptor-mediated endocytosis of the lysosomal acid lipase secreted by cultured human fibroblasts. J Lipid Res 1982; 23:114–123.
111. Brown MS, Sobhani MK, Brunschede GY, Goldstein JL. Restoration of a regulatory response to low density lipoprotein in acid lipase-deficient human fibroblasts. J Biol Chem 1976; 251:3277–3286.
112. Goldstein JL, Dana SE, Faust JR, Beaudet AL, Brown MS. Role of lysosomal acid lipase in the metabolism of plasma low density lipoproteins. Observations in cultured fibroblasts from a patient with cholesteryl ester storage disease. J Biol Chem 1975; 250:8487–8495.
113. Van Cong N, Weil D, Hors-Cayla MC, Gross MS, Heuertz S, Foubert C, Frezal J. Assignment of the genes for human lysosomal acid lipases A and B to chromosomes 10 and 16. Hum Genet 1980; 55:375–381.
114. Koch G, Lalley PA, McAvoy M, Shows TB. Assignment of *LIPA*, associated with human acid lipase deficiency, to human chromosome 10 and comparative assignment to mouse chromosome 19. Somat Cell Genet 1981; 7:345–358.
115. Meyers WF, Hoeg JM, Demosky SJ, Herbst JJ, Brewer HB. The use

of parenteral hyperalimentation and elemental formula feeding in the treatment of Wolman disease. Nutr Res 1985; 5:423–429.
116. Poznansky MJ, Hutchison SK, Davis PJ. Enzyme replacement therapy in fibroblasts from a patient with cholesteryl ester storage disease. FASEB J 1989; 3:152–156.
117. Sandersleben JV, Hanichen T, Fiebiger I, Brem G. Lipidspeicherkrankheit vom Typ der Wolmanschen Erkrankung des Menschen beim Foxterrier. Tierarztl Praxis 1986; 14:253–263.
118. Schubert WK, Partin J, Schiff L, Hoyumpa A. Clofibrate therapy in cholesterol ester storage disease: reduction of serum cholesterol, serum bile acids and liver lipid content. Gastroenterology 1969; 56:1221.
119. Marosvari I. Wolman disease in twins. Acta Paediatr Hung 1985; 26:61–64.
120. Sundaravalli N, Bhaskar Raju B, Prema A, Pushpa V, Nedunchelian N, Shetty MVK, Sudarsanam D. Wolman's disease. Indian Pediatr 1986; 23:950–953.
121. Pastor Bevia E, Pedraz Garcia C, Heras de Pedro MI, Garcia Parron A, Escudero Bueno G, Benito Zaballos MF, Salzar Villalobos V. Enfermedad de Wolman: aportacion de tres casos. An Esp Pediatr 1987; 26:301–304.
122. Vargas Torcal F, Gomez Garcia A, Cuevas J, Young EP. Enfermedad de Wolman. An Esp Pediatr 1987; 27:195–198.
123. Gatti R, Lombardo C, Filocamo M, Borrone C, Porro E. Comparative study of 15 lysosomal enzymes in chorionic villi and cultured amniotic fluid cells. Early prenatal diagnosis in seven pregnancies at risk for lysosomal storage diseases. Prenat Diag 1985; 5:329–336.
124. Gross MS, Van Cong N, Hors-Cayla MC, Weil D, Heuertz S, Foubert C. Les lipases acides et les mutations responsables des maladies de Wolman et de surcharge a esters du cholesterol. Ann Genet 1983; 26:10–16.

PART 12

Inherited Abnormalities in Mitochondrial Fatty Acid Oxidation

Paul M. Coates, Ph.D.
Daniel E. Hale, M.D.

The first well-documented disorders of fatty acid oxidation were described in the mid-1970s in patients with skeletal muscle weakness or exercise-induced rhabdomyolysis and abnormalities in muscle fatty acid metabolism associated with muscle carnitine deficiency[1] or carnitine palmityltransferase (CPT) deficiency.[2] Shortly thereafter, the syndrome of systemic carnitine deficiency was reported[3]; in this disorder, plasma, muscle, and liver carnitine levels are low, and fatty acid metabolism in muscle and sometimes liver is impaired. Characterization of another group of inborn errors of mitochondrial fatty acid oxidation began in 1982–1983 with the description of medium-chain acyl-CoA dehydrogenase (MCAD) deficiency[4–7] in patients with disorders of fasting adaptation. Subsequently, long-chain acyl-CoA dehydrogenase (LCAD) deficiency[8] and short-chain acyl-CoA dehydrogenase (SCAD) deficiency[9–11] were described, and a defect in the cellular uptake of carnitine has now been identified in several patients.[12] In this discussion, we review the pathway of fatty acid oxidation and then describe the clinical, laboratory, pathologic, and metabolic findings in patients with disorders of fatty acid oxidation, for the most part resulting from deficiency of each of the acyl-CoA dehydrogenases. Detailed description of this pathway and its genetic defects is provided elsewhere.[13,14]

FASTING ADAPTATION AND FATTY ACID OXIDATION

Successful adaptation to the fasting state requires the actions of several biochemical pathways, the interactions of many tissues, and the regulation of these processes by various hormones.[15–17] In the immediate postprandial period, nutrients absorbed from the gut are stored in many tissues, a process regulated primarily by insulin. During the postabsorptive state, insulin levels fall, resulting in the activation of the glycogenolytic pathway to yield glucose-6-phosphate. In the liver, glucose-6-phosphate can be dephosphorylated and released into the blood stream, whereas muscle glycogen can be used only endogenously, since glucose-6-phosphatase activity is not expressed in muscle tissue. As fasting is further prolonged and insulin levels decline further, the liver gluconeogenic pathway is activated. Substrates for gluconeogenesis include amino acids, derived from muscle protein catabolism, and lactate and pyruvate, derived from glycolysis. The mobilization of amino acids is enhanced by growth hormone. Increased gluconeogenesis ensures a constant supply of glucose for those organs and tissues that require glucose, especially brain and red blood cells. However, the capacity for gluconeogenesis is limited, and prolonged muscle catabolism threatens the ability of the organism to obtain nutrients; hence, as fasting in prolonged, fat becomes the primary metabolic fuel.

Most of the stored metabolic fuel is in the form of fat. This fat is stored principally in adipose tissue as triglyceride, with the component fats consisting mainly of palmitate (16:0) and oleate (18:1). When insulin reaches a very low concentration, fats are released from adipose tissue, a process that is facilitated by cortisol. Fats may be used by both skeletal and cardiac muscle directly to meet energy needs. They are metabolized in the liver (and kidney) to acetyl-CoA with the consequent production of both reducing equivalents (nicotinamide-adenine dinucleotide [NADH]) and energy (adenosine triphosphate [ATP]). All three compounds enhance gluconeogenesis and promote the disposal of ammonia (ureagenesis) resulting from the use of amino acids as gluconeogenic precursors. While acetyl-CoA derived from fatty acid oxidation may enter the tricarboxylic acid cycle, approximately 90 percent enters the ketogenic pathway, resulting in the formation of the ketone bodies acetoacetate and 3-hydroxybutyrate.[13] These ketones may be used by muscle; perhaps more importantly, the brain can derive 25 to 40 percent of its energy needs from ketones after a period of adaptation. Thus, the overall scheme of fasting adaptation is the provision of glucose for those tissues that have an absolute requirement for it; the provision of an alternative fuel for those tissues that can utilize fat in place of glucose; and the provision of an auxiliary fuel (ketones) for both muscle and brain.

Fatty Acid Oxidation

Because fats are the major source of fuel during fasting, the biochemical pathways for fatty acid oxidation are most active under these conditions.[18,19] Fats released by adipose tissue are taken up by the liver and other tissues in a concentration-dependent manner (Fig. 1). Once inside the cell, they are activated by an ATP-dependent acyl-CoA ligase to the respective coenzyme A (CoA) ester. Long-chain fatty acids (i.e., more than 10 carbons in length) are activated in the cytosol and may enter the pathways for triglyceride, phospholipid, or cholesteryl ester synthesis. Alternatively, they may enter either the peroxisomal or the mitochondrial beta-oxidation pathways. Under fasting conditions, fatty acids are directed primarily toward mitochondrial beta-oxidation. Long-chain acyl-CoA esters must be transported across the inner mitochondrial membrane via a transport system consisting of carnitine palmityltransferase I (CPT I), which substitutes carnitine for the CoA; a translocase that transports the carnitine ester across the membrane; and CPT II, which replaces the carnitine with CoA within the mitochondrion. Shorter-chain fatty acids (i.e., 10 or fewer carbons) enter the mitochondria directly as free acids and are activated to form CoA esters within the matrix.

Once inside the mitochondrion, the acyl-CoA ester undergoes sequential removal of a two-carbon moiety (acetyl-CoA) from the carboxyl terminal end of the molecule. The removal of each acetyl-CoA requires the consecutive action of four enzymes[20]: acyl-CoA dehydrogenase, enoyl-CoA hydratase, 3-hydroxyacyl-CoA dehydrogenase, and 3-ketoacyl-CoA thiolase (Fig. 2).

Acyl-CoA dehydrogenase inserts a double bond between the second (alpha) and third (beta) carbons of the acyl-CoA, forming an enoyl-CoA and generating electrons that are transferred to a unique electron acceptor, electron transfer flavoprotein (ETF). In turn, reduced ETF is oxidized by ETF: ubiquinone oxidoreductase (ETF dehydrogenase) and coenzyme Q, with the ultimate transfer of electrons to the electron transport chain. Three acyl-CoA dehydrogenases have been identified which differ in their specificity for the chain length of the acyl-CoA. The second reaction in beta-oxidation involves hydration of the enoyl-CoA to form L-3-hydroxyacyl-

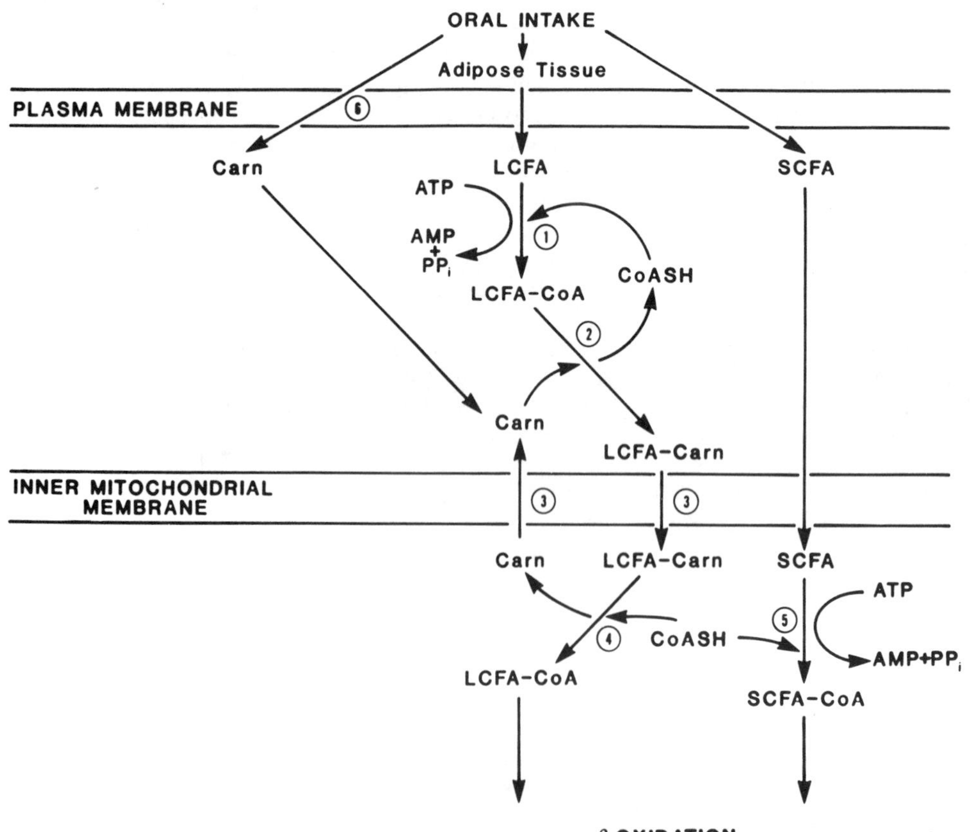

FIGURE 1 Pathway of fatty acid entry, activation, mitochondrial uptake, beta-oxidation, and carnitine uptake. Numbers indicate the sequence of reactions. 1, Fatty acid activation by acyl-CoA synthase to form acyl-CoA esters; 2, fatty acyl-CoA transesterification to carnitine by carnitine palmityltransferase I (CPT I) prior to mitochondrial translocation; 3, carnitine translocase; 4, re-esterification of acylcarnitine to acyl-CoA by CPT II; 5, intramitochondrial acyl-CoA synthase for medium- and short-chain fatty acids; 6, plasma membrane carnitine transport system.

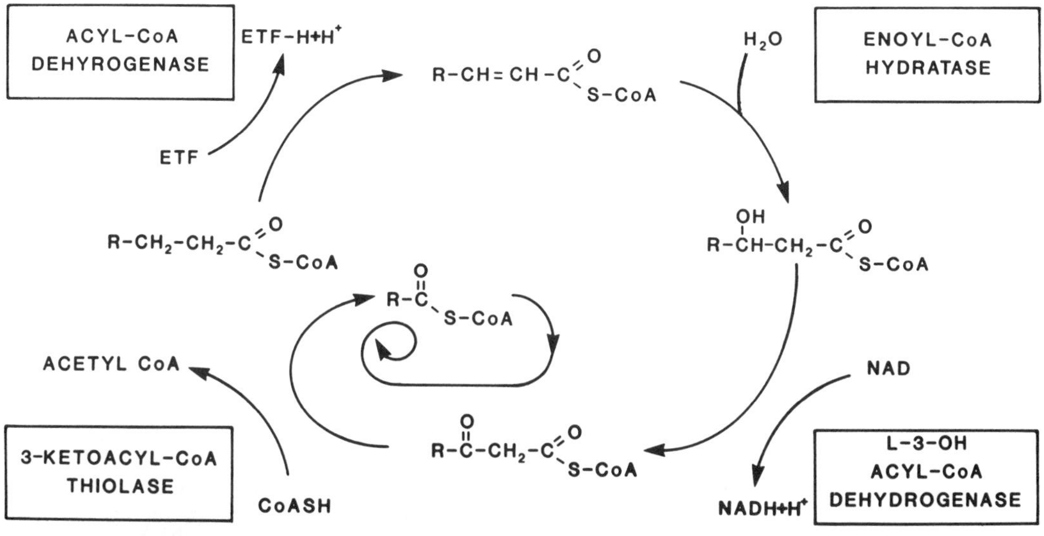

FIGURE 2 Spiral of fatty acyl-Coa beta-oxidation in mitochondria. An acyl-CoA enters the spiral, whereupon acyl-CoA dehydrogenase inserts a double bond, forming an enoyl-CoA and transferring electrons to electron transfer flavoprotein (ETF). Enoyl-CoA hydratase adds water across the double bond to form a 3-hydroxyacyl-CoA, which is oxidized by an NAD-linked 3-hydroxyacyl-CoA dehydrogenase to form a 3-ketoacyl-CoA. In the presence of free coenzyme A (CoASH), 3-ketoacyl-CoA thiolase cleaves the alpha, beta-bond to yield acetyl-CoA and an acyl-CoA moiety, now two carbons shorter, which can re-enter the spiral.

CoA catalyzed by enoyl-CoA hydratase(s). The third reaction is oxidation of the hydroxy group to a keto group in an NAD^+-dependent reaction. Two 3-hydroxyacyl-CoA dehydrogenases have been identified that differ in their chain-length specificity. The final reaction, catalyzed by 3-ketoacyl-CoA thiolase(s), is cleavage of the alpha, beta bond in the presence of reduced CoA, to form acetyl-CoA and an acyl-CoA now two carbons shorter than the original substrate (e.g., palmityl-CoA, with 16 carbons, yields acetyl-CoA and myristyl-CoA, with 14 carbons). Acyl-CoA compounds can cycle through beta-oxidation as many times as it is possible to generate acetyl-CoA fragments (e.g., palmityl-CoA can make as many as seven cycles through beta-oxidation). As the molecule becomes shorter, it will be recognized preferentially by enzymes with different chain-length specificity.

Odd-chain acyl-CoA compounds are oxidized by the same series of reactions described above, until the three-carbon moiety, propionyl-CoA, is formed, which is degraded by the biotin-dependent enzyme, propionyl-CoA carboxylase.

Unsaturated acyl-CoA compounds are also oxidized by the same series of reactions, until the double bond is reached.[21] Further oxidation requires the activity of two additional enzymes, 3 cis, 2 trans-enoyl-CoA isomerase and 2,4-dienoyl-CoA reductase, followed by enoyl-CoA hydratase and the remainder of the beta-oxidation pathway.

The peroxisomes also perform beta-oxidation[22] but use a slightly different sequence of events and preferentially oxidize very long chain fatty acids (more than 20 carbons). The activation of these fatty acids requires a unique peroxisomal acyl-CoA ligase. The acyl-CoA is then dehydrogenated by an acyl-CoA oxidase instead of the acyl-CoA dehydrogenase in mitochondria. The peroxisomal enoyl-CoA hydratase and 3-hydroxyacyl-CoA dehydrogenase functions are present in a single protein (the bifunctional enzyme). The peroxisomal 3-ketoacyl-CoA thiolase performs the same function as the mitochondrial enzyme, but it is genetically distinct.

Pathways for Fatty Acid Disposal

The recent description of defects in fatty acid oxidation has focused attention on alternative pathways for fatty acid utilization and disposal. In the face of a defect in fatty acid oxidation, there is an accumulation of acyl-CoA intermediates within the cytosol and/or the mitochondrial matrix. In addition to peroxisomal beta-oxidation (discussed above), there are at least four additional mechanisms available for the disposition of acyl-CoA esters[14]: (1) thioester cleavage of the CoA ester to yield the free acid; (2) transesterification of the CoA ester with carnitine via carnitine acyltransferase(s); (3) conjugation of the CoA esters with glycine via glycine *N*-acylase; and (4) microsomal omega- and (omega-1)-oxidation to yield dicarboxylic acids and (omega-1) hydroxy fatty acids. The net effect of these alternative pathways is the formation of intermediates that can be readily excreted from the cell and ultimately in the urine, at the same time that intramitochondrial pools of CoA are conserved. The relative contribution of each of these mechanisms to the disposal of abnormal fatty acids is not known.

Regulation of Fatty Acid Oxidation

The regulation of fatty acid oxidation in mammalian tissues by hormones, competing substrates, cofactors, and diet has been reviewed extensively elsewhere.[13,19,20] The primary regulator of hepatic fatty acid oxidation and ketogenesis during fasting is the plasma concentration of free fatty acids, although there are other regulatory points. In the transition from the fed to the fasted state, the liver converts from an organ of glucose uptake and fatty acid synthesis to one of glucose production, fatty acid oxidation, and ketogenesis.

Hormonal control of fatty acid oxidation is exerted at the level of substrate mobilization from adipose tissue and by indirect effects on the activity of CPT I. Insulin inhibits lipolysis in adipose tissue, thereby decreasing the level of free fatty acids available for oxidative metabolism; it also stimulates acetyl-CoA carboxylation and lipogenesis in the liver, in turn increasing tissue levels of malonyl-CoA, an inhibitor of CPT I, thereby inhibiting fatty acid oxidation. Glucagon stimulates hepatic fatty acid oxidation indirectly by inhibiting acetyl-CoA carboxylase, which in turn reduces tissue levels of malonyl-CoA, thereby promoting fatty acid oxidation. In the fed state, in which the glucagon-to-insulin ratio is low, the liver directs fatty acid metabolism toward synthesis. Under these conditions, oxidation of fatty acids is suppressed by the high tissue levels of malonyl-CoA. In the fasting state, elevation of the glucagon-to-insulin ratio suppresses malonyl-CoA synthesis and consequently directs fatty acids toward mitochondria for oxidation.

GENETIC DEFECTS IN FATTY ACID OXIDATION

General Clinical Features and Laboratory Findings

At least three intramitochondrial defects in fatty acid oxidation have been characterized,[4-11] in addition to defects in cell membrane carnitine transport[12] and in the transesterification of acyl-CoA.[2,23] With the exception of MCAD deficiency, few patients with the other defects have yet been identified. In the following discussion, we will emphasize the features that should arouse concern about a defect in fatty acid oxidation (Table 1). It will be followed by a description of the individual defects.

TABLE 1
Features of Fatty Acid Oxidation Defects*

1. **History**
   - Prompted by fasting
   - Episodic Reye-like disease
   - Progressive obtundation
   - Similarly affected siblings
   - Family history of Reye syndrome or SIDS
2. **Physical Examination**
   - Obtundation
   - Muscle weakness
   - Hepatomegaly
   - Cardiomegaly, cardiomyopathy
   - Developmental delay
   - Seizures
3. **Laboratory Evaluation†**
   - Hypoglycemia
   - Hypoketonemia
   - Dicarboxylic aciduria
   - Mild hyperammonemia
   - Modestly elevated liver enzymes
   - Low plasma and tissue carnitine levels
   - Increased urinary carnitine excretion

*Not all patients with fatty acid oxidation defects express all of these features.

†These laboratory findings may be evident only at the time of an episode.

Because fats are important metabolic fuels, primarily during fasting, a defect is likely to be manifested when food intake is decreased or interrupted, as in the case of a viral gastroenteritis, or when energy demands are higher, as occurs with fever. The inability to arouse the child or persistent vomiting often precipitates the hospital visit. Additional evidence suggesting a fatty acid oxidation defect includes previous similar episodes in the proband or a history of irritability or difficulty in arousing the child after a normal overnight fast. Since most of these defects are inborn errors of metabolism, a careful family history may demonstrate that other siblings had catastrophic illnesses in the first years of life. The potential diagnoses given to these siblings may have included sudden infant death syndrome (SIDS), Reye's syndrome, or unexplained hypoglycemia.

In most cases, the clinical features at the time of presentation are not specific to defects in fatty acid oxidation. Obtundation and/or coma is often the most prominent feature. Evidence of incipient shock (tachycardia, low blood pressure) may be found and may reflect either dehydration secondary to persistent vomiting or cardiac malfunction secondary to disordered energy metabolism. Cardiac enlargement on chest radiograph has been seen in some patients. Hepatomegaly may be present; in most cases in which liver biopsy has been performed, the hepatic enlargement has resulted from significant fatty infiltration of the liver. Muscle weakness and hypotonia have been found on initial examination of some patients and have persisted even after the patient has recovered from the acute episode. Occasionally, developmental delay and seizures have been identified. Obviously, the physical abnormalities reflecting the precipitating illness (e.g., otitis media) may also be noted.

Because the historical and clinical features of fatty acid oxidation disorders are relatively nonspecific, the clinical laboratory often provides the first clues to disordered energy metabolism (Table 2). The most important diagnostic specimens are those collected at the time of presentation. The two most rapidly available tests are also two of the most useful—a blood glucose measurement and an analysis of the urine for the presence of ketones. Blood glucose can be quickly measured using a chemically treated plastic strip (Chemstrip bG) and the appropriate electronic reader (Accuchek II). Blood glucose measurements should always be checked by obtaining a serum sample. A blood glucose level of less than 50 mg per deciliter suggests a defect in energy metabolism, whereas a blood glucose level greater than 100 mg per deciliter tends to rule out such a defect. A blood glucose in the 50 to 100 mg per deciliter range is not helpful without additional laboratory information. The presence of "large ketones" in the urine when the blood sugar is less than 50 mg per deciliter is evidence of normal fatty acid mobilization and oxidation. Trace or small ketones when a child is hypoglycemic is not an adequate response and may suggest a problem.

Ideally, blood should also be obtained at the time of presentation for the determination of the hormones regulating fasting adaptation (growth hormone, cortisol, insulin) and for

TABLE 2
Laboratory Evaluation of a Potential Defect in Fatty Acid Oxidation

1. Emergency Room Evaluation

   If **blood glucose** is low (≤50 mg/dl), then test **urine ketones**. If "absent" or "trace," then process blood and urine.

2. Secondary Evaluation

   Blood hormones: insulin, cortisol, growth hormone
   Blood metabolites: lactate, pyruvate, alanine, free fatty acids, beta-hydroxybutyrate, free and total carnitine, glucose
   Urine metabolites: drug screen, metabolic screen, organic acids, acylglycines, free and total carnitine, acylcarnitine profile

metabolites known to change in normal fasting (free fatty acids, lactate, pyruvate, alanine, 3-hydroxybutyrate, carnitine). The first urine should be saved and evaluated for organic acid content and sent for metabolic screen. Specimens obtained when the child is well and fed are far less likely to be informative in considering a disorder of fatty acid oxidation than those obtained when the child is acutely ill or fasting. If appropriate studies are not obtained at the time of presentation, then a carefully monitored fasting study may be necessary to adequately evaluate fasting adaptation. Many children with defects in fatty acid oxidation excrete significant quantities of dicarboxylic acids, acylglycine conjugates, and acylcarnitines in their urine. Not surprisingly, the circulating levels of free fatty acids are high, as are the levels of growth hormone and cortisol. Insulin levels should be low or undetectable. A number of other biochemical abnormalities have been found in some patients. These include elevations of lactate, ammonia, uric acid, serum glutamic-oxaloacetic transaminase, serum glutamic-pyruvic transaminase, and myoglobin. The mechanisms leading to these changes remain speculative but probably reflect a failure of intracellular energy production.

Medium-Chain Acyl-CoA Dehydrogenase Deficiency

This disorder has emerged as the most frequently diagnosed defect in fatty acid oxidation. Hence, much of what is known about the clinical, biochemical, and molecular aspects of fatty acid oxidation disorders has been learned from the study of medium-chain acyl-CoA dehydrogenase (MCAD) deficiency.

Clinical Presentations. Since the first patients with MCAD deficiency were described in 1982–1983,[4–7] more than 100 patients have been identified[14] (D.E. Hale and P.M. Coates: unpublished observations). The disease is most frequently characterized by recurrent episodes of illness, generally provoked by fasting, in children within the first 2 years of life. The child presents with vomiting and lethargy that may progress to coma. Hypoglycemia, although often present, is not an absolute feature of MCAD deficiency; frequently, patients can be ill in spite of normal glucose levels, suggesting that clinical symptoms may be caused by increased levels of fatty acids or their metabolites. Between episodes, patients with MCAD deficiency can appear normal, with no muscle weakness or exercise intolerance.

There is considerable variation in the clinical presentation of MCAD deficiency, even within the same family. Sudden infant death syndrome,[24] recurrent Reye's syndrome,[25,26] and episodic hypoglycemic coma[27] have all been described as presentations of MCAD deficiency; patients have also been described who are completely asymptomatic.[28,29] The children may have only one episode of illness or multiple recurrences; in some cases they appear to be asymptomatic. The earliest onset of symptoms was at 1 week of age. The greatest frequency of presentation occurs between 5 and 24 months of age. There is no report of first symptoms after age 6 years. Furthermore, there appears to be less recurrent illness after this age, and symptoms requiring hospitalization are rare in the second decade. Since the disorder has only recently been defined, the long-term course is not yet clear and the effects of pregnancy on affected females are yet to be determined.

The mortality rate is significant.[14] In the first year of life, 13 percent died with their first episode; after 12 months of age, 43 percent died with their first episode. It should be noted that three children first identified with MCAD deficiency at 2, 5, and 6 months of age died during an intercurrent illness between 26 and 30 months of age. There appears to be a period between 15 and 26 months of age during which mortality is extremely high (59 percent).

Approximately one-third of families identified with this disorder have had one or more unexplained sibling deaths. In a few of these, the diagnosis of MCAD deficiency was made post mortem.[24,29,30] If a sibling carried the diagnosis of either Reye's syndrome or SIDS, attempts should be made to obtain clinical and autopsy information, since that child may have had the cerebral edema and fatty liver commonly encountered in MCAD deficiency. Postmortem diagnosis either by specific enzyme assay or by acylcarnitine measurement may be possible if tissue has been stored frozen.

Laboratory Investigations. The initial laboratory studies usually include serum electrolytes, glucose, ammonia, transaminases, and urinalysis. Although there may be a mild metabolic acidosis, a large anion gap is unusual and, if present, often indicates superimposed lactic acidosis. Hypoglycemia (less than 50 mg per deciliter) is usually present, but normal or borderline glucose levels have been observed in lethargic patients with MCAD deficiency, suggesting that the central nervous system manifestations are not due entirely to hypoglycemia. Therefore, the diagnosis of MCAD deficiency should not be excluded on this basis alone. Hypoketosis, particularly in the face of hypoglycemia, is often noted. Ammonia levels in the blood are usually only mildly elevated (80 to 120 μg per deciliter) but have been observed as high as 430 μg per deciliter. There is often a mild (two- to four-fold) elevation in serum transaminases.

These findings alone give sufficient cause to proceed with more specific diagnostic testing, including gas chromatography–mass spectrometry (GC-MS) analysis of organic acids, carnitine assays, acylcarnitine analysis, and specific enzyme assay. Except for the enzyme assay, the other studies can be obtained relatively quickly, so that early decisions regarding patient management and the exclusion of other disorders from the differential diagnosis can be made.

When mitochondrial beta-oxidation is limited by MCAD deficiency, partially oxidized medium-chain fatty acids, such as octanoic acid and cis-4-decenoic acid, may accumulate and have been identified in plasma from MCAD-deficient patients.[31] Alternative pathways,[32] such as omega- and (omega-l)-oxidation and peroxisomal beta-oxidation, become involved, resulting in the production of medium-chain dicarboxylic acids, chiefly adipic ($C_{6:0}$), suberic ($C_{8:0}$), dehydrosuberic ($C_{8:1}$), sebacic ($C_{10:0}$), and dehydrosebacic ($C_{10:1}$) acids. The corresponding (omega-l)-hydroxy acids (5-hydroxyhexanoate and 7-hydroxyoctanoate) also may be present in the urine of these patients. Among the most specific findings are the glycine conjugates, suberylglycine, hexanoylglycine, and phenylpropionylglycine.[33] Unlike diseases such as methylmalonic aciduria and isovaleric acidemia, the concentrations of abnormal urinary metabolites in MCAD deficiency vary greatly, depending upon the nutritional status of the patient. Dicarboxylic acid excretion itself is not diagnostic of MCAD deficiency; it is commonly seen in other diseases (such as diabetic ketoacidosis) or following the administration of medium-chain triglycerides (MCT). In the latter setting, only saturated dicarboxylic acids are excreted, in contrast to both saturated and unsaturated forms seen in MCAD deficiency.[26] Furthermore, the relative concentrations of the C_6, C_8, and C_{10} dicarboxylic acids differ between MCAD deficiency and MCT feeding; in MCAD deficiency, these tend to be present with C_6 greater than C_8 greater than C_{10}, whereas the reverse is usually found in the urine of patients fed MCT.[34]

An affected child who is not symptomatic at the time of testing and is receiving normal dietary intake typically has low total plasma carnitine levels. Urinary free carnitine relative to creatinine may also be reduced and associated with a relative increase in acylcarnitines. In many children with MCAD deficiency, the ratio of urinary acylcarnitine to free carnitine (normally 4 or less) is significantly increased, even though absolute carnitine excretion (in micromoles per kilogram per 24 hours) is frequently decreased. These reductions parallel the reported concentrations of carnitine in tissues. Six untreated cases of MCAD deficiency (including three cases originally described as having systemic carnitine deficiency) were characterized by tissue levels of carnitine reduced to 16 to 42 percent of normal in liver and 16 to 25 percent of normal in muscle.[14] The identification of acylcarnitine species excreted by MCAD-deficient children[35,36] is often of greater value in diagnosis than is the measurement of total or even esterified carnitine levels and, in some instances, is more sensitive and specific than capillary GC-MS analysis of urinary organic acids. The child with MCAD deficiency has a characteristic acylcarnitine profile, including hexanoylcarnitine, octenoylcarnitine, octanoylcarnitine, and decenoylcarnitine, and there may be very little signal corresponding to the normal species, acetylcarnitine. This latter observation is consistent with the reduced capacity to produce acetyl-CoA in this beta-oxidation defect.

The primary pathologic findings in MCAD-deficient patients include hepatic light microscopic and ultrastructural changes, but alterations have been observed in other tissues. Cerebral edema is noted post mortem in most cases.[7,29,36,37] Hepatic light microscopic alterations in MCAD deficiency are essentially limited to steatosis, which may be either macro- or microvesicular in nature.[37] In some cases, the microvesicular fat accumulation has been indistinguishable from that seen in Reye's syndrome, but ultrastructural studies have clearly demonstrated that the generalized mitochondrial changes characteristic of Reye's syndrome were not present. Specifically, the matrix swelling and rarefaction commonly seen in hepatic mitochondria of patients with Reye's syndrome have not been observed in mitochondria from patients with MCAD deficiency. Increased matrix density and intracristal widening, seen in some patients, give the mitochondria a condensed appearance; occasionally, crystalloids have been observed in the matrix, associated with an increased number of cristae and with enlargement and abnormal shape of the mitochondria.[37]

Nature of the Enzyme Defect in MCAD Deficiency. The specific enzyme defect[14] has been demonstrated in cultured skin fibroblasts, peripheral mononuclear leukocytes, liver, and muscle. Several methods have been used in different laboratories to measure MCAD and other acyl-CoA dehydrogenase activities. Using an assay based upon reduction of the natural electron acceptor, ETF[28,37,38] (D.E. Hale and P.M. Coates: unpublished observations), MCAD activity measured with octanoyl-CoA as substrate has been generally less than 10 percent of control levels in fibroblasts from MCAD-deficient patients (Table 3). Comparable results have been obtained using the tritium-release assay,[39] the artificial dye reduction assay,[6] and the single ion monitoring GC-MS method.[4]

Dehydrogenase activities toward other acyl-CoA compounds have been measured in cells from MCAD-deficient patients. LCAD activity measured against palmityl-CoA as substrate is normal. By contrast, dehydrogenase activity toward butyryl-CoA as substrate is reduced to 50 percent of control levels in cells from MCAD-deficient patients.[6,28,40] These data suggest that MCAD has considerable activity toward short-chain acyl-CoA compounds; this has been confirmed by the use of a monospecific antibody directed against MCAD, which completely inhibits octanoyl-CoA dehydrogenation and 50 percent of the activity toward butyryl-CoA in control cells.[41]

Table 3 further demonstrates that cells from parents of MCAD-deficient patients have intermediate levels of MCAD activity using octanoyl-CoA as substrate, consistent with their being heterozygous for an autosomal recessive trait. The mean residual enzyme activity is 49.5 percent of control levels, ranging from 35 to 67 percent; there has been no overlap between heterozygote levels and either control or affected levels of MCAD activity. This has important ramifications in terms of genetic counseling and diagnosis (see below).

Biochemical and Molecular Aspects. Human liver MCAD is a homotetramer,[42] with each subunit containing 1

TABLE 3
Acyl-CoA Dehydrogenase Activities in Fibroblasts and Leukocytes from Patients with MCAD Deficiency, Their Parents, and Controls

Subjects (n)	Palmityl-CoA	Octanoyl-CoA	Butyryl-CoA
Patients (64)	2.20 ± 0.30*	0.24 ± 0.12	0.97 ± 0.14
Parents (25)	2.15 ± 0.21	2.04 ± 0.32	1.53 ± 0.12
Controls (142)	2.19 ± 0.22	4.17 ± 0.37	2.20 ± 0.24

*nmol of electron transfer flavoprotein reduced per minute per milligram of protein, mean ± standard deviation.

mol of flavin adenine dinucleotide (FAD). The human MCAD subunit is synthesized on cytoplasmic ribosomes as a 50,000 dalton precursor, with a leader peptide sequence of 4,000 daltons; the mature enzyme subunit, once translocated to the mitochondrial matrix, has a molecular weight of 46,000 daltons.[40,43] Among 13 human MCAD-deficient cultures, in which residual enzyme activity toward octanoyl-CoA ranged from 6 to 13 percent of control levels, the MCAD precursor was synthesized and processed to the mature MCAD, and both were indistinguishable in size from the corresponding precursor and mature forms of MCAD in control cells.[40] These data suggest that the mutation(s) causing MCAD deficiency, at least in these 13 patients, is likely to be a point mutation affecting the catalytic activity of the enzyme. There is a single report of a 4-amino acid insertion in the leader peptide of MCAD, resulting in a failure of mitochondrial uptake of the enzyme, thereby causing MCAD deficiency.[44] Matsubara et al[45] have cloned the cDNAs encoding rat and human MCAD and have assigned the human gene to the short arm of chromosome 1, band p31.

Management and Treatment. Because of the nature of this particular metabolic defect, situated in the middle of a pathway that, at least in liver, is generally activated only under conditions of fasting stress, the management of MCAD-deficient patients includes the avoidance of fasting, even though some patients tolerate fasting well. Once it has been recognized that the patient has a disorder of fatty acid oxidation, the frequency of further episodes may be reduced by ensuring regular and adequate caloric intake with a diet moderately high in carbohydrate.

Some patients with MCAD deficiency have been able to withstand repeated fasting insults; as long as these episodes are appropriately treated with intravenous glucose administration (8 to 10 mg per kilogram per minute), the long-term outlook for many patients is good.[14] Because there are considerable differences among patients in their ability to tolerate fasting, it is important to tailor recommendations about maximum interval between meals to the individual patient.

L-Carnitine supplementation has been advocated in the management of patients with MCAD deficiency, by analogy with the use of glycine and L-carnitine supplementation in isovaleric acidemia.[46,47] The primary defect in both disorders is enzymatic. Hence, supplementation with carnitine, as with glycine in isovaleric acidemia, does not correct the enzyme abnormality and therefore is not expected to ameliorate the failure of fasting ketogenesis. On the other hand, carnitine represents a useful conjugation pathway for the removal of potentially toxic intermediates that accumulate under conditions of fasting stress in patients with MCAD deficiency, as suggested by the enhanced excretion of medium-chain acylcarnitines following carnitine administration.

Counseling, Family Screening, and Prenatal Diagnosis. MCAD deficiency has emerged as a common cause of clinical disease resembling Reye's syndrome, especially in the first 2 years of life,[48] and it has been implicated in cases of SIDS,[49] but accurate estimates of its frequency in the population have not been made. Its approximate frequency in the United Kingdom, based upon several indirect lines of evidence, is between 1:10,000 and 1:25,000 (M.J. Bennett: personal communication), making MCAD deficiency a common hereditary metabolic disorder, with heterozygotes present in the population at an estimated frequency of 1 to 2 percent.

Asymptomatic siblings of patients with MCAD deficiency should be tested. Urinary acylcarnitines (hexanoyl- and octanoylcarnitine) following oral administration of a test dose of L-carnitine (100 mg per kilogram p.o.) or acylglycines (hexanoylglycine and phenylpropionylglycine) have become important indicators of this enzyme defect.[33,47] Neither acylcarnitine nor acylglycine analysis, however, will discriminate between heterozygotes and normals. Enzyme activity can be measured in leukocytes or fibroblasts[28]; this has the advantage that heterozygous individuals can be distinguished from controls as well as from those with MCAD deficiency. Among 11 siblings of five MCAD-deficient patients, three were identified with MCAD deficiency, four with heterozygote levels of enzyme activity, and four with control levels.[28] Given that the frequency of heterozygotes may approach 1 percent and that the disease carries the potential for sudden death, attention should also be given to the screening of siblings of the parents and to extending the screening to unrelated spouses of those siblings if the latter are found to be heterozygotes.

Prenatal diagnosis of MCAD deficiency has been reported[50] and should be considered as an option for the early detection of an affected fetus. It is likely that prenatal diagnosis will rarely be sought for the purpose of pregnancy termination, since disease associated with this defect is often preventable by appropriate management and intervention during episodes of fasting stress, but there may well be families in which parents feel unable to cope with bringing up a second affected child.

Long-Chain Acyl-CoA Dehydrogenase Deficiency

Clinical Presentations. Fourteen patients have been identified with long-chain acyl-CoA dehydrogenase (LCAD) deficiency since the defect was described by Hale et al in three infants in 1985[8,51,52] (D.E. Hale and P.M. Coates: unpublished observations). This disorder shares some features in common with MCAD deficiency, including recurrent episodes of vomiting, coma, and hypoglycemia brought on by fasting or a viral prodrome; hypoketosis with medium-chain dicarboxylic aciduria; low plasma and tissue carnitine levels; and micro- and macrovesicular steatosis of the liver. By contrast, however, LCAD-deficient children typically have had a more severe illness with an earlier mean age of onset (5.5 months versus 13 months), and with a striking involvement of cardiac and skeletal muscle not seen in patients with MCAD deficiency. Four patients died during their first episode, one patient died during a recurrence, and another patient, who was badly damaged in the initial episode, died of aspiration pneumonia at age 5 years. Three have significant psychomotor deficiency resulting from their initial episode. Two young children whose impaired fasting adaptation was recognized early and in whom serious decompensation has been avoided are thriving at 10 months and 1 year of age. One patient, age 21 years, is healthy and asymptomatic. Two other patients (females, 24 and 27 years) have significant muscle pain and myoglobinuria reminiscent of the muscular form of carnitine palmityltransferase deficiency (see below).

One of these had the onset of her symptoms at age 8 years and the other had symptoms starting at age 18 years.

Laboratory Investigations. Upon fasting or when clinically ill, these patients are hypoglycemic, hypoketotic, and acidotic, and they have abnormal liver function tests and hyperuricemia. In two of these patients, serum CPK was elevated during periods of fasting stress. The urinary organic acid profile reveals reduced or absent ketones and dicarboxylic aciduria. In addition to the C_6-C_{10} dicarboxylic aciduria typical of MCAD-deficient patients, there was evidence for the excretion of longer-chain (C_{12} and C_{14}) dicarboxylic acids in two patients.[51] Suberylglycine, hexanoylglycine, and phenylpropionylglycine excretion have not been observed in LCAD deficiency.[8,33] As in MCAD deficiency, patients with LCAD deficiency have had a secondary carnitine deficiency; muscle, liver, and plasma carnitine levels in one patient were all low,[8] and plasma carnitine levels in other patients have been low. Urinary carnitine excretion is low when these patients are ill; short-chain acylcarnitines, chiefly acetylcarnitine, are the major excretion products.[14,47] This latter finding is in contrast to the urinary carnitine ester profiles of patients with other defects in mitochondrial metabolism, in which the predominant acylcarnitine corresponds to the acyl-CoA derivative that accumulates proximal to the metabolic block[14]; it is likely that long-chain acylcarnitines are not readily excreted by the kidney. Hepatic light microscope alterations[37] include panlobular steatosis, with both macrovesicular and microvesicular droplets, portal fibrosis, and absence of necrosis or cholestasis. Liver from one patient had electron microscopic findings similar to those seen in MCAD deficiency, namely mitochondrial matrix density with widening of the intracristal space.

Nature of the Enzyme Defect in LCAD Deficiency. The enzyme defect has been demonstrated in cultured fibroblasts from ten patients and in leukocytes from four of them (Table 4). Using an ETF-based assay with palmityl-CoA as substrate, cells from the patients had less than 10 percent of control levels of LCAD activity. In spite of the marked clinical heterogeneity in this small group of patients, there were no apparent differences among them in residual LCAD activity. It should be noted that the enzyme defect could be detected in liver of one patient,[8] but the assay of LCAD in liver should be done at low protein concentrations, since high concentrations obscure the LCAD defect by as-yet-unknown mechanisms (D.E. Hale: unpublished observations).

Parents' fibroblasts and leukocytes had approximately 50 percent of control LCAD activity (Table 4), consistent with heterozygosity for an autosomal trait. Four asymptomatic siblings of two of these patients have been screened: one had normal LCAD activity and three had activities within the heterozygote range.

Biochemical and Molecular Aspects. Rat liver LCAD[53] has a native molecular weight of 180,000 by gel filtration; it is a homotetramer with a subunit molecular weight of 45,000, each containing 1 mol of FAD. Its purification from human sources has not been reported, and there are as yet no data regarding the molecular aspects of LCAD deficiency.

Treatment and Counseling. As is the case with MCAD deficiency, management should be aimed at avoiding fasting, maintaining a high carbohydrate intake, frequent feeding, and treating episodes of illness with intravenous glucose. The role of carnitine supplementation in this disorder has not been assessed systematically. It is possible that MCT feeding might provide a route for administering calories, since medium-chain fatty acids enter the beta-oxidation spiral below the metabolic block. Obviously, this should be attempted only after ruling out a defect of medium-chain fatty acid oxidation, such as MCAD deficiency.

Currently, the only way to make the diagnosis of LCAD deficiency is to measure acyl-CoA dehydrogenase activities in fibroblasts or leukocytes.[8] Given that it is a life-threatening illness, diagnosis should be made as early as possible, so that appropriate modifications of formula and feeding schedule can be made. Asymptomatic siblings can be tested by measurement of LCAD activity in fibroblasts and leukocytes. As noted earlier, acyl-CoA dehydrogenase activities can be readily measured in cultured amniotic fluid cells.[50] It should therefore be possible to carry out the prenatal diagnosis of LCAD deficiency, but this has not yet been attempted.

TABLE 4
Acyl-CoA Dehydrogenase Activities in Fibroblasts and Leukocytes from Patients with LCAD Deficiency, Their Parents, and Controls

Subjects (n)	Palmityl-CoA	Octanoyl-CoA	Butyryl-CoA
Patients (10)	0.31 ± 0.21*	3.89 ± 0.41	2.08 ± 0.31
Parents (11)	1.19 ± 0.27	4.06 ± 0.49	2.20 ± 0.14
Controls (142)	2.19 ± 0.22	4.17 ± 0.37	2.20 ± 0.24

*nmol of electron transfer flavoprotein reduced per minute per milligram of protein, mean ± standard deviation.

Short-Chain Acyl-CoA Dehydrogenase Deficiency

Clinical Presentations and Laboratory Findings. Short-chain acyl-CoA dehydrogenase (SCAD) deficiency has been reported in only a few patients, and the clinical and laboratory findings are variable. Amendt et al[10] reported a female infant (Neonate II) who began to vomit and became lethargic and hypertonic in the newborn period, with hypoglycemia, acidosis, and hyperammonemia. Organic acid analysis showed lactic acidosis, ketosis and increased butyrate, and ethylmalonate and adipate excretion. On day five, she had fixed, dilated pupils and no spontaneous movement, and a brain scan showed little blood flow. She died on day six.

Coates et al[11] described a female infant of unrelated parents whose early postnatal life was complicated by poor feeding and frequent emesis. During the first year of life, she exhibited poor weight gain, developmental delay, progressive skeletal muscle weakness, hypotonia, and microcephaly. Skeletal muscle biopsy was unremarkable except for minor generalized lipid accumulation in type 1 fibers. She never had episodes of hypoglycemia, rarely had organic aciduria, had low-normal plasma carnitine levels, but had 50 percent of control levels of muscle carnitine, 75 percent of which was esterified. She responded poorly to a fat-restricted diet supplemented with L-carnitine. Developmental testing at 21 months revealed significant motor, cognitive developmental, and language delay. Increasing difficulty with poor oral intake necessitated insertion of a gastrostomy tube at 23 months. At 32 months, she showed a significant weight gain and overall improvement in strength.

Turnbull et al[9] reported a 46-year-old woman with no previous neuromuscular disorders who presented with persistent weakness in the left arm and in both legs which was exacerbated by mild exertion. Neurologic examination revealed a proximal myopathy, which was confirmed by electromyography. Serum creatine kinase was normal. There was excess neutral lipid in type 1 fibers of skeletal muscle, but no other abnormalities were detected. Muscle carnitine levels were low (25 percent of control) with an increased proportion of acylcarnitine to free carnitine. Plasma carnitine levels were low normal. The major urinary metabolite was ethylmalonate; fasting was not associated with hypoglycemia and blood ketone body levels were elevated. Her muscle weakness did not respond to treatment with either carnitine or prednisolone.

Pathologic Findings. In two cases, these were limited to muscle and included lipid vacuolization, especially in type 1 fibers.[9,11] One case[10] had cerebral edema, hepatosplenomegaly with fatty changes, cholestasis, and focal hepatocellular necrosis.

Nature of the Enzyme Defect in SCAD Deficiency. With butyryl-CoA as substrate, cultured skin fibroblasts from three patients[9,10] had 50 percent of control levels of enzyme activity, all of which was inhibited by incubation of the cells with anti-MCAD antibody. These data demonstrated that they had a specific SCAD deficiency and provided further evidence for the overlapping substrate specificity of MCAD. Cultured fibroblasts from the parents of one patient had intermediate levels of SCAD, consistent with their being heterozygous for an autosomal trait.[11] Studies of cells from members of the other families were not done.

Skeletal muscle SCAD activity in one case, measured with butyryl-CoA as substrate,[9] was 25 percent of control levels; acyl-CoA dehydrogenase activities toward longer-chain substrates (octanoyl-, decanoyl-, dodecanoyl-, and palmityl-CoA) were well within normal limits. SCAD activity in her fibroblasts, however, was normal.[10,11]

Biochemical and Molecular Aspects. Human liver SCAD[42] is a homotetramer, with a subunit molecular weight of 41,000; each subunit contains 1 mol of FAD. Ozasa et al[54] reported the molecular cloning and nucleotide sequence of cDNA encoding rat liver SCAD, but these studies have not yet been performed in human material. The gene for human SCAD has been assigned to chromosome 12.[55]

Counseling. Currently, the only way to make the diagnosis of SCAD deficiency is to measure acyl-CoA dehydrogenases directly, ideally in the presence of an antibody that inhibits the activity of MCAD toward the short-chain substrate, butyryl-CoA. Limited data indicate that heterozygotes for SCAD deficiency can be detected; hence, testing of family members should be possible. Likewise, prenatal diagnosis of SCAD deficiency is theoretically possible, but it has not yet been attempted.

Carnitine Palmityltransferase Deficiency

Two distinct presentations of carnitine palmityltransferase (CPT) deficiency have been reported. The first description of CPT deficiency by DiMauro and DiMauro[2] was in a patient with episodic muscle weakness and myoglobinuria; since that time, 40 patients have been reported, most of whom have presented in late childhood or adulthood. Their CPT deficiency has been demonstrated in muscle, liver, leukocytes, platelets, and fibroblasts.[56] A distinct clinical presentation, with hypoglycemia and hypoketosis, was reported in two children under one year of age[23,57]; neither of them had skeletal muscle abnormalities, but in both cases, fibroblast CPT activity was markedly reduced.

Carnitine Transport Defect

Several patients have been described[12,58–60] with clinical and laboratory evidence of a fatty acid oxidation disorder, with extremely low plasma and tissue carnitine levels, which was ameliorated by carnitine supplementation. Clinically, some of them have resembled patients with MCAD deficiency, presenting early in life with episodes of hypoketotic hypoglycemia brought on by fasting. Unlike patients with MCAD deficiency, they did not excrete significant amounts of dicarboxylic acids or unusual acylglycines or acylcarnitines in urine. Some of these patients have presented later in life (2 years or older) with cardiomyopathy. Still others have had both presentations, that is, one or more episodes of hypoketotic hypoglycemia in infancy and later development of cardiomyopathy (C.A. Stanley, D.E. Hale, and P.M. Coates: unpublished observations).

In all cases, patients have had plasma carnitine levels less than 10 μM, with muscle and liver carnitine levels less than 5 percent of control. Treatment with carnitine has frequently resulted in significant clinical improvement. Detailed studies[12] of carnitine transport in fibroblasts from one of these patients demonstrated virtually absent carnitine uptake, which appeared to reflect a defect in transport of carnitine in muscle and kidney.

OTHER DEFECTS IN FATTY ACID OXIDATION

Defects of other enzymes have been identified which have a considerable impact on flux through the beta-oxidation pathway. Abnormalities in the structure and function of electron transfer flavoprotein (ETF) and of ETF dehydrogenase have been associated with a spectrum of disorders (multiple acyl-CoA dehydrogenation defects, ethylmalonic-adipic aciduria, glutaric aciduria type II) in which the dehydrogenation of numerous substrates (fatty acyl-CoA isovaleryl-CoA, isobutyryl-CoA, 2-methyl branched-chain acyl-CoA, glutaryl-CoA, and sarcosine) is impaired.[61–63] Deficiency of HMG-CoA lyase affects ketone body formation from acetyl-CoA and has been associated with a Reye's syndrome–like disease,[64,65] which in some respects resembles MCAD deficiency.[13] Acetoacetyl-CoA thiolase deficiency[66,67] has been demonstrated in several patients with metabolic acidosis and significant ketosis, occasionally associated with hypoglycemia.

Unexplained Defects in Fatty Acid Oxidation

Within the last few years, patients have been reported who have many clinical and laboratory features consistent with a defect in fatty acid oxidation but have been shown not to have an acyl-CoA dehydrogenase deficiency. Given the complexity of the beta-oxidation spiral (Fig. 2), the fact that the other enzymes in the pathway—enoyl-CoA hydratases, 3-hydroxyacyl-CoA dehydrogenases, and 3-ketoacyl-CoA thiolases—have been proven or suggested to exist in multiple forms with different chain length specificity, and the fact that the complete oxidation of unsaturated fatty acids requires additional enzyme-mediated steps, it would not be surprising to find defects elsewhere in fatty acid oxidation.

Bennett et al[68] reported a patient with a defect in fibroblast short-chain fatty acid oxidation whose clinical and laboratory findings were remarkably like those described for patients with SCAD deficiency described by Amendt et al,[10] but her fibroblasts had normal SCAD activity.[11]

Patients have been described who have many of the features of LCAD deficiency, including fasting intolerance, dicarboxylic aciduria, and muscle weakness, but who excrete hydroxydicarboxylic acids in their urine[69-72] (D.E. Hale: unpublished observations). The specific location of the hydroxyl group, reported to be in the 3-position of the long- chain acids excreted by these patients, may be an important clue to the site of their enzyme defect, either primary or secondary, at the level of 3-hydroxyacyl-CoA dehydrogenase.[73]

REFERENCES

1. Engel AG, Angelini C. Carnitine deficiency of human skeletal muscle with associated lipid storage myopathy: a new syndrome. Science 1973; 179:899–901.
2. DiMauro S, DiMauro PMM. Muscle carnitine palmityltransferase deficiency and myoglobinuria. Science 1973; 182:929–931.
3. Karpati G, Carpenter S, Engel AG, Watters G, Allen J, Rothman S, Klassen G, Mamer OA. The syndrome of systemic carnitine deficiency: clinical, morphologic, biochemical, and pathophysiologic features. Neurology 1975; 25:16–24.
4. Kolvraa S, Gregersen N, Christensen E, Hobolth N. In vitro fibroblast studies in a patient with C_6-C_{10}-dicarboxylic aciduria: evidence for a defect in general acyl-CoA dehydrogenase. Clin Chim Acta 1982; 126:53–67.
5. Divry P, David M, Gregersen N, Kolvraa S, Christensen E, Collet JP, Dellamonica C, Cotte J. Dicarboxylic aciduria due to medium chain acyl CoA dehydrogenase defect. A cause of hypoglycemia in childhood. Acta Paediatr Scand 1983; 72:943–949.
6. Rhead WJ, Amendt BA, Fritchman KS, Felts SJ. Dicarboxylic aciduria: deficient [$^{1-14}$C] octanoate oxidation and medium-chain acyl-CoA dehydrogenase in fibroblasts. Science 1983; 221:73–75.
7. Stanley CA, Hale DE, Coates PM, Hall CL, Corkey BE, Yang W, Kelley RI, Gonzales EL, Williamson JR, Baker L. Medium-chain acyl-CoA dehydrogenase deficiency in children with non-ketotic hypoglycemia and low carnitine levels. Pediatr Res 1983; 17:877–884.
8. Hale DE, Batshaw ML, Coates PM, Frerman FE, Goodman SI, Singh I, Stanley CA. Long-chain acyl coenzyme A dehydrogenase deficiency: an inherited cause of nonketotic hypoglycemia. Pediatr Res 1985; 19:666–671.
9. Turnbull DM, Bartlett K, Stevens DL, Alberti KGMM, Gibson GJ, Johnson MA, McCulloch AJ, Sherratt HSA. Short-chain acyl-CoA dehydrogenase deficiency associated with a lipid-storage myopathy and secondary carnitine deficiency. N Engl J Med 1984; 311:1232–1236.
10. Amendt BA, Greene C, Sweetman L, Cloherty J, Shih V, Moon A, Teel L, Rhead WJ. Short-chain acyl-CoA dehydrogenase deficiency: clinical and biochemical studies in two patients. J Clin Invest 1987; 79:1303–1309.
11. Coates PM, Hale DE, Finocchiaro G, Tanaka K, Winter SC. Genetic deficiency of short-chain acyl-coenzyme A dehydrogenase in cultured fibroblasts from a patient with muscle carnitine deficiency and severe skeletal muscle weakness. J Clin Invest 1988; 81:171–175.
12. Treem WR, Stanley CA, Finegold DN, Hale DE, Coates PM. Primary carnitine deficiency due to a failure of carnitine transport in kidney, muscle and fibroblasts. N Engl J Med 1988; 319:1331–1336.
13. Stanley CA. New genetic defects in mitochondrial fatty acid oxidation and carnitine deficiency. Adv Pediatr 1987; 34:59–88.
14. Roe CR, Coates PM. Acyl-CoA dehydrogenase deficiencies. In: Scriver CR, et al, eds. The metabolic basis of inherited disease. 6th ed. New York: McGraw Hill, 1988: 889.
15. Cahill GF, Herrera MG, Morgan AP, Soeldner JS, Steinke J, Levy PL, Reichard GA, Kipnis DM. Hormone-fuel interrelationships during fasting. J Clin Invest 1966; 45:1751–1769.
16. Cahill GF. Starvation in man. Clin Endocrinol Metab 1976; 5:397–415.
17. Kaye R, Davidson MH, Williams ML, Kumagai M, Picou DM. The response of blood glucose, ketones, and plasma nonesterified fatty acids to fasting and epinephrine injection in infants and children. J Pediatr 1961; 59:836–847.
18. McGarry JD, Foster DW. Regulation of hepatic fatty acid oxidation and ketone body production. Ann Rev Biochem 1980; 49:395–420.
19. Bremer J, Osmundsen H. Fatty acid oxidation and its regulation. In: Numa S, ed. Fatty acid metabolism and its regulation. Amsterdam: Elsevier, 1984; 113.
20. Schulz H. Oxidation of fatty acids. In: Vance DE, Vance JE, eds. Biochemistry of lipids and membranes. Menlo Park, CA: Benjamin/ Cummings, 1985:116.
21. Schulz H, Kunau WH. Beta-oxidation of unsaturated fatty acids: a revised pathway. Trends Biochem Sci 1987; 12:403–406.
22. Hashimoto T. Comparison of enzymes of lipid β-oxidation in peroxisomes and mitochondria. In: Fahimi HD, Sies H, eds. Peroxisomes in biology and medicine. Berlin: Springer-Verlag, 1987: 87.
23. Damaugre F, Bonnefont JP, Mitchell G, Nguyen-Hoang N, Pelet A, Rimoldi M, DiDonato S, Saudubray JM. Hepatic and muscular presentations of carnitine palmitoyl transferase deficiency: two distinct entities. Pediatr Res 1988; 24:308–311.
24. Howat AJ, Bennett MJ, Variend S, Shaw L. Deficiency of medium chain fatty acylcoenzyme A dehydrogenase presenting as the sudden infant death syndrome. Br Med J 1984; 288:976.
25. Glasgow AM, Eng G, Engel AG. Systemic carnitine deficiency simulating recurrent Reye syndrome. J Pediatr 1980; 96:889–891.
26. Taubman B, Hale DE, Kelley RI. Familial Reye-like syndrome: a presentation of medium-chain acyl-coenzyme A dehydrogenase deficiency. Pediatrics 1987; 79:382–385.
27. Colle E, Mamer OA, Montgomery JA, Miller JD. Episodic hypoglycemia with ψ-hydroxy fatty acid excretion. Pediatr Res 1983; 17:171–176.
28. Coates PM, Hale DE, Stanley CA, Corkey BE, Cortner JA. Genetic deficiency of medium-chain acyl coenzyme A dehydrogenase: studies in cultured skin fibroblasts and peripheral mononuclear leukocytes. Pediatr Res 1985; 19:671–676.
29. Duran M, Hofkamp M, Rhead WJ, Saudubray JM, Wadman SK. Sudden child death and "healthy" affected family members with medium-chain acyl-coenzyme A dehydrogenase deficiency. Pediatrics 1986; 78:1052–1057.
30. Roe CR, Millington DS, Maltby DA, Wellman RB. Post-mortem recognition of inherited metabolic disorders from specific acylcarnitines in tissue in cases of sudden infant death. Lancet 1987; i:512.
31. Duran M, Mitchell G, De Klerk JBC, De Jager JP, Hofkamp M, Bruinvis L, Ketting D, Saudubray JM, Wadman SK. Octanoic acidemia and octanoylcarnitine excretion with dicarboxylic aciduria due to defective oxidation of medium-chain fatty acids. J Pediatr 1985; 107:397–404.
32. Gregersen N. The acyl-CoA dehydrogenation deficiencies. Scand J Clin Lab Invest 1985; 45(Suppl 174):1–60.
33. Rinaldo P, O'Shea JJ, Coates PM, Hale DE, Stanley CA, Tanaka K. Medium chain acyl-CoA dehydrogenase deficiency: diagnosis by stable isotope dilution analysis of urinary *N*-hexanoylglycine and 3-phenylpropionylglycine. N Engl J Med 1988; 319:1308–1313.

34. Mortensen PB, Gregersen N. Medium-chain triglyceride medication as a pitfall in the diagnosis of non-ketotic C_6-C_{10}-dicarboxylic acidurias. Clin Chim Acta 1980; 103:33–37.
35. Roe CR, Millington DS, Maltby DA, Bohan TP, Kahler SG, Chalmers RA. Diagnostic and therapeutic implications of medium-chain acylcarnitines in the medium-chain acyl-CoA dehydrogenase deficiency. Pediatr Res 1985; 19:459–464.
36. Roe CR, Millington DS, Maltby DA, Kinnebrew P. Recognition of medium-chain acyl-CoA dehydrogenase deficiency in asymptomatic siblings of children dying of sudden infant death or Reye-like syndromes. J Pediatr 1986; 108:13–18.
37. Treem WR, Witzleben CA, Piccoli DA, Stanley CA, Hale DE, Coates PM, Watkins JB. Medium-chain and long-chain acyl CoA dehydrogenase deficiency: clinical, pathologic and ultrastructural differentiation from Reye's syndrome. Hepatology 1986; 5:1270–1278.
38. Frerman RE, Goodman SI. Fluorometric assay of acyl-CoA dehydrogenases in normal and mutant human fibroblasts. Biochem Med 1985; 33:38–44.
39. Amendt BA, Rhead WJ. Catalytic defect of medium-chain acyl-coenzyme A dehydrogenase deficiency. Lack of both cofactor responsiveness and biochemical heterogeneity in eight patients. J Clin Invest 1985; 76: 963–969.
40. Ikeda Y, Hale DE, Keese SM. Coates PM, Tanaka K. Biosynthesis of variant medium chain acyl-CoA dehydrogenase in cultured fibroblasts from patients with medium chain acyl-CoA dehydrogenase deficiency. Pediatr Res 1986; 20:843–847.
41. Hale DE, Finocchiaro G, Coates PM, Tanaka K. Substrate chain length specificity of the residual enzyme activity in medium chain acyl-CoA dehydrogenase (MCAD) deficient cells: study using specific antibodies. Pediatr Res 1986; 20:329A.
42. Finocchiaro G, Ito M, Tanaka K. Purification and properties of short chain acyl-CoA, medium chain acyl-CoA, and isovaleryl-CoA dehydrogenases from human liver. J Biol Chem 1987; 262:7982–7989.
43. Ikeda T, Tanaka K. Immunoprecipitation and electrophoretic analysis of four human acyl-CoA dehydrogenases and electron transfer flavoprotein using antibodies raised against the corresponding rat enzymes. Biochem Med Metab Biol 1987; 37:329–334.
44. Strauss AW, Chu T, Eftimi R, Kelly DP. Mitochondrial protein uptake requirements: mutational analysis of the transit peptide. Pediatr Res 1988; 23:334A.
45. Matsubara Y, Kraus JP, Yang-Feng TL, Francke U, Rosenberg LE, Tanaka K. Molecular cloning of cDNAs encoding rat and human medium-chain acyl-CoA dehydrogenase and assignment of the gene to human chromosome 1. Proc Natl Acad Sci USA 1986; 83:6543–6547.
46. Roe CR, Millington DS, Maltby DA, Kahler SG, Bohan TP. L-Carnitine therapy in isovaleric acidemia. J Clin Invest 1984; 74:2290–2295.
47. Roe CR, Millington DS, Maltby DA. Diagnostic and therapeutic implications of acylcarnitine profiling in organic acidurias associated with carnitine insufficiency. In: Borum PR, ed. Clinical aspects of human carnitine deficiency. New York: Pergamon Press, 1986:97.
48. Reye's syndrome and aspirin: epidemiological associations and inborn errors of metabolism. Lancet 1987; ii:429–431.
49. Sudden infant death and inherited disorders of fat oxidation. Lancet 1986; ii:1073–1075.
50. Bennett MJ, Allison F, Pollitt RJ, Manning NJ, Gray RGF, Green A, Hale DE, Coates PM. Prenatal diagnosis of medium-chain acyl-CoA dehydrogenase deficiency in family with sudden infant death. Lancet 1987; i:440–441.
51. Naylor EW, Mosovich LL, Guthrie R, Evans JE, Tieckelmann H. Intermittent non-ketotic dicarboxylic aciduria in two siblings with hypoglycemia: an apparent defect in β-oxidation of fatty acids. J Inherited Metab Dis 1980; 3:19–24.
52. Schwenk WF, Hale DE, Haymond MW. Decreased fasting free fatty acids with L-carnitine in children with carnitine deficiency. Pediatr Res 1988; 23:491–494.
53. Ikeda Y, Okamura-Ikeda K, Tanaka K. Purification and characterization of short-chain, medium-chain, and long-chain acyl-CoA dehydrogenases from rat liver mitochondria. Isolation of the holo- and apoenzymes and conversion of the apoenzyme to the holoenzyme. J Biol Chem 1985; 260:1311–1325.
54. Ozasa H, Ikeda I, Finocchiaro G, Matsubara Y, Tanaka K. Molecular cloning and nucleotide sequence of cDNA encoding rat liver short chain acyl-CoA dehydrogenase. Am J Hum Genet 1987; 1:A232.
55. Barton DE, Yang-Feng TL, Finocchiaro G, Ozasa H, Tanaka K, Francke U. Short chain acyl-CoA dehydrogenase (ACADS) maps to chromosome 12 (q22-qter) and electron transfer flavoprotein (ETFA) to 15 (q23-q25). Cytogenet Cell Genet 1987; 46:577.
56. Angelini C, Trevisan C, Isaya G, Pegolo G, Vergani L. Clinical varieties of carnitine and carnitine palmityltransferase deficiency. Clin Biochem 1987; 20:1–7.
57. Bougneres PF, Saudubray JM, Marsac C, Bernard O, Odievre M, Girard J. Fasting hypoglycemia resulting from hepatic carnitine palmitoyl transferase deficiency. J Pediatr 1981; 98:742–746.
58. Chapoy PR, Angelini C, Brown WJ, Stiff JE, Shug AL, Cederbaum SD. Systemic carnitine deficiency—a treatable inherited lipid-storage disease presenting as Reye's syndrome. N Engl J Med 1980; 303:1389–1394.
59. Tripp ME, Katcher ML, Peters HA, Gilbert EF, Arya S, Hodach RJ, Shug AL. Systemic carnitine deficiency presenting as familial endocardial fibroelastosis. A treatable cardiomyopathy. N Engl J Med 1981; 305:385–391.
60. Waber LJ, Valle D, Neill C, DiMauro S, Shug A. Carnitine deficiency presenting as familial cardiomyopathy: a treatable defect in carnitine transport. J Pediatr 1982; 101:700–705.
61. Gregersen N, Kolvraa S, Rasmussen K, Christensen E, Brandt NJ, Ebbesen F, Hansen FH. Biochemical studies in a patient with defects in the metabolism of acyl-CoA and sarcosine: another possible case of glutaric aciduria type II. J Inherited Metab Dis 1980; 3:67–72.
62. Amendt BA, Rhead WJ. The multiple acyl-coenzyme A dehydrogenation disorders, glutaric aciduria type II and ethylmalonic-adipic aciduria. Mitochondrial fatty acid oxidation, acyl-coenzyme A dehydrogenase, and electron transfer flavoprotein activities in fibroblasts. J Clin Invest 1986; 78:205–213.
63. Frerman FE, Goodman SI. Deficiency of electron transfer flavoprotein or electron transfer flavoprotein: ubiquinone oxidoreductase in glutaric acidemia type II fibroblasts. Proc Natl Acad Sci USA 1985; 82:4517–4520.
64. Schutgens RBH, Heymans H, Ketel A, Veder HA, Duran M, Ketting D, Wadman SK. Lethal hypoglycemia in a child with a deficiency of 3-hydroxy-3-methylglutarylcoenzyme A lyase. J Pediatr 1979; 94:89–91.
65. Robinson BH, Oei J, Sherwood WG, Slyper AH, Heininger J, Mamer OA. Hydroxymethylglutaryl CoA lyase deficiency: features resembling Reye syndrome. Neurology 1980; 30:714–718.
66. Hartlage P, Eller G, Carter L, Roesel A, Hommes F. Mitochondrial acetoacetyl-CoA thiolase deficiency. Biochem Med Metab Biol 1986; 36:198–206.
67. Yamaguchi S, Orii T, Sakura N, Miyazawa S, Hashimoto T. Defects of biosynthesis of mitochondrial acetoacetyl-CoA thiolase in cultured fibroblasts from a boy with 3-ketothiolase deficiency. J Clin Invest 1988; 81:813–817.
68. Bennett MJ, Gray RGF, Isherwood DM, Murphy N, Pollitt RJ. The diagnosis and biochemical investigation of a patient with a short-chain fatty acid oxidation defect. J Inherited Metab Dis 1985; 8(Suppl 2):135–136.
69. Glasgow AM, Engel AG, Bier DM, Perry LW, Dickie M, Todaro J, Brown BI, Utter MF. Hypoglycemia, hepatic dysfunction, muscle weakness, cardiomyopathy, free carnitine deficiency and long-chain acylcarnitine excess responsive to medium chain triglyceride diet. Pediatr Res 1983; 17:319–326.
70. Riudor E, Ribes A, Boronat M, Sabado C, Dominguez C, Ballabriga A. A new case of C_6-C_{14}-dicarboxylic aciduria with favourable evolution. J Inherited Metab Dis 1986; 9 (Suppl 2):297–299.
71. Pollitt RJ, Losty H, Westwood A. 3-Hydroxydicarboxylic aciduria: a distinctive type of intermittent dicarboxylic aciduria of possible diagnostic significance. J Inherited Metab Dis 1987; 10(Suppl 2):266–269.
72. Kelley RI, Morton DH. 3-Hydroxyoctanoic aciduria: identification of a new organic acid in the urine of a patient with non-ketotic hypoglycemia. Clin Chim Acta 1988; 175:19–26.
73. Hale DE, Thorpe C, Braat K, Wright JH, Roe CR, Coates PM, Hashimoto T, Glasgow, AM. The L-3-hydroxyacyl-CoA dehydrogenase deficiency. In: Tanaka K, Coates PM, eds. Fatty acid oxidation: clinical, biochemical, and molecular aspects. New York: Alan R. Liss, 1990: 503.

PART 13

Alpha$_1$-Antitrypsin Deficiency

David H. Perlmutter, M.D.

Homozygous PiZZ alpha$_1$-antitrypsin (alpha$_1$-AT) deficiency is an autosomal recessive disorder associated with reduction in serum concentrations of alpha$_1$-AT (10 to 15 percent of normal concentrations), premature development of pulmonary emphysema, and, in some cases, chronic liver disease. This deficiency is the most common metabolic cause of emphysema in adults and liver disease in children and the most common metabolic disease for which children undergo liver transplantation.[1] The incidence and prevalence of this deficiency depend on the population under study. In the most extensively studied population, the Swedish population, the incidence of the deficiency is approximately 1 in 1,639 live births.[2] Data from eight separate studies suggest that the prevalence of alpha$_1$-AT deficiency in the United States is 1 in approximately 2,000 individuals.[3] It especially affects Caucasians of Northern European ancestry [4,5] but also occurs in Maoris in New Zealand[6] and Iranians.[7] The deficiency was not identified in population studies in black Africans in Zaire.[8]

The availability of more sophisticated molecular techniques in recent years has allowed a greater understanding of the pathogenesis of alpha$_1$-AT deficiency, but several critical issues still need to be resolved. First, the relationship between molecular pathology, cellular pathology, and plasma deficiency is not clearly understood. The PiZ allele is characterized by two amino acid substitutions[9-11] encoded by two nucleotide substitutions.[12,13] One of these substitutions, alanine for valine at residue 213, is also present in 20 to 25 percent of individuals with the normal M_1 haplotype and therefore is not likely by itself to be involved in the defect. It is not known how the other substitution, lysine for glutamate at residue 342, results in a selective decrease in rate of secretion with accumulation of the abnormal alpha$_1$-AT molecule in the endoplasmic reticulum. Second, the mechanism for tissue injury in liver is not known. Third, there is wide variability in the incidence and severity of emphysema, even when cigarette smoking is taken into consideration. The factors that determine this variability have not been identified.

Although orthotopic liver transplantation is available for treatment of liver disease in alpha$_1$-AT deficiency, and protein replacement therapy for treatment of emphysema has been licensed by the Food and Drug Administration, a more detailed understanding of the three aforementioned pathogenetic issues will be necessary for the development of alternative rational therapeutic approaches. Herein I discuss these issues in the context of our current knowledge of the structure and function of alpha$_1$-AT, and the pathophysiology, clinical diagnosis, and treatment of homozygous PiZZ alpha$_1$-AT deficiency.

STRUCTURE OF ALPHA$_1$-ANTITRYPSIN

A single ~12.2-kb gene on human chromosome 14q31-32.3 encodes a 52-kDa single-chain glycoprotein alpha$_1$-AT.[14-16] There is a "sequence-related gene" ~12 kb downstream from this gene.[15,17] Since there is no evidence that the sequence-related gene is expressed, it is considered a pseudogene.

The alpha$_1$-AT gene (Fig. 1) is organized in seven exons and six introns.[18,19] The first three exons and a short 5′ segment of the fourth exon code for 5′ untranslated regions of the alpha$_1$-AT mRNA. The first two exons and a short 5′

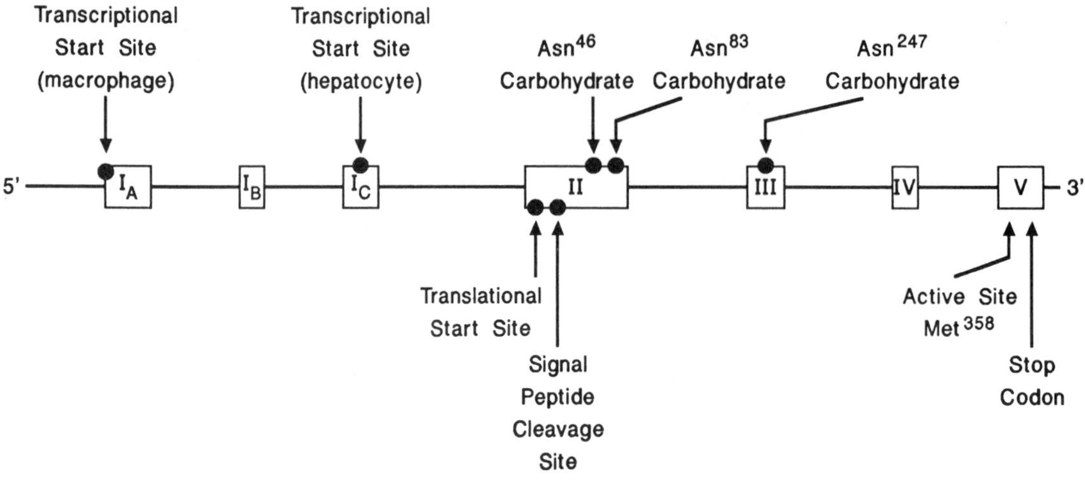

FIGURE 1 Schematic representation of the human alpha$_1$-AT gene (not drawn to scale).

segment of the third exon are included in the primary transcript in macrophages but not in hepatocytes, accounting for a slightly longer mRNA. There may be, in fact, two mRNA species in macrophages from certain donors and under certain physiologic conditions, depending on alternative post-transcriptional splicing pathways involving one of the two most 5′ exons. Most of the fourth exon and the remaining three exons encode the protein sequence of alpha$_1$-AT. There is a 72-base sequence that constitutes the 24 amino acid amino terminal signal sequence. There are three sites for asparagine-linked carbohydrate attachment, residues 46, 83, and 247. All three are used for post-translational glycosylation. The active site, so-called P_1 residue, met 358, is encoded within the seventh exon (exon V).

Gene Family. Alpha$_1$-AT shares molecular structural and functional characteristics with other members of the "serpin" supergene family (Fig. 2), including antithrombin III,[20] alpha$_1$-antichymotrypsin,[21] C1 inhibitor,[22,23] alpha$_2$-antiplasmin,[24] protein C inhibitor,[25] heparin co-factor II,[26,27] plasminogen activator inhibitors I and II,[28,29] ovalbumin,[30] angiotensinogen,[28] and corticosteroid-binding globulin.[31] These genes share 25 to 40 percent primary structural homology with higher degrees of regional homology in functional domains. With the exception of ovalbumin and angiotensinogen, each serpin gene encodes a single chain glycoprotein. Each serpin functions as a suicide inhibitor by forming an equimolar complex with a specific target protease. Therefore, it is thought that these genes are derived from a common ancestral gene. Since the positions of introns are not conserved among members, the evolution of the family is considered an example of evolution by intron-exon shuffling.[32]

A comparison of alpha$_1$-AT with other members of the serpin supergene family has led to several novel concepts of the structure and function of alpha$_1$-AT. For instance, the domain that contains the reactive site residue is conserved among the serpins, but the critical so-called P_1 residue is different and constitutes the specificity of the inhibitor. This concept led to the discovery of alpha$_1$-AT$_{\text{Pittsburgh}}$, a variant in which the P_1 residue of alpha$_1$-AT, met 358, is replaced by arg 358. In this variant alpha$_1$-AT functions as a thrombin inhibitor, and a severe bleeding diathesis results.[33] The aminoterminal tail of alpha$_1$-AT and the other serpins is also considered an important domain on the basis of structure-function relationships. It is variable in length in individual serpins, relatively lacking in order, exteriorly located, and accessible for cleavage. Angiotensin I and II are cleaved from this domain of angiotensinogen, and the heparin-binding site occupies this region of antithrombin III. Third, the carboxy-terminal fragment of alpha$_1$-AT and the other serpins bears important structural and functional characteristics. There is a much higher degree of sequence homology among serpins in the carboxy terminus. A small fragment at this terminus is cleaved during formation of the inhibitory complex with serine protease. The carboxy-terminal fragment of alpha$_1$-AT may possess the chemotactic activity of the molecule[34,35] and may be the proximate mediator of regulation of alpha$_1$-AT gene expression in macrophages.[36]

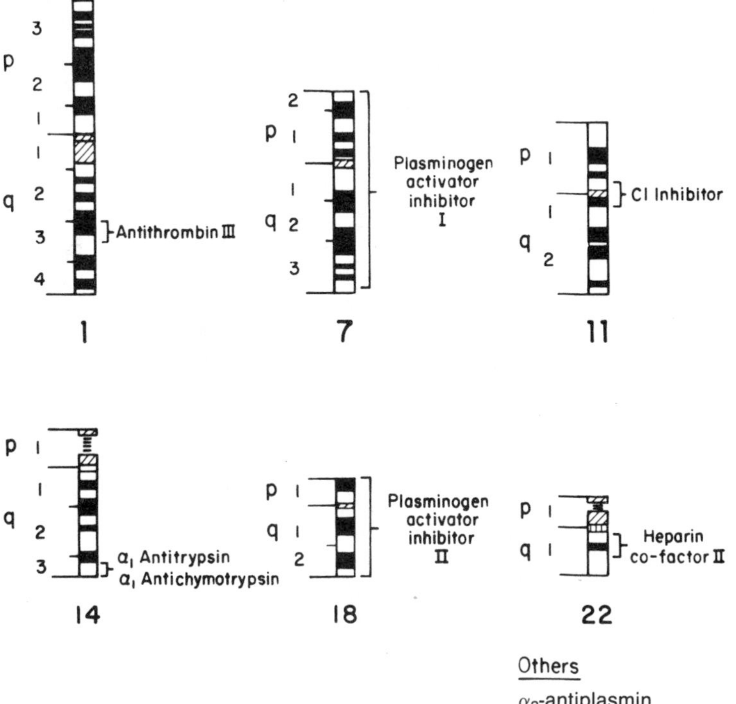

FIGURE 2 Chromosomal localization of serpins. Brackets indicate the extent of possible localization based on current studies. Localization of serpins listed under "others" has not yet been reported.

The Pi System for Classification of Structural Variants of Alpha$_1$-AT. Variants of alpha$_1$-AT in humans are classified according to the Pi, or protease inhibitor, phenotype system as defined by agarose electrophoresis or isoelectric focusing of plasma in polyacrylamide at acid pH.[37] The Pi classification assigns a letter to variants, according to migration of the major isoform, using alphabetic order from anode to cathode, or from low to high isoelectric point. For example, the most common normal variant migrates to an intermediate isoelectric point, designated M. Individuals with the most common severe deficiency have an alpha$_1$-AT allelic variant that migrates to a high isoelectric point, designated Z.

In recent years it has become possible to identify greater polymorphic variation of alpha$_1$-AT by restriction fragment length and direct DNA sequence analysis. Using these techniques in addition to isoelectric focusing, more than 75 allelic variants have been reported.[38]

Normal Allelic Variants. The most common normal variant of alpha$_1$-AT is termed M_1 (Table 1) and is found in 65 to 70 percent of Caucasians in the United States.[39] A restriction fragment length polymorphism may further subdivide individuals with the classic M_1 allele.[40] The normal M_3 allele, which differs from M_1 by a single base change,[38] is found in approximately 10 percent of the same population. The M_2 allele, characterized by an additional base change from the M_3 sequence, occurs in 15 to 20 percent of the United States' Caucasian population.[41,42] There are many rare normal allelic variants with allelic frequencies of less than 0.1 percent.[42] In each case these variants are associated with serum concentrations of and functional activity for alpha$_1$-AT within the normal range.

Null Allelic Variants. Alpha$_1$-AT variants in which alpha$_1$-AT is not detectable in serum are rare. All the reported individuals with homozygous Pi null alpha$_1$-AT phenotypes have developed emphysema between the ages of 20 and 30 years.[43-47] There has been no evidence of liver injury in individuals with this defect who have been examined in detail.[47,48] Potential molecular mechanisms for the null phenotype have been identified by DNA sequence analysis of three null alleles.[49-51] In two cases single base deletions in different locations within the coding sequence result in frameshift mutations, premature stop codons, and absence of alpha$_1$-AT mRNA.[49,50] In a third case, two bases are deleted in the carboxy-terminal region of the alpha$_1$-AT coding sequence. This deletion predicts a frameshift/stop mutation and synthesis of a truncated protein.[51] In fact, when expressed in mouse hepatoma cells, cDNA from this individual directs the synthesis of a truncated protein.[52]

Dysfunctional Variants. Only one dysfunctional variant of alpha$_1$-AT has been described, alpha$_1$-AT$_{Pittsburgh}$.[33] This variant was identified in a 14-year-old boy who died from an episodic bleeding disorder. A single amino acid substitution, met to arg at residue 358, converted alpha$_1$-AT from an elastase inhibitor to a thrombin inhibitor. The episodic nature of the illness was attributed to changes in the synthesis of the mutant protein during the host response to acute inflammation and tissue injury, the acute-phase response.

Deficiency Variants. The Z allele is the deficient variant most commonly associated with clinical disease. Individuals with homozygous PiZZ alpha$_1$-AT deficiency have serum concentrations of inhibitor that are approximately 10 to 15 percent of normal. As mentioned above, this deficiency is associated with pulmonary emphysema, chronic liver disease, and hepatocellular carcinoma.

It is now known that there is a selective defect in secretion of alpha$_1$-AT in *Xenopus* oocytes injected with RNA from liver of PiZZ individuals and in human blood monocytes from individuals with PiZZ. The abnormal protein accumulates

TABLE 1
Allotypic Variants of Alpha$_1$-Antitrypsin

	Defect		Clinical Disease	
			Liver	Lung
Normal Variants				
M_1			–	–
M_1 (ala 213)	Single base substitution	Val 213–ala 213	–	–
M_3	Single base substitution	Glu 376–asp 376	–	–
M_2	Two base substitutions	Glu 376–asp 376 Arg 101–his 101	–	–
Deficient Variants				
Z	Single base substitution M_1 (ala 213)	Glu 342–lys 342	+	+
S	Single base substitution	Glu 264–val 264	–	–
$M_{Heerlen}$	Single base substitution	Pro 369–leu 369	–	+
$M_{Procida}$	Single base substitution	Leu 41–pro 41	–	+
M_{Malton}	?Single base deletion	?Phe 52	?+	+
M_{Duarte}	Unknown	Unknown	?+	+
Null Variants				
$Null_{Granite\ Falls}$	Single base deletion	Tyr 160	–	+
$Null_{Bellingham}$	Single base deletion	Lys 217	–	+
$Null_{Mattawa}$	Single base insertion	Phe 353	–	+
$Null_{Hong\ Kong}$	Dinucleotide deletion	Leu 318	–	+
Dysfunctional Variants				
Pittsburgh	Single base substitution	Met 358–arg 358	–	–

inside the cell (Fig. 3).[53–55] Microsome- supplemented cell-free translation studies suggest that the nascent protein encoded by PiZZ liver RNA may be translocated into the lumen of the endoplasmic reticulum (ER) with approximately the same efficiency as that encoded by PiMM liver RNA.[56] Electron microscopic studies of liver from these individuals suggest that the abnormal protein accumulates in the ER.[57] They therefore suggest that the defect in PiZZ cells affects transport of newly synthesized alpha$_1$-AT from ER to Golgi.

It is not known, however, how the substitution of lys for glu at residue 342 in the alpha$_1$-AT coding sequence of the PiZ allele results in a defect in transport form ER to Golgi. The substitution does not appear to occur in a region that is important to post-translational processing or modification, including glycosylation. Thus, it has been suggested that the PiZ substitution results in an abnormality in folding, or tertiary structure, of the newly synthesized alpha$_1$-AT protein. Unfortunately, studies of the tertiary structure of alpha$_1$-AT have been difficult to incorporate into further understanding of the secretory defect for several reasons. First, it has only been possible to crystallize alpha$_1$-AT in a form that is modified at the reactive site peptide bond (met 358–ser 359) by formation of a complex with serine protease chymotrypsin.[58] In this form, the met 358 and ser 359 are arranged on strands at opposite ends of the molecule, implying that there is a major structural rearrangement of the inhibitor during modification. Second, it has not been possible to study the tertiary structure of alpha$_1$-AT or other proteins during post-translational transport and processing. Nevertheless, based on studies of the modified alpha$_1$-AT molecule,[58] Loebermann et al suggested that glu 342, which is replaced by lys in the Z variant, is in a strategic position to affect the conformation of alpha$_1$-AT during the formation of a complex with serine protease. The crystal structure also predicts a salt bridge between glu 342 and lys 290 in the PiM allele. Substitution of lys for glu at 342 in the PiZ allele would prevent formation of this salt bridge. However, recent site-directed mutagenesis studies show that the glu 342–lys 290 salt bridge is not required for appropriate secretion of alpha$_1$-AT.[58] Therefore, it is likely that the substitution of lysine for glutamate at residue 342 has other important effects on the folding of alpha$_1$-AT in PiZZ individuals.

There are several possible ways in which an alteration in conformation of alpha$_1$-AT might affect its secretion. For example, an alteration in folding might preclude the interaction of alpha$_1$-AT with another protein that ordinarily facilitates its secretion, such as a receptor or a key glycosylating enzyme. Despite relatively extensive investigation, however, there is no evidence for a receptor that binds alpha$_1$-AT.[60–62] Alternatively, an alteration in folding might expose an epitope on alpha$_1$-AT that is recognized by another protein, and the consequent protein-protein interaction is responsible for specific intracellular retention of alpha$_1$-AT. In fact, several recent observations suggest that misfolded proteins are selectively retained within the endoplasmic reticulum by interaction with members of the heat shock/stress protein family. First, two members of the stress protein family, glucose-regulated proteins grp 78 and grp 94, are known to be localized to the ER.[63,64] Second, one of these, grp 78, binds loosely and transiently to secretory proteins before assembly or folding is complete and binds tightly to misfolded proteins that accumulate within the ER.[65] It

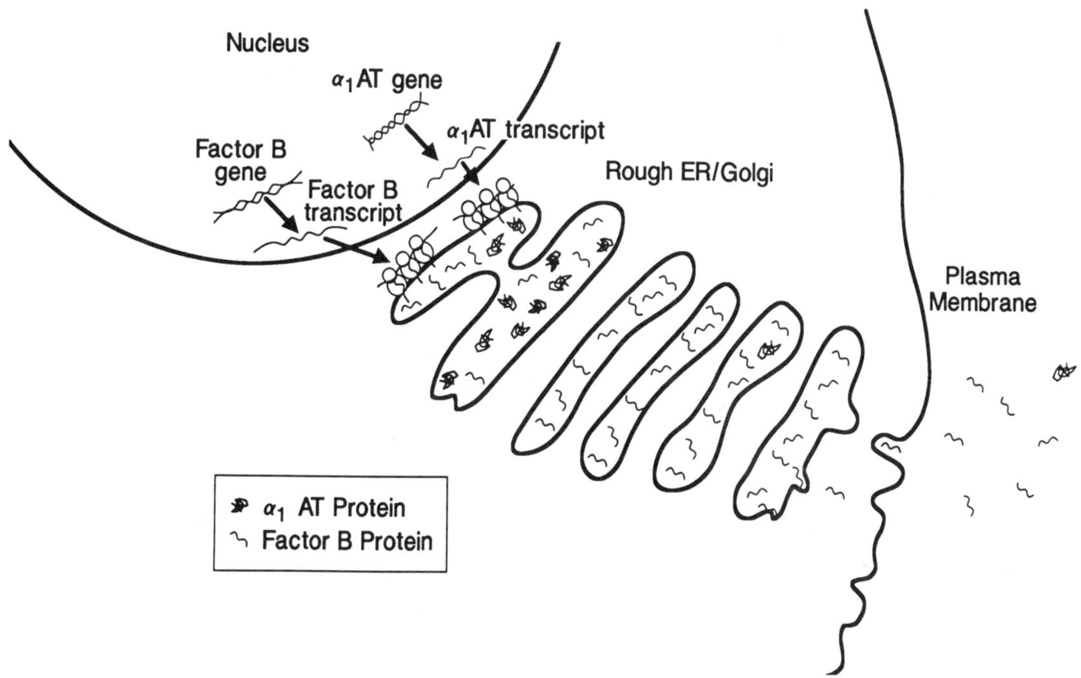

FIGURE 3 Schematic representation of the intracellular accumulation of alpha$_1$-AT in monocytes from individuals with homozygous PiZZ alpha$_1$-AT deficiency. Factor B is a complement protein secreted by monocytes and representing a normal control in experiments that elucidate this defect. (Adapted from Perlmutter DH, et al. Induction of the stress response in alpha$_1$-antitrypsin deficiency. Trans Assoc Am Phys 1988; ci:33–41.)

has also been shown that synthesis of stress proteins, the so-called stress response, is activated by the presence of misfolded, or denatured proteins, within the cell. There is a marked increase in levels of stress proteins in cells that accumulate misfolded proteins during treatment with amino acid analogues.[66] Expression of stress protein hsp 70 is induced in *Xenopus* oocytes by microinjection of proteins in denatured form, but not by injection of the same proteins in native form.[67] Finally, synthesis of specific ER-localized stress proteins may be activated by the presence of misfolded proteins within that specific intracellular compartment.[68]

With these considerations in mind, we recently examined the possibility that these stress proteins are induced in cells of PiZZ individuals inside which the mutant alpha$_1$-AT molecule accumulates. These studies show that synthesis of heat shock/stress proteins hsp 70, hsp 90, and ubiquitin is markedly increased in monocytes from PiZZ individuals with liver disease and slightly increased in PiZZ individuals with emphysema, but not increased in PiZZ individuals without evidence of tissue injury. There is also an increase in the expression of genes encoding the stress proteins in livers of PiZZ individuals relative to that of PiMM individuals. Induction of the stress response is confined to cells that synthesize and therefore retain alpha$_1$-AT within the cell. Furthermore, there is preliminary evidence that alpha$_1$-AT binds to one of the stress proteins within the monocytes of PiZZ individuals.[69]

Recognition and binding of the abnormally folded alpha$_1$-AT molecule by a stress protein in the ER could represent a secondary mechanism by which the cell attempts to protect itself. Paradoxically, this binding might accentuate the primary defect by favoring intracellular retention of alpha$_1$-AT. Alternatively, the interaction between PiZ alpha$_1$-AT and a putative stress-induced ER protein could represent the primary defect in this genetic disorder. According to this "primary defect" hypothesis, the nucleotide substitution that affects the PiZ allele is localized to a domain that is ordinarily involved in a transient and loose association with the stress-induced ER protein, and this substitution results in greater relative retention within the ER by producing tighter, more stable binding. These potential mechanisms are currently being investigated.

The alpha$_1$-AT S variant is the most common deficiency variant, having an allelic frequency in the United States Caucasian population of 0.02 to 0.03.[42] It is not associated with clinical disease, even though serum levels of alpha$_1$-AT are reduced to 50 to 60 percent of normal. There is a single base substitution, glu 264–val 264, encoded by a single nucleotide substitution, in the S allele.[18] It is not yet clear how this substitution is related to the reduction in serum alpha$_1$-AT concentrations. At one time it was reported that the S variant was associated with an unstable RNA due to incorrect post-transcriptional splicing.[70] More recent studies of this allelic variant suggest that there is an unstable protein, especially when underglycosylated.[71]

There are several other alleles associated with alpha$_1$-AT deficiency, but they are extremely rare. The $M_{Heerlen}$ and $M_{Procida}$ alleles are characterized by single base substitutions (proline 369–leucine 369, and leucine 41–proline 41, respectively), low serum concentrations of alpha$_1$-AT, and pulmonary emphysema.[72-74] Two other rare deficiency alleles, M_{Malton} and M_{Duarte}, are associated with low serum concentrations of alpha$_1$-AT and emphysema.[75,76] In single individuals with these alleles, hepatocyte alpha$_1$-AT globule and liver disease have been reported.[77,78]

FUNCTION

Alpha$_1$-AT is an inhibitor of serine proteases in general, but its most important targets are neutrophil elastase and cathepsin G, proteases released by activated neutrophils. Several lines of evidence suggest that inhibition of neutrophil elastase is the major physiologic function of alpha$_1$-AT. First, individuals with alpha$_1$-AT deficiency are susceptible to premature development of emphysema, a lesion that may be induced in experimental animals by instillation of excess amounts of neutrophil elastase.[79-85] In fact, these observations have led to the concept that destructive lung disease may result from perturbations of the net balance of elastase and alpha$_1$-AT within the local environment of the lung.[86] Second, the kinetics of association of alpha$_1$-AT and neutrophil elastase are more favorable, by several orders of magnitude, than those for alpha$_1$-AT and any other serine protease.[87] Third, alpha$_1$-AT constitutes greater than 90 percent of the neutrophil elastase inhibitory activity in the one body fluid that has been examined, pulmonary alveolar lavage fluid.[86]

Alpha$_1$-AT acts competitively by allowing its target enzymes to bind directly to a substrate-like region within the carboxy-terminal region of the inhibitor molecule. This reaction between enzyme and inhibitor is essentially second order, and the resulting complex contains one molecule of each of the reactants. A peptide bond in the inhibitor is hydrolyzed during formation of the enzyme-inhibitor complex. However, hydrolysis of this reactive-site peptide bond does not proceed to completion. An equilibrium, nearly unity, is established between complexes in which the reactive-site peptide bond of alpha$_1$-AT is intact (native inhibitor) and those in which this peptide bond is cleaved (modified inhibitor). The complex of alpha$_1$-AT and serine protease is a covalently stabilized structure, resistant to dissociation by denaturing compounds including sodium dodecyl sulfate and urea. The interaction between alpha$_1$-AT and serine protease is suicidal in that the modified inhibitor is no longer able to bind and/or inactivate enzyme. During complex formation and hydrolysis of the reactive site peptide bond, an ~4 kDA carboxy-terminal fragment of the inhibitor may be released. It is not known, however, whether this peptide fragment is actually released under physiologic conditions, since it remains attached to the modified alpha$_1$-AT by tenacious hydrophobic association during isolation.[88,89]

The net functional activity of alpha$_1$-AT in complex biologic fluids may be modified by several factors. First, the reactive-site methionine of alpha$_1$-AT may be oxidized and thereby rendered inactive as an elastase inhibitor.[90,91] The relationship of oxidation to the net biologic activity of alpha$_1$-AT in vivo is not fully understood. However, alpha$_1$-AT is oxidatively inactivated in vitro by activated neutrophils[92-94] and by oxidants released by alveolar macrophages of cigarette smokers.[95] Second, the functional activity of alpha$_1$-AT may be modified by proteolytic inactivation. A metallo-protease secreted by mouse macrophages,[96] a human neutrophil-derived metallo enzyme,[97] thiol-protease cathepsin L,[98] and *Pseudomonas* elastase[99] represent examples of proteases that have been shown to cleave and inactivate alpha$_1$-AT. Moreover, secreted products of rabbit alveolar macrophages have been shown to modify alpha$_1$-AT functional activity by proteolytic inactivation.[100]

Although alpha$_1$-AT from the plasma[101] or liver[102] of individuals with PiZZ alpha$_1$-AT deficiency is functionally active, there may be a decrease in its specific elastase inhibitory capacity. Ogushi and colleagues have shown that the kinetics of association with neutrophil elastase and the stability of complexes with neutrophil elastase were significantly decreased for alpha$_1$-AT from PiZZ plasma.[103] There was no decrease in functional activity of alpha$_1$-AT from PiSS individuals.

Several recent studies suggest that alpha$_1$-AT has functional activities other than inhibition of serine protease. The carboxy-terminal fragment of alpha$_1$-AT, which can be generated during formation of a complex with serine protease or during proteolytic inactivation by thiol- or metalloproteases such as macrophage elastase or *Pseudomonas* elastase, is a potent neutrophil chemoattractant.[34,35] The chemotactic response is equivalent to that elicited by formylmethionyl-leucyl-phenylalanine. The carboxy-terminal fragment of alpha$_1$-AT may also be responsible for an increase in synthesis of alpha$_1$-AT in human monocytes and macrophages when incubated with exogenous neutrophil elastase.[36]

EXPRESSION OF ALPHA$_1$-AT

The predominant site of synthesis of plasma alpha$_1$-AT is the liver. This is most clearly shown by conversion of plasma alpha$_1$-AT to donor phenotype after orthotopic liver transplantation.[104,105] It is synthesized in human hepatoma cells as a 52 kDa precursor, undergoes post-translational, dolichol phosphate–linked glycosylation at three asparagine residues and also undergoes tyrosine sulfation.[60,61,106] It is secreted as a 55-kDa native single-chain glycoprotein with a half-time for secretion of 35 to 40 minutes.

Tissue-specific expression of alpha$_1$-AT in human hepatoma cells is directed by structural elements within a 750-nucleotide region upstream of the hepatocyte transcriptional start site in exon Ic (Fig. 4).[107–109] There are at least three interesting structural motifs within this region. First, a weak enhancer element is localized in the most 5′ aspect. Second, a hepatocyte-specific transcriptional element is located within residues −137 to −37. This element has two domains: a proximal domain with homology to the alpha and beta chains of fibrinogen and a distal domain bearing homology with haptoglobin. Third, there is a strong enhancer element located approximately 200 nucleotides upstream of the transcriptional start site, but the element is not specific for hepatocyte transcription. This element also has several domains: in the center there is an 8-nucleotide sequence similar to the canonical core enhancer; distally there are 11 bases homologous with those flanking haptoglobin; proximally there are 10 bases identical to the binding site for transcription factor AP-1. Similar AP-1 binding sequences have been identified in the 5′ flanking region of metallothioneins I and IIa, sv40, retinol-binding protein, collagenase, and stromelysin. AP-1 is also thought to be one of the transcription factors that mediate the effects of phorbol esters and thereby of protein kinase C activation.[110–112] It represents a complex of several different proteins, including proteins encoded by the proto-oncognenes C-jun and C-fos.[113,114] There are also at

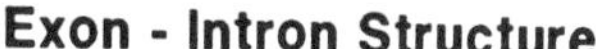

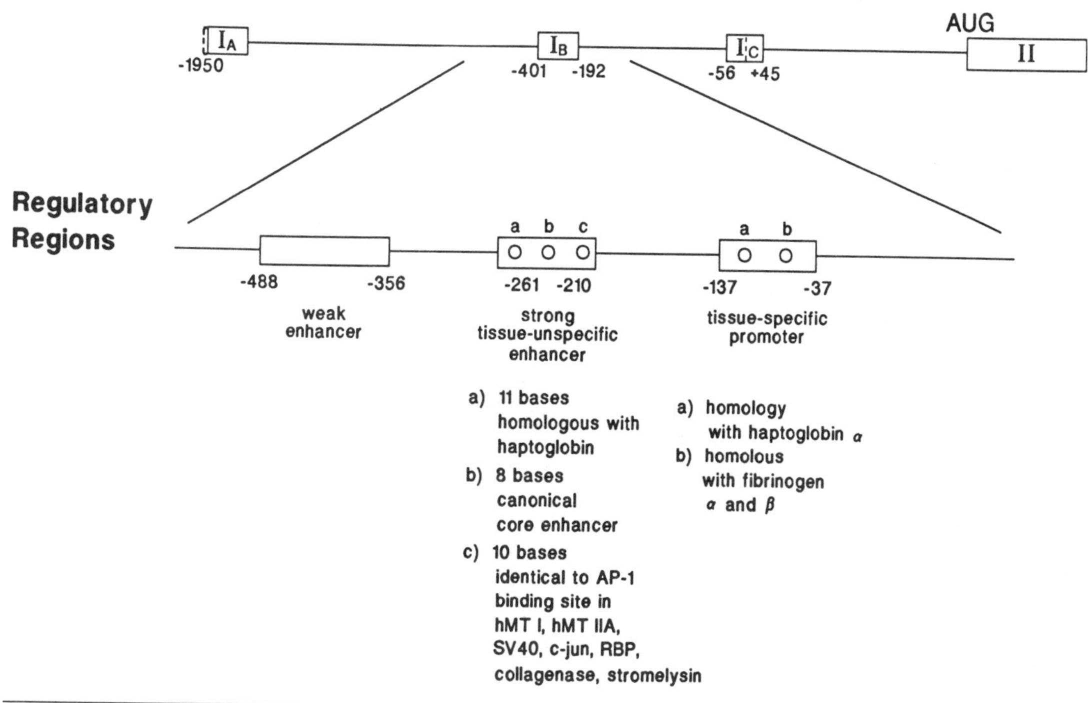

FIGURE 4 Schematic representation of the upstream noncoding region of the alpha$_1$-AT gene (not drawn to scale).

least two distinct trans-acting factors that bind to the proximal element to determine hepatocyte-specific transcription.[108,109,115]

Plasma concentrations of alpha$_1$-AT increase three-to fourfold during the host response to inflammation/tissue injury.[116,117] The source of this additional alpha$_1$-AT has always been considered the liver, and so alpha$_1$-AT is known as a positive "hepatic acute phase reactant." In contrast to other hepatic acute-phase reactants, synthesis of alpha$_1$-AT in human hepatoma cells (HepG2, Hep3B) is not regulated by the acute-phase mediators interleukin-1 or tumor necrosis factor.[118,119] Recently, we have shown that another monokine, interferon $\beta 2$ (IFN$\beta 2$)/interleukin-6, does mediate an increase in expression of alpha$_1$-AT in HepG2 and Hep3B cells.[120] IFN$\beta 2$ was originally described on the basis of its antiviral activity and its capacity to induce proliferation of B lymphocytes.[121] It is now known to elicit many changes in hepatic acute-phase gene expression and probably constitutes much of the activity previously termed hepatocyte-stimulating factor.[122] Thus, IFN$\beta 2$ is likely to be the physiologic mediator of the acute-phase response of alpha$_1$-AT. In this respect, it is similar to fibrinogen, a hepatic acute-phase gene with promoter sequences homologous with those of alpha$_1$-AT[115] and a gene that may be a target of protein kinase C activation.[123] Plasma concentrations of alpha$_1$-AT also increase during oral contraceptive therapy and pregnancy. Nominal changes in plasma alpha$_1$-AT levels follow administration of the synthetic androgen danazol.[124]

Alpha$_1$-AT is also synthesized and secreted in primary cultures of human blood monocytes and bronchoalveolar and breast milk macrophages.[125] The cellular defect in homozygous PiZZ alpha$_1$-AT deficiency, the selective defect in secretion of alpha$_1$-AT, is expressed in monocytes and macrophages from deficient individuals.[53,54] It is now thought that transcription of the alpha$_1$-AT gene in macrophages starts ~2 kb upstream from the start site used in hepatocytes.[126,127] Although the same polypeptide is synthesized in the two cell types, a slightly longer mRNA transcript may be present in macrophages, depending on alternative post-transcriptional splicing of two upstream short open-reading frames.[127]

Expression of alpha$_1$-AT in monocytes and macrophages is profoundly influenced by products generated during inflammation (Fig. 5). Bacterial lipopolysaccharide (LPS) mediates a five- to 10-fold increase in synthesis of alpha$_1$-AT in mononuclear phagocytes, predominantly increasing the translation efficiency of alpha$_1$-AT mRNA.[128,129] The translational regulation of alpha$_1$-AT by LPS therefore involves a mechanism analogous to that of the yeast gene GCN4 during amino acid starvation and that of the human ferritin gene in response to iron. The analogy to yeast GCN4 is interesting in that both macrophage alpha$_1$-AT mRNA and GCN4 mRNA have multiple short open-reading frames with initiation codons in the upstream untranslated regions.[130,131] These sequences have recently been shown to control the translation of the yeast GCN4 gene product both under basal conditions and in response to amino acid starvation.[132] A sequence within the 5′ untranslated region of the human ferritin gene is responsible for translational regulation of that gene by iron.[133–135]

Expression of alpha$_1$-AT in human macrophages is also regulated by a novel tissue-specific mechanism, whereby elastase directly regulates the synthesis of its inhibitor.[36] In nanomolar concentrations, neutrophil or pancreatic elastase mediates a dose- and time-dependent increase in steady-state levels of alpha$_1$-AT mRNA and in the rate of synthesis of alpha$_1$-AT in human monocytes and bronchoalveolar macrophages. The response requires enzymatically active elastase and is dependent on the presence of alpha$_1$-AT, either endogenous or exogenous in origin. Thus, regulation of alpha$_1$-AT expression may require the formation of an elastase–alpha$_1$-AT complex. The regulatory phenomenon could be mediated by the 4-kDa carboxy-terminal fragment cleaved during complex formation or by an epitope on the 51-kDa modified inhibitor newly exposed by virtue of the conformational change that accompanies complex formation.

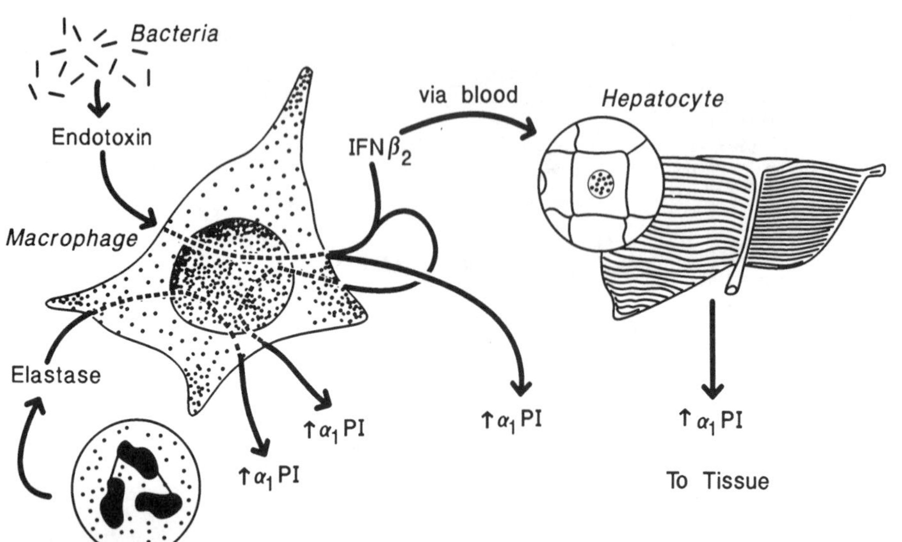

FIGURE 5 Schematic representation of the regulatory factors that affect alpha$_1$-AT expression in human macrophages and hepatocytes.

Macrophages, which represent the first line of host defense at epithelial linings, may therefore control the expression of alpha$_1$-AT on the basis of the net balance of elastase and "anti-elastase" in the local microenvironment.

IFNβ2 also regulates synthesis of alpha$_1$-AT in human monocytes and macrophages.[120] There is an increase in steady-state levels of alpha$_1$-AT mRNA and in synthesis of alpha$_1$-AT in monocytes incubated in the presence of recombinant IFNβ2. This autocrine, or paracrine, pathway is distinct from that of LPS: the effect of IFNβ2 is blocked by antibody to IFNβ2 but not by antibody to the lipid A moiety of LPS or by polymyxin B; the effect of LPS is blocked by antibody to lipid A or by polymyxin B but not by antibody IFNβ2. This monokine is the only well-characterized and highly purified factor known to regulate alpha$_1$-AT expression in a tissue-nonspecific fashion.

None of these factors that regulate synthesis of alpha$_1$-AT has an effect on the rate of post-translational processing and/or secretion of alpha$_1$-AT. In monocytes from normal PiMM individuals, the effects of LPS, elastase, or IFNβ2 are reflected by the appearance of greater alpha$_1$-AT in the extracellular fluid but with the same kinetics as control PiMM monocytes. In monocytes from deficient PiZZ individuals, there is, however, greater intracellular accumulation of the abnormal alpha$_1$-AT molecule under the influence of the regulatory factors.[36,128,136] Hence, these regulating factors tend to exaggerate the intrinsic defect in secretion of alpha$_1$-AT that characterizes the homozygous PiZZ alpha$_1$-AT deficiency.

Alpha$_1$-AT mRNA has been isolated from multiple tissues in transgenic mice,[109,126,137] but it has not been possible to distinguish whether such alpha$_1$-AT mRNA is in ubiquitous tissue macrophages or other cell types. We have recently demonstrated synthesis and secretion of alpha$_1$-AT in a human colonic adenocarcinoma cell line (Caco2) that differentiates into a villous enterocyte.[138] Alpha$_1$-AT mRNA in Caco2 cells and human jejunal epithelium is 1.6 kb corresponding to the size of alpha$_1$-AT mRNA in human hepatoma cells but smaller than the 1.8 kb alpha$_1$-AT mRNA in human monocytes and macrophages.[139] These data indicate that alpha$_1$-AT is expressed in small intestine by a cell type other than the macrophages, probably the enterocyte. Synthesis and secretion of alpha$_1$-AT in Caco2 cells are similar to those in HepG2 cells as shown by metabolic labeling experiments. Alpha$_1$-AT is synthesized as a 52-kDa precursor polypeptide, converted to its mature, fully glycosylated 55-kDa form intracellularly, and the native protein secreted with a half-time of 37 minutes. It is secreted at both the basolateral and luminal membranes, as shown by pulse-chase labeling of Caco2 cells cultured in polarized orientation on nitrocellulose filters. Expression of alpha$_1$-AT in Caco2 enterocytes is not affected by soluble factors that regulate expression of alpha$_1$-AT in macrophages and hepatocytes. However, expression of alpha$_1$-AT increases markedly in Caco2 cells as they differentiate into enteric villus-type cells.

CLEARANCE AND DISTRIBUTION

The half-life of alpha$_1$-antitrypsin in plasma is approximately 5 days.[140,142] It is estimated that the daily production rate of alpha$_1$-AT is 34 mg per kilogram body weight with 33 percent of the intravascular pool of alpha$_1$-AT degraded daily. Several physiologic factors may affect the rate of alpha$_1$-AT catabolism: desialylated alpha$_1$-AT is cleared from the circulation in minutes,[142,143] probably via hepatic asialoglycoprotein receptor-mediated endocytosis; rate of alpha$_1$-AT clearance may increase during the host response to inflammation.[144] There is a slight increase in the rate of clearance of radiolabeled PiZZ alpha$_1$-AT compared with PiMM alpha$_1$-AT when infused into PiMM individuals, but this difference does not account for the decrease in serum levels of alpha$_1$-AT in deficient individuals.[144,145]

Alpha$_1$-AT diffuses into most tissues and is found in most body fluids.[146] The concentration of alpha$_1$-AT in lavage fluid from the lower respiratory tract is approximately equivalent to that in serum.[86] Alpha$_1$-AT is also found in feces, and increased fecal concentrations of alpha$_1$-AT correlate with inflammatory lesions of the bowel.[147-149] In each case it has been assumed that the alpha$_1$-AT was derived from serum. Local sites of synthesis, such as macrophages and epithelial cells, may also make important contributions to the alpha$_1$-AT pool in these tissues and body fluids.

LIVER DISEASE

Soon after homozygous PiZZ alpha$_1$-AT deficiency was described, an association with premature development of emphysema was discovered.[150] Eriksson noticed that some of the individuals with emphysema also had cirrhosis of the liver,[151] but an association between alpha$_1$-AT deficiency and liver disease was first clearly established by Sharp et al in 1969.[152] Sharp also noticed the distinctive histopathologic features of inclusion bodies in the ER of liver cells in these children.[153]

The most important study of liver disease in alpha$_1$-AT deficiency has been conducted by Sveger, who prospectively screened 200,000 newborn infants in Sweden.[2] One hundred and twenty-seven PiZZ infants were identified and have been followed clinically since that time (Fig. 6). These infants were evaluated clinically at age 6 months. Fourteen of the 127 PiZZ infants had prolonged obstructive jaundice (group I). Nine of these infants had severe liver disease and five mild liver disease by clinical and laboratory criteria. Eight other PiZZ infants (group II) had minimal abnormalities in serum bilirubin, serum transaminases, and hepatic size. Approximately 50 percent of the remaining infants (group III) had abnormal serum transaminases.

Sveger has recently collated data regarding the clinical outcome for these infants at 12 years of age.[154] Three children from the group with prolonged obstructive jaundice (group I) died from liver disease before reaching 8 years of age. One group I child died from an unrelated cause. Fifty percent of the remaining children from group I had abnormal serum transaminases at 12 years of age. These children were otherwise not affected clinically by liver disease. Of the children from groups II and III re-examined at 12 years of age, 15 percent had abnormal serum transaminases. One child from this group died in an accident. This study therefore indicates that at least 75 percent of prospectively identified PiZZ children have no evidence of liver injury by 12 years of age. Other studies of the incidence, prevalence, or prognosis of liver disease in alpha$_1$-AT deficiency[155-165] cannot be compared to the

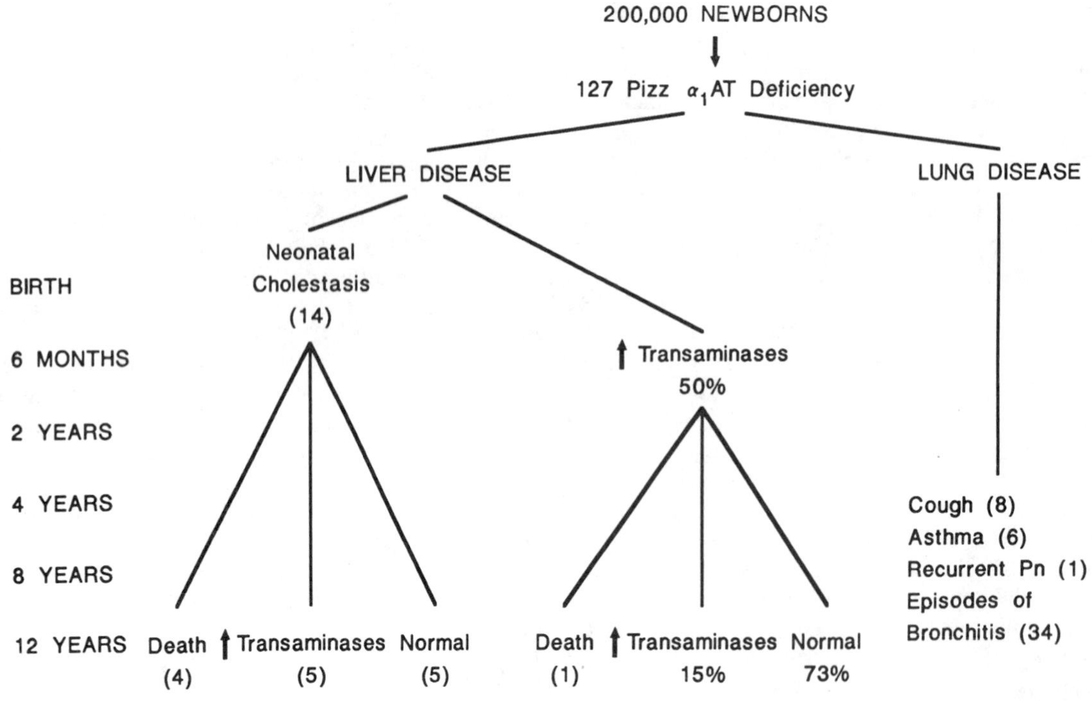

FIGURE 6 Summary of the results of a prospective nationwide study conducted in Sweden by Sveger.[2,154]

Sveger study in that these studies involve PiZZ populations in which there is a bias in ascertainment; i.e., the studies include only children referred to a specialty clinic.

Homozygous PiZZ alpha$_1$-AT deficiency now appears to be the most common metabolic disease to cause the neonatal hepatitis syndrome[155,166] and the most common metabolic disease for which children undergo liver transplantation in the United States.[1] Adults with homozygous PiZZ alpha$_1$-AT deficiency have a significantly higher risk for cirrhosis and primary liver cancer than the general population.[167] There is also a higher prevalence of heterozygous PiMZ alpha$_1$-antitrypsin phenotype than PiMM phenotype among adults with chronic active hepatitis or cirrhosis.[168,169]

Liver involvement usually is first noticed in the first 2 months of life because of persistent jaundice. Serum transaminases are slightly elevated. The liver may be enlarged. These infants are then generally admitted to hospital with a diagnosis of "neonatal hepatitis syndrome." Many infants have minimal clinical liver disease but persistent serum transaminase abnormalities for the first few years of life. Approximately 10 percent of such infants have moderate to severe clinical liver disease with complications of liver synthetic dysfunction (bleeding diathesis, ascites, feeding difficulties, and poor growth) occurring during the first few years of life. A small number of infants are initially recognized because of a cholestatic clinical syndrome, characterized by pruritus, hypercholesterolemia, and a striking paucity of intrahepatic bile ducts on histopathologic examination.[156] Fulminant liver failure is rarely observed in early infancy.[170] It is often impossible to distinguish affected infants from those with other known medical, or even surgical, causes of neonatal hepatitis by routine clinical criteria.

Liver disease associated with alpha$_1$-AT deficiency may also be first discovered in late childhood or early adolescence when the affected individual presents with abdominal distention from hepatosplenomegaly and/or ascites or presents with upper intestinal bleeding due to esophageal variceal hemorrhage. In some of these cases there is a history of unexplained prolonged obstructive jaundice in the neonatal period. In others there is no evidence of any previous liver injury even when the neonatal history is carefully reviewed. Although many of these children have progressive hepatic decompensation necessitating liver transplantation, a few lead relatively uncomplicated lives for several years despite moderate to severe liver synthetic dysfunction.

Diagnosis is established by a serum alpha$_1$-antitrypsin phenotype determination in isoelectric focusing or agarose electrophoresis at acid pH. The phenotype should be determined in all cases of neonatal hepatitis or unexplained chronic liver disease in older children. Serum concentrations of alpha$_1$-AT may be helpful but are occasionally misleading. For instance, serum alpha$_1$-AT concentrations may increase during the host response to inflammation, even in homozygous PiZZ individuals, giving a false impression of the severity of the deficiency state.

The distinctive histologic feature of homozygous PiZZ alpha$_1$-AT deficiency, periodic acid-Schiff–positive, diastase-resistant globules in the ER of hepatocytes, will substantiate the diagnosis. The presence of these globules should not be interpreted as diagnostic for alpha$_1$-AT deficiency. Similar structures are occasionally observed in PiMM individuals with other liver diseases.[171–173] The globules are eosinophilic, round to oval, and 1 to 40 microns in diameter. They are most prominent in periportal hepatocytes.[57,156,174–176] They may also be seen in Kupffer cells and cells that have the appearance of bile duct epithelial origin.[174,177] There may also be evidence of variable degrees of hepatocellular necrosis, inflammatory cell infiltration, periportal fibrosis, and/or cirrhosis.

Several theoretical explanations for the pathogenesis of liver injury in deficient individuals have been discussed in the literature. In one theory, accumulation of alpha$_1$-antitrypsin in the ER of liver cells is thought to be directly related to liver injury.[70] Evidence supporting the "accumulation theory" of liver injury includes the absence of histologic changes in liver of individuals with rare Pi null variants, defects in synthesis of alpha$_1$-AT (see above). However, careful diagnostic evaluation for liver disease has been conducted in only a few Pi null individuals. One potential pathophysiologic consequence of intracellular accumulation of an abnormally folded protein is induction of the heat shock/stress response. In our recent studies the heat shock/stress response was fully activated in cells of deficient individuals with liver disease but not in those of deficient individuals with emphysema, deficient individuals without tissue injury, PiMM individuals with liver disease of other etiologies, or individuals with deficiency of the PiS type (see above). There are several possible explanations for activation of this response to especially affect the subpopulation of PiZZ individuals with liver disease. These individuals may have a slower rate of removal, or degradation, of accumulated alpha$_1$-AT than PiZZ individuals who develop emphysema or PiZZ individuals who do not develop tissue injury. Alternatively, there may be an intrinsic difference in the function and/or activation of the stress protein system in this subset of the PiZZ population. It is also possible that cells which synthesize alpha$_1$-AT in these individuals are exposed to higher, or more sustained, concentrations of factors that up-regulate the expression of alpha$_1$-AT and thereby accentuate the accumulation of abnormal alpha$_1$-AT molecules in the ER. It will now be important to determine if the chronic expression of stress proteins disturbs cellular metabolism in a way that causes liver injury and/or inflammation.

An alternative but less likely possibility is that liver damage is a consequence of diminished serum concentrations of alpha$_1$-AT, rendering the liver susceptible to proteolytic attack. If this were the case one might expect to see even more severe liver injury in Pi null individuals and to see an incidence and prevalence of liver disease similar to that of emphysema. Udall et al have suggested that the liver of alpha$_1$-AT deficient neonates may be especially susceptible to proteolytic attack during the neonatal period in which there is enhanced intestinal permeability to macromolecules.[178] These investigators then reported that breast-fed alpha$_1$-AT–deficient infants had less severe liver disease than their bottle-fed counterparts, and suggested that the alpha$_1$-AT present in breast milk provides the protective effect.[164] Unfortunately, the study was retrospective and interpretation limited by bias in ascertainment of patients. Furthermore, there is no evidence that breast milk alpha$_1$-AT is present or functionally active in the intestinal lumen or that there are increased levels of alpha$_1$-AT–protease complexes in the intestinal fluid or portal circulation of breast-fed as compared with bottle-fed infants. Furthermore, if breast-fed deficient infants absorb more alpha$_1$-AT–protease complexes than free protease, they might be theoretically expected to sustain greater liver injury. Complexes of alpha$_1$-AT and protease have chemotactic activity.[34,35] Complexes may also mediate an increase in the expression of the alpha$_1$-AT gene in macrophages and thereby cause greater intracellular accumulation of the abnormal alpha$_1$-AT molecule in macrophages from deficient individuals.[36]

PULMONARY EMPHYSEMA

The incidence and prevalence of emphysema in alpha$_1$-AT deficiency has not been studied prospectively. Autopsy studies suggest that 60 to 65 percent of individuals with homozygous PiZZ alpha$_1$-AT deficiency develop clinically significant lung injury.[179] There are numerous anecdotal reports of smoking PiZZ individuals who do not have any symptoms of lung disease or evidence of pulmonary function abnormalities until the seventh or eighth decade of life. (JA Pierce: personal communication). The typical individual with lung disease is male and a cigarette smoker. There is insidious onset of dyspnea in the third to fourth decade of life. Approximately 50 percent of these individuals develop cough and recurrent lung infections. The disease progresses to a severe limitation of air flow. There is a reduction in the forced expiratory volume, increase in total lung capacity, and reduction in diffusing capacity. Chest radiographs demonstrate hyperinflation with marked lucency at the lung bases.[180] Histopathologic studies demonstrate panacinar emphysema, more prominent in the lower lung.[180,181]

The destructive effect of cigarette smoking on the outcome of lung disease in alpha$_1$-AT deficiency has been demonstrated in many studies. Actuarial studies suggest that cigarette smoking reduces median survival by over 20 years in deficient individuals.[182] The rate of decline in forced expiratory volume is four times greater in smoking than in nonsmoking deficient individuals.[183]

OTHER CLINICAL DISORDERS

Many other clinical diagnoses have been reported in individuals with alpha$_1$-AT deficiency.[184-192] None of these diagnoses has been shown to have a specific association with alpha$_1$-AT deficiency when subjected to careful analysis. An interesting association between the Z allele and rheumatoid arthritis was suggested by studies in two rheumatology clinics,[193,194] but further studies have not been conducted. The obvious relationship between protease-inhibitor balance and destructive inflammatory disease of synovial tissues make this a provocative subject for more detailed investigation.

TREATMENT

The most important treatment for alpha$_1$-AT deficiency is avoidance of cigarette smoking. Cigarette smoking markedly accelerates the destructive lung disease associated with alpha$_1$-AT deficiency, reduces the quality of life, and significantly shortens the longevity of these individuals.[182,183,195] These facts need to be presented to the families of affected pediatric patients in an unambiguous manner. Although it is not usually an issue that arises in the pediatric gastrointestinal and liver clinic, it may be necessary to carefully monitor the smoking habits of the family and, during interval visits, re-emphasize the important effect of smoking on outcome for deficient individuals.

Liver disease associated with alpha$_1$-AT deficiency has been treated by orthotopic liver transplantation. In a study of 250 pediatric patients who underwent liver transplantation with cyclosporine and predisone treatment in Pittsburgh from 1980 to 1986, there were 29 children with alpha$_1$-AT deficiency. Five of these 29 died during the follow-up period.[1,196] This represents a 75 to 80 percent survival, slightly higher than the overall 69.2 percent 5-year survival in children who have undergone liver transplantation. Five of the surviving patients still have chronic complications from transplantation. These results did not appear to be affected by the severity of liver disease at the time of transplantation, since 80 percent had ascites and 59 percent had experienced variceal hemorrhage. Nevertheless, it should be noted that even individuals with alpha$_1$-AT deficiency and moderate to severe liver dysfunction may have relatively low rates of progression of disease. A selective group of these patients may, therefore, not require transplantation as urgently as patients with other forms of liver disease. Deficient individuals with mild liver dysfunction do not necessarily have a poor prognosis, as demonstrated by Sveger (see above), and therefore should not be considered for transplantation until there is evidence for progressive deterioration. Because it is not known whether extrahepatic alpha$_1$-AT synthesis is an important factor in the development of emphysema, or whether alpha$_1$-AT synthesis by Kupffer cells that repopulate the donor liver is an important factor in the development of liver disease, it is not known whether deficient individuals who have undergone liver transplantation are susceptible to emphysema or recurrent liver disease.

Most alpha$_1$-AT–deficient children with liver disease are not candidates for alternative surgical interventions. However, there are rare specific clinical situations in which a portacaval or splenorenal shunt might be considered, e.g., a child with only mild liver synthetic dysfunction and mild parenchymal liver injury, but severe portal hypertension. Several children with severe liver disease and alpha$_1$-AT deficiency have survived 10 to 15 years after shunt surgery before requiring liver transplantation (J Folkman: personal communication). Moreover, previous hepatobiliary surgery is not a statistically significant risk factor for poor outcome of subsequent liver transplantation surgery.[197]

There have been trials of pharmacologic therapy for alpha$_1$-AT deficiency. Patients have been given synthetic androgens, danazol or stanazolol, because of the dramatic effects of the same agents in individuals with hereditary angioedema,[198] a deficiency of the homologous serine proteinase inhibitor C1 inhibitor, and because danazol was initially found to increase serum levels of alpha$_1$-AT in PiZZ individuals.[199] However, further evaluation has demonstrated that danazol increases serum levels of alpha$_1$-AT in only half of deficient individuals, and the magnitude of the effect is small.[200] If the effect of the pharmacologic agent is at the level of synthesis of alpha$_1$-AT, this type of therapy has the theoretical drawback of causing greater intracellular accumulation of the mutant alpha$_1$-AT and thereby the potential pathophysiologic consequence of intracellular retention of misfolded protein (see above).

Patients with alpha$_1$-AT deficiency and emphysema have also undergone replacement therapy with purified plasma alpha$_1$-AT. Twenty-one PiZZ and Pi null individuals were treated for 6 months with weekly infusions of purified alpha$_1$-AT.[201,202] There was improvement in serum concentrations of alpha$_1$-AT and concentrations of alpha$_1$-AT and neutrophil elastase inhibitory capacity in bronchoalveolar lavage fluid. There were no significant side effects during these trials. Although this study demonstrates only biochemical efficacy, purified plasma alpha$_1$-AT has been licensed for use in alpha$_1$-AT–deficient individuals with established emphysema because it is thought that data regarding clinical efficacy are virtually impossible to collect. This form of therapy is designed for individuals with established and progressive emphysema. Protein replacement therapy is not being considered for individuals with liver disease, since there is little information to support the notion that deficient serum levels of alpha$_1$-AT are mechanistically related to liver injury. There are several theoretic drawbacks to protein replacement therapy; e.g., there may be greater influx of neutrophils into the target organs, since the carboxy-terminal fragment of alpha$_1$-AT possesses chemoattractant properties[34,35]; there may be greater intracellular accumulation of the mutant alpha$_1$-AT during protein replacement therapy if feedback regulation of alpha$_1$-AT synthesis is mediated by the complex of alpha$_1$-AT and elastase or by a fragment of alpha$_1$-AT exposed during complex formation or limited proteolysis.[36] The potential for oxidative inactivation of plasma-derived alpha$_1$-AT may be ultimately addressed by the use of sequence-modified recombinant alpha$_1$-AT.[94,203-205] However, therapy with recombinant alpha$_1$-AT will be possible only if high levels of expression of the fully glycosylated and therefore more stable form of the molecule can be achieved.

Gene replacement therapy for alpha$_1$-AT deficiency has been discussed in the literature.[206,207] For the near future considerations have been confined to somatic gene therapy. Ethical concerns and the potential for insertional mutagenesis have precluded current consideration of germ-line gene therapy for human disease. Construction of retroviral vectors with the coding sequence and appropriate regulatory sequence elements of the "foreign" gene has permitted stable tissue-specific expression in vivo.[206,209] The alpha$_1$-AT gene in a retroviral vector has been inserted into mouse fibroblasts[210] and these fibroblasts transplanted into the peritoneal cavities of nude mice.[211] The product of the transferred gene, human alpha$_1$-AT, was detected in sera and bronchial washings for up to 4 weeks. Other genes have been expressed after transplantation into several different sites,[212] including transplantable human epidermal cells.[213] Nevertheless, there are still major obstacles to be overcome before gene replacement becomes acceptable for treatment of human disease: appropriate level of expression, stability of expression, physiologic regulation of expression, and absence of undesirable effects on expression of other genes. Even more important for alpha$_1$-AT deficiency is the problem of concomitant expression of the endogenous mutant allele. Furthermore, in this case, expression of the transferred normal allele may exacerbate the intrinsic cellular defect by establishing competition with the product of the mutant allele for components of the secretory pathway (see above). Several novel ideas for functional inactivation or induction of mutations in specific cognate genes have been proposed,[214-216] but little is known about the effects of such manipulations, even in experimental animals. Expression of the defective alpha$_1$-AT gene, therefore, makes gene replacement a much less attractive possibility for therapy of this deficiency. Alternative strategies for at least partial correction of this defect may result from a more detailed understanding of the intracellular fate of the abnormal alpha$_1$-AT molecule (see above).

GENETIC COUNSELING

Restriction fraction length polymorphisms detected with synthetic oligonucleotide probes[217-220] and family studies[221] allow prenatal diagnosis of alpha$_1$-AT deficiency. Nevertheless, it is not clear how prenatal diagnosis for this deficiency should be used and how families should be counseled regarding the diagnosis. Data reviewed above indicate that 70 to 75 percent of individuals with alpha$_1$-AT deficiency do not have evidence of liver disease at age 12 years and that nonsmoking PiZZ individuals may not develop emphysema or even pulmonary function abnormalities until ages 60 to 70. These data could support a counseling strategy in which amniocentesis and abortion are discouraged. The only other data on this subject suggest that there is a 78 percent chance that a second PiZZ child will have serious liver disease if the older sib had serious liver disease.[163] This study, however, is retrospective and heavily influenced by bias in ascertainment of patients. The issue will not be resolved until studied prospectively, as, for example, in the Swedish population.[2,153]

Similar issues have discouraged interest in the development of mass screening programs for diagnosis of alpha$_1$-AT deficiency. Although the incidence of the deficiency is relatively high for an inborn error of metabolism, 1 in 1,600 to 1,700 live births in many regions,[2,3] and avoidance of cigarette smoking can have a major effect on the outcome of the disorder, screening has not been initiated because many individuals may be clinically unaffected and because diagnosis of this deficiency in asymptomatic children has the potential for significant negative psychological effects (T. Sveger: unpublished observations).

Acknowledgments

I am indebted to Ronald G. Crystal and Tomas Sveger for sharing manuscripts in press, to James P. Keating and Harvey R. Colten for critical review of this chapter, and to Joyce L. Thomas for secretarial assistance. The studies were supported in part by the friends of Shaun Harrington, the friends of Clifford Hoffman, by an American Gastroenterological Association/Industry (Merck, Sharp and Dohme) Research Scholar Award, by an RJR Nabisco Research Scholar Award, by an American Heart Association Established Investigator Award, and by US PHS HL37784.

REFERENCES

1. Gartner JC, Zitelli BJ, Malatack JJ, Shaw BW, Iwatsuki S, Starzl TE. Orthotopic liver transplantation in children: two-year experience with 47 patients. Pediatrics 1984; 74:140–145.
2. Sveger T. Liver disease in α_1-antitrypsin deficiency detected by screening of 200,000 infants. N Engl J Med 1976; 294:1316–1321.
3. Silverman EK, Miletich JP, Pierce JA, Sherman LA, Broze GJ, Campbell EJ. Alpha-l-antitrypsin deficiency: prevalence estimation from direct population screenings. Am Rev Respir Dis; in press.
4. Fagerhol MK. Serum Pi types in Norwegians. Acta Pathol Microbiol Scand 1967; 70:421–426.
5. Pierce JA, Eradio B, Dew TA. Antitrypsin phenotypes in St. Louis. JAMA 1975; 231:609–612.
6. Janus ED, Joyce PR, Sheat JM, Carrell RW. Alpha-l-antitrypsin variants in New Zealand, NZ Med J 1975; 82:289–291.
7. Kellerman G, Walter H. Investigations on the population genetics of alpha-l-antitrypsin polymorphism. Humangenetik 1970; 10:145–150.
8. Vanderville D, Martin J-P, Ropartz C. Alpha-l-antitrypsin polymorphism in a Bantu population. Humangenetik 1974; 21:33–38.
9. Jeppsson J-O. Amino acid substitution Glu-Lys in α_1-antitrypsin PiZ. FEBS Lett 1976; 65:195–197.
10. Yoshida L, Lieberman J, Gaidulis L, Ewing C. Molecular abnormality of human α_1-antitrypsin variant (PiZ) associated with plasma activity deficiency. Proc Natl Acad Sci USA 1976; 73:1324–1328.
11. Owen MC, Carrell RW. α_1-antitrypsin: sequence of the Z variant tryptic peptide. FEBS Lett 1976; 79:247–249.
12. Kidd VJ, Wallace RB, Itakura K, Woo SLC. α_1- antitrypsin deficiency detection by direct analysis of the mutation of the gene. Nature (London) 1983; 304:230–234.
13. Nukiwa T, Satoh K, Brantly ML, Ogushi F, Fells GA, Courtney M, Crystal RG. Identification of a second mutation in the protein-coding sequence of the Z-type alpha-l-antitrypsin gene. J Biol Chem 1981; 34:15989–15994.
14. Pearson SJ, Tetri P, George DL, Francke U. Activation of human α_1-antitrypsin gene in rat hepatoma x human fetal liver cell hybrids depends on presence of human chromosome 14. Somatic Cell Mol Genet 1983; 9:567–592.
15. Lai EC, Kao F-T, Law ML, Woo SLC. Assignment of the α_1-antitrypsin gene and sequence-regulated gene to human chromosome 14 by molecular hybridization. Am J Hum Genet 1983; 35:385–392.
16. Rabin M, Watson M, Kidd V, Woo SLC, Breg WR, Ruddle FH. Regional location of α_1-antichymotrypsin and α_1-antitrypsin genes on human chromosome 14. Somatic Cell Mol Genet 1986; 12:209–214.
17. Kidd VJ, Woo SLC. Molecular analysis of the serine proteinase inhibitor gene family. In: Barrett AJ, Salvesen G, eds. Proteinase inhibitors. Amsterdam: Elsevier Science, 1986: 421.
18. Long GL, Chandra T, Woo SLC, Davie EW, Kurachi K. Complete nucleotide sequence of the cDNA for human α_1-antitrypsin and the gene for the S variant. Biochemistry 1984; 23:4828–4837.
19. Perlino E, Cortese R, Ciliberto G. The human α_1-antitrypsin gene is transcribed from two different promoters in macrophages and hepatocytes. EMBO J 1987; 6:2767–2771.
20. Hunt LT, Dayhoff MO. A surprising new protein super family containing ovalbumin, antithrombin III and alpha-l-proteinase inhibitor. Biochem Biophys Res Commun 1980; 95:864–871.
21. Chandra T, Stackhouse K, Kidd VJ, Robson KJH, Woo SLC. Sequence homology between human αl-antichymotrypsin and antithrombin III. Biochemistry 1983; 22:4496–5001.
22. Bock SC, Skriver K, Nielsen E, Thogerson H-C, Wiman B, Donaldson DH, Eddy RL, Marrinan J, Radziejewska E, Huber R, Shows TB, Magnusson S. Human Cl inhibitor: primary structure, cDNA cloning and chromosomal localization. Biochemistry 1986; 25:4294–4301.
23. Davis AE, Whitehead AS, Harrison RA, Dauphinais A, Bruns GAP, Cicardi M, Rosen FS. Human inhibitor of the first component of complement Cl: characterization of cDNA clones and localization of the gene to chromosome 11. Proc Natl Acad Sci USA 1986; 83:3161–3165.
24. Holmes WE, Nelles L, Lijnen HR, Collen D. Primary structure of human α_2-antiplasmin, a serine protease inhibitor. J Biol Chem 1987; 262:1659–1664.
25. Suzuki K, Deyashiki Y, Nishioka J, Kurachi K, Akira M, Yamamoto S, Hashimoto S. Characterization of a cDNA for human protein C inhibitors: a new member of the plasma serine protease inhibitor super family. J Biol Chem 1987; 262:611–616.
26. Ragg H. A new member of the plasma protease inhibitor gene family. Nucleic Acids Res 1986; 14:1073–1088.
27. Inhorn RC, Tollefsen DM. Isolation and characterization of a partial cDNA clone for heparin cofactor II. Biochem Biophys Res Comm 1986; 137:431–436.

28. Ye RD, Wun T-C, Sadler JE. cDNA cloning and expression in *Escherichia* coli of a plasminogen activator inhibitor from human placenta. J Biol Chem 1987; 262:3718–3725.
29. Webb AC, Collins KL, Snyder SE, Alexander SJ, Roswenwasser LJ, Eddy RL, Shows TB, Auron PE. Human monocyte Arg-Serpin cDNA. Sequence, chromosomal assignment and homology to plasminogen activator-inhibitor. J Exp Med 1987; 166:77–94.
30. Doolittle RF, Angiotensinogen is related to the antitrypsin-antithrombin-ovalbumin family. Science 1983; 222:417–419.
31. Hammond GL, Smith CL, Goping IS, Underhill DA, Harley MJ, Reventos J, Musto NA, Gunsalus GL, Bardin CW. Primary structure of human corticosteroid binding globulin, deduced from hepatic and pulmonary cDNAs, exhibits homology with serine proteinase inhibitors. Proc Natl Acad Sci USA 1987; 84:5153–5157.
32. Carrell RW, Travis J. α_1-antitrypsin and the serpins: variation and countervariation. Trends Biol Sci 1985; 10:20–24.
33. Owen MC, Brennan SO, Lewis JH, Carrell RW. Mutation of antitrypsin to antithrombin: α_1-antitrypsin Pittsburgh (358 Met — Arg), a fatal bleeding disorder. N Engl J Med 1983; 309:694–698.
34. Banda MJ, Rice AG, Griffin GL, Senior RM. αl-proteinase inhibitor is a neutrophil chemoattractant after proteolytic inactivation by macrophage elastase. J Biol Chem 1988; 263:4481–4484.
35. Banda MJ, Rice AG, Griffin GL, Senior RM. The inhibitory complex of human αl-proteinase inhibitor and human leukocyte elastase is a neutrophil chemoattractant. J Exp Med 1988; 167:1608–1615.
36. Perlmutter DH, Travis J, Punsal PI. Elastase regulates the synthesis of its inhibitors, αl-proteinase inhibitor, and exaggerates the defect in homozygous PiZZ αl-proteinase inhibitor deficiency. J Clin Invest 1988; 81:1774–1780.
37. Pierce JA, Eradio BG. Improved identification of antitrypsin phenotypes through isoelectric focusing with dithioerythritol. J Lab Clin Med 1979; 94:826–831.
38. Brantly M, Nukiwa T, Crystal RG. Molecular basis of αl-antitrypsin deficiency. Am J Med 1988; 84:13–31.
39. Carrell RW, Jeppsson J-O, Laurell C-B, Brennan SO, Owen MC, Vaughan L, Boswell DR. Structure and variation of human αl-antitrypsin. Nature (London) 1982; 298:329–334.
40. Nukiwa T, Brantly M, Ogushi F, Fells G, Satoh K, Stier L, Courtney M, Crystal RG. Characterization of the M1 (ala 213) type of αl-antitrypsin, a newly recognized common "normal" αl-antitrypsin haplotype. Biochemistry 1987; 26:5259–5267.
41. Kueppers F, Christopherson MJ. Alpha-l-antitrypsin: further genetic heterogeneity revealed by isoelectric focusing. Am J Hum Genet 1978; 30:359–365.
42. Dykes D, Miller S, Polesky H. Distribution of αl-antitrypsin variants in a US white population. Hum Hered 1984; 34:308–310.
43. Talamo RC, Langley CE, Reed CE, Makino S. Alpha-l-antitrypsin deficiency: a variant with no detectable α-l-antitrypsin. Science 1973; 181:70–71.
44. Schandevyl W, Hennebert A, Leblanc G, de Coster A, Yernault JC, Acheten G, Ledoux M, Buneaux JJ. Alpha-l-antitrypsin deficiency of Pi00 type and connective tissue defect. In: Martin J-P. L'alpha-l-antitrypsin et le systeme Pi. Paris: INSERM, 1975: 97.
45. Ohashi A, Watanabe Y, Nakai H, Inokuma S. Familial cases of α-l-antitrypsin deficiency (PI NULL Type). Nippon Naika Gakkai Zasshi 1978; 67:50–56.
46. Garver RI, Mornex J-F, Nukiwa T, Brantly M, Courtney M, LeCocq J-P, Crystal RG: Alpha-l-antitrypsin deficiency and emphysema caused by homozygous inheritance of non-expressing alpha-l-antitrypsin genes. N Engl J Med 1986; 314:762–766.
47. Muensch H, Gaidulis L, Kueppers F, So SY, Escano G, Kidd VJ, Woo SLC. Complete absence of serum alpha-l-antitrypsin in conjunction with an apparently normal gene structure. Am J Hum Genet 1986; 38:898–907.
48. Feldmann G, Martin J-P, Sesboue R, Ropartz C, Perelman R, Nathanson M, Scringe P, Benhamou J-P. The ultrastructure of hepatocytes in alpha-l-antitrypsin deficiency with the genotype Pi—. Gut 1975; 16:796–799.
49. Nukiwa T, Takahashi H, Brantly M, Courtney M, Crystal RG. αl-antitrypsin Null $_{\text{granite falls}}$, a nonexpressing αl-antitrypsin gene associated with a frameshift stop mutation in a coding exon. J Biol Chem 1987; 262:11999–12004.
50. Satoh K, Nukiwa T, Brantly M, Garver RI, Courtney M, Hofker M, Crystal RG. Emphysema associated with complete absence of alpha-l-antitrypsin in serum and the homozygous inheritance of stop codon in an αl-antitrypsin coding exon. Am J Hum Genet 1988; 42:77–83.
51. Hardick C, Sifers R, Carlson J, Kidd V, Woo SLC. A null allele of the human α-l-antitrypsin gene is caused by a frameshift mutation. Am J Hum Genet 1986; 39:A202.
52. Sifers RN, Brashears-Macatee S, Kidd VJ, Muensch H, Woo SLC. A frameshift mutation results in a truncated α_1-antitrypsin that is retained within the rough endoplasmic reticulum. J Biol Chem 1988; 263:7330–7335.
53. Perlmutter DH, Kay RM, Cole FS, Rossing TH, Van Thiel DH, Colten HR. The cellular defect in αl-proteinase inhibitor deficiency is expressed in human monocytes and in xenopus oocytes injected with human liver mRNA. Proc Natl Acad Sci USA 1985; 82:6918–6921.
54. Mornex J-F, Chytil-Weir A, Martinet Y, Courtney M, LeCocq JP, Crystal RG. Expression of the alpha-l-antitrypsin gene in mononuclear phagocytes of normal and alpha-l-antitrypsin-deficient individuals. J Clin Invest 1986; 77:1952–1961.
55. Foreman RC, Judah JD, Colman A. Xenopus oocytes can synthesize but do not secrete the Z variant of human α-l-antitrypsin. FEBS Lett 1984; 168:84–88.
56. Verbanac KM, Heath EC. Biosynthesis, processing and secretion of M and Z variant human α-l-antitrypsin. J Biol Chem 1986; 261:9979–9989.
57. Feldmann G, Bignon J, Chahinian P, Degott C, Benhamou J-P. Hepatocyte ultrastructural charges in α-l-antitrypsin deficiency. Gastroenterology 1974; 67:1214–1224.
58. Loebermann H, Tokuoka R, Deisenhofer J, Huber R. Human α-l-proteinase inhibitor. Crystal structure analysis of two crystal modifications: molecular model and preliminary analysis of the implications for function. J Mol Biol 1984; 177:531–556.
59. Foreman RC. Disruption of the lys 290-glu 342 salt bridge in human α-l-antitrypsin does not prevent in its synthesis and secretion. FEBS Lett 1987; 216:79–82.
60. Lodish HF, Kong N, Snider M, Strous GJAM. Hepatoma secretory proteins migrate from rough endoplasmic reticulum to Golgi at characteristic rates. Nature (London) 1983; 304:80–83.
61. Lodish HF, Kong N. Glucose removal from N-linked oligosaccharides is required for efficient maturation of certain secretory glycoproteins form the rough endoplasmic reticulum to the Golgi complex. J Cell Biol 1984; 98:1720–1729.
62. Lodish HF, Kong N, Hirani S, Rasmussen J. A vesicular intermediate in the transport of hepatoma secretory proteins from the rough endoplasmic reticulum to the Golgi complex. J Cell Biol 1987; 104:221–230.
63. Munro S, Pelham HRB. An HSP 70-like protein in ER: identity with the 78 kD glucose-regulated protein and immunoglobulin heavy chain binding protein. Cell 1986; 46:291–300.
64. Mazzarella RA, Green MJ. ERp99, an abundant, conserved glycoprotein of the endoplasmic reticulum, is homologous to the 90-kDA heat shock protein (hsp90) and the 94-kDa glucose regulated protein (grp 94). J Biol Chem 1987; 262:8875–8883.
65. Hendershot L, Bole D, Kearney JF. The role of immunoglobulin heavy chain binding protein in immunoglobulin transport. Immunol Today 1987; 8:111–113.
66. Kelly PM, Schlesinger MJ. The effect of amino acid analogues and heat shock on gene expression in chicken embryo fibroblasts. Cell 1978; 15:1277–1286.
67. Anathan J, Goldberg AL, Voellmy R. Abnormal proteins serve as eukaryotic stress signals and trigger the activation of heat shock genes. Science 1986; 232:522–524.
68. Kozutsumi K, Segal M, Normington K, Gething M-J, Sambrook J. The presence of misfolded proteins in the endoplasmic reticulum signals the induction of glucose regulated proteins. Nature (London) 1988; 332:462–464.
69. Perlmutter DH, Schlesinger M, Pierce JA, Punsal PI, Schwartz AL. Synthesis of stress proteins is increased in individuals with homozygous PiZZ α_1-antitrypsin deficiency and liver disease. J Clin Invest 1989; 84:1555–1561.
70. Carrell RW. α_1-antitrypsin: molecular pathology, leukocytes and tissue damage. J Clin Invest 1986; 77:1427–1431.
71. Curiel D, Chytl A, Stier L, Crystal RG. Mechanism of S-type α_1-antitrypsin deficiency: retroviral gene transfer demonstrates the gene mutation causes a preglycosylation processing abnormality. Clin Res 1988; 36:591A.

72. Kramps JA, Brouwers JW, Maesen F, Dijkman JH. PiM $_{heerlen}$, a PiM allele resulting in very low α_1-antitrypsin serum levels. Hum Genet 1981; 59:104–107.
73. Hofker MH, Nukiwa T, Van Paassen HMB, Nelen M, Frants RR, Klasen EC, Crystal RG. A Pro— Leu substitution in codon 369 in the α_1-antitrypsin deficiency variant PiM $_{heerlen}$. Am J Hum Genet 1987; 41:A220.
74. Takahashi H, Nukiwa T, Ogushi F, Brantly M, Courtney M, Crystal RG. Identification and molecular analysis of a new variant of α_1-antitrypsin characterized by marked reduction of serum levels. Am Rev Respir Dis 1987; 135:A292.
75. Sproule BJ, Cox DW, Hsu K, Salkie ML, Herbert FA. Pulmonary function associated with the M malton deficient variant of alpha-1-antitrypsin. Am Rev Respir Dis 1983; 127:237–240.
76. Cox DW, Billingsley GD, Smyth S. Rare types of α_1-antitrypsin associated with deficiency. In: Arnaud A, ed. Electrophoresis. Berlin: Walter de Gruyter, 1981: 507.
77. Reid CL, Wiener GJ, Cox DW, Richter JE, Geisinger KR. Diffuse hepatocellular dysplasia and carcinoma associated with M malton variant of α_1-antitrypsin. Gastroenterology 1987; 93:181–187.
78. Crowley JJ, Sharp HL, Freier E, Ishak KG, Schow P. Fatal liver disease associated with α_1-antitrypsin deficiency PiM/PiM duarte. Gastroenterology 1987; 93:242–244.
79. Gross P, Pfitzer EA, Tolker E, Babyak MA, Kaschak M. Experimental emphysema. Arch Environ Health 1965; 11:50–58.
80. Janoff A, Sloan B, Weinbaum G, Damiano V, Sandhaus RA, Elias J, Kimbel P. Experimental emphysema induced with purified human neutrophil elastase: tissue localization of the instilled protease. Am Rev Respir Dis 1977; 115:461–478.
81. Senior RM, Tegner H, Kuhn C, Ohlsson K, Starcher BC, Pierce JA. The induction of pulmonary emphysema with human leukocyte elastase. Am Rev Respir Dis 1977; 116:469–475.
82. Marco V, Moss B, Meranze DR, Weinbaum G, Kimbel P. Induction of experimental emphysema in dogs using leukocyte homogenates. Am Rev Respir Dis 1971; 104:595–598.
83. Hayes JA, Korthy A, Snider GL. The pathology of elastase-induced panacinar emphysema in hamsters. J Pathol 1975; 117:1–14.
84. Janoff A, White T, Carp H, Harel S, Dearing R, Lee D. Lung injury induced by leukocytic proteases. Am J Pathol 1979; 97:111–129.
85. Karlinsky JB, Snider GL. Animal models of emphysema. Am Rev Respir Dis 1978; 117:1109–1133.
86. Gadek JE, Fells GA, Zimmerman RL, Rennard SI, Crystal RG. Antielastase of the human alveolar structures. Implications for the protease-antiprotease theory of emphysema. J Clin Invest 1981; 68:889–898.
87. Travis J, Salvesen GS. Human plasma proteinase inhibitors. Annu Rev Biochem 1983; 52:655–709.
88. Carrell RW, Owen M, Brennan S, Vaughan L. Carboxy terminal fragment of human α_1-antitrypsin from hydroxylamine cleavage: homology with antithrombin III. Biochem Biophys Res Commun 1979; 91:1032–1037.
89. Morris M, Odani S, Ikenaka T. Characterization of a peptide released during the reaction of human α_1-antitrypsin and bovine chymotrypsin. J Biochem 1979; 86:915–921.
90. Lieberman J. Elastase, collagenase, emphysema and alpha-1-antitrypsin deficiency. Chest 1976; 70:62–67.
91. Carp H, Janoff A. Possible mechanisms of emphysema in smokers: in vitro suppression of serum elastase inhibitory capacity by fresh cigarette smoke and its prevention by antioxidants. Am Rev Respir Dis 1978; 118:617–621.
92. Carp H, Janoff A. In vitro suppression of serum elastase inhibitory capacity by reactive oxygen species generated by phagocytosing polymorphonuclear leukocytes. J Clin Invest 1979; 63:793–797.
93. George PM, Vissers MCM, Travis J, Winterbourn CC, Carrell RW. A genetically engineered mutant of α_1-antitrypsin protects connective tissue from neutrophil damage and may be useful in lung disease. Lancet 1984; ii:1426–1428.
94. Ossanna PJ, Test ST, Matheson NR, Regiani S, Weiss SJ. Oxidative regulation of neutrophil elastase-alpha-1-proteinase inhibitor interactions. J Clin Invest 1986; 72:1939–1951.
95. Hubbard RC, Ogushi F, Fells GA, Cantin AM, Jallat S, Courtney M, Crystal RG. Oxidants spontaneously released by alveolar macrophages of cigarette smokers can inactivate the active site of α_1-antitrypsin, rendering it ineffective as an inhibitor of neutrophil elastase. J Clin Invest 1987; 80:1289–1295.
96. Banda MJ, Clark EJ, Werb Z. Limited proteolysis by macrophage elastase inactivates human α_1-proteinase inhibitor. J Exp Med 1980; 152:1563–1570.
97. Desrochers PE, Weiss SJ. Proteolytic inactivation of alpha-1-proteinase inhibitor by a neutrophil metallo-proteinase. J Clin Invest 1988; 81:1646–1650.
98. Johnson DA, Barrett AJ, Mason RW. Cathepsin L inactivates α_1-proteinase inhibitor by cleavage in the reactive site region. J Biol Chem 1986; 261:14748–14751.
99. Morihara K, Tsuzuki H, Oda K. Protease and elastase of *Pseudomonas aeruginosa*: inactivation of human plasma α_1-proteinase inhibitor. Infect Immunol 1979; 24:188–193.
100. Banda MJ, Clark EJ, Werb Z. Regulation of alpha-1-proteinase inhibitor function by rabbit alveolar macrophages: evidence for proteolytic rather than oxidative interaction. J Clin Invest 1985; 75:1758–1762.
101. Miller RR, Kuhlenschmidt MS, Coffee CJ, Kuo I, Glew RH. Comparison of the chemical, physical and survival properties of normal and Z-variant α_1-antitrypsin. J Biol Chem 1976; 251:4751–4757.
102. Bathurst IC, Travis J, George PM, Carrell RW. Structural and functional characterization of the abnormal Z α_1-antitrypsin isolated from human liver. FEBS Lett 1984; 177:179–183.
103. Ogushi F, Fells GA, Hubbard RC, Straus SD, Crystal RG. Z-type α_1-antitrypsin is less competent than M1-type α_1-antitrypsin as an inhibitor of neutrophil elastase. J Clin Invest 1987; 89:1366–1374.
104. Hood JM, Koep L, Peters RF, Schröter GPJ, Weil R, Redeker AG, Starzl TE. Liver transplantation for advanced liver disease with α_1-antitrypsin deficiency. N Engl J Med 1980; 302:272–276.
105. Alper CA, Raum D, Awdeh ZL, Petersen BH, Taylor PD, Starzl TE. Studies of hepatic synthesis in vivo of plasma proteins including orosomucoid, transferrin, alpha-1-antitrypsin, C8, and factor B. Clin Immunol Immunopathol 1980; 16:84–88.
106. Liu M-C, Yu S, Sy J, Redman CM, Lipmann F. Tyrosine sulfation of proteins from human hepatoma cell line HepG2. Proc Natl Acad Sci USA 1985; 82:7160–7164.
107. Ciliberto G, Dente L, Cortese R. Cell-specific expression of a transfected human α_1-antitrypsin gene. Cell 1985; 41:531–540.
108. DeSimone V, Ciliberto G, Hardon E, Paonessa G, Palla F, Lundberg L, Cortese R. Cis- and trans-acting elements responsible for the cell specific expression of the human α_1-antitrypsin gene. EMBO J 1987; 6:2759–2766.
109. Sifers RN, Carlson JA, Clift SM, DeMayo FJ, Bullock DW, Woo SLC. Tissue-specific expression of the human α_1-antitrypsin gene in transgenic mice. Nucleic Acid Res 1987; 15:1459–1475.
110. Angel P, Imagawa M, Chiu R, Stein B, Imbra RJ, Rahmsdorf HJ, Jonat C, Herrlich P, Karin M. Phorbol ester-induced genes contain a common cis element recognized by a TPA-modulated trans-acting factor. Cell 1987; 99:729–839.
111. Bohmann D, Bos TJ, Admon A, Nishimura T, Vogt PK, Tijan R. Human proto-oncogene c-jun encodes a DNA binding protein with structural and functional properties of transcription factor AP-1. Science 1987; 238:1386–1392.
112. Angel P, Allegretto EA, Okino ST, Hattori K, Boyle WJ, Hunter T, Karin M. Oncogene jun encodes a sequence-specific transactivator similar to AP-1. Nature (London) 1988; 332:166–171.
113. Rauscher FJ, Sambucetti LC, Curran T, Distel RJ, Spiegelman BM. Common DNA binding site for fos protein complexes and transcription factor AP-1. Cell 1988; 52:471–480.
114. Franza BR, Rauscher FJ, Josephs SF, Curran T. The Fos complex and Fos-related antigens recognize sequence elements that contain AP-1 binding sites. Science 1988; 239:1150–1153.
115. Courtois G, Morgan JG, Campbell LA, Fourel G, Crabtree GR. Interaction of a liver-specific nuclear factor with the fibrinogen and α_1-antitrypsin promoters. Science 1987; 238:688–692.
116. Aronsen K-F, Ekelund G, Kindmark C-O, Laurell C-B. Sequential changes of plasma proteins after myocardial infarction. Scand J Clin Lab Invest 1972; 29 (suppl 24):127.
117. Dickson I, Alper CA. Changes in serum proteinase inhibitor levels following bone surgery. Clin Chem Acta 1974; 54:381–385.
118. Perlmutter DH, Goldberger G, Dinarello CA, Mizel SB, Colten HR. Regulation of class III major histocompatibility complex gene products by interleukin-1. Science 1986; 232:850–852.
119. Perlmutter DH, Dinarello CA, Punsal PI, Colten HR. Cachectin/tumor necrosis factor regulated hepatic acute-phase gene expression. J Clin Invest 1986; 78:1349–1354.

120. Perlmutter DH. Distinct mediators and mechanisms regulate human acute phase gene expression. In: Pardue ML, Feramisco JR, Lindquist S, eds. Stress-induced proteins. New York: Alan R. Liss, Inc, 1989: 257.
121. Sehgal PB, May LT. Human β2-interferon. J Interfer Res 1987; 7:521–537.
122. Gauldie J, Richards C, Harmish D, Landsdorp P, Baumann H. Interferon $\beta 2/\beta$-cell stimulatory factor type 2 shares identity with monocyte-derived hepatocyte-stimulating factor and regulates the major acute phase protein response in liver cells. Proc Natl Acad Sci USA 1987; 84:7251–7255.
123. Evans E, Courtois GM, Kilian PL, Fuller GM, Crabtree GR. Induction of fibrinogen and a subset of acute phase response genes involves a novel monokine which is mimicked by phorbol esters. J Biol Chem 1987; 262:10850–10854.
124. Laurell C-B, Rannevik G. A comparison of plasma protein changes induced by danazol, pregnancy and estrogens. J Clin Endocrinol Metab 1979; 49:719–925.
125. Perlmutter DH, Cole FS, Kilbridge P, Rossing TH, Colten HR. Expression of the α_1-proteinase inhibitor gene in human monocytes and macrophages. Proc Natl Acad Sci USA 1985; 82:795–799.
126. Kelsey GD, Povey S, Bygrave AE, Lovell-Badge RH. Species- and tissue-specific expression of human alpha-l-antitrypsin in transgenic mice. Genes Dev 1987; 1:161–171.
127. Perlino E, Cortese R, Ciliberto G. The human α-l-antitrypsin gene is transcribed from two different promoters in macrophages and hepatocytes. EMBO J 1987; 6:2767–2771.
128. Barbey-Morel C, Pierce JA, Campbell EJ, Perlmutter DH. Lipopolysaccharide modulates the expression of α_1-proteinase inhibitor and other serine proteinase inhibitors in human monocytes and macrophages. J Exp Med 1987; 166:1041–1054.
129. Perlmutter DH, Punsal PI. Distinct and additive effects of elastase and endotoxin on α_1-proteinase inhibitor and other serine proteinase inhibitor expression in macrophages. J Biol Chem; 1988; 263:16499–16503.
130. Thireos B, Driscoll Penn M, Greer H. 5′ untranslated sequences are required for the translational control of a yeast regulatory gene. Proc Natl Acad Sci USA 1984; 81:5096–5100.
131. Hinnebusch AG. Evidence for translational regulation of the activator of general amino acid control in yeast. Proc Natl Acad Sci USA 1984; 81:6442–6446.
132. Mueller PP, Hinnebusch AG. Multiple upstream AUG codons mediate translational control of GCN4. Cell 1986; 45:201–207.
133. Hentze MW, Rouault TA, Caughman SW, Dancis A, Harford JB, Klausner RD. A cis-acting element is necessary and sufficient for translational regulation of human ferritin expression in response to iron. Proc Natl Acad Sci USA 1987; 84:6730–6734.
134. Hentze MW, Caughman SW, Rouault TA, Barriocanal JG, Dancis A, Harford JB, Klausner RD. Identification of the iron-responsive element for translational regulation of human ferritin mRNA. Science 1987; 238:1570–1573.
135. Aziz N, Munro HN. Iron regulates ferritin mRNA translation through a segment of cis 5′ untranslated region. Proc Natl Acad Sci USA 1987; 84:8478–8482.
136. Takemura S, Rossing TH, Perlmutter DH. A lymphokine regulates expression of alpha-l-proteinase inhibitor in human monocytes and macrophages. J Clin Invest 1986; 77:1207–1213.
137. Carlson JA, Rogers BB, Sifers RN, Hawkins HK, Finegold MJ, Woo SLC. Multiple tissues express alpha-l-antitrypsin in transgenic mice and man. J Clin Invest 1988; 82:26–36.
138. Pinto M, Robine-Leon S, Appay M-D, Kedinger M, Triadou N, Dussaulx E, Lacroix B, Simon-Assmann P, Haffen K, Fogh J, Zweibaum A. Enterocyte-like differentiation and polarization of the human colon carcinoma cell line Caco-2 in culture. Biol Cell 1983; 47:323–330.
139. Perlmutter DH, Alpers DH, Daniels JD. Expression of the αl-antitrypsin gene in a human intestinal epithelial cell line. J Biol Chem 1989; 264:9485–9490.
140. Makino S, Reed CE. Distribution and elimination of exogenous alpha-l-antitrypsin. J Lab Clin Med 1970; 75:742–746.
141. Laurell C-B, Nosslin B, Jeppsson J-O. Catabolic rate of α_1-antitrypsin of Pl type M and Z in man. Clin Sci Mol Med 1977; 52:457–461.
142. Jones EA, Vergalla J, Steer CJ, Bradley-Moore PR, Vierling JM. Metabolism of intact and desialylated α_1-antitrypsin. Clin Sci Mol Med 1978; 55:139–148.
143. Jeppsson J-O, Laurell C-B, Nosslin B, Cox DW. Catabolic rate of Pl types S, and M malton and of asialylated M-protein in man. Clin Sci Mol Med 1978; 55:103–107.
144. Koj A, Regoeczi E. Effect of experimental inflammation on the synthesis and distribution of antithrombin III and α_1-antitrypsin in rabbits. Br J Exp Pathol 1978; 59:473–481.
145. Glaser CB, Karic L, Fallat RJ, Stockert R. Plasma survival studies in rat of the normal and homozygote deficient forms of α_1-antitrypsin. Biochem Biophys Acta 1977; 495:87–95.
146. Gadek JE, Crystal RG. α_1-antitrypsin deficiency. In: Stanbury JB, Wyngaarden JB, Fredrickson DS, Goldstein JL, Brown MS, eds. The metabolic basis of inherited disease. 5th ed. New York: McGraw-Hill, 1983: 1450.
147. Thomas DW, Sinatra FR, Merritt RJ. Random fecal alpha-l-antitrypsin concentration in children with gastrointestinal disease. Gastroenterology 1981; 80:776–782.
148. Hill RE, Hercz A, Corey ML, Gilday DL, Eng B, Hamilton JR. Fecal clearance of α_1-antitrypsin: a reliable measure of enteric protein loss in children. J Pediatr 1981; 99:416–418.
149. Florent C, L'Hirondel C, Desmazures C, Aymes C, Bernier JJ. Intestinal clearance of α_1-antitrypsin: a sensitive measure for detection of protein-losing enteropathy. Gastroenterology 1981; 81:777–780.
150. Laurell C-B, Eriksson J. The electrophoretic β_1-globulin pattern of serum in α_1-antitrypsin deficiency. Scand J Clin Lab Invest 1963; 15:132–140.
151. Eriksson S. Studies in α_1-antitrypsin deficiency. Acta Med Scand [Suppl] 1965; 432:1–85.
152. Sharp HL, Bridges RA, Krivit W, Freier ER. Cirrhosis associated with alpha-l-antitrypsin deficiency: a previously unrecognized inherited disorder. J Lab Clin Med 1969; 73:934–939.
153. Sharp HL. Alpha-l-antitrypsin deficiency. Hosp Pract 1971; 6:83–96.
154. Sveger T. The natural history of liver disease in α_1-antitrypsin deficient children. Acta Paediatr Scand 1988; 77:847–851.
155. Moroz SP, Cutz E, Cox DW, Sass-Kortsak A. Liver disease associated with alpha-l-antitrypsin deficiency in childhood. J Pediatr 1976; 88:19–25.
156. Hadchouel M, Gautier M. Histopathologic study of the liver in the early cholestatic phase of alpha-l-antitrypsin deficiency. J Pediatr 1976; 89:211–215.
157. Odievre M, Martin J-P, Hadchouel M, Alagille D, Thaler MM. Alpha-l-antitrypsin deficiency and liver disease in children: phenotypes, manifestations and prognosis. Pediatrics 1976; 57:226–231.
158. McPhie JL, Binnie S, Brunt PW. α_1-antitrypsin deficiency and infantile liver disease. Arch Dis Child 1976; 51:584–588.
159. Hirschberger M, Stickler GB. Neonatal hepatitis and alpha-l-antitrypsin deficiency: the prognosis in five patients. Mayo Clin Proc 1977; 52:241–245.
160. Nemeth A, Strandvik B. Natural history of children with alpha-l-antitrypsin deficiency and neonatal cholestasis. Acta Paediatr Scand 1982; 71:993–999.
161. Nemeth A, Strandvik B. Liver disease in children with alpha-l-antitrypsin deficiency without neonatal cholestasis. Acta Paediatr Scand 1982; 71:1001–1005.
162. Nebbia G, Hadchouel M, Odievre M, Alagille D. Early assessment of evolution of liver disease associated with α_1-antitrypsin deficiency in childhood. J Pediatr 1983; 102:661–665.
163. Psacharopoulos HT, Mowat AP, Cook PJL, Carlile PA, Portmann B, Rodeck CH. Outcome of liver disease associated with α_1-antitrypsin deficiency (PiZ). Arch Dis Child 1983; 58:882–887.
164. Udall JN, Dixon M, Newman AP, Wright JA, James B, Block KJ. Liver disease in α_1-antitrypsin deficiency. A restrospective analysis of the influence of early breast- vs bottle-feeding. JAMA 1985; 253:2679–2682.
165. Ghishan FK, Greene HL. Liver disease in children with PiZZ α_1-antitrypsin deficiency. Hepatology 1988; 8:307–310.
166. Cottrall K, Cook PJL, Mowat AP. Neonatal hepatitis syndrome and alpha-l-antitrypsin deficiency: an epidemiological study in Southeast England. Postgrad Med J 1974; 50:376–380.
167. Eriksson S, Carlson J, Velez R. Risk of cirrhosis and primary liver cancer in alpha-l-antitrypsin deficiency. N Engl J Med 1986; 314:736–739.
168. Hodges JR, Millward-Sadler GH, Barbatis C, Wright R. Heterozygous MZ alpha-l-antitrypsin deficiency in adults with chronic active hepatitis and cryptogenic cirrhosis. N Engl J Med 1981; 304:357–360.
169. Carlson J, Eriksson S. Chronic 'cryptogenic' liver disease and malignant hepatoma in intermediate alpha-l-antitrypsin deficiency identified by a PiZ-specific monoclonal antibody. Scand J Gastroenterol 1985; 20:835–842.

170. Ghishan FK, Gray GF, Green HL. α_1-antitrypsin deficiency presenting with ascites and cirrhosis in the neonatal period. Gastroenterology 1983; 85:435–438.
171. Palmer PE, Christopherson WM, Wolfe HJ. Alpha-l-antitrypsin, protein marker in oral contraceptive-associated hepatic tumors. Am J Clin Pathol 1977; 68:736–739.
172. Reintoft I, Hagerstrand I. Demonstration of α_1-antitrypsin in hepatomas. Arch Pathol Lab Med 1979; 103:495–498.
173. Qizilbash A, Young-Pong O. Alpha-l-antitrypsin liver disease differential diagnosis of PAS-positive, diastase-resistant globules in liver cells. Am J Clin Pathol 1983; 79:697–702.
174. Yunis EJ, Agostini RM, Glew RH. Fine structural observations of the liver in α_1-antitrypsin deficiency. Am J Clin Pathol 1976; 82:265–286.
175. Blenkinsopp WK, Haffenden GP. Alpha-l-antitrypsin bodies in liver. J Clin Pathol 1977; 30:132–137.
176. Hultcrantz R, Mengarelli S. Ultrastructural liver pathology in patients with minimal liver disease and α_1-antitrypsin deficiency: a comparison between heterozygous and homozygous patients. Hepatology 1984; 4:937–945.
177. Rosenthal P, Liebman WM, Thaler MM. Alpha-l-antitrypsin deficiency and severe infantile liver disease. Am J Dis Child 1979; 133:1195–1196.
178. Udall JN, Bloch KJ, Walker WA. Transport of proteases across neonatal intestine and development of liver disease in infants with α_1-antitrypsin deficiency. Lancet 1982; ii:1441–1443.
179. Eriksson S. Alpha-l-antitrypsin deficiency and liver cirrhosis in adults. Acta Med Scand 1987; 221:461–467.
180. Guenter CA, Welch MH, Russell TR, Hyde RM, Hammarsten JF. The pattern of lung disease associated with alpha-l-antitrypsin deficiency. Arch Intern Med 1968; 122:254–259.
181. Thurlbeck WM, Henderson JA, Fraser RG, Bates DV. Chronic obstructive disease. A comparison between clinical, roentgenologic, functional and morphologic criteria in chronic bronchitis, emphysema, asthma and bronchiectasis. Medicine 1970; 49:81–98.
182. Larsson C. Natural history and life expectancy in severe alpha-l-antitrypsin deficiency, PiZ. Acta Med Scand 1978; 204:345–351.
183. Janus ED, Phillips NT, Carrell RW. Smoking, lung function and α_1-antitrypsin deficiency. Lancet 1985; i:152–154.
184. Moroz SP, Cutz E, Balfe JW, Sass-Kortsak A. Membranoproliferative glomerulonephritis in childhood cirrhosis associated with alpha-l-antitrypsin deficiency. Pediatrics 1976; 57:232–238.
185. Strife CF, Hug G, Chuck G, McAdams AJ, David CA, Kline JJ. Membranoproliferative glomerulonephritis and α_1-antitrypsin deficiency in children. Pediatrics 1983; 71:88–92.
186. Miller F, Kuschner M. Alpha-l-antitrypsin deficiency, emphysema, necrotizing angiitis and glomerulonephritis. Am J Med 1969; 46:615–619.
187. Viraben R, Massip P, Dicostanzo B, Mathieu C. Necrotizing panniculitis with alpha-l-antitrypsin deficiency. J Am Acad Dermatol 1986; 14:684–687.
188. Freeman HJ, Weinstein WM, Shnitka TK, Crockford PM, Herbert FA. Alpha-l-antitrypsin deficiency and pancreatic fibrosis. Ann Intern Med 1976; 85:73–76.
189. Novis BH, Young GO, Bank S, Marks IN. Chronic pancreatitis and alpha-l-antitrypsin deficiency. Lancet 1975; ii:748–749.
190. Ray MB, Zumwalt R. Islet-cell hyperplasia in genetic deficiency of alpha-l-proteinase inhibitor. Am J Clin Pathol 1986; 85:681–687.
191. Andre F, Andre C, Lambert R, Descos F. Prevalence of alpha-l-antitrypsin deficiency in patients with gastric or duodenal ulcers. Biomedicine 1974; 21:222–224.
192. Klasen EC, Polanco I, Biemond I, Vazquez C, Pena AS. Alpha-l-antitrypsin and coeliac disease in Spain. Gut 1984; 21:948–950.
193. Cox DW, Huber O. Rheumatoid arthritis and alpha-l-antitrypsin. Lancet 1976; i:1216–1217.
194. Arnaud P, Galbraith RM, Faulk WP, Ansell BM. Increased frequency of the MZ phenotype of alpha-l-protease inhibitor in juvenile chronic polyarthritis. J Clin Invest 1977; 60:1442–1444.
195. Tobin MJ, Cook PJL, Hutchison DCS. Alpha-l-antitrypsin deficiency: the clinical and physiological features of pulmonary emphysema in subjects homozygous for P_1 type Z. Br J Dis Chest 1983; 77:14–27.
196. Esquivel CO, Iwatsuki S, Gordon RD, Marsh WW, Konery B, Makowka L, Tzakis AG, Todo S, Starzl TE. Indications for pediatric liver transplantation. J Pediatr 1987; 111:1039–1045.
197. Cuervas-Mons V, Rimola A, Van Thiel DH, Gavaler JS, Schade RR, Starzl TE. Does previous abdominal surgery alter the outcome of pediatric patients subjected to orthotopic liver transplantation? Gastroenterology 1986; 90:853–857.
198. Gelfand JA, Sherins RJ, Alling DW, Frank MM. Treatment of hereditary angioedema with danazol: reversal of clinical and biochemical abnormalities. N Engl J Med 1976; 295:1444–1448.
199. Gadek JE, Fulmer JD, Gelfand JA, Frank MM, Petty TL, Crystal RG. Danazol-induced augmentation of serum α_1-antitrypsin levels in individuals with marked deficiency of this anti-protease. J Clin Invest 1980; 66:82–87.
200. Wewers MD, Gadek JE, Keogh BA, Fells GA, Crystal RG. Evaluation of danazol therapy for patients with PiZZ alpha-l-antitrypsin deficiency. Am Rev Respir Dis 1986; 134:476–480.
201. Wewers MD, Casolaro A, Sellers SE, Swayze SC, McPhaul KM, Wittes JJ, Crystal RG. Replacement therapy for alpha-l-antitrypsin deficiency associated with emphysema. N Engl J Med 1987; 316:1055–1062.
202. Wewers MD, Casolaro A, Crystal RG. Comparison of alpha-l-antitrypsin levels and antineutrophil elastase capacity of blood and lung in a patient with the alpha-l-antitrypsin phenotype null-null before and during alpha-l-antitrypsin augmentation therapy. Am Rev Respir Dis 1987; 135:539–543.
203. Cabezon T, DeWilde M, Herion P, Loriau R, Bollen A. Expression of human α_1-antitrypsin cDNA in the yeast *Saccharomyces cerevisiae*. Proc Natl Acad Sci USA 1984; 81:6594–6598.
204. Courtney M, Jallat S, Tessier L-H, Benavente A, Crystal RG, Lecocq J-P. Synthesis in *E. coli* of α_1-antitrypsin variants of therapeutic potential for emphysema and thrombosis. Nature (London) 1985; 313:149–151.
205. Matheson NR, Gibson HL, Hallewell R, Barr PJ, Travis J. Recombinant DNA-derived forms of human α_1-proteinase inhibitor: studies on the alanine 358 and cysteine 358 substituted mutants. J Biol Chem 1986; 261:10404–10409.
206. Ledley FD. Somatic gene therapy for human disease. J Pediatr 1987; 110:167–174.
207. Ledley FD, Woo SLC. Molecular basis of α_1-antitrypsin deficiency and its potential therapy by gene transfer. J Inherited Metab Dis 1986; 9(suppl 1):85–91.
208. Dzierzak EA, Papayannopoulou T, Mulligan RC. Lineage-specific expression of human β-globin gene in murine bone marrow transplant recipients reconstituted with retrovirus-transduced stem cells. Nature (London) 1988; 331:35–41.
209. Weatherall DJ. The slow road to gene therapy. Nature (London) 1988; 331:13–14.
210. Garver RL, Chytil A, Karlsson S, Fells GA, Brantly ML, Courtney M, Kantoff PW, Nienhuis AW, Anderson WF, Crystal RG. Production of glycosylated physiologically normal human α_1-antitrypsin by mouse fibroblasts modified by insertion of a human α_1-antitrypsin cDNA using a retroviral vector. Proc Natl Acad Sci USA 1987; 84:1050–1054.
211. Garver RI, Chytil A, Courtney M, Crystal RG. Clonal gene therapy: transplanted mouse fibroblast clones express human α_1-antitrypsin gene in vivo. Science 1987; 237:762–764.
212. Selden RF, Skoskiewicz MJ, Howie KB, Russell PS, Goodman HM. Implantation of genetically engineered fibroblasts into mice: implications for gene therapy. Science 1987; 236:714–718.
213. Morgan JR, Barrandon Y, Green M, Mulligan RC. Expression of an exogenous growth hormone gene by transplantable human epidermal cells. Science 1987; 237:1476–1479.
214. Herskowitz I. Functional inactivation of genes by dominant negative mutations. Nature (London) 1987; 379:219–222.
215. Thomas KR, Capecchi MR. Site-directed mutagenesis by gene targeting in mouse embryo-derived stem cells. Cell 1987; 51:503–512.
216. Thomas KR, Capecchi MR. Introduction of homologous DNA sequence into mammalian cells induces mutations in the cognate gene. Nature (London) 1986; 324:34–38.
217. Kidd VJ, Wallace RB, Itakura K, Woo SLC. α_1-antitrypsin deficiency detection by direct analysis of the mutation in the gene. Nature (London) 1983; 304:230–234.
218. Kidd VJ, Golbus MS, Wallace RB, Itakura K, Woo SLC. Prenatal diagnosis of α_1-antitrypsin deficiency by direct analysis of the mutation site in the gene. N Engl J Med 1984; 310:639–642.
219. Cox DW, Woo SLC, Mansfield T. DNA restriction fragments associated with α_1-antitrypsin deficiency indicate a single origin for deficiency allele PiZ. Nature (London) 1985; 316:79–81.
220. Cox DW, Mansfield T. Prenatal diagnosis of α_1-antitrypsin deficiency and estimates of fetal risk for disease. J Med Genet 1987; 24:52–59.
221. Nukiwa T, Brantly M, Garver R, Paul L, Courtney M, LeCocq J-P, Crystal RG. Evaluation of "at risk" alpha-l-antitrypsin genotype SZ with synthetic oligonucleotide gene probes. J Clin Invest 1986; 77:528–537.

PART 14

Disorders of Bile Acid Synthesis

Kenneth D.R. Setchell, Ph.D.

For several decades, bile acids have been implicated in the pathogenesis of liver disease; however, their exact role in initiating or perpetuating liver injury is difficult to discern. Nonspecific alterations in serum, urinary, and biliary bile acid composition are found in infants and children with neonatal cholestasis. However, until recently it has proved difficult to determine whether such changes are primary or secondary to cholestatic conditions. Largely as a consequence of advances in technology,[1] specific inborn errors in bile acid biosynthesis have been recently recognized[2] that appear to be causal in the pathogenesis of the idiopathic and familial forms of neonatal hepatitis.[3-6] Although the exact genetic basis of these defects remains to be established, the deficiency in activity of specific enzymes involved in bile acid synthesis results in diminished production of primary bile acids that are essential for promoting bile flow[7] with the concomitant production of atypical bile acids with the potential for causing liver injury. This discussion outlines the normal pathways for bile acid synthesis, highlights the differences in bile acid metabolism in early life, and outlines the features of inborn errors in bile acid synthesis.

CHEMISTRY

The bile acids are a group of compounds that belong to the steroid class.[8] Structurally they consist of a four-ringed, cyclopentanoperhydrophenanthrene nucleus (ABCD rings) with a side chain, most commonly of five carbon atoms in length, terminating in a carboxylic acid (Fig. 1); they are therefore acidic steroids. A great variety of bile acids can be found in biologic fluids, and significant species differences exist with regard to the synthesis and metabolism of the bile acids.[9] In humans, the principal bile acids synthesized by the liver[10] have hydroxy groups substituted in the nucleus at the carbon positions C-3, C-7, and C-12, but additional reactions involving hydroxylations, epimerization, and oxidoreduction also take place, leading to a complex array of structures. Although many of the products of these reactions may be of negligible quantitative importance in health, during the diseased state they may constitute a relatively large proportion of the total bile acid pool.[1] Additionally, during early development it is apparent that these alternative pathways for bile acid synthesis and metabolism become quantitatively important, as is evident from the findings of relatively high proportions of bile acids hydroxylated at the C-1, C-2, C-4, and C-6 positions of the nucleus.[11,12]

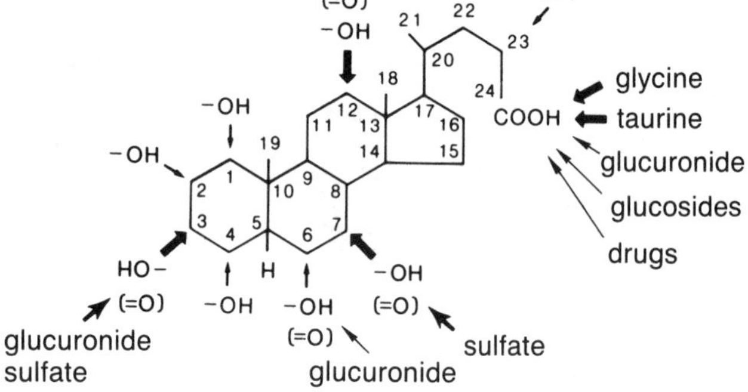

FIGURE 1 Chemical structure of the bile acid (5β-cholanoic acid) nucleus indicating the numbering system for each carbon atom and the various positions of the substituent groups for the majority of bile acids found in normal and pathophysiologic conditions (the size of the arrows indicates the relative quantitative importance of each substituent group).

The two principal bile acids synthesized by the liver and referred to as the "primary" bile acids,[10] are cholic acid (3α, 7α, 12α-trihydroxy-5β-cholanoic acid) and chenodeoxycholic acid (3α, 7α-dihydroxy-5β-cholanoic acid). These bile acids are extensively conjugated to the amino acids glycine and taurine to yield the corresponding glyco- and tauro-conjugates.[13] To a lesser extent, conjugation to glucuronic acid to form glucuronide ethers[14] and esters[15] and sulfuric acid to form sulfate conjugates[16] also occurs. More recently, bile acid conjugates of glucosides,[17,18] *N*-acetylglucosaminides,[19] and drugs[20] have also been recognized (Fig. 1).

The bile acids perform several important functions. They represent one of the major catabolic pathways for the elimination of cholesterol from the body.[10] More importantly, from the standpoint of hepatobiliary disease, bile acids provide the primary driving force for the promotion and secretion of bile[7]; they are therefore essential to the development of the biliary excretory route for the elimination of many endogenous and exogenous toxic substances, such as bilirubin, xenobiotics, and drug metabolites. Within the intestinal lumen, the detergent action of bile acids facilitates the absorption of fats and the fat-soluble vitamins, and the importance of this role becomes apparent in chronic cholestasis, where fat malabsorption and fat-soluble vitamin deficiency present significant clinical management problems.

Physiologically the normal bile acid pool size is 2 to 4 g, but the effectiveness of this pool is increased by an efficient enterohepatic recycling (10 to 12 times per day) stimulated by postprandial gallbladder contraction.[21] Conservation of the bile acid pool occurs by an efficient reabsorption, principally from the small intestine, and an effective hepatic extraction from the portal venous circulation, so that each day less than 5 percent of the pool is lost in the stools.[22] This bile acid loss is compensated for by hepatic synthesis of bile acids; therefore, in the steady state determination of fecal bile acid excretion will provide an estimate of daily bile acid synthesis rates.[22]

PATHWAYS FOR BILE ACID SYNTHESIS

The biochemical pathways for bile acid synthesis in the adult have been relatively well defined and are reviewed in detail elsewhere.[10] Much of this information has been derived from in vitro and in vivo studies of precursor-to-product relationships in various animal species, most notably the rat and rabbit, and from studies of pathologic disorders affecting bile acid production.[10] This discussion therefore serves to indicate only the salient features of the pathways. Because cholesterol is a C_{27} sterol, its conversion to the two primary bile acids, cholic and chenodeoxycholic acids, requires several major alterations to the molecule (Fig. 2). These include (1) the introduction of additional hydroxy groups at positions C-7 (for both chenodeoxycholic and cholic) and C-12 (for cholic acid); (2) epimerization of the 3β-hydroxy group; (3) reduction of the Δ^5 bond; (4) reduction in length of the side chain from C_8 to C_5, with the formation of a terminal carboxylic acid, and (5) conjugation to the amino acids, glycine and taurine.

In the major pathway for bile acid synthesis from cholesterol, there are at least nine principal reactions, each catalyzed by distinct enzymes located in various subcellular fractions within the hepatocyte (Table 1).

Step 1: Cholesterol 7α-Hydroxylase

The first step in bile acid synthesis involves the introduction of a hydroxy group at the C-7 position of the nucleus, (Fig. 3),[23] a reaction catalyzed by the microsomal enzyme, cholesterol 7α-hydroxylase.[24]

A vast literature exists on the role of cholesterol 7α-hydroxylase in bile acid synthesis that cannot be covered within the scope of this review, and the reader is directed to several excellent reviews.[10,24] This step is potentially the most important since it is rate-limiting for bile acid synthesis[25] and is subject to negative feedback regulation by the flux of bile acids returning to the liver. This was readily demonstrated from studies in rats where biliary drainage led to a 10-fold increase in cholesterol 7α-hydroxylase activity[26,27] and taurochenodeoxycholic acid infusion restored the activity to normal in this animal model.[28] Likewise, cholestyramine administration also increases the activity of cholesterol 7α-hydroxylase.

The fact that cholesterol 7α-hydroxylase regulates overall bile acid synthesis is of clinical importance from the standpoint of treatment of metabolic defects involving enzymes in the pathway, as is discussed later.

Step 2: 3β-Hydroxysteroid Dehydrogenase/Isomerase

The conversion of 7α-hydroxycholesterol to 7α-hydroxy-4-cholesten-3-one is catalyzed by a microsomal 3β-

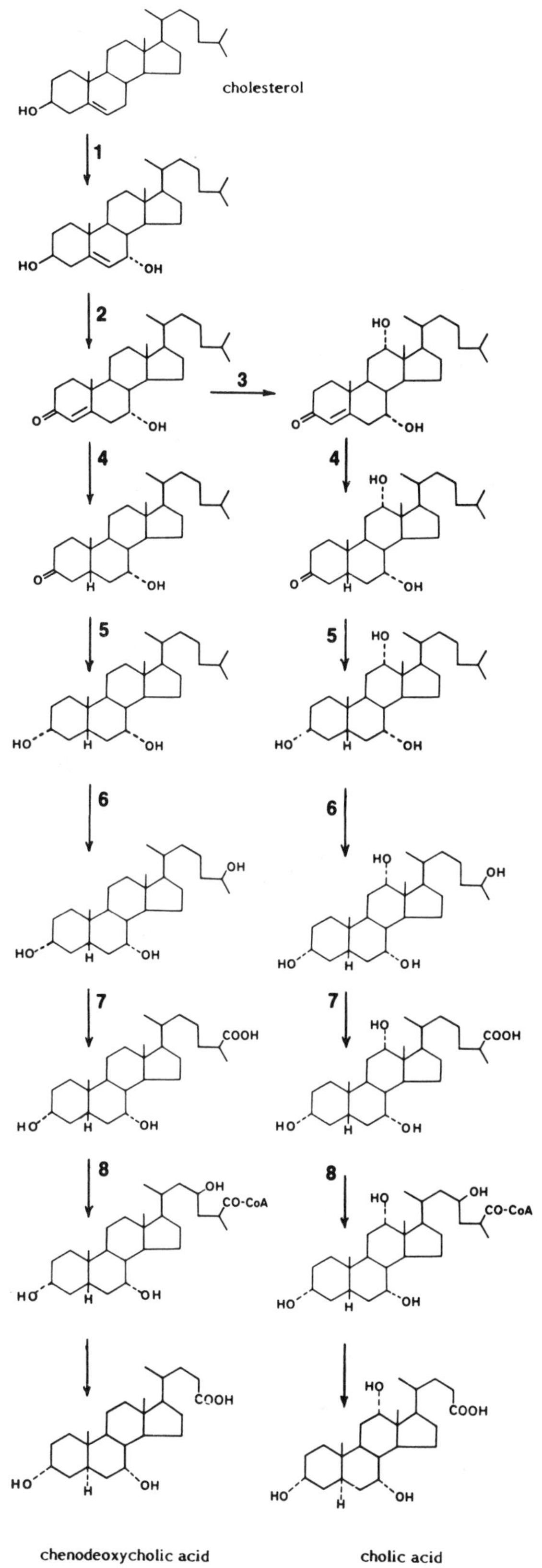

cholesterol

chenodeoxycholic acid

cholic acid

FIGURE 2 The classical biochemical pathway for primary bile acid synthesis from cholesterol indicating the principal steps to cholic and chenodeoxycholic acid formation. Each numbered reaction is catalyzed by individual hepatic enzymes listed in Table 1.

TABLE 1
Key Reactions Involved in the Formation of Bile Acids from Cholesterol

	Structural Change	Enzyme	Subcellular Location
Step 1	C-7 hydroxylation	7α-Hydroxylase	Microsomal
Step 2	Oxidation 3β-OH→3-oxo and $\Delta^5 \to \Delta^4$	3β-HSD/isomerase	Microsomal
Step 3	C-12 hydroxylation (cholic acid only)	12α-Hydroxylase	Microsomal
Step 4	Reduction of $\Delta^4 \to 5\beta$(H)	Δ^4-3-Oxosteroid 5β-reductase	Cytosolic
Step 5	Reduction of 3-oxo→3α-OH	3α-HSD	Cytosolic
Step 6	Side-chain hydroxylation at C-26	26-Hydroxylase	Mitochondrial
Step 7	Side-chain oxidation→C-26 COOH	Alcohol/acetaldehyde dehydrogenase	Cytosolic
Step 8	(i) Formation of CoA derivative	Fatty acid β-oxidation system	Peroxisomal
	(ii) Hydroxylation at C-24	Fatty acid β-oxidation system	Peroxisomal
	(iii) β-Oxidation	Fatty acid β-oxidation system	Peroxisomal
Step 9	Conjugation to amino acids	CoA ligase/amino acid acyltransferase	Microsomal and peroxisomal

hydroxysteroid dehydrogenase/isomerase enzyme (Fig. 4), and considerable effort has gone into understanding the mechanism of this relatively complex two-step reaction[29,30] involving oxidation of the 3β-hydroxy group and isomerization of the Δ^5 bond.

It is possible that 7α-hydroxy-5-cholesten-3-one is formed as the intermediate compound, but all attempts to isolate it have proved unsuccessful. It would appear that a single highly specific enzyme of molecular weight 46 kDa is responsible for catalyzing this reaction[31] and that the mechanism differs from the analogous reaction common to steroid hormone synthesis.

Step 3: 12α-Hydroxylation

The conversion of 7α-hydroxy-4-cholesten-3-one into 7α, 12α-dihydroxy-4-cholesten-3-one is catalyzed by cytochrome P-450–dependent microsomal 12α-hydroxylase (Fig. 5). This reaction is responsible for diverting sterol intermediates into the cholic acid pathway. The enzyme also shows specificity toward 5α-cholestane-3α,7α-diol and 7α-hydroxycholesterol in rabbits.

Studies in rats have shown that the introduction of a C-26 hydroxy group appears to prevent subsequent 12α-hydroxylation and that thyroid hormone inhibits its activity while stimulating microsomal C-26 hydroxylase activity.[32,33] It is probable that both enzymes may be of importance in regulating the synthesis of cholic acid in rats.[33] This, however, is not the case for humans, in whom the introduction of a C-26 hydroxy group has no inhibitory effect upon the microsomal 12α-hydroxylase activity and thyroid hormone has only a small influence upon the cholic-to-chenodeoxycholic acid ratio. These differences serve to highlight species variations that need to be considered in the use of animal models for humans. Other factors influencing microsomal 12α-hydroxylase include bile acid feeding,[34,35] which has an inhibitory effect, and cholestyramine administration, which increases the ratio of cholic-to-chenodeoxycholic acid[36] probably because of an interruption of the normal return of bile acids to the liver. Similarly, biliary drainage[25] and starvation[37] increase its activity. The fact that there appears to be no correlation between 12α-hydroxylase activity and the ratio of biliary cholic-to-chenodeoxycholic acids in humans[38] indicates that other factors, such as the extent of enterohepatic recycling, intestinal metabolism, and absorption, are important in regulating the relative proportions of intermediates that are diverted to each pathway.

Step 4: Δ^4-3-Oxosteroid 5β-Reductase

A soluble NADPH-dependent Δ^4-3-oxosteroid 5β-reductase enzyme is responsible for catalyzing the reaction that leads to the saturation of the Δ^4-bond and the formation of the 5β-(H) configuration at the AB ring junction[39,40] that is common to the majority of bile acids found in most animal species, including humans (Fig. 6).

Little is known of the factors regulating the activity of this enzyme, although when it was originally isolated and partially purified,[37,38] it was shown to have specificity toward the C_{19} and C_{21} 3-oxo-4-ene steroids. It is probable, however, that there are several enzymes with different substrate specificities.

Step 5: 3α-Hydroxysteroid Dehydrogenase

Conversion of 7α-hydroxy-5β-cholestan-3-one and 7α, 12α-dihydroxy-5β-cholestan-3-one by reduction into the respective 3α-hydroxy-analogues (Fig. 7) takes place in the cytosolic fraction under the influence of a NADPH-dependent 3α-hydroxysteroid dehydrogenase enzyme.[39–41]

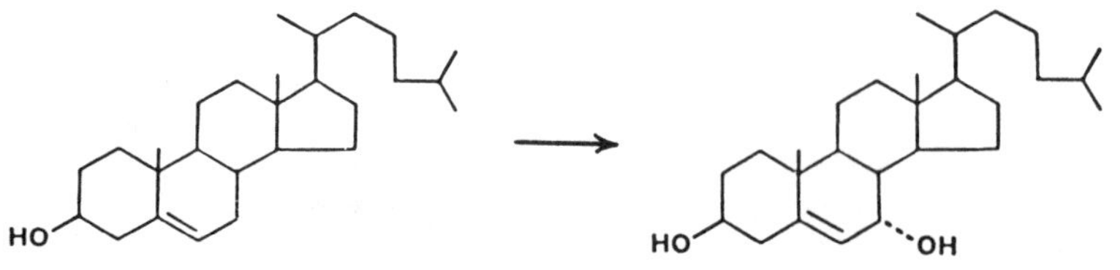

HO → HO OH

FIGURE 3 Step 1: cholesterol 7α-hydroxylase.

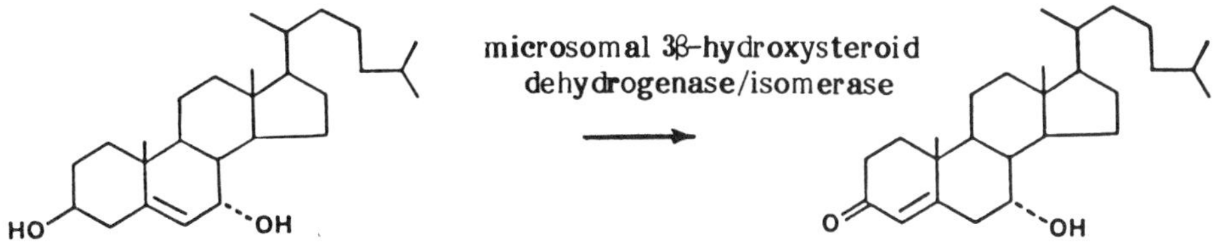

7α-hydroxycholesterol

7α-hydroxy-4-cholesten-3-one

FIGURE 4 Step 2: changes to the AB rings of the steroid nucleus.

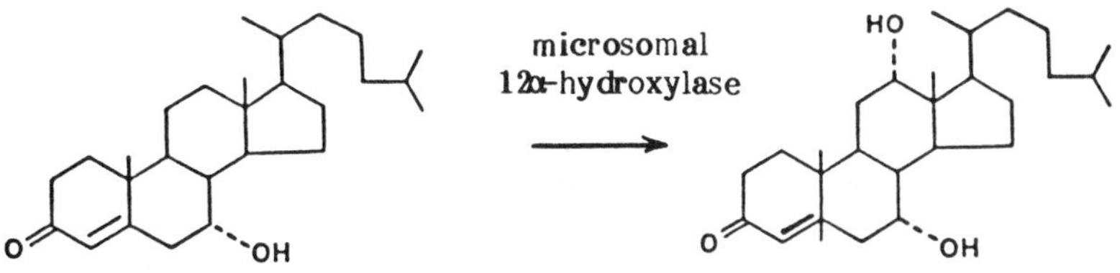

FIGURE 5 Step 3: Introduction of 12α-hydroxy group in pathway to cholic acid synthesis.

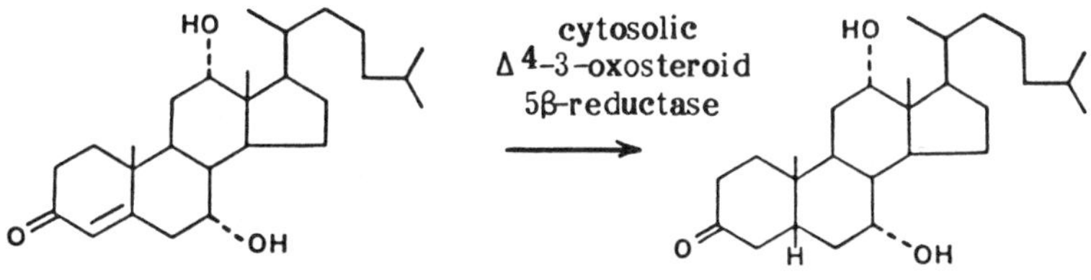

Δ 4-3-oxo group

3-oxo-5β(H)

FIGURE 6 Step 4: saturation of the steroid ring.

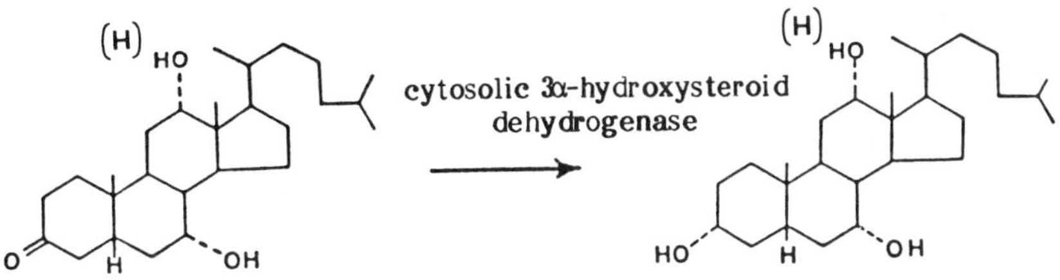

FIGURE 7 Step 5: reduction of the steroid A-ring to yield the 3α-hydroxy-5β(H) structure that is common to most bile acids found in biologic fluids of humans.

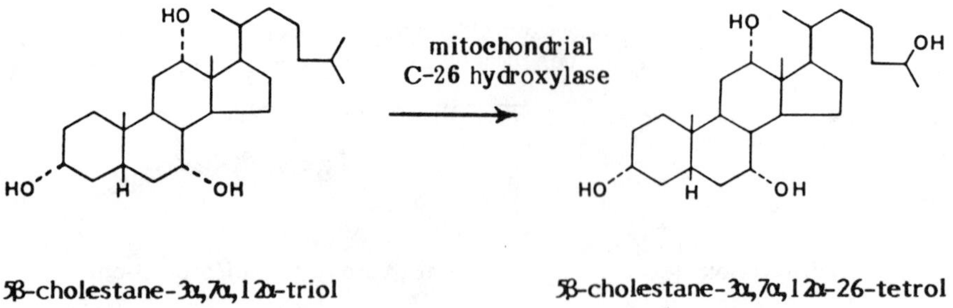

mitochondrial C-26 hydroxylase

5β-cholestane-3α,7α,12α-triol

5β-cholestane-3α,7α,12α-26-tetrol

FIGURE 8 Step 6: first step in the oxidation of the side chain: introduction of a C-26 hydroxyl group.

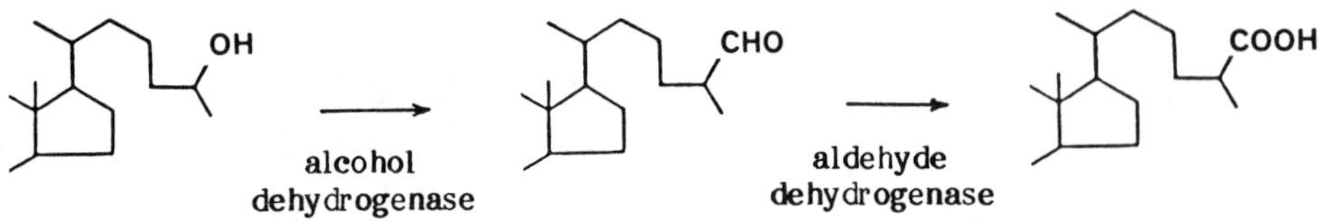

alcohol dehydrogenase

aldehyde dehydrogenase

FIGURE 9 Step 7: side-chain oxidation-formation of C_{27}-cholestanoic acids.

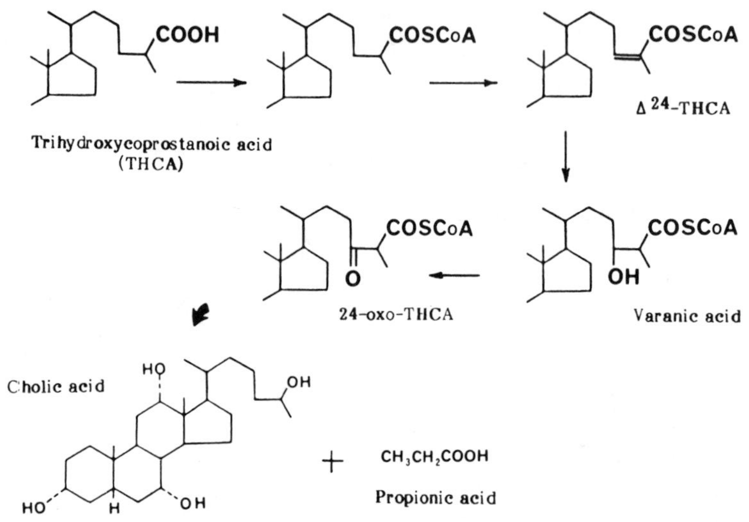

Trihydroxycoprostanoic acid (THCA)

Δ 24-THCA

Varanic acid

24-oxo-THCA

Cholic acid

+ CH_3CH_2COOH

Propionic acid

FIGURE 10 Sequence of reactions involved in the peroxisomal side-chain oxidation of cholestenoic acids to yield the C_{24}-cholanoic acid nucleus. The same sequence of reactions occurs for 3α,7α-dihydroxy-5β-cholestanoic acid (DHCA).

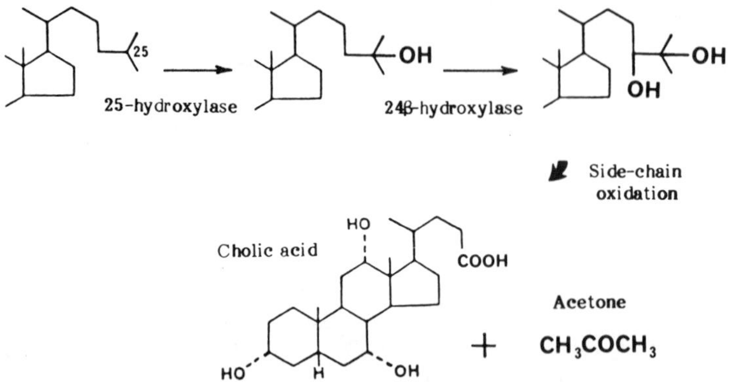

25-hydroxylase

24β-hydroxylase

Side-chain oxidation

Cholic acid

Acetone

+ CH_3COCH_3

FIGURE 11 The C-25 hydroxylation pathway leading to the formation of cholic acid in humans.

Step 6: C-26 Hydroxylase

The mechanism by which oxidation of the C_{27} sterol side chain occurs has been the subject of extensive study. Under normal conditions it would appear that the first step involves the introduction of a hydroxy group at the C-26 position (Fig. 8).

This reaction can occur in both the microsomal and mitochondrial fractions[10]; for humans, the mitochondrial C-26 hydroxylase appears quantitatively the more important. The mitochondrial C-26 hydroxylation has been shown to be stereospecific, involving hydroxylation of the 25-pro-S methyl group to yield the 26-hydroxylated product with a 25(R) configuration. On the other hand, the microsomal C-26 hydroxylation seems to involve the formation of the 25(S) product. The mitochondrial C-26 hydroxylase exhibits a broad substrate specificity but is particularly active toward 5β-cholestan-3α,7α-diol, 5β-cholestan-3α,7α,12α-triol and 7α-hydroxy-4-cholesten-3-one.[42,43] The reaction involves a cytochrome P-450 species,[44] and the enzyme can be induced by phenobarbital treatment or by starvation.

Although the microsomal C-26 hydroxylase (also cytochrome P-450 dependent) is of minor quantitative importance in humans, compared with the mitochondrial enzyme it has a higher substrate specificity in the rat.[42] The microsomal fraction of rat liver, however, hydroxylates other positions in the side chain, i.e., C-23, C-24 (α and β), and C-25, with the latter being as efficient as C-26 hydroxylation.[45]

Step 7: Formation of Cholestanoic Acids

The oxidation of the C-26 hydroxylated intermediates into the respective cholestanoic acids takes place rapidly in two steps[46] with the formation of the aldehyde as the intermediate (Fig. 9). After purification of the enzymes responsible for these reactions, it was concluded that they were identical to the hepatic ethanol dehydrogenase and aldehyde dehydrogenase enzymes (Fig. 9).[47-50]

Step 8: Oxidation of Side Chain

Oxidation of the side chain of the cholestanoic acid intermediates has been shown to involve reactions analogous to those responsible for the mitochondrial β-oxidation of fatty acids with the formation of 24α-hydroxylated and CoA derivatives and subsequent release of propionic acid (Fig. 10).[51] In the rat a microsomal system was also demonstrated,[52] but more recently it has become recognized that the peroxisomal fraction has the highest capacity for oxidation of 3α,7α,12α-trihydroxy-5β-cholestan-26-oic acid into cholic acid,[53] and it is probable that the subcellular fractions isolated in early studies of this reaction were contaminated with peroxisomes. Although in all of these studies it has not been possible to isolate a Δ^{24} intermediate, the involvement of a desaturase and a hydratase has been proven from labeled studies.[10,52]

Step 9: Conjugation of Bile Acids

After synthesis of cholic and chenodeoxycholic acids, amidation with the amino acids glycine and taurine occurs to yield the glyco- and tauro-conjugates. This reaction involves a CoA ligase and an amino acid acyltransferase.[54,55]

A microsomal bile acid CoA ligase first leads to the formation of a bile acid—CoA thioester that acts as the substrate for the cytosolic bile acid CoA:amino acid *N*-acyltransferase enzyme to conjugate with the amino acid.[56] In the normal adult the ratio of glycine-to-taurine conjugated bile acids is 3:1,[13] but this can be altered by an increased availability of taurine as occurs during taurine feeding[57] or in early life[12] where hepatic taurine stores are high[58] because of selective placental transfer.[59] The specificity of the conjugating enzymes has been studied and found to be influenced by the length and the structure of the side chain. For example, nor-bile acids (C_{23}) with a four-carbon side chain are not amidated while homo-bile acids (C_{25}) are poor substrates for the conjugating enzyme.[60]

Conjugation of bile acids in the steroid rings is a further important pathway that significantly increases the polarity of the molecule, thereby facilitating renal excretion. A sulfotransferase enzyme catalyzes the formation of bile acid sulfates,[61] most commonly at the C-3 position, but C-7 and C-12 sulfates are also found.[62] This enzyme shows sex-dependent differences in rats,[63] and its activity has been shown to be relatively low in the fetus compared with the adult.[64] This is evident from the finding of relatively small proportions of bile acid sulfates in fetal bile.[12]

Glucuronidation of bile acids is a further important pathway,[65] and a number of glucuronyl transferase enzymes catalyze the formation of both glucuronide ethers (ring conjugation) and esters (side-chain carboxyl conjugates).[15] The affinity of this conjugation system is relatively specific; for example, short-chain bile acids are preferentially glucuronidated,[66] while bile acids possessing a 6α-hydroxy group tend to form the 6-0-ethers.[67]

Several other conjugation pathways for bile acids have been recently recognized. Glucosides[17,18] and *N*-acetylglucosaminides[19] of nonamidated and glycine- and taurine-conjugated bile acids have been found in normal human urine,[18] and quantitative excretion (1 μmol per day) approximates that of bile acid glucuronides.[68] While a microsomal glucosyltransferase from human liver has been isolated and characterized,[69] and this reaction can occur in extrahepatic tissue, the mechanism of formation of the *N*-acetylglucosaminides remains to be established, although it is possible that intestinal microorganisms may play a role in their formation.

The identification of bile acid conjugates of fluorouracil highlights the fact that drug interactions with hepatic conjugation enzymes can take place and may possibly play a role in the development of drug-induced cholestasis. Following the administration of this chemotherapeutic agent, one of the major metabolites found in the bile was the 2-fluoro-β-alanine conjugate of cholic acid.[20]

Alternative Pathways for Bile Acid Synthesis

The simplified view of the pathways for bile acid synthesis described above lead to the widely held assumption that the sequence of reactions occurs in an orderly manner, with side-chain oxidation taking place after completion of the changes to the steroid nucleus. Significant advances in methods of studying biosynthetic pathways have made it evident that multiple and alternative pathways coexist.[70,71] This is particularly evident in early life and in pathologic conditions of cholestasis. Perhaps the most contentious issue has involved the relative importance of alternative pathways for primary bile acid synthesis and, in particular, those involved in side-chain oxidation.

As detailed above, side-chain oxidation proceeds with an initial C-26 hydroxylation and release of propionic acid; however, an alternative pathway (Fig. 11) involving prior C-25 hydroxylation and release of acetone has been described, and the relative quantitative importance of these two pathways has been controversial.[72] The available evidence provides overwhelming support for the C-26 hydroxylation pathway being the major pathway for bile acid synthesis in normal humans. This includes the finding of a rapid and complete conversion of 5β-cholestane-3α,7α,12α,26-tetrol and trihydroxycoprostanic acid (THCA) to cholic acid versus the incomplete conversion of the 25-hydroxylated tetrol[73,74] and lack of appreciable accumulation of 25-hydroxylated intermediates in Zellweger's syndrome.[75] Evidence in support of the 25-hydroxylation pathway being the major pathway for humans derives from the findings of Salen et al who showed that when radiolabeled THCA was administered to a healthy individual, the specific activity of cholic acid was about 20 percent of the radiolabeled precursor, suggesting that 80 percent of cholic acid bypassed the C-26 hydroxylation pathway in favor of C-25 hydroxylation.[76] These results could be artifactual and arise from methodologic difficulties of achieving equilibrium, or because of prior metabolism of the administered precursor. In a recent study the quantitative importance of the C-25 hydroxylation pathways was assessed in vivo by measuring the production of [^{14}C] acetone following prior labeling of the cholesterol pool with [26-^{14}C] cholesterol.[77] These elegant studies concluded that in the adult rat the C-25 hydroxylation pathway accounted for less than 2 percent of the total bile synthesis,[77] while for humans this value was less than 5 percent.[78]

An alternative pathway for chenodeoxycholic acid synthesis[79] that is seemingly important in early life involves side-chain shortening prior to nuclear modifications, reactions that are initiated via a cholesterol C-26 hydroxylase (Fig. 12). In this pathway, 26-hydroxycholesterol is converted to 3β-hydroxy-5-cholenoic acid, lithocholic acid, and finally to chenodeoxycholic acid.[80-85]. Although this pathway may be of minor importance in the adult, it probably accounts for the increased levels of 3β-hydroxy-5-cholenoic and lithocholic acids in early life and in severe cholestatic conditions.

The synthesis of *allo*-(5α-H) bile acids warrants discussion. In many lower vertebrates *allo*-bile acids are the major species of bile acids.[9] However, in humans they are normally present in relatively small proportions and are generally believed to result from bacterial metabolism of 3-oxo-5β-bile acids during the course of their enterohepatic circulation. Studies of rodents have indicated that *allo*-bile acids may also be derived from 5α-cholestanol,[86,87] which can be efficiently 7α-hydroxylated in rat liver[88] and subsequently converted to 7α-hydroxy-5α-cholestan-3-one and then to 5α-cholestane-3α,7α-diol.[89] The 12α-hydroxylase enzyme shows a high specificity toward the 5α-sterols[90-92] and 5α-cholestane-3α,7α,12α-triol is readily formed from 5α-cholestane-3α,7α-diol, and then converted to *allo*-cholic acid in the bile fistula rat.[89]

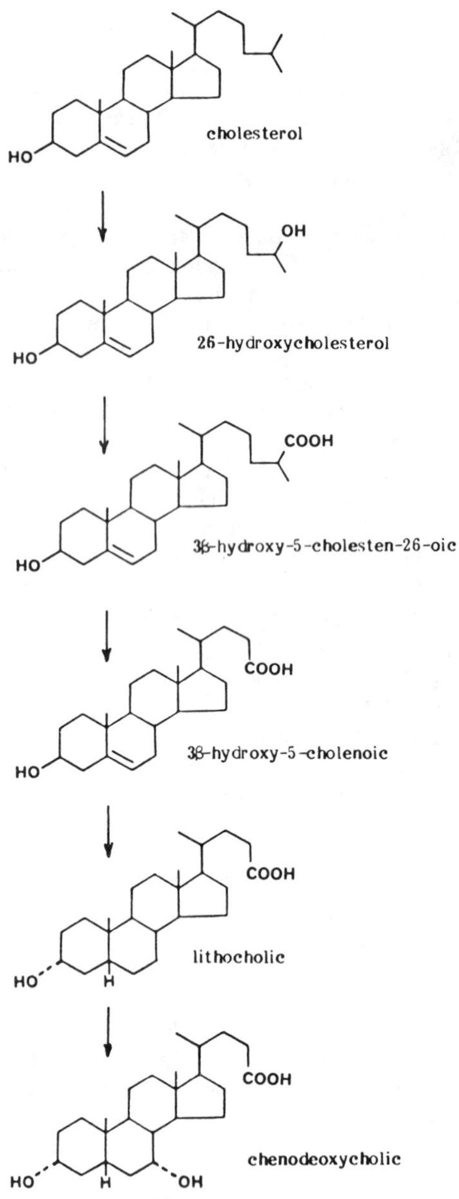

FIGURE 12 The Yamasaki pathway to chenodeoxycholic acid synthesis. Side-chain oxidation precedes changes to the nucleus.

A further mechanism for the formation of *allo*-bile acids involves their direct conversion from 7α-hydroxy-4-cholesten-3-one and 7α,12α-dihydroxy-4-cholesten-3-one by the action of an active Δ^4-3-oxosteroid 5α-reductase. This reaction has been demonstrated in rats, where the enzyme shows a three- to fourfold higher activity in female compared with male rats,[93] but no sex differences have been demonstrated for humans. Indeed, the quantitative importance of this reaction in humans is uncertain, but recently large amounts of *allo*-bile acids were present in patients with a deficiency in the bile acid^4-3-oxosteroid 5β-reductase enzyme.[5,6] It is probable, therefore, that in humans the substrate specificity of the 5β-reductase is so much higher than the corresponding 5α-reductase, that 5β-bile acids are preferentially formed from the corresponding 3-oxo-4-ene sterol intermediates. Only in the absence of this reaction does the 5α-reductase become quantitatively important.

Finally, it should also be realized that intestinal microflora play an important role in bile acid metabolism[94] and in the maintenance of the integrity of the enterohepatic circulation. Lithocholic (3α-hydroxy-5β-cholanoic acid) and deoxycholic (3α, 12α-dihydroxy-5β-cholanoic) acids are the principal bile acids referred to as the "secondary" bile acids. Both are formed following the deconjugation and 7α-dehydroxylation of the primary bile acids, conjugated chenodeoxycholic and cholic acids. Lithocholic acid is relatively insoluble and is consequently poorly absorbed from the intestinal lumen. It is found in relatively high proportions in the meconium[95] and amniotic fluid[96,97] but is barely detectable in fetal bile.[12] In severe cholestatic conditions, deoxycholic acid levels in the serum become undetectable, and this bile acid appears to be a useful marker of the extent of impairment of the enterohepatic circulation. Alternatively, elevations in the serum unconjugated bile acid concentrations,[98] particularly of secondary bile acids, will reflect increased bacterial activity as occurs in bacterial overgrowth of the small bowel.[99,100] On the other hand, severe cholestasis frequently results in elevations in lithocholic acid, generally as the sulfate conjugate,[101] indicating that under this condition lithocholic acid is a primary product of hepatic synthesis. Synthesis is presumed to take place via the Yamasaki pathway[79] discussed earlier, i.e., oxidation of 3β-hydroxy-5-cholenoic acid, which has been documented to occur in experimental animals.[84]

BILE ACID SYNTHESIS DURING EARLY DEVELOPMENT

Until recently, knowledge of hepatic bile acid synthesis and metabolism during human development was limited, although ontogenic studies have been carried out in several animal species.[64,102–108] Detailed analytic studies of human fetal gallbladder bile[12,109] and in vitro studies of hepatic subcellular fractions[110,111] have been carried out that have led to an appreciation that significant qualitative and quantitative differences occur with regard to bile acid synthesis and metabolism between the developing and adult livers. Since biliary excretion is the principal route for bile acid secretion, the analysis of gallbladder bile permits a direct means of assessing hepatic synthesis and secretion.

The earliest studies of human fetal gallbladder bile were performed approximately 20 years ago using methodology less advanced than is currently available but nevertheless established that primary bile acid synthesis was relatively well developed during early gestation.[112,113] These early studies showed that the concentration of chenodeoxycholic acid was greater than cholic acid in midgestation and that these primary bile acids were conjugated mainly to taurine.[112,113] These findings were recently corroborated and extended using improved methodology,[12,109] and they confirmed that pathways for primary bile acid synthesis were developed as early as the twelfth week of gestation. The observation that chenodeoxycholic acid concentrations exceed those of cholic acid at this stage of human development, and the relatively low total biliary bile acid concentration markedly contrasts the biliary bile acid composition of the full-term infant or the adult, where cholic acid is the predominant bile acid.[114,115] These differences are also found in amniotic fluid examined at different times during gestation.[97] The reason for these differences is unclear, but several possibilities may account for these data. Cholic acid synthesis may be reduced in early life as a consequence of a relative immaturity in hepatic 12α-hydroxylase activity. However, in vitro studies appear to indicate that 12α-hydroxylase activity is reasonably well developed at this stage of gestation.[116] Preferential clearance of cholic acid by metabolism to more polar C-1, C-2, C-4, or C-6 tetrahydroxy bile acids would lead to a relative increase in the proportion of chenodeoxycholic acid. Recent studies indicate, however, that tetrahydroxy bile acids constituted less than 2 percent of the total biliary bile acids of the human fetus.[12] The most likely explanation is that alternative pathways for the synthesis of chenodeoxycholic acid predominate during early life; a biosynthetic pathway involving the side chain hydroxylation of cholesterol prior to nuclear modification has been described that leads to chenodeoxycholic acid synthesis via 3β-hydroxy-5-cholenoic and lithocholic acids.[79–87] If this pathway is quantitatively important, significant amounts of these monohydroxy bile acids would be expected, and although these are barely detectable in fetal bile,[12] relatively high proportions can be found in meconium.[95]

The most obvious feature of bile acid synthesis and metabolism during development is the relatively large proportion of a complex array of bile acids not typically found in adult bile[11] (Fig. 13). Interestingly, the profile of biologic fluids of the newborn and fetus[12,109] resembles that observed for adult patients with severe cholestasis.[117,118] Analysis of human fetal gallbladder bile[12,109] and in vitro incubations of hepatic subcellular fractions with radiolabeled bile acids have served to confirm the quantitative importance of several hepatic hydroxylation pathways including C-6 and C-1 hydroxylation.[110,111] Hyocholic acid (3α,6α,7α-trihydroxy-5β-cholanoic acid) is a major biliary bile acid of the fetus, and concentrations often exceed cholic acid concentrations[12] while a series of C-1 hydroxy isomers can also be found.[12,109]

1β-Hydroxylation has been demonstrated in vitro by human fetal microsomes,[110] and several C-1 hydroxylated bile acid isomers have been found in the urine of healthy adults [117] and infants[119], in meconium,[2,95,120] and in biologic fluids from patients with liver disease.[118,121] Recently a novel and previously unknown hydroxylation pathway, C-4 hydroxylation, was revealed that was suggested to be unique to early human development.[12,122] 3α,4β,7α-Trihydroxy-5β-cholanoic acid accounted for 5 to 15 percent of the total biliary bile acids in early gestation, raising questions regarding the physiologic importance of this metabolic pathway.

Secondary bile acids can be found in fetal bile but only in very small proportions. This is consistent with the lack of bacterial flora in the fetal gut and the maternal fetal placental transport of secondary bile acids that has been demonstrated in vivo[104,106] and in vitro.[123]

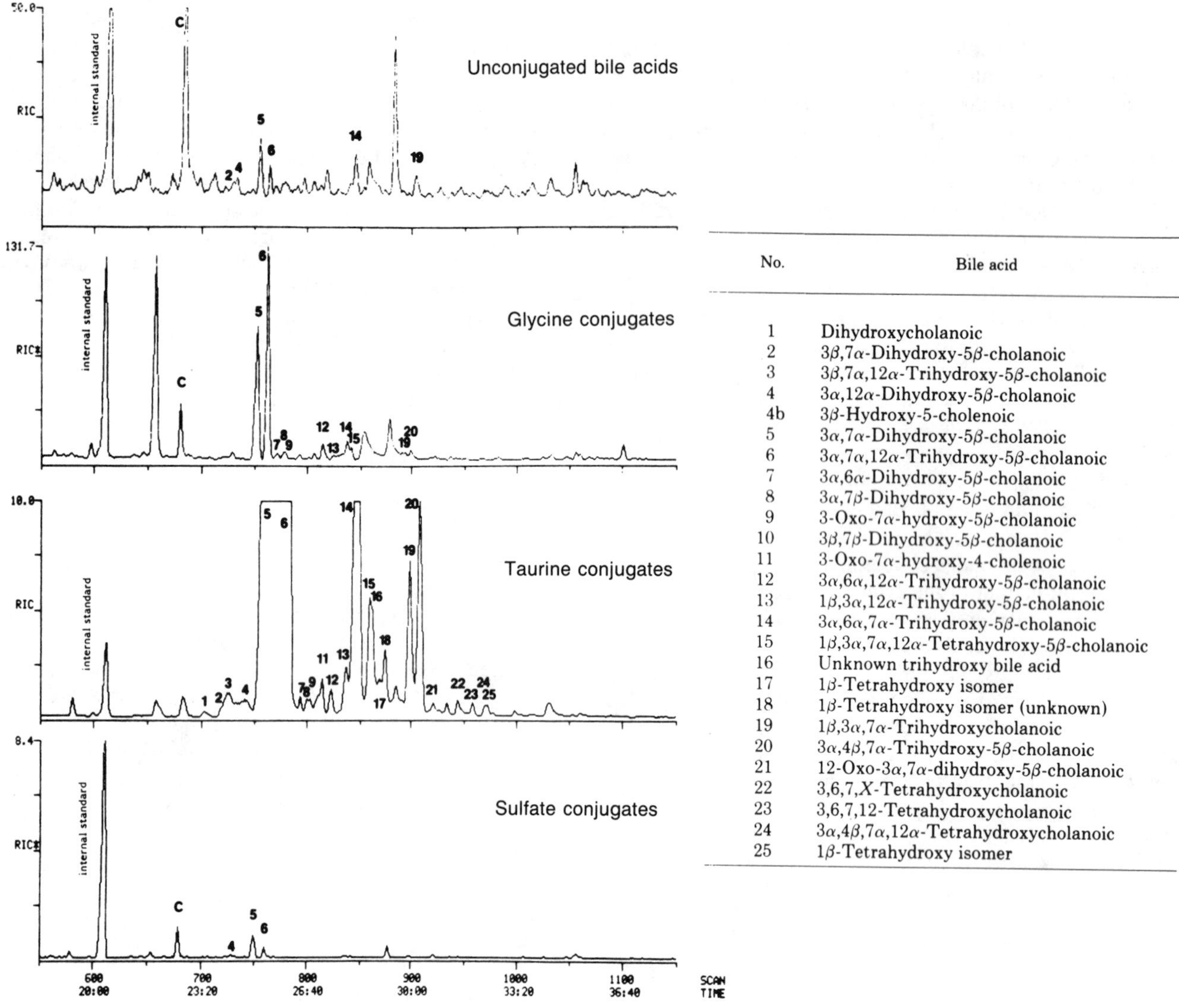

No.	Bile acid
1	Dihydroxycholanoic
2	3β,7α-Dihydroxy-5β-cholanoic
3	3β,7α,12α-Trihydroxy-5β-cholanoic
4	3α,12α-Dihydroxy-5β-cholanoic
4b	3β-Hydroxy-5-cholenoic
5	3α,7α-Dihydroxy-5β-cholanoic
6	3α,7α,12α-Trihydroxy-5β-cholanoic
7	3α,6α-Dihydroxy-5β-cholanoic
8	3α,7β-Dihydroxy-5β-cholanoic
9	3-Oxo-7α-hydroxy-5β-cholanoic
10	3β,7β-Dihydroxy-5β-cholanoic
11	3-Oxo-7α-hydroxy-4-cholenoic
12	3α,6α,12α-Trihydroxy-5β-cholanoic
13	1β,3α,12α-Trihydroxy-5β-cholanoic
14	3α,6α,7α-Trihydroxy-5β-cholanoic
15	1β,3α,7α,12α-Tetrahydroxy-5β-cholanoic
16	Unknown trihydroxy bile acid
17	1β-Tetrahydroxy isomer
18	1β-Tetrahydroxy isomer (unknown)
19	1β,3α,7α-Trihydroxycholanoic
20	3α,4β,7α-Trihydroxy-5β-cholanoic
21	12-Oxo-3α,7α-dihydroxy-5β-cholanoic
22	3,6,7,X-Tetrahydroxycholanoic
23	3,6,7,12-Tetrahydroxycholanoic
24	3α,4β,7α,12α-Tetrahydroxycholanoic
25	1β-Tetrahydroxy isomer

FIGURE 13 Reconstructed total ion current chromatograms following GC-MS analysis of the methyl ester–trimethylsilyl ether derivatives of bile acids isolated according to their mode of conjugation from human fetal bile using lipophilic anion exchange chromatography. GC-MS conditions were as follows: GC column, 30 meters × 0.4 mm inner diameter; DB-1 fused silica; temperature-programmed operation 225 to 295°C with increments of 2°C per minute following initial and final isothermal periods of 5 and 20 minutes, respectively; mass spectrometry performed in electron impact ionization (70 eV) mode with repetitive scanning, 2 seconds per cycle, of the GC effluent; internal standard, coprostanol; C, residual cholesterol in sample. Bile acids were identified from their mass spectra and retention indices.

The principal bile acid conjugation reaction of the fetal liver involves amidation with taurine (Fig. 14). In fetal bile, 85 percent of the total biliary bile acids are taurine conjugates,[12] markedly contrasting the pattern for adult bile where the glycine-to-taurine ratio is approximately 3:1.[13] This reflects the increased accumulation and availability of taurine in the fetal liver[58] resulting from selective placental transport.[59]

Bile acid sulfates, which are generally increased in cholestatic conditions in adults,[101,117,124-126] are virtually absent in early gestation.[12] This probably reflects an immaturity in the bile acid sulfotransferase enzyme in early life or may be a consequence of additional and preferential metabolism of bile acids by hydroxylation. By contrast, lithocholic acid sulfate and 3β-hydroxy-5-cholenoic acid sulfate are found in relatively large proportions in the meconium[95] and amniotic fluid.[96,97,127]

Meconium has also been shown to contain a series of short-chain bile acids that are monohydroxylated.[128-130] These compounds possess a steroid nucleus of 20-, 21- and 22-carbon atoms and are predominantly found as the glucuronide or sulfate conjugates.[66,130] In contrast to the monohydroxy-C_{24} bile acids that are cholestatic, the major short chain bile acid, etianic acid (3α-hydroxy-5β-androstan-17β-carboxylic acid) produces a marked choleresis in the rat[66] indicating how

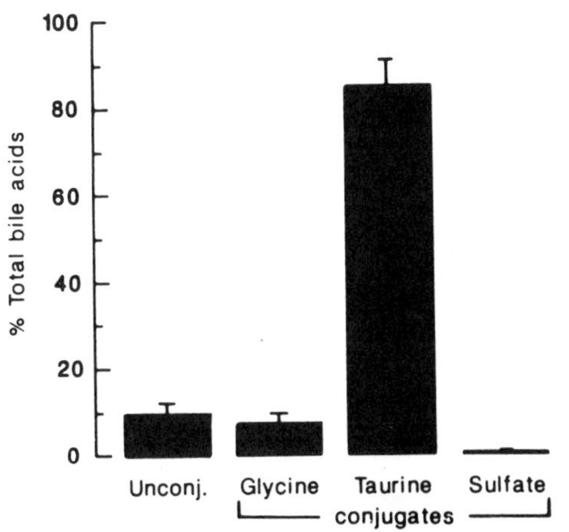

FIGURE 14 Histogram showing the relative proportions (mean ±SD) of unconjugated and conjugated bile acids found in human fetal bile during early gestation (weeks 16 to 19). (From Setchell et al.[12])

relatively small changes in the steroid nucleus are associated with marked differences in physiologic properties. The origin of these short-chain bile acids is unknown, but their close similarity in structure to steroid hormones might indicate that they may be metabolic products of steroid hormones formed during pregnancy.

INBORN ERRORS IN BILE ACID SYNTHESIS

The earliest defect in bile acid synthesis to be reported was the lipid-storage disease of cerebrotendinous xanthomatosis.[131] Later the cerebrohepatorenal syndrome of Zellweger[132] was described, which should be considered as a metabolic defect secondary to organelle dysfunction. Studies of these defects have greatly increased our understanding of normal pathways for bile acid synthesis. During the last 5 years and largely as a consequence of improvements in analytical techniques,[1] two new defects in bile acid synthesis associated with familial neonatal hepatitis syndromes have been described,[3-6] and further inborn errors may be found in the future.

Disorders in Bile Acid Metabolism Affecting Side-Chain Oxidation

Cerebrotendinous Xanthomatosis

Cerebrotendinous xanthomatosis (CTX) is a rare inherited lipid storage disease, first described by Van Bogaert et al,[131] that has an estimated prevalence of 1:70,000. Characteristic features of the disease include progressive neurologic dysfunction, dementia, ataxia, cataracts, and the presence of xanthomatous lesions in the brain and tendons. Biochemically the disease can be distinguished from other conditions involving xanthomatous deposits by (1) a significantly reduced synthesis of primary bile acids; (2) an elevated biliary, urinary, and fecal excretion of bile alcohol glucuronides; (3) a low plasma cholesterol concentration with deposition of cholesterol and cholestanol in the tissues; and (4) a markedly elevated level (10- to 100-fold) of cholestanol. Elegant studies by Salen and co-workers[133,134] demonstrated the metabolic defect to result from an impairment in oxidation of the cholesterol side-chain and that chenodeoxycholic acid synthesis is reduced to a greater extent than cholic acid synthesis.[135-137]

Controversy has existed over the exact nature of the biochemical defect in CTX, but the primary defect would appear to be due to a deficiency in mitochondrial C_{27}-steroid-26-hydroxylase (Fig. 15).

Evidence in support of this contention is derived from the findings that (1) the mitochondrial fraction of the liver from a patient with CTX was shown to be completely devoid of

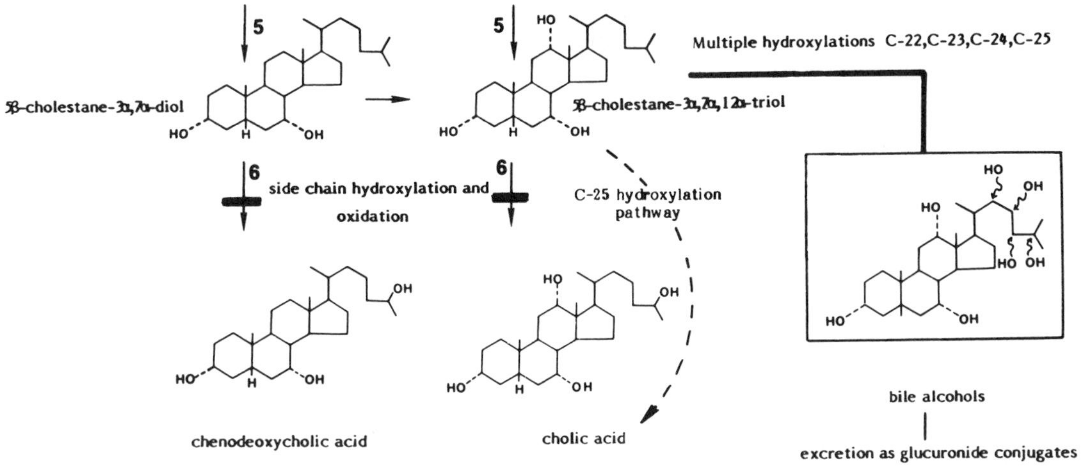

FIGURE 15 Metabolic defect in cerebrotendinous xanthomatosis (CTX) resulting in diminished primary bile acid synthesis and excessive production of bile alcohols.

26-hydroxylase activity[138]; (2) the amounts of 5β-cholestane-3α,7α,12α-triol, the substrate for this enzyme, in liver homogenates was 50-fold greater than normal[138]; (3) the serum of patients with CTX has no detectable or markedly reduced levels of 26-hydroxycholesterol compared with normal[139]; (4) intravenous administration of radiolabeled precursors showed that only those precursors having a C-26 hydroxy group were converted to cholic acid;[138] (5) the spectrum of bile alcohol glucuronides resulting from the biochemical defect are extensively polyhydroxylated in the side chain at all positions except C-26.

To explain the findings of greatly increased amounts of 5β-cholestane-3α,7α,12α, 25-tetrol, Salen et al[136] proposed a deficiency in microsomal 24(S)-hydroxylation; this reaction normally yields 5β-cholestane-3α,7α,12α, 24, 25-pentol. Studies using this radiolabeled cholestanepentol have shown it can be converted to cholic acid, indicating an alternative pathway to the classical C-26 hydroxylation pathway for cholic acid synthesis,[72,133] but the quantitative importance of this pathway in health is relatively minor.[78] If the primary defect in CTX is a deficiency in 24(S)-hydroxylase, this would not explain the greatly reduced synthesis of chenodeoxycholic acid,[140] which in humans is synthesized via the C-26 hydroxylation pathway. A deficiency in C-26 hydroxylase on the other hand would lead to elevations in 5β-cholestane-3α,7α-diol and 7α-hydroxy-4-cholesten-3-one,[141] thus making them more available for 12α-hydroxylation and preferential conversion to cholic acid via the C-25 hydroxylation pathway.[142] Interestingly, microsomal 12α-hydroxylase activity has been shown to be threefold higher in patients with CTX.[137]

Irrespective of the exact nature of the defect, the impaired oxidation of the cholesterol side chain results in accelerated cholesterol synthesis and metabolism that leads to greatly increased production and excretion of bile alcohol glucuronides.[134,143-148] These bile alcohols have the common 5β-cholestane-3α,7α,12α-triol nucleus with additional hydroxy groups in the side chain, specifically at the C-22, C-23, C-24, and C-25 positions (Fig. 12). The major bile alcohol excreted in bile and feces is the 5β-cholestane-3α,7α,12α,25-tetrol,[134,145,148,149] while the more polar 5β-cholestane-3α,7α,12α,23,25-pentol predominates in urine.[146,148,150] It has been suggested that the difference in these patterns could be due either to more efficient renal excretion of the more polar pentol or as a result of renal C-23 hydroxylation of 5β-cholestane-3α,7α,12α,25-tetrol.[148,149] The virtual absence of bile alcohols with a C-26 hydroxy group would further support the primary defect to be due to a deficiency in hepatic C-26 hydroxylase.

The elevation in a 5α-cholestan-3β-ol (cholestanol) in the nervous system of CTX patients first observed by Menkes et al[15] and the high plasma concentrations of this sterol[136] are unique features of the disease. An elevated plasma cholestanol-to-cholesterol ratio has been proposed as a means of diagnosis,[152] but it should be realized that this is not specific to CTX because elevations may also occur in liver disease. The origins of the increased cholestanol may be from elevations in the precursor sterol, 4-cholesten-3-one; hepatic microsomes prepared from CTX patients have been shown to produce three times more 4-cholesten-3-one than similar preparations from healthy controls.[153] Using pulse-labeling techniques Salen et al[153] showed that 4-cholesten-3-one would yield labeled cholestanol, while the corresponding 7α-hydroxy intermediate was converted to bile acids. An alternative and novel pathway for the formation of cholestanol that did not involve the 7α-hydroxy intermediates was proposed by the late Skrede and co-workers.[154,155] It was suggested that hepatic rather than intestinal 7α-dehydroxylation occurred to produce a cholesten-4, 6-dien-3-one intermediate. Circumstantial evidence in support of this pathway would include (1) the increased cholesterol 12α-hydroxylase activity found in CTX because of reduced bile acid feedback, (2) the increased availability of 7α-hydroxylated intermediates, and (3) the observation that cholestyramine treatment, which stimulates cholesterol 7α-hydroxylase activity, leads to increased cholestanol output in CTX, whereas the opposite response occurs during chenodeoxycholic acid feeding. The neurologic dysfunction observed in CTX appears to be a manifestation of cholestanol deposition in the tissues.

Peroxisomal Disorders

The peroxisomes are ubiquitous subcellular organelles that were first recognized in the cytoplasm of the mouse kidney cells.[156] They were originally thought to have limited function, but later were recognized to play a key role in the β-oxidation of fatty acids.[157] They have since been shown to be responsible for as many as 40 enzyme reactions, including the peroxisomal synthesis of cholesterol,[158] and are essential for the biosynthesis of primary bile acids.[53,159]

Genetic defects involving peroxisomes include the cerebrohepatorenal Zellweger's syndrome[132] and related diseases. These conditions may be classified into three main groups according to the extent of peroxisomal dysfunction (Table 2).

The syndromes in which there is a generalized impairment in numerous peroxisomal functions as a consequence of a markedly reduced or undetectable number of peroxisomes include Zellweger's syndrome,[132,160,161] infantile Refsum's disease,[162] neonatal adrenoleukodystrophy,[163] hyperpipecolic acidemia,[164] and rhizomelic chondrodysplasia punctata,[165] and these conditions share many similarities in their clinical

TABLE 2
Peroxisomal Disorders

A. Genetic diseases with a general impairment of numerous peroxisomal functions and reduced or undetectable peroxisome numbers
   1. Cerebrohepatorenal (Zellweger's) syndrome[132,160,161]
   2. Infantile Refsum's disease[162]
   3. Neonatal adrenoleukodystrophy[163]
   4. Hyperpipecolic acidemia*[164]
   5. Rhizomelic chondrodysplasia punctata*[165]

B. Genetic diseases with generalized impairment of peroxisomal function but normal number of peroxisomes
   1. Pseudo-Zellweger's syndrome[166]

C. Genetic diseases with a single enzyme defect and a normal number of peroxisomes
   1. X-linked adrenoleukodystrophy[163]
   2. Adult Refsum's disease*[167]
   3. Acatalasemia[168]

*The number of peroxisomes has not been documented in these disorders. (From Setch KDR, Street JM. Inborn errors of bile acid synthesis. Semin Liver Dis 1987; 7:85–99.)

presentation and neurologic manifestation. These include severe hypotonia, psychomotor retardation, hepatomegaly, simian crease, craniofacial dysmorphism, and failure to thrive.[169] Pseudo-Zellweger's syndrome,[166] a condition in which there is a generalized impairment in peroxisomal dysfunction but a normal number of peroxisomes, shows many clinical and pathologic similarities to Zellweger's syndrome.

Only those disorders with a generalized impairment of peroxisomal function have been found to have abnormal bile acid synthesis reflected by an accumulation of bile acid precursors.[2] Although both the mitochondrial and microsomal fractions have been shown to convert 3α,7α,12α-trihydroxy-5β-cholestan-26-oic acid into cholic acid, it is the peroxisomal fraction that has the highest capacity for this reaction.[53] For this reason, elevated levels of trihydroxycoprostanic and dihydroxycoprostanic acids are consistently found in biologic fluids of patients with Zellweger's syndrome, neonatal adrenoleukodystrophy, and pseudo-Zellweger's syndrome, and in infantile Refsum's disease (Fig. 16). Interestingly these long-chain C_{27} bile acids are not found in rhizomelic chondrodysplasia punctata,[165] and there appear to have been no studies of bile acid metabolism in hyperpipecolic acidemia[164] and acatalasemia.[168]

The presence of other bile acid precursors is not uncommon in these conditions, and it is possible that earlier descriptions of increased proportions of bile acid precursors in children with intrahepatic biliary atresia may have been due to the failure to recognize milder variants of the Zellweger's syndrome.[170,171] The in vivo and in vitro capacity of the liver to convert bile acid precursors into cholic and chenodeoxycholic by patients with Zellweger's syndrome was studied by Kase et al.[53,75,172] Tritiated 7α-hydroxy-4-cholesten-3-one was rapidly converted to dihydroxycoprostanic acid (DHCA) and THCA but only slowly converted to cholic and chenodeoxycholic acids with only 10 percent conversion after 48 hours, while cholic acid and chenodeoxycholic acid pool sizes and synthesis rates were markedly reduced. These data confirm that there is a deficiency in side-chain cleavage of the cholestanoic precursors and highlight the important role of the peroxisome in bile acid synthesis.[173] Frequently levels of DHCA are lower than THCA—this condition may be accounted for by alternative pathways for the formation of chenodeoxycholic acid, or because of transformation by 12α-hydroxylation to THCA.[174] Despite the reported low bile acid synthesis rate,[75] many studies have shown normal or increased serum levels of primary bile acids in patients with peroxisomal disorders. This may be a consequence of impaired hepatic uptake of bile acids because of generalized hepatic dysfunction.

In addition to DHCA, THCA, and varanic acid (the C-24 hydroxylated derivative of THCA), other atypical bile acids have been identified in the Zellweger's syndrome. A C_{29}-dicarboxylic acid is a major component of the serum[175,176] and although not always present it can account for up to 40 percent of the total serum bile acids in Zellweger's syndrome and infantile Refsum's disease.[75,175,177-180] The biosynthetic pathway leading to the production of this unusual bile acid is uncertain. Administration of tritiated 5β-cholestane-3α,7α,12α-triol and THCA to a patient with Zellweger's syndrome showed only a slow conversion to the C_{29} bile acid, however, its accumulation in serum may be accounted for by its relatively poor renal clearance and biliary excre-

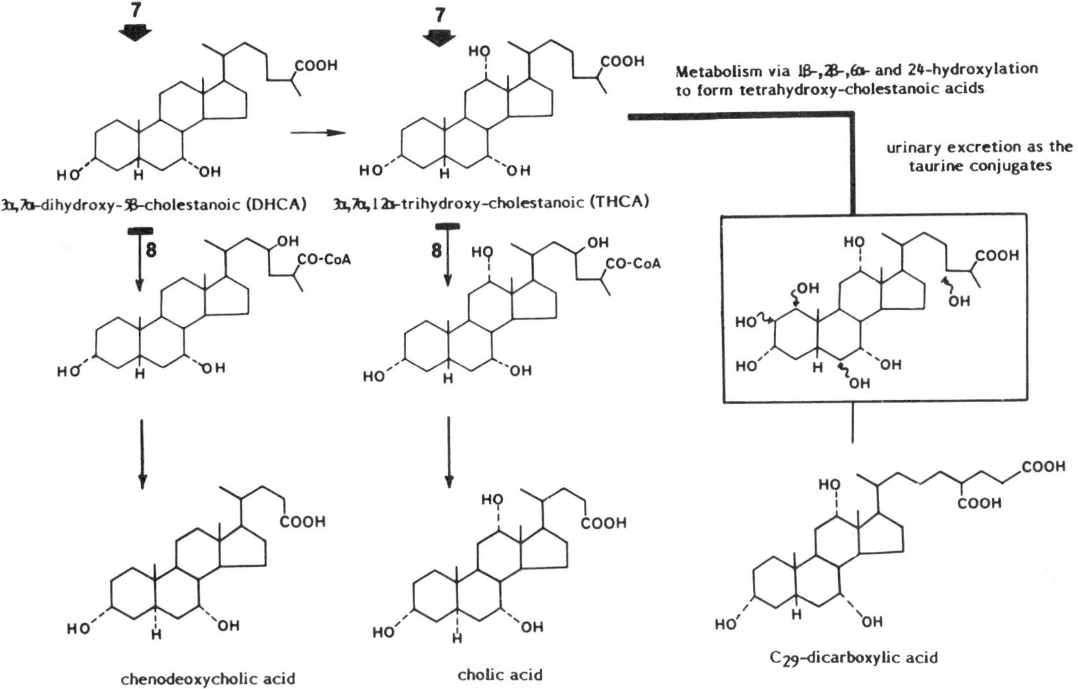

FIGURE 16 Biochemical abnormalities occurring in the cerebrohepatorenal Zellweger's syndrome resulting in diminished bile acid synthesis and increased production of long-chain cholestanoic acids.

tion. Monohydroxy C_{27} bile acids also found in the serum of patients with Zellweger's syndrome include 3α-hydroxy-5β-cholestan-26-oic and 3β-hydroxy-5-cholesten-26-oic acids.[175,181] In contrast to other cholestatic conditions only low concentrations of 3β-hydroxy-5-cholenoic acid have been reported in the serum and urine of three patients with Zellweger's syndrome.[175]

Perhaps not surprisingly, in view of the predominance of 1β- and 6α-hydroxylation pathways in early life,[12,109] the urine of these patients generally contains large proportions of 1β- and 6α-hydroxylated tetrahydroxycholestanoic acids that are mainly conjugated with taurine.[179] These probably arise from metabolism of the accumulated THCA and DHCA[75] as a means of facilitating the excretion of these bile acid intermediates. These rather specific metabolites provide a useful means of diagnosing Zellweger's and pseudo-Zellweger's syndrome when fast atom bombardment–mass spectrometry (FAB-MS) is employed, since the spectra revealed an intense ion of *m/z* (mass-to-charge ratio) 572 corresponding to the presence of taurine conjugated tetrahydroxycholestanoic acids.[179]

Disorders in Bile Acid Metabolism Involving Changes to the Steroid Nucleus

Until recently there had been no reports of defects in bile acid synthesis affecting early steps in the conversion of cholesterol to cholic and chenodeoxycholic acids, nor had any defect been associated with neonatal hepatitis syndromes. In the last 2 years, however, two new metabolic defects were described, a 3β-hydroxysteroid dehydrogenase/isomerase deficiency[3,4] and a Δ^4-3-oxosteroid-5β-reductase deficiency.[5,6] In both instances these defects were associated with familial giant cell hepatitis and neonatal cholestasis.

3β-Hydroxysteroid Dehydrogenase/Isomerase Deficiency

In this first metabolic defect to be described involving early steps in the bile acid biosynthetic pathway, the affected patient was the fifth child born to Saudi-Arabian parents who were first cousins. This infant was the third to be affected by progressive liver disease from birth; the previous infants had both died within the first few years following similar clinical histories. Jaundice, pale stools, and dark urine were noted on the third day of life and by 3 months of age biochemical indices of liver function were consistent with cholestasis, hepatocellular damage, and fat-soluble vitamin malabsorption, however, initial studies failed to detect cholic or chenodeoxycholic acids in the plasma leading to speculation of an inborn error. Consent for a liver biopsy was denied, but liver biopsies of the previous two siblings revealed a cholestasis, an aggressive hepatitis, and the presence of giant cells and fibrosis.

Analysis of the urine from this patient by gas chromatography–mass spectrometry (GC-MS) indicated the presence of a series of methoxylated trimethylsiloxy derivatives of methylcholenoates (unsaturated bile acids) that were artifacts of the sample work-up and led to suspicion of the presence of bile acids having an allylic hydroxy group.[4] Direct analysis of the urine by FAB-MS confirmed the presence of large amounts (equivalent to approximately 10 mg per day excretion) of (unsaturated) dihydroxy- and trihydroxy-cholenoates as the sulfate and glyco-sulfate conjugates.[3,4] This negative ion FAB-MS spectrum was unique and significantly different from the spectra typically observed for cholestatic patients in which primary bile acid synthesis is unimpaired.[2] Milder methods of hydrolysis of these acid labile bile acid conjugates led to their identification by GC-MS as having structures consistent with 3β,7α-dihydroxy-5-cholenoic and 3β,7α,12α-trihydroxy-5-cholenoic acids. These findings indicated a defect in bile acid synthesis. In the major pathway of bile acid synthesis from cholesterol, 7α-hydroxycholesterol is oxidized to 7α-hydroxy-4-cholesten-3-one, a reaction that is catalyzed by a microsomal 3β-hydroxysteroid-Δ^5-steroid dehydrogenase/isomerase enzyme (step 2 in the pathway). This reaction did not take place in this infant, presumably because of an absence of the enzyme, and this resulted in the failure to synthesize primary bile acids with the concomitant production and accumulation of increased quantities of 3β-hydroxy-Δ^5 sterol intermediates that subsequently undergo side-chain oxidation to yield C_{24} bile acids retaining the nuclear structure of 7α-hydroxycholesterol (Fig. 17). These findings confirm that oxidation of the cholesterol side chain can occur prior to completion of the reactions involved in modification of the steroid ring structure.

A 3β-hydroxysteroid Δ^5 steroid dehydrogenase/isomerase is also involved in the synthesis of the steroid hormones, but it has been shown that different enzymes are responsible for these reactions.[31] This is apparent from the fact that steroid hormone synthesis and metabolism were unaffected in this infant.

The mechanism of cholestasis and liver injury in this condition is speculated to be the result of this metabolic error, occuring because of either the failure to synthesize adequate amounts of primary bile acids that are essential to the promotion and secretion of bile or the increased production of unusual bile acids with hepatotoxic potential. The monohydroxy bile acid 3β,hydroxy-5-cholenoic acid has been shown to be markedly cholestatic in the rat and hamster[182] and, although 3β,7α-dihydroxy-5-cholenoic acid did not cause cholestasis in the hamster,[85] the finding may be explained by its metabolism to chenodeoxycholic acid in this species, a conversion that did not take place in this infant. It is still possible, therefore, that in humans these 3β-hydroxy-Δ^5 bile acids may be hepatotoxic.

Δ^4-3-Oxosteroid 5β-Reductase Deficiency

As a consequence of continued application of the technique of FAB-MS for screening abnormalities in urinary bile acid excretion[2] a further inborn error in bile acid synthesis was recognized.[5,6] This involved the Δ^4-3-oxosteroid 5β-reductase catalyzed conversion of the intermediates 7α-hydroxy-4-cholesten-3-one and 7α,12α-dihydroxy-4-cholesten-3-one into the corresponding 3-oxo-5β(H) structures (Fig. 6). The defect was identified in monochorionic male twins that were born with a marked cholestasis; a previous sibling (brother) also born with neonatal hepatitis had died of liver failure at 4 months of age. Liver functions tests revealed an

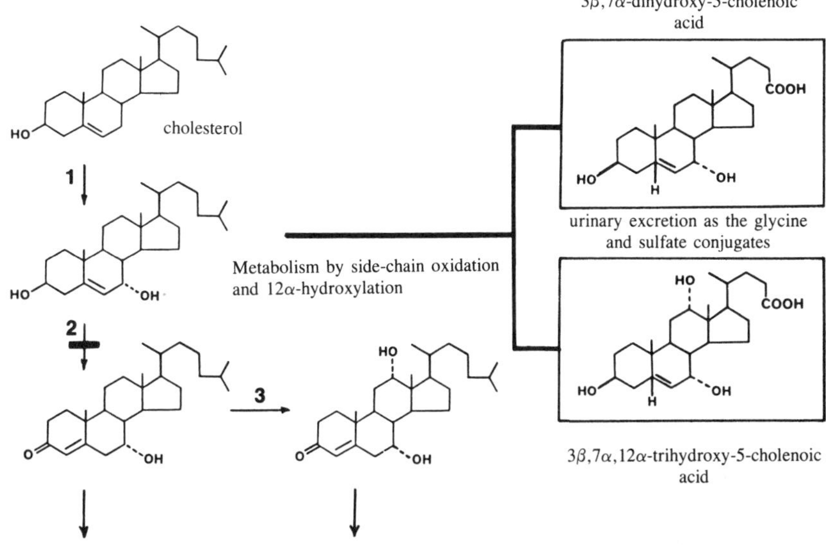

FIGURE 17 Biochemical defect involving a deficiency in the activity of 3β-hydroxysteroid dehydrogenase/isomerase enzyme catalyzing early changes (step 2) in the pathway for bile acid synthesis from cholesterol.

elevation in serum aminotransferase levels, marked conjugated hyperbilirubin, and coagulopathy. Liver biopsies revealed marked lobular disarray as a result of giant cell and pseudoacinar transformation of hepatocytes, hepatocellular and canalicular bile stasis, and extramedullary hematopoiesis. On electron microscopy, bile canaliculi were small and sometimes slitlike in appearance and showed few or absent microvilli containing a variable amount of electron-dense material.[5]

Initial screening of the urine of both infants using the FAB-MS technique indicated the presence of elevated amounts of bile acids having molecular weights consistent with taurine conjugates of hydroxy-oxo-cholenoic and dihydroxy-oxo-cholenoic acids. GC-MS analysis of the urine samples following extraction, solvolysis, hydrolysis, and derivatization of bile acids[183] confirmed the predominance of two major components that were identified as 3-oxo-7α-hydroxy-4-cholenoic and 3-oxo-7α,12α-dihydroxy-4-cholenoic acids. Urinary bile acid excretion was elevated in both infants compared with healthy newborn infants of a similar age[5] and consistent with a cholestatic condition. Quantitatively the Δ^4-3-oxo bile acids composed 75 to 92 percent of the total urinary bile acids. Gallbladder bile contained only traces (less than 2 μM) of bile acids and because urinary excretion represented the major route for bile acid loss, estimates of bile acid synthesis rates from daily urinary output indicated markedly reduced total bile acid synthesis rates (less than 3 mg per day) compared with reported data for newborn infants[184] or adults.[185] Serum bile acids were elevated in both infants. Chenodeoxycholic acid was the major serum bile acid identified, however, there were relatively high concentrations of *allo*-chenodeoxycholic and *allo*-cholic acids (approximately 30 percent of total bile acids) and lesser amounts (6 to 10 percent) of the Δ^4-3-oxo bile acids in the serum. These findings highlight that compartmentalization of different bile acids can occur that may necessitate the simultaneous analysis of different biologic fluids to confirm diagnosis of the specific biochemical defect.

These biochemical findings indicated a defect in bile acid synthesis affecting the conversion of the 3-oxo-Δ^4 intermediates to the corresponding 3α-hydroxy-5β(H)-structures (Fig. 18). This conversion is catalyzed by a NADPH-dependent Δ^4-3-oxosteroid-5β reductase enzyme[39-41] to yield the saturated 3-oxo-C_{27} intermediates. An apparent inactivity or deficiency of this enzyme in these twins explains the failure to form adequate amounts of cholic and chenodeoxycholic acids and the concomitant production of the Δ^4-3-oxo cholenoic acids and *allo*-bile acids.

In the normal pathway of bile acid synthesis, side-chain oxidation occurs following the nuclear alterations.[10] The finding of *allo*-bile acids and bile acids having a Δ^4-3-oxo structure in plasma and urine further indicates that pathways exist whereby side-chain oxidation may precede the nuclear changes. The occurrence of significant concentrations of *allo*-bile acids in these patients lends support for an active hepatic Δ^4-3-oxosteroid 5α-reductase catalyzing the conversion of the Δ^4-3-oxo sterol intermediates to the corresponding 3α-hydroxy-5α(H)-structures.

As with the earlier-described defect it can be speculated that cholestasis resulted either because of the lack of synthesis of adequate amounts of primary bile acids, which provide a major driving force for bile secretion, or because of the accumulation of Δ^4-3-oxo- and *allo*-bile acids, which may be hepatotoxic. The unique morphologic findings in these patients poses the intriguing question of whether maturation of the canalicular membrane and transport system for bile acid secretion requires a threshold concentration of primary bile acids in early development. It should be pointed out that from limited experience to date, increased production of Δ^4-3-oxo bile acids in patients with liver disease appears indicative of a poor clinical prognosis.[6,186]

Other Disorders of Bile Acid Metabolism

A brief description of a single case of a deficiency in the C_{24} steroid-7α-hydroxylase enzyme was reported by Javitt et

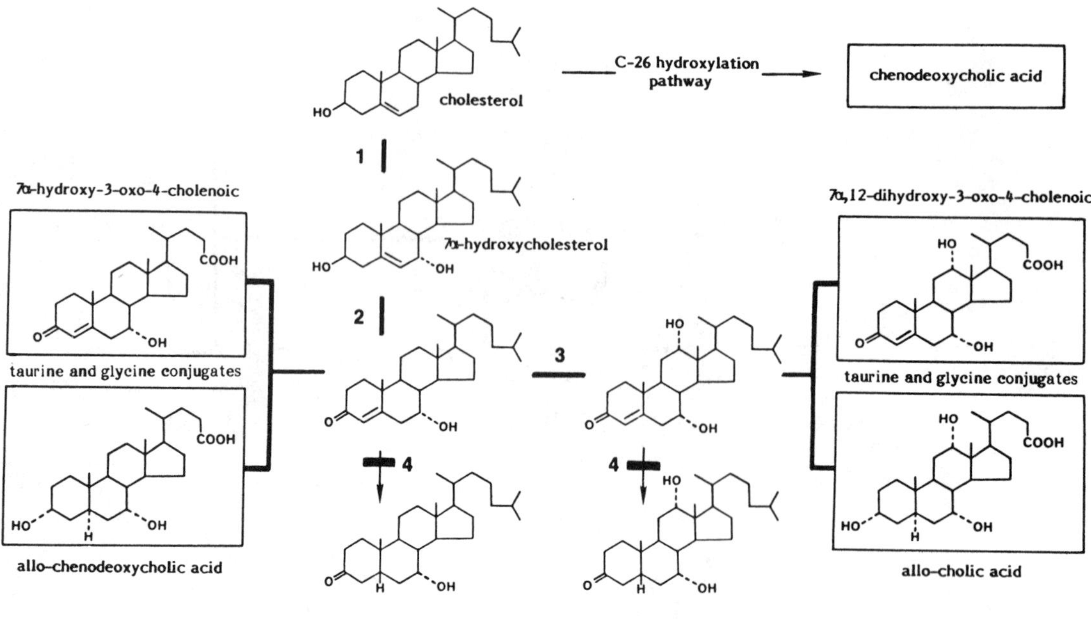

FIGURE 18 Biochemical defect involving a deficiency in the activity of the Δ^4-3-oxosteroid 5β-reductase enzyme responsible for catalyzing early changes (step 4) in the pathway for bile acid synthesis from cholesterol.

al.[187] The patient was a 6-year-old female with cholestasis from birth. Serum bile acid concentration was markedly elevated (229 μmol per liter) of which 3β-hydroxy-5-cholenoic acid reportedly account for 10 percent of the total bile acids. [16,17,22,23-$^3H_4$]3β-Hydroxy-5-cholenoic acid was administered intravenously and compared with normal humans and hamsters; only a minor conversion (3 percent) to chenodeoxycholic acid was reported. This was used as supportive evidence for an absence of the cytochrome P-450 dependent microsomal C_{24}-steroid-7α-hydroxylase enzyme involved in the Yamasaki pathway for chenodeoxycholic acid synthesis from this unsaturated monohydroxy bile acid.

A defect in 12α-hydroxylase was also claimed in a 10-year-old girl who from the age of 3 years had steatorrhea but had chronic constipation (bowel movements occurring once every 3 to 6 weeks) and celiac disease. Evidence in support of this bile acid defect was based upon the finding of reduced total biliary bile acid concentrations of which cholic acid accounted for 17 percent of the total bile acids, and a markedly reduced cholic acid synthesis rate. These findings were supported by the failure to show 12α-hydroxylase activity in a wedge biopsy of liver tissue. The authors speculated that in the absence of other explanations the marked constipation may be associated with a congenital bile acid deficiency.[189]

Methods for Studying Bile Acid Metabolism and Their Application to the Diagnosis of Inborn Errors in Bile Acid Synthesis

A battery of techniques is available for the measurement of bile acids in biologic fluids, and these have been compiled and extensively reviewed in the fourth volume of the book series *The Bile Acids*[1] and elsewhere.[190,192] Technologic advances have meant that techniques such as paper, thin-layer, and packed column gas chromatography have largely become superseded by extremely sensitive and specific assays. Immunoassay[193] and bioluminescence[194] techniques will continue to be commonplace in the future because of their high-sensitivity, precision and suitability for handling large numbers of samples. However, the limited information that these single-assay procedures yield make them generally unsuitable for detecting specific inborn errors in bile acid metabolism.

High-performance liquid chromatography (HPLC) heralded a new era in bile acid analysis, and the technique—now extensively employed—is clearly a useful tool.[192,195] Limitations of HPLC include restricted sensitivity, particularly where ultraviolet absorption is used as the detection technique, so that it is best suited to the direct analysis of the principal amidated species of biliary bile acids but has little value in detecting low levels of bile acids in serum. Improvements in sensitivity are possible by pre- or post-column reactions.[192,195] Recent advances in mass spectrometry now permit the HPLC column to be coupled directly to the mass spectrometer, which then serves as a specific HPLC detector,[196] and this technique will undoubtedly prove to be a useful tool for metabolic profiling.

Accurate identification of inborn errors in metabolism requires techniques that afford detailed metabolic profiles and GC-MS will continue to be the principal confirmatory tool.[191,197,198] Because of the high cost, the technical difficulty, and the time-consuming nature of bile acid analysis by GC-MS, the technique is outside the scope of most routine clinical laboratories. For this reason the diagnosis of patients with inborn errors in bile acid synthesis has proved to be difficult

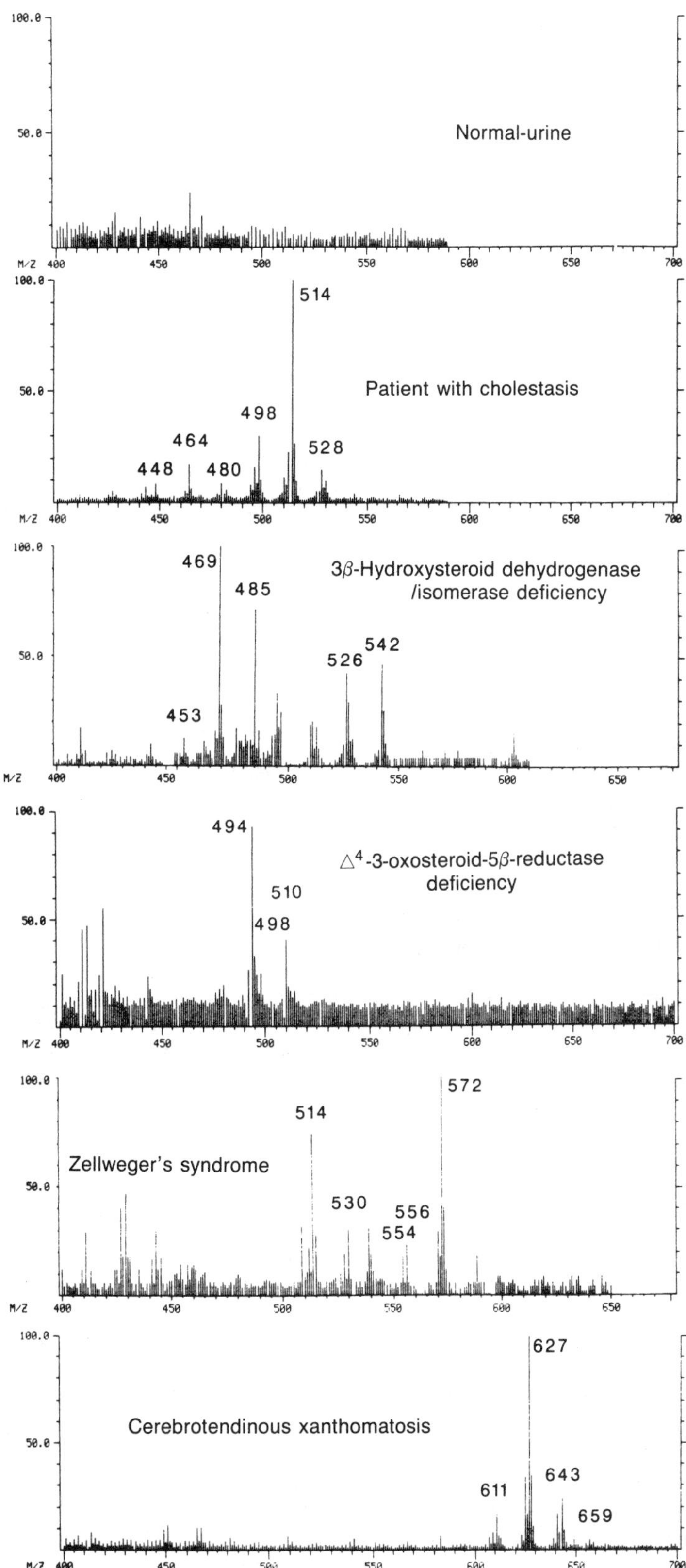

FIGURE 19 Negative-ion FAB-MS mass spectra recorded from the analysis of urine from (1) healthy individual; (2) patient with cholestatic liver disease not resulting from any defect in primary bile acid synthesis; (3) a patient with deficiency in 3β-hydroxysteroid dehydrogenase/isomerase enzyme; (4) patient with a deficiency in the Δ^4-3-oxosteroid 5β-reductase enzyme; (5) a patient with cerebrotendinous xanthomatosis; (6) patient with Zellweger's syndrome. The origins of the ions in these spectra are detailed elsewhere,[2,3,5,179] and the profiles are relatively specific for each defect.

and probably accounts for low reported incidence of such metabolic defects.

One of the most significant advances to have taken place in mass spectrometry was the introduction of FAB-MS, which simplified and extended the scope of mass spectrometry. By this technique nonvolatile compounds can be analyzed directly in biologic samples or simple extracts, thereby circumventing the need for extensive and time-consuming sample pretreatments. Intact bile acid conjugates are ideally suited to FAB-MS[2,179,191,197,198] and mass spectra can be generated from small microliter volumes of urine that indicate the presence of steroid and bile acids conjugates. The technique is rapid and simple and involves spotting the sample onto the tip of a probe containing a drop of glycerol. The probe is introduced into the ion-source of the instrument and a beam of fast atoms is directed at the target containing the sample. Negative ions generated by the ionization process are recorded and a mass spectrum generated.

In healthy individuals, urinary bile acid excretion is of negligible quantitative importance and consequently the mass spectrum obtained is unremarkable and shows largely background ions and the presence of steroid hormone metabolites. In cholestatic conditions, urinary bile acid excretion increases and bile acid conjugates can be readily detected in the negative ion mass spectrum as single intense ions corresponding to the $[M-H]^-$ ions (Fig. 19). In the absence of an inborn error in bile acid synthesis, ions appear that correspond to the glyco- and tauro-conjugates of the primary bile acids, cholic and chenodeoxycholic acids. A list of ions relative to bile acid conjugates has been published elsewhere.[2] In the case of an inborn error in bile acid synthesis a unique FAB-MS profile will be obtained revealing ions corresponding in mass to the accumulated intermediates and/or their metabolites in the biosynthetic pathway proximal to the enzyme block. Because of the inability of FAB-MS to distinguish positional or stereo isomers of bile acid conjugates, positive identification of the structures requires analysis by GC-MS after prior hydrolysis to cleave the conjugate moiety and derivatization. FAB-MS is thus a complementary technique that permits the rapid and definitive screening of urine samples for inborn errors in bile acid synthesis, and because of its simplicity a case could be made for screening for defects in bile acid synthesis in all patients who present in the first weeks of life with unresolved neonatal cholestasis. Only then will a better indication of the incidence of these metabolic defects be determined.

New Perspectives for Treatment of Inborn Errors of Bile Acid Synthesis

Experience in the treatment of inborn errors in bile acid synthesis is somewhat limited, largely because until recently these disorders were rarely recognized, previously unknown, or poorly understood.[2]

The cerebrohepatorenal (Zellweger's) syndrome, because of the multiple congenital abnormalities, is a fatal autosomal recessive disease in which death occurs in most patients within the first few months of life. The primary defect in Zellweger's syndrome may involve the assembly of the peroxisomes, since it is possible to have peroxisomal enzyme activity in the absence of peroxisomes.[199] Clofibrate, a hypolipidemic drug, causes a marked proliferation in hepatic peroxisomes in rats[200] and an increase in the activity of the peroxisomal β-oxidation of fatty acids.[157,201] Clofibrate treatment over periods of 3 to 6 weeks in two infants with Zellweger's syndrome was ineffectual; no obvious change in the clinical status or the progression of the disease was reported and its use was not recommended.[199]

For the more specific defects in bile acid metabolism recently associated with familial neonatal hepatitis and cholestasis, the experience to date suggests that untreated these infants have a poor prognosis with progression of the disease to cirrhosis and death. Oral bile acid administration has been suggested as a potential therapy for patients with these inborn errors.[3,5,6] The rationale for this approach is that oral bile acid administration would (1) provide a stimulus for bile-flow, (2) inhibit endogenous synthesis of bile acids, thereby preventing the further accumulation of potentially hepatotoxic bile acids that are produced in response to the enzyme deficiency, and (3) improve growth by improving fat absorption.

Oral bile acid therapy has been shown to be effective in the treatment of cerebrotendinous xanthomatosis, but this condition is not manifest by hepatic abnormalities. Long-term treatment with chenodeoxycholic acid (750 mg per day) lowers plasma cholestanol concentrations to within the normal range,[202,203] markedly reduces the urinary excretion of bile alcohols,[2,146,204] and improves the clinical condition.[203] Similar suppression of endogenous synthesis of cholestanol and bile alcohols occurs with cholic acid administration,[204] but it should be noted that ursodeoxycholic acid has proved ineffective.[203,204]

The improvement in the biochemical and clinical status of these patients is attributed to the marked suppression in endogenous bile acid synthesis mediated by the negative feedback of administered primary bile acids on hepatic cholesterol 7α-hydroxylase, the rate-limiting enzyme for bile acid synthesis and/or HMG-CoA reductase, the rate-controlling enzyme for cholesterol synthesis.[135,202] Of potential concern in the use of chenodeoxycholic acid is the increase in hepatic enzyme concentrations and symptoms of diarrhea that have been documented when the drug is used for gallstone dissolution.[205] However, in a study of 17 patients with CTX treated with chenodeoxycholic acid, none of these side effects were reported.[203] Nevertheless, chenodeoxycholic acid therapy is not to be recommended for patients with neonatal hepatitis and cholestasis.

The effectiveness of oral bile acid therapy has been investigated in both the Δ^4-3-oxosteroid 5β-reductase deficiency and the 3β-hydroxysteroid dehydrogenase deficiency recently described and associated with neonatal hepatitis and cholestasis. In both instances, previous siblings in these families had died of cirrhosis and liver failure.

In twin boys with Δ^4-3-oxosteroid 5β-reductase deficiency, a combination of cholic acid and ursodeoxycholic acid (100 mg per day of each bile acid) was given orally in solution.[6] Cholic acid was used as a means of suppressing endogenous bile acid synthesis that otherwise leads to the accumulation of the potentially hepatotoxic Δ^4-3-oxo- and *allo*-bile acids. Ursodeoxycholic acid was incorporated because of its potent choleretic action and recently described beneficial effects on improving indices of liver function in adults with other liver diseases.[206-208] By means of this approach, complete suppression of Δ^4-3-oxo and *allo*-bile acids occurred in these patients and total bilirubin levels returned to normal after 6 months of therapy. Significant normalization in the bile cannalicular structure was also noted after bile acid therapy. Both infants continued to grow and have survived to beyond 2 years of age, although a previous brother had died, untreated, at age 4 months. Measurements of bile acids in biologic samples from these patients after 1 year of therapy showed the presence of cholic and chenodeoxycholic acids and virtual absence of Δ^4-3-oxo bile acids. These findings can be explained by intestinal bacterial conversion of Δ^4-3-oxo bile acids into the corresponding 3α-hydroxy-5β(H) analogues once biliary secretion and an enterohepatic circulation were restored by bile acid therapy.

Comparable biochemical and clinical results have also been found in an infant with a 3β-hydroxysteroid dehydrogenase/isomerase deficiency,[209] similarly treated with bile acids. Suppression of endogenous synthesis of bile acids with the 3β-hydroxy-5-ene structure resulting from the enzyme deficiency occurred by feeding chenodeoxycholic acid (125 mg per day) and indices of hepatic function normalized. The finding of cholic and chenodeoxycholic acids was also attributed to the bacterial conversion of the 3β-hydroxy-5-ene C_{24} bile acids into the conventional 3α-hydroxy-5β-primary bile acids during their enterohepatic cycling.

Thus, although the use of oral bile acid therapy in inborn errors in bile acid synthesis is largely experimental and the long-term effects are uncertain, the limited experience with this approach is promising. It appears that at the very least it may offer stabilization of the progression of liver disease, allowing these infants to survive and grow to a point at which alternative treatments may be more appropriately performed.

Note: Since completion of this text, a patient was discovered with a 3β-hydroxysteroid dehydrogenase/isomerase deficiency. This defect was identified in a jaundiced 10-year-old boy with chronic hepatitis.[210] Investigations revealed a conjugated hyperbilirubinemia and elevated transaminases. Liver biopsy demonstrated cholestasis, numerous binucleate hepatocytes, occasional necrotic hepatocytes with variable portal tract inflammation, and fibrosis. FAB-MS and GC-MS of the urine, serum, and bile revealed no detectable cholic or chenodeoxycholic acid but instead high levels of $3\beta,7\alpha$-dihydroxy-5-cholenoic and $3\beta,7\alpha,12\alpha$-trihydroxy-5-cholenoic acids that accounted for more than 90 percent of the total bile acids in these fluids. Oral bile acid therapy with chenodeoxycholic acid (250 mg per day) resulted in increased appetite and activity, and within 4 weeks, total bilirubin levels normalized. This recent finding indicates that inborn errors in bile acid synthesis may cause severe late-onset chronic liver disease and confirms the potential of oral bile acid therapy in the treatment of these conditions.

REFERENCES

1. Setchell KDR, Kritchevsky D, Nair PP. In: Setchell KDR, Kritchevsky D, Nair PP, eds. The bile acids. Vol 4. Methods and applications. New York: Plenum Press, 1988.
2. Setchell KDR, Street JM. Inborn errors of bile acid synthesis. Semin Liver Dis 1987; 7:85–99.
3. Clayton PT, Leonard JV, Lawson AM, Setchell KDR, Andersson S, Egestad B, Sjövall J: Familial giant cell hepatitis associated with synthesis of 3β, 7α-dihydroxy- and 3β, 7α, 12α-trihydroxy-5-cholenoic acids. J Clin Invest 1987; 79:1031–1038.
4. Clayton PT, Lawson AM, Setchell KDR, Andersson S, Egestad B, Sjövall J: A new inborn error of bile acid biosynthesis. In: Paumgartner G, Stiehl A, Gerok W, eds. Bile acids and the liver. Lancaster, UK: MTP Press Ltd, 1987: 259.
5. Setchell KDR, Suchy FJ, Welsh MB, Zimmer-Nechemias L, Heubi J, Balistreri WF. Δ^4-3-Oxosteroid 5β-reductase deficiency described in identical twins with neonatal hepatitis—a new inborn error in bile acid synthesis. J Clin Invest 1988; 82:2135–2146.
6. Setchell KDR, Suchy FJ, Welsh MB, Zimmer-Nechemias L, Balistreri WF. A new inborn error in bile acid synthesis— Δ^4-3-oxosteroid 5β-reductase deficiency described in identical twins with neonatal hepatitis. Proceedings of the X International Bile Acid Meeting, Trends in Bile Acid Research, June 9–11, 1988, pp 197–206.
7. Boyer JL. New concepts of mechanisms of hepatic bile formation. Physiol Rev 1980; 60:303–326.
8. Klyne W. The chemistry of the steroids. London: Methuen and Co, Ltd, 1957.
9. Haslewood GAD. In: The biological importance of bile salts. Amsterdam: North Holland Publishing Co, 1978.
10. Björkhem I. Mechanism of bile acid biosynthesis in mammalian liver. In: Danielsson H, Sjövall J, eds. Sterols and bile acids. BV Amsterdam: Elsevier Science Pub, 1985: 231.
11. Lester R, St Pyrek J, Little JM, Adcock E. Diversity of bile acids in the fetus and newborn infant. J Pediatr Gastroenterol Nutr 1983; 2:355–364.
12. Setchell KDR, Dumaswala R, Colombo C, Ronchi M. Hepatic bile acid metabolism during early development revealed from the analysis of human fetal gall-bladder bile. J Biol Chem 1988; 263:16637–16644.
13. Sjövall J. Dietary glycine and taurine conjugation in man. Proc Soc Exp Biol Med 1959; 100:676–678.
14. Back P, Spaczynski K, Gerok W. Bile salt glucuronides in urine. Hoppe-Seyler's Physiol Chem 1974; 355:749–752.
15. Shattuck KE, Radominska-Pyrek A, Zimniak P, Adcock EW, Lester R, St. Pyrek J. Metabolism of 24-norlithocholic acid in the rat: formation of hydroxyl- and carboxyl-linked glucuronides and effect on bile flow. Hepatology 1986; 6:869–873.
16. Palmer RH. Formation of bile acid sulfates: a new pathway of bile acids metabolism in humans. Proc Natl Acad Sci 1967; 58:1047–1050.
17. Matern H, Matern S. Formation of bile acid glucosides and dolichyl phosphoglucose by microsomal glucosyltransferases in liver, kidney and intestine of man. Biochim Biophys Acta 1987; 921:1–6.
18. Marschall H-U, Egestad B, Matern H, Matern S, Sjövall J. Evidence for bile acid glucosides as normal constituents in human urine. FEBS Letts 1987; 213:411–414.
19. Marschall H-U, Egestad B, Matern H, Matern S, Sjövall J. N-acetylglucosaminides. A new type of bile acid conjugate in man. J Biol Chem 1989; 264:12989–12993.
20. Sweeny DJ, Barnes S, Heggie GD, Diasio RB. Metabolism of 5-fluorouracil to an N-cholyl-2-fluoro-β-alanine conjugate: previously unrecognized role for bile acids in drug conjugation. Proc Natl Acad Sci 1987; 84:5439–5443.
21. LaRusso NF, Korman MG, Hoffman NE, Hofmann AF. Dynamics of the enterohepatic circulation of bile acids. Postprandial serum concentrations of conjugates of cholic acid in health, cholecystectomized patients, and patients with bile acid malabsorption. N Engl J Med 1974; 291:689–691.
22. Setchell KDR, Street JM. Fecal bile acids. In: Setchell KDR, Kritchevsky D, Nair PP, eds. The bile acids. Vol 4. Methods and applications, New York: Plenum Press, 1988: 441.
23. Danielsson H, Einarsson K. Further studies on the formation of the bile acids in the guinea pig. Acta Chem Scand 1964; 18:831–832.
24. Myant NB, Mitropoulos KA. Cholesterol 7α-hydroxylase. J Lipid Res 1977; 18:135–153.
25. Danielsson H, Einarsson K, Johansson G. Effect of biliary drainage on individual reactions in the conversion of cholesterol to taurocholic acid. Bile acids and steroids 180. Eur J Biochem 1967; 2:44–49.
26. Thomason JC, Vars HM. Biliary excretion of cholic acid and cholesterol in hyper-, hypo- and euthyroid rats. Proc Soc Exp Biol Med 1953; 83:246–248.
27. Eriksson S. Biliary excretion of bile acids and cholesterol in bile fistula rats; bile acids and steroids. Proc Soc Exp Biol Med 1957; 94:578–582.

28. Bergstrom S, Danielsson H. On the regulation of bile acid formation in the rat liver. Acta Physiol Scand 1958; 43:1–7.
29. Green K, Samuelsson B. Mechanisms of bile acid biosynthesis studies with 3α-H^3 and 4β-H^3-cholesterol. Bile acids and steroids. J Biol Chem 1964; 239:2804–2808.
30. Björkhem I. On the mechanism of the enzymatic conversion of cholest-5-ene-3β, 7α-diol into 7α-hydroxycholest-4-en-3-one. Eur J Biochem 1969; 8:337–344.
31. Wikvall K. Purification and properties of a 3β-hydroxy-Δ^5-C_{27}-steroid oxidoreductase from rabbit liver microsomes. J Biol Chem 1981; 256:3376–3380.
32. Mitropoulos KA, Suzuki M, Myant NB, Danielsson H. Effects of thyroidectomy and thyroxine treatment on the activity of 12α-hydroxylase and of some components of microsomal electron transfer chains in rat liver. FEBS Lett 1968; 1:13–15.
33. Björkhem I, Danielsson H, Gustafsson J. On the effect of thyroid hormone on 26-hydroxylation of C_{27}-steroids in rat liver. FEBS Lett 1973; 31:20–22.
34. Danielsson H. Influence of dietary bile acids on formation of bile acids in rat. Steroids 1973; 22:667–676.
35. Ahlberg J, Angelin B, Björkhem I, Einarsson K, Gustafsson JA, Rafter J. Effects of treatment with chenodeoxycholic acid on liver microsomal metabolism of steroids in man. J Lab Clin Med 1980; 95:188–194.
36. Angelin B, Björkhem I, Einarsson K, Ewerth S. Cholestyramine treatment reduces postprandial but not fasting serum bile acid levels in humans. Gastroenterology 1982; 83:1097–1101.
37. Johansson G. Effect of cholestyramine and diet on hydroxylations in the biosynthesis and metabolism of bile acids. Eur J Biochem 1970; 17:292–295.
38. Björkhem I, Eriksson M, Einarsson K. Evidence for a lack of regulatory importance of the 12α-hydroxylase in formation of bile acids in man: an in vivo study. J Lipid Res 1983; 24:1451–1456.
39. Bérsèus O. Conversion of cholesterol to bile acids in rats: purification and properties of the Δ^4-3-ketosteroid 5β-reductase and a 3α-hydroxysteroid dehydrogenase. Eur J Biochem 1967; 2:493–502.
40. Bérsèus O. Studies on the conversion of cholesterol into bile acids (Thesis) Opuscula Medica 1967; suppl 6.
41. Bérsèus O, Björkhem I. Enzymatic conversion of a Δ^4-3-ketosteroid into a 3α-hydroxy-5β steroid: mechanism and stereochemistry of hydrogen transfer form NADPH. Bile acids and steroids 190. Eur J Biochem 1967; 2:503–507.
42. Björkhem I, Gustafsson J. Omega-hydroxylation of steroid side-chain in biosynthesis of bile acids. Eur J Biochem 1973; 36:201–212.
43. Björkhem I, Gustafsson J. Mitochondrial omega-hydroxylation of cholesterol side chain. J Biol Chem 1974; 249:2528–2535.
44. Okuda K, Weber P, Ullrich V. Photochemical action spectrum of the co-inhibited 5β-cholestan-3α,7α,12α-triol 26-hydroxylase system. Biochem Biophys Res Commun 1977; 74:1071–1076.
45. Cronholm T, Johansson G. Oxidation of 5β-cholestan-3α, 7α, 12α-triol by rat liver microsomes. Eur J Biochem 1970; 16:373–381.
46. Masui T, Herman R, Staple E. the oxidation of 5β-cholestan-3α, 7α, 12α, 25-tetrol to 5β-cholestan-3α, 7α, 12α-triol-26-oic acid via 5β-cholestane-3α, 7α, 12α-triol-26-al by rat liver. Biochim Biophys Acta 1966; 117:266–268.
47. Okuda K, Takigawa N. The dehydrogenation of 5β-cholestane-3α, 7α, 12α, 26-tetrol by rat liver. Biophys Acta 1969; 176:873–879.
48. Okuda K, Takigawa N. Separation of 5β-cholestane-3α, 7α, 12α, 26-tetrol oxidoreductase, and acetaldehyde-NAD oxidoreductase from the soluble fraction of rat liver by gel filtration. Biochem Biophys Res Commun 1968; 33:788–793.
49. Okuda K, Takigawa N. Rat liver 5β-cholestane-3α, 7α, 12α, 26-tetrol dehydrogenase as a liver alcohol dehydrogenase. Biochim Biophys Acta 1970; 222:141–148.
50. Okuda K, Higuchi E, Fukuba R. Horse liver 3, 7, 12-trihydroxy-5-cholestan-26-al dehydrogenase as a liver aldehyde dehydrogenase. Biochim Biophys Acta 1973; 293:15–25.
51. Masui T, Staple E. The formation of bile acids from cholesterol. The conversion of 5β-cholestane-3α, 7α-triol-26-oic acid to cholic acid via 5β-cholestane-3α, 7α, 12α, 24-xi-tetrol-26-oic acid I by rat liver. J Biol Chem 1966; 241:3889–3893.
52. Gustafsson J. Biosynthesis of cholic acid in rat liver. 24-Hydroxylation of 3α, 7α, 12α-trihydroxy-5β-cholestanoic acid. J Biol Chem 1975; 250:8243–8247.
53. Kase F, Björkhem I, Pedersen JI. Formation of cholic acid from 3α, 7α, 12α-trihydroxy-5β-cholestanoic acid by rat liver peroxisomes. J Lipid Res 1983; 24:1560–1567.
54. Killenberg PG. Measurement and sub-cellular distribution of choloyl-CoA synthetase and bile acid - CoA: amino acid N-acyltransferase activates in rat liver. J Lipid Res 1978; 19:24–31.
55. Killenberg PG. Bile acid—CoA: amino acid N-acyltransferase. Methods Enzymol 1981; 77:308–313.
56. Lim WC, Jordan TW. Sub-cellular distribution of hepatic bile acid-conjugating enzymes. Biochem J 1981; 197:611–618.
57. Hardison WGM. Hepatic taurine concentration and dietary taurine as regulators of bile acid conjugation with taurine. Gastroenterology 1978; 75:71–75.
58. Sturman JA, Gaull GE. Taurine in the brain and liver of the developing human and monkey. J Neurochemistry 1975; 25:831–835.
59. Stegink LK, Reynolds WA, Pitkin RM, Cruikshank DP. Placental transfer of taurine in the rhesus monkey. Am J Clin Nutr 1981; 34:2685–2692.
60. Czuba B, Vessey DA. The effect of bile acid structure on the activity of bile acid-CoA: glycine/taurine-N-acetyltransferase. J Biol Chem 1982; 257:8761–8765.
61. Chen LJ, Bolt RJ, Admirand WH. Enzymatic sulfation of bile salts. Partial purification and characterization of an enzyme from rat liver that catalyzed the sulfation of bile salts. Biochim Biophys Acta 1977; 480:219–227.
62. Loof L, Hjerten S. Partial purification of a human liver sulphotransferase active towards bile salts. Biochim Biophys Acta 1980; 617:192–204.
63. Barnes S, Burhol PG, Zander R, Haggstrom G, Settine RL, Hirschowitz BI. Enzymatic sulfation of glycochenodeoxycholic acid by tissue fractions from adult hamsters. J Lipid Res 1979; 20:952–959.
64. Watkins JB, Goldstein E, Coryer R, Brown ER, Eraklis A. Sulfation of bile acids in the fetus. In: Presig R, Bircher J, eds. The liver, quantitative aspects of structure and function. Gstaad: Edito Cantor Aulendorf, 1974: 249.
65. Back P. Bile acid glucuronides II isolation of a chenodeoxycholic acid glucuronide from plasma in intrahepatic cholestasis. Hoppe-Seylers Z Physiol Chem 1976; 357:213–217.
66. Little JM, Pyrek JSt, Lester R. Hepatic metabolism of 3α-hydroxy-5β-etianic acid (3α-hydroxy-5β-androstan-17β-carboxylic acid) in the rat. J Clin Invest 1983; 71:73–80.
67. Radominska-Pyrek A, Zimmiak P, Irshaid YM, Lester R, Tephly TR, Pyrek JST. Glucuronidation of 6α-hydroxy bile acids by human liver microsomes. J Clin Invest 1987; 80:234–241.
68. Almé B, Sjövall J. Analysis of bile acid glucuronides in urine. Identification of 3α, 6α, 12α-trihydroxy-5-β-cholanoic acid. J Steroid Biochem 1980; 13:907–916.
69. Matern H, Matern S, Gerok W. Formation of bile acid glucosides by a sugar nucleotide-independent glucosyltransferase isolated from human liver microsomes. Proc Natl Acad Sci 1984; 81:7036–7040.
70. Vlahcevic ZR, Schwartz CC, Gustafsson J, Halloran LG, Danielsson H, Swell L. Biosynthesis of bile acids in man. Multiple pathways to cholic and chenodeoxycholic acid. J Biol Chem 1980; 255:1925–2933.
71. Swell L, Gustafsson J, Schwartz CC, Halloran LG, Danielsson H, Vlahcevic ZR. An in vivo evaluation of the quantitative significance of several potential pathways to cholic and chenodeoxycholic acids from cholesterol in man. J Lipid Res 1980; 21:455–466.
72. Shefer S, Cheng FW, Dayal B, Hauser S, Tint GS, Salen G, Mosbach EH. A 25-hydroxylation pathway of cholic and biosynthesis in man and rat. J Clin Invest 1986; 57:897–903.
73. Hanson RF, Staples AB, Williams GC. Metabolism of 5β-cholestane-3α, 7α, 12α, 26-tetrol and 5β-cholestane-3α, 7α, 12α, 25-tetrol into cholic acid in normal human subjects. J Lipid Res 1979; 20:489–493.
74. Hanson RF, Williams GC. Metabolism of 3α, 7α, 12α-trihydroxy-5β-cholenstan-26-oic acid in normal subjects with an intact enterohepatic circulation. J Lipid Res 1977; 656–658.
75. Kase BF, Pedersen JI, Strandvik B, Björkhem I. In vivo and in vitro studies on formation of bile acids in patients with Zellweger's syndrome. J Clin Invest 1985; 76:2392–2402.
76. Salen G, Batta AK, Tint GS, Dayal B, Shefer S. The transformation of 3α, 7α, 12α-trihydroxycoprostanoic acid to cholic acid in humans. In: Paumgartner G, Stiehl A, Gerok W, eds. Bile acids and cholesterol in health and disease. Lancaster, UK: MTP Press Limited, 1983: 91.
77. Duane WC, Björkhem I, Hamilton JN, Mueller SM. Quantitative importance of the 25-hydroxylation pathway for bile acid biosynthesis in rat. Hepatology 1988; 8:613–618.

78. Duane WC, Pooler PA, Hamilton JN. Bile Acid Synthesis in Man. In vivo activity of the 25-hydroxylation pathway. J Clin Invest 1988; 82:82–85.
79. Yamasaki K. Alternative biogenetic pathways of C24-bile acids with special reference to chenodeoxycholic acid. Kawasaki Med J 1978; 4:227–264.
80. Wachtel N, Emerman S, Javitt NB. Metabolism of cholest-5-ene-3β, 26-diol in the rat and hamster. J Biol Chem 1968; 243:5207–5212.
81. Anderson KE, Kok E, Javitt NB. Bile acids synthesis in man: metabolism of 7α-hydroxycholesterol-^{14}C and 26-hydroxycholesterol-^{3}H. J Clin Invest 1972; 51:112–117.
82. Krisans SK, Thompson SL, Pena LA, Kok E, Javitt NB. Bile acid synthesis in rat liver peroxisomes: metabolism of 26-hydroxycholesterol to 3β-hydroxy-5-cholenoic acid in the hamster. J Lipid Res 1985; 26:1324–1332.
83. Mitropoulos KA, Myant NB. The formation of lithocholic acid, chenodeoxycholic acid and α- and β-muricholic acids from cholesterol incubated with rat liver mitochondria. Biochem J 1968; 103:472–479.
84. Kok E, Burstein S, Javitt NB, Gut M, Byon CY. Bile acid synthesis. Metabolism of 3β-hydroxy-5-cholenoic acid in the hamster. J Biol Chem 1981; 256:6155–6159.
85. Kulkarni B, Javitt NB. Chenodeoxycholic acid synthesis in the hamster: a metabolic pathway via 3β, 7α-dihydroxy-5-cholen-24-oic acid. Steroids 1982; 40:581–589.
86. Karavolas HJ, Elliott WH, Hsia SL, Doisy Jr. EA, Matschiner JT, Thayer SA, Doisy EA. Bile acids. XXII. Allocholic acid, a metabolite of 5α-cholestan-3β-ol in the rat. J Biol Chem 1965; 240:1568–1577.
87. Hofmann AF, Mosbach EH. Identification of allodeoxycholic acid as the major component of gallstones induced in the rabbit by 5α-cholestan-3β-ol. J Biol Chem 1964: 239:2813–2821.
88. Shefer S, Hauser S, Mosbach EH. 7α-hydroxylation of cholestanol by rat liver microsomes. J Lipid Res 1968; 9:328–333.
89. Björkhem I, Gustafsson J. On the conversion of cholestanol into allocholic acid in rat liver. Eur J Biochem 1971; 18:207–213.
90. Ali SS, Elliott WH. Bile acids. LI. Formation of 12α-hydroxyl derivatives and companions from 5α-sterols by rabbit liver microsomes. J Lipid Res 1976; 17:386–392.
91. Mui MM, Elliott WH. Bile acids. XXXII. Allocholic acid, a metabolite of allochenodeoxycholic acid in bile fistula rats. J Biol Chem 1971; 246:302–304.
92. Blaskiewicz RJ, O'Neil GJ Jr, Elliott WH. Bile acids. XLI. Hepatic microsomal 12α-hydroxylation of allocheodeoxycholate to allocholate. Proc Soc Exp Biol Med 1974; 146:92–95.
93. Björkhem I, Einarsson K. Formation and metabolism of 7α-hydroxy-5α-cholestan-3-one and 7α, 12α-dihydroxy-5α-cholestan-3-one in rat liver. Eur J Biochem 1970; 13:174–179.
94. Hylemon PB. Metabolism of bile acids in intestinal microflora. In: Danielsson H, Sjövall J, eds. Sterols and bile acids. BV Amsterdam: Elsevier Science, 1985: 331.
95. Back P, Walter K. Developmental pattern of bile acid metabolism as revealed by bile acid analysis of meconium. Gastroenterology 1970; 78:671–676.
96. Shoda J, Mahara R, Osuga T, Tohma M, Ohnishi S, Miyazaki H, Tanaka N, Matsuzaki H, Tanaka N, Matsuzaki Y. Similarity of unusual bile acids in human umbilical cord blood and amniotic fluid from newborns and sera and urine from adults patients with cholestatic liver disease. J Lipid Res 1988; 29:847–858.
97. Nakagawa M, Setchell KDR. Bile acid metabolism in early life—studies of amniotic fluid. J Lipid Res 1989; in press.
98. Setchell KDR, Lawson AM, Blackstock EJ, Murphy GM. Diurnal changes in serum unconjugated bile acids in normal man. Gut 1982; 23:637–642.
99. Lewis B, Panveliwalla D, Tabaquali S, Wootton IDP. Serum bile acids in the stagnant-loop syndrome. Lancet 1969; i:219–220.
100. Setchell KDR, Harrison DL, Gilbert JM, Murphy GM. Serum unconjugated bile acids: qualitative and quantitative profiles in ileal resection and bacterial overgrowth. Clin Chim Acta 1985; 152:297–306.
101. Bartholomew TC, Summerfield JA, Billing BH, Lawson AM, Setchell KDR. Bile acid profiles in human serum and skin interstitial fluid and their relationship to pruritus studies by gas chromatography-mass spectrometry. Clin Sci 1982; 63:65–73.
102. Danielsson H, Rutter WJ. The metabolism of bile acids in the developing rat liver. Biochem J 1968; 7:346–352.
103. Smallwood RA, Lester R, Piasecki GJ, Klein PD, Greco R, Jackson BT. Fetal bile salt metabolism: II. Hepatic excretion of endogenous bile salt and of a taurocholate load. J Clin Invest 1972; 51:1388–1397.
104. Little JM, Smallwood RA, Lester R, Piasecki GJ, Jackson BT. Bile salt metabolism in the primate fetus. Gastroenterology 1975; 69:1315–1320.
105. Ravi Subbiah MT, Marai L, Dinh DM, Penner JW. Sterol and bile acid metabolism during development I. Studies on the gallbladder and intestinal bile acids of newborn and fetal rabbit. Steroids 1977; 29:83–92.
106. Sewell RB, Hardy KJ, Smallwood RA, Hoffman NE. Fetal bile salt metabolism: placental transport of taurocholate in sheep. Am J Physiol 1980; 239:G354–G357.
107. Suchy FJ, Balistreri WF, Breslin JS, Dumaswala R, Setchell KDR, Garfield SA. Absence of an acinar gradient for bile acid uptake in developing rat liver. Pediatr Res 1987; 21:417–421.
108. Haber LR, Vaupshas V, Vitullo BB, Seemayer TA, de Belle RC. Bile acid conjugation in organ culture of human fetal liver. Gastroenterology 1978; 74:1214–1223.
109. Colombo CC, Zuliani G, Ronchi M, Breidenstein J, Setchell KDR. Biliary bile acid composition of the human fetus in early gestation. Pediatr Res 1987; 21:197–200.
110. Gustafsson J, Andersson S, Sjövall J. Bile acid metabolism during development: metabolism of taurodeoxycholic acid in human fetal liver. Biol Neonate 1985; 47:26–31.
111. Gustafsson J, Andersson S, Sjövall J. Bile acid metabolism during development: metabolism of lithocholic acid in human fetal liver. Pediatr Res 1987; 21:99–103.
112. Poley JR, Dower JC, Owen CA, Stickler GB. Bile acids in infants and children. J Lab Clin Med 1964; 63:838–846.
113. Sharp HL, Peller J, Carey JB, Krist W. Primary and secondary bile acids in meconium. Pediatr Res 1971; 5:274–279.
114. Bongiovanni AM. Bile acid content of gallbladder of infants, children and adults. J Clin Endocrinol Metab 1965; 25:678–685.
115. Encrantz JC, Sjövall J. On the bile acids in duodenal contents of infants and children. Clin Chim Acta 1959; 4:793–799.
116. Gustafsson J. Bile acid biosynthesis during development: hydroxylation of C_{27}-sterols in human fetal liver. J Lipid Res 1986; 27:801–806.
117. Almé B, Bremmelgaard A, Sjövall J, Thomasson P. Analysis of metabolic profiles of bile acids in urine using a lipophilic anion exchanger and computerized gas-liquid chromatography-mass spectrometry. J Lipid Res 1977; 18:359–362.
118. Bremmelgaard A, Sjövall J. Bile acid profiles in urine of patients with liver diseases. Eur J Clin Invest 1979; 9:341–348.
119. Strandvik B, Wikström S-Å. Tetrahydroxylated bile acid in healthy human newborns. Eur J Clin Invest 1982; 12:301–305.
120. Tohma M, Mahara R, Takeshita H, Kurosawa T, Ikegawa S, Nittono H. Synthesis of 1β-hydroxylated bile acids and identification of 1β, 3α, 7α-trihydroxy- and 1β, 3α, 7α, 12α-tetrahydroxy-5β-cholanoic acids in human meconium. Chem Pharm Bull (Tokyo) 1985; 33:3071–3073.
121. Bremmelgaard A, Sjövall J. Hydroxylation of cholic, chenodeoxycholic, and deoxycholic acids in patients with intrahepatic cholestasis. J Lipid Res 1980; 21:1072–1081.
122. Dumaswala R, Setchell KDR, Iida T, Goto J, Nambara T. Identification of 3α, 4β, 7α-trihydroxy-5β-cholanoic acid in human bile reflecting on new pathway in bile acid metabolism in man. J Lipid Res 1989; 30:847–856.
123. Dumaswala R, Setchell KDR, Suchy FJ. A specific transport mechanism for bile acids exists on the brush border membrane of the human placental syncytiotrophoblast. (Abstract) Pediatr Res 1988; 23:302.
124. Stiehl A. Bile salt sulphates in cholestasis. Eur J Clin Invest 1974; 4:59–63.
125. Makino I, Shinozaki K, Nakagawa S, Mashimo K. Measurement of sulfated and non-sulfated bile acids in human serum and urine. J Lipid Res 1974; 15:132–138.
126. Stiehl A, Raedsch R, Rudolph G, Gundert-Remy U, Senn M. Biliary and urinary excretion of sulfated, glucuronidated and tetrahydroxylated bile acids in cirrhotic patients. Hepatology 1985; 5:492–495.
127. Délèze G, Paumgartner G, Karlaganis G, Giger W, Reinhard M, Sidiropoulos D. Bile acid pattern of human amniotic fluid. Eur J Clin Invest 1978; 8:41–45.
128. St Pyrek J, Sterzycki R, Lester R, Adcock E. Constituents of human meconium: II. Identification of steroidal acids with 21 and 22 carbon atoms. Lipids 1982; 17:241–249.

129. St Pyrek J, Lester R, Adcock EW, Sanghvi AT. Constituents of human meconium-I. Identification of 3-hydroxy-etianic acids. J Steroid Biochem 1983; 18:341–351.
130. Street JM, Balistreri WF, Setchell KDR. Bile acid metabolism in the perinatal period—excretion of conventional and atypical bile acids in meconium. Gastroenterology (Abstract) 1986; 90:1773.
131. Van Bogaert L, Scherer HJ, Epstein E. Une forme cerebrale de la cholesterinoise generalisée. Paris: Masson et Cie, 1937.
132. Bowen P, Lee CSN, Zellweger H, Lindenberg R. A familial syndrome of multiple congenital defects. Bull Johns Hopkins Hosp 1964; 114:402–414.
133. Salen G, Shefer S, Cheng FW, Dayal B, Batta AK, Tint GS. Cholic acid biosynthesis. The enzyme defect in cerebrotendinous xanthomatosis. J Clin Invest 1979; 63:38–44.
134. Setoguchi T, Salen G, Tint GS, Mosbach EH. A biochemical abnormality in cerebrotendinous xanthomatosis. Impairment of bile acid biosynthesis associated with incomplete degradation of the cholesterol side chain. J Clin Invest 1974; 53:1393–1401.
135. Salen G, Grundy SM. The metabolism of cholestanol, cholesterol and bile acids in cerebrotendinous xanthomatosis. J Clin Invest 1973; 52:2822–2835.
136. Salen G. Cholestanol deposition in cerebrotendinous xanthomatosis—a possible mechanism. Ann Intern Med 1971; 75:843–851.
137. Salen G, Shefer S, Tint GS, Nicolau G, Dayal B, Batta AK. Biosynthesis of bile acids in cerebrotendinous xanthomatosis. Relationship of bile acid pool sizes and synthesis rates to hydroxylations at C-12, C-25 and C-26. J Clin Invest 1985; 76:744–751.
138. Oftebro H, Björkhem I, Skrede S, Schreiner A, Pedersen JI. Cerebrotendinous xanthomatosis. A defect in mitochondrial 26-hydroxylation required for normal biosynthesis of cholic acid. J Clin Invest 1980; 65:1418–1430.
139. Javitt NB, Kok E, Cohen B, Burstein S. Cerebrotendinous xanthomatosis: reduced serum 26-hydroxycholesterol. J Lipid Res 1982; 23:627–630.
140. Salen G, Shefer S. Mosbach EH, Hauser S, Cohen BI, Nicolau G. Metabolism of potential precursors of chenodeoxycholic acid in cerebrotendinous xanthomatosis (CTX). J Lipid Res 1979; 20:22–30.
141. Björkhem I, Oftebro H, Skrede S, Pedersen JI. Assay of the intermediates in bile acid biosynthesis using isotope dilution—mass spectrometry: hepatic levels in the normal state and in cerebrotendinous xanthomatosis. J Lipid Res 1981; 22:191–200.
142. Oftebro H, Björkhem I, Skormer FC, Pedersen JI. Cerebrotendinous xanthomatosis: defective liver mitochondrial hydroxylation of chenodeoxycholic precursors. J Lipid Res 1981; 22:632–640.
143. Shefer S, Dayal B, Tint GS, Salen G, Mosbach EH. Identification of pentahydroxy bile alcohols in cerebrotendinous xanthomatosis: characterization of 5β-cholestane-3α,7α,12α,24,25-pentol and 5β-cholestane-3α,7α,12α,23,25-pentol. J Lipid Res 1975; 16:280–286.
144. Hoshita T, Yasuhara M, Kihira K, Kuramoto T. Identification of (23S)-5β-cholestane-3α, 7α, 12α, 23, 25-pentol in cerebrotendinous xanthomatosis. Steroids 1976; 27:657–664.
145. Hoshita T, Yasuhara M, Une M, Kibe A, Itoga E, Kito S, Kuramoto T. Occurrence of bile alcohol glucuronides in bile of patients with cerebrotendinous xanthomatosis. J Lipid Res 1980; 21:1015–1021.
146. Wolthers BG, Volmer M, Van der Molen J, Koopman BJ, de Jager AE, Waterreus RJ. Diagnosis of cerebrotendinous xanthomatosis (CTX) and effect of chenodeoxycholic acid therapy by analysis of urine using capillary gas chromatography. Clin Chim Acta 1983; 131:53–65.
147. Karlaganis G, Karlaganis V, Sjövall J. Bile alcohol glucuronides in urine: secondary metabolites of intermediates formed in the formation of bile acids from cholesterol? In: Paumgartner G, Stiehl A, Gerok W, eds. Bile acids and cholesterol in health and disease. Lancaster, UK: MTP Press Ltd, 1983: 119.
148. Shimazu K, Kuwabara M, Yoshii M, Kihira K, Takeuchi H, Nakano I, Ozawa S, Onuki M, Hatta Y, Hoshita T. Bile alcohol profiles in bile, urine and feces of a patient with cerebrotendinous xanthomatosis. J Biochem 1986; 99:477–483.
149. Hoshita T. Bile alcohols and primitive bile acids. In: Danielsson H, Sjövall J, eds. Sterols and bile acids. Amsterdam: Elsevier, 1985: 279.
150. Yasuhara M, Kuramoto T, Hoshita T, et al. Identification of 5β-cholestane-3α,7α,12α,23-tetrol, 5β-cholestane-3α,7α,12α,24α-tetrol and 5β-cholestane-3α,7α,12α,24β-tetrol in cerebrotendinous xanthomatosis. Steroids 1978; 31:333–345.
151. Menkes JH, Schimschock JR, Swanson PD. Cerebrotendinous xanthomatosis. Arch Neurol 1968; 19:47–63.
152. Koopman BJ, Van der Molen JC, Wolthers BG, de Jager AEJ, Waterreus RJ, Gips CH. Capillary gas chromatographic determination of cholestanol/cholesterol ratio in biological fluids. Its potential usefulness for the follow-up of some liver diseases and its lack of specificity in diagnosing CTX (cerebrotendinous xanthomatosis). Clin Chim Acta 1984; 137:305–315.
153. Salen S, Shefer S, Tint GS. Transformation of 4-cholesten-3-one and 7α-hydroxy-4-cholesten-3-one into cholestanol and bile acids in cerebrotendinous xanthomatosis. Gastroenterology 1984; 87:276–283.
154. Skrede S, Björkhem I, Buchmann MS, Hopen G, Fausa O. A novel pathway for biosynthesis of cholestanol with 7α-hydroxylated C_{27}-steroids as intermediates, and its importance for the accumulation of cholestanol in cerebrotendinous xanthomatosis. J Clin Invest 1985; 75:448–455.
155. Skrede S, Buchmann MS, Björkhem I. Hepatic 7α-dehydroxylation of bile acid intermediates, and its significance for the pathogenesis of cerebrotendinous xanthomatosis. J Lipid Res 1988; 29:157–164.
156. Rhodin J. Correlation of ultrastructural organization and function in normal and experimentally changed proximal tubule cells of the mouse kidney. (Doctoral thesis) Karolinska Institute, Stockholm, Akitbolaget, Godvil, 1954.
157. Lazarow PB, DeDuve C. A fatty acyl-CoA oxidizing system in rat liver peroxisomes; enhancement by clofibrate, a hypolipidemic drug. Proc Natl Acad Sci USA 1976; 73:2043–2046.
158. Thompson SL, Burrows R, Laub RJ, Krisans SK. Cholesterol synthesis in rat liver peroxisomes. Conversion of mevalonic acid to cholesterol. J Biol Chem 1987; 262:17420–17425.
159. Prydz K, Kase BF, Björkhem I, Pedersen JI. Formation of chenodeoxycholic acid from 3α,7α-dihydroxy-5β-cholestanoic acid by rat liver peroxisomes. J Lipid Res 1986; 27:622–628.
160. Goldfischer S, Moore CL, Johnson AB, Spiro AJ, Valsamis MP, Wisniewski HK, Ritch RH, Norton WT, Rapin I, Gartner LM. Peroxisomal and mitochondrial defects in the cerebrohepatorenal syndrome. Science 1973; 182:62–64.
161. Kelly RI. The cerebrohepatorenal syndrome of Zellweger, morphological and metabolic aspects. Am J Med Genet 1983; 16:503–17.
162. Poll-The BT, Saudubray JM, Ogier H, Schutgens RBH, Wanders RJA, Schrakamp G, Van Den Bosch H, Trijbels JMF, Poulos A, Moser HW, van Eldere J, Eyssen HJ. Infantile Refsum's disease: biochemical findings suggesting multiple peroxisomal dysfunction. J Inher Metab Dis 1986; 9:169–174.
163. Goldfischer SJ, Collins J, Rapin I, Coltoff-Schiller B, Chang C-H, Nigro M, Black VH, Javitt NB, Moser HW, Lazarow PB. Peroxisomal defects in neonatal onset and X-linked adrenoleukodystrophies. Science 1985; 227:67–70.
164. Burton BK, Reeds SP, Remy WT. Hyperpipecolic acidemia: Clinical and biochemical observations in two male siblings. J Pediatr 1983; 99:729–734.
165. Heymens HS, Oorthuys JWE, Nelck G, Wanders RJA, Schutgens RBH. Rhizomelic chondrodysplasia punctata: another peroxisomal disorder. N Engl J Med 1985; 313:187–188.
166. Goldfischer S, Collins J, Rapid I, Neumann P, Neglia W, Spiro AJ, Ishii T, Roels F, Vamecq J. VanHoof F. Pseudo-Zellweger syndrome: deficiencies in several peroxisomal oxidative activities. J Ped 1986; 108:25–32.
167. Moser HW, Moser AE, Singh I, O'Neill BP. Adrenoleukodystrophy: survey of 303 cases: biochemistry, diagnosis and therapy. Ann Neurol 1984; 16:628–641.
168. Aebi HE, Wyss SR. Acatalasemia. In: Stanbury JB, Wyngaarden JB, Fredrickson DS, eds. The metabolic basis of inherited disease. New York: McGraw-Hill, 1978: 1792.
169. Schutgens RB, Heymans HSA, Wanders RJA, van den Bosch HVD, Tager JM. Peroxisomal disorders: a newly recognized group of genetic diseases. Eur J Pediatr 1986; 144:430–440.
170. Hanson RF, Isenberg JN, Williams GC, Hachey D, Szczepanik P, Klein PD, Sharp HL. The metabolism of 3α, 7α, 12α-trihydroxy-5β-cholestan-26-oic acid in two siblings with cholestasis due to intrahepatic bile duct anomalies. J Clin Invest 1975; 56:577–587.
171. Eyssen H, Parmentier G, Compernolle F, Boon J, Eggermont E. Trihydroxy coprostanic acid in duodenal fluid of two children with intrahepatic bile duct anomalies. Biochim Biophys Acta 1972; 273:212–221.
172. Kase BJ, Björkhem I, Haga P, Pedersen JI. Defective peroxisomal cleavage of the C_{27}-steroid side chain in the cerebro-hepato-renal syndrome of Zellweger. J Clin Invest 1985; 75:427–435.

173. Björkhem I, Kase BF, Pedersen JI. Role of peroxisomes in the biosynthesis of bile acids. Scan J Clin Lab Invest 1985; 177:23–31.
174. Hanson RF. The formation and metabolism of 3α, 7α-dihydroxy-5β-cholestan-26-oic acid in man. J Clin Invest 1971; 50:2051–2055.
175. Parmentier GG, Janssen GA, Eggermont EA, Eyssen HJ. C_{27} Bile acids in infants with coprostanic acidemia and occurrence of a 3α, 7α, 12α-trihydroxy-5β-C_{29} dicarboxylic bile acid as a major component in their serum. Eur J Biochem 1979; 102:173–183.
176. Janssen G, Toppet S, Parmentier G. Structure of the side chain of the C_{29} dicarboxylic bile acid occurring in infants with coprostanic acidemia. J Lipid Res 1982; 23:456–465.
177. Eyssen H, Eggermont E, van Eldere J, Jaeken J, Parmentier G, Janssen G. Bile acid abnormalities and the diagnosis of cerebro-hepatorenal syndrome (Zellweger syndrome). Acta Paediatr Scand 1985; 74:539–544.
178. Délèze G, Björkhem I, Karlaganis G. Bile acids and bile alcohols in two patients with Zellweger (cerebro-hepato-renal) syndrome. J Pediatr Gastroenterol Nutr 1986; 5:701–710.
179. Lawson AM, Madigan MJ, Shortland D, Clayton PT. Rapid diagnosis of Zellweger syndrome and infantile Refsum's disease by fast atom bombardment-mass spectrometry of urine bile acids. Clin Chim Acta 1986; 161:221–231.
180. Clayton PT, Lake BD, Hall NA, Shortland DB, Carruthers RA, Lawson AM. Plasma bile acids in patients with peroxisomal dysfunction syndromes: Analysis by capillary gas chromatography–mass spectrometry. Eur J Pediatr 1987; 146:166–173.
181. Janssen G, Parmentier G. A further study of the bile acids in infants with coprostanic acidemia. Steroids 1981; 37:81–89.
182. Javitt N, Emerman S. Effect of sodium taurolithocholate on bile flow and bile acid excretion. J Clin Invest 1968; 47:1002–1014.
183. Setchell KDR, Matsui A. Serum bile acid analysis: the application of liquid-gel chromatographic techniques and capillary column gas chromatography and mass spectrometry. Clin Chim Acta 1983; 127:1–17.
184. Watkins JB, Ingall D, Szczepanik P, Klein PD, Lester R. Bile-salt metabolism in the new born. Measurement of pool size and synthesis by stable isotope technique. N Engl J Med 1973; 288:431–434.
185. Hofmann AF, Cummings SA. Measurement of bile acid and cholesterol kinetics in man by isotope dilution: principles and applications. In: Barbara L, Dowling RH, Hofmann AF, Roda E, eds. Bile acids in gastroenterology. Lancaster, UK: MTP Press, 1982: 75.
186. Clayton PT, Patel E, Lawson AM, Carruthers RA, Tanner MS, Strandvik B, Egestad B, Sjövall J. 3-Oxo-Δ^4 bile acids in liver disease. Lancet 1988; 4:1283–1284.
187. Javitt NB, Kok E, Gut M, Rajagopalan I, Budai K. Neonatal cholestasis: Identification of a metabolic error in bile acid synthesis. (Abstract) Pediatr Res 1986; 200.
188. Iser JH, Dowling RH, Murphy GM, Ponz de Leon M, Mitropoulos KA. Congenital bile salt deficiency associated with 28 years of intractable constipation. In: Paumgartner G, Stiehl A, eds. Bile acid metabolism in health and disease. Lancaster, UK: MTP Press, 1977: 231.
189. Dowling RH. Bile acids in constipation and diarrhoea. In: Barbara L, Dowling RH, Hofmann AF, Roda E, eds. Bile acids in gastroenterology. Lancaster, UK: MTP Press, 1982: 157.
190. Street JM, Trafford DJH, Makin HLJ. The quantitative estimation of bile acids and their conjugates in human biological fluids. J Lipid Res 1983; 24:491–511.
191. Setchell KDR, Lawson AM. The bile acids. In: Lawson AM, ed. Clinical biochemistry principles, methods, applications. Vol 1, Mass spectrometry. Berlin: Walter de Gruyter, 1988: 54.
192. Street JM, Setchell KDR. Chromatographic methods for bile acid analysis. Biomedical Chromatography 1988; 263:16637–16644.
193. Roda A, Roda E, Festi D, Colombo C. Immunological methods for serum bile acid analysis. In: Setchell KDR, Kritchevsky D, Nair PP. eds. The bile acids. Vol 4, Methods and applications. New York: Plenum Press, 1988: 269.
194. Scholmerich J, Roda A, DeLuca M. Bioluminescence assays using immobilized enzymes in bile acid analysis. In: Setchell KDR, Kritchevsky D, Nail PP, eds. The bile acids. Vol 4, Methods and applications. New York: Plenum Press, 1988: 315.
195. Nambara T, Goto J. High-performance liquid chromatography. In: Setchell KDR, Kritchevsky D, Nail PP, eds. The bile acids. Vol 4, Methods and applications. New York: Plenum Press, 1988: 43.
196. Setchell KDR, Vestal C. Thermospray ionization liquid chromatography-mass spectrometry (LC-MS)—a new and highly specific technique for the analysis of bile acids. J Lipid Res 1989; 30:1459–1469.
197. Lawson AM, Setchell KDR. Mass spectrometry of bile acids. In: Setchell KDR, Kritchevsky D, Nair PP, eds. The bile acids. Vol 4, Methods and applications. New York: Plenum Press, 1988: 167.
198. Sjövall J, Lawson AM, Setchell KDR. Mass spectrometry of bile acids. In: Law JH, Rilling HC, eds. Methods in enzymology. Vol 3. London: Academic Press, 1985: 63.
199. Lazarow PB, Black V, Shio H, Fujiki Y, Harjra AK, Datta NS, Bangara BS, Dancis J. Zellweger syndrome: biochemical and morphological studies on two patients treated with clofibrate. Pediatr Res 1985; 19:1356–1364.
200. Hess R, Staubli W, Riess W. Nature of the hepatomegalic effect produced by ethyl-chlorphenoxy-isobutyrate in the rat. Nature 1965; 208:856–858.
201. Lazarow PB. Three hypolipidemic drugs increase hepatic palmitoyl enzyme A oxidation in rat. Science 1977; 197:580–581.
202. Salen G, Meriwether TW, Nicolan G. Chenodeoxycholic acid inhibits increased cholesterol and cholestanol synthesis in patients with cerebrotendinous xanthomatosis. Biochem Med 1975; 14:57–74.
203. Berginer VM, Salen G, Shefer S. Long-term treatment of cerebrotendinous xanthomatosis with chenodeoxycholic acid. N Engl J Med 1984; 311:1649–1652.
204. Koopman BJ, Wolthers BG, Vander Molen JC, Waterreus RJ. Bile acid therapies applied to patients suffering from cerebrotendinous xanthomatosis. Clin Chim Acta 1985; 152:115–122.
205. Bachrach WH, Hofmann AF. Ursodeoxycholic acid in the treatment of cholesterol cholelithiasis. Dig Dis Sci 1982; 27:833–856.
206. Leuschner U, Leuschner M, Sieratzki J, Kurtz W, Hubner K. Gallstone dissolution with ursodeoxycholic acid in patients with chronic active hepatitis and two years follow-up. A pilot study. Dig Dis Sci 1985; 30:642–649.
207. Hofmann AF, Popper H. Ursodeoxycholic acid for primary biliary cirrhosis. (Letter) Lancet 1987; ii:398–399.
208. Poupon R, Chretien Y, Poupon RE, Ballet F, Calmus Y, Darvis F. Is ursodeoxycholic acid an effective treatment for primary biliary cirrhosis? Lancet 1987; i:834–836.
209. Ichimiya H, Egestad B, Nazer H, Gunasekaran T, Clayton PT, Sjövall J. Bile acids and alcohols in an infant with hepatic 3β-hydroxy-Δ^5-steroid dehydrogenase deficiency: effect of chenodeoxycholic acid treatment. Presented at 2nd International Symposium on Mass Spectrometry in Health and Life Sciences, San Francisco, 1989, p 12.
210. Setchell KDR, Flick R, Watkins JB, Piccoli DA. Chronic hepatitis in a 10-yr-old due to an inborn error in bile acid synthesis—diagnosis and treatment with oral bile acid. American Gastroenterology Association, May 13–16, San Antonio, TX, 1990.

PART 15

Wilson's Disease

Randi G. Pleskow, M.D.
Richard J. Grand, M.D.

Wilson's disease is a rare autosomal recessive disorder of copper metabolism. Kinnear Wilson described the entity in 1912 and considered it to be a degenerative disorder of the central nervous system (CNS) associated with asymptomatic cirrhosis.[1] In 1921, Hall reported the hepatic symptoms and introduced the name *hepatolenticular degeneration*.[2] It is now generally accepted that the disorder is related to excessive accumulations of copper in the liver, CNS, kidneys, cornea, skeletal system, and other organs. The prevalence of the disorder is one in 30,000 world wide, with a carrier frequency of one in 90.[3] Wilson's disease frequently presents in childhood, although the diagnosis may not be confirmed until adulthood.

PATHOPHYSIOLOGY

Although Wilson's disease has been recognized as an entity for more than 60 years, the basic biochemical defect is still unknown. Wilson's disease is a disorder of copper balance in which the biliary excretion of copper is inadequate.[4] Copper is an essential trace element required in a number of enzyme systems. The main dietary sources of copper include liver, kidney, shellfish, chocolate, dried beans, peas, and unprocessed wheat. Under normal circumstances, 50 percent of ingested copper is unabsorbed and lost in the feces,[5] and 30 percent is lost through the skin.[6] A negligible amount normally is excreted in the urine. The 20 percent remaining is critically balanced for homeostasis. A number of studies have addressed the question of whether there is an increase in copper absorption from the gastrointestinal (GI) tract in Wilson's disease. Studies measuring the peak copper concentration in blood following an oral dose of radiocopper have shown no difference between Wilson's disease and control patients.[7] Most investigators agree that the biliary excretion of copper is impaired in patients with Wilson's disease.[4,8] One elegant study used radiocopper to evaluate the abnormal biliary excretion of copper. The radioisotope was given orally 18 hours before cholecystectomy to two women, one with Wilson's disease the other without. The specific activities and concentrations of copper were measured in bile and in subcellular fractions of liver. In the patient with Wilson's disease, the lysosomal concentration of copper was greater, whereas the biliary concentration of copper was lower than in the control subject. From this study and other data it has been concluded that the basic biochemical defect lies in the excretion of copper from the lysosomes into the bile.[9]

Attention has also been given to the role that ceruloplasmin may play in the pathogenesis of the disease. Ceruloplasmin is a blue-colored alpha$_2$-globulin with a molecular mass of 132 kDa. It is produced exclusively in the liver, but its role in copper metabolism is unknown. Typically, in Wilson's disease, there is a deficiency of ceruloplasmin in serum or plasma. However, 5 to 25 percent of patients with Wilson's disease have normal levels of ceruloplasmin[3] owing primarily to the acute phase response associated with active liver disease. Low levels are found in heterozygotes who have no manifestation of the disease.[10] The etiology of the decreased level of ceruloplasmin is unknown. Both apo-ceruloplasmin and the number of atoms of copper per ceruloplasmin molecule are normal in Wilson's disease, but the synthetic rate of the protein is reduced.[3] Techniques using the cloned ceruloplasmin gene[11] indicate that both a reduced rate of transcription and a decreased level of ceruloplasmin mRNA are present in patients with Wilson's disease. However, ceruloplasmin mRNA was found in one patient who had no detectable serum ceruloplasmin. Hence, a translational or post-translational defect, in addition to the transcriptional defect, may underlie the abnormality in ceruloplasmin levels in Wilson's disease.[12]

Iyengar et al studied cholecystokinin-stimulated biliary secretions in Wilson's disease patients and in control patients. Using Sephadex chromatography, they isolated in controls a high molecular weight copper-containing substance that was absent in Wilson's disease samples, that was protease-resistant, and that increased with an increase in dietary copper in control patients. This high molecular weight protein cross-reacted with antibodies to human plasma ceruloplasmin; no such cross-reactivity was found in samples from patients with Wilson's disease. The authors postulated that the high molecular weight substance was ceruloplasmin or a ceruloplasmin-like protein. The copper bound in this protease-resistant protein was not reabsorbed by the intestine but instead was successfully excreted in the feces.[13]

The role of ceruloplasmin in the normal biliary excretion of copper and other mechanisms of hepatic copper excretion, as well as abnormalities in Wilson's disease, require further study. A genetic or cellular defect in the processing of ceruloplasmin, however, is unlikely to explain completely the pathogenesis of Wilson's disease. Furthermore, the gene for ceruloplasmin is on chromosome 3, while the Wilson's disease gene has been linked to the esterase D locus on chromosome 13.[14]

CLINICAL MANIFESTATIONS

The clinical manifestations of Wilson's disease usually are related to hepatic or CNS involvement (Table 1). The present-

TABLE 1
Manifestations of Wilson's Disease

Hepatic
Acute hepatitis
Chronic active hepatitis
Cirrhosis
Fulminant hepatic failure
Central Nervous System
Neurologic
Psychiatric
Ophthalmologic
Miscellaneous
Hemolytic anemia
Endocrinologic
Renal
Skeletal
Cardiac
Cholelithiasis

ing features are variable, and clinical disease is rarely present before 5 years of age. Most of the manifestations are related to deposition of copper in specific organs. In Sternlieb's series,[15] the initial clinical manifestations were hepatic in 42 percent, neurologic in 34 percent, psychiatric in 10 percent, hematologic or endocrinologic in 12 percent, and renal in 1 percent (Table 2). Approximately 25 percent of patients present with more than one organ involved.[15] Of 50 cases reviewed by Walshe, 31 had hepatic and 17 had neurologic presentations.[16] In the pediatric age group, it is common for the hepatic manifestions to precede the neurologic manifestations by many years.

Hepatic Manifestations

Manifestations of liver disease are greatly varied. Wilson's disease may present as an acute self-limited hepatitis. There may be full recovery, and the patient is thought to have had viral hepatitis. Young patients especially may present with a clinical and histologic picture similar to that of chronic active hepatitis. Neurologic dysfunction and Kayser-Fleischer rings may not be found,[18-19] and serum ceruloplasmin may be normal.[20] One series reviewed 17 patients, ages 7 to 21 years, with Wilson's disease, all of whom had a picture similar to that of chronic active hepatitis.[17] Serum ceruloplasmin was normal in three (all three had severe hepatic failure),

TABLE 2
Presenting Symptoms of Wilson's Disease

	Sternlieb and Scheinberg[15]	Walsh[16]
Hepatic	42%	62%
CNS		34%
Neurologic	34%	
Psychiatric	10%	
Hematologic and endocrinologic	12%	
Renal	1%	

At presentation more than one organ was involved in 25 percent.

Kayser-Fleischer rings were present in nine patients, and neurologic dysfunction was present in three patients. Cirrhosis was present on initial biopsy in 15 patients, and four patients died in 3 weeks of fulminant hepatic failure despite D-penicillamine treatment. Another five patients died within 2 years, mostly secondary to complications of their liver disease.

Perman et al assessed the accuracy of three findings—serum ceruloplasmin, 24-hour urinary copper excretion, and hepatic copper concentration—in differentiating Wilson's disease from chronic active hepatitis.[19] Of 45 patients evaluated, 20 had idiopathic chronic active hepatitis and 25 had Wilson's disease, all in the pediatric age group. Serum ceruloplasmin was decreased in 25 percent of patients with idiopathic chronic active hepatitis and normal in 28 percent of patients with Wilson's disease. The majority of patients with normal ceruloplasmin were symptomatic. Urinary copper excretion over 24 hours was elevated in five of 18 patients with idiopathic chronic active hepatitis, and four of these had values greater than 100 μg per 24 hours. In all the patients with Wilson's disease who had urine collections, the values were elevated. In one presymptomatic patient, the value was only 68 μg per 24 hours (normal, 48 ± 16). In six of nine patients with chronic active hepatitis studied, hepatic copper concentrations were elevated, but none was greater than 300 μg per gram of dry liver. In contrast, all nine patients with Wilson's disease who were biopsied had hepatic copper levels greater than 400 μg per gram of dry weight. On the basis of this study, determination of serum ceruloplasmin or urinary copper excretion alone is insufficient to make the diagnosis of Wilson's disease. The investigators concluded that hepatic copper content was the most reliable test for differentiating idiopathic chronic active hepatitis from Wilson's disease in pediatric patients.[19]

Liver disease may present as a fulminant hepatitis that can progress within weeks to hepatic failure, ascites, renal insufficiency, and death.[21-23] Without a history of Wilson's disease or hepatic or neurologic disease in the family, it is difficult to distinguish fulminant Wilson's disease from hepatic failure of other causes. McCullough et al found that, in general, patients with fulminant Wilson's disease were younger than those with idiopathic hepatic failure. Although seven of nine patients with Wilson's disease did have Kayser-Fleischer rings,[24] it should be noted that such rings may not yet be present when liver disease appears. Also, the rings are not pathognomonic for Wilson's disease; other forms of chronic liver disease may be associated with them (Table 3).[25] Patients with idiopathic fulminant hepatic failure may have decreased ceruloplasmin as well,[26] probably secondary to decreased hepatic synthetic function.[19,26] McCullough's group also reported elevated 24-hour urinary copper excretion in patients with idiopathic fulminant hepatitis; this may be explained by release of copper by the necrotic liver cells. They also found that patients with Wilson's disease tended to have higher copper levels in the serum, urine, and liver; lower elevations of transaminase levels; higher bilirubin values; and lower hemoglobin values than patients with other forms of hepatic failure.[24]

Patients presenting with fulminant hepatic failure have a particularly poor outcome even if the diagnosis of Wilson's disease is made. Treatment with oral D-penicillamine is often

TABLE 3
Conditions Associated with Kayser-Fleischer Rings

Wilson's disease
Chronic active hepatitis
Primary biliary cirrhosis
Cryptogenic cirrhosis
Intrahepatic cholestasis

successful but may be limited by renal failure.[27] Several studies have shown that adding D-penicillamine to peritoneal dialysis solution was not beneficial.[28-30] However, Rakela and associates reported on a patient with Wilson's disease presenting with acute hepatic failure, hemolysis, and anuric renal failure in whom postdilution hemofiltration and continuous arteriovenous hemofiltration with oral D-penicillamine allowed removal of more than 95,000 μg of copper, with nearly 80,000 μg removed by postdilution hemofiltration alone.[31] Finally, patients with Wilson's disease may present with features of cirrhosis including portal hypertension, ascites, varices, and hypoalbuminemia. In contrast to other causes of cirrhosis, there have been few reported cases of hepatocellular carcinoma evolving from Wilson's disease with cirrhosis.[32,33]

Central Nervous System Involvement

When Wilson initially described hepatolenticular degeneration, he thought the CNS damage was limited to the basal ganglia, especially the putamen.[1] It is now known that CNS involvement is more extensive, and a wide spectrum of neurologic findings ensues. Neurologic manifestations have been reported to occur as early as 6 years of age,[3] but more typically they begin in the second to third decade of life and are usually associated with the presence of Kayser-Fleischer rings. The onset of neurologic symptoms is gradual, and severity progresses without treatment. CNS damage in Wilson's disease is limited almost exclusively to the motor system, with the sensory system being spared. Common first neurologic symptoms are tremor, inco-ordination, dystonia, and difficulty with fine motor tasks such as dressing oneself and writing.[34] Later, other manifestations such as masklike facies, drooling, dysarthria, rigidity, and gait disturbances may become apparent. The patient often becomes highly frustrated, since the intellect is unchanged. Older patients are frequently misdiagnosed as having a pure psychiatric disorder or neurologic disease such as multiple sclerosis or a basal ganglia disorder.[34]

Computed tomography (CT) of the head may be helpful in the diagnosis (Table 4). CT findings are more apt to be present in patients with neurologic involvement but may also be abnormal in patients who are asymptomatic or have only hepatic involvement. In one study of 60 patients with Wilson's disease, 73 percent had ventricular dilatation, 63 percent cortical atrophy, 55 percent brain stem atrophy, 45 percent basal ganglia hypodensity, and 10 percent posterior fossa atrophy; in 18 percent findings were normal.[35] Cavitation of the putamen has also been described.[35,36] The CT abnormalities apparently do not represent actual copper deposition, since this would be expected to show as hyperdense areas. Rather, the changes are likely to be secondary to the damage that copper deposition causes. The hypodense areas, along with areas of generalized atrophy, are fairly characteristic of Wilson's disease.[35] The severity of the CT abnormalities does not correlate with clinical symptoms[37] and is also of little prognostic value, since patients with extensive involvement often do quite well.[35] Harik reported on one patient whose CT worsened despite clinical improvement.[37] Using sensory evoked potentials (somatosensory, brain stem auditory, and pattern-reversal visual evoked potentials) in patients with Wilson's disease, a high incidence of abnormalities was found in Wilson's disease patients with neurologic involvement but not in either asymptomatic patients or those with only hepatic involvement. The investigators also concluded that other basal ganglia diseases do not have such abnormalities, and therefore this may be a useful method of differentiating Wilson's disease from other disorders.[38] Magnetic resonance imaging (MRI) seems to be even more useful than CT in characterizing neurologic abnormalities. Cases have been reported in which the CT scan was normal, but the MRI scan was abnormal. A number of cases have shown more extensive involvement on MRI than on CT.[39] The hypodense areas seen on CT appear as areas of increased intensity on MRI, suggesting that edema may produce the CT abnormality.[40]

Neurologic symptoms may actually worsen during treatment. Of 20 D-penicillamine–treated patients recently reported, six experienced an initial neurologic deterioration. Three subsequently improved, but three did not recover. The authors speculate that with vigorous initial treatment, an excessive amount of copper is liberated from the liver and deposited in the brain. They propose that this may be prevented with gradual introduction of therapy.[34]

Psychiatric Manifestations

Psychiatric manifestations may be quite dramatic in patients with Wilson's disease. These include poor school performance, anxiety, depression, compulsive behavior, phobias, aggressive outbursts, neurosis, and even psychosis.[41,42] Affected patients are frequently labeled with erroneous psychiatric diagnoses before the diagnosis of Wilson's disease is made. It is sometimes difficult to distinguish the symptoms due to excessive copper deposition from those secondary to the individual's reaction to having a chronic disease. This is particularly an issue in adolescent patients, and psychological intervention is often helpful.

TABLE 4
Head CT Scan Findings in Wilson's Disease

Ventricular dilatation	73%
Cortical atrophy	63%
Brain stem atrophy	55%
Basal ganglia hypodensity	45%
Posterior fossa atrophy	10%
Normal	18%

Adapted from Williams and Walshe.[35]

Ophthalmologic Manifestations

Ophthalmologic manifestations of Wilson's disease have received considerable attention, since their presence may help lead to the diagnosis before any laboratory result is available. Kayser-Fleischer rings are usually present in patients with neurologic findings but are also frequently present in those with only hepatic manifestations, as well as in some asymptomatic patients.[43] Kayser first described the ring in a patient thought to have multiple sclerosis,[44] and several years later Fleischer reported an association of the ring with cirrhosis.[45] The Kayser-Fleischer ring may have a variable color depending upon the color of the iris. It has been described as a golden brown, brownish green, greenish yellow, bronze, or tannish green discoloration in the zone of Descemet's membrane in the limbic region of the cornea. It can sometimes be seen with the naked eye, but a slit-lamp examination is mandatory. The rings begin to form superiorly and then inferiorly and finally extend laterally to complete the ring.

The rings consist of copper granules; however, they represent only a small fraction of the total corneal copper content. The bulk of copper deposition is in the stromal layer, but no color change is seen in any of the corneal layers except in Descemet's membrane. Copper is initially taken up by the aqueous humor and diffuses into the cornea. Movement of water-soluble substances such as copper is a function of the evaporation of tears from the surface of the cornea. Evaporation is less at the superior poles and somewhat less at the inferior poles. Therefore, since the solvent flow is less in these areas, copper deposition is first seen there. Likewise, with treatment, the rings fade in the reverse order in which they appear.[46] Kayser-Fleischer rings are not specific for Wilson's disease. They have been seen in patients with chronic active hepatitis,[47,48] primary biliary cirrhosis,[49] and cryptogenic cirrhosis[48,50] and in children with chronic intrahepatic cholestasis (see Table 3).[41]

Sunflower cataracts are seen less frequently than Kayser-Fleischer rings and, when present, are accompanied by Kayser-Fleischer rings.[46] They can be seen with an ophthalmoscope as a greenish gray or golden disc in the anterior capsule of the lens with spokes radiating toward the lens periphery.[52] Most of these cataracts resolve with therapy, and they do not affect vision.[46]

Cardiac Manifestations

Although Wilson's disease is a multisystem disorder, there have been few studies evaluating the cardiac manifestations. One study of 53 patients showed electrocardiographic (ECG) abnormalities in 34 percent, including left ventricular hypertrophy, ST depression, T-wave inversion, premature ventricular contractions, sinoatrial block, and atrial fibrillation.[53] Thirteen percent of patients had arrhythmias, whereas 40 control patients of similar age all had normal ECGs. Of these Wilson's disease patients, 19 percent had mild asymptomatic orthostatic hypotension. Response to a Valsalva maneuver (as a test for normal autonomic functioning) was abnormal in six of 18 patients with Wilson's disease who were able to perform the maneuver.[53] Autopsy reports have shown cardiac hypertrophy, fibrosis, small vessel sclerosis, and myocardial inflammatory cell infiltrates, although gross abnormalities are not impressive. Pathologic findings did not correlate with myocardial copper content, which may be low or high. Several cases of sudden death are reported, presumably secondary to cardiac arrhythmia that may or may not be related to Wilson's disease.[54]

Renal Manifestations

Renal involvement is a widely recognized complication of Wilson's disease. It is characterized by proximal tubular dysfunction as indicated by aminoaciduria, glycosuria, increased excretion of uric acid and calcium, as well as a decrease in filtration rate and effective renal blood flow.[55,56] There is an acidification defect that is likely a distal tubular dysfunction in which patients are unable to acidify urine to a pH of less than 5.2 despite an acid load. Usually, however, patients are able to maintain normal or nearly normal plasma pH levels despite this renal tubular defect.[57-59]

Renal stones were reported in seven of 45 patients (16 percent) studied. Four of the seven patients with stones were discovered either before or simultaneously with the diagnosis of Wilson's disease. In the same study, microscopic hematuria was found in five of seven patients with stones and 19 of 47 patients with Wilson's disease without stones.[57] The histopathologic changes in renal biopsies are not impressive. Scheinberg and Sternlieb reported elevated copper concentrations in the kidney at autopsy in eight patients with untreated Wilson's disease.[60] Rubeanic acid staining has demonstrated granules, presumed to be copper, within the tubular epithelium.[61] Renal function has been shown to improve with penicillamine therapy.[62-64]

Skeletal Manifestations

A wide variety of skeletal changes are observed in patients with Wilson's disease. These include osteoporosis, rickets, osteomalacia, spontaneous fractures, osteochondritis dissecans, and osteoarthritis.[65,66] Bone demineralization is the most common abnormality seen. Renal defects causing hypercalciuria and hyperphosphaturia with resultant hypocalcemia and hypophosphatemia are the main etiology of demineralization.[67,68] Other factors include dystonic contractures and immobilization. Chronic liver disease itself has been shown to cause skeletal abnormalities.[69] Patients in the pediatric age group rarely have significant skeletal changes on radiograph.

Other Manifestations

Hemolysis is a recognized complication of Wilson's disease. It may precede other clinical manifestations of the disease and be short-lived or may progress to anemia and be the first recognized abnormality of the disease. Hemolysis may occur secondary to an oxidative injury to red blood cell membranes from excess copper,[70] but the exact mechanism remains unknown.

As a consequence of hemolysis as well as cirrhosis, cholelithiasis may complicate Wilson's disease. The stones are a mixed type containing both cholesterol and pigment. Gallstones should be looked for in patients with Wilson's disease; likewise, in a child with gallstones, Wilson's disease should be considered in the differential diagnosis.[71]

NATURAL HISTORY

Deiss et al have devised a valuable staging system that explains many of the confusing findings in Wilson's disease.[62] Revisions of the scheme are also available.[3] In stage I, a progressive accumulation of copper occurs in the cytosol of the hepatocytes. The process continues until all hepatic binding sites for copper are saturated. This stage is asymptomatic and usually occurs before age 5 years. In stage II, copper in the hepatocyte is redistributed from the cytosol to the lysosomes and, at the same time, copper is released from the liver. If this release occurs gradually, the patient remains asymptomatic. If the redistribution is rapid, hepatic necrosis may occur, and the patient may become symptomatic from liver disease. In addition, rapid release of copper into the blood may result in hemolytic anemia. If these complications resolve, the patient becomes asymptomatic again. In stage III, copper continues to be stored in the lysosomes, and varying degrees of fibrosis or cirrhosis develop. In this stage, accumulation of copper also occurs in other tissues, i.e., brain, cornea, kidney, or skeleton. Patients may remain asymptomatic for years if the liver and brain deposition of copper progresses slowly. If the accumulation occurs rapidly, then liver, and/or CNS disease becomes apparent in a short time (stage IV). Stage V occurs when treatment is begun before the patient succumbs to hepatic failure or irreversible brain damage.[72]

LIVER PATHOLOGY

None of the liver specimens were normal from more than 260 patients with Wilson's disease analyzed by Sternlieb and Scheinberg; even a specimen from a 3½-year-old boy was abnormal.[3] Characteristic histologic findings are present but by no means pathognomonic.

Fat deposition is one of the earliest changes seen in the liver biopsy. Fine lipid droplets composed of triglycerides are dispersed throughout the cytoplasm.[73,74] As the disease progresses, these lipid droplets increase in size until hepatic steatosis is manifested. In early stages, electron microscopy shows the mitochondria to be of varying shapes and sizes. The matrix density is increased, with vacuolated and crystalline inclusions. Inner and outer mitochondrial membranes, which are normally opposed, become separated and the intercristal spaces expand. Peroxisomes, which are involved in cellular lipid metabolism, may become enlarged with a granular, flocculant matrix of varying density rather than with the homogeneous matrix seen in normal peroxisomes.[75] As the hepatic lesion progresses, there is collagen deposition and eventually development of fibrosis. Histology indistinguishable from that of idiopathic chronic active hepatitis may develop, as well as hepatic necrosis (Fig. 1). If the patient does not succumb, cirrhosis develops. Once cirrhosis is established, the fatty changes, as well as those changes seen in the mitochondria and peroxisomes, disappear. The electron microscopic findings are then relatively normal except for excessive amorphous or globular copper-containing lipofuscin granules and lipid-containing lysosomes.[76]

A high copper content is found normally in the fetal and neonatal liver.[77] The etiology is not known, but it is postulated that immaturity of bile excretion plays a role in this increased copper level.[78] Some of the copper binds to a sulfhydryl-rich protein, known as copper-associated or copper-binding protein, which is bound in hepatic lysosomes.[79] This lysosomal copper may be stained by orcein.[80] Between the third and sixth month of life, hepatic copper levels fall to within the normal adult range and these orcein-positive granules are no longer seen in the normal liver. In children older than 6 months of age, orcein-positive granules are found only in abnormal conditions, including Wilson's disease, biliary atresia, paucity of intrahepatic ducts, primary biliary cirrhosis, sclerosing or chronic cholangitis, cirrhosis, and primary hepatic tumors (Table 5). Orcein-positive granules are not seen in acute liver disease. In contrast to Wilson's disease, the orcein-positive granules in other disease states are found mainly at the periphery of the liver lobules.[81] In Wilson's disease, these granules are widespread in some lobules but may be completely absent in others.[81,82] Not all the livers from patients with Wilson's disease contain stainable copper-associated protein. In the early stages of the disease, when the liver copper concentration is highest, the copper is distributed diffusely in the cytoplasm and is absent from the lysosomes[82] and therefore is not stainable. In the later stages of the disease, copper is redistributed to the lysosomes; then copper may be stained by rubeanic acid and copper-associated protein by orcein.[76] However, histochemical techniques cannot completely confirm a diagnosis of Wilson's disease. Confirmation is dependent on quantitative measurement of hepatic copper content. Other disorders associated with elevated hepatic copper concentrations are listed in Table 5.

DIAGNOSIS

The diagnosis of Wilson's disease may be made readily when the classic triad of hepatic disease, neurologic involvement, and Kayser-Fleischer rings is present. However, in the absence of this triad, the diagnosis begins with a high index of suspicion, especially in children. No single test can con-

TABLE 5
Conditions Associated with Elevated Hepatic Copper Concentration

Normal infant less than 6 months of age
Cholestasis syndromes
Biliary atresia
Paucity of intrahepatic ducts
Sclerosing cholangitis
Primary biliary cirrhosis
Indian childhood cirrhosis
Primary hepatic tumors
Wilson's disease

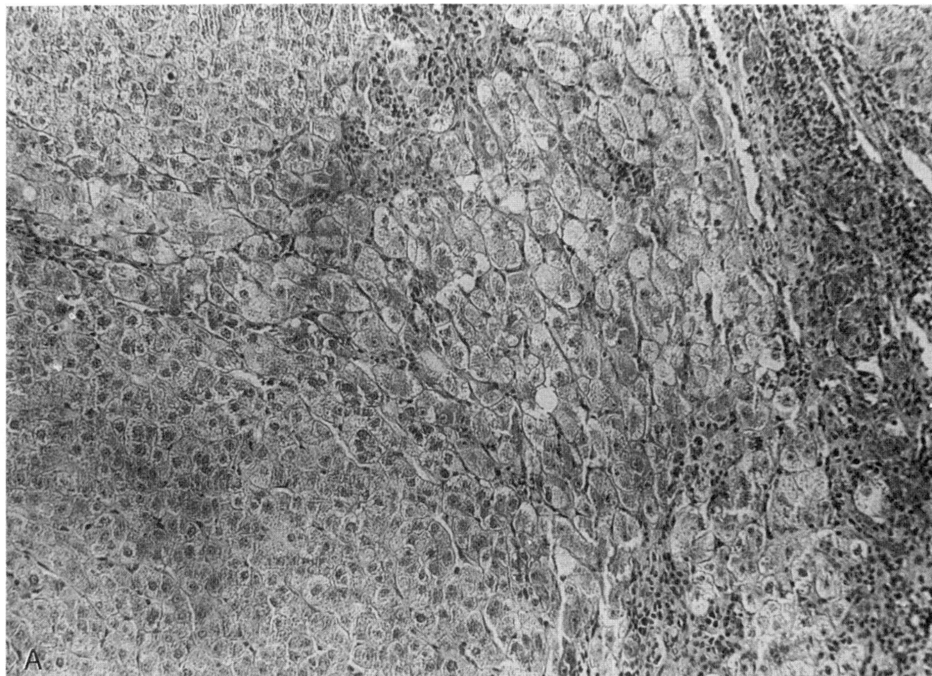

FIGURE 1 *A*, Wedge biopsy showing a broad band of fibrous tissue at the right margin. There is an intense portal inflammatory response with round cells spilling across the limiting plate into the lobule. There is considerable hepatocellular necrosis with marked variations in cell size and some fat as well as pigment deposition.

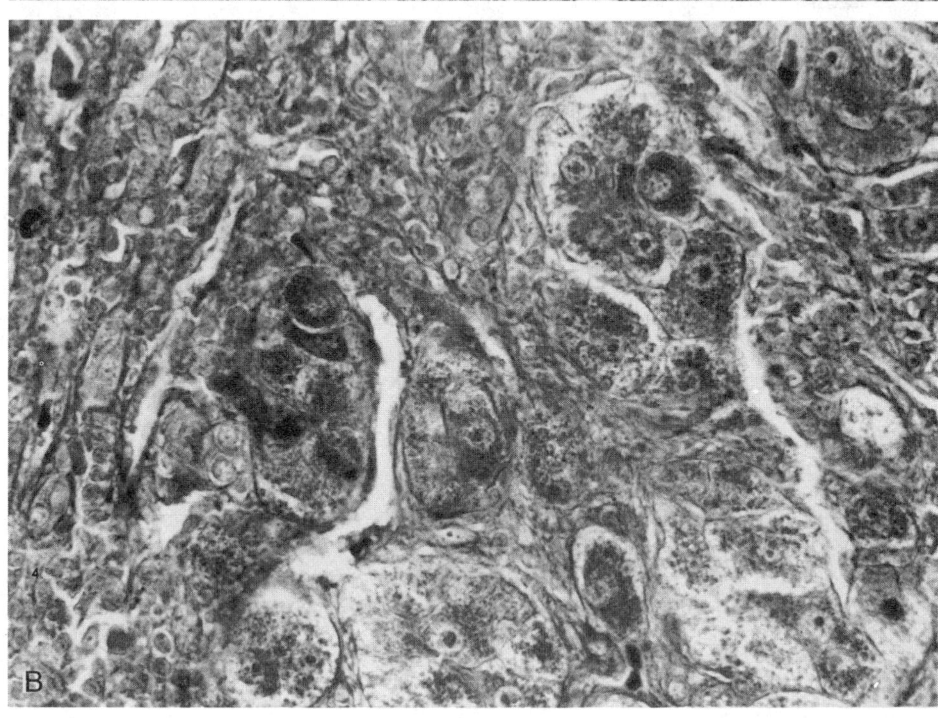

B, High-power view showing irregularities in cell size, hepatocellular necrosis, pigment deposition, and bile duct proliferation. The limiting plate has been distorted as shown by interdigitation of connective tissue and hepatocellular elements. Inflammatory cells are seen crossing the limiting plate into the lobule. (From Grand and Vawter.[99])

firm the diagnosis with 100 percent accuracy (Table 6). Rather, it is clinical and family history, the physical examination, and certain key laboratory investigations that collectively may establish the diagnosis.

A majority of children and adolescents with Wilson's disease have decreased serum ceruloplasmin values, and at least 75 percent of those presenting with hepatic manifestations have low values. Decreased values may also be seen in a number of other conditions, including malnutrition, protein-losing enteropathy, nephrotic syndromes, severe hepatic insufficiency,[3] and hereditary hypoceruloplasminemia,[83] as well as being a normal occurrence in the neonate.[84] Ceruloplasmin may be elevated during acute hepatitis as a consequence of the acute phase response or during estrogen therapy or pregnancy (Table 7).[85] Difficulty in diagnosis also arises in 10 percent of heterozygotes who have low serum ceruloplasmin

TABLE 6
Diagnosis of Wilson's Disease

- Clinical information
- Family history
- Kayser-Fleischer rings
- Laboratory tests
  - Hematologic
  - Liver function
  - Copper
    - Serum copper—less than 20 μg/dl
    - Urinary copper—greater than 100 μg/24 hour
    - Hepatic copper—greater than 250 μg/gram dry weight of liver
    - Radiocopper uptake

TABLE 8
Conditions Associated with Elevated Urinary Copper Excretion

- Primary biliary cirrhosis
- Chronic active hepatitis
- Fulminant hepatic failure
- Cholestasis syndromes
  - Biliary atresia
  - Paucity of intraheptic ducts
  - Sclerosing cholangitis

levels but no manifestations of Wilson's disease.[26] Therefore, serum ceruloplasmin should not be used as the sole determinant in diagnosing the disease.

Urinary copper excretion, which is normally less than 40 μg per 24 hours, is usually greater than 100 μg per 24 hours in persons with Wilson's disease and may be greater than 5,000 μg per 24 hours with a fulminant presentation.[24] The urine collections must be obtained in copper-free containers. Abnormal urinary copper excretion is not specific for Wilson's disease, since it may be elevated in patients with primary biliary cirrhosis,[86] chronic active hepatitis,[19] fulminant hepatitis, and cholestasis (Table 8).[26] Urinary copper excretion is a good measurement to follow during treatment of patients with Wilson's disease.

Kayser-Fleischer rings should always be looked for by slit-lamp examination, but they are not always present and are by no means pathognomonic for Wilson's disease (see Table 3).[47-51] They may be helpful when considering the possibility of treatment noncompliance, as in a patient whose Kayser-Fleischer rings have faded and then returned.

A liver biopsy should be performed whenever possible. Microscopic and ultrastructural analyses are valuable; measurements of quantitative hepatic copper concentrations are mandatory. Normal hepatic copper concentration is less than 50 μg per gram of dry weight of liver.[87] Patients with Wilson's disease generally have values greater than 250 μg per gram of dry liver, and values may be greater than 1,000 μg per gram of dry liver. A normal hepatic copper concentration rules out the diagnosis of Wilson's disease. While an elevated value confirms the diagnosis in the proper clinical setting, elevated values may be seen in other conditions (see Table 5).[88-90] These can usually be distinguished by other techniques.

If the diagnosis is still uncertain, the rate of incorporation of radiocopper into ceruloplasmin may be determined. Following a fast of 8 hours, a dose of 2.0 mg of radiocopper is administered orally. The concentration of radiocopper is measured in the serum 1, 2, 4, 24, and 48 hours later. The radiocopper rises in the 1-hour and 2-hour samples and then falls. In normal individuals, the serum concentration rises again to a higher level in the 24-hour or 48-hour sample, representing incorporation into ceruloplasmin. However, in patients with Wilson's disease, even those with normal ceruloplasmin levels, the secondary rise is not achieved. This test is also helpful in identifying heterozygotes,[91] except for those with low serum ceruloplasmin concentrations.

Asymptomatic relatives, especially siblings of patients with Wilson's disease, should be screened. They should have a careful physical examination, including slit-lamp examination, and measurement of serum ceruloplasmin concentration, hepatic transaminase levels, and 24-hour urinary copper excretion. If these are all normal, the diagnosis is excluded. However, if even one test is abnormal, a liver biopsy should be performed and samples sent for quantitative copper determination and histologic examination. In general, liver disease in the pediatric age group should be considered Wilson's disease until proven otherwise.

TABLE 7
Conditions Associated with Altered Ceruloplasmin Concentrations

- **Decreased**
  - Malnutrition
  - Protein-losing enteropathy
  - Nephrotic syndrome
  - Hepatic insufficiency
  - Hereditary hypoceruloplasminemia
  - Neonates
  - Menkes' syndrome
  - Wilson's disease
  - Heterozygosity for Wilson's disease
- **Elevated**
  - Estrogen therapy
  - Infection/inflammation
  - Pregnancy

TREATMENT

For many years, early diagnosis of Wilson's disease had little clinical significance. In 1951, Denny-Brown and Porter[92] as well as Cumings[93] introduced dimercaprol (BAL) as an effective treatment for Wilson's disease. However, the daily painful intramuscular injections made BAL impractical. In 1956, Walshe drastically changed the outcome of patients with Wilson's disease by showing that D-penicillamine is an effective treatment.[94] Wilson's disease is fatal if untreated, but successful outcome is achieved with effective pharmacologic therapy. The Food and Drug Administration approved D-penicillamine as effective and safe for Wilson's disease in 1963. In 1968, Sternlieb and Scheinberg showed its effectiveness also in asymptomatic patients (Table 9).[95]

TABLE 9
Treatment of Wilson's Disease

Dietary restriction of copper
D-Penicillamine
Triethylene tetramine (Trientine)
Zinc
Orthotopic liver transplantation

Penicillamine is a sulfur-containing amino acid that is a metabolite of penicillin, which chelates copper and then is excreted in the urine. When initiating therapy, a very small dose should be used; the dose should then be gradually increased to 1 g daily and administered orally in four divided doses 30 to 45 minutes before meals or 2 or more hours after eating. In young children, the dose is 20 mg per kilogram of body weight.[3] It has been shown that penicillamine is better absorbed in the absence of food.[96] Patients should also receive 25 mg of pyridoxine three times a week because of potential antipyridoxine effects of penicillamine.[97] As a consequence of treatment, urinary copper excretion may be more than 5,000 μg in a 24-hour period. However, this decreases with time; after months to years of therapy, it can be as low as 600 μg in a 24-hour period.[62] Usually there is a dramatic improvement in symptoms within weeks of beginning therapy. If there is no improvement, the daily dose of penicillamine may be raised to 1.5 to 2 g per day, although one must consider faulty patient compliance as a possible cause of poor response. Most patients become clinically asymptomatic or nearly so within months of beginning treatment, but some may not show significant functional improvement before 1 year. As a consequence of therapy, liver function tests improve and hepatic concentration of copper decreases. The neurologic manifestations occasionally initially worsen[34] but generally improve, although dysarthria associated with masklike facies may not disappear.[32] Kayser-Fleischer rings may disappear or fade partially.

Falkner and associates reported a 10-year-old child who had advanced liver cirrhosis and whose repeated liver biopsy was practically normal 27 months after starting penicillamine therapy. Initial biopsy as well as the one obtained following treatment was obtained by laparotomy, and multiple samples were taken to decrease sampling error.[98] This report is unusual in showing virtually complete reversal of liver pathology. Most other studies have shown improvement in liver biopsy findings with decreased portal fibrosis, inflammation, and necrosis, but not normalization.[99-101] The patient's compliance with therapy is best assessed using sequential determinations of 24-hour urinary copper excretion. In addition, Sternlieb and Scheinberg recommend the assessment of free serum copper. This is accomplished by spot determinations of total serum copper and ceruloplasmin concentrations. A factor of three is then multiplied by the ceruloplasmin value, and that value is subtracted from the total serum copper level. A resulting figure not greater than 20 indicates compliance.

Undesirable side effects of penicillamine therapy may occur within the first 3 weeks of treatment in 20 percent of patients. These include fever, skin rash, lymphadenopathy, granulocytopenia, and thrombocytopenia.[102] Other reactions that may occur later include nephrotoxicity with proteinuria or even nephrotic syndrome,[103] lupus-like syndrome,[104] Goodpasture's syndrome (which was fatal in three patients),[105] elastosis perforans serpiginosa,[106,107] and pemphigoid lesions of the mouth, vagina, and skin.[108,109] A penicillamine dermatopathy may occur in patients receiving more than 2 g of penicillamine for several months. Penicillamine interferes with cross-linking of collagen and elastin and leads to a weakening of the subcutaneous tissue, so that bleeding into the subcutaneous tissue may occur with even slight trauma.[3,107] Sternlieb and Scheinberg recommend that treatment of these reactions include discontinuation of penicillamine to allow the reaction to resolve. Two to 3 days before reinstituting therapy they begin 20 to 30 mg of prednisone (0.5 mg per kilogram of body weight). Penicillamine should be introduced in a much lower dose and gradually increased. Once penicillamine is tolerated, the prednisone may be withdrawn.[3] If the reaction was severe, one may not wish to attempt this but to institute other decuprinizing agents (Table 9).

Death has occurred as early as 8 months following discontinuation of D-penicillamine in a patient who had become asymptomatic with treatment and then was noncompliant. There are several reports of death within 1 year of stopping therapy in noncompliant patients. This raises the question of the exact mechanisms of D-penicillamine action. A patient who has been decuprinized with therapy should not succumb to death after just 8 months of copper reaccumulation (as initial copper accumulation takes more than 5 years in stage I). Scheinberg and associates suggest that penicillamine may form a nontoxic complex with copper. When penicillamine treatment is suddenly stopped, there may be a sudden dissociation of this complex and massive amounts of copper may be released, accounting for the rapid hepatic decompensation that occurs in suddenly noncompliant patients. The first sign of relapse after stopping penicillamine is a silent rise in serum transaminase levels.[108] The rise may be low compared with the amount of ongoing hepatic injury. Bilirubin becomes elevated later, and there is a decrease in serum albumin concentration, elevation in free serum copper levels,[3] and an elevation in 24-hour urinary excretion of copper. The urinary copper excretion is rarely greater than 1,000 μg in patients taking penicillamine regularly. It may be greater than 2,000 μg in a patient who has been noncompliant and then begins taking penicillamine again before urine collection.[108]

In 1969, Walshe introduced triethylene tetramine dihydrochloride (Trientine) as an alternative chelating agent to penicillamine for a patient who had developed an immune complex nephritis after 6 years of penicillamine treatment.[110] Cupriuresis, as great as or greater than that achieved with penicillamine, may be achieved with Trientine.[111] Walshe also reported 20 patients treated with Trientine because of intolerable side effects from penicillamine. These side effects included immune complex nephritis, dermatologic involvement, and bone marrow toxicity. These patients were followed for 14 months to 10 years. Half were very ill at the time of diagnosis. Eight had received little penicillamine since the side effects had developed. Eight other patients were asymptomatic and remained so on Trientine. The remaining four patients had residual neurologic symptoms on penicillamine, and these resolved on Trientine. Most patients have complete recovery of the side effects seen with penicillamine, although at least one patient with elastosis perforans serpiginosa did not improve with Trientine. Two other patients with penicillamine-induced lupus did not improve upon discontinuation of penicillamine and introduction of Trientine. Walshe reports that iron deficiency anemia may develop in patients treated with Trientine, especially women. This resolves with daily iron supplements.[112] Both penicillamine and Trientine have been reported to be safe during pregnancy, and eight healthy infants have been born to women treated with Trientine throughout pregnancy.[113] Trientine is given orally in divided doses of 1 to 1.5 g daily, 1 hour before or 2 hours after meals. In children less than 10 years of age, 0.5 g (approximately 20 mg per kilogram) daily is recommended.[114]

Zinc, a known antagonist of copper absorption, has been introduced as a possible alternative treatment for Wilson's disease in patients previously successfully treated with penicillamine. Smith and Larson, in 1946, reported on the antagonistic effects of zinc on copper balance in rats.[115] A decrease in liver copper content secondary to zinc supplementation in sheep was reported in 1954.[116] Patients with sickle cell anemia treated with zinc had been observed to develop copper deficiency.[117] In 1961, the role of zinc in producing negative copper balance in Wilson's disease was first described.[118] Several patients subsequently demonstrated clinical improvement when treated with zinc alone.[118–120]

Copper is absorbed mainly in the proximal small intestine.[121] Its absorption is increased in the presence of chelating agents, a high-protein diet, anions, and L-amino acids. Fiber, bile, ascorbic acid, and zinc inhibit its absorption. Once copper crosses the intestinal brush border, it binds to metallothionein in the cytosol of the enterocytes. Zinc, copper, cadmium, glucagon, glucocorticoids, and bacterial infections induce the synthesis of intestinal metallothionein.[122] Metallothionein has a higher affinity for copper than for zinc,[123] and the copper that is methallothionein-bound cannot pass the serosa but is sloughed with the intestinal cells into the lumen. Therefore, copper levels in stool are increased in patients treated with zinc.[124]

Hill and associates reported on the use of varying dosage schedules of zinc acetate in 14 patients with Wilson's disease. Most (13) of these patients were previously decuprinized with penicillamine. All the decuprinized patients were maintained in a negative to neutral copper balance during treatment with zinc.[125] Since the balance studies were not long-term, the question of gradual reaccumulation of body copper is raised.[126] Van Caillie-Bertrand et al described two children with Wilson's disease who were clinically stable after treatment with penicillamine and were then treated with zinc sulfate, 150 mg three times a day as a loading dose followed by a maintenance dose of 100 mg three times a day.[127] Liver function tests remained normal after 3 years of treatment. Serum copper values continued to fall, and urinary copper was low, as expected, since copper loss with zinc treatment is through the intestine. Of great concern were the measured hepatic copper contents; in one patient the liver copper content fell, but in the other patient it rose threefold. The latter patient also had an increase in urinary copper excretion after a challenge dose of D-penicillamine following the 3-year treatment with zinc.

TABLE 10
Indications for Orthotopic Liver Transplantation in Wilson's Disease

Fulminant hepatic failure
Cirrhosis with decompensation
Progression of hepatic dysfunction despite treatment

From Sternlieb.[129]

Although zinc seems to be a basically safe medication, long-term effects are not known and efficacy is unproven. Lymphocyte response to phytohemagglutinin, chemotaxis, and bacterial phagocytosis were reduced in normal males receiving 150 mg of zinc twice a day for six weeks.[128] More information is needed concerning the long-term effects of zinc therapy in Wilson's disease before it can be recommended in place of penicillamine or Trientine, even in a decuprinized patient. Regardless of what decuprinizing agent one uses, a low copper diet should be advised in all patients with Wilson's disease (Table 9).

Orthotopic liver transplantation has been performed in several patients with Wilson's disease (Table 10). Sternlieb defined three groups of patients who should be considered for liver transplants[129]: (1) patients presenting with a clinical picture of fulminant hepatitis, often an adolescent or young patient; (2) patients with findings of severe hepatic decompensation who have not improved after 2 to 3 months of adequate chelation therapy as well as therapy for hepatic failure; (3) patients who have been effectively treated but have developed severe progressive hepatic insufficiency acutely after stopping penicillamine. Reports on those Wilson's disease patients surviving liver transplants have demonstrated extremely favorable outcome. Tests of copper status, including serum ceruloplasmin, serum copper, and 24-hour urinary copper excretion, normalize within 1 to 2 months.[130] There are several reports of improvement of neurologic symptomatology following transplantation. Polson and associates describe two patients, one who preoperatively had continued worsening of neurologic manifestations despite penicillamine treatment and the other who had continued worsening of hepatic as well as neurologic symptoms. In both patients, recovery of neurologic function occurred but was slow.[131]

The findings that clinical and laboratory abnormalities normalize following liver transplantation support the now-accepted theory that the metabolic defect of Wilson's disease is localized within the liver.

REFERENCES

1. Wilson SAK. Progressive lenticular degeneration: a familial nervous disease associated with cirrhosis of the liver. Brain 1912; 34:295–509.
2. Hall HC. La degenerescence hepatico-lenticulaire malade de Wilson-pseudo-sclerose. Paris: Mason and Cie, 1921.
3. Scheinberg IH, Sternlieb I. Wilson's disease. Philadelphia: WB Saunders, 1984.
4. Frommer DJ. Defective biliary excretion of copper in Wilson's disease. Gut 1974; 15:125–129.
5. Strickland GT, Becker WM, Leu ML. Absorption of copper in homozygotes and heterozygotes for Wilson's disease and controls: isotope tracer studies with^{67} copper-^{64}copper. Clin Sci 1972; 43:617–625.

6. Jacob RA, Sandstead HH, Munoz JM, Klevay LM, Milne DB. Whole body surface loss of trace metals in normal males. Am J Clin Nutr 1981; 34:1379–1383.
7. Sternlieb I, Scheinberg IH. Radiocopper in diagnosing liver disease. Semin Nucl Med 1972; 2:176–188.
8. Gibbs K, Walshe JM. Biliary excretion of copper in Wilson's disease. Lancet 1980 ii:538–539.
9. Sternlieb I, Van den Hamer CJA, Morell AG, Alpert S, Gregoriadis G, Scheinberg IH. Lysosomal defect of hepatic copper excretion in Wilson's disease (hepatolenticular degeneration). Gastroenterology 1973; 64:99–105
10. Gibbs K, Walshe JM. A study of the ceruloplasmin concentrations found in 75 patients with Wilson's disease. Their kinships and various control groups. Q J Med 1979; 48:447–463.
11. Koschinsky ML, Funk WD, Vanoost BA, MacGillivray RTA. Complete cDNA sequence of human preceruloplasmin. Proc Natl Acad Sci USA 1986; 83:5086–5090.
12. Czaja MJ, Weiner FR, Schwarzenberg SJ, Sternlieb I, Scheinberg IH, VanThiel DH, LaRusso NF, Giambrone MA, Kirschner R, Koschinsky ML, MacGillivray RTA, Zern MA. Molecular studies of ceruloplasmin deficiency in Wilson's disease. J Clin Invest 1987; 80:1200–1204.
13. Iyengar V, Brewer GJ, Dick RD, Owyang C. Studies of cholecystokinin-stimulated biliary secretions reveal a high molecular weight copper-binding substance in normal subjects that is absent in patients with Wilson's disease. J Lab Clin Med 1988; 111:267–274.
14. Frydman MB, Bonne-Tamir LA, Farrer PM, Conneally A, Magazanik A, Asknel S, Goldwitch Z. Assignment of the gene for Wilson's disease to chromosome 13. Linkage to the esterase D locus. Proc Natl Acad Sci USA. 1985; 82:1819–1821.
15. Sternlieb I, Scheinberg IH. Wilson's disease. In: Wright R, Alberti KGM, Karran S, Millward-Sadler GH, eds. Liver and biliary disease: pathophysiology, diagnosis, management. London: WB Saunders, 1979: 774.
16. Walshe JM. Wilson's disease, a review. In: Peisach J, Aisen P, Blumberg WE, eds. The biochemistry of copper, New York: Academic Press, 1966: 475.
17. Scott J, Gollan JL, Samounan S, Sherlock S. Wilson's disease presenting as chronic active hepatitis. Gastroenterology 1978; 74:645–651.
18. Slovis TL, Dubois RS, Rodgerson DO, Silverman A. The varied manifestations of Wilson's disease. J Pediatr 1971; 78:578–584.
19. Perman JA, Werlin SL, Grand RJ, Watkins JB. Laboratory measures of copper metabolism in the differentiation of chronic active hepatitis and Wilson's disease in children. J Pediatr 1979; 94:564–568.
20. Sternlieb I, Scheinberg IH. Chronic hepatitis as a first manifestation of Wilson's disease. Ann Intern Med 1972; 76:59–64.
21. Roche-Sicot J, Benhamou JP. Acute intravascular hemolysis and acute liver failure associated as a 1st manifestation of Wilson's disease. Ann Intern Med 1977; 86:301–303.
22. Adler R, Matinovski V, Heuser ET, Presser DH, Robinson RG. Fulminant hepatitis: a presentation of Wilson's disease. Am J Dis Child 1977; 131:870–872.
23. Doering EG III, Savage RA, Dittmer TE. Hemolysis, coagulation defects, and fulminant hepatic failure as a presentation of Wilson's disease. Am J Dis Child 1979; 133:440–441.
24. McCullough AJ, Fleming CR, Thistle JL, Baldus WP, Ludwig J, McCall JT, Dickson ER. Diagnosis of Wilson's disease presenting as fulminant hepatic failure. Gastroenterology 1983; 84:161–167.
25. Fleming CR, Dickson ER, Wahner HW, Hollenhorst RW, McCall JT. Pigmented corneal rings in non-Wilsonian liver disease. Ann Intern Med 1977; 86:285–288.
26. Walshe JM, Briggs J. Ceruloplasmin in liver disease; a diagnostic pitfall. Lancet 1962; ii:263–265.
27. Vielhauer W, Eckardt V, Hollermuller KH, Luth JB, Schulle B, Prellwitz W, Sonntag W. D-Penicillamine in Wilson's disease presenting as acute liver failure with hemolysis. Dig Dis Sci 1982; 27:1126–1129.
28. DeBont B, Moulin D, Stein F, VanHoof F, Lauwerys R. Peritoneal dialysis with D-penicillamine in Wilson's disease. J Pediatr 1985; 107:545–547.
29. Hamlyn AN, Gollan JL, Douglas AP, Sherlock S. Fulminant Wilson's disease with hemolysis and renal failure: copper studies and assessment of dialysis regimens. Br Med J 1977; 2:660–662.
30. Rector WG Jr, Uchida T, Kanel GC, Redeker AG, Reynolds TB. Fulminant hepatic and renal failure complicating Wilson's disease. Liver 1984; 4:341–347.
31. Rakela J, Kurtz SB, McCarthy JT, Ludwig J, Ascher NL, Bloomer JR, Claus PL. Fulminant Wilson's disease treated with posdilution hemofiltrations and orthotopic liver transplantation. Gastroenterology 1986; 90:2004–2007.
32. Kamakura K, Kimura S, Igarashi S, Fujiwara K, Toshitsugu O. A case of Wilson's disease with hepatoma. J Jpn Soc Int Med 1975; 64:232–238.
33. Terao H, Itakura H, Nakota K, Kano K, Muro T, Furukawa R, Kusumoto M, Munehisa T, Mogataki S, Ishii N, Koji T, Hirama M. An autopsy case of hepatocellular carcinoma in Wilson's disease. Acta Heptol Jpn 1982; 23:439–445.
34. Starosta-Rubinstein S, Young A, Kluin K, Hill G, Aisen AM, Gabrielsen T, Brewer GJ. Clinical assessment of 31 patients with Wilson's disease. Correlations with structural changes on magnetic resonance imaging. Arch Neurol 1987; 44:365–370.
35. Williams FJB, Walshe JM. Wilson's disease. An analysis of the cranial computerized tomographic appearances found in 60 patients and the changes in response to treatment with chelating agents. Brain 1981; 104:735–752.
36. Selekler K, Kansu T, Zileli T. Computed tomography in Wilson's disease. Arch Neurol 1981; 38:727–728.
37. Harik SI, Donovan Post MJ. Computed tomography in Wilson's disease. Neurology 1981; 31:107–110.
38. Chu N-S. Sensory evoked potentials in Wilson's disease. Brain 1986; 109:491–507.
39. Lawler GA, Pennock JM, Steiner RE, Jenkins WJ, Sherlock S, Young IR. Nuclear magnetic resonance (NMR) imaging in Wilson's disease. J Comput Assist Tomogr 1983; 7:1–8.
40. Aisen AM, Martel W, Gabrielsen TO, Glazer GM, Brewer G, Young AB, Hill G. Wilson disease of the brain: MR imaging. Radiology 1985; 157:137–141.
41. Scheinberg IH, Sternlieb I, Richman J. Psychiatric manifestations in patients with Wilson's disease. Birth Defects original article series. Vol. IV. Bergsma D, Scheinberg IH, Sternlieb I, eds. New York: The National Foundation—March of Dimes, 1968: 85.
42. Goldstein NP, Ewert MA, Randall RV, Gross JB. Psychiatric aspects of Wilson's disease (hepatolenticular degeneration). Results of psychometric tests during long-term therapy. Am J Psychiatry 1968; 124:1555–1561.
43. Werlin SL, Grand RJ, Perman JA, Watkins JB. Diagnostic dilemmas of Wilson's disease: diagnosis and treatment. Pediatrics 1978; 62:47–51.
44. Kayser B, Ueber einen Fall Von angeborener grunlicher Verfarbung der Cornea. Klin Monatsbl Augenheilkd 1902; 40:22–25.
45. Fleisher B. Die periphere braun-grunliche Hornhautverfarbung. Als symptom einer eigenartigen allgemeiner Krankung. Munch Med Wochenschr 1909; 56:1120–1123.
46. Wiebers DO, Hollenhurst RW, Goldstein NP. The ophthalmologic manifestations of Wilson's disease. Mayo Clin Proc 1977; 52:409–416.
47. Fleming CR, Dickson ER, Wahner HW, Holenhorst RW, McCall JT. Pigmented corneal rings in non-Wilsonian liver disease. Ann Intern Med 1977; 86:285–288.
48. Frommer D, Morris J, Sherlock S, Abrams J, Newman S, Kayser-Fleischer-like rings in patients without Wilson's disease. Gastroenterology 1977; 72:1331–1335.
49. Fleming CR, Dickson ER, Hollenhorst RW, Goldstein NP, McCall JT, Baggenstoss AH., Pigmented corneal rings in a patient with primary biliary cirrhosis. Gastroenterology 1975; 69:220–225.
50. Rimola A, Bruguera M, Rodes J. Kayser- Fleischer-like rings in a cryptogenic cirrhosis. Arch Intern Med 1978; 138:1857–1858.
51. Jones EA, Rabin L, Buckley CH, Webster GK, Owens D. Progressive intrahepatic cholestasis of infancy and childhood. A clinicopathological study of a patient surviving to the age of 18 years. Gastroenterology 1976; 71:675–682.
52. Herron BE. Wilson's disease. Ophthalmol Semin 1976; 1:63–69.
53. Kuan P. Cardiac Wilson's disease. Chest 1987; 91:579–583.
54. Factor SM, Cho S, Sternlieb I, Scheinberg IH, Goldfischer S. The cardiomyopathy of Wilson's disease. Myocardial alterations in 9 cases. Virchows Arch 1982; 397:301–311.
55. Bearn AG, Yu TF, Gutman AB. Renal function in Wilson's disease. J Clin Invest 1957; 36:1107–1114.
56. Leu ML, Strickland GT, Gutman RA. Renal function in Wilson's disease: response to penicillamine therapy. Am J Med Sci 1970; 260:381–398.

57. Wiebers DO, Wilson DM, McLeod RA, Goldstein NP. Renal stones in Wilson's disease. Am J Med 1979; 67:249–254.
58. Fulop M, Sternlieb I, Scheinberg IH. Defective urinary acidification in Wilson's disease. Ann Intern Med 1968; 68:770–777.
59. Wilson DM, Goldstein NP. Bicarbonate excretion in Wilson's disease (hepatolenticular degeneration). Mayo Clin Proc 1974; 49:394–400.
60. Scheinberg IH, Sternlieb I. Metabolism of trace metals. In: Bundy PK, ed. Duncan's Disease of Metabolism. 6th ed. Vol 2, Endocrinology and Nutrition, Philadelphia: WB Saunders 1969: 550.
61. Reynolds ES, Tannen RL, Tyler HR. The renal lesion in Wilson's disease. Am J Med 1966; 40:518–527.
62. Deiss A, Lee GR, Cartwright GE. Hemolytic anemia in Wilson's disease. Ann Intern Med 1970; 73:413–418.
63. Elsas LJ, Hayslett JP, Spargo BH, Durant JL, Rosenberg LE. Wilson's disease with reversible renal tubular dysfunction: correlation with proximal tubular ultrastructure. Ann Intern Med 1971; 75:427–433.
64. Walshe JM. Effect of penicillamine on failure of renal acidification in Wilson's disease. Lancet 1968; i: 775–778.
65. Finby N, Bearn AG. Roentgenographic abnormalities of the skeletal system in Wilson's disease (hepatolenticular degeneration). Am J Roentgenol 1958; 79:603–611.
66. Mindelzun R, Elkin M, Scheinberg IH, Sternlieb I. Skeletal changes in Wilson's disease. A radiological study. Radiology 1970; 94:127–132.
67. Strickland GT, Leu M-L. Wilson's disease. Clinical and laboratory manifestations in 40 patients. Medicine 1975; 54:113–137.
68. Golding DN, Walshe JM. Arthropathy of Wilson's disease. Study of clinical and radiological features in 32 patients. Ann Rheum Dis 1977; 36:99–111.
69. Paterson CR, Losowsky MS. The bones in chronic liver disease. Scand J Gastroenterol 1967; 2:293–300.
70. Schouwink G. De hepato-cerebral degenerati. Met een onderozoek van de zinkstofwisseling; academisch proefshrift. Amsterdam: van der Wiel, Arnhem, 1961.
71. Rosenfield N, Grand RJ, Watkins JB, Ballantyne TVN, Levey R. Cholelithiasis and Wilson's disease. J Pediatr 1978; 92:210–213.
72. Dobyns WB, Goldstein NP, Gordon H. Clinical spectrum of Wilson's disease (hepatolenticular degeneration). Mayo Clin Proc 1979; 54:35–42.
73. Scheinberg IH, Sternlieb I. The liver in Wilson's disease. Gastroenterology 1959; 37:550–564.
74. Sternlieb I. Mitochrondrial and fatty changes in hepatocytes of patients with Wilson's disease. Gastroenterology 1968; 55:354–367.
75. Sternlieb I, Quintana N. The peroxisomes of human hepatocytes. Lab Invest 1977; 36:140–149.
76. Goldfischer S, Sternlieb I. Changes in the distribution of hepatic copper in relation to the progression of Wilson's disease (hepatolenticular degeneration). Am J Pathol 1968; 53:883–901.
77. Epstein O. Liver copper in health and disease. Postgrad Med 1983; 59 (suppl 4):88–94.
78. Shenker S, Dawber NH, Schmid R. Bilirubin metabolism in the fetus. J Clin Invest 1964; 43:32–39.
79. Nakanuma Y, Karino T, Ohta G. Orcein positive granules in the hepatocytes in chronic intrahepatic cholestasis. Virchows Arch 1979; 382:21–30.
80. Sipponen P. Orcein positive hepatocellular material in longstanding biliary diseases. I. Histochemical characteristics. Scand J Gastroenterol 1976; 11:545–552.
81. Sumithran E, Looi LM. Copper binding protein in liver cells. Hum Pathol 1985; 16:677–682.
82. Goldfischer S, Popper H, Sternlieb I. The significance of variations of copper in liver disease. Am J Pathol 1980; 99:715–730.
83. Edwards CQ, Williams DM, Cartwright GE. Hereditary hypoceruloplasminemia. Clin Genet 1979; 15:311–316.
84. Scheinberg IH, Cook CD, Murphy JA. The concentration of copper and ceruloplasmin in maternal and infant plasma at delivery. J Clin Invest 1954; 33:963.
85. Sternlieb I. Diagnosis of Wilson's disease. Gastroenterology 1978; 74:787–789.
86. Dickson ER, Fleming CR, Ludwig J. Primary biliary cirrhosis. Prog Liver Dis 1979; 6:487–502.
87. Smallwood RA, Williams HA, Rosenoer VM, Sherlock S. Liver copper levels in liver disease: studies using neutron activation analysis. Lancet 1968; ii:1310–1313.
88. Evans J, Newman S, Sherlock S. Liver copper levels in intrahepatic cholestasis of childhood. Gastroenterology 1978; 75:875–878.
89. Tanner MS, Portmann B, Mowat AP, Williams R, Pandit AN, Mills CF, Brewer I. Increased hepatic copper concentration in Indian childhood cirrhosis. Lancet 1979; i:1203–1205.
90. Maggiore G, DeGiacomo C, Sessa F, Burgio GR. Idiopathic hepatic copper toxicosis in a child. J Pediatr Gastroenterol Nutr 1987; 6:980–983.
91. Sternlieb I, Scheinberg IH. The role of radiocopper in the diagnosis of Wilson's disease. Gastroenterology 1979; 77:138–142.
92. Denny-Brown D, Porter H. The effect of BAL (2,3-dimercaptopropanol) on hepatolenticular degeneration (Wilson's disease). N Engl J Med 1951; 245:922–925.
93. Cumings JN. The effect of BAL in hepatolenticular degeneration. Brain 1951; 74:10–22.
94. Walshe JM. Penicillamine, a new oral therapy for Wilson's disease. Am J Med 1956; 21:487–495.
95. Sternlieb I, Scheinberg IH. Prevention of Wilson's disease in asymptomatic patients. N Engl J Med 1968; 278:352–359.
96. Bergstrom RF, Kay DR, Harkcom TM, Wagner JG. Penicillamine kinetics in normal subjects. Clin Pharmacol Therapeut 1981; 30:404–413.
97. Jaffe I, Altman K, Merryman P. The antipyridoxine effect of penicillamine in man. J Clin Invest 1964; 43:1869–1873.
98. Falkner S, Samuelson G, Sjolin S. Penicillamine-induced normalization of clinical signs and liver morphology and histochemistry in a case of Wilson's disease. Pediatrics 1970; 45:260–268.
99. Grand RJ, Vawter GF. Juvenile Wilson's disease. Histologic and functional studies during penicillamine therapy. J Pediatr 1975; 87:1161–1170.
100. Sternlieb I, Feldman G. Effects of anticopper therapy on hepatolenticular mitochondria in patients with Wilson's disease. Gastroenterology 1976; 71:457–461.
101. Marecek Z, Heyrovsky A, Volek V. The effect of long term treatment with penicillamine on the copper content in the liver in patients with Wilson's disease. Acta Hepatol Gastroenterol 1975; 22:292–296.
102. Sternlieb I, Scheinberg IH. Penicillamine therapy in hepatolenticular degeneration. JAMA 1964; 189:748–754.
103. Adams DA, Goldman R, Maxwell MH, Latta H. Nephrotic syndrome associated with penicillamine therapy of Wilson's disease. Am J Med 1964; 36:330–336.
104. Walshe JM. Penicillamine and the SLE syndrome. J Rheumatol 1981; 8(suppl 7):155–160.
105. Sternlieb I, Bennett B, Scheinberg IH. D-Penicillamine induced Goodpasture's syndrome in Wilson's disease. Ann Intern Med 1975; 82:673–676.
106. Pass F, Goldfischer S, Sternlieb I. Scheinberg IH. Elastosis perforans serpiginosa during penicillamine therapy for Wilson's disease. Arch Dermatol 1973; 108:713–715.
107. Steinlieb I, Fisher M, Scheinberg IH. Penicillamine-induced skin lesions. J Rheumatol 1981; 8(suppl 7):149–154.
108. Scheinberg IH, Jaffe ME, Steinlieb I. The use of Trientine in preventing the effects of interrupting penicillamine therapy in Wilson's disease. N Engl J Med 1987; 371:209–213.
109. Eisenberg E, Ballow M, Wolfe SH, Krutchkoff DJ, Tanzer JM. Pemphigus-like mucosal lesions: a side effect of penicillamine therapy. Oral Surg Oral Med Oral Pathol 1981; 51:409–414.
110. Walshe JM. Management of penicillamine nephropathy in Wilson's disease: a new chelating agent. Lancet 1969; ii:1401–1402.
111. Walshe JM. Copper chelation in patients with Wilson's disease. A comparison of penicillamine and triethylene tetramine dihydrochloride. Q J Med 1973; 42:441–452.
112. Walshe JM. Treatment of Wilson's disease with Trientine (triethylene tetramine)dihydrochloride. Lancet 1982; i:643–647.
113. Walshe JM. The management of pregnancy in Wilson's disease treated with Trientine. Q J Med 1986; 58:81–87.
114. Trientine for Wilson's disease. Med Lett Drugs Ther 1986; 28:67.
115. Smith SE, Larson EJ. Zinc toxicity in rats: antagonist effects of the copper and liver. J Biol Chem 1946; 163:29–38.
116. Dick AT. Studies on the accumulation and storage of copper in crossbred sheep. Autr J Agric Res 1954; 5:511–514
117. Brewer GJ, Schoomaker EB, Leichtman DA, Kruckeberg WC. The use of pharmacological doses of zinc in the treatment of sickle cell anemia. Prog Clin Biol Res 1977; 14:241–258.
118. Hoogenraad TV, Van Den Hamer CJ, Koevoet R, de-Ruyter- Korver EG. Oral zinc in Wilson's disease. Lancet 1978; ii:1262.

119. Hoogenraad TV, Koevoet R, de-Ruyter-Korver EG. Oral zinc sulphate as long term treatment in Wilson's disease (hepatolenticular degeneration). Eur Neurol 1979; 18:205–211.
120. Hoogenraad TU, Van Den Hamer CJA. Three years of continuous oral zinc therapy in 4 patients with Wilson's disease. Acta Neurol Scand 1983; 67:356–364.
121. Sternlieb I. Gastrointestinal copper absorption in man. Gastroenterology 1967; 52:1038–1041.
122. Cousins RJ. Absorption, transport and hepatic metabolism of copper and zinc: special reference to metallothionein and ceruloplasmin. Physiol Rev 1985; 65:238–309.
123. Menard MP, McCormick CC, Cousins RJ. Regulation of intestinal metallothionein biosynthesis in rats by dietary zinc. J Nutr 1981; 111:1353–1361.
124. Brewer GJ, Hill GM, Prasad AS, Cossack ZT. Oral zinc therapy for Wilson's disease. Ann Intern Med 1983; 99:314–319.
125. Hill GM, Brewer GJ, Prasad AS, Hydrick CR, Hartmann DE. Treatment of Wilson's disease with zinc. I. Oral zinc therapy regimens. Hepatology 1987; 7:522–528.
126. Lipsky MA, Gollan JL. Treatment of Wilson's disease: in D-penicillamine we trust—What about zinc? Hepatology 1987; 17:593–595.
127. Van Caillie-Bertrand M, Degenhart HJ, Visser HKA, Sinaasappel M, Bouquet J. Oral zinc sulphate for Wilson's disease. Arch Dis Child 1985; 60:656–659.
128. Chandra RK. Excessive intake of zinc impairs immune responses. JAMA 1984; 252:1443–1446.
129. Sternlieb I. Wilson's disease: indications for liver transplants. Hepatology 1984; 4:15S–17S.
130. Sokol RJ, Francis PD, Gold SH, Ford DM, Lum GM, Ambruso DR. Orthotopic liver transplantation for acute fulminant Wilson's disease. J Pediatr 1985; 107:549–552.
131. Polson RJ, Rolles K, Calne RY, Williams R, Marsden D. Reversal of severe neurological manifestations of Wilson's disease following orthotopic liver transplantation. Q J Med 1987; 244:685–691.

PART 16

Familial Intrahepatic Cholestasis: An Overview

Caroline A. Riely, M.D.

The infant who presents with jaundice between the ages of 6 weeks and 3 months poses a daunting diagnostic challenge to the clinician. Once indirect hyperbilirubinemia secondary to breast-milk jaundice has been excluded, the physician begins a diagnostic search aimed at demonstrating the presence of an intrinsic liver disease, such as biliary atresia, or a secondary effect on the liver from some extrahepatic disease, such as *Escherichia coli* urinary tract infection. After all the usual suspects have been excluded, there remains a small group of well-described but poorly understood syndromes collectively known as familial intrahepatic cholestasis.[1] These disorders are listed in Table 1. Several of them are described in detail in other chapters in this book. The intent of this chapter is to provide a diagnostic overview of these syndromes, to illustrate their similarities and differences, and to demonstrate how these characteristics may be used to aid in the differential diagnosis of these fascinating disorders.

TABLE 1
The Familial Intrahepatic Cholestatic Syndromes

Alagille's syndrome
Nonsyndromatic paucity of the interlobular bile ducts
Byler's syndrome
Norwegian cholestasis
North American Indian cholestasis
Benign recurrent intrahepatic cholestasis

The label *familial intrahepatic cholestatic syndrome* is restricted to disorders that meet the following requirements: The liver disease is characterized by intrahepatic cholestasis, out of proportion to hepatitis or hepatic failure (at least initially); the disorders occur in family groupings and are presumed to be genetic in etiology; and the pathogenic mechanisms are so far unexplained. In a sense, this is a wastebasket diagnosis, into which disorders are placed only if they cannot be more completely categorized. One hopes that expanding knowledge will decrease the number of disorders in this wastebasket as more diseases become understood and their pathogeneses fully characterized. Indeed, the defects in several newly described disorders of bile acid metabolism associated with familial intrahepatic cholestasis, as well as in the peroxisomal disorder known as Zellweger's syndrome, have recently been characterized; these disorders will not be included in this discussion.[2-4] And by convention, certain other incompletely understood inherited diseases that may present with cholestasis in infants, either frequently ($alpha_1$-antitrypsin deficiency) or rarely (cystic fibrosis), are not included in this group of disorders. Unhappily, surprisingly little progress in understanding the disorders that constitute familial intrahepatic cholestasis has been made in the last 2 years. The challenge to solve these mysteries of nature remains unmet.

INDIVIDUAL SYNDROMES

Alagille's Syndrome

Although infantile cholestasis with paucity of interlobular bile ducts had been reported as early as 1950,[5] it was Alagille who first noted the association with cardiac disease and odd facies.[6] His tremendous experience with this syndrome has recently been reviewed.[7] The hallmark of this disorder is extrahepatic organ involvement. Most obvious is the heart, with 85 percent of patients having congenital heart disease, ranging from peripheral pulmonary artery stenosis, the typical lesion, through more complex defects such as tetralogy of Fallot. Vertebral anomalies, primarily "butterfly" vertebrae, are seen in 87 percent of affected patients. The typical eye anomaly is posterior embryotoxon, an abnormality of the anterior chamber.[8] This finding, a subtle one the detection of which should be left to an ophthalmologist, occurs in 88 percent of affected individuals, as contrasted with up to 8 to 10 percent of normals. The face is striking and, in Alagille's series, typical in 95 percent of affected patients. The unusual facies, coupled with an abnormally high, hoarse voice, makes for an unforgettable clinical impression; once encountered, it is easy to recognize again by simply talking to an affected patient.

Other organs can also be affected, although less frequently or prominently. Anomalies of the kidneys have reported,[9] and as many as three out of four patients investigated with kidney biopsy by Alagille had mesangiolipidosis of the kidney.[7] We have encountered a deforming bland arthritis (see Fig. 1), and this has also been reported by others.[10] Mental retardation has been reported in a minority of patients. Some affected individuals have had problems with impulse control and personality, perhaps related to the chronic illness or to the subtle neurologic deficits associated with vitamin E malabsorption.[11]

Scattered reports suggest that the extrahepatic bile duct, as well as the intrahepatic bile ducts, may also be abnormal. Several typical patients have had biliary atresia.[1,12] Endoscopic retrograde cholangiography in older patients has shown beading and narrowing of the bile ducts suggestive of sclerosing cholangitis.[13] At autopsy, one patient had a fibrotic, narrowed extrahepatic bile duct.[1]

Not only is there variation in the organs affected but there is also variation in the severity of the dysfunction. Thus, affected patients may have liver disease that is detectable only biochemically or, alternatively, debilitating and unremitting cholestasis with failure to thrive. This variability leads to diagnostic confusion. For example, patients with mild cholestasis may be referred first to the cardiologist. Also, as is true of the other familial intrahepatic cholestatic syndromes, a period of observation may be necessary to confirm the diagnosis by watching the evolution of the disease over time.

The outcome of affected patients has been debated. In Alagille's group, only 26 percent of patients died, 19 percent of deaths due to liver disease. A larger proportion (29 percent) died of congenital heart disease. The largest proportion died of infection.[7] One would wonder if these deaths were due to infection associated with liver disease, such as spontaneous bacterial peritonitis. which was responsible for the death at age 18 of one of our patients. In our much smaller series, Alagille's syndrome was not as benign as we initially thought, and 4 out of 10 died precociously, the oldest at age 39 years from subacute bacterial endocarditis complicating dialysis-dependent chronic renal failure.[1] One of our patients died of malignancy, presumably cholangiocarcinoma, and there is an increasing number of reports of hepatic malignancy complicating this syndrome.[14]

Nonsyndromatic Paucity of the Interlobular Bile Ducts

It has become evident that there exists a small group of patients with intrahepatic cholestasis in infancy and a paucity of interlobular bile ducts who do not have the multiple organ involvement typical of Alagille's syndrome. At least at presentation, their liver disease is superimposible on that of Alagille's syndrome. This disorder is rare, affecting 28 percent of all patients with interlobular bile duct paucity in Alagille's experience.[7] As our understanding of liver disease in childhood improves, some patients with identifiable disease other than familial intrahepatic cholestasis are recognized within this group. For example, Alagille found that almost a quarter of the patients labeled as having nonsyndromatic paucity had either alpha$_1$-antitrypsin deficiency or congenital rubella.[7]

For the patients who remain in this group after all other liver diseases have been excluded, the prognosis is thought to be worse than that for typical Alagille's syndrome, although in a minority the disease has resolved spontaneously.[15,16] Within this group, fewer patients have a positive family history. A similar histologic picture associated with a progressive course has been reported in adults.[17] Given the heterogeneity within this group of patients, it seems safe to speculate that it does not represent one single defect, but rather the result of a variety of injuries.

Byler's Syndrome

Like nonsyndromatic paucity of the interlobular bile ducts, and unlike Alagille's syndrome, the patients included under this diagnostic heading probably include a heterogeneous group of etiologies. Indeed, the patients recently reported with defects in bile acid metabolism[3,4] would previously have been classed in this group, which consists of a fairly large number of similar patients defined as follows: no other organ involvement, a progressive form of intrahepatic cholestasis, and frequently affected siblings. The first reports were published in 1965, originally in patients descended from an Amish immigrant to the United States named Byler.[18] Although this disorder has now been reported from around the world, particularly in societies in which consanguinity is common, the original name is still applied because it evokes the typical syndrome and because we have no better understanding of its etiology as of yet.[19]

In this disorder there is pronounced cholestasis, demonstrated by the pruritus, jaundice, and elevation in the total serum bile acid level, and by bile plugs on biopsy, without the other typical biochemical hallmarks of cholestasis. In affected patients, the serum level of gamma-glutamyl transpeptidase (GGTP) is normal, or close to normal, as are the levels of 5′-nucleotidase and cholesterol.[20] Although elevated, the level of alkaline phosphatase is not as high as in other forms of cholestasis. Recent investigation has shown that the level of GGTP in liver is normal, despite the absence of an elevation in serum.[21] Thus, Byler's syndrome is a unique form of cholestasis, characterized by unusual laboratory results.

After beginning with bouts of jaundice, the usual course for patients affected with Byler's syndrome is a progressively downhill one. Cholelithiasis is common, and pancreatitis has been reported. These patients develop portal hypertension, with varices seen on endoscopy or ultrasonography, but rarely experience upper gastrointestinal (GI) hemorrhage. Instead, patients usually die, often but not invariably in childhood, of hepatic failure with coagulopathy, ascites, or hepatic encephalopathy, usually within 1 year of the onset of these complications. Liver transplant is appropriate for affected patients, who should be treated aggressively with fat-soluble vitamins in order to minimize the deficiency states. Possible beneficial effects from bile acid feeding with ursodeoxycholic acid, as have been found in other forms of cholestasis, are under investigation. An interesting report of four affected patients suggests that external biliary diversion of a part of the bile flow results in dramatic improvement of the cholestasis, suggesting the presence of a toxin, perhaps a toxic bile acid, in bile.[22] As is the case in other forms of childhood liver disease, hepatic malignancy may develop.[23]

Norwegian Cholestasis

This relapsing form of intrahepatic cholestasis has been reported from Norway and in children of Norwegian extraction in Minnesota, as well as from Australia.[24-26] Bouts of typical cholestasis associated with giant cell transformation of the liver begin early in life. Later, lymphedema of the lower extremities develops. The prognosis for affected individuals is better than in the other forms of intrahepatic cholestasis, although fibrosis or cirrhosis may develop.[16]

North American Indian Cholestasis

This recently described syndrome is restricted thus far to members of a tribe of native North Americans from a remote part of Quebec.[27] As infants, these children have a bout of neonatal hepatitis with jaundice and giant cell transformation on biopsy. The jaundice resolves, but the children are left with cholestasis and go on to develop progressive liver disease, characterized by severe portal hypertension with variceal hemorrhage, usually leading to death in childhood. Affected children have prominent telangiectasias on their cheeks. Like other forms of familial intrahepatic cholestasis, the pathogenic mechanisms are unknown, but in this syndrome there is prominent thickening of the pericanalicular ectoplasm, suggesting a defect in the microfilament web that is responsible for "milking" bile from the liver.

Benign Recurrent Intrahepatic Cholestasis

Benign recurrent intrahepatic cholestasis (BRIC) is a form of relapsing cholestasis that was first reported in 1959.[28] There are no accompanying extrahepatic manifestations. The first attack comes in childhood but rarely in infancy. During attacks, patients are highly symptomatic, with severe pruritus followed by jaundice associated weight loss and abdominal pain.[29] What precipitates attacks is unclear, although pregnancy does seem to be a precipitant.[30] BRIC may be related to cholestasis of pregnancy, a condition thought to be due to an inherited sensitivity to estrogens.[31] Patients affected with BRIC do not have progressive liver disease and are normal clinically and biochemically between attacks.

DIFFERENTIAL DIAGNOSIS

Characteristics in Common

The common hallmarks that allow us to group these disparate syndromes together are listed in Table 2. Affected patients come to medical attention in childhood, usually because they become symptomatic or because their liver disease is detected on screening, perhaps of members of an affected family. In Alagille's syndrome, rare individuals experience no symptoms and are identified in adulthood when a child is investigated.[9]

All patients have cholestasis. By strict definition, this means that they have elevations in the total serum bile acid level. Disorders of bile acid metabolism that result in the presence of abnormal bile acids in the absence of one or both of the major primary bile acids are not considered to be members of this group of diseases, although new sophisticated techniques of bile acid characterization may uncover some abnormalities of bile acid metabolism in this group in the future.[32] Most patients experience pruritus, often intolerable, as a major symptom of their disease. In very young infants, the only sign may be jaundice, and the child may die before pruritus, which is not manifested by infants younger than 4 to 6 months old, begins. Interestingly, resolution of pruritus may presage the onset of hepatic failure, followed by death, particularly in patients with Byler's syndrome. Jaundice, often mistakenly thought to be necessary to make a diagnosis of cholestasis, is usually present, but not invariably, and may resolve while the pruritus persists. In affected patients, the cholestasis is often intermittent. In Byler's syndrome and

TABLE 2
Familial Intrahepatic Cholestatic Syndromes: Characteristics in Common

Onset in infancy or childhood
Cholestasis, often with remissions and relapses
Clinical: pruritus, jaundice
Biochemical: ↑ serum bile acids, alkaline phosphatase
Hepatomegaly, usually modest
Malabsorption of fat-soluble vitamins, with attendant rickets, retinopathy, neuropathy
Liver biopsy—possible findings:
Paucity of the interlobular bile ducts
Giant cells
Potential for malignant transformation, either hepatocellular carcinoma or adenocarcinoma of the bile ducts
Positive family history of disease in parents or siblings, or a history of parental consanguinity

BRIC, bouts of jaundice may follow infections. In Alagille's syndrome, the cholestasis may resolve with age.

Hepatomegaly is present at the disease onset, although it is usually not massive, such as that seen in storage diseases. Malabsorption of fats, associated with the diminished intraluminal bile acid concentrations, is frequent, although it may be subclinical. Many, if not most, of these patients suffer from deficiencies of the fat-soluble vitamins, most notably vitamins D and E. The associated deficiency states have been only recently recognized and the importance of their treatment emphasized.[11]

Hepatic histology is very varied within this group of disorders. Nevertheless, certain findings may be found in any of these syndromes. A paucity of the interlobular bile ducts, much like the marked ductopenia seen in primary biliary cirrhosis in adults, or in the vanishing bile duct syndrome after liver transplantation, is the histology characteristic of Alagille's syndrome and of nonsyndromatic paucity. Scattered reports confirm that this finding also occurs, although much less frequently, in the other forms of familial intrahepatic cholestasis. Interestingly, the ductopenia in these disorders is not associated with the portal zone inflammatory infiltrate characteristic of primary biliary cirrhosis, although cholangitis has been reported to precede ductopenia in Alagille's syndrome. Thus, it is evident that ductopenia is a nonspecific histologic finding. It would seem likely that the paucity of interlobular bile ducts is not the cause of the cholestasis, but more likely the result. Another possible common histologic feature is the presence of giant cell transformation of the liver. This is particularly prominent in North American Indian cholestasis and Norwegian cholestasis, but scattered giant cells can be found in biopsies from the other disorders also, particularly if the biopsy is done early in life.

Another characteristic common to several forms of familial intrahepatic cholestasis is the propensity for malignant transformation of the liver. Hepatic malignancies, either hepatocellular carcinoma or adenocarcinoma of the bile ducts, have been reported in patients with Alagille's syndrome and Byler's syndrome. It would seem wise to screen all affected individuals periodically with imaging (ultrasonography or liver spleen scintigraphy) and alpha-fetoprotein measurements. This malignant potential is shared by all forms of chronic liver disease but is most common in patients with tyrosinemia.

Finally, by definition all forms of familial intrahepatic cholestasis share a positive family history. Disease in several members of a sibship has been reported for all of these syndromes. There is frequent consanguinity among parents of children with Byler's syndrome. The affected North American Indians come from an isolated and inbred tribe. Patients with Alagille's syndrome may have an affected parent, although often the disorder is subclinical. When present, a positive family history is strongly suggestive of these syndromes. The absence of affected family members does not rule out familial intrahepatic cholestasis.

Distinguishing Characteristics

Although similar in many ways, the familial intrahepatic cholestatic syndromes have many distinguishing features (Table 3), differences that probably are important clues to

TABLE 3
Familial Intrahepatic Cholestatic Syndromes: Characteristics Useful in Differential Diagnosis

	Alagille's Syndrome	Nonsyndromatic Paucity	Byler's Syndrome	Norwegian	North American Indian	Benign Recurrent Intrahepatic Cholestasis
Birth weight	Low	Low	Normal	High	—	—
Age at onset	Usually <3 months up to age 3 years	<3 months	Usually <3 months up to age 10 years	<3 months	<3 months	1–15 years
Associated anomalies	Heart, eyes, bones, kidneys	None	None	Lymphedema	Telangiectasia of cheeks	None
Biliary tract anomalies	Biliary atresia, sclerosing cholangitis	—	—	—	—	—
Laboratory results						
Cholesterol	↑↑	↑	Normal	↑	Normal	↑
Gamma-glutamyl transpeptidase	↑	↑	Normal	↑	↑	—
Sweat chloride	Normal	—	↑	—	—	—
Liver histology						
Early	↓ No. bile ducts	↓ No. bile ducts	Cholestasis	Giant cells	Giant cells	Cholestasis
Late	Biliary cirrhosis	Biliary cirrhosis	Fibrosis	Portal fibrosis	Cirrhosis	Cholestasis
Course						
Outcome	Often improves	Progressive	Progressive	Often benign	Progressive	Benign
Gastrointestinal bleeding	Rare	—	Rare	Rare	Common	Never
Hepatic failure	Rare	Occurs	Common	Rare	Occurs	Never
Cholelithiasis	Rare	Rare	Common	—	—	—
Response to biliary diversion	None	—	Good	—	—	—
Inheritance						
Autosomal	Dominant	—	Recessive	Recessive	Recessive	—

— = not known or not reported; ↑ = increased; ↓ = decreased.

their underlying pathophysiologic mechanisms, if only we could interpret them. For example, the normal birth weight of patients with Byler's syndrome implies normal intrauterine development and an abnormality that is active only after birth. On the other hand, the usual small birth weight of patients with Alagille's syndrome suggests an intrinsic defect with prenatal effects. Interestingly, patients with Norwegian cholestasis have been reported to be large for gestational age at birth.

The age at onset of symptoms may also be helpful in the differential diagnosis. The most common age of presentation for patients with Alagille's syndrome is within the first 3 months of life, and this diagnosis should always be considered in the differential diagnosis of neonatal jaundice, along with biliary atresia and alpha$_1$-antitrypsin deficiency. Other patients with Alagille's syndrome develop symptoms later, perhaps as late as age 3 years. Byler's syndrome is less well defined and has a wider span of age of presentation. Again, the most common time of onset is before the age of 3 months. But new cases may appear later, perhaps as late as ages 5 to 10 years. Norwegian cholestasis also presents in the neonatal period, although the typical lymphedema begins later in life. Patients with North American Indian cholestasis have a bout of neonatal jaundice, which may be subclinical, followed by resolution, only to present later in life with severe portal hypertension. It is rare for a patient with benign recurrent intrahepatic cholestasis to present before the age of 1 year, and new onset of disease has been reported up until age 15. In familial intrahepatic cholestasis, the clinical characteristics of the liver disease provide few distinguishing features, at least at presentation. It is the presence or absence of anomalies outside of the liver which is most helpful in differential diagnosis. As discussed previously, Alagille's syndrome has associated anomalies, particularly of the heart, eyes, bones, and kidney, that strongly suggest the correct diagnosis. The coincidence of this cholestatic liver disease with these anomalies in diverse organ systems demonstrates that this is not simply a disease of bile formation alone, but is perhaps a defect in some integral structural protein. Nonsyndromatic paucity, Byler's syndrome, and BRIC have no associated anomalies that might be helpful in diagnosis. The lymphedema of Norwegian cholestasis is a useful diagnostic sign but is unfortunately usually not present at the time of initial presentation. The cheek telangiectasias, "paper money" skin, of children with North American Indian cholestasis may be helpful in making this diagnosis.

The abnormalities of the biliary tract occasionally associated with Alagille's syndrome are of interest. Thus, neonates thought to have biliary atresia should be evaluated for this form of familial intrahepatic cholestasis. It is unclear whether the sclerosing cholangitis–like picture also seen in Alagille's syndrome is present at its onset. It is not associated with any symptoms, such as abdominal pain or cholangitis, and is detected only with cholangiography.

Laboratory results can be helpful in the differential diagnosis of familial intrahepatic cholestasis. Patients with Alagille's syndrome may have very high levels of cholesterol, with dramatic xanthomata. An interesting characteristic of Byler's syndrome, one that probably has pathogenic significance, is the lack of significant elevation in GGTP or 5′-nucleotidase. The level of these enzymes may be minimally raised, but never into the usual range seen in cholestasis, be it familial intrahepatic cholestasis or bile duct obstruction. Finally, an elevated level of sweat chloride has been reported in some patients with Byler's syndrome.[33] This is not a common finding but may be helpful if present. Sweat chloride levels are not reported to be elevated in forms of cholestasis other than cystic fibrosis.

Hepatic histopathology can be both helpful and confusing. The numerous similarities between syndromes are discussed above. Their differences are real but are difficult to appreciate if only one biopsy specimen is available. The striking finding in both Alagille's syndrome and nonsyndromatic paucity is ductopenia, often with a very bland-appearing portal triad that is simply missing bile ducts. If a careful study of the ratio of bile duct to portal triads is done by counting many microscopic fields, a ratio in normals of 0.9 to 1.8 bile ducts per triad is found. In Alagille's syndrome the ratio is decreased to 0 to 0.4 duct per triad. This finding is not unique to these two syndromes but is certainly most striking here.

The other diagnostic features of histopathology are less distinctive. Patients with Byler's syndrome have a progressive fibrosis that results in fine fibrous tissue spreading throughout the lobule, without forming distinct fibrous bands clearly outlining nodules. This is in contrast to patients with Alagille's syndrome, in whom cirrhosis, when it develops, has a typical pattern of secondary biliary cirrhosis with smooth-contoured bands of fibrosis bridging portal areas and outlining nodules. Patients with Norwegian cholestasis may show progressive portal fibrosis. The giant cell transformation seen early in the course of North American Indian cholestasis is striking but resolves as the patients become older.

Observation of the course of disease over time is very helpful in leading to the correct diagnosis in any one individual. This diagnostic tool is granted only to those with patience, and it can be difficult to explain to the family of a sick infant that final confirmation of diagnosis rests with simply watching. Nevertheless, this is an important tool, particularly in dealing with this frustrating group of diseases of unknown etiology. In Alagille's syndrome, the severity of the cholestasis is usually evident within the first few months after presentation. Thus, patients who are severely affected are so shortly after presentation. As age increases, the severity of the cholestasis tends to abate. Byler's syndrome tends to be more insidious. The cholestasis often improves and may even disappear clinically after the initial presentation. It recurs within months to years and may continue to come in "attacks" without any clear precipitant. Ultimately, the cholestasis becomes permanent. Norwegian cholestasis is also characterized by "attacks" of jaundice. In affected North American Indians, the cholestasis is most severe in infancy. Although pruritus and cholestatic laboratory tests may persist, jaundice fades in these patients and it is not evident that they have progressive disease until they present with variceal hemorrhage due to portal hypertension. Portal hypertension occurs in Alagille's and Byler's syndromes, but associated complications are rare.

Choledocholithiasis is more common in all forms of liver disease than among normal individuals. Within the familial intrahepatic cholestatic syndromes, symptomatic biliary tract disease due to stones is most common in patients with Byler's syndrome, who also have been reported to have pancreatitis, occasionally with acute attacks. Choledocholithiasis is not reported as a problem in the other forms of familial intrahepatic cholestasis, although gallstones are known to be more frequent in patients with a past history of cholestasis of pregnancy, which may be considered to be one of this group of syndromes.[34]

Progression to death in hepatic failure is the usual outcome in Byler's syndrome, usually by 4 to 5 years after the disease onset. The range of duration for the course of this illness is wide, with some patients dying within months of diagnosis and some patients living into adolescence and young adulthood. A minority of patients with Alagille's syndrome (2 out of 21 deaths in Alagille's series) die of hepatic failure, which occurs principally in infants who are severely affected from the neonatal period. Late deaths in this syndrome may be secondary to portal hypertension and its complications. Nonsyndromatic paucity of the intralobular bile ducts also progresses to death with hepatic failure or portal hypertension, usually more rapidly than in patients with classic Alagille's syndrome.

Because no effective therapy for these syndromes has yet been devised, it is not possible to use response to therapy to provide diagnostic clues. The one exception is a difference between Alagille's syndrome and Byler's syndrome in the response to biliary diversion. In their report of 6 patients treated by diverting about 50 percent of bile drainage to the outside, Whitington and Whitington reported success, with resolution of cholestasis, in the four patients with Byler's syndrome but not in the two with Alagille's syndrome. Confirmation of this interesting observation is awaited.

Finally, the pattern of inheritance may be useful in differentiating these syndromes. Alagille's syndrome appears in subsequent generations and in sibships, suggesting inheritance

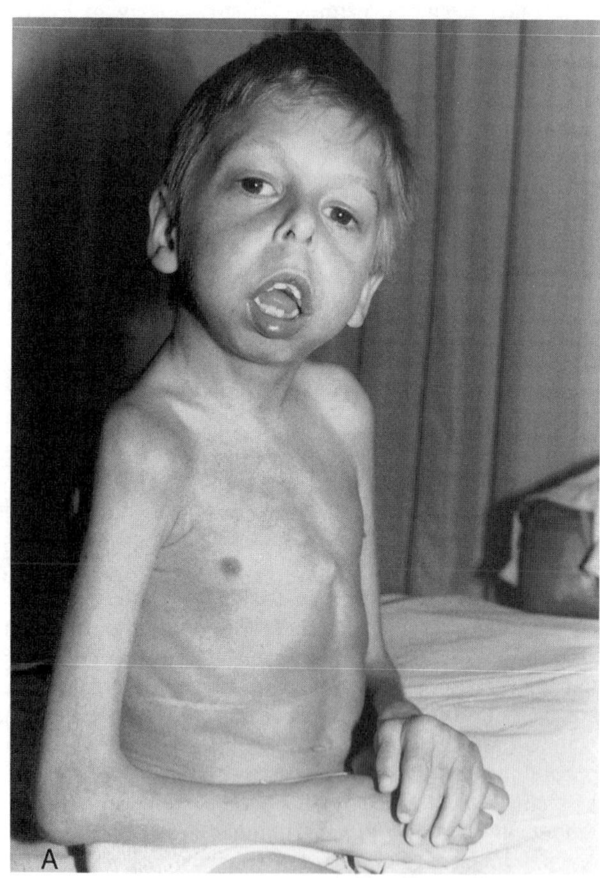

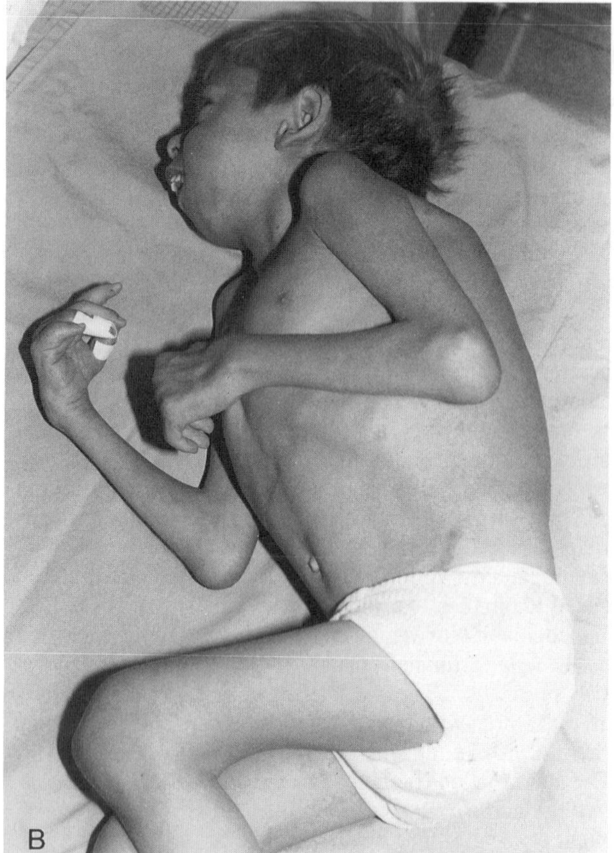

FIGURE 1 Deforming arthritis complicating Alagille's syndrome. This 10-year-old boy presented at birth with a heart murmur, presumed to be due to peripheral pulmonic stenosis. At age 9 weeks jaundice was noted. Exploratory laparotomy demonstrated intrahepatic and extrahepatic biliary atresia, and he underwent cholecystohepatoenterostomy. Although his jaundice faded 7 months after surgery, he developed severe xanthomata with high serum cholesterol levels (up to 3,400 mg per deciliter). With increasing age, his bilirubin and cholesterol values have improved and his pruritus and xanthomata have resolved. Arthritis with limitation of motion and deformed joints but without erythema or tenderness was first noted at age 18 months. Multiple serologic tests, including rheumatoid factor and antinuclear antibody, have been negative. Despite the improvement in his liver disease, he has had severe growth failure, weighing 12 kg at age 11 years.[1] *A*, Face, upper torso, and hands. Although his face is unusual in appearance, it is not typical for Alagille's syndrome. His hands are deformed, with multiple swollen joints. *B*, Multiple joint contractures. Contractures, with severe limitation of motion in elbows, hips, and knees, are evident, as is his failure to thrive.

as an autosomal dominant. The wide variability in the expression of this disorder also suggests autosomal dominant inheritance. Byler's syndrome is more common in sibships and in children of consanguineous parents. For example, families from North Africa, where consanguinity is common, are well represented in the ranks of those affected with Byler's syndrome. Both Norwegian and North American Indian forms of cholestasis are inherited as autosomal recessive disorders.

A Case in Point

The differences among the familial intrahepatic cholestatic syndromes as displayed in Table 3 are oversimplified. For any individual patient, the differential diagnosis may be quite difficult. For example, the patient illustrated in Figure 1 presented a diagnostic dilemma, one that is still incompletely resolved. He was small for dates at birth and had a murmur compatible with peripheral pulmonic stenosis. Exploratory laparotomy performed at age 2 months in assessment of jaundice and acholic stools failed to demonstrate a normal extrahepatic bile duct and he underwent a gallbladder Kasai procedure. His jaundice cleared slowly, but did eventually; however, he developed severe hypercholesterolemia with widespread xanthomata. Over time, these too resolved, initially in response to cholestyramine, but later remained improved without binding-resin therapy.

The course of the cholestasis in this patient made it evident that his was not a usual case of biliary atresia. The marked hypercholesterolemia that resolved over time, associated with his low birth weight and cardiac murmur, made a diagnosis of Alagille's syndrome likely. Interestingly, several patients with biliary atresia and typical Alagille's syndrome have been reported since this child's birth. His face, although unusual, was not typical, however, and posterior embryotoxon was not found on several eye examinations. To further complicate matters he developed a severe deforming arthritis that was atypical for rheumatoid arthritis. Careful perusal of the literature revealed that this finding had been previously reported in Alagille's syndrome, although clearly it must be rare, as it was not reported in Alagille's series of 80 cases.

What is the correct diagnosis for this patient? Observation over 11 years has demonstrated cholestasis, initially severe, then resolving. This disease course, together with his typical heart murmur and atypical, but reported, joint disease, make Alagille's syndrome the most likely diagnosis. He is, however, quite atypical. Given his extrahepatic disorders, none of the other familial intrahepatic cholestatic syndromes seems likely. Perhaps he has an unusual syndrome of defective bile acid metabolism. This seems unlikely, given his longevity and extrahepatic involvement.

This case demonstrates the diagnostic problems that persist in evaluating infants and children with prolonged cholestasis. A thorough knowledge of these syndromes and a prolonged period of observation can help make the diagnosis. But exact diagnostic accuracy will be available only when the pathogenic mechanisms and the defective enzymes or structural proteins are identified. At that time the diagnostic wastebasket of familial intrahepatic cholestasis can be discarded.

REFERENCES

1. Riely CA. Familial intrahepatic cholestatic syndromes. Semin Liver Dis 1987; 7:119–133.
2. Schutgens RB, Heymans HSA, Wanders RJA, et al. Peroxisomal disorders: a newly recognized group of genetic diseases. Eur J Pediatr 1986; 144:430–440.
3. Clayton PT, Leonard JV, Lawson AM, et al. Familial giant cell hepatitis associated with synthesis of 3β, 7α-dihydroxy- and $3\beta,7\alpha,12\alpha$-trihydroxy-5-cholenoic acids. J Clin Invest 1987; 79:1031–1038.
4. Setchell KDR, Suchy FJ, Welsh MB, et al. Δ^4-3-oxosteroid 5β-reductase deficiency described in identical twins with neonatal hepatitis. J Clin Invest 1988; 82:2148–2157.
5. Ahrens EH Jr, Harris RC, MacMahon HE. Atresia of the intrahepatic bile ducts. Pediatrics 1951; 8:628–647.
6. Alagille D, Habib EC, Thomassin N. L'atrésie des voies biliaires intra-hépatiques avec voies biliaires extra-hépatiques perméables chez l'enfant. A propos de 25 observations. J Paris Pediatr 1969; 301–318.
7. Alagille D, Estrada A, Hadchouel M, et al. Syndromic paucity of interlobular bile ducts (Alagille syndrome or arteriohepatic dysplasia): review of 80 cases. J Pediatr 1987; 110:195–200.
8. Riely CA, Cotlier E, Jensen PS, Klatskin G. Arteriohepatic dysplasia: a benign syndrome of intrahepatic cholestasis with multiple organ involvement. Ann Intern Med 1979; 91:520–527.
9. Labrecque DR, Mitros FA, Nathan RJ, et al. Four generations of arteriohepatic dysplasia. Hepatology 1982; 2:467–474.
10. Berman MD, Ishak KG, Schaefer EF, et al. Syndromatic hepatic ductular hypoplasia (arteriohepatic dysplasia). A clinical and hepatic histologic study of three patients. Dig Dis Sci 1981; 26:485–497.
11. Sokol RJ, Guggenheim MA, Fannaccone ST, et al. Improved neurologic function after long-term correction of vitamin E deficiency in children with chronic cholestasis. N Engl J Med 1985; 313:1580–1586.
12. Kocoshis SA, Cottrill CM, O'Connor WN, et al. Congenital heart disease, butterfly vertebrae, and extrahepatic biliary atresia: a variant of arteriohepatic dysplasia? J Pediatr 1981; 99:436–439.
13. Gorelick FS, Dobbins JW, Burrell M, Riely CA. Biliary tract abnormalities in patients with arteriohepatic dysplasia. Dig Dis Sci 1982; 27:815–820.
14. Rabinovitz M, Imperial JC, Schade RR, Van Thiel DH. Hepatocellular carcinoma in Alagille's syndrome: a family study. J Pediatr Gastroenterol Nutr 1989; 8:26–30.
15. Alagille D. Cholestasis in the first three months of life. Prog Liver Dis 1979; 6:471–485.
16. Mowat AP. Hepatitis and cholestasis in infancy: intrahepatic disorders. In: Liver disorders in childhood. Boston: Butterworths, 1987.
17. Ludwig J, Wiesner RH, LaRusso NF. Idiopathic adulthood ductopenia. A cause of chronic cholestatic liver disease and biliary cirrhosis. J Hepatol 1988; 7:193–199.
18. Clayton RJ, Iber FL, Reubner BH, McKusick VA. Byler's disease: fatal familial intrahepatic cholestasis in an Amish kindred. J Pediatr 1965; 67:1026–1028.
19. Odievre M, Gautier M, Hadchouel M, Alagille D. Severe familial intrahepatic cholestasis. Arch Dis Child 1973; 48:806–812.
20. Maggiore G, Bernard O, Riely CA, et al. Normal serum gamma-glutamyltransferase activity identifies groups of infants with idiopathic cholestasis with poor prognosis. J Pediatr 1987; 111:251–252.
21. Chobert MN, Bernard O, Bulle F, et al. High hepatic gamma-glutamyltransferase (gamma-GT) activity with normal serum gamma-GT in children with progressive indiopathic cholestasis. J Hepatol 1989; 8:22–25.
22. Whitington PF, Whitington GL. Partial external diversion of bile for the treatment of intractable pruritus associated with intrahepatic cholestasis. Gastroenterology 1988; 95:130–136.
23. Dahms BB. Hepatoma in familial cholestatic cirrhosis of childhood. Arch Pathol Lab Med 1979; 103:30–33.
24. Aagenaes O. Hereditary recurrent cholestasis with lymphoedema—two new families. Acta Paediatr Scand 1974; 63:465–471.
25. Sharp HL, Krivit W. Hereditary lymphedema and obstructive jaundice. J Pediatr 1971; 78:491–496.
26. Danks SM, Campbell PE, Smith AL, Rogers J. Prognosis of babies with neonatal hepatitis. Arch Dis Child 1977; 52:368–372.
27. Weber AM, Tuchweber B, Yousef I, et al. Severe familial cholestasis in North American Indian children; a clinical model of microfilament dysfunction? Gastroenterology 1981; 81:653–662.

28. Summerskill WHJ. The syndrome of benign recurrent cholestasis. Am J Med 1965; 38:298–305.
29. Eriksson S, Larsson C. Familial benign chronic intrahepatic cholestasis. Hepatology 1983; 3:391–398.
30. De Pagter AGF, Van Berge Henegouwen GP, ten Bokkel Huinink JA, Brandt K-H. Familial benign recurrent intrahepatic cholestasis. Interrelation with intrahepatic cholestasis of pregnancy and from oral contraceptives? Gastroenterology 1976; 71:202–207.
31. Reyes H. The enigma of intrahepatic cholestasis of pregnancy: lessons from Chile. Hepatology 1982; 2:87–96.
32. Setchell KDR, Street JM. Inborn errors of bile acid systhesis. Semin Liver Dis 1987; 7:85–99.
33. Hillemeier AC, Hen J, Riely CA, et al. Meconium peritonitis and increasing sweat chloride determinations in a case of familial progressive intrahepatic cholestasis. Pediatrics 1982; 69:325–327.
34. Samsioe G, Johnson P, Gustafson A. Studies in cholestasis of pregnancy. VI. Fatty acid composition of glycero-phospholipids before and after delivery. Acta Obstet Gynecol Scand 1977; 56:31–35.

PART 17

Disorders of Peroxisomal Metabolism

Richard I. Kelley, M.D., Ph.D.

Zellweger's syndrome and a rapidly expanding spectrum of related peroxisomal diseases have recently emerged as major identifiable causes of liver disease in the pediatric population. Because of the wide range of associated nonhepatic abnormalities in these disorders and the often initially silent nature of the progressive liver disease, many patients with peroxisomal diseases are coming to the attention of the gastroenterologist from a variety of different hospital clinics, where they may have been followed for many months or years. Thus, acquiring a thorough understanding of the clinical and metabolic characteristics of peroxisomal disorders has become essential for practicing gastroenterologists.

The cerebrohepatorenal syndrome of Zellweger is by far the best known of the genetic disorders of peroxisomal metabolism. Although Zellweger's syndrome was first described as an autosomal recessive, multiple congenital anomaly syndrome in 1964,[1] the discovery in 1973[2] that hepatic and renal cells of patients with Zellweger's syndrome were devoid of recognizable peroxisomes and had dysfunctional mitochondria refocused attention on Zellweger's syndrome as a possible metabolic disorder. As a result, the last 15 years have witnessed the redefinition of Zellweger's syndrome as the prototypic "metabolic malformation syndrome" and the development of a new field of biochemical genetics, with the result that now almost a dozen clinical disorders have been identified or redescribed as diseases of the peroxisome. In some, such as classic Zellweger's syndrome and neonatal adrenoleukodystrophy (ALD), the entire peroxisome and most of its associated biochemical functions appear to be lost or severely diminished. In others, such as X-linked ALD and primary (type I) hyperoxaluria, only a single peroxisomal enzyme appears to be deficient. Overall, the discovery and biochemical characterization of these peroxisomal experiments of nature have substantially increased our understanding of the importance of the peroxisome in human metabolism. In this chapter, we review the principal metabolic functions of the peroxisomes and the major clinical disorders associated with an apparent primary deficiency of peroxisomal metabolism. Guides to the diagnosis and treatment of the peroxisomal disorders are also presented.

STRUCTURE AND FUNCTION OF NORMAL PEROXISOMES

Tissue Distribution and Characteristics of Peroxisomes

Peroxisomes are ubiquitous subcellular organelles defined by DeDuve[3] as small (0.1 to 0.1 μm), dense, subcellular particles bounded by a single membrane and containing the enzymatic machinery for the evolution and consumption of hydrogen peroxide. Similar peroxidative organelles in plants host the important glyoxylate cycle and related carbohydrate pathways and are known as glyoxysomes. The term *microbodies* is commonly used to refer to both organelles.[4,5]

Although large (0.5 to 1.5 μm) and more conspicuous peroxisomes were first identified only in hepatocytes (Fig.1) and renal proximal tubular cells, essentially all mammalian cells except erythrocytes have since been found to contain peroxisomes or smaller (0.1 to 0.2 μm) versions of the same organelle, which are called *microperoxisomes*. Hepatocytes and renal tubular cells have the greatest abundance of peroxisomes, which may constitute as much as 1 percent of the cell mass, whereas the collective volume of peroxisomes in muscle, fibroblasts, and neuronal tissue is at least an order of magnitude lower.[6,7] In most tissues, peroxisomes appear as round or ovoid organelles with a finely granular matrix, bounded by a single membrane, and stainable by a catalase detecting reaction with diaminobenzidine. By electron microscopy, the membrane is trilaminar but is thinner than the trilaminar single membrane of lysosomes and lacks the clear zone found subjacent to the lysosomal membrane. The

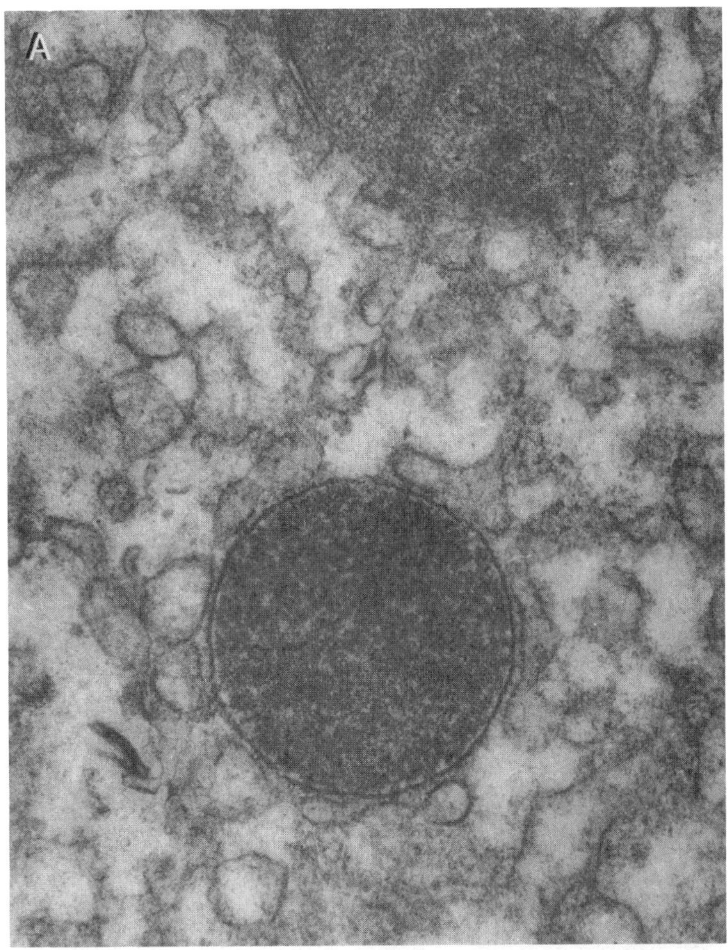

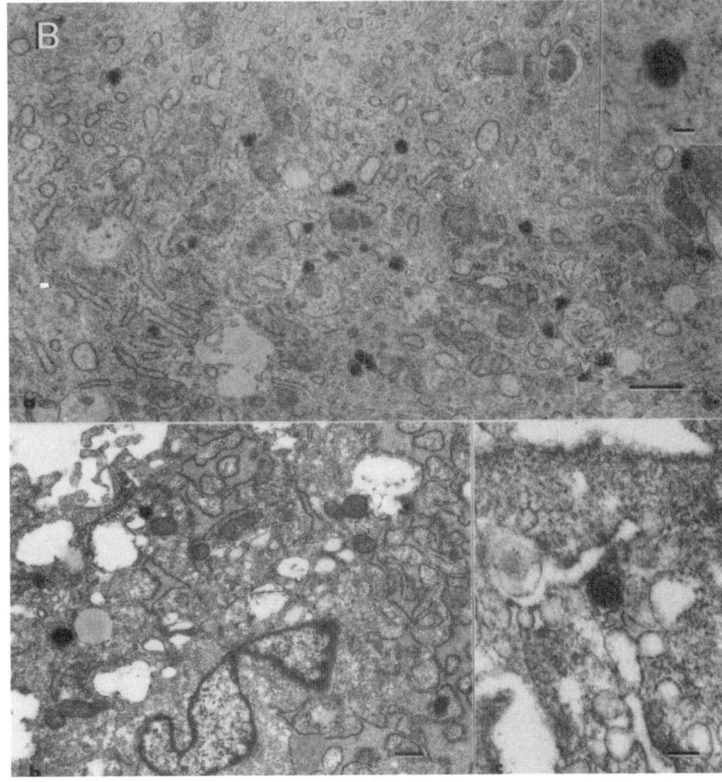

FIGURE 1 *A*, Electron micrograph of a normal human liver peroxisome showing a heterogeneous matrix surrounded by a single membrane. Human peroxisomes lack dense "nucleoids" present in the peroxisomes of most other vertebrate species. *B*, Electron micrographs of fibroblasts incubated in a medium for the demonstration of peroxisomal catalase by the deposition of an electron-dense reaction product. *Top*, Normal human fibroblast containing several peroxisomes with variable staining (*inset*: magnification to show heterogeneous distribution of catalase staining). *Bottom*, Electron-dense small peroxisomes in the cytoplasm of fibroblasts from a patient with Zellweger's syndrome. (Courtesy of Sydney Goldfischer, M.D.)

larger peroxisomes of most species contain a dense, crystalline-like "nucleoid" core believed to contain urate oxidase, because species that lack urate oxidase, such as humans and birds, also lack peroxisomal cores. An important characteristic of hepatic peroxisomes of some species is proliferation induced by a variety of unusual lipids, such as trans-unsaturated fatty acids, by clofibrate, a hypolipidemic drug, and by thyroxine.[8,9]

Peroxisomes appear to be independent organelles with a biogenesis separate from other subcellular organelles and compartments.[10] As yet, there is no evidence for specific peroxisomal DNA encoding the synthesis of peroxisomal proteins. Rather, the organelle most likely begins as a microperoxisome, formed by fission of a mature peroxisome, which then grows through spontaneous assembly of peroxisome-specific membrane components and importation of targeted peroxisomal proteins synthesized on free polyribosomes. It is this proposed mechanism of biogenesis that may be defective in Zellweger's syndrome and related generalized disorders of the peroxisome.

Peroxisomes are mostly randomly distributed in hepatocytes, but often occur closely juxtaposed to the endoplasmic reticulum (ER), from which peroxisomes were once thought to arise by budding, or sometimes preferentially surrounding glycogen or triglyceride deposits.[11] This close association with ER is denoted structurally by a dense thickening (the marginal plate) of the segment of the peroxisomal membrane paralleling the ER.[6,12,13] Moreover, in tissues with a high rate of fatty acid beta-oxidation, there is a nonrandom association of peroxisomes with mitochondria, usually separated by an intercalated bilayer of ER.[11] An extreme structural specialization of peroxisomes occurs in the cells of sebaceous glands, where the peroxisomal compartment exists as an extensive, interconnected filamentous network believed to subserve the synthesis of the unusual waxes and ether-lipids of sebum.[14] Coreless, filamentous tails and interperoxisomal connections have also been found by careful serial sectioning of rat liver[15] and may be common, if variable, features of the peroxisomal space.

Metabolic Pathways of the Peroxisome

Once thought to be merely vestigial in higher organisms, the vertebrate peroxisome is now known to contain a remarkable variety of highly specialized and essential enzymatic systems for synthetic and degradative metabolism of, largely, lipids and amino acids (Table 1).[4] From a clinical biochemical viewpoint, the most important of these functions are (1) beta-oxidation of very long chain fatty acids (VLCFA), (2) synthesis of bile acids, (3) synthesis of plasmalogens, (4) oxidase-mediated oxidation of amino acids, and (5) catalatic and peroxidatic decomposition of hydrogen peroxide by catalase. In addition, peroxisomes appear to have a role in the alpha oxidation of phytol-derived phytanic acid and, in some species, in the synthesis of highly specialized biochemicals such as waxy esters and pheromones.[16] For some processes, such as beta-oxidation of fatty acids, a complete pathway exists in the peroxisome, whereas for others, such as bile acid or plasmalogen synthesis, only one or two essential steps of the pathway are unique to the peroxisome.

TABLE 1
Major Metabolic Functions of the Peroxisome

Beta-oxidation of fatty acids
Beta-oxidation of dicarboxylic acids
Alpha-oxidation of phytanic acid
Synthesis of ether lipids (e.g., plasmalogens)
Synthesis of bile acids
Synthesis of waxy esters
Oxidation of D- and L-amino acids
Oxidation of L-α-OH-acids (e.g., 2-OH-phytanate)
Amino acid transamination
Oxidative catabolism of polyamines
Catabolism of purines
Catalatic and peroxidatic decomposition of hydrogen peroxide

Peroxisomal Fatty Acid Oxidation

Although fatty acid beta-oxidation was first recognized as a function of peroxisomes (glyoxysomes) of germinating seedlings in 1969,[17] it was not until 1978 that a complete ensemble of beta-oxidative enzymes functionally similar to those of mitochondria was documented in mammalian peroxisomes (Fig. 2).[18] However, despite identical stereochemistry and evolutionary homology of most of the peroxisomal and mitochondrial beta-oxidation enzymes,[19] the rate-limiting enzymes and the organelles' substrate specificities are distinctly different. The first step of beta oxidation in the peroxisome is carried out by a single, hydrogen peroxide–generating acyl-CoA oxidase with a broad specificity for all but short chain (C4-C8) fatty acids.[20] In contrast, three separate acyl-CoA dehydrogenases—short, medium, and long chain ACD—catalyze the degradation of fatty acids in mitochondria. In addition, peroxisomes contain an unusual monomeric enzyme, the "bifunctional enzyme," which alone sequentially catalyzes the enoyl-CoA hydratase and 3-OH-acyl-CoA dehydrogenase activities carried out by two separate enzymes in mitochondria. All three primary peroxisomal beta-oxidation enzymes have been isolated and characterized in pure form from rat liver and their corresponding structural genes sequenced.[19-21]

From a physiologic standpoint, mitochondria are most important in the conversion of dietary fatty acids—palmitate, oleate, linoleate, and stearate—into acetyl-CoA for energy metabolism, ketogenesis, and various synthetic pathways. Peroxisomes, on the other hand, appear to specialize in the beta-oxidation of VLCFA (longer than C22),[22] certain unsaturated fatty acids,[23,24] dicarboxylic acids,[25] branched-chain fatty acids, and a variety of xenobiotic acids, such as phenyl-substituted fatty acids.[26] The end products of beta-oxidation—acetyl-CoA in mitochondria versus acetyl-carnitine and octanyl-carnitine in peroxisomes—as well as the fate of the extracted reducing equivalents—coupled to ATP synthesis in mitochondria versus lost to hydrogen peroxide and its exergonic reactions in peroxisomes—also differ. Lastly, the total capacity of peroxisomal, but not mitochondrial, beta-oxidation can be substantially amplified in some species by exposure to preferred substrates or drugs, such as clofibrate and related hypolipidemic drugs,[8,9] which also cause perox-

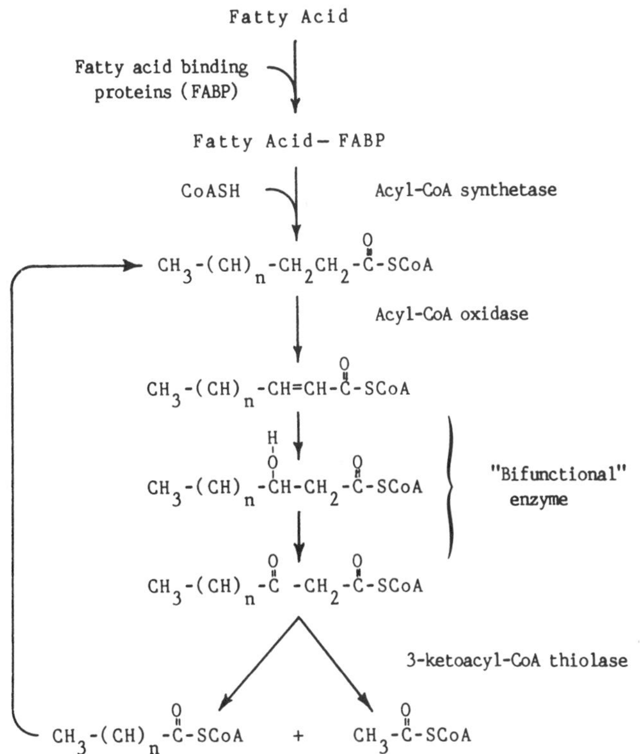

FIGURE 2 Pathway for peroxisomal beta-oxidation of fatty acids. Medium-chain, long-chain, and very long chain fatty acids are chain-shortened by two carbons for each cycle of beta-oxidation down to an 8- or 6-carbon fatty acid. The acetate units and remnant fatty acids leave the peroxisome as carnitine esters via the action of acetylcarnitine and octanylcarnitine transferases.

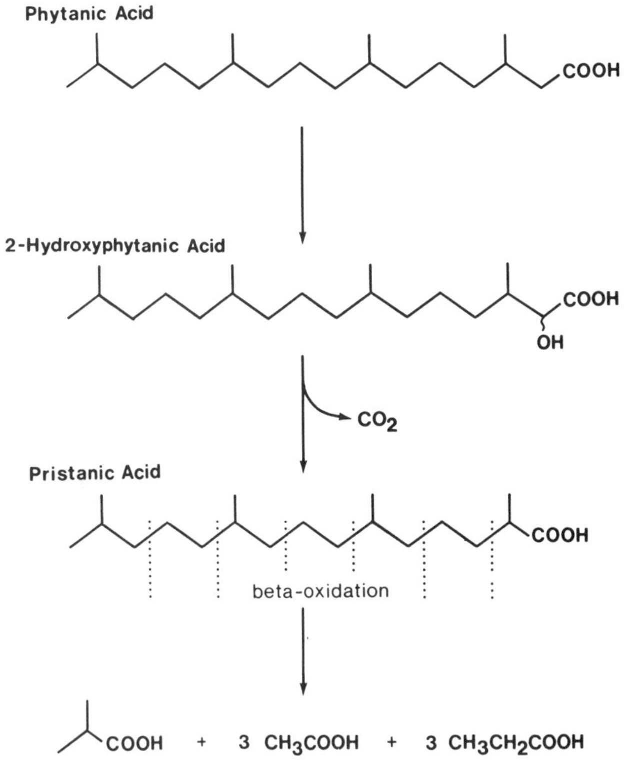

FIGURE 3 Sequence of alpha-oxidation of phytanic acid. Unlike beta-oxidation of straight-chain fatty acids, the reaction is not dependent on coenzyme A, and the first step may be a direct hydroxylation, rather than dehydrogenation, followed by hydration.

isomal proliferation. As will be described later, it is the deficiency of this highly specialized system for beta-oxidation that is responsible for several of the clinically most important biochemical markers for peroxisomal disease, such as increased levels of very long chain fatty acids and bile acid precursors.

Phytanic Acid Oxidation

Phytanic acid (3,7,11,15-tetramethylhexadecanoic acid) is a polyisoprenoid branched-chain fatty acid produced by oxidation of the free phytol chain of chlorophyll (Fig. 3). In the human diet, free phytol is concentrated in green vegetables, vegetable fats, and animal fats, but preformed phytanic acid occurring in animal and fish fats may be the largest source of phytanic acid.[27] Dietary phytanic acid must undergo further alpha-oxidation to pristanic acid (2,6,10,14-tetramethylpentadecanoic acid) before it can be fully catabolized by peroxisomal and mitochondrial beta-oxidative systems, although terminal omega-oxidation probably activates a small portion of phytanic acid for beta-oxidation from the omega end.[28]

Alpha-oxidation of phytanic acid begins with a direct hydroxylation of the alpha-carbon of the free acid by phytanic acid oxidase, yielding L-2-OH-phytanate.[29] The L-2-hydroxy acid is then further oxidized by a peroxisomal L-2-OH-acid oxidase to 2-oxophytanic acid before alpha-cleavage to CO_2 and pristanic acid.[30] Because there is no synthesis of 2-OH-phytanic acid from phytanic acid in tissues of patients with adult Refsum's disease,[31] the primary defect causing adult Refsum's disease is presumed to be a deficiency of phytanic acid oxidase itself. It is less clear for Zellweger's syndrome and related generalized peroxisomal diseases in which a block in phytanic acid metabolism occurs. Although a deficiency of a peroxisomal phytanic acid oxidase is suspected in Zellweger's syndrome, infantile Refsum's disease, and neonatal ALD because of their almost universally increased levels of phytanic acid, experimental evidence indicates that phytanic acid oxidation may be largely a mitochondrial activity, at least in rat liver.[32] However, it has also been shown that most oxidation of L-2-OH-phytanic acid to 2-oxophytanic acid occurs in the peroxisomal fraction of rat kidney.[30] Although deficient peroxisomal processing of phytanic acid is almost certainly responsible for the increased levels of phytanic acid in the generalized peroxisomal disorders, conclusive identification of the deficient peroxisomal enzymes or factors awaits further study.

Bile Acid Synthesis

Bile acids are synthesized from cholesterol by a complex series of cytochrome P-450–dependent ring hydroxylations of the cholesterol steroid nucleus, followed by a final beta-oxidative cleavage of a propionate group from the branched C20-C27 side chain of cholesterol (Fig. 4). Normally, only the final end-products of bile acid synthesis, cholic acid and chenodesoxycholic acid, occur in bile or other body fluids in any significant amount. However, in 1972, Eyssen and colleagues[33] reported that the duodenal fluid of infants with a Zellweger's-like syndrome contained unusually large amounts of the bile acid intermediates, dihydroxycoprostanic acid (DHCA) and trihydroxycoprostanic acid (THCA). Until then, DHCA and THCA had been known to be abundant acids only in the bile of certain primitive vertebrates, such as the alligator. In addition, a previously unknown C29-dicarboxylic bile acid has been found to be substantially increased in the blood of patients with Zellweger's syndrome.[34] The finding of increased levels of DHCA and THCA in Zellweger's syndrome and the discovery that hepatocytes of Zellweger's syndrome are devoid of peroxisomes have focused attention on the possible role of peroxisomes in the conversion of DHCA and THCA into their respective C24 bile acids, chenodeoxycholic acid and cholic acid.[34,35]

Although bile acid ring hydroxylations most likely take place in the microsomal compartment, experimental evidence now argues that cleavage of the cholesterol side chain, the final step in the synthesis of bile acids, occurs largely if not exclusively in the peroxisome. This conclusion has been reached both from careful subcellular fractionation studies in rat liver[35] and from the evidence that essentially all patients with Zellweger's syndrome and related generalized peroxisomal deficiency syndromes have elevations of THCA, DHCA, and C29-dicarboxylic bile acids.[36] Moreover, recent studies of the bile acids of patients with deficiencies of only one of the three peroxisomal beta-oxidation enzymes (discussed below) suggest that peroxisomal bifunctional enzyme and 3-ketoacyl-CoA thiolase, but not peroxisomal acyl-CoA oxidase, participate in cholesterol side chain cleavage. The initial beta-hydroxylation of the cholesterol side chain is now thought to be mediated either by a P-450–type cytochrome hydroxylase or by an acyl-CoA oxidase distinct from the VLCF acyl-CoA oxidase. Also important with regard to the peroxisomal metabolism of bile acids has been the discovery of an immunologically and physiologically distinct isozyme of hydroxymethylglutaryl (HMG) CoA reductase in peroxisomes.[37] In ER, HMG-CoA reductase catalyzes the synthesis of mevalonate from HMG and serves as the rate-limiting step of cholesterol biosynthesis.[38] The presence in peroxisomes of this essential enzyme of cholesterol biosynthesis suggests that peroxisomes may synthesize a pool of cholesterol with metabolic fates different from those of cholesterol synthesized in the ER.

Ether-Lipid Biosynthesis

In contrast to conventional phospholipids, which contain two fatty acyl groups ester-linked to a glycerophosphoryl backbone, plasmalogens are phospholipids with one acyl group ester-linked to the second carbon and an unusual, alpha-unsaturated long-chain alcohol ether-linked to the first carbon. Plasmalogens are major components of membrane structural phospholipid in all cells and constitute up to 90 percent of ethanolamine phospholipids in myelin.[39] Platelet-activating factor (alkyl-, acetyl-glycerophosphorylcholine)

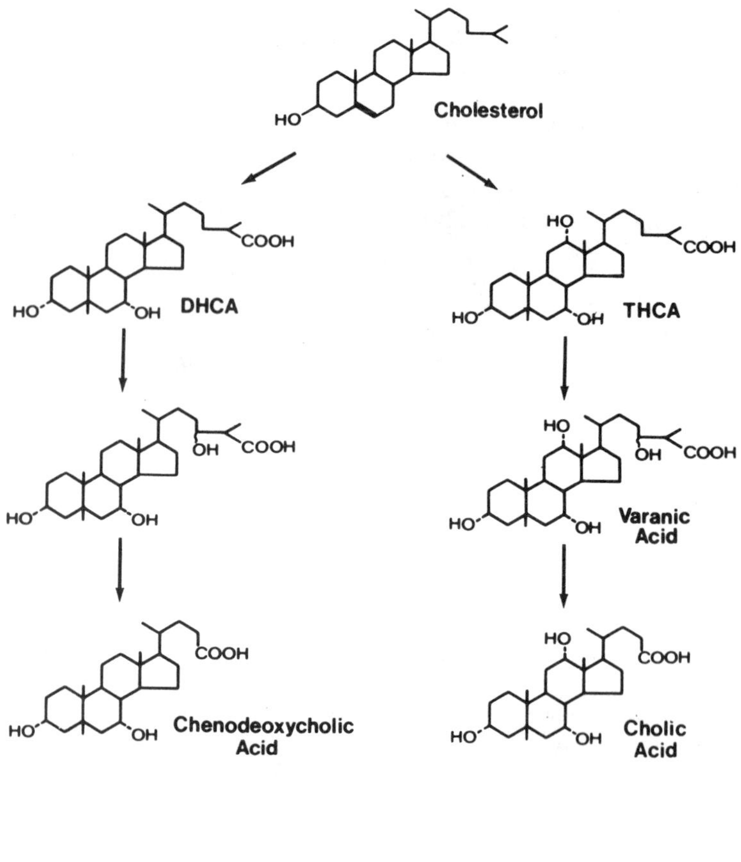

FIGURE 4 Conversion of cholesterol to bile acids via beta-oxidation of the C22-C27 side chain: DHCA = 3α,7αdihydroxy-5β-cholestanoic acid; THCA = 3α,7α,12α-tri-hydroxy-5β-cholestanoic acid; varanic acid = 3α,7α,12α,24γ-tetrahydroxy-5β-cholestanoic acid; chenodeoxycholic acid = 3α,7α-dihydroxy-5β-cholanoic acid; cholic acid = 3α,7α,12α-trihydroxy-5β-cholanoic acid. The levels of both THCA and DHCA are markedly increased in most patients with a generalized peroxisomal disease.

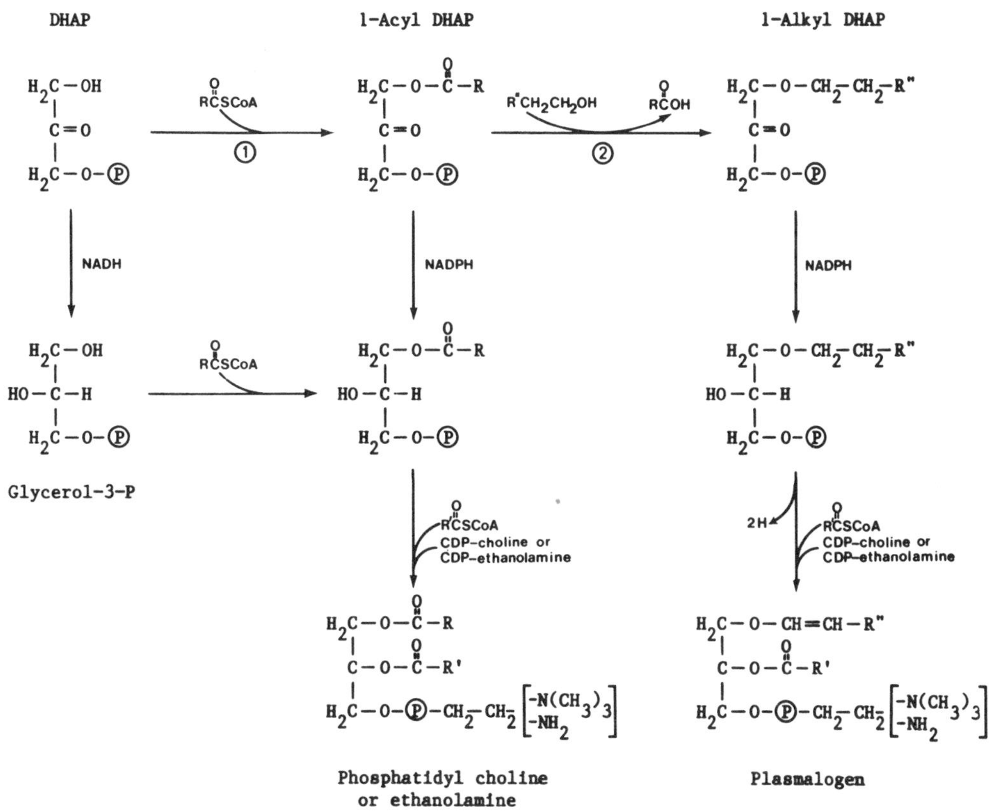

FIGURE 5 Pathway for biosynthesis of glycerol-ether lipids. DHAP acyl-transferase and alkyl DHAP synthase, which catalyze the first two steps (labeled *1* and *2*) in the synthesis of plasmalogens, are located in the peroxisome, whereas other reactions take place in the microsomes or mitochondria or both. DHAP = dihydroxyacetone phosphate.

also is an ether-lipid, the only one known to have a specific biochemical function.[40]

The first two steps of ether-lipid biosynthesis (DHAP acyltransferase and alkyl-DHAP synthase, Fig. 5) have been shown to take place in the peroxisome.[41] The product of these initial reactions, 1-alkyl-glycerol-3-phosphate, is then transferred to the ER, where alpha-beta desaturation of the alcohol takes place and enzymes for normal ester-lipid biosynthesis complete the formation of plasmalogens. There is also evidence that acyl-CoA reductase, which catalyzes the synthesis of the long-chain alcohols incorporated into plasmalogens, is a peroxisomal enzyme and derives its reducing equivalents from NADPH generated through the action of a peroxisomal form of isocitrate dehydrogenase.[42]

Catabolism of Pipecolic Acid and Other Amino Acids

Pipecolic acid (2-piperidine-carboxylic acid), a cyclic imino acid and homologue of proline, is synthesized in animals via a minor pathway of lysine catabolism, then further oxidized sequentially to alpha-aminoadipic acid and glutaric acid (Fig. 6).[43] The initial and probably rate-limiting step in the conversion of L-pipecolic acid to alpha-aminoadipic acid is catalyzed by an FAD-dependent, L-pipecolic acid oxidase.[44] Although both D- and L-forms of pipecolic acid occur in nature, only the L-isomer appears to be synthesized in animals and only L-pipecolic acid accumulates to any significant degree in patients with peroxisomal deficiency syndromes.[45]

Although L-pipecolic acid has been shown experimentally to meet most criteria for an endogenously synthesized CNS neurotransmitter and to have strong inhibitory effects on selected central nervous system (CNS) neurons,[46] it is not clear what, if any, physiologic role pipecolic acid plays in the CNS. The rates of synthesis and oxidation of pipecolic acid, its tissue distribution, and even its subcellular localization appear to vary considerably among different vertebrate animals. In most mammals, formation of pipecolic acid contributes to less than 1 percent of lysine degradation in the liver,[47] where the alternative saccharopine pathway of lysine metabolism (see Fig. 6) appears to predominate. In contrast, conversion to L-pipecolic acid may be the major catabolic fate of L-lysine in rat brain.[48] More interesting, perhaps, is that while the peroxisome is the site of L-pipecolic acid oxidation to L-alpha-aminoadipic acid in man and other primates,[49,50] mitochondria but not peroxisomes appear to contain this activity in rabbits and rats.[50] Such differences in subcellular enzyme localization are unusual but not unprecedented and may reflect evolutionary flexibility of enzyme targeting mediated by cellular gene-splicing strategies.

Interestingly, D-pipecolic acid, which is not abnormally elevated in Zellweger's syndrome, appears to be oxidized only in peroxisomes in the rat and other animals.[51]

Metabolism of Hydrogen Peroxide

In mitochondria, the oxidation of a substrate by an NAD- or FAD-dependent dehydrogenase is followed by transfer of the extracted electrons to the electron transport (respiratory) chain and thence eventually to oxygen to form water. In contrast, in the peroxisome, reducing equivalents are transferred directly to molecular oxygen through the action of one of the flavin-dependent peroxisomal oxidases to form hydrogen peroxide.[5] The large amounts of hydrogen peroxide generated by the many different peroxisomal oxidases would be cytotoxic without mechanisms for its safe decomposition within the peroxisome. Catalase, which is one of the most abundant proteins in liver,[52] serves this function and decomposes hydrogen peroxide by either a *catalatic* mechanism:

$$2\ H_2O_2 \rightarrow 2\ H_2O + O_2$$

or a *peroxidatic* process:

$$H_2O_2 + RH_2 \rightarrow R + 2\ H_2O$$

Most oxidase-generated hydrogen peroxide appears to be degraded in situ by the peroxidatic mechanism.[53] Although the absolute level of catalase activity in Zellweger's syndrome cells is normal, most of the enzyme is found in the cytoplasmic compartment and not in the particulate, i.e., peroxisome-containing, fraction.[54]

The hydrogen peroxide–generating reactions of peroxisomal oxidases are highly exergonic and, unlike mitochondrial dehydrogenation reactions, are unconstrained by respiratory control and the synthesis of ATP. This exothermic nature of peroxisomal respiration may contribute to the heat-producing capacity of specialized tissues such as brown fat, in which cold adaptation causes a marked proliferation of peroxisomes.[55]

PEROXISOMAL DISEASES

Generalized Disorders of Peroxisomal Metabolism (Table 2)

The nomenclature of the three syndromes now classified as generalized disorders of peroxisomal metabolism—Zellweger's syndrome, infantile Refsum's disease, and neona-

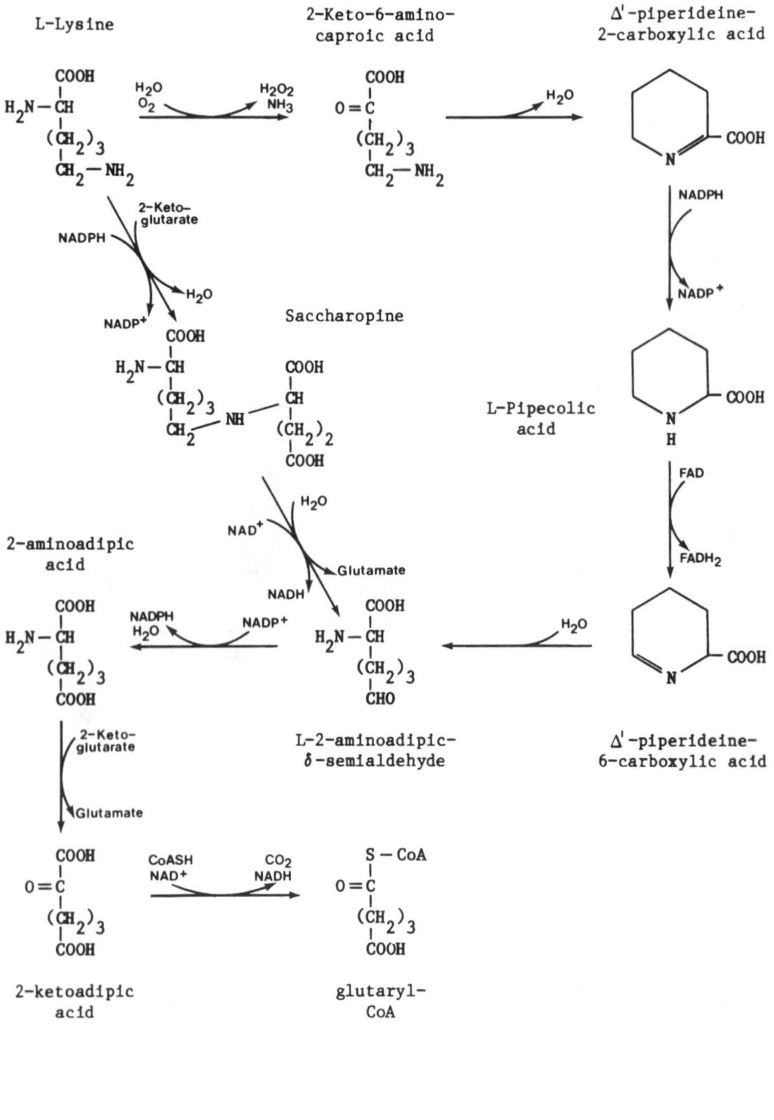

FIGURE 6 Biosynthesis of pipecolic acid and its relationship to the dual pathways for lysine catabolism to glutaryl-CoA.

TABLE 2
Classification of Peroxisomal Diseases

I. **Absence or decreased abundance of hepatic peroxisomes**
Cerebrohepatorenal Zellweger's syndrome
Neonatal adrenoleukodystrophy
Infantile Refsum's disease

II. **Deficiencies of more than one peroxisomal enzymatic pathway but intact peroxisomes**
Rhizomelic chondrodysplasia punctata

III. **Deficiency or absence of single peroxisomal enzyme**
Acyl-CoA oxidase deficiency ("pseudo-neonatal ALD")
Peroxisomal bifunctional enzyme deficiency
Peroxisomal 3-ketoacyl-CoA thiolase deficiency ("pseudo-Zellweger's syndrome")
X-linked ALD (VLCF acyl CoA ligase deficiency)
Hyperoxaluria type I (alanine:glyoxylate aminotransferase deficiency)
Adult Refsum's disease
Acatalasemia

TABLE 3
Major Clinical Characteristics of Zellweger's Syndrome

Craniofacial	Midface hypoplasia, mongoloid facies, hypertelorism, narrow papebral fissures, inner epicanthal folds, anteverted nares, high narrow forehead, large fontanels
Skeletal	Clinodactyly, camptodactyly, equinovarus deformity, joint contractures
Neurologic	Severe hypotonia; absent Moro, suck, and grasp reflexes, complex seizure disorder (often neonatal), profound psychomotor retardation, degenerative neurologic disease
Sensory	Optic atrophy, salt-and-pepper retinopathy, cataracts, glaucoma, Brushfield spots, blindness (often congenital), nystagmus, sensorineural deafness
Hepatic	Hepatomegaly ± splenomegaly, prolonged or persistent jaundice, signs of portal hypertension, coagulopathy
Other	Cryptorchidism, hypospadias, patent ductus arteriosus, septal defects, single palmar creases

tal ALD—reflects more the type of specialists who described the first patients than the characteristic biochemistry or pathology of these overlapping syndromes. Only recently has evidence appeared that most patients with the diagnosis of infantile Refsum's disease have a genetic defect that is allelic with a single Zellweger's syndrome complementation group[56,57] and that several different genetic defects are manifest as Zellweger's syndrome.[57] Furthermore, although there appear to be at least four different complementation groups for "classic" Zellweger's syndrome, the majority of patients fall into one large complementation group encompassing the full clinical spectrum from severe Zellweger's syndrome to neonatal ALD.[57] The specific primary biochemical defects causing these three syndromes are now being worked out and, when known, should clarify the confusing and somewhat arbitrary nomenclature of the generalized disorders of peroxisomal metabolism. However, because most of the existing clinical literature views Zellweger's syndrome, infantile Refsum's disease, and neonatal ALD as separate clinical entities, they are discussed individually here, notwithstanding their often overlapping clinical and biochemical features.

Zellweger's Syndrome

Zellweger's syndrome was first delineated in 1967 as a typical, multiple congenital anomaly syndrome by Passarge and McAdams,[58] who suggested the descriptive term "cerebrohepatorenal" syndrome. Subsequently, Opitz and colleagues[59] presented a comprehensive study of the pathology of Zellweger's syndrome, while several more recent review articles[60,61] have discussed the syndrome in light of its emerging complexity of biochemical abnormalities.

The majority of patients with Zellweger's syndrome are diagnosed as newborns or young infants, based on a relatively stereotypical phenotype, summarized in Table 3, and a variety of anatomic and histologic abnormalities (Table 4).

In the early months, the most noticeable abnormalities that suggest the diagnosis of Zellweger's syndrome are the characteristic facial appearance (Fig. 7), profound hypotonia, and absent neonatal reflexes. A typical infant with the syndrome has a high forehead with widely open metopic suture, widely spaced and upslanting palpebral fissures, underdeveloped supraorbital ridges, triangular mouth, and low-set, abnormally shaped ears. The appearance is often reminiscent of Down's syndrome. However, because most of the craniofacial and other dysmorphic characteristics of Zellweger's syndrome are individually relatively nonspecific, the diagnosis of Zellweger's syndrome is often missed at birth. Hepatocellular disease is usually less apparent during the first 3 months than later but may be evident as hypertransaminasemia, coagulopathy, or hepatomegaly alone.[62,63] Other important and somewhat more specific clues to the diagnosis of Zellweger's syndrome are glomerulocystic kidney disease,[64] abnormal calcification of the patella and other apophyseal cartilage ("chondrodysplasia punctata"),[65] cerebral dysgenesis,[66,67] and pigmentary retinopathy.[68] Structural abnormalities of the heart, mostly septal defects and conotruncal malformations, are also common. Seizures, which occur in more than 70 percent, are often severe and difficult to treat. Because of the severity of the cerebral malformations, most infants with Zell-

TABLE 4
Major Anatomic and Histologic Abnormalities of Zellweger's Syndrome

Neurologic	Cerebral/cerebellar neuronal migration defects, microgyria, pachygyria, olivary dysplasia, septo-optic dysplasia, agenesis of corpus callosum, dysmyelination, demyelination
Liver	Fibrosis progressing to cirrhosis, intrahepatic biliary dysgenesis and stasis, absent peroxisomes, abnormal mitochondria, iron storage (early), lipid storage (late)
Renal	Cortical glomerulocystic disease, hydronephrosis, abnormal lobulation
Skeletal	Chondrodysplasia punctata (nonrhizomelic), osteoporosis, retarded skeletal maturation, bell-shaped chest (secondary to hypotonia)
Other	Pancreatic islet cell hyperplasia, thymic hypoplasia, diGeorge's sequence

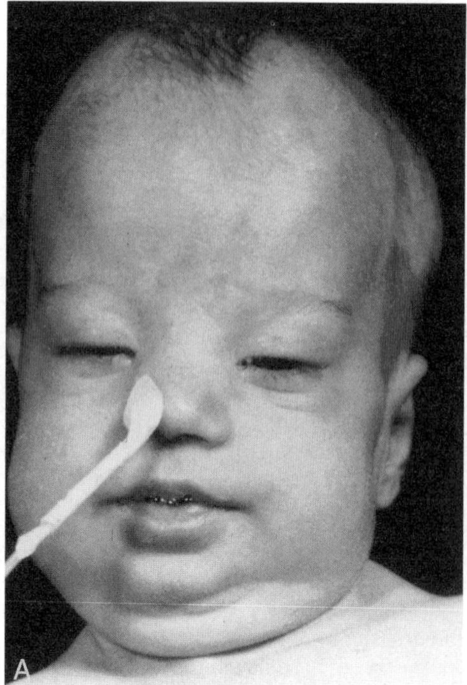

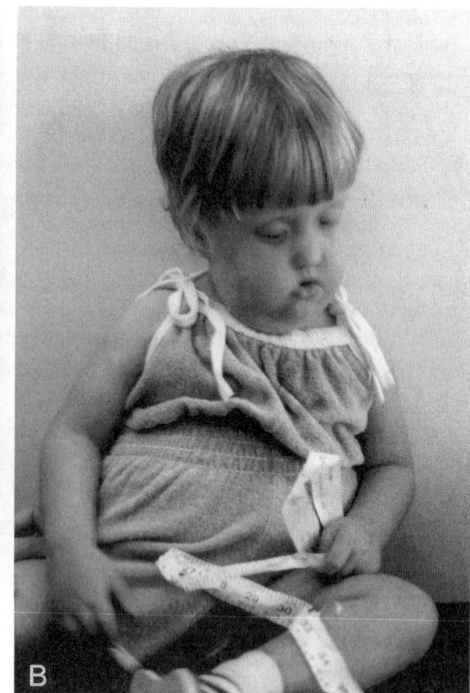

FIGURE 7 Facial appearance of patients with Zellweger's syndrome, *A*, at birth, and *B*, at 3 years. Note in *B* the postural evidence of persistent, severe hypotonia.

weger's syndrome achieve no development milestones and die within a few weeks or months of birth from seizures, apnea, aspiration, or pneumonia. Those patients who survive the first 6 months may show a slight degree of neurologic development and improved muscular tone, but often eventually succumb to chronic hepatocellular disease and progressive cirrhosis, if not the complications of their severe neurologic disease. Patients who were diagnosed with classic Zellweger's syndrome as neonates yet have survived for more than 2 years are known but are rare.[69] Detailed compilations of the clinical characteristics of patients with Zellweger's syndrome have been published by Heymans[70] and Wilson and colleagues.[71]

Although glomerulocystic disease of the kidney can be anatomically quite severe, renal glomerular or tubular insufficiency, apart from mild generalized aminoaciduria and proteinuria, is uncommon. Similarly, the diagnostically important chondrodysplasia punctata affects mostly apophyseal cartilage, such as the patella, and does not itself cause dwarfing. Other unexplained abnormalities with little obvious clinical consequence include islet cell hyperplasia, thymic hypoplasia, and siderosis.[58]

The CNS disease of Zellweger's syndrome is notable for the coexistence of congenital developmental abnormalities and acquired degenerative changes.[66,67,72] The most common CNS malformations are cerebral and cerebellar heterotopias, pachymicrogyria, and olivary hypoplasia. Partial agenesis of the corpus callosum, hypoplasia of the cerebellar vermis, and septo-optic dysplasia are also common but more variable. Another unusual characteristic of the brains of patients with Zellweger's syndrome is increased brain water and correspondingly increased brain weight. In addition to these abnormalities, most of which can be attributed to defective neuronal migration, myelin synthesis is qualitatively abnormal and, in longer-surviving individuals, a demyelinating process that resembles that of X-linked ALD occurs.[73,74] When active demyelination is present (most commonly in the centrum semiovale, corpus callosum, occipital white matter, and cerebellum), macrophages with vacuolar lipid inclusions and "angulate" lysosomes are found. These storage macrophages are essentially the same as those found in the degenerating white matter of patients with X-linked ALD.[75] The recognition of the existence of an ALD-like white matter disease in Zellweger's syndrome led to the discovery that patients with Zellweger's syndrome, like those with X-linked ALD, have increased concentrations of VLCFAs both in the CNS and systemically.[76-78]

Lethal or potentially lethal liver disease is almost universal in patients with Zellweger's syndrome who survive the neonatal period.[62,63,79-83] Although the liver disease is often minimal during first few months of life, and may even be absent, some combination of lobular disarray, focal hepatocytic necrosis, portal fibrosis or cirrhosis, intracellular and intracanalicular cholestasis, and increased iron storage can usually be demonstrated on biopsy (Fig. 8). Foamy, lipid-filled hepatocytes, biliary dysgenesis, multinucleated giant cells, and focal areas of parenchymal collapse are also found, but less commonly. By electron microscopy and histochemistry (for the marker enzyme catalase), peroxisomes have been undetectable in the liver of almost all classic Zellweger's syndrome patients.[2,79,80] Abnormally shaped and dark-staining mitochondria with tubular cristae and paracrystalline inclusions as well as scattered lipid-storage macrophages with angulate lysosomes are also often found (Fig. 9).[81] The chemical composition of the lamellar lipid material causing the distortion of lysosomes is not known but is suspected to be very long chain fatty acids. Except for scattered cellular necrosis, the histology of most hepatocytes is surprisingly normal, particularly in older infants, despite the progression of fibrosis and cirrhosis. By the age of 6 months, advanced cirrhosis and its many sequelae usually dominate the clinical picture. A rapid progression from giant cell transformation without fibrosis to hepatocyte necrosis to cirrhosis in 3 to 4 months has been documented by serial biopsy in several patients. The cause of cirrhosis in Zellweger's syndrome is not known, but increased levels of compounds such as hydrogen peroxide and unsaturated VLCFAs, which have aberrant metabolism in a peroxisome-deficient liver, have been proposed as hepatotoxins.

In addition to a variety of diagnostically useful anatomic and histologic abnormalities, there are now available several laboratory tests for diagnosis of defective peroxisomal metabolism, listed in Table 5 and discussed in more detail in following sections. All these peroxisomal abnormalities can usually be demonstrated in an infant with Zellweger's syndrome, and their documentation in the proper clinical setting often obviates the need to demonstrate absent or severely diminished peroxisomes by liver biopsy. Other less specific but relatively common and sometimes useful biochemical abnormalities are also listed in Table 5.

TABLE 5
Laboratory Abnormalities Common in Zellweger's Syndrome

Abnormalities of Peroxisomal Metabolism	
Increased levels of:	very long chain fatty acids (p,u,t)
	di- and trihydroxycoprostanic acids (p,u)
	pipecolic and hydroxypipecolic acids (p,u)
	phytanic and pristanic acids (p,t)
	dicarboxylic and epoxydicarboxylic acids (p,u)
Decreased levels of:	plasmalogens, platelet-activating factor (p,t)
	phytanic acid oxidase (t)
	peroxisomal fatty acid beta-oxidation (t)
	particulate catalase (t)
Associated Biochemical Abnormalities	
Increased levels of:	serum transaminases, bilirubin
	serum iron and iron saturation (early months)
	CSF protein (variable, late)
	threonine (p,u)
	urine amino acids (generalized aminoaciduria)
	p-OH-phenyllactate (u)
Decreased levels of:	cholesterol (p)
	prothrombin, other coagulation factors (p)

p = plasma; u = urine; t = tissues/fibroblasts.

Infantile Refsum's Disease

Infantile Refsum's disease was first described in 1982 by Scotto and colleagues as a syndrome of developmental retardation, pigmentary retinopathy, sensorineural hearing loss, and mildly to moderately increased plasma levels of phytanic acid.[84] Although infantile Refsum's disease differs clinically from Zellweger's syndrome, both histologic evidence of absent liver peroxisomes and recent fibroblast complementation studies suggest that infantile Refsum's disease is actually a mild form of Zellweger's syndrome, as originally suggested by Poulos et al.[85]

The first patients with infantile Refsum's disease described in the literature lacked the characteristic facial appearance of Zellweger's syndrome, except for a few, mild craniofacial abnormalities such as epicanthal folds, anteverted nares, and midfacial hypoplasia. Unlike patients with classic Zellweger's syndrome, who rarely achieve any psychomotor development, those with infantile Refsum's disease have walked and even have acquired some language skills.[86,87] Similarly, hypotonia

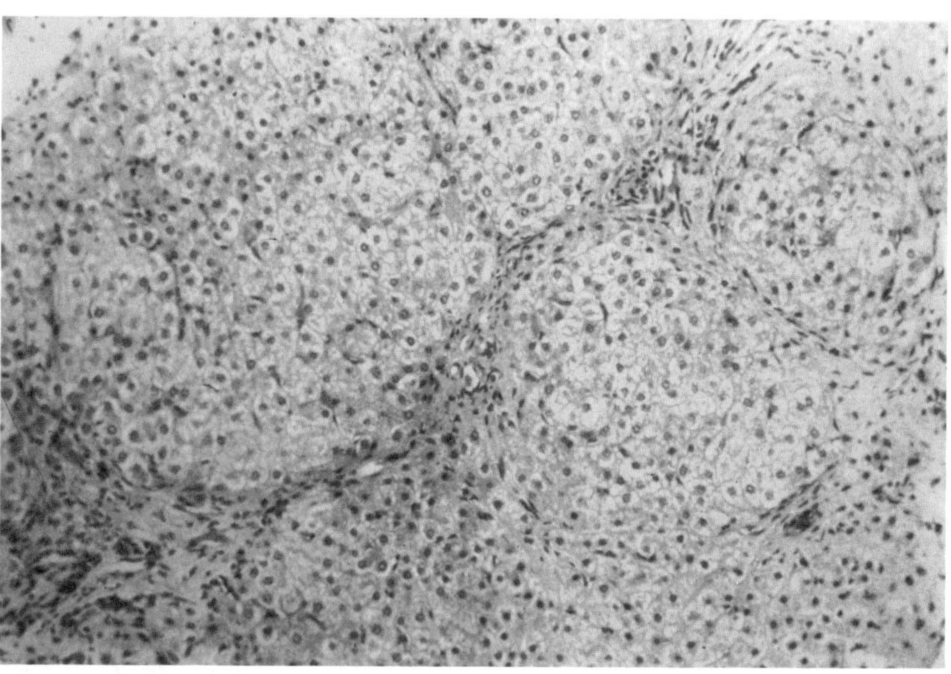

FIGURE 8 Liver histology in Zellweger's syndrome at 6 months showing lobular disorganization and early bridging fibrosis. (Courtesy of H. Moser, M.D.)

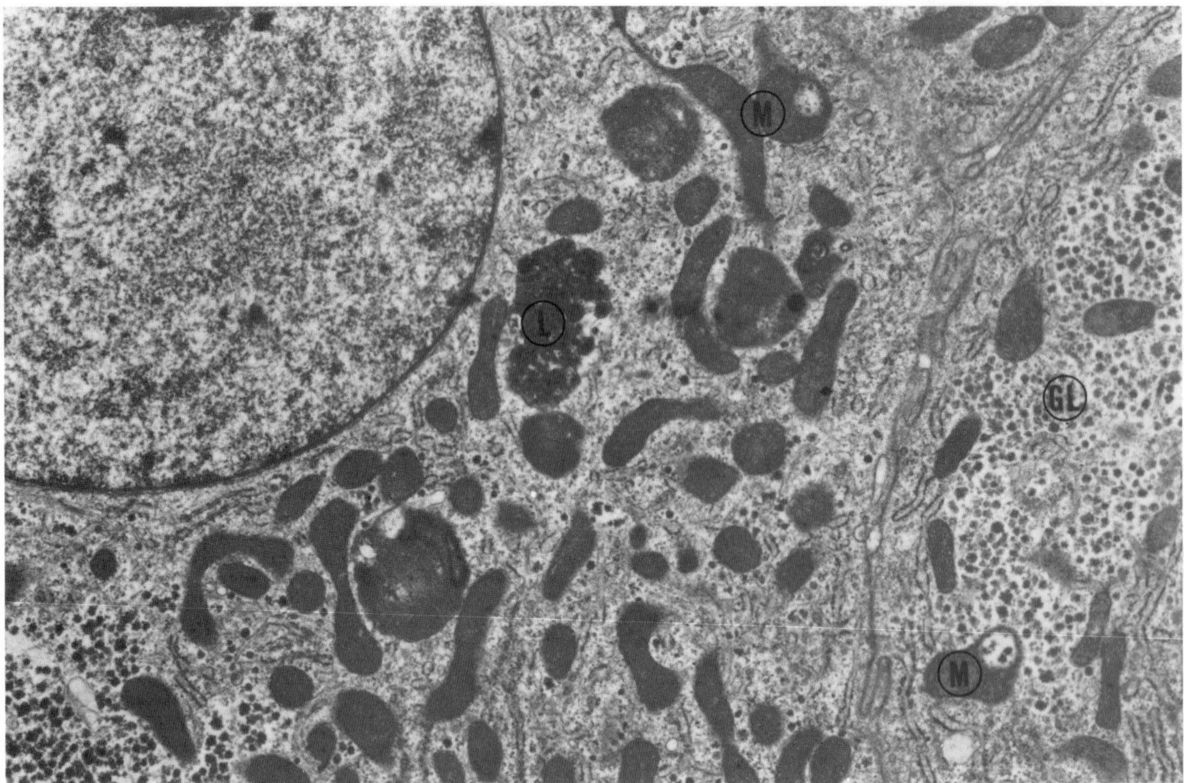

FIGURE 9 Liver ultrastructure in Zellweger's syndrome. Mitochondria (M) with bizarre shapes and dense matrices are seen together with normal lysosomes (L) and glycogen (GL). The mitochondrial abnormalities probably arise secondary to the peroxisomal defect, as many patients with Zellweger's syndrome have normal-appearing mitochondria. (Courtesy of Sydney Goldfischer, M.D.)

is less severe in infantile Refsum's disease, and a few patients have shown improving or normal muscle tone and brisk deep tendon reflexes beyond infancy. On the other hand, pigmentary retinopathy, macular degeneration, and sensorineural hearing loss are progressive such that, because of their longer survival, most patients with infantile Refsum's disease become blind and deaf by 2 years of age, and some earlier.

Liver disease is much less prominent in infantile Refsum's disease than it is in Zellweger's syndrome. Levels of serum transaminases and bilirubin are usually normal or only minimally increased and hepatomegaly not as common. Nevertheless, major complications of hepatic disease, such as cerebral and gastrointestinal (GI) hemorrhages secondary to coagulopathy, have occurred.[86] Both intrinsic liver disease and malabsorption of vitamin K secondary to defective bile-acid synthesis probably contribute to the coagulopathy. Associated vitamin A and vitamin E deficiencies are also common and may exacerbate visual and neurologic degeneration. Histologically, the livers of infantile Refsum's disease patients lack the lobular disorganization and biliary dysgenesis typical of Zellweger's syndrome, but progressive fibrosis apparently is common. Morphologically recognizable peroxisomes are absent or at most represented by small numbers of catalase-positive microperoxisomes.[88] Hepatocytes and especially Kupffer cells often have inclusions of lipid vacuoles and leaflets similar to the lipid inclusions of X-linked and neonatal ALD. In addition, unusual hepatocytic glycogen inclusions, only infrequently seen in Zellweger's syndrome, appear to be relatively common in infantile Refsum's disease. In the only patient with infantile Refsum's disease to come to autopsy, a 12-year-old boy,[89] advanced micronodular cirrhosis was found. Other important pathologic abnormalities in that patient included hypoplastic adrenals without degenerative changes, extensive infiltrates of lipid-storage macrophages in the lymph nodes, severe hypoplasia of the cerebellar granule layer, and severe degenerative changes in the retina and cochlea.

In addition to the full spectrum of peroxisomal biochemical abnormalities—increased levels of VLCFA, phytanic acid, pipecolic acid, and bile acid intermediates and depressed levels of erythrocyte plasmalogens—infantile Refsum's disease patients commonly have persistently low levels of serum cholesterol and alpha- and beta-lipoproteins.[86] Because plasmalogens and their precursors can be assimilated from the diet, erythrocyte plasmalogen levels, which are very low in infants with Zellweger's syndrome, may increase and even normalize over a period of 6 to 12 months after birth. Nevertheless, when assayed in liver or fibroblasts, tissue levels and rates of synthesis of plasmalogens are consistently depressed.[86]

Neonatal Adrenoleukodystrophy

Between 1978 and 1982, several reports were published describing a total of 11 infants and young children of both sexes who suffered from a constellation of CNS, adrenal, and biochemical abnormalities almost identical to that of childhood (X-linked) ALD.[90,91] However, the apparent autosomal recessive inheritance of the disorder, its connatal presentation, and a variety of associated systemic abnormalities uncharacteristic of X-linked ALD suggested that this new "neonatal" ALD was a genetically distinct disorder. The observation that some infants with neonatal ALD resembled patients with Zellweger's syndrome then led to the discovery of multiple defects of peroxisomal metabolism and absent or severely diminished peroxisomes on liver biopsy in a number of these patients. Several review articles have described in detail the full spectrum of clinical and biochemical abnormalities in neonatal ALD.[91–93]

As in Zellweger's syndrome, most infants with neonatal ALD are severely hypotonic at birth and develop myoclonic seizures in the newborn period or during the first few weeks of life. Dysmorphic features may be limited to midfacial hypoplasia, epicanthal folds, and simian creases or may be absent altogether (Fig. 10). Psychomotor development is globally retarded and few patients achieve a mental age greater than 2 years. Growth is usually moderately to severely retarded, although some patients have had normal linear growth. In addition, nystagmus, pigmentary retinopathy, optic atrophy, limited vision, and deafness further handicap most of these children. After many months or years of slow psychomotor development, children with neonatal ALD begin to lose skills and enter a phase lasting over several months or years during which complete neurologic deterioration to a terminal vegetative state ensues.

The diagnosis of neonatal ALD is often unsuspected until autopsy, when the findings of demyelination and adrenal atrophy suggest the diagnosis of a form of ALD. However, in contrast to the purely acquired CNS defects of X-linked ALD, signs of prenatal CNS maldevelopment such as dysmyelination, polymicrogyria, and cerebral and cerebellar heterotopias similar to those of Zellweger's syndrome are found at autopsy. In addition, infiltrates of macrophages filled with lamellar lipid inclusions are often found throughout the nervous system and the reticuloendothelial system. The main difference between the CNS disease of neonatal ALD and that of patients classified as having Zellweger's syndrome and infantile Refsum's disease is the greater degree of demyelination in the children with neonatal ALD.

Unlike Zellweger's syndrome, but more like infantile Refsum's disease, hepatic disease is usually clinically silent or mild in neonatal ALD. Typically, only limited fibrosis or early cirrhosis is found by biopsy or at autopsy.[91,92] By electron microscopy, hepatic peroxisomes are severely reduced in both number and size but are usually not undetectable as they are in Zellweger's syndrome and most infantile Refsum's disease patients. Renal cysts and punctate cartilage calcification are absent in neonatal ALD, an apparent distinction between neonatal ALD and Zellweger's syndrome when the presence of demyelination and frank adrenal atrophy are used as primary criteria for the diagnosis of neonatal ALD.[91]

Most patients with neonatal ALD manifest all of the peroxisomal biochemical abnormalities characteristic of Zellweger's syndrome, although the measured level of activity of some enzymes, such as phytanic acid oxidase and dihydroxyacetone phosphate acyltransferase, may be somewhat higher. Similarly, the plasma levels of VLCFA are often lower than in Zellweger's syndrome and may be limited to increases of only saturated VLCFA.[91] Although not understood, the elevation of saturated but not monounsaturated VLCFA is a biochemical pattern that appears to distinguish neonatal ALD from Zellweger's syndrome when strict pathologic criteria are used for diagnosis.[91]

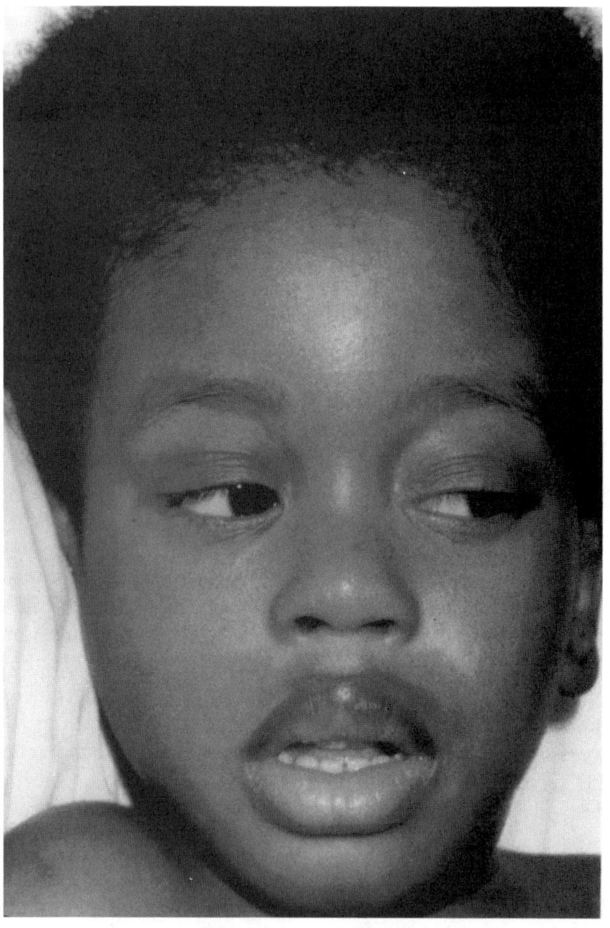

FIGURE 10 Facial appearance of a young child with neonatal adrenoleukodystrophy. Dysmorphic features are few but include a low nasal bridge and mild ptosis.

Hyperpipecolic Acidemia

Three separate reports have described infants with progressive neurodegenerative disease and hyperpipecolic acidemia, who, for a variety of reasons, were not considered to meet criteria for the diagnosis of Zellweger's syndrome.[94–96] Although these patients are often grouped separately in reviews of peroxisomal disorders, recent studies of cultured fibroblasts or autopsy tissues from these patients have shown that all of them also had increased levels of VLCFA.[97] Accordingly, because of apparent deficiencies of at least two metabolically unrelated peroxisomal enzyme systems, these cases should be reclassified as examples of neonatal ALD or other generalized peroxisomal disorders rather than cases of isolated hyperpipecolic acidemia. Although there are several as yet unreported patients who are suspected to have isolated hyperpipecolic acidemia (R. Kelley, S. Mihalik, P.

Auborg: unpublished observations), and who differ clinically from Zellweger's syndrome, infantile Refsum's disease, or neonatal ALD, none has yet been proven enzymatically to have a deficiency of either D-pipecolic acid oxidase or L-pipecolic acid oxidase, both of which appear to be peroxisomal enzymes in humans.[50]

Molecular Defects and Clinical Relatedness of the Generalized Peroxisomal Disorders

Biochemically, Zellweger's syndrome and infantile Refsum's disease are almost indistinguishable,[85,86,88,98] except for differences attributable to age, such as high levels of pipecolic acid and phytanic acid in infantile Refsum's disease. Recognizable peroxisomes are usually undetectable in liver biopsy specimens of these two syndromes, and particulate catalase, a marker for intact peroxisomes, is very low in cultured fibroblasts.[99] The principal enzymes of peroxisomal beta-oxidation—acyl-CoA oxidase, bifunctional protein, and 3-ketoacyl-CoA thiolase—are typically absent by immunoblotting techniques, but their synthesis and rapid cytoplasmic degradation can sometimes be demonstrated by immunologic methods.[100,101] Of special importance is that cell-fusion experiments, using restoration of plasmalogen synthesis as a marker for in vitro genetic complementation between cell lines, have shown that most Zellweger's syndrome and infantile Refsum's disease fibroblast lines do not complement.[56,57] Because of these results and because the two diseases do not occur within the same sibship, Zellweger's syndrome and infantile Refsum's disease are now thought to be different molecular defects occurring at the same genetic locus.

Working on the hypothesis that the primary defect in Zellweger's syndrome is the peroxisomal equivalent of I-cell disease, in which there is a defect of importation of targeted enzymes into lysosomes, Santos, Lazarow, and co-workers[102] demonstrated that some Zellweger's syndrome fibroblasts contain membranous elements that may be "empty" peroxisomes. The apparently defective biogenesis of peroxisomes in Zellweger's syndrome and infantile Refsum's disease may be tissue-specific or toxic in nature, because some patients have been found to have relatively normal-appearing peroxisomes in fibroblasts,[103] albeit reduced in number. As yet, however, the primary genetic defect has not been determined for any Zellweger's syndrome or infantile Refsum's disease patient. No consistent biochemical abnormalities have been found in obligate heterozygotes for any of these syndromes.

Diseases Caused by a Deficiency of a Single Peroxisomal Beta-Oxidation Enzyme

Childhood X-Linked Adrenoleukodystrophy

The degradation of VLCFAs begins with their activation to corresponding co-enzyme A thioesters by a specific VLCF acyl-CoA synthetase (ligase). The VLCF acyl-CoA esters are then degraded by successive cycles of beta-oxidative cleavage of two-carbon acetyl-CoA units mediated by three peroxisome-specific enzymes: acyl-CoA oxidase, bifunctional enzyme, and 3-ketoacyl-CoA thiolase (see Fig. 2). The cause of reduced VLCFA oxidation in X-linked ALD has recently been identified as an apparently isolated deficiency of peroxisomal VLCF acyl-CoA synthetase activity.[104–106] Whether the enzyme itself or an associated factor is the actual genetic lesion remains to be determined. There appear to be no other peroxisomal biochemical abnormalities in X-linked ALD, and hepatic peroxisomes are normal in both size and number.

Childhood X-linked ALD, one of the sudanophilic leukodystrophies also called "Schilder's disease," is a rare but well-known disorder with varying presentations from early childhood to late adult years.[107] When onset is between 5 and 10 years of age, X-linked ALD usually begins with a combination of behavioral, gait, and auditory disturbances and ends fatally after several years of devastating global neurologic degeneration, with or without adrenal insufficiency. In adults, in whom a milder form of ALD is known as *adrenomyeloneuropathy* (AMN), peripheral nerve dysfunction and adrenal insufficiency predominate over relatively mild CNS disturbances. Occasionally, clinically unaffected older adults with classic biochemical findings are discovered within pedigrees of cases of typical X-linked ALD or AMN.

In contrast to the multiple congenital abnormalities characteristic of neonatal ALD, all of the neurologic and endocrinologic defects of X-linked ALD are acquired, usually beginning no earlier than 4 or 5 years of age. Nevertheless, diagnostic elevations of VLCFA in plasma and other tissues in X-linked ALD are present at birth.[107] Moreover, because of its mode of inheritance, X-linked ALD is also often manifest to a milder degree clinically and biochemically by carrier females.[108,109] Although X-linked ALD offers an excellent opportunity to understand the mechanism by which increased levels of VLCFA affect the CNS and steroid-secreting organs, very little is known at this time about the pathogenesis of VLCFA-associated CNS degeneration or endocrine dysfunction in either neonatal or X-linked ALD.

Acyl-Coenzyme A Oxidase Deficiency—"Pseudo-neonatal Adrenoleukodystrophy"

Two siblings who were severely hypotonic at birth and developed myoclonic seizures in the first week of life, but who lacked the dysmorphic appearance and other malformations characteristic of Zellweger's syndrome,were found by Poll-The and colleagues[110] to have an apparently isolated deficiency of peroxisomal acyl-CoA oxidase. VLCFA were elevated in plasma and fibroblasts to the same degree as in typical Zellweger's syndrome, but all other biochemical markers of peroxisomal dysfunction, including levels of bile acid intermediates, were normal. The children showed some psychomotor development in the first 2 years despite, at the same time, progressive sensorineural deafness and tapetoretinal degeneration. By the age of 2 years, global neurologic deterioration, extensive white matter degeneration, and laboratory evidence of adrenal insufficiency had developed. The children continued to deteriorate, and both died in a vegetative state by 4 years of age. There was no clinical or biochemical evidence of liver disease during life and liver histology by closed biopsy was notable only for somewhat increased peroxisomal size and variability and some lipoid deposits in hepatocytes. Cirrhosis or fibrosis was not found. Isolated acyl-CoA oxidase deficiency was documented by enzymatic assay of fibroblasts and by immunologic methods[110] but has not yet been confirmed as the primary genetic defect by molecular or heterozygote studies.

Peroxisomal Bifunctional Enzyme Deficiency

A patient with a deficiency of peroxisomal bifunctional enzyme has recently been described.[111] At birth, the affected infant was severely hypotonic, macrocephalic, and neurologically depressed but lacked hepatosplenomegaly, dysmorphic facies, or other clinical characteristics of Zellweger's syndrome. Myoclonic seizures were first seen at 3 hours of age and were resistant to standard anticonvulsant therapy. Funduscopic, renal ultrasonography, and skeletal radiographic examinations were normal at birth, but both visual and auditory evoked responses were very abnormal. A brain biopsy at the age of 6 weeks disclosed Zellweger's-like polymicrogyria with subjacent cerebral heterotopias. The infant died from an acute infection at 5½ months, having shown no psychomotor development from birth. At autopsy, central white matter demyelination, severe adrenal atrophy, microscopic glomerular cysts, mild hepatic portal fibrosis, and a normal abundance of hepatic peroxisomes were documented. Plasma levels of pipecolic acid and phytanic acid and red cell levels of plasmalogens were all normal, but plasma levels of bile acid intermediates and VLCFA were substantially increased. The absence of peroxisomal bifunctional enzyme, but not peroxisomal thiolase or acyl-CoA oxidase, was demonstrated by immunoblot analysis.

Peroxisomal 3-Ketoacyl-CoA Thiolase Deficiency—"Pseudo-Zellweger's Syndrome"

Several patients with many clinical, anatomic, and histologic characteristics of Zellweger's syndrome have been found by liver biopsy to have, rather than absent peroxisomes, abundant normal to larger than normal peroxisomes.[112,113] Like patients with Zellweger's syndrome, these children were severely hypotonic at birth, lacked normal neonatal reflexes, and usually developed myoclonic seizures at or shortly after birth. Typical Zellweger's-like CNS dysgenesis and renal polycystic disease also were present, but chondrodysplasia punctata and cirrhosis were absent. Moreover, unlike typical Zellweger's syndrome, adrenal atrophy was advanced, and ALD-like "balloon cells" and "cytoplasmic clefts" of the inner adrenal cortex were quite prominent in one infant dying at 11 months. Because of the strong resemblance of these patients to those with Zellweger's syndrome, the name "pseudo-Zellweger's syndrome" often has been used for this disorder.

Of the usual spectrum of metabolic abnormalities found in Zellweger's syndrome, only those that reflect a deficiency of peroxisomal beta-oxidation, i.e., increased levels of VLCFA and bile acid precursors (DHCA and THCA), were abnormal in the pseudo-Zellweger's syndrome patients. As a result, a more detailed study of the enzymes of peroxisomal beta-oxidation was undertaken by Schram et al.[114] They discovered that a single enzyme, peroxisomal 3-ketoacyl-CoA thiolase, appeared to be deficient in liver tissue from the original children reported by Goldfischer and colleagues.[112] However, confirmation of peroxisomal 3-ketoacyl-CoA thiolase deficiency as the primary genetic defect in these patients awaits further enzymologic and genetic studies. Although the original case study[112] reported mildly increased plasma levels of pipecolic acid, quantitation of this imino acid by more accurate isotope dilution methods showed normal levels at the age of 3 months.[98]

Characteristically, infants with peroxisomal thiolase deficiency show virtually no psychomotor development and, in most respects, follow the same clinical course as infants with classic Zellweger's syndrome. Pseudo-Zellweger's syndrome is an intriguing disorder that, because of its apparently isolated enzymatic defect, will likely shed more light on the role of peroxisomal beta-oxidation in overall cellular lipid metabolism than Zellweger's syndrome, which is biochemically much more complex.

Pathophysiology of Zellweger's Syndrome and Other Disorders with Abnormal Peroxisomal Beta-Oxidation

The important discovery that an apparently isolated deficiency of peroxisomal 3-ketoacyl-CoA thiolase is associated with a clinical disorder that is an excellent phenocopy for Zellweger's syndrome[112,114] provides insight into the pathogenesis of the various systemic abnormalities in the peroxisomal diseases. All of the primary disorders of peroxisomal beta-oxidation except X-linked ALD (wherein VLCFA are not activated to CoA esters) are associated with neuronal migration defects, hypotonia, abnormal reflexes, and seizures. This suggests that prenatal elevations of VLCFA-CoA esters may be the proximate cause of the congenital CNS abnormalities. However, because polycystic kidneys and the craniofacial features of Zellweger's syndrome may occur only in patients who have a deficiency of one of the terminal enzymes of peroxisomal beta-oxidation (bifunctional enzyme and 3-ketoacyl-CoA thiolase), or who lack peroxisomes entirely, then either the increased levels of bile acid intermediates or the increased levels of unsaturated or 3-hydroxy-VLCF-acyl-CoA compounds may be key to craniofacial and renal maldevelopment. Similarly, the development of chondrodysplasia punctata may be dependent on deficient plasmalogen synthesis, which appears to be the biochemical common ground shared by Zellweger's syndrome and rhizomelic chondrodysplasia punctata, described below.

The elevation of DHCA and THCA inpatients having peroxisomal thiolase or bifunctional enzyme deficiency, but not acyl-CoA oxidase deficiency, also raises several questions about the conversion of cholesterol to bile acids via a beta-oxidative side-chain cleavage reaction. If the proposed enzyme deficiencies for acyl-CoA oxidase, bifunctional enzyme, and peroxisomal thiolase deficiency syndrome are genetically correct and functionally significant, then there may be a separate acyl-CoA oxidase in the peroxisome for initiating beta-oxidation of the cholesterol side chain. Alternatively, mitochondrial beta-oxidation or a microsomal or peroxisomal P-450 hydroxylase may catalyze the initial beta-hydroxylation of the cholesterol side chain.

Other Disorders of Peroxisomal Metabolism

Rhizomelic Chondrodysplasia Punctata

Although named for its severe rhizomelic chondrodystrophy and diffuse epiphyseal and extraepiphyseal punctate calcification, rhizomelic chondrodysplasia punctata (RCDP) is better described as an autosomal recessive, multiple congenital malformation syndrome with major nonskeletal abnormalities in the CNS (neuronal migration defect, seizures, deafness), eye (cataracts, blindness, corneal defects), and skin (ichthyosis).[115] All children with RCDP have severe growth retardation and profound mental deficiency, and most die before 1 year of age from respiratory insufficiency or complications of the CNS disease.

Recognizing that the punctate cartilage calcification of RCDP resembles that of Zellweger's syndrome, Heymans and colleagues[116] tested patients with RCDP for abnormalities of peroxisomal metabolism and discovered that both plasmalogen synthesis and phytanic acid oxidation were severely deficient. The most severe depression in the plasmalogen pathway was in the level of alkyl-DHAP synthase,the second enzyme of peroxisomal plasmalogen synthesis, which was reduced to less than 10 percent of normal. Phytanic acid oxidase activity was equally depressed. Plasma levels of phytanic acid in RCDP patients have on average been higher than those of age-matched Zellweger's patients and may even reach the high levels characteristic of adult Refsum's disease in the rare longer-surviving patients with RCDP.[117]

Because levels of intermediates of phytanic acid oxidation are not increased,the defect in phytanic acid oxidation in RCDP is presumed to be limited to the initial alpha-hydroxylation step, as in adult Refsum's disease. Plasma levels of pipecolic acid, VLCFA, and bile acids are normal in RCDP, and liver and renal disease have also been absent.[117] Although one RCDP patient was reported to have reduced numbers of hepatic peroxisomes, others have had normally sized and abundant peroxisomes.[116] The mechanism by which combined deficiencies of two apparently unrelated peroxisomal biochemical pathways arises is unclear. Because both alkyl-DHAP synthase and phytanic acid oxidase appear to be membrane-limited enzymes, a primary abnormality of the peroxisomal membrane is possible. Interestingly, although VLCFA oxidation appears to be normal in RCDP, the peroxisomal thiolase exists largely in an unprocessed, higher molecular weight precursor form,[117] which further suggests that the primary defect in RCDP may involve specific enzyme-processing (importing) functions of the peroxisomal membrane. As yet, neither autosomal dominant (Conradi-Hunerman syndrome) nor X-linked recessive chondrodysplasia punctata has been found to have structural or biochemical peroxisomal abnormalities.

Heredopathia Atactica Polyneuritiformis—Adult Refsum's Disease

In contrast to infantile Refsum's disease, the adult form of the disease is usually not evident clinically until the second or third decade. The major abnormalities in adult Refsum's disease, all of which are acquired and progressive, include pigmentary retinopathy, sensorineural deafness, cerebellar ataxia, polyneuritis, ichthyosis, and cardiac conduction abnormalities.[119–121] A mild epiphyseal dysplasia may also occur in some patients. Although clinical hepatic disease is absent, ultrastructural changes in the liver have been found to include excessive hepatocytic deposits of lipofuscin, vacuoles containing various types of lipoid accumulations, and an apparent deficiency of rough endoplasmic reticulum.[121] Vacuolization of renal tubular cells and structural abnormalities of their mitochondria have been reported and related to mild to moderate degrees of proximal renal tubular insufficiency in adult Refsum's disease. Biochemically, Refsum's disease is characterized by increased levels of free and esterified phytanic acid in the blood and tissues and a corresponding absence of phytanic acid oxidase activity as measured in fibroblasts and other solid tissues.[31] All other peroxisomal functions appear to be normal. Because of many years of accumulation of phytanic acid before diagnosis, levels of phytanic acid in plasma at the time of diagnosis of adult Refsum's disease are often greater than 1,000 μg per milliliter, compared with typical plasma levels of 10 to 200 μg per milliliter in Zellweger's syndrome, infantile Refsum's disease, or RCDP.[85,122] The disorder, which is one of the rarest inborn errors of metabolism, is inherited as an autosomal recessive genetic trait.

Stabilization and even partial reversal of the complications of adult Refsum's disease can be achieved by restriction of dietary phytanic acid combined with direct elimination of accumulated phytanic acid by plasmapheresis, if necessary.[123,124] Although phytanic acid oxidase activity segregates with mitochondria in rats,[32] because abnormally low phytanic acid oxidase activity occurs in all disorders with absent or severely reduced numbers of peroxisomes, and because subcellular location of an enzymatic activity may vary among different species, some role of the peroxisomes in the alpha-hydroxylation of phytanic acid in man is likely. Hence, adult Refsum's disease is often provisionally classified as a peroxisomal disease.

Primary Hyperoxaluria—Alanine: Glyoxylate Aminotransferase Deficiency

Primary (type I) hyperoxaluria is a disease characterized by excessive oxalate synthesis, precipitation of calcium oxalate in the kidney, and subsequent progressive nephrocalcinosis.[125] Renal insufficiency usually develops during the first decade and may be followed by extrarenal calcification of the joints and, especially, myocardium. Except for some patients for whom pharmacologic doses of pyridoxine can substantially reduce the synthesis and excretion of oxalate, renal failure is inevitable. Although most of the oxalic acid in primary hyperoxaluria is produced by the liver, the liver is not subject to oxalate deposition or otherwise clinically diseased. Hepatic and peroxisomal ultrastructure is normal, apart from a mild to moderate increase in lipofuscin deposits.[126]

Danpure et al[127,128] recently have shown that type I hyperoxaluria is caused by deficient reclamation of glyoxylate, most of which is normally transaminated to glycine by alanine:glyoxylate aminotransferase (AGT). A deficiency of this pyridoxine-dependent enzyme causes glyoxylate instead to be further oxidized to the metabolic end-product oxalate.

AGT has for many years been known to be located exclusively within the peroxisome,[129] and its deficiency appears to be the only peroxisomal defect in primary hyperoxaluria. Interestingly, hyperoxaluria does not occur in Zellweger's syndrome, in which tissue levels, although not subcellular distribution, of AGT are normal.[130] Apparently, location of AGT in the cytoplasm does not impair its function as a transaminase. Because the AGT-deficient liver is the major source of oxalate, there have been several attempts to treat late-stage primary hyperoxaluria with combined kidney-liver transplantation, the long-term efficacy of which in the surviving patients remains to be determined.

Acatalasemia

Catalase is present in all peroxisomes at high concentrations and serves the vital function of peroxidatic and catalatic disposal of hydrogen peroxide produced, among other sources, by the many peroxisomal oxidases.[5,9] Catalase is also present in the cytosol of erythrocytes, which lack recognizable peroxisomes. Acatalasemia is a rare, autosomal recessive disorder first identified in patients with progressive oral gangrene and characterized biochemically by a complete absence of enzymatically and, in some patients, immunologically detectable catalase in erythrocytes.[131,132] Because the only pathology associated with human acatalasemia is oral gangrene,[131] catalase in other tissues is presumed to be at least partially active, but this has so far not been studied in detail. Although the pathogenesis of oral gangrene in this disorder is not fully understood and only a minority of patients have any recognizable pathology, one theory holds that erythrocyte catalase detoxifies hydrogen peroxide produced by bacteria that invade superficial mucosal capillaries.[132] In the absence of catalase, tissue destruction by bacterial hydrogen peroxide proceeds unchecked and encourages further invasion of bacteria.

DIAGNOSIS AND TREATMENT OF PEROXISOMAL DISORDERS

Clinical Problems Suggesting a Peroxisomal Disease

Even though children with Zellweger's syndrome, infantile Refsum's disease, or neonatal ALD are almost invariably considered abnormal at birth because of an abnormal appearance, hypotonia, or simply an abnormal neurologic examination, the diagnosis of a peroxisomal disorder is often delayed for many months. For example, the not uncommon neonatal history of a difficult breech delivery, severe connatal hypotonia, and abnormal neonatal reflexes characteristic of Zellweger's syndrome is often misdiagnosed as perinatal asphyxia before clinical evidence of liver disease, pigmentary retinopathy, or degenerative neurologic process at a later time suggests a different diagnosis. The initial clinical impression of birth injury is often reinforced by the frequent occurrence of myoclonic seizures during the newborn period. Alternatively, the finding of a combination of salt-and-pepper retinopathy and psychomotor retardation in many of these children may lead to a mistaken diagnosis of congenital rubella or other prenatal infection. Cockayne syndrome, Leber's congenital amaurosis, and Usher's syndrome are other diagnoses commonly given to the more mildly affected patients with prominent pigmentary retinopathy and an extinguished electroretinogram. For these children, it is usually the appearance of an unexpected abnormality for the diagnosis being carried, such as cirrhosis or frank neurologic deterioration, that leads to a re-evaluation and the ultimate diagnosis of a peroxisomal disorder. Table 6 lists some of the diagnoses most commonly considered or given to patients with generalized peroxisomal disorders. The clinician should consider the possibility of an underlying peroxisomal disorder when consulted about a patient with any of these diagnoses. There are a number of clinical abnormalities that are especially important clues for the diagnosis of a peroxisomal disorder, as summarized in Table 7.

Gastroenterologists are not uncommonly the first to suggest the diagnosis of a peroxisomal disease when consulted about a neurologically handicapped child who has unexpectedly been found to have hepatomegaly, hepatic dysfunction, or simply persistently elevated serum transaminases. GI bleeding secondary to a coagulopathy or varices or both is another common cause for involvement of the GI specialist. More than once, the combination of hypotonia, neurologic deterioration, hepatomegaly, and evidence by liver biopsy of lipid inclusions in the Kupffer cells has been misdiagnosed as Niemann-Pick disease or other lysosomal lipidosis in a child with neonatal ALD or infantile Refsum's disease who has marked VLCFA storage in macrophages. In these cases, careful electron microscopic examination of the storage material should differentiate the lipoid globules with associated birefrigent lamellar lipid structures characteristic of the peroxisomal diseases from the lipid inclusions of the lysosomal sphingolipidoses.

Other, diverse routes have led to the diagnosis of a peroxisomal disease. The finding of either chondrodysplasia punctata (without rhizomelic shortening) or characteristic glomerular polycystic kidney disease in the newborn with consistent neurologic signs is virtually diagnostic of Zellweger's syndrome. In the older, more mildly affected child without

TABLE 6
Differential Diagnosis of Zellweger's Syndrome, Infantile Refsum's Disease, and Neonatal Adrenoleukodystrophy

Down's syndrome; other chromosomal disorders
Congenital hepatic fibrosis/polycystic kidneys
Hypotonic cerebral palsy
Congenital infection (TORCH) syndrome
Rhizomelic chondrodysplasia punctata
Lowe's oculocerebrorenal syndrome
Usher's syndrome
Leber's congenital amaurosis
Cockayne's syndrome
Septo-optic dysplasia (deMorsier's syndrome)
Meckel's syndrome (encephalosplanchnocystica)

TABLE 7
Clinical and Pathologic Characteristics of the Peroxisomal Disorders of Infancy and Early Childhood

Metabolite Level	Zellweger's Syndrome	Infantile Refsum's Disease	Neonatal Adrenoleuko-dystrophy	Acyl-CoA Oxidase Deficiency	Bifunctional Enzyme Deficiency	Peroxisomal Thiolase Deficiency	Rhizomelic Chondrodysplasia Punctata
Abnormal facies	+++	+	+	–	–	+++	+++
Congenital hypotonia	+++	++	++	+++	+++	+++	–
Neonatal seizures	+++	+	++	+	+	++	+
Psychomotor retardation	+++	++	++	++	+++	+++	+++
Pigmentary retinopathy	++	+++	+++	++	++	+++	–
Sensorineural deafness	+	++	++	++	++	++	–
Absent or diminished hepatic peroxisomes	+++	+++	+	–	–	–	–
Hepatic fibrosis/cirrhosis	+++	+	+	–	+/–	–	–
Coagulopathy	+++	++	++	–	–		
Adrenal lipid inclusions and/or atrophy	+	+	++	+++	+++	+++	–
Polycystic kidneys	+++	–	–	–	+/–	+	–
Epiphyseal/apophyseal calcific stippling	++	–	–	–	–	+	+++
Growth retardation	+++	++	++	–	+	+	+++
Mean survival (yr)	0.6	>5	3.0	4	1	0.9	1.0

– = absent; + = mild or occasional; ++ = moderate or common; +++ = severe or universal.

renal or skeletal lesions, neurosensory defects—optic atrophy, pigmentary retinopathy, extinguished electroretinogram, and deafness—are the most common problems that should lead to the consideration of a peroxisomal disease. Less commonly, hepatomegaly, prolonged jaundice, coagulopathy, GI bleeding, or other evidence of chronic liver disease in a neurologically abnormal older child will be the cause for testing for a generalized peroxisomal disorder.

In general, a patient with any two of the major diagnostic criteria listed in Table 8 should lead the clinician to serious consideration of a generalized disorder of peroxisomal metabolism or one of the single-enzyme defects of peroxisomal beta-oxidation, which can closely mimic Zellweger's syndrome, infantile Refsum's disease, or neonatal ALD.

Laboratory Evaluation of Patients with Peroxisomal Disorders

Although a definitive diagnosis of a generalized peroxisomal disorder at one time required demonstration of abnormal or absent peroxisomes by liver biopsy, now the diagnosis can in most cases be unambiguously established by measurement of specific peroxisomal metabolites and enzymes in plasma, erythrocytes, fibroblasts, and other tissues, as outlined in Tables 9 and 10. Nevertheless, whenever the diagnosis of a peroxisomal disease is entertained for a patient who is to have a liver biopsy, a portion of the biopsy specimen should be processed for study of peroxisomal ultrastructure and specific staining.

In general, the measurement of VLCFA levels in plasma, which is now available in several laboratories, is a good screening test for a generalized disorder of peroxisomal metabolism, X-linked ALD, or other defect of peroxisomal beta-oxidation.[77] The most important measurements in plasma are the absolute level of C26 VLCFA and the ratio of C26 to C22 VLCFAs, both of which are markedly elevated in Zellweger's and related syndromes. VLCFA abnormalities can even be detected in autopsy tissues preserved in formalin for many years. If RCDP is the diagnosis under consideration,

TABLE 8
Major Diagnostic Criteria for a Generalized Peroxisomal Disorder

Abnormal peroxisomal enzyme or metabolite level
Characteristic facial appearance
Evidence of cerebral dysgenesis
Hepatic fibrosis/cirrhosis, cholestasis, biliary dysgenesis
Polycystic (cortical) kidney disease
Extinguished electroretinogram, optic atrophy, pigmentary retinopathy
Sensorineural hearing loss
Punctate calcification of cartilage

TABLE 9
Tests for Evaluation of Peroxisomal Metabolism

Plasma	VLCFAs, phytanic acid, pipecolic acid, bile acid intermediates
Erythrocytes	Plasmalogens
Urine	Pipecolic acid; long-chain, odd-carbon, and epoxy dicarboxylic acids; bile acid intermediates
Fibroblasts or tissues	VLCFAs, VLCFA beta-oxidation rate, phytanic acid oxidase, plasmalogen content, plasmalogen synthesis, DHAP acyl-transferase, alkyl-DHAP synthase, sedimentable catalase, peroxisomal size and abundance

TABLE 10
Peroxisomal Metabolites in the Peroxisomal Disorders of Infancy and Early Childhood

Metabolite Level	Zellweger's Syndrome	Infantile Refsum's Disease	Neonatal Adrenoleuko-dystrophy	Acyl-CoA Oxidase Deficiency	Bifunctional Enzyme Deficiency	Perox. Thiolase Deficiency	Rhizomelic Dysplasia Punctata
Increased very long chain fatty acids	+++	+++	+++	+++	+++	+++	–
Increased urinary pipecolic acid*	+++	+/–	+/–	–	–	–	–
Increased plasma pipecolic acid*	+	+++	+++	–	–	–	–
Decreased red cell plasmalogens†	+++	+/–	+/–	–	–	–	+++
Increased plasma phytanic acid‡	+	+++	++	–	–	–	++
Increased plasma bile acid intermediates	+++	+++	+++	–	++	+++	–

*Age-related increase of plasma pipecolate level and decrease of urine pipecolate level are largely dependent on normal maturation of proximal renal tubular iminoglycine transport function between birth and 6 months of age.
†May increase to normal levels by age 6 months from dietary intake of plasmalogens.
‡Normal levels at birth; increases are age- and diet-dependent.

then the measurement of plasmalogens in erythrocyte cell membranes or their synthesis in cultured fibroblasts and a plasma phytanic acid level are required. False-negative results are uncommon, and more detailed testing of plasma or fibroblasts is not usually required to rule out Zellweger's syndrome, neonatal ALD, infantile Refsum's disease, RDCP, or X-linked ALD. There have been only a few cases of autopsy-confirmed neonatal ALD in which plasma levels of VLCFA were only high-normal but subsequent studies in cultured fibroblasts were diagnostic of a multiple peroxisomal deficiency syndrome. Also, it is important to recognize that specimens obtained post mortem or from patients with severe hepatic disease or sepsis may have abnormal elevations of VLCFA or pipecolic acid. As expected for a newly delineated group of diseases, the clinical spectrum of peroxisomal diseases continues to widen, and new variants, particularly those with partial deficiencies, probably remain to be described.

When plasma levels of VLCFA are increased in a patient suspected to have a generalized peroxisomal disorder, additional metabolite measurements are needed to help define the disorder. When all or most other peroxisomal metabolite levels (pipecolic acid, plasmalogens, phytanic acid, bile acid intermediates) are abnormal, then Zellweger's syndrome, infantile Refsum's disease, or neonatal ALD is the diagnosis. On the other hand, if plasma levels of pipecolic acid and plasmalogen metabolism in fibroblasts are normal in a Zellweger's-like patient or the nondysmorphic, severely hypotonic patient with elevated VLCFA, then one of the isolated defects of peroxisomal beta-oxidation is likely, i.e., acyl-CoA oxidase deficiency,[110] bifunctional enzyme deficiency,[111] or peroxisomal thiolase deficiency.[112] The clinical distinction between X-linked ALD and one of the other isolated peroxisomal beta-oxidation defects is usually not a question. Despite the often severe adrenal atrophy present in patients with pseudo-Zellweger's syndrome, neonatal ALD, and infantile Refsum's disease, adrenal insufficiency is rarely evident clinically but can sometimes be demonstrated by provocative tests of adrenal function.[91,92]

Because renal tubular immaturity limits pipecolic acid transport (via the iminoglycine transport system) in newborns, some infants with Zellweger's syndrome may have normal or nearly normal plasma pipecolic acid levels but diagnostically increased urinary pipecolic acid levels. Conversely, after maturation of imino acid transport, previously diagnostic urinary levels of pipecolic acid may revert to normal at the same time that plasma levels become diagnostically increased. In addition, because red cell plasmalogens may normalize with age from dietary sources, specific assay of plasmalogen synthesis in fibroblasts, leukocytes, or thrombocytes may be necessary in some cases.

Prenatal diagnosis of peroxisomal diseases is possible both by traditional amniotic cell culture and by newer chorionic villus biopsy technique. Measurement of VLCFA, plasmalogen synthesis, and phytanic acid oxidase are commonly performed and reliable.[133–135] In addition, assay of VLCFA oxidation and measurement of particulate (i.e., peroxisomal) catalase versus soluble catalase can be performed on amniocytes and cultured chorionic villous cells as back-up tests.[136,137] Although there is little experience with prenatal diagnosis of the single-enzyme defects of peroxisomal beta-oxidation, it is likely that these will be detectable by measurement of VLCFA levels and lignoceric acid (C24:0) oxidation rates in prenatally obtained specimens. The absence of a peroxisomal beta-oxidation enzyme also can be detected by immunoblot analysis, whereas, except for acyl-CoA oxidase deficiency, direct enzyme assay of tissues would be technically difficult because of the presence of much greater quantities of homologous mitochondrial enzyme activities. Of course, immunoblot analysis can be normal if a defect in a peroxisomal beta-oxidation enzyme does not change the stability or electrophoretic character of the enzyme. Finally, because prenatal diagnosis of most of the peroxisomal disorders involves the determination of metabolite and enzyme activity levels that are secondarily abnormal, rather than the measurement of the primary genetic defect, which is unknown in most cases, it is important to measure more than one diagnostic metabolite or enzyme level and also to have evidence of the feasibility of a tissue biochemical diagnosis documented by prior studies on the proband's fibroblasts or other tissues.

Treatment of Peroxisomal Disorders

General Measures

Zellweger's Syndrome, Infantile Refsum's Disease, and Neonatal Adrenoleukodystrophy. Treatment of peroxisomal disorders is mostly supportive. For the more severe, generalized peroxisomal disorders, neurologic deficits appear to be dictated largely by primary brain malformations and, as such, are irreversible. Even if the postnatal demyelination and CNS degeneration that occur in the generalized peroxisomal disorders could in some way be prevented, it is unlikely that any of the classically affected patients would achieve even a marginal level of function.

Supportive therapy for longer-surviving children with generalized peroxisomal deficiency syndromes should address at least four main areas: (1) nutrition, (2) seizures and other neurologic disabilities, (3) progressive liver disease, and (4) sensory and/or communication deficits.

Nutrition. Growth retardation in Zellweger's syndrome, infantile Refsum's disease, and neonatal ALD is highly common but not universal. Nutritional efforts to improve growth may be beneficial if significant malabsorption exists. Most often, however, even intensive nutritional therapy does little to ameliorate the growth retardation, which appears to be intrinsic in most cases and not caused by inadequate nutrition. In the more severely affected children, swallowing dysfunction and gastroesophageal reflux are common problems that require medical attention, including nasogastric or gastrostomy feeding for many patients.

Neurologic. Seizures are most typically myoclonic and often respond poorly to traditional one- or two-drug anticonvulsant therapy. More severely affected infants are not infrequently in a state of unremitting status epilepticus. Some of the newer benzodiazepines, such as chlorazepate, have been effective for some patients, but experience with them is limited and the variable liver disease complicates the use of most anticonvulsants. Apnea, primary or secondary to seizures, is almost universal in Zellweger's syndrome and is one of the more common causes of death.

Liver Disease. Liver disease is rapidly progressive in classic Zellweger's syndrome but more variably progressive in patients with milder forms of generalized peroxisomal disease. Early in the course of Zellweger's syndrome, the only therapy needed for liver disease may be pharmacologic amounts of vitamin K to ameliorate (but not usually cure) a coagulopathy and special dietary measures to minimize the complications of fat malabsorption. Later, the expected complications of cirrhosis and end-stage liver disease emerge—variceal bleeding, ascites, hepatic encephalopathy, deteriorating seizure control, multiple hepatic synthetic deficiencies, and delayed drug metabolism—and may require intensive clinical management in some patients.

Adrenal Atrophy. Although adrenal atrophy can be severe in neonatal ALD and infantile Refsum's disease, and ACTH levels are often increased, specific therapy for adrenal insufficiency is rarely required. In X-linked ALD, however, clinically significant adrenal insufficiency is common, especially among adults with the milder AMN form of the disease, and requires appropriate adrenal steroid replacement therapy. Addison's disease may be the only sign of X-linked ALD in the older child or adult for many years before neurologic problems emerge.

Sensory. For patients with neonatal ALD or infantile Refsum's disease phenotypes, who occasionally may achieve a developmental level of 2 or 3 years, visual and auditory deficiencies often become important management issues. The use of hearing aids may enable some patients to make surprising gains in communication skills and interactions with others. Even the use of sign language by severely hearing- and speech-impaired patients is known. Apparently poor cognitive development in these children should not automatically be attributed solely to their congenital and acquired CNS defects if auditory and visual deficits remain unaided.

Other Peroxisomal Disorders. Because of its rarity, there is much less experience with the care of children with RCDP than the generalized peroxisomal disorders. While liver disease is absent in RCDP, seizures, respiratory insufficiency, and recurrent pneumonia are common management problems. Despite often excellent care, most RCDP patients die before 1 year of age from the complications of respiratory insufficiency. Growth retardation in long-term survivors is severe and, of course, not specifically treatable. Treatment of the single enzyme defects of peroxisomal beta-oxidation varies. Patients with peroxisomal thiolase deficiency have the neurologic problems of Zellweger's syndrome but, except for defective bile acid synthesis, appear to lack significant liver disease. Patients with isolated defects of acyl-CoA oxidase or peroxisomal bifunctional enzyme require therapy for the same range of neurologic and sensory deficits found in neonatal ALD, but clinically significant liver disease has been absent in the few reported cases. However, as older, more mildly affected variants of these newer peroxisomal diseases are found, liver disease may yet emerge as a clinical problem.

Specific Metabolic Therapies

In part because of the often excellent response of patients with adult Refsum's disease to dietary restriction of phytanic acid and phytol, a number of attempts have been made to treat patients with Zellweger's or related peroxisomal syndromes by correction of one or more of the characteristic biochemical abnormalities. Specifically, diets to limit the intake of pipecolic acid, phytanic acid, and very long chain fatty acids have been given to several patients with Zellweger's syndrome or infantile Refsum's disease.[71,138,139] No therapy, however, has been clearly beneficial despite sometimes substantial improvement in the metabolite levels. In one patient with infantile Refsum's disease treated with a low phytanic acid diet, phytanic acid levels normalized and VLCFA levels improved, but the abundance of hepatic lamellar lipid inclusions continued to increase.[139] Batyl alcohol, an octadecyl ether of glycerol that can be converted to plasmalogens in the microsomes, has also been given as a dietary supplement. Although red cell plasmalogen levels rose to normal on batyl alcohol supplements, there was no definite clinical improvement.[138]

Other therapies without obvious benefit have included adrenal steroids and treatment with clofibrate, theoretically to increase peroxisomal numbers.[140]

Despite the poor results of metabolic therapies for the peroxisomal disorders, there remains the possibility that extended trials of this nature may affect the course of sensory or other neurologic deterioration in some of the more mildly affected, longer-surviving patients if treatment is begun before degenerative neurologic changes have advanced.[141] For example, the use of VLCFA-restricted diets supplemented with triolein has been successful in lowering plasma levels of saturated VLCFA in X-linked ALD, and, for some patients with the later-onset variant, AMN, nerve conduction velocities have improved on VLCFA-lowering diets (H. Moser: unpublished observation). On the other hand, attempts at partial enzyme reconstitution by bone marrow transplantation for X-linked ALD have not delayed progression of the disease despite, in some, successful bone marrow engraftment and improved VLCFA levels.[142]

REFERENCES

1. Bowen P, Lee CSN, Zellweger H, Lindenberg R. A familial syndrome of multiple congenital defects. Bull Johns Hopkins Hosp 1964; 114:402–414.
2. Goldfischer S, Moore CL, Johnson AB, Spiro AJ, Valsamis MP, Wisniewski HK, Ritch RH, Norton WT, Rapin I, Gartner LM. Peroxisomal and mitochondrial defects in the cerebro-hepato-renal syndrome. Science 1973; 182:62–64.
3. DeDuve C. Evolution of the peroxisome. Ann Ny Acad Sci 1969; 168:369–381.
4. Novikoff PM, Novikoff AB. Microperoxisomes. J Histochem Cytochem 1973; 21:963–966.
5. Tolbert NE. Metabolic pathways in peroxisomes and glyoxisomes. Ann Rev Biochem 1981; 50:133–157.
6. Bock P, Kramar R, Pavelka M. Peroxisomes and related particles in animal tissues. In: Berkeley MA, Beermann W, Franke WW, Rudkin G, Sitte P, eds. Cell biology monographs. Vol 7. New York: Springer-Verlag, 1980.
7. Hruban Z, Vigil EL, Slesers A, Hopkins E. Microbodies: constituent organelles of animal cells. Lab Invest 1972; 27:184–191.
8. Svoboda DJ, Azarnoff DL. Response of hepatic microbodies to a hypolipidemic agent, ethyl chlorophenoxyisobutyrate (CPIB). J Cell Biol 1966; 30:442–450.
9. Hawkins JM, Jones WE, Bonner FW, Gibson GG. The effect of peroxisome proliferators on microsomal, peroxisomal, and mitochondrial enzyme activities in the liver and kidney. Drug Metab Rev 1987; 18:441–515.
10. Lazarow PB, Fujuki Y. Biogenesis of peroxisomes. Ann Rev Cell Biol 1985; 1:489–530.
11. Hruban Z, Rechcigl M. Microbodies and related particles. Morphology, biochemistry, and physiology. Int Rev Cytol 1969; Suppl 1.
12. Gorgas K, Zaar K. Peroxisomes in sebaceous glands. III. Morphological similarities of peroxisomes with smooth endoplasmic reticulum and Golgi stacks in the circumanal gland of the dog. Anat Embryol 1984; 169:9–20.
13. Zaar K, Vokl A, Fahimi HD. Association of isolated bovine kidney cortex peroxisomes with endoplasmic reticulum. Biochim Biophys Acta 1987; 897:135–142.
14. Gorgas K. Peroxisomes in sebaceus glands. V. Complex peroxisomes in the mouse preputial gland: serial sectioning and three-dimensional reconstruction studies. Anat Embryol 1984; 169:261–274.
15. Gorgas K. Serial section analysis of mouse hepatic peroxisomes. Anat Embryol 1985; 172:21–32.
16. Kolattukudy PE, Bohnet S, Rogers L. Diesters of 3-hydroxy fatty acids produced by the uropygial glands of female mallards uniquely during the mating season. J Lipid Res 1987; 28:582–585.
17. Beevers H. Glyoxysomes of castor bean endosperm and their relation to gluconeogenesis. Ann NY Acad Sci 1969; 168:313–324.
18. Lazarow PB. Rat liver peroxisomes catalyse the β-oxidation of fatty acids. J Biol Chem 1977; 253:1522–1528.
19. Hijikata M, Ishii N, Kagamiyama H, Osumi T, Hashimoto T. Structural analysis of cDNA for rat peroxisomal 3-ketoacyl-CoA thiolase. J Biol Chem 1987; 262:8151–8156.
20. Osumi T, Hashimoto T, Ui N. Purification and properties of acyl-CoA oxidase from rat liver. J Biochem (Tokyo) 1980; 87:1735–1746.
21. Hashimoto T. Individual peroxisomal beta-oxidation enzymes. Ann NY Acad Sci 1982; 386:5–12.
22. Singh I, Moser AE, Goldfischer S, Moser HW. Lignoceric acid is oxidized in the peroxisome: implications for the Zellweger cerebro-hepato-renal syndrome and adrenoleukodystrophy. Proc Natl Acad Sci USA 1984; 81:4203–4207.
23. Neat CE, Thomassen MS, Osmundsen H. Induction of peroxisomal beta-oxidation in rat liver by high fat diets. Biochem J 1980; 186:369–371.
24. Bremer J, Norum KR. Metabolism of very-long-chain monounsaturated fatty acids (22:1) and the adaptation to their presence in the diet. J Lipid Res 1982; 23:243–256.
25. Mortensen PB, Kolvraa S, Gregersen N, Rasmussen K. Cyanide-insensitive and clofibrate enhanced beta-oxidation of dodecanedioic acid in rat liver. Biochim Biophys Acta 1982; 713:393–397.
26. Yamada J, Ogawa S, Horie S, Watanabe T, Suga T. Participation of peroxisomes in the metabolism of xenobiotic acyl compounds: comparison between peroxisomal and mitochondrial β-oxidation of ω-phenyl fatty acids in rat liver. Biochim Biophys Acta 1987; 921:292–301.
27. Steinberg D, Mize CE, Avigan J, Fales HM, Eldjarn L, Try K, Stokke O, Refsum S. Studies on the metabolic error in Refsum's disease. J Clin Invest 1967; 46:313–322.
28. Bilimoria JD, Clemens ME, Gibberd FB, Whitelaw MN. Metabolism of phytanic acid in Refsum's disease. Lancet 1982; ii:194–196.
29. Avigan J, Steinberg D, Gutman A, Mize CE, Milne WA. Alpha-decarboxylation, an important pathway for degradation of phytanic acid in animals. Biochem Biophys Res Commun 1966; 24:838–844.
30. Draye J-P, van Hoof F, de Hoffmann E, Vamecq J. Peroxisomal oxidation of L-2-hydroxyphytanic acid in rat kidney cortex. Eur J Biochem 1987; 167:573–578.
31. Eldjarn L, Stokke O, Try K. Alpha-oxidation of branched chain fatty acids in man and its failure in patients with Refsum disease showing phytanic acid accumulation. Scand J Clin Invest 1966; 18:694–695.
32. Skjeldal OH, Stokke O. The subcellular localization of phytanic acid oxidase in rat liver. Biochim Biophys Acta 1987; 921:38–42.
33. Eyssen H, Parmentier G, Compernolle F, Boon J, Eggermont E. Trihydroxycoprostanic acid in the duodenal fluid of two children with intrahepatic bile duct anomalies. Biochim Biophys Acta 1972; 273:212–221.
34. Parmentier GG, Janssen GA, Eggermont EA, Eyssen HJ. C27 bile acids in infants with coprostanic acidemia and occurrence of a 3α, 7α, 12α, trihydroxy 5β-C29 dicarboxylic bile acid as a major component in their serum. Eur J Biochem 1979; 102:173–183.
35. Bjorkhem I, Kase F, Pedersen JI. Role of peroxisomes in the synthesis of bile acids. Scand J Clin Lab Invest 1985; 45(Suppl 177):23–31.
36. Schutgens RBH, Heymans HSA, Wanders RJA, van den Bosch H, Tager J. Peroxisomal disorders: a newly recognized group of genetic diseases. Eur J Pediatr 1986; 144:430–440.
37. Keller G-A, Barton MC, Shapiro DJ, Singer SJ. 3-hydroxy--3-methylglutaryl-coenzyme A reductase is present in peroxisomes in normal rat liver cells. Proc Natl Acad Sci USA 1985; 82:770–774.
38. Brown MS, Goldstein JL. Multivalent feedback regulation of HMG CoA reductase, a control mechanism coordinating isoprenoid synthesis and cell growth. J Lipid Res 1980; 21:505–517.
39. Snyder F, ed. Ether lipids. New York: Academic Press, 1972.
40. Hanahan DJ, Demopoulos CA, Liehr J, Pinckard RN. Identification of platelet activating factor isolated from rabbit basophils as acetyl glyceryl ether phosphorylcholine. J Biol Chem 1980; 255:5514–5516.
41. Hajra AK, Burke CL, Jones CL. Subcellular localization of acyl coenzyme A: dihydroxyacetone phosphate acyltransferase in rat liver peroxisomes (microbodies). J Biol Chem 1979; 254:10896–10900.
42. Bishop JE, Hajra AK. Mechanism and specificity of formation of long chain alcohols by developing rat brain. J Biol Chem 1981; 256: 9542–9550.
43. Rothstein M, Miller LL. The conversion of lysine to pipecolic acid in the rat. J Biol Chem 1954; 211:851–858.
44. Meister A, Radhakrishnan AN, Buckley SD. Enzymatic synthesis of L-pipecolic acid and L-proline. J Biol Chem 1958; 229:789–800.

45. Lam S, Hutzler J, Dancis J. L-Pipecolaturia in Zellweger syndrome. Biochim Biophys Acta 1986; 882:254–257.
46. Takahama K, Miyata T, Hashimoto T, Yoshiro O, Hitoshi T, Kase Y. Pipecolic acid. A new type of L-amino acid possessing bicuculline-sensitive action in the mammalian brain. Brain Res 1982; 239:295–298.
47. Ghadimi H, Chou WS, Kesner L. Biosynthesis of saccharopine and pipecolic acid from L- and DL-^{14}C-lysine by human and dog liver in vitro. Biochem Med 1971; 5:56–66.
48. Chang YF. Lysine metabolism in rat brain: the pipecolic acid forming pathway. J Neurochem 1978; 30:347–354.
49. Wanders RJA, Romeyn GJ, van Roermund CWT, Schutgens RBH, van den Bosch H, Tager JM. Identification of L-pipecolate oxidase in human liver and its deficiency in the Zellweger syndrome. Biochem Biophys Res Commun 1988; 154:33–38.
50. Mihalik SJ, Rhead WJ. L-Pipecolic acid oxidation in the rabbit and cynomolgus monkey: evidence for differing organellar locations and cofactor requirements in each species. J Biol Chem 1989; in press.
51. Zaar K, Angermuller S, Volkl A, Fahimi HD. Pipecolic acid is oxidized by renal and hepatic peroxisomes. Implications for Zellweger's cerebro-hepato-renal syndrome (CHRS). Exp Cell Res 1986; 164:267–271.
52. De Duve CP, Bauduin P. Peroxisomes (microbodies and related particles). Physiol Rev 1966; 46:323–357.
53. Chance B, Oshino N. Kinetics and mechanisms of catalase in peroxisomes of the mitochondrial fraction. Biochem J 1971; 122:225–233.
54. Wanders RJA, Kos A, Roest B, Meijer AJ, Schrakamp G, Heymans HSA, Tegelaers WHH, van den Bosch H, Schutgens RBH, Tager JM. Activity of peroxisomal enzymes and intracellular distribution of catalase in Zellweger syndrome. Biochem Biophys Res Commun 1984; 123:1054–1061.
55. Negergaard J, Alexson S, Cannon B. Cold adaptation in the rat: increased brown fat peroxisomal beta-oxidation relative to maximal mitochondrial oxidative capacity. Am J Physiol 1980; 239:C208–C216.
56. Brul S, Westerveld A, Stijland A, Wanders RJA, Schram AW, Heymans HSA, Schutgens RBH, van den Bosch H, Tager JM. Genetic heterogeneity in the cerebro-hepato-renal (Zellweger) syndrome and other inherited disorders with a generalized impairment of peroxisomal functions. A study using complementation analysis. J Clin Invest 1988; 81:1710–1715.
57. Roscher AA, Hoefler S, Hoefler G, Paschke E, Paltauf G, Moser AB, Moser HW. Genetic and phenotypic heterogeneity in disorders of peroxisome biogenesis: a complementation study involving cell lines from 19 patients. Pediatr Res 1989; 26:67–72.
58. Passarge E, McAdams AJ. Cerebro-hepato-renal syndrome. A newly recognized hereditary disorder of multiple congenital defects, including sudanophilic leukodystrophy, cirrhosis of the liver, and polycystic kidneys. J Pediatr 1967; 71:691–702.
59. Opitz JM, ZuRhein GM, Vitale L, Shahidi NT, Howe JJ, Chou SM, Shanklin DR, Sybers HD, Dood AR, Gerritsen T. The Zellweger syndrome (cerebro-hepato-renal syndrome). Birth Defects OAS 1969; V(2):144–158.
60. Kelley RI. Review: the cerebrohepatorenal syndrome of Zellweger, morphologic and metabolic aspects. Am J Med Gen 1983; 16:503–517.
61. Schutgens RBH, Heymans HSA, Wanders RJA, van den Bosch H, Tager JM. Review. Peroxisomal disorders: a newly recognized group of genetic diseases. Eur J Pediatr 1986; 144:430–440.
62. Carlson BR, Weinberg AG. Giant cell transformation in cerebrohepatorenal syndrome. Arch Pathol Lab Med 1978; 102:596–599.
63. Mooi WJ, Dingemans KP, van den Bergh Weerman MA, Jobsis AC. Ultrastructure of the liver in the cerebrohepatorenal syndrome of Zellweger. Ultrastruct Pathol 1983; 5:135–144.
64. Bernstein J, Brough AJ, McAdams AJ. The renal lesion in syndromes of multiple congenital malformations. The cerebrohepatorenal syndrome; Jeune asphyxiating thoracic dystrophy; tuberous sclerosis; Meckel syndrome. Birth Defects OAS 1974; X(4):35–43.
65. Poznanski AK, Nosanchuk JS, Baublis J, Holt JF. The cerebro-hepato-renal syndrome (CHRS) (Zellweger's syndrome). AJR 1970; 109:313–322.
66. Mei Liu H, Bangaru BS, Kidd J, Boggs J. Neuropathological considerations in cerebro-hepato-renal syndrome (Zellweger's syndrome). Acta Neuropathol (Berl) 1976; 34:115–123.
67. Volpe JJ, Adams RD. Cerebro-hepato-renal syndrome of Zellweger: an inherited disorder of neuronal migration. Acta Neuropathol (Berl) 1972; 20:175–198.
68. Cohen SMZ, Brown FR, Martyn L. Moser HW, Chen W, Kistenmacher M, Punnett H, Grover W, de la Cruz ZC, Chan NR, Green WR. Ocular histopathologic and biochemical studies of the cerebrohepatorenal syndrome (Zellweger's syndrome) and its relationship to neonatal adrenoleukodystrophy. Am J Ophthalmol 1983; 96:488–501.
69. Bleeker-Wagemaker EM, Oorthuys JWE, Wanders RJA, Schutgens RBH. Long term survival of a patient with cerebro-hepato-renal (Zellweger) syndrome. Clin Genet 1986; 29:160–164.
70. Heymans HS. Cerebro-hepato-renal (Zellweger) syndrome. Clinical and biochemical consequences of peroxisomal dysfunction. Thesis, University of Amsterdam, 1984.
71. Wilson GN, Holmes RG, Custer J, Lipkowitz JL, Stover J, Datta H, Hajra A. Zellweger syndrome: diagnostic assays, syndrome delineation, and potential therapy. Am J Med Genet 1986; 24:69–82.
72. Powers JM, Tummons RC, Moser AB, Moser HW, Huff DS, Kelley RI. Neuronal lipidosis and neuronal axonal dystrophy in cerebro-hepato-renal (Zellweger) syndrome. Acta Neuropathol 1987; 73:333–343.
73. Agamanolis DP, Robinson HB Jr, Timmons GD. Cerebro-hepato-renal syndrome. Report of a case with histochemical and ultrastructural observations. J Neuropathol Exp Neurol 1976; 35:226–246.
74. Vuia O, Hager H, Rupp H, Koch F. The neuropathology of a peculiar form of cerebro-renal syndrome in a child. Neuropaediatrie 1973; 4:322–337.
75. Schaumberg HH, Powers JM, Raine CS, Suzuki K, Richardson EP. Adrenoleukodystrophy: a clinical and pathological study of 17 cases. Arch Neurol 1975; 32:577–591.
76. Brown FR, McAdams AJ, Cummins JW, Konkol R, Singh I, Moser AB, Moser HW. Cerebro-hepato-renal (Zellweger) syndrome and neonatal adrenoleukodystrophy: similarities in phenotype and accumulation of very long chain fatty acids. Johns Hopkins Med J 1982; 151:344–361.
77. Moser AE, Singh I, Brown FR, Solish GI, Kelley RI, Benke PJ, Moser HW. The cerebrohepatorenal (Zellweger) syndrome. Increased levels and impaired degradation of very-long-chain fatty acids and their use in prenatal diagnosis. N Engl J Med 1984; 310:1141–1146.
78. Poulos A, Sharp P, Singh H, Johnson D, Fellenberg A, Pollard A. Detection of a homologous series of C26-C38 polyenoic fatty acids in the brain of patients without peroxisomes (Zellweger's syndrome). Biochem J 1986; 235:607–610.
79. Endres W, Müller-Hocker J, van der Ende A, Schutgens RBH, Bise K, Hubner G, Wadman SK. Cerebro-hepato-renal syndrome of Zellweger: absence of liver peroxisomes, hypocatalasia, and renal excretion of pipecolic and trihydroxycoprostanoic acids. Eur J Pediatr 1981; 135:331–336.
80. Govaerts L, Monnens L, Tegelaers W, Trijbels F, van Raay-Selten A. Cerebro-hepato-renal syndrome of Zellweger: clinical symptoms and relevant laboratory findings in 16 patients. Eur J Pediatr 1982; 139:125–128.
81. Muller-Hocker J, Bise K, Endres W, Hubner G. Zür morphologie und diagnostik des Zellweger Syndroms. Virchows Arch[A] 1981; 393:103–114.
82. Pfeifer U, Sandage K. Licht- und Elektronenmikroskopische Leberbefunde beim Cerebro-Hepato-Renalen Syndrom nach Zellweger (Peroxisomen-Defizienz). Virchovs Archiv [A] 1979; 384:269–284.
83. Challa VK, Geisinger KR, Burton BK. Pathologic alterations in the brain and liver in hyperpipecolic acidemia. J Neuropathol Exp Neurol 1983; 42:627–638.
84. Scotto JM, Hadchouel M, Odievre M, Laudat M-H, Saudubray J-M, Dulac O, Beucler I, Beaun P. Infantile phytanic acid storage disease, a possible variant of Refsum's disease: three cases, including ultrastructural studies of the liver. J Inherited Metab Dis 1982; 5:83–90.
85. Poulos A, Sharp P, Whiting M. Infantile Refsum's disease (phytanic acid storage disease): a variant of Zellweger's syndrome? Clin Genet 1984; 26:579–586.
86. Budden SS, Kennaway NG, Buist NRM, Poulos A, Weleber RE. Dysmorphic syndrome with phytanic acid oxidase deficiency, abnormal very-long-chain fatty acids, and pipecolic acidemia: studies in four children. J Pediatr 1986; 108:33–89.
87. Poulos A, Whiting MJ. Identification of 3-alpha, 7-alpha, 12-alpha, trihydroxy-5-beta-cholestan-26-oic acid, an intermediate in cholic acid synthesis, in the plasma of patients with infantile Refsum's disease. J Inherited Metab Dis 1985; 8:13–17.
88. Roels F, Cornels A, Poll-The BT, Aubourg P, Ogler H, Scotto J, Saudubray JM. Hepatic peroxisomes are deficient in infantile Refsum

disease: a cytochemical study of 4 cases. Am J Med Genet 1986; 25:257–271.

89. Torvik A, Torp S, Kase BF, Ek J, Skjeldal O, Stokke O. Infantile Refsum's disease: a generalized peroxisomal disorder. Case report with postmortem examination. J Neurol Sci 1988; 85:39–53.
90. Ulrich J, Herschkowitz N, Heitz P, Sigrist T, Baerlocher P. Adrenoleukodystrophy. Preliminary report of a connatal case. Light and electron microscopical, immunohistochemical and biochemical findings. Acta Neuropathol 1978; 43:77–83.
91. Kelley RI, Datta NS, Dobyns WB, Hajra AK, Moser AB, Noetzel MJ, Zackai EZ, Moser HW. Neonatal adrenoleukodystrophy: new cases, biochemical studies, and differentiation from Zellweger and related peroxisomal polydystrophy syndromes. Am J Med Genet 1986; 23:869–901.
92. Aubourg P, Scotto J, Rocchiccioli F, Feldmann-Pautrat D, Robain O. Neonatal adrenoleukodystrophy. J Neurol Neurosurg Psychiatry 1986; 49:77–86.
93. Vamecq J, Draye JP, van Hoof F, Mission JP, Evrard P, Verellen G, Eyssen HJ, van Eldere J, Schutgens RBH, Wanders RJA, Roels F, Goldfischer SL. Multiple peroxisomal enzymatic deficiency disorders. A comparative biochemical and morphological study of Zellweger cerebro-hepato-renal syndrome and neonatal adrenoleukodystrophy. Am J Pathol 1986; 125:524–535.
94. Gatfield PD, Taller E, Hinton GG, Wallace AC, Abdelnour GM, Haust MD. Hyperpipecolatemia: a new metabolic disorder associated with neuropathy and hepatomegaly: a case study. Can Med Assoc J 1968; 99:1215–1233.
95. Burton BK, Reed SP, Remy WT. Hyperpipecolic acidemia. Clinical and biochemical observations in two male siblings. J Pediatr 1982; 99:729–734.
96. Thomas GH, Haslam RHA, Batshaw ML, Capute AJ, Neidengard L, Ransom JL. Hyperpipecolic acidemia associated with hepatomegaly, mental retardation, optic nerve dysplasia, and progressive neurologic disease. Clin Gen 1975; 8:376–382.
97. Wanders RJA, van Roermund CWT, van Wijland MJA, Schutgens RBH, Tager JM, van den Bosch H, Thomas GH. Peroxisomes and peroxisomal functions in hyperpipecolic acidemia. J Inherited Metab Dis 1988; 11(suppl 2):161–164.
98. Kelley R. Unpublished observations.
99. Wanders RJA, Schutgens RBH, Schrakamp G, van den Bosch H, Tager JM, Schram AW, Hashimoto T, Poll-The BT, Saudubray JM. Infantile Refsum disease: deficiency of catalase containing particles (peroxisomes), alkyldihydroxyacetone phosphate synthase and peroxisomal β-oxidation enzyme proteins. Eur J Pediatr 1986; 145:172–175.
100. Suzuki Y, Orii T, Mori M, Tatibana M, Hashimoto T. Deficient activities and proteins of peroxisomal beta-oxidation enzymes in infants with Zellweger syndrome. Clin Chim Acta 1986; 156:191–196.
101. Chen WW, Watkins PW, Osumi T, Hashimoto T, Moser HW. Peroxisomal beta-oxidation enzyme proteins in adrenoleukodystrophy: distinction between X-linked and neonatal adrenoleukodystrophy. Proc Natl Acad Sci USA 1987; 84:1425–1428.
102. Santos MJ, Imanaka T, Shio H, Small GM, Lazarow PB. Peroxisomal membrane ghosts in Zellweger syndrome—aberrant organelle assembly. Science 1988; 239:1536–1538.
103. Arias JA, Moser AB, Goldfischer SL. Ultrastructural and cytochemical demonstration of peroxisomes in cultured fibroblasts from patients with peroxisomal deficiency disorders. J Cell Biol 1985; 100:1789–1792.
104. Hashimi M, Stanley W, Singh I. Lignoceroyl-CoASH ligase: enzyme defect in fatty acid β-oxidation in X-linked adrenoleukodystrophy. FEBS Lett 1986; 86:247–250.
105. Wanders RJA, van Roermund CWT, van Wijland MJA, Schutgens RBH, Heikoop J, van den Bosch H, Schram AW, Tager JM. Peroxisomal fatty acid β-oxidation in relation to the accumulation of very long chain fatty acids in cultured skin fibroblasts from patients with Zellweger syndrome and other peroxisomal disorders. J Clin Invest 1987; 80:1778–1783.
106. Wanders RJA, van Roermund CWT, van Wijland MJA, Schutgens RBH, Schram AW, Tager JM, van den Bosch H, Schalkwijk C. X-linked adrenoleukodystrophy: identification of the primary defect at the level of a deficient peroxisomal very-long chain fatty acyl-CoA synthetase using a newly developed method for the isolation of peroxisomes from fibroblasts. J Inherited Metab Dis 1988; 11(suppl 2):173–177.
107. Moser HW, Moser AE, Singh I, O'Neill BP. Adrenoleukodystrophy: survey of 303 cases: biochemistry, diagnosis and therapy. Ann Neurol 1984; 16:628–641.
108. Moser HW, Moser AE, Trojak JE, Supplee SW. Identification of female carriers for adrenoleukodystrophy. J Pediatr 1983; 103:54–59.
109. O'Neill BP, Moser HW, Saxena KM, Marmion LC. Adrenoleukodystrophy: clinical and biochemical manifestations in carriers. Neurology 1984; 34:798–801.
110. Poll-The BT, Roels F, Ogier H, Scotto J, Vamecq J, Schutgens RBH, Wanders RJA, van Roermund CWT, Wijland MJA, Schram AW, Tager JM, Saudubray JM. A new peroxisomal disorder with enlarged peroxisomes and a specific deficiency of acyl-CoA oxidase (pseudo-neonatal adrenoleukodystrophy). Am J Hum Genet 1988; 42:422–434.
111. Watkins PA, Chen WW, Harris CJ, Hoefler G, Hoefler S, Blake DC, Balfe A, Kelley RI, Moser AB, Beard ME, Moser HW. Peroxisomal bifunctional enzyme deficiency. J Clin Invest 1989; 83:771–777.
112. Goldfischer SL, Collins J, Rapin I, Neumann P, Neglia W, Spiro AJ, Ishii T, Roels F, Vamecq F, van Hoof F. Pseudo-Zellweger syndrome: deficiencies in several peroxisomal oxidative capacities. J Pediatr 1986; 108:25–32.
113. RJA Wanders. Personal communication.
114. Schram AW, Goldfischer SL, van Roermond CWT, Brouwer-Kelder EM, Collins J, Hashimoto T, Heymans HSA, van den Bosch H, Schutgens RBH, Tager JM, Wanders RJA. Human peroxisomal 3-oxoacyl-coenzyme A thiolase deficiency. Proc Natl Acad Sci USA 1987; 84:1494–1496.
115. Spranger JW, Opitz JM, Bidder U. Heterogeneity of chondrodysplasia punctata. Humangenetik 1974; 11:190–212.
116. Heymans HSA, Oorthuys JWE, Nelck G, Wanders RJA, Dingemans KP, Schutgens RBH. Peroxisomal abnormalities in rhizomelic chondrodysplasia punctata. J Inherited Metab Dis 1986; 9(suppl 2):329–331.
117. Hoefler G, Hoefler S, Watkins PW, Chen WW, Moser AB, Baldwin B, McGillivary B, Charrow J, Friedman JM, Rutledge L, Hashimoto T, Moser HW. Biochemical abnormalities in rhizomelic chondrodysplasia punctata. J Pediatr 1988; 112:726–733.
118. Webber KO, Datta NS, Hajra AK. Properties of the enzymes catalysing the biosynthesis of lysophosphatide and its ester analog in cultured fibroblasts from Zellweger syndrome patients and normal controls. Arch Biochem Biophys 1987; 254:611–620.
119. Refsum S. Heredopathia atactica polyneuritiformis: a familial syndrome not hitherto described. Acta Psychiatr Neurol Scand (Suppl) 1946:38:1–303.
120. Gibberd FB, Billimoria JD, Goldman JM, Clemens E, Evans R, Whitelaw MN, Retsas S, Sherratt RM. Heredopathia atactica polyneuritiformis: Refsum's disease. Acta Neurol Scand 1985; 72:1–17.
121. Kolodny EH, Hass WK, Lane B, Drucker WD. Refsum's disease. Report of a case including electron microscopic studies of the liver. Arch Neurol 1965; 12:583–596.
122. Poulos A, Sharp P, Fellenberg AJ, Danks DM. Cerebro-hepato-renal (Zellweger) syndrome, adrenoleukodystrophy, and Refsum's disease: plasma changes and skin fibroblast phytanic acid oxidase. Hum Genet 1985; 70:172–177.
123. Moser HW, Braine H, Pyeritz RE, Ullman D, Murray C, Asbury AK. Therapeutic trial of plasmapheresis in Refsum disease and in Fabry disease. Birth Defects OAS 1980; XVI:491–497.
124. Eldjarn L, Try K, Stokke O, Munthe-Kaas AW, Refsum S, Steinberg D, Avigan J, Mize C. Dietary effects on serum phytanic acid levels and on clinical manifestations in heredopathia atactica polyneuritiformis. Lancet 1966; i:691–693.
125. Williams HE, Smith LH. Primary hyperoxaluria. In: Stanbury JB, Wyngaarden JB, Fredrickson DS, eds. The metabolic basis of inherited disease. New York: McGraw-Hill, 1983:204.
126. Iancu TC, Danpure CJ. Primary hyperoxaluria type I: ultrastructural observations in liver biopsies. J Inherited Metab Dis 1987; 10:330–338.
127. Danpure CJ, Jennings PR. Peroxisomal alanine: glyoxylate aminotransferase deficiency in primary hyperoxaluria type 1. FEBS Lett 1986; 201:20–24.
128. Danpure CJ, Jennings PR, Watts RW. Enzymological diagnosis of primary hyperoxaluria type 1 by measurement of hepatic alanine: glyoxylate amino-transferase activity. Lancet 1987; i:289–291.
129. Noguchi T, Takada Y. Peroxisomal localization of alanine:glyoxylate aminotransferase in human liver. Arch Biochem Biophys 1979; 196:645–647.

130. Wanders RJA, Van Roermund CWT, Westra R, Schutgens RBH, van der Ende MA, Tager JM, Monnens LAH, Baadenhuysen H, Govaerts L, Przyrembel H, Wolff ED, Blom W, Huijmans JGM, van Laerhoven FGM. Alanine glyoxylate aminotransferase and the excretion of oxalate and glycollate in hyperoxaluria type I and the Zellweger syndrome. Clin Chim Acta 1987; 165:311–319.
131. Takahara S. Progressive oral gangrene probably due to a lack of catalase in the blood (acatalasemia). Lancet 1952; ii:1011.
132. Aebi HE, Wyss SR. Acatalasemia. In: Stanbury JB, Wyngaarden JB, Fredrickson DS, eds. The metabolic basis of inherited disease. 3rd ed. New York: McGraw-Hill, 1983:1792.
133. Schutgens RBH, Schrakamp G, Wanders RJA, Heymans HSA, Moser HW, Moser AB, Tager JM, van den Bosch H, Aubourg P. The cerebro-hepato-renal (Zellweger) syndrome: prenatal detection based on impaired biosynthesis of plasmalogens. Prenatal Diag 1985; 5:337–344.
134. Rocchiccioli F, Aubourg P, Choiset A. Immediate prenatal diagnosis of Zellweger syndrome by direct measurement of very long chain fatty acids in chorionic villus cells. Prenatal Diag 1987; 7:349–354.
135. Hajra AK, Datta NS, Jackson LG, Moser AB, Moser HW, Larsen JW, Powers J. Prenatal diagnosis of Zellweger cerebro-hepato-renal syndrome. N Engl J Med 1985; 312:445–446.
136. Wanders RJA, van Wijland MJA, van Roermund CWT, Schutgens RBH, van den Bosch H, Tager JM, Nijenhuis A, Tromp A. Prenatal diagnosis of Zellweger syndrome by measurement of very long chain fatty acid (C26:0) beta-oxidation in cultured chorionic villous fibroblasts: implications for early diagnosis of other peroxisomal disorders. Clin Chim Acta 1987; 165:303–310.
137. Wanders RJA, Schrakamp G, van den Bosch H, Tager JM, Schutgens RBH. A prenatal test for the cerebro-hepato-renal (Zellweger) syndrome by demonstration of the absence of catalase-containing particles (peroxisomes) in cultured amniotic fluid cells. Eur J Pediatr 1986; 145:136–138.
138. Holmes RD, Wilson GN, Hajra AK. Oral ether-lipid therapy in patients with peroxisomal disorders. J Inherited Metab Dis 1987; 10(suppl 2):239–241.
139. Robertson EF, Poulos A, Sharp P, Manson J, Wise G, Jaunzems A, Carter R. Treatment of infantile phytanic acid storage disease: clinical, biochemical and ultrastructural findings in two children treated for 2 years. Eur J Pediatr 1988; 148:133–144.
140. Bjorkhem I, Blomstrand S, Glaumann H, Stradvik B. Unsuccessful attempts to induce peroxisomes in two cases of Zellweger disease by treatment with clofibrate. Pediatr Res 1985; 19:590–593.
141. Moser AB, Borel J, Odone A, Naidu S, Cornblath D, Sanders DB, Moser HW. A new dietary therapy for adrenoleukodystrophy. Biochemical and preliminary clinical results. Ann Neurol 1987; 21:240–247.
142. Moser HW, Brown FR, Tutschka PJ, Brown FR, Moser AB, Yeager AM, Singh I, Mark SA, Kumar AAJ, McDonnell JM, White CL, Maumenee IH, Green WR, Powers JM, Santos GW. Bone marrow transplant in adrenoleukodystrophy. Neurology 1984; 34:1410–1417.

PART 18

Reye's Syndrome

James E. Heubi, M.D.

DEFINITION

Reye's syndrome is a disease characterized by a severe noninflammatory encephalopathy and fatty degeneration of the viscera. The condition typically affects children of all ages after a prodromal illness. Liver dysfunction is transient, and morbidity relates to cerebral edema and its complications. The cause of Reye's syndrome is unknown, and treatment is empiric with specific emphasis on measures to relieve intracranial hypertension. Mortality is approximately 30 percent. If the child survives the acute illness, hepatic and cerebral pathology are generally reversed; however, a small proportion of children have long-term neurologic sequelae related to cerebral hypoxia.

HISTORY

In 1963, the Australian investigators Reye, Morgan, and Baral described the clinicopathologic features of the disease that is now recognized as Reye's syndrome.[1] An American investigative team, led by Johnson, described the illness in North Carolina youngsters.[2] Over the next 25 years more than 3,000 cases have been reported to the Centers for Disease Control in the United States, and cases have been identified in countries throughout the world. In recent years, there has been a marked decline in the reported cases; however, the case fatality rate remains approximately 30 percent.

Clinical and Pathologic Features

The clinical and laboratory features of the illness are relatively specific. Typically the child initially has an uncomplicated respiratory illness (approximately 60 percent), varicella (approximately 30 percent), or gastroenteritis (approximately 10 percent). As the child is beginning to improve from the prodromal illness (usually 3 to 5 days from onset), pernicious emesis begins. Low-grade fever may be present, but usually patients are afebrile. Children with a varicella prodrome may still have active cutaneous lesions. Initially, patients are well oriented but irritable and lethargic. The progression of sensorial changes is variable (Table 1). Some patients remain lethargic only to variable degrees (grades I and II) with no progression to unconsciousness. It is exceedingly likely that these patients will recover uneventfully, and this group may account for as many as three-fourths of all cases.[4] Some patients progress to a hyperexcitable state (agitated delirium), during which they become disoriented and are intermittently out of contact with their environment (grade

TABLE 1
Clinical Stages of Reye's Syndrome*

	Grade	Symptoms
Mild	1	Quiet, responds to commands
	2	Lethargic, stuporous, thick speech
	3	Agitated delirium, intermittently out of contact with environment
Severe	4	Coma: decorticate/decerebrate posturing, hyperpnea, hyperpyrexia
	5	Coma: flaccid paralysis, apnea

*Based upon the coma grading system of Bobo et al.[3]

III coma). Further progression to deeper comatose states (grades IV and V) may transpire over a few hours to 48 hours or longer. Seizure activity is rare in mildly affected patients but may occur in subjects in deeper levels of coma. The encephalopathy typically persists for 24 to 96 hours, and gradual improvement in neurologic function occurs in survivors. With the widespread use of barbiturates for treatment of cerebral edema, the progression of coma and its resolution are dictated more by the drug's effects than by the natural course of the disease. In patients with permanent neurologic sequelae, return to a static level of function may require weeks. The characteristic presentation of Reye's syndrome, including a well-demarcated prodromal illness followed by vomiting and variable degrees of neurologic impairment, occurs in the overwhelming majority of children (Fig. 1). However, in infants less than 1 year of age, sensorial changes may be much less distinct; hypoglycemia and coma may be even more pronounced and a clear history of vomiting obscure.

The physical findings at presentation are largely limited to neurologic signs. Variable lethargy, combativeness, or coma is present. No focal neurologic findings are observed unless brain stem herniation has already occurred. Pupillary light and deep tendon reflexes are symmetric, with findings dependent upon coma grade. Pathologic reflexes (Babinski) are commonly found. Patients are rarely icteric at presentation, and the liver is usually normal in size or only mildly enlarged.

At the time of presentation, most patients have had multiple episodes of emesis, and the serum glutamic-oxalo-acetic transaminase (SGOT [AST]) and serum glutamic-pyruvic transaminase (SGPT [ALT]) are 3 to 30 times normal. (Most authorities consider the onset of Reye's syndrome to coincide with the onset of emesis.) During the course of the illness, the SGOT and SGPT may continue to rise despite clinical improvement or fall in the face of clinical deterioration. In most cases they return to normal 7 to 14 days after presentation (Fig. 1). The height of SGOT and SGPT elevation is not predictive of clinical severity or outcome of the disease. Serum ammonia concentrations are variable at presentation. Comatose subjects universally have elevated venous or arterial ammonia concentrations ranging from 2 to 20 times normal. In contrast, noncomatose patients may

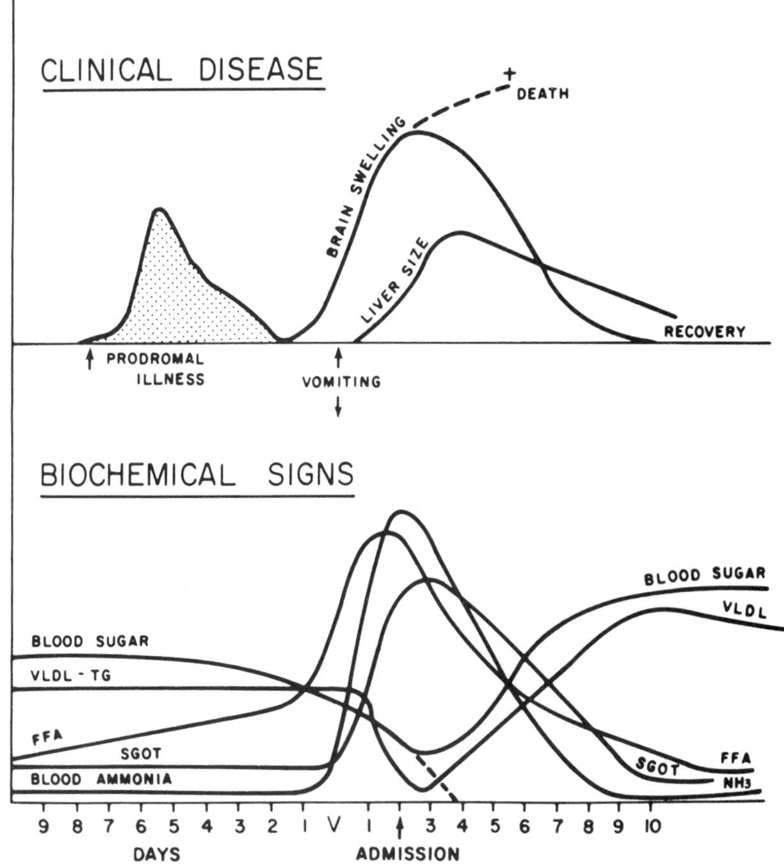

FIGURE 1 Clinical and laboratory findings in Reye's syndrome. (From Partin JC. Hepatic encephalopathy in Reye's syndrome. Pediatr Ann 1977; 6:101–114.)

have normal or mildly to moderately elevated (two to five times normal) ammonia concentrations.[5] With recovery, ammonia concentrations normalize over 2 to 5 days. Admission serum NH_3 may be predictive of disease severity and outcome. Numerous investigators have suggested that an initial serum NH_3 greater than five times normal in comatose subjects predicts death or a poor outcome.[6–8] Noncomatose subjects with serum NH_3 greater than twice normal and a prothrombin time prolonged greater than 3 seconds are likely to progress to deeper coma grades (five of seven cases).[5] The serum glucose may be normal but frequently is reduced in infants and normalizes with intravenous fluid therapy. The serum bilirubin rarely exceeds 1 mg per deciliter at presentation unless superimposed shock is present. The prothrombin time is usually only modestly prolonged (1 to 3 seconds over control), but occasionally significant prolongation (3 to 10 seconds) is present. The serum electrolytes are generally normal except that serum CO_2 may be reduced. The BUN and creatinine may be mildly elevated, indicative of mild dehydration. A mixed metabolic acidosis–respiratory alkalosis may be present in comatose subjects. Typical serum amino acid patterns are observed with elevations of alanine, glutamine, alpha-amino-n-butyrate, and lysine.[9] Marked elevations of serum free fatty acids and reductions in very low density lipoproteins (VLDL) are present. Recently, investigators have identified serum dicarboxylic acids and urinary dicarboxylic acid, including adipic, suberic, and subacic acids, in children with Reye's syndrome.[10,11] Cerebrospinal fluid findings include fewer than eight white blood cells (WBC) per cubic millimeter with normal protein and glucose concentrations. If hypoglycemia is present, hypoglycorrhachia may be present.

Percutaneous liver biopsy confirms the diagnosis of Reye's syndrome. On gross examination the liver is pale or yellow instead of the normal tan or brown color. Liver histology, histochemistry, and ultrastructural pathology are quite specific for Reye's syndrome.[12,13] Examination of the hematoxylin and eosin–stained sections reveals normal or swollen hepatocytes with centrally located nuclei, insignificant inflammation, rare cellular necrosis, and no cholestasis (Fig. 2*A*). Lipid histochemical studies reveal abundant small droplets of fat in hepatocytes in a panlobular distribution (Fig. 2*B*). Histochemical studies of mitochondrial enzymes (succinic acid dehydrogenase) allow demonstration of a variable reduction in enzyme activity in the lobule, with preservation of activity in periportal areas. In contrast, cytosolic enzyme (DPNH) activity is normal. The mitochondrial alterations, which are considered pathognomonic of the disease, include matrix expansion, loss of matrix density and dense bodies, and irregularities of the limiting membrane (Fig. 2*C*). Additional ultrastructural findings include lipid accumulation, glycogen depletion, increased numbers of peroxisomes, and decreased numbers of mitochondria.[14]

Histopathologic alterations are found in additional tissues. Fatty change is found in the collecting ducts of the kidney, heart, pancreas, and muscle. Cerebral edema is manifested by flattened gyri and narrowed sulci. There is no significant inflammatory change in the brain or meninges. Microscopic changes are generally considered secondary to cerebral edema and hypoxic neural injury. Blebs and vesicles are found in myelin sheaths. Astrocyte swelling may be present. Ultrastructural studies of brain biopsies have shown mitochondrial alterations like those found in liver, only in neurons.[15,16]

DIFFERENTIAL DIAGNOSIS

The differential diagnosis of Reye's syndrome is dependent in part upon the age of the patient and the presence or absence of coma. The clinical diagnosis of Reye's syndrome in older subjects can be readily made when multiple criteria are present (based on criteria formulated by the Centers for Disease Control [CDC]) including (1) a prodromal illness, (2) acute onset of persistent vomiting 3 to 7 days after the prodromal illness with or without changes in sensorium, (3) SGOT and SGPT at least three times normal with normal or elevated serum NH_3 but no jaundice, (4) cerebrospinal fluid containing 8 or fewer WBC per cubic millimeter, (5) microvesicular fatty metamorphosis of the liver, and (6) no other reasonable explanation for the illness. The sequence of events in which a prodromal illness is followed by vomiting, serum transaminase elevation, and hyperammonemia with development of agitated delirium and coma is stereospecific for Reye's syndrome. For comatose patients of all ages, meningitis, viral encephalitis, toxin- or drug-induced coma (especially by acetaminophen or salicylate), hypoxic encephalopathy and anoxic liver damage, centrilobular necrosis with shock and encephalopathy, and hepatic failure due to hepatitis must be considered. In most of these circumstances, historic facts and additional laboratory determinations (as indicated by history) can effectively satisfy the practitioner that these conditions are not present.

For the noncomatose patient, the differential diagnosis includes anicteric hepatitis A or B, Epstein-Barr viral hepatitis, cytomegaloviral hepatitis, varicella hepatitis, and drug-induced hepatitis (acetaminophen or salicylate). All of the above conditions can be excluded by appropriate serologies, serum drug levels, and close attention to the history of the antecedent prodromal illness.

Infants less than 1 year of age usually have significant encephalopathy (grade III or IV). Consideration must be given to inborn errors of metabolism. Hypoglycemia or hepatic encephalopathy may prompt medical attention in infants with galactosemia, hereditary fructose intolerance, or even glycogen storage disease; however, serum bilirubin may be elevated in the former two conditions and hepatomegaly is prominent in all. In recent years, a number of conditions have been identified in infants and children initially believed to have recurrent Reye's syndrome. Inborn errors of ureagenesis, including ornithine transcarbamylase (OTC) deficiency and carbamyl phosphate synthetase deficiency, may mimic Reye's syndrome. Affected males with OTC deficiency usually present in the newborn period with extreme hyperammonemia, and Reye's syndrome is not considered. Heterozygote females with OTC deficiency commonly present with recurrent episodes of life-threatening hyperammonemia, orotic aciduria, and characteristically elevated serum glutamine and reduced serum citrulline concentrations. Liver histology may reveal microvesicular fatty change; however, mitochondrial morphology is normal or distinctly different from Reye's syndrome.[17] Multiple defects in fatty acid metabolism may mimic Reye's syndrome. Systemic carnitine deficiency, car-

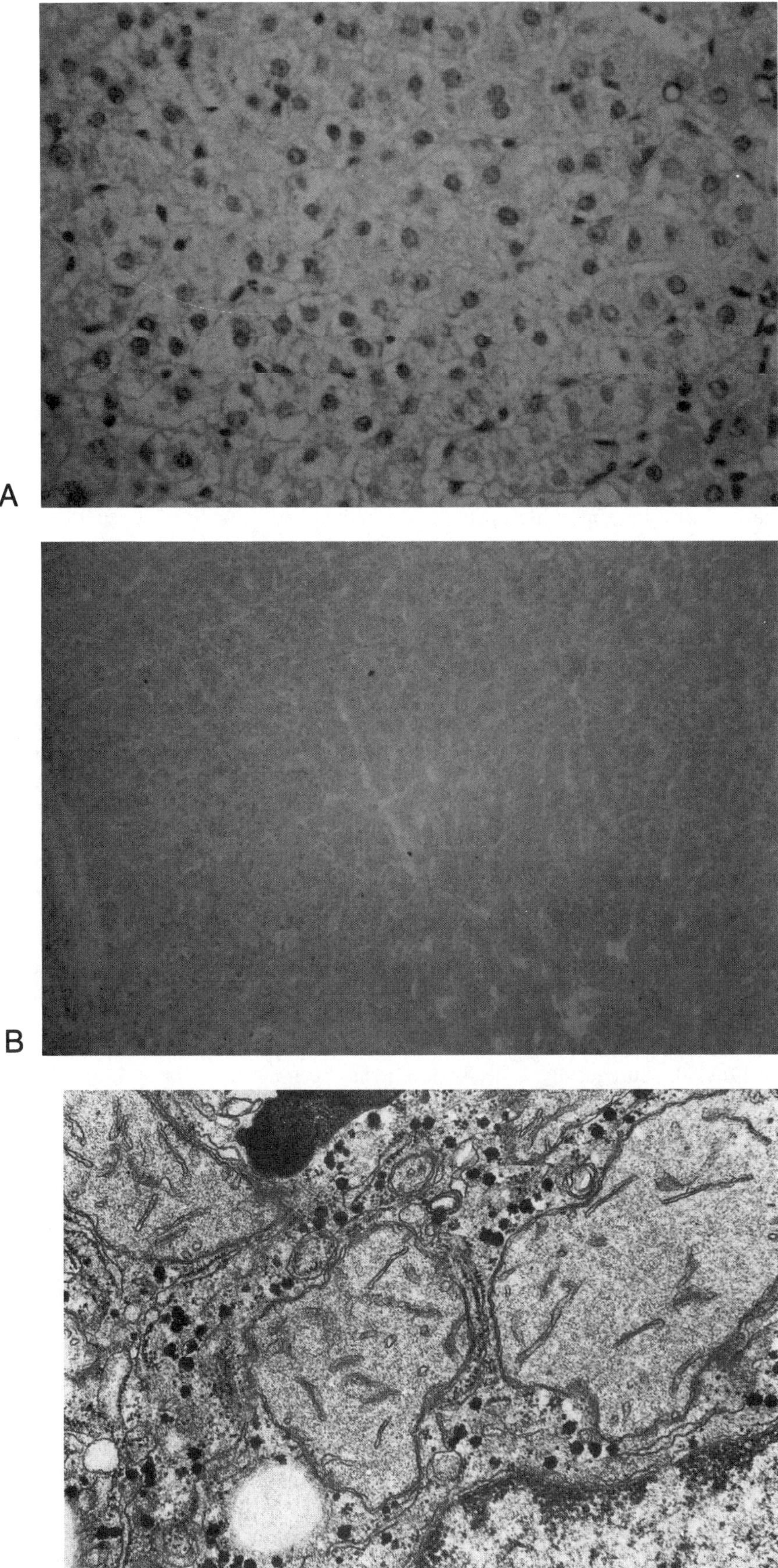

FIGURE 2 Histology, enzyme histochemistry, and ultrastructural pathology of Reye's syndrome. *A*, Hematoxylin and eosin–stained section of a percutaneous liver biopsy showing absence of significant necrosis and cholestasis with mildly increased hepatocyte size and centrally located nuclei. *B*, Sudan IV–stained section of liver biopsy showing small to moderate droplet lipid distributed throughout the lobule with a gradient from central to portal areas. *C*, Electron micrograph showing enlargement and irregularity of mitochondrial membrane with reduction in density of the matrix and loss of dense bodies.

nitine palmitoyl transferase deficiency, and medium-chain and long-chain acyl CoA dehydrogenase deficiencies commonly present with recurrent episodes of lethargy, seizures, coma, and hepatomegaly. Hypoglycemia, mild elevations of serum AST and ALT, hyperammonemia, acidosis, reduced serum carnitine, ketopenia, and dicarboxylic aciduria are common. Liver histology may reveal microvesicular or macrovesicular fatty change with mitochrondrial alterations different from those of Reye's syndrome.[18] Additional organic acidemias, including beta-hydroxy-beta-methylglutaric acidemia and isovaleric acidemia, are phenotypically similar to Reye's syndrome. The recurrent nature of attacks, young age, family history, and disease-specific biochemical perturbations generally suggest metabolic disease rather than Reye's syndrome in these clinical circumstances.

EPIDEMIOLOGY AND DEMOGRAPHY

Reye's syndrome almost exclusively affects infants and children. Few well-documented cases have been reported in adults. Over 10 years of surveillance in Ohio from 1966 to 1976, the median age of affected children was found to be 5 to 6 years.[19] Despite recent reductions in incidence, the median age remains between 5 and 9 years (34 percent of cases from December 1, 1985 to November 30, 1986). Males and females are equally affected. Affected children are predominantly white, and the disease is relatively uncommon in black children. Cases more commonly originate in rural areas, followed by suburban and urban areas. Remarkable regional differences in disease incidence have been found in the United States. Pacific states, Nevada, and most South Atlantic and east south central states tend to have low incidence rates for Reye's syndrome. Several mountain, west north central, and east north central states have high incidence rates.[20] A voluntary surveillance system for Reye's syndrome was begun by the CDC in 1968. Initial yearly incidence rates were between 11 and 83 cases. Between 1974 and 1983, an increase in reporting frequency was observed. In 1978–79 236 cases were reported, and a peak of 555 cases was reported in 1979–80. Subsequently, a steady decline has been noted, with only 91 cases reported in 1984–85 and 101 cases in 1985–86.[21] Over recent years there has been a trend toward diagnosis in earlier coma stages.[22] Nationwide, the incidence of Reye's syndrome has ranged from 0.15 to 0.88 cases per 100,000 children under age 18 years. In a 5-year retrospective study in Ohio from 1973 to 1977, the incidence rate was 2.8 to 4.7 cases per year per 100,000 children less than age 18 years in the absence and presence of influenza B epidemics, respectively.[19] Prospective surveillance in Michigan in 1973–74 resulted in an incidence of 2.4 cases per 100,000 during a 7-month influenza B epidemic.[23] More recently, in a prospective study in Cincinnati in 1980–81, when influenza A was prevalent, the incidence of liver biopsy–proven cases of Reye's syndrome was 3.5 cases per 100,000 population less than 17 years of age.[4] If CDC criteria had been utilized to establish the diagnosis of Reye's syndrome rather than biopsy confirmation, a frequency of 5.6 cases per 100,000 population under age 17 years would have been observed. Noncomatose cases accounted for more than three-fourths of all cases in the Cincinnati study, suggesting that the prevalence of noncomatose cases is likely to be much higher than previously recognized. Despite high community awareness and aggressive surveillance efforts since the year 1980 to 1981, the total number of cases in Cincinnati has continued to decline. This parallels the striking decline in cases noted nationwide. Many authorities have attributed the recent decline in incidence to a decreasing use of aspirin, but proof of a causal relationship between aspirin usage and Reye's syndrome is still lacking (see below). Little information is available on the annual incidence of Reye's syndrome in other countries except the British Isles. From 1981 to 1983, there were 110 cases of Reye's syndrome reported to the Public Health Laboratory Service Communicable Disease Surveillance Center (PHLS CDC). In 1983–1984, approximately 81 cases were reported; thereafter, there were 40 to 50 cases per year during 1984 to 1986 and only 13 cases reported in the first 7 months surveillance in 1986–87 (Susan Hall: personal communication). In a retrospective study based upon cases identified in Australia between 1973 and 1982, Orlowski et al reported a declining incidence of Reye's syndrome.[24] The foregoing information suggests that there may be a global decline in the incidence of Reye's syndrome.

PATHOGENESIS

Despite intensive study of Reye's syndrome since its description in 1963, the pathogenesis of the disease remains poorly defined. As outlined in Figure 3, a proposed schema of the pathogenesis is illustrated that summarizes our knowledge regarding clinical observations and their potential roles in Reye's syndrome. It is evident that a series of cascading events transpires during the course of Reye's syndrome. Two hypotheses are possible: (1) A primary injury to the mitochondria of multiple organs including liver, brain, and muscle produces the multiple observed abnormalities of Reye's syndrome. (2) A primary hepatic injury may lead to the metabolic consequences that produce the biochemical abnormalities and encephalopathy. It seems most likely that these hypotheses are not mutually exclusive, and elements of both may be used to explain the pathogenesis of Reye's syndrome.

Morphologic, morphometric, and biochemical studies have confirmed the presence of structural and functional alterations in mitochondria of patients with Reye's syndrome. Reduced numbers of pleomorphic, enlarged mitochondria with disrupted cristae, electron-lucent matrices and reduced dense bodies are characteristic and pathognomonic of the hepatic pathology of Reye's syndrome.[12,13] Hepatic mitochondrial enzymes involved in ureagenesis, gluconeogenesis, and the citric acid cycle are reduced, whereas enzymes localized to the hepatic cytosol are normal.[25] Indirect evidence of mitochondrial injury derives from the identification of dicarboxylic acids in serum and urine of affected children.[10,11] These organic acids are typically produced if mitochondrial beta-oxidation is compromised or overwhelmed by the influx of fatty acids. As a compensatory mechanism, peroxisomes metabolize fatty acids, but the end products—sebacic (C_{10}), suberic (C_8), and adipic (C_6) acids—are formed because beta-oxidation cannot proceed beyond 6-carbon chain lengths. Morphologic and biochemical study of the brain in

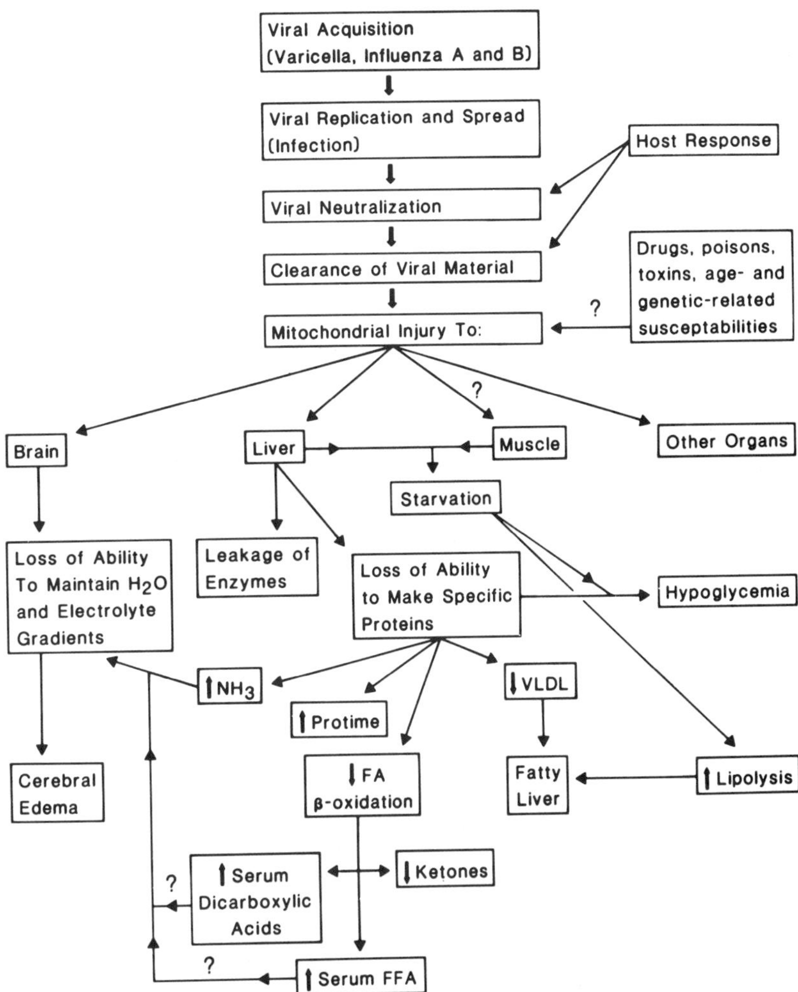

FIGURE 3 Proposed schema of the pathogenesis of Reye's syndrome. Question marks denote areas in which the role of certain factors is currently uncertain but may be of importance in the pathogenesis of the disease. (From Heubi JE. Reye's syndrome: current concepts. Hepatology 1987; 7:155–164; © by Williams & Wilkins.)

Reye's syndrome has been extremely limited, since tissue must be studied while subjects are still alive to yield useful information. Since the end result of Reye's syndrome is cerebral edema and death, postmortem studies do not allow elucidation of the pathogenic changes of the disease in evolution. Studies of brain tissue obtained at the time of decompressive craniectomy have proved helpful, but results must be interpreted with caution, since this tissue was obtained after the child had developed such severe cerebral edema that decortication was required to save the patient's life. From these studies, tissue analysis has revealed astrocytic swelling and myelin blebs. Mitochondrial morphologic alterations have been found only in neurons; however, mitochondrial enzyme activities are not reduced.[15,16,26] Two concurrent mechanisms of cerebral injury may explain the findings. An initial neuron mitochondrial lesion may be followed by astrocyte swelling that may be secondary to hyperammonemia.

Biochemical derangements caused by hepatic injury associated with primary mitochondrial alteration may be significant contributors to the pathogenesis of the disease. Hyperammonemia results from excess nitrogen load secondary to protein catabolism and reductions in the intramitochondrial urea cycle enzymes ornithine transcarbamylase and carbamylphosphate synthetase. Hyperammonemia correlates with severity of ultimate coma grade and death with Reye's syndrome as well as likelihood of progression to deeper coma grades in noncomatose subjects.[5–8] Graded infusions of ammonium acetate lead to progressive alteration in consciousness in young primates related to intracranial hypertension with astrocytic swelling but no neuronal pathology.[27] Infants dying in hyperammonemic coma have astrocytic swelling with cerebral edema, whereas recurrent bouts of hyperammonemia lead to cerebral atrophy in infants. Patients dying of liver failure and portosystemic encephalopathy have gross cerebral edema with swollen astrocytes. Hyperammonemia does not appear to initiate the encephalopathy of Reye's syndrome, since at the onset of emesis (which most authorities believe is the onset of Reye's syndrome), when only lethargy may be present, most patients do not have hyperammonemia.[5] However, hyperammonemia may be an important compounding factor coupled with the primary mitochondrial injury.

The role of fatty acids in the pathogenesis of Reye's syndrome has long been the subject of debate. Excessive lipolysis with impaired hepatic metabolism of the liberated fatty acids is characteristic of all coma grades of Reye's syndrome. Elevated concentrations of serum free fatty acids are present even in mild cases, but the concentrations are not directly proportional to severity of coma grade.[27] Coincident with elevated serum free fatty acids and ketopenia, dicarboxylic acids are found in urine and serum. Infusions of short-chain fatty acids in animals lead to increased intracranial pressure, encephalopathy, and mild elevations of serum ammonia concentrations. Fatty acids of varying chain lengths are capable of uncoupling oxidative phosphorylation and inhibiting beta-oxidation in isolated liver mitochondria. Nonesterified fatty acids can induce mitochondrial swelling in vitro and reduce mitochondrial and cellular transport functions. Dicarboxylic acids of C_6 to C_{10} chain length have been identified in urine, and increased concentrations of other short-chain dicarboxylic acids have been found in the sera of patients with Reye's syndrome. Dicarboxylic acids are commonly encountered in urine from patients with inborn errors of metabolism involving the beta-oxidative pathway. The clinical presentation of these subjects is very similar to that of children with Reye's syndrome, and the pathogenesis of their encephalopathies may have common origins. Whether dicarboxylic acidemia is secondary to mitochondrial dysfunction or is intimately involved in the pathogenesis of Reye's syndrome remains undefined.[28]

Despite considerable debate regarding the role of aspirin in the pathogenesis of Reye's syndrome, its role remains undefined (see below for discussion regarding aspirin and Reye's syndrome). Aspirin usage commonly precedes the onset of Reye's syndrome, and salicylate concentrations are higher on admission in affected children than in community-based controls. No correlation has been found between salicylate concentrations and coma grade.[29] Since children who have died after salicylate intoxication have cerebral edema and hepatic microvesicular fatty change without necrosis, interest in salicylates in the pathogenesis of Reye's syndrome has been generated.[30] Salicylates uncouple mitochondrial respiration, impair ATP formation, and induce mitochondiral swelling. Salicylates and salicyl compounds may potentiate Ca^{2+}-induced damage to the inner mitochondrial membrane. Multiple hypothetical considerations for the role of aspirin in the pathogenesis have been raised, including compromising of mitochondrial function directly by uncoupling oxidative phosphorylation, increasing the CoA load to the mitochondrion for oxidation, and displacing bound fatty acids and dicarboxylic acids from serum albumin.[28] In the animal model of Reye's syndrome developed by Davis et al, Balb/c mice injected with influenza A/Lee virus and given aspirin, the aspirin-treated mice had no increased mortality over the non–aspirin-exposed animals.[31]

Additional factors have been considered in the pathogenesis of Reye's syndrome. These include endotoxin, interferon, and tumor necrosis factor. Their roles in the pathogenesis remain poorly defined. Based upon available evidence, it appears that a primary mitochondrial injury initiates multiple metabolic disturbances. Synergistically, the metabolic perturbations and the underlying mitochondrial injury lead to the pathophysiology. Since no good animal model for Reye's syndrome has been developed despite extensive efforts, many of the proposed hypotheses cannot be tested.

ETIOLOGY

The cause of Reye's syndrome remains unknown despite many years of study. An antecedent viral illness usually precedes the onset of the disease. An upper respiratory illness is part of the prodrome of Reye's syndrome in 60 to 70 percent of cases, while varicella accounts for 20 to 30 percent of the prodromes and diarrheal illnesses account for 5 to 15 percent. Influenza A and B and varicella have been most thoroughly investigated. A temporal relationship has been shown between epidemics of influenza A and B and Reye's syndrome in 1973–74, 1976–77, 1977–78, 1979–80, and 1981–81. Seasonal variations in the incidence of Reye's syndrome associated with varicella have been observed. The disease almost exclusively affects children, but rare adult cases have been described. Siblings are infrequently affected and the study of the role of genetic factors in the disease has largely been unrewarding.

Even in the report of Reye et al, there were suggestions that an environmental toxin might be implicated in the etiology of the disease. However, subsequent investigations have been largely unrewarding. Although a variety of agents including salicylates, valproic acid, the unripe fruit of the Akee tree, margosa oil, chlordane, pyrrolizidine, camphor, methylbromides, and hornet stings may produce conditions phenotypically similar to Reye's syndrome, none has sufficiently similar laboratory, histopathologic, or ultrastructural pathology findings to make them serious candidates as the cause of the disease.

Some agents require specific attention, since a number of investigators have found them to be particularly good candidates as causative agents. Based upon clustering of cases of Reye's syndrome in an area of pesticide spraying in Canada and a history of contact with pesticides among children with Reye's syndrome, a relationship between pesticides and or their emulsifiers was suggested.[32] No studies have shown accumulation of these materials in either the serum or tissues of affected subjects. Animal studies have been performed to evaluate the possible role of emulsifiers in the etiology of Reye's syndrome. When mice were infected with encephalomyocarditis virus and exposed to emulsifiers, hepatic fatty change occurred, minimal alterations in AST were observed, and increased mortality was noted compared with controls. Emulsifier-treated mice infected with influenza B had increased mortality and increased serum NH_3 compared with control groups who were either infected with influenza A or treated with emulsifier alone.[33,34] None of these models produced sufficiently similar changes to those observed with Reye's syndrome to be seriously considered as a model for the disease. Another agent, aflatoxin B, was found in the blood and urine from several children with Reye's syndrome; however, follow-up studies failed to show significant differences between amounts found in affected children and controls.

The relationship between Reye's syndrome and antecedent aspirin exposure has been recognized for years. Results of studies by Linnemann et al in the 1970s indicated that 95 percent of biopsy-proven cases of Reye's syndrome had prior aspirin exposure.[35] A series of case-control studies has increased concern regarding a link between aspirin and Reye's syndrome. In a study of seven children with Reye's syndrome reported in 1980, Starko et al found that a greater proportion of affected children than controls were exposed to aspirin.[36] A two-part study from Michigan reported that 24 of 25 patients with Reye's syndrome received aspirin compared to 34 of 46 controls during 1979–80 whereas 12 of 12 patients with Reye's syndrome received aspirin compared with 13 of 29 controls in 1980–81.[37] Between December 1978, and March, 1980, 97 cases of Reye's syndrome were studied and compared with 156 control subjects in Ohio.[38] Aspirin was ingested by 97 percent of patients with Reye's syndrome compared with 71 percent of controls. A third study conducted by the CDC designed to minimize flaws of previous studies confirmed the findings of the antecedent studies. Twenty-seven cases of Reye's syndrome were identified; aspirin was ingested in 96 percent, compared to 38 percent among 140 controls from four different populations.[39]

Two additional lines of study have suggested a circumstantial relationship between Reye's syndrome and prior aspirin exposure. Patients with connective tissue disease who are chronically treated with aspirin appear to be at increased risk over the general population for development of Reye's syndrome. Secondly, results of surveys from Michigan, Ohio, and Houston and nationwide have shown a decline in aspirin usage among children, which parallels the decline in the reported cases of Reye's syndrome.[40,41] The role of aspirin in the etiology of Reye's syndrome may be questioned on at least two points. The causality of the relationship between the decline in aspirin usage and the incidence of Reye's syndrome in the United States has been recently questioned because of studies from Australia. On that continent, the disease has largely disappeared in the face of long-term usage of paracetamol (acetaminophen) in preference to aspirin.[25] Secondly, in an animal model recently developed by Davis et al that closely mimics Reye's syndrome, mortality of affected animals is not increased by aspirin exposure with concentrations as high as 68 mg per deciliter.[31]

TREATMENT

Early recognition, before the development of serious neurologic signs, and treatment with an intravenous glucose-electrolyte solution results in a better outcome than any other treatment currently available for Reye's syndrome. All physicians and nursing personnel (especially in emergency rooms, clinics, and private offices) should be familiar with the cardinal presenting symptoms of Reye's syndrome. Public awareness programs have also been highly effective in enhancing parental awareness and have improved efforts to identify early (noncomatose) cases. In any child with varicella who repeatedly vomits or any child who begins vomiting after recovery from an acute respiratory illness, Reye's syndrome should be suspected and a physical examination and measurement of SGOT or SGPT should be performed. If the SGOT or SGPT is elevated greater than three times normal with or without neurologic symptoms, the child should be hospitalized for careful observation and treatment with intravenous fluids containing 10 percent glucose, 40 to 60 mEq per square meter per day, of sodium, and 40 to 60 mEq per square meter per day of potassium at a rate of 1,500 to 1,800 cc per square meter per day. Appropriate additional laboratory studies should be obtained including serum bilirubin, prothrombin time, plasma ammonia, blood glucose, electrolytes, blood urea nitrogen, serum salicylate, and serum and urine analyses for both metabolic and toxic screens. Appropriate serologies should be obtained to exclude hepatitis A or B, Epstein-Barr virus, and cytomegalovirus. The need to perform a lumbar puncture should be determined by the managing physician. The necessity of a liver biopsy to establish the diagnosis of Reye's syndrome in noncomatose patients is difficult to determine with certainty. The risk of liver biopsy (approximately 1 per 100 for significant bleeding) may be greater than the derived benefit from the procedure, since most noncomatose patients recover uneventfully with intravenous glucose-electrolyte solutions and observation. If the plasma ammonia is not greater than 2 1/2 times normal and the prothrombin times is prolonged no more than 3 seconds, the patient has only a 5 percent likelihood of progression to deeper coma grades.[5] Usually within 48 to 96 hours, the vomiting subsides, the appetite returns and the child may be discharged from the hospital.

If the child is comatose (greater than grade II coma), a lumbar puncture with examination of the cerebrospinal fluid is mandatory to exclude infection. All comatose patients should be hospitalized in an intensive care setting in which there is 24-hour nursing care available. It is highly preferable to have in-house medical staff available on a 24-hour basis. Intravenous fluids should be administered using 10 percent glucose-electrolyte solutions at a rate of 1,200 to 1,500 cc per square meter per day. Urine output, specific gravity, and Clinitest level should be monitored using an indwelling Foley catheter. Parenteral vitamin K (5 mg) should be given and a percutaneous liver biopsy performed to confirm the diagnosis of Reye's syndrome. Early elective endotracheal intubation is wide in most cases. Administration of paralyzing agents such as Pavulon may be necessary to allow effective ventilation. It is desirable to keep the pCO_2 between 20 and 25 mm Hg. Mechanical ventilation is indicated as coma depth increases and when agents such as barbiturates are considered in the management. All comatose patients should have an intracranial pressure (ICP) monitoring device inserted. Multiple devices are available, including intraventricular cannulae, Richmond bolts, and epidural transducers. The device to be used depends upon the neurosurgical consultant's preference. It is also wise to obtain a continuous measurement of mean arterial pressure (MAP) through an arterial line. By simultaneously measuring the intracranial pressure and mean arterial pressure, one can ensure an adequate cerebral perfusion pressure (CPP). CPP (MAP−ICP) should optimally exceed 50 to 60 mm Hg. To optimize CPP, the environment should be quiet and the head of the bed raised 30 degrees. A cooling blanket should be used if necessary to maintain normothermia. Hypothermia has not been shown to be of any benefit. Maintenance of the P_{CO_2} between 20 and 25 mm Hg with the aid of mechanical ventilation and paralyzing agents is useful. Cerebral dehydrating agents are useful on a short-term basis. Glycerol, urea, and mannitol have been used. Most centers prefer mannitol in doses of 0.25 to 1.0 gm per kilogram every 4 to 6 hours. Dexamethasone has not been useful for management of cerebral edema in Reye's syndrome.[42] If the patient still has uncontrollable intracranial hypertension despite the foregoing measures, barbiturate therapy should be considered. Initial loading with 3 to 5 mg per kilogram of pentobarbital is recommended with subsequent hourly doses of 1 to 3 mg per kilogram to maintain a serum pentobarbital level at 2.5 to 4.0 mg per deciliter.[4] It is essential that serum levels be monitored carefully because systemic hypotension is exceedingly common with the dosages usually employed. If the mean arterial pressure declines so that cerebral perfusion is compromised or the serum barbiturate level exceeds 4.0 mg per deciliter, doses should be withheld. After achievement of good control of ICP, pentobarbital can be weaned after 24 hours of stable measurements with rapid return of normal neurologic function in children without residual effects and slower recovery in those with permanent neurologic impairment. The overwhelming majority of patients are managed successfully with the techniques described; however, in a very small percentage of patients cerebral perfusion is still compromised despite the clinician's best efforts. In the situation in which all other modes of therapy have failed, decompressive craniectomy may be lifesaving.[44] No specific guidelines for patient selection can be offered, and permanent neurologic sequelae are likely to be frequent, since this therapy is necessitated when it is realized that the patient has already sustained a period of cerebral hypoperfusion during the time period when the clinician has attempted more conventional forms of therapy. Most of these children require long periods to recover to a stable neurologic condition with attendant needs for rehabilitation.

Additional treatment modalities have been used including exchange transfusion, peritoneal dialysis, total body washout, and carnitine administration. None has proven value over the supportive techniques described above.[42]

Hepatic enzymes (SGOT, SGPT) generally normalize within 2 weeks of the onset of Reye's syndrome. If a liver biopsy is not performed, hepatic enzyme measurements should be repeated until they are normal. No biochemical measures obtained during the course of hospitalization are particularly helpful in determining short-term or long-term prognosis. If patients have persistent neurologic dysfunction, prolonged rehabilitation may be necessary. These usually include occupational and physical therapy and remedial educational programs.

OUTCOME

The nationwide case fatality rates for Reye's syndrome reported to the CDC from 1974 to 1986 have varied from 26 to 42 percent.[21] Case fatality rates are directly related to the admitting coma grade and the highest grade of coma attained during the course of the illness. In recent years with the use of barbiturate coma, it has been more difficult to assess maximum depth of coma, but all subjects placed in drug-induced coma are grade III or greater. At selected centers with many cases of Reye's syndrome, results are superior to those reported by the CDC. One such example is Cincinnati. Since 1969, more than 280 cases have been treated with an overall mortality of 7 percent and significant neurologic sequelae in 3 percent. No patients with Reye's syndrome admitted with grade I or II coma have died, and few have had any neurologic residual. A progressive decline in survival has been observed with patients in coma grades III to V on admission, 25 percent of whom have died. Only 7 percent of patients admitted with grade III coma died, whereas 28 percent in grade IV and 100 percent in grade V coma on admission died.[45] Follow-up neuropsychologic examinations in survivors have suggested that survivors admitted in coma grade III and IV may have a variety of sequelae ranging from obvious psychomotor retardation with neurologic deficits to more subtle perceptual abnormalities. These deficits appear to be correlated with duration of coma and peak depth of coma. Additional clinical observations have suggested that prognosis in terms of both mortality and neuropsychologic impairment is considerably worse for infants less than 1 year of age than for older subjects. No deficits have been observed in children admitted in coma grades I and II.[46]

REFERENCES

1. Reye RDK, Morgan G, Baral J. Encephalopathy and fatty degeneration of the viscera: a disease entity in childhood. Lancet 1963; ii:749–752.
2. Johnson GM, Scurletis TD, Carroll NB. A study of sixteen fatal cases of encephalitis-like disease in North Carolina children. NC Med J 1963; 24:464–473.
3. Bobo RC, Schubert WK, Partin JC, et al. Reye syndrome: treatment by exchange transfusion with special reference to the 1974 epidemic in Cincinnati, Ohio. J Pediatr 1975; 87:881–886.
4. Lichtenstein PK, Heubi JE, Daugherty CC, et al. Grade I Reye's syndrome: a frequent cause of vomiting and liver dysfunction after varicella and upper-respiratory-tract infection. N Engl J Med 1983; 309:133–139.
5. Heubi JE, Daugherty CC, Partin JS, et al. Grade I Reye's syndrome—outcome and predictors of progression to deeper coma grades. N Engl J Med 1984; 311:1539–1542.
6. Roe CR, Schonberger LB, Gelbach SH, et al. Enzymatic alterations in Reye's syndrome: prognostic implications. Pediatrics 1975; 55:119–126.
7. Huttenlocher PR. Reye's syndrome: relationship of outcome to therapy. J Pediatr 1972; 80:845–850.
8. Fitzgerald JF, Clark JH, Angelides AG, et al. The prognostic significance of peak ammonia levels in Reye syndrome. Pediatrics 1982; 70:997–1000.
9. Hilty MD, Romshe CA, Delamater PV. Reye's syndrome and hyperaminoacidemia. J Pediatr 1974; 84:362–365.
10. Tonsgard JH. Urinary dicarboxylic acids in Reye syndrome. J Pediatr 1985; 107:79–84.
11. Tonsgard JH. Serum dicarboxylic acids in patients with Reye syndrome. J Pediatr 1986; 109:440–445.
12. Bove KE, McAdams AJ, Partin JC, et al. The hepatic lesion in Reye's syndrome. Gastroenterology 1975; 69:685–697.
13. Partin JC, Schubert WK, Partin JS. Mitochondrial ultrastructure in Reye's syndrome (encephalopathy and fatty degeneration of the viscera). N Engl J Med 1971; 285:1339–1343.
14. Daugherty CC, Gartside PS, Heubi JE, et al. A morphometric study of Reye's syndrome. Correlation of reduced mitochondrial numbers and increased mitochondrial size with clinical manifestations. Am J Pathol 1987; 129:313–326.
15. Partin JC, Partin JS, Schubert WK, et al. Brain ultrastructure in Reye's syndrome (encephalopathy and fatty alteration of the viscera). J Neuropathol Exp Neurol 1975; 34:425–444.
16. Partin JS, McAdams AJ, Partin JC, et al. Brain ultrastructure in Reye's syndrome II. J Neuropathol Exp Neurol 1978; 37:796–819.
17. Zimmerman A, Bachmann C, Colombo J-P. Ultrastructural pathology in congenital defects of the urea cycle: ornithine transcarbamylase and carbamyl phosphate synthetase deficiency. Virchows Arch [B] 1981; 393:321–331.
18. Treem WR, Witzleben CA, Piccoli DA, et al. Medium-chain and long-chain Acyl CoA dehydrogenase deficiency: clinical, pathologic and ultrastructural differentiation from Reye's syndrome. Hepatology 1986; 6:1270–1278.
19. Sullivan-Bolyai JZ, Marks JS, Johnson D, et al. Reye's syndrome in Ohio, 1973–77. Am J Epidem 1980; 112:629–638.
20. Sullivan-Bolyai JZ, Corey L. Epidemiology of Reye syndrome. Epidemiol Rev 1981; 3:1–26.
21. Centers for Disease Control. MMWR 1987; 36:689–691.
22. Hurwitz ES, Nelson DB, David C, et al. National surveillance for Reye syndrome: a five-year review. Pediatrics 1982; 70:895–900.

23. Corey L, Rubin RJ, Thompson TR, et al. Influenza B-associated Reye's syndrome: incidence in Michigan and potential for prevention. J Infect Dis 1977; 135:398–407.
24. Orlowski JP, Gillis J, Kilham HA. A catch in the Reye. Pediatrics 1987; 80:638–642.
25. Brown RE, Forman DT. The biochemistry of Reye's syndrome. Crit Rev Clin Lab Sci 1982; 17:247–297.
26. Robinson BH, Taylor J, Cutz E, et al. Reye's syndrome: preservation of mitochondrial enzymes in brain and muscle compared with liver. Pediatr Res 1978; 12:1045–1047.
27. Voorhies TM, Ehrlich ME, Duffy TE, et al. Acute hyperammonemia in the young primate: physiologic and neuropathologic correlates. Pediatr Res 1983; 17:970–975.
28. Heubi JE, Partin JC, Partin JS, Schubert WK. Reye's syndrome: current concepts. Hepatology 1987; 7:155–164.
29. Partin JS, Schubert WK, Partin JC, et al. Serum salicylate concentrations in Reye's syndrome. A study of 130 biopsy-proven cases. Lancet 1982; i:191–194.
30. Starko KM, Mullick FG. Hepatic and cerebral pathology findings in children with fatal salicylate intoxication: further evidence for a causal relation between salicylate and Reye's syndrome. Lancet 1983; 1:326–329.
31. Davis LE, Green CL, Wallace JM. Influenza B virus model of Reye's syndrome in mice. Ann Neurol 1985; 18:556–559.
32. Crocker JFS, Ozere RL. The incidence and etiology of Reye's syndrome in Eastern Canada. In: Crocker JFS, ed. Reye's syndrome II. New York: Grune and Stratton, 1979: 3.
33. Crocker JFS, Rozee KR, Ozere RL, et al. Insecticide and viral interaction as a cause of fatty visceral changes and encephalopathy in the mouse. Lancet 1974; ii:22–24.
34. Crocker JFS, Renton KW, Lee SH, et al. Biochemical and morphological characteristics of a mouse model of Reye's syndrome induced by the interaction of influenza B virus and a chemical emulsifier. Lab Invest 1986; 54:32–40.
35. Linnemann CC Jr, Shea L, Partin JC, et al. Reye's syndrome: epidemiologic and viral studies, 1963–1974. Am J Epidemiol 1975; 101:517–526.
36. Starko KM, Ray CG, Dominquez LB, et al. Reye's syndrome and salicylate use. Pediatrics 1980; 66:859–864.
37. Waldman RJ, Hall WN, McGee H, et al. Aspirin as a risk factor in Reye's syndrome. JAMA 1982; 247:3089–3094.
38. Halpin TJ, Holtzhauer FJ, Campbell RJ, et al. Reye's syndrome and medication use. JAMA 1982; 248:687–691.
39. Hurwitz ES, Barrett MJ, Bregman D, et al. Public Health Service study of Reye's syndrome and medications. JAMA 1987; 257:1905–1911.
40. Remington PL, Rowley D, McGee H, et al. Decreasing trends in Reye syndrome and aspirin use in Michigan, 1979 to 1984. Pediatrics 1986; 77:93–98.
41. Arrowsmith JB, Kennedy DL, Kuritsky JN, Faich GA. National patterns of aspirin use and Reye syndrome reporting, United States, 1980 to 1985. Pediatrics 1987; 79:858–863.
42. DeVivo DC. Reye syndrome. Neurol Clin North Am 1985; 3:95–115.
43. Marshall LF, Shapiro HM, Rauscher A, Kaufman NM. Pentobarbital therapy for intracranial hypertension in metabolic coma. Crit Care Med 1978; 6:1–5.
44. Shaywitz BA, Lister G, Duncan CC. What is the best treatment for Reye's syndrome? Arch Neurol 1986; 43:730–731.
45. Heubi JE. The changing face of Reye's syndrome in Cincinnati. In: Pollack JD, ed. Reye's syndrome IV. Bryan OH: National Reye's Syndrome Foundation, 1984: 60.
46. Brunner RL, O'Grady DJ, Partin JC, Schubert WK. Neuropsychological consequences of Reye's syndrome. J Pediatr 1979; 95:706–711.

PART 19

Neonatal Iron Storage Disease

David A. Piccoli, M.D.
Camillus L. Witzleben, M.D.
John B. Watkins, M.D.

Goldfischer et al described two cases of severe neonatal liver disease associated with prominent stainable iron in the parenchymal cells of a number of visceral organs and reviewed 10 similar previously reported cases.[1] Several reports of similar cases have subsequently appeared, and more than 50 cases have been described.[2-8] The clinicopathologic picture is now referred to as perinatal hemochromatosis, or neonatal iron storage disease. Since large stainable iron stores can be found in the liver in some infants with no liver disease,[8] it is important to emphasize that, by definition, in neonatal iron storage disease, (1) iron is stored in *multiple* organs and (2) there is severe liver disease present at or shortly after birth. It must also be kept in mind that since the designation is based on a phenotype of unknown etiology, more than one disease may actually be included under this name.[8] No biochemical defect has been identified, and the diagnosis is made on the basis of the phenotype.

PATHOLOGY AND PATHOGENESIS

The characteristic hepatic histopathology includes, in addition to the stainable iron in hepatocytes, diffuse fibrosis with loss of normal architecture and prominent proliferation of bile duct elements. Hepatocyte giant cell transformation may be prominent. Central vein alterations have been said to be characteristic.[9]

No consistent lesions other than excessive iron stores are found in other viscera. The excess stainable iron may be present in only a few or in many organs.[8,10] Pancreas, heart, and thyroid are perhaps most commonly involved, but virtually all viscera except lymph nodes and spleen have shown such storage.

The significance of the stored iron is unclear. It may play a pathogenetic role in the liver disease, it may be an indirect biochemical marker, it may reflect the time of onset and the severity of the liver disease, or it may represent some combination of these possibilities. Attempts to remove the iron stores have not been beneficial.[5]

Fetoplacental iron uptake is marked in the third trimester of gestation in normal human infants,[11] and iron is transported against a concentration gradient. The regulation of the iron transport is modulated by fetal, placental, and maternal factors.[12] In several reported cases of neonatal iron storage disease, there have been antemortem elevations of transferrin saturation and ferritin.[5,6,13] However, in vitro studies of ferritin or transferrin receptor synthesis in fibroblasts of patients have revealed no abnormality. There has been no consistent pattern of abnormality in iron storage or metabolism in the parents of affected patients, although in one family there was increased hepatocellular ferritin in a child who died,[2] and the mother and a sibling had increased serum transferrin and undetectable ferritin. In another family, the father of two affected infants was found to have HLA-A3–associated adult-onset hemochromatosis.[13]

Any discussion of the pathogenesis of neonatal iron storage disease must recognize that in the absence of a known etiology or consistent biochemical defect, it is possible that the observed clinicopathologic picture is the end stage of more than one disorder, i.e., that neonatal iron storage disease may in fact be the end result of more than one disease.[8]

GENETICS AND INHERITANCE

Many cases are sporadic, but the majority of series have reported some sibling pairs with the phenotype of perinatal hemochromatosis, and an autosomal recessive mode of inheritance has been postulated.[1,5,8] In other pedigrees an autosomal co-dominant inheritance has been postulated.[7] However, one report of three affected siblings from two fathers suggested an autosomal dominant inheritance,[2] in which both mother and one surviving child have undetectable ferritin and increased serum transferrin. As noted, in one family the father of two infants who died with the phenotype had HLA-A3–associated primary adult-onset hemochromatosis.[12]

CLINICAL MANIFESTATIONS

The clinical picture is characterized by severe progressive hepatic insufficiency, which may be evident in utero. Hepatic damage may occur at as early as 16 weeks' gestation.[6] Severe fetal hepatic dysfunction is suggested by intrauterine hydrops evident on fetal ultrasonography, and by the large number of stillborn infants seen in the late second trimester and beyond. Intrauterine growth retardation and premature birth are common.[7] A number of these children are born with anemia and non–immune-mediated hydrops. Since both hepatic disease and hepatic iron deposition can occur in other disorders, the diagnosis can be made only in the absence of hemolysis, chronic transfusions, and syndromes associated with hemosiderosis.

The affected infants have a coagulopathy and hypoalbuminemia in addition to edema or anasarca. Some patients also have respiratory and renal insufficiency. Disseminated intravascular coagulation (DIC) is uncommon, and both the fibrinogen and the fibrin split products are low. Analysis of the vitamin K–dependent clotting factors demonstrates the hepatic synthetic defect, with relatively normal levels of Factor VIII (unless DIC or sepsis has ensued), and the coagulopathy is refractory to vitamin K therapy. Local bleeding (e.g., cephalhematoma or marked intrapartum ecchymoses) or gastrointestinal bleeding from either a mucosal or variceal source may occur.

Conjugated hyperbilirubinemia may be present early and is typically progressive. The magnitude is frequently greater than that seen in biliary atresia and derives from defects in conjugation and excretion, as well as from the increased load of tissue hemoglobin seen in bruised infants. Transaminase elevation may be minimal (owing to the decreased mass of viable hepatocytes). Hepatosplenomegaly and portal hypertension may be present, with associated hypersplenism.

Respiratory distress and renal failure are secondary to the decrease in perfusion and oncotic pressure. In one case, intrinsic renal disease with microscopic renal cysts has been reported.[5] Serous effusions and ascites may be present.

The differential diagnosis in a newborn with significant hepatic dysfunction includes common viral infections such as cytomegalovirus, herpesvirus, echovirus, coxsackievirus, adenovirus, and hepatitis B. Bacterial sepsis, syphilis, and toxoplasmosis must be considered. Specific testing should be performed for galactosemia, hereditary fructose intolerance, hereditary tyrosinemia, alpha$_1$-antitrypsin deficiency, and cystic fibrosis. Urine and serum organic acids should be analyzed for defects of intermediary metabolism. A family history of other idiopathic stillborn or neonatal deaths suggests an inherited disorder of some type, and a careful review of the medical records, including autopsies, may suggest this specific diagnosis.

The majority of infants with perinatal hemochromatosis die in the first days or weeks of life, but a few rare survivors have been identified.[2,14] It has been common for the diagnosis to be first made at the autopsy of the first affected child.

DIAGNOSIS

If the diagnosis is suspected on the basis of historical, clinical, and/or laboratory criteria, transferrin saturation and ferritin levels should be determined. A liver biopsy may be difficult to perform in infants with perinatal hemochromatosis owing to the relative complications of a coagulopathy, thrombocytopenia, and ascites. When done, histologic examination typically shows marked loss of hepatocytes, fibrosis, loss of architecture, bile ductule increase, and significant iron accumulation. Hepatocyte giant cell transformation may or may not be present. Such severe subacute and chronic liver disease, although nonspecific, is only rarely seen in the neonate with more clearly defined diseases.[8]

The demonstration of increased iron stores in other organs is very important in diagnosing perinatal hemochromatosis. Evidence of increased iron stores can be obtained through a magnetic resonance scan of the abdomen. Histologic evaluation and iron staining of the minor salivary glands on the lower lip may provide information about extrahepatic iron storage.[15]

So far as we are aware, prenatal diagnosis has not yet been satisfactorily performed, although information that might facilitate this is potentially available through in utero magnetic resonance imaging or in utero venous umbilical cord blood sampling. The disorder should be suspected when hydrops is detected by fetal ultrasonography in the absence of hemolytic anemia. Genetic counseling is important prior to the initiation of subsequent pregnancies.

PROGNOSIS

Perinatal hemochromatosis is usually fatal. Few well-documented survivals have been reported.[2,14] Postnatal chelation therapy has not altered the outcome of the disease.[5,13] Attempts to deplete maternal iron or deliver the infant early have not proved successful. Several infants have been successfully transplanted with good outcome.[16] In considering prognosis and genetic counseling, it must be emphasized that in the absence of a specific biochemical marker, it is possible that the phenotype represents the end stage of a number of different disorders.[8]

REFERENCES

1. Goldfischer S, Grotsky HW, Chang CH, Berman EL, Richert RR, Karmarkar SD, Roskamp JO, Morecki R. Idiopathic neonatal iron storage involving the liver, pancreas, heart, and endocrine and exocrine glands. Hepatology 1981; 1:58–64.
2. Jacknow G, Johnson D, Freese D, Smith C, Burke B. Idiopathic neonatal iron storage disease. Lab Invest 1983; 48:7P.
3. Kurnetz R, Yang SS, Holmes R, Harrison DD. Neonatal jaundice and coagulopathy. J Pediatr 1985; 107:982–987.
4. Blisard KS, Bartow SA. Neonatal hemochromatosis. Hum Pathol 1986; 17:376–383.
5. Jonas MM, Kaweblum YA, Fojaco R. Neonatal hemochromatosis: failure of deferoxamine therapy. J Pediatr Gastroenterol Nutr 1987; 6:984–988.
6. Silver MM, Beverley DW, Valberg LS, Cutz E, Phillips MJ, Shaheed WA. Perinatal hemochromatosis. Clinical, morphologic, and quantitative iron studies. Am J Pathol 1987; 128:538–554.
7. Knisely AS, Magid MS, Dische MR, Cutz E. Neonatal hemochromatosis. Birth Defects 1987; 23:75–102.
8. Witzleben CL, Uri A. Perinatal hemochromatosis: entity or end result? Hum Pathol 1989; 20:335–340.
9. Knisely AS, O'Shea PA, Mroczek E, Taylor S. Distinctive features of hepatic pathology in 20 cases of neonatal hemochromatosis. Lab Invest 1988; 58:49A.
10. Witzleben CL, Uri AK. Neonatal hemochromatosis. (Letter) Am J Gastroenterol 1988; 83:1429.
11. Pribilla W, Bothwell TH, Finch CA. Iron transport to the fetus in man. In: Wallerstein RO, Mettier SR, eds. Iron in clinical medicine. Berkeley: University of California Press; 1958: 58.
12. Okuyamo T, Tawada T, Furuya H, Villee CA. The role of transferrin and ferritin in the fetal-maternal-placental unit. Am J Obstet Gynecol 1985; 152:344–350.
13. Glista BA, Bautista A, Prudencio M, Desposito F. Neonatal iron storage disease. (Abstract) Pediatr Res 1986; 20:410A.
14. Colletti RB, Clemmons JJ. Familial neonatal hemochromatosis with survival. J Pediatr Gastroenterol Nutr 1988; 7:39–45.
15. Knisely AS, O'Shea PA, Stocks JF, Dimmick JE. Oropharyngeal and upper respiratory tract mucosal-gland siderosis in neonatal hemochromatosis: an approach to biopsy diagnosis. J Pediatr 1988; 113:871–874.
16. Esquivel CO, Marino IR, Fioravanti V, Van Thiel DH. Liver transplantation for metabolic disease of the liver. Gastroenterol Clin of North Am 1988; 17:167–175.

PART 20

Cholestasis Associated with Parenteral Nutrition

Richard H. Sandler, M.D.
Ronald E. Kleinman, M.D.

In 1971 Peden et al first noted the association of cholestatic liver disease and parenteral nutrition (PN) in a preterm infant.[1] Since then many reports have confirmed an association between PN and liver disease in both children[2-7] and adults,[8-10] although whether this is a causal relationship remains controversial.[11-13] After catheter-related complications, cholestatic liver disease is now the second most common reason for premature discontinuation of PN in infants and children.[14] The incidence of PN-associated cholestasis (PNAC) varies widely depending upon the clinical circumstances, with estimates ranging from 7 to 57 percent.[8,15-18] Possible reasons for the variations in reported incidence rates include differences in sample size, diagnostic criteria, patient age, concurrent enteral feeding practices, underlying disease, and the composition of PN solutions. The peak prevalence occurs in ill premature infants on PN for extended periods of time (Fig. 1).

PATHOGENESIS

Patients on PN often have underlying conditions that cause or are associated with liver and biliary tract disease, so it is difficult to ascertain the degree to which PN itself is an independent risk factor for PNAC. In fact, no single etiology has been shown responsible for PNAC. Although possible causes including toxicity or deficiency of components of PN solutions have been proposed, associations have also been

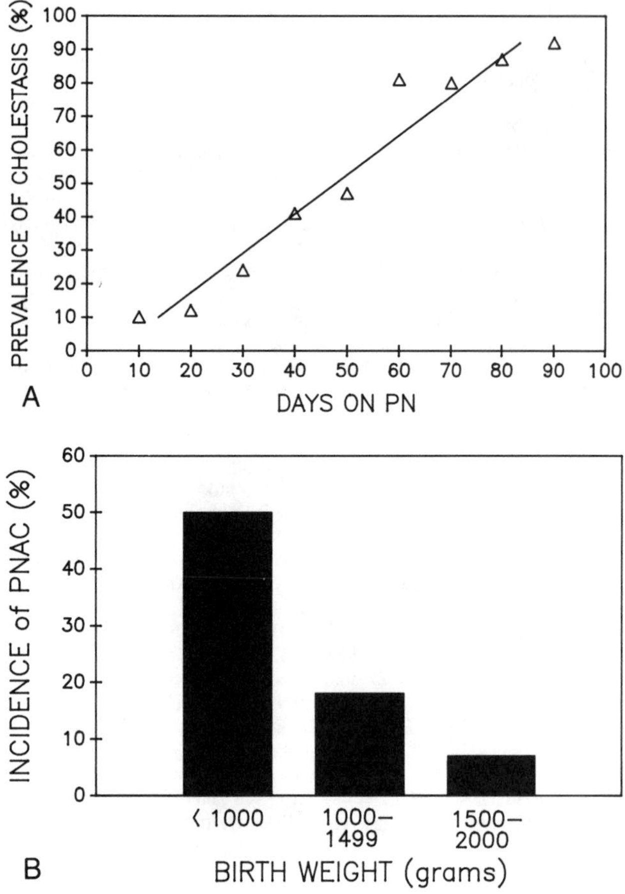

FIGURE 1 Prevalence of parenteral nutrition–associated cholestasis (PNAC). *A*, Prevalence of cholestasis in 62 premature infants on parenteral nutrition (PN), showing a direct relationship between prevalence and number of days on PN in this study population. *B*, Cholestasis incidence in 62 premature infants on PN, demonstrating an inverse relationship to birth weight. (Data from Beale et al.[15])

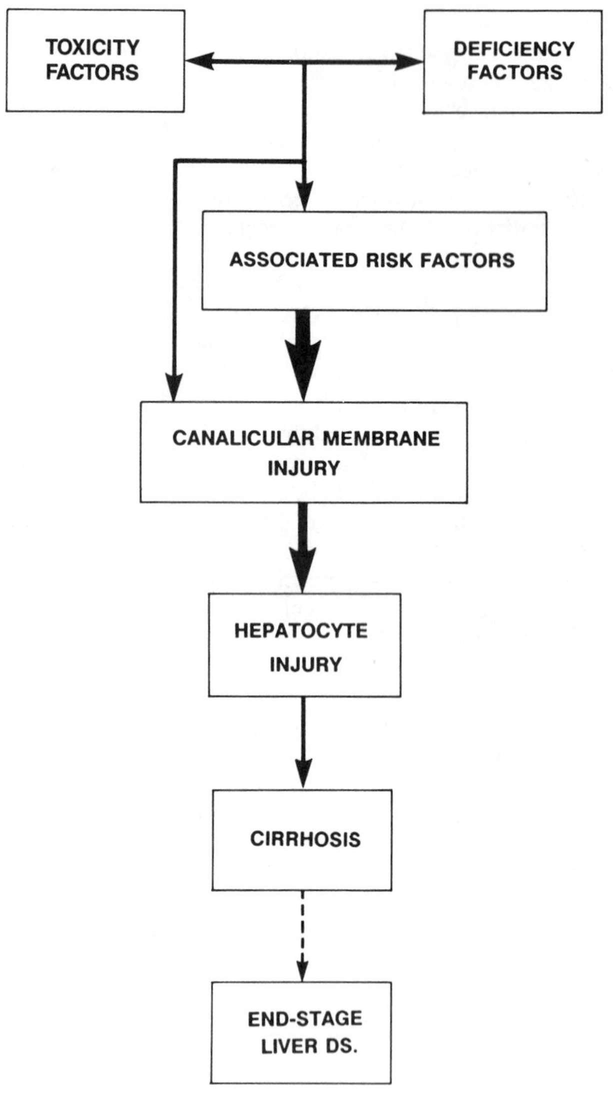

FIGURE 2 Pathogenesis of PNAC.

noted with prematurity, lack of enteral feeding, infections, surgery, and other clinical conditions (Fig. 2).

TOXICITY OF PARENTERAL NUTRITION COMPONENTS

Carbohydrates and Energy Load

Glucose infusions have been shown to decrease bile flow in animals,[19-21] and hepatic dysfunction has been associated with infusion of excessive calories in adults[22-26] and infants.[8,16,27] The source of calories (carbohydrate versus fat) does not seem to make a difference.

Amino Acids

Direct infusion of amino acids may lead to hyperaminoacidemia[28] and hyperaminoaciduria.[29] Animal studies have demonstrated a cholestatic effect of amino acids in vivo[19] and in vitro.[30-32] Similar findings have been reported in human studies.[16,23,33-36] Human infants receiving 3.6 gm per kilogram per day of protein (versus 2.3 gm per kilogram per day) showed an earlier rise and higher peak direct bilirubin levels, but the incidence of PNAC was similar in both groups of infants.[16]

Individual amino acids may also be hepatotoxic. Tryptophan[37] and methionine-cycloleucine,[38] have been associated with decreased bile flow. Alanine may cause decreased taurocholate uptake as demonstrated in isolated hepatocytes, perhaps leading to decreased taurine and increased glycine bile acid conjugation.[31] The latter may result in a higher risk of cholestasis (as discussed below under Amino Acids). Several enzymatic pathways of amino acid metabolism have not matured in the low birth weight infant, including those of phenylalanine, threonine, and the sulfur-containing amino acids methionine and cysteine.[39] Because the components of most commercially available amino acid solutions have been developed for adults, their use in premature infants and young neonates may provoke metabolic dysfunction.

Excess homocystine has been shown to cause hepatocellular damage with iron deposition in rat hepatocytes and Kupffer cells,[40] while increased cystine (dicysteine) may lead to cholestasis and histologic changes of PNAC including periportal necrosis, bile duct proliferation, portal fibrosis, and triaditis.[41] Necrosis and cirrhosis of the rat liver from cystine have also been documented.[42] Methionine has been shown to cause hepatocellular injury in neonatal rats,[43,44] an effect that may be preventable with arginine and glycine supplementation.[45] Elevated serum levels of methionine have been documented in infants on PN, perhaps resulting from blockage of the trans-sulfuration pathway, increased production by remethylation of homocystine, or impairment of the final oxidation of sulfur-containing amino acids.[46,47] Finally, tryptophan and (to a lesser extent tyrosine) photo-oxidation products are hepatotoxic,[48–50] and this effect may be facilitated by riboflavin.[50,51] Merritt et al performed intraperitoneal injections of different amino acids for 1 week to weanling and suckling rat pups.[48] Cholestatic changes (as suggested by the serum cholyglycine level) were only seen in pups under 12 days old. Cholestasis was dependent on the tryptophan dose, was not seen with other amino acids, and was reduced when the amino acid solutions were protected from light.

Lipids

Impaired bilirubin excretion has been noted in adults receiving high doses of intravenous lipids.[52,53] Lipofuscin, a Kupffer cell pigment, has been associated with intravenous lipid and may be partially responsible for the Kupffer cell hyperplasia seen in many infants with PNAC.[54,55] Cottonseed oil–containing lipid emulsions were associated with cholestasis and severe hepatic injury.[56–58] However, currently available lipid emulsions do not contain cottonseed oil and have not been associated with PNAC when 1 to 2 g per kilogram per day of lipid were administered.[16,23,24,35,56,59–62] Some authors have suggested that current lipid suspensions may actually help prevent PNAC when used to replace glucose calories by reducing the carbohydrate load.[25,63]

Trace Minerals

There is little evidence that trace mineral toxicity has an important role in the pathogenesis of PNAC. Copper and manganese are normally excreted in the bile and might become hepatotoxic in the setting of physiologic or PN-associated cholestasis.[59] Tungsten excess induces sulfite oxidase deficiency in experimental animals,[64] which might contribute to decreased oxidation of sulfur-containing amino acids and possibly PNAC (see the above discussion of possible hepatotoxicity of sulfur-containing amino acids).

PARENTERAL NUTRITION DEFICIENCIES THAT MAY CONTRIBUTE TO PATHOGENESIS

Amino Acids

Amino acid deficiency leading to PNAC was first suggested by Touloukian and Seashore in 1975, when they hypothesized that relative lack of an amino acid such as taurine, important in bile acid conjugation in neonates, may lead to PNAC.[65] In the absence of taurine, glycine conjugates predominate (as they do later in life), producing a hepatotoxic bile acid composition in the immature infant. Conflicting preliminary evidence exists on the importance of PN taurine supplementation for premature infants. For example, in an uncontrolled study of 40 infants and children on PN supplemented with taurine for 5 to 21 days, the incidence of PNAC was lower than that previously seen in several centers.[66] Conversely, in a randomized very short term (10 day) study of 20 preterm infants, Cooke et al reported that PN taurine supplementation did not appear to lower the incidence of PNAC.[67] Finally, glutathione deficiency can occur in rats on PN.[68] If that is also true for humans, then a deficiency of this tripeptide could be of significance since glutathione may help maintain normal bile flow and protect the liver from hepatotoxic injury.[54]

Miscellaneous Deficiencies

Choline and carnitine are absent from currently available PN solutions. Both are important in fat metabolism, and there is sketchy evidence that this absence may contribute to hepatic steatosis. For example, adults on PN have lower serum choline levels than control patients fed hospital food,[69] and although there is no direct evidence in human neonates, newborn rats may have increased choline requirements.[70] Choline deficiency in rats results in hepatic steatosis,[71] perhaps because of decreased synthesis of phosphatidylcholine. The latter is a phospholipid necessary for lipoprotein biosynthesis, and with decreased lipoprotein production triglycerides may accumulate in the liver, leading to steatosis.[72]

Low carnitine levels have been documented in both neonates[73] and adults[74] on PN. Although carnitine is synthesized from methionine and lysine in muscle and liver, production may be limited in premature infants and neonates.[75] Carnitine is required for the complete oxidation of long-chain fatty acids by the mitochondria. Deficiency may lead to hepatic and muscular steatosis.[76] However, at least one recent study of four adult patients with PNAC and carnitine deficiency failed to show improvement in the liver fat content, liver structure, and liver function tests despite supplementation with carnitine and a return to normal of blood and hepatic carnitine concentrations.[77]

Deficiency of the trace minerals selenium[78] or molybdenum may play a role in the development of PNAC. Molybdenum is a component of sulfite oxidase, an enzyme important in the oxidative degradation of sulfur-containing amino acids,[79] and low concentrations of molybdenum have been found in the livers of premature infants.[80] As mentioned above, sulfur-containing amino acids may be hepatotoxic.

CLINICAL ASSOCIATIONS THAT MAY CONTRIBUTE TO PATHOGENESIS

Prematurity appears to be an important, although not an independent risk factor for the development of PNAC (see Fig. 1*B*).[2,15,18,27,60,65,81] Immaturity of the enterohepatic circulation of bile acids has been implicated in the pathogenesis of PNAC in premature infants.[82] Normal bile flow depends on adequate synthesis, conjugation, secretion, and recirculation of bile acids,[83,84] with bile acid secretion being the rate-limiting step.[82,85,86] Human and animal data suggest that neonates have decreased[82,87] or altered[88,89] biosynthesis of bile acids. Diminished bile acid secretion,[90,91] decreased bile acid pool size,[54] hypofunctioning of the gallbladder,[92] decreased intraluminal concentrations of bile acids,[93,94] lowered intestinal reabsorption of bile acids,[95] and decreased hepatic extraction of bile acids from portal blood[96] have all been documented in the premature infant. These deficiencies are common in very immature infants and improve with increased gestational age.[82] Finally, certain secondary bile acids, such as lithocholate, have been shown to cause cholestasis and hepatic cell necrosis.[97] The ability to detoxify secondary bile acids such as lithocholate via sulfation may be decreased in the neonate, as suggested by the finding of reduced hepatic bile salt sulfotransferase activity in neonatal rats.[98]

Lack of enteral feedings appears to be an independent risk factor for the development of PNAC,[2,5,15,17,18,80,99-101] mediated by decreased hormonal stimulation of bile flow,[102-105] diminished hormonal stimulation of hepatobiliary development, and/or an increase in toxic bile acid formation. Marked differences exist in serum cholecystokinin, glucagon, enteroglucagon, gastrin, motilin, gastric inhibitory polypeptide (GIP), and secretin in enterally fed, compared with parenterally nourished, neonates.[102-104] Improvement of PNAC has been shown in a rat model using cholecystokinin-octapeptide,[106] and in a premature infant treated with a cholecystokinin analogue.[107]

Lack of enteral nutrition has also been shown to decrease gut motility in animals and humans.[108-110] Decreased motility could lead to increased residence time in the colon of primary bile acids such as chenodeoxycholic acid, affording greater opportunity for conversion by bacteria to secondary bile acids such as lithocholate. Lithocholate is increased in the serum of both infants[111] and adults[112] with PNAC, and has been shown to be hepatotoxic in some animal models[97] but not in others.[113]

Infection has been implicated as a cause of cholestasis in patients either on[2,8,15-17,114,115] or off[116-124] PN. Infants with necrotizing enterocolitis have as much as sevenfold increased risk of PNAC.[2,55,125-127] Bacterial overgrowth of the bowel, a well-known complication of short bowel syndrome, may play a role in the development of PNAC by increasing lithocholate production.[112] Improvement of PNAC with metronidazole therapy provides indirect support for intestinal bacteria playing a role in the development of PNAC.[128-131] Abdominal surgery,[132] short bowel,[133] inflammatory bowel disease,[112,129,134,135] and hematologic malignancies[135] are among the other clinical entities reported to be associated with PNAC, although antibiotics, chemotherapy, and radiotherapy are clearly confounding factors.

CLINICAL MANIFESTATIONS

Diagnosis and Laboratory Findings

The diagnosis of PNAC rests on identification of the typical disease course, including use of PN for over 1 to 2 weeks, the presence of risk factors, and characteristic biochemical and histologic findings. Patients on PN may have hepatomegaly from increased hepatic glycogen and/or fat storage. In the absence of cholestasis, hepatomegaly alone in this setting is not associated with progressive liver disease.[136,137]

A detailed discussion of the diagnostic approach to cholestasis is provided elsewhere in this book. The diagnostic armamentarium includes the history and physical examination, laboratory tests, and radiologic imaging techniques such as ultrasonography and hepatobiliary scintigraphy (Fig. 3). Attention should be directed toward eliminating alternative etiologies for cholestasis, including infections, hepatitis, congestive heart failure, hepatic vein thrombosis, biliary sludge (with or without cholelithiasis), extrahepatic biliary atresia, choledochal cyst, or liver diseases caused by alpha$_1$-antitrypsin deficiency, cystic fibrosis, tyrosinemia, or panhypopituitarism. Liver biopsy, although often not required to make the diagnosis of PNAC in the proper setting, can be performed to aid diagnostic and prognostic accuracy.

PNAC causes characteristic biochemical changes in the serum. An elevated conjugated bilirubin (greater than 1.5 mg per deciliter or greater than 40 percent of total bilirubin) is probably the most clinically important biochemical indicator, especially as measured by a diazo reaction utilizing ethyl anthranilate.[35,49,62,63,138-140] Total bilirubin is of more limited value, given the many other reasons for its elevation in ill infants and children.[141] Similarly, total serum alkaline phosphatase is often elevated in this population by the bone isoenzyme, especially in the context of nutritional compromise.[142] Total serum bile acids or cholic acid conjugates such as sulfated lithocholic acid may provide an early sign of PNAC,[58,60,111,114,138,143] although this suggestion is controversial.[144] Although some authors have proposed using gamma-glutamyl transpeptidase[145] or 5′-nucleotidase,[138] neither has proved to be any more sensitive than conjugated bilirubin as an early indicator of PNAC.[146]

Indicators of compromised hepatic synthetic function, such as a decreased serum albumin or a prolonged prothrombin time, are ominous signs of impending hepatic failure. However, other explanations should be sought for these findings, such as excessive protein loss or vitamin K deficiency.

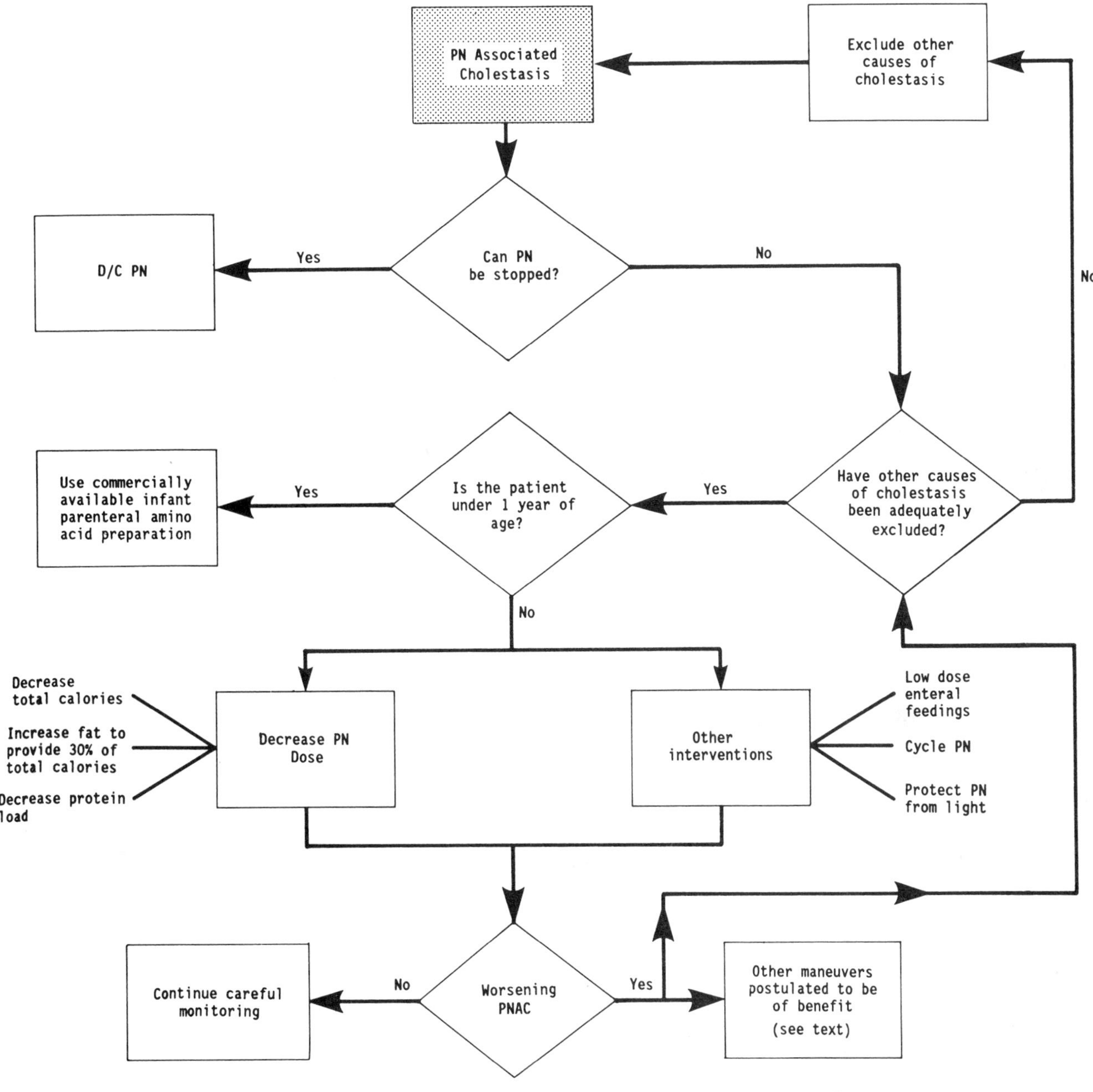

FIGURE 3 Management algorithm for PNAC.

Hyperammonemia in infants with PNAC may relate to protein overload and/or hepatocellular damage.[47]

Pathology

Light Microscopy

The histologic changes seen in adults[62,147] and infants[18,55,81,125,132,148–150] with PNAC are characteristic but nonspecific. Cholestasis in hepatocytes, canaliculi, and Kupffer cells are a consistent finding (Fig. 4). Cholestasis is most severe in the centrilobular region; relatively little bile plugging is seen in portal bile ducts or periportal hepatocytes. The degree of histologic cholestasis may not correlate with the serum bilirubin values.[125]

Steatosis is one of the most common histologic findings, correlating most strongly with calorie load rather than lipid infusion burden.[21,151,152] Kupffer cell hyperplasia, ballooned hepatocytes, and lobular disarray are noted in most biopsies, with sinusoidal fibrosis and focal necrosis being somewhat less common. Persistent extramedullary hematopoiesis is usually seen in infants. Portal zone changes include mild to moderate inflammation and periportal fibrosis in most patients, with variable bile duct proliferation and occasional bridging fibrosis. Periportal inflammatory infiltrate is most often lymphocytic, but neutrophils and eosinophils can be

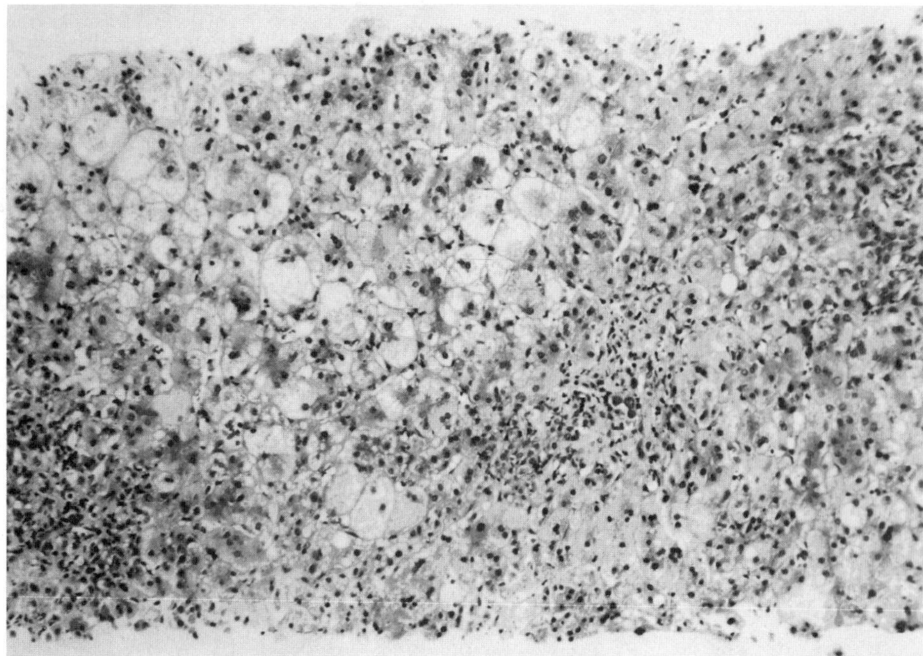

FIGURE 4 Light microscopy of a patient with PNAC shows nonspecific periportal inflammation and mild lobular disarray, with ballooning of hepatocytes, microvesicular steatosis, and focal pseudoacinar arrangement of hepatocytes. Cholestasis is present within canaliculi, hepatocytes, Kupffer cells, and occasional bile ducts. (Courtesy of Antonio Perez, M.D., Department of Pathology, Children's Hospital, Boston.)

present. Kupffer cells[78] and periportal hepatocytes[125] show variable amounts of lipofuscin, seen as yellow-brown, periodic acid-Schiff–positive diastase resistant granules. Occasionally bile duct hyperplasia and cholestasis can mimic extrahepatic obstruction.[55,153] Although it is a relatively uncommon occurrence, PNAC can progress to cirrhosis.[18,55,81,149,150]

Electron Microscopy

Several typical, but not diagnostic, ultrastructural changes are seen with PNAC.[55,125,148,149] Most common are increased glycogen, lysosomal particles with cholesterol-like crystals, and nonspecific mitochondrial changes such as enlargement with abundant matrix and peripheral displacement of cristae. Numerous collagen fibers are found in the perisinusoidal spaces of Disse when fibrosis is present.

COMPLICATIONS AND PROGNOSIS

Complications that have been linked with PNAC include hepatocellular injury and biliary tract disease. There has been a single case report of hepatocellular carcinoma in a 6-month-old infant after prolonged PN.[154] Signs of hepatocellular disease usually resolve after discontinuation of PN, although histologic evidence of injury can be found many months later.[55] Liver disease sometimes progresses to cirrhosis,[18,55,81,149,150] and in a few patients to liver failure if PN is continued in the face of severe PNAC.[55,127,132,147,155] Biliary tract complications of PNAC include acalculous cholecystitis, biliary sludge, and cholelithiasis.[10,155-162] Acalculous cholecystitis presents as acute cholecystitis without evidence of gallstones. The observation that acalculous cholecystitis might be a complication of PN was first reported in 1972,[163] and was later confirmed by other investigators.[157-159,164,165] Delay in diagnosis is common, leading to increased morbidity and mortality from gallbladder perforation and bile peritonitis.

Biliary sludge may be an important intermediate stage before stone formation appears, contributed to in part by gallbladder hypomotility of patients on PN.[155,156,166] From 12 to 40 percent of children on long-term PN develop biliary sludge or cholelithiasis, with the higher percentage seen in patients with ileal disorders or resection.[157,167] Hemolytic anemia and prolonged use of furosemide also appear to increase the risk of gallstone formation.[168,169] Both pigmented and cholesterol stones have been found in these patients.[157] Although surgery has been recommended for cholecystitis in this setting, the increased morbidity and mortality in these often ill patients is cause for concern.[170]

TREATMENT

The approach to prevention and treatment of PNAC includes decreasing known or suggested risk factors, changing the PN dose or components, and possibly using medical and/or surgical interventions that might be of benefit (see Fig. 3). When biochemical evidence of cholestasis or hepatocellular injury is discovered, appropriate efforts to exclude other causes of liver disease are first undertaken. After PNAC has been diagnosed (usually by exclusion), then the single most effective intervention is discontinuation of the PN, since rapid improvement of PNAC usually occurs after the PN is stopped.[17,55,134] If PN can not be discontinued, then efforts should be made to ensure that the patient is receiving appropriate amounts of protein, carbohydrate, and calories. Low-dose enteral feedings,[156,171] cycling of the PN for 12 hours a day,[172,173] and protection of the PN from light[48-51] may be helpful. Patients under 1 year of age may be placed on commercially available amino acid solutions formulated for young infants, although the data supporting their efficacy are preliminary.[66,174,175]

If PNAC becomes more severe despite the above maneuvers, a re-evaluation of the diagnosis is necessary. If PNAC remains as the diagnosis, more speculative interventions can be attempted. These include use of choleretics such as barbiturates[176–178] and ursodeoxycholic acid (UDCA)[179]; carnitine, choline, or other supplementation of the PN[66,67,126]; metronidazole or other antibiotics[129–131,159]; hormonal stimulation of bile flow and gallbladder function with cholecystokinin analogues[106,107]; glucagon, which may reduce hepatic steatosis[180]; or irrigation of the biliary tree.[181,182] Other unproven measures include the use of bowel prokinetic agents that may help decrease toxic secondary bile acid formation; removal or reduction of PN copper,[56] manganese,[56] or tungsten[64]; or lowering of PN bisulfite antioxidants.[171] Most children progressing to end-stage liver disease from PNAC also have short bowel syndrome. Present criteria for liver transplantation commonly preclude the procedure for children with major disease in two organ systems (e.g., liver and bowel), but recent trends are moving toward liberalization of these criteria.

CONCLUSIONS

Liver disease commonly occurs in infants and children on parenteral nutrition. Much research must be done to unravel the complex web of possible etiologies. Although many preventive and therapeutic interventions have been proposed, large prospective trials are needed to demonstrate the efficacy and the safety of these measures. Meanwhile, careful attention to the details of PN indications, dosing, and monitoring should significantly reduce the incidence and morbidity of this disorder.

REFERENCES

1. Peden VH, Witzleben CL, Skelton MA. Total parenteral nutrition. (Letter) J Pediatr 1971; 78:180–181.
2. Bell RL, Ferry GD, Smith EO, Shulman RJ, Christensen BL, Labarthe DR, Wills CA. Total parenteral nutrition-related cholestasis in infants. J Parenter Enteral Nutr 1986; 10:356–359.
3. Merritt RJ. Cholestasis associated with total parenteral nutrition. J Pediatr Gastroenterol Nutr 1986; 5:9–22.
4. Sax HC, Bower RH. Hepatic complications of total parenteral nutrition. J Parenter Enteral Nutr 1988; 12:615–618.
5. Hughes CA, Talbot IC, Ducker DA, Harran MJ. Total parenteral nutrition in infancy: effect on the liver and suggested pathogenesis. Gut 1983; 24:241–248.
6. Balistreri WF, Novak DA, Farrell MK. Bile acid metabolism, total parenteral nutrition, and cholestasis. In: Lebenthal E, ed. Total parenteral nutrition: indications, utilization, complications and pathophysiological considerations. New York: Raven Press, 1986; 319.
7. Baker SS, Dwyer E, Queen P. Metabolic derangements in children requiring parenteral nutrition. J Parenter Enteral Nutr 1986; 10:279–281.
8. Kubota A, Okada A, Nezu R, Kamata S, Imura K, Takagi Y. Hyperbilirubinemia in neonates associated with total parenteral nutrition. J Parenter Enteral Nutr 1988; 12:602–606.
9. Baker AL, Rosenberg IH. Hepatic complications of total parenteral nutrition. Am J Med 1987; 82:489–497.
10. Klien S, Nealon WH. Hepatobiliary abnormalities associated with total parenteral nutrition. Semin Liver Dis 1988; 8:237–246.
11. Jeejeebhoy KN. Hepatic manifestations of total parenteral nutrition: need for prospective investigation. Hepatology 1988; 8:428–429.
12. Wolfe BM, Walker BK, Shaul DB, Wong L, Ruebner BH. Effect of total parenteral nutrition on hepatic histology. Arch Surg 1988; 123:1084–1090.
13. MacFadyen BV, Dudrick SJ, Baquero G, Gum ET. Clinical and biological changes in liver function during intravenous hyperalimentation. J Parenter Enteral Nutr 1979; 3:438–441.
14. Sheard NF, Kleinman RE, TPN cholestasis in premature infants: the role of parenteral nutrition solutions. Pediatr Ann 1987; 16:243–252.
15. Beale EF, Nelson RM, Bucciarelli RL, Donnelly WH, Eitzman DV. Intrahepatic cholestasis associated with parenteral nutrition in premature infants. Pediatrics 1979; 64:342–347.
16. Vileisis R, Inwood RJ, Hunt CE. Prospective controlled study of parenteral nutrition associated cholestatic jaundice: effect of protein intake. J Pediatr 1980; 96:893–897.
17. Rodgers BM, Hollenbeck IL, Donnelly WH, Talbert JL. Intrahepatic cholestasis with parenteral alimentation. Am J Surg 1976; 131:149–155.
18. Pereira GR, Sherman MS, DiGiacoma J, Ziegler M, Roth K, Jacobowski D. Hyperalimentation-inducted cholestasis. Increased incidence and severity in premature infants. Am J Dis Child 1981; 135:842–847.
19. Zahavi I, Shaffer EA, Gall DG. Total parenteral nutrition–associated cholestasis: acute studies in infant and adult rabbits. J Pediatr Gastroenterol Nutr 1985; 4:622–627.
20. Mashima Y. Effect of calorie overload on puppy livers during parenteral nutrition. J Parenter Enteral Nutr 1979; 3:139–145.
21. Keim NL. Nutritional effects of hepatic steatosis induced by parenteral nutrition in rats. J Parenter Enteral Nutr 1987; 11:18–22.
22. Stein TP, Mullen JL. Hepatic fat accumulation in man with excess parenteral glucose. Nutr Res 1985; 5:1347–1351.
23. Lowry SF, Brennan MF. Abnormal liver function during parenteral nutrition: relation to infusion excess. J Surg Res 1979; 26:300–307.
24. Wagner WH, Lowry AC, Silberman H. Similar liver function abnormalities occur in patients receiving glucose-based and lipid-based parenteral nutrition. Am J Gastroenterol 1983; 78:199–202.
25. Meguid MM, Akahoshi MP, Jeffers S, Hayashi RJ, Hammond WG. Amelioration of metabolic complications of conventional total parenteral nutrition. A prospective randomized study. Arch Surg 1984; 119:1294–1298.
26. Greenlaw CW. Liver enzyme elevation with total parenteral nutrition. Drug Intell Clin Pharmacol 1980; 14:702–709.
27. Hirai Y, Sanada Y, Fujiwara T, Hasegawa S, Kuwabara N. High calorie infusion-induced hepatic impairments in infants. J Parenter Enteral Nutr 1979; 3:146–150.
28. Heird WC, Driscoll JM Jr, Schullinger JN, Grebin B, Winters RW. Intravenous alimentation in pediatric patients. J Pediatr 1972; 80:351–372.
29. Lloyd-Still JD, Shwachman H, Filler RM. Intravenous hyperalimentation in pediatrics. Dig Dis 1972; 17:1043–1052.
30. Graham MF, Tavill AS, Halpin TC, Louis LN. Inhibition of bile flow in the isolated perfused rat liver by a synthetic parenteral amino acid mixture: associated net amino acid fluxes. Hepatology 1984; 4:69–73.
31. Blitzer BL, Ratoosh SL, Donovan CB. Amino acid inhibition of bile acid uptake by isolated rat hepatocytes: relationship to dissipation of transmembrane Na gradient. Am J Physiol 1983; 245:G399–G403.
32. Bucuvalas JC, Goodrich AL, Blitzer BL, Suchy FJ. Amino acids are potent inhibitors of bile acid uptake by liver plasma membrane vesicles isolated from suckling rats. Pediatr Res 1985; 19:1298–1304.
33. Riely CA, Fine PL, Boyer JL. Progressively rising serum bile acids—a common effect of parenteral nutrition (Abstract). Gastroenterology 1979; 77:34A.
34. Sankaran K, Berscheid B, Verma V, Zakhary G, Tan L. An evaluation of total parenteral nutrition using Vamin and Aminosyn as protein base in critically ill preterm infants. J Parenteral Enteral Nutr 1985; 9:439–442.
35. Black DD, Suttle EA, Whitington PF, Whitington GL, Korones SD. The effect of short-term total parenteral nutrition on hepatic function in the human neonate: a prospective randomized study demonstrating alteration of hepatic canalicular function. Pediatrics 1981; 99:445–449.
36. Merritt RJ, Shah PH, Hack SL, Henton D, Smith T, Thomas DW, Sinatra FR. Treatment of protracted diarrhea of infancy. Am J Dis Child 1984; 138:770–774.

37. Merritt RJ, Sinatra FR, Henton DH. Cholestatic effect of tryptophan and its metabolites in suckling rat pups. (Abstract) Pediatr Res 1982; 16:171A.
38. Preisig R, Rennert O. Biliary transport and cholestatic effect of amino acids. (Abstract) Gastroenterology 1977; 73:1240.
39. Rigo J, Senterre J. Parenteral nutrition in the very-low-birth-weight infant. In: Kretchmer N, Minkowski A, eds. Nutritional adaptation of the gastrointestinal tract of the newborn. New York: Raven Press, 1983; 191–205.
40. Klavins JV. Pathology of amino acid excess. Effects of administration of excessive amounts of sulphur containing amino acids: homocystine. Br J Exp Pathol 1963; 44:507–515.
41. Klavins JV. Pathology of amino acid excess. Effects of administration of excessive amounts of sulphur containing amino acids: L-cystine. Br J Exp Pathol 1963; 44:516–519.
42. Earle DP Jr, Smull K, Victor J. Effects of excess dietary cysteic acid, DL-methionine, and taurine on the rat liver. J Exp Med 1942; 75:317–323.
43. Stekol JA, Szaran J. Pathological effects of excessive methionine in the diet of growing rats. J Nutr 1962; 77:81–90.
44. Phillips MJ, Oda M, Mak E, Fisher MM, Jeejeebhoy KN. Microfilament dysfunction as a possible cause of intrahepatic cholestasis. Gastroenterology 1975; 69:48–58.
45. Klavins JV, Peacocke IL. Pathology of amino acid excess III. Effects of administration of excessive amounts of sulfur-containing amino acids: methionine with equimolar amounts of glycine and arginine. Br J Exp Pathol 1964; 45:533–547.
46. Zarif MA, Pildes RS, Szanto PB, Vidyasagar D. Cholestasis associated with administration of L-amino acids and dextrose solutions. Biol Neonate 1976; 29:66–76.
47. Poley R. Liver and nutrition: hepatic complications of total parenteral nutrition. In: Lebenthal E, ed. Textbook of gastroenterology and nutrition in infancy. New York: Raven Press 1981: 743.
48. Merritt RJ, Sinatra FR, Henton DH, Neustein H. Cholestatic effect of intraperitoneal administration of tryptophan to suckling rat pups. Pediatr Res 1984; 18:904–907.
49. Grant JP, Cox LE, Kleinman LM, Maher MM, Pittman MA, Tangrea JA, Brown JH, Cross E, Beazley RM, Jones ES. Serum hepatic enzyme and bilirubin elevations during total parenteral nutrition. Surg Gynecol Obstet 1977; 145:573–580.
50. Nixon TB, Wang RJ. Formation of photoproducts lethal for human cells in culture by daylight, fluorescent light and bilirubin light. Photochem Photobiol 1977; 26:589–593.
51. Bhatia J, Stegnink LD, Ziegler EE. Riboflavin enhances photooxidation of amino acids under simulated clinical conditions. J Parenter Enteral Nutr 1983; 7:277–279.
52. Salvian AJ, Allardyce DB. Impaired bilirubin secretion during total parenteral nutrition. J Surg Res 1980; 28:547–555.
53. Allardyce DB. Cholestasis caused by lipid emulsions. Surg Gynecol Obstet 1982; 154:641–647.
54. Sinatra FR. Development of hepatobiliary function: potential role in the development of total parenteral nutrition-associated cholestasis. In: Gross I, Hill H, Shapiro L (eds). Infant nutrition: development and disease. Mead Johnson Symposium on Perinatal and Developmental Medicine 1989; 31:32.
55. Dahms BB, Halpin TC. Serial liver biopsies in parenteral nutrition-associated cholestasis of early infancy. Gastroenterology 1981; 81:136–144.
56. Sinatra F. Does total parenteral nutrition produce cholestasis? In: Neonatal cholestasis. Proceedings of the 87th Ross Conference on Pediatric Research. Columbus, Ohio: Ross Laboratories, 1984: 85.
57. Hakansson I. Experience in long-term studies on nine intravenous fat emulsions in dogs. Nutr Dieta 1968; 10:54–76.
58. Edgren B, Hallberg D, Hakansson I, Meng HC, Wretlind A. Long-term tolerance study of two fat emulsions for intravenous nutrition in dogs. Am J Clin Nutr 1964; 14:28–36.
59. Farrell MK, Balistreri WF, Suchy FJ. Serum sulfated lithocholate as an indicator of cholestasis during parenteral nutrition in infants and children. J Parenter Enter Nutr 1982; 6:30–33.
60. Sondheimer JM, Bryan H, Andrews W, Forstner GG. Cholestatic tendencies in premature infants on and off parenteral nutrition. Pediatrics 1978; 62:984–989.
61. Tulikoura I, Huikuri K. Morphological fatty changes and function of the liver, serum free fatty acids, and triglycerides during parenteral nutrition. Scand J Gastroenterol 1982; 17:177–185.
62. Sheldon GF, Petersen SR, Sanders R. Hepatic dysfunction during hyperalimentation. Arch Surg 1978; 113:504–508.
63. Watters DA, Chamroonkul S, Griffith CD, Blundell G, Amos A, Gove LF, Saunders JH, Eastwood MA. Changes in liver function tests associated with parenteral nutrition. J R Coll Surg Edin 1984; 29:339–344.
64. Johnson JL, Rajagopalan KV. Human sulfite oxidase deficiency. Characterization of the molecular defect in a multicomponent system. J Clin Invest 1976; 58:551–556.
65. Touloukian RJ, Seashore JH. Hepatic secretory obstruction with total parenteral nutrition in the infant. J Pediatr Surg 1975; 10:353–360.
66. Heird WC, Dell RB, Helms RA, Greene HL, Ament ME, Karna P, Storm MC. Amino acid mixture designed to maintain normal plasma amino acid patterns in infants and children requiring parenteral nutrition. Pediatrics 1987; 80:401–408.
67. Cooke RJ, Whitington PF, Kelts D. Effect of taurine supplementation on hepatic function during short-term parenteral nutrition in the premature infant. J Pediatr Gastroenterol Nutr 1984; 3:234–238.
68. Heyman MD, Tseng HC, Thaler MM. Total parenteral nutrition decreases hepatic glutathione concentrations in weanling rats. (Abstract) Hepatology 1984; 3:234–238.
69. Sheard NF, Tayek JA, Bistrian BR, Blackburn GL, Zeisel SH. Plasma choline concentrations in humans fed parenterally. Am J Clin Nutr 1986; 43:219–224.
70. Zeisel SH, Wurtman RJ. Developmental changes in rat blood choline concentration. Biochem J 1981; 198:565–570.
71. Zeisel SH. Dietary choline: Biochemistry, physiology and pharmacology. Ann Rev Nutr 1981; 1:95–121.
72. Lombardi B. Pathogenesis of fatty liver. Fed Proc 1965; 24:1200–1205.
73. Schiff D, Chan G, Seccombe D, Hahn P. Plasma carnitine levels during intravenous feeding of the neonate. J Pediatr 1979; 95:1043–1046.
74. Bowyer BA, Fleming CR, Ilstrup D, Nelson J, Reek S, Burnes J. Plasma carnitine levels in patients receiving home parenteral nutrition. Am J Clin Nutr 1986; 43:85–91.
75. Shenai J, Borum P. Tissue carnitine reserves of newborn infants. Pediatr Res 1984; 18:679–681.
76. Chapoy PR, Angelini C, Brown WJ, Stiff JE, Shug AL, Cederbaum SD. Systemic carnitine deficiency—a treatable inherited lipid-storage disease presenting as Reye's syndrome. N Engl J Med 1980; 303:1389–1394.
77. Bowyer BA, Miles JM, Haymond MW, Fleming CR. L-carnitine therapy in home parenteral nutrition patients with abnormal liver tests and low plasma carnitine concentrations. Gastroenterology 1988; 94:434–438.
78. Berger HM, Den Ouden AL, Calame JJ. Pathogenesis of liver damage during parenteral nutrition: is lipofuscin a clue? Arch Dis Child 1985; 60:774–776.
79. Johnson JL, Rajagopalan KV. Purification and properties of sulfite oxidase from human liver. J Clin Invest 1976; 58:543–550.
80. Meinel B, Bode JC, Koenig W, Richter FW. Contents of trace elements in the human liver before birth. Biol Neonate 1979; 36:225–232.
81. Benjamin DR. Hepatobiliary dysfunction in infants and children associated with long-term total parenteral nutrition. A clinico-pathologic study. Am J Clin Pathol 1981; 76:276–283.
82. Balistreri WF, Heubi JE, Suchy FJ. Immaturity of the enterohepatic circulation in early life: Factors predisposing to physiologic maldigestion and cholestasis. J Pediatr Gastroenterol Nutr 1983; 2:346–354.
83. Hofmann AF. The enterohepatic circulation of bile acids. Clin Gastroenterol 1977; 6:3–24.
84. Boyer JL. New concepts of the mechanisms of hepatocyte bile formation. Physiol Rev 1980; 60:303–326.
85. Forker EL. Mechanisms of hepatic bile formation. Ann Rev Physiol 1977; 39:323–347.
86. Jones RS, Meyers WC. Regulation of hepatic biliary secretion. Annu Rev Physiol 1979; 41:67–82.
87. Li JR, Subbiah MTR, Kottke BA. Hepatic 3-hydroxy-3-methyl-glutaryl Coenzyme A reductase activity and cholesterol 7-alpha-hydroxylase activity in neonatal guinea pig. Steroids 1979; 34:47–51.
88. Back P, Walter K. Developmental pattern of bile acid metabolism as revealed by bile acid analysis of meconium. Gastroenterology 1980; 78:671–676.
89. Lester R, St Pyrek J, Little JM, Adcock EW. Diversity of bile acids in the fetus and newborn infant. J Pediatr Gastroenterol Nutr 1983; 2:355–364.
90. Graham TO, Van Thiel DH, Little JM, Lester R. Synthesis of taurocho-

late by rate fetal liver in organ culture: effects of cortisol in vitro. Am J Physiol 1979; 237:E177–E184.
91. Little JM, Richey JE, Van Thiel DH, Lester R. Taurocholate poll size and distribution in the fetal rat. J Clin Invest 1979; 63:1042–1049.
92. Denehy C, Ryan JP. Age related changes in gallbladder motility. (Abstract) Fed Proc 1982; 41:1491.
93. Norman A, Strandvik B, Ojamae O. Bile acids and pancreatic enzymes during absorption in the newborn. Acta Paediatr Scand 1972; 61:571–576.
94. Watkins JB, Szczepanik P, Gould JB, Klein P, Lester R. Bile salt metabolism in the human premature infants. Preliminary observations of pool size and synthesis rate following prenatal administration of dexamethasone and phenobarbital. Gastroenterology 1975; 69:706–713.
95. de Belle RC, Vaupshas V, Vitullo BB, Haber LR, Shaffer E, Mackie GG, Owen H, Little JM, Lester R. Intestinal absorption of bile salts: immature development in the neonate. J Pediatr 1979; 94:472–476.
96. Suchy FJ, Bucuvalas JC, Goodrich AL, Moyer MS, Blitzer BL. Taurocholate transport and Na^+-K^+-ATPase activity in fetal and neonatal rat liver plasma membrane vesicles. Am J Physiol 1986; 251:G655–G673.
97. Gadcz TR, Allan RN, Mack E, Hofmann AF. Impaired lithocholate sulfation in the rhesus monkey: a possible mechanism for chenodeoxycholate toxicity. Gastroenterology 1976; 70:1125–1129.
98. Balistreri WF, Zimmer L, Suchy FJ, Bove KE. Bile salt sulfotransferase: alterations during maturation and noninducibility during substrate ingestion. J Lipid Res 1984; 25:228–235.
99. Nakai H, Landing BH. Factors in the genesis of bile stasis in infancy. Pediatrics 1961; 27:300–307.
100. Rager R, Finegold MJ. Cholestasis in immature newborn infants: Is parenteral alimentation responsible? J Pediatr 1975; 86:264–269.
101. Greenberg G, Wolman S. Christofides N, Bloom SR, Jeejeebhoy KN. Effect of total parenteral nutrition on gut hormone release in humans. Gastroenterology 1981; 80:988–993.
102. Aynsley-Green A. Plasma hormone concentrations during enteral and parenteral nutrition in the human newborn. J Pediatr Gastroenterol Nutr 1983; 2(suppl 1):108–112.
103. Lucas A. Endocrine aspects of enteral nutrition. In: Kleinberger G, Deutsch E, eds. New aspects of clinical nutrition. Proceedings of the 4th Congress of the European Society of Parenteral and Enteral Nutrition (ESPEN), Vienna, September 27–29, 1982. Basel: Karger, 1983: 581.
104. Lucas A, Bloom SR, Aynsley-Green A. Metabolic and endocrine consequences of depriving preterm infants of enteral nutrition. Acta Paediatr Scand 1983; 72:245–249.
105. Bloomer JP, Barrett PVD, Rodkley FL. Studies on the mechanism of fasting hyperbilirubinemia. Gastroenterology 1971; 61:479–487.
106. Innis SM. Effect of cholecystokinin-octapeptide on total parenteral nutrition-induced changes in hepatic bile secretion and composition in the rat. J Pediatr Gastroenterol Nutr 1986; 5:793–798.
107. Schwartz JB, Merritt RJ, Rosenthal P, Diament M, Sinatra FR, Ramos A. Ceruletide to treat neonatal cholestasis. (Letter) Lancet 1988; i:1219–1220.
108. Gleghorn EE, Merritt RJ, Henton D, Sinatra FR. Changes in gastrointestinal motility with total parenteral nutrition not associated with bacterial overgrowth (Abstract). Clin Res 1985; 33:118A.
109. Levinson S, Bhasker M, Morin R, Snape WJ Jr. Effects of intraluminal and intravenous nutrients on colonic motility. (Abstract) Gastroenterology 1983; 84:1229.
110. Weisbroot NW, Copeland EM, Thor PJ, Dudrick SJ. Small bowel motility during intravenous hyperalimentation in the dog. (Abstract) Gastroenterology 1975; 68:154.
111. Farrell MK, Gilster S, Balistreri WF. Serum bile acids: an early indicator of parenteral nutrition-associated liver disease. (Abstract) Gastroenterology 1984; 86:1074.
112. Fouin-Fortunet H, Le Quernec L, Erlinger S, Lerebours E, Colin R. Hepatic alterations during total parenteral nutrition in patients with inflammatory bowel disease: a possible consequence of lithocholate toxicity. Gastroenterology 1982; 82:932–937.
113. Gratton F, Weber AM, Tuchweber B, Morazain R, Roy CC, Yousef IM. Effect of chronic administration of taurolithocholate on bile formation and liver ultrastructure in the rat. Liver 1987; 7:130–137.
114. Manginello FP, Javitt NB. Parenteral nutrition and neonatal cholestasis. J Pediatr 1979; 94:296–298.
115. Roger R, Finegold MJ. Cholestasis in immature newborn infants: Is parenteral alimentation responsible? J Pediatr 1975; 86:264–269.
116. Bernstein J, Brown AK. Sepsis and jaundice in early infancy. Pediatrics 1962; 29:873–882.
117. Hamilton JR, Sass-Korstak A. Jaundice associated with severe bacterial infection in young infants. J Pediatr 1963; 63:121–132.
118. Abernathy CO, Utili R, Zimmerman HJ. Immaturity of the biliary excretory system predisposes neonates to intrahepatic cholestasis. Med Hypotheses 1979; 5:641–647.
119. Nolan JP. The role of endotoxin in liver injury. Gastroenterology 1975; 69:1346–1353.
120. Utili R, Abernathy CO, Zimmerman HJ. Mini-review: Endotoxin effects on the liver. Life Sci 1977; 20:553–568.
121. Utili R, Abernathy CO, Zimmerman HJ. Cholestatic effects of *Escherichia coli* endotoxin on the isolated perfused rat liver. Gastroenterology 1976; 70:248–253.
122. Utili R, Abernathy C, Zimmerman H. Inhibition of Na^+, K^+-ATPase by endotoxin: a possible mechanism for endotoxin-induced cholestasis. J Infect Dis 1977; 136:583–587.
123. Minuk GY, Rascanin N, Sarjeant ES, Pai CH. Sepsis and cholestasis: the in vitro effects of bacterial products on 14C-taurocholate uptake by isolated rat hepatocytes. Liver 1986; 6:199–204.
124. Alverdy JC, Aoys E, Moss GS. Total parenteral nutrition promotes bacterial translocation from the gut. Surgery 1988; 104:185–190.
125. Bernstein J, Chang CH, Brough AJ, Heidelberger KP. Conjugated hyperbilirubinemia in infancy associated with parenteral alimentation. J Pediatr 1977; 90:361–367.
126. Cooper A, Betts JM, Pereira GR, Ziegler MM. Taurine deficiency in the severe hepatic dysfunction complicating total parenteral nutrition. J Pediatr Surg 1984; 19:462–466.
127. Hodes JE, Grosfeld JL, Weber TR, Schreiner RL, Fitzgerald JF, Mirkin LD. Hepatic failure in infants on total parenteral nutrition (TPN): Clinical and histopathologic observations. J Pediatr Surg 1982; 17:463–468.
128. Freund HR, Muggia-Sullam M, LaFrance R, Enrione EB, Popp MB, Bjornson HS. A possible beneficial effect of metronidazole in reducing TPN-associated liver function derangements. J Surg Res 1985; 38:356–363.
129. Capron JP, Gineston JL, Herve MA, Braillon A. Metronidazole in prevention of cholestasis associated with total parenteral nutrition. Lancet 1983; i:446–447.
130. Lambert JR, Thomas SM. Metronidazole prevention of serum liver enzyme abnormalities during total parenteral nutrition. J Parenter Enteral Nutr 1985; 9:501–503.
131. Elleby H, Solhaug JH. Metronidazole, cholestasis and total parenteral nutrition. Lancet 1983; i:1161.
132. Postuma R, Trevenen CL. Liver disease in infants receiving total parenteral nutrition. Pediatrics 1979; 63:110–115.
133. Stanko RT, Nathan G, Mendelow H, Adibi SA. Development of hepatic cholestasis and fibrosis in patients with massive loss of intestine supported by prolonged parenteral nutrition. Gastroenterology 1987; 92:197–202.
134. Bengoa JM, Hanauer SB, Sitrin MD, Baker AL, Rosenberg IH. Pattern and prognosis of liver function test abnormalities during parenteral nutrition in inflammatory bowel disease. Hepatology 1985; 5:79–84.
135. Naji AA, Anderson FH. Cholestasis associated with parenteral nutrition develops more commonly with hematologic malignancy than with inflammatory bowel disease. (Letter) J Parenter Enteral Nutr 1984; 8:325.
136. Balistreri WF, Novak DA, Farrell. Bile acid metabolism, total parenteral nutrition, and cholestasis. In: Lebenthal E, ed. Total parenteral nutrition: Indications, utilization, complications and pathophysiological considerations. New York: Raven Press, 1986: 319.
137. Alpers DH, Sabesin S, Fatty liver, biochemical and clinical aspects. In: Schiff L, Schiff ER, eds. Diseases of the liver. Philadelphia: JB Lippincott, 1987: 949.
138. Whitington PF. Cholestasis associated with total parenteral nutrition in infants. Hepatology 1985; 5:693–696.
139. Killenberg PG, Stevens RD, Wildermann RF, Wildermann NM. The laboratory method as a variable in the interpretation of serum bilirubin fractionation. Gastroenterology 1980; 78:1011–1015.
140. Lindor KD, Fleming CR, Abrams AA, Hirschkorn MA. Liver function values in adults receiving total parenteral nutrition. JAMA 1979; 241:2398–2400.
141. Odell GB. Neonatal hyperbilirubinemia. New York: Grune & Stratton, 1980.
142. Glasgow JFT. Evaluation of liver function. In: Chandra RK, ed. The liver and biliary system in infants and children. Edinburgh: Churchill Livingstone, 1979: 80–123.
143. Kaplowitz N, Kok E, Javitt NB. Post prandial serum bile acid for the

detection of hepatobiliary disease. JAMA 1973; 225:292–293.

144. Beckett GJ, Glass EJ, Callaghan MO, Elton RA, Hume R. Measuring bile-salt concentrations lacks clinical value for detecting hepatic dysfunction in infants receiving parenteral nutrition. Clin Chem 1985; 31:1168–1171.

145. Naji AA, Andersen FH. Sensitivity and specificity of liver function tests in the detection of parenteral nutrition-associated cholestasis. J Parenteral Enteral Nutr 1985; 9:307–308.

146. Cartlidge PH, Rutter N. Gamma-glutamyltransferase in the newborn. Early Hum Dev 1987; 15:213–216.

147. Bowyer BA, Fleming CR, Ludwig J, Petz J, McGill DB. Does long-term home parenteral nutrition in adult patients cause chronic liver disease? J Parenter Enteral Nutr 1985; 9:11–17.

148. Phillips MJ, Poucell S, Patterson J, Valencia P. The liver: An atlas and text of ultrastructural pathology. New York: Raven Press, 1987: 101.

149. Cohen C, Olsen MM. Pediatric total parenteral nutrition, liver histopathology. Arch Pathol Lab Med 1981; 105:152–156.

150. Kibort PM, Ulich TR, Berquist WE, Lewin KJ, Ament ME. Hepatic fibrosis and cirrhosis in children on long-term total parenteral nutrition. (Abstract) Gastroenterology 1982; 82:1099.

151. Wolfe RR, Allsop JR, Burke JF. Glucose metabolism in man: response to intravenous glucose infusion. Metabolism 1979; 28:210–220.

152. Sax HC, Talamini MA, Brackett K, Fischer JE. Hepatic steatosis in total parenteral nutrition: failure of fatty infiltration to correlate with abnormal serum hepatic enzyme levels. Surgery 1986; 100:697–704.

153. Body JJ, Bleiberg H, Bron D, Maurage H, Bigirimana V, Heimann R. Total parenteral nutrition-induced cholestasis mimicking large duct obstruction. Histopathology 1982; 6:787–792.

154. Patterson K, Kapur SP, Chandra RS. Hepatocellular carcinoma in a noncirrhotic infant after prolonged parenteral nutrition. J Pediatr 1985; 106:797–800.

155. Vargas JH, Amend ME, Berquist WE. Long-term home parenteral nutrition in pediatrics: ten years of experience in 102 patients. J Pediatr Gastroenterol Nutr 1987; 6:24–32.

156. Messing B, Bories C, Kunstlinger F, Bernier JJ. Does total parenteral nutrition induce gallbladder sludge formation and lithiasis? Gastroenterology 1983; 84:1012–1019.

157. Roslyn JJ, Berquist WE, Pitt HA, Mann LL, Kangarloo H, DenBesten L, Ament ME. Increased risk of gallstones in children receiving total parenteral nutrition. Pediatrics 1983; 71:784–789.

158. Roslyn JJ, Pitt HA, Mann LL, Ament ME, DenBesten L. Gallbladder disease in patients on long-term parenteral nutrition. Gastroenterology 1983; 84:148–154.

159. Messing B, DeOliveira FJ, Galian A, Bernier JJ. Cholestasis during total parenteral nutrition: demonstration of facilitating factors and association with gallbladder lithiasis. Gastroenterol Clin Biol 1982; 6:740–747.

160. Pitt HA, King W 3rd, Mann LL, Roslyn JJ, Berquist WE, Ament ME, DenBesten L. Increased risk of cholelithiasis with prolonged total parenteral nutrition. Am J Surg 1983; 145:106–112.

161. Hill GL, Mair WSJ, Goligher JC. Gallstones after ileostomy and ileal resection. Gut 1975; 16:932–936.

162. Dowling RH, Bell GD, White J. Lithogenic bile in patients with ileal dysfunction. Gut 1971; 13:415–420.

163. Andersen JL, Acalculous cholecystitis. A possible complication of parenteral hyperalimentation. Report of a case. Med Ann DC 1972; 41:448–450.

164. Petersen SR, Sheldon GF. Acute acalculous cholecystitis: a complication of hyperalimentation. Am J Surg 1979; 138:814–815.

165. Saldana RL, Stein CA, Kopelmann AE. Gallbladder distension in ill premature infants. Am J Dis Child 1983; 137:1179–1180.

166. Cano N, Cicero F, Ranieri F, Martin J, DiCostanzo J. Ultrasonographic study of gallbladder motility during total parenteral nutrition. Gastroenterology 1986; 91:313–317.

167. King DR, Ginn-Pease ME, Lloyd TV, Hoffman J, Hohenbring K. Parenteral nutrition with associated cholelithiasis: another iatrogenic disease of infants and children. J Pediatr Surg 1987; 22:593–596.

168. Boyle RJ, Rumner TE, Volberg FM. Cholelithiasis in a 3 week old small premature infant. Pediatrics 1983; 71:967–969.

169. Whitington PF, Black DD. Cholelithiasis in premature infants treated with parenteral nutrition and furosemide. J Pediatr 1980; 97:647–649.

170. Roslyn JJ, Pitt HA, Mann L, Fonkalgrud EW, DenBester L. Parenteral nutrition induced gallbladder disease: a reason for early cholecystectomy. Am J Physiol 1984; 148:58–63.

171. Merritt RJ. Cholestasis associated with total parenteral nutrition. J Pediatr Gastroenter Nutr 1986; 5:9–22.

172. Ternullo SR, Burkart GJ. Experience with cyclic hyperalimentation in infants. (Abstract) J Parenter Enter Nutr 1979; 3:516.

173. Maini B, Blackburn GL, Bistrian BR, Flatt JP, Page JG, Bothe A, Benotti P, Rienhoff HY. Cyclic hyperalimentation: An optimal technique for preservation of visceral protein. J Surg Res 1976; 20:515–525.

174. Helms RA, Christensen ML, Mauer EC, Storm MC. Comparison of a pediatric versus standard amino acid formulation in preterm neonates requiring parenteral nutrition. J Pediatr 1987; 110:466–470.

175. Winters RW, Heird WC, Dell RB, Nicholson JF. Plasma amino acids in infants receiving parenteral nutrition. In: Greene HL, Holliday MA, Munro HN, eds. Clinical nutrition update; amino acids. Chicago: American Medical Association, 1977: 147.

176. South M, King A. Parenteral nutrition-associated cholestasis: recovery following phenobarbitone. J Parenter Enteral Nutr 1987; 11:208–209.

177. Gleghorn EE, Merritt RJ, Subramanian N, Ramos A. Phenobarbital does not prevent total parenteral nutrition-associated cholestasis in noninfected neonates. J Parenter Enteral Nutr 1986; 10:282–283.

178. Berger HM. Phenobarbital therapy and parenteral nutrition. (Letter) J Parenter Enteral Nutr 1987; 11:331.

179. Sandler RH, Maller ES, Meyers AF, Snyder JD, Kleinman RE. Use of ursodeoxycholic acid (UDCA) for children with severe liver disease from total parenteral nutrition (TPN): report of three cases. (Abstract) Pediatr Res 1989; 25:124.

180. Li SJ, Nussbaum MS, McFadden DW, Gapen CL, Dayal R, Fischer JE. Addition of glucagon to total parenteral nutrition (TPN) prevents hepatic steatosis in rats. Surgery 1988; 104:350–357.

181. Cooper A, Ross AJ III, O'Neill JA, Bishop HC, Templeton JM Jr, Ziegler MM. Resolution of intractable cholestasis associated with total parenteral nutrition following biliary irrigation. J Pediatr Surg 1985; 20:772–774.

182. Enzenauer RW, Montrey JS, Baria PJ, Woods J. Total parenteral nutrition cholestasis: a cause of mechanical biliary obstruction. Pediatrics 1985; 76:905–908.

PART 21

Vascular Disorders Involving the Liver

James A. O'Neill Jr., M.D.

The various disorders of the vascular tree that relate to the liver may be categorized as congenital and acquired. In the congenital group, a variety of vascular tumors and hamartomas are encountered. The prime consideration in the acquired category is portal hypertension in its various forms.

CONGENITAL VASCULAR TUMORS AND HAMARTOMAS

Many hemangiomas of the liver are localized lesions that are small enough to be of no clinical significance. They do not appear to have long-term malignant potential. At times, however, large localized hemangiomas, even though benign, present as abdominal masses of such size that hepatic resection is in order. In addition, some of these lesions have a tendency to rupture and bleed spontaneously into the abdomen. Schwartz and Husser have recently described a series of adults with localized hemangiomas and other pathologic variants of hemangioma that necessitated resection.[1] The same general considerations are true in childhood, as it is not possible to predict which lesions will demonstrate growth and which will remain static in size. About 20 percent of patients with vascular lesions of the liver also have cutaneous hemangiomas that usually display parallel rates of growth. Hemangiomas of a localized nature are invariably benign, but, on rare occasions in older children and adults, transformation to hemangioendotheliosarcoma occurs.

At times, hemangiomatous malformations exist throughout the entire liver, in which case the pathology is invariably hemangioendothelioma. These lesions are rarely localized, and patients who have them present with massive hepatomegaly and progressive congestive heart failure. Although occasional patients demonstrate spontaneous regression when treated with digitalis alone, the majority, particularly those who present within the first 6 months of life, present significant clinical problems. The typical presentation is one of massive hepatomegaly, severe congestive heart failure, cutaneous hemangiomas that demonstrate progressive growth, and, frequently, marked thrombocytopenia.[2,3] In our experience, females have this problem more often than males.

Diagnosis

Whether patients have localized hemangiomas or generalized hemangioendotheliomatosis, the typical clinical picture mentioned above and the co-existence of cutaneous hemangiomas are strong indications that the hepatic lesion is vascular in nature. Although serum alpha-fetoprotein is frequently elevated in infants with vascular lesions of the liver, it is not specific and may indicate the presence of hepatoblastoma just as well. Radiologic studies are the most helpful ones. Plain films of the chest and abdomen may demonstrate widespread calcification within the liver. Although calcification may be noted with malignant hepatoblastoma, it is not distributed in the same pattern as generalized hemangioendotheliomatosis calcification. Although abdominal ultrasonography may confirm that the pathology is in the liver it is not necessarily specific to the type of pathology present. On real-time ultrasonography there may be indications of aortic and portal venous enlargement as well as enlargement of the hepatic veins indicative of arteriovenous shunting within the liver, but this, too, is not specific, as it may be noted as well in patients who have malignant lesions. The various types of radionuclide studies have not been helpful to us except perhaps as an indication that the process may be localized rather than generalized. We have found other studies such as arteriography to be more specific in this regard. However, in the last 5 years we have tended to use arteriography for therapeutic reasons only, as described below, and have replaced this study for diagnostic purposes with computed tomographic (CT) scanning. Our method of utilizing CT for diagnosis and follow-up of patients with infantile hemangioendothelioma of the liver has been described by Mahboubi et al.[5] The CT is performed first without contrast and then with bolus contrast injection. Three image patterns have been seen in our patients with hepatic hemangioendothelioma that have not been noted in patients with hepatoblastoma or hepatocellular carcinoma. The unenhanced CT of the liver shows areas of diminished density that occupy almost the entire liver, and in most of these patients only minimal normal liver tissue is seen. Following bolus injection of intravenous contrast material, a pattern of contrast enhancement leading from the periphery toward the center of the lesion is seen, followed shortly by enhancement in the center of some of the lesions and, finally, after a 10-minute delay, essentially complete isodense filling of the liver is seen.

Treatment

For localized hemangiomas of the liver, we have preferred to perform exploration and either biopsy or resection in order to be certain of the nature of the lesion. All such patients have been symptomatic and have presented with large abdominal masses. Since the chance of malignancy in an infant under the age of 1 year of age who presents with a large hepatic mass is close to 80 percent, we have not thought that simple observation should be performed, even though we have had a strong suspicion of benign hemangioma from the pattern of the CT. There simply has not been sufficient experience with this study to permit a specific preoperative histologic diagnosis. On rare occasions, we have found it beneficial to use hepatic arteriography and hepatic artery embolization in order to reduce the size and vascularity of some localized lesions preoperatively. In our series of more than 30 patients with localized benign hemangiomas of the liver treated by resection, there has not been any mortality.

The management of widespread multinodular hemangiomas or hemangioendotheliomas of the liver is much more difficult. We have found that the clinical course of these patients is quite variable. Unfortunately, even though these lesions are histologically benign, mortality has been reported to be as high as 70 percent. Death usually results from high-output cardiac failure secondary to extensive arteriovenous shunting within the tumor. Respiratory failure, hepatic failure, disseminated intravascular coagulation, and marked hemorrhage may be contributory to mortality despite replacement with blood products, platelets, and aggressive treatment of cardiac failure. Surgical resection is not an option because of the diffuse nature of the lesions in both lobes of the liver.

One of the first forms of treatment used in patients like this was radiation therapy.[6] Doses have ranged from 350 to 1,500 cGy. It is difficult to evaluate the value of radiotherapy, but most people who have dealt with this lesion have not found it to contribute significantly to the welfare of these patients. However, it has been difficult to be certain about this, since these patients have usually been treated with a number of other agents at the same time because of the critical nature of their disorder. Five of our 16 patients with widespread hepatic hemangioendotheliomatosis were treated with radiotherapy, and we were not able to demonstrate any specific benefit.[2] In addition, one of our patients with hepatic hemangioendothelioma treated with radiotherapy developed fatal leukemia 12 years later.

Chemotherapy has also been used but with mixed success. We treated one patient with doxorubicin with no effect. We, as well as others, have used cyclophosphamide with some suggestion that it may have induced regression.

In 1970, Touloukian first reported the use of prednisone in a patient with hepatic hemangioendothelioma during infancy, basing his use of the drug on the 1967 report by Zarem and Edgerton of successful treatment of juvenile hemangiomas of the skin with prednisone in several patients.[7,8] We have found prednisone therapy in association with treatment of the congestive heart failure to be quite helpful and have used steroids as the initial treatment in all patients over the last 10 years. We have found that most hemangiomas tend to progress during the first year of life, only to regress thereafter. The steroids appear to accelerate the rate of involution of hepatic hemangioendothelioma in our experience, but not in all patients.

In 1967, deLorimier et al reported the use of hepatic artery ligation in a patient with extensive hepatic hemangiomatosis.[9] This method of treatment of giant hemangioma of the liver with heart failure was also found to be beneficial by Laird et al, Moazam et al, and others.[10,11] However, once again, hepatic artery ligation did not always produce resolution of the process, and some patients died from the procedure because the performance of hepatic artery ligation in an infant with a huge liver, severe respiratory impairment, uncontrollable heart failure, and a coagulopathy is a surgical undertaking with high associated mortality. We have also used hepatic artery ligation in the past with improvement in congestive heart failure and resolution of the hepatic hemangioendothelioma.

Hepatic artery ligation has been replaced by us and others with selective hepatic arteriography and embolization with polyvinyl sponge particles, silicone balloons, and, more recently, wire coils.[12] We use this procedure only in patients who have failed treatment with steroids.

We have found that occasional patients are resistant even though successful occlusion of the hepatic artery has been accomplished. We believe that this is because we have been able to demonstrate that in some patients the primary vascular supply to the tumor is via the portal vein rather than the hepatic artery.[2]

The protocol that we recommend for patients suspected to have hepatic hemangioendotheliomatosis is as follows: After obtaining plain chest and abdominal radiographs and ultrasonography of the liver, CT with contrast is performed in order to differentiate hepatic hemangioma or hemangioendothelioma from hepatoblastoma. The presence of alphafetoprotein is more indicative of a malignant than a benign lesion, but is not specific. Once the diagnosis of hepatic hemangioendothelioma is made, we recommend the use of prednisone for patients who have massive hepatomegaly, congestive heart failure, and respiratory impairment. If symptoms progress despite steroid therapy, hepatic arteriography and embolization are performed, but if hepatic arteriography demonstrates portal venous flow to be the primary source of blood supply to the tumor, hepatic artery occlusion is unlikely to help. It is under these circumstances that we would resort to either radiotherapy or cyclophosphamide or both. For the rare patients who do not respond to this complete sequence of treatment, the only therapy we can envision at this time is transplantation of the liver. Fortunately, the majority of patients have resolution of symptoms and involution of the process. We recommend ultrasound follow-up at 6-month intervals thereafter, since we have seen one patient successfully treated with prednisone who later developed hemangioendotheliosarcoma.[13] Although the tumor was located throughout both lobes of the liver initially, the malignant process was localized in the left lobe of the liver in this patient.

PORTAL HYPERTENSION

Portal hypertension is a sporadic problem of childhood that presents a significant clinical challenge. The etiologies, approaches, and timing of approaches to management of children with portal hypertension are different from those same considerations in adults. In adults, the prime cause of portal hypertension is some form of cirrhosis, whereas a common etiology in childhood is extrahepatic portal obstruction, usually due to portal vein thrombosis (Table 1). However, increasing numbers of children are now surviving initial operation for biliary atresia so that the incidence of cirrhosis in childhood is rising. Portal hypertension in childhood may be categorized as follows in their relative order of frequency:

TABLE 1
Etiology of Portal Hypertension

Extrahepatic
Subhepatic—portal vein thrombosis due to a congenital anomaly or acquired from omphalitis, umbilical venous catheter, splenic vein thrombosis due to portal phlebitis
Suprahepatic (Budd-Chiari syndrome)—hepatic venous or inferior vena caval obstruction due to a congenital anomaly or acquired from trauma, tumor, clotting disorders, oral contraceptive drugs, primary pulmonary hypertension

Intrahepatic
Cirrhosis acquired from viral hepatitis, biliary atresia, metabolic diseases, mucoviscidosis, alpha$_1$-antitrypsin deficiency, congenital hepatic fibrosis, and other disorders

extrahepatic portal hypertension due to portal vein thrombosis, intrahepatic portal hypertension due to parenchymal liver disease, splenic vein thrombosis, and suprahepatic venous obstruction (Budd-Chiari syndrome).

Patients with extrahepatic portal hypertension generally have no definitive history, but occasionally a history of oomphalitis, umbilical rash and infection, or use of an umbilical venous catheter during the neonatal period is obtained. Those patients who present with bleeding esophageal varices related to cirrhosis or intrahepatic portal hypertension usually have a history of viral hepatitis, biliary atresia, neonatal jaundice, metabolic disease, or cystic fibrosis. It is much more common to obtain a history suggestive of etiology in patients with intrahepatic portal hypertension than in those with portal vein thrombosis.

Clinical Presentation

The most common presenting problem we have seen in a series of 42 children with portal hypertension over the last 15 years was upper gastrointestinal (GI) bleeding, which occurred in 80 percent of the patients. Pinkerton et al reported this same finding in 70 percent of his patients.[14] In our patients with cirrhosis, the onset of bleeding ranged from 1.5 to 5 years, with a mean of 3 years, whereas patients with extrahepatic portal hypertension presented with bleeding between 3 and 7 years of age, with a mean of 4.5 years. In addition, the intensity of the bleeding tended to be more severe in patients with cirrhosis than in those with portal vein occlusion. Children with intrahepatic portal hypertension generally also have disorders of coagulation when they present with bleeding. Bloody vomitus and tarry stools are characteristic of serious bleeding, whereas tarry stools in the absence of hematemesis generally indicate slow and lesser degrees of bleeding. Clatworthy and Boles, among others, have shown in their extensive series of patients that splenomegaly in the absence of any other signs or symptoms is the presenting feature of portal hypertension in approximately 25 percent of children with this problem.[15] Hypersplenism manifested by thrombocytopenia and neutropenia may become evident in those who have splenomegaly associated with portal vein thrombosis for several years. However, it is of interest that bleeding and infection related to the thrombocytopenia and neutropenia are distinctly rare. For this reason splenectomy is not indicated for hypersplenism alone, since many patients develop spontaneous portosystemic collaterals and gradually have resolution of the hypersplenism; the same is true of those patients who have shunt procedures performed. Clinically evident ascites is generally a later manifestation of cirrhosis and end-stage liver disease, but it is of interest that Clatworthy and Boles first described ascites as a presenting sign of portal hypertension in infants with acute portal venous obstruction.[15] This latter condition was found to be a transient early phenomenon clearing after a year or so.

Upper GI hemorrhage following an upper respiratory infection is characteristic of patients with portal vein thrombosis, but it does not appear to be causally related to initiating hemorrhage in patients with cirrhosis. It has clearly been demonstrated that aspirin administration to patients with portal hypertension tends to produce hemorrhage, so its use is contraindicated.

Enlargement of the liver as a clinical finding is generally seen only in patients with intrahepatic portal hypertension, since the liver in patients with portal vein thrombosis is normal.

Diagnosis

When a child suspected of having portal hypertension presents with hemorrhage, initial laboratory studies should include complete blood count with platelet and differential white blood cell counts, electrolytes, glucose, liver function tests, and coagulation studies. Patients with cirrhosis tend to have disordered coagulation, electrolyte disturbances, and mild abnormalities of liver function tests. In contrast, the child with portal vein thrombosis usually has normal liver function tests and mild manifestations of hypersplenism, although coagulation studies are usually normal.

Conventional chest radiographs should be performed in order to rule out aspiration of blood in children who have suffered extensive upper GI hemorrhage. In controlled situations, we perform a barium esophagram, as it is capable of accurately demonstrating the presence of esophageal varices 70 percent of the time. We perform endoscopy on all patients with upper GI hemorrhage using a flexible scope, attempting to visualize the esophagus, stomach, and duodenum. This technique appears to be 95 percent accurate in demonstrating varices when they are the cause of bleeding.

Liver-spleen scan with technetium is useful for evaluating hepatic function and perfusion. Ultrasonography and CT may also be used for this purpose. We have deferred the use of angiography until surgical intervention is contemplated. The goal of angiographic evaluation of patients with portal hypertension is to determine the site of portal venous obstruction if present, the anatomy and distribution of collaterals, the dynamics of portal flow, and the adequacy of available portal tributaries for shunting procedures. Celiac and superior mesenteric arteriography followed through the venous phase is our preference for patients with cirrhosis or other forms of intrahepatic portal hypertension. In these instances, the spleen is generally not so large that it traps contrast material to the extent that it does not permit adequate opacification of the portal venous tree. Superior mesenteric arteriography generally demonstrates the superior mesenteric vein and the central portions of the portal and splenic veins clearly enough to determine their size and adequacy for shunting. However, in those instances of extrahepatic portal hypertension due to portal or splenic vein thrombosis associated with extensive splenomegaly, even selective splenic arteriography may not be sufficient to adequately visualize the splenic and associated veins.

Our preference under these circumstances is splenoportography, which we have performed under either heavy sedation or general anesthesia without any problem.[16] It is important to demonstrate normal coagulation parameters prior to performing percutaneous puncture of the spleen for performance of splenoportography. We prefer to evaluate all patients who are going to require operation with arteriography or splenoportography, but on rare emergent occasions we have not been able to perform such studies ahead of time. In these rare instances, we have performed operative mesenteric venography with a single exposure film, as this sort of study is capable of adequately demonstrating at least the superior mesenteric and portal veins, but not the splenic vein. In patients with extrahepatic portal hypertension, we have also found splenoportography to be helpful in that this procedure permits measurement of splenic pulp pressure, which, when elevated in excess of 300 mm of saline, indicates portal hypertension. We have found that the only reliable method of demonstrating splenic vein thrombosis is splenoportography.

The Budd-Chiari syndrome, which is hepatic vein thrombosis or suprahepatic caval obstruction, is exceedingly rare in childhood but when encountered is best studied by means of transjugular hepatic venography.[17]

Percutaneous needle biopsy has been helpful in those patients thought to have intrahepatic forms of portal hypertension, again provided that adequate precautions have been taken regarding evaluation of the patient's coagulation status. This technique, combined with contrast radiography of the portal venous tree, has generally been capable of determining the cause of the patient's portal hypertension and has served as a guide to treatment.

Treatment

Extrahepatic Portal Hypertension

Emergency management of these patients, who first present with upper GI hemorrhage, includes blood and blood component replacement as required, bed rest, sedation, and nasogastric suction. Generally this is sufficient to stop bleeding in the majority of instances, but occasionally bleeding is persistent and may require placement of a Sengstaken-Blakemore tube. An additional measure to control bleeding is intravenous administration of vasopressin with an infusion rate of 0.1 to 0.2 units per milliliter per kilogram per minute titrated according to the patient's pulse rate and skin circulation. Once bleeding has been controlled, the dose is tapered. Although vasopressin was initially infused into the superior mesenteric artery as described by Baum and Nusbaum, we now prefer intravenous administration of this drug, as it appears to be just as effective and certainly simpler to administer in this fashion.[18] Operative intervention during an acute bleeding episode in patients with extrahepatic portal hypertension is rarely required. As shown by Fonkalsrud, approximately 25 percent of patients with portal vein thrombosis develop spontaneous venous collaterals sufficient to permit long-term nonoperative management.[19] This leaves 75 percent of patients who require some form of operative treatment.

We prefer to operate on an elective or semielective basis, so intravenous infusion of vasopressin has been extremely helpful in terms of carrying patients through bleeding episodes in order to allow for preoperative preparation. Some patients with extrahepatic portal hypertension are unshuntable either because they are considered to be too small and not to have adequate venous channels for construction of a shunt or because they have sufficient degrees of portal phlebitis to have suffered occlusion of widespread areas within the portal tree. We also believe that patients with active portal phlebitis are poor candidates for shunting procedures, as they have a tendency to clot their shunts as well. Occasional patients who have failed various shunting procedures may also reach a nonshuntable state. For these various reasons, over time a number of operative procedures have been developed to directly attack bleeding varices; unfortunately, these nonshunt procedures generally fail in our experience and that of others.[17] Since bleeding invariably recurs following the performance of splenectomy alone in patients with portal vein thrombosis, this approach is no longer used. Transesophageal ligation of varices and the Sugiura procedure, which involves esophageal transection, splenectomy, and extensive devascularization of the lower esophagus and stomach, do appear to be adequate temporizing measures, but we have found that rebleeding invariably occurs.[20,21] In our hands, the best temporizing direct approach has been transabdominal ligation of the varices associated with gastric devascularization. We have also found that in the occasional patient in whom no shunt procedure is possible, esophagogastrectomy with total esophagectomy and colon interposition is capable of providing a good long-term result. If total esophagectomy is not performed, bleeding eventually recurs. It should be emphasized that nonshunt procedures should be performed only when there is no other alternative. In 1979, Terblanche et al and subsequently others reported success with endosclerosis performed at the time of endoscopy.[22] We have found this procedure to be particularly useful in patients with cirrhosis, but on long-term follow-up, bleeding has recurred in our patients, in many instances because of the presence of varices in the stomach which are not amenable to injection therapy. Other temporizing measures that we have used include splenic artery ligation and partial splenic embolization.

A variety of shunt procedures are available for patients with extrahepatic portal hypertension, but generally portacaval shunt is not possible, since that vein is not patent in most patients. We prefer to temporize in patients with extrahepatic portal hypertension for two reasons. First, some patients may form sufficient spontaneous collaterals to have resolution of hemorrhage over time. Second, as originally suggested by Clatworthy, shunts have a higher rate of patency if they can be constructed of veins larger than 1.0 cm in diameter.[23] Even though vascular techniques have improved since his original reports, permitting smaller shunts to remain open, such shunts may not carry sufficient flow to adequately decompress the portal tree for long periods of time. Originally we and most others preferred the central splenorenal shunt with splenectomy, but since it has become known that splenectomy may be followed by overwhelming infection, we have preferred other types of shunting procedures. These include the Clatworthy cavomesenteric shunt, the H-type interposition mesocaval shunt with autogenous internal jugular vein, and the distal splenorenal shunt described by Warren and Zeppa.[23-25] On occasion, makeshift shunts have been devised in patients with venous abnormalities or absent kidneys. Martin has described a method of performing portacaval shunting in patients with extrahepatic portal hypertension, but we have not found this to be feasible in most instances.[26] Since recurrent postoperative bleeding has been less of a problem in patients in whom we have performed either cavomesenteric or interposition H-graft mesocaval shunts as described by Drapanas, we have preferred these procedures.[24]

Recently, we have attempted to perform selective distal splenorenal shunting without splenectomy when technically feasible, since it is designed to preserve portal flow to the liver while shunting varices into the systemic venous tree via the spleen and its distal vein, thus theoretically having a lesser incidence of portal encephalopathy associated with it. The exact incidence of this latter problem, while originally suggested to be high by Voorhees and Price, has not been borne out in the experience of most individuals, including ourselves.[27,28] The selective distal splenorenal shunt of Warren and Zeppa is more technically demanding, and when it fails, bleeding episodes may be much more severe. Because of the variability of the anatomy and pathology of the portal tree in patients with extrahepatic portal hypertension, it is important to have a variety of shunt procedure options available. Additionally, technical factors are the key to the achievement of a successful shunt procedure. We strongly believe that prophylactic shunt procedures should not be performed in patients with portal vein thrombosis who have not previously bled.

Intrahepatic Portal Hypertension

Although children with portal vein thrombosis can generally be helped through several bleeding episodes until they are large enough for successful shunting to be accomplished, this is generally not the case in children with cirrhosis and intrahepatic portal hypertension, since they usually bleed at an earlier age and with greater intensity as time progresses. If this is permitted to continue, additional degrees of liver damage may occur. When a patient with bleeding esophageal varices related to cirrhosis presents initially, supportive therapy is initiated and we prefer to use sclerotherapy and infusion of vasopressin as initial therapeutic measures (Table 2). If gastric varices are thought to be present from endoscopic evaluation, injection of the esophageal varices is performed. If bleeding continues, the options include transthoracic or transabdominal ligation of varices in young children or shunt procedures in children who are believed to be of sufficient size for a successful shunt to be performed. We prefer to perform early elective shunts once a pattern of recurrent bleeding has been established, but on occasion we have had to perform emergency shunt procedures during episodes of uncontrollable exsanguinating. Although we have used endosclerosis, variceal ligation, and the Sugiura procedure in

TABLE 2
Various Options in the Management of Portal Hypertension

Direct (temporizing procedures or for unshuntable patients)
Injection sclerotherapy
Transthoracic ligation of esophageal varices
Transabdominal ligation of gastroesophageal varices
Sugiura procedure
Tanner gastric division, esophagogastrectomy
Total esophagectomy with colon replacement
Splenic artery ligation or embolization
Splenectomy
Indirect (definitive procedures)
End-to-side portacaval shunt
Side-to-side portacaval shunt
Central splenorenal shunt with splenectomy
Cavomesenteric shunt (Clatworthy procedure)
H-graft interposition cavomesenteric shunt
Selective distal splenorenal shunt without splenectomy
Makeshift shunts

patients with cirrhosis, all of these patients have rebled in time.

The shunt procedures that we have used have included end-to-side portacaval, side-to-side portacaval, central splenorenal, interposition H-graft mesocaval, cavomesenteric, and selective distal splenorenal shunts. The most effective procedure for prevention of recurrent bleeding has been a portacaval shunt because it has provided the largest-caliber anastomosis in small subjects. Although we have succeeded with the interposition H-graft mesocaval shunt, it has generally taken some time to adapt to higher flow, and decompression of the portal tree has taken longer than with either the portacaval or central splenorenal shunts.

Splenic Vein Thrombosis

This entity has been best managed by splenectomy and disconnection of all collaterals from the spleen to the stomach and esophagus. However, occasional patients have had both splenic vein and associated portal vein thrombosis, and even though splenectomy has been successful initially, portosystemic shunting has eventually been required if it was not performed initially.

Suprahepatic Portal Hypertension

This syndrome may result from obstruction of the hepatic veins anywhere from the afferent branch of a lobule to the entry of the inferior vena cava into the right atrium. This results in hepatic congestion, fibrosis, and ascites. This may also be due to tumors, clotting disorders, trauma, administration of oral contraceptive drugs, or even primary pulmonary hypertension. Takeuchi et al have reported a procedure for resection of congenital webs from the supradiaphragmatic inferior vena cava.[29] If the suprahepatic venous obstruction is accessible, it may be treated either directly by approaching the obstruction or alternately by side-to-side portacaval shunt.

Results of Treatment

We have now treated more than 30 patients with extrahepatic portal hypertension. Ten of these patients required direct attacks on the varices with variceal ligation, the Sugiura procedure, splenic artery ligation, or colon interposition. As a reflection of the efficacy of these procedures, every one of these patients rebled and all but one required reoperation. On the other hand, 29 of these patients have had indirect treatment in the form of various shunt procedures; although nine of these patients had rebleeding, only a single patient has required reoperation, and there have not been any deaths in this series of patients. A single patient had the complication of chylous ascites postoperatively, which required peritoneovenous shunt, but bleeding did not recur. A single patient with splenic vein thrombosis and associated portal vein thrombosis responded very well for 5 years to splenectomy alone but then rebled and required an H-graft interposition mesocaval shunt, and he has since done well.

Sixteen patients have now been treated for intrahepatic forms of portal hypertension. Four of these patients have had either variceal ligation or the Sugiura procedure. All four rebled, and there were five reoperations in this group of four patients. Shunt procedures of various types have been performed on all 16 patients, with one reoperation. Bleeding recurred in eight of the shunted patients, but only one required reoperation. As expected in any series of patients with cirrhosis and progressive liver disease, there have been nine deaths among the 16 patients with inrahepatic forms of portal hypertension. We have not encountered any patients with the Budd-Chiari syndrome.

Injection sclerotherapy has been used extensively in our series of patients over the last 5 years. Although it has been effective initially in most patients, two patients have required emergency shunt procedures, and it is of interest that virtually all of the remaining patients have eventually rebled. We believe that this is because the overwhelming majority of our patients have had associated gastric varices.

Despite the fact that Voorhees and Price reported portal encephalopathy on long-term follow-up of their patients, neither Boles nor we ourselves have noted this problem over long periods of follow-up.[17,27,28] It certainly is a potential problem, however. For this reason, the selective distal splenorenal shunt would theoretically appear to be preferable for the management of patients requiring portosystemic shunt.

REFERENCES

1. Schwartz S, Husser WC. Cavernous hemangioma of the liver. A single institution report of 16 cases. Ann Surg 1987; 205:456–465.
2. Holcomb GW, O'Neill JA, Mahboubi S, Bishop HC. Experience with hepatic hemangioendothelioma in infancy and childhood. J Pediatr Surg 1988; 23:661–666.
3. Dargeon HW, Adiao AC, Pack GT. Hemangioma with thrombocytopenia. J Pediatr 1959; 54:285–295.
4. Jackson C, Greene HL, O'Neill JA, Kirchner S. Hepatic hemangioendothelioma. Angiographic appearance and apparent prednisone responsiveness. Am J Dis Child 1977; 131:74–77.
5. Mahboubi S, Sunaryo FP, Glassman MS, Patel K. Computed tomography in the management and follow-up of infantile hemangioendothelioma of the liver in infants and children. J Comp Tomogr 1987; 11:370–375.
6. Rotman M, John M, Stowe S, Inamdar S. Radiation treatment of pediatric hepatic hemangiomatosis and coexisting cardiac failure. N Engl J Med 1980; 302:852.
7. Touloukian RJ. Hepatic hemangioendothelioma during infancy: pathology, diagnosis and treatment with prednisone. Pediatrics 1970; 45:71–76.
8. Zarem HA, Edgerton MT. Induced resolution of cavernous hemangiomas following prednisolone therapy. Plast Reconstr Surg 1967; 39:76–83.
9. deLorimier AA, Simpson EB, Baum RS, Carlsson E. Hepatic artery ligation for hepatic hemangiomatosis. N Engl J Med 1967; 277:333–337.
10. Laird WP, Friedman S, Koop CE, Schwartz GJ. Hepatic hemangiomatosis. Successful management by hepatic artery ligation. Am J Dis Child 1976; 130:657–659.
11. Moazam F, Rodgers BM, Talbert JL. Hepatic artery ligation for hepatic hemangiomatosis of infancy. J Pediatr Surg 1983; 18:120–123.
12. Burke DR, Verstandig A, Edwards O, Meranze SG, McLean GK, Stein EJ. Infantile hemangioendothelioma: angiography features and factors determining efficacy of hepatic artery embolization. Cardiovasc Intervent Radiol 1986; 9:154–157.
13. Kirchner SG, Heller RM, Kasselberg AG, Greene HL. Infantile hepatic hemangioendothelioma with subsequent malignant degeneration. Pediatr Radiol 1981; 11:42–45.
14. Pinkerton JA, Holcomb GW, Foster JH. Portal hypertension in children. Ann Surg 1972; 175:870–883.
15. Clatworthy HW, Boles ET. Extrahepatic portal bed block in children: pathogenesis and treatment. Ann Surg 1959; 150:371–383.
16. Foster JH, Conkle DM, Crane JM, Burko H. Splenoportography, an assessment of its value and risk. Ann Surg 1975; 179:773–780.
17. O'Neill JA. Portal hypertension in childhood. In: Dean RH, O'Neill JA, eds. Vascular disorders of childhood. Philadelphia: Lea & Febiger, 1983: 142.
18. Baum S, Nusbaum M. The control of gastrointestinal hemorrhage by selective mesenteric arterial infusion of vasopressin. Radiology 1971; 98:479–505.
19. Fonkalsrud EW. Surgical management of portal hypertension in childhood. Long-term results. Arch Surg 1980; 115:1042–1045.
20. Crile G. Transesophageal ligation of bleeding esophageal varices. Arch Surg 1950; 61:654–660.
21. Sugiura M, Futagawa S. Further evaluation of the Sugiura procedure in the treatment of esophageal varices. Arch Surg 1977; 112:1317–1321.
22. Terblanche J, Northover JM, Bornman P, Kahn D, Barbezat GO, Sellars SL, Saunders SJ. A prospective evaluation of injection sclerotherapy in the treatment of acute bleeding from esophageal varices. Surgery 1979; 85:239–245.
23. Clatworthy HW, Wall T, Watman RN. A new type of portal-to-systemic venous shunt for portal hypertension. Arch Surg 1955; 71:588–596.
24. Drapanas T. Interposition mesocaval shunt for treatment of portal hypertension. Ann Surg 1972; 176:435–446.
25. Warren WD, Zeppa R, Fomon JJ. Selective transplenic decompression of gastroesophageal varices by distal splenorenal shunt. Ann Surg 1967; 166:437–455.
26. Martin LW. Changing concepts of management of portal hypertension. J Pediatr Surg 1972; 7:559–562.
27. Voorhees AP, Price JB. Extrahepatic portal hypertension: retrospective analysis of 127 cases and associated clinical implications. Arch Surg 1974; 108:338–341.
28. Boles ET, Birken G. Extrahepatic portal hypertension in children. Long-term evaluation. Chir Pediatr 1983; 24:23–29.
29. Takeuchi J, Takada A, Hasumura Y, Matsuda Y, Ikegami F. Budd-Chiari syndrome associated with obstruction of the inferior vena cava. Am J Med 1971; 51:11–20.

PART 22

Systemic Conditions Affecting the Liver

Christopher B. O'Brien, M.D.

Hepatic involvement by systemic disease in children is not uncommon. Frequently, it is expressed in liver histologic findings as a nonspecific, spotty portal inflammation. Some portal tracts are involved, whereas others are not. In a similar fashion, there can be focal areas of necrosis with associated Kupffer cell hyperplasia. Sometimes scattered steatosis may be evident. This pattern is termed a *reactive hepatitis*. Liver granulomas are also frequent hepatic manifestations of systemic disease outside the liver.

Occasionally, the associated hepatic dysfunction may be the presenting manifestation of an occult disease occurring outside the liver and shows a specific histologic pattern on liver biopsy. This discussion is organized by organ system involved in the primary disease process or by the general class of disease.

THE LIVER IN HEART DISEASE

The clinical syndrome depends upon whether shock is present along with the existence and severity of any underlying congenital heart disease.[1] There are two major presentations depending upon the speed at which the cardiac decompensation develops: acute hepatic ischemia and a more chronic hepatic congestion. Each has different clinical manifestations, opposite patterns of serum liver enzyme abnormalities, and unique histologic findings on liver biopsy.[2] The histologic picture also depends upon the relative balance of the right- and left-sided heart dysfunction. Right-sided heart failure results in a rise in the pressure of the inferior vena cava.[3] This produces distention of the hepatic veins. This in turn leads to sinusoidal *congestion* and hemorrhage, with pressure necrosis of the hepatocytes in acinar zone 3. Left-sided heart failure, in contrast, produces zone 3 liver cell hypoxia leading to necrosis and *collapse* of the reticulin framework, but without swollen sinusoids.[4]

Acute Hepatic Ischemia

This term is probably more descriptive of the pathophysiology present than the more traditional term *acute ischemic hepatitis*. The term *hepatitis* is a misnomer, implying an infectious causation. Acute cardiac decompensation frequently results in liver damage through both right- and left-sided chamber dysfunction. The consequence of left ventricular failure is frequently hypoxia and a decreased cardiac output. Hypoperfusion of the liver with poorly oxygenated blood is a consequence. Combined right ventricular failure results in circulatory stasis within the liver. In addition, there is elevation of the pressure within the sinusoid, resulting in acute pressure necrosis on the hepatocyte.[5]

Clinical Presentation. The child's initial presentation often can simulate an acute viral hepatitis. Tender hepatomegaly is almost uniformly present on physical examination. This finding resolves over a short period of time with improvement in the function of the heart.[1] Blood studies reveal serum transaminases routinely in the thousands; there is often a marked hyperbilirubinemia, and the prothrombin time is typically greatly prolonged.[6]

Differential Diagnosis. This involves a search for viral etiologies, drug-induced hepatotoxicity, and, less frequently, sudden, complete common bile duct obstruction. These include hepatitis A, B, C (non-A, non-B, NANB), D (delta), cytomegalovirus and Epstein-Barr virus serologies, along with a serum and urine toxicology screen.

Histology. Biopsy of the liver reveals centrizonal,[7] focal necrosis with acidophilic hepatocytes. Scant inflammation, usually consisting of polymorphonuclear leukocytes, is present. There can be hemorrhage outside the sinusoids into the hepatocytes. Focal collapse of the perivenular reticulin infrastructure with preservation of the overall acinar architecture is characteristic.

Prognosis. This can be good, and the sine qua non of the diagnosis is the prompt improvement and complete normalization of the serum enzymes during correction of the acute cardiac problem. If the patient has pre-existing liver disease or cirrhosis, then fulminant hepatic failure may ensue.[4]

Chronic Hepatic Congestion

Clinical Presentation. The chronic sequel of congenital heart disease tends to be manifestations of right ventricular failure. The more common presentation is the insidious onset of mildly abnormal serum liver function tests. Tender hepatomegaly is generally present on physical examination early in the clinical course. But with time, cardiac fibrosis follows. The liver then becomes firm and nontender.

Histology. There is a nutmeg pattern on the surface attributable to engorged and hemorrhagic perivenular areas alternating with the paler midzonal regions. Histologically, acinar zone 3 congestion with sinusoidal dilatation and loss of hepatocytes is prominent.[8] If heart failure continues, the hepatic veins show phlebosclerosis with a linkage of the perivenular zone by fibrotic bands that show little inflammation (i.e., reverse lobulation).[9] True cirrhosis is not present.

Prognosis. Prognosis is that of the underlying heart disease.[1]

SARCOIDOSIS AND THE LIVER

Definition and Immunopathogenesis

Sarcoidosis is a chronic multisystem disorder of unknown etiology. There appears to be an aberrant immune response to an unknown stimulus, resulting in the activation and proliferation of helper T cells without a concomitant increase in suppressor T cells.[10] This T-cell proliferation is maintained by the continued release of interleukin 2, the T-cell growth factor.[11] These activated helper T cells release lymphokines that attract and activate monocytes. This causes lymphocytic and monocytic infiltrate. Noncaseating epithelioid granulomas form in the involved tissues.

Sarcoidosis is uncommon in children. A study of 400 patients with sarcoidosis found only 8.5 percent of the patients to be children or adolescents.[12] However, patients as young as 6 months old have been reported.[13]

Clinical Manifestations

All organs in the body can be affected. Most commonly involved are the lung, lymph nodes, and liver. Two subsets of pediatric sarcoidosis exist. Children less than 5 years old tend to have only joint involvement, uveitis, and skin rash.[14] Children ages 8 to 15 years almost always have lung involvement, with the liver, spleen, skin, and eye (uveitis) involved in 30 to 40 percent of cases. Liver involvement, when present, is most frequently asymptomatic, and evidence of synthetic failure, portal hypertension, or ascites is rare. The liver is most often normal in size and texture on palpation.

Hepatic Histology

Liver biopsy reveals granulomas, most often located in the periportal region. They tend to be large and well formed. There is a central zone of eosinophilic necrosis without caseation, encircled by large, basophilic epitheloid cells with an outside rim of lymphocytes and macrophages. Sometimes multinucleated giant cells (nuclei can have either central or peripheral location) are present. The reticulin framework is seen on special stains, in contrast to hepatic tuberculosis. Healing results in an acellular collection of hyaline-like material encircled by fibrosis.[15] (See Tables 1 and 2 for other causes of hepatic granulomas.)

TABLE 1
Infectious Systemic Diseases Associated with Hepatic Granulomas in Children

Viral	**Parasitic**
Cytomegalovirus	Ascariasis
Mononucleosis	Strongyloidiasis
Bacterial	Toxoplasmosis
Actinomycosis	**Fungal**
Histoplasmosis	Aspergillosis
Brucellosis	Candidiasis
Mononucleosis	Cryptococcosis
Tularemia	Histoplasmosis
Listeriosis	**Other**
Nocardiosis	Q fever
Mycobacterial	Syphilis
Tuberculosis	

Modified from MacSween.[15]

TABLE 2
Other Systemic Diseases Associated with Hepatic Granulomas in Children

Chronic granulomatous disease of childhood
Hypogammaglobulinemia
Sarcoidosis
Drug-induced
Allopurinol
Phenytoin
Procarbazine
Sulfonamides

Modified from MacSween.[15]

Treatment

The results of adrenocorticoid administration on liver function and the histologic appearance are unclear. Some authors report improvement, whereas others believe that therapy is ineffective.[5]

CYSTIC FIBROSIS

See Chapter 29, Part 2.

THE LIVER IN ENDOCRINE DISEASES

Thyroid

Hepatic physiology and cellular synthetic activity are under direct control by the thyroid hormones: T_4 (thyroxine) and T_3 (triiodothyrinine). On a molar basis, T_3 is several times more potent than T_4. The liver is the major organ responsible for the peripheral conversion of T_4 to T_3.[16]

Hyperthyroidism. This is associated with abnormal serum liver function tests in 15 to 75 percent of patients.[17] The alkaline phosphatase is most typically elevated, but the bilirubin and transaminases may also be moderately increased.[18] Overt clinical jaundice rarely occurs and is thought to be secondary to high-output heart failure due to the hyperthyroidism. Hepatic histologic findings appear normal on light microscopy. Electron microscopy shows enlarged mitochondria, glycogen depletion, and hypertrophied smooth endoplasmic reticulum.[19]

Hypothyroidism. In congenital hypothyroidism (cretinism), a persistent unconjugated hyperbilirubinemia is found and may persist for several weeks after the initiation of thyroid replacement.[20]

Adrenal Cortex

Cushing's syndrome is often seen to result in steatosis on liver biopsy.[21]

Pancreas

Juvenile Type 1 (Insulin-Dependent) Diabetes Mellitus. During periods of adequate blood glucose control, there tends to be no clinical evidence of liver disease. With diabetic ketoacidosis or during episodes of uncontrolled diabetes, hepatomegaly is often present on physical examination. The edge is tense and tender secondary to the massive influx of glycogen into the liver. Histology demonstrates washed-out, fuzzy hepatocytes secondary to glycogen deposition with vacuolated (glycogenated) nuclei.

NUTRITIONAL LIVER DISEASE

Parenteral Nutrition

Liver disease is frequently encountered in infants receiving total parenteral nutrition (TPN). Although the overall incidence is estimated to be approximately 30 percent,[22,23] it rises to approach 100 percent in premature infants maintained on TPN for longer than 90 days.[24,25] In addition to the duration of TPN, other risk factors include low birth weight, presence of sepsis, other pre-existing types of liver disease, and recent surgery. (See Chapter 28, Part 20.)

Clinical Manifestations. The time course of the hepatic injury can be divided into early and late disease.[24,26] Early disease, which is predominantly cholestatic, occurs about 2 to 3 weeks after the start of TPN and is characterized by an increase in the conjugated bilirubin and the 5′-nucleotidase. If the TPN is stopped at this point, the bilirubin returns promptly to normal and the late form of the liver disease does not occur. However, if it is necessary to continue the TPN, then transaminases progressively rise after about 6 to 8 weeks. With continued TPN, signs of hepatic dysfunction develop and permanent hepatic damage including fibrosis and cirrhosis finally results.[24,27]

Proposed Theories. There have been many theories proposed to explain the mechanism of TPN-induced liver disease. Most of the earlier theories have been disproven by improvements in the composition of the present TPN solutions.[24]

More recently, investigators have believed that either amino acid excess, deficiency, or imbalance could result in neonatal liver disease. Carnitine and taurine are nonessential amino acids that are usually not added to TPN solutions. A relative deficiency of carnitine would lead to inadequate fatty acid oxidation.[28] Similarly, neonates who become deficient in taurine are unable to form taurocholic acid and have decreased bile flow with cholestasis.[29]

On the other hand, Vileisis et al found that infants receiving TPN solutions with a high protein concentration developed cholestatic jaundice earlier and achieved a significantly greater peak direct bilirubin than those receiving low-protein concentrations.[22]

Watkins et al suggested that hepatic canalicular excretory function is not well developed and demonstrated a diminished bile acid pool and bile acid synthetic rate in these infants.[33] Fouin-Fortunet et al noted that elevated levels of lithocholic acid (a hepatotoxic bile acid) were found only in children who developed TPN-associated liver disease.[30]

Finally, Rager and Finegold have suggested that fasting, with the lack of the normal gastrointestinal stimuli (including cholecystokinin secretion) for bile formation and bile flow, may be the primary mechanism involved.[31]

Histology. Cholestasis is a universal finding on liver biopsies. The portal areas become edematous and expanded with increased fibrous tissue. This can progress to portal-portal bridging. Bile duct proliferation occurs in the severely involved cases. Almost all children show a pericholangitis consisting of granulocytes and mononuclear cells.

Prognosis and Treatment. The best treatment is prevention by limiting the duration of TPN support in the high-risk situations mentioned earlier. Once abnormal serum liver function tests are noted, TPN should be stopped if at all possible. Some research suggests that the simultaneous administration of oral intake, if at all possible, or intravenous cholecystokinin (CCK) may prevent the onset of this complication. The chance for return toward normal liver function and histology is dependent upon the duration of the TPN and the amount of damage sustained.

Obesity

On biopsy, the liver shows macrovesicular fatty change in acinar zone 3. Rarely, the liver can show changes of steatohepatitis.[32] This was thought until recently to be a disease

TABLE 3
Systemic Diseases Associated with Steatosis of the Liver in Children

Microvesicular
Drug hepatotoxicity
Vitamin A
Tetracycline
Valproic acid
Salicylates (Reye's syndrome)
Metabolic
Congenital hyperammonemia syndromes and urea cycle disorders
Zellweger's syndrome (cerebrohepatorenal syndrome)
Disorders of fatty acid oxidation
Macrovesicular
Drug hepatotoxicity
Methotrexate
Fetal alcohol syndrome
Adrenocorticosteroids
Nutritional
Obesity
Kwashiorkor
Metabolic
Abetalipoproteinemia
Galactosemia
Glycogen storage diseases (especially type 1)
Tyrosinemia
Wilson's disease
Homocystinurea

Modified from Sherlock.[5]

seen only in adult patients. However, Moran et al reported three obese children who presented with mild abdominal pain and abnormal serum liver function tests. On liver biopsy, the patients had macrovesicular steatosis and scattered polymorphonuclear leukocytes with early portal-portal bridging fibrosis. This can mimic alcoholic hepatitis.

Kwashiorkor Syndrome

The liver in these children on biopsy demonstrates extensive, acinar zone 1, macrovesicular steatosis. (See Table 3 for other causes of steatosis in children; see also Chapter 41, Part 2.)

THE LIVER IN CONNECTIVE TISSUE DISEASES

The connective tissue diseases rarely affect the liver. The presence of significant histologic change has not, for the most part, been documented.

Juvenile Rheumatoid Arthritis (JRA or Still's Disease)

Secondary to JRA Alone. The acute, febrile, systemic type of JRA occasionally results in mild abnormalities of serum liver function tests, particular the transaminases.[33] Histologic examination of the liver demonstrates a mild, nonspecific, reactive change.[34,35]

Secondary to Drugs Used to Treat. See Chapter 28, Part 6.

Salicylates. Overt liver disease, however, is more frequently associated with the drugs used for treatment of the juvenile rheumatoid arthritis. Salicylate therapy is the treatment most frequently given and implicated in drug toxicity of two different types. The first is a toxic hepatitis characterized by transaminase elevation. Some authors find this to be common, with 25 to 65 percent of their patients demonstrating abnormal serum liver function.[36,37] Female children are more frequently involved than are male children. The aspartate aminotransferase (AST) is often twice the alanine aminotransferase (ALT). There is minimal alkaline phosphatase and 5′-nucleotidase elevation. Although frequently mild, the hepatitis can be severe with a prolonged prothrombin time and encephalopathy.[38] Liver biopsies in this group of patients show focal necrosis and a lymphocytic infiltrate of the portal regions.[33]

If there is only mild transaminase elevation with no prolongation of the prothrombin time, the salicylates can be maintained. The serum liver function tests of most patients in this group return to normal despite continuation of therapy. Marked elevation of the transaminases associated with prolongation of the prothrombin time mandate a termination of the salicylate therapy.

The second and much more rare complication is the development of Reye's syndrome (see Chapter 28, Part 18).[39]

Methotrexate. Methotrexate has also been occasionally administered for juvenile rheumatoid arthritis unresponsive to conventional therapy. Some hepatotoxicity has been demonstrated.[40]

Systemic Lupus Erythematosus

Typically, serum liver function tests are normal in children with systemic lupus erythematosus. Some investigators, however, have found poorly characterized hepatic functional abnormalities on more sophisticated testing (i.e., fasting serum bile acid levels and the Bromsulphalein excretion test).[41] Although more serious forms of liver disease have been reported, it is not clear what contribution hepatitis C (NANB) played in those patients.

Similar to juvenile rheumatoid arthritis, Reye's syndrome has been reported in children with systemic lupus erythematosus treated with aspirin.[42]

Finally, it must be emphasized that the autoimmune form of chronic active hepatitis ("lupoid" hepatitis) is not part of the multiorgan involvement in systemic lupus erythematosus. There is recent confirmation that the two diseases are immunologically discrete entities.[43]

HEMATOLOGIC DISEASES

Sickle Cell Anemia

Liver disease associated with sickle cell anemia is frequently multifactorial.[44] The first process is often a posttransfusion, acquired, chronic viral hepatitis. The viruses most frequently involved are hepatitis C (NANB) and hepatitis B. The spectrum of liver involvement is the same as in those children without sickle cell anemia.

The second process is specific for sickle cell anemia. This is characterized by markedly increased direct and indirect bilirubin, a prolonged prothrombin time, but only mild to moderate transaminase elevation. The child may even be mildly transaminase elevation. The child may even be mildly encephalopathic.[45] Liver biopsy demonstrates the characteristic findings of sickled erythrocytes within the sinusoids. This is most prominent around the perivenular area. Sinusoidal congestion results, and prominent zone 2 necrosis and cholestasis (including bile plugs) are present. In contrast to chronic passive congestion (see heart disease section earlier), the sinusoidal engorgement is panacinar and not just zone 3. There is Kupffer cell hyperplasia. These phagocytes can be seen to contain phagocytosed erythrocytes and ceroid. There can be "capillarization" of the sinusoids. This is a pathologic basement membrane that forms and produces functional obstruction of the fenestrations of the hepatocytes. There is steatosis related to the underlying anemia.[9]

The Kupffer cells also phagocytize hemosiderin. This stems from the massive number of transfusions that some of these patients receive. Secondary hemosiderosis requiring iron chelation therapy has been reported and can be found in any child requiring chronically a considerable number of blood transfusions.[46]

Finally, calcium bilirubinate pigment gallstones form in 50 to 66 percent of children by their late teens.

Hemolytic Disease of the Newborn

See Chapter 28, Part 8.

Hodgkin's Disease

There are three forms of jaundice associated with Hodgkin's disease. The first is due to tumor cell infiltration and destruction of the portal triads.[47] The second form is Hodgkin's infiltration and resultant obstruction of the major bile ducts. The third form of jaundice associated with Hodgkin's disease is unexplained. Children can have intermittent episodes of jaundice, often occurring prior to the diagnosis of Hodgkin's disease. Histology demonstrates only cholestasis with some nonspecific Kupffer cell hyperplasia.[48]

GRAFT-VERSUS-HOST DISEASE

There are multiple causes of hepatic dysfunction after bone marrow transplantation. Sources of liver damage include a graft-versus-host response, opportunistic infections, posttransfusion virus-induced chronic hepatitis, radiation hepatitis, veno-occlusive disease (azathioprine), and other drug-induced injury in this patient population. Some series find the incidence of graft-versus-host disease (GVHD) to be approximately 80 percent in long-term survivors after allogeneic bone marrow transplantation.[49] (See Chapter 27, Part 7.)

Clinical Presentation. Clinical features of acute GVHD are skin, gastrointestinal tract, and liver disease. Jaundice is manifested in approximately 50 percent of children who develop acute GVHD. The chronic form of GVHD is marked by generalized failure to thrive, with lachrymal and salivary gland injury, skin involvement, and chronic, unremitting liver injury.

Autoimmune Antibodies. Autoimmune antibodies that can be present include antinuclear, anti-smooth muscle, antimitochondrial, anti-liver kidney microsome, and antiepidermal antibodies. Native anti-DNA, anti-extractable nuclear antigen, anticentromere, and anti-salivary gland duct antibodies are not usually present.[53]

Histology. Classic features on liver histology include extensive bile duct disruption and dropout with cytologic aberration of the bile duct epithelium.[50] In addition, there is frequently cholestasis, piecemeal necrosis, and invasion of the vascular endothelium by lymphocytes ("endothelialitis"). The portal inflammation often appears minimal compared to the degree of bile duct damage.[51]

Veno-occlusive disease is often a complicating factor in this group of patients, ensuing in almost 20 percent of a recently described series.[52] The evidence points to pretransplantation chemotherapy and radiation as predisposing factors.[53]

INFLAMMATORY BOWEL DISEASE

Steatosis is found in up to 50 percent of patients with inflammatory bowel disease. Chronic hepatitis associated with inflammatory bowel disease (IBD) was described in the past. In older textbooks this was termed "pericholangitis." Since the advent of endoscopic retrograde cholangiopancreatography (ERCP), it is now apparent that many of these cases were simply the hepatic manifestations of primary sclerosing cholangitis. MacSween believes that this term should no longer be used.[54] (See Chapter 27, Parts 13 and 14.)

Finally, a nonspecific hepatitis has also been reported in children with inflammatory bowel disease. Again, it will be interesting to find out what percentage of the patients with chronic hepatitis thought secondary to IBD actually had drug-induced hepatotoxicity or hepatitis C (NANB).

Drug-induced Hepatotoxicity

Sulfasalazine has also been reported to cause hepatotoxicity in this group of patients.

Primary Sclerosing Cholangitis

This disease is being reported with greater frequency since the use of endoscopic retrograde pancreatography. About three-quarters of the patients have associated ulcerative colitis. There is some suggestion that treatment with ursodiol may be efficacious in improving symptoms and serum liver function tests in this group of patients.[55] It should be noted, however, that all patients studied to date have been adults.

REFERENCES

1. Sivan Y, Nutman J, Zeevi B, Berant M, Levinsky L, Schonfeld T. Acute hepatic failure after open-heart surgery in children. Pediatr Cardiol 1987; 8:127–130.
2. Mace S, Borkat G, Liebman J. Hepatic dysfunction and cardiovascular abnormalities. Occurrence in infants, children and young adults. Am J Dis Child 1985; 139:60–65.
3. Mercado H, Castellanor AW. Wedged hepatic venous pressure in congenital heart disease. Angiology 1979; 30:182–191.
4. Arcieli JM, Moore GW, Hutchins GM. Hepatic morphology in cardiac dysfunction: a clinicopathologic study of 1,000 subjects at autopsy. Am J Pathol 1981; 104:159–166.
5. Sherlock S. Diseases of the liver and biliary system. 8th ed. Oxford: Blackwell Scientific Publications, 1989.
6. Gibson PR, Dudley FJ. Ischemic hepatitis: clinical features, diagnosis and prognosis. Aust N Z J Med 1984; 14:822–825.
7. Shiraki K. Hepatic cell necrosis in the newborn. A pathologic study of 147 cases, with particular reference to congenital heart disease. Am J Dis Child 1970; 119:395–400.
8. Bras G, Brandt KH. Vascular disorders. In: MacSween RN, Anthony PP, Scheuer PJ, eds. Pathology of the liver. 2nd ed. Edinburgh: Churchill Livingstone, 1987:478.
9. Kanel GC, Ucci AA, Kaplan MN, Wolfe HJ. A distinctive hepatic lesion associated with heart failure. Am J Clin Pathol 1980; 73:235–239.
10. Spurzem JR, Saltini C, Crystal RG. Functional significance of anti-T-lymphocyte antibodies in sarcoidosis. Am Rev Respir Dis 1988; 137:600–605.

11. Muller-Quernheim J, Kronke M, Strausz J, Schykowski M, Ferlinz R. Interleukin-2 receptor gene expression by bronchopulmonary lavage lymphocytes in pulmonary sarcoidosis. Am Rev Respir Dis 1989; 140:82–88.
12. Tonitrova NS. [Sarcoidosis in children and adolescents (author's trans)]. Z Erkr Atmungsorgane 1977; 149:P283–285.
13. Esteban-Zurron I, Carmona-Valera JA, Gimenez-Abadia MA, Cabrerizo-Portero D, Lucas-Moreno JM, Castro-Garcia FJ, Peris-Mencheta MD. [Sarcoidosis in childhood. Presentation of a case in a very young child.] An Esp Pediatr 1985; 23:44–50.
14. Hoover KL, Kahn JA, Giangiacomo J. Pediatric ocular sarcoidosis. Surv Ophthalmol 1986; 30:215–282.
15. MacSween RN. Liver pathology associated with diseases of other organs. In: MacSween RN, Anthony PP, Scheuer PJ, eds. Pathology of the liver. 2nd ed. Edinburgh: Churchill Livingstone, 1987:646.
16. Van Thiel DA. The liver and the endocrine system. In: Arias IM, Jokoby WB, Popper H, Schachter D, Shafritz DA, eds. The liver: biology and pathology. 2nd ed. New York: Raven Press, 1988: 1007.
17. Ashkar FS, Miller R, Smoak WM, Gilson AJ. Liver disease in hyperthyroidism. South Med J 1971; 64:462–465.
18. Beckett GJ, Kellett HA, Gow SM, Hussey AJ, Hayes JD, Toft AD. Subclinical liver damage in hyperthyroidism and in thyroxine replacement therapy. Br Med J 1985; 291:427.
19. Dooner HP, Parada J, Aliaga C, Hohl C. The liver in thyrotoxicosis. Arch Intern Med 1967; 120:25–32.
20. Weldon AP, Danks DM. Congenital hypothyroidism and neonatal jaundice. Arch Dis Child 1972; 47:469–471.
21. Soffer LJ, Iannaccone A, Gagrilove JL. Cushing's syndrome: a study of 50 patients. Am J Med 1961; 30:129–146.
22. Vileisis RA, Inwood RJ, Hunt CE. Prospective controlled study of parenteral nutrition–associated cholestatic jaundice: effect of protein intake. J Pediatr 1980; 96:893–897.
23. Postuma R, Trevenen CL. Liver disease in infants receiving total parenteral nutrition. Pediatrics 1979; 63:110–115.
24. Beale EF, Nelson RM, Bucciarelli RL, Donnelly WH, Eitzman DV. Intrahepatic cholestasis associated with parenteral nutrition in premature infants. Pediatrics 1979; 64:342–347.
25. Benjamin DR. Hepatobiliary dysfunction in infants and children associated with long-term total parenteral nutrition. A clinico-pathologic study. Am J Clin Pathol 1981; 76:276–283.
26. Beckett GJ, Glass EJ, Callaghan MO, Elton RA, Hume R. Measuring bile-salt concentrations lacks clinical value for detecting hepatic dysfunction in infants receiving parenteral nutrition. Clin Chem 1985; 31:1168–1171.
27. Rogers BM, Hollenbeck JI, Donnelly WH, Talbert JL. Intrahepatic cholestasis with parenteral alimentation. Am J Surg 1976; 131:149–155.
28. Grant JP, Cox CE, Kleinman LM, Maher MM, Pittman MA, Tangrea JA, Brown JH, Gross E, Beazley RM, Jones RS. Serum hepatic enzyme and bilirubin elevations during parenteral nutrition. Surg Gynecol Obstet 1977; 145:573–580.
29. Watkins JB, Szczepanik P, Gould JB, Klein P, Lester R. Bile salt metabolism in the human premature infant. Gastroenterology 1975; 69:706–713.
30. Fouin-Fortunet H, Le-Quernec L, Erlinger S, Lerebours E, Colin R. Hepatic alterations during TPN in patients with inflammatory bowel disease: a possible consequence of lithocholate toxicity. Gastroenterology 1982; 82:932–937.
31. Rager R, Finegold MJ. Cholestasis in immature newborn infants: is parenteral alimentation responsible? J Pediatr 1975; 86:264–269.
32. Moran JR, Ghishan FK, Halter SA, et al. Steatohepatitis in obese children. A cause of chronic liver dysfunction. Am J Gastroenterol 1983; 78:374.
33. Rachelefsky GS, Kar NC, Coulson A, Sarkissian E, Stiehm ER, Paulus HE. Serum enzyme abnormalities in juvenile rheumatoid arthritis. Pediatrics 1976; 58:730–736.
34. Schaller J. The liver and arthritis. J Pediatr 1971; 79:139–141.
35. Schaller J, Beckwith B, Wedgwood RJ. Hepatic involvement in juvenile rheumatoid arthritis. J Pediatr 1970; 77:203–210.
36. Russell AS, Sturge RA, Smith MA. Serum transaminases during salicylate therapy. Br Med J 1971; 2:428–429.
37. Athreya BH, Moser G, Cecil HS, Myers AR. Aspirin- induced hepatotoxicity in juvenile rheumatoid arthritis. A prospective study. Arthritis Rheum 1975; 18:347–352.
38. Makela AL, Lang H, Korpela P. Toxic encephalopathy with hyperammonaemia during high-dose salicylate therapy. Acta Neurol Scand 1980; 61:146–156.
39. Remington PL, Shabino CL, McGee H, Preston G, Sarniak AP, Hall WN. Reye's syndrome and juvenile rheumatoid arthritis in Michigan. Am J Dis Child 1985; 139:870–872.
40. Truckenbrodt H, Hafner R. Methotrexate therapy in juvenile rheumatoid arthritis: a retrospective study. Arthritis Rheum 1986; 29:801–807.
41. Altomonte L, Zoli A, Sommella L, Palumbo P, Greco AV, Magaro M. Concentration of serum bile acids as an index of hepatic damage in systemic lupus erythematosus. Clin Rheumatol 1984; 3:209–212.
42. Hansen JR, McCray PB, Bale JF, Corbett AJ, Flanders DJ. Reye's syndrome associated with aspirin therapy for systemic lupus erythematosus. Pediatrics 1985; 76:202–205.
43. Gurian LE, Rogoff TM, Ware AJ, Jordan RE, Combes B, Gilliam JN. The immunologic diagnosis of chronic active 'auto-immune' hepatitis: distinction from systemic lupus erythematosus. Hepatology 1985; 5:397–402.
44. Mills LR, Mwakyusa D, Milner PF. Histopathologic features of liver biopsy specimens in sickle cell disease. Arch Pathol Lab Med 1988; 112:2904.
45. Buchanan GR, Glader BE. Benign course of extreme hyperbilirubinemia in sickle cell anemia: analysis of six cases. J Pediatr 1977; 91:21–24.
46. Cohen A, Schwartz E. Iron chelation therapy in sickle cell anemia. Am J Hematol 1979; 7:69–76.
47. Cavalli G, Casali AM, Lambertini F, Busachi C. Changes in the small biliary passages in the hepatic localization of Hodgkin's disease. Virchows Arch 1979; 384:295–306.
48. Perra DR. Cholestasis associated with extrabiliary Hodgkin's disease: report of three cases and review of four others. Gastroenterology 1974; 67:680.
49. Rouquette-Gally AM, Boyeldieu D, Prost AC, Gluckman E. Autoimmunity after allogenic bone marrow transplantation. A study of 52 long-term surviving patients. Transplantation 1988; 46:238–240.
50. Shulman HM, Sharma P, Amos D, Fenster LF, McDonald GB. A coded histologic study of hepatic graft-versus-host disease after human bone marrow transplantation. Hepatology 1988; 8:463–470.
51. Snover DC, Weisdorf ASA, Ramsay NK, McGlave P, Kersey JH. Hepatic graft versus host disease: a study of the predictive value of liver biopsy in diagnosis. Hepatology 1984; 4:123–130.
52. Kojima S, Matsuyama K, Kodera Y. Bone marrow transplantation for hepatitis-associated aplastic anemia. Acta Haematol 1988; 79:7–11.
53. Dulley FL, Kanfer EJ, Appelbaum FR, Amos D, Hill RS, Buckner CD, Shulman HM, McDonald GB, Thomas ED. Veno-occlusive disease of the liver after chemoradiotherapy and autologous bone marrow transplantation. Transplantation 1987; 43:870–873.
54. MacSween RN. Primary sclerosing cholangitis. In: Anthony PP, MacSween RN, eds. Recent advances in histopathology No. 12. Edinburgh: Churchill Livingstone, 1984:158.
55. Podda M, Ghezzi C, Battezzati PM, Bertolini E, Crosignani A, Petroni ML, Zuin M. Ursodeoxycholic acid for chronic liver disease. J Clin Gastroenterol 1988; 10:S25–S31.

PART 23

Chronic Hepatitis

Joseph F. Fitzgerald, M.D.

Chronic hepatitis is a continuous inflammatory hepatopathy that is capable of progression to cirrhosis, liver failure, and death. This process may be initiated by viral infections, defective metabolism, and unknown factors that incite overreaction of immune responsiveness. There are not clinical, biochemical, serologic, or morphologic findings that are pathognomonic of chronic hepatitis. The diagnosis depends on fulfillment of predefined criteria that are arbitrary at best.

Reports of individuals who were afflicted with chronic inflammation of the liver, which was associated with hyperproteinemia and fluctuating icterus, appeared in the medical literature in the fourth and fifth decades of this century.[1,2] The common components of "chronic hepatitis" were outlined in the presentation of Kunkel et al in 1951[3] when they described young women who had an active hepatopathy and accompanying hypergammaglobulinemia, fever, arthralgias, acne, and amenorrhea. Their observations were expanded in 1956,[4] and thereafter women so affected were often referred to as "Kunkel girls." Good[5] observed in 1956 that adolescent females with the manifestations described by Kunkel had an increased number of plasma cells in their portal and periportal zones on microscopic examination of liver biopsies. The appellation "plasma cell hepatitis" was applied briefly to these patients in the history of this disease. The observation of MacKay et al[6] in the same year had a more lasting effect. These investigators found a positive lupus erythematosus cell preparation in a significant number of Kunkel girls. Subsequent immunoserologic findings were thought to have definite etiologic significance. There must have been male patients with chronic hepatitis during this period who did not have autoimmune features or nonspecific immune markers and who did not have an excessive number of plasma cells in their biopsies. The picture became clearer with the discovery of a serologic marker for hepatitis B virus (HBV) infection in the late 1960s. Several reports convincingly established that HBV infection could become chronic and could progress to cirrhosis and death.[7-9] It thus became evident that there are two major groups of patients with chronic hepatitis: one group consisting equally of males and females who have serologic support for chronic HBV disease and a second group, composed mainly of females, who have autoimmune clinical features and nonspecific immune markers in their blood. Two separate reports of pediatric patients with autoimmune chronic hepatitis appeared in the 1970s.[10,11]

DEFINITION

Recognition that standard clinical methodology lacks the preciseness for documentation of chronic liver disease has resulted in increased dependence on duration of illness as a criterion for chronicity. Acute hepatopathies are usually self-limited. Splenomegaly, ascites, encephalopathy, spider nevi, and palmar erythema may accompany an acute insult to the liver,[12] and up to 40 percent of patients with chronic hepatitis experience an abrupt onset of symptoms.[13] Even autoimmune markers such as anti–smooth muscle antibody (ASMA), antimitochondrial antibody (AMA), and antinuclear antibody (ANA), which are so intimately associated with chronic active hepatitis (CAH), may be found in patients with toxic hepatitis, acute viral hepatitis, and extrahepatic obstruction.[14-19] The histologic features that are so important in establishing the diagnosis of CAH may be seen in slowly resolving acute viral hepatitis,[20] and histologic features of acute viral infection such as "ballooning" degeneration, acidophilic cell necrosis, and Kupffer cell hyperplasia may be seen in patients with clinically severe CAH.[21,22] The presence of cirrhosis establishes unequivocally the diagnosis of CAH; however, sampling error may miss this lesion.[22,23]

The above led to dependence on duration of illness as a criterion for chronicity. Clinical and laboratory confirmation of continued hepatic inflammation for at least 10 weeks excludes self-limited acute hepatitis in most instances and supports chronicity.[24] Continuous activity for 6 months establishes unequivocally the unresolving nature of the inflammatory process[25] and fulfills the international criteria for chronic disease.[26,27] Strict adherence to an arbitrary time requirement for the establishment of chronicity, however, diminishes the diagnostic value of clinical, biochemical, immunologic, and histologic findings.[24] The onset of illness is uncertain, more often that not, which may needlessly delay therapy.[28,29] The presence of hypoalbuminemia, marked hypergammaglobulinemia, nonspecific immunoserologic tests (e.g., ANA, ASMA, AMA, or anti–liver kidney microsomal antibody), and ascites in a patient with disease of less than 6 months' duration could justify therapeutic intervention, even though the international criteria for chronicity are not completely fulfilled.

Satisfaction of the time criterion for chronicity does not equate with CAH. The International Association for the Study of Liver, in conjunction with the World Health Organization, recognizes two distinct forms of *chronic hepatitis* based on histologic findings.[26,30] Chronic persistent hepatitis (CPH) is characterized by limitation of the inflammatory round cell infiltrate to the portal tract with no, or minimal, periportal necrosis. Moderate to severe periportal necrosis supports an aggressive process (i.e., CAH).[30] The former is a benign process that does not require therapeutic intervention.

Evaluation of the intraobserver error and sampling variability in the diagnosis of CAH by percutaneous needle biopsy has demonstrated that the consistency of grading the type

TABLE 1
Classification of Chronic Hepatitis

HBsAg-positive chronic hepatitis
HBsAg-negative chronic hepatitis
Autoimmune chronic active hepatitis
Primary biliary cirrhosis
Infectious agents
Non-A, non-B hepatitis viruses
Epstein-Barr virus
Cytomegalovirus
Metabolic/genetic disturbances
Wilson's disease
Alpha$_1$-antitrypsin deficiency
Cystic fibrosis

and degree of hepatic inflammation is 90 percent.[24] Reproducibility of morphologic interpretation by the same observer is 94 percent, and sampling error in assessment of the severity of the necrosis and inflammation is trivial.[23]

ETIOLOGY

Chronic hepatitis is the histologic expression of a variety of distinct disease states. The most pivotal differentiating marker is the presence of hepatitis B surface antigen (HBsAg). This allows the initial segregation of patients into those that are HBsAg-positive and those that are HBsAg-negative (Table 1). The latter group can be further divided into autoimmune, infectious, and metabolic causes. Strong indirect support for the existence of chronic non-A, non-B (NANB) hepatitis was presented by Tabor et al in 1980.[31] The imminent availability of an assay for the identification of circulating antibodies to a major etiologic virus of human NANB hepatitis may identify the true etiology of a number of cases of HBsAg-negative chronic hepatitis.[32] Progression of Epstein-Barr virus and cytomegalovirus hepatitis to CAH has not been demonstrated. CAH has developed in an infant infected with human immunodeficiency virus,[33] but the finding of serologic markers for HBV in both blood and liver suggest that the chronic hepatopathy is due to HBV infection rather than human immunodeficiency virus infection.

Metabolic causes of HBsAg-negative CAH include homozygous protease-inhibitor ZZ (PiZZ) alpha$_1$-antitrypsin deficiency liver disease and Wilson's disease. Heterozygous PiMZ alpha$_1$-antitrypsin deficiency has been found in adults with CAH and cryptogenic cirrhosis.[34]

PATHOGENESIS

The mechanisms involved in the pathogenesis of CAH are incompletely understood, although there is an increasing body of evidence which implicates cellular autoimmune reactions. Early studies demonstrated a common sensitization of peripheral blood lymphocytes, which were obtained from patients with chronic hepatitis, directed against human liver-specific lipoprotein (LSP). This sensitization was less prominent in patients with chronic hepatitis who had received immunosuppressive treatment.[35] Mieli-Vergani et al[36] presented immunologic data in 1979 indicating that lymphocytes from patients with HbsAg-negative CAH generated a cytotoxic response to autologous hepatocytes that were isolated from percutaneous liver biopsies. This cytotoxicity appeared to correlate with disease activity, and it disappeared during immunosuppressive therapy. The addition of excess purified LSP to their microcytotoxicity assay blocked the reaction, indicating that LSP was the major target antigen.

Simultaneous investigations of immunoregulatory function, which was accomplished by measuring in vitro proliferative responses and immunoglobulin synthesis, suggested that suppressor T-cell function was deficient in patients with CAH.[37-41] Nouri-Aria et al[42] detected a severe defect in concanavalin-induced suppressor T-cell activity in 22 patients with HBsAg-negative autoimmune CAH and 26 patients with HBsAg-positive CAH. They found normal values in 21 patients with "autoimmune" hepatitis in whom remission had been induced with prednisolone. They further observed that suppressor T-cell activity was greatly improved when lymphocytes from patients with autoimmune CAH were preincubated with low-dose prednisolone in vitro. No clear effect of prednisolone could be demonstrated when the cells were obtained from patients with HBsAg-positive CAH. Their results suggested that a fundamental difference might exist in the nature of the suppressor T-cell defect in autoimmune and HBsAg-positive forms of CAH. They suggested that suppressor T cells were not deficient in number in autoimmune CAH but that they existed in a functionally defective form and that prednisolone pretreatment stimulated a differentiation step.[42]

Activated suppressor T cells accumulate at the site of hepatocyte injury in patients with chronic HBV infection.[43] This observation would seem to support the importance of lymphocyte-mediated cytolytic mechanisms in the tissue-damaging process. The ratio of helper to suppressor T-lymphocyte subpopulations in the peripheral blood is increased in patients with "autoimmune" CAH,[44] and the ratio of helper to suppressor subpopulations of the mononuclear cell infiltrate in the liver is also greater in patients with autoimmune CAH compared with patients with HBsAg-positive CAH.[45] Interestingly, there is no difference in the helper-to-suppressor ratio in the intrahepatic mononuclear cell infiltrate between patients with autoimmune CAH and those with resolving chronic HBV disease, manifested by the presence of antibody to hepatitis Be antigen (anti-HBe) in their serum.[46]

Lymphocytes from patients with autoimmune CAH generated T-lymphocyte migration inhibitory factors when they were incubated with LSP.[46] These factors were not generated by the lymphocytes of control patients or patients with HBsAg-positive CAH. The generation of T-lymphocyte inhibitory factor activity by T cells from autoimmune CAH patients was suppressed when these cells were co-cultured with T cells from normal subjects or patients with HBsAg-positive CAH but was unaffected when cocultured with T cells from other patients with autoimmune CAH.[46]

These results are consistent with a hypothesis that a defect exists in the specific suppressor T-cell population that controls the immune response to LSP. The loss of T-cell tolerance to LSP cannot be secondary to chronic liver disease, since it is not found in patients with HBsAg-positive CAH, nor is it likely to be a nonspecific consequence of an autoimmune process, since it was not observed in patients with autoimmune thyroid disease.[41] The observation that HBsAg-positive CAH patients had T cells that maintained tolerance to LSP emphasizes the disease specificity of the defect in autoimmune CAH. The presence of an LSP-specific suppressor T-cell defect, uninfluenced by disease activity or treatment, may be of fundamental importance in the pathogenesis of autoimmune CAH. The development of autoimmune CAH, its response to corticosteroid treatment, and the high relapse rate that occurs when steroids are withdrawn, would fit the hypothesis that the disease is triggered in genetically susceptible individuals by agents, including viruses and drugs, that produce a helper T-cell response against an autoantigen that is present in LSP preparations and is expressed on the liver cell membrane.[46] This autoimmune response is then perpetuated by an LSP-specific suppressor T-cell defect and amplified by a generalized suppressor cell defect. The latter may be ameliorated by corticosteroid therapy, but persistence of the LSP-specific defect allows the majority of patients to remount a vigorous autoimmune response when corticosteroid support is withdrawn.[46] Sera from 12 of 13 patients with untreated CAH studied by Larcher et al[47] contained antibodies to LSP. The titer of anti-LSP correlated with the degree of piecemeal necrosis on hepatic biopsy, but not with the degree of the abnormality of standard biochemical tests of liver function or serum immunoglobulin concentrations. The titer of anti-LSP fell as liver damage improved with the institution of immunosuppressive therapy.

Hepatitis B core antigen (HBcAg) is an important target for T-cell cytotoxicity in HBsAg-positive CAH, and it has been demonstrated on the surface of isolated hepatocytes using polyclonal and monoclonal antibodies. This suggests that only hepatocytes with active viral replication that are expressing determinants associated with the inner capsid of HBV are subject to T-cell cytolysis.[48] Patients with HBsAg-positive CAH have a reduced helper T-cell subpopulation.[49] HBV may also infect lymphocytes per se, producing a selective immunodeficiency that results in persistent infection with relatively little hepatocyte damage.[50] Hafez et al[51] found a decreased total T-cell number and a decreased helper-to-suppressor ratio in 19 children with HBsAg-positive CPH. They also noted an increased incidence of HLA-A1 antigen in this patient population compared with 60 normal subjects matched for age and sex. They suggested that genetic influencing of the helper-to-suppressor ratio might affect susceptibility to chronicity in HBV disease.

Patients with autoimmune CAH have been found to have antibodies directed against several normal components of the hepatocyte membrane such as the liver membrane antigen,[52] LSP,[53] and the hepatic asialoglycoprotein receptor known as hepatic lectin.[54] All 14 children with autoimmune CAH studied by Mieli-Vergani et al[55] had circulating antibodies to LSP, as did seven of eight with primary sclerosing cholangitis. In vitro microcytotoxicity assays have shown that patients with autoimmune CAH generate killer (K) lymphocytes that are cytotoxic to autologous hepatocytes. The cytotoxicity is mediated by antibodies to LSP.[36] These patients have increased numbers of circulating activated T-helper cells[56] and decreased antigen-specific and non–antigen-specific T-suppressor function.[46,57,58]

Whether defective suppressor T-cell function is a primary or a secondary phenomenon is unclear, but the former seems likely, since both patients and their HLA haplotype-identical first-degree relatives have defective T-suppressor function.[59] Mieli-Vergani et al[55] found that the number of T lymphocytes bearing HLA-IL2R was markedly increased in autoimmune CAH, irrespective of disease duration, suggesting either a persisting impairment of regulating mechanisms that possibly derive from genetic influences or the presence of a perpetual activating stimulus, or both. The majority of the HLA IL2R–positive T lymphocytes in children with autoimmune CAH express the helper phenotype.[56]

CLINICAL FEATURES

Chronic hepatitis is often insidious in its presentation. Approximately 30 percent of children with chronic HBV disease are asymptomatic, and they are identified by routine screening for HBV infection.[60] Chronic persistent hepatitis is qualitatively similar to acute hepatitis, and symptoms of fatigue, malaise, abdominal pain, and weight loss may precede or accompany the physical signs of icterus, dark urine, light stools, and fever. A mildly tender and enlarged liver may be found. Splenomegaly is unusual, and evidence of advanced liver disease (e.g., ascites, spider nevi, palmar erythema, and encephalopathy) is lacking.

Patients with CAH display more prominent clinical features (Table 2). Subjective complaints can include fatigue, weakness, nausea, and right upper abdominal quadrant discomfort. Objective findings may include fever, icterus, hepatomegaly, splenomegaly, spider nevi, and ascites. Extrahepatic features such as acne, amenorrhea, arthritis, dermatitis, pleurisy, colitis, thyroiditis, parotitis, thrombophlebitis, and diabetes mellitus may accompany autoimmune CAH.[61] A Coombs-positive hemolytic anemia and a tendency toward disseminated intravascular coagulation may be noted.[61] A nonspecific nephritis, indistinguishable from systemic lupus erythematosus, may be observed. Patients with CAH may rarely be encephalopathic at the time of presentation.

TABLE 2
Clinical Features in 38 Children with HBsAg-Negative Chronic Active Hepatitis

Feature	Number
Jaundice	31
Hepatomegaly	29
Malaise	23
Splenomegaly	21
Spider angiomas	11
Arthralgia and/or arthritis	8
Ascites	7
Pruritus	7
Amenorrhea	6
Skin rash	4
Hepatic coma	2
Ulcerative colitis	2
Clubbing	1
Lymphadenopathy	1
Hematuria	1
Thyroiditis	1

The presenting clinical features of 57 children with chronic hepatitis were reviewed by Odievre et al in 1983.[62] Twenty-one of these children had CPH and 36 had CAH by hepatic biopsy. Eighteen of the 21 children with CPH were HBsAg-positive compared with 7 of 36 with CAH. Thirteen of 21 with CPH displayed hepatomegaly, compared with 34 of 36 with CAH. Splenomegaly was noted in 7 of 21 with CPH and 23 of 36 with CAH. The children with CPH were usually asymptomatic and exhibited minimal persistent or recurrent elevations of the aminotransferase levels.

LABORATORY INVESTIGATION

Investigation of patients with chronic liver disease, as with acute liver disease, should be progressive rather than "shotgun." A tiered investigation is outlined on Table 3. Initial laboratory studies should include a complete blood count, platelet count, reticulocyte count, total and fractionated serum bilirubin, aspartate aminotransferase (AST/SGOT), alanine aminotransferase (ALT/SGPT), gamma-glutamyltransferase (GGT), and prothrombin time, to assess hepatic synthetic function. The serum alkaline phosphatase level is of limited value in children owing to the increased levels that accompany bone growth. A picture that suggests hepatocellular dysfunction, manifested by significant elevations of the aminotransferase levels with minimal or no elevation of the GGT, supports a diagnosis of hepatitis. The establishment of chronicity is often difficult, as indicated previously. Chronicity is supported by physical findings such as a firm liver with irregular contour, which is palpable primarily in the epigastrium, splenomegaly, and ascites. Additional findings of chronic liver disease include spider angiomata, muscle wasting, and a low serum albumin.

The next test in sequence is to search for serologic markers of persistent HBV infection (HBsAg, HBeAg, anti-HBc IgM, and IgG). Sjögren and Hoofnagle[63] have demonstrated that 99 percent of patients with HBeAg-positive chronic HBV disease are positive for anti-HBc-IgM.

Elimination of chronic HBV disease leads to the second major tier of tests. Other infectious causes can be eliminated by searching for serologic support for non-A, non-B (NANB) hepatitis,[33] Epstein-Barr virus, and cytomegalovirus. Wilson's disease is excluded by measuring the serum ceruloplasmin and 24-hour urinary copper excretion. Slit-lamp examination of the eyes for Kayser-Fleischer rings and "sunflower" cataracts should be performed. Cystic fibrosis is excluded by measuring the sweat electrolytes. Alpha$_1$-antitrypsin deficiency is excluded by measuring the serum alpha$_1$-antitrypsin content and by performing protease-inhibitor (Pi) phenotyping. Heterozygous MZ alpha$_1$-antitrypsin deficiency has been found in adults with CAH and cryptogenic cirrhosis.[34] A protein electrophoretogram allows one to detect hypoalbuminemia, often seen in advanced liver disease, a depressed alpha$_1$-globulin fraction associated with alpha$_1$-antitrypsin deficiency, and hypergammaglobulinemia, which is almost universally found with autoimmune CAH. Autoimmune CAH and primary biliary cirrhosis (PBC) are accompanied by the presence of high titers of non-organic-specific autoantibodies. An elevated titer of AMA occurs in 11 to 35 percent of patients with HBsAg-negative CAH and 83 to 100 percent of cases of PBC.[64] ASMA is found in 61 to 86 percent of patients with HBsAg-negative CAH and 32 to 49 percent of patients with PBC.[64] ANA is found frequently in both disease processes. The results of non-organ-specific antibody determinations at the time of diagnosis in 38 children with HBsAg-negative CAH are presented in Table 4. Elevated titers of non-organ-specific antibodies support the diagnosis of autoimmune CAH. Differentiation of CAH from primary biliary cirrhosis may be difficult in the adolescent female, although antimitochondrial antibodies are less frequently positive in CAH and are usually of lower titer.[65]

Anatomic evaluation has a definite place in the assessment of patients with chronic liver disease. A standard liver-spleen scan provides a permanent record of the dimensions of these organs for future comparisons. Fasting abdominal ultrasonography and hepatobiliary scintigraphy may be needed to exclude cholelithiasis, acute or chronic gallbladder dysfunction,

TABLE 3
Evaluation of Chronic Hepatitis

Initial
- Complete blood cell count (CBC)
- Bilirubin with fractions
- Aspartate aminotransferase (AST/SGOT)
- Alanine aminotransferase (ALT/SGPT)
- Gamma-glutamyltransferase (GGT)
- Prothrombin time
- Protein electrophoresis

Specific
- HBsAg; anti-HBc IgM and IgG; HBeAg and anti-HBe
- CMV inclusion cytology
- Monospot; EBV panel
- Alpha$_1$-antitrypsin level/protease inhibitor (Pi) phenotyping
- Ceruloplasmin
- Determination of copper excretion in a 24-hour urine collection
- Sweat iontophoresis

Autoimmune studies
- Antinuclear antibody titer
- Anti-smooth muscle antibody titer
- Antimitochondrial antibody titer
- Anti-liver-kidney microsomal antibody (LKMA) titer (where available)

Anatomic evaluation
- Liver-spleen scan
- Fasting abdominal ultrasonography
- Technetium ^{99m}Tc hepatobiliary scintigraphy
- Percutaneous liver biopsy

TABLE 4
Non-Organ-Specific Autoantibodies in 38 Children with HBsAg-Negative Chronic Active Hepatitis

	Number of Patients	
	Total	Positive
Antinuclear antibody	35	24
Anti-smooth muscle antibody	18	14
Antimitochondrial antibody	18	2

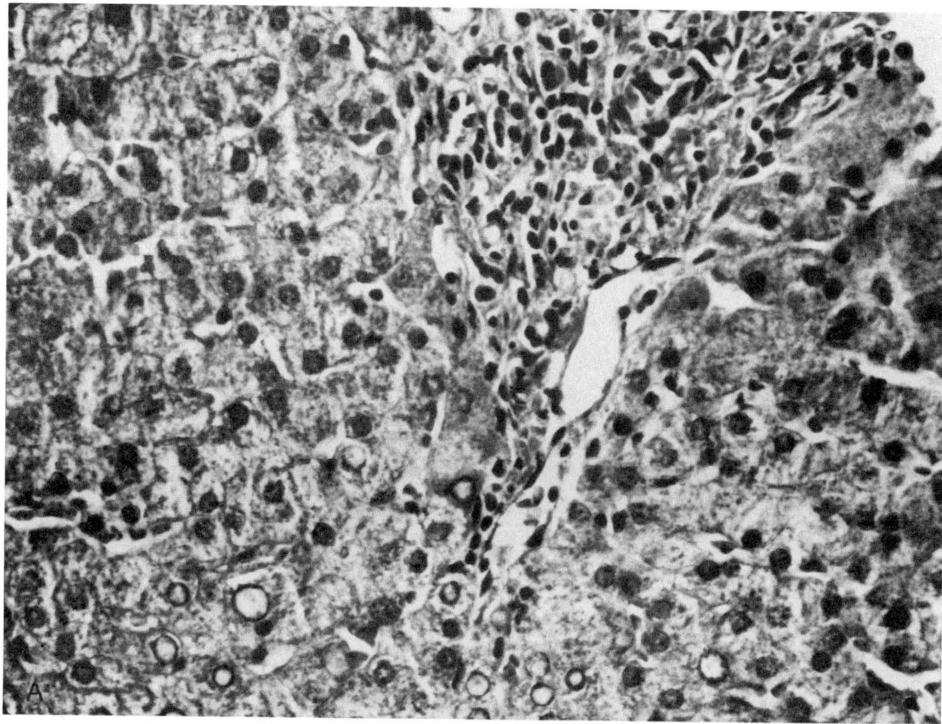

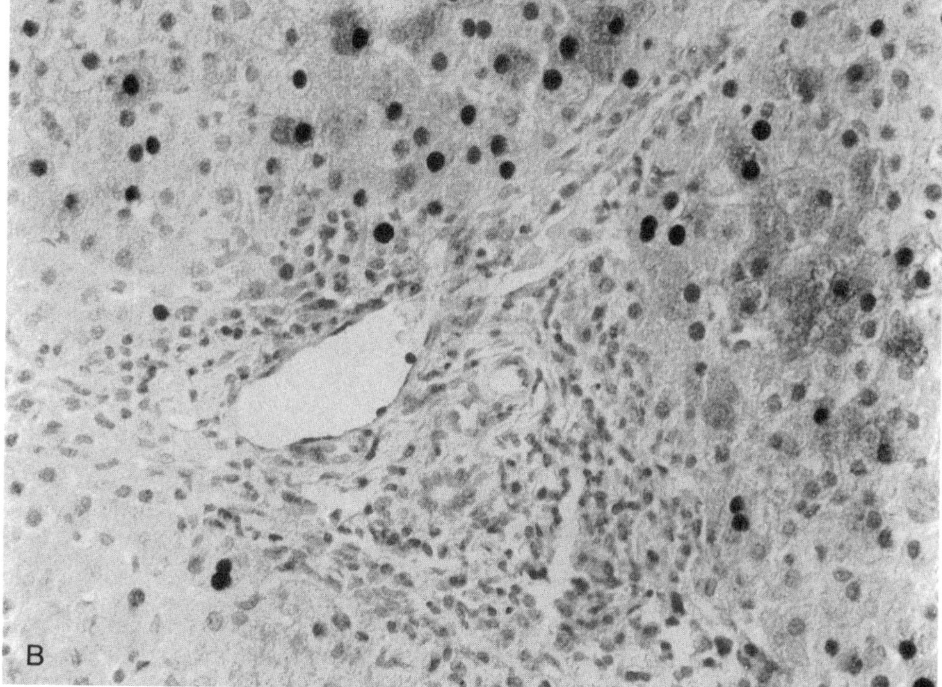

FIGURE 1 *A*, Chronic persistent hepatitis. Inflammatory cells infiltrate and expand the portal zone without disrupting the limiting plate or invading the hepatic lobule. Normal hepatic architecture is preserved (hematoxylin and eosin, ×200). *B*, Immunohistochemical stain of a hepatic biopsy from a 3-year-old girl with HBsAg-positive chronic persistent hepatitis revealing an inflammatory infiltrate expanding a portal zone with a sharp limiting plate. The dense intracytoplasmic material is HBsAg (×200).

cystic dilation of the extrahepatic biliary tree, and intra- or extrahepatic obstruction in the occasional patient with significant elevation of GGT activity.

Differentiation of CPH from CAH ultimately relies on microscopic examination of liver tissue. Immunohistochemical studies for HBcAg and HBsAg should be performed on all biopsies. The histologic picture of CPH is that of expansion of the portal tracts with a chronic inflammatory infiltrate while retaining preservation of the normal hepatic architecture (Fig. 1). Piecemeal necrosis is mild or absent. The distinction between CPH and minimal-lesion CAH is often difficult.[66] There is a risk of sampling error, as stated previously, and some portal tracts in CAH may fail to show the typical features of CAH. This probably explains some of the reported instances of transition from CPH to CAH on subsequent biopsy. The histologic picture of CPH is not specific; it represents only one of many causes of portal inflammation.

Early definitions of CAH emphasized the importance of piecemeal necrosis at the margins of the portal tracts as the initial lesion (Fig. 2). Boyer and Klatskin[67] emphasized the

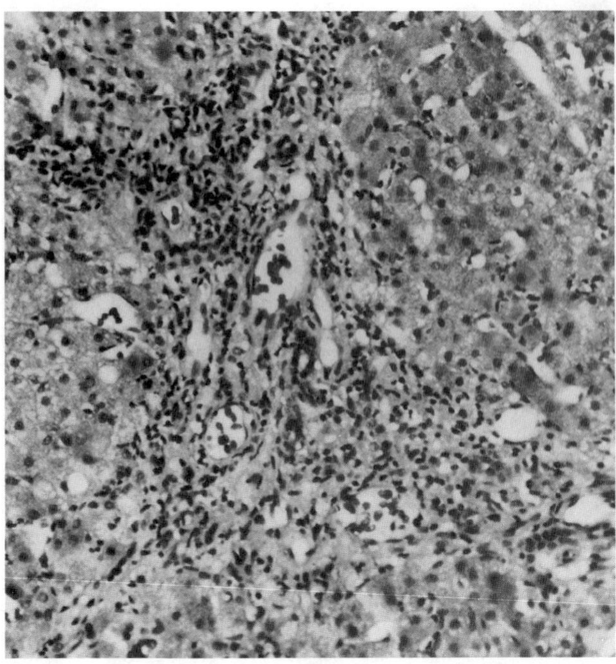

FIGURE 2 Chronic active hepatitis. Inflammatory activity totally disrupts the portal zone limiting plate. Periportal ("piecemeal") necrosis is manifest as inflammatory cells entrap periportal hepatocytes (hematoxylin and eosin, ×400).

association of bridging hepatic necrosis with the subsequent development of cirrhosis (Fig. 3). Bridging hepatic necrosis is a process of confluent hepatocellular necrosis linking the vascular structures of the hepatic lobules. Both processes (i.e., piecemeal necrosis and bridging hepatic necrosis) are probably important in disease progression. Advanced CAH is an active cirrhosis with portoportal fibrous bridging and division of the hepatic lobule into pseudolobules by fibrous septae. Both are readily apparent on the Mallory trichrome stain. A significant number of patients have evidence of cirrhosis on their initial biopsy.[68,69]

Studies conducted by Okuno et al[70] and Cooksley and colleagues[71] reinforced the importance of bridging hepatic necrosis in the development of cirrhosis. Only 4 of 40 patients in the former and none of 19 patients in the latter study who did *not* have bridging necrosis on their initial biopsy progressed to cirrhosis. Cooksley et al[71] presented additional data on 50 patients who had bridging necrosis on their initial biopsy. Seventeen were HBsAg-positive. They were followed for a median period of 36 months; there was one death due to hepatic failure and 7 of 36 had cirrhosis on repeat biopsies.

TREATMENT

CPH does not require therapy. Since this diagnosis depends on subjective interpretation of the degree of inflammation and periportal necrosis on a single hepatic biopsy, however, it is wise to monitor the patient and perform a second biopsy if necessary in order to increase the certainty of the benign diagnosis. There is support for an opinion that the finding of piecemeal necrosis alone (i.e., without bridging hepatic necrosis) may not require the initiation of immunosuppressive therapy, as noted previously.

Early studies of patients with HBsAg-negative CAH documented unrelenting progression to death within 3 years if the disease was untreated.[72,73] These early observations led to prescription of corticosteroids in the hope of suppressing the inflammation and halting the progress to cirrhosis and death. Azathioprine was introduced to the therapeutic strategy in the mid-1970s.[74] Azathioprine appears to augment the corticosteroid effect, which allows reduction of the steroid requirement and the unwanted steroid side effects. This combination therapy has been used successfully in children.[29,62]

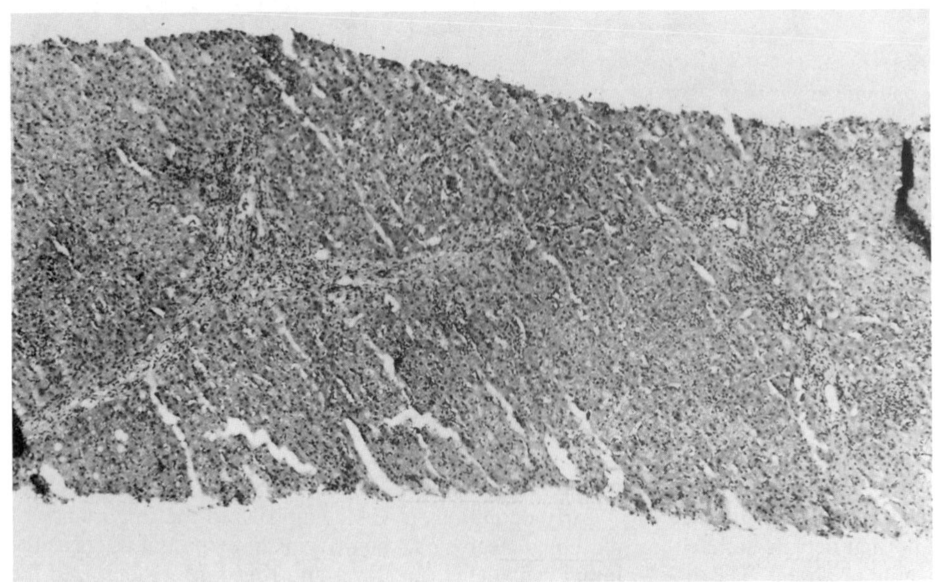

FIGURE 3 Chronic active hepatitis. Inflammatory cells connect adjacent portal areas, resulting in confluent hepatocellular (bridging) necrosis. This represents a precirrhotic lesion (hematoxylin and eosin, ×100).

I initially treat patients with HBsAg-negative CAH with prednisone in a dosage of 2 mg per kilogram per day (up to 60 mg).[11,28,62,75] It is provided in a single morning dose. Remission is defined as a resolution of symptoms and signs of active liver disease and a reduction in the aminotransferase levels (AST/SGOT and ALT/SGPT) to less than 2.5-fold elevated. An alternate-day treatment strategy (i.e., 2 mg per kilogram on alternate mornings) can be instituted when clinical and biochemical remissions are attained. This can often be accomplished after 4 to 6 weeks of therapy. The prednisone is then reduced by 5-mg increments every 4 weeks, with careful monitoring of the patient's clinical and biochemical status. Clinical and/or biochemical relapse dictates return to a daily steroid program. An alternate-day program may be reinstituted when tapering of the daily dose has been successful. A typical course of therapy lasts 12 to 18 months. Azathioprine is not routinely prescribed but is added when clinical and biochemical remission is not achieved with prednisone alone or when frequent relapses prevent reduction of the steroid dosage. A single daily dose of 1.0 to 1.5 mg per kilogram is administered. The hemogram and platelet count must be monitored closely in the early course of azathioprine therapy. The azathioprine is discontinued when the prednisone is tapered to 5 mg on alternate days. Gastrointestinal (GI) upset, skin rashes, leukopenia, and thrombocytopenia are early manifestations of azathioprine toxicity.[24] These abate with reduction in dosage or discontinuation of the medication. Azathioprine has been found to be an idiopathic hepatotoxin with the potential for combined cholestatic and hepatocellular injury in humans.[76]

It has been our policy to examine hepatic histology early in the course of therapy to confirm remission and 4 to 6 weeks after therapy has been discontinued. Our experience to date is that a rise in the serum aminotransferase values accompanies histologic relapse, which parallels the experience in adults reported from the Mayo Clinic.[77] It may be that frequent histologic reassessment will be deemed unnecessary in the future.

Monitoring the fasting serum cholylglycine level provides additional information regarding the completeness of remission, since the level appears to correlate well with the histologic picture.[78–80] Patients who have cirrhosis on their initial biopsy are more likely to experience a relapse and demonstrate continued need for immunosuppressive therapy.[28,29,81,82]

I have encountered an occasional patient similar to the one reported by Maggiore et al[83] who presented insidiously with liver failure. Evaluation excluded chronic HBV disease, Wilson's disease, alpha$_1$-antitrypsin deficiency disease, and cystic fibrosis. High titers of non–organ-specific antibodies supported a diagnosis of autoimmune CAH. The prothrombin time was prolonged and failed to correct with the administration of parenteral vitamin K and fresh-frozen plasma. The initiation of immunosuppressive therapy resulted in dramatic clinical and biochemical response. The prothrombin time corrected, and percutaneous liver biopsy was consistent with chronic aggressive liver disease.

The majority of patients with chronic HBV disease have CPH, although some clearly have aggressive disease. Proper management of these patients remains controversial. Immunosuppressive therapy, as outlined above, was initially prescribed. Bortolotti et al[84] reviewed the courses of 16 children with HBsAg-positive CAH. Two had cirrhosis on their initial biopsies. Eleven of the 16 received immunosuppressive therapy, and only one achieved a complete and protracted remission. Two of the five untreated patients achieved complete remission after 2 and 3 years of follow-up, respectively. Why the five patients were not treated is unclear, and the study was not prospective or controlled. Lam et al[85] actually concluded that prednisolone had a deleterious effect on adult patients with HBsAg-positive CAH. Prednisolone initiated an early transient decrease in the serum bilirubin concentrations, but it tended to delay the remissions that occurred in all control patients. The death rate and the frequency of complications were increased in the patients who received prednisolone. They subsequently provided histologic data that they believed supported their earlier conclusion.[86] The steroid-treated patients more frequently demonstrated persistence of piecemeal necrosis, more lipofuscin and iron in Kupffer cells, and increased quantities of both HBcAg and HBsAg in their hepatocytes. Portal inflammation and fibrosis were unaffected. Neither study was above criticism. Conn et al[87] pointed out in an editorial accompanying the second report form the Hong Kong co-workers that their design lent itself to unintentional bias, yet they concluded that corticosteroids seem to induce little or no improvement in patients with HBsAg-positive CAH and that they might be detrimental.

Burrell et al[88] pointed out that recent immunologic data seem to suggest that there are different mechanisms for hepatocyte injury accompanying chronic HBV infection: one associated with viral replication and the other dependent on immunologic factors. Persistent viral replication correlates with continued presence of HBeAg in the blood, although active liver disease has been documented in patients who are HBeAg-negative.[88] Sagnelli et al[89] found that prednisolone alone or combined with azathioprine did not modify the course of HBeAg-positive patients but did have a definite positive effect in HBeAg-negative patients. Azathioprine alone was ineffective in both patient groups. Giusti et al[90] retrospectively analyzed the course of 139 Italian children with HBsAg-positive CAH. All children were observed for at least 1 year. Thirty-eight of the 139 were treated with prednisone (or prednisolone), 78 were treated with prednisone (or prednisolone) and azathioprine, and 23 were untreated. The untreated patients deteriorated more frequently than those treated with steroid therapy alone or with combination therapy. Remission or improvement was observed more frequently in the treated patients. There was no reference to the HBeAg status of the patients in the report. They concluded that corticosteroid and combination therapy were not deleterious and were possibly beneficial in children with HBsAg-positive CAH.

Various small clinical trials that were designed to evaluate the effect of antiviral agents in the management of HBsAg/HBeAg-positive CAH have been published. Neither human leukocyte interferon[91] nor adenine arabinoside[92–94] has been found to be effective in clearing HBsAg from the serum or eradicating HBV from hepatocytes. Fattovich et al[95] have presented data that suggest that long-term levamisole may be beneficial in chronic HBeAg-positive CAH. Ten patients treated with levamisole demonstrated a tendency toward normalization of their aminotransferase activities and suppression of HBV replication. Japanese investigators concluded from a prospective controlled study of 43 patients with HBeAg-positive CAH that immunomodulation by corticosteroid therapy withdrawal followed by treatment with adenine arabinoside was more effective than treatment with adenine arabinoside alone.[96] This report supported the observation of Scullard et al[97] that patients with HBsAg-positive CAH who had a history of recent steroid therapy seemed to respond better to antiviral therapy.

Optimal management of NANB CAH is unclear. A preliminary report suggests that long-term, low-dose alpha-interferon therapy may be effective in controlling the disease activity.[98] I have successfully suppressed the active component of the disease in an adolescent male hemophiliac with NANB CAH with prednisone and azathioprine. Interestingly, the aminotransferase levels did not respond to prednisone alone. It is hoped that the anticipated clarification of this disease entity which should follow the discovery of Kuo et al[32] will lead to cleaner management data.

SUMMARY

CAH was a fatal illness when I developed a special interest in this disease process more than 20 years ago. Aggressive management has a dramatic effect on the course of patients with autoimmune CAH. We have been successful in weaning virtually all of our patients from immunosuppressive therapy over varying periods of time. Recent immunologic studies provide us with theories that may account for the differences noted in the response to immunosuppressive therapy between patients with HBsAg-positive CAH and patients who are HBsAg-negative, and between subgroups in both major classes. The role of antiviral agents in the routine management of HBsAg/HBeAg-positive and NANB virus chronic active liver disease awaits further study, as does the role of other immunosuppressive therapeutic options (e.g., methotrexate, cyclosporine, and OKT-3) in the management of both HBsAg-positive and HBsAg-negative CAH. Although it is true that we have only scratched the surface in our understanding of this malady (or group of maladies), I have witnessed the gain of tremendous insight over the past 20 years, and I expect that our understanding will continue to increase. Chronic hepatitis is now considered a manageable rather than a fatal disease.

REFERENCES

1. Cullinan ER. Idiopathic jaundice (often recurrent) associated with subacute necrosis of the liver. St Barth Hosp Rep 1936; 69:55–142.
2. Amberg S. Hyperproteinemia associated with severe liver damage. Proc Staff Meet Mayo Clin 1942; 17:360–362.
3. Kunkel HG, Ahrens EH Jr, Eisenmenger WJ, Bongiovanni AM, Slater RJ. Extreme hypergammaglobulinemia in young women with liver disease of unknown etiology. (Abstract) J Clin Invest 1951; 30:654.
4. Bearn AG, Kunkel HG, Slater RJ. The problem of chronic liver disease in young women. Am J Med 1956; 21:3–15.
5. Good RA. Plasma cell hepatitis and extreme hypergammaglobulinemia in adolescent females. (Abstract) Am J Dis Child 1956; 92:508–509.
6. MacKay JR, Taft LI, Cowling DC. Lupoid hepatitis. Lancet 1956; ii:1323–1326.
7. Bulkley BH, Heizer WD, Goldfinger SE, Isselbacher KJ. Distinctions in chronic active hepatitis based on circulating hepatitis-associated antigen. Lancet 1970; ii:1323–1326.
8. Dudley FJ, Scheuer PJ, Sherlock S. Natural history of hepatitis-associated antigen-positive chronic liver disease. Lancet 1972; ii:1388–1393.
9. Sherlock S. Chronic hepatitis. Gut 1974; 15:581–597.
10. Dubois RS, Silverman A. Treatment of chronic active hepatitis in children. Postgrad Med J 1974; 50:386–391.
11. Arasu TS, Wyllie R, Hatch TF, Fitzgerald JF. Management of chronic aggressive hepatitis in children and adolescents. J Pediatr 1979; 95:514–522.
12. Mistilis SP, Blackburn CRB. Acute chronic hepatitis. Am J Med 1970; 48:484–495.
13. Schalm SW, Korman MG, Summerskill WHJ, Czaja AJ, Bagenstoss AH. Severe chronic active liver disease: prognostic significance of initial morphologic patterns. Am J Dig Dis 1977; 22:973–980.
14. Doniach D, Roitt IM, Walker JG, Sherlock S. Tissue antibodies in primary biliary cirrhosis, active chronic (lupoid) hepatitis, cryptogenic cirrhosis and other liver diseases and their clinical implications. Clin Exp Immunol 1966; 1:237–262.
15. Golding PL, Smith M, Williams R. Multisystem involvement in chronic liver disease: studies on the incidence and pathogenesis. Am J Med 1973; 55:772–782.
16. Walker JG. Immunological tests in liver diseases. Ann Clin Biochem 1970; 7:93–96.
17. Ludwig RN, Doedhar SD, Brown CH. Autoimmune tests in chronic active disease of the liver. Cleveland Clin Q 1971; 38:105–112.
18. Klatskin G, Kantor FS. Mitochondrial antibody in primary biliary cirrhosis and other diseases. Ann Intern Med 1972; 77:533–541.
19. Lam KC, Mistilis SP, Perrott N. Positive tissue antibody tests in patients with prolonged extrahepatic biliary obstruction. N Engl J Med 1972; 286:1400–1401.
20. Czaja AJ, Wolf AM. Chronic active liver disease (CALD) with acute viral features (AVF): to treat or not to treat? (Abstract) Gastroenterology 1978; 74:1023.
21. Schalm SW, Korman MG, Summerskill WHJ, Czaja AJ, Baggenstoss AH. Severe chronic active liver disease: prognostic significance of initial morphologic patterns. Am J Dig Dis 1977; 22:973–980.
22. Scheuer PJ. Liver biopsy in the diagnosis of cirrhosis. Gut 1970; 11:275–278.
23. Soloway RD, Baggenstoss AH, Schoenfield LJ, Summerskill WJH. Observer error and sampling variability tested in evaluation of hepatitis and cirrhosis by liver biopsy. Am J Dig Dis 1971; 16:1082–1086.
24. Czaja AJ. Current problems in the diagnosis and management of chronic active hepatitis. Mayo Clin Proc 1981; 56:311–323.
25. Boyer JI. Chronic hepatitis: a perspective on classification and determinants of prognosis. Gastroenterology 1976; 70:1161–1171.
26. Nomenclature, diagnostic criteria, and diagnostic methodology for diseases of the liver and biliary tract. Fogarty Int Center Proc 1976; 22:1–11.
27. Summerskill WHJ. Chronic hepatitis—1975. (Editorial) Am J Dig Dis 1975; 20:1087–1090.
28. Fitzgerald JF. Chronic hepatitis. (Editorial) J Pediatr 1984; 104:893–895.
29. Maggiore G, Bernard O, Hadchouel M, Hadchouel P, Odievre M, Alagille D. Treatment of autoimmune chronic active hepatitis in childhood. J Pediatr 1984; 104:839–844.
30. DeGroote J, Desmet VJ, Gedigk P, Korb G, Popper H, Poulsen H, Scheuer PJ, Schmid M, Thaler H, Uehlinger E, Wepler W. A classification of chronic hepatitis. Lancet 1968; ii:626–628.
31. Tabor E, Seeff LB, Gerety RJ. Chronic non-A, non-B hepatitis carrier state. N Engl J Med 1980; 303:140–143.
32. Kuo G, Choo Q-L, Alter HJ, Gitnick GL, Redeker AG, Purcell RH, Miyamura T, Dienstag JF, Alter MJ, Stevens CE, Tegtmeier GE, Bonino F, Colombo M, Lee W-S, Kuo C, Berger K, Shuster JR, Overby LR, Bradley DW, Houghton M. An assay for circulating antibodies to a major etiologic virus of human non-A, non-B hepatitis. Science 1989; 244:362–364.
33. Thung SN, Gerber MA, Benkov KJ, Guttenberg M, Gordon RE. Chronic active hepatitis in a child with human immunodeficiency virus infection. Arch Pathol Lab Med 1988; 112:914–916.
34. Hodges JR, Millward-Sadler GH, Barbatis C, Wright R. Heterozygous MZ alpha-1-antitrypsin deficiency in adults with chronic active hepatitis and cryptogenic cirrhosis. N Engl J Med 1981; 304:557–560.
35. Ortono L, Laghi V, Cauda R, Nervo P. Lymphocyte transformation test with rabbit liver specific lipoprotein (RLSP) in chronic active hepatitis. Clin Exp Immunol 1979; 38:231–234.

36. Mieli-Vergani G, Vergani D, Jenkins PJ, Portmann B, Mowat AP, Eddleston ALWF, Williams R. Lymphocyte cytotoxicity to autologous hepatocytes in HBsAg-negative chronic active hepatitis. Clin Exp Immunol 1979; 38:16–21.
37. Hodgson HJF, Wands JR, Isselbacher KJ. Alteration in suppressor cell activity in chronic active hepatitis. Proc Natl Acad Sci USA 1978; 75:1549–1553.
38. Tremolada F, Fattovich G, Panebianco G, Ongaro G, Realdi G. Suppressor cell activity in viral and non-viral chronic active hepatitis. Clin Exp Immunol 1980; 40:89–95.
39. Kakuma S, Yata K, Kashio T. Immunoregulatory T-cell function in acute and chronic liver disease. Gastroenterology 1980; 79:613–619.
40. Chisari FV, Castle KL, Xavier C, Anderson DS. Functional properties of lymphocyte subpopulations in hepatitis B virus infection. I. Suppressor cell control of T lymphocyte responsiveness. J Immunol 1981; 126:38–44.
41. Coovadia HM, McKay IR, D'Apice AJF. Suppressor cells assayed by three different methods in patients with chronic active hepatitis and systemic lupus erythematous. Clin Immunol Immunopathol 1981; 18:268–275.
42. Nouri-Aria KT, Hegarty JE, Alexander GJM, Eddleston ALWF, Williams R. Effect of corticosteroids on suppressor-cell activity in "autoimmune" and viral chronic active hepatitis. N Engl J Med 1982; 307:1301–1304.
43. Pape GR, Rieber EP, Eisenburg J, Hoffmann R, Balch CM, Paumgartner G, Riethmuller G. Involvement of the cytotoxic/suppressor T-cell subset in liver tissue injury of patients with acute and chronic liver diseases. Gastroenterology 1983; 85:657–662.
44. Thomas HC, Brown D, LaBrooy J, Epstein O. T cell subsets in autoimmune and HBV-induced chronic liver disease, HBs antigen carriers with normal histology and primary biliary cirrhosis: a review of the abnormalities and the effects of treatment. J Clin Immunol 1982; 2:57S–60S.
45. Montano L, Aranguibel, Boffill M, Goodall AH, Janossy G, Thomas HC. An analysis of the composition of the inflammatory infiltrate in autoimmune and hepatitis B virus-induced chronic liver disease. Hepatology 1983; 3:292–296.
46. Vento S, Hegarty JE, Bottazzo G, Macckia E, Williams R, Eddleston ALWF. Antigen specific suppressor cell function in autoimmune chronic active hepatitis. Lancet 1984; i:1200–1204.
47. Larcher VF, Macdonald A, Vegmente A, Mowat AP, Eddleston ALWF, Williams R. Antibodies to liver-specific lipoprotein in children with chronic liver disease due to "autoimmune" chronic active hepatitis, cystic fibrosis, and alpha-l-antitrypsin deficiency. J Pediatr Gastroenterol Nutr 1984; 3:728–733.
48. Naumov NV, Mondelli M, Alexander GJM, Tedder RS, Eddleston ALWF, Williams R. Relationship between expression of HBV antigens in isolated hepatocytes and autologous lymphocyte cytotoxicity in patients with chronic HBV infection. Hepatology 1984; 4:63–68.
49. Mazzetti M, Stefanini GF, Mazzeo V, Baraldini M, Cononica GW, Marini E, Miglio F, Gasbarrini G, Lee WM. Alterations in helper-specific circulating T lymphocytes and in the autologous mixed lymphocyte reaction in chronic hepatitis B. J Gastroenterol 1987; 82:130–134.
50. Pontisso P, Poon MC, Tiollais P, Brechot C. Detection of hepatitis B virus DNA in mononuclear blood cells. Br Med J 1984; 288:1563–1566.
51. Hafez M, Abdalla A, El-Shennawy F. Immune regulation dysfunction in chronic persistent hepatitis. Dis Markers 1988; 6:15–21.
52. Hopf U, Meyer zum Buschenfeld KH, Arnold W. Detection of a liver-membrane autoantibody in HBsAg-negative chronic active hepatitis. N Engl J Med 1976; 294:578–582.
53. Jensen DM, McFarlane IG, Portmann BS, Eddleston ALWF, Williams R. Detection of antibodies directed against a liver-specific membrane lipoprotein in patients with acute and chronic active hepatitis. N Engl J Med 1978; 299:1–7.
54. McFarlane BM, McSorley CG, Vergani D, McFarlane IG, Williams R. Serum autoantibodies reacting with the hepatic asialoglycoprotein receptor protein (hepatic lectin) in acute and chronic liver disorders. J Hepatol 1986; 3:196–205.
55. Mieli-Vergani G, Lobo-Yeo A, McFarlane BM, McFarlane IG, Mowat AP, Vergani D. Different immune mechanisms leading to autoimmunity in primary sclerosing cholangitis and autoimmune chronic active hepatitis of childhood. Hepatology 1989; 9:198–203.
56. Lobo-Yeo A, Alviggi L, Mieli-Vergani G, Portmann B, Mowat AP, Vergani D. Preferential activation of helper/inducer T lymphocytes in autoimmune chronic active hepatitis. Clin Exp Immunol 1987; 67:95–104.
57. Kashio P, Motta R, Kakumu S. Lymphocyte suppressor cell activity in acute and chronic liver disease. Clin Exp Immunol 1981; 44:459–466.
58. Nouri-Aria K, Lobo-Yeo A, Vergani D, Mieli-Vergani G, Eddleston ALWF, Mowat AP. T suppressor cell function and number in children with liver disease. Clin Exp Immunol 1985; 61:283–289.
59. Nouri-Aria KT, Donaldson PT, Hegarty JE, Eddleston ALWF, Williams R. HLA A1-B8-DR3 and suppressor cell function in first degree relatives of patients with autoimmune chronic active hepatitis. J Hepatol 1985; 1:235–241.
60. Bortolotti F, Calzia R, Vegnente A, Cadrobbi P, Rugge M, Armigliato M, Marazzi MG, Iorio R, Crivellaro C, Piscopo R, Realdi G. Chronic hepatitis in childhood: the spectrum of the disease. Gut 1988; 29:659–664.
61. Fitzgerald JF. Chronic hepatitis. Sem Liv Dis 1982; 2:282–290.
62. Odievre M, Maggiore G, Homberg J-C, Saadoun F, Courouce A-M, Yvart J, Hadchouel M, Alagille D. Seroimmunologic classification of chronic hepatitis in 57 children. Hepatology 1983; 3:407–409.
63. Sjögren M, Hoofnagle JH. Immunoglobulin M antibody to hepatitis B core antigen in patients with chronic type B hepatitis. Gastroenterology 1985; 89:252–258.
64. Kurki P, Miettinen A, Linder E, Pikkarainen P, Vioristo M, Salaspuro MP. Different types of smooth muscle antibodies in chronic active hepatitis and primary biliary cirrhosis: their diagnostic and prognostic significance. Gut 1980; 21:878–884.
65. Czaja AJ, Dickson ER. Severe chronic active liver disease (CALD) and primary biliary cirrhosis (PBC): reliability of clinical differentiation. (Abstract) Gastroenterology 1980; 79:1011.
66. Scheuer PJ. Histology in chronic hepatitis. Ann Acad Med 1980; 9:182–184.
67. Boyer JL, Klatskin G. Pattern of necrosis in acute viral hepatitis. Prognostic value of bridging (subacute hepatic necrosis). N Engl J Med 1970; 283:1063–1071.
68. Cook GC, Mulligan R, Sherlock S. Controlled trial of corticosteroid therapy in active chronic hepatitis. Q J Med 1971; 40:159–185.
69. Murray-Lyon IM, Stern RB, Williams R. Controlled trial of prednisone and azathioprine in active chronic hepatitis. Lancet 1973; i:735–737.
70. Okuno T, Ou O, Ueda T, Iwai M, Nakajima E, Ogasawara T, Okanoue T, Takino T, Mori K. [Prognistic significance of bridging hepatic necrosis in chronic active hepatitis: a follow-up study.] Nippon Naika Gakkai Zasshi 1983; 72(4):416–422.
71. Cooksley WGE, Bradbear RA, Robinson W, Harrison M, Halliday JW, Powell LW, Ng H-S, Seah C-S, Okuda K, Scheuer PJ, Sherlock S. The prognosis of chronic active hepatitis without cirrhosis in relation to bridging necrosis. Hepatology 1986; 6:345–348.
72. Geall MG, Schoenfield LJ, Summerskill WHJ. Classification and treatment of chronic active liver disease. Gastroenterology 1968; 55:724–729.
73. Soloway RD, Summerskill WHJ, Baggenstoss AH, Geall MG, Gitnick GL, Elveback LR, Schoenfield LJ. Clinical, biochemical and histological remission of severe chronic active liver disease: a controlled study of treatments and early prognosis. Gastroenterology 1972; 63:820–833.
74. Summerskill WHJ, Korman MG, Ammon HV, Baggenstoss AH. Prednisone for chronic active liver disease: dose titration, standard dose, and combination with azathioprine compared. Gut 1975; 16:876–883.
75. Fitzgerald JF. Chronic active hepatitis. In: Gellis S, Kagan B, eds. Current Pediatric Therapy, Philadelphia: WB Saunders, in press.
76. DePinho RA, Goldberg CS, Lefkowitch JH. Azathioprine and the liver. Gastroenterology 1984; 86:162–165.
77. Czaja AJ, Wolf AM, Baggenstoss AH. Laboratory assessment of severe chronic active liver disease during and after corticosteroid therapy: correlation of serum transaminase and gamma globulin levels with histologic features. Gastroenterology 1981; 80:687–692.
78. Korman MG, Hofmann AF, Summerskill WHJ. Assessment of activity in chronic active liver disease: serum bile acids compared with conventional tests and histology. N Engl J Med 1974; 290:1399–1402.
79. Jones MB, Weinstock S, Koretz RL, Lewin KJ, Higgins J, Gitnick GL. Clinical value of serum bile acid levels in chronic hepatitis. Dig Dis Sci 1981; 26:978–983.
80. Monroe PS, Baker Al, Schneider JF, Krager PS, Klein PD, Schoeller D. The aminopyrine breath test and serum bile acids reflect histologic severity in chronic hepatitis. Hepatology 1982; 2:317–322.
81. Vegnente A, Larcher VF, Mowat AP, Portmann B, Williams R. Duration of chronic active hepatitis and the development of cirrhosis. Arch Dis Child 1984; 59:330–335.
82. Czaja AJ, Davis GL, Ludwig J, Taswell HF. Complete resolution of

inflammatory activity following corticosteroid treatment of HBsAg-negative chronic active hepatitis. Hepatology 1984; 4:622–627.
83. Maggiore G, Bernard O, Hadchouel M, Alagille D. Life-saving immunosuppressive treatment in severe autoimmune chronic active hepatitis. J Pediatr Gastroenterol Nutr 1985; 4:655–658.
84. Bortolotti F, Cadrobbi P, Crivellaro C, Bertaggia A, Alberti A, Realdi G. Chronic hepatitis type B in childhood: longitudinal study of 35 cases. Gut 1981; 22:499–504.
85. Lam KC, Lai CL, Ng RP, Trepco C, Wu PC. Deleterious effect of prednisolone in HBsAg-positive chronic active hepatitis. N Engl J Med 1981; 304:380–386.
86. Wu PC, Lai CL, Lam KC, Ho J. Prednisolone in HBsAg-positive chronic active hepatitis: histologic evaluation in a controlled prospective study. Hepatology 1982; 2:777–783.
87. Conn HO, Maddrey WC, Soloway RD. The detrimental effects of adrenocorticosteroid therapy in HBsAg-positive chronic active hepatitis: fact or artifact? Hepatology 1982; 2:885–887.
88. Burrell CJH, Gowans EJ, Rowland R, Hall P, Jilbert AR, Marmion BP. Correlation between liver histology and markers of hepatitis B virus replication in infected patients: a study by *in situ* hybridization. Hepatology 1984; 4:20–24.
89. Sagnelli E, Piccinino F, Manzello G, Felaco FM, Filippini P, Malo G, Pasquale G, Izzo CM. Effect of immunosuppressive therapy on HBsAg-positive chronic active hepatitis in relation to presence or absence of HBeAg and anti-HBe. Hepatology 1983; 3:690–695.
90. Giusti G, Piccinino F, Sagnelli E, Ruggiero G, Galanti B, Gallo C. Immunosuppressive therapy of HBsAg-positive active hepatitis in childhood: a multicentric retrospective study on 139 patients. J Pediatric Gastroenterol Nutr 1988; 7:17–21.
91. Schalm SW, Heijtink RA. Spontaneous disappearance of viral replication and liver cell inflammation in HBsAg-positive chronic active hepatitis: results of a placebo vs. interferon trial. Hepatology 1982; 2:791–794.
92. Bassendine MF, Chadwick RG, Salmeron J, Shipton U, Thomas HC, Sherlock S. Adenine arabinoside therapy in HBsAg-positive chronic liver disease: a controlled study. Gastroenterology 1981; 80:1016–1022.
93. Hoofnagle JH, Minuk GY, Dusheiko GM, Schafer DF, Johnson R, Straus S, Jones EA, Gerin JL, Ishak K. Adenine arabinoside 5′-monophosphate treatment of chronic type B hepatitis. Hepatology 1982; 2:784–788.
94. Hoofnagle JH, Hanson RG, Minuk GY, Pappas SC, Schafer DF, Dusheiko GM, Straus SE, Popper H, Jones EA. Randomized controlled trial of adenine arabinoside monophosphate for chronic type B hepatitis. Gastroenterology 1984; 86:150–157.
95. Fattovich G, Brollo L, Pontisso P, Pornaro E, Rugge M, Alberti A, Realdi G. Levamisole therapy in chronic type B hepatitis. Results of a double-blind randomized trial. Gastroenterology 1986; 91:692–696.
96. Yokosuka O, Omata M, Imazeki F, Hirota K, Mori J, Uchiumi K, Ito Y, Okuda K. Combination of short-term prednisolone and adenine arabinoside in the treatment of chronic hepatitis B. A controlled study. Gastroenterology 1985; 89:246–251.
97. Scullard GH, Pollard RB, Smith JL, Sacks SL, Gregory PB, Robinson WS, Merigan TC. Antiviral treatment of chronic hepatitis B virus infection. I. Changes in viral markers with interferon combined with adenine arabinoside. J Infect Dis 1981; 6:772–783.
98. Hoofnagle JH, Mullen KD, Jones BD, Rustgi V, Bisceglie AD, Peters M, Waggoner JG, Park Y, Jones EA. Treatment of chronic non-A, non-B hepatitis with recombinant human alpha interferon. N Engl J Med 1986; 315:1575–1578.

PART 24

Cirrhosis

M. Michael Thaler, M.D.

DEFINITION

What is cirrhosis? In broadest terms, cirrhosis represents the end-stage of *any* chronic liver disease. Liver damage caused by infectious, autoimmune, toxic, or dysmorphic factors may initiate a repetitive sequence of cell injury and repair. Given time, this circular process leads to a self-sustained pathophysiologic disorder of the liver called *cirrhosis,* superimposed on or supplanting the original disease process. The clinicopathologic manifestations of the cirrhotic state, regardless of primary etiology, reflect the dynamic interplay among cell injury (necrosis), repair response (fibrogenesis), and restoration of lost liver cell mass (regeneration), which brings a chronic liver disorder to the point of irreversibility. That point may be reached when intrahepatic blood distribution channels are permanently *distorted* by cross-linked fibrous tissue and *compressed* by regenerative elements, resulting in inadequate distribution of essential nutrients and metabolites to hypoperfused areas of the liver acinus.[1] Current understanding of mechanisms involved in the pathogenesis of cirrhosis is summarized below.

PATHOGENESIS

Any agent, organism, or structural anomaly that interferes with essential components of hepatocellular metabolism may elicit loss of cell viability. Dying liver cells are gradually enmeshed in a matrix of connective tissue secreted by themselves and other parenchymal cell types. A contractile fibrous network gradually begins to interfere with sinusoidal blood flow, resulting in accelerated cellular dropout in underperfused or inadequately drained lobular areas. Diminution of the parenchymal cell mass or total metabolic capacity eventually reaches the threshold required to unleash the liver's unique compensatory growth response. Nodular foci of

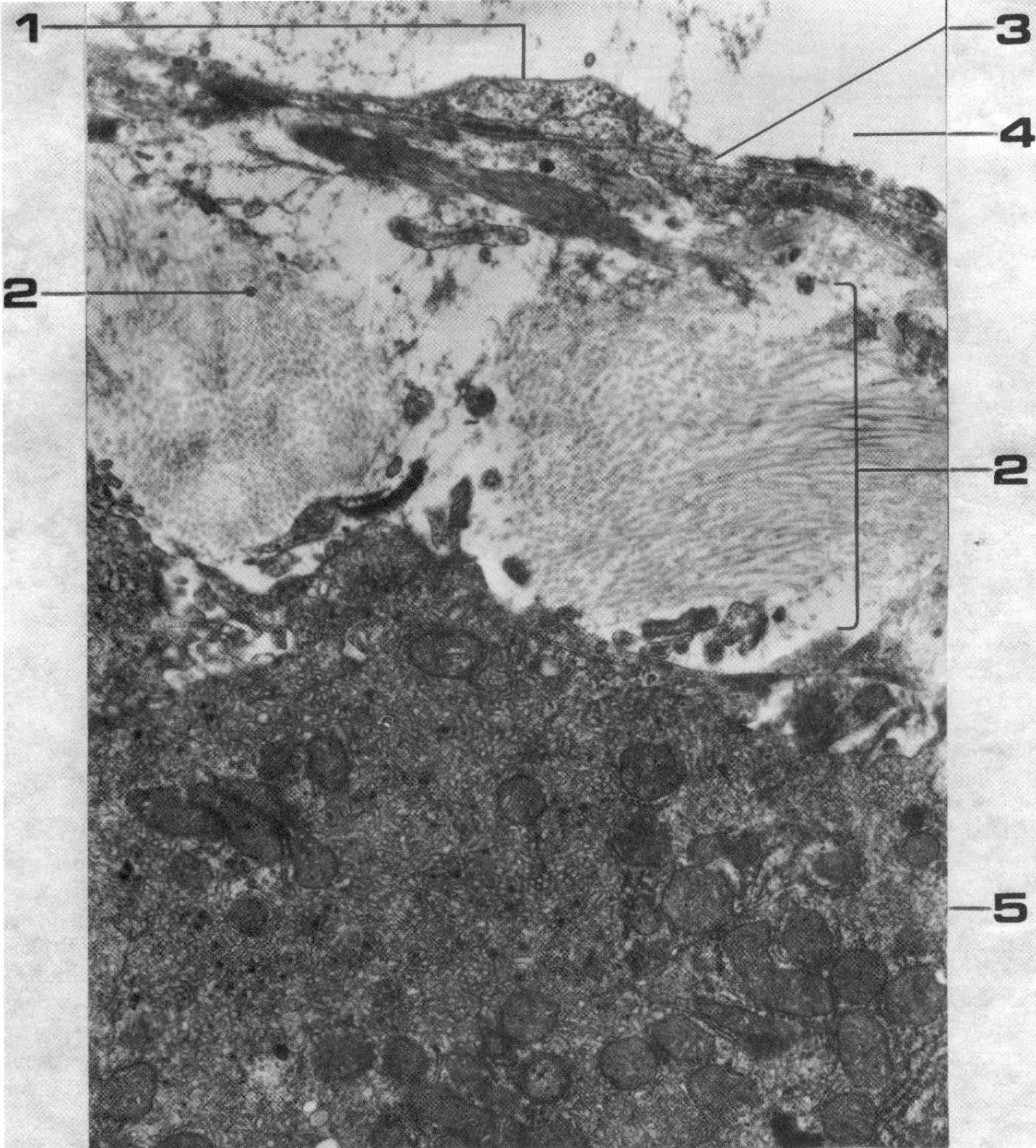

FIGURE 1 Rat liver cell showing deposition of collagen in the space of Disse after treatment with alcohol. *1*, Endothelial cells; *2*, collagen fibers in the space of Disse; *3*, sinusoidal basement membrane; *4*, sinusoidal space; *5*, cytoplasm (×18,000).

proliferating liver cells burgeon inside lobules, stretching the surrounding connective tissue lattice. Scar and nodule distort and compress the interlobular portal vein and hepatic artery branches. Thus, the primary disease process (e.g., Wilson's disease) initiates a circle of cell injury, fibrosis, and regeneration driven by microcirculatory insufficiency after the initiating event has abated.

Liver cells respond to any kind of injury with deposition of collagen in the space of Disse (Fig. 1). Initially, this incomplete fibrous barrier does not interfere with exchange of essential nutrients and metabolites between sinusoidal blood and liver cell surfaces. With continued exposure to a pathogen or toxin, as occurs in chronic infection or intake of an hepatotoxic agent, a thick basement "membrane" begins to blanket the sinusoidal surface, blocking contact between the blood stream and liver cells lining the sinusoids. This "capillarization" of sinusoids results in the formation of portal-to-central fibrous septa, providing conduits for shunts between the terminal branches of the portal vein and hepatic artery and the centrally positioned hepatic vein radicals (Fig. 2).[3]

Shunting blood away from the parenchyma accentuates the cell injury and promotes progressive distortion of lobular architecture with fibrous tissue and regenerative nodules. The resulting compression of venous drainage produces a nearly

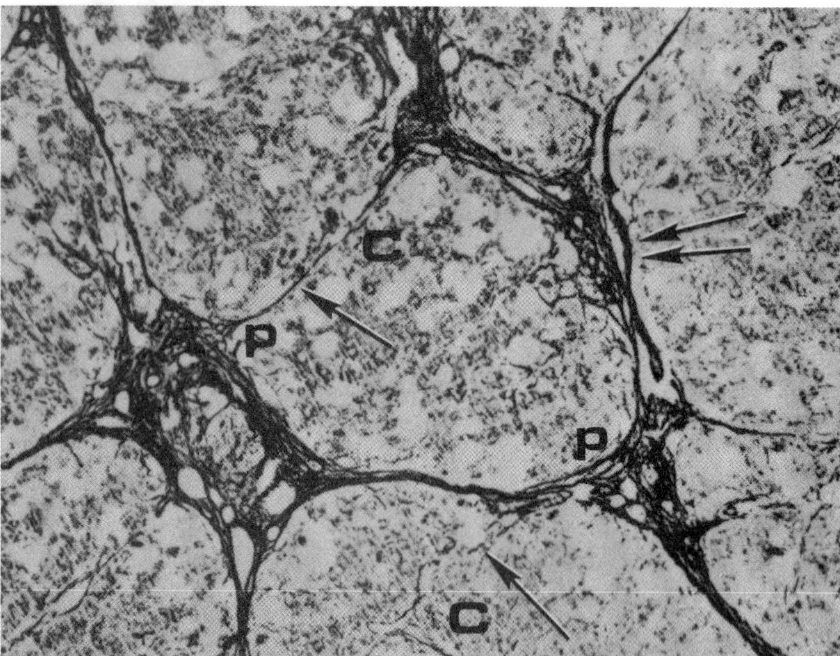

FIGURE 2 "Capillarization" of sinusoids. The initial step toward irreversibility in the development of cirrhosis is formation of a continuous connective tissue sinusoidal "membrane" (*arrow*) that effectively directs the flow of blood from the portal vein and hepatic artery in the portal zone (P) to central vein terminal branches (C). Portal-to-portal connective tissue bridges (*double arrows*) are also in evidence (reticulin stain, ×70).

10-fold reduction in total portal blood flow through the liver and forces development of extrahepatic portal-systemic collateral channels.[4] At the sinusoidal level, portal hypertension is augmented by arterioportal anastomoses forming in the capillarized septa.

In summary, cirrhosis is a progressive deterioration in liver structure and function due to the combined effects of necrosis in hypoperfused regions of the liver lobule, replacement of dying liver cells with scar tissue, deformation of lobular architecture with nodules containing actively replicating hepatocytes, and permanent distortion of the intrahepatic vascular network. Ongoing necrosis and self-perpetuation of the pathologic process are the inevitable results.

MECHANISMS OF FIBROGENESIS AND REGENERATION

Investigations of factors and control mechanisms responsible for fibrogenesis and liver regeneration are beginning to reveal molecular reactions to hepatocellular injury that determine the development and self-propagation of the cirrhotic state. Knowledge of these repair processes is a prerequisite for prophylactic strategies that may prevent progression of most chronic liver diseases to cirrhosis.

Hepatocytes and endothelial cells are induced to synthesize collagen when confronted by inflammatory cells activated by toxins, infectious agents, or antigens. Activated T lymphocytes and macrophages release several incompletely characterized factors known collectively as cytokines. In addition, fat-storing cells (also known as Ito cells) located in the space of Disse become active producers of collagen in response to various stressful conditions, and fibroblasts secrete collagen in periportal tracts when stimulated by extrahepatic biliary obstruction, periportal inflammation (pericholangitis), and viral infections (for a review, see reference 5).

The extracellular matrix formed around injured hepatocytes contains the surface glycoprotein fibronectin, which forms covalent bonds with collagen and fibrin and attracts collagen-forming cells to sites of hepatocellular damage. Both injury and regeneration also stimulate the deposition of a pericellular basement membrane composed of laminin, a disulfide cross-linked polymeric glycoprotein that plays an important part in liver morphogenesis and organization of liver plates. Laminin is not detected in normal human liver sinusoids but appears in basement membranes lining sinusoids undergoing capillarization.[6]

In cirrhosis and precirrhotic liver disease, hepatocytes synthesize stromal matrix proteins (collagens type I and IV, and fibronectin); Ito cells produce collagens type I, III, and IV, fibronectin, and laminin; and endothelial and cholangiolar cells synthesize type IV collagen and laminin.[5]

The phenomenon of liver regeneration remains unexplained, despite intensive efforts over five decades to identify the exact physiologic mechanisms involved. A variety of hormones with defined effects on intermediary metabolism stimulate liver cell growth but do not initiate it. Regenerative activity following partial hepatectomy in rats has been enhanced with insulin, glucagon, growth hormone, adrenocorticotropic hormone (ACTH), cortisol, thyroxine, estrogen, and vasopressin.

Several peptide "growth factors" have been identified in serum of partially hepatectomized rats or extracted from the regenerating liver remnant, but none has been conclusively linked with the regenerative process in vivo. Among the most promising candidates for an essential role in compensatory hepatic hyperplasia are the transforming growth factors al-

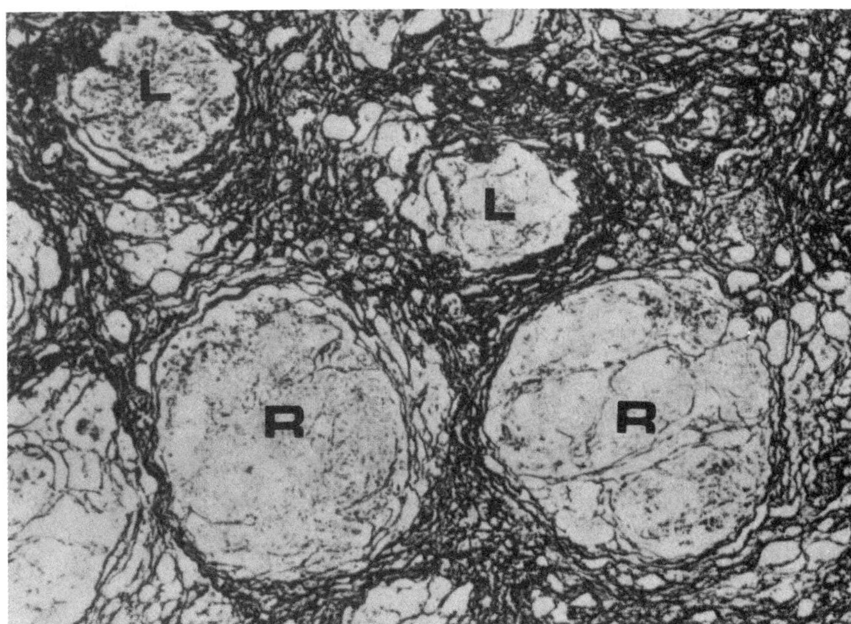

FIGURE 3 Micronodular cirrhosis. Advanced stage of the process initiated with sinusoidal capillarization shown in Figure 2. Thick wavy bands of condensed collagen surround regenerating lobules (R) and collapsing lobules (L) (reticulin stain, ×70).

pha and beta (TGF-alpha and TGF-beta).[7] Both are synthesized in the liver, increase during liver regeneration, and have been purified to homogeneity. TGF-alpha appears to act via the epidermal growth factor receptor to stimulate liver cell growth, whereas TGF-beta may provide the inhibitory signal required to stop hepatocellular replication when total liver cell mass has been restored. TGF-alpha has been found in ascites fluid from cirrhotic patients. Of particular interest in relation to cirrhosis is a report that fibroblasts induced by TGF-beta synthesized collagen and stimulated formation of capillary loops (angiogenesis) when injected into newborn mice.[8] These preliminary results raise the intriguing possibility that TGF-beta may play a role in both fibrogenesis and regenerative activity as a regulator of the repair process.

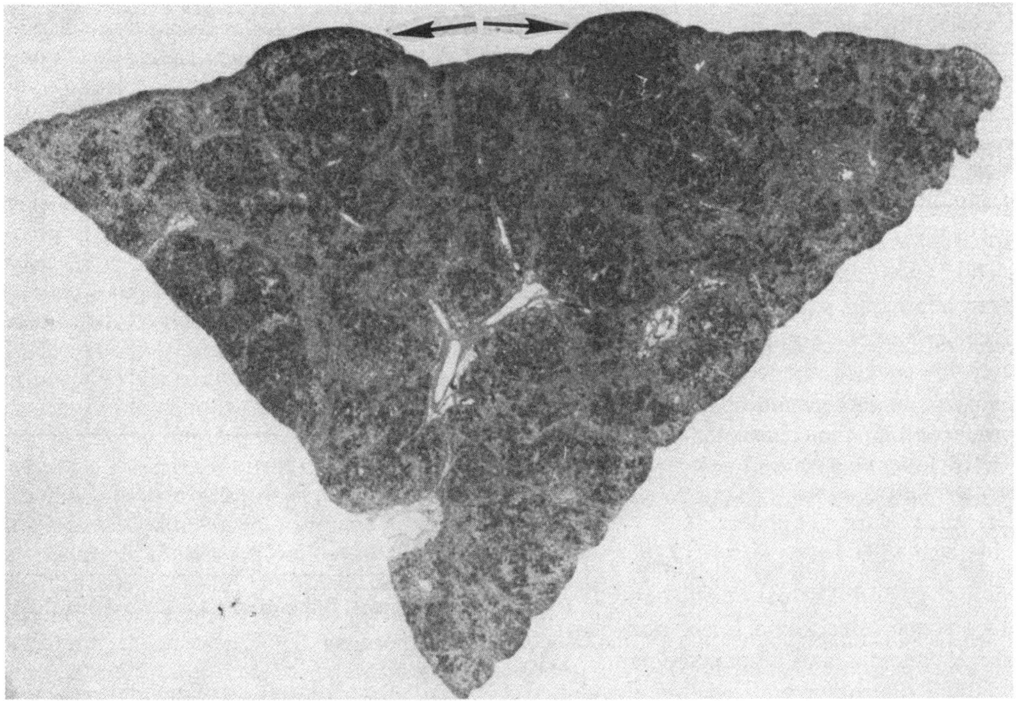

FIGURE 4 Micronodular cirrhosis. Wedge liver biopsy from an infant with end-stage cirrhosis (see Fig. 8). Two surface nodules (*arrows*) suggest "hobnailed" appearance of the liver exterior. Dense, lightly stained fibrous bands course randomly through the darker parenchyma, outlining regenerative nodules and remaining islands of surviving hepatocytes (postnecrotic scarring). Note irregularity of the cut surfaces, especially evident at the right edge, reflecting condensation of connective tissue (Masson trichrome, ×20).

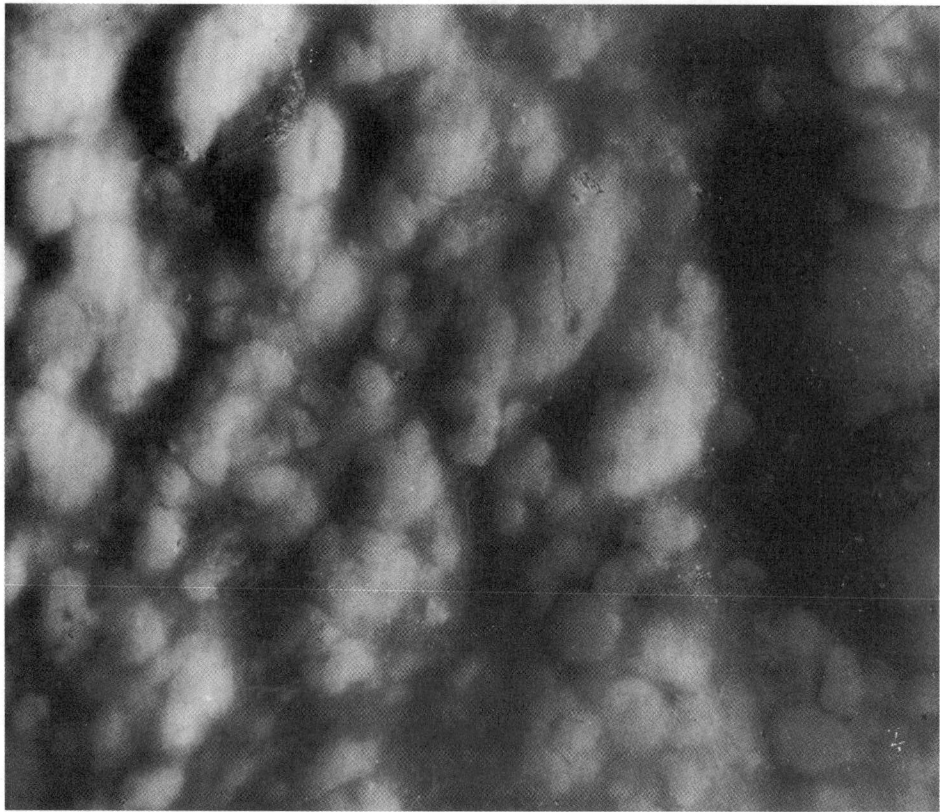

FIGURE 5 Macronodular cirrhosis. Liver surface showing coarse, irregularly shaped nodules and nodes measuring 1 cm or greater in cross section. Dark plaques of scar tissue separate the protruding tumor-like regenerative structures that compress and distort the remnants of the original lobular architecture and vascular network, detectable as a fine mesh (×9).

CLASSIFICATIONS OF CIRRHOSIS

Several classifications of cirrhosis based on morphologic, histologic, clinical, or etiologic criteria have been proposed. None provides logical guidelines for a practical approach to the individual patient, because the gross and microscopic features observed in liver biopsies correlate poorly with the clinical course, and the primary etiology is only tangentially related to the injury-repair-injury circle that sustains the cirrhotic state (see Pathogenesis). The gross morphologic appearance of the liver reflects patterns of collagen deposition as the disease process evolves. Initially, perilobular and interlobular bands of connective tissue delineate single lobules (Fig. 2). As lobules collapse and are replaced with fibrous and regenerating tissue, a crop of *micronodules* is generated (Figs. 3 and 4). The micronodular phase advances to *mixed* cirrhosis as ongoing cell death and repair processes create increasingly dysfunctional versions of the original parenchymal architecture. Eventually, the entire surface of the liver becomes corrugated with randomly distributed tumor-like protrusions of *macronodular* cirrhosis (Fig. 5). Nodules up to several centimeters in cross section begin to predominate several years after onset of the cirrhotic process.[2]

Histologic patterns of collagen deposition reflect the original zones of inflammation and necrotic collapse. When periportal deposits of fibrous tissue predominate but the lobular structure is still preserved, the cirrhosis is often described as "biliary" (Fig. 6). Distortion of the lobular architecture by irregular bands of fibrous tissue and displacement of portal and central zone structures by condensation of liver stroma are characterized as "postnecrotic" cirrhosis (see Fig. 4).

Since cirrhosis is the end result of liver cell injury from any cause, and the structural sequelae only rarely indicate the primary disease process, the gross and microscopic appearance of cirrhotic subtypes may not correlate with etiology. The small, uniformly sized nodules of micronodular cirrhosis are frequently observed in the *early* stages of extrahepatic biliary atresia, Indian childhood cirrhosis, venous outflow obstruction, and hemochromatosis. A mix of larger and smaller nodules (mixed cirrhosis) develops in later phases of these disorders. Macronodular patterns are observed in advanced stages of inflammatory hepatitides and in chronic metabolic disorders such as Wilson's disease and $alpha_1$-antitrypsin deficiency.[9]

In dealing with chronic liver disease in young patients, characterization of the primary disease process is of paramount importance for counseling purposes. Most inherited metabolic defects and congenital biliary malformations present in infancy or early childhood. These conditions can be associated with characteristic clinical evolutionary patterns. In contrast, the course of idiopathic or self-inflicted disorders that predominate in adults is less predictable (e.g., chronic active hepatitis, primary biliary cirrhosis, alcoholic cirrhosis). For this reason, a classification based on etiology (Table 1) provides information especially useful in guiding the diagnostic investigation of pediatric patients with chronic liver disease.

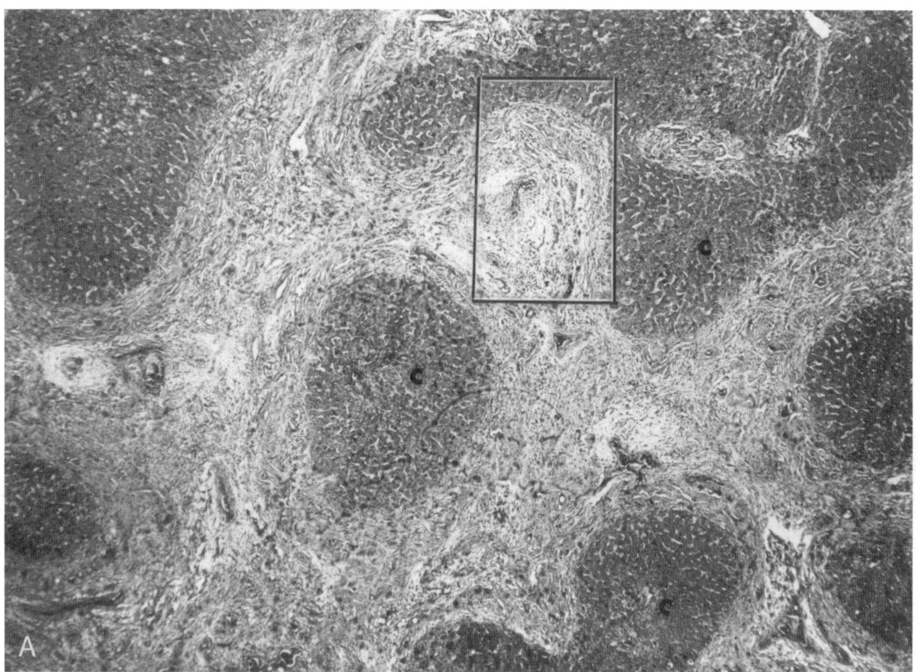

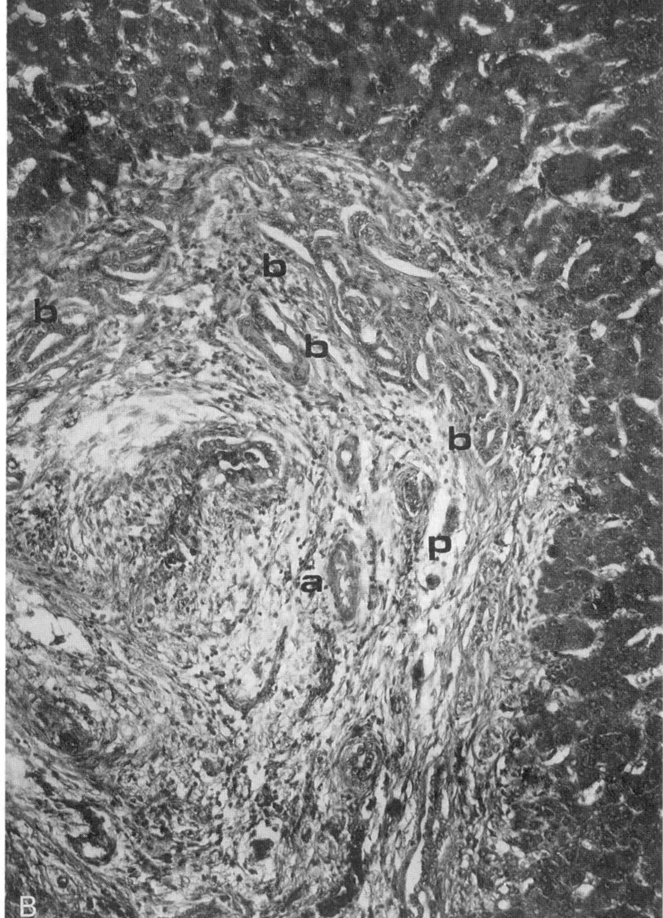

FIGURE 6 *A*, Biliary cirrhosis. Liver from a 2-month-old infant with extrahepatic biliary atresia. Dense bands of collagen surround lobules in which central veins (c) are normally located (Masson trichrome, ×80.) *B*, Higher magnification of area enclosed within black borders in *A*. Many proliferating bile ducts (b) are embedded within the fibrous tissue. Normal sinusoidal pattern of the parenchyma (dark-staining peripheral area) indicates that the parenchymal islands represent pseudolobules, not regenerating nodules. a = hepatic arteriole; p = portal vein.

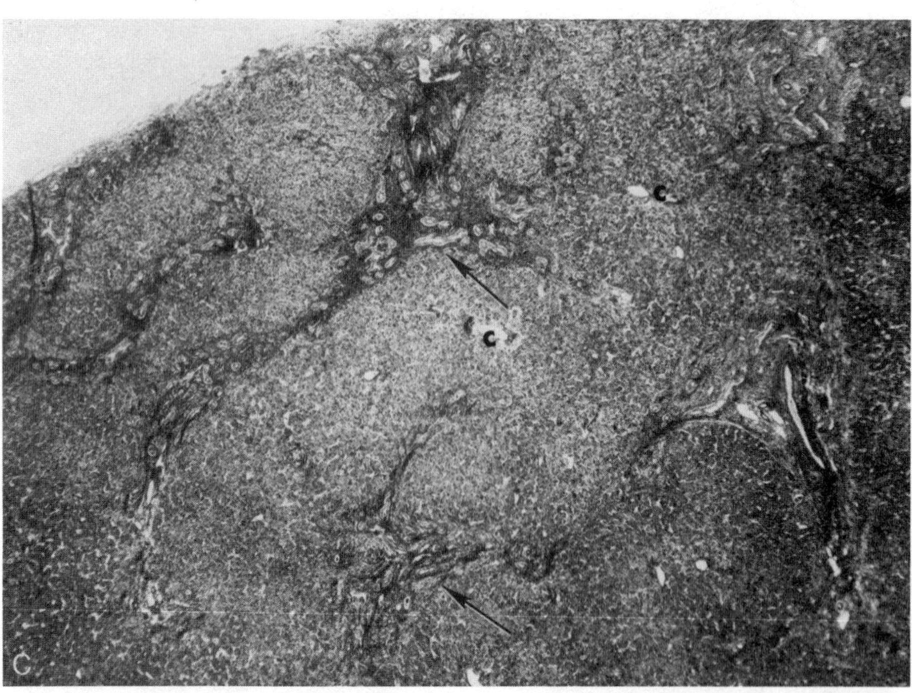

FIGURE 6 *Continued C*, Liver from the same patient at age 18 years. The abundant fibrous tissue observed in *A* has disappeared, leaving numerous proliferating bile ducts (*arrows*), but the relationship between portal and central zone structures has been preserved. The patient has a functioning Roux-en-Y choledochojejunostomy. Portal hypertension is the main clinical sequela of extrahepatic biliary atresia in this case. c = central vein (Masson trichrome, ×80).

CLINICOPATHOLOGIC FEATURES OF CIRRHOSIS

The clinical manifestations of cirrhosis in the individual patient depend on the equilibrium between injury and repair. The primary disease determines the type, severity, and rate of progression of hepatocellular damage and hence plays a major role in the clinical expression of the cirrhotic state. In situations in which injury progresses more rapidly than repair, patients present with signs of hepatocellular failure, with ascites and bleeding disorders due to inadequate synthesis of albumin and clotting factors, severe jaundice reflecting an inability to form or secrete bile, and encephalopathy as the result of failure to detoxify neurotoxic metabolites such as ammonia. When the repair processes of fibrogenesis and regeneration predominate and hepatocellular damage has been contained or arrested, portal hypertension and gastrointestinal hemorrhage constitute the main clinical problem.

According to these principles, disorders associated with modest liver cell damage may persist in a precirrhotic condition for many years. Such milder liver diseases produce focal necrotic lesions that heal by scarring but cause loss of functional liver mass insufficient to induce a generalized regenerative response. More extreme or prolonged pathologic states induce zonal necrosis in the poorly perfused areas of the liver acinus (zone 3), leading to formation of portocentral fibrous connections or bridges. This type of bridging produces shunting of sinusoidal blood along newly formed fibrous septa, as described above (see Fig. 2). The lobule-sized islands of parenchyma delineated by connective tissue consist of pre-existing liver cells or regenerating elements, depending on the extent of losses sustained by the functional liver cell mass (see Figs. 2 and 3). Regenerative activity in such cases may proceed slowly, causing gradual expansion of nodules within demarcation lines established by portocentral or portal-portal bridges, with gradual deformation of lobular architecture and compression of the terminal blood vessels (micronodular cirrhosis) (see Fig. 4). Removal of the primary disease agent (e.g., copper in Wilson's disease) may arrest the injury-repair sequence, especially in cases in which regenerative activity has not progressed to the stage of permanent interference with intrahepatic blood flow. For this reason, the presence of extensive fibrous tissue deposits without accompanying regenerative nodules in representative liver biopsies may be consistent with a potentially reversible precirrhotic state.

The importance of the distinction between fibrosis and cirrhosis becomes evident in young infants with cholestasis due to extrahepatic biliary obstruction. Atretic or cystic malformations of the common bile duct stimulate copious deposition of connective tissue in periportal lobular areas, forming portal-portal bridges that divide the parenchyma into lobule-sized pseudonodules (Fig. 6*A*). Unless accompanied by extensive inflammation and necrosis, the fibrous tissue is strikingly reduced by condensation or resorption, and the normal relationship between portal zone blood vessels and central veins is preserved after bile flow is surgically established (Fig. 6*B*).[10]

Major truncation of the functional liver cell mass triggers an active proliferative response in the remaining viable

TABLE 1
Diseases Associated with Cirrhosis

Disease	Usual Clinical Presentation	Treatment
Disorders Presenting in Infancy		
Metabolic disorders		
Alpha$_1$-antitrypsin deficiency	Cholestasis, portal hypertension	Liver transplant
Fructosemia	Hepatomegaly, liver failure	Dietary exclusion of fructose
Galactosemia	Hepatomegaly, liver failure	Dietary exclusion of milk products
Gaucher's disease	Hepatomegaly	None
Glycogen storage disease, type III	Hepatomegaly, rare liver disease	Dietary control
Glycogen storage disease, type IV	Hepatomegaly, liver failure	Transplantation
Niemann-Pick disease, type D	Hepatomegaly, liver failure	Liver transplant
Trihydroxycoprostanic acidemia	Cholestasis, liver disease	Liver transplant (?)
Tyrosinosis	Hepatomegaly, liver failure	Liver transplant
Acid esterase deficiency (Wolman's disease)	Hepatomegaly, liver failure	Liver transplant
Infections		
Viral hepatitides		
Cytomegalovirus	Hepatomegaly, cholestasis	Acyclovir
Herpes simplex	Jaundice, liver failure	Acyclovir
Rubella	Hepatomegaly, cholestasis	None
Hepatitis B ± delta virus	Hepatomegaly, fulminant liver failure	Immunization at birth
Hepatitis C (post-transfusion)	Hepatomegaly, cholestasis	?Interferon alpha
Syphilis	Hepatomegaly, cholestasis	Penicillin
Bacterial infections		
Neonatal sepsis	Hepatomegaly, jaundice	Antibiotics
Ascending cholangitis	Cholestasis, fever	Antibiotics
Biliary malformations		
Atresia of the common bile duct	Cholestasis, portal hypertension	Liver transplant
Arteriohepatic dysplasia (Watson-Alagille syndrome)	Cholestasis	Supportive therapy
Intrahepatic biliary hypoplasia	Cholestasis	Supportive therapy, liver transplant
Choledochal cyst	Recurrent cholestasis	Surgical correction
Vascular lesions		
Congestive heart failure	Hepatomegaly	Treatment of heart failure
Congestive pericarditis	Hepatomegaly, ascites	Pericardiectomy
Hepatic venous outflow obstruction		
Budd-Chiari syndrome	Ascites, hepatomegaly	Portacaval shunt, liver transplant
Congenital venocaval web	Ascites, hepatomegaly	Angioplasty, membranotomy
Veno-occlusive liver disease	Portal hypertension	Symptomatic treatment (?shunt)
Toxic and nutritional disorders		
Solvents (e.g., carbon tetrachloride)	Cholestasis, liver failure	Liver transplant
Natural toxins (mushrooms, aflatoxin)	Liver failure, cholestasis	Liver transplant
Total parenteral alimentation	Cholestasis	Enteral diet, liver transplant
Hypervitaminosis A	Portal hypertension	Discontinue vitamin A intake
Idiopathic disorders		
Cerebrohepatorenal syndrome (Zellweger's syndrome)	Hepatomegaly, jaundice	?Liver transplant
Familial intrahepatic cholestasis (Byler's disease)	Cholestasis, liver failure	Liver transplant
Neonatal (giant cell) hepatitis	Hepatomegaly, cholestasis	Supportive therapy, ?liver transplant
Disorders Presenting in Children and Adolescents		
Inherited metabolic disorders		
Cystic fibrosis	Portal hypertension, cholestasis	Sclerotherapy, vascular shunt
Hemochromatosis	Hepatomegaly	Chelation therapy, venesection
Hepatic porphyria	Usually quiescent	Hematin, venisection
Histiocytosis X	Hepatomegaly	Chemotherapy
Indian childhood cirrhosis	Hepatomegaly, cholestasis, ascites	?Chelation (copper), ?liver transplant
Hepatolenticular degeneration (Wilson's disease)	Hepatomegaly, cholestasis, liver failure	Chelation (penicillamine)
Infectious and inflammatory diseases		
Chronic active hepatitis	Cholestasis, ascites	Steroid hormones, liver transplant
Chronic hepatitis B ± delta	Cholestasis, ascites	?Liver transplant
Chronic hepatitis C (post-transfusion)	Cholestasis, chronic liver disease	?Liver transplant, interferon alpha
Primary sclerosing cholangitis	Cholestasis, hepatomegaly	Liver transplant
Ulcerative colitis	Cholestasis	Treatment of primary disease
Biliary malformations		
Choledochal cyst	Recurrent cholestasis	Choledochojejunostomy
Congenital hepatic fibrosis	Portal hypertension	Sclerotherapy, vascular shunt
Intrahepatic cystic biliary dilatation (Caroli's disease)	Recurrent cholangitis	?Liver transplant
Toxic, nutritional, and idiopathic disorders		
Hepatotoxic drugs (e.g., methotrexate)	Cholestasis, hepatomegaly	Discontinue drug, ?liver transplant
Malnutrition	Variable	Dietary or intake correction

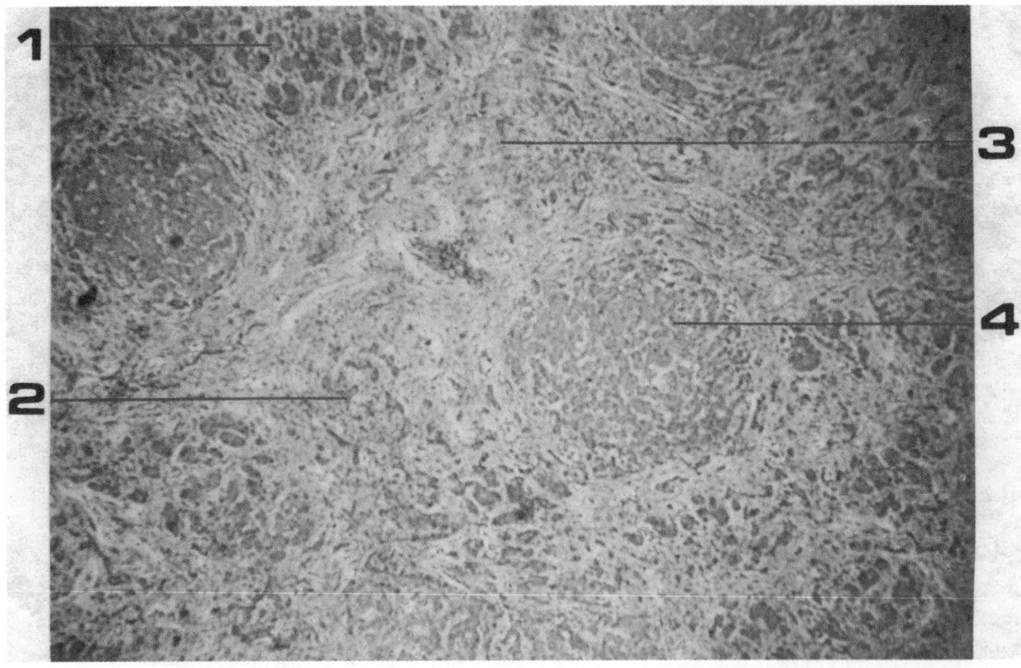

FIGURE 7 Subacute hepatic necrosis. Extensive distortion of lobular architecture, with lobular fragmentation (1), zonal necrosis (2), fibrosis (3), and active regeneration (4) (hematoxylin and eosin, ×50).

hepatocytes. Destruction of several adjoining lobules combined with active formation of regenerative nodules leads to a grossly distorted parenchyma, with broad bands of connective tissue carrying portal zone structures as remnants of collapsed lobules, and nodules varying greatly in size (macronodular or postnecrotic cirrhosis). This morphology is often observed in the terminal stages of chronic active hepatitis or subacute hepatic necrosis due to viral hepatitis (Fig. 7).

CLINICAL PATTERNS OF CIRRHOSIS

As previously indicated, cirrhosis manifests itself clinically in combinations of two characteristic pathologic patterns: failure of hepatocellular functions and portal hypertension. Depending partly on primary etiology, partly on age, and partly on co-existing disease, the patient may present with quiescent, asymptomatic illness, usually discovered in the course of investigation for another disorder *(compensated or quiescent cirrhosis)*; with chronic liver disease proceeding to complications such as ascites, severe cholestasis, or encephalopathy *(decompensated cirrhosis)*; with gastrointestinal bleeding *(portal hypertension with compensated cirrhosis)*; or with gastrointestinal (GI) bleeding combined with other features of liver disease *(portal hypertension with decompensated cirrhosis)*.

Compensated Cirrhosis

Cirrhosis may exist for many years in a quiescent or compensated state. The illness has no historical antecedents and is often discovered incidentally. In such fully compensated cases, the only physical abnormality may be a firm, enlarged liver, often accompanied by a palpable spleen. Liver function tests may remain in the normal range, with the exception of elevated serum alkaline phosphatase levels or slightly increased serum transaminase levels. Further investigation, including liver biopsy, may reveal Wilson's disease, alpha$_1$-antitrypsin deficiency, or evidence of hepatitis B infection, but in most instances compensated cirrhosis remains cryptogenic.

Decompensated Cirrhosis

Overtly apparent cirrhosis can take the form of hepatic parenchymal or vascular decompensation, or a combination of both. Infants with decompensated cirrhosis fail to thrive; children exhibit stunted growth and suffer from anorexia, muscle weakness, and fatigue. Jaundice is present in most instances of hepatocellular failure. The appearance of jaundice in a patient with previously quiescent or compensated cirrhosis is a sign of serious deterioration in the balance between injury and repair. Generally, patients with parenchymal decompensation also present with signs of increased resistance to intrahepatic blood flow due to active regenerative activity intended to replace the lost liver cell mass. Such patients will display, in addition to jaundice, subtle edema, mild to moderate ascites, esophageal varices, and hypersplenism. Commonly present are anemia, steatorrhea, and digital clubbing. Intermittent fever and abdominal right upper quadrant or epigastric pain occur occasionally.

Patients whose underlying disease involves the biliary tree (*biliary cirrhosis*) have a history of severe cholestasis (jaundice, pruritus, dark urine, light stools) that may progress to cirrhosis over months or years. Infants with extrahepatic

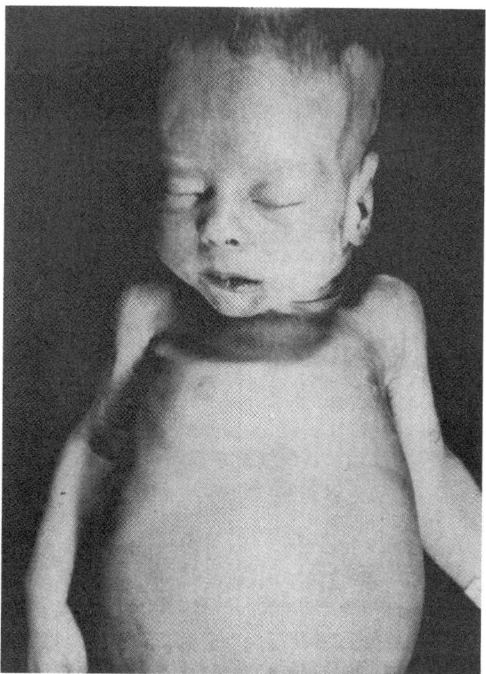

FIGURE 8 Infant with decompensated cirrhosis. Signs of end-stage liver disease include abdominal distention due to ascites, periorbital edema, dystrophic upper extremities, and ecchymoses on chin and left shoulder. The liver biopsy from this patient is shown in Figure 4.

biliary atresia invariably develop hepatocellular and vascular decompensation, unless the obstacle to bile flow is removed prior to permanent distortion of the intrahepatic blood vessels. After infancy, biliary cirrhosis may develop in cystic fibrosis as a result of biliary stasis and recurrent cholangitis. A much rarer cause of biliary cirrhosis, originally named after an Amish family (Byler's disease), progresses in all instances to liver failure and massive GI hemorrhage.

As indicated previously, infants or children with inherited metabolic diseases develop signs of liver disease, e.g., hepatomegaly, cholestasis, or ascites, long before cirrhosis supervenes. The list includes alpha$_1$-antitrypsin deficiency, Wilson's disease, tyrosinosis, and miscellaneous, less frequently encountered entities (Table 1). As the disease process evolves, dying liver cells are replaced by an irregular network of connective tissue (*postnecrotic cirrhosis*). This type of cirrhosis is more likely to progress to hepatocellular failure than is the biliary variety and is less frequently associated with cholestasis. Idiopathic antecedents of postnecrotic cirrhosis in infants include neonatal hepatitis and fatal neonatal cirrhosis (Fig. 8).[11] Chronic active hepatitis is the leading cause of postnecrotic cirrhosis in older children.[12]

Congestive or "Cardiac" Cirrhosis

Increased pressure in the right atrium due to heart failure, constrictive pericarditis, and congenital cardiac malformations is transmitted to the hepatic veins, causing chronic congestion of centrilobular areas (zone 3) of the liver (postsinusoidal portal hypertension). Sinusoids entering the terminal central vein radicals are distended and engorged with blood (Fig. 9). The combination of portal hypertension and sluggish blood flow results in focal hemorrhage and necrosis in central areas and then gradual replacement with fibrous bands. These central-to-central bridges are responsible for reversed lobulation, a histologic pattern characteristic of "cardiac cirrhosis."

Identical microscopic changes occur in patients with hepatic outflow obstruction due to Budd-Chiari syndrome,[13] usually associated with clotting disorders such as polycythemia

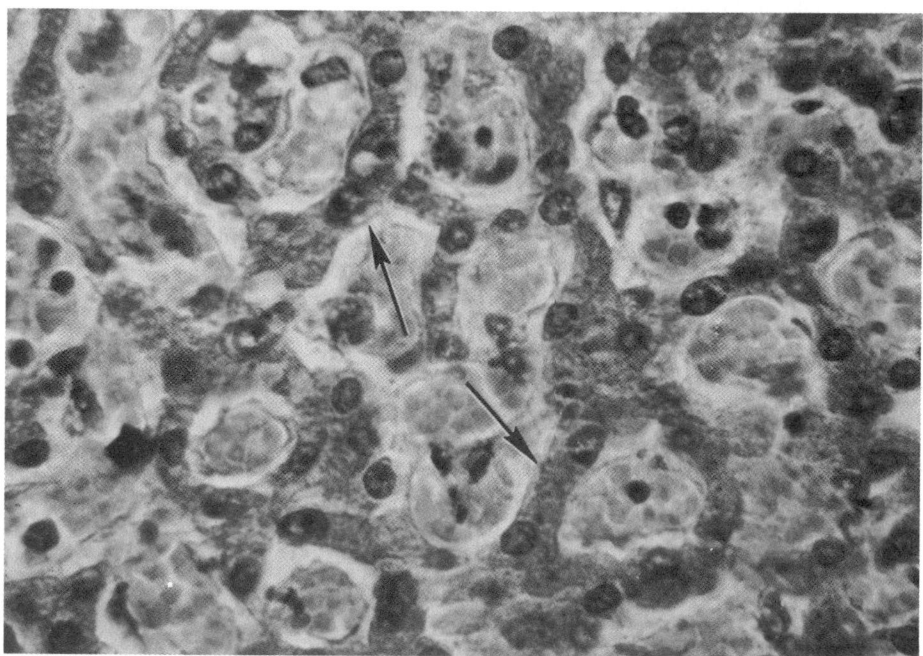

FIGURE 9 Congestive cirrhosis. Engorged central zone sinusoids. Liver cell plates (*arrows*) are compressed by intrasinusoidal hypertension (×450).

or congenital webs in the inferior vena cava above the liver. Veno-occlusive disease acquired from ingestion of pyrrolizidine alkaloids in bush teas[14] or produced by chemoradiotherapy of bone marrow transplant recipients[15] is a relatively common cause of congestive cirrhosis caused by intrahepatic venous outflow obstruction.

The liver is enlarged, smooth, and *tender* in all types of congestive cirrhosis. Splenomegaly develops as the portal pressure increases. Ascites is present in most patients with established postsinusoidal portal hypertension.

The diagnosis of congestive cirrhosis is based on percutaneous liver biopsy findings showing the characteristic centrizonal congestion, with central-to-central bridging in chronic cases. Relief of venous obstruction may be possible and is amenable to surgical correction by shunting or balloon angioplasty.[16] Patients with lesions causing intrahepatic postsinusoidal portal hypertension have received liver transplants.[17]

SYSTEMIC AND EXTRAHEPATIC MANIFESTATIONS OF CIRRHOSIS

Chronic liver disease of every type and etiology is associated with complex abnormalities of fluid compartmentalization, multiple nutritional and malabsorptive disorders, and a general susceptibility to systemic bacterial infections. The pathogenesis and clinical aspects of these manifestations are discussed elsewhere in this text.

Decompensated cirrhosis involves many systems. Gastrointestinal, hematologic, pulmonary, cardiovascular, cutaneous, endocrine, neurologic, and metabolic manifestations develop as cirrhosis progresses.

Gastrointestinal lesions associated with cirrhosis include esophageal and rectal varices due to portal hypertension, gastroesophageal reflux due to ascites, gastritis, peptic ulcer, and gallstones. The combination of varices and lower gastroesophageal sphincter incompetence increases the danger of severe hemorrhage from an eroded variceal vein.

Anemia occurs in the majority of children with cirrhosis, reflecting many possible causes: GI blood loss, dilutional factors, hemolysis associated with hypersplenism or red cell antibodies, and macrocytic anemia due to folic acid deficiency. Anemia may also result from hidden bleeding due to deficient production of coagulation factors synthesized by the liver, particularly prothrombin, Factor VII, and Factor IX. Bone marrow depression occurs following chronic blood loss combined with malnutrition. Iron depletion in a hypoplastic bone marrow or hemosiderin deposition and excess iron storage in the liver may complicate the course.[18]

Pulmonary function may be seriously compromised in children with cirrhosis. Exertional dyspnea is evident in patients with hepatosplenomegaly and ascites, but it is also observed in patients with reduced arterial oxygen saturation, which may be sufficiently severe to produce cyanosis. The hypoxemia is due to intrapulmonary arteriovenous shunts, reduced diffusion capacity, ventilation-perfusion mismatch, and portopulmonary venous collaterals connecting esophageal varices with the pulmonary veins. The specific mechanisms responsible for these changes in pulmonary perfusion are only partially understood. Clubbing of fingertips is present in all cases with chronic dyspnea and pulmonary hypoperfusion. Right-to-left shunting is demonstrable in such cases by peripheral venous contrast echocardiography and pulmonary angiography.[19]

Cardiovascular adjustments associated with chronic liver disease become prominent in cirrhosis. Mainly, cardiac output is increased in the presence of decreased peripheral resistance. Patients often appear flushed and warm to the touch, with a full pulse and high-output cardiac murmurs.

The *skin* in cirrhosis commonly displays spider angiomata and convoluted arterioles, especially prevalent on the upper torso, believed to be related to hormonal abnormalities. Palmar erythema is also present occasionally but is not specific for cirrhosis.

Endocrine abnormalities observed in adults with cirrhosis have been associated mainly with alcohol intake. Delayed pubescence is observed in teenagers with chronic liver disease. Disturbances of menstruation are common in young girls with cirrhosis.

Encephalopathy develops in cirrhosis as hepatocellular decompensation progresses.

Electrolyte abnormalities are usually present, the most prevalent being hypokalemia. Low serum potassium is due to a combination of frequent vomiting and secondary hypoaldosteronism. The use of diuretics to clear edema or ascites contributes to potassium loss. Hyponatremia is also common, reflecting poorly understood dilutional mechanisms. Decreased serum albumin levels are usually present in malnourished patients with decompensated cirrhosis.

PHYSICAL FINDINGS

The physical signs of cirrhosis develop from features commonly associated with all chronic liver diseases superimposed on manifestations of the primary pathologic process. Disorders affecting bile drainage or secretion are invariably characterized by early, progressive cholestasis manifesting as jaundice, pruritus, steatorrhea, and xanthomata, with sequelae of longstanding vitamin D or E deficiency appearing later in the course. Atretic and hypoplastic malformations of the extrahepatic or intrahepatic bile ducts and inherited defects of bile acid metabolism, such as trihydroxycoprostanic acidemia[20] and, most probably, familial intrahepatic cholestasis (Byler's disease),[21] are examples of severely cholestatic conditions presenting in early infancy.

In contrast to rapid development of severe cholestasis in primary biliary dysfunctional states, the clinical presentation of inborn errors of metabolism or chronic inflammatory liver diseases varies with the degree of hepatocellular injury (necrosis) and effectiveness of compensatory or repair mechanisms. Thus, inherited defects causing acute liver failure, such as galactosemia, the acute form of tyrosinemia and, less uniformly, hereditary fructose intolerance, appear in early infancy with signs of hepatocellular failure (jaundice, hepatomegaly, bleeding disorders, ascites, vomiting, and failure to thrive).

When the primary process responsible for parenchymal damage is less aggressive or proceeds more slowly, the development of clinical signs pointing to liver disease and eventual transition to cirrhosis can be insidious. Several important inherited causes of chronic liver disease in infants, children, and adolescents belong in the latter category, including alpha$_1$-antitrypsin deficiency, cystic fibrosis, Wilson's disease, and glycogen storage disease, type III. Similarly, chronic inflammatory states such as chronic active hepatitis and hepatopathy associated with ulcerative colitis may advance to irreversibility without readily detectable signs or symptoms. A percutaneous liver biopsy is an important diagnostic and prognostic tool in such quiescent cases, revealing the degree of inflammatory and necrotic activity, the extent and pattern of "postnecrotic" scarring, and diagnostic features of the primary disease process, e.g., the periodic acid-Schiff–positive granules observed in alpha$_1$-antitrypsin deficiency, copious copper deposits in Wilson's disease, and lesions of piecemeal necrosis strongly suggestive of chronic active hepatitis.

Portal hypertension is a constant component of both types of cirrhosis (biliary and postnecrotic), usually manifesting earlier and with greater severity in the biliary variety. The first indication of a cryptogenic liver illness may be massive hemorrhage from esophageal varices or, less frequently, from hemorrhoids. Rapid decompensation of a chronic liver disease is occasionally precipitated by GI variceal bleeding. The physical examination is usually confirmatory of a chronic disorder involving the liver in a patient with quiescent or fully compensated cryptogenic cirrhosis. Palpation of the abdomen reveals either a shrunken liver not detectable below the costal margin or an enlarged, firm liver with an irregular-edge and an anomalous lobar configuration. Detection of a palpable spleen or retrograde flow in the periumbilical venous plexus virtually confirms the presence of portal hypertension when associated with a shrunken or enlarged liver. Ascites is difficult to detect in small children with enlarged abdominal organs, but its presence may be elicited in advanced cases by demonstration of shifting dullness.

The sudden appearance or exacerbation of jaundice in a child with a compensated or quiescent chronic liver illness usually heralds impending hepatocellular failure and a shift in the cirrhotic equilibrium (injury versus repair) to the left. Other physical signs indicating movement toward cirrhosis include ascites, peripheral edema, behavioral changes suggestive of encephalopathy, unexplained bruises, progressive idiopathic anemia, and the characteristic smell of fecal breath (fetor hepaticus).

DIAGNOSIS

The advent of liver transplantation has revolutionized our approach to diagnosis of chronic liver diseases, shifting the emphasis from what it is to how serious it is, how much worse it is going to become, and when. As is strikingly apparent from Table 1, the majority of disorders associated with cirrhosis or intractable liver disease represent currently acceptable indications for a liver transplant. This fact lends urgency to the diagnosis of cirrhosis, redefined in practical terms as a condition dictating replacement of the patient's liver with a new one.

The current emphasis on transplantation as standard therapy for cirrhosis reflects the general failure of other medical or surgical measures to arrest the progression of cirrhosis or to improve the quality of life for these chronically ill children. In this light, the primary concern of a clinician faced with an infant or child with chronic liver disease is to determine the degree of functional decompensation and the severity of portal hypertension. The standard laboratory tests providing useful information include serum albumin, prothrombin time, and blood ammonia determinations. Deterioration of

TABLE 2
Disease-Specific Diagnostic Tests

Metabolic Disorders	Diagnostic Tests
Alpha$_1$-antitrypsin deficiency	Serum antitrypsin activity; P*i* phenotyping
Cystic fibrosis	Sweat electrolytes (Na, Cl)
Fructosemia	Fructose-l-phosphate aldolase E measurement (liver) Fructose-1,6-diphosphatase measurement (liver)
Galactosemia	Galactose-l-phosphate uridyl transferase measurement (liver)
Gaucher's disease	Glucocerebrosidase measurement (leukocytes)
Niemann-Pick disease	Sphingomyelinase measurement (leukocytes, liver)
Glycogen storage, type III	Debrancher enzyme (amylo-1,6-glucosidase) measurement (leukocytes, liver)
Glycogen storage, type IV	Brancher enzyme (amylo-1,4--1,6-transglucosidase) measurement (leukocytes, liver)
Trihydroxycoprostanic acidemia	Trihydroxycoprostanic acid measurement (bile, serum, urine)
Tyrosinosis	Succinylacetone (serum, urine)
Wilson's disease	Copper concentration (liver)
Wolman's disease (acid esterase deficiency)	Acid esterase measurement (leukocytes, liver)
Porphyria(s)	Porphyrin excretory pattern (urine)
Infections	
Viral hepatitides	
Cytomegalovirus	Virus isolation; serum conversion; specific antibody
Herpes simplex	Virus isolation, immunofluorescent antibody (liver)
Congenital rubella	Virus isolation; specific antibody
Hepatitis B ± delta	Hepatitis B surface antigen; delta-specific antibody
Hepatitis C	Immunoassay for viral protein
Syphilis (congenital)	*Treponema pallidum* (skin)

these indices signals the need for investigation according to a fixed protocol intended to evaluate the patient's "credentials" for a liver transplant.

The essential diagnostic procedures involved are a percutaneous liver biopsy (preferably performed with a Trucut needle) and Doppler ultrasonography of the abdominal cavity. The liver biopsy establishes the presence of cirrhosis in terms of histologic criteria and may indicate the underlying disease process. Ultrasonography is useful in confirmation of ascites, detection of hepatic and biliary cysts and vascular lesions, estimation of relative size and blood flow through the liver and spleen, and, most importantly, determination of patency and dimensions of the portal vein. A blocked portal vein is a contraindication to liver transplantation.

The primary disease or defect can be established with precision in most infants with chronic liver disease due to inherited errors of metabolism or structural anomalies of the bile ducts. The tests and procedures related to each condition are listed in Table 2. Valid and timely predictions of clinical evolution and outcome can often be made with a specific diagnosis in hand, allowing transplantation to occur while the patient is optimally prepared for surgery.

REFERENCES

1. Goresky CA, Huet PM, Marleau O, et al. Blood tissue exchange in cirrhosis of the liver. In: Tygstrup N, Orlandi F, eds. Methods and fields of research. Amsterdam: Elsevier, 1987: 143.
2. Popper M. Pathologic aspects of cirrhosis. A review. Am J Pathol 1977; 228–264.
3. Schaffner F, Popper M. Capillarization of hepatic sinusoids in man. Gastroenterology 1963; 44:239–242.
4. McIndoe AH. Vascular lesions of portal cirrhosis. Arch Pathol 1928; 5:23.
5. Biagini G, Ballandini G. Liver fibrosis and intracellular matrix. Review. J Hepatol 1989; 8:115.
6. Hahn G, Wick G, Pencev D, et al. Distribution of basement membrane proteins in normal and fibrotic human liver: collagen type IV, laminin and fibronectin. Gut 1980; 21:63–71.
7. Fausto N, Mead JE. Regulation of liver growth: protooncogenes and transforming growth factors. Lab Invest 1989; 60:4.
8. Roberts AB, Sporn MB, Assoian RK, et al. Transforming growth factor type B: rapid induction of fibrosis and angiogenesis *in vivo* and stimulation of collagen formation *in vitro*. Proc Natl Acad Sci 1986; 83:4167–4171.
9. Fauerholdt L, Schlichting P, Christensen E, et al. Conversion of micronodular cirrhosis into macronodular cirrhosis. Hepatology 1983; 3:928.
10. Thaler MM, Gellis SS III. Progression and regression of cirrhosis in biliary atresia. Am J Dis Child 1968; 116:271.
11. Thaler MM. Fatal neonatal cirrhosis: entity or end result? A comparative study of 24 cases. Pediatrics 1964; 33:721.
12. Silverman A, Roy CC, eds. Chronic active hepatitis. In: Pediatric clinical gastroenterology. 3rd ed. St. Louis: CV Mosby, 1983: 685.
13. Taneja A, Mitra SK, Moghe PD, et al. Budd-Chiari syndrome in childhood secondary to inferior vena caval obstruction. Pediatrics 1979; 63:808–812.
14. Fox DW, Hart MC, Bergeson PS, et al. Pyrrolizidine (Senecio) intoxication mimicking Reye syndrome. J Pediatr 1978; 93:980–982.
15. Shulman HM, McDonald GB, Matthews D, et al. An analysis of hepatic veno-occlusive disease and centrilobular hepatic degeneration following bone marrow transplantation. Gastroenterology 1980; 79:1178.
16. Prandi D, et al. Side-to-side portocaval shunt in the treatment of Budd-Chiari syndrome. Gastroenterology 1975; 68:127.
17. Putnam CW, et al. Liver transplantation for Budd-Chiari syndrome. JAMA 1976; 236:1142.
18. Sheehy TW, Berman A. The anemia of cirrhosis. J Lab Clin Med 1960; 56:72–82.
19. Keren G, Boichis H, Swas TS, et al. Pulmonary arteriovenous fistulae in hepatic cirrhosis. Arch Dis Child 1983; 58:302.
20. Hanson RF, Isenberg JN, Williams GC, et al. The metabolism of 3α, 7α, 12α-trihydroxy-5β-cholestan-26-oic acid in 2 siblings with cholestasis due to intrahepatic bile duct anomalies: an apparent inborn error of cholic acid synthesis. J Clin Invest 1975; 56:577.
21. De Vos R, De Wolf-Peters C, Desmet V, et al. Progressive intrahepatic cholestasis (Byler's disease): case report. Gut 1975; 16:1225.

PART 25

Liver Transplantation

Ronald E. Kleinman, M.D.
Jay P. Vacanti, M.D.

We have now completed the first quarter century of human liver transplantation. Widespread acceptance of this procedure was significantly enhanced in 1983 when a consensus conference sponsored by the National Institutes of Health recommended broader application of liver transplantation.[1] The impact of this consensus conference has been felt throughout the United States, where the number of centers performing more than five liver transplants per year has increased dramatically. Improvements in surgical technique and postoperative care have clearly contributed to the improvement in outcome following liver transplantation. In addition, perhaps the major factor leading to improved survival was the introduction of cyclosporine as a component of the immunosuppressive regimen for liver graft recipients.

Although the first recipient of a human liver to survive for an extended period of time underwent transplantation in 1967, 1-year survival could be expected for only four of ten patients undergoing liver transplantation between 1963 and 1979. Since that time, various centers have reported 3- to 5-year actuarial survival rates of 65 to 80 percent. With improved survival, the variety of disorders of the liver considered appropriate for transplantation has expanded considerably. Although there are several liver diseases that affect both children and adults, most liver transplants during infancy and childhood involve disorders unique to this age group, such as extrahepatic biliary atresia, inborn errors of metabolism, and intrahepatic biliary hypoplasia. We have evaluated and transplanted pediatric patients with disorders from all the major categories of liver disease. In addition to performing the operation, a successful liver transplant program must incorporate careful procedures for evaluation of transplant candidates, ongoing assessment and support of patients prior to transplantation, and the extremely complex and intensive postoperative support, including immunosuppression and its attendant complications. Recipients of liver grafts are candidates for lifetime immunosuppression and thus are subject to continuing expert medical care for life by the transplant team.

HISTORY AND RECENT DEVELOPMENTS

From 1967 to 1980 liver transplantation was done almost exclusively by Starzl, first in Colorado and later in Pittsburgh, and in England by Calne at Cambridge. Immunosuppression was achieved in most patients with the combination of prednisone and azathioprine or cyclophosphamide. Antilymphocyte globulin and thoracic duct drainage were sometimes used as adjuncts to immunosuppressive therapy. Survival beyond 2 years was achieved in only 20 percent of patients, few of whom were children. Our own experience with liver transplantation began in January, 1984, as part of The Boston Center for Liver Transplantation. Personnel, experience, protocols, and data have been shared in a joint effort of four Boston hospitals performing liver transplantation, both in adults and in children. Permission to proceed was granted by the State of Massachusetts with the understanding that there could be no reduction in pre-existing hospital services and that data were to be periodically reviewed by the Massachusetts Department of Public Health.[2] At the present time there are more than 75 centers in the United States with programs in orthotopic liver transplantation.

A liver transplantation program requires enormous resources because of the requirement for support from multiple medical services, including anesthesia, blood bank, social services, psychiatry, nutrition support, and clinical laboratories. The average charges for a patient undergoing liver transplantation, including the pretransplant evaluation and continuing postoperative care, is approximately $150,000, with a range from $50,000 to over $500,000. Since 1983 much of this cost has been borne by third-party payers. Significant expenses remain, however, for the parents of children in the liver transplant program. These include the considerable costs of living near the hospital for the 2 weeks to 6 months or longer that the patients are hospitalized following transplantation and the cost of immunosuppressive medications following liver transplantation.

A comparison of the results of liver transplantation and conventional treatment is compromised by different criteria for selection of candidates and diagnosis of hepatic reserve and by differing availability of resources, including donor organs. In our experience, the risk of dying after undergoing liver transplantation is approximately equal to the risk of dying while waiting for a transplant. The longest survival following an orthotopic liver graft is more than 20 years.[3] Patients have married, and several recipients have carried pregnancies successfully to term.

The quality of life for most patients appears to be excellent at 1 or more years following transplantation. Psychometric testing of adult patients[4] using tests measuring cognitive capacity, psychiatric status, and social functioning did not reveal any neuropsychological impairment. The psychiatric status of these patients appears to be comparable to that observed in patients with other chronic illnesses, such as Crohn's disease. These patients exhibit some degree of depression, social withdrawal, disruption of personality integration, and difficulties with social conformity. The most common problems noted in social functioning were impairment of sleep and rest.

For pediatric patients, one of the most positive outcomes of liver transplantation has been accelerated growth.[5,6] In our own experience, more than half of the patients achieve accelerated height velocity and improvements in height and weight in spite of the use of immunosuppressive doses of prednisone to prevent rejection. The greater percentage of pediatric patients exhibit catch-up growth after 1 year following transplantation when doses of prednisone are reduced.

Although survival has improved considerably for pediatric patients following liver transplantation, the smallest patients remain doubly disadvantaged. Patients weighing less than 12 kg have a higher incidence of vascular obstruction following transplantation and a lower survival rate (approximately 60 percent). It is this group for whom organs are also the most difficult to obtain, although newer techniques such as reduction hepatectomy and the use of organs from anencephalic donors may increase the availability of organs for this group of patients. The latter source is currently the subject of intense ethical debate that is unlikely to be resolved soon. A number of states have recently passed "required request laws," which mandate that, under appropriate circumstances, the next of kin be made aware of the possibility for organ donation.[7] In conjunction with this effort, many people are now declaring their intent to donate organs as part of a living will before death. Nevertheless, availability of donor livers is still a major limiting factor in transplantation. It has been estimated that 2 percent of all hospital deaths are potential liver donors and that many of these potential donors are not being identified.[8–10]

TABLE 1
Progressive Hepatic Decompensation

I. Diminished hepatic synthetic function
   A. Prolongation of prothrombin time unresponsive to vitamin K administration
   B. Hypoalbuminemia
   C. Hyperammonemia

II. Symptomatic portal hypertension
   A. Ascites
   B. Recurrent variceal bleeding
   C. Encephalopathy

III. Growth failure

SELECTION OF PATIENTS

Candidates for transplantation should have a well-defined chronic, progressive, and irreversible liver disorder manifested in one of the ways listed in Table 1.

No single test of liver function can determine when chronic liver disease has reached an irreversible state and will then continue to progress to hepatic failure. A history of ascites, an indirect bilirubin of greater than 6 mg per deciliter, and a cholesterol of less than 100 mg per deciliter, along with a partial thromboplastin time of greater than 20 seconds following vitamin K administration, have been considered signs of intractable and irreversible liver dysfunction.[11]

It has been suggested, although not confirmed, that survival following transplantation is not related to clinical status prior to transplantation. In our own experience, patients with multiple organ dysfunction before transplant have a lower survival following transplantation. Many centers, including our own, prioritize candidates for liver transplantation according to their clinical status before transplant, with the sickest patients receiving the highest priority. Because of the scarcity of organs, when a donor liver becomes available, the recipient is often chosen on the basis of size compatibility with the donor liver. Although major blood group compatibility is a consideration, because of the urgent need for an organ, we and others have transplanted across A-B-O blood groups with little or no difference in survival compared with major blood group–matched organs. No attempt is made to match minor blood groups or histocompatibility antigens.[12] Tissue matching does not appear to be an important consideration in liver transplantation, and although hyperacute rejection of the liver has been demonstrated in an animal model, it appears to occur rarely in the clinical setting.

Because there are many children with chronic liver disease who follow a stable and relatively uncomplicated course for extended periods of time, knowledge of the clinical course of specific disorders is helpful in timing the liver transplant. In addition, knowledge of an individual patient's course is imperative, and, therefore, the patient's primary physician must be included in the selection process when possible.

There are several contraindications to liver transplantation. Advance cardiac or pulmonary disease and concomitant severe hypoxemia due to right-to-left shunting may exclude a patient from receiving a liver graft. Patients with chronic disease of both the liver and lung, such as cystic fibrosis, have received liver transplants, although for the most part these are patients with minimal lung disease.[13] For patients with severely compromised pulmonary function, liver-lung transplants have been performed.

Extrahepatic malignancy or metastatic hepatobiliary malignancy is a stronger contraindication to liver transplantation. In the rare patient with a slow-growing tumor such as a fibrolamellar hepatocarcinoma diffusely involving the liver, but not extending beyond the liver capsule, transplantation is often the only possible life-saving procedure. In the majority of patients, however, rapid growth or spread beyond the liver capsule precludes liver transplantation because of the poor results in these patients.[14] For patients with hepatocellular carcinoma, histologic confirmation of the diagnosis, assessment of extent of involvement within the liver, and assessment of metastatic involvement are essential. Patients with malignancies or with conditions in which malignancies commonly complicate the underlying disease process, such as hereditary tyrosinemia, must be told that if malignancy is found beyond the liver capsule at the time of exploration, the operation will not continue. In these circumstances another potential recipient should be available at the time of transplantation so that the donor organ can be used if spread of the malignant process has been underestimated in the pretransplant evaluation.

Patients with infection must also be considered carefully before transplantation is undertaken. Sepsis must be controlled before transplantation takes place. Viremia is also a contraindication to transplantation, although patients with subclinical cytomegalovirus or other viral infections have successfully undergone transplantation. The effect of immunosuppression is often to activate these infections and produce hepatocellular necrosis in the post-transplant period. Indications and contraindications for transplantation in hepatitis B surface antigen–positive patients are still not completely defined. Recurrence of infection may be reduced if patients are transfused with hyperimmune globulin intraoperatively.

Pretransplant Evaluation

The pretransplant evaluation has the following objectives: (1) to define the patient's disorder; (2) to define the patient's present medical status; (3) to determine eligibility and priority for transplantation; (4) to arrange for appropriate interim supportive care. This requires the efforts of a multidisciplinary team, which includes transplant surgeon, hepatologist, transplant nurse-coordinator, radiologist, pathologist, psychologist, social worker, immunologist, and other medical subspecialists determined by the patient's clinical condition. During the evaluation the patients become acquainted with the hospital and with the medical and surgical team. An assessment of the metabolic and nutritional effects of the liver disorder is necessary to determine if optimum medical and surgical therapy has been applied to the particular condition. If not, recommendations for such therapy may be provided to determine the progressive and irreversible nature of the patient's liver disorder. Blood group typing is performed so that an A-B-O–compatible donor can be sought, if possible, and the blood bank can be organized to provide up to 100 liters of blood, sometimes necessary during the transplant surgery. Pulmonary function studies and neurologic and psychometric evaluation may be necessary in individual cases.

Because conditions such as biliary atresia often are complicated by vascular anomalies, an anatomic evaluation of the liver and vascular supply may be helpful. Ultrasonography of the right upper quadrant provides an estimate of the size of and blood flow through the portal vein. We have observed a progressive reduction in the diameter of the portal vein in one of our patients followed serially with ultrasonographic evaluation of the right upper quadrant. Thus the timing of transplantation may be influenced if this phenomenon is observed in other patients.

Patients with chronic diseases of the liver frequently suffer from major compromise of both psychosocial and motor development, usually as a direct consequence of the severity of their liver disease. Thus, the emotional preparation of both patient and family is an important facet of the pretransplant evaluation. Once initiated, hepatic transplantation becomes a lifelong process. Pediatric patients must have a supportive family that understands and accepts the nature of the transplantation process. The family must be able to tolerate the uncertainty inherent in waiting for an organ to become available and the intensive medical therapy of the post-transplant period. A patient should be prepared for surgery, which may occur at an unpredictable time, last from 7 to 24 hours, and require from 2 weeks to more than 6 months in the hospital. Arrangements should be made for the patient and family to remain in the vicinity of the transplantation center for several weeks to several months after discharge depending on the complications that arise following transplantation. Once the pretransplant evaluation has been completed, candidates are placed on a priority call.

Organ donation and procurement are currently handled on a regional basis. The regional organ bank is connected to the United Network for Organ Sharing (UNOS), which is currently developing a national integrated program for procurement and disbursement of donor organs. Patients are listed with the local organ bank according to a weighted score determined in part by severity of liver dysfunction and need for hospital support prior to receiving a liver transplant. In all cases, regional needs are met first before organs are shared nationally. In some cases it may be also 1 year before the appropriate donor organ becomes available, so the primary physician should be aware of the need for continued outpatient monitoring of the candidate.

Candidates for Transplantation

For the most part, pediatric candidates for liver transplantation have had chronic disorders of the liver. There is considerable heterogeneity in the clinical courses of most of the liver disorders that present in infancy and childhood. Approximately one-third of children with biliary atresia lead relatively normal lives after hepatic portoenterostomy, but the remainder undergo progressive liver destruction over varying time intervals.[15,16] Infants with syndromes of extrahepatic biliary hypoplasia are often clinically indistinguishable from those with extrahepatic biliary atresia. In the absence of cirrhosis, however, these patients have a different clinical course, tending toward stable inactive disease after infancy that is compatible with a relatively normal adolescence.

Inborn errors of metabolism are the second most common group of liver disorders for which children have been transplanted.[17] Alpha$_1$-antitrypsin deficiency is the most common inborn metabolic disorder of the liver in infants, but only 15 to 20 percent of those affected develop serious chronic liver disease. Even in those severely affected, the course of liver involvement is highly variable, with some patients progressing rapidly during the first year of life toward liver failure and others entering remission until the early adolescent years. Thus, those disorders for which children most often require a liver graft may have similar presentations but varying clinical courses, emphasizing the need for careful evaluation and selection of liver graft recipients and timing of the transplant operation.

Hereditary tyrosinemia type I is an example of a lethal metabolic disorder. Patients develop liver failure during infancy or progressive hepatic compromise with portal hypertension and commonly hepatocellular carcinoma. The replacement of the liver corrects the enzyme deficiency, with decreased excretion of urinary succinyl acetone and succinyl acetoacetate in many patients.[18] In some patients, however, renal tubular dysfunction continues despite successful liver transplantation. Thus, correcting a specific enzyme defect by orthotopic liver transplantation may not correct defects in other affected organs. The concomitant presence of hepatomas in many patients with metabolic liver disease also raises the issue of the advisability of transplantation for primary hepatic malignancies in childhood. Patients with hepatic malignancies found incidentally at the time of surgery tend to have a lower incidence of tumor recurrence following transplantation.[19]

Those patients for whom the primary indication for transplantation is hepatic malignancy have a very poor outcome, with 2-year survival of approximately 30 percent, owing largely to recurrence of the tumor.[20] Despite the overall grim prognosis for these patients, we and others continue to evaluate and in some cases perform transplants for patients with hepatic malignancy, including bile duct malignancy, confined entirely to the liver. We currently have several patients who are tumor-free 2 years after transplantation.

Because of the involvement of multiple organs, unique approaches to transplantation have been taken in patients with conditions such as familial hypercholesterolemia. Orthotopic transplantation of the liver and heart from the same donor has been performed in a patient with severe familial hypercholesterolemia.[21] The combined transplantation of both liver and kidney is another example of such an approach for patients with metabolic disease involving multiple organs.[22] In a few cases fetal liver cells have been transplanted into patients with Fabry's disease, with both objective and subjective improvement in clinical symptoms although with very short-term follow-up.[23]

Although most patients receive liver grafts for chronic disorders, orthotopic liver transplantation has been performed for patients with acute fulminant hepatic failure in the setting of a chronic disorder such as Wilson's disease.[24] In general, transplantation for fulminant hepatic failure following a recently acquired hepatic disorder has a poorer outcome than transplantation for chronic disorders. However, patients who are transplanted with acute hepatic failure due to infectious hepatitis A, B, or non-A, non-B, the acute fulminant hepatitis of Wilson's disease, or drug-induced hepatic failure have a higher survival rate (30 percent) following transplantation than with other modes of therapy.[25]

Growth failure and bone disease are prominent features of a majority of patients considered for liver transplantation. In addition, recurrent sepsis, variceal hemorrhage, and encephalopathy complicate the courses of many of these infants and children. Although age has not appeared to influence outcome following transplantation in a reported series of patients,[11] our own experience is that the smallest patients (those less than 12 kg), who are also usually the youngest patients, have a lower actuarial survival following the transplant operation. The usual reasons for graft failure in these very small patients include vascular thrombosis following transplantation, rejection, and primary graft nonfunction. Up to 40 percent of patients less than 12 kg experience arterial thrombosis in the immediate post-transplant period.[26] For patients who experience graft failure, retransplantation is an option. The shortage of donors severely limited the ability to retransplant many of these patients, and we have successfully managed a number of patients with compromised blood flow to the new liver with retransplantation.

The vast majority of patients with biliary atresia are first treated with hepatoportoenterostomy. Although the transplant operation is more difficult in patients who have had a prior hepatoportoenterostomy, this has not influenced survival following the operation, and we continue to advocate that all patients with biliary atresia diagnosed in the first 10 weeks of life undergo hepatoportoenterostomy and that transplantation be considered only if this operation fails. In addition to the altered anatomy created by the hepatoportoenterostomy, patients with biliary atresia, as mentioned above, often have vascular anomalies that further complicate the transplant operation.

OPERATIVE PREPARATION AND ANESTHETIC MANAGEMENT

With regionalization of transplantation centers, patients must be rapidly mobilized for the operative procedure when a donor organ becomes available. Patients who are not in the hospital must be notified, usually through a portable paging system, and arrangements for transportation must be set far in advance so that the patient may be delivered to the hospital by the quickest possible route. Upon arrival at the hospital, a preoperative assessment of the patient's physical condition is made and an intravenous infusion of cyclosporine is initiated at a dose of 2 mg per kilogram over 2 to 4 hours. Patients are brought to the operating room in advance of beginning the actual operative procedure so that peripheral and central intravenous catheters may be placed for monitoring fluid replacement and drug administration. Hemodilution from extensive fluid loss and subsequent transfusion changes the requirements for a number of anesthetic medications and increases the need for extremely intensive patient monitoring.

Once the hepatectomy begins, coagulation and fluid balance must be carefully monitored. For patients with longstanding disease, the development of extensive collateral circulation, adhesions from prior surgery such as hepatoportoenterostomy, and the coagulopathy imposed by the chronic liver disease often lead to heavy blood loss and subsequent fluid replacement. We have used an average of 40 units of packed red blood cells, fresh frozen plasma, and platelets in patients less than 12 kg in weight and 60 units in patients more than 12 kg. Packed red cells must be as fresh as possible in order to diminish the chances of massive hemolysis with subsequent hyperkalemia. The availability of rapid infusion systems[27] may be mandatory to preserve hemodynamic stability under conditions of massive blood loss. In addition, a cell-saver device may be used to decrease the extraordinary demand on the blood bank during the operation.

At the beginning of the anhepatic phase, the potential for a sudden reduction in blood pressure occurs with cross-clamping of the inferior vena cava. In older patients this may be obviated by venovenous bypass. In all patients, intensive monitoring of hemodynamic parameters and rapid replacement of fluid to maintain blood pressure are essential. With orthotopic replacement of the liver and re-establishment of circulation, marked changes in serum potassium, sodium, and calcium occur. Metabolism of citrate and lactate from transfused solutions may produce initial acidemia and then ultimately alkalosis.

Particular care must be taken to maintain euthermia during the period of revascularization.[28] This may be extremely difficult at a time when the liver must remain chilled in order to preserve optimal function following revascularization. The reduction of coagulation factors, with the exception of Factor VIII, and elevation of fibrinolytic split products produce a coagulopathy similar to disseminated intravascular coagulation.[29] Standard monitoring of coagulation during the operative procedure includes repeated measurements of platelets, partial thromboplastin time, and prothrombin time and the use of thromboelastographic tracings. The thromboelastogram examines whole blood clotting time and may be particularly useful because of the ease and speed with which this test can be performed.[30] During the final phase of the operative procedure, with return of blood flow through the inferior vena cava, hepatic artery, and portal circulation, the rise in systemic blood pressure may be particularly pronounced, along with changes in acid-base status.[31]

Improvements in organ procurement and preservation have also contributed to improvement in survival. The donor must have had a good urine output with cardiovascular stability; prolonged ischemia, hypotension, or asystole excludes a potential donor. In addition, there can have been no pre-existing trauma to the liver, diabetes, hypertension, acute systemic infection, or malignancy other than primary brain tumor. Criteria for brain death must be explicit and decisions made expeditiously, since the liver is damaged by warm ischemia.

Donor Operation

Most often the donor hepatectomy is now performed in the context of a multiorgan harvest. The techniques for many teams harvesting heart, heart-lung, liver, and kidneys are now well established.[32] Pancreatic transplantation is assuming a greater role in the treatment of diabetes. Efforts are now underway in several centers surgically to allow the transplantation of both organs from a single donor.

Special concerns for a pediatric harvest include delicate fluid and electrolyte management, good temperature regulation, avoidance of hypothermia during the donor harvest, and hemodynamic stability during the harvest procedure. The donor operation is carried out through a long midline incision from the sternal notch to the pubis. Both hemidiaphragms are incised to allow wide exposure in the thorax as well as in the abdomen. The liver is inspected for swelling, firmness, and viability. The porta is first examined for the presence of a replaced left hepatic artery off the left gastric artery (which occurs in about 19 percent of cases) or a replaced right hepatic artery arising from the superior mesenteric artery (present in about 20 percent of normal cases). Rarely, both situations occur in the donor. This arterial inflow must be carefully preserved.

The porta hepatis is dissected to isolate the celiac access down to the aorta. The aorta is isolated through the diaphragmatic hiatus immediately above the celiac access for cross-clamping at the time of perfusion, and the bile duct is then isolated down to the duodenum and the portal vein is dissected down to its retropancreatic origin from the confluence of the splenic, coronary, and superior mesenteric veins. The pancreas is divided for ready access to this. The triangular ligaments are taken down, allowing the dome of the liver to lie free, and the inferior vena cava above the liver is isolated. The diaphragmatic attachments of the right lobe of the liver are then dissected, and the right adrenal vein is identified and ligated before division. The inferior vena cava below the liver is isolated above the take-off of the renal veins. The right colon is mobilized so that the inferior vena cava and the aorta above their bifurcations are both isolated for perfusion and drainage.

At this point the other teams mobilize the kidneys and heart. After placement of the perfusion cannulas, the heart is isolated, perfused, and removed after the aorta is clamped above the celiac axis. The superior mesenteric artery is ligated and the liver is cold-perfused. Many groups continue to advocate precooling the liver with lactated Ringer's solution through the splenic vein before the aortic perfusion. The University of Wisconsin (UW) solution seems to afford much greater protection to the cold-preserved liver.[33] Early experimental results in many institutions support its major advantage over Eurocollins solution (Table 2). Specifically, it relies on a hetastarch for its osmotic pressure as opposed to albumin, and it relies on lactobionate instead of glucose or dextrose as a carbohydrate source for the cold-preserved hepatocytes. Its use has allowed up to 20 hours of preservation of livers before implantation, as opposed to the previous limit of 6 to 8 hours using Eurocollins solution. In our short experience, the incidence of primary graft nonfunction in the small infant has decreased dramatically.

Recipient Operation

The recipient operation is timed in relation to the donor operation to minimize the cold preservation time of the liver. In adults, this total time has increased safely to 20 hours, but

TABLE 2
Preservation Fluids

Eurocollins (mM/L)		University of Wisconsin Solution	
KH_2PO_4	15	K lactobionate	100 mM
K_2HPO	42	$NaKH_2PO_4$	25 mM
KCl	15	Adenosine	5 mM
$NaHCO_3$	10	$MgSO_4$	5 mM
Glucose	194	Glutathione	3 mM
pH	7.0	Raffinose	30 mM
mOsm/L	355	Allopurinol	1 mM
		Insulin	100 U/L
		Bactrim	0.5 ml/L
		Hydroxyethol starch	5 g/dl
		Na	30 mM
		K	120 mM
		OSM	320–330 mOSm/L
		pH	7.4

Adapted from Jamieson NV, Sundberg R, Lindell S, Southard JH, Belzer FO. A comparison of cold storage solution for hepatic preservation using the isolated perfused rabbit liver. Cryobiology 1988; 25:300–310.

we have not tested this in small children because of our prior high incidence of primary graft nonfunction. We have now also routinely employed either exchange transfusion in very small babies or plasmapheresis in larger infants and children in those situations in which marked coagulopathy from hepatic synthetic dysfunction has been a problem. This aggressive approach has led to less blood loss during the recipient hepatectomy. We routinely place a double-lumen Broviac catheter into the right neck before the recipient hepatectomy begins. We also prepare infants and children for venovenous bypass if we are concerned that adequate collaterals have not formed. We perform venovenous bypass in the infants using a circuit and pump similar to those used for extracorporeal membrane oxygenation. The venous outflow from the patient to the pump is both from the inferior vena cava, accessed by means of the femoral vein, and from the cut end of the portal vein. In small babies the blood is returned to the heart via the right internal jugular vein. We have employed this rarely, but it has been lifesaving in circumstances of acute hepatic failure.

The recipient hepatectomy is performed through a large subcostal transverse incision (Fig. 1). This allows free access to the upper abdomen and lower abdomen in small infants. The Buchwalder retractor is used to optimize our exposure. Loop magnification and headlights are essential for accurate dissection as well as placement of the graft. Most often the recipient hepatectomy is performed in the presence of prior surgery, since most children have biliary atresia and have undergone a Kasai portoenterostomy. This dissection is tedious, time-consuming, and associated with greater blood loss than the unoperated abdomen. However, it can be done safely and accurately. The Roux-en-Y limb of intestine is dissected free from the porta. If its length is not sufficient or adhesions have made it unusable, one must remove it and construct a new intestinal limb for children with biliary atresia. The inferior vena cava above and below the liver, the hepatic artery down to the level of the gastroduodenal artery and beyond, and the portal vein are dissected free.

Once the new liver has been inspected and found usable, clamps are placed and the native liver is removed. The retroperitoneum and diaphragm are inspected and all bleeding points are controlled before placement of the new liver. The three venous anastomoses are performed and vascular inflow is established. The liver is relatively hypoxemic but vascularizes as the arterial anastomosis is constructed. The preferred reconstruction of the artery is shown (Fig. 1). A patch of aorta can be anastomosed to the common hepatic artery at the level of the gastroduodenal artery. This patch can include the superior mesenteric artery as well. We have found this reconstruction to be superior to an aortic conduit in unusual vascular situations, as has been previously described. Once satisfactory vascular inflow is established, the biliary reconstruction is performed. In the case of biliary atresia, a Roux-en-Y limb is anastomosed side to end with the donor bile duct. The gallbladder is removed. A Silastic biliary stent is placed through the intestinal limb into the bile duct for drainage. As shown, wide drainage is achieved and the abdomen closed.

Because of the extreme donor scarcity in small infants, several groups are now looking into reduction hepatectomy and using either the anatomic left lobe or the left lateral seg-

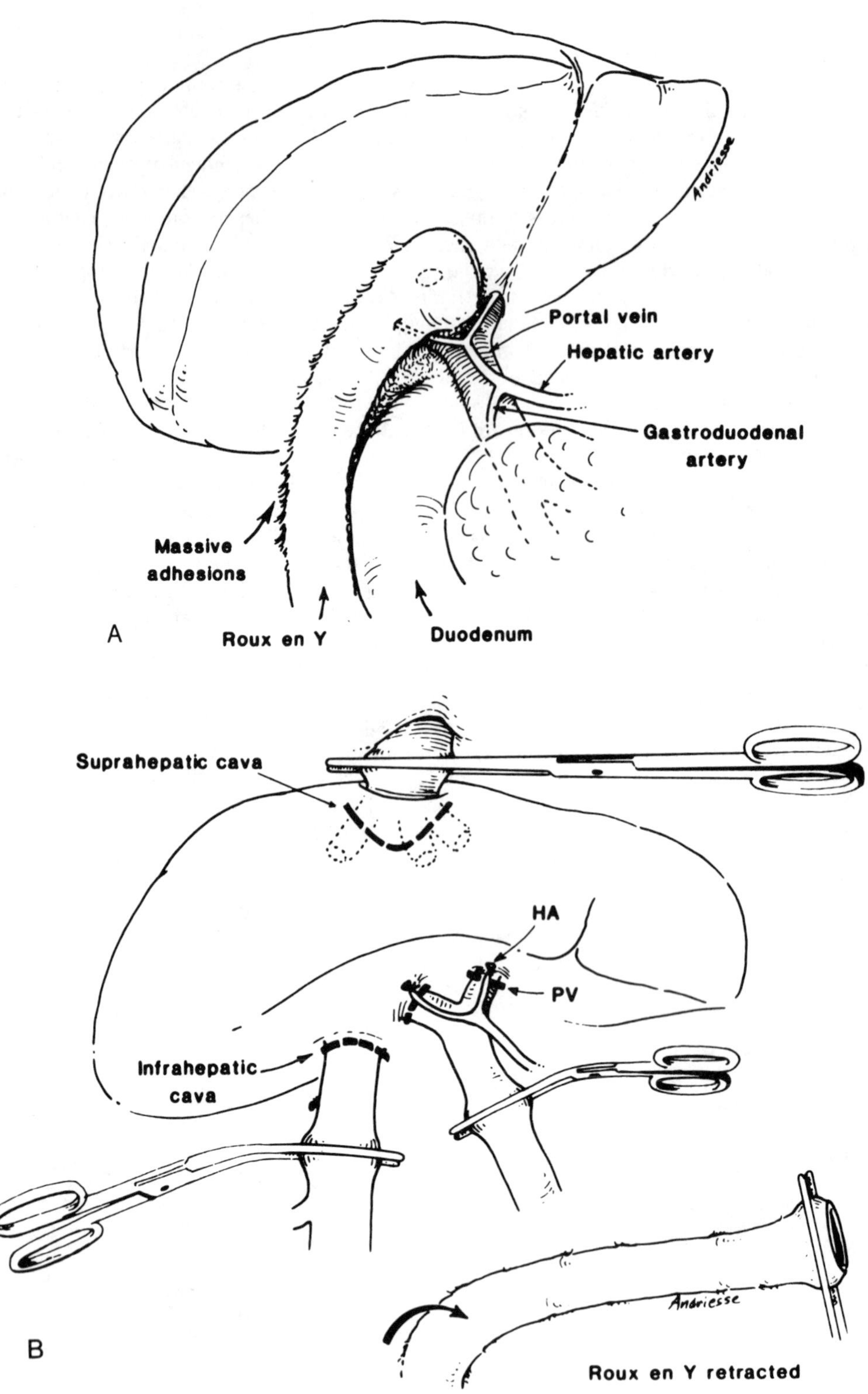

FIGURE 1 Details of recipient operation for pediatric liver transplantation. *A*, Recipient hepatectomy in biliary atresia showing massive adhesions in the porta hepatis. *B*, Lines of resection in removing the native liver.

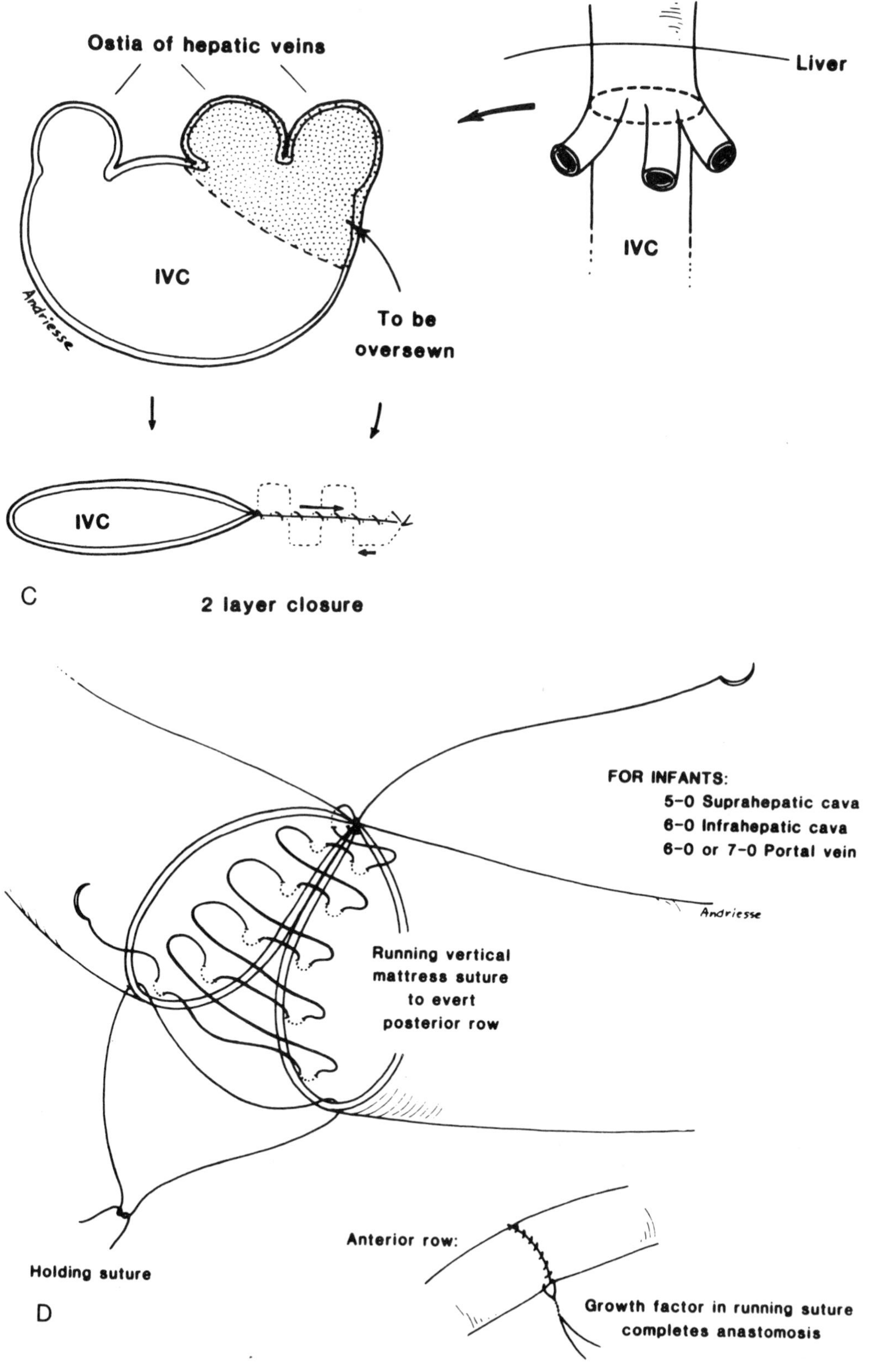

FIGURE 1 *Continued. C,* Technique of tailoring suprahepatic caval cuff for anastomosis. *D,* Running vertical mattress suture technique for venous anastomosis.

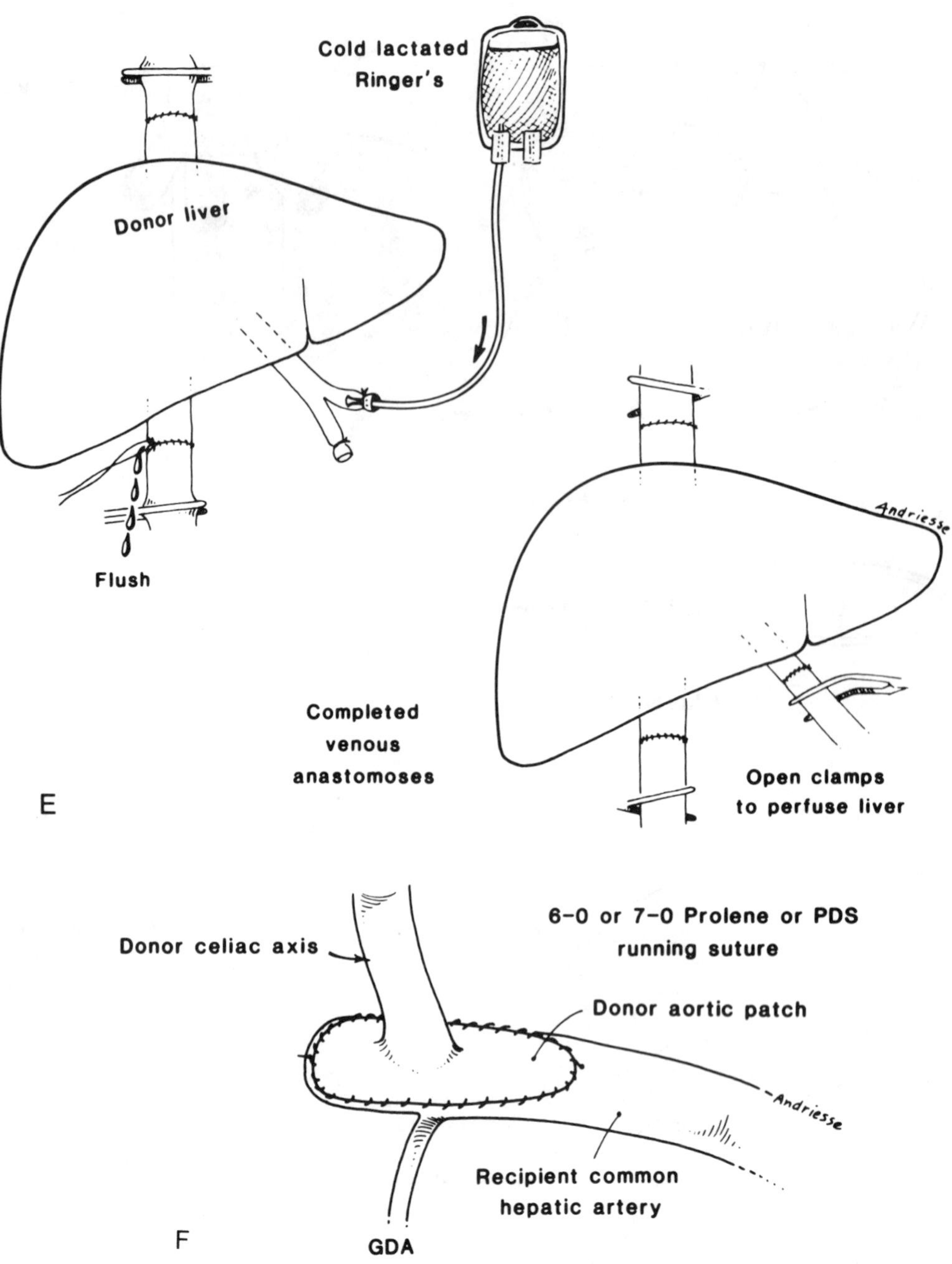

FIGURE 1 *Continued. E,* Flush of donor liver prior to completion of infrahepatic caval anastomosis and then completion of that anastomosis and portal venous anastomosis. *F,* Preferred arterial reconstruction.

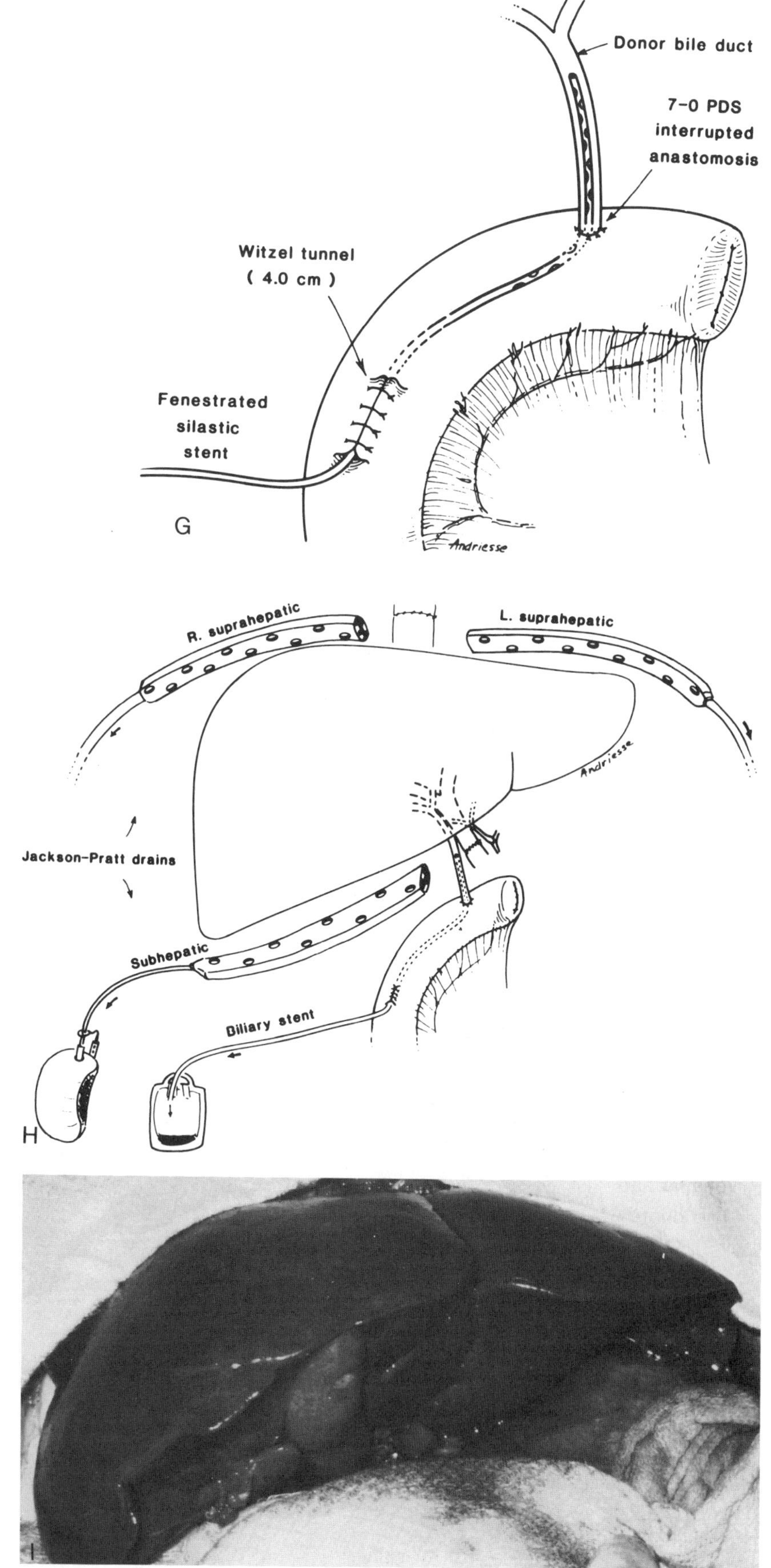

FIGURE 1 *Continued. G,* End-to-side choledochojejunostomy for children with biliary atresia: bile duct reconstruction using Roux-en-Y limb. *H,* Detail of donor liver after completion of implantation, showing drain positions. *I,* Photograph of newly transplanted liver, which is now well perfused.

ment (Fig. 2). Early reports[34,35] have shown sufficient promise to make this an alternative in the situation of small infants for whom whole organ grafts are not available.

In summary, several improvements in operative management in the last 5 years have led to improving survival in small children requiring liver transplantation. These include better preservation fluids, techniques for venovenous bypass in small children, the use of plasmapheresis or exchange transfusion immediately prior to transplantation, and reduction hepatectomy in the setting of donor scarcity.

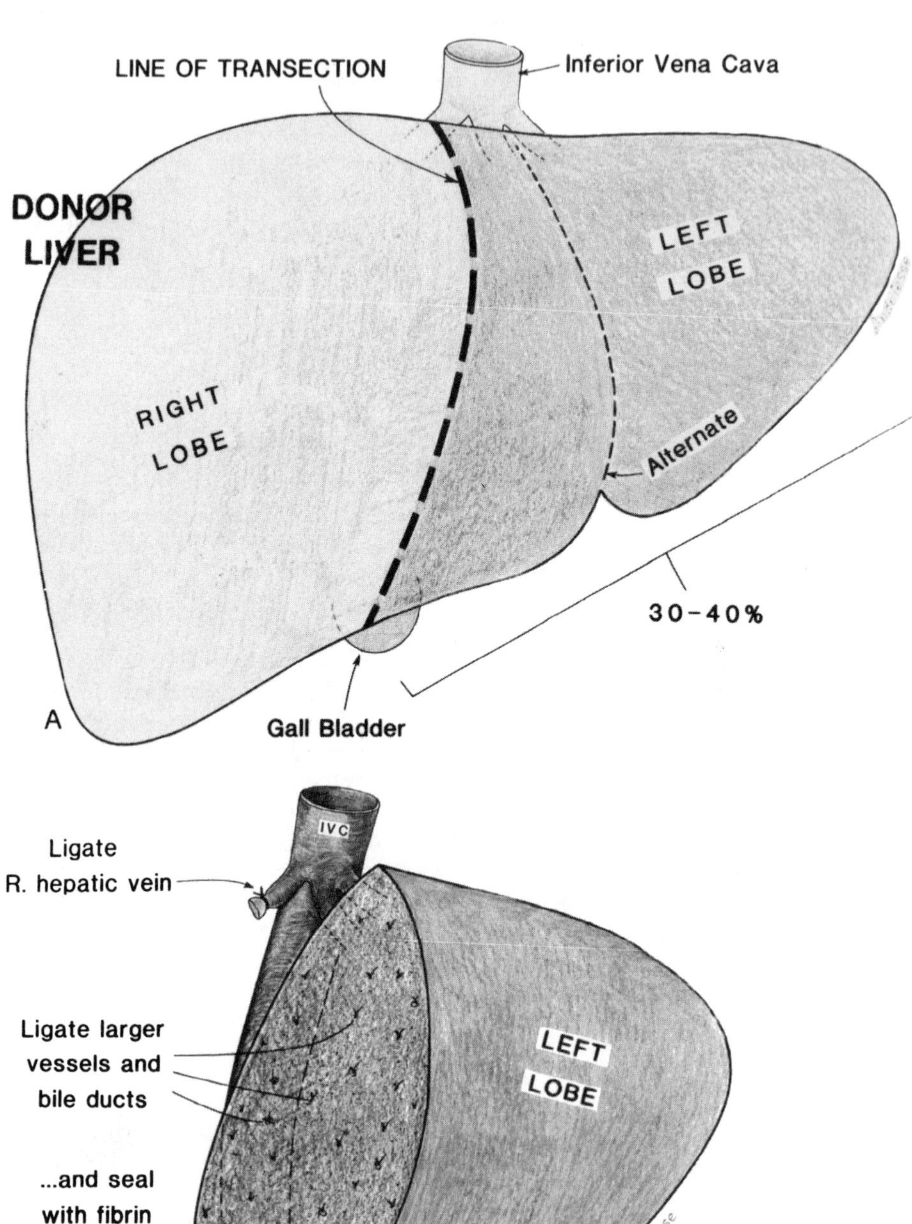

FIGURE 2 Reduced size allograft for transplantation in small infants. *A*, Lines of resection for implantation of reduced size allograft. One line of transection is through the demarcation between the anatomic right lobe and the left lobe. The dotted line is at the level of the left lateral segment. *B*, The completed transection. The raw surface is handled by suture ligation of visible open vessels and bile ducts and then application of fibrin sealant.

Postoperative Complications and Management

Hypertension

The most common medical complication in our patients following liver transplantation has been hypertension. This has occurred in 90 percent of our recipients within the first 2 months following the operation. The pathogenesis of post-transplant hypertension is probably multifactorial. It has been observed in patients not treated with cyclosporine and in patients undergoing cardiac or renal transplantation. Occasionally hypertension is severe enough to precipitate hypertensive encephalopathy. Multiple antihypertensive medications may be necessary, including diuretic therapy, angiotensin-converting enzyme inhibitors such as captopril, or vasodilators such as hydralazine. The prevalence of hypertension often declines with increasing time from the operative procedure, and often at 2 years following transplantation antihypertensive medications are no longer needed.

Infections

Infections are the second most common complication that we have seen in our series of patients. The risk of developing infection following transplantation is related to the presence of infection and the repeated use of antibiotics before transplantation, to contamination of the donor liver, to the immunization status of the graft recipient, and, perhaps most important, to the immunocompetence of the graft recipient. In some cases, the underlying liver disease may have been caused by an infectious agent, such as hepatitis B, cytomegalovirus (CMV), Epstein-Barr (EB) virus, or human immunodeficiency virus. Some of these same viral infections may be present in the recipient as subclinical infections identified only by serologic evidence of humoral immunity to one or another of the viral antigens. In both cases immunosuppression may lead to reactivation of the infection following transplant with devastating effects, both on the graft and on other organ systems of the recipient. Primary infections with these viral agents occur when the recipient acquires the infection as a result of the transplantation procedure itself, often as a result of transplantation of an organ or transfusion of blood that contain a virus such as CMV.

Chronic liver disease is often complicated by recurrent gram-negative infections. This is particularly true for chronic biliary tract disease. Patients with biliary atresia who have had a portoenterostomy often have episodes of recurrent cholangitis. The use of multiple, different antibiotics for prolonged periods of time directly correlates with the emergence of resistant organisms that may be exceptionally difficult to treat following transplantation, when the patient is immunosuppressed. In particular it is these patients who often develop life-threatening septicemia due to resistant gram-negative bacteria or opportunistic organisms, such as fungi.

If a patient has not had the standard live viral immunizations for measles, mumps, and rubella and at least 1 month remains before transplantation, we recommend giving these routine immunizations. Unfortunately, immunization for varicella is not available in the United States. No live viral vaccine should be given to patients within 1 month of transplantation. In addition to standard immunizations, influenza, *Haemophilus influenzae* B, and pneumococcal vaccine should be given prior to transplant and then yearly following the transplant.

The donor liver should be cultured during the transplant procedure for bacterial contamination and for subclinical viral infections. In the perioperative period prophylactic antibiotics are provided to cover gram-negative bacilli, *Staphylococcus aureus*, and anaerobic bacteria. Perioperative cultures of bile, tracheal aspirate, intraperitoneal drainage, the nasal mucosa, and stool are part of routine surveillance for potentially life-threatening infections. The signs of infection following transplantation may be very difficult to discern and even more difficult to differentiate from other complications such as rejection. Fever, increasing white blood count, and worsening liver functions may be signs of infection or of other complications such as rejection. The source of infection following transplantation may be in virtually any organ system.

Liver transplant recipients appear to be especially predisposed to oral, pharyngeal, and systemic candidiasis.[36] Dehiscence of the biliary anastomosis or operative trauma to the intestine has been identified in many of the patients developing disseminated candidal infections. Patients with biliary tract obstruction or obstruction of the hepatic artery or portal vein may also develop bacteremia, seeding from ischemic abscesses within the liver. This complication is almost universal in those patients with vascular obstruction to the liver and must be recognized promptly. Although retransplantation may be necessary, percutaneous drainage of the abscess with ultrasound guidance has been performed, allowing the successful treatment of these lesions with systemic antibiotics.[37]

After initial perioperative coverage with broad-spectrum antibiotics, antibiotic coverage is directed at specific infectious complications that develop. Once oral intake is not restricted and gastrointestinal (GI) function is not disturbed, oral nystatin may reduce the incidence of oral-pharyngeal candidiasis. Although protective isolation may be possible in some transplant centers, it is not known if isolation alone without filtered laminar flow systems and rigorous disinfection of foods, skin, and mucosa reduces the incidence of infection in the immunocompromised host.[38]

CMV and EB virus infections may be treated by reducing immunosuppression and using specific viral chemotherapeutic agents, such as acyclovir, or the investigational agent dihydroxyphenylglycol. The use of high-titer anti-CMV immune globulin is currently being studied in the pretransplant period to reduce reactivation of CMV infection following transplantation. Zoster immune globulin should be administered along with acyclovir following exposure to varicella. Hyperimmune or monoclonal immune globulin is given during or immediately after surgery to hepatitis B surface antigen–positive patients undergoing transplantation.

As we noted, vascular thrombosis is a major complication occurring in up to 40 percent of patients who weigh less than 12 kg. With deteriorating liver functions in the first week following transplantation, compromise of blood flow to the liver should be suspected. This can be evaluated with Doppler ultrasonography, CT scan, or angiography. The absence of flow through both the portal vein and hepatic artery indicates the urgent need for retransplantation. With the presence of blood flow through one or the other vessel the patient may be treated expectantly, observed for ischemic abscesses and bile duct integrity, and retransplanted only if liver functions progressively deteriorate. Anticoagulants are not routinely used in the absence of vascular obstruction. If obstruction does occur, an antiplatelet agent such as salicylic acid may be of benefit.

Pulmonary complications following liver transplant are common. Infection, hemodynamic instability, surgical technique, and chemotherapeutic agents used in immunosuppression may all result in respiratory compromise. Dysmotility of the right hemidiaphragm due to injury or denervation of the diaphragm may result in pulmonary insufficiency and atelectasis. We have successfully treated one patient with prolonged diaphragmatic dysfunction with the negative-pressure respirator. Pulmonary infections, particularly with opportunistic organisms, contribute to morbidity following surgery. Both azathioprine and cyclosporine may produce interstitial pneumonitis and noncardiogenic pulmonary edema.[39]

GI bleeding is another major complication affecting patients following transplantation.[40] Ulcers, gastritis, bleeding from the enterostomy site, and bleeding from varices in patients who develop portal vein thrombosis are the most frequent GI complications. Perforation or fistula formation, usually at the site of a biliary anastomotic leak, is a less frequent but serious GI complication. Because of immunosuppression, the presentation of these complications may be subtle. Pancreatitis may arise as a result of pancreatotoxic immunosuppressive agents or severe malnutrition. In the early period after liver transplantation, patients are in a state of hypercatabolism with increased tissue breakdown.[41] Careful attention to nutritional requirements is extremely important for healing and rehabilitation following the operation. Patients are initially supported with parenteral nutrition and then with enteral nutrition as intestinal function returns following the surgery.

Seizures are the most common neurologic complication following transplantation. In a series of adult patients, 25 percent developed seizures, half of them within the first week after surgery.[42] Cyclosporine has been implicated in the development of seizures, particularly in conjunction with hypomagnesemia and hypocholesterolemia. In addition, central nervous system infection, air embolus, and vascular accidents must be considered in all of these patients. Cerebral abscess is an almost inevitably fatal disorder.

Primary graft nonfunction is a generic term indicating that a transplanted liver, once reperfused, is unable to function satisfactorily. If retransplantation is not performed urgently, death results. Damage can occur from instability in the donor, inadequate preservation, or reperfusion injury. The role of vascular thrombosis in primary graft nonfunction is controversial. We believe that damage to the microcirculation or hepatic swelling from rejection or fluid overload may cause high vascular resistance and lead to retrograde occlusion of arterial inflow in some cases of arterial thrombosis. Whatever the initiating event, we have the distinct impression that use of UW solution has dramatically decreased the incidence of primary graft nonfunction.

Rejection

In spite of the introduction of cyclosporine, which dramatically diminishes the incidence of both early and late rejection, rejection remains a major obstacle in liver transplantation. The clinical manifestations of rejection are nonspecific and variable in both severity and timing. Although hyperacute rejection has been described, it appears to be a rare phenomenon. Furthermore, graft acceptance and patient survival between A-B-O–incompatible donor and recipient do not appear to differ from those A-B-O–matched donors and recipients.[43] Alloantibodies are commonly found in the serum of recipients of A-B-O–mismatched organs.[44] These antibodies may be produced by B lymphocytes transplanted with the graft or by the recipient's B cells. The significance of these antibodies remains to be determined. The hemolysis and anemia that may be seen in some of these patients are generally self-limited but occasionally may be prolonged. This phenomenon is usually controlled by the immunosuppressive agents used to control rejection.

In cases in which drug-induced immunosuppression is inadequate, plasmapheresis may be useful. Fever, enlargement of the liver, and elevation of serum transaminases, bilirubin, and alkaline phosphatase with deterioration of hepatic synthetic function may all herald rejection. Edema of the liver and poor uptake of radioisotope are observed when CT scans and radionuclide studies are done during these episodes. As mentioned above, it is important to determine that ischemia from vascular obstruction, infection, and/or drug toxicity is not responsible for the deterioration in liver function.

Liver biopsy may be useful for histologic examination and for culture. The characteristic histologic features of rejection include portal and lobular infiltration by lymphocytes, degeneration of biliary epithelium with progression to paucity of bile ducts and endothelialitis of both venules and arterioles. Polymorphonuclear leukocytes may be seen within the bile duct epithelia along with epithelial ballooning, degeneration, and cholestasis. With severe rejection or chronic rejection, obliterative endarteritis, hepatocellular necrosis with fibrosis or cirrhosis and infiltration of portal triads with polymorphonuclear leukocytes, eosinophils, and lymphocytes, and absence of bile ducts are common features.[45]

The absence of bile ducts within the first 3 months following transplantation has been labeled the acute vanishing bile duct syndrome.[46] This appears to be an irreversible phenomenon of rejection similar to that seen in graft-versus-host disease and primary biliary cirrhosis. The absence of most interlobular bile ducts together with fever, jaundice, and marked elevation of serum bilirubin and alkaline phosphatase that persists despite antirejection treatment indicate the need for retransplantation. Some of these patients, including one of our own, have redeveloped this lesion in the second graft.

IMMUNOSUPPRESSION

Both helper and cytotoxic T lymphocytes, recognizing class I and class II alloantigens, play an important role in graft rejection.[47] In humans but not in all mammalian species, vigorous rejection of the orthotopic liver graft is the rule in the absence of active immunosuppression. Williams, in an early report of 26 liver transplants, described the rapid failure of a liver graft in a patient who received no immunosuppressive therapy.[48] Although the rapidity of rejection and the relevance of pre-existing immunity to donor histocompatibility antigens for liver grafts and for the transplantation of the kidney or heart may differ, a combination of immunosuppressive agents has been standard therapy for all liver graft recipients.

Modern immunosuppressive therapy for liver grafts usually involves the use of several different agents, each of which interrupts the elaboration of the rejection reaction at a different point. In simplified form, class II foreign human leukocyte antigens are present on the surface of cells in the donor graft. Circulating T-helper cells recognize these antigens and are activated, both by the interaction with antigen and by soluble mediators from activated macrophages. Interleukin-1 (IL-1), a macrophage product, also causes activation of T-helper cells. These activated T-helper cells, which produce IL-2, are necessary for the progression of the rejection response. Cytotoxic lymphocytes, which begin to differentiate after encountering class I antigens, are stimulated by IL-2, which promotes their differentiation and proliferation. The further elaboration of cytokines by activated cytotoxic T cells and T-helper cells, recruits macrophages, granulocytes, B cells, and natural killer T cells in the graft site.[49] Although it is clear that the T-helper cell is necessary and responsible for amplification of the rejection phenomenon, it is not clear whether T-helper cells or cytotoxic T cells are primarily responsible for effecting rejection.

Since the introduction of cyclosporine for liver transplants was reported in 1979, it, in combination with other agents including corticosteroids, azathioprine, and monoclonal or polyclonal antilymphocyte globulin, has been the mainstay of immunosuppressive therapy.

Glucocorticoids

The mechanism of glucocorticoid-induced immunosuppression is controversial. Although ineffective in preventing liver rejection when used alone, corticosteroids may act synergistically with the other previously mentioned agents to diminish rejection. Proliferating antigen-activated lymphocytes are decreased in number after exposure to corticosteroids, which are known to activate suppressor cells. Both of these actions may be important in ameliorating the active immune response to the heterologous liver graft. In addition to lymphopenia, corticosteroid administration in humans produces redistribution of circulating peripheral lymphocytes, preferentially removing the helper-inducer (CD-4) lymphocyte subset from the circulating intravascular lymphocyte pool. Other effects of corticosteroids, especially on the production of interleukins, may explain the synergy between corticosteroids and other agents such as cyclosporine.

The adverse effects of prolonged high-dose corticosteroids use in children are well known and are not reviewed here. Because of the synergism between corticosteroids and cyclosporine, the dose of corticosteroid can be decreased in a relatively short period of time and the drug administered at low dose in an alternate-day regimen to markedly reduce the toxicity. During the first post-transplant week, doses of 60 to 100 mg of intravenous prednisone or its equivalent are administered daily and then tapered to 5 to 20 mg per day. Episodes of rejection and treated with intravenous boluses of high-dose corticosteroid.

Antilymphocyte Globulin

Polyclonal antilymphocyte globulin (ALG), produced in animals, has been used with conflicting results as an adjunct immunosuppressive agent in hepatic, renal, and cardiac transplants in humans. Owing to differences in purity and potency among preparations of ALG, its efficacy in promoting long-term survival of renal allograft recipients is controversial. The experience in pediatric liver recipients is limited and therefore anecdotal. In general, ALG has been reserved for treatment of acute rejection unresponsive to glucocorticosteroids and cyclosporine. ALG has been extensively studied and causes a reduction in circulating T cells by an unknown mechanism. Side effects of the drug include all of the adverse effects of systemic administration of heterologous serum and can be serious enough to limit its use.

An important recent development is the use of monoclonal anticytotoxic/inducer T-cell antibodies, produced by murine plasmacytomas. These antibodies selectively destroy host cells active in rejection and theoretically eliminate the adverse effects of irrelevant antibodies found in polyclonal ALG. The pan-T monoclonal antibody, OKT-3, has proved to be the most effective of these monoclonal antibodies investigated to date. In a multicenter controlled trial, OKT-3 reversed rejection episodes more effectively than did corticosteroids.[50] Current trials are in progress to evaluate the use of monoclonal antibodies as initial immunosuppressive therapy in place of cyclosporine. The repeated use of these antibodies is limited by the development of host antibodies against the OKT-3 antibody. A number of other monoclonal antibodies that react only with activated lymphoblasts, are currently being evaluated. Antibodies aimed at specific T-cell subsets that can be used in sequence or combination and thereby avoid the development of antimonoclonal antibodies by the host are goals for the future.[51]

Azathioprine

Until the late 1970s, the combination of azathioprine and prednisone was the principal regimen used to suppress rejection following liver transplantation. The high failure rate in the first year after transplantation of livers and cadaveric kidneys dampened enthusiasm for liver transplantation. Since the advent of cyclosporine, azathioprine has become an adjunct immunosuppressant in most centers and is used as initial therapy or when toxicity precludes the further use of cyclosporine. Azathioprine is similar to its parent compound, 6-mercaptopurine, which affects purine nucleotide synthesis and metabolism. Oral doses of the drug vary from 1 to 5 mg per kilogram per day. Doses must be lowered when the drug is used together with allopurinol. The most common toxic effect of azathioprine is myelosuppression; it has also caused severe hepatitis and cholestasis.

Cyclosporine

Cyclosporine is metabolized in the liver via the cytochrome P-450 microsomal enzyme system. It is not clear whether these metabolites are able to enhance immunosuppression or produce toxic complications. A variety of techniques are available to measure cyclosporine in biologic fluids. Fifty to 60 percent of cyclosporine in the systemic circulation is bound to erythrocytes. Another 4 to 9 percent is bound to lymphocytes, and the remainder is found in the plasma fraction, virtually all of which is bound to plasma proteins. Trough levels of cyclosporine are usually measured for therapeutic decisions, with measurements on whole blood samples running four to six times the levels detected in serum. Two principal techniques are available for measurement of levels, radioimmunoassay (RIA) and high-pressure liquid chromatography (HPLC). RIA depends upon antibody recognition of the cyclosporine molecule and its metabolites. Recently an RIA utilizing monoclonal antibodies specific for the parent molecule has been developed for use on whole blood samples.[52] HPLC can also recognize and measure the parent molecule. Measurements by polyclonal RIA are four to five times higher than by HPLC on the same biologic fluid. The therapeutic range for trough cyclosporine levels by RIA range from 50 to 250 ng per milliliter for serum.[53]

Cyclosporine is eliminated principally by excretion through bile. Less than 10 percent of cyclosporine is excreted through the kidney.[54] The absorption of cyclosporine through the GI tract is quite variable, as reflected by systemic drug levels measured after oral administration. Graft recipients receive cyclosporine by the intravenous route intraoperatively and in the immediate postoperative period, then by a combination of oral and intravenous administration, and finally by oral administration. Our experience and that of others has been that oral requirements for cyclosporine are significantly higher in pediatric patients than in adult patients. Intravenous doses are usually 4 to 6 mg per kilogram per day, and oral doses vary from 15 to as high as 35 mg per kilogram per day for some of our pediatric patients. Dosing must be individualized to minimize side effects such as nephrotoxicity. Once bile flow is completely internalized, drug absorption frequently improves.

TABLE 3
Adverse Effects of Cyclosporine

Nephrotoxicity
Hepatotoxicity
Hirsutism
Tremors and seizures
Gingival hyperplasia
Hypertension
Hemolytic anemia
Thrombocytopenia
Lymphoma

A number of other drugs are known to affect cyclosporine concentrations in the systemic circulation. Decreased serum concentrations are seen with concurrent use of phenytoin, phenobarbital, rifampin, isoniazid, and trimethoprim. In contrast, ketoconazole, erythromycin, and methylprednisolone increase serum concentrations. Finally, the nephrotoxicity of cyclosporine may be potentiated by other known nephrotoxic medications, such as aminoglycosides. A list of the most common adverse effects of cyclosporine is found in Table 3.

Cyclosporine may produce hepatotoxicity with histopathology similar to rejection. Hepatotoxicity rapidly reversed in patients receiving cyclosporine for immunosuppression following renal transplantation with lowering of cyclosporine dose or change from cyclosporine to azathioprine. Toxicity in this study occurred as late as 13 months following transplantation.[55]

LONG-TERM MANAGEMENT

The majority of pediatric patients who survive transplantation encounter fewer and fewer complications with increasing time from the procedure. Survival curves plateau by 2 years following the procedure with very little mortality after that period of time. As we mentioned previously, the majority of patients grow and develop at an accelerated rate compared with their pretransplant status. The average cyclosporine dose for our patients is 8 to 21 mg per kilogram per day and prednisone 0.5 to 1 mg per kilogram per day by 1 year after transplantation. The long-term requirement for immunosuppression and the consequences of prolonged immunosuppression have not been determined. Voluntary discontinuation of immunosuppressant has resulted in graft rejection in the Starzl experience. Repeat transplantation has been required in as many as one-third of children since the introduction of cyclosporine, and a few patients have required more than two transplants. Most of these have been done in the first postoperative month. Recipient hepatectomy and replacement are technically easier, but 1-year survival is lower than in the overall group.[56]

It may be difficult to separate chronic rejection from other causes of hepatic dysfunction, including recurrence of the original disease.[57] Thus, for some diseases in which specific serologic or biochemical markers do not exist, such as primary sclerosing cholangitis, it may be difficult to separate disease recurrence from allograft rejection or even from graft-versus-host disease. Recurrence of original liver disease after transplantation is a particular concern for patients with malignancies and viral-induced hepatitis. Diagnosing the recurrence of some of these entities may be further compromised because of modifications of the clinicopathologic features by immunosuppression. Although recurrence of inborn errors of metabolism has not been identified, the clinical expression of these genetic errors in extrahepatic sites may become apparent only over several years.

SUMMARY

Liver transplantation remains the only hope for survival for infants and children with end-stage liver disease. Survival following transplantation has improved over the past 25 years from 20 percent to better than 80 percent for some groups of recipients. Enhanced survival with high quality of life following transplantation is a result of improved transplant care, improved surgical techniques, and more effective immunosuppression. The lack of donor organs and toxicity from nonspecific immunosuppressive therapy remain major obstacles to even more favorable results. Current efforts to improve organ preservation, understand rejection, develop specific immunotherapy, and promote organ donation hold much promise for the future.

REFERENCES

1. Salans LB, Roth HP, Kraut JR, et al. National Institutes of Health Consensus Development Conference Statement. Liver Transplantation, June 20-23, 1983. Hepatology 1984; 4:107S–110S.
2. Vacanti JP, Lillehei CW, Jenkins RL, Donahoe PK, Cosimi AB, Kleinman RE, Grand RJ, Cho SI. Liver transplantation in children: The Boston Center Experience in the first 30 months. Transplant Proc 1987; 19:3261–3266.
3. Starzl TE, Iwatsuki S, Van Thiel DH, Gartner CJ, Zitelli BJ, et al. Evolution of liver transplantation. Hepatology 1982; 2:614–636.
4. Van Thiel DH, Tarter R, Gavaler JS, Potanko WM, Schade RR. Liver transplantation in adults: an analysis of cost and benefits at the University of Pittsburgh. Gastroenterology 1986; 90:211–216.
5. Spolidoro JVN, Berquist WE, Pehlivanoglu E, et al. Growth acceleration in children after orthotopic liver transplantation. J Pediatr 1988; 112:41–44.
6. Urbach AH, Gartner JC Jr, Malatack JJ, et al. Linear growth following pediatric liver transplantation. Am J Dis Child 1987; 141:547–549.
7. Novick AC, Epstein F. The need for mandatory organ-donor request. Cleve Clin J Med 1987; 54:163–164.
8. Van Thiel DH, Shade RR, Hakala TR, et al. Liver procurement for orthotopic liver transplantation: an analysis of the Pittsburgh experience. Hepatology 1984; 4:66S–72S.
9. Stuart F. Need, supply and legal issues related to organ transplantation in the United States. Transplant Proc 1984; 16:87–94.
10. Tolle SW, Bennett WM, Kickam DH, Benson LA. Responsibilities of primary physicians in organ donation. Ann Intern Med 1987; 106:740–744.
11. Malatack JJ, Schaid DJ, Urbach AH. Choosing a pediatric recipient for orthotopic liver transplantation. J Pediatr 1987; 4:479–489.
12. Gordon RD, Iwatsuk IS, Esquivel CO, et al. Liver transplantation across A-B-O blood groups. Surgery 1986; 2:342–348.
13. Cox KL, Ward RL, Furginele TL, et al. Orthotopic liver transplantation in patients with cystic fibrosis. Pediatrics 1987; 80:571–574.
14. O'Grady JG, Polson RJ, Rolles K, Calne RY, Williams R. Liver transplantation for malignant disease. Results in 93 consecutive patients. Ann Surg 1988; 207:373–379.
15. Alagille D. Extrahepatic biliary atresia. Hepatology 1984; 4:7S–10S.
16. Kobayashi A, Itabashi F, Ohbe Y. Long term prognosis in biliary atresia after hepatic portoenterostomy: analysis of 35 patients who survive beyond 5 years of age. J Pediatr 1984; 105:243–246.
17. Esquivel CO, Iwatsuki S, Gordon RD, et al. Indications for pediatric liver transplantation. J Pediatr 1987; 111:1039–1045.
18. Tachman M, Freese DK, Sharp HL, et al. Contribution of extrahepatic tissues to biochemical abnormalities in hereditary tyrosinemia type I: study of 3 patients after liver transplantation. J Pediatr 1987; 110:399–403.
19. Starzl TE, Zitelli BJ, Shaw BW Jr, et al. Changing concepts of liver replacement for hereditary tyrosinemia and hepatoma. J Pediatr 1985; 106:604–606.
20. Bismuth H, Ericzon BG, Rolles K, Castaing D, Otte JB, Ringe B, Sloof M. Hepatic transplantation in Europe. First report of the European Liver Transplant Registry. Lancet 1987; ii:674.
21. Starzl TE, Bhanson HT, Hardesty RL, et al. Heart-liver transplantation in a patient with familial hypercholesterolemia. Lancet 1984; i:1382–1383.
22. Shaw BW, Hakala T, Rosenthal JT, et al. Combination donor hepatectomy and nephrectomy and early functional results of allographs. Surgery 1982; 155:321–325.
23. Touraine JL, Malik MC, Broot H, et al. Maladie de Fabry: deux malade ameliores par la greffe de cellules de foie foetal. Nouv Press Med 1979; 8:1499–1503.
24. Sokol RJ, Francis PD, Gold SH. Orthotopic liver transplantation for acute fulminant Wilson disease. J Pediatr 1985; 107:549–552.
25. Peleman RR, Gavaler JS, Van Thiel DH, et al. Orthotopic liver transplantation for acute and subacute hepatic failure in adults. Hepatology 1987; 7:484–489.
26. Wozney P, Zayko AB, Bron KM, et al. Vascular complications after liver transplantation. Am J Radiol 1986; 147:657–663.
27. Rosenblatt R. A new method for massive fluid resuscitation in the trauma patient. Anesth Analg 1983; 62:613–616.
28. Aldrete JA, Clapp HW, Starzl TE. Body temperature changes during organ transplantation. Anesth Analg 1970; 49:384–388.
29. Owen CA Jr, Rettke SR, Bowie EJW, et al. Hemostatic evaluation of patients undergoing liver transplantation. Mayo Clin Proc 1987; 62:761–772.
30. Kangy G, Martin DJ, Marquez J, et al. Intraoperative changes in blood coagulation and thromboelastographic monitoring in liver transplantation. Anesth Anal 1985; 64:888–896.
31. Shiao J, Hasosheng B, Zicheng M, Chrongrong G. Anesthesia in orthotopic liver transplantation. Anesthetists 1981; 30:153–157.
32. Wood RR, Shaw BW Jr. Multiple organ procurement. In: Cerilli G, ed. Organ transplantation and replacement. New York: Lippincott, 1988: 322.
33. Kalayoglu M, Sollinger HW, Stratton RJ, et al. Extended preservation of the liver for clinical transplantation. Lancet 1988; i:617–619.
34. Broelsch CE, Emond JC, Thistlewaite JR, Rouch DA, Whitington PF, Lichtor JL. Liver transplantation with reduced-size donor organs. Transplantation 1988; 45:519–524.
35. Strong R, Ong TH, Pillay P. A new method of segmental orthotopic liver transplantation in children. Surgery 1988; 104:104–107.
36. Schroter GPJ, Maholescher M, Putnam CW, et al. Fungus infections after liver transplantation. Ann Surg 1977; 186:115–122.
37. Hoffer SA, Teele RL, Lillehei CW, Vacanti JP. Infected bilomas and hepatic artery thrombosis in infant recipients of liver transplants. Interventional radiology and medical therapy as an alternative to retransplantation. Radiology 1988; 169:435–438.
38. Nauseef WM, Maki DG. A study of the value of simple protective isolation in patients with granulocytopenia. N Engl J Med 1981; 304:448–453.
39. Kroka MJ, Cortese DA. Pulmonary aspects of chronic liver disease and liver transplantation. Mayo Clin Proc 1985; 60:407–418.
40. Koep LJ, Starzl TE, Weil R. Gastrointestinal complications of hepatic transplantation. Transplant Proc 1979; 11:257–261.
41. Shanbhogue RLK, Bistrian BR, Jenkins RL, et al. Increased protein catabolism without hypermetabolism after human orthotopic liver transplantation. Surgery 1987; 101:146–149.
42. Adams DH, Benson B, Honigsberger L, et al. Neurological complications following liver transplantation. Lancet 1987; 949–951.
43. Iwatsuki S, Iwiki Y, Kano T, et al. Successful transplantation form cross-matched positive donors. Transplant Proc 1981; 13:286–288.
44. Ramsey G, Musbacher J, Starzl TE, Lindsay GD. Isohemagglutinins of graft origin after A-B-O unmatched liver transplantation. N Engl J Med 1984; 311:1167–1170.
45. Snovar DC, Freese DK, Sharp HL, et al. Liver allograph rejection. Am J Surg Pathol 1987; 1:1–10.
46. Ludwig J, Wiesner RH, Batts KP, Perkins JD, Krom RAF. The acute vanishing bile duct syndrome (acute irreversible rejection) after orthotopic liver transplantation. Hepatology 1987; 7:4176–4183.
47. Bach FH, Sachs DH. Current concepts: immunology. Transplantation immunology. N Engl J Med 1987; 317:489–492.
48. Williams R, Smith M, Shilkin KB, et al. Liver transplantation in man. The frequency of rejection, biliary tract complications and recurrence

of malignancy based on an analysis of 26 cases. Gastroenterology 1973; 64:1026–1048.
49. Tilney NL, Strom TB, Kupiec-Weglinski JW. Humoral and cellular mechanisms in acute allograft injury. J Pediatr 1987; 1116:1000–1003.
50. Ortho Multicenter Transplant Study Group. A randomized clinical trial of OKT-3 monoclonal antibody for acute rejection of cadaveric renal transplants. N Engl J Med 1985; 313:337–342.
51. Delmonico FL, Cosimi AB. Monoclonal antibody treatment of human allograft recipients. Surg Gynecol Obstet 1988; 166:89–98.
52. Ball PE, Munzer H, Keller HP, Abisch E, Rosenthaler J. Specific ^3H radioimmunoassay with a monoclonal antibody for monitoring cyclosporine in blood. Clin Chem 1988; 34:257–260.
53. Kahan BD. The pivotal role of the liver in immunosuppression by cyclosporine. Viewpoints on digestive diseases. 1987; 19(2).
54. Maurer G, Loosli HR, Shreirer E, et al. Disposition of cyclosporine in several animal species and man. I. Structural elucidation of its metabolites. Drug Metab Dispos 1984; 12:120–126.
55. Klintmalm GBG, Iwatsuki S, Starzl TE. Cyclosporine A. Hepatotoxicity in 66 renal allographed recipients. Transplantation 1981; 32:488–489.
56. Gartner JC, Zitelli BJ, Malatack JJ, et al. Orthotopic liver transplantation in children: two year experience with 47 patients. Pediatrics 1984; 47:140–145.
57. Van Thiel DH, Gavaler JS. Recurrent disease in patients with liver transplantation. Hepatology 1987; 7:181–183.

PART 26

Disorders of the Intrahepatic Bile Ducts

David A. Piccoli, M.D.
Camillus L. Witzleben, M.D.

As noted in the introduction to the following part of this chapter, Disorders of the Extrahepatic Bile Ducts, many disorders are now recognized as involving both intrahepatic and extrahepatic ducts, and the reader should refer to the index for the location of specific duct disorders.

EMBRYOLOGY OF THE INTRAHEPATIC DUCTS

The intrahepatic ducts develop primarily by a process of differentiation from the hepatocytes at the margins of the portal tracts. This differentiation results in the formation of the so-called ductal plate, which takes place in a centripetal fashion beginning from the hilus,[1] through a process termed by Desmet *remodeling*. After completion of this process, the ductal plate disappears, leaving only the centrally located highly differentiated interlobular duct. The ductal plates make their first appearance in the seventh to eighth weeks of gestation,[2] and a few persisting elements of the plates may be present at or beyond term.[1] Persistence of the ductal plate in the postnatal liver, accompanied by an increase in portal tract fibrous tissue, creates a lesion known as the ductal plate malformation,[3] biliary dysgenesis,[4] or congenital hepatic fibrosis.[5] This lesion is found in combination with renal abnormalities (usually cysts) in a number of heritable conditions in which there is actual or potential cystic dilatation of the biliary ducts (see below, discussion of cystic duct disease). In addition to these heritable disorders, Desmet[1] has suggested that persistence of the ductal plate can also be associated with extrahepatic biliary atresia (EHBA), which is not heritable and not associated with renal disease (see discussion of extrahepatic biliary atresia in Part 27 of this chapter). The interlobular ducts formed from the differentiation and remodeling of the ductal plate are joined by intrahepatic extensions of the extrahepatic ducts (themselves derived from the cephalic portion of the hepatic diverticulum) to complete the bile duct system. The physiologic and biochemical factors governing the differentiation and remodeling of the ductal plate (e.g., the role of bile secretion, the role of the surrounding connective tissue, the role of the concomitantly developing basement membrane, and the role of the portal tract vasculature) are essentially unknown at present. Understanding these factors may well be the key to understanding the genesis of a number of duct paucity conditions and a number of the cystic diseases of the liver.

INTRAHEPATIC BILE DUCT CYSTIC CONDITIONS

Cystic diseases of the intrahepatic bile ducts present a wide range of disorders. They include both sporadically occurring and heritable conditions, and extend from lesions typically discovered incidentally to frank malignancies. A modified classification scheme[6] is presented in Table 1. The distinction between communicating and noncommunicating cysts is clinically significant, because when duct cysts communicate with the biliary tree, they have a greater likelihood of causing clinical disease. Communicating duct cysts can be associated with cholangitis, stone formation, and (relatively uncommonly) neoplasia. Noncommunicating duct cysts are usually asymptomatic, but if sufficiently large may present as an abdominal mass or biliary obstruction.

This discussion focuses on heritable diseases associated with intrahepatic duct cysts. For a discussion of so-called isolated or sporadic cysts the reader is referred elsewhere.[6] Other nonheritable intrahepatic duct cysts, which are frequently associated with choledochal cysts, are discussed in Part 27 of this chapter.

In considering cystic intrahepatic bile ducts, it is necessary to be familiar with the so-called ductal plate malforma-

TABLE 1
Hepatic Cysts of Duct Origin

"Solitary"
"Polycystic" (heritable; lesions in other viscera)
  Noncommunicating cysts (adult polycystic disease—ADPKD)*
  Communicating cysts
    With ductal plate malformation
      Autosomal recessive polycystic kidney disease (ARPKD)†
      Congenital hepatic fibrosis (CHF)†
      Malformation syndromes
      Congenital hepatic fibrosis-nephronophthisis
    Without ductal plate malformation
      "Simple" Caroli's disease
  "Hepatic" polycystic disease‡
  "Systemic biliary dilatation" (nonheritable, no other visceral lesions, type V choledochal cyst)
    With choledochal cyst
    Without choledochal cyst

*A percentage of cases of ADPKD have the ductal plate malformation and communicating duct cysts.
†Congenital hepatic fibrosis and ARPKD may be different presentations of the same disorder.
‡Existence of this is speculative.

tion, also called congenital hepatic fibrosis or biliary dysgenesis. This consists of plates or cisternae of duct elements characteristically found at the circumference of the portal tracts and is associated with increased portal tract fibrous tissue (Fig. 1). The prominent duct elements should not be confused with the proliferating duct elements commonly seen as a response to a variety of hepatic insults, including mechanical obstruction. Jorgensen[3] recognized the similarity between these portal tracts and those seen in fetal life, and coined the term *ductal plate malformation* to signify that the lesion represents an arrest in the development of normal portal tract and bile duct structures, or, as characterized by Desmet,[1] a disruption of the normal "remodeling" of the embryonic bile duct and portal tract structures into their mature forms. Although most commonly associated with heritable disorders, the ductal plate persistence can be seen in at least one apparently acquired disorder, EHBA.[1] The relevance of this lesion to cystic bile ducts lies in the fact that the abnormal ducts have larger diameters than normal ducts and seem to have a propensity to become dilated.

Discussions of intrahepatic duct cystic dilatation must include mention of Caroli's disease. Many radiologists and clinicians classify virtually all patients with intrahepatic duct dilatation as having Caroli's disease. We believe this usage is imprecise and inadequately specific in view of the genetic and pathologic information that has accumulated since Caroli's original papers. Caroli actually described two "forms" of "congenital dilatation of the segmental intrahepatic biliary tree."[7] In the more common of these, there were portal tract lesions that appear from his description to be what we now call the ductal plate malformation. In the other form, there were no histologic abnormalities other than the duct ectasia. Both forms were associated with renal disease, and both could be seen in the same family. The vast majority of reported cases of Caroli's disease described since Caroli's report appear to have been associated with the ductal plate malformation, and thus appear to be examples of what we now know as congenital hepatic fibrosis or autosomal recessive polycystic kidney disease (ARPKD), which was formerly termed

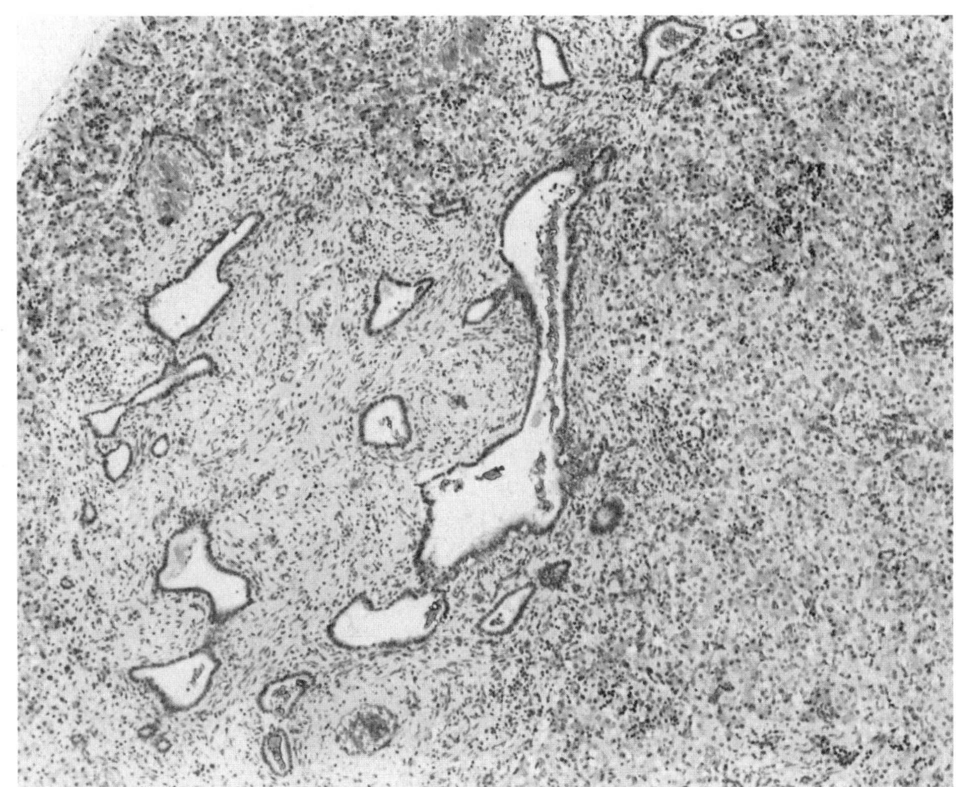

FIGURE 1 Ductal plate malformation in patient with autosomal recessive polycystic kidney disease/congenital hepatic fibrosis (ARPKD/CHF). The abnormal duct structures are typically peripheral in the tracts, tend to be dilated, and have angular shapes. These ducts communicate proximally and distally with the bile drainage system. The same (or highly similar) portal tract lesions are also seen in a number of malformation syndromes (see text) (hematoxylin and eosin, original magnification ×20).

infantile polycystic disease (IPCD), with prominent duct dilatation. In addition, this may rarely be found in autosomal dominant polycystic kidney disease (ADPKD). It has, however, been suggested that there is a group of cases distinct from ADPKD, congenital hepatic fibrosis (CHF), and ARPKD by virtue of the level of ducts involved, which should be called Caroli's disease.[1,8] Alternatively, the term Caroli's disease could be restricted to cases with no portal tract abnormality other than segmental duct dilatation, as in the "simple" form described by Caroli.[7]

HERITABLE INTRAHEPATIC BILE DUCT CYSTIC DISEASE (ADPKD/ARPKD/CHF)

The major heritable conditions characterized by intrahepatic bile duct cysts are ADPKD, also called "adult polycystic disease," and ARPKD, which was formerly termed infantile polycystic disease. The latter is intimately related to, if not identical with, CHF. There are also a number of heritable malformation syndromes characterized by potential bile duct cysts and renal disease. The ductal plate malformation is seen in all of these conditions (least commonly in ADPKD). Whenever the ductal plate malformation is the basis for the cysts, the cysts communicate proximally and distally with the biliary tree. Renal cysts of tubular origin or other renal developmental lesions are typically present in all these conditions. The renal lesions tend to be dissimilar in the different clinical conditions.

As will be discussed, it is unclear whether or not ARPKD and CHF are different disorders or different clinical manifestations of the same disorder. We will focus primarily on the clinical entity of CHF, because the hepatic manifestations predominate.

Congenital Hepatic Fibrosis and Autosomal Recessive Polycystic Kidney Disease

The term *congenital hepatic fibrosis* was coined by Kerr et al.[5] The disorder is composed of a characteristic hepatopathology, cystic disease of the kidneys, portal hypertension, and an increased risk of ascending cholangitis. In many pedigrees the disease appears to be inherited in an autosomal recessive manner.[9,10]

Pathology of CHF and ARPKD

The hepatic lesion of ductal plate malformation is found in all cases of CHF-ARPKD. The renal lesion when identified in infancy is characterized by radially arranged tubular cysts occupying most of the large externally smooth renal mass with widely spaced glomeruli (Fig. 2). The longer patients survive, the less characteristic the renal lesions become, since the cysts become more rounded, and in some cases with survival beyond the neonatal period, it may be difficult on examination of biopsies to correctly classify the lesion.[11] The pathogenesis of the renal lesion has not been determined.

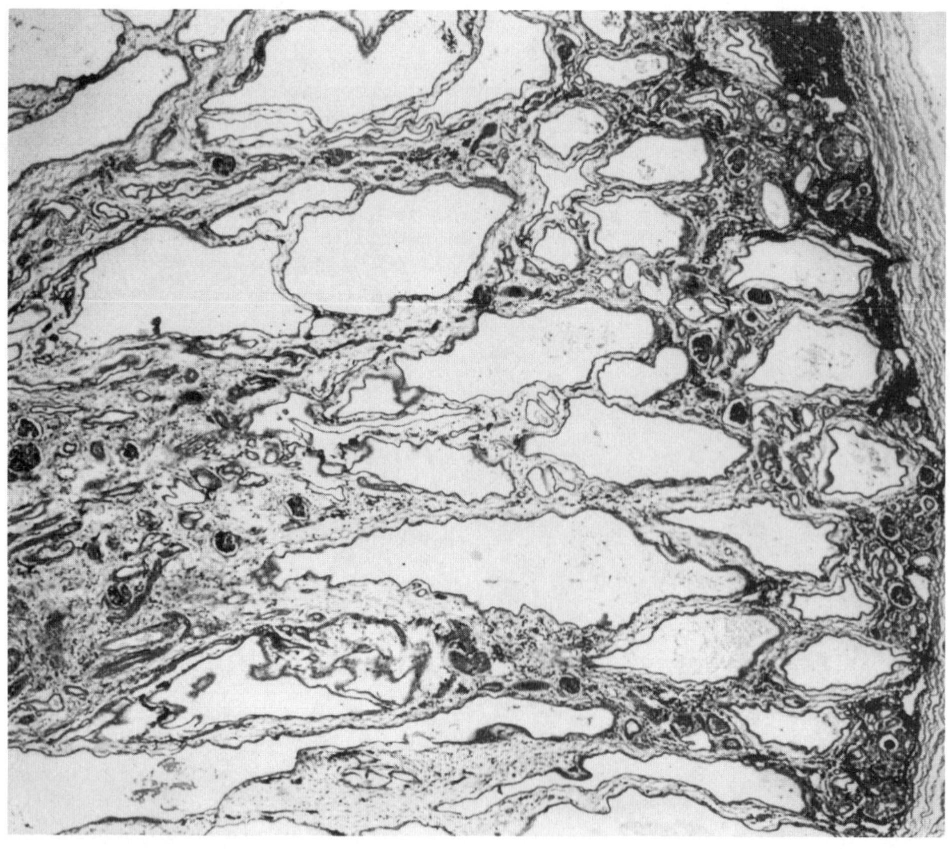

FIGURE 2 Light micrograph of renal cortex of newborn patient with infantile (recessive) ARPKD. Numerous elongated radially arranged cysts are present. Intervening parenchyma is essentially normal. In patients with longer survival, the cysts tend to become rounded and less distinctive. The relation of the clinical entities of ARPKD and congenital hepatic fibrosis (CHF) to each other is a matter of debate (see text) (hematoxylin and eosin, original magnification ×10).

Relationship Between CHF and ARPKD

The relationship of ARPKD to CHF is controversial. The hepatic conditions in both lesions are essentially similar, as they all consist of the ductal plate malformation. The renal lesions, which consist of tubular cysts in both, classically differ markedly in both pathology and clinical severity. In newborn patients with ARPKD, the renal lesions are diffuse and prominent clinically, whereas in patients who exhibit the clinical picture of CHF the renal lesions are often not as evident in early life and are minor. However, with long survival, in patients with ARPKD the lesions become increasingly similar. This could suggest that the two conditions are actually one disorder with the apparent differences being related in part to the length of survival of the patients. Evidence contrary to this unitary point of view lies in the observation that the clinicopathologic presentations tend to "breed true" within a given family (suggesting genetic differences between disorders),[12] although variability has been described in some families.[13] Similar controversies exist between age and genetic predisposition when both the hepatic and the renal lesions are examined morphometrically or reviewed relative to the frequency of carcinoma. Thus, there is evidence both for and against the pathogenic identity of CHF and ARPKD that can be resolved only by further study. For the purpose of this presentation, they will be treated as a single entity, with different clinicopathologic presentations.

Clinical Presentation of CHF and ARPKD

The clinical manifestations of CHF-ARPKD vary in large part according to the age at first presentation. The renal disease predominates in neonates and infants (ARPKD), whereas the hepatic-related disease predominates in older children and adults (CHF). The clinical profile has been divided into four groups at presentation: perinatal, neonatal, infantile, and juvenile groups,[12] but these subdivisions appear to have no genetic or pathogenetic implications, and in our view serve no useful purpose.

Renal Disease in ARPKD

The renal disease may vary from an incidental finding in older children to a major cause of early mortality. In infants who present with the renal manifestations of infantile polycystic disease the kidneys are enlarged and severely dysfunctional. They may be palpable on examination, and an abdominal radiograph will demonstrate bilaterally enlarged kidneys. Excretory urography may only poorly visualize the collecting system. The nephrogram (characteristic of the neonatal presentation) demonstrates a radiolucent mottled parenchyma attributable to the cystic changes of the nephrons. Many infants with ARPKD will develop uremia and chronic renal failure. Respiratory distress occurs from compression exerted by the enlarged kidneys, fluid retention, congestive heart failure, concomitant pulmonary hypoplasia, or pneumonia. Progressive renal failure and hypertension may occur over the first few weeks or months of life, and mortality is high. In these children the hepatic fibrosis may be progressive but is rarely a clinically important factor. There have been uncommon reports of patients at autopsy with the clinical picture of congenital hepatic fibrosis who had normal kidney structure and function.[14]

Renal Disease in CHF

Palpable kidneys are often noted at initial evaluation in association with arterial hypertension.[9,15] The intravenous pyelogram demonstrates enlarged kidneys and tubular ectasia with alternating dense and radiolucent streaks radiating from the medulla to the cortex. Renal dysfunction is present in approximately 20 percent of patients, as evidenced by decreased maximal concentrating capacity, an elevated serum BUN, and a chronic mild metabolic acidosis.[9,15,16] Even in some patients with an initially normal IVP, there may be an evolution to the typical radiographic findings in later life and in most cases cysts are present on pathologic evaluation.[17]

Hepatic Disease in CHF

Portal Hypertension. In the older patients with CHF-ARPKD, the most significant abnormality is portal hypertension. The precise pathogenesis is unknown, but is thought to be associated with the hepatic fibrosis and/or portal vein abnormalities. Clinically, hematemesis or melena is the presenting sign in 30 to 70 percent of patients from pediatric and mixed population studies.[9,15] In children, the age for presentation of hematemesis may be as early as the first year of life,[18] but it usually ranges from 5 to 13 years. Firm or hard hepatomegaly is present in nearly all patients, often with a prominent left lobe, and this is usually one of the presenting findings. Splenomegaly occurs in the majority, accompanied by hypersplenism with thrombocytopenia. Splenic pressure is elevated, and naturally occurring splenorenal or gastrorenal shunts are occasionally documented. Portal vein abnormalities are characteristic, and duplication of the intrahepatic branches is common.[9,19] Occasionally, portal vein thrombosis is documented.

Biliary Lesions and Ascending Cholangitis. Dilatation of the intrahepatic ducts is common in this condition,[9,20] as is an increased risk for cholangitis.[9,12,14,21–25] The cholangitis may be occult, acute, or chronic in nature, and contributes significantly to both the morbidity and mortality of CHF.

Vascular Abnormalities. In addition to the duplication of the intrahepatic portal venous system, other vascular abnormalities and congenital heart disease[26] are recognized associations. These include cerebral,[27] hepatic, splenic, and renal aneurysms[28] and cerebellar hemangioma. Pulmonary arteriovenous fistulas are reported following portosystemic shunting,[29] but this is unlikely to be due to the CHF alone.

Diagnosis of CHF and ARPKD

The diagnosis in a patient with hepatomegaly or portal hypertension is suggested based on clinical and radiographic observations. The liver is usually enlarged and quite firm, with a prominent left lobe. The spleen, and occasionally the kidneys, is also palpable. In the majority of patients the biochemical parameters of hepatic synthetic function are normal. A mild elevation of the transaminases may exist in some cases, but the bilirubin is usually normal. The white blood count, sedimentation rate, and globulin level should be determined as evidence of chronic cholangitis. An elevated blood urea nitrogen (BUN), creatinine, or decreased creatinine clearance provides evidence for renal involvement. The initial radiographic evaluation should be ultrasonography with Doppler evaluation of the portal vasculature. Evidence of portal hypertension, splenomegaly, and intense hepatic echogenicity supports the diagnosis. Evidence of duplication of the intrahepatic vasculature is also confirmatory. The renal sonogram may show increased size and echogenicity of the kidneys. An intravenous pyelogram will confirm the diagnosis in most cases, but it may not be necessary.

Percutaneous liver biopsy will show ductal plate malformation in the great majority of patients, although a few older ones will have hepatic fibrosis without obvious biliary dysgenesis. It is important to culture all liver specimens for bacterial pathogens, in addition to evaluating the tissue for evidence of cholangitis. Particularly in the older patients, the demonstration (by biopsy or otherwise) of cystic renal disease is helpful in establishing the diagnosis.

Therapy for CHF

Portosystemic shunting is the treatment of choice, as there is a low incidence of postoperative encephalopathy or hyperammonemia.[9] Prospective trials of other alternative approaches such as sclerotherapy or pharmacologic management of varices are not yet available. Nevertheless, the presence of spontaneous portosystemic shunts in some children suggests that sclerotherapy may be beneficial if it can be shown to hasten the development of hemodynamically significant shunts without surgery. If surgery is selected as the treatment for portal hypertension, the type of shunt should be carefully chosen to prevent the limitation of options for either hepatic or renal transplantation in later life.

Prolonged cholangitis is a major complication and has been responsible for hepatic failure and death. Therefore, unexplained fever or serologic evidence of inflammation, even in the absence of fever, warrants a diagnostic liver biopsy and aspirate for culture.[21] It should be remembered that any manipulation of the extrahepatic biliary tree carries an increased risk of infection in patients with abnormal ducts or bile stasis.[30] In cases of refractory cholangitis, surgical management and external or internal drainage may be necessary to resolve the hepatobiliary infection.[30] In patients with stasis and refractory cholangitis a choleretic agent may significantly augment therapy. Dehydrocholic acid has been used with antibiotic therapy,[31] and in the future there may be a role for ursodeoxycholic acid, a potent choleretic, in the therapy of this disorder.

Prognosis for CHF

In general, the prognosis for those older children who present with CHF is favorable. The limitations are those imposed by complications of the disease, namely portal hypertension, cholangitis, and occasionally, renal failure. Chronic renal failure is usually limited to patients with a presentation in infancy. As noted, portal hypertension is usually successfully managed and rarely complicated by hepatic encephalopathy. Ascending cholangitis with sepsis and hepatic failure is a major cause of death in most series.[9,15,24] In those patients with chronic cholangitis and/or progressive hepatic dysfunction, liver transplantation may prove to be the optimal therapy.

Congenital Hepatic Fibrosis-Nephronophthisis

In this heritable disorder, there is a combination of hepatic lesions having some similarity to congenital hepatic fibrosis with severe tubulointerstitial renal disease.[32,33] Its relation to the previously discussed disorders is not clear, since the renal lesions differ considerably from those seen in the previously discussed disorders, and since even the hepatic lesion sometimes does not show a completely typical ductal plate malformation.

Autosomal Dominant Polycystic Kidney Disease

"Adult" polycystic disease can be anatomically identified even in fetal life. It is important to recognize for its genetic implications, even though the functional significance of the finding is not apparent until beyond childhood. The hepatic lesions are primarily duct cysts that are readily demonstrated ultrasonographically. Cysts increase in size from childhood until 40 to 50 years of age. They are recognized and are perhaps present at an earlier age in women than in men. Commonly, the cysts in this condition are dilated ductal elements that are not demonstrated to communicate with the distal biliary tree. However, there may also be portal tract lesions consistent with the (communicating) ductal plate malformation in a percentage of patients.[34] This finding and the recent localization of the gene for ADPKD to chromosome 16 suggest that unrecognized interrelationships may still exist between this condition and CHF-ARPKD, even though the loci for the two disorders are not allelic.[35,36]

The renal lesion consists of cysts that appear to arise from multiple areas along the nephron and increase in size with age, eventuating in the kidneys and becoming large cystic reniform masses with inadequate numbers of functioning nephrons.[37]

Cysts may also be found in other organs, including spleen, pancreas, thyroid, ovary, endometrium, seminal vesicles, and epididymis, and cerebral artery aneurysms are present in 15 percent of cases.[35]

Hepatic Polycystic Disease

Some evidence from studies of medicolegal autopsies and occasional families suggests that a polycystic liver disease may exist that occurs in the absence of renal disease and is dominantly inherited.[38] Although detailed pathologic studies or family studies are insufficient to definitely confirm the existence of such an entity, this is a possibility worth investigating.

OTHER MALFORMATION SYNDROMES

The potential for bile duct cyst formation is also present in a number of malformation syndromes of which the ductal plate malformation is a part. Landing has demonstrated morphometric differences between some of these syndromes and ARPKD and CHF.[39] These syndromes are said to include Meckel's syndrome, Ivemark's syndrome, Zellweger's syndrome, Jeune's syndrome, Elejalde's syndrome, glutaric aciduria syndrome type II, Majewski's syndrome, Robert's syndrome, Saldino-Noonan syndrome, Smith-Lemli-Opitz syndrome, and trisomy 1 and 13 syndromes,[40] as well as other unclassified syndromes.[41] Most are heritable conditions. It is interesting that most also have cystic renal disease, usually renal dysplasia, as a component. The pathogenetic implications of this coexistence of renal and hepatic cysts in these malformation syndromes and in ADPKD and CHF-ARPKD is not clear, particularly since the renal disease varies considerably in character among the various conditions.

BILE DUCT PAUCITY—INTRODUCTION

Decrease in ductal number (paucity) is one of the most significant abnormalities of the intralobular bile ducts in children.[42] Bile duct paucity can be defined *only* histologically. In patients at or beyond 37 weeks gestational age, paucity is present when histologic examination demonstrates that the ratio of ducts to portal tracts is less than 0.9. In determining this ratio, it should be kept in mind that (1) bile ductules should not be included in the counting, (2) counts must involve sufficient portal tracts to be representative of the liver as a whole, and (3) this ratio is not applicable in premature infants.[43] The standard for the number of portal tracts required is 20, although some authors suggest that as few as five portal tracts may be sufficient.[43] Since 20 portal tracts are obtainable only on an operative wedge biopsy or with multiple needle biopsies, we are willing to make, or at least strongly suggest, the diagnosis of paucity with a smaller sample number if additional supporting evidence is present (e.g., phenotypic features of syndromic bile duct paucity).

Because there is little conclusive evidence (precise knowledge) of the factors that influence the development, viability, and maintenance of the intrahepatic bile ducts, it is not possible to formulate a genuinely coherent classification of the duct paucity conditions. For example, in some situations, there is an active destruction of previously existing ducts; in others, paucity is associated with a primary disease. For this reason, the disorders outlined in Table 2 are more a list of conditions than a true classification.

TABLE 2
Disorders with Bile Duct Paucity

I. Syndromic Bile Duct Paucity (SBDP)—Alagille's Syndrome
II. Nonsyndromic Bile Duct Paucity
  A. Idiopathic
  B. Associated with primary disease
    1. Metabolic
      Alpha$_1$-antitrypsin deficiency
      Hypopituitarism
      Cystic fibrosis
      Trihydroxycoprostanic acid excess
    2. Chromosomal
      Down's syndrome
      Chromosomal abnormalities
    3. Infectious
      Congenital cytomegalovirus infection
      Congenital rubella infection
      Congenital syphilis
      Hepatitis B
    4. Immunologic
      Graft-versus-host disease
      Chronic hepatic allograft rejection
      Primary sclerosing cholangitis
    5. Other
      Zellweger's syndrome
      Ivemark's syndrome

In many instances of primary disease-paucity association, a causal relationship has not been established.

Syndromic Bile Duct Paucity—Alagille's Syndrome

Syndromic bile duct paucity (SBDP), defined by paucity and the presence of specific extrahepatic findings, is a diagnosis that has both genetic and prognostic implications.[44-49] Also known as Alagille's syndrome, Watson-Alagille syndrome, arteriohepatic dysplasia, syndromic intrahepatic biliary hypoplasia, intrahepatic biliary atresia, intrahepatic biliary dysgenesis, and syndromic paucity of the interlobular bile ducts, it is increasingly recognized as an important and relatively common cause of neonatal jaundice and cholestasis in older children.

Definition

SBDP is characterized by a marked reduction in the number of the interlobular bile ducts and cholestasis, occurring in association with cardiac, musculoskeletal, ocular, facial, renal, and neurodevelopmental abnormalities.

The condition was recognized independently by Watson and Miller[50] and by Alagille and co-workers.[44] It is a familial disease with a wide variability in its clinical spectrum, even within individual pedigrees. The list of abnormalities associated with the syndrome has steadily increased since the initial descriptions, but the principal manifestations have remained essentially unchanged.

Incidence and Inheritance

The incidence of Alagille's syndrome has been estimated at 1 per 100,000 births[51] with an equal sex incidence.[48] The family history is positive for related clinical features in 15 percent. Numerous studies have demonstrated family pedigrees with an autosomal dominant inheritance pattern, low penetrance, and markedly variable expression.[44,46,50,52-54] Other studies have suggested an autosomal recessive inheritance.[55] A large number of cases appear to be sporadic, although this may be the result of subclinical expression in first-degree relatives. Although a patient with arteriohepatic dysplasia and a deletion in chromosome 20 has been reported,[56] final resolution of the inheritance of this disorder must await the definition of a consistent genetic marker.

Hepatic Pathology

Although it was originally considered that patients with this condition had a diminution in the number of interlobular bile ducts from earliest life, a number of reports have established that the portal tract–to–bile duct ratio may not be clearly abnormal at birth.[57–60] The ducts that are present are typical histologically and immunohistochemically.[61] In some cases, there may be increased numbers of ductules, especially when there is portal inflammation.[61,62] This latter finding is particularly important, since on occasion it has been misinterpreted as EHBA. Both clinicians and pathologists must keep this possible error in mind when evaluating neonates with cholestasis who functionally exhibit the findings of biliary obstruction.

Characteristically, intralobular ducts are lost over a variable period of months or even years,[57–60] and the condition becomes definable in morphologic terms. As with any infantile cholestatic condition, hepatocyte giant cells may be present. Histologic cholestasis may be prominent early, but tends to disappear in older cases. Ultrastructural studies have demonstrated apparent retention of bile in hepatocytes at the level of the Golgi, unusually large amounts of intercellular bile, and relatively normal bile canaliculi. These features are different from those seen in other infantile cholestatic conditions,[63] and this may be diagnostically useful. Because these findings are not absolute, however, sampling errors and possible inexperience of observers make this a tenuous basis for diagnostic differentiation in all but the most experienced hands.[64]

Several groups have described a reduction in the number of portal tracts in this condition.[65,66] The portal tracts may or may not show an inflammatory infiltrate, and early in life there is minimal or no fibrosis.[65] Hashida and Yunis have described epithelial degeneration, concentric mesenchymal layering around ducts, edema, and lymphatic and vascular dilatation in the portal tracts.[65] They also emphasize perisinusoidal (as opposed to portal) fibrosis as an early finding.

A particularly interesting feature of SBDP is the lack of invariable progression to secondary biliary cirrhosis despite the absence of ducts and the subsequent retention of potential irritants and toxins, including bile acids and copper. This paradoxical natural history is not unique to SBDP. It is rare, for example, for graft-versus-host–related duct paucity to lead to biliary cirrhosis. This dichotomy between prolonged retention of bile elements and relatively uncommon development of progressive liver disease represents an interesting experiment of nature. Progressive liver disease and significant fibrosis do, however, develop in 10 to 20 percent of patients.[67] The development of hepatocellular carcinoma is rare.[68–70] In cases that have come to transplantation,[65] there have been observed to be an irregular distribution of fibrosis, with the greatest severity near the hilus. It has been emphasized that the end-stage lesion is different from secondary biliary cirrhosis.[65] There is currently no way of predicting which individual case will develop significant morphologic liver disease.

The pathogenesis of the duct paucity in SBDP is unknown. On the basis of the previously mentioned ultrastructural studies, it has been proposed that the patients have an inability to secrete bile.[63] Although there is morphologic and functional evidence that bile is secreted for some time in these patients,[64,65] it is theoretically possible that a failure or abnormality of bile secretion is a critical element in the duct loss in SBDP. Another possible pathogenesis that has been postulated is an abnormality in vascular anlage.

There are anecdotal cases reported where biliary atresia and syndromic paucity coexist in the same patient, and the two disorders have been reported in different members of the same family.[71] We have seen no convincing clinicopathologic evidence for this coexistence (i.e., there is no convincing demonstration of extrahepatic pathology characteristic of EHBA[72] despite radiologic evidence of small bile ducts) and suggest that most reports actually describe SBDP with reduced bile flow and histologic bile ductule increase.

Nonhepatic Pathology

Structural lesions, gross and/or microscopic, have been found in many other organs and systems in SBDP, including the heart, eyes, kidneys, skeletal system, and genitalia.[44,45,48,73] Functional abnormalities are seen in others (e.g., CNS).

Genitourinary lesions that have been described in patients with SBDP include solitary kidney,[74,75] infantile polycystic kidney disease,[75] nephrolithiasis, renal failure and tubulointerstitial nephropathy,[76,77] bifid pelvis,[50] reduplicated ureters,[78] renal artery stenosis,[52] hypogonadism, testicular atrophy, ectopic kidneys,[50] and delayed puberty.[45] In many patients, a characteristic "lipidosis"[52,73,76,79–81] involves the glomeruli most prominently and apparently reflects prolonged elevations of serum cholesterol. With the exception of this lipidosis and the tubulointerstitial nephritis, the other genitourinary abnormalities seem to be developmental.

The relationship of the hepatic disease to other systemic manifestations is unclear. It is not evident how a prenatal abnormality of liver structure or function could account for those extrahepatic findings present at birth, such as butterfly vertebrae and posterior embryotoxon.

There have been several reported cases of hepatic malignancy in patients with Alagille's syndrome, in both the presence[69] and absence of cirrhosis,[67] including three of four siblings in one kinship who developed hepatocellular carcinoma.[82] A nodular hamartoma resembling focal nodular hyperplasia was seen in one patient with end-stage cirrhosis.[83]

Clinical Manifestations

SBDP usually presents in the first 3 months of life in symptomatic patients.[46] It is one of the more common etiologies of cholestasis and jaundice in the neonatal period and must be distinguished from biliary atresia and nonsyndromic bile duct paucity. In older children, SBDP may present as a chronic hepatic disease. Adults are commonly undiagnosed until a related child with syndromic paucity is identified.

The extreme variability of the clinical manifestations and the incomplete penetrance of the syndrome obscure the diagnosis. Some patients demonstrate progressive pruritus, cirrhosis, or liver failure, resulting in liver transplantation. Others have few or no symptoms and remain undiagnosed as adults.

Although most patients present with hepatic manifestations, the associated cardiac disease generally accounts for the majority of the early mortality.[45,46] The cardiac lesions vary from a common clinically insignificant peripheral pulmonary artery stenosis to major intracardiac anomalies. The diagnosis is made when characteristic or compatible liver histology is accompanied by the major extrahepatic findings of the syndrome: chronic cholestasis, characteristic facies, cardiac murmur, vertebral anomalies, and posterior embryotoxon.

Hepatic Manifestations. The majority of symptomatic patients present in infancy and will have manifestations of hepatic disease ranging from mild cholestasis and pruritus to progressive liver failure. There is extreme variability in the extent of the hepatic disease, even within families. It is not uncommon to identify a relative with the syndrome who is anicteric and clinically well. The severity of the disease in the parent is of no prognostic value as to severity in relatives or in subsequent children.[54] The degree of hepatic disease does not correlate with the severity of the other systemic manifestations such as cardiac disease.

Hepatomegaly, with a firm or normal consistency, is recognized in nearly all patients.[45] Splenomegaly is rare in infancy, but appears in one-third to two-thirds by the second decade.[45,46,84]

The most common laboratory abnormalities are elevations of serum bile acids, conjugated bilirubin, alkaline phosphatase, and gamma-glutamyl transpeptidase, which suggest a defect in biliary excretion in excess of the abnormalities in hepatic metabolism or synthesis. There are elevations of the serum aminotransferases, up to 10-fold, which may persist throughout childhood. In general, however, metabolic regulation of transamination, urea synthesis, glucose homeostasis, and protein synthesis are well maintained.

Jaundice is present in the majority of symptomatic patients, and presents as a conjugated hyperbilirubinemia in the neonatal period. In half of these infants it is persistent, resolving only in later childhood. Jaundice commonly is noted during intercurrent illnesses, but the magnitude of the hyperbilirubinemia is minor compared with the degree of cholestasis. Cholestasis is manifest by pruritus and elevations in serum bile acid concentrations. This pruritus is among the most severe in any chronic liver disease. It is rarely present before 3 to 5 months of age,[45,46] but is seen in nearly all children by the third year of life even in those who are anicteric.[45,84,85]

The presence of severe cholestasis results in the formation of xanthomas, characteristically on the extensor surfaces of the fingers, the palmar creases, nape of the neck, popliteal fossa, buttocks, and around inguinal trauma sites. The lesions persist throughout childhood but may gradually disappear after 10 years of age.[86] The timing for the formation of xanthomas relates to the severity of the cholestasis and correlates with a serum cholesterol greater than 500 mg per deciliter. Hypercholesterolemia and hypertriglyceridemia may be profound, reaching levels exceeding 1,000 mg per deciliter and 2,000 mg per deciliter respectively, with the expected abnormalities in lipoproteinemia. The incidence of atheromata is unknown, but they are reported in a child as young as 4 years of age found at autopsy to have extensive aortic and endocardial fat deposition.[46]

Diminished bile salt excretion and low intraluminal bile salt concentrations result in ineffective solubilization and absorption of dietary lipid, essential fatty acids, and fat-soluble vitamins. The deficiency of fat-soluble vitamins has profound systemic effects. Coagulopathy (vitamin K deficiency), rickets (vitamin D deficiency), retinopathy (vitamin E and A deficiency), and a peripheral neuropathy and myopathy (vitamin E deficiency) may occur.[87] Deficiency in essential fatty acids correlates with fat malabsorption, reduced thromboxane B_2 synthesis, and eicosanoid production.[88]

Growth failure is a common feature (50 to 90 percent) during childhood with delayed pubertal development. This is thought to be the result of caloric deprivation from fat malabsorption, the intrinsic vertebral and skeletal abnormalities, and perhaps a secondary abnormality in endocrine function as demonstrated by elevated growth hormone levels with diminished somatomedin production.[44] Hepatic synthetic function is usually well preserved. Serum albumin and ammonia are normal as is the prothrombin time with adequate vitamin K supplementation. Nevertheless, progression to cirrhosis and hepatic failure, initially reported to be uncommon, are recognized with increasing frequency.

Cardiovascular Manifestations. A wide range of cardiovascular abnormalities has been reported in patients with syndromic paucity.[45] The most common lesions are pulmonary artery stenoses at various sites in the proximal and distal tree, commonly at bifurcations.[50] The entire pulmonary vascular tree may be hypoplastic, either alone or in association with other cardiovascular lesions. Among these, tetralogy of Fallot is the most common (7 to 9 percent). Other lesions include truncus arteriosus,[50] secundum atrial septal defect, patent ductus arteriosus,[75] ventriculoseptal defects, and pulmonary atresia.[75] Systemic vascular anomalies, including coarctation of the aorta, renal artery stenosis, and small carotid arteries occur sporadically.[44,50,52] Although the majority of cardiac and vascular lesions are of no hemodynamic consequence, significant lesions do occur, and in some series have been the predominant cause of early death.[45,46] Accordingly, it is advisable to seek formal diagnosis for any murmur in a patient with hepatic disease. Doppler cardiography is usually sufficient in structural cardiac disease, but cardiac catheterization or digital subtraction arteriography may be necessary for diagnosis in some cases.[89]

Characteristic Facies. Characteristic facies are described in the original reports of SBDP. These consist of a prominent forehead, moderate hypertelorism with deep set eyes, a small pointed chin, and a saddle or straight nose that in profile may be in the same plane as the forehead.[45] The facies may be present at birth, but in general become more obvious with increasing age. The usefulness of the facies as a major criterion for diagnosis of Alagille's syndrome has been challenged because of interobserver differences. It has been suggested that these facies are a common result of early and chronic cholestasis,[90] but the constellation of findings and the finding of typical facies in asymptomatic parents may be striking.

Vertebral and Musculoskeletal Abnormalities. Vertebral abnormalities are described in the initial reports of this syndrome.[45] These lesions are characterized by failure of the fusion of the anterior arches of the vertebrae, producing a butterfly appearance on x-ray film, which is of no structural consequence (Fig. 3). Although these abnormalities are present from birth, they are often unrecognized at the time of evaluation for neonatal hepatitis, only to be identified on spine films taken later. Other associated skeletal abnormalities include: an abnormal narrowing of the adjusted interpeduncular space in the lumbar spine in half of the patients,[45,91] a pointed anterior process of C1 and spina bifida occulta,[92] fusion of the adjacent vertebrae, hemivertebrae,[75] and the presence of a bony connection between ribs.[50] The fingers may seem short, and the thumbs broad. Digital clubbing may be evident.[46]

Ocular Abnormalities. A number of abnormalities have been described in SBDP, but many are secondary to chronic vitamin deficiencies. The primary defects include posterior embryotoxon (prominent Schwalbe's line), which can be identified at birth (Fig. 4), and Axenfeld's anomaly (iris strands to the posterior embryotoxon). Posterior embryotoxon has been reported in up to 89 percent of patients,[45] but is not specific, as it occurs in 10 to 15 percent of the general population. Other ocular findings have included exotropia, ectopic pupil, band keratopathy, choroidal folds, and anomalous optic discs.[93] Retinal pigmentary changes are identified in many patients with cholestasis, but they are not specific for the syndrome and are attributed to fat-soluble vitamin deficiencies.[45]

Central and Peripheral Nervous System Abnormalities. Significant mental retardation (IQ less than 80) is a prominent feature in the initial reports of syndromic paucity.[44,49] More recent estimates are lower, perhaps owing to better recognition of the syndrome, the identification of less severely affected individuals, or more aggressive nutritional management. Current studies emphasize the impact of chronic liver disease on brain development regardless of etiology[94,95] and focus on the role of vitamin E therapy and aggressive nutritional management with intervention programs to optimize outcome. No controlled trials are yet available to fully evaluate these claims.

Diagnosis—Clinical Criteria

The specific diagnosis of SBDP can only be established by the clinical phenotype. Alagille has recently proposed revised diagnostic criteria of this disorder based on the presence of five major abnormalities. In addition to proper hepatic histopathology, the major criteria are chronic cholestasis, characteristic facies, cardiac murmur, vertebral abnormalities, and posterior embryotoxon.[45] The frequency of these abnormalities from two series is shown in Table 3.[45,46]

Since all patients with significant bile duct paucity will manifest some degree of chronic cholestasis, Alagille recommends the use of the other four criteria (facies, murmur, vertebral anomalies, and posterior embryotoxon) to define the syndrome.[45] In 36 percent of patients, all four features were present. Another 52 percent had three of the four features and 12 percent had only two features. Based on these data, Alagille has recommended that the diagnosis can be made with cholestasis and two of the other four abnormalities. The

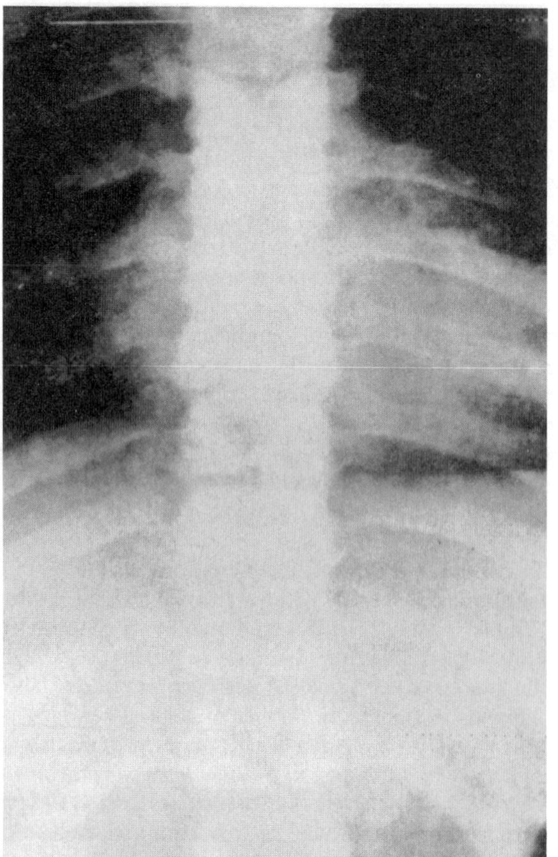

FIGURE 3 Butterfly vertebrae.

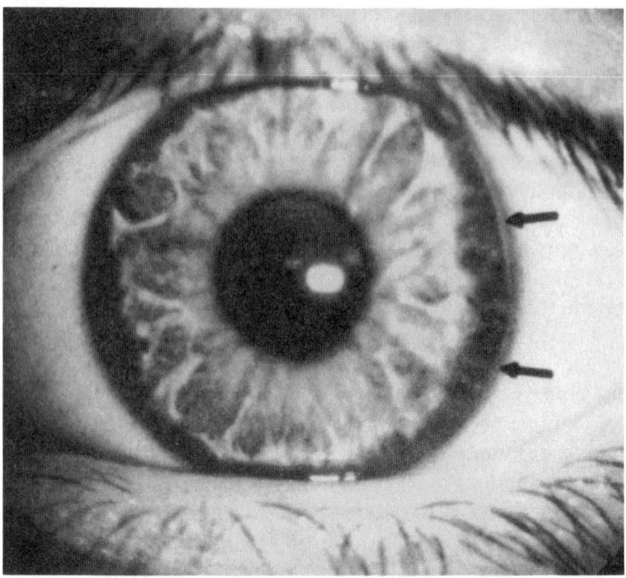

FIGURE 4 Posterior embryotoxon.

TABLE 3
Frequency of Diagnostic Abnormalities in Patients with Syndromic Bile Duct Paucity

	Alagille[45] (n = 80)		DePrettere[46] (n = 27)	
Chronic cholestasis	73/80	91%	25/27	93%
Characteristic facies	76/80	95%	19/27	70%
Cardiac murmur	68/80	85%	26/27	96%
Vertebral abnormalities	70/80	87%	6/18	33%
Embryotoxon	55/62	88%	9/16	56%

need for more specific criteria is evidenced by the frequency of embryotoxon in the general population (10 percent), the subjective assessment of the facies, the potential difficulties in assigning a pathologic basis to a mild systolic flow murmur, and the incidence of cardiac disease both in biliary atresia (10 percent) and in congenital rubella. In difficult cases, a family history of related disease is helpful.

In the majority of patients, the hepatic manifestations of the disease dominate the clinical picture. Patients may present with neonatal hepatitis, jaundice, pruritus, cholestasis, or cardiac disease, or they may be identified as asymptomatic siblings (or parents). The syndrome must be distinguished from other etiologies of neonatal hepatitis and from extrahepatic obstructions such as biliary atresia (see Part 27 of this chapter). The usual evaluation will include an initial laboratory evaluation to identify other etiologies, followed by a sonogram, nuclear scintiscan, liver biopsy, and possible operative cholangiogram.

An infant with SBDP usually has an elevated conjugated bilirubin and moderately elevated levels of the aminotransferases. The gamma-glutamyl transpeptidase, alkaline phosphatase, serum bile acids, and cholesterol may be dramatically elevated, but none of these findings aids in the discrimination of SBDP from biliary atresia or other causes of extrahepatic obstruction.

Although no evidence of mechanical extrahepatic obstruction in SBDP exists, differentiation from biliary atresia can be difficult.[45,50,96] Sonographic examination may not identify the extrahepatic tree owing to diminished gallbladder size, and it is rarely diagnostic. Diagnostic tools that may definitively demonstrate patency of the extrahepatic biliary tree include ^{99m}Tc-DISIDA and similar scintiscans,[46] and radiologic cholangiography via either endoscopic retrograde cholangiopancreatography (ERCP), percutaneous transhepatic cholangiography (PTC),[97] gallbladder, or operative cholangiography. A technetium-labeled scintiscan may show excretion into the duodenum in some patients with SBDP, but in others will not demonstrate communication (as is also seen in biliary atresia).[98]

The liver biopsy is the most useful preoperative study for the discrimination of SBDP from EHBA. Difficulties in histologic diagnosis may arise early in infancy, however, because bile ductule proliferation[62] may obscure duct paucity or because some ducts may in fact be present early in life (see above). In very young infants in whom the percutaneous liver biopsy is not diagnostic, it may be helpful to delay exploration for 1 to 2 weeks and repeat the biopsy (while recognizing that the success of therapy for EHBA is correlated with surgery before 60 days of life).[99] An operative wedge biopsy should be obtained if laparotomy is undertaken. An intraoperative cholangiogram performed by an experienced surgeon must be attempted and carefully interpreted prior to the construction of a portoenterostomy. The extrahepatic bile ducts are anatomically normal and patent in Alagille's syndrome, but may be so narrow that an operative cholangiogram will fail to identify a patent system. Because operative cholangiography alone may result in an incorrect diagnosis of biliary atresia in up to 20 percent of cases,[50,96] a careful preoperative search should be performed for the syndromic features. Hepatoportoenterostomy is inappropriate in SBDP and may increase morbidity.[45,96] The correct diagnosis is also important for the genetic implications.

In older children, striking abnormalities are seen in fasting bile acid levels, serum lipids, gamma-glutamyl transferase, and alkaline phosphatase. Bile acids in severe disease may be elevated 100-fold. The conjugated bilirubin is commonly moderately elevated. The magnitude of the hyperbilirubinemia is usually less than that of the bile acid elevation, and jaundice may disappear during childhood despite persistently elevated bile acids. Most patients have elevated levels of triglyceride and cholesterol, which in severe cases may be from 1,000 to 2,000 mg per deciliter. Moderate elevations of the aminotransferases are common, although to lesser values than the gamma-glutamyl transferase. In the majority of patients, the hepatic synthetic and metabolic functions are normal. Prothrombin time following parenteral vitamin K is usually normal. There may be deficiencies in substances requiring bile acids for absorption, such as vitamins A, D, E, and K and essential fats.

Treatment

Infants with intrahepatic cholestasis may have significant fat malabsorption. Since one-half of the calories in infant formulas may be from fat, this defect contributes significantly to overall caloric deprivation. Medium-chain triglycerides are hydrolyzed and absorbed in the absence of bile salt micelle formation, and thus are a significant caloric additive. Optimal diets include increased amounts of medium-chain triglycerides and optimization of the carbohydrate and protein intake. Essential fatty acids may also be malabsorbed, resulting in clinically evident deficiency. This has resulted in acral lesions resembling porphyria, which have responded to parenteral supplementation of essential fatty acids.

Fat-soluble vitamin deficiency is present to a variable degree in most patients with bile duct paucity. Oral or parenteral supplementation is necessary for prevention of vitamin deficiencies. Further exacerbation of these deficiencies may be caused by therapy for cholestasis, such as phenobarbital or cholestyramine. Oral or intramuscular vitamin K corrects the coagulopathy in most patients, and its failure to do so may herald significant synthetic dysfunction. Aggressive therapy should be maintained in patients with clinical bleeding or evidence of significant hypersplenism. Rickets is seen in patients unless supplemented with oral or intramuscular vitamin D. Early evidence of elevated serum alkaline phosphatase may be obscured, and serum levels of vitamin D should be checked at frequent intervals.

Deficiency of vitamins E and A may result in significant neurologic abnormalities including cerebellar ataxia, peripheral neuropathy, abnormalities of extraocular movement, and retinopathy.[87,100] Vitamin E may be the most difficult to adequately supplement. In addition, the serum level must be corrected for the serum lipid level in children with marked cholestasis. Currently, supplementation with oral or intramuscular preparations may be required to prevent or treat this disorder. Vitamin A levels should also be monitored, and oral or intramuscular replacement given as indicated. However, measurement of liver concentrations of vitamin A provides a more accurate indication of vitamin A status because serum levels of retinol and plasma retinol binding protein are still normal when hepatic stores of vitamin A are depleted.

Pruritus is the most significant symptom for many children. Antihistamines may provide some relief, and care should be taken to keep the skin hydrated with emollients. Fingernails must be trimmed. Cholestyramine relieves pruritus in children who can be convinced to take sufficient amounts, but some children develop a severe acidosis on this therapy.[101] Phenobarbital appears to have little effect on either jaundice or on pruritus, although it has a proven effect enhancing bile salt independent bile formation. Ultraviolet therapy may give temporary relief of pruritus in some cases.[102] Ursodeoxycholic acid is a potent choleretic, and preliminary reports suggest that it may have a dramatic effect in reducing symptomatic cholestasis.

Prognosis

The outcome of SBDP is highly variable and is most directly related to the severity of the hepatic and the cardiac lesions, with mortality equally attributable to these two organs. Complex congenital cardiac disease is a major cause of early mortality, while hepatic complications account for most of the later morbidity and mortality. These data are reflected in a recent follow-up study, which reports a mortality rate of 26 percent (21 of 80) in 10 years, with only four deaths attributable to hepatic disease (portal hypertension in two and hepatic failure in two). Therapeutic options have been discussed in previous sections and are directed toward specific complications of the prolonged cholestasis or the cardiovascular manifestations. In those with progressive liver failure, transplantation has been successful.

Introduction to Nonsyndromic Bile Duct Paucity

Nonsyndromic bile duct paucity is the term used to designate all instances of paucity except those occurring in Alagille's syndrome (arteriohepatic dysplasia, or SBDP). It includes all nonsyndromic cases either with or without an associated primary disease. Thus defined, it covers such a great range of disorders that it is inappropriate to talk of a prognosis for nonsyndromic paucity generally. In those cases associated with a primary disorder, the principal determinant of outcome is usually the primary disease itself. In reviewing reports of supposed nonsyndromic paucity, it should also be kept in mind that there has been an inappropriate tendency to identify progressive intrahepatic cholestasis with paucity in the absence of histologic proof of paucity.

Only a few series of nonsyndromic cases have been published (earlier series of paucity probably include both syndromic and nonsyndromic cases, since the syndrome has only relatively recently been recognized). Kahn et al[58] and Alagille et al[103] have reported series based on histologic criteria. In the series of Kahn et al, of 17 patients with nonsyndromic paucity, nine were associated with well-defined primary diseases, including Down's syndrome, hypopituitarism, cystic fibrosis, alpha$_1$-antitrypsin deficiency, cytomegalovirus infection, and Ivemark's syndrome (in addition to these, other disorders, including trihydroxycoprostanic acid deficiency, rubella, chromosomal abnormalities, graft-versus-host disease, rejection of allograft livers, primary sclerosing cholangitis, and possibly Zellweger's syndrome have also been associated with paucity).[42] In the remaining eight cases in the series of Kahn, the paucity was apparently primary or idiopathic (i.e., not associated with any defined disease). The nonsyndromic cases had the clinical and general histopathologic picture of "neonatal hepatitis." One of the most striking features, in the series of Kahn, was that all the nonsyndromic patients had paucity before the age of 90 days, whereas syndromic cases did not have paucity before 90 days of age. Their nonsyndromic cases also differed from their syndromic cases in that there was more portal fibrosis and less portal inflammation in the nonsyndromic cases. The clinical course of the patients with nonsyndromic paucity without underlying disease was not outlined in detail, but progressive liver disease was uncommon. Several aspects of this series deserve comment.

Most authors, ourselves included, have seen histologic paucity in at least occasional syndromic patients before the age of 90 days, so this cannot be taken as an absolute criterion. Also, the frequency of nonsyndromic paucity in this series (23 cases in 10 years) is higher than we have appreciated in our institution. It should also be noted that this study was conducted using needle-biopsy specimens, and there is some lack of agreement as to how many portal tracts must be evaluated to obtain a statistically accurate estimate of bile duct numbers. As previously mentioned, in evaluating liver biopsies for paucity, it must be recognized, as pointed out by Kahn et al, that in premature infants a bile duct–to–portal tracts ratio of less than 0.9 may be normal.[43]

Alagille et al[103] describe 24 patients with nonsyndromic paucity who were classified into two groups—group I presenting in the first few weeks of life with cholestasis and group II presenting later. The groups differ histologically, with group I having portal inflammation, giant cell change, and minimal fibrosis, and group II having more portal fibrosis and inflammation in relation to paucity. The outcome of these two groups is highly variable, as one-half developed biliary cirrhosis and 38 percent died from hepatic failure. About one-third are anicteric with only biochemical evidence of hepatic disease. Rubella was identified in one patient. It is of note that only 60 percent of these patients were screened for alpha$_1$-antitrypsin deficiency, but 29 percent of those tested had protease inhibitor Z (PiZ). Overall, therefore, it is not clear how many of the cases in this series were truly sporadic or idiopathic, and how many were associated with primary diseases.

Nonsyndromic Paucity with Primary Disease

Detailed discussions of the various primary diseases are presented elsewhere in this text so the discussion here is limited to the pathogenesis of paucity in the few primary conditions in which this pathogenesis is either partially understood or can be plausibly hypothesized.

In terms of paucity associated with well-defined primary diseases, it should be noted that (1) in virtually all of these, paucity is reported in only a small percentage of patients with the diseases, and (2) many of the diseases (e.g., trihydroxycoprostanic acid excess, Ivemark's syndrome) are themselves rare. From these facts it is evident that a causal association between duct paucity and a number of these disorders is not well established.

Bile Duct Paucity in Graft-Versus-Host Disease

Bile duct injury, sometimes eventuating in duct paucity, is one of the most distinctive hepatic lesions in graft-versus-host disease (GVHD). This injury is presumably the basis for the disappearance of ducts and potential paucity that occurs in some patients. It is unusual to find hepatic GVH lesions in the absence of cutaneous manifestations of GHVD. The duct manifests injury by epithelial "atypia," vacuolization, variable staining of nuclei and cytoplasm, and regeneration. Frank necrosis of epithelium can be seen on occasion. Accompanying the epithelial injury, there is often a lymphocytic infiltrate, sometimes with macrophages intermixed. On occasion there is close proximity of lymphocytes and ducts and even invasion of the ducts by lymphocytes. In any single biopsy, however, it is not uncommon for the injury to be out of proportion to the inflammatory infiltrate, and the presence of endothelialitis may be useful in indicating that the epithelial lesions reflect GVHD.[104] Centrilobular cholestasis is frequently present, and is particularly intense when duct paucity has developed. The duct injury and paucity may be patchy (focal). Detailed reconstruction studies[105] have suggested that the injury begins in relatively small ducts (± 30 microns in diameter). When duct paucity is present in a patient with bone marrow transplant, or when there is prominent active duct destruction in such a patient, the diagnosis is quite straightforward, particularly in the absence of cytomegalovirus (CMV) infection. Reports of duct ultrastructure, which are uncommon, have described a number of rather nonspecific changes involving duct epithelium and basement membrane, as well as close contacts between epithelial cells and lymphocytes.[106,107] Immunohistochemical studies reveal increased numbers of $HNK1^+$ (killer) cells, leu 3^+ cells, and expression of HLA-DR (MHC class II) positivity by the epithelial cells.[105,108,109] The latter is not found in normal liver but is found in a variety of conditions affecting the bile ducts, many of which have been speculated to have an immune-related pathogenesis (see above). The precise role and importance of these alterations in ducts in GVHD in the genesis of the duct lesions remains to be determined, but the effects may be mediated through the action of cytotoxic lymphocytes, as appears to be the situation in mucocutaneous GVHD.[110]

It is interesting to note that despite the rather common occurrence of bile duct injury in GVHD, including a number of cases with paucity of ducts, it is uncommon to find reports of cirrhosis, biliary or otherwise, in GVHD.[111,112] At least superficially, this seems analogous to the similarly infrequent development of progressive liver disease in SBDP.

Bile Duct Paucity in Liver Allograft Rejection

Bile duct injury is a significant element of the rejection of hepatic allografts,[104,113-116] and evidence of extensive damage (i.e., involving greater than 50 percent of ducts) in a biopsy from a transplanted liver is regarded as strong evidence of acute rejection.[113] This damage is manifested by a variety of histologic features, including vacuolization of epithelial lining cells, variations in nuclei in these cells, and infiltration of the ducts by inflammatory cells. The latter are most commonly lymphocytes, but neutrophils or eosinophils are not uncommon and may occasionally predominate. Active duct injury is accompanied by a lymphocytic or mixed portal infiltrate beyond the ducts. In a full-blown or classic case of cellular (acute) rejection, so-called endothelialitis (together with duct injury and portal inflammatory infiltrate) forms the third element of a triad diagnostic for rejection.[113] Ultrastructural studies[116] have demonstrated similarities of the duct lesions in hepatic allograft rejection and those seen in both primary biliary cirrhosis and chronic GVHD. These lesions include point contacts between inflammatory cells and duct epithelial cells, a variety of subcellular alterations in epithelial cells extending to the point of degeneration, and basement membrane thickening. It should be noted that substantially similar ultrastructural changes may also be seen in primary sclerosing cholangitis[106,107] and EHBA.[72] If sufficiently severe, the injury may result in duct loss to the point of paucity. Focal or transient paucity is not clinically or prognostically significant, but widespread persistent paucity is an ominous prognostic finding.[113] In hepatic allograft rejection it is characteristic for portal tracts that have lost their ducts to show minimal or no inflammatory infiltrate. This probably speaks to the role of the infiltrating cells in the pathogenesis of the duct injury and loss. There is evidence that the inflammation and/or the duct injury are immunologically determined.

It has been demonstrated[117,118] that following transplantation, HLA-DR (class II) antigens become expressed on bile duct epithelium (and on other hepatic cell types as well). This same phenomenon is also seen in a variety of other human disorders, including GVHD, primary sclerosing cholangitis, primary biliary cirrhosis, extrahepatic obstruction,[105,108,109,119] and some experimental conditions.[120] A possible scenario is that portal tract cells normally expressing class II antigens are initially affected in transplantation and rejection and that these cells then induce expression of class II antigens by the duct epithelial cells (either by the action of activated T cells or the presence of lymphokines), rendering these previously nonexpressive duct cells targets for immune-mediated injury. Although interest in class II antigen has tended to focus on DR, there have been suggestions that DQ is actually more significant. Opinions differ regarding whether class I disparities between donor and recipient are significant in the duct loss.[121,122]

Bile Duct Paucity in Cytomegalovirus Infection

It is well known that hepatic CMV infection can involve the bile ducts. A few cases have been described in which the association of CMV infection and bile duct loss was such that it seems reasonable to postulate that CMV-related duct injury can result in duct loss and/or paucity.[123,124]

PRIMARY SCLEROSING CHOLANGITIS

Primary sclerosing cholangitis (PSC) is a rare disorder that is increasingly recognized in children. It is characterized by a generalized beading and stenosis of the biliary tree in the absence of choledocholithiasis, accompanied by histologic abnormalities of the bile ducts. It may occur in patients who are otherwise well but is often associated with ulcerative colitis.[125] Secondary sclerosing cholangitis describes similar bile duct changes when a clearly predisposing factor such as choledocholithiasis or biliary surgery has been identified.

Histopathology

The histopathology of the extrahepatic biliary tree in childhood PSC has not been described, although it is reasonable to assume that it resembles that seen in adults.[126] In our experience with pediatric patients, examination of the liver will in a number of cases reveal findings highly suggestive of this diagnosis.[127] We have also observed that hepatic pathology may precede unequivocal cholangiographic abnormalities. This discordance suggests that in children, intrahepatic disease may precede extrahepatic disease. PSC may be present years before the development of inflammatory bowel disease.[127]

In our material, duct obliteration and periductal fibrosis have been rare findings on liver biopsy. On the other hand, we have found a combination of prominent duct proliferation with portal inflammation (typically polymorphonuclear leukocytes), and variable portal fibrosis (up to and including cirrhosis) in the absence of histologic cholestasis or hepatocyte lesions, is sufficiently characteristic of PSC to warrant diagnostic studies to examine the integrity of the extrahepatic tree.[127] A variety of less specific hepatic histopathologic pictures can be present in both children and adults, including, but not limited to, a picture resembling chronic active hepatitis.[126,128–132] One series of childhood cases showed only rare histologic cholestasis but consistent orcein positivity.[129] In one interesting series of neonatal PSC, the histopathology was characterized by duct loss.[133] The ultrastructural features in children are, in our experience, nonspecific and generally resemble those seen in EHBA,[134] in adults with PSC, and in primary biliary cirrhosis and GVHD.[135]

Etiology

The precise cause of PSC is not known. Because PSC is closely associated with ulcerative colitis,[125] it has been suggested that an altered mucosal barrier leads to portal bacteremia or the absorption of toxic metabolites and bile acids. A viral etiology has been suggested, analogous to the reovirus-induced cholangitis seen in mice and postulated for human infants.[136] Hepatic disease may be compounded by a defect in excretion of bile acids or metals, such as copper, which accumulates in PSC. More recent studies have focused on the role of genetic and immunologic factors. PSC has been reported in sets of siblings and in a mother-son pair.[137,138] Additionally, there is a reported increase in the frequency of HLA-B8 and HLA-DR3 in patients with PSC.[139] HLA-B8 is also associated with other autoimmune disorders. Autoantibodies against colon and bile duct epithelium and immune complexes have been identified in PSC.[140–143] PSC may also be caused by toxins. Intra-arterial infusion of fluoroideoxyuridine chemotherapy resulted in a 17 percent incidence of PSC.[144] Although PSC is probably an immunologically mediated disease, it may be initiated by some toxic or infectious agent in genetically susceptible individuals.

Clinical Features

The peak incidence of PSC occurs in the third and fourth decades, with a male predominance. Chronic ulcerative colitis is present in 50 to 75 percent or adults with PSC.[145] It is relatively rare in childhood, but is increasingly recognized in the younger age group.[128,129,146–150] Of interest, several of these reports have included children with various immunodeficiencies.[151–154] PSC has been seen in infancy.[52] It may precede by years the onset of ulcerative colitis.[127]

The clinical presentation is highly variable. Usually, the onset of PSC is insidious. Patients may have hepatomegaly, hepatitis, intermittent jaundice, pruritus, idiopathic fevers, abdominal pain, or weight loss. Some present with advanced liver disease and cirrhosis, or with frank suppurative cholangitis.

Diagnosis

The diagnosis should be considered in any child with liver abnormalities and inflammatory bowel disease. An elevated alkaline phosphatase or gamma-glutamyl transferase suggests the disorder. Commonly, the serum cholylglycine is elevated markedly out of proportion to the bilirubin. The serum transminases may be elevated, and in chronic progressive disease there may be evidence of hepatic synthetic dysfunction. There is an association with HLA-B8 and HLA-DR3. Additionally, a number of autoantibodies have been identified that may have some clinical usefulness. Elevations of both IgG and IgM are seen in some patients. As noted, certain liver biopsy findings are highly suggestive of the disease.

The advent of ERCP in children has greatly enhanced visualization of the biliary tree. ERCP in children has replaced percutaneous transhepatic or intraoperative cholangiography as the optimal diagnostic technique.[129,155] The diagnostic findings are multiple irregular stricturing and dilatation of the intrahepatic and extrahepatic bile ducts, which give it a characteristic appearance of beading. In some cases only the intrahepatic or the extrahepatic bile ducts may be abnormal. However, with serial cholangiograms the majority of patients with disease limited to the intrahepatic ducts will progress to involvement of the extrahepatic ducts.[156]

Therapy

There is at present no significant therapy for PSC in adults. A large number of treatments have been studied with only limited success.[157] Antibiotics, corticosteroids, cytotoxic drugs, and cholestyramine have been used. Trials are underway for antifibrinogenic agents and choleretics such as ursodeoxycholic acid. In some patients, transhepatic or endoscopic balloon dilatation is useful for major strictures.[158] At the present time, liver transplantation is the definitive therapy for PSC. In fact, PSC is currently the most common indication for liver transplantation at some centers.[159] In adults, early liver transplantation may be preferable. In one series, 10 percent of patients transplanted for PSC had unrecognized cholangiocarcinoma, despite a recognized disease duration of only 1 to 7 years.[160] Chemical and radiologic abnormalities have rarely recurred in patients transplanted for PSC (2 percent of one series), but these changes are similar to those seen following histologically proven rejection for other disorders.[36]

General therapy for chronic cholestasis includes caloric and fat-soluble vitamin supplementation and antipruritic agents. Cholangitis can occur spontaneously, but it is more common after manipulation of the biliary tract.

Prognosis

No long-term studies of pediatric patients with PSC have been completed. Chronic cholestasis may lead to cholelithiasis and recurrent biliary infections. In adults, the course is usually one of slow progression to cirrhosis, portal hypertension, and death from liver failure, generally with 7 years of diagnosis.[49,51] Cholangiocarcinoma develops in 10 to 15 percent of adult patients with PSC.[161]

REFERENCES

1. Desmet V. Pathology of cholangiopathies. Conference on mechanisms and management of pediatric hepatobiliary disease. Arlington, 1988:61.
2. Boris Reubner. Personal communication.
3. Jorgensen M. The ductal plate malformation. Acta Pathol Microbiol Scand 1977; (suppl A)257.
4. Bernstein J. Hepatic involvement in hereditary renal syndromes. Birth Defect Orig Art Series 1987; 21:115–130.
5. Kerr DNS, Harrison CV, Sherlock S, et al. Congenital hepatic fibrosis. Q J Med NS 1961; 30:91–117.
6. Witzleben CL. Cystic diseases of the liver. In: Zakim D, Boyer TD, eds. Hepatology, a textbook of liver disease. Philadelphia: WB Saunders, 1982:1193.
7. Caroli J, Soupault R, Kossakowski J, et al. La dilatation polykystique congenitale des voies biliares intra-hepatiques: essai de classification. Sem Hop Paris 1958; 14:496.
8. Desmet VJ. Intrahepatic bile ducts under the lens. J Hepatol 1985; 1:545–559.
9. Alvarez F, Bernard O, Brunelle F, Hadchouel M, Leblanc A. Odievre M, Alagille D. Congenital hepatic fibrosis in children. J Pediatr 1981; 99:370–375.
10. Pereira Lima J, da Silveira TR, Geyer G, Grigoletti Scholl J. Congenital hepatic fibrosis: a family study. J Pediatr Gastroenterol Nutr 1984; 3:626–629.
11. Lieberman E, Madrigal-Salinas L, Gwin J, et al. Infantile polycystic disease of the kidneys and liver: clinical, pathological and radiologic correlations and comparisons with congenital hepatic fibrosis. Medicine 1971; 50:277.
12. Blyth H, Ockenden BG. Polycystic kidneys and liver presenting in childhood. J Med Genet 1971; 8:257.
13. Gang D, Herrin J. Infantile polycystic disease of the liver and kidneys. (Abstract) Lab Invest 1980; 42:3.
14. Williams R, Scheuer PJ, Heard BE. Congenital hepatic fibrosis with an unusual pulmonary lesion. J Clin Pathol 1964; 17:135–142.
15. Kerr DN, Okonkwo S, Choa RG. Congenital hepatic fibrosis: the long term prognosis. Gut 1978, 19:514–520.
16. Anand SK, Chan JC, Lieberman E. Polycystic disease and hepatic fibrosis in children, renal function studies. Am J Dis Child 1975; 129:810–813.
17. Kerr DNS, Warrick CK, Hart-Mercer J. A lesion resembling medullary sponge in patients with congenital hepatic fibrosis. Clin Radiol 1962; 13:85–91.
18. Fiorillo A, Migliorati R, Vajro P, Caldore M, Vecchione R. Congenital hepatic fibrosis with gastrointestinal bleeding in early infancy. Clin Pediatr 1982; 21:183–185.
19. Odievre M, Chaumont P, Montagne JP, Alagille D. Anomalies of the intrahepatic portal venous system in congenital hepatic fibrosis. Radiology 1977; 122:427–430.
20. Bouquien H, Delumeau G, Lenne Y, et al. Cited in Murray-Lyon IM, Shilkin KB, Laws JW, et al. Non-obstructive dilatation of the intrahepatic biliary tree with cholangitis. Q J Med 1972; 41:477.
21. Alvarez F, Hadchouel M, Bernard O. Latent chronic cholangitis in congenital hepatic fibrosis. Eur J Pediatr 1982; 139:203–205.
22. Howlett SA, Shulman ST, Ayoub EM, Alexander RA, Donnelly WH, Cerda JJ. Cholangitis complicating congenital hepatic fibrosis. Am J Dig Dis 1975; 20:790–795.
23. Lam SK, Wong KP, Chan PK, Ngan H, Todd D, Ong GB. Fatal cholangitis after endoscopic retrograde cholangiopancreatography in congenital hepatic fibrosis. Aust NZ J Surg 1978; 48:199–202.
24. Murray Lyon IA, Shilkin KB, Laws JS, Illing RC, Williams R. Cholangitis complicating congenital hepatic fibrosis. Gut 1972; 13:319.
25. Sanchez C, Gonzalez E, Garau J. Trimethoprim-sulfamethoxazole treatment of cholangitis complicating congenital hepatic fibrosis. Pediatr Infect Dis 1986; 5:360–363.
26. Naveh Y, Roguin N, Ludatscher R, Auslaender L, Schramek A, Aharon M. Congenital hepatic fibrosis with congenital heart disease, a family study with ultrastructural features of the liver. Gut 1980; 21:799–807.
27. King K, Genta RM, Giannella RA, Weesner RE. Congenital hepatic fibrosis and cerebral aneurysm in a 32-year-old woman. J Pediatr Gastroenterol Nutr 1986; 5:481–484.
28. Murray-Lyon IM, Shilkin KB, Laws JW, Illing RC, Williams R. Non-obstructive dilatation of the intrahepatic biliary tree with cholangitis. Q J Med 1972; 164:477.
29. Maggiore G, Borgna Pignatti C, Marni E, Abbati G, Magrini U. Pulmonary arteriovenous fistulas: an unusual complication of congenital hepatic fibrosis. J Pediatr Gastroenterol Nutr 1983; 2:183–186.
30. Dusol M Jr, Levi JU, Glasser K, Schiff ER. Congenital hepatic fibrosis with dilation of intrahepatic bile ducts. A therapeutic approach. Gastroenterology 1976; 71:839–843.
31. Stillman AE, Earnest DL, Woolfenden JM. Hepatobiliary scintigraphy for cholestasis in congenital hepatic fibrosis, diagnosis and treatment. Am J Dis Child 1985; 139:41–45.
32. Boichis H, Passwell J, David R, et al. Congenital hepatic fibrosis and nephronophthisis: a family study. Q J Med 1973; 42:221.
33. Witzleben CL, Sharp AR. "Nephronophthisis-congenital hepatic fibrosis": an additional hepatorenal disorder. Human Pathol 1982; 13:728–733.
34. Grunfeld JP, Albouze G, Junger P, et al. Liver changes and complications in adult polycystic disease. Adv Nephrol 1985; 14:1.
35. Reeder S, Breuning M, Davies K, et al. A highly pleomorphic DNA marker linked to adult polycystic kidney disease on chromosome 16. Nature 1985; 37:542–544.
36. Wirth B, Zerves K, Fischbach M, et al. Autosomal recessive and dominant forms of polycystic kidney disease are not allelic. Human Genet 1987; 77:221–222.
37. Kissane JM. Congenital malformations. In: Heptinstall RH, ed. Pathology of the kidney. 2nd ed. Boston: Little Brown, 1974:69.
38. Karhumen P, Tenhu M. Adult polycystic liver and kidney diseases are separate entities. Clin Genet 1986; 30:29.
39. Landing BH, Wells TR, Claireaux AE. Morphometric analysis of liver lesions in cystic diseases of childhood. Hum Pathol 1980; 11(suppl):549.

40. Bernstein J, Stickler G, Neel I. Congenital hepatic fibrosis: evolving morphology. Acta Pathol Microbiol Immunol Scand 1988; 4(suppl):17–26.
41. Miranda D, Schinella R, Finegold M. Familial renal dysplasia. Microdissection studies in siblings with associated central nervous system and hepatic malformations. Arch Pathol 1972: 93:483.
42. Witzleben CL. Bile duct paucity ("intrahepatic atresia"). Perspect Pediatr Pathol 1982; 7:185–201.
43. Kahn E, Markowitz J, Aiges H, Daum F. Human ontogeny of the bile duct to portal space ratio. Hepatology 1989; 10:21–23.
44. Alagille D, Odievre M, Gautier M, Dommergues JP. Hepatic ductular hypoplasia associated with characteristic facies, vertebral malformations, retarded physical, mental, and sexual development, and cardiac murmur. J Pediatr 1975; 86:63–71.
45. Alagille D, Estrada A, Hadchouel M, Gautier M, Odievre M. Dommergues JP. Syndromic paucity of interlobular bile ducts (Alagille syndrome or arteriohepatic dysplasia): review of 80 cases. J Pediatr 1987; 110:195–200.
46. Deprettere A, Portmann B, Mowat AP. Syndrome paucity of the intrahepatic bile ducts: diagnostic difficulty; severe morbidity throughout early childhood. J Pediatr Gastroenterol Nutr 1987; 6:865–871.
47. Deutsch J, Smith AL, Danks DM, Campbell PE. Long term prognosis for babies with neonatal liver disease. Arch Dis Child 1985; 60:447–451.
48. Mueller RF. The Alagille syndrome (arteriohepatic dysplasia). J Med Genet 1987; 24:621–626.
49. Odievre M, Hadchouel M, Landrieu P, Alagille D, Eliot N. Long term prognosis for infants with intrahepatic cholestasis and patent extrahepatic biliary tract. Arch Dis Child 1981; 56:373–376.
50. Watson GH, Miller V. Arteriohepatic dysplasia: familial pulmonary arterial stenosis with neonatal liver disease. Arch Dis Child 1973; 48:459–466.
51. Danks DM, Campbell PE, Jack I, Rogers J, Smith AL. Studies of the aetiology of neonatal hepatitis and biliary atresia. Arch Dis Child 1977; 52:360–367.
52. LaBrecque DR, Mitros FA, Nathan RJ, Romanchuk KG. Judisch GF, El Khoury GH. Four generations of arteriohepatic dysplasia. Hepatology 1982; 2:467–474.
53. Riely CA, LaBrecque DR, Ghent C, Horwich A, Klatskin G. A father and son with cholestasis and peripheral pulmonic stenosis: a distinct form of intrahepatic cholestasis. J Pediatr 1978; 92:406–414.
54. Shulman SA, Hyams JS, Gunta R, Greenstein RM, Cassidy SB. Arteriohepatic dysplasia (Alagille syndrome): extreme variability among affected family members. Am J Med Genet 1984; 19:325–332.
55. Mueller RF, Pagon RA, Pepin MG, Haas JE, Kawabori I, Stevenson JG, Stephan MJ, Blumhagen JD, Christie DL. Arteriohepatic dysplasia: phenotypic features and family studies. Clin Genet 1984; 25:323–331.
56. Byrne JL, Harrod MJ, Friedman JM, Howard-Peebles PN. del(20p) with manifestations of arteriohepatic dysplasia. Am J Med Genet 1986; 24:673–678.
57. Dahms BB, Petrelli M, Wyllie R, Henoch MS, Halpin TC, Morrison S, Park MC, Tavill AS. Arteriohepatic dysplasia in infancy and childhood: a longitudinal study of six patients. Hepatology 1982; 2:350–358.
58. Kahn E, Daum F, Markowitz J, Teichberg S, Duffy L, Harper R, Aiges H. Nonsyndromatic paucity of interlobular bile ducts: light and electron microscopic evaluation of sequential liver biopsies in early childhood. Hepatology 1986; 6:890–901.
59. Ghishan FK, LaBrecque DR, Mitros FA, Younoszai MK. The evolving nature of "infantile obstructive cholangiopathy". J Pediatr 1980; 97:27–32.
60. Levin SE, Zarvos P, Milner S, Schmaman A. Arteriohepatic dysplasia: association of liver disease with pulmonary arterial stenosis as well as facial and skeletal abnormalities. Pediatrics 1980; 66:876–883.
61. Witzleben CL, Steigman C. Unpublished observations.
62. Novotny NM, Zetterman RK, Antonson DL, Vanderhoof JA. Variation in liver histology in Alagille's syndrome. Am J Gastroenterol 1981; 75:449–450.
63. Valencia-Mayoral P, Weber J, Cutz E, Edwards VD, Phillips MJ. Possible defect in the bile secretory apparatus in arteriohepatic dysplasia (Alagille's syndrome): a review with observations on the ultrastructure of liver. Hepatology 1984; 4:691–698.
64. Witzleben CL, Finegold M, Piccoli DA, Treem WR. Bile canalicular morphometry in arteriohepatic dysplasia. Hepatology 1987; 7:1262–1266.
65. Hashida Y, Yunis EJ. Syndromatic paucity of interlobular bile ducts: hepatic histopathology of the early and endstage liver. Pediatr Pathol 1988; 8:1–15.
66. Hadchouel M, Hugon RN, Gautier M. Reduced ratio of portal tracts to paucity of intrahepatic bile ducts. Arch Pathol Lab Med 1978; 102:402.
67. Perrault J. Paucity of interlobular bile ducts: getting to know it better. (Editorial) Dig Dis Sci 1981; 26:481–484.
68. Adams PC. Hepatocellular carcinoma associated with arteriohepatic dysplasia. Dig Dis Sci 1986; 31:438–442.
69. Kaufman SS, Wood RP, Shaw BW Jr, Markin RS, Gridelli B, Vanderhoof JA. Hepatocellular carcinoma in a child with the Alagille syndrome. Am J Dis Child 1987; 141:698–700.
70. Ong E, Williams SM, Anderson JC, Kaplan PA. MR imaging of a hepatoma associated with Alagille syndrome. J Comput Assist Tomogr 1986; 10:1047–1049.
71. Alagille D. Intrahepatic biliary atresia (hepatic ductular hypoplasia). In: Berenberg SR, ed. Liver diseases in infancy and childhood. Baltimore: Williams & Wilkins, 1976:129.
72. Witzleben CL, Buck BE, Schnaufer L, Brzosko WJ. Studies on the pathogenesis of biliary atresia. Lab Invest 1978; 38:525.
73. Riely CA, Cotlier E, Jensen PS, Klatskin G. Arteriohepatic dysplasia: a benign syndrome of intrahepatic cholestasis with multiple organ involvement. Ann Intern Med 1979; 91:520–527.
74. Oestreich AE, Sokol RJ, Suchy FJ, Heubi JE. Renal abnormalities in arteriohepatic dysplasia and nonsyndromic intrahepatic biliary hypoplasia. Ann Radiol (Paris) 1983; 26:203–209.
75. Greenwood RD, Rosenthal A, Crocker AC, Nadas AS. Syndrome of intrahepatic biliary dysgenesis and cardiovascular malformations. Pediatrics 1976; 58:243–247.
76. Hyams JS, Berman MM, Davis BH. Tubulointerstitial nephropathy associated with arteriohepatic dysplasia. Gastroenterology 1983; 85:430–434.
77. Tolia V, Dubois RS, Watts FB Jr, Perrin E. Renal abnormalities in paucity of interlobular bile ducts. J Pediatr Gastroenterol Nutr 1987; 6:971–976.
78. Flick AL. Arteriohepatic dysplasia: a 16 year follow up during treatment with cholestyramine. West J Med 1982; 136:62–65.
79. Chung Park M, Petrelli M, Tavill AS, Hall PW 3d, Henoch MS. Dahms BB. Renal lipidosis associated with arteriohepatic dysplasia (Alagille's syndrome). Clin Nephrol 1982; 18:314–320.
80. Russo PA, Ellis D, Hashida Y. Renal histopathology in Alagille's syndrome. Pediatr Pathol 1987; 7:557–568.
81. Pokorny W, Wagner IU, WeiBenbacher G, Wimmer M. Gallengangshypoplasie-syndrom mit charakteristischer Facies, PulmonalgefaBanomalien und fakultativ anderen MiBbildunger. Klin Padiat 1976; 188:255–262.
82. Rabinowitz M, Imperial JC, Schade RR, Van Thiel DH. Hepatocellular carcinoma in Alagille's syndrome: a family study. J Pediatr Gastro Nutr 1989; 8:26–30.
83. Nishikawa A, Mori H, Takahashi M, Ojima A, Shimokawa K, Furuta T. Alagille's syndrome, A case with a hamartomatous nodule of the liver. Acta Pathol Jpn 1987; 37:1319–1326.
84. Mowat AP. Hepatitis and cholestasis in infancy: intrahepatic disorders. In: Mowat AP, ed. Liver diseases in childhood. 2nd ed. London: Butterworth, 1987:66.
85. Collins DM, Shannon FT, Campbell CB. Bile acid metabolism in mild arteriohepatic dysplasia. Aust NZ J Med 1981; 11:48–51.
86. Weston CF, Burton JL. Xanthomas in the Watson Alagille syndrome. J Am Acad Dermatol 1987; 16:1117–1121.
87. Alvarez F, Landrieu P, Laget P, Lemonnier F, Odievre M, Alagille D. Nervous and ocular disorders in children with cholestasis and vitamin A and E deficiencies. Hepatology 1983; 3:410–414.
88. Dupont J, Amedee Manesme O, Alagille D, Chambaz J, Pepin D. Eicosanoid synthesis in Alagille syndrome. (Letter) N Engl J Med 1986; 314:718.
89. Brindza D, Moodie DS, Wyllie R, Sterba R. Intravenous digital subtraction angiography to assess pulmonary artery anatomy in patients with the Alagille syndrome. Cleveland Clin Q 1984; 51:493–497.
90. Sokol RJ, Heubi JE, Balistreri WF. Intrahepatic "cholestasis facies": is it specific for Alagille syndrome? J Pediatr 1983: 103:205–208.
91. Rosenfield NS, Kelley MJ, Jensen PS, Cotlier E, Rosenfield AT, Riely CA. Arteriohepatic dysplasia: radiologic features of a new syndrome. AJR 1980; 135:1217–1223.
92. Berman MD, Ishak KG, Schaefer EJ, Barnes S, Jones EA. Syndro-

matic hepatic ductular hypoplasia (arteriohepatic dysplasia): a clinical and hepatic histologic study of three patients. Dig Dis Sci 1981; 26:485–497.

93. Romanchuk KG, Judisch GF, LaBrecque DR. Ocular findings in arteriohepatic dysplasia (Alagille's syndrome). Can J Ophthalmol 1981; 16:94–99.

94. Sokol RJ, Guggenheim MA, Iannaccone ST, et al. Improved neurologic function after long-term correction of vitamin E deficiency in children with chronic cholestasis. N Eng J Med 1985; 313:1580–1586.

95. Stewart SM, Uauy R, Kennard BD, Waller DA, Benser M, Andrews WS. Mental development and growth in children with chronic liver disease of early and late onset. Pediatrics 1988; 82:168–172.

96. Markowitz J, Daum F, Kahn EI, Schneider KM, So HB, Altman RP, Aiges HW, Alperstein G, Silverberg M. Arteriohepatic dysplasia, I. Pitfalls in diagnosis and management. Hepatology 1983; 3:74–76.

97. Carty H. Percutaneous transhepatic fine needle cholangiography in jaundiced infants. Ann Radiol 1978; 21:149–154.

98. Summerville DA, Marks M, Treves ST. Hepatobiliary scintigraphy in arteriohepatic dysplasia (Alagille's syndrome), a report of two cases. Pediatr Radiol 1988; 18:32–34.

99. Hitch DC, Shikes RH, Lilly JR. Determinants of survival after Kasai's operation in biliary atresia using actuarial analysis. J Ped Surg 1979; 14:310–314.

100. Sokol RJ, Bove KE, Heubi JE, et al. Vitamin E deficiency during chronic childhood cholestasis—presence of sural nerve lesion prior to 1½ years of age. J Pediatr 1983; 103:197–204.

101. Sharp HL, Carey JB, White JG, et al. Cholestyramine therapy in patients with a paucity of intrahepatic bile ducts. J Pediatr 1967; 71:723–736.

102. Person JR. Ultraviolet A (UV-A) and cholestatic pruritus. Arch Dermatol 1981; 117:684.

103. Alagille D. Cholestasis in children. In : Alagille D, Odievre M, eds. Liver and biliary tract disease in children. New York: John Wiley & Sons, 1979:185.

104. Snover DC, Freese DK, Sharp HL, Bloomer JR, Najarian JS, Ascher NL. Liver allograft rejection. An analysis of the use of biopsy in determining outcome of rejection. Am J Surg Pathol 1987; 11:1–10.

105. Tanaka M, Umihara J, Chiba S, Ishikawa E. Intrahepatic bile duct injury following bone marrow transplantation. Analysis of pathological features based on three-dimensional and histochemical observation. Acta Pathol Jpn 1986; 36:1793–1806.

106. Bernuau D, Feldmann G, Degott C, Gisselbrecht C. Ultrastructural lesions of bile ducts in primary biliary cirrhosis. A comparison with the lesions observed in graft versus host disease. Hum Pathol 1981; 12:782–793.

107. Bernuau D, Gisselbrecht C, Devergie A, Feldmann G, Gluckman E, Marty M, Boiron M. Histological and ultrastructural appearance of the liver during graft versus host disease complicating bone marrow transplantation. Transplantation 1980; 29:236–244.

108. Dilly SA, Sloane JP. An immunohistological study of human hepatic graft-versus-host disease. Clin Exp Immunol 1985; 62:545–553.

109. Miglio F, Pignatelli M, Mazzeo V, Baraldini M, Steffanini GF, Guardigli G, Bandini G, Ricci P, Gasbarrini G. Expression of major histocompatibility complex class II antigens on bile duct epithelium in patients with hepatic graft-versus-host disease after bone marrow transplantation. J Hepatol 1987; 5:182–189.

110. Sale GE, Gallucci BB, Schubert MM, Sullivan KM, Thomas ED. Direct ultrastructural evidence of target-directed polarization by cytotoxic lymphocytes in lesions of human graft-versus-host disease. Arch Pathol Lab Med 1987; 111:333–336.

111. Yau JC, Zander AR, Srigley JR, Verm RA, Stroehlein JR, Korinek JF, Vellekoop L, Dicke KA. Chronic graft-versus-host disease complicated by micronodular cirrhosis and esophageal varices. Transplantation 1986; 41:129–130.

112. Knapp AB, Crawford JM, Rappeport JM, Gollan JL. Cirrhosis as a consequence of graft-versus-host disease. Gastroenterology 1987; 92:513–519.

113. Snover DC, Weisdorf SA, Ramsay NK, McGlave PH, Kersey JH. Hepatic graft versus host disease. a study of the predictive value of liver biopsy in diagnosis. Hepatology 1984; 4:123–130.

114. Snover DC, Sibley RK, Freese DK, Sharp HL, Bloomer JR, Najarian JS, Ascher NL. Orthotopic liver transplantation: a pathological study of 63 serial liver biopsies from 17 patients with special reference to the diagnostic features and natural history of rejection. Hepatology 1984; 4:1212–1222.

115. Demetris AJ, Lasky S, Van T gy of hepatic transplantation. A immunosuppressed with cyclospo 1985; 118:151–161.

116. Vierling JM, Fennel RH Jr. Histopatho hepatic allograft rejection: evidence of prog lobular bile ducts. Hepatology 1985; 5:1076–

117. Takacs L, Szende B, Monostori E, Rot A, Lapis I. Expression of HLA-DR antigens on bile duct cel transplant. Lancet 1983; ii:1500.

118. Demetris AJ, Lasky S, Van Thiel DH, Starzl TE, Whit duction of DR/IA antigens in human liver allografts. Transp 1985; 40:504–509.

119. Chapman RWG, Marborgh BA, Rhodes JM, Summerfield DR, Sche PJ, Sherlock S. Primary sclerosing cholangitis: a review of its clinical features, cholangiography and hepatic histology. Gut 1980; 21:870–877.

120. Takacs L, Szende B, Rot A, Diamanstein T. Expression of MHC class II antigens on bile duct epithelium in experimental graft versus host disease. Clin Exp Immunol 1985; 60:449–456.

121. Betts K, Moore S, Perkins S, Wiesner R, et al. Influence of positive lymphocyte crossmatch and HLA mismatching on vanishing bile duct syndrome in human liver allografts. Transplantation 1988; 45:376–379.

122. Donaldson P, O'Grady J, Portmann B, David H, et al. Evidence for an immune response to HLA class I antigens in the vanishing bile duct syndrome after liver transplantation. Lancet 1987; ii:945–948.

123. Finegold MJ, Carpenter RJ. Obliterative cholangitis due to cytomegalovirus: a possible precursor of paucity of intrahepatic bile ducts. Hum Pathol 1982; 13:662.

124. Oppenheimer E, Esterly J. Cytomegalovirus infection. A possible cause of biliary atresia. (Abstract) Am J Pathol 1973; 71:2.

125. Schrumpf E, Fausa O, Kolmannskog F, Elgjo K, et al. Sclerosing cholangitis in ulcerative colitis—a follow-up study. Scand J Gastroenterol 1982; 17:33–39.

126. LaRusso NF, Wiesner RH, Ludwig J, MacCarty RL. Primary sclerosing cholangitis. N Engl J Med 1984; 310:899–903.

127. Witzleben CL, Piccoli DA, Widzer S, Conard K, Watkins JB. Pediatric sclerosing cholangitis. (Abstract) 1988; Lab Invest 58:104.

128. Classen M, Gotze H, Richter HJ, Bender S. Primary sclerosing cholangitis in children. J Pediatr Gastroenterol Nutr 1987; 6:197–202.

129. el-Shalrawi M, Wilkinson M, Portmann B, Mieli-Vergani G, Chong SKF, Williams R, Mowat A. Primary sclerosing cholangitis in childhood. Gastroenterology 1987; 92:1226–1235.

130. Chapman RWG, Arborgh BAM, Rhodes JM, et al. Primary sclerosing cholangitis: a review of its clinical features, cholangiography, and hepatic histology. Gut 1980; 21:870–877.

131. Lefkowitch JH. Primary sclerosing cholangitis. Arch Intern Med 1982; 142:1157–1160.

132. Wiesner RH, LaRusso NF. Clinicopathologic features of the syndrome of primary sclerosing cholangitis. Gastroenterology 1980; 79:200–206.

133. Amedee-Manesme O. Bernard O, Brunelle F, Hadchouel M, Polonovski C, Baudon JJ, Beguet P, Alagille D. Sclerosing cholangitis with neonatal onset. J Pediatr 1987; 111:225–229.

134. Witzleben CL, Schnaufer L. Morphogenesis of porta epithelial injury in EHBA. (Abstract) Lab Invest 1987; 56:88.

135. Chlumsky A, Chlumsky J, Krtek V, Jirkovska A, Pirk F, Skala I. Primary sclerosing cholangitis. Light and electron microscopy of hepatic tissue in two cases. Pathol Res Pract 1985; 179:487–492.

136. Bangaru B, Morecki R, Glaser JH, Gartner LM, Horwitz MS. Comparative studies of biliary atresia in the human newborn and reovirus-induced cholangitis in weanling mice. Lab Invest 1980; 43:456–462.

137. Quigley EMM, LaRusso NF, Ludwig J, MacSween RNM, et al. Familial occurrence of primary sclerosing cholangitis and chronic ulcerative colitis. Gastroenterology 1983; 85:1160–1165.

138. Silber GH, Finegold MJ, Wagner ML, Klish WJ. Sclerosing cholangitis and ulcerative colitis in a mother and her son. J Pediatr Gastroenterol Nutr 1987; 6:147–152.

139. Chapman RW, Varghese Z, Gaul R, Patel G, et al. Association of primary sclerosing cholangitis with HLA-B8. Gut 1983; 13:38–41.

140. Mieli-Vergani G, Lobo-Yeo A, McFarlane BM, McFarlane IG, Mowat AP, Vergani D. Different immune mechanisms leading to autoimmunity in primary sclerosing cholangitis and autoimmune chronic active hepatitis of childhood. Hepatology 1989; 9:198–203.

141. Chapman RW, Selby W, Shepherd H, Sherlock S, et al. Serum anticolon antibodies, ulcerative colitis and sclerosing cholangitis. Gut 1983; 24:474.

, et al. Elevat-
g cholangitis.

rlock S, Jewell
ary sclerosing

erg DA, Leong
ter continuous
202:176–181.
Diagnosis and
ver Dis 1985;

ing cholangitis

rosing cholan-

HL. Sclerosing
e. Clin Pediatr

of the primary
986; 99:155–158.

150. Johnson DA, Cattau EL Jr, Hancock JE. Pediatric primary sclerosing cholangitis. Dig Dis Sci 1986; 31:773–777.
151. Record CO, Eddleston ALW, Shilkin KB, Williams R. Intrahepatic sclerosing cholangitis associated with a familial immunodeficiency. Lancet 1973; ii:18–20.
152. DiPalma JA, Strobel CT, Farrow JG. Primary sclerosing cholangitis associated with hyperimmunoglobulin M immunodeficiency (dysgammaglobulinemia). Gastroenterology 1986; 91:464–468.
153. Ben-Dov D, Weinberg G, Auslaender L. Sclerosing cholangitis associated with familial combined immunodeficiency in a 1-year-old infant. Isr J Med Sci 1985; 21:391–393.
154. Naveh Y, Mendelsohn H, Spira G, Auslaender L, Mandel H, Berant M. Primary sclerosing cholangitis associated with immunodeficiency. Am J Dis Child 1983; 137:114–117.
155. Allendorph M, Werlin SL, Geenen JE, Hogan WJ, Venu RP, Stewart ET, Blank EL. Endoscopic retrograde cholangiopancreatography in children. J Pediatr 1987; 110:206–211.
156. LaRusso NF, Wiesner RH, Ludwig J. Is primary sclerosing cholangitis a bad disease? Gastroenterology 1987; 92:2031–2033.
157. Lindor KD, Wiesner RH, LaRusso NF. Recent advances in the management of primary sclerosing cholangitis. Semin Liver Dis 1987; 7:322–327.
158. May GR, Bender CE, LaRusso NF, Wiesner RH. Nonoperative dilatation of dominant strictures in primary sclerosing cholangitis. AJR 1985; 145:1061–1064.
159. Krom RA, Wiesner RH, Rettke SR, Ludwig J, Southorn PA, Hermans PE, Taswell HF. The first 100 liver transplantations at the Mayo Clinic. Mayo Clin Proc 1989; 64:84–94.
160. Marsh JW, Iwatsuki S, Makowka L, Esquivel CO, Gordon RD, Todo S, Tzakis A, Miller C, Van Thiel D, Starzl TE. Orthotopic liver transplantation for primary sclerosing cholangitis. Ann Surg 1988; 207:21–25.
161. Wee A, Ludwig J, Coffey RJ, et al. Hepatobiliary carcinoma associated with primary sclerosing cholangitis and chronic ulcerative colitis. Hum Pathol 1985; 16:719–726.

PART 27

Disorders of the Extrahepatic Bile Ducts

David A. Piccoli, M.D.
Camillus L. Witzleben, M.D.

The division between this part of Chapter 28 and the preceding part, Disorders of Intrahepatic Bile Ducts, is considerably artificial, since many of the disorders in this chapter potentially affect both the intrahepatic and extrahepatic bile ducts. The reader should refer to the index to determine where a particular disorder is discussed.

EMBRYOLOGY OF THE EXTRAHEPATIC BILE DUCTS

The extrahepatic biliary system (and presumably some of the larger intrahepatic ducts) develops from the cephalic portion of the hepatic diverticulum during the fourth to sixth weeks of gestation. These ductal elements establish continuity with the bile canaliculi through the interlobular ducts, which in turn arise from a differentiation of hepatocytes into the so-called ductal plate (see Part 26 of this chapter).

EXTRAHEPATIC BILIARY ATRESIA

Definition

Extrahepatic biliary atresia (EHBA) is characterized by the destruction or absence of portions of the extrahepatic biliary system at a point (or points) between the liver hilus and the duodenum with attendant complete obstruction to bile flow. The obstruction to flow, if not relieved, inevitably results in secondary biliary cirrhosis. The clinical phenotype of biliary atresia may be subdivided into two groups: (1) patients with isolated biliary atresia, and (2) those with situs inversus and polysplenia syndrome. Biliary atresia may also be divided into anatomic types: type 1, atresia of the common bile duct and a patent proximal system, type 2, atresia involving the hepatic duct but with patent proximal ducts, and type 3, atresia involving the right and left hepatic ducts at the porta hepatis.

These clinical and anatomic subdivisions have clinical and prognostic implications.[1]

The term *intrahepatic biliary atresia*, which actually refers to intrahepatic bile duct paucity (see Part 26 of this chapter), should not be confused with EHBA. These two problems rarely, if ever, coexist in a single patient.

Pathology and Pathogenesis

With the introduction of the portoenterostomy as a therapy for EHBA, it became possible to study the histopathology of the extrahepatic biliary tree in detail (from excised specimens) at an earlier stage of the disorder than had been possible. Studies of the excised remnants of the biliary tree demonstrate a range of histopathology, from active inflammation and evident degeneration of duct epithelium through more chronic inflammation with an increase in number of small duct and glandular elements, to frank scarring (Fig. 1).[2] In many cases a combination of these features is present. The epithelial injury, inflammation, and fibrosis are associated with complete obliteration of the lumen of one or both hepatic ducts, or of the common bile duct for varying lengths, because of either fibrosis and/or complete loss (absence) of duct structure. A great variety of patterns of lumen obliteration or duct loss have been reported. Our data have not shown multiple areas of obstruction separated by patent areas. When inflammation is present, the porta hepatis is typically the site of the most active inflammation. Occasionally, bile is prominent in the porta hepatis, but more often it is inconspicuous, suggesting that the proximal inflammation and duct injury are not necessarily a secondary effect of an absent distal lumen with bile retention locally. The relative absence of bile pigment at this time may reflect an absence of hepatocyte excretory activity. The gallbladder is often absent; when present, it often has chronic inflammation and fibrosis, with a variable loss of the mucosal epithelium and muscularis.

Definition of the histopathology of the biliary tree early in life is important because the presence of "active" disease involving the extrahepatic biliary tree appears to argue that EHBA is usually not a failure of development. Rather, it is an acquired lesion, probably beginning late in fetal life. However, biliary atresia may coexist with unequivocal malformations, most notably with the polysplenia syndrome or hyposplenia,[3-6] and it has been suggested that cases of EHBA with associated malformations may begin very early in intrauterine life. Schweizer[7] has suggested that in such cases the secondary effects of the atresia may be particularly far advanced early in postnatal life, and there may be a poor response to hepatoportoenterostomy. It has also been suggested that cases of very early onset may be associated with the persistence of the ductal plate.[8] Thus, it is possible that there is more than one type of biliary atresia and that more than one etiology or pathogenesis may lead to a final common lesion. In our experience with cases of EHBA with and without the polysplenia syndrome, we have not been able to discern any qualitative difference in the inflammatory-destructive lesions, which are present in both.

With the demonstration of an active pathology, possibly reflecting a primary insult to the biliary tree, it was anticipated that an etiologic agent might be detectable in either the serum or the excised tissues. The search for such agents has proved to be frustrating. For the majority of viruses, serologic and electron microscopic studies have been negative. Studies for hepatitis A and B have been negative.[2,9] Infants with EHBA and their mothers were found to have an increase in antibody titers to reovirus type 3 by Glaser et al,[10,11] although this has not been confirmed by others.[12,13] Moreover, in neonatal mice, reovirus type 3 can cause bile duct lesions similar to those caused by EHBA.[14] In human infants, it has been extremely difficult to identify evidence of virus infection in the liver. Morphologic evidence of reovirus has been reported only extremely rarely.[15,16] It is possible that both the temporal course of the infection and the duration of virus persistence are such that by the time clinical disease has developed, the virus has disappeared. This is supported by the fact that it is even difficult to demonstrate the virus in the extrahepatic biliary tree in the murine model of injury.[17] Further attempts to search for evidence of reovirus and other viruses in the biliary tracts of patients with EHBA are clearly necessary.

Other causes of EHBA must be considered. There are several reports of the incidence of biliary atresia in twins, in one or both.[18-21] One report of EHBA in only one of HLA identical twins suggests an environmental rather than genetic etiology. Biliary atresia is more common in Japan than in the United States, but in Hawaii it is more common in Chinese than Japanese or Caucasian individuals.[22] Rarely, biliary atresia has been reported to occur in subsequent children within a family.[23]

The descriptions and comments above have been primarily directed toward the lesions of the extrahepatic ducts in EHBA. The question of lesions of the intrahepatic ducts in this condition is even more obscure. Some authors have emphasized that destructive lesions of the intrahepatic ducts exist in EHBA at or before the time of portoenterostomy.[24] More important, in most patients with portoenterostomies who have satisfactory bile drainage, there has been a gradual disappearance of intrahepatic ducts. The phenomenon was recognized before surgical intervention was available and was attributed to secondary effects of the prolonged obstruction. However, observation of the same phenomenon after portoenterostomy has led to the concept that the basic pathogenetic process actually involves both the intrahepatic and extrahepatic bile ducts, with the process continuing and gradually obliterating the intrahepatic tree. Other investigators suggest that this loss of intrahepatic ducts is the result of repeated episodes of cholangitis following portoenterostomy. The issue of the long-term fate of the intrahepatic ducts in EHBA is an important one, since it bears heavily on the ultimate utility of hepatoportoenterostomy.

Patients with EHBA and polysplenia syndrome have clearly definable congenital anomalies.[4] These are a complex of "bilateral left-sidedness," usually with bilobed lungs on both sides, abdominal heterotaxia and situs ambiguous, and multiple spleens. There is a 50 to 70 percent incidence of gastro-

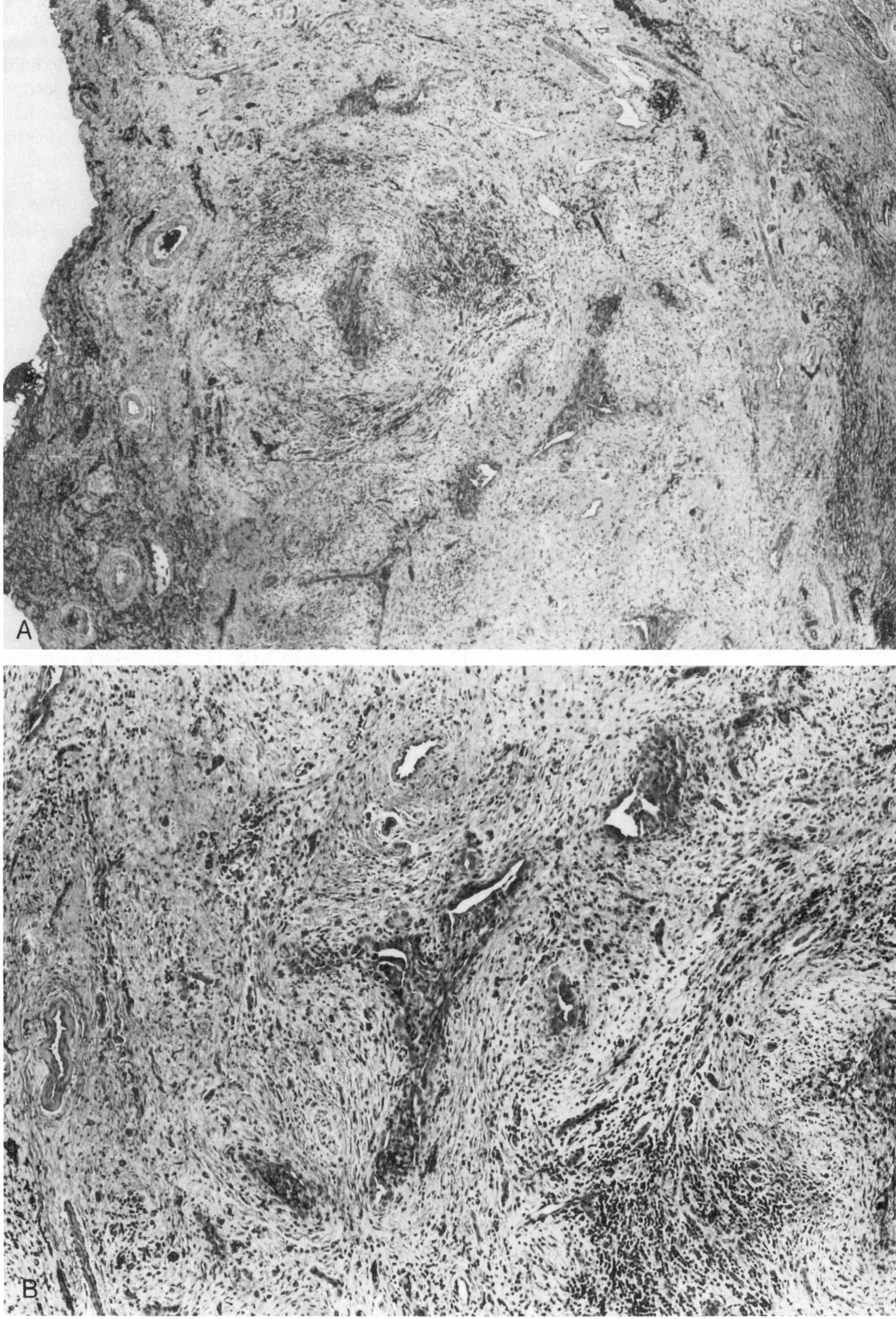

FIGURE 1 Light micrographs of porta hepatis removed from patient with extrahepatic biliary atresia (EHBA) during portoenterostomy. *A*, Illustration of fibrosis, loss of normal large ducts, and inflammation in relation to the small duct remnants. *B*, Illustration of epithelial injury and loss in the duct remnants (original magnifications ×10 and ×20, respectively).

intestinal malformations associated with this syndrome, including biliary atresia, tracheoesophageal fistula, esophageal atresia, duodenal atresia, jejunal atresia, and malrotation of the intestines. A number of congenital anomalies have been reported near the liver, including azygous continuation of the inferior vena cava, a preduodenal portal vein, and hepatic arterial abnormalities.[3,4,6,25] It is presumed that these abnormalities and the associated biliary atresia occur early in the development of the fetus, and thus are different in character and etiology from the majority of cases of EHBA, although we have not seen persistence of the ductal plate in the cases of polysplenia with EHBA that we have examined. The local vascular abnormalities seen in this group of patients have a direct impact on the technical difficulties encountered in liver transplantation, where hepatic arterial, portal venous, and biliary enteric anastomoses must be constructed.

Clinical Course

Findings at Presentation in Early Infancy

It is often difficult to pinpoint the onset of the clinical disease in EHBA. The unconjugated physiologic jaundice of infancy may seem to merge into a conjugated hyperbilirubinemia recognized 2 to 6 weeks later, with dark urine and acholic stools. Although complete disruption of the extrahepatic biliary tree is demonstrated at cholangiography, the serum conjugated bilirubin in most infants will be 7 mg per deciliter or less. Because these babies appear clinically well in early infancy, the importance of this mild jaundice may not be recognized. Jaundice present at two weeks of age may no longer be physiologic and warrants investigation.

There are no historical factors, physical findings, or laboratory studies that adequately identify all cases of biliary atresia. Infants with biliary atresia are usually full-term babies with a normal gestational history, who appear healthy despite the onset of jaundice. This description is in contrast to many cases of neonatal hepatitis. Appetite and weight gain are initially normal. In some cases the acholic stools are noted from birth, but commonly the stools become progressively more pale during the first weeks of life.

Hepatomegaly is present early in infants with biliary atresia. The liver may be quite large, and is usually firm or hard to palpation. In patients with polysplenia syndrome, the midline liver may be appreciated only in the hypogastrium. Splenomegaly is commonly present. Cardiac anomalies are common in the polysplenia syndrome, and this group represents the majority of cardiac murmurs found in EHBA. Although the signs of chronic hepatic failure are rare at the time of diagnosis, they may be seen as early as 3 months of age.

The total serum bilirubin is commonly 6 to 12 mg per deciliter at the time of diagnosis, and 50 to 80 percent is conjugated. In the majority of patients this value remains fairly constant during the first weeks of disease. Any neonate with a conjugated bilirubin greater than 2.0 mg per deciliter or 15 percent of the total bilirubin should have a structural evaluation and close clinical observation.

At the time of the initial evaluation, the serum aminotransferases are usually elevated, although sometimes only to levels twice normal. The alkaline phosphatase is also usually elevated, and the gamma-glutamyl transpeptidase can be markedly elevated early in the course of disease.[26-28] Hepatic synthetic function and the serum albumin are normal early in life. A mild coagulopathy may exist secondary to prolonged fat malabsorption, which should resolve rapidly with the administration of parenteral vitamin K.

Findings Later in Infancy and Childhood

In infants in whom the diagnosis has been delayed, or in children in whom the surgery has failed to provide adequate drainage, there is a marked progression of hepatic disease. The bilirubin progressively increases to as high as 30 mg per deciliter, and the skin has a greenish hue. The liver is enlarged and firm, and splenomegaly invariably ensues. Cirrhosis and hepatic synthetic dysfunction occur, with hypoalbuminemia and ascites. Coagulopathy occurs owing to a decreased synthesis of clotting factors (as well as fat malabsorption) and is exacerbated by hypersplenism and thrombocytopenia. Portal hypertension is uniformly present, and esophageal variceal hemorrhage may be intractable.

In cases of progressive disease, cachexia and fat malabsorption result in a severe failure to thrive, even in those in whom an aggressive nutritional regimen is attempted. A supplementation of fat-soluble vitamins is necessary to prevent rickets and neuropathy. Profound pruritus may occur, which is commonly resistant to medical therapy. In untreated infants the mean expected survival is about 11 months, and in children with a failure of hepatoportoenterostomy the life expectancy (prior to transplantation) is from 6 months to several years; rarely, a child survives into the second decade.[29] Death occurs from chronic hepatic failure, usually complicated by massive gastrointestinal hemorrhage, or overwhelming bacterial infection (pneumonia or peritonitis).

Differential Diagnostic Evaluation

In any infant with a suspected conjugated hyperbilirubinemia, it is important to immediately investigate infectious, metabolic, and structural etiologies for which early therapy will alter the outcome of the disease. The evaluation of neonatal cholestasis is outlined elsewhere in this book, and has been reviewed extensively.[30-33] After consideration of bacterial and viral infectious etiologies, and of critical metabolic disorders such as galactosemia, a structural evaluation should be performed. Rarely, a metabolic disease and biliary atresia may be present together.[34,35]

No single biochemical test has been able to provide a discrimination between biliary atresia and the other causes of conjugated hyperbilirubinemia. Candidate tests, alone or in conjunction with a functional assessment of biliary excretion, have included gamma-glutamyl transpeptidase,[27,36] and lipoprotein-X,[28,37] but each lacks the sensitivity and specificity to be used generally for screening or diagnosis.[26]

An abdominal sonogram will identify choledochal cysts and other causes of extrahepatic obstruction leading to ductal dilatation, such as cholelithiasis. Since there is usually no ductal dilatation in EHBA, either the extrahepatic tree will not be visualized or portions will appear to have a normal caliber. In many cases, a remnant gallbladder will be identified, although at operation this may be filled only with white bile. Some investigators have monitored the contractility of the gallbladder to aid in the evaluation of biliary atresia.[38] Doppler evaluation may show significant portal hypertension or identify vascular malformations, as in the polysplenia syndrome. In infants with polysplenia, ultrasonography frequently is the diagnostic examination, as hepatic anomalies, vascular malformations, and multiple spleens are evident. In the polysplenia syndrome, the position of the liver is difficult to determine, and identification of the right margin of the liver, which may be quite small, should be performed before attempting percutaneous biopsy. Sonographic estimation of ascites is useful, because it is a relative contraindication to percutaneous liver biopsy.

If the sonogram is not diagnostic for a structural lesion, the patency of the extrahepatic biliary system may be demonstrated by a nuclear scintiscan. ^{99}Tc-labeled diisopropyl iminodiacetic acid (DISIDA) scintigraphy has been extremely useful in infants.[39,40] This agent, and other derivatives of iminodiacetic acid, have excellent hepatic uptake and biliary secretion. Evidence of radioactivity in the duodenum proves the patency of the extrahepatic biliary system and eliminates biliary atresia from consideration. Unfortunately, no evidence of excretion may be seen in both biliary atresia and neonatal hepatitis, and further evaluation must be pursued. Other diagnostic studies may provide useful information. The ratio of the hepatic to cardiac pools of DISIDA early in the scan is increased in neonatal hepatitis compared with biliary atresia.[41] Alternatively, assay of the duodenal contents for bile by drainage[42,43] or the string test for evidence of radioactive tracer following a scintiscan[44] may demonstrate patency of the extrahepatic system.

If the sonogram is nondiagnostic and the nuclear scintiscan does not demonstrate patency, a further diagnostic evaluation is necessary.[45] The percutaneous liver biopsy may predict the correct diagnosis in up to 94 percent of cases.[33] The critical pathologic finding is the presence of bile duct proliferation. Although not pathognomonic, this proliferation, especially when combined with a polymorphonuclear exudate and histologic cholestasis in a completely obstructed neonate, is highly suggestive of mechanical obstruction and warrants a laparotomy and cholangiogram. The most likely confusing disorder is alpha$_1$-antitrypsin deficiency, which should be ruled out before laparotomy.

Preoperative and Operative Cholangiography, Surgical Exploration

In selected cases, preoperative cholangiography has been used to evaluate these infants. Both endoscopic retrograde cholangiopancreatography (ERCP)[46,47] and percutaneous gallbladder puncture[48] have been shown to delineate the extrahepatic biliary system. Percutaneous transhepatic cholangiography (PTC) is unlikely to be successful, because the intrahepatic biliary system is not dilated.

Surgical exploration is necessary when continuity of the extrahepatic system cannot be demonstrated by scintiscan, and liver histology is compatible with biliary atresia. In general, the approach is to perform an operative cholangiogram through the gallbladder, which may be small or atretic. Care must be taken to ensure adequate filling of the intrahepatic biliary system. Intrahepatic biliary hypoplasia (nonsyndromic and syndromic bile duct paucity) may be mistaken for biliary atresia.[49] The preoperative percutaneous biopsy is useful for the discrimination of these two disorders, since bile duct paucity is seen in the former disease and bile duct proliferation in the latter one. It is important to recognize, however, that cases of eventual paucity may show proliferation at some time in their course (see Part 26 of this chapter). Others have advocated methylene blue cholangiography under direct visualization, which has been reported to improve the ability to discriminate "biliary hypoplasia" from biliary atresia.[50] If the extrahepatic system cannot be demonstrated via an operative cholangiogram, a careful dissection to the porta hepatis is completed.

Therapeutic Surgical Options

The surgical approach depends on the preference of the surgeon and the extrahepatic anatomy. The majority of cases do not have patent extrahepatic bile ducts, so the Kasai hepatoportoenterostomy or one of its modifications is generally performed. The porta hepatis is dissected and the surface of the liver is cut to expose an area through which bile may drain. In most cases, this is then anastomosed to a Roux-en-Y jejunal limb. Some surgeons have advocated this approach even for "correctable" forms of biliary atresia.[51] Modifications of the initial procedure are numerous, but in general they are designed to decompress the Roux-en-Y and to decrease the risk of ascending cholangitis, by lengthening and/or interrupting the jejunal conduit (see below). More than 20 variants of the classic hepatic portoenterostomy have been devised in order to improve the efficacy of the operation.[52] In the minority of patients with favorable anatomy, some surgeons have advocated performing a hepatoportocholecystostomy to decrease the likelihood of cholangitis. In rare correctable biliary atresia, with patent common hepatic and cystic ducts, a cholecystojejunostomy has been advocated, although long-term results have not been impressive.

The major long-term postoperative problems are a failure to drain bile and ascending cholangitis. To improve the likelihood of bile drainage, choleretics such as phenobarbital and bile acids and bile acid binding resins have been given.[53] To decrease bile duct inflammation and destruction, and to improve bile flow, corticosteroids have been administered postoperatively,[54,55] with varied results.

One-fourth to one-half of patients (depending on age and surgical center) will not have adequate bile drainage following surgery. In these patients in whom the initial operation was unsuccessful, some surgeons have advocated reoperation, which may have up to a 40 percent rate of success at reestablishing bile drainage.[56] The results are more favorable if the initial operation established adequate, although temporary, bile drainage.[57,58] In patients who have had an operative procedure, controversy remains about the increased risk for subsequent transplantation.[59] In patients who previously established drainage but subsequently had a relapse of jaundice, cholangitis is the major cause, although nonbiliary tract disease and scar formation at the porta hepatis are frequent etiologies.[60]

Ascending cholangitis is a frequent and serious complication of a successful operation, occurring in 50 to 100 percent of patients.[61–65] In attempts to decrease this problem, surgical modifications have been tried including: (1) increasing the length of the Roux-en-Y limb to greater than 30 to 40 cm,[66] (2) exteriorizing the Roux limb resulting in drainage into an ostomy, with distal refeeding of bile into the Roux limb,[64] (3) construction of a valved conduit,[67,68] and (4) antibiotic instillation into the conduit. Medical approaches to the problem have included: (1) choleretics to improve flow and drainage, (2) administration of postoperative intravenous antibiotics, and (3) long-term prophylactic oral antibiotics. Although temporary exteriorization of the conduit has been attempted for control of cholangitis, several studies have shown no effect, and there is a marked increase in morbidity, including a required reoperation within months for closure.[69]

Success of Operation

A number of attempts have been made to predict the success of the hepatoportoenterostomy in individual patients. Good results depend in part on the age of the patient at the time of operation. A number of series have shown that results are dramatically better before 56 to 70 days of age.[55,70] The luminal size of the major biliary branches in the resected specimen has been suggested to correlate with outcome.[71]

The outcome may be closely related to bile drainage and resolution of jaundice.[72] When the operative approach includes exteriorization of the bilioenteric conduit, it is possible to monitor the bile flow from the liver. Bile is collected and measured to monitor drainage in these patients. To further these observations, Matsuo et al[73] performed endoscopy through the jejunal limb and visualized the portal anastomosis. The best outcome was correlated with visually evident bile draining from distinct bile duct orifices, the poorest outcome with no visible drainage.

Long-term results have been evaluated in several series.[1,55,74,75] Occasional patients have survived with a high quality of life into the third decade.[76] The most significant predictive factor is resolution of jaundice.[70,77] In patients who remained jaundiced, all died or underwent transplantation by 8 years of age. In contrast, in jaundice-free children the survival was 90 percent at 10 years of age.[55] In different series it is apparent that the long-term survival rates vary greatly according to the age at operation, the skill of the surgical team, and the approach to the management of cholangitis.[61,78]

The resolution of jaundice dose not necessarily follow from the establishment of satisfactory bile flow.[63] One-fourth of patients may have good bile flow despite persistent jaundice. Cholangitis and shortened red cell life span may be factors in this dichotomy.

Cholangitis

The most common complication of a hepatoportoenterostomy is cholangitis, which occurs in 50 to 100 percent of infants. It occurs most commonly during the first 2 years following surgery. The diagnosis is best made in a febrile infant by the demonstration of an organism by liver culture, or by hepatic histology compatible with cholangitis.[79,80] Unfortunately, biopsy is necessary because infants will have a number of nonspecific febrile episodes that may be clinically indistinguishable from cholangitis, and no single laboratory value can accurately predict the disorder. The combination of an increased bilirubin and erythrocyte sedimentation rate is suggestive of cholangitis but may not be present early in the disease. Even a positive blood culture may arise from multiple sources.[81] Thus, when cholangitis is clinically suspected, a liver biopsy should be performed for culture and histologic examination if the patient is clinically stable. The majority of organisms identified are gram-negative rods (including *Pseudomonas*), although some gram-positive cocci, *Haemophilus influenzae* and *Candida*, have been identified.[79,80,82] Since many of these organisms are hospital-acquired, the identification of the antibiotic resistance pattern is crucial for optimal therapy. Many antibiotics have poor penetration into the biliary system, and at the current time an optimal initial combination therapy should include a cephalosporin and an aminoglycoside, pending culture results.[79]

Because cholangitis can cause either temporary or permanent damage, aggressive therapy is fully justified. In refractory cases, long-term intravenous antibiotics may be necessary, and an investigation should be undertaken to determine whether there is either an infected bile lake or an abscess, which may resolve only after definitive drainage.[83,84]

Because of the magnitude of damage from cholangitis, chronic oral antibiotic prophylaxis has been advocated. Despite adequate penetration into the biliary system, prophylactic trimethoprim-sulfamethoxazole therapy has not been demonstrated to have a significant effect on the rate of cholangitis.[85]

In some patients who initially appear to do well, there is a progressive loss of bile ducts evident on biopsy, and jaundice recurs. It is believed that some of the ongoing biliary damage is due to chronic cholangitis, which has not been adequately detected or treated.

Portal Hypertension

Portal hypertension occurs in many cases in the first months of life, and is commonly present at the time of diagnosis. Abnormal intrahepatic vasculature occurs with an evidently reduced number of portal veins in the second month of age, and this may be responsible for causing an early persinusoidal block.[86] Although hepatic fibrosis may occasionally resolve postoperatively,[77] it may progress throughout childhood, even in children with low serum bilirubin levels. The majority of patients develop portal hypertension, with ongoing hepatic inflammation. Splenomegaly, variceal hemorrhage, and return of jaundice may occur. By 5 years of age, 40 to 80 percent of children have varices demonstrable by endoscopy,[65,87] and it is probable that a higher percentage have elevated portal pressures. Portal hypertension may also result in severe varices at the stoma site of Roux-en-Y exteriorization,[68] and in colonic varices.[88] Although portal hypertension may be due to intrahepatic disease in most patients with biliary atresia, portal vein thrombosis has been demonstrated in 20 percent of patients post-Kasai with portal hypertension.[87] This is probably due in part to surgical complications and/or sepsis and cholangitis. Furthermore, the caliber of the portal vein may progressively decrease in patients with a failed operation.[89] This finding has significance for possible portosystemic shunt options but is critical in the pretransplant evaluation, as the portal vein provides most of the blood flow to the graft.

Before liver transplantation was available, patients with severe bleeding required portosystemic shunts. Currently, as with other etiologies of portal hypertension, a shunt should be avoided if liver transplantation is anticipated. Pharmacologic treatment with beta-blocking agents has been suggested in children. Endoscopic sclerotherapy has been successful in the maintenance of these patients.[90,65] Splenic embolization has been used in selected cases.[91]

Biliary atresia is the most common indication for transplantation in the pediatric population.[92,93] The results of transplantation in this group have been excellent, despite the fact that these infants have had one or more major operations in the hepatic fossa, with a rearrangement of the biliary, enteric, and (in shunt patients) vascular structures at the porta hepatis. Furthermore, in patients in whom the initial diagnosis has been significantly delayed and cirrhosis is demonstrated at the time of initial evaluation, some surgeons have advocated liver transplantation as the initial therapy.[94]

Chronic Hepatic Failure

Chronic hepatic failure and synthetic dysfunction may occur in patients following portoenterostomy. Previously, death was inevitable from synthetic dysfunction, bleeding, or infection. Rare cases of acute hepatic infarction late in the course of biliary atresia may be due to vascular compromise.[95] More recently, advances in liver transplantation have markedly altered this course of disease and have significantly improved the long-term outcome. A major restriction on the success of transplantation had been the limited availability of appropriately sized organs, a problem significantly reduced by the technical success of reduced-size organ grafting.[96,97]

CHOLEDOCHAL CYST

Choledochal cysts are one component of a complex involving dilatation of the extrahepatic and intrahepatic bile ducts. A more accurate term is "congenital segmental cystic dilatation of the biliary ductal system."[98]

Choledochal cysts were classified into anatomic types by Alonzo-Lej et al,[99] and those initial groups have been expanded and subdivided.[100,101] The most common type (type I) is a congenital cystic dilatation of the common bile duct without associated intrahepatic ductal dilatation. Type II is a diverticular malformation of the common bile duct, and type III is a choledochocele associated with an ampullary obstruction. The type IV malformation has multiple cysts of the intrahepatic or extrahepatic ducts, or both. Type V has single or multiple intrahepatic cysts. Further subdivisions of these five types have been made by several authors.[101,102]

Pathogenesis/Pathology

The incidence of choledochal cysts varies dramatically among different populations, with a markedly higher incidence in the Far East. The female-to-male ratio is 2–5:1.[103–107] Choledochal cyst is usually an isolated anomaly and is not associated with congenital malformations of other organs. This suggests that it is probably not due to an early gestational event.

The pathogenesis of choledochal cysts continues to be a matter of speculation and debate.[108] Pathogenetic theories must include an explanation of in utero development of at least some cysts.[103,109] Kato and co-workers have suggested that reflux of pancreatic enzymes in the fetus is responsible for destruction of the biliary mucosa,[110] but theories that involve injuries of a local nature do not account for the frequent systemic dilatation of bile duct elements seen in association with choledochal cysts. Regarding the pathogenesis of choledochal cysts, there is clinical evidence suggesting that more than one "type" of choledochal cyst may exist[111]; therefore, no single pathogenesis may be involved in all cases. Todani and colleagues[113] have identified a subset of choledochal cysts with cylindric dilatation of the choledochus, with some differences of anatomy and associated liver findings compared with the majority of cysts. Theories of pathogenesis have included congenital weakness of the wall, primary mucosal abnormality, reflux, and obstruction of the duct system. The association of abnormalities at the junction of the pancreatic and common ducts with choledochal cysts has suggested that pancreatic reflux may be important in the pathogenesis of choledochal cysts.[110] Moreover, there is a high incidence of stenosis (of varying severity) of the choledochus associated with these cysts.[112,113] Further support for the reflux hypothesis comes from Iwai and co-workers, who demonstrated that sphincter function was absent at the anomalous pancreaticobiliary junction.[114]

It is important to recognize, as originally described from Japan, that many, if not all, choledochal cysts are simply one manifestation of a tendency for a "systemic" dilatation of the bile duct system (i.e., there is a high incidence of actual or potential dilatation of intrahepatic bile ducts in cases of choledochal cyst).[110,115] Despite this tendency toward intrahepatic duct dilatation, the lack of heritability, of renal lesions, and of portal tract abnormalities argues against consideration of choledochal cyst as a type of "polycystic disease."

Histologically, most choledochal cysts have a largely fibrous wall with or without a mild mononuclear inflammation. There may be scant fragments of muscle in the fibrous tissue. Often there is no epithelium lining the cysts, but variable lengths of biliary (columnar) or a single cell layer of markedly flattened epithelium may be found. Other pathologic features that may be present in a small number of cases include prominent inflammation, stone formation (8 percent), perforation, or an epithelial malignancy. The most common malignancies are adenocarcinoma (73 to 84 percent), undifferentiated anaplastic carcinoma (7 percent), squamous carcinoma (4 percent), and adenoacanthoma (4 percent).[101,106,116–118] The malignancy associated may involve the extraheptatic ducts, the pancreatic ducts, the gallbladder, or the liver. On occasion, malignancy has developed after a prolonged interval following complete cyst excision,[119-121] but in general, total cyst excision seems to significantly decrease the development of malignancy.

Clinical Presentation

Occasionally, the choledochal cyst is detected in utero by prenatal ultrasonography.[103,122-124] Classically, choledochal cysts present with a triad of pain, abdominal mass, and jaundice.[99] This triad appears in only a minority of patients with choledochal cysts.[104,106,125] In many patients the presenting symptoms may be quite nonspecific. Neonates or infants in the first year may present with chronic or intermittent jaundice. In the neonate, the picture of acholic stools, conjugated hyperbilirubinemia, and hepatomegaly must be differentiated from other causes of obstructive hyperbilirubinemia. In two series of children, the most common symptoms and signs were jaundice (52 to 90 percent), vomiting (53 percent), abdominal pain (42 to 68 percent), acholic stools (36 to 37 percent), and hepatomegaly (36 to 63 percent), with the classic triad seen in only 11 to 17 percent.[104,111]

In older patients there may be abdominal pain, digestive complaints, or mild intermittent jaundice. An abdominal mass is palpable in about 24 percent of patients.[104] Intermittent biliary stasis can result in ascending cholangitis, cholelithiasis, pancreatitis, rupture of the cyst, progressive biliary cirrhosis, portal hypertension, hepatic failure, or malignant transformation of the cyst itself.[118] Some cases have been identified fortuitously in asymptomatic adults.[126]

Diagnosis

The laboratory findings are similar to those seen in patients with chronic biliary obstruction. Elevations of the alkaline phosphatase and gamma-glutamyl transferase levels are seen in 70 percent, and a conjugated hyperbilirubinemia is seen in 56 percent. Elevated serum amylase and lipase or an increased urinary amylase clearance would suggest an associated pancreatitis secondary to ductal obstruction. Pancreatitis occurs in up to 34 percent of adults.[121] Mild transaminase elevations are seen in 70 percent.[104] Secondary biliary cirrhosis, which occurs in up to 26 to 30 percent,[104] may result in significant hepatic synthetic compromise as evidenced by abnormalities of serum albumin or coagulation studies. Secondary biliary cirrhosis develops largely in older patients, but has been seen under 1 year of age.[104]

The most useful diagnostic study is abdominal ultrasonography,[122] which correctly identifies the lesion in 80 to 100 percent of cases.[104,122] Occasionally the diagnosis is made on routine prenatal ultrasonography.[122] An upper gastrointestinal barium examination identifies the lesion in a smaller number of patients.[104]

In selected cases, a technetium-labeled scintiscan (^{99m}Tc-DISIDA) will contribute to the diagnosis. In cases of suspected dilatation of the intrahepatic ducts a PTC will delineate the anatomy. For patients with distal biliary obstruction, or when a choledochocele is suspected, an ERCP is the diagnostic study of choice. This approach permits definition of the anatomy[127] and the relationship of the common to the pancreatic ducts, and in older patients it may be useful to exclude the presence of carcinoma in the dependent portion of the duct preoperatively. In smaller patients, where ERCP is technically difficult, or when the capability for specialized studies is not available, an intravenous contrast CT cholangiogram may serve to delineate the anatomy.[104] The success of this approach may be limited by the requirement for adequate hepatic uptake of the contrast agent and normal renal function.

Treatment

A detailed recommendation of operative procedures based on the classification of the cysts has been published by Todani et al.[101] In all cases surgical resection with removal of the entire cyst is recommended whenever possible, and this approach appears to result in a lower incidence of postoperative jaundice, obstruction, cholangitis, stone formation, reoperation, and subsequent malignancy.[101,104-106,108,122,128-132]

Risk of Malignancy

The incidence of cancer in adults with choledochal cysts is reported as high as 17.5 to 28 percent, with an even greater risk (19 to 50 percent) for those whose initial surgery included an enteric drainage procedure.[106,118,121] In patients with an enteric drainage procedure, the carcinoma also appeared at an earlier age (mean 30 years) compared with those whose primary carcinomas occurred within the choledochal cyst (mean 50 years).[118] This may in part be due to enhanced susceptibility of the cyst wall to mutagens.[133,134] Carcinoma may appear in the first decade of life. Nearly one-half of cancers are intrahepatic, so that the risk is not eliminated by cyst excision alone.[120,121] When malignancy does occur, the prognosis overall is extremely poor; gallbladder tumors have the best prognosis.[135]

Prognosis

A general estimate of the long-term prognosis depends on the initial hepatic damage, the success of the biliary drainage, the development of cholangitis, the presence of intrahepatic cystic dilatations or lithiasis, the amount of residual choledochal cyst, and the development of malignancy. Chronic obstruction predisposes to a high infection rate and may result in a biliary cirrhosis and portal hypertension,[136] which may regress following successful drainage.[137]

OTHER DUCTAL ANOMALIES

A number of biliary tract malformations other than choledochal cysts have been described. Among the more common of these are *accessory bile ducts*, which are extranumerary ducts usually arising in the right lobe of the liver and entering one of the normal extrahepatic ducts or the cystic duct. It is uncertain whether these are the only means of drainage of the hepatic segments from which they originate. Other accessory ducts may provide abnormal communications between various elements of the extrahepatic biliary duct system (e.g., between left and right hepatic ducts). Closely related are the so-called cholecystohepatic ducts (sinuses of Luschka). These are abnormal duct elements that arise in the liver and enter the wall of the gallbladder. It appears that these do not enter the lumen of the gallbladder but may pass through the wall to enter one of the normal extrahepatic duct elements. These accessory ducts are common,[138-140] and are usually of no physiologic importance, although rarely they provide the sole route of egress of bile from the liver. Recognition of biliary tract anomalies and their precise details, either before or at the time of surgery, is of major importance.

Other biliary tract anomalies that have been described include duplication or partial division by a septum of the common duct,[138] heterotopic gastric tissue,[141] agenesis of the common duct,[142] and congenital bronchobiliary fistula (usually between the right main stem bronchus and the bile duct system within the left lobe of the liver).[143-146] Apparent stenosis and localized atresia, as well as duplication of the common duct have been reported in association with duodenal atresia.[147]

The short choledochus syndrome involves abnormal insertion of the bile duct high in the duodenum.[148-150] In some cases, it appears that the common duct is actually an elongated cystic duct.[149] Symptoms are unusual, but duodenal ulcer or gastritis may occur. Malignancy was found in one case.[151]

ISOLATED STRICTURE OF THE EXTRAHEPATIC BILE DUCTS

Stricture of the bile ducts, much less common in children than in adults, may occur as a result of surgical or blunt trauma,[152,153] or as the sequela of inflammation with or without stones. On occasion, bile duct stricture may occur in a child without evident cause, in which case it is said to be "congenital."[154] However, the implication that these idiopathic cases develop in utero is, so far as we know, unsubstantiated. These idiopathic strictures occur most commonly at the bifurcation of the hepatic ducts.[155] Strictures may also occur at the ampulla of Vater. In some cases this is secondary to chronic relapsing pancreatitis.[156] For distal and ampullary strictures, operative sphincteroplasty is the therapeutic procedure of choice, although in some older children endoscopic sphincterotomy may be successful in relieving obstruction. Choledochoenterostomy may be necessary for more proximal strictures that cannot be repaired primarily.

PERFORATION OF THE BILE DUCTS

Spontaneous perforation of the extrahepatic bile duct is a rare condition that occurs within the first few months of life. The most common site of perforation is the point at which the cystic and common hepatic ducts join to form the common duct.[157] Bile may leak into the peritoneal cavity and produce a sterile bile peritonitis, with subsequent pseudocyst formation.

The pathogenesis of spontaneous perforation is unclear. Typically, no anatomic obstruction or narrowing of the duct system can be found. Suggested etiologies include pancreatic reflux,[157] distal common duct obstruction,[158] and a ruptured choledochal cyst.[159] The tendency for the perforation to occur at a particular point along the extrahepatic tree suggests that a unique susceptibility may exist to a variety of processes including a developmental defect,[158] pressure following functional obstruction,[160] vascular or infectious insults, or the result of bile reflux.[157,161-163] At surgery, a large saclike structure is frequently found in the tissue adjacent to the perforation. This structure apparently represents the loculation of bile by an inflammatory and fibrosing response, and should not be confused with a choledochal cyst.

Perforation secondary to pigment gallstones also occurs at the junction of the cystic and common bile ducts.[164] This finding supports the hypothesis that there is an intrinsic weakness of the duct wall at that site. Alternatively, stones located at this site may have developed as a consequence of a previous spontaneous perforation complicated by stasis and infection.

Clinical Manifestation

Infants usually are asymptomatic for the first few weeks of life. There may be progressive abdominal distention, vomiting, jaundice, discolored stools, and occasionally associated failure to gain weight. A mild hyperbilirubinemia occurs in some, but the transaminases are usually normal. In some infants progressive abdominal distention is followed by bile peritonitis. Ultrasonography will show fluid in the peritoneal cavity, but may otherwise be nondiagnostic.[165] Occasionally loculated fluid or a stone is present.[164] A ^{99m}Tc-labeled scintiscan (e.g., DISIDA scan) will demonstrate tracer draining into the peritoneal cavity.[166] Paracentesis in infants with ascites will demonstrate bile-stained fluid.

Therapy

Surgical therapy is required, and several options have been suggested as the treatment of choice. Simple drainage may be successful in some cases; however, the bile duct may remain obstructed in these cases. Primary anastomosis may be possible. If a distal obstruction is identified by operative cholangiography, a cholecystoenterostomy is usually performed. This has been complicated in some cases by cholangitis, which may be decreased by the construction of a Roux-en-Y limb.

REFERENCES

1. Hayes DM, Kimura K, ed. Biliary atresia: the Japanese experience. Cambridge, MA: Harvard University Press, 1980:22.
2. Witzleben CL, Buck BE, Schnaufer L, Brzosko WJ. Studies on the pathogenesis of biliary atresia. Lab Invest 1978; 38:525.

3. Paddock RJ, Arensman RM. Polysplenia syndrome: spectrum of gastrointestinal congenital anomalies. J Pediatr Surg 1982; 17:563–566.
4. Chandra R. Biliary atresia and other structural anomalies in the congenital polysplenia syndrome. J Pediatr 1974; 80:649–655.
5. Peoples WM. Polysplenia: a review of 146 cases. Pediatr Cardiol 1983; 3:35–38.
6. Abramson SJ, Berdon WE, Altman RP, Amodio JB, Levy J. Biliary atresia and non-cardiac polysplenic syndrome: US and surgical considerations. Radiology 1987; 163:377–379.
7. Schweizer P. Long term results and prognosis after hepatic portoenterostomy for the treatment of biliary atresia. In: Waldschmidt J, Charrissis G, Schier F, eds. Cholestasis in neonates. Munich: W Zuckschwerdt, 1988:88.
8. Desmet V. Pathology of cholangiopathies. Conference on Mechanisms and Management of Pediatric Hepatobiliary Disease. Arlington, 1988:61.
9. Balistreri W, Tabor E, Drucker J, Gerety R. Serologic markers of hepatitis A (HAV) and B (HBV) in biliary atresia (BA) and neonatal hepatitis. Pediatr Res 1979; 12:429.
10. Glaser JH, Balistreri WF, Morecki R. The role of reovirus type 3 in persistent infantile cholestasis. J Pediatr 1984; 105:912.
11. Glaser JH, Morecki R. Reovirus type 3 and neonatal cholestasis. Semin Liver Dis 1987; 7:100–107.
12. Brown WR, Sokol RJ, Levin MJ, Silverman A, Tamaru T, Lilly JR, Hall RJ, Cheney M. Lack of correlation between infection with reovirus 3 and extrahepatic biliary atresia or neonatal hepatitis. J Pediatr 1988; 113:670–676.
13. Dussaix E, Hadchouel M, Tardieu M, Alagille D. Biliary atresia and reovirus type 3 infection. N Engl J Med 1984; 311:658.
14. Phillips PA, Keast D, Papadimitriou JM, Walters MN, Stanley M. Chronic obstructive jaundice induced by reovirus type 3 in weanling mice. Pathology 1969; 1:193.
15. Morecki R, Glaser J, Johnson A, Kress Y. Detection of reovirus type 3 in the porta hepatis of an infant with extrahepatic biliary atresia: ultrastructural and immunocytochemical study. Hepatology 1984; 4:1137–1142.
16. Phillips M, Poucell S, Patterson J, Valencia-Mayoral P. The liver. An atlas and text of ultrastructural pathology. New York: Raven Press, 1987.
17. Bangaru B, Morecki R, Glaser J. Comparative studies of biliary atresia in the human newborn and reovirus induced cholangitis in weanling mice. Lab Invest 1980; 456–463.
18. Strickland AD, Shannon K, Coln CD. Biliary atresia in two sets of twins. J Pediatr 1985; 107:418–420.
19. Hyams JS, Glaser JH, Leichtner AM, Morecki R. Discordance for biliary atresia in two sets of monozygotic twins. J Pediatr 1985; 107:420–422.
20. Moore TC, Hyman PE. Extrahepatic biliary atresia in one human leukocyte antigen identical twin. Pediatrics 1985; 76:604–605.
21. Werlin SL. Extrahepatic biliary atresia in one of twins. Acta Pediatr Scand 1981; 70:943.
22. Witzleben CL. Bile duct paucity ("intrahepatic atresia"). Perspect Pediatr Pathol 1982; 7:185–201.
23. Lachaux A, Descos B, Plauchu H, Wright C, Louis D, Raveau J, Hermier M. Familial extrahepatic biliary atresia. J Pediatr Gastroenterol Nutr 1988; 7:280–283.
24. Haas J. Bile duct and liver pathology in biliary atresia. World J Surg 1978; 2:561.
25. Yamagiwa I, Ohta M, Obata K, Washio M. Case report of biliary atresia associated with preduodenal portal vein, ventricular septal defect and bilobed spleen. Z Kinderchir 1988; 43:108–109.
26. Sinatra FR. The role of gamma-glutamyl transpeptidase in the preoperative diagnosis of biliary atresia. J Pediatr Gastroenterol Nutr 1985; 4:167–168.
27. Fung KP, Lau SP. Gamma-glutamyl transpeptidase activity and its serial measurement in differentiation between extrahepatic biliary atresia and neonatal hepatitis. J Pediatr Gastroenterol Nutr 1985; 4:208–213.
28. Tazawa Y, Yamada M, Nakagawa M, Tada K, Konno T, Ohi R, Kasai M. Significance of serum lipoprotein-X and gamma-glutamyltranspeptidase in the diagnosis of biliary atresia. A preliminary study in 27 cholestatic young infants. Eur J Pediatr 1986; 145:54–57.
29. Ohi R, Chiba T, Mochizuki I, et al. Long-term follow-up of patients with biliary atresia. Conference on mechanisms and management of pediatric hepatobiliary disease. Arlington, VA, 1988; 96.
30. Balistreri WF. Neonatal cholestasis. J Pediatr 1985; 106:171–184.
31. Riely CA. Familial intrahepatic cholestatic syndromes. Semin Liver Dis 1987; 7:119–133.
32. Watkins JB, Katz AJ, Grand RJ. Neonatal hepatitis: a diagnostic approach. Adv in Pediatr 1977; 24:399–454.
33. Ferry DG, Selby ML, Udall J, Finegold M, Nichols B. Guide to early diagnosis of biliary obstruction in infancy. Review of 143 cases. Clin Pediatr 1985; 24:305–311.
34. Nord KS, Saad S, Joshi VV, McLoughlin LC. Concurrence of α_1-antitrypsin deficiency and biliary atresia. J Pediatr 1987; 111:416–418.
35. Adam G, Brereton RJ, Agrawal M, Lake BD. Biliary atresia and meconium ileus associated with Niemann-Pick disease. J Pediatr Gastroenterol Nutr 1988; 7:128–131.
36. Manolaki AG, Larcher VF, Mowat AP, Barrett JJ, Portmann B, Howard ER. The pre-laparotomy diagnosis of extrahepatic biliary atresia. Arch Dis Child 1983; 58:591–594.
37. Poley JR, Caplan DB, Magnani HN, Alaupovic P, Smith EI, Campbell DB, Bhatia M, Burdelski M, Bojanovski D. Quantitative changes of serum lipoprotein-X after cholestyramine administration in infants with cholestatic biliary tract and liver disease. Eur J Clin Invest 1978; 8:397–404.
38. Weinberger E, Blumhagen JD, Odell JM. Gallbladder contraction in biliary atresia. AJR 1987; 149:401–402.
39. Dick MC, Mowat AP. Biliary scintigraphy with DISIDA. A simpler way of showing bile duct patency in suspected biliary atresia. Arch Dis Child 1986; 61:191–192.
40. Spivak W, Sarkar S, Winter D, Glassman M, Donlon E, Tucker KJ. Diagnostic utility of hepatobiliary scintigraphy with ^{99m}Tc-DISIDA in neonatal cholestasis. J Pediatr 1987; 110:855–861.
41. el Tumi MA, Clarke MB, Barrett JJ, Mowat AP. Ten minute radiopharmaceutical test in biliary atresia. Arch Dis Child 1987; 62:180–184.
42. Greene HL, Helinek GL, Moran R, O'Neill JA. A diagnostic approach to prolonged obstructive jaundice by 24-hour collection of duodenal fluid. J Pediatr 1979; 95:412–414.
43. Rosenthal P, Liebman WM, Sinatra FR, Perman JA, Thaler MM. String test in evaluation of cholestatic jaundice in infancy. J Pediatr 1985; 107:253–255.
44. Rosenthal P, Miller JH, Sinatra FR. Hepatobiliary scintigraphy and the string test in the evaluation of neonatal cholestasis. J Pediatr Gastroenterol Nutr 1989; 8:292–296.
45. Tolia V, Dubois RS, Kagalwalla A, Fleming S, Dua V. Comparison of radionuclear scintigraphy and liver biopsy in the evaluation of neonatal cholestasis. J Pediatr Gastroenterol Nutr 1986; 5:30–34.
46. Heyman MB, Shapiro HA, Thaler MM. Endoscopic retrograde cholangiography in the diagnosis of biliary malformations in infants. Gastrointest Endosc 1988; 34:449–453.
47. Guelrud M, Jaen D, Torres P, Mujica C, Mendoza S, Rivero E, Romer H, Avila B, Viera L. Endoscopic cholangiopancreatography in the infant: evaluation of a new prototype pediatric duodenoscope. Gastrointest Endosc 1987; 33:4–8.
48. Treem WR, Grant EE, Barth KH, Kremers PW. Ultrasound guided percutaneous cholecystocholangiography for early differentiation of cholestatic liver disease in infants. J Pediatr Gastroenterol Nutr 1988; 7:347–352.
49. Markowitz J, Daum F, Kahn EI, Schneider KM, So HB, Altman RP, Aiges HW, Alperstein G, Silverberg M. Arteriohepatic dysplasia, I. Pitfalls in diagnosis and management. Hepatology 1983; 3:74–76.
50. Schwartz MZ. An alternate method for intraoperative cholangiography in infants with severe obstructive jaundice. J Pediatr Surg 1985; 20:440–442.
51. Lilly JR, Hall RJ, Vasquez-Estevez J, Karrer F, Shikes RH. The surgery of "correctable" biliary atresia. J Pediatr Surg 1987; 22:522–525.
52. Hayes DM, Kimura K, eds. Biliary atresia: the Japanese experience. Cambridge, MA: Harvard University Press, 1980:64.
53. Vajro P, Couturier M, Lemonnier F, Odievre M. Effects of postoperative cholestyramine and phenobarbital administration on bile flow restoration in infants with extrahepatic biliary atresia. J Pediatr Surg 1986; 21:362–365.
54. Karrer FM, Lilly JR. Corticosteroid therapy in biliary atresia. J Pediatr Surg 1985; 20:693–695.
55. Ohi R, Hanamatsu M, Mochizuki I, Chiba T, Kasai M. Progress in the treatment of biliary atresia. World J Surg 1985; 9:285–293.
56. Hata Y, Uchino J, Kasai Y. Revision of porto-enterostomy in congenital biliary atresia. J Pediatr Surg 1985; 20:217–220.

57. Ohi R, Hanamatsu M, Mochizuki I, Ohkohchi N, Kasai M. Reoperation in patients with biliary atresia. J Pediatr Surg 1985; 20:256–259.
58. Freitas L, Gauthier F, Valayer J. Second operation for repair of biliary atresia. J Pediatr Surg 1987; 22:857–860.
59. Millis JM, Brems JJ, Hiatt JR, Klein AS, Ashizawa T, Ramming KP, Quinones-Baldrich WJ, Busuttil RW. Orthotopic liver transplantation for biliary atresia. Evolution of management. Arch Surg 1988; 123:1237–1239.
60. Takemoto H, Inomata Y, Matsukawa Y, Tanaka K, Satomura K, Ozawa K. Icteric flare-up in patients with biliary atresia after hepatic portoenterostomy. Z Kinderchir 1988; 43:92–94.
61. Houwen RH, Zwierstra RP, Severijnen RS, Bouquet J, Madern G, Vos A, Bax NM. Prognosis of extrahepatic biliary atresia. Arch Dis Child 1989; 64:214–218.
62. Canty TG, Self TW, Collins DL, Bonaldi L. Recent experience with a modified Sawaguchi procedure for biliary atresia. J Pediatr Surg 1985; 20:211–216.
63. Chiba T, Mochizuki I, Hanamatsu M, Ohi R, Kasai M. Studies on the changes of serum bilirubin level after surgery in biliary atresia. Tohoku J Exp Med 1985; 146:17–25.
64. Matory YL, Miyano T, Suruga K. Hepaticportoenterostomy as surgical therapy for biliary atresia. Surg Gynecol Obstet 1985; 161:541–545.
65. Ohi R, Mochizuki I, Komatsu K, Kasai M. Portal hypertension after successful hepatic portoenterostomy in biliary atresia. J Pediatr Surg 1986; 21:271–274.
66. Lally KP, Kanegaye J, Matsumura M, Rosenthal P, Sinatra F, Atkinson JB. Perioperative factors affecting the outcome following repair of biliary atresia. Pediatrics 1989; 83:723–726.
67. Reynolds M, Luck SR, Raffensperger JG. The valved conduit prevents ascending cholangitis: a follow-up. J Pediatr Surg 1985; 20:696–702.
68. Andrews HG, Zwiren GT, Caplan DB, Ricketts R. Biliary atresia: an evolving perspective. South Med J 1986; 79:581–584.
69. Burnweit CA, Coln D. Influence of diversion on the development of cholangitis after hepatoportoenterostomy. J Pediatr Surg 1986; 21:1143–1146.
70. Pett S, Pelham A, Tizard J, Barnes N, Mieli-Vergani G, Mowat AP, Williams R, Rolles K, Calne R. Pediatric liver transplantation: Cambridge/King's series, December 1983 to August 1986. Transplant Proc 1987; 19:3256–3260.
71. Chandra RS, Altman RP. Ductal remnants in extrahepatic biliary atresia: a histopathologic study with clinical correlation. J Pediatr 1978; 93:196.
72. Suruga K, Miyano T, Arai T, Ogawa T, Sasaki K, Deguchi E. A study of patients with long-term bile flow after hepatic portoenterostomy for biliary atresia. J Pediatr Surg 1985; 20:252–255.
73. Matsuo S, Yoshiie K, Ikeda K. Endoscopic evaluation of the porta hepatis in patients with biliary atresia. Endoscopy 1985; 17:54–59.
74. Altman RP. Long-term results after the Kasai procedure. In: Daum F, ed. Extrahepatic biliary atresia. New York: Marcel Dekker, 1983:91.
75. Kobayashi A, Itavashi F, Ohbe Y. Long-term prognosis in biliary atresia after hepatic portoenterostomy: analysis of 35 patients who survived beyond 5 years of age. J Pediatr 1984; 10:243–246.
76. Kasai M. Advances in treatment of biliary atresia. Jpn J Surg 1983; 13:265–276.
77. Dessanti A, Ohi R, Hanamatsu M, Mochizuchi I, Chiba T, Kasai M. Short term histological liver changes in extrahepatic biliary atresia with good postoperative bile drainage. Arch Dis Child 1985; 60:739–742.
78. McClement JW, Howard ER, Mowat AP. Results of surgical treatment for extrahepatic biliary atresia in United Kingdom 1980-2. Survey conducted on behalf of the British Paediatric Association Gastroenterology Group and the British Association of Paediatric Surgeons. Br Med J [Clin Res] 1985; 290:345–347.
79. Ecoffey C, Rothman E, Bernard O, Hadchouel M, Valayer J, Alagille D. Bacterial cholangitis after surgery for biliary atresia. J Pediatr 1987; 111:824–829.
80. Piccoli DA, Mohan P, McConnie RM. Cholangitis post-Kasai: diagnostic value of blood cultures and liver biopsy. (Abstract). Pediatr Res 1986; 20:247.
81. Kuhls TL, Jackson MA. Diagnosis and treatment of the febrile child following hepatic portoenterostomy. Pediatr Infect Dis 1985; 4:487.
82. Chen CC, Chang PY, Chen CL. Refractory cholangitis after Kasai's operation caused by candidiasis: a case report. J Pediatr Surg 1986; 21:736–737.
83. Werlin SL, Sty RJ, Starshak RJ, Glicklich M, Nathan R. Intrahepatic biliary tract abnormalities in children with corrected extrahepatic biliary atresia. J Pediatr Gastroenterol Nutr 1985; 4:537–541.
84. Gleghorn EE, Rosenthal P, Vachon L, Diament M. Long-term external catheter biliary drainage for recurrent cholangitis after hepatoportoenterostomy. J Pediatr Gastroenterol Nutr 1986; 5:485–488.
85. Mowat AP. Liver disorders in childhood. London: Butterworth 1987.
86. Ohuchi N, Ohi R, Takahashi T, Kasai M. Postoperative changes of intrahepatic portal veins in biliary atresia—a 3-D reconstruction study. J Pediatr Surg 1986; 21:10–14.
87. Gautier M, Vallayer J, Odievre M, Alagille D. Histological liver evaluation 5 years after surgery for extrahepatic biliary atresia. A study of 20 cases. J Pediatr Surg 1984; 19:263.
88. Berezin S, Yu WY, San Filippo JA, Newman LJ. Colonic variceal bleeding in a child. J Pediatr Surg 1985; 20:88–89.
89. Hernandez-Cano AM, Geis JR, Rumack CH, Stellin GP, Lilly JR. Portal vein dynamics in biliary atresia. J Pediatr Surg 187; 22:519–521.
90. Stellen GP, Lilly JR. Esophageal endosclerosis in children. Surgery 1985; 98:970–975.
91. Kumpe DA, Rumack CM, Pretorius DH, Stoecker TJ, Stellin GP. Partial splenic embolization in children with hypersplenism. Radiology 1985; 155:357–362.
92. Gordon RD, Shaw BW Jr, Iwatsuki S, Esquivel CO, Starzl TE. Indications for liver transplantation in the cyclosporine era. Surg Clin North Am 1986; 66:541–556.
93. Esquivel CO, Iwatsuki S, Gordon RD, March WW Jr, Koneru B, Makowka L, Tzakis AG, Todo S, Starzl TE. Indications for pediatric liver transplantation. J Pediatr 1987; 111:1039–1045.
94. Lilly JR, Hall RJ. Liver transplantation and Kasai operation in the first year of life: therapeutic dilemma in biliary atresia. J Pediatr 1987; 110:561–562.
95. Gartner JC Jr, Jaffe R, Malatack JJ, Zitelli BJ, Urbach AH. Hepatic infarction and acute liver failure in children with extrahepatic biliary atresia and cirrhosis. J Pediatr Surg 1987; 22:360–362.
96. Broelsch CE, Emond JC, Thistlethwaite JR, Rouch DA, Whitington PF, Lichtor JL. Liver transplantation with reduced-size donor organs. Transplantation 1988; 45:519–524.
97. Ong TH, Lynch SV, Pillay SP, Balderson GA, Wall DR, Shepherd R, Cleghorn G, et al. Reduced-size orthotopic liver transplantation in children: an experience with seven cases. Transplant Proc 1989; 21:2443–2444.
98. Glenn F, McSherry CK. Congenital segmental cystic dilatation of the biliary ductal system. Ann Surg 1973; 177:705.
99. Alonzo-Lej F, Revor WB, Pessagno DJ. Congenital choledochal cyst with a report of 2, and an analysis of 94 cases. Surg Gynecol Obstet Internat Abst Surg 1959; 108:1–30.
100. Longmire WP Jr, Mandiola SA, Gordon HE. Congenital cystic disease of the liver and biliary system. Ann Surg 1971; 174:711.
101. Todani T, Watanabe Y, Narusue M, et al. Congenital bile duct cysts. Classification, operative procedures and review of thirty-seven cases including cancer arising from choledochal cyst. Am J Surg 1977; 134:263.
102. Greene FL, Brown JJ, Rubinstein P, Anderson MC. Choledochocele and recurrent pancreatitis. Diagnosis and surgical management. Am J Surg 1985; 149:306–309.
103. Howell C, Templeton J, Weiner S, et al. Antenatal diagnosis and early surgery for choledochal cyst. J Pediatr Surg 1983; 18:387–393.
104. Sherman P, Kolster E, Davies C, Stringer D, Weber J. Choledochal cysts: heterogeneity of clinical presentation. J Pediatr Gastrointest Nutr 1986; 5:867–872.
105. Robertson JF, Raine PA. Choledochal cyst: a 33-year review. Br J Surg 1988; 75:799–801.
106. Yamaguchi M. Congenital choledochal cyst. Analysis of 1,433 patients in the Japanese literature. Am J Surg 1980; 140:653–657.
107. Klotz D, Cohn BD, Kottmeier PK. Choledochal cyst; diagnostic and therapeutic problems. J Pediatr Surg 1973; 8:271.
108. Spitz L. Choledochal cyst. Surg Gynecol Obstet 1978; 147:444–452.
109. Wiedman MA, Tan A, Martinez CJ. Fetal sonography and neonatal scintigraphy of a choledochal cyst. J Nucl Med 1985; 26:893–896.
110. Kato T, Hebiguchi T, Matsuda K, et al. Action of pancreatic juice on the bile duct: pathogenesis of congenital choledochal cyst. J Pediatr Surg 1981; 16:146–151.
111. Barlow B, Tabor E, Blanc WA, Santulli TV, Harris RC. Choledochal cyst: a review of 19 cases. J Pediatr 1976; 89:934–940.
112. Babbitt DP. Congenital choledochal cysts: New etiological concept

based on anomalous relationships of the common bile duct and pancreatic bulb. Ann Radiol 1969; 12:231.
113. Todani T, Watanabe Y, Fujii T, et al. Cylindrical dilatation of the choledochus: A special type of congenital bile duct dilatation. Surgery 1985; 98:964.
114. Iwai N, Tokiwa K, Tsuto T, Yanagihara J, Takahashi T. Biliary manometry in choledochal cyst with abnormal choledochopancreatico ductal junction. J Pediatr Surg 1986; 21:873–876.
115. Todani T, Watanabe Y, Fujii T, et al. Congenital choledochal cyst with intrahepatic involvement. Arch Surg 1984; 119:1038.
116. Flanigan DP. Biliary cysts. Ann Surg 1975; 182:635.
117. Todani T, Tabuchi K, Watanabe Y, et al. Carcinoma arising in the wall of congenital bile duct cysts. Cancer 1979; 44:1134.
118. Todani T, Watanabe Y, Toki A, Urushihara N. Carcinoma related to choledochal cysts with internal drainage operations. Surg Gynecol Obstet 1987; 164:61–64.
119. Takiff H, Stone M, Fonkalsrud E. Choledochal cysts: results of primary surgery and need for re-operation in young patients. Am J Surg 1985; 150:141.
120. Gallagher P, Millis R, Mitchinson M. Congenital dilatation of the intrahepatic ducts with cholangiocarcinoma. J Clin Pathol 1972; 25:804.
121. Adson MA. Choledochal cyst experience: Comment. Ann Surg 1987; 205:539–540.
122. O'Neill JA Jr, Templeton JM Jr, Schnaufer L, Bishop HC, Ziegler MM, Ross AJ III. Recent experience with choledochal cyst. Ann Surg 1987; 205:533–539.
123. Frank JL, Hill MC, Chirathivat S, Sfakianakis GN, Marchildon M. Antenatal observation of a choledochal cyst by sonography. AJR 1981; 137:166.
124. Dewbury KC, Aluwihare AP, Birch SJ, Freeman NV. Prenatal ultrasound demonstration of a choledochal cyst by sonography. Br J Radiol 1980; 53:906.
125. Saing H, Tam PKH, Lee JMH, Pe-Nyum. Surgical management of choledochal cysts: a review of 60 cases. J Pediatr Surg 1985; 20:443–448.
126. Ramage AA, Tedesco FJ, Schuman BM. Asymptomatic choledochal cyst. Am J Gastroenterol 1985; 80:816–818.
127. Cheney M, Rustad DG, Lilly JR. Choledochal cyst. World J Surg 1985; 9:244–249.
128. O'Neill JA, Clatworthy HW. Management of choledochal cysts: a fourteen-year follow up. Am Surg 1971; 37:230–237.
129. Caudle SO, Dimler M. The current management of choledochal cyst. Am Surg 1986; 52:76–80.
130. Tan KC, Howard ER. Choledochal cyst: a 14-year surgical experience with 36 patients. Br J Surg 1988; 75:892–895.
131. Lilly JR. The surgical treatment of choledochal cyst. Surg Gynecol Obstet 1979; 149:36–42.
132. Todani T, Narushe M, Watanabe Y, Tabuchi K, Okajima K. Management of congenital choledochal cyst with intra-hepatic involvement. Ann Surg 1978; 187:272–280.
133. Fortner JG. An appraisal of the pathogenesis of primary carcinoma of the extrahepatic duct. Surg 1958; 43:563.
134. Ohkawa H, Sawaguchi S, Yamazaki Y, et al. Experimental analysis of the ill effect of anomalous pancreaticobiliary ductal unions. J Pediatr Surg 1982; 17:7–13.
135. Kinoshita H, Nagata E, Hirohashi K, et al. Carcinoma of the gallbladder with an anomalous connection between the choledochus and pancreatic duct. Report of 10 cases and review of the literature in Japan. Cancer 1984; 54:762–769.
136. Kim SH. Choledochal cyst: survey by the Surgical Section of the American Academy of Pediatrics. J Pediatr Surg 1981; 16:402–407.
137. Yeong ML, Nicholson GI, Lee SP. Regression of biliary cirrhosis following choledochal cyst drainage. Gastroenterology 1982; 82:332–335.
138. Goor DA, Ebert PA. Anomalies of the biliary tree. Report of a repair of an accessory bile duct and review of the literature. Arch Surg 1972; 104:302–309.
139. Stokes TL, Old L. Cholecystohepatic duct. Am J Surg 1978; 135:703–705.
140. Kihne MJ, Schenken JR, Moor BJ, Karrer W. Persistent cholecystohepatic ducts. Arch Surg 1980; 115:972–974.
141. Kalman PG, Stone RM, Phillips MJ. Heterotopic gastric tissue of the bile duct. Surgery 1981; 89:384–386.
142. Markle GB. Agenesis of the common bile duct. Arch Surg 1981; 116:350–352.
143. Weitzman JJ, Cohen SR, Woods LO, Chadwick DL. Congenital bronchobiliary fistula. J Pediatr 1968; 73:329–334.
144. Sane SM, Sieber WK, Girdany BR. Surgery 1971; 679:599–608.
145. Neuhauser EBD, Elkin M, Landing B. Congenital direct communication between biliary system and respiratory tract. Am J Dis Child 1959; 83:654.
146. Waggett IN, Sane SM, Sieber WK, Girdany BR. Surgery 1971; 69:599–608.
147. Reid IS. Biliary tract abnormalities associated with duodenal atresia. Arch Dis Child 1973; 48:952–957.
148. Lehmann H, Popken H, Schlaak B. The short choledochus syndrome. Case report and retrograde endoscopic visualization of the biliary system. Acta Hepato-Gastro 1978; 25:158–161.
149. Selembier Y. Les choledoques "courtes". La Nouvelle Presse Medicale 1977; 6:2977–2984.
150. Lindner HH, Pena VA, Ruggeri RA. A clinical and anatomical study of anomalous terminations of the common bile duct into the duodenum. Ann Surg 1976; 184:626–632.
151. Guivarc'h, cited in Lindner HH, Pena VA, Ruggeri RA. A clinical and anatomical study of anomalous terminations of the common bile duct into the duodenum. Ann Surg 1976; 184:626–632.
152. Smith R. Strictures of the bile ducts. Prog Surg 1971; 9:157–175.
153. Kendall RS, Chapoy PR, Busuttil RW, Kolodny M, Ament ME. Acquired bile duct stricture in childhood related to blunt trauma. Am J Dis Child 1980; 134:851–854.
154. Chapoy PR, Kendall RS, Fonkalsrud E, Ament ME. Congenital stricture of the common hepatic duct: an unusual case without jaundice. Gastroenterology 1981; 80:380–383.
155. Alagille P, Odievre M. Maladies du foie et des voces biliares chez l'enfant. Flam Med Sci (Fr) 1978; 11:142.
156. Holcomb GW, O'Neill JA, Holcomb GW. Cholecystitis, cholelithiasis and common duct stenosis in children and adults. Ann Surg 1980; 191:626–634.
157. Johnston JH. Spontaneous perforation of the common bile duct in infancy. Br J Surg 1961; 48:532.
158. Lilly J, Weintraub W, Altman P. Spontaneous perforation of the extrahepatic bile ducts and bile peritonitis in infancy. Surgery 1974; 75:664.
159. Chen WJ, Chang C, Hung W. Congenital choledochal cyst: with observations on rupture of the cyst and intrahepatic ductal dilatation. J Pediatr Surg 1973; 10:537.
160. Andersson D, Helin I, Nettelblad SC, Cederlund CG. Spontaneous perforation of the extrahepatic bile ducts in an infant. Pediatrics 1982; 70:601–603.
161. Lloyd DA, Mickel RE. Spontaneous perforation of the extrahepatic ducts in neonates and infants. Br J Surg 1980; 67:621–623.
162. Hyde GA. Spontaneous perforation of bile ducts in early infancy. Pediatrics 1965; 35:453–457.
163. Howard ER, Johnston DJ, Mowat AP. Spontaneous perforation of common bile duct in infants. Arch Dis Child 1976; 51:883.
164. Descos B, Bernard O, Brunelle F, Valayer J, Feldmann D, Hadchouel M, Alagille D. Pigment gallstones of the common bile duct in infancy. Hepatology 1984; 4:678–683.
165. Bahia JO, Boal DK, Karl SR, Gross GW. Ultrasonographic detection of spontaneous perforation of the extrahepatic bile ducts in infancy. Pediatr Radiol 1986; 16:157–159.
166. Fawcett HD, Hayden CK, Swischuk LE, Lobe TE. Spontaneous extrahepatic biliary duct perforation in infancy. J Can Assoc Radiol 1986; 37:206–207.

PART 28

Gallbladder Disease

Eldon A. Shaffer, M.D., FRCPC, F.A.C.P., F.A.C.G.

GALLSTONE DISEASE

Epidemiology

An estimated 20 to 25 million adults in North America are afflicted with gallstones, the most common cause of biliary tract disease in this age group.[1] In Canada, calculous disease of the biliary tract is also a major health hazard, accounting for about 130,000 admissions to hospital and 80,000 cholecystectomies annually.[2] In the United States, the clinical frequency, based on the Framingham study,[3] suggests that 12 million females and 6 million males harbor gallstones. About 800,000 new cases of cholelithiasis develop each year; approximately half of these ultimately undergo surgery, cholecystectomy being the third most common major operation.

Cholelithiasis has been considered less common in infancy and childhood.[4] The first case of gallstones in a child was published by Gibson in 1874. At autopsy he found concretions in the gallbladder and common duct of an 18-year-old boy whose chief symptoms had been abdominal pain, vomiting, and acholic feces. By 1928, 228 cases had been reported.[5] Even into the 1980s, individual cases were still being reported, mostly in small series.[6,7] Gallstones have even been detected in utero[8] and in neonates.[9] The incidence of gallbladder disease in children and adolescents appears to be rising according to hospitalization figures from Sweden.[10] In North America, 4 percent of cholecystectomies are performed on patients below the age of 20.[11,12]

Epidemiology, "the study of disease occurrence in human populations," is crucial to understanding disease causation.[13] Accurate information on the frequency of gallstone disease in adults and particularly children is fragmentary. Estimates of occurrence and information about associated factors in adults have come primarily from clinical and autopsy studies, which contain both selection and detection bias.[14] The fact that gallstone disease is frequently asymptomatic[15] tends to underestimate the true frequency and obscure real associations.

Incidence refers to the rate of development of new cases over a given period. The incidence of biliary tract disease is generally considered to be rising both in the Western world and in Japan,[16] but other studies have suggested that there may be no real increase over the last 30 years[17] or perhaps even a decrease.[18] Large increases in biliary operations have occurred over the last 30 years on both sides of the Atlantic, but the number of cholecystectomies is still six times higher in North America than in western Europe.[16] Such large differences in the rates at which surgery is performed may reflect either a heightened tendency to disease, improved diagnostic expertise, or better health care delivery. Conversely, this could imply that therapeutic usefulness has been exceeded and eventually may lead to excess mortality. Thus, the true frequency of cholelithiasis cannot be gleaned from surgical rates, which reflect the indications for treatment and not necessarily the prevalence of biliary disease.[16,19]

Prevalence describes the number of people who have gallstones at a certain point in time and is best determined by performing a random diagnostic survey (ultrasonography being more accurate and safer than oral cholecystography) of an unselected population. This allows inclusion of both symptomatic and asymptomatic cases. The true prevalence has been examined in adult Caucasians (Fig. 1) and Pima Indians (Fig. 2). These surveys reveal that women have gallstones more frequently than men and that the frequency of gallstones increases with age in both sexes. In North American Indians[20–22] and Chileans,[23] prevalence in females increases from 10 percent in teenagers to 70 percent by the forties. In males, the corresponding figures are lower at 1 to 2 percent and 25 percent, respectively. By 60 years of age, 70 percent of male Pima Indians have gallstones. Gallstone disease may not be common in young white children, but its prevalence increases markedly with puberty, particularly in girls (Fig. 3). This is the time at which cholesterol saturation of bile rises, preceding the development of gallstones (see Fig. 2). Gallbladder surgery is most commonly performed in middle age, although stone formation likely occurred years earlier.

International differences, at least from autopsy studies, abound (Table 1). The frequency rates vary from epidemic proportions in American Indians to virtual nonexistence in the Masai tribe of sub-Sahara Africa. Marked differences exist even within the boundaries of one country, such as India, perhaps related to socioeconomic and dietary factors. Only limited information is available on the type of stone found. Cholesterol gallstones predominate in modern Western civilization and are increasing in Japan as they acquire life-styles associated with Western cultures, whereas pigment stones are more common in other Asian populations.

In children, cholelithiasis is clearly linked to chronic hemolytic states.[4] The prevalence of gallstones in sickle cell disease is 17 to 29 percent in children and increases with age.[25,26] Parity, obesity, and a positive family history are all risk factors for cholesterol gallstones in adolescence.[6,7,10] The frequency of cholecystitis/cholelithiasis is the same in both sexes until puberty but rises throughout childhood, particularly in adolescent girls[10] (Fig. 3). The prevalence remains higher in women than in men during the fertility period and after the menopause.[21,27,28] The association between gallstone disease and the fertility period, pregnancy, and exogenous female sex hormones has long been suspected, but most

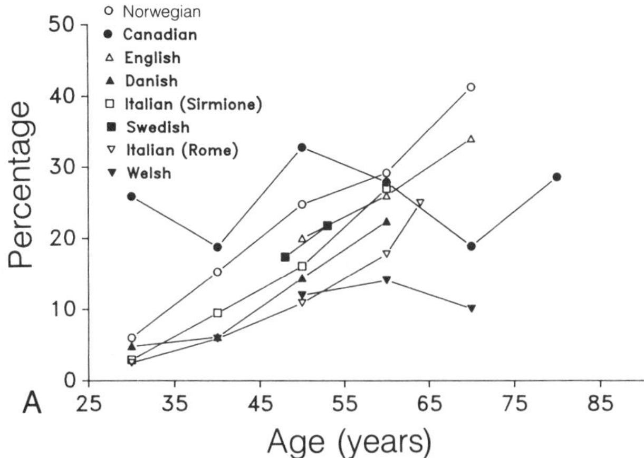

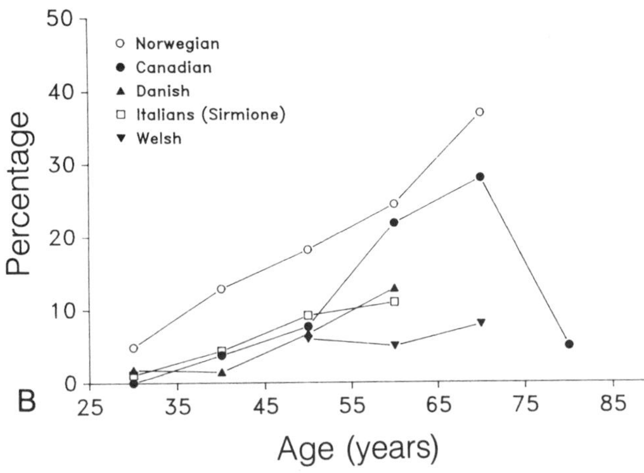

FIGURE 1 Prevalence of gallstones in European and Canadian adults of white origin. Both women (*A*) and men (*B*) demonstrate an age-specific increase in frequency of gallstones as demonstrated by surveys using ultrasonography or oral cholecystography. Gallstones were more prevalent in females and increased with age in both sexes.

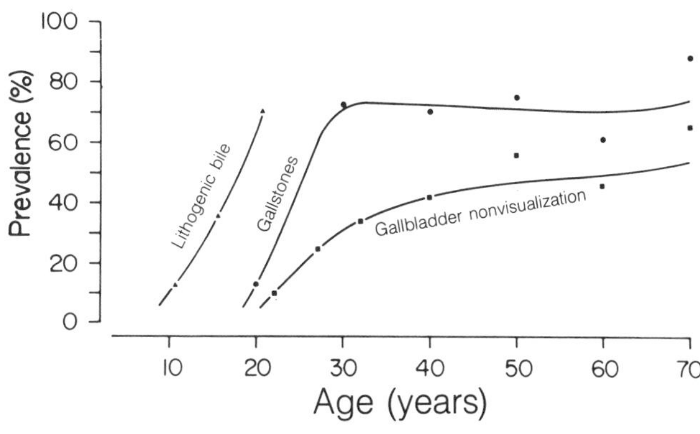

FIGURE 2 Natural history of gallstone disease in female Pima Indians. The first event, the development of lithogenic bile containing excess cholesterol, occurred during the teens. The prevalence of gallstones rose rapidly from age 20 to 30 years, followed several years later by nonvisualization on oral cholecystography. (From Bennion et al.[20])

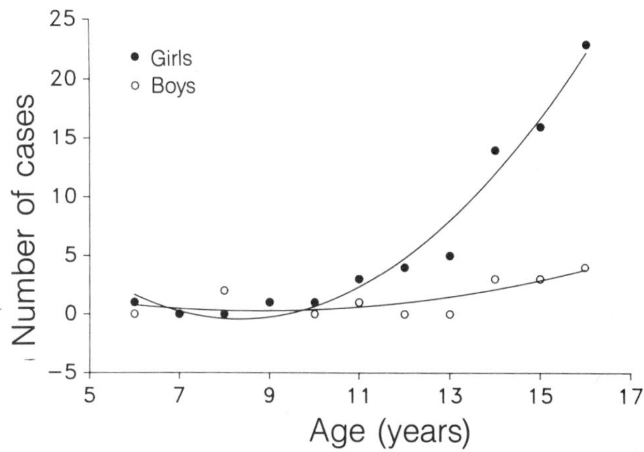

FIGURE 3 Incidence of gallbladder disease according to age and sex of 89 hospitalized Swedish patients under 16 years of age.[10] For boys there was a slow increase with age. Girls had a similar slow increase until 10 to 11 years, after which the rise became exponential.

TABLE 1
Frequency of Gallstone Disease in Different Countries (Autopsy Studies)

Very Common (30–70%)	Common (10–30%)	Intermediate (< 10%)	Rare (~0%)
American Indians	United States (whites)	United States (blacks)	East Africa
United States	Canada (whites)	China	Canada (Eskimos)
Canada	Russia	Japan	Indonesia
South America	United Kingdom	Thailand	West Africa
Sweden	Australia	Northern India	Southern India
Chile	Norway	Greece	
Czechoslovakia	Western Europe	Southeast Asia	
	South Africa (whites)	Portugal	

Modified from Shaffer and Small.[16]

studies have encompassed clinical gallstones only, which may be biased by diagnostic suspicion.[14] In point-prevalence studies, gallstone disease was associated with young age at menarche, abortions, and multiple childbirths.[29] The younger age at menarche suggests that gallstone disease is associated with the length of the fertility period. One compounding factor may be the close relationship between obesity and early menarche.[30] Pregnancy is also a risk factor in young women.[31] The importance of oral contraceptives has been controversial.[29] The association may be changing with the introduction of low-dose estrogen and progestin.

The generally accepted risk factors for development of cholelithiasis[32,33] are best classified according to gallstone type: pigment versus cholesterol (Table 2). These putative risk factors have been largely derived from studies in adults. Some also apply to childhood and adolescence.

Natural History of Gallstone Disease

Gallstone disease is a frequent problem in Western countries, with between one-fifth of men and one-third of women eventually developing cholelithiasis. Fortunately, the attendant mortality is low, with only 6,000 deaths annually in the United States. From an economic perspective, the approximately 500,000 cholecystectomies performed each year represent 2.5 percent of all health-care costs in the United States.[34] This financial burden is likely to increase as ultrasonographic examinations of the abdomen, done for other indications such as nonspecific dyspepsia, identify gallstones more frequently. The result will be an increased number of clinically "silent" gallstones. In the pediatric age group, questions of management become more perplexing with the advent of new therapies (such as medical dissolution and

TABLE 2
Risk Factors for Gallstones

	Adult		Child	
Factor	Pigment Stone	Cholesterol Stone	Pigment Stone	Cholesterol Stone
Demography				
Race	Asian	American Indian Northern European White	— —	American Indian
Female sex	?	++	—	++
Age	+	++	—	Adolescence
Familial	?	++	Hemoglobinopathies	+
Diet	+	Obesity (high calorie) Low fiber High animal fats Polyunsaturated fats Weight reduction	—	Obesity — — —
Gallbladder stasis	+ Total parenteral nutrition	++ Reduced meal frequency Vagotomy Pregnancy	— Total parenteral nutrition	— Reduced meal frequency
Female sex hormones				
Parity	—	+	—	++
Fertility period	—	Early menarche	—	Early menarche
Oral contraceptives	—	+	—	+
Estrogens		+		
Associated diseases				
Definite	Hemolytic anemia Biliary infections Chronic hemolysis Alcoholic cirrhosis Biliary parasites Strictures, foreign bodies in biliary tree Sclerosing cholangitis Erythropoietic protoporphyria	Ileal disease or loss Cystic fibrosis Primary biliary cirrhosis Diabetes mellitus	Hemolytic anemia Sickle-cell thalassemia	Cystic fibrosis Ileal disease Congenital defects in bile salt synthesis
Probable	Hyperparathyroidism Somatostatinoma Pheochromocytoma	Hypertriglyceridemia		
Drugs	Clofibrate			

++ = definite; + = probable; ? = questionable; — = unknown.

lithotripsy), which provide alternatives to cholecystectomy. Hence, there is an ever-increasing need to determine the natural history of gallstone disease.

The *silent gallstone* by definition does not cause biliary pain or biliary tract disease such as acute cholecystitis or cholangitis. Rather, it is detected incidentally during investigation of another problem, such as ultrasonography for nonspecific dyspeptic symptoms.

Most studies on the natural history of cholelithiasis have contained inaccuracies: failing to differentiate symptomatic from asymptomatic patients, loosely defining biliary tract symptoms and complications, and providing variable follow-up (Table 3). For years, clinicians assumed that about 50 percent (51 of Comfort's[36] 112 cases in Table 3) would develop symptoms or complications over 10 to 20 years—hence the belief that all gallstones require cholecystectomy. Actually 30 had "indigestion" (a nonspecific symptom), whereas 21 (19 percent) experienced "colic" and 5 (4 percent) became jaundiced (true biliary symptoms). Subsequent studies have confirmed that about 23 percent of individuals with silent gallstone disease develop biliary pain or a biliary complication.[37] A unique study by Gracie and Ransohoff[38] examined the fate of gallstones that had been discovered incidentally 24 years earlier on a pre-employment oral cholecystogram (Table 3). Of 123 persons, biliary pain developed in 16, and three of these experienced a biliary tract complication: two had acute cholecystitis and one pancreatitis. None died. When complications arose, they were more likely to occur after a prior episode of biliary colic. Similarly, biliary tract pain was more likely to recur if there had been a previous attack within 12 months. The higher probability of biliary pain in the National Cooperative Gallstone Study[39] likely reflects frequency of follow-up: an office visit with a specific questionnaire every 3 to 4 months. Certainly the risk of a major complication requiring nonelective cholecystectomy was low in both studies, 2.5 to 4 percent. Further support comes from ultrasound surveys. When gallstones are detected, most people (70 to 80 percent) have no biliary symptoms.[27,40–43] No comparable studies are available in children.

Such a large number of asymptomatic gallstones creates an enormous potential for inappropriate intervention. Cholecystectomy rates in North America have been three to four times higher than those in England and Wales,[44] despite evidence that gallstone prevalence is similar in both countries (see Fig. 2). The difference in operating rates has been ascribed to supply factors such as greater surgical manpower in North America rather than patient demand for intervention. Thus the indications for cholecystectomy may be rather arbitrary and often unnecessary. Because of the benign nature of symptomatic gallstones, expectant management is advisable.[45]

Symptomatic gallstones imply biliary pain without complications (acute cholecystitis or cholangitis). Persons who already have had biliary pain have a more ominous prognosis (Table 3). In the National Cooperative Gallstone Study, the placebo group contained a subgroup of 112 patients who had experienced biliary pain within the last 12 months.[39] Sixty-nine percent developed biliary pain within the next 2 years, and 6 percent required cholecystectomy. The lifetime risk for a biliary complication beyond 2 years presumably is higher; perhaps half of those with further biliary pain develop a major complication.

TABLE 3
Reports on the Natural History of Gallstone Disease*

Study	Number of Patients	Years of Follow-up	Biliary Tract Pain (%)	Yearly Incidence (% per Year)	Major Complications (%)	Comment	Type of Study
Silent gallstones							
Comfort et al (Ann Surg 1948; 128:931–937)	112	10–20	19	~1	?4	Gallstones found incidentally at surgery	Retrospective
Lund (Ann Surg 1960; 151:153–162)	34	5–20	33	Symptoms developed within 5 years	20	Hospital survey	Retrospective
Wenckert and Robertson (Gastroenterology 1966; 50:376–381)	781	11	35	3.2	18	Survey based on finding an abnormal cholecystogram	Retrospective
Newman et al (Am J Gastroenterol 1968; 50:476–496)	191	2–22 (5)	?	2.2	?	Clinical survey of "patients without pain"	Retrospective
Gracie and Ransohoff (N Engl J Med 1982; 307:798–800)	123	11–24	13	2%—0–4 years 1%—5–9 years 0.5%—9–14 years 0%—thereafter	2.5	Male university faculty; truly "silent" cholecystographic screen of healthy population	Retrospective
Symptomatic (painful) gallstones							
Thistle et al (Ann Intern Med 1984 101:171–175)	193	2	31	22	4	No biliary pain within last 12 months	Prospective (National Cooperative Gallstone Study)
	112	2	69			Biliary pain within last 12 months	

*Adapted from Shaffer.[35]

Classification of Gallbladder and Bile Duct Stones

In any individual, sets of stones possess a unique composition and virtually an identical appearance on cross section, indicating a similar history of growth. Stones can be divided into two major categories (Table 4)[46]:

1. *Cholesterol stones* contain more than 50 percent cholesterol with a variable amount of proteins (including glycoproteins) and calcium salts (such as calcium bilirubinate, calcium hydroxyapatite, and calcium carbonate). Few stones are pure cholesterol; most contain rings of protein and calcium salts.
2. *Pigment stones* are complex mixtures of several insoluble calcium salts that are not normal constituents of bile.
   a. *Black*: primarily a covalently linked, linear polymer of bilirubin or other pyrroles. The large amount of calcium salts, as phosphates and carbonates, accounts for 50 percent of these stones being radiopaque on plain radiographic films. Less than 10 percent cholesterol is present in most. These small stones are very hard and lustrous black like coal and do not possess rings.
   b. *Brown*: predominantly amorphous calcium bilirubinate and calcium salts of fatty acids. Cholesterol content may be somewhat higher at 10 to 30 percent. The relatively high cholesterol and fatty acid soap content produces a soft, soap-like consistency.

PIGMENT GALLSTONES

Epidemiology

Black Pigment Stones

Black pigment stones account for up to 25 percent of gallstones found at cholecystectomy in the United States.[3,47] There is no female predominance. In North America, blacks and whites have an equal incidence. Elsewhere, black pigment stones account for 20 percent of gallbladder stones in India, 9 percent in Japan (and rising), but virtually none in South America.

The risk is increased in patients with hemolysis or alcoholic cirrhosis and in the older age group. Age appears to be a major factor, particularly in chronic hemolysis. Black pigment stones with sickle hemoglobinopathy occur in 14 percent of children below 10 years, increases to 36 percent in 10- to 20-years-olds, and reaches 50 percent by age 22 and 60 to 85 percent by 33 years.[25,26,48]

Long-term intravenous parenteral nutrition predisposes to black pigment gallstone disease in infants. In adult patients on total parenteral nutrition, biliary sludge appears in the gallbladder by 4 to 6 weeks, and then gallstones develop within months if treatment is continued.[49,50] Biliary sludge is a sediment of cholesterol crystals plus bilirubin granules embedded in a matrix of mucous gel. This precipitate differs from

TABLE 4
Classification of Cholesterol and Pigment Gallstones

Characteristics	Cholesterol Stones	Black Pigment Stones	Brown Pigment Stones
Color	Pale yellow-white ± surface brownish	Black, "tarry" (can be dark brown)	Brown to orange
Consistency	Hard Crystalline ± laminated Central dark nucleus	Hard, shiny Crystalline	Soft-"earthy", greasy 50% amorphous Rest crystalline, inorganic salts Laminated
Number, size, and shape	Multiple: 2–25 mm faceted, smooth Solitary: 2–4 cm (~10%) round, smooth	Multiple: < 5 mm irregular or smooth	Multiple: 10–30 mm Round, smooth Molded when in ducts
Composition	Cholesterol monohydrate > 50% Other: Glycoprotein Calcium salts	Pigment polymer~40% Calcium salts (phosphates, carbonates) ~15%* Cholesterol (2%) Unmeasured (30%)*	Calcium bilirubinate~60% Calcium fatty acid soaps (palmitate and stearate) ~15%* Cholesterol (15%) Unmeasured (10%)*
Radiodensity	Lucent	50% opaque (alpha $CaCO_3$ content)	Lucent
CT scan (Hounsfield units)	<20–60	>140	60–140
Location in biliary system	Gallbladder ± common duct	Gallbladder Intrahepatic ducts	Common duct
Clinical associations	Metabolic No infection No inflammation	Hemolysis Cirrhosis Total parenteral nutriton (TPN)	Infection Infestation Inflammation

*Can be much higher to 66%.
Adapted in part from Trotman and Soloway.[46]

classic black pigment stones because of the high cholesterol content yet lacks the fatty acid content and clinical setting to be classified as a forerunner of brown pigment stones.

Black pigment stones are not associated with bacterial infections of the biliary tract and tend to form primarily in the gallbladder.

Brown Pigment Stones

These stones represent a major health problem in the Orient, particularly in rural areas. Most are associated with biliary infection or infestation (*Ascaris lumbricoides*, *Clonorchis sinensis*, or *Opisthorchis viverrini*) and lead to chronic cholangitis and eventually cholangiocarcinoma.

In the West, brown pigment stones are extremely rare but have been linked to retained suture material following cholecystectomy, biliary stricture, and sclerosing cholangitis—that is, a foreign body or chronic biliary obstruction. Brown pigment stones represent the majority of "recurrent" gallstones, stones that reform more than 18 to 20 months after cholecystectomy.

Brown pigment stones account for more than 20 percent of gallbladder stones found in parts of China, perhaps associated with the traditional rice and vegetable–based diet. They are uncommon in Mongolia, where a meat-based diet is consumed. In Japan, brown pigment stones have decreased from 90 percent in 1935 to 20 percent in 1978, concomitant with an increase in cholesterol stones and the adoption of a Western diet.[51,52] Like black pigment stones, they are a disease of advanced age, although Orientals may first present in their thirties.

The location of brown stones within the biliary system is also unusual. They develop in the intra- and extrahepatic bile ducts, often in the absence of gallbladder stones. There is a slight difference in composition, depending upon the site of formation. Intrahepatic brown pigment stones contain more cholesterol and less bilirubin than extrahepatic stones.[53]

Pathogenesis

Black Pigment Stones

Black pigment stones occur because of a superabundance of unconjugated bilirubin in bile: from increased bilirubin secretion secondary to hemolysis, incomplete conjugation of bilirubin, or deconjugation (either nonenzymatically or from bacterial or other enzymes) during transit through the biliary tree.[54] Monoconjugated bilirubin may also contribute to the pigment as a co-precipitant[55] and as a source of unconjugated bilirubin, being transformed by spontaneous (nonenzymatic) hydrolysis. When the solubility of bile is exceeded, the excess unconjugated bilirubin precipitates as calcium bilirubinate. Calcium bilirubinate then polymerizes, binds to mucin produced by the gallbladder mucosa, and is retained. The black color results from the structure of this highly cross-linked polymer. The varied oxidative states of the repeat units produce various colors that collectively absorb light throughout the physical spectrum.

Formation of black pigment stones in the gallbladder therefore requires bile supersaturated with unconjugated bilirubin and available free calcium. Increased bilirubin is produced and excreted in hemolytic states, but excessive bilirubin in bile is not solely responsible. Chronic hemolysis exists in all sickle hemoglobinopathy patients, yet only 50 percent develop gallstones by age 20. The rate of hemolysis may change, but the concentrations of unconjugated bilirubin in bile, although increased, are similar in sickle hemoglobinopathy subjects with and without gallstones. Additional pathogenetic factors must be necessary: calcium salts and mucin acting as a nidus to initiate stone growth[56] or the sickling process leading to stasis by damaging the gallbladder wall and impairing emptying.[57] In cirrhosis, the reduction in bile salt secretion may affect pigment solubility and calcium binding. Excess unconjugated (or free) bilirubin could also result from increased enzymatic hydrolysis of the conjugated bilirubin excreted in bile.[58] Enhanced beta-glucuronidase activity may originate from bacteria present in infected bile, enzymes released from damaged epithelial cells in the biliary system, from white blood cells, or from decreased inhibition of this enzyme (e.g., decreased D-glucaric acid in bile from a protein-deficient diet). Increased pH from defective acidification of bile by the gallbladder also may affect calcium and bilirubin solubility[59]; an alkaline bile increases the available free calcium.

These stones become radiopaque when significant quantities of calcium carbonates and phosphates are present. About 15 to 20 percent of all gallstones in the Western world are radiopaque. Two-thirds are pigment stones and the remainder cholesterol stones. Conversely, 80 percent of radiolucent gallstones are cholesterol and the rest calcium bilirubinate. Rarely, pure calcium carbonate or calcium phosphate stones occur.

Calcium bilirubinate is present as microcrystals in black stones but is amorphous (without structure) in brown stones. Mucin provides a variable meshwork for the precipitation of solids in bile. This may be particularly important for black pigment stones, but mucin forms only a minimal network in brown pigment stones.

Brown Pigment Stones

Brown pigment stones follow tissue or bacterial enzyme breakdown of bilirubin glucuronide to form amorphous calcium bilirubinate. They are almost uniformly associated with infection, primarily *Escherichia coli* and other bacteria. This produces beta-glucuronidase, which deconjugates bilirubin glucuronide and phospholipase A_1, which splits off fatty acids from lecithin. Ductal precipitation of calcium bilirubinate, the calcium slats of fatty acid (as calcium palmitate and stearate), and some cholesterol produces soft, greasy stones that are shaped by the duct system. Bacteria and their glycocalyx may contribute to the precipitation and adhesion of bilirubin pigment.[60]

Treatment

Understanding the pathogenesis of pigment stone formation leads to rational therapy. The treatment of choice for black pigment stones is cholecystectomy, since these stones do not recur even though hemolysis progresses, as in sickle cell disease. When black pigment stones develop in association with cirrhosis, the severity of the liver disease may preclude a safe cholecystectomy.

Brown pigment stones differ. Their problem represents stasis and continued infection and infestation. In the West, treatment is endoscopic retrograde cholangiopancreatography (ERCP) with sphincterotomy, fracture by lithotripsy (when necessary), and basket retrieval. Radiologic and choledochoscopic (peroral or percutaneous) techniques also can retrieve stones, avoiding surgery. Stones may recur and require a choledochojejunostomy or even a hepatojejunostomy with a subcutaneous access limb for repeated percutaneous instrumentation to remove recurring stones. For hepatolithiasis, management should be directed at an early attempt to provide adequate biliary drainage and aggressive removal of recurrent stones. If the disease is segmental, regional hepatic resection may be curative.

There is no effective oral medication for either black or brown pigment stones. Shock wave lithotripsy can fracture rings of calcium salts in cholesterol stones, allowing dissolution of the more central cholesterol layers by oral bile acids. Lithotripsy can also safely fragment brown pigment stones in the common duct when removal by ERCP techniques is not possible. In the future, contact solvents, such as a combination of mono-octanoin with a calcium-binding agent such as ethylene glycol tetra-acetic acid, may prove effective.

CHOLESTEROL GALLSTONES

Pathogenesis

Cholesterol gallstone formation is the end stage of a long process.[16]

Chemical Stage

Bile becomes supersaturated with cholesterol. The liver (not the gallbladder) is the source of abnormal or supersaturated bile containing excess cholesterol, more than can be solubilized by bile salts and lecithin. Supersaturated bile may develop as early as puberty and is often associated with obesity; 8 to 12 years later the stone appears (see Fig. 2). The liver produces supersaturated bile by either a decreased secretion of bile salts, increased secretion of cholesterol, or both (Table 5). In obese patients, the basic defect is excessive cholesterol secretion. In the average patient with gallstones, there is also a reduced bile salt pool and decreased bile salt secretion.[16] Under these circumstances, bile salt synthesis is inappropriate; the liver should sense that a decreased pool is cycling through the enterohepatic circulation and increase bile salt synthesis, which would then restore the pool size and secretion rate to normal.

Physical Stage

Cholesterol precipitates as microcrystals. Cholesterol, a sterol insoluble in water, is solubilized in aqueous bile by bile salts (acting as biologic detergents) and lecithin as *mixed micelles*. Lecithin enlarges micelles, providing greater solubilizing capacity than simple micelles of bile salts.[61] Biliary cholesterol is also carried as small *unilamellar vesicles* of lecithin and cholesterol.[62] The limits of cholesterol solubility have been expressed as a triangular phase diagram (Fig. 4). The micellar solubilizing capacity of bile is quite limited.[63] Excess cholesterol may be held only temporarily in supersaturated micelles. Cholesterol also is transported as phospholipid vesicles. These *multilamellar vesicles*, several micrometers in size, are thermodynamically more stable than smaller unilamellar vesicles, which are metastable. In fact, vesicles solubilize cholesterol much more efficiently than mixed micelles and carry a major portion of the cholesterol in bile.[62,64] This occurs because many molecules of bile salts and lecithin are necessary to transport cholesterol, whereas the cholesterol-to-lecithin ratio in vesicles is about 1:1. The proportion of cholesterol carried in vesicles versus micelles depends upon (1) the bile salt concentration—at low concentrations most cholesterol is in vesicles, and (2) the cholesterol-to-phospholipid ratio—when the ratio is sufficiently high, the carrying capacity is exceeded. In dilute hepatic bile, cholesterol is transported in vesicles primarily with phospholipids, not bile salts. Conversely, in concentrated gallbladder bile, cholesterol is carried mainly in mixed micelles of bile salts and phospholipids. Hence, those gallbladder biles that contain a higher proportion of cholesterol in vesicles and a high

TABLE 5
Pathophysiologic Basis for Formation of Bile Saturated with Cholesterol

Secretory Defect	Mechanism	Examples
Decreased bile salt secretion	Reduced bile salt pool	
Excessive bile salt loss	Malabsorption decreases bile salt pool; synthesis cannot fully compensate	Ileal resection, disease (e.g., Crohn's disease) or bypass; cystic fibrosis with steatorrhea; congenital transport defect
Defective bile salt synthesis	a. Depressed synthesis b. Oversensitive bile salt synthesis (depressed relative to small bile salt pool)	Congenital defects of bile salt synthesis; primary biliary cirrhosis; type IIb hyperlipoproteinemia
Increased cholesterol secretion	Excessive cholesterol synthesis, tissue mobilization, or increased dietary intake	Obesity, drugs (sex hormones, clofibrate); type IV hypolipoproteinemia, American Indians
Both		Most gallstone patients

cholesterol-to-lecithin ratio are more likely to precipitate cholesterol. These two forms (micelles versus vesicles) and the proportion of cholesterol to lecithin may explain the uncoupling among the three biliary lipids at low bile salt secretion rates, as discussed elsewhere.

The second stage of cholesterol gallstone formation therefore consists of a change in the gallbladder bile from a liquid supersaturated with cholesterol to a two-phase system of aqueous bile plus solid crystals of cholesterol. Nucleation involves the aggregation of molecules into a critical cluster in which the aggregation rate exceeds the dissolution rate. Two processes are possible: *homogeneous nucleation*, in which crystallization occurs without foreign material, and *heterogeneous nucleation*, in which crystallization takes place on a foreign surface (e.g., desquamated epithelial cell, protein, calcium salts, precipitated bile acids, or a foreign body).[33] If the abnormal bile is labile with a great excess of cholesterol in a clear solution (i.e., above the metastable zone, say at point X in Figure 4), cholesterol precipitates spontaneously. Such homogeneous nucleation requires cholesterol monomers to automatically coalesce into a cluster of sufficient size to permit continuous crystal growth without the influence of other solids. The degree of cholesterol supersaturation present in the bile of experimental animals or in humans is not sufficient thermodynamically to promote homogeneous nucleation without the influence of other solids or factors. Heterogeneous nucleation can occur at a lesser degree of cholesterol supersaturation (e.g., the shaded metastable zone in Figure 4) and depends on the presence of additional substance(s) that facilitate the nucleation of cholesterol by lowering the threshold for crystal formation. This phase diagram, however, does not completely take into account the fact that there are two major transport forms of cholesterol in bile: cholesterol-phospholipid vesicles and mixed bile salt-phospholipid-cholesterol micelles. Inability to predict accurately the physiochemical state of human bile (i.e., vesicle/micelle ratio) does not detract from the fact that vesicles are important in initiating the nucleation of cholesterol crystals.[65]

Rapid aggregation of cholesterol-phospholipid vesicles is crucial for the crystallization of biliary cholesterol.[66,67] Small unilamellar vesicles (70 to 100 nm) form first. These vesicles fuse and aggregate, enlarging to 3,000 nm. Calcium enhances this aggregation. Eventually cholesterol microcrystals appear within fields of clustered vesicles.[68] The rate of cholesterol crystal formation is directly related to the amount of cholesterol transported in vesicles.[69] Further crystal growth originates from vesicles supersaturated with cholesterol, not from micelles.

If nucleation of cholesterol crystals is the second key event[70] (the first being the formation of bile with excess cholesterol), then what is the foreign surface on which hetero-

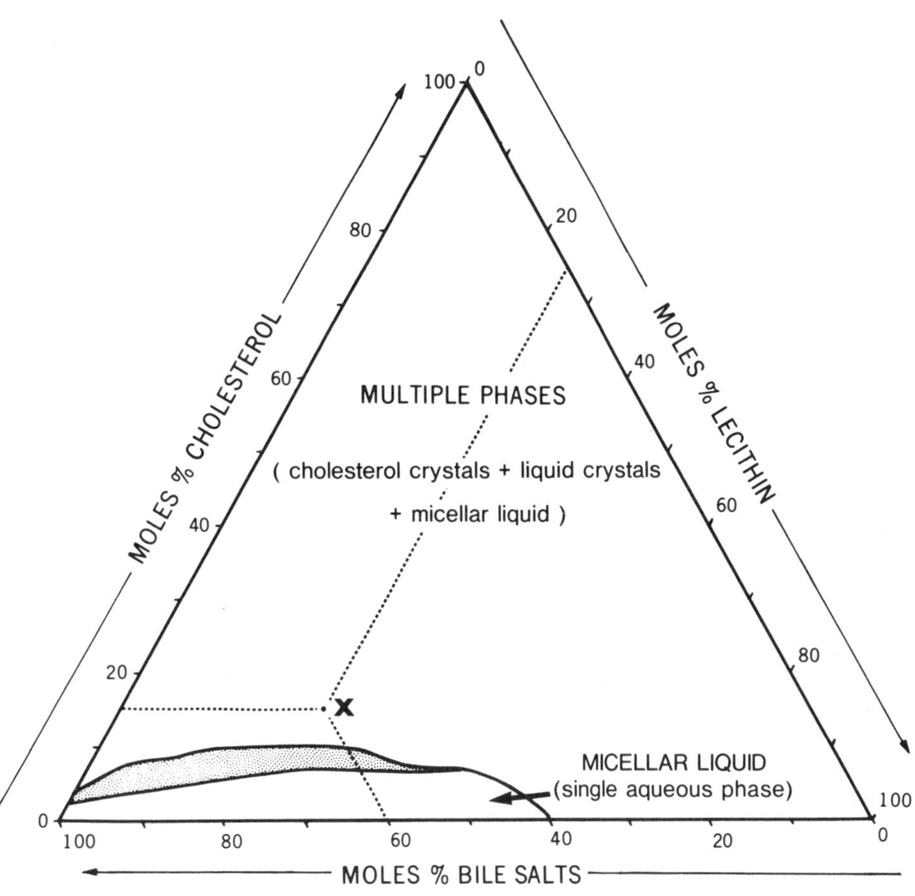

FIGURE 4 Triangular phase diagram for expressing relative molar concentrations of salts, lecithin, and cholesterol in a set water content (here 10 percent) by weight per volume. The relation between the three constituents can be shown as a single point. Point X, for example, is 60 percent bile salts (i.e., bile salt concentration is 60 percent of the sum of all three lipids), 25 percent lecithin, and 15 percent cholesterol. The equilibrium limits for micellar solubility are denoted by the micellar liquid zone in the left lower portion. The clear portion represents that bile composition in which the micellar solution is unsaturated with cholesterol. The shaded micellar area is supersaturated yet unstable (or metastable); although clear initially, cholesterol soon nucleates, causing bile to become turbid. Above the solid line is a labile zone in which supersaturated mixed micelles and unilamellar vesicles can only transiently solubilize the excess cholesterol that spontaneously precipitates. (From Shaffer.[33])

geneous nucleation occurs? One strong candidate is mucin. In gallstone disease, excess amounts of mucin are produced by the gallbladder epithelium.[71] The ability of mucin to promote nucleation relates to its hydrophobic domains, which bind phospholipid and cholesterol.[72,73] The appearance of biliary sludge precedes gallstone formation in some patients.[49] Biliary sludge consists of mucous gel, hydrophobic bile pigments, cholesterol-lecithin vesicles, and solid cholesterol crystals.[50] The organic matrix of cholesterol gallstones also contains a macromolecular complex of mucin and bilirubin. Cholesterol crystals therefore may nucleate in the mucous gel that adheres to the epithelial surface of the gallbladder rather than in the bulk aqueous phase of the bile.[74] Mucus, however, may be a nonspecific agent and not the factor causing rapid (within 1 to 2 days) nucleation.[75] Calcium salts, trace materials, and pigment have been excluded as pronucleating agents. Even the origin of the nucleating agent is in doubt. Initially, gallbladder bile was identified as the origin rather than hepatic bile.[77] Recently, a relatively small protein has been isolated from hepatic bile, indicating that the source is the liver.[78]

The primary event creates the center of the stone. Once crystallization begins, the process can self-perpetuate by heterogeneous nucleation. The center may therefore hold the key to pathogenesis and in cholesterol gallstones is frequently pigmented (see Table 2). The composition of the pigmented centers of cholesterol gallstones differs from that of black pigment stone nidus,[76] but a protein-pigment complex could provide the surface for heterogeneous nucleation.

A deficiency of one or more antinucleating agents is also possible. Apolipoproteins A-I and A-II prolong nucleating time,[79] perhaps interacting with lipid vesicles to inhibit their aggregation. These apolipoproteins are present in normal bile but also have been found in bile that nucleates rapidly.

Gallstone Growth

Gallstones grow at about 1 to 2 mm per year,[80] being present many years (5 to 20) before symptoms lead to cholecystectomy. Gallstones do not continually form in the gallbladder but probably nucleate as crops of stones that then grow at the same rate. The basis for this is the retention and aggregation of cholesterol microcrystals. Retention occurs locally in the gallbladder. Mucin accumulates, forming a colloidal gel that entraps cholesterol microcrystals and creates a scaffold for the further addition of crystals.

Gallbladder stasis with impaired contractility has been demonstrated experimentally as an early pathogenetic event, even before cholesterol crystals appear.[81] Gallbladder motility worsens once stones develop. Some but not all patients with cholelithiasis have impaired emptying.[82] Such biliary stasis has been associated with prolonged parenteral hyperalimentation (forming biliary sludge), pregnancy, and use of sex hormones (progesterone being the likely culprit).[83]

In early childhood, bile is quite unsaturated with respect to cholesterol[84] consistent with the rarity of cholelithiasis in the 1- to 4-year-old age group. Biliary cholesterol saturation in children is even lower than in healthy young adults.[85] In the first weeks of life, the bile salt pool expands and is maintained during childhood at a size that actually exceeds that in adults when corrected for differences in body size. In contrast, the Pima Indians, who are at high risk for cholesterol gallstone formation, have developed abnormal biliary lipid composition by age 9 to 12 years.[20] No earlier studies are available, but conceivably the defect could date back to infancy. Puberty in white and Pima females is associated with a rise in endogenous estrogens and the use of oral contraceptives, which reduce the bile salt pool and increase cholesterol secretion and saturation.[20] This explains the increased frequency of gallstones during adolescence and the resistance to stone formation in childhood.

MANIFESTATIONS OF CHOLELITHIASIS

Gallstone disease indicates the presence of a macroscopic solid phase either as gallstones or sludge in the biliary tract, usually the gallbladder. *Gallbladder disease* indicates defective function and/or morphologic changes (inflammation, fibrosis) of the gallbladder. This commonly is associated with stones in the gallbladder; the one exception is acalculous cholecystitis, a rare occurrence in adults but not children.

Asymptomatic Gallstones

Cholelithiasis indicates the presence of gallstones but not necessarily any symptoms. Most are clinically silent. Indeed, 66 to 80 percent of adults with gallstones detected on epidemiologic screening surveys are asymptomatic and remain so when followed for up to 6 years.[86]

A wide variety of "dyspeptic" symptoms (fat intolerance, flatulence, bloating, postprandial fullness, heartburn, nausea, vomiting, and vague discomforts) have been attributed incorrectly to gallstones. All are nonspecific. None represents true biliary pain. In nonulcer dyspepsia and the irritable bowel syndrome,[87] cholelithiasis is often considered yet rarely causes such symptoms.

Biliary Colic

True biliary symptoms occur when stones obstruct the cystic or common bile ducts, resulting in sudden distention of the gallbladder and/or biliary tract. "Colic" is a poor term, as the pain does not increase and decrease periodically. Rather, the pain comes on suddenly, quickly becomes severe, remains steady for 1 to 3 hours, and then gradually disappears over 30 to 90 minutes, leaving a vague ache. The duration may be less than 1 hour but is not as brief as 15 to 30 minutes. Although biliary colic can follow a fatty or spicy meal, there is no causal relation; attacks can occur anytime, day or night.

Biliary colic, although variable in location, characteristically is located in the epigastrium or right upper quadrant. Mediated by the splanchnic nerves, the pain may radiate to the back (interscapular area), right scapula, or tip of the shoulder, down an arm, or into the neck like angina. Pain may be confined to the back. Analgesics are required for relief. Episodes of pain occur irregularly, separated by painfree periods lasting days to years. Severity also varies in intensity.

As with other forms of visceral pain, movement does not aggravate the pain of biliary colic. The patient is usually restless and may exhibit vasomotor features such as sweating and pallor. Nausea and vomiting may accompany a severe attack. Fever and rigors are absent.

During an attack and often soon after the pain disappears, findings consist of right upper abdominal or epigastric tenderness, perhaps with some guarding. There are no overt peritoneal signs. Often the examination is completely normal.

Laboratory tests, including the white blood cell count, are usually normal. In 10 to 20 percent, there may be a transient, mild elevation of serum bilirubin, alkaline phosphatase, aminotransferase, or gamma-glutamyl transpeptidase.

Between attacks, the patient feels well. Over longer periods, the activity of the disease remains fairly constant.[39] If the patient is having frequent attacks, this pattern is likely to continue.

Pain lasting more than 6 to 12 hours, especially if accompanied by persistent vomiting or fever, suggests another process such as cholecystitis or pancreatitis. Conversely, abdominal pain and bloating relieved by defecation indicate an irritable bowel syndrome.

Diagnosis

Plain abdominal roentgenography identifies the 15 percent or more of stones that have a high calcium content. Ultrasonography is the most sensitive and specific method to detect gallstones (as echogenic objects that cast an acoustic shadow), sludge (echogenic material that layers but does not produce an acoustic shadow), or a thickened gallbladder wall, which indicates inflammation.[88] If the ultrasound examination is normal or the gallbladder is not identified (suggesting a shrunken and diseased gallbladder, when not obscured by intestinal gas or ascites), then oral cholecystography should be performed in suspected cases. Oral cholecystography has been a good technique for over 60 years but is slightly less accurate than ultrasonography and requires more preparation. Oral cholecystography, however, will determine gallbladder function (i.e., it fills and concentrates the radiographic agent excreted in bile) and the type of stone (calcified or not, although this requires a preliminary plain film). It better defines the number of stones than does ultrasonography. Hence, cholecystography is essential when selecting patients for nonoperative therapy such as bile acid dissolution. Persistent nonopacification after 2 days of receiving an oral contrast agent is 95 percent diagnostic for gallbladder disease. Other tests, such as ERCP or percutaneous gallbladder puncture, are secondary and carry risks.[88]

Management

Expectant. In the treatment of asymptomatic adults with gallstones, expectant management is now increasingly accepted as superior to elective cholecystectomy as far as both mortality and costs are concerned.[45] Even diabetes mellitus, a traditional indication for prophylactic cholecystectomy, is best managed expectantly in the absence of biliary symptoms.

Medical. In the nonsurgical approach to cholelithiasis, two principles are clear: (1) None of these regimens is approved for children. (2) Individuals with truly silent gallstones require neither medical nor surgical treatment.

Dissolution Therapy with Oral Bile Acids. Two bile acids are capable of reducing cholesterol saturation of bile and dissolving gallstones: chenodeoxycholic acid and ursodeoxycholic acid.

Chenodeoxycholic acid is moderately effective in selected cases. Complete dissolution occurs by 2 years in approximately 40 percent of patients with radiolucent gallstones and a functioning gallbladder. Success rate increases to 60 percent if criteria are restricted to small stones (well below 1.5 cm in diameter) with a smooth surface, and to 80 percent for tiny, radiolucent stones that float on oral cholecystography. The buoyancy of floating stones indicates a high cholesterol content with little calcium.[89-91] The National Cooperative Gallstone Study virtually destroyed the use of chenodeoxycholic acid, as only 14 percent of patients experienced complete dissolution on 750 mg per day of chenodeoxycholic acid.[92] The poor results likely reflected the low dose chosen, the ideal being 15 mg per kilogram of body weight per day. Because of the potential for hepatotoxicity (although reversible), diarrhea (usually dose-related), and possibly even atherogenesis from elevated low-density lipoprotein cholesterol,[93] chenodeoxycholic acid therapy has limited appeal.

Ursodeoxycholic acid has been used for many years in Japan as an aphrodisiac and digestive. This 7-beta-hydroxy epimer of chenodeoxycholic acid is normally present in only trace amounts in human bile. The effective dose, 8 to 13 mg per kilogram per day, is best given at bedtime to enrich hepatic secretions at a time when the enterohepatic circulation becomes limited owing to fasting. In contrast to chenodeoxycholic acid, ursodeoxycholic acid has no known adverse effects and appears quite safe. It does not cause diarrhea, hepatic dysfunction, or increased serum cholesterol. Unlike chenodeoxycholic acid, ursodeoxycholic acid does not suppress bile acid synthesis and may reduce cholesterol absorption from the intestine. Ursodeoxycholic acid desaturates bile by decreasing the hepatic secretion of cholesterol. Dissolution occurs via formation of vesicles rather than micelles. Ursodeoxycholic acid may also dissolve gallstones somewhat faster than chenodeoxycholic acid but has a higher incidence of stone calcification, which would preclude any benefit from further use of this bile acid. Its efficacy is similar to that of chenodeoxycholic acid, approaching 80 percent in ideal cases with small, noncalcified, floating stones.[91,94-96] Both agents improve nonspecific, dyspeptic symptoms.[96]

Combination therapy with chenodeoxycholic acid and ursodeoxycholic acid may be effective. Preliminary evidence suggests that combination therapy with 6 to 8 mg per kilogram per day of each bile acid dissolves gallstones more rapidly. Ursodeoxycholic acid adds a hepatoprotective effect; chenodeoxycholic acid makes it cheaper!

The indications for bile acid therapy are generally limited to asymptomatic or minimally symptomatic patients with small, radiolucent gallstones, particularly if they float. Less than 30 percent of all patients with gallstones are suitable, however. Further, the compliance necessary for a 1- to 2-year course of oral bile acids and the high recurrence rate (50 percent by 5 years) following dissolution have dampened enthusiasm for bile acid therapy. Other novel, although not yet fully evaluated, therapeutic modalities follow.

Shock-Wave Fragmentation of Gallstones (Lithotripsy). The principle of extracorporeal shock waves to fragment kidney stones has been applied to both gallbladder and common duct stones.[97] Shock waves are a strong form of sound waves yet contain multiple frequencies that provide higher energy and greater tissue penetration.[98] These single pressure pulses require a medium in which to propagate, unlike electromagnetic waves. Wave propagation is determined by the acoustic impedance of the media and by changes at any interface between two different media. For example, a sound wave in water would be completely reflected at a metal surface.

Most body components have an acoustic impedance similar to that of water. Soft tissues that are more than 70 percent water do not absorb the shock waves. Gallstones differ in their impedance and therefore absorb energy as the wave reflects from the surfaces of entry and exit. The absorbed energy creates a primary fissure that subsequently serves as an interface to liberate shock-wave energy, eventually displacing a discrete fragment from the stone surface. The stone may fragment along pre-existing microfissure lines. An indirect mechanism may be the formation and the violent collapse of microscopic gas bubbles in the liquid bile adjacent to the stone. This cavitation effect would act on the stone surface.

There are three major techniques to generate shock waves: spark gap, piezoelectric, and electromagnetic sources. In the first, a high-voltage generator discharges, creating sparks between underwater electrodes. This suddenly vaporizes water and creates a pressure wave that is transmitted via a water bag applied to the patient's body. Under ultrasound guidance, the pressure wave is then focused onto the gallstone. The piezoelectric shock-wave generator uses multiple piezoceramic crystal elements arranged in a mosaic dish and submerged in water. Several hundred to several thousand elements generate converging shock waves. Discharge of a capacitor produces crystal deformation, which induces a pressure wave in the adjacent water. The wave energy for a piezoelectric generator is lower than that of the other two devices, requiring a larger surface area for shock-wave generation and the need for more shock waves. The third system, the electromagnetic shock-wave generator, is an elongated water-filled shock tube. A voltage is discharged into an electromagnetic coil located at the base, which generates a pressure wave by means of a metal membrane. The resultant plane wave is then transmitted along the tube and focused by an acoustic lens.

Up to 1,600 or more shock-wave discharges are delivered within 30 to 120 minutes, being triggered by the R wave of the patient's electrocardiogram. With the newer-generation lithotripters, pain is minimal and requires only minor analgesia. The resultant stone fragments are either ejected from the gallbladder or dissolved by the concomitant use of ursodeoxycholic acid plus chenodeoxycholic acid (7 to 8 mg per kilogram of each, given with the evening meal). Bile acid therapy is initiated 1 week before shock-wave treatment and continued for up to 3 months.[97]

Inclusion criteria involve (1) a history of biliary colic, (2) a solitary radiolucent stone (diameter less than 3 cm) or up to three lucent stones with similar total volumes, (3) a functioning gallbladder or oral cholecystography, and (4) clear detection of stones by ultrasonography without obstacles such as lung or bone. Exclusion criteria are acute cholecystitis, gastroduodenal ulcer, acute pancreatitis, cystic or vascular aneurysms in the shock-wave path, coagulopathy, and pregnancy.

Preliminary reports are enticing. There have been no adverse effects, except for gross hematuria in 3 to 9 percent, the occasional development of acute pancreatitis, and episodes of biliary colic in about one-third before fragments disappeared. The true success rate has not been accurately determined in control studies, but up to 30 percent of patients experience complete disappearance within 2 months after lithotripsy, rising to 60 at 4 to 8 months and 91 percent after 1 year. The initial experience shows it to be safe and quite effective. Unfortunately, only 15 to 25 percent of patients are suitable for stone fragmentation. The best candidates are single, relatively small stones (less than 2 cm). There are only anecdotal reports in children.

Direct Contact Solvents—Methyl Tertiary Butyl Ether. Methyl tertiary butyl ether possesses a high capacity for solubilizing cholesterol and has been directly instilled into the gallbladder to rapidly dissolve gallstones.[99] Catheters are advanced percutaneously through the liver into the gallbladder, and the solvent is infused after aspirating the bile. Frequent cycles of infusion and aspiration can dissolve gallstones within hours. This procedure involves obvious risks, particularly the transhepatic placement of the catheter. Further, methyl tertiary butyl ether can produce nausea, vomiting, and duodenitis. Like other treatments, dissolution may be incomplete, leading to early recurrence. In general, use of direct contact solvents should be reserved for highly selected patients who are unfit for surgery.

Prevention and Treatment of Gallstone Recurrence

Gallstones recur in 50 percent of patients by 5 years following bile acid dissolution. The figure could be even higher after lithotripsy. Gallstone recurrence can be approached by either primary prevention or therapeutic intervention at any of three of its pathogenetic stages: hepatic secretion of supersaturated bile, nucleation of cholesterol crystals, and/or gallbladder stasis. Prophylaxis would involve elimination of the risk factors. For young children in whom a specific etiologic factor can usually be identified, this may be possible in some cases (e.g., children temporarily on total parenteral nutrition) but not others (e.g., chronic hemolysis, ileal resection, or cystic fibrosis). In adolescents, risk factors are less clear (e.g., racial background, female sex), but some are correctable, like obesity or use of oral contraceptives. Therapeutic intervention to reduce cholesterol saturation of bile has not been overwhelmingly successful in trials to date. Neither low-dose bile acids nor dietary manipulation with a low-cholesterol, high-fiber diet has been effective. Simvastatin, a competitive inhibitor of HMG-CoA reductase and hence cholesterol synthesis, lowers cholesterol saturation of bile. The value of a HMG-CoA reductase inhibitor remains to be seen. Use of acetylsalicylic acid to impair prostaglandin synthesis and thus to inhibit mucin hypersecretion (part of the second phase of gallstone formation) is also possible. The same applies to maneuvers that might improve gallbladder emptying. The latter would certainly be an asset in shock-wave therapy when evacuation of stone fragments becomes important.

Cholecystectomy. All children with cholelithiasis should be considered for elective cholecystectomy even if asymptomatic, as the natural history of gallstone disease in this age group is unknown. Expectant management certainly is not a good option for those with symptoms; most experience recurrent attacks.[39,86] For children medically unfit or unwilling to undergo surgery, lithotripsy or contact solvent dissolution may be a reasonable alternative.

CALCULOUS CHOLECYSTITIS

Chronic Cholecystitis

Some degree of chronic inflammation inevitably accompanies cholelithiasis. Calculous obstruction of the cystic duct produces biliary colic and if prolonged leads to acute cholecystitis. Biliary colic may be associated with a gallbladder that appears normal or possesses minimal round cell infiltration and fibrosis. Conversely, symptoms may be minimal while gallbladder scarring is marked.

The clinical features are those of either biliary colic or a previous episode of acute cholecystitis which resolved leaving the organ chronically inflamed.

Diagnosis

A plain film of the abdomen, ultrasonography, and oral cholecystography are the principal methods to detect gallstones. If the gallbladder is fibrotic and shrunken, visualization by these techniques may be difficult. Demonstration of calculi confirms biliary tract disease but does not necessarily relate symptoms to the presence of stones. Imaging the gallbladder with a nuclear medicine scan sometimes helps in difficult cases. Cholescintigraphy with ^{99m}Tc-iminodiacetic acid derivatives should normally demonstrate gallbladder filling. Nonvisualization in suspected cases of acute cholecystitis is diagnostic.[100] The test is much less sensitive in chronic cholecystitis,[88] in which the gallbladder commonly fills. If no filling occurs, then biliary tract disease is likely.

Acalculous biliary pain or *chronic acalculous cholecystitis* implies true biliary colic but without demonstrable gallstones. Gallbladder contraction in response to CCK has been invoked to determine if the abdominal pain can be related to abnormal gallbladder emptying, as determined by cholecystography or cholescintigraphy. A positive CCK-provocation test reproduces the biliary pain and is associated with impaired gallbladder evacuation. Despite sporadic reports, there is no convincing evidence that these tests have diagnostic value.[101–103] The entity remains poorly defined.

Treatment

Cholecystectomy is the definitive treatment, particularly for children. In elective cases without significant systemic disease (e.g., diabetes mellitus or cystic fibrosis) or cirrhosis, the risk of surgery is low, with mortality on the order of 0.1 to 0.2 percent. Cholecystectomy does not disturb fat absorption, as adequate bile salt output into the duodenum is maintained.[16] The situation may differ when bile salt malabsorption is associated with cholesterol gallstone formation. With ileal dysfunction or loss (e.g., Crohn's disease or necrotizing enterocolitis) or cystic fibrosis, gallbladder storage function becomes more important. After an overnight fast in which the gallbladder fills, the breakfast meal initiates the largest dump of bile into the duodenum. Subsequent meals have lesser outputs. Following cholecystectomy, meal-induced bile entry is less effective, especially if the bile salt pool is significantly reduced by malabsorption.

Acute Cholecystitis

The gallbladder becomes acutely inflamed with transmural edema in acute cholecystitis. Cholelithiasis is present in 90 percent of adult cases; 10 percent are acalculous. In young children, gallstones are less common.

The initial event is thought to be obstruction of the cystic duct. The basis for the inflammatory response is not clear. Simple ligation of the cystic duct in an experimental animal causes only resorption of gallbladder contents without an inflammatory response. There may be a mechanical component from distention and ischemia, chemical mediators from the release of lysolecithins or prostaglandins, and/or a bacterial infection. An enzyme present in the gallbladder mucosa, phospholipase A, hydrolyzes biliary lecithin, producing lysolecithin.[104] Lysolecithin increases the synthesis of prostaglandin (PGE_2) by the gallbladder mucosa. Prostaglandins then change the gallbladder from an absorbing to a secreting epithelium[105,106] and also stimulate mucus production.[71] With obstruction of the cystic duct, increased fluid secretions increase intraluminal pressure, creating a vicious circle—distention, mucosal damage, phospholipase release increasing lysolecithin, more prostaglandin synthesis, greater secretion, increased distention—culminating in inflammation. The last component, bacterial infection, probably does not contribute even though enteric bacteria are commonly cultured. Acute cholecystitis is a chemical inflammation.

The mucosa exhibits an acute inflammatory response. With the cystic duct obstructed, the gallbladder becomes distended with bile, an inflammatory exudate, or, when severe, pus. The gallbladder wall can go on to necrosis and perforation. If resolution occurs, the mucosal surface heals and the wall scars, but the gallbladder may not function (i.e., fill with contrast agent) on oral cholecystography. Should the inflammation subside but the cystic duct remain obstructed, the lumen becomes distended with a clear mucoid fluid (termed *hydrops of the gallbladder*). The hydropic gallbladder is evident as a right upper quadrant mass that is not tender. Cholecystectomy is indicated.

Presentation in both children and adults is with acute abdominal pain and tenderness, with onset like an episode of biliary colic (Table 6). There may be a previous history of biliary colic. The pain can develop almost anywhere in the abdomen. Unlike biliary colic, it persists for more than 6 to 12 hours. The visceral pain of cystic duct obstruction is replaced by parietal pain as the gallbladder becomes inflamed. The pain worsens and localizes in the right upper quadrant. Anorexia and vomiting are common. Fever is usually low grade and not associated with rigors.

TABLE 6
Comparison of Biliary Colic to Acute Cholecystitis

Characteristics	Biliary Colic	Acute Cholecystitis
Pain	Constant	Constant
Duration	Hours	Hours to days
Vomiting	Yes	Yes
Onset	Rapid	Variable
Jaundice	No	Later (20%)
Tenderness	RUQ	RUQ
Fever	No	Yes
Leukocytosis	Minimal	Marked
Resolution	Spontaneous	Spontaneous (>66%)

RUQ = right upper quadrant.

There is characteristically tenderness in the right upper quadrant. During palpation of the right upper quadrant, a deep breath worsens the pain and the inspiratory effort suddenly ceases (Murphy's sign). Tenderness or hyperesthesia in the area of the right scapula (Boa's sign) is less common. More severe cases exhibit peritoneal signs: guarding and local rebound tenderness. A reflex paralytic ileus may be present. Patients ill with such parietal pain are reluctant to move. An enlarged gallbladder can be palpated in one-third of cases, particularly with the first attack; later it scars and becomes contracted. Guarding also obscures this finding. If chronic hemolysis is a factor in pigment stone formation, the spleen may be enlarged.

Jaundice with mild hyperbilirubinemia and elevated liver enzymes (including aminotransferase) occur in about 20 percent, even in the absence of common duct stones. The higher the bilirubin level, the more likely is choledocholithiasis. Leukocytosis is common. The amylase can be mildly elevated (to 1,000 μ per deciliter) without pancreatitis. If higher, suspect a common duct stone.

Diagnosis

Ultrasound diagnosis comes from detecting the stone(s) and a thickened gallbladder wall and eliciting tenderness over the sonographically identified gallbladder (the ultrasonographic Murphy's sign). Another important imaging test is cholescintigraphy.[100] Nonvisualization of the gallbladder at 1 hour is highly accurate for acute cholecystitis; a normal scan virtually eliminates acute cholecystitis.[88] False positives occur with prolonged fasting or use of total parenteral nutrition and marked hepatocellular disease. Late visualization by 1 to 4 hours sometimes happens in chronic cholecystitis.

Management

Treatment is surgical and in the hospital. The patient may require rehydration, observation, and analgesia. Antibiotics are used even without overt suppuration, as bile is quite likely to become infected in severe cases. Surgery becomes indicated if the disease progresses within the first 24 hours; an enlarging, inflammatory mass develops in the right hypochondrium; peritonitis becomes generalized; or complications such as an empyema and perforation supervene. In mild or resolving acute cholecystitis, cholecystectomy can be either delayed (2 to 3 months after remission) or performed early (not as an emergency but sometime during the current admission). Early cholecystectomy is becoming the treatment of choice.

Complications of Acute Calculous Cholecystitis

Acute cholecystitis normally resolves spontaneously, usually within 3 days. In about one-third of cases, the inflammation progresses to necrosis, perforation, or empyema (Fig. 5). If pain, tachycardia, fever, peritoneal signs, and leukocytosis worsen or persist, features of a secondary infection (empyema or cholangitis) supervene, or a perforation is suspected, then urgent surgery becomes mandatory.[107]

Empyema is suppurative cholecystitis with an intraluminal abscess—an inflamed gallbladder containing pus. It results from persistent obstruction of the cystic duct and progression of the acute inflammatory process. Systemic features of a bacteremia—hectic fever, chills, prostration, and marked leukocytosis—all indicate the need for urgent surgery. When empyema affects the elderly, the presentation is often indolent, painless, and afebrile yet carries a high mortality.[108]

Perforation occurs when unresolved inflammation leads to

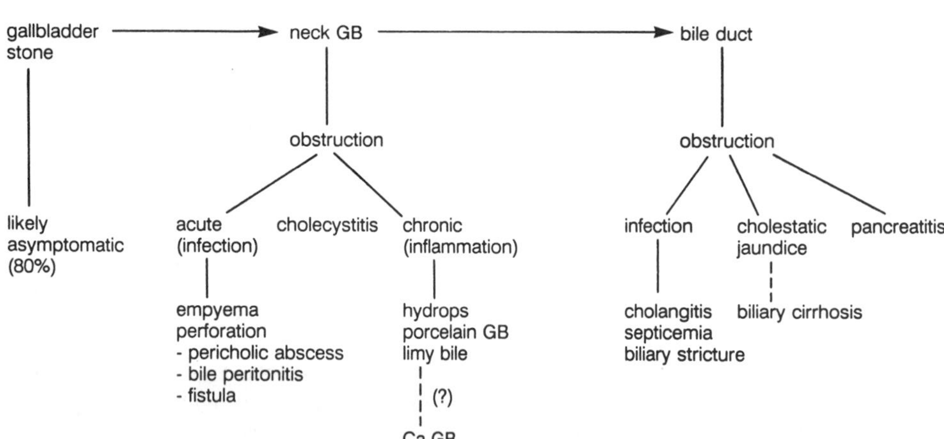

FIGURE 5 Potential complications of cholelithiasis. Migration of the stone in the gallbladder to impact in the neck of the gallbladder or the bile duct can cause obstruction and result in complications. Cystic duct obstruction produces cholecystitis. Common duct obstruction can produce cholangitis, cholestatic jaundice, and/or pancreatitis. Chronic calculous cholecystitis may be associated with the development of carcinoma of the gallbladder in certain races. Chronic bile duct obstruction leads to secondary biliary cirrhosis.

gangrene, often in the fundus of the gallbladder, which is relatively avascular. Localized perforation results in a pericholecystic abscess. The leakage is contained but produces a palpable mass with peritoneal signs in the right upper quadrant. Free perforation with bile peritonitis is fortunately uncommon, as the mortality rate reaches 30 percent. With perforation, the enlarged gallbladder, which sometimes is associated with acute cholecystitis, disappears, and the pain temporarily resolves. Acute peritonitis supervenes. In both localized and free perforations, surgical drainage of the abscess is essential. When possible, cholecystectomy should also be performed. Antibacterial therapy and general support are also necessary. Finally, gallstones can erode into an adjacent loop of bowel, creating a cholecystoenteric fistula. Migration of the stone into the small bowel can then produce obstruction at the ileocecal sphincter (*gallstone ileus*). Plain films show air in the biliary system and features of a distal small bowel obstruction.

Limy bile occurs when prolonged biliary tract obstruction causes loss of the pigment material from bile and precipitation of calcium salts in the lumen. Complete obstruction of the cystic duct or common duct from any cause, benign or malignant, results in "white bile." In most instances, a gallstone obstructs the cystic duct. Bilirubin is deconjugated and then metabolized to colorless compounds. Absorption of organic compounds also contributes to the formation of white bile. The hydropic gallbladder then secretes calcium into the lumen, opacifying the bile and causing "milk of calcium" or "limy" bile. In another complication of calculous cholecystitis, calcium accumulates in the wall of the gallbladder, producing a *porcelain gallbladder.* The mural calcifications are easily identified on plain radiographs of the abdomen. The porcelain gallbladder results from acute, recurrent, inflammatory episodes involving the gallbladder. Although most of these patients have had recurrent acute cholecystitis in the past, the porcelain gallbladder per se produces no symptoms. Yet up to 50 percent of patients develop carcinoma of the gallbladder, making prophylactic cholecystectomy a necessity.

Choledocholithiasis (Common Duct Stones)

Ductal stones are classified according to their site of origin. *Primary stones* are formed in the bile ducts, whereas *secondary stones* originate in the gallbladder and then migrate into the common bile duct.[109] In the Western world, virtually all cholesterol stones and most pigment stones are secondary when the gallbladder is intact.[110,111] Thus, over 85 percent of patients with common duct stones also have stones in the gallbladder. *Residual stones* are those missed at the time of cholecystectomy. *Recurrent stones* develop more than 2 years after surgery. Although cholesterol stones predominate in the gallbladder and in the common duct, the proportion of pigment material in ductal stones rises with time after cholecystectomy. Nonabsorbable suture material is often found in the centers of these recurrent stones, perhaps acting as a nidus for their formation.[111] About 40 percent of all common duct stones are of pigment, much higher than the frequency of pigment stones among gallbladder stones.[110] Stasis and infection are the basic ingredients. Bacterial deconjugation of bilirubin accompanied by mucin or bacterial biofilm which agglomerates the precipitated pigment leads to earthy, brown stones. Primary ductal stones therefore develop proximal to a stricture or in conjunction with a congenital anomaly (e.g., a choledochal cyst or Caroli's disease).

Choledocholithiasis may present without symptoms or with biliary colic, obstructive jaundice, cholangitis, or pancreatitis (Fig. 5). Little is known about the asymptomatic state, which presumably exists some time before the obstructive features supervened. The rate of onset of the obstruction, whether or not it is complete, and any bacterial contamination of bile determine the resulting syndrome.

Biliary colic results from sudden obstruction of the common duct causing increased pressure, up to 25 to 30 cm H_2O, which is the maximum secretory pressure of bile.[112]

Cholangitis consists of bacterial infection and obstruction involving the bile ducts: pus under pressure. Any condition producing biliary tract obstruction is liable to cause bacterial infection of bile within the bile ducts: most commonly a common duct stone or biliary stricture following surgery, less likely a neoplastic obstruction. This difference relates to the high-grade obstruction with neoplasms, the intermittency of obstruction with a stone or inflammatory stricture which allows retrograde ascent of bacteria, and the prior surgical manipulation in post-traumatic strictures that may have introduced bacterial contamination. Unknown is how the mucosal defense mechanism is actually bridged or the route of bacteria invasion. Certainly bile is an excellent culture medium and the biliary tree empties unprotected into the duodenum, which periodically contains bacteria. The normal barrier to bacteria in the duodenum must be broken to allow ascent in a ductal system compromised by stasis. The infection is usually an enteric organism such as *E. coli* or *Klebsiella* or an anaerobe such as *Bacteroides*.

Obstruction and infection permit regurgitation of ductal bacteria into hepatic venous blood, causing a bacteremia with chills and spiking fevers. Upper abdominal pain ensues. The third component of "Charcot's triad," jaundice, results from the mechanical obstruction plus intrahepatic cholestasis due to sepsis. Pain and fever are very common, jaundice less so. Most patients appear toxic and febrile. Abdominal tenderness is evident. A tender, enlarged liver may suggest secondary hepatic abscesses. Hypotension, confusion, and a septic picture predominate.

Leukocytosis and abnormal liver biochemistry are common. Blood cultures reveal the causative microorganism. Ultrasonography often reveals dilated ducts, but cholangiography, either by endoscopy from below or percutaneous transhepatic catheterization from above, is necessary to localize the site and cause.

Management of cholangitis in the very ill necessitates decompression of the biliary system. In the past, laparotomy was the only recourse. Now, endoscopic surgery (ERCP) and percutaneous transhepatic catheterization are quite feasible. Good antibiotic coverage is essential; in milder cases, this alone may resolve the episode. Endoscopic sphincterotomy with extraction of a common duct stone or placement of stents through a stricture or a cholangiocarcinoma can be quite effective in those unfit for surgery. Most come to common bile duct exploration with removal of the stone and perhaps the gallbladder if still present, plus provision for adequate biliary drainage. To eliminate any narrowing, sphincteroplasty, choledochoduodenostomy, or a Roux-en-Y choledochojejunostomy may be necessary. A T tube may be left as a decompression vent and as a route to the common duct for diagnostic (e.g., cholangiography) or therapeutic maneuvers (e.g., basket extraction or contact solvent infusion for retained stones).

Obstructive jaundice with conjugated hyperbilirubinemia results from bile duct obstruction. Such cholestasis with impaired bile formation may develop rapidly if the gallbladder is absent or too diseased to temporarily decompress the obstructed biliary system by its absorptive and storage functions. This is often the case with choledocholithiasis in which jaundice can develop within a day. Obstruction of the common bile duct below the entry of the cystic duct may cause the gallbladder to dilate and present as an abdominal mass. With gallstones, the gallbladder may be fibrotic and unable to dilate. Besides, choledocholithiasis does not usually cause complete obstruction. The basis for "Courvoisier's law" is thus reasonable but far from perfect: the presence of a palpable, nontender gallbladder in a jaundiced patient suggests that the biliary obstruction is secondary to a malignancy in the distal common duct or periampullary region. Neoplasia presents gradually with pruritus and jaundice, often without pain and usually unassociated with biliary colic or cholangitis.

Obstruction produces dilation of the biliary tree which can be readily detected by ultrasonography or computed tomography scan. Dilatation may not be evident acutely. If dilated ducts are detected, either an ERCP or a transhepatic cholangiogram reveals the diagnosis. Without dilated ducts, either a liver biopsy in cases of suspected hepatocellular disease or an ERCP is performed.

Chronic obstruction produces steatorrhea from deficient bile salts, impaired absorption of the fat-soluble vitamins (A, D, E, and K), pruritus, and xanthomas. Eventually, after 3 months to 5 years of constant or intermittent obstruction, *secondary biliary cirrhosis* develops. Serum bilirubin, alkaline phosphatase, 5′-nucleotidase, and gamma-glutamyl transpeptidase all rise within hours of a complete obstruction. Alkaline phosphatase synthesis in the canalicular membrane increases secondary to the retained bile salts. The other components are retained products that normally are excreted in bile. Complete obstruction produces light, clay-colored stools, termed "acholic" because they lack bile. Relieving the obstruction normalizes these values, often within 2 weeks if the onset was recent.

Management

The primary therapy of choledocholithiasis is surgery, emergently for cholangitis that is unresponsive to medical therapy and electively for most common duct stones. Increasingly, new techniques are replacing common duct exploration at laparotomy in selected cases:

ERCP. Endoscopic retrograde cholangiopancreatography is not only an important diagnostic tool for biliary tract disease but provides access to remove stones via balloons or baskets.[113] In high-risk patients, biliary stents can temporarily control cholangitis. Endoscopic sphincterotomy assists in stone removal and, combined with mechanical lithotripsy, can extract multiple large stones. Endoscopic lithotripsy to fragment large stones has employed laser, ultrasonic, or electrohydraulic techniques. ERCP can also place a nasobiliary cannula for direct infusion of solvents. Percutaneous transhepatic stone removal is particularly feasible for retained stones if a T tube has been in place. In general, the technique used depends on the expertise available.

Mono-octanoin. Since bile acids require weeks for stone dissolution, new contact solvents with high capacities for solubilizing cholesterol are being evaluated. Mono-octanoin, a medium-chain monoglyceride synthesized from vegetable oil, is an excellent cholesterol solvent when modified. The emulsified oil buffered to a pH of 7.4 is infused at a rate of 3 to 7 ml per hour by a precision pump with a 12- to 15-ml manometer in line to prevent biliary pressure from rising above the hepatic secretory pressure of bile (~30 cm H_2O). Access to the bile duct with its radiolucent stone(s) is gained by a T tube, percutaneous transhepatic catheter, or nasobiliary tube inserted at ERCP. Despite reports of 50 to 86 percent complete dissolution, critical analysis reveals treatment to be unequivocally successful in only 26 percent and a valuable adjunct to interventional treatment in another 8 percent.[114] In 9 percent, mono-octanoin was discontinued because of side effects such as abdominal pain, nausea, vomiting, and diarrhea. Even chemical cholangitis has been reported. Use of this direct-contact solvent should be limited to cholesterol stones "retained" after cholecystectomy. Most "recurrent" stones are primary duct stones composed predominantly of calcium bilirubinate. These brown pigment stones do not dissolve. Large and lucent, they are difficult to distinguish radiologically from cholesterol stones, perhaps partly explaining the poor results with mono-octanoin. Thus, contact solvent dissolution of retained bile duct calculi is second-line therapy compared to mechanical extraction.

Extracorporeal Shock-Wave Lithotripsy. For stones too large to be removed endoscopically, fragmentation has been an asset.[115] Nasobiliary catheters are placed to visualize the common duct by injecting contrast medium because ultrasonography is less accurate. After shock-wave lithotripsy, fragments either pass spontaneously or are extracted endoscopically. Extracorporeal shock-wave lithotripsy has even been used for retained stones in a cystic duct remnant.

NONCALCULOUS GALLBLADDER DISEASE

Gallstone disease is undoubtably the most common condition affecting the gallbladder, but a variety of important acalculous diseases also affect the gallbladder, particularly in children.[116] Acalculous diseases of the gallbladder may be classified in general terms (Table 7). Specific examples follow.

Congenital Abnormalities

Congenital anomalies of the gallbladder result from embryonic maldevelopment and are of most interest to the surgeon attempting to identify the biliary anatomy at cholecystectomy. There are numerous variations for the cystic duct and artery.

TABLE 7
Acalculous Diseases of the Gallbladder

Congenital
Anomalies of size, shape, and position
Anatomic abnormality of the cystic duct
Congenital absence of the gallbladder
Duplication of the gallbladder
Aberrant gastric mucosa
Inflammatory (acalculous cholecystitis)
Primary—no apparent cause
Secondary
Infectious agents: bacterial, viral, parasitic
Trauma, surgery, burns
Chronic inflammatory process (sclerosing, Crohn's)
Ischemic (SLE)
Degenerative (cholecystosis)
Cholesterolosis
Adenomyosis
Neoplastic
Adenoma
Carcinoma
Sarcoma
Metastatic carcinoma

SLE = systemic lupus erythematosus.

Agenesis of the gallbladder is rare. Although associated with stone formation, the basis is obscure, as these patients do not produce bile containing excess cholesterol.[117]

Gallbladders that "float" on a long mesentery can undergo torsion, presenting with features similar to acute cholecystitis. Children and elderly women seem prone to torsion of the gallbladder.[118]

Most congenital defects of the biliary system are related to abnormalities in the original budding process of the hepatic diverticulum or to failure of the duct system to vacuolize during embryogenesis. The result is accessory bile ducts and cystic lesions of the ducts. A variety of cystic and atretic lesions can involve the cystic duct, common duct, or hepatic duct system.

Acute Acalculous Cholecystitis

Chronic acalculous cholecystitis is also termed "acalculous biliary pain" or "biliary dyskinesia," as noted earlier. Here the morphologic features of inflammation are modest and, if present, consist of chronic changes. In contrast, acute acalculous cholecystitis is acute inflammation of the gallbladder without gallstones. Over 3 percent of all gallbladders removed for acute cholecystitis contain no stones.[119] In children, more than half of cases lack gallstones. Acute acalculous cholecystitis in children has been associated with an intercurrent infection: viral gastroenteritis, bacterial enteric infections (e.g., salmonellosis, shigellosis, *E. coli* infection), streptococcal infection, and pneumonia. No definitive infectious agent, however, has been identified. It may also accompany metabolic, vascular, traumatic, malignant, or congenital diseases. There is often a congenital anomaly of the biliary, vascular, or ductal systems. Stagnation of bile has been implicated, particularly as the entity occurs soon after surgery and while the patient is on total parenteral nutrition.[120] Spasm of the sphincter of Oddi, perhaps from the postoperative use of opiates, could accentuate biliary stasis. If sporadic, sphincter spasm would permit reflux of pancreatic contents or bacteria, leading to chemical inflammation and infected bile. Conversely, the gallbladder vascular bed may be overly reactive to a systemic illness or other event, weakening the mucosal defense mechanisms and allowing biliary contents like lysolecithin to damage the gallbladder wall. In children, congenital narrowing or inflammation of the cystic duct or external compression from an enlarged lymph node could produce obstruction.[121,122]

The clinical presentation is similar to that of acute cholecystitis in which the gallbladder harbors a stone. The difference lies in the setting, e.g., the postoperative or posttraumatic patient or the sick child on total parenteral nutrition. The cardinal findings of fever, a tender mass, or jaundice may be obscured in these ill patients. Leukocytosis and abnormal liver biochemistry may not help.

Diagnosis is often made at laparotomy performed for an acute abdominal condition. With a high degree of clinical suspicion, the diagnosis can be obtained by cholescintigraphy or ultrasonography. Cholescintigraphy will demonstrate failure of the radionuclide to visualize the gallbladder but good hepatic uptake and entry into the duodenum. On ultrasonography there is mural thickening, a distended gallbladder, sludge within the lumen, and the halo sign of subserosal edema. No stone is evident.

Prompt cholecystectomy is the best therapy. Prognosis depends upon any underlying condition.

Acute Hydrops of the Gallbladder

Idiopathic distention of the gallbladder occurs independently of obvious obstruction or inflammatory disease. Gallstones are not present; the gallbladder is not acutely inflamed; bile is sterile, and the extrahepatic bile ducts are normal in size. Age of onset ranges from early infancy to adolescence. Boys are more commonly affected than girls.

The cause is unknown. Half of patients who undergo surgery have evidence of enlarged mesenteric lymph nodes. There is also a temporal relationship to a preceding infectious illness, especially streptoccal and staphylococcal disease. Leptospirosis may also be causal. Acute dilation has been associated with the mucocutaneous lymph node (Kawasaki) syndrome,[123] Sjögren's disease,[124] and systematic sclerosis.[125] The disease has also occurred as a complication of the nephrotic syndrome, familial Mediterranean fever, and leukemia. The importance of cystic duct narrowing or obstruction or a congenital abnormality is unclear. Acute distention conceivably may result from impaired emptying or increased mucous secretion by the gallbladder. The common denominator appears to be a preceding infectious illness with inflammation of the cystic duct and enlargement of an adjacent lymph node leading to cystic duct obstruction and gallbladder distention. In some, stenosis or hypoplasia of the cystic duct can be identified.

Onset is acute with crampy abdominal pain, nausea, and vomiting. Localization and description of the pain may be difficult for younger children. The pain generally becomes continuous and more intense. There is frequently a preceding history of a febrile illness compatible with the mucocutaneous lymph node syndrome. Examination reveals upper abdominal tenderness, particularly on the right. A mass may also be palpable in the right upper quadrant. Fever is absent or slight and jaundice uncommon.

Ultrasonography reveals a massive, echo-free gallbladder with normal bile ducts. Cholecystography will not visualize the gallbladder.

In the past, surgery was frequently performed and revealed a large, distended gallbladder. Cholecystectomy was then usually performed. The advent of ultrasonography provided a reliable preoperative diagnosis. Treatment has become nonoperative, with emphasis placed on managing the intercurrent illness through supportive care and adequate hydration. Prognosis is excellent. Spontaneous resolution occurs within a few weeks, and gallbladder function returns to normal. Aspiration of the gallbladder under ultrasonography or drainage via cholecystostomy occasionally may be considered if rupture appears imminent. As full recovery is anticipated, surgery should be avoided whenever possible.

Cholecystoses

Cholesterolosis consists of deposits of cholesterol esters and triglycerides within submucosal macrophages and in epithelial cells. The submucosal cholesterol deposits produce a fine yellow reticular pattern on a red background of mildly inflamed mucosa, appearing like a strawberry—hence the term "strawberry gallbladder." There is no etiologic association with bile supersaturated with cholesterol, and bile acid therapy does not reverse the changes. Some of the cholesterol deposits protrude like polyps. Occasionally these polyps break off and form a nidus for cholesterol gallstones, which develop in 10 to 15 percent. The pathogenesis of cholesterolosis is unrelated to that for cholesterol gallstones, which form secondarily. Rather, the basis for the mucosal disease may relate to increased hepatic synthesis of cholesterol or methyl sterols, which are precursors to cholesterol. These free sterols may then transfer from bile to the gallbladder mucosa to be esterified and deposited.[126] Whether or not symptoms develop is uncertain. Some come to cholecystectomy.

Adenomyosis is characterized by hyperplasia of the mucosa, particularly the muscularis, and by deep clefts termed Rokitanski-Aschoff sinuses. The cause is unknown but has been attributed to muscular dysfunction in which excessive intraluminal pressure creates the sinuses. The meaning of any biliary-like symptoms is moot.

Neoplasms of the Gallbladder

Carcinoma of the gallbladder is uncommon, although it carries a poor prognosis. Gallstones are present in 80 percent of cases, an association that accounts for the higher prevalence in women and certain racial groups. Unknown is whether or not gallstones lead to the development of carcinoma of the gallbladder or are innocent bystanders. Although gallstones may be a factor, the risk of developing carcinoma of the gallbladder in persons with cholelithiasis is likely overestimated, being more on the order of 0.5 percent.[127] This risk is too low to advocate prophylactic cholecystectomy in people with asymptomatic gallstones. The situation differs for native Americans, in whom the risk of gallbladder carcinoma rises to 5 percent of women by age 85 years, the same as for carcinoma of the lung in heavy cigarette smokers. Carcinoma of the gallbladder is not a problem in childhood.

Benign tumors are more common, particularly as adenomas. Adenomatous gallbladder polyps have been described in the Peutz-Jeghers syndrome.[128] Other benign tumors are extremely rare.

REFERENCES

1. Strom BL, West SL. The epidemiology of gallstone disease. In: Cohen S, Soloway RD, eds. Gallstones. New York: Churchill Livingstone, 1985:1.
2. Fisher MM. Perspectives on gallstones. In: Fisher MM, Goresky CA, Shaffer EA, Strasberg SM, eds. Gallstones. New York: Plenum, 1979:1.
3. Friedman GD, Kannel WB, Dawber TR. The epidemiology of gallbladder disease: observations in Framingham study. J Chronic Dis 1966; 19:273–292.
4. Strauss RG. Cholelithiasis in childhood. Am J Dis Child 1969; 117:689–692.
5. Potter AH. Gallbladder disease in young subjects. Surg Gynecol Obstet 1928; 46:795–808.
6. Grace N, Rodgers B. Cholecystitis in childhood. Clinical observations based on 30 surgically treated cases. Clin Ped 1977; 16:179–181.
7. Takiff H, Fonkalsrud EW. Gallbladder disease in childhood. Am J Dis Child 1984; 138–565–568.
8. Kingensmith WC, Cioffi-Ragan DT. Fetal gallstones. Radiology 1988; 167:143–144.
9. Brill PW, Winchester P, Rosen MS. Neonatal cholelithiasis. Pediatr Radiol 1982; 12:285–288.
10. Nilsson S. Gallbladder disease and sex hormones. Acta Chir Scand 1966; 132:275–279.
11. Calabrese C, Pearlman DM. Gallbladder disease below the age of 21 years. Surgery 1971; 70:413–415.
12. Honore LH. Cholesterol cholelithiasis in adolescent females. Arch Surg 1980; 114:62–64.
13. Friedman GD. Primer of epidemiology. New York: McGraw-Hill, 1974.
14. Sackett DL. Bias in analytical research. J Chron Dis 1979; 32:51–63.
15. Jorgensen T. Abdominal symptoms and gallstone disease: an epidemiological investigation. Hepatology 1989; 9:856–860.
16. Shaffer EA, Small DM. Gallstone disease: pathogenesis and management. Curr Probl Surg 1976; 13:1–72.
17. Balzer K, Goebell H, Breuer N, Ruping KW, Leder LD. Epidemiology of gallstones in a German industrial town (Essen) from 1940–1975. Digestion 1986; 33:189–197.
18. Norrby S, Fagerberg G, Sjodahl R. Decreasing incidence of gallstone disease in a defined Swedish population. Scand J Gastroenterol 1986; 21:158–162.
19. Opit LJ, Greenhill S. Prevalence of gallstones in relation to differing treatment rates for biliary disease. Br J Prev Soc Med 1974; 28:268–272.
20. Bennion LJ, Knowler WC, Mott DM, Spangnola AM, Bennett PH. Development of lithogenic bile during puberty in Pima Indians. N Engl J Med 1979; 300:873–876.
21. Sampliner RE, Bennett PH, Comess LJ, Rose FA, Burch TA. Gallbladder disease in Pima Indians: demonstration of high prevalence and early onset by cholecystography. N Engl J Med 170; 283:1358–1364.
22. Williams CN, Johnston JL, Weldon KLM. Prevalence of gallstones and gallbladder disease in Canadian Micmac Indian women. Can Med Assoc J 1977; 117:758–760.
23. Covarrubios C, Valdivieso V, Nervi F. Epidemiology of gallstone disease in Chile. In: Capocaccia L, Ricci G, Angelico F, Angelico M, Attili AF, eds. Epidemiology and prevention of gallstone disease. Lancaster, England: MTP Press, 1984:26.
24. Capocaccia L, Ricci G. Epidemiology of gallstone disease. Ital J Gastroenterol 1985; 17:215–218.

25. Bond LR, Hatty SR, Horn MEC, Dick M, Meire HB, Bellingham AJ. Gallstones in sickle cell disease in the United Kingdom. Br J Med 1987; 295:234–236.
26. Schubert TT. Hepatobiliary system in sickle cell disease. Gastroenterology; 186; 90:2013–2021.
27. Barbara L, Sama C, Labate AMM, Taroni F, Rusticale AG, Festi D, Sapio C, Roda E, Banterle C, Puci A, Formentini F, Colasanti S, Nardin F. A population study on the prevalence of gallstone disease: the Sirmione Study. Hepatology 1987; 7:913–917.
28. Jorgensen T. Prevalence of gallstones in a Danish population. Am J Epidemiol 1987; 126:912–921.
29. Jorgensen T. Gallstones in a Danish population: fertility period, pregnancies, and exogenous female sex hormones. Gut 1988; 29:433–439.
30. Garn SM, LaBelle M, Rosenberg KR, Hawthorne BN. Maturation timing as a factor in female fatness and obesity. Am J Clin Nutr 1986; 43:879–883.
31. Lee SS, Wasiljew BK, Lee M-J. Gallstones in women younger than thirty. J Clin Gastroenterol 1987; 9:65–69.
32. Bennion LJ, Grundy SM. Risk factors for the development of cholelithiasis in man. N Engl J Med 1978; 299:1161–1167, 1221–1227.
33. Shaffer EA. Gallstones: current concepts of pathogenesis and medical dissolution. Can J Surg 1980; 6:517–532.
34. Glenn F. Silent gallstones. Ann Surg 1981; 193:251–225.
35. Shaffer E. Gallstone formation, dissolution and asymptomatic cholelithiasis. Ann Coll Phys Surg Can 1985; 18:309–315.
36. Comfort MW, Gray HK, Wilson JM. The silent gallstone: a ten to twenty year follow-up of 112 cases. Ann Surg 1948; 128:931–937.
37. Gracie WA, Ransohoff DF. Natural history and expectant management of gallstone disease. In: Cohen S, Soloway RD, eds. Gallstones. New York: Churchill Livingstone, 1985:27.
38. Gracie WA, Ransohoff DF. The natural history of silent gallstones. The innocent gallstone is not a myth. N Engl J Med 1982; 307:798–800.
39. Thistle JL, Cleary PA, Lachin JM, Tyor MP, Hersh T. The natural history of cholelithiasis: the National Cooperative Gallstone Study. Ann Intern Med 1984; 101:171–175.
40. Rome Group for the Epidemiology and Prevention of Cholelithiasis (GREPCO). Prevalence of gallstone disease in Italian female population. Am J Epidemiol 1984; 119:796–805.
41. Barbara L. Epidemiology of gallstones: Sermione Study. In: Capocaccia L, Ricci G, Angelico F, Attili AF, eds. Epidemiology and prevention of gallstone disease. Lancaster, England: MTP Press, 1984:22.
42. Pixley F, Wilson D, McPherson K, Mann J. Effect of vegetarianism on development of gallstones in women. Br Med J 1985; 291:11–12.
43. Jorgensen T. Abdominal symptoms and gallstone disease: an epidemiological investigation. Hepatology 1989; 9:856–860.
44. McPherson K, Strong PM, Epstein A, Jones L. Regional variations in the use of common surgical procedures: within and between England and Wales, Canada, and the United States of America. Soc Sci Med 1981; 15A:273–288.
45. Ransohoff DF, Gracie WA, Wolfenson LB, Neuhauser D. Prophylactic cholecystectomy or expectant management for silent gallstones: a decision analysis to assess survival. Ann Intern Med 1983; 99:199–204.
46. Trotman BW, Soloway RD. Pigment gallstone disease: summary of the National Institutes of Health—International Workshop Hepatology 1982; 1:879–884.
47. Trotman BW, Soloway RD. Pigment vs cholesterol cholelithiasis: clinical and epidemiological aspects. Am J Dig Dis 1975; 20:735–740.
48. Sarnaik S, Slovis TL, Corbett DP, Emami A, Whitten CF. Incidence of cholelithiasis in sickle-cell anemia using the ultrasonic gray-scale technique. J Pediatrics 1980; 96:1005–1008.
49. Messing B, Bories C, Kunstlinger F, Bernier JJ. Does total parenteral nutrition induce gallbladder sludge formation and lithiasis? Gastroenterology 1983; 84:1012–1019.
50. Lee SP, Maher K, Nicholls JF. Origin and fate of biliary sludge. Gastroenterology 1988; 94:170–176.
51. Nakayama F, Miyaka H. Changing state of gallstone disease in Japan. Composition of the stones and treatment of the condition. Am J Surg 1970; 120:794–799.
52. Masuda H, Nakayama F. Composition of bile pigment in gallstones and bile and their etiological significance. J Lab Clin Med 1979; 93:353–360.
53. Yamashita N, Yanagisawa J, Nakayama F. Composition of intrahepatic calculi. Etiological significance. Dig Dis Sci 1988; 33:449–453.
54. Ostrow JD. The etiology of pigment gallstones. Hepatology 1984; 4:2155–2225.
55. Trotman BW, Nair CR, Bernstein SE. Monoconjugated bilirubin is a major component of hemolysis-induced gallstones in mice. Hepatology 1988; 8:919–929.
56. Cahalane MJ, Neubrand MW, Carey MC. Physical-chemical pathogenesis of pigment gallstones. Semin Liver Dis 1988; 8:317–328.
57. Everson GT, Nemeth A, Kourourian S, Zogg D, Leff NB, Dixon D, Githens JH, Pretorius D. Gallbladder function is altered in sickle cell hemoglobinopathy. Gastroenterology 1989; 96:1307–1316.
58. Maki T. Pathogenesis of calcium bilirubinate gallstones. Ann Surg 1966; 164:90–100.
59. Rege RV, Moore EW. Pathogenesis of calcium-containing gallstones. Canine ductular bile, but not gallbladder bile is supersaturated with calcium carbonate. J Clin Invest 1986; 77:21–26.
60. Stewart L, Smith AL, Pellegrini CA, Motson RW, Way LW. Pigment gallstones form as a composite of bacterial microcolonies and pigment solids. Ann Surg 1987; 206:242–250.
61. Carey MC, Small DM. Micelle formation by bile salts: physical-chemical and thermodynamic considerations. Arch Intern Med 1972; 130:506–527.
62. Somjen G, Gilat T. Contribution of vesicular and micellar carriers to cholesterol transport in human bile. J Lipid Res 1985; 26:699–704.
63. Carey MC, Small DM. The physical chemistry of cholesterol solubility in bile. Relationship to gallstone formation and dissolution in man. J Clin Invest 1978; 61:998–1026.
64. Pattinson NR, Chapman BA. Distribution of biliary cholesterol between mixed micelles and nonmicelles in relation to fasting and feeding in humans. Gastroenterology 1986; 91:697–702.
65. Schriever CE, Jungst D. Association between cholesterol-phospholipid vesicles and cholesterol crystals in human gallbladder bile. Hepatology 1989; 9:541–546.
66. Kibe A, Dudley MA, Halpern Z, Lynn MP, Breuer AC, Holzbach RT. Factors affecting cholesterol monohydrate crystal nucleation time in model systems of supersaturated bile. J Lipid Res 1985; 26:1102–1111.
67. Halpern Z, Dudley MA, Lynn MP, Nadler JM, Breuer AC, Holzbach RT. Vesicle aggregation in model systems of supersaturated bile: relation to crystal and lipid composition of the vesicular phase. J Lipid Res 1986; 27:295–306.
68. Halpern Z, Dudley MA, Kibe A, Lynn MP, Breuer AC, Holzbach RT. Rapid vesicle formation and aggregation in abnormal human biles. A time-lapse video-enhanced contrast microscopy study. Gastroenterology 1985; 90:875–885.
69. Harvey PRC, Somjen G, Gilat T, Gallinger S, Strasberg SM. Vesicular cholesterol in bile. Relationship to protein concentration. Biochim Biophys Acta 1988; 958:10–18.
70. Holan KR, Holzbach RT, Hermann RE, Cooperman AM, Claffey WJ. Nucleation time: a key event in the pathogenesis of cholesterol gallstone disease. Gastroenterology 1979; 77:611–617.
71. Lee SP, LaMonte JT, Carey MC. Role of gallstone mucus hypersecretion in the evolution of cholesterol gallstone: studies in a prairie dog. J Clin Invest 1981; 67:1712–1723.
72. Smith BF, LaMonte JT. Hydrophobic binding properties of bovine gallbladder mucin. J Biol Chem 1984; 257:12170–12177.
73. Smith BF. Human gallbladder mucin binds biliary lipids and promotes cholesterol crystal nucleation in model bile. J Lipid Res 1987; 28:1088–1097.
74. Carey MC, Cahalane MJ. Whither biliary sludge? Gastroenterology 1988; 95:508–523.
75. Harvey PRC, Rupar CA, Gallinger S, Petrunka CN, Strasberg SM. Quantitative and qualitative comparison of gallbladder mucous glycoprotein from patients with and without gallstones. Gut 1985; 27:374–381.
76. Malet PF, Williamson CE, Trotman BW, Soloway RD. Composition of pigmented centers of cholesterol gallstones. Hepatology 1986; 5:477–481.
77. Burnstein MJ, Ilson RG, Petrunka CN, Taylor RD, Strasberg SM. Nucleation of cholesterol monohydrate crystals from hepatic and gallbladder bile of patients with cholesterol gallstones. Gut 1983; 24:836–844.
78. Groen AK, Stout JPJ, Drapers JAG, Hoek JF, Grijm R, Tytgat GN. Cholesterol and nucleation—influencing activity in t-tube bile. Hepatology 1988; 8:347–352.
79. Holzbach RT, Kibe A, Thiel E, Howell JH, Marsh M, Hermann RE. Biliary proteins. Unique inhibitors of cholesterol nucleation in human gallbladder bile. J Clin Invest 1984; 73:35–45.
80. Mok HYI, Druffel ERM, Rampone WM. Chronology of cholelithia-

sis. Dating gallstones from atmosphere radiocarbon produced by nuclear bomb explosion. N Engl J Med 1986; 314:1075–1077.

81. Fridhandler TM, Davison JS, Shaffer EA. Defective gallbladder contractility in the ground squirrel and prairie dog during the early stages of cholesterol gallstone formation. Gastroenterology 1983; 85:830–836.
82. Pomeranz IS, Shaffer EA. Abnormal gallbladder emptying in a subgroup of patients with gallstones. Gastroenterology 1985; 88:787–791.
83. Shaffer EA, Taylor PJ, Logan K, Gadomski S, Corenblum B. The effect of a progestin on gallbladder function in young women. Am J Obstet Gynecol 1984; 148:504–507.
84. Von Bergmann J, Von Bergmann K, Hadorn B, Paumgartner G. Biliary lipid composition in early childhood. Clin Chim Acta 1975; 64:241–246.
85. Heubic JE, Soloway RD, Balistreri WF. Biliary lipid composition in healthy and diseased infants, children, and young adults. Gastroenterology 1982; 82:1265–1269.
86. Schoenfield LJ, Carulli N, Dowling RH, Sama C, Wolpers C. Asymptomatic gallstones: definition and treatment. Gastroenterol Int 1989; 2:25–29.
87. Talley NJ, Phillips SF. Non-ulcer dyspepsia: potential causes and pathophysiology. Ann Intern Med 1988; 108:865–879.
88. Health and policy committee, American College of Physicians. How to study the gallbladder. Ann Intern Med 1988; 109:752–754.
89. Thistle JL, Hofmann AF, Ott BJ, Stephens DH. Chemotherapy for gallstone dissolution. Efficacy and safety. JAMA 1978; 239:1041–1046.
90. Tangedhal T, Carey WD, Ferguson DR, Forsythe S, Williams M, Paradis K, Hightower NC. Drug and treatment efficacy of chenodeoxycholic acid in 97 patients with cholelithiasis and increased surgical risk. Dig Dis Sci 1983; 28:545–551.
91. Hofmann AF. Medical treatment of cholesterol gallstones by bile desaturating agents. Hepatology 1984; 4:199S–208S.
92. Schoenfield LJ, Lachin JM, The Steering Committee, The National Cooperative Gallstone Study Group. Chenodiol (chenodeoxycholic acid) for dissolution of gallstones: the National Cooperative Gallstone Study: a controlled trial of efficacy and safety. Ann Inter Med 1981; 95:257–282.
93. Schoenfield LJ, Grundy SM, Hofmann AF, Lachin JM, Thistle JL, Tyor MP. The National Cooperative Gallstone Study viewed by its investigators. Gastroenterology 1983; 84:644–655.
94. Tokyo Cooperative Gallstone Study Group. Efficacy and indications of ursodeoxycholic acid treatment for dissolving gallstones. A multicenter double-blind trial. Gastroenterology 1980; 78:542–548.
95. Bachrach WH, Hofmann AF. Ursodeoxycholic acid in the treatment of cholesterol cholelithiasis. Dig Dis Sci 1982; 27:833–856.
96. Meredith TJ, Williams GV, Maton PN, Murphy GM, Saxton HM, Dowling RH. Retrospective comparison of "cheno" and "urso" in the medical treatment of gallstones. Gut 1982; 23:382–389.
97. Sackmann M, Delius M, Sauerbruch T, Holl J, Weber W, Ippisch E, Hagelauer U, Wess O, Hepp W, Brendel W, Paumgartner G. Shockwave lithotripsy of gallbladder stones. N Engl J Med 1988; 318:393–397.
98. Ferrucci JT, Delius M, Burhenne HJ. Biliary lithotripsy. Chicago: Year Book Medical Publishers, 1988.
99. Thistle JL, May GR, Bender CE, Williams HJ, LeRoy AJ, Nelson PE, Peine CJ, Petersen BT, McCullough ME. Dissolution of cholesterol gallbladder stones by methyl tert-butyl ether administered by percutaneous transhepatic catheter. N Engl J Med 1989; 320:633–693.
100. Paré P, Shaffer EA, Rosenthall L. Nonvisualization of the gallbladder by ^{99m}Tc-HIDA cholescintigraphy as evidence of cholecystitis. Can Med Assoc J 1978; 118:384–386.
101. Goldberg HI. Cholecystokinin cholecystography. Semin Radiol 1976; 11:175–179.
102. David GB, Berk RN, Scheible FW, Witztum KF, Gilmore IT, Strong RM, Hofmann AF. Cholecystokinin cholecystography, sonography, and scintigraphy: detection of chronic acalculous cholecystitis. AJR 1982; 139:1117–1121.
103. Brugge WR, Brand DL, Atkins HL, Lane BP, Abel WG. Gallbladder dyskinesia in chronic acalculous cholecystitis. Dig Dis Sci 1985; 31:461–467.
104. Thornell E. Mechanisms in the development of acute cholecystitis and biliary pain. A study on the role of prostaglandins and effects of indomethacin. Scand J Gastroenterol 1982; 17(Suppl 76):1–31.
105. Neiderhiser D, Thornell E, Bjorck S, Svanik J. The effect of lysophosphatidylcholine on gallbladder function in the cat. J Lab Clin Med 1983; 101:699–707.
106. Thornell E. Jivegard L, Bukhave K, Rask-Madsen J, Svanik J. Prostaglandin E_2 formation by the gallbladder in experimental cholecystitis. Gut 1986; 27:370–373.
107. Jones RS. A review of surgery for gallstone disease. Semin Liver Dis 1983; 3:157–161.
108. Thornton JR, Heaton KW, Espiner HJ, Eltringham WK. Empyema of the gallbladder: a complication in the natural history of acute cholecystitis. Gut 1983; 24:1183–1185.
109. DenBesten L, Doty JE. Pathogenesis and management of choledocholithiasis. Surg Clin North Am 1981; 61:893–906.
110. Bernhoft RA, Pellegrini CA, Motson RW, Way LW. Composition and morphologic and clinical features of common duct stones. Am J Surg 1984; 148:77–85.
111. Whiting MJ, Watts JMcK. Chemical composition of common duct stones. Br J Surg 1985; 73:229–232.
112. Cole MJ, Shaffer EA. Determinants of biliary secretory pressure: the effects of two different bile acids. Can J Physiol Pharmacol 1988; 66:1303–1307.
113. Vennes JA. Management of calculi in the common duct. Semin Liver Dis 1983; 3:162–171.
114. Palmer KR, Hofmann AF. Intraductal mono-octanoin for the direct dissolution of bile duct stones: experience in 343 patients. Gut 1985; 27:196–202.
115. Sauerbruch T, Stern M. Fragmentation of bile duct stones by extracorporeal shock waves. A new approach to biliary calculi after failure of routine endoscopic measures. Gastroenterol 1989; 95:146–152.
116. Williamson RCN. Acalculous disease of the gallbladder. Gut 1988; 29:860–872.
117. Ahlberg J, Angelin B, Einaisson K, Leijd B. Biliary lipid composition and bile acid kinetics in patients with agenesis of the gallbladder with a note on the frequency of this anomaly. Acta Chir Scand 1978; (suppl) 482:15–20.
118. Greenwood RK. Torsion of the gallbladder. Gut 1963; 4:27–29.
119. Glenn F. Acute acalculous cholecystitis. Ann Surg 1979; 189:458–465.
120. Thurston WA, Kelly EN, Silver MM. Acute acalculous cholecystitis in a premature infant treated with parenteral nutrition. Can Med Assoc J 1985; 135:332–334.
121. Traynelis VC, Hrabovsky EE. Acalculous cholecystitis in the neonate. Am J Dis Child 1985; 139:893–895.
122. Ternberg JL, Keating JP. Acute acalculous cholecystitis. Complications of other illnesses in childhood. Arch Surg 1978; 110:543–547.
123. Slovis TL, Hight DW, Philippart AI, Subois RS. Sonography in the diagnosis and management of hydrops of the gallbladder in children with mucocutaneous lymph node syndrome. Pediatrics 1980; 65:789–794.
124. Tanaka K, Shemada M, Hattori M, Utsunomiya T, Oya N. Sjogren's syndrome with abnormal manifestations of the gallbladder and central nervous system. J Pediatr Gastroenterol Nutr 1985; 4:148–151.
125. Coperman PWM, Medd WE. Diffuse systemic sclerosis with abnormal liver and gallbladder. Br Med J 1967; 3:353–354.
126. Tilvis RS, Aro J, Strandberg TE, Lempiner M, Miettinen TA. Lipid composition of bile and gallbladder mucosa in patients with acalculous cholesterolosis. Gastroenterology 1982; 82:607–615.
127. Gracie WA, Ransohoff DF. Natural history and expectant management of gallstone disease. In: Cohen S, Soloway DR, eds. Gallstones. New York: Churchill Livingstone, 1985:27.
128. Foster DR, Foster DBE. Gallbladder polyps in Peutz-Jeghers syndrome. Postgrad Med J 1980; 56:373–376.

CHAPTER 29

The Pancreas

PART 1

Congenital Anomalies

Hinda Kopelman, M.D., FRCPC

Congenital anomalies of the pancreas are often discovered incidentally at endoscopy, surgery, or autopsy. Less frequently they are associated with important clinical manifestations requiring recognition and intervention. Because they are usually the result of alterations in organ development, they are best appreciated in the context of a brief review of the embryology of the pancreas.

The human pancreas is first recognizable in the fourth week of gestation as two outpouchings of the endodermal lining of the duodenum. The dorsal bud rapidly grows away from the duodenum into an elongated structure that will form the tail, body, and part of the head of the developed pancreas. The ventral outpouching is divided into right and left portions; the left normally atrophies, whereas the right grows more slowly and is pulled posteriorly by its connection to the common bile duct as the duodenum rotates. This ventral primordium eventually fuses with the dorsal pancreatic bud to create the remainder of the head of the pancreas and the uncinate process (Fig. 1).

Each of the two pancreatic primordia possesses its own ductal system. The ventral duct, arising from the common bile duct, anastomoses with the dorsal duct to form the main pancreatic duct of Wirsung and usually preserves its association with the bile duct by opening into a common duodenal papilla, the ampulla of Vater. The duct of the dorsal bud arises directly from the duodenal wall and becomes the accessory pancreatic duct of Santorini, commonly patent in the mature pancreas.

Understanding the dual embryologic origin of the pancreas is important because of the disruption that may occur during the development, migration, and fusion of the two pancreatic buds and their ductal systems. Such errors are thought to account for a number of congenital anomalies of the pancreas, including pancreatic ductal anomalies, annular and ectopic pancreas, and agenesis, hypoplasia, and dysplasia of the pancreas. These congenital abnormalities will be discussed with respect to current understanding of their pathogenesis, clinical presentation, diagnosis, and management.

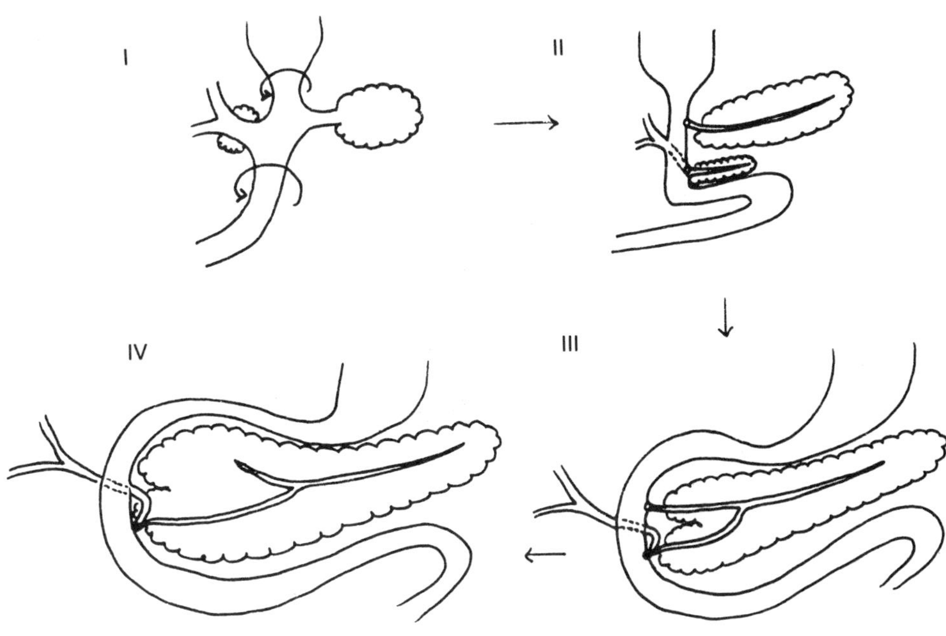

FIGURE 1 *I*, The pancreas originates as a dorsal bud and two ventral pancreatic buds. The left ventral pancreatic bud atrophies. *II*, Rotation of the stomach and duodenum with elongation of the duodenum and common bile duct has carried the right ventral pancreas around posteriorly to approximate the dorsal pancreas. *III*, Fusion of the right ventral bud with its dorsal partner completes the head and uncinate process of the pancreas. *IV*, The accessory duct and its papilla regress. The main pancreatic duct is formed from the fusion of ventral and dorsal ducts and empties into the ampulla of Vater.

ANNULAR PANCREAS

This relatively uncommon congenital anomaly was first reported in 1818 and only later received its name because of the presence of histologically normal pancreatic tissue surrounding the duodenum in a ringlike fashion.

Pathogenesis

Theories suggested to explain the development of this anomaly include hypertrophy of normal pancreatic tissue, fusion of heterotopic pancreatic rests, failure of the left ventral bud to atrophy, and failure of free rotation of pancreatic tissue of the right ventral outpouching. The last is the most accepted theory to date: As the left ventral bud atrophies, the tip of the right primordium becomes adherent to the anterior duodenum. As the duodenum rotates and the ventral bud migrates toward its dorsal partner, pancreatic tissue is drawn around the duodenum, forming the annulus.[1] This theory not only adequately accounts anatomically for the most common variants of annular pancreas but is also supported by most fetal evidence reported.[2]

Annular pancreas in children is associated with a number of other congenital malformations (Table 1), suggesting that the defect of annular pancreas is due to an early embryologic malformation. Evidence suggesting a genetic etiology is supported by the high incidence of Down's syndrome in pediatric patients with annular pancreas. Down's syndrome occurred in 30 of 146 reported pediatric cases (21 percent) in one literature review.[3] In addition, three reports of familial annular pancreas[4–6] suggest that in a small proportion of cases, this anomaly may be transmitted as a genetically dominant trait.

Clinical Presentation

Symptomatic annular pancreas may present at any age from birth, including premature birth, through adult life. In a review of 281 cases in the English literature,[3] approximately 50 percent occurred in the pediatric age group, and, of these, 86 percent presented in neonates. The age at presentation is clearly determined by the degree of duodenal obstruction and by coexistent anomalies. In one study of pediatric annular pancreas,[7] approximately half the infants had complete obstruction of the duodenum, and three-fourths had other associated congenital anomalies.

When annular pancreas results in high gastrointestinal (GI) obstruction, polyhydramnios in utero and vomiting of feeds from birth are typical. The obstruction may not be secondary to extrinsic compression of the duodenum by the pancreatic tissue ring, as frequently an associated intrinsic duodenal obstruction exists.[8]

In children presenting with symptoms attributable to annular pancreas beyond the neonatal period, and in adults, complete obstruction is unlikely. Partial obstruction may give rise to recurrent vomiting. Less frequently, annular pancreas is detected in an individual presenting with peptic ulceration.[9] Partial obstruction by the annulus, leading to chronic gastric antral distention and increased gastric acid secretion, may contribute to peptic ulceration. Kiernan et al[3] reported that the most frequent major complaint among adults presenting with annular pancreas was pain (69 percent); peptic ulcer was noted in 19 percent, and hematemesis in 10 percent. In comparison, hematemesis occurred in only 0.7 percent of pediatric patients with annular pancreas.[3]

Although jaundice was described in half the neonates presenting with annular pancreas in one study,[7] a literature review by Kiernan et al[3] noted only one case of possible common bile duct obstruction from the pancreatic annulus.

TABLE 1
Incidence of Congenital Anomalies Associated with Annular Pancreas

Anomaly	Pediatric Cases (n = 146)	Adult Cases (n = 135)
Down's syndrome	30	0
Intestinal malrotation	29	2
Intrinsic duodenal obstruction	28	11
Cardiac defects	27	2
Meckel's diverticulum	9	1
Imperforate anus	8	0
Duodenal bands	7	1
Spinal defects	3	0
Cryptorchidism	2	0
Other	8	1

Modified from Kiernan et al.[3]
In some cases of annular pancreas there were no associated anomalies, whereas in others more than one anomaly were present.

Diagnosis

In neonates, the typical appearance of a "double bubble" effect on supine and upright plain abdominal films with the absence of distal small bowel gas suggests a high GI obstruction, requiring urgent operative relief. The differential diagnosis includes duodenal atresia/stenosis, duodenal web, Ladd's bands, and volvulus associated with anomalies of intestinal rotation.

In children beyond the neonatal period and in adults, barium studies demonstrate a smooth symmetric filling defect and proximal duodenal luminal dilatation, with or without partial gastric outlet obstruction (Fig. 2).

Definitive diagnosis is made at laparotomy. The annular pancreas can be recognized as a band of pinkish white tissue, 0.8 to 5.0 cm in diameter, involving the second portion of the duodenum in 85 percent of cases and usually proximal to the ampulla of Vater. Its tissue surrounds the duodenum, firmly attaches to it, and often grows into the duodenal wall.

Management

Surgical intervention is mandatory in cases of pancreatic annulus with obstruction. However, direct division of the annular ring is not recommended[3,7,8]; such attempts may be technically difficult, if not impossible, owing to the frequent intramural invasion of pancreatic tissue; division of the pancreatic tissue and its duct[10] is associated with a high risk of pancreatic peritonitis, postoperative pancreatitis, pancreatic fistulas, and late fibrosis; the frequent association of intrinsic duodenal obstruction by stenosis, atresia, or web[11]

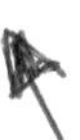

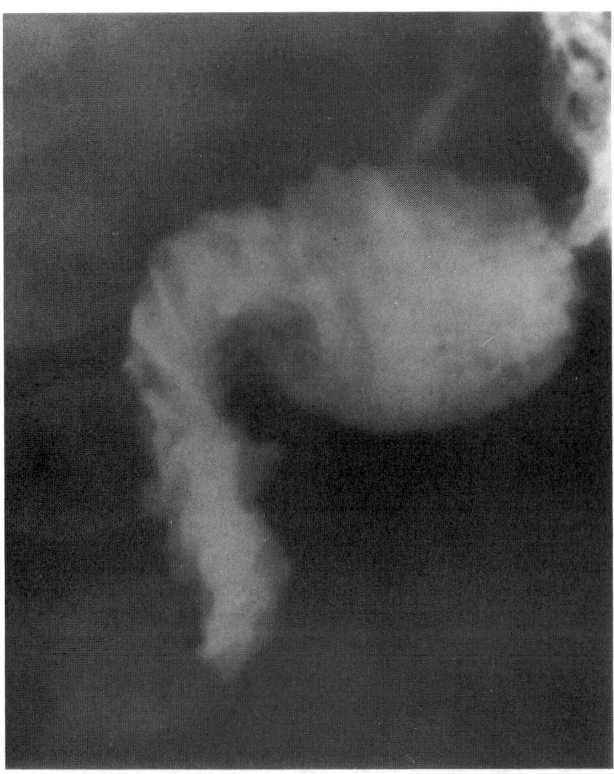

FIGURE 2 Barium study demonstrating a fixed filling defect of the duodenum with proximal dilatation due to annular pancreas in a 21-month-old child.

accounts for the high morbidity and rate of reoperation for incomplete relief of obstruction when this approach was used.

The recommended surgical approach is a bypass operation, preferably duodenoduodenostomy. Duodenojejunostomy is a second alternative. Gastroenterostomy, associated with a significant risk of stomal or anastomotic ulceration unless combined with vagotomy, is discouraged in the pediatric population.

ECTOPIC PANCREAS

Variously referred to as heterotopic, accessory, or aberrant pancreas, ectopic pancreas is defined as the presence of pancreatic tissue lacking anatomic and vascular continuity with the main body of the pancreas.

Pathogenesis

Although heterotopia is generally thought to occur secondary to an antenatal event, it is unlikely that a single embryologic mechanism can account for all presentations of this anomaly. Theories regarding the pathogenesis of ectopic pancreas have included the following: in situ errors of pluripotent endodermal stem cell differentiation; multiple ventral pancreatic buds with failure of atrophy and subsequent growth and sequestration of pancreatic tissue; adhesion of embryonic pancreatic cells to neighboring structures during elongation and rotation of the gut and pancreatic primordia; and budding of pancreatic tissue from the embryonic anlagen or from pancreatic ducts de novo, with attachment to the gut wall and separation from the main pancreas during elongation of the GI tract.

Clinical Presentation

The incidence of ectopic pancreas has been examined in both autopsy and surgical series. Most series place the autopsy rate at 1 to 2 percent[12,18] and the rate of recognition at the time of laparotomy at 0.2 percent.[13] In children, the incidence is far less than the numbers reported from autopsy series would suggest. Furthermore, among a group of patients with ectopic pancreas in the stomach, only 2 percent were children.[14] These lower incidences probably reflect the decreased likelihood of detection of ectopic tissue during radiographic, endoscopic, or surgical exploration alone and the far lower incidence of these interventions in the pediatric population. While this may change with the increased use of double-contrast radiography and endoscopy in children, the higher autopsy numbers do suggest that ectopic pancreatic tissue is rarely symptomatic enough by itself to prompt evaluation. This was confirmed by a study of 212 nonautopsy cases.[15]

Because of the close developmental association of the embryonic pancreatic primordial buds to the foregut, it is not surprising that 70 to 90 percent of pancreatic ectopia occurs in the upper GI tract.[15,16] Most pancreatic ectopia in the upper GI tract is found in the gastric antrum. However, pancreatic ectopia has been reported to occur throughout the GI tract. In one study,[15] 5 percent occurred in Meckel's diverticula, 1 percent in the ileum, and 4 percent outside the GI tract itself. Extraintestinal sites have included the liver, gallbladder, omentum, lungs, and umbilicus, although this list may not be exhaustive.

In most cases, this congenital anomaly is an incidental finding and requires no further investigation or management. The most common clinical symptoms that have been attributed to ectopic pancreas include abdominal (especially epigastric) pain, dyspepsia, and GI bleeding. Although a causal relationship between the ectopic tissue and these symptoms is often questionable in the absence of other pathology, this finding cannot be completely dismissed.

There are several case reports of aberrant pancreatic tissue causing serious clinical problems. Massive upper GI bleeding[17] has been reported in association with ectopic pancreas secondary to inflammation and ulceration of the tissue or adjacent structures. Partial pyloric obstruction by ectopic tissue in the gastric antrum has been described, as well as obstruction of the ampulla of Vater, the intestine, and the biliary tree. It has been reported as a cause of cholecystitis, intussusception, and jejunal atresia. Pancreatitis in the ectopic tissue and severe inflammation with necrosis of adjacent structures have been reported.[18] Several cases of cancer occurring in ectopic pancreatic tissue have been described.[19]

Diagnosis

Although definitive diagnosis is made histologically, the majority of cases occurring in the gastric antrum have a unique radiographic and endoscopic appearance that often

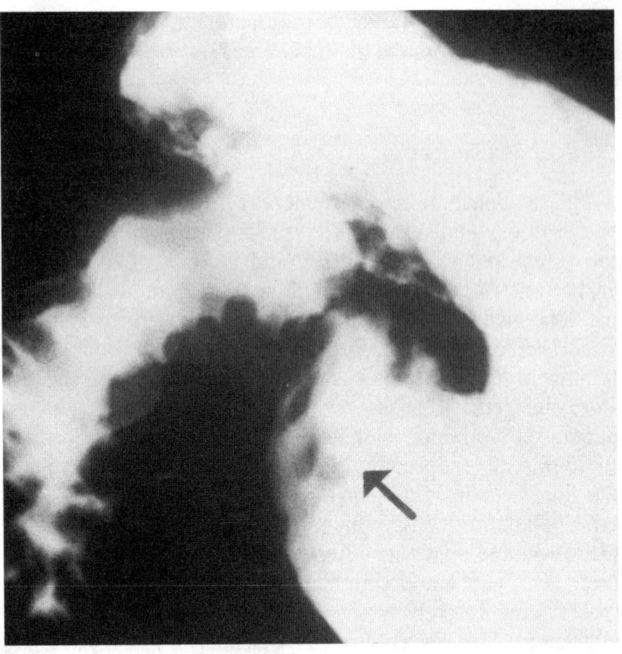

FIGURE 3 Typical radiographic appearance of ectopic pancreas (*arrow*) in the antrum of the stomach. Note the surrounding halo and central umbilication, which contains barium.

makes possible a diagnosis in the absence of surgical excision and pathologic confirmation. Radiographically and endoscopically, ectopic pancreas is recognizable as a well-defined dome-shaped filling defect, usually less than 1 cm, often along the greater curvature of the antrum or in the prepyloric region, with a central umbilication (Fig. 3). While similar in appearance to leiomyomas, these latter are often located more proximally in the fundus and are larger in size. Mucosal biopsy yields normal gastric mucosa because the nodules are submucosal or subserosal in location. Pathologic examination of ectopic pancreatic tissue usually reveals normal pancreatic lobules with all the elements of pancreatic ducts, acini, and islets of Langerhans. Occasionally, only widely separated pancreatic ductal structures are evident.

Management

Management remains somewhat controversial. Because this abnormality is largely asymptomatic and rarely associated with clinical pathology, the incidental finding of such a lesion, especially when characteristic, does not necessarily warrant surgical excision. However, in the complicated situations, when clinical symptoms may be associated with its presence or when its appearance is difficult to differentiate from other lesions such as leiomyoma or carcinoid, excision may be indicated.

PANCREATIC AGENESIS, HYPOPLASIA, AND DYSPLASIA

Although complete agenesis of the pancreas is rare and usually incompatible with life, varying degrees of partial agenesis, dysplasia, and hypoplasia do occur, and their recognition may have important clinical implications for diagnosis and management.

Pathogenesis

The spectrum of entities, including complete and partial agenesis of the pancreas, is believed to arise from a primary defect in early embryonic organogenesis. In partial agenesis, histologically normal pancreatic tissue is formed, but the size and shape of the gland are limited by the lack of development of structures arising from one of the pancreatic primordia. It is more commonly due to dorsal pancreatic agenesis. This condition should not be confused with the entities of pancreatic hypoplasia and dysplasia in which the pancreas has developed normally in size and shape but has suffered severe disruption of the normal process of cellular differentiation. In pancreatic hypoplasia, replacement of much of the exocrine epithelial structures with fatty tissue and reduction in the number of smaller ducts and their terminal differentiation are characteristic. In dysplasia, the parenchyma is disorganized, with dilated primitive ducts surrounded by fibromuscular collars.

The occurrence of this diverse group of disorders in chromosomal trisomy syndromes[20] and in siblings[21] suggests that some may be genetic in origin. However, an early intrauterine insult may account for both the failure of normal differentiation and the presence of dysplastic and degenerative pathologic features in some cases.[22]

Clinical Presentation

The clinical manifestations of these disorders may be attributable to both exocrine and endocrine pancreatic dysfunction.

Agenesis. Case reports of congenital absence of the pancreas, confirmed at autopsy, describe infants with significant intrauterine growth retardation, insulin-dependent hyperglycemia, and decreased survival beyond the neonatal period.[23,24] The intrauterine growth retardation is due to the lack of fetal insulin and its important trophic effects in utero.[23] The hyperglycemia differs from juvenile diabetes mellitus in its lack of associated hyperglucagonemia. These infants would also be expected to suffer from severe failure to thrive postnatally, with associated diarrhea, hypoalbuminemia, and anemia, as a result of exocrine pancreatic insufficiency and malabsorption. One case report of such a living infant with both endocrine and exocrine insufficiency attributed to functional pancreatic agenesis may not represent true agenesis, as no radiologic, surgical, or autopsy evidence was available to confirm the diagnosis.[25]

Cases of partial pancreatic agenesis, sometimes referred to in the literature as congenital short pancreas, are unlikely to be symptomatic with either endocrine or exocrine pancreatic insufficiency, because of the presence of adequate tissue to maintain normal function. The patients have been reported to present in adult life with abdominal or back pain. The finding of partial pancreatic agenesis has not always been clearly linked to the presenting symptoms and therefore may be simply an incidental finding. However, the possibility of an association between it and the development of recurrent or chronic pancreatitis has been raised.[26,27]

Hypoplasia and Dysplasia. Individuals with pancreatic hypoplasia or dysplasia that is severe enough to reduce the functional exocrine tissue to less than 2 to 5 percent of normal manifest exocrine pancreatic insufficiency and malabsorption but can be differentiated from partial agenesis because of the presence of normal tissue size at radiologic examination, at surgery, or at autopsy. These individuals may have endocrine tissue adequate to maintain euglycemia unless they are very severely affected.

The association of pancreatic hypoplasia and dysplasia with other congenital anomalies has taken many forms, including the Schwachman-Diamond syndrome,[28] sideroblastic bone marrow dysfunction in association with pancreatic dysfunction,[29] Johanson-Blizzard syndrome,[30,31] and a number of syndromes of variable involvement of hepatic, renal, and pancreatic dysplasia.[32,33]

Diagnosis

Definitive anatomic diagnosis of pancreatic agenesis, complete or partial, can be made at surgery or autopsy. However, useful diagnostic aids in the past have included angiography, selenomethionine scanning, and endoscopic retrograde cholangiopancreatography (ERCP). More recently, these have been replaced or complemented by abdominal sonography and computed tomography (CT). The latter has been useful in diagnosing dorsal pancreatic agenesis when findings at ERCP were misleading and incorrectly suggested the diagnosis of pancreas divisum.[34] In addition, abdominal CT can be helpful in detecting pancreatic hypoplasia because of the altered tissue density secondary to fatty replacement of exocrine structures.

Functional diagnosis in pancreatic aplasia, hypoplasia, and dysplasia syndromes is of prime clinical importance, as it dictates management strategies. The documentation of significant fat malabsorption on a 72-hour fecal fat balance study, an abnormally low circulating immunoreactive trypsinogen level, or an abnormal bentiromide test all confirm the absence of sufficient pancreatic exocrine secretion to maintain normal digestion. Although differentiation among agenesis, hypoplasia, and dysplasia of the pancreas requires anatomic studies, patients with any of these disorders and functional pancreatic insufficiency require similar forms of medical management.

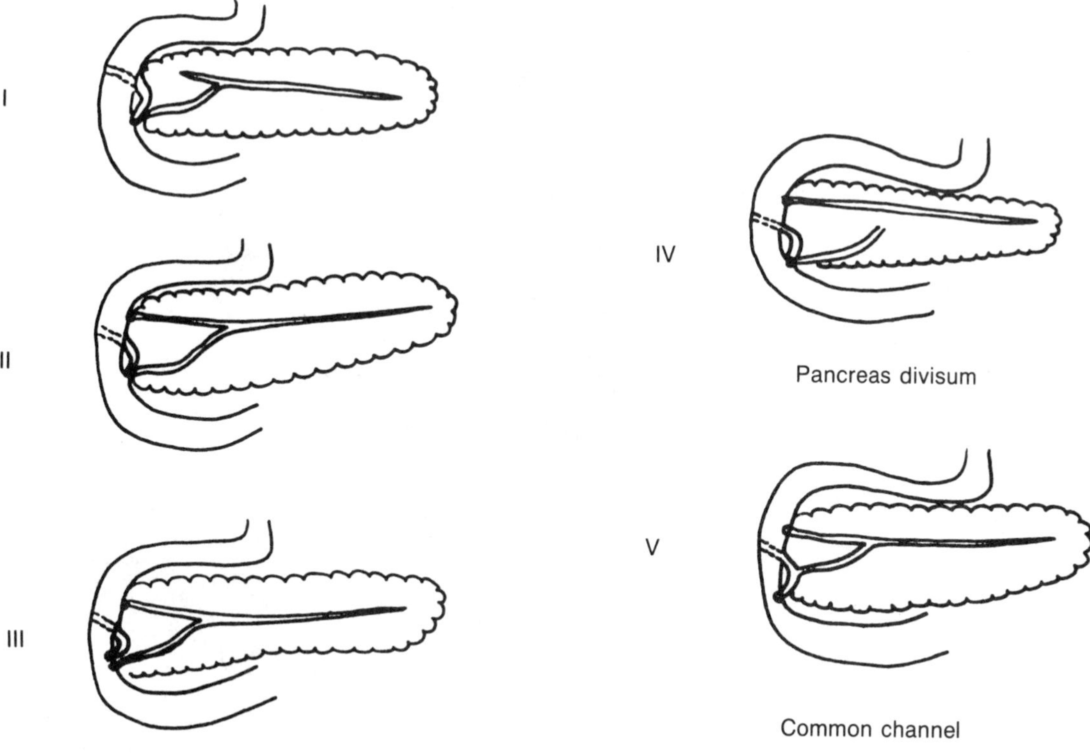

FIGURE 4 Five of the more common ductal anatomic variants are diagrammed. *I*, In the most common variant, seen in 40 to 50 percent of individuals, the main pancreatic duct (Wirsung) enters the duodenum together with the common bile duct at the ampulla of Vater. The accessory pancreatic duct (Santorini) has regressed. *II*, In the second most common variant, the accessory duct of Santorini persists and enters the duodenum proximal to the ampulla of Vater through the accessory ampulla. This occurs in approximately 35 percent of cases. *III*, In 5 percent of individuals, the main pancreatic duct enters the duodenum separately from the common bile duct. The accessory duct and ampulla may or may not be present. *IV*, Pancreas divisum occurs in 5 to 10 percent of individuals when main and accessory pancreatic ducts do not communicate. *V*, In 5 to 10 percent of individuals, the main pancreatic duct enters the common bile duct 5 to 15 mm before the ampulla of Vater, creating a common channel of pancreaticobiliary secretion.

The absence of functional insufficiency does not exclude the diagnosis of partial aplasia, hypoplasia, or dysplasia of milder degree. In this instance, quantitative stimulated pancreatic secretion studies can assess the degree of pancreatic exocrine tissue reserve compared to normal.

In patients with hyperglycemia, the diagnosis of pancreatic agenesis or severe hypoplasia should be entertained when glucagon levels and responses are blunted, in contrast to the excesses seen typically in patients with hyperglycemia due to insulin-dependent diabetes mellitus.

Management

Patients with documented functional pancreatic exocrine insufficiency require aggressive oral supplementation with pancreatic enzymes and fat-soluble vitamins and provision of a high-energy diet containing balanced protein, carbohydrate, and fat. When well-managed, pancreatic insufficiency should not contribute to growth failure. Endocrine insufficiency requires the introduction of insulin in all patients with agenesis but less frequently in those with partial aplasia, hypoplasia, or dysplasia of the pancreas.

DUCTAL ANOMALIES

Normal embryologic fusion of the two pancreatic primordia and their ductal systems leads to a number of common variations in the anatomy of the pancreatic ductal system (Fig. 4). However, only two of these common variants have been implicated in the pathogenesis of clinical disease: pancreas divisum and anomalous junction of the common bile duct.

Pancreas Divisum

Pancreas divisum refers to the congenital abnormality resulting from incomplete fusion of dorsal and ventral pancreatic ductal systems. It is the most common congenital anomaly of the pancreas. Controversy surrounds the contention that it is a treatable cause of acute recurrent pancreatitis.

Pathogenesis

In pancreas divisum, the dorsal pancreatic duct functions as the main drainage system for the bulk of the pancreatic tissue but opens into the relatively smaller accessory papilla. Some have suggested that during pancreatic stimulation and secretion, increased pressure within this ductal system and an associated anatomic or functional stenosis at the accessory papilla account for the development of acute and recurrent pancreatitis in these individuals, who lack an alternate pancreatic outflow tract.

Clinical Presentation

The importance of pancreas divisum in clinical disease was first highlighted when it was identified in 25 percent of adult patients with documented pancreatitis not due to alcohol or biliary tract disease.[35] This figure was far greater than the 5 to 10 percent incidence of this anatomic variant noted in most autopsy or endoscopic series.[36] However, the argument for a causal relationship between the anatomic finding and clinical symptomatology has met with controversy.[36]

The true incidence of clinical pancreatic symptoms with this anomaly remains unknown. The spectrum of clinical findings that have been suggested to be causally linked to this congenital anomaly or variant includes recurrent attacks of documented acute pancreatitis and intermittent or continuous epigastric pain, often radiating to the back, in the absence of hyperamylasemia.[37] No evidence supports a causal relationship between pancreas divisum and chronic pancreatitis, although the two do occur together.

No reports of the natural history of symptomatic patients with pancreas divisum have been published. For the most part, these individuals are thought to maintain normal pancreatic parenchyma and ductal structure, with neither spontaneous resolution nor severe progression to chronic pancreatitis.[37] However, a report of patients with pancreas divisum and dorsal pancreatic fibrosis but normal ventral pancreatic tissue[38] may represent the potential for more advanced pathology within the spectrum of clinical presentations.

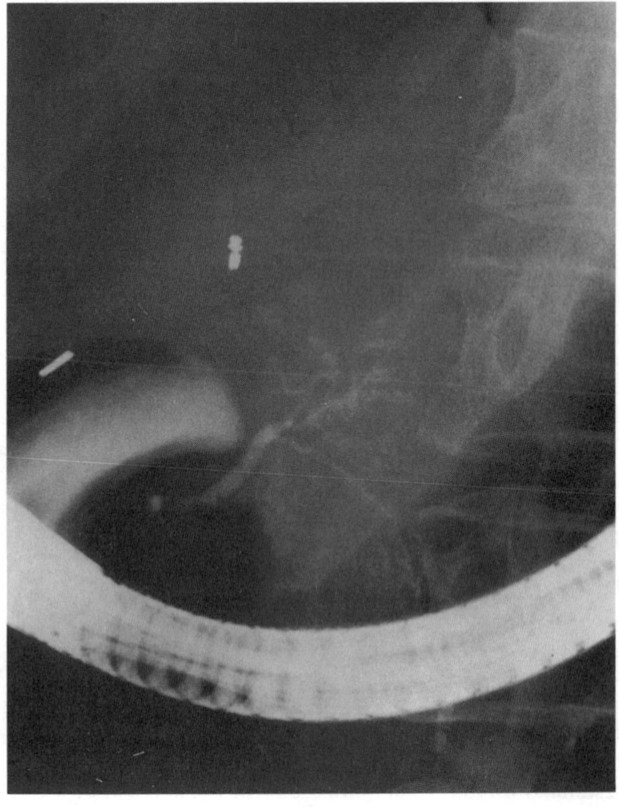

FIGURE 5 Pancreas divisum suggested by this endoscopic retrograde cholangiopancreatogram demonstrating a short duct of Wirsung confined to the head of the pancreas and ending in terminal arborizations with no filling of the duct draining the body and tail of the pancreas. (Courtesy of Dr. Jabbari, Montreal General Hospital, Division of Gastroenterology.)

A number of reports have described the occurrence of pancreas divisum in the pediatric population.[39-43] The ages of the children at the time of presentation ranged from 5 to 18 years. As in adults, these children presented with acute and recurrent pancreatitis; a number had pancreatic pseudocysts at the time of diagnosis. In one series of 25 children with acute recurrent pancreatitis, 16 percent were found to have pancreas divisum and no other explanation for their recurrent attacks of pancreatitis.[40,42]

Diagnosis

Diagnosis of pancreas divisum depends on ERCP, which has been successfully performed in children without undue complications.[39-43] Typically, cannulation of the ampulla of Vater fails to demonstrate the normal pancreatic ductal configuration. Instead, a short duct of Wirsung, confined to the head of the gland, ends in fine terminal arborizations and there is no filling of the main pancreatic duct (Fig. 5). The duct of Wirsung may even be completely absent in approximately 5 percent of cases. To confirm the diagnosis, the accessory papilla should be cannulated in order to visualize the normal dorsal duct of Santorini, draining the remainder of the gland. This is not always technically possible, although some skilled endoscopists using newer catheters have reported success in at least 90 percent of cases.[36] Alternatively, the accessory duct can be cannulated at laparotomy in the tail of the pancreas and pancreas divisum confirmed by operative pancreatogram.

Proponents of pancreas divisum as a cause of symptoms have suggested that the patients most likely to benefit from surgical intervention are those with anatomic or functional obstruction of the accessory papilla.[44] Attempts at manometric measurements of sphincter pressure[45] and sphincter size and sonographic documentation of duct dilatation during secretin stimulation[46] have been proposed in adults. To date there have been no reports of their use in children.

Management

Because of the controversy surrounding pancreas divisum as a clinical problem, the approach to management also remains controversial.[37,47] Conservative medical approaches are not usually associated with spontaneous improvement or resolution; pharmacologic attempts to alter functional stenosis of the accessory papilla have been unsuccessful; and trials of oral pancreatic enzyme supplements, advocated to treat chronic pancreatic pain by suppressing pancreatic exocrine secretion,[48] have not decreased symptoms. These approaches should, however, be considered on an individual basis.

Endoscopic balloon dilatation, papillotomy, and stenting have all been attempted. They are technically difficult, may precipitate pancreatitis, and are commonly associated with restenosis. Sphincteroplasty involving the accessory papilla is the preferred surgical approach. It is often combined with sphincteroplasty of the main papilla and should be performed when pancreatic inflammation is minimal. It has been associated with a definite but limited success rate. The best results have been achieved in individuals presenting with acute recurrent pancreatitis, in the absence of chronic pancreatitis, and with objective evidence of accessory papilla stenosis.[44] In refractory cases, distal pancreatic resections with or without distal drainage into a Roux-en-Y loop of intestine have been carried out. Although this may result in pain relief in some cases, it is rarely advocated as the procedure of choice.

Common Channel Syndrome

Anomalous junctions of the common bile duct and the main pancreatic duct are frequently encountered anatomic variants (see Fig. 4) and have been implicated in the pathogenesis of choledochal cysts and pancreatitis.

Pathogenesis

The presence of a long common channel with the pancreaticobiliary junction located outside the duodenal wall has been associated with both the development of pancreatitis and the pathogenesis of choledochal cysts.[49-52] Animal models that recreate the anatomy of a long common channel have implicated reflux of pancreatic juice into the bile duct in the pathogenesis of choledochal cyst. In addition, the finding of very high amylase values in the choledochal cyst fluid at surgery has corroborated this concept. The occurrence of pancreatitis associated with anomalous junctions of the pancreaticobiliary tree is presumably due to the reflux of bile into the pancreatic duct; bile is a known experimental initiator of intense pancreatitis. Reflux of ductal contents in either direction apparently occurs owing to the absence of the sphincter of Oddi, which normally prevents this at the intraduodenal junction of the two ductal systems; it may also be related to the angle between the two systems at their junction.

Clinical Presentation

More than half of all cases of choledochal cyst present before the age of 10 years. The classic presentation is that of abdominal pain, usually right upper quadrant pain, jaundice, and a palpable right upper quadrant mass. Fever and vomiting may often be present, Occasionally, cholangitis and severe sepsis may occur. The occurrence of elevated serum amylase values is not uncommon. The abdominal pain that is invariably present may be due to concomitant pancreatitis, in addition to possible cholangitis.

Diagnosis

Abdominal sonography is often diagnostic of choledochal cyst but can be aided by CT, nuclear scanning of the biliary tree, and ERCP. As the use of these techniques has increased, so has the diagnosis of choledochal cyst. Recognition of the presence of a long common channel can be made only by ERCP or at the time of laparotomy and intraoperative cholangiography.

Management

Management of choledochal cyst should include complete resection of the extrahepatic cyst in addition to the creation of a Roux-en-Y hepatojejunostomy. Complications of cholangitis with recurrent stenosis requiring reoperation and an increased incidence of occurrence of carcinoma in any residual cyst mucosa[53] have discouraged the use of simple drainage procedures.

REFERENCES

1. Laughlin EH, Keown ME, Jackson JE. Heterotopic pancreas obstructing the ampulla of Vater. Arch Surg 1983; 118:979-980.
2. Ikeda Y, Irving IM. Annular pancreas in a fetus and its three-dimensional reconstruction. J Pediatr Surg 1984; 19:160-164.
3. Kiernan PD, ReMine SG, Kiernan PC, ReMine WH. Annular pancreas. Arch Surg 1980; 115:46-50.
4. Jackson LG, Apostolides P. Autosomal dominant inheritance of annular pancreas. Am J Med Genet 1978; 1:319-321.
5. Montgomery RC, Poindexter MH, Hall GH, Leigh JE. Report of a case of annular pancreas of the newborn in two consecutive siblings. Pediatrics 1971; 48:148-149.
6. MacFadyen UM, Young ID. Annular pancreas in mother and son. Am J Med Genet 1987; 27:987-988.
7. Merrill JR, Raffensperger JG. Pediatric annular pancreas: twenty years experience. J Pediatr Surg 1976; 11:921-925.
8. Ravitch MM. The pancreas in infants and children. Surg Clin North Am 1975; 377-385.
9. Johnston DWB. Annular pancreas: a new classification and clinical observations. Can J Surg 1978; 21:241-244.
10. Heyman RL, Whelan TJ Jr. Annular pancreas: demonstration of the annular duct on cholangiography. Ann Surg 1967; 165:3.
11. Elliot GB, Klinen MR, Elliot KA. Pancreatic annulus: a sign or a cause of duodenal obstruction? Can J Surg 1968; 11:357-364.
12. Strobel CT, Smith LE, Fonkalsrud EW, Isenberg JN. Ectopic pancreatic tissue in the gastric antrum. J Pediatr 1978; 92:586-588.
13. Barbosa JdeC, Dockerty MB, Waugh JM. Pancreatic heterotopia: review of the literature and report of 41 authenticated surgical cases of which 25 were clinically significant. Surg Gynecol Obstet 1946; 82:527-542.
14. Palmer ED. Aberrant pancreatic tumours. Medicine 1951; 30:83-96.
15. Dolan RV, ReMine WH, Dockerty MB. The fate of heterotopic pancreatic tissue: a study of 212 cases. Arch Surg 1974; 109:762-765.
16. Pearson S. Aberrant pancreas: review of the literature and report of three cases, one of which produced common and pancreatic duct obstruction. Arch Surg 1951; 63:168-184.
17. Clark RE, Teplick SK. Ectopic pancreas causing massive upper GI hemorrhage. Gastroenterology 1975; 69:1331-1333.
18. Fan S, O'Brian DS, Borger JA. Ectopic pancreas with acute inflammation. J Pediatr Surg 1982; 17:86-87.
19. Hickman DM, Frey CF, Carson JW. Adenocarcinoma arising in gastric heterotopic pancreas. West J Med 1981; 135:57-62.
20. Warkany J, Pasarge E, Smith LB. Congenital malformations in autosomal trisomy syndromes. Am J Dis Child 1966; 112:502-517.
21. Winter WE, Maclaren NK, Riley WJ, Toskes PP, Andres J, Rosenbloom AL. Congenital pancreatic hypoplasia: a syndrome of exocrine and endocrine pancreatic insufficiency. J Pediatr 1986; 109:465-468.
22. Lumb G, Beautyman W. Hypoplasia of the exocrine tissue of the pancreas. J Pathol Bacteriol 1952; 64:679-686.
23. Lemons JA, Ridenour R, Orsini EN. Congenital absence of the pancreas and intrauterine growth retardation. Pediatrics 1979; 64:255-257.
24. Dourov N, Buyl-Strouvens ML. Agenesie du pancreas. Arch Fr Pediatr 1969; 26:641.
25. Howard CP, Go VLW, Infante AJ, Perrault J, Gerich GE, Haymond MW. Longterm survival in a case of functional pancreatic agenesis. J Pediatr 1980; 97:786-789.
26. Gilinsky NH, Del Favero G, Cotton PB, Leer WR. Congenital short pancreas: a report of two cases. Gut 1985; 26:304-310.
27. Bretagne JF, Darnault P, Raoul JL, Gadron Y, Gosselin M, Cousin P, Gastard J. Calcifying pancreatitis of a congenital short pancreas: a case report with successful endoscopic papillotomy. Am J Gastroenterol 1987; 82:1314-1317.
28. Shwachman H, Diamond L, Oski F, Khaw K. The syndrome of pancreatic insufficiency and bone marrow dysfunction. J Pediatr 1964; 65:645-663.
29. Pearson H, Lobel J, Kocoshis S, Naiman J, Windmiller J, Lammi A, Hoffman R, Marsh J. A new syndrome of refractory sideroblastic anemia with vacuolization of marrow precursors and exocrine pancreatic dysfunction. J Pediatr 1979; 95:976-984.
30. Johanson A, Blizzard R. A syndrome of congenital aplasia of the alae nasai, deafness, hypothyroidism, dwarfism, absent permanent teeth, and malabsorption. J Pediatr 1971; 79:982-987.
31. Moeschler JB, Polak MJ, Jenkins JJ, Amato RSS. The Johanson Blizzard syndrome: a second report of full autopsy findings. Am J Med Genet 1987; 26:133-138.
32. Yeoh GPS, Bannatyne PM, Russell P, Storey B. Combined renal and pancreatic dysplasia in the newborn. Pathology 1985; 17:653-657.
33. Bernstein J, Chandra M, Creswel J, Kahn E, Malouf NN, McVicar M, Weinberg AG, Wybel RE. Renal-hepatic-pancreatic dysplasia: a syndrome reconsidered. Am J Med Genet 1987; 26:391-403.
34. Shah KK, DeRidder PH, Schwab RE, Alexander TJ. CT diagnosis of dorsal pancreatic agenesis. J Comput Assist Tomogr 1987; 11:170-171.
35. Cotton PB. Congenital anomaly of pancreas divisum as a cause of obstructive pain and pancreatitis. Gut 1980; 21:105-114.
36. Delhaye M, Engelholm L, Cremer M. Pancreas divisum: congenital anatomical variant or anomaly? Gastroenterology 1985; 89:951-958.
37. Warshaw AL. Pancreas divisum: a case for surgical treatment. Adv Surg 1987; 21:93-110.
38. Blair AJ, Russell CG, Cotton PB. Resection for pancreatitis in patients with pancreas divisum. Ann Surg 1984; 200:590-594.
39. Blustein PK, Gaskin K, Filler R, Ho C, Connon J. Endoscopic retrograde cholangiopancreatography in pancreatitis in children and adolescents. Pediatrics 1981; 68:387-393.
40. Cotton PB, Laage NJ. ERCP in children. Arch Dis Child 1982; 57:131-136.
41. Yedlin ST, Dubois RS, Philippart AI. Pancreas divisum: a cause of pancreatitis in childhood. J Pediatr Surg 1984; 19:793-794.
42. Forbes A, Leung JWC, Cotton PB. Relapsing acute and chronic pancreatitis. Arch Dis Child 1984; 59:927-934.
43. Wagner CW, Golladay ES. Pancreas divisum and pancreatitis in children. Am Surg 1988; 22-26.
44. Warshaw AL, Richter JM, Schapiro RH. The cause and treatment of pancreatitis associated with pancreas divisum. Ann Surg 1983; 198:443-452.
45. Geenen JE, Hogan WJ, Dodds WJ, Stewart ET, Arrdorfer RC. Intraluminal pressure recording from the human sphincter of Oddi. Gastroenterology 1980; 78:317-324.
46. Warshaw AL, Simeone J, Schapiro RH, Hedberg SE, Mueller PE, Ferruci JT. Objective evaluation of ampullary stenosis with ultrasonography and pancreatic stimulation. Am J Surg 1985; 149:65-72.
47. Harig JM, Hogan WJ. Pancreas divisum: a case against surgical treatment. Adv Surg 1987; 21:111-126.
48. Slaff J, Jacobson D, Tillman CR, Curington C, Toskes P. Protease specific suppression of pancreatic exocrine secretion. Gastroenterology 1984; 87:44-52.
49. Kato O, Hattori K, Suzuki T, Tachio F, Yuasa T. Clinical significance of anomalous pancreaticobiliary union. Gastrointest Endosc 1983; 29:94-98.
50. Todani T, Watanabe Y, Fujii T, Vemura S. Anomalous arrangement of the pancreaticobiliary ductal system in patients with a choledochal cyst. Am J Surg 1984; 147:672-676.
51. Rattner DW, Schapiro RH, Warshaw AL. Abnormalities of pancreatic and biliary ducts in adult patients with choledochal cysts. Arch Surg 1983; 118:1068-1074.
52. Okada A, Oguchi Y, Kamata S, Ikeda Y, Kawashima Y, Saito R. Common channel syndrome: diagnosis with ERCP and surgical management. Surgery 1983; 93:634-642.
53. Lilly JR. The surgical treatment of choledochal cyst. Surg Gynecol Obstet 1979; 149:36.

PART 2

Cystic Fibrosis

Gordon Forstner, M.D., FRCPC
Peter R. Durie, B.Sc., M.D., FRCPC

GENERAL FEATURES

Cystic fibrosis (CF) is an inherited disease that affects many secreting epithelial tissues but is principally recognized by pulmonary and pancreatic failure. It was first separated from other "celiac" syndromes and the relationship between the pancreatic and lung lesions clarified by Fanconi et al[1] in Germany and Anderson[2] in the United States. The demonstration of pancreatic insufficiency was the key to the clinical diagnosis until di Sant'Agnese et al[3] showed that patients secreted sweat containing high concentrations of sodium chloride. The one essential finding for diagnosis continues to be that of a high sweat sodium or chloride. In 1950, Gibbs et al[4] showed that steatorrhea was not seen in all patients. Since then it has gradually become apparent that the clinical expression of the disease may be quite variable.

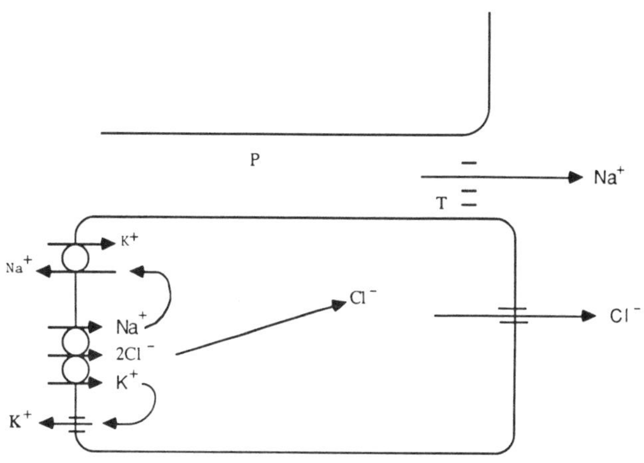

FIGURE 1 The ion channel hook-up of a typical epithelial cell biologically engineered to produce a net secretion of chloride through the epithelial membrane into the lumen. Sodium follows chloride, but through a paracellular route, in response to the electrical gradient set up by chloride. Note that chloride moves "down hill," because the three basal channels cause it to accumulate internally. Na+ = sodium; K+ = potassium; Cl− = chloride; P = paracellular route; T = tight junction. The circles in the basolateral membrane denote coupled ion transporters.

ETIOLOGY AND PATHOGENESIS

The electrolyte abnormalities in sweat are evidence of a secretory lesion that probably affects all epithelial cells. Quinton[5] initially showed that chloride permeation was defective in the sweat duct, and this work was quickly followed by evidence of a similar defect in the respiratory tract epithelium.[6] Subsequent work in the isolated secretory coil of the sweat gland,[7] respiratory epithelium,[8] and isolated secretory cells in culture[9] has revealed that apical chloride channels are present but unresponsive to regulatory pathways involving cyclic AMP. Patch clamp techniques have recently been used to show that specific chloride channels that open in the presence of the catalytic subunit of cyclic AMP–dependent protein kinase and ATP in normal cells do not do so in cells cultured from CF patients.[10]

Currently, therefore, the key defect in CF appears to involve the activation of a regulatory protein that controls the opening or "gating" of an apical plasma membrane chloride channel. Apical chloride channels are important elements in the secretion of sodium chloride by epithelial cells[11] (Fig. 1). In these cells basolateral membrane transport processes give rise to the intracellular accumulation of chloride ion to levels exceeding its electrochemical potential in the cell exterior. When the apical chloride channel opens, the electrochemical gradient causes chloride to exit through the apical membrane, generating a lumen-negative voltage that stimulates sodium exit through paracellular tight junctions. Secretion of water follows the movement of sodium and chloride. Defective apical chloride channels should therefore lead to a diminished secretory volume. This is the case in the pancreas, where secretin normally stimulates ductal secretion via a cyclic AMP–mediated response,[12] probably involving the activation of an apical chloride channel.[13] In patients with CF, secretin-induced secretion of chloride, bicarbonate, and fluid is deficient even when the pancreatic acini appear to be spared.[14] Secretagogues such as cholera toxin and vasoactive intestinal peptide (VIP), which stimulate secretion via cyclic AMP–responsive chloride channels, induce a pronounced secretory response in the intestine. These channels appear to be defective in CF.[15]

Many of the manifestations of CF are consistent with a general lack of success in maintaining the luminal hydration of macromolecules. Mucous secretions in the bronchi and intestine are viscid and inspissated, and crypts are distended with secretions as if fluid flow were insufficient to wash them outward. The glands that are affected earliest, such as the pancreas and vas deferens, appear to be vulnerable to flow-related problems because of the tortuosity and length of their ducts or the high protein concentration of their secretions. Measurements of protein in CF meconium suggest relative dehydration,[16] and pancreatic juice protein is hyperconcentrated even in CF patients in whom the pancreas seems other-

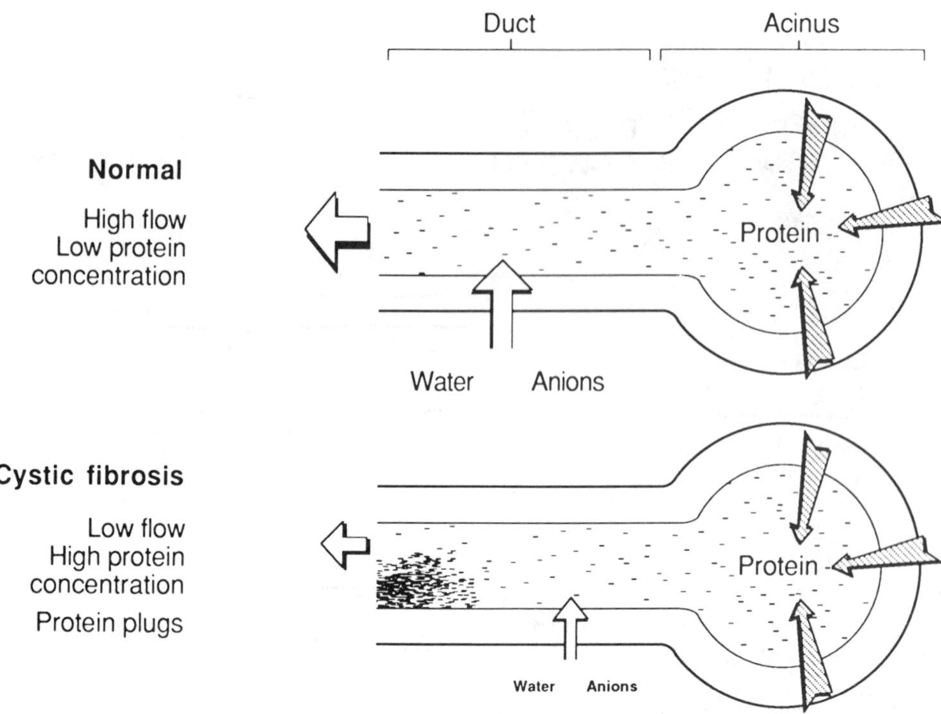

FIGURE 2 Pancreatic pathophysiology in cystic fibrosis (CF). When ductal water flow is reduced owing to decreased anion secretion, the protein concentration in the duct rises. High concentrations of protein favor microprecipitation and plugging of duct lumina.

wise to be spared.[17] Therefore, good, although not conclusive, evidence supports the hypothesis that CF develops primarily as a result of plugging of ducts and glands by macromolecules that have gelled or precipitated in concentrated secretions. Figure 2 depicts a likely scenario in pancreatic ductules in which pancreatic secretions become concentrated owing to the failure of chloride and bicarbonate secretion. The hypothesis predicts that the disease will affect tissues with special solvation problems.

PATHOLOGY

Almost all lesions in the disease have an obstructive element in which a duct or air passage is blocked by intraluminal mucus and other proteins. The pulmonary and pancreatic lesions affect health most dramatically, but hepatic, reproductive, and intestinal tissues are significantly affected by obstructive lesions (Table 1).

The Lung

The lung is not affected before it expands at birth and encounters surface hydration problems. Mucous plugging in terminal bronchioles is the earliest feature. Clearance of secretions is chronically impaired. Chronic infection develops at the level of the terminal bronchiole, and gradually the gland is destroyed by bronchiectasis, emphysema, and atelectasis. Curiously, *Staphylococcus aureus* is frequently cultured from the lung in the early stages as if the viscid surface proteins encouraged selective colonization. With antibiotic treatment, *Pseudomonas* species become resident.

The Gastrointestinal Tract and Appendages

In contrast to the lung, the pancreas appears to be affected in utero, since acinar growth is arrested.[18] At birth, intralobular ductules are plugged with mucus, and many are dilated. Acinar cells may still be relatively intact at this stage, although atrophic, but, in time, acinar and proximal ductal cells disappear and are replaced by fibrous tissue and fat. Endocrine elements are relatively preserved. Islets may even appear to be increased in histologic sections because of the contracted intervening glandular elements. Islets begin to disappear as patients reach adolescence.

The Intestine

The intestine may also be affected in utero when the low flow rate of intestinal contents makes it especially vulnerable to solvation problems. Rubbery masses of meconium can accumulate at the level of the terminal ileum, resulting in meconium ileus. Histologic sections invariably reveal crypts distended and filled with mucus. Meconium protein is high at birth,[19] suggesting hyperconcentration of solids. In later life episodes of intermittent intestinal obstruction with inspissated fecal content are common.

The characteristic hepatic feature is a focal biliary cirrhosis in which small biliary ducts are obstructed by eosinophilic material in a rather patchy pattern throughout the liver.[20]

The gallbladder in infants with meconium ileus is often atrophic and filled with mucus rather than bile, and the cystic duct is occluded. Hypofunctioning of the gallbladder continues to be frequent as children mature, possibly owing to poor filling through the cystic duct.

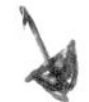

TABLE 1
The Pathology of Cystic Fibrosis

Organ	Physiologic Changes	Pathology
Lung	Distal airway obstruction, glandular hyperplasia; mucous hypersecretion	Early—terminal bronchiolar plugging; peribronchiolar inflammation Late—mucous casts; atelectasis, bronchiectasis, emphysema, cor pulmonale
Pancreas	Decreased volume and increased concentration of secretions	Early—duct plugging, dilatation, acinar atrophy Late—fibrous and fatty replacement, packing and loss of islets
Intestine	Concentrated secretions, mucus altered—hyperglycosylated and hypersulfated	Meconium plug, distal ileum; crypt dilatation; meconium peritonitis; distal intestinal obstruction syndrome; constipation
Liver	Reduced bile salt secretion, increased circulating bile salt concentration	Bile ductular hyperplasia, eosinophilic plugging of intrahepatic bile duct, focal biliary cirrhosis Late—multilobular cirrhosis
Gallbladder	Reduced bile salt pool; lithogenic bile	Cystic duct occlusion, hypoplastic gallbladder, gallstones
Salivary glands	High calcium concentration	Inspissated mucus in intercalated ducts, mild inflammation
Epididymis and vas deferens		Absent—fibrous replacement

The Reproductive Tracts

The vas deferens is occluded in virtually all adult male patients. The earliest lesion appears to be intraluminal plugging by inspissated material,[20] quickly followed by ductal atrophy and obliteration by fibrous tissue. Almost 100 percent of males are sterile. Increased viscosity of cervical mucus has been described, but perhaps because the cervical os is relatively large or the secretory flow is sufficient to prevent obstruction, pathology is minimal. Healthy CF females successfully conceive and carry pregnancies to term.

Other Systems

Renal stones occur occasionally. Uric acid stones are iatrogenic, secondary to the large amount of purine in pancreatic supplements. Hyperoxaluria is common, as in other malabsorptive disorders, but the incidence of oxalate stones is not high, perhaps because the urinary calcium concentration is relatively low.

INHERITANCE

CF is inherited as an autosomal recessive trait with highest incidence in Caucasians. In whites in northern Europe, England, Ireland, North America, Australia, and New Zealand, the incidence is between 1 in 2,000 and 1 in 3,000 live births. Elsewhere a declining incidence is found that is proportional to the degree of racial intermixing. The disease is almost unknown in Japan, India, the Middle East, China, and black Africa. In recent years, new cases have been observed in a number of countries such as Mexico and Pakistan where the incidence was previously thought to be low, suggesting that diagnostic and reporting deficiencies are a problem in some nations.

There is no good test for the heterozygote, but on the basis of a homozygote incidence of 1 in 2,000, the carrier frequency ought to be about 5 percent. This is an extremely high incidence for a gene that was lethal in childhood until recent times. It is much too high to be explained by random mutation and is not compatible with extraordinary amplification within a founding population, since there is little evidence of gene dilution throughout the Caucasian world. Some survival advantage for heterozygotes may exist. Perhaps the unresponsive chloride channel has protected infants from the effect of cyclic AMP–dependent toxigenic diarrhea,[21] as this illness must have carried off normal infants regularly in the past.

The gene has recently been localized to the long arm of chromosome 7 in region q22,[22,23] and a complete description of the gene seems imminent at writing. DNA polymorphism probes are available, which permit homozygote identification in utero by examination of amniotic cell DNA, provided that one affected sibling has been identified. Recent evidence suggests that some genetic heterogeneity is present. Preservation of pancreatic function in some patients appears to have resulted from at least three different mutations, all of which are significantly different from the mutational event underlying pancreatic insufficiency.[24]

PROGNOSIS

In most patients the outcome of the disease depends entirely on the pulmonary complications. These begin, often insidiously, as a chronic pulmonary infection caused by the plugging of small airways by thick, viscid secretions and lead eventually to widespread destruction of terminal bronchioles, bronchiectasis, atelectasis, and emphysema with associated respiratory failure, hemoptysis, and cor pulmonale. Death results from respiratory failure or overwhelming pulmonary infection. The median survival for patients in Canada is 28 years for males and 19 years for females. There is no explanation for the great discrepancy between sexes. Girls appear to do almost as well as boys until the early teens but subsequently worsen at a much faster rate.

Gastrointestinal (GI) factors may play an important role in determining overall prognosis, because both male and female patients who lack sufficient pancreatic disease to produce steatorrhea have remarkably well-preserved pulmonary function, at least into the third decade.[25]

PANCREATIC DISEASE

The classification of pancreatic disease in CF can be confusing. Patients who have steatorrhea obviously have pancreatic insufficiency and should be so classified. Those who absorb fat normally are less easily classified. They are often said to have normal pancreatic function but, when tested, may function at less than the normal level. Nevertheless, it is useful to continue to consider the patients who lack steatorrhea as a single group because their overall prognosis appears to be different from that of CF patients with steatorrhea, and they may be genetically distinct. Since *pancreatic insufficiency* has often been used synonymously with fat malabsorption, we think the term is worth preserving to designate patients who have steatorrhea. The term *pancreatic sufficiency* can then be used to designate patients who are able to digest and absorb fat normally, although the term is an operational one, restricted to fat assimilation, and it does not imply that another function such as the ability to secrete zymogens is necessarily normal.

Figure 3 summarizes these concepts. Approximately 85 percent of patients have pancreatic insufficiency. Of the pancreatic sufficient patients, approximately half have subnormal zymogen secretion on pancreatic stimulation.

Pancreatic Insufficiency (Patients with Steatorrhea)

Pathology

Pancreatic damage begins in utero and first appears as an arrest of acinar development.[18,20] At birth intralobular ductules are filled with mucus, and many are dilated. Acini are still relatively intact, although there is evidence of early atrophy and there are variable degrees of interstitial fibrosis. By the end of the first year of life, advanced acinar destruction is always present, and exocrine elements are progressively replaced by fibrous tissue and fat.[26] With time, ductules and acini disappear. Endocrine elements are relatively preserved, but as patients grow older there is islet cell loss and the gland becomes completely replaced by a fibroadipose stroma. Pancreatic calcification, a late complication of chronic pancreatitis, is unusual but is seen in older patients with CF. Macroscopic cysts over 3 mm in diameter were found in 2 percent of patients screened by ultrasonography.[27]

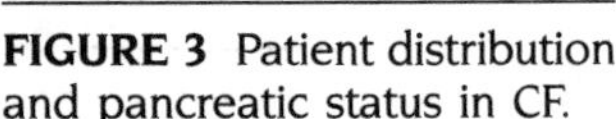

FIGURE 3 Patient distribution and pancreatic status in CF.

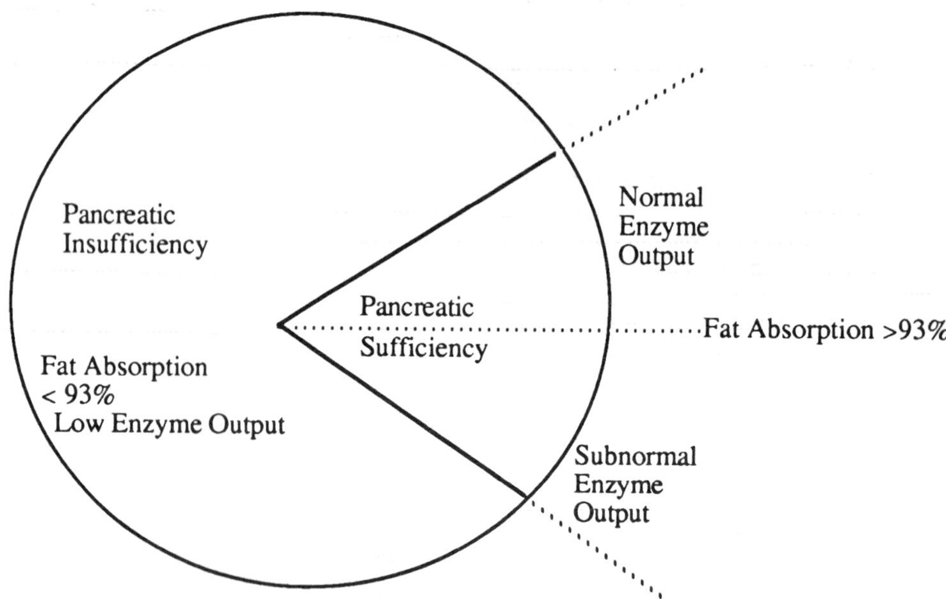

Clinical Features

The traditional stereotype of a CF child with thin, wasted limbs and buttocks, protuberant abdomen, finger clubbing, ravenous appetite, persistent cough, and loose, foul, greasy, frequent stools applies to a relatively small number of patients at diagnosis. Steatorrhea is usually present, but the stool pattern frequently seems normal to parents, and stools are often not watery or explosive. If, as is frequently the case in the first few months, chest complications are absent or mild, increased appetite may compensate for stool energy losses and patients may thrive. However, when chest problems become severe or the infant suffers from an additional malady such as esophageal reflux or esophagitis, reduced oral intake leads to a rapid and profound weight loss. In addition to wasting, skeletal growth may be slowed and short stature may develop over a comparatively brief period.

Hypoalbuminemia, edema, and anemia are dramatic complications, frequently seen together in infants under the age of 6 months, with a peak incidence at 3 to 4 months.[28] Affected patients are almost always untreated and often undiagnosed. The cause appears to be profound maldigestion and malnutrition, often aggravated by an inadequate caloric intake due to a poor supply of breast milk or intercurrent illness. Anemia has been attributed to low iron-binding globulin secondary to inadequate protein intake. Vitamin E levels are low, and hemolysis due to vitamin E deficiency may contribute. Soy protein has been incriminated because of its low digestibility, but the syndrome occurs in infants on all formulae and also in those who are breast fed. Patients improve rapidly with pancreatic supplementation and adequate caloric intake.

Rectal prolapse occurs in 20 percent of patients and usually develops between 1 and 2.5 years of age. In almost half the cases the episodes of prolapse precede[29] and should suggest the diagnosis.

Deficiencies of fat-soluble vitamins are common biochemically but rare clinically. At birth, bruising and intracranial or GI bleeding due to vitamin K deficiency have been reported.[30] It is common to find evidence of vitamin E deficiency,[31] but clinical sequelae are unusual. Ophthalmoplegia, absent deep tendon reflexes, hand tremors, ataxia, and positive rombergism are being reported with increasing frequency in late adolescent and adult patients with CF,[32,33] suggesting that clinical vitamin E deficiency is a late sequela of suboptimally treated pancreatic insufficiency. Most patients with clinical vitamin E deficiency have had significant cholestasis as well. Diminished intraluminal concentration of bile salts may possibly exacerbate vitamin E malabsorption. Overt rickets is very rare, but in older children with prolonged malnutrition, bony demineralization is not uncommon, and in some patients 25-hydroxyvitamin D levels may be low.[34] Vitamin B_{12} may be malabsorbed in untreated patients owing to formation of R-binder complexes.[35] Megaloblastic anemia has not been reported, presumably because pancreatic supplements facilitate vitamin B_{12}–intrinsic factor binding. Lindemans et al[36] found instead that patients on a standard treatment regimen often had elevated serum vitamin B_{12} levels. Patients also had increased transcobalamin II and R-binder levels, possibly as the result of associated hepatic disease. Most patients with pancreatic insufficiency have low plasma and tissue levels of linoleic acid, but symptomatic essential fatty acid deficiency is rare.

Biochemical evidence of insulin deficiency becomes more frequent with increasing age as pancreatic islets disappear and can be demonstrated in one-third of patients.[37,38] Clinically significant diabetes mellitus is generally mild and easily controlled with small doses of insulin. The immunoreactive insulin response to glucose is delayed and diminished, even before glucose intolerance can be demonstrated. The enteroinsular axis functions appropriately. Enhanced basal and oral glucose–stimulated gastric inhibitory peptide levels are found once carbohydrate intolerance develops.[39]

In addition, a number of intestinal complications, meconium ileus, distal intestinal obstruction syndrome, rectal prolapse, and cholelithiasis are strongly correlated with pancreatic insufficiency.

Diagnosis

In our clinic approximately 60 percent of patients are diagnosed before the age of 1 year, 85 percent before the age of 5 years. Failure to thrive, frequent foul stools, rectal prolapse, or the triad of hypoalbuminemia, edema, and anemia in an infant should suggest the diagnosis, especially when a history of respiratory complaints is present. Edema may produce low sweat chloride concentrations, even with adequate secretory stimulation.[40] It is wise, therefore, to repeat a negative sweat test once edema subsides.

Pancreatic insufficiency can usually be diagnosed by looking at the stool smear, which is loaded with neutral fat droplets. Deficient secretion of pancreatic enzymes may be suspected from a low random or 24-hour stool chymotrypsin activity.[41] Serum levels of pancreatic trypsinogen are often increased before the age of 8 years, but subnormal values become established thereafter.[42] Most patients with steatorrhea have low plasma para-aminobenzoic acid (PABA) levels or decreased urinary excretion of PABA following the administration of *N*-benzoyl-L-tyrosyl-PABA.[43] Quantitative determination of 3- or 5-day fecal fat excretion with a known fat intake establishes the presence of steatorrhea. Fecal fat excretion is surprisingly variable, amounting to as much as 80 percent of intake in some patients, with a mean of 38 percent.[44]

The only truly definitive test for pancreatic insufficiency continues to be the documentation of low enzyme output from the pancreas following stimulation by secretin and cholecystokinin. Patients with steatorrhea all had a lipase output with stimulation that was less than 1.5 percent of the average for controls.[45]

Paradoxically, pancreatic insufficiency in very early infancy is associated with elevated levels of serum trypsinogen. Screening for high serum trypsinogen values in heel-prick blood samples appears to detect the majority of patients with CF, including those with pancreatic sufficiency.[46,47] Neonatal screening shortens the mean time of diagnosis from 1.5 years to 7 weeks and, when combined with a follow-up trypsinogen assay and sweat test, is capable of identifying at least 90 percent of patients.[48]

Treatment

All patients should receive regular supplementation with pancreatic enzymes. Enteric-coated, acid-resistant microspheres that release their pancreatic enzymes at a pH of 5.5 to 6.0 have largely replaced capsules containing pancreatic extract powders, because the number of capsules required for symptomatic relief is greatly reduced. A reasonable starting dose is three to four capsules per meal, one with each snack. If steatorrhea remains a significant problem, the number of capsules may be increased to approximately double this level. It seems reasonable to take the capsules at regular intervals through the meal.

It is uncommon to correct the steatorrhea completely. Low duodenal and jejunal pH resulting from inadequate neutralization of gastric acid inactivates pancreatic lipase and interferes with lipolysis as a result of bile salt precipitation.[49] In one study, when pancreatic extracts were supplemented with cimetidine and bicarbonate to inhibit and neutralize gastric acid secretion, absorption improved significantly, but stool fat excretion fell to less than 7 percent of intake in only three of 45 tests.[50] Enteric-coated microspheres have improved this performance, but patients often remain steatorrheic in spite of high levels of enzyme supplementation.[51,52] One should recall that the response to pancreatic supplementation depends on the amount of fat in the diet.[50] Patients taking large amounts of fat daily may require one or two additional capsules with meals and snacks. A few patients are refractory to the acid-resistant preparations; some may possibly have high gastric acid output that prevents neutralization of duodenal and upper jejunal secretions to the degree required for pancreatic enzyme release.[53] Oral taurine supplementation (30 mg per kilogram per day) has been report ed to benefit some refractory patients.[54] Most of the lipase activity in the postprandial duodenum of patients with pancreatic insufficiency comes from lingual lipase, which does not require bile salts for activation and is active at a lower pH than pancreatic lipase.[55] Acid lipases of this nature might be ideal ingredients of pancreatic supplements.

Pancreatic Sufficiency (Patients Without Steatorrhea)

Pathology

In perhaps one-fifth of all patients with CF, the relentless progression of pancreatic disease either does not occur or seems to be retarded for one or two decades. Pancreatic morphology has been studied in relatively few of these cases, but the available evidence suggests that many have considerable pancreatic damage. Large portions of the pancreas are often atrophic and in areas of relative preservation there are irregular plugging of the large and small ducts and variable amounts of fibrous tissue.[56,57] In approximately 50 percent of these patients, however, pancreatic enzyme secretion is within the normal range, suggesting that pathologic damage is minimal.

Clinical Features

The outstanding feature of pancreatic-sufficient patients is their relative freedom from pulmonary disease.[25] Figure 4 summarizes the difference in the rates of deterioration of the

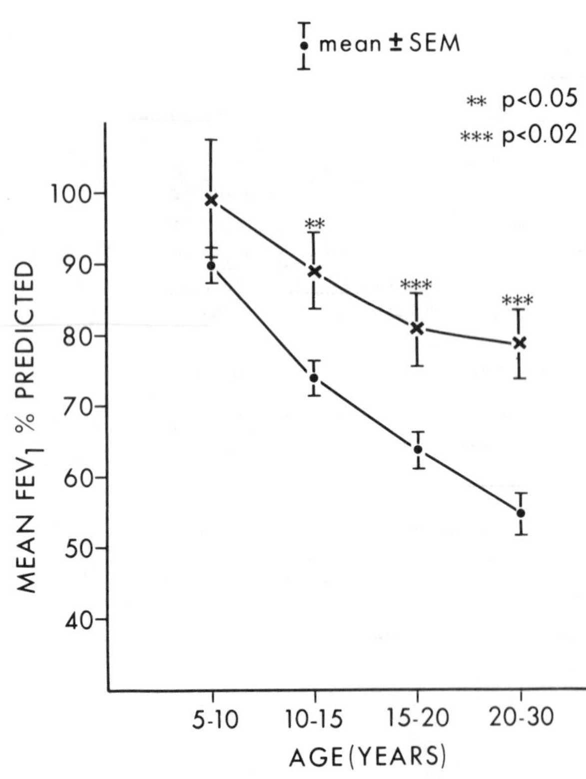

FIGURE 4 One-second forced expiratory volume (FEV_1) fell more rapidly with age in patients with pancreatic insufficiency than it did in patients with pancreatic sufficiency.

1-second forced expiratory volume in pancreatic-sufficient and insufficient patients and shows progressive deterioration in the patients with pancreatic insufficiency, with minimal change in the pancreatic-sufficient group. Similar results were obtained with a variety of other pulmonary function tests. Colonization of the lung by *Pseudomonas aeruginosa* and *Pseudomonas cepacia* is also reduced compared with pancreatic-insufficient patients.[58] Not surprisingly, the overall prognosis for these patients is much better than that for patients with pancreatic insufficiency. Between 1970 and 1982, 123 deaths from CF occurred in Toronto; only three patients had pancreatic sufficiency.

There is no doubt that pancreatic-sufficient patients have CF. Diagnostic DNA markers have correctly identified our pancreatic-sufficient patients in studies of families with more than one affected sibling.[59] The mean sweat chloride estimation is lower than that of patients with pancreatic insufficiency but well above the normal range. The mean age at presentation in our initial series[25] was 5 years, considerably later than that of patients with pancreatic insufficiency. Whereas 90 percent of steatorrheic patients are diagnosed by 6 years of age, the 90 percent diagnostic range is not achieved in pancreatic-sufficient patients until age 20.

Approximately one-quarter of our patients presented with respiratory symptoms, 75 percent exhibited some evidence of clinical chest disease, 39 percent had clubbing, 30 percent had nasal polyps, and 4 percent had a rectal prolapse, which suggests that this complication is not completely res-

TABLE 2
Intestinal Complications of Cystic Fibrosis

Likely Age	Condition
At birth	Meconium ileus
0–2 years	Rectal prolapse
After 10 years	Distal intestinal obstruction syndrome Constipation Gastroesophageal reflux Pneumatosis intestinalis

tricted to patients with pancreatic insufficiency. In general, pancreatic-sufficient patients appear to be better off nutritionally. Males with pancreatic sufficiency have significantly greater weight relative to height than their male pancreatic-insufficient counterparts, but it is not yet clear whether pancreatic-sufficient females enjoy a similar advantage.[58]

Eight percent of the group had acute pancreatitis. This is the only complication of CF that appears to be exclusively restricted to patients with pancreatic sufficiency,[57] almost certainly because they are the only patients with sufficient surviving pancreatic tissue after the first few years of life to generate an active inflammatory response.

Diagnosis

Patients with pancreatic sufficiency are diagnosed most commonly as the result of a routine trypsinogen screening or a sweat chloride test performed for respiratory symptoms or because of a family history of CF. Occasionally metabolic alkalosis, rectal prolapse, loose stools, or an unexplained attack of pancreatitis may prompt investigation.

INTESTINAL TRACT DISEASE

Table 2 lists intestinal complications of CF.

Pathology

The intestinal mucosa is not damaged irreversibly by CF. Villous structure and absorptive cells are generally normal in appearance. Disaccharidase activities may even be increased. Surface and crypt mucus is often increased. Some crypts may be greatly distended and even cystlike, as if obstructed. At birth and throughout life the lumen contains masses of rubbery, green-black meconium, which adhere tightly to the intestinal surface. Undegraded proteins, particularly albumin, are the major constituents. The meconium protein content at birth is approximately six to eight times that of normal meconium.[19]

Meconium Ileus

Approximately 10 to 15 percent of patients with CF present at birth or shortly thereafter with signs and symptoms of small bowel obstruction. The cause is a plug of meconium in the terminal ileum, which is acquired in utero as perhaps the first overt manifestation of diminished pancreatic function. Typically no meconium is passed and there is progressive abdominal distention. Rubbery, firm loops of bowel may be visible or palpable, and the rectal examination is unproductive. A history of polyhydramnios may be obtained. Almost all patients with meconium ileus develop pancreatic insufficiency, although exceptions have been recorded.[60]

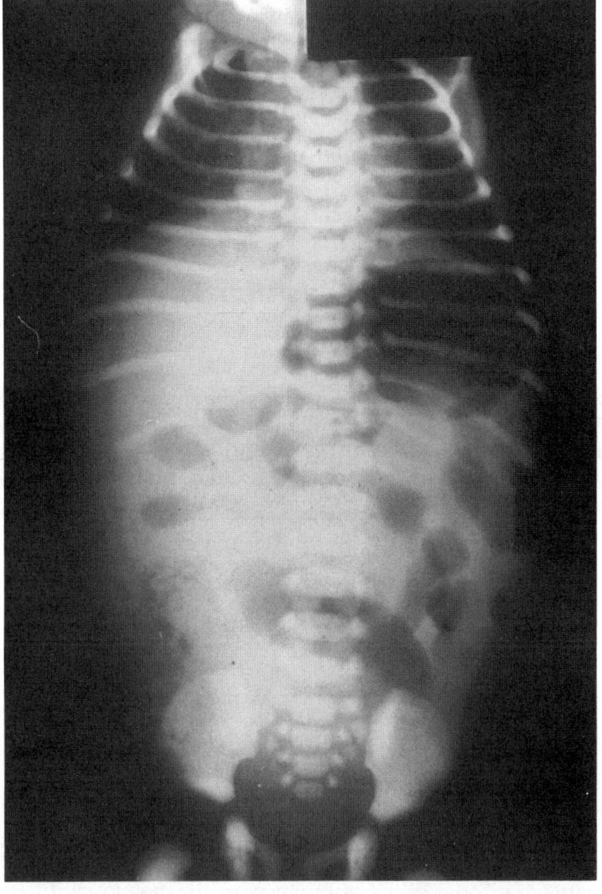

FIGURE 5 Meconium ileus. A plain roentgenogram of the abdomen shows multiple gas-filled loops, displaced by meconium in the right lower quadrant. Multiple small bubbles of gas are conspicuous within the meconium. No air is in the rectum.

The radiologic findings are characteristic (Fig. 5). In addition to air-fluid levels and distended loops of small bowel, small bubbles of gas are trapped in the meconium of the distal small bowel, giving a ground-glass appearance. A barium enema demonstrates a small collapsed microcolon. Half of the cases of meconium ileus are complicated by volvulus, atresia, and/or meconium peritonitis. Atresia and meconium peritonitis usually result from intrauterine events associated with volvulus or extravasation of meconium through a perforation. Intraperitoneal calcification may be apparent on plain radiographs. Meconium pseudocysts may appear in the inflammatory reaction, ascites may develop, and an infectious peritonitis may occur if the perforation does not close.

Meconium ileus is almost always associated with CF, but rare reports of the condition have appeared in association with stenosis of the pancreatic duct,[61] with partial pancreatic aplasia,[62] and with a normal GI tract.[63] Approximately one-third of patients with meconium peritonitis and one-fifth of patients with atresia of the small bowel[64] are said to have CF.

Most patients can be relieved of their intestinal obstruction with diatrizoate (Gastrografin) or Hypaque enemas. The major hazard is that these hypertonic solutions may cause a dangerous loss of fluid and electrolyte into the bowel. Infants ought to be supported with continuous intravenous fluids during the procedure. Colonic perforation has been reported[65] but is rare. Gastrografin enemas are contraindicated for complicated meconium ileus. The surgical approach to meconium ileus usually involves removal of the plug with irrigation at the time of surgery. If there is atresia or peritonitis, a limited resection should be performed. The immediate survival of these patients has continued to improve from decade to decade and is now more than 90 percent in many centers. Beyond the first year of life their outlook, in contrast to what was previously thought, is the same as that for other patients with the disease.

Rectal Prolapse

Rectal prolapse occurs in 18.5 percent of patients and usually develops between 1 and 2.5 years of age. Onset after age 5 years is rare. In almost half of their cases, Stern et al reported that episodes of prolapse preceded the diagnoses.[29] Kulczycki and Shwachman initially emphasized the importance of rectal prolapse as a presenting symptom in CF.[66] A history of rectal prolapse is equally important. In the Cleveland series of 112 patients, 20 patients who were not diagnosed with CF until after 4 years of age had not had a prolapse for at least 1 year before diagnosis.

Rectal prolapse has a tendency to spontaneously resolve. Patients who have not received pancreatic supplements often improve dramatically when they receive them. However, if episodes of rectal prolapse develop while the patient is on pancreatic supplements, dietary and supplement manipulation rarely improves the situation.[29] With time, children learn to reduce the prolapsed mucosa themselves and the significance of the problem seems to fade. Approximately 10 percent of patients require surgical correction, usually for repeated episodes that are either painful or a nuisance.

Distal Intestinal Obstruction Syndrome (Meconium Ileus Equivalent)

Later in life about 10 percent of patients with CF[67] suffer from recurrent complaints attributable to partial or complete bowel obstruction. Almost all patients have pancreatic insufficiency, although occasional exceptions occur.[68] Although inspissated intraluminal masses play an etiologic role, the resemblance to meconium ileus is somewhat tenuous and the term *distal intestinal obstruction syndrome* (DIOS)[69] is preferred. DIOS is most commonly a chronic condition produced by partial bowel obstruction. Large fecal masses can be palpated in the abdomen, particularly in the cecal area. These masses may persist for many months in spite of the daily passage of several stools. Intermittent abdominal distention and cramping occur, and the appetite may be reduced, with weight loss. Between exacerbations, patients may be symptom-free, but some complain of constant insidious abdominal pain. At times, attacks seem to be precipitated by specific factors, such as the sudden withdrawal of pancreatic supplements, immobilization, or respiratory tract infection. Rarely the putty-like obstructive masses in the right colon and terminal ileum precipitate acute obstructive episodes with ileus and vomiting. Holsclaw et al[70] found that 1 percent of patients with CF presented with intussusception, presumably with an adherent fecal mass as the lead point. In 22 episodes in 19 patients, only two required intestinal resection. The common site for the intussusception was ileocolic. DIOS is not more common in patients who present with meconium ileus.[71]

Episodes of DIOS are usually responsive to medical management but tend to recur. In chronic cases it is important to ensure adequate pancreatic replacement therapy because the failure to digest intraluminal protein is a major cause of constipation and obstruction. A diet that is high in roughage and a mild laxative, such as mineral oil, may be sufficient to relieve the patient. In acute obstructive episodes, characterized by clear evidence of small bowel obstruction, such as vomiting or air-fluid levels throughout the small intestine, a nasogastric tube should be introduced and the impaction should be cleared with enemas. Most centers use 10 percent *N*-acetylcysteine as a mucus-clearing agent. Even though the masses are not particularly mucoid, this agent seems to be sufficiently irritating to dislodge the fecal plugs. *N*-Acetylcysteine may be introduced by mouth, by D-tube, or by Miller-Abbot tube, depending upon the indication. Gastrografin enemas may be used as a last resort. In the absence of signs of acute small bowel obstruction, chronic intractable symptoms may be relieved for surprisingly long periods by intestinal lavage with 5 to 6 liters of a balanced isotonic polyethylene glycol–salt solution (Golytely) delivered orally or through a nasogastric tube.[72] Although this approach may at first sight seem overzealous, it has in our experience as well as that of others,[68] been greeted with excellent acceptance by patients who have failed to find relief with laxatives and mucolytics. Repeated lavage is well tolerated and can be administered at home by the patient. Surgery is reserved for the rare patients with intussusception that cannot be relieved by enema and for the even more unusual patient with clear evidence of an obstructive mass that cannot be removed by the persistent application of conservative measures.

CONSTIPATION

Older patients with CF suffer from a very high incidence of abdominal cramping and decreased stool frequency. Many of these patients also have chronic DIOS, but constipation appears to be about three times more frequent.[73] The most characteristic radiologic finding is copious fecal material throughout the colon. These patients respond to an initial regimen of enemas, followed by long-term oral laxatives. Some may benefit from intermittent GI lavage.

PNEUMATOSIS INTESTINALES

Intramural intestinal gas probably develops from dissection of air along vascular sheaths and is generally seen in patients with advanced pulmonary disease. Forty-one cases were identified from autopsy records of 491 patients at the Children's Hospital in Boston.[74] Air collects initially in the colonic wall, forming submucosal cysts. When more than half of the colon is involved, linear collections of air appear in the mucosa and subserosal air cysts are present. The air is not a threat, but it is a reminder of the ominous prognosis of the pulmonary disease.

GASTROESOPHAGEAL REFLUX

Esophagitis and esophageal stricture (Fig. 6) occur secondary to esophageal reflux, usually in the absence of any evidence of hiatal hernia.[75] Chronic pulmonary disease and multiple medications are probable predisposing factors. Patients are usually older children or adolescents. Of 68 patients over the age of 5 years studied by Scott et al,[76] regurgitation and heartburn were experienced by more than 20 percent, while of 23 asymptomatic siblings of the same age, none had regurgitation and only one had heartburn. Twenty-four-hour esophageal pH recording is the most sensitive test for confirming the diagnosis. Gastroesophageal reflux should always be considered as the cause of anorexia, weight loss, or unexplained anemia in an adolescent with CF. Esophagitis may be severe. Feigelson et al[77] reported an endoscopic incidence of 76 percent in 37 patients with marked respiratory problems who were part of a systematic prospective study.

HEPATOLOGY

Pathology

Severe liver disease is uncommon,[78,79] but microscopic evidence of small bile duct obstruction is found in 50 percent of autopsied cases.[80] The earliest lesion, seen in patients dying of meconium ileus, consists of bile ductular hyperplasia

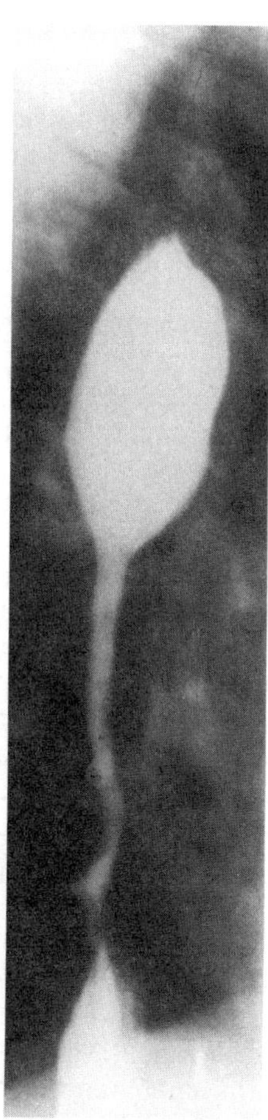

FIGURE 6 Elongated esophageal stricture secondary to chronic peptic esophagitis in an adolescent patient with chronic esophageal reflux. The stricture was 10 cm in length beginning at the esophagogastric junction and was associated with profound dysphagia and weight loss.

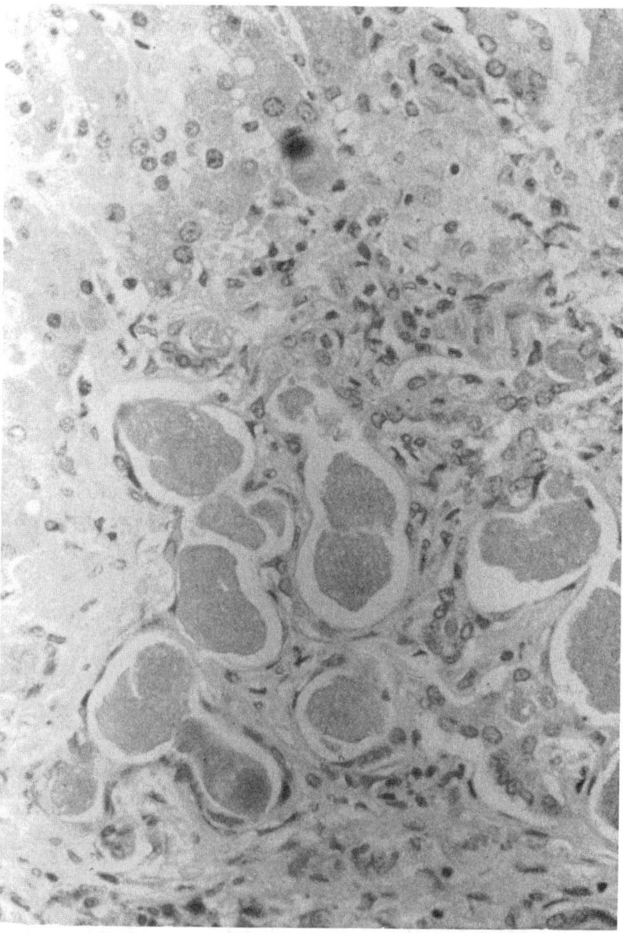

FIGURE 7 A portal area from the liver biopsy of a CF patient with focal biliary cirrhosis displays marked eosinophilic plugging of bile ductules. Bile ductules are increased in number and their cells are flattened. Fibrous tissue and numbers of inflammatory cells are increased.

TABLE 3
Clinical Hepatobiliary Problems in Cystic Fibrosis

Prolonged neonatal jaundice
Hepatomegaly
Hepatosplenomegaly
Variceal hemorrhage
Massive splenic enlargement
Decompensated cirrhosis
Cholelithiasis
Extrahepatic bile duct obstruction
Pancreatic fibrosis compressing common bile duct
Malignant cholangiocarcinoma

within portal tracts. Focal biliary cirrhosis is highly characteristic of CF and consists of eosinophilic plugging of small ductules in portal tracts (Fig. 7) with ductule dilatation and flattening of bile ductular cells, surrounded in a patchily inconsistent manner by a chronic inflammatory reaction and an increase in fibrous tissue. Large intra- and extrahepatic ducts may be distended with inspissated mucus. Significantly, parenchymal architecture and liver cell integrity are well preserved.

Centrilobular fatty infiltration is probably the most common finding in liver biopsy samples. It may be related to fat malabsorption and malnutrition. Increased prominence of Ito cells has been reported.[81] No specific electron microscopic abnormalities have been identified. Micronodular cirrhosis, complicated by portal hypertension, occurs in 2 to 5 percent of older children and adolescents with CF.[78,79]

In approximately 25 percent of cases the gallbladder is hypoplastic and filled at autopsy with transparent grey mucus. Esterly and Openheimer found microscopic changes in 19 of 44 cases consisting of numerous epithelium-lined mucosal multiloculated cysts.[82] There was no evidence of inflammation. In a majority of the abnormal gallbladders there was no bile as the result of cystic duct obstruction. Gallbladder lesions are seen at birth and, as with the pancreas, appear to evolve in utero.

Clinical Features

Clinical hepatobiliary problems associated with CF are listed in Table 3.

Neonatal Jaundice

Prolonged cholestatic jaundice in the neonatal period is reportedly a complication of CF, but the case rests on a few scattered reports[83-85] and there is a strong possibility that these represent the co-existence of other conditions with CF. CF should nevertheless be considered in the differential diagnosis of neonatal jaundice. Meconium ileus is said to be a predisposing factor, but the incidence in infants with meconium ileus is less than 1 percent.[86] There is no distinguishing clinical presentation. The onset may be delayed to the second or third week. Stools can be pale, suggesting biliary atresia, and both liver and spleen are often palpable. The serum bilirubin is predominantly direct, with minor to moderate elevation of transaminases. Jaundice usually resolves by the twelfth week. Investigations should include a search for other causes of neonatal jaundice as well as liver biopsy. The diagnosis is one of exclusion.

Hepatomegaly

Isolated hepatomegaly may be due to steatosis. Patients are undernourished, and pulmonary disease is frequently well advanced. The liver is smooth, soft, and only moderately enlarged. Liver function is not deranged, although fasting bile salt levels may be increased. Steatosis is not alarming per se, but it should alert one to the possibility of a precarious nutritional state, and rigorous efforts should be made to correct the deficiency. In older patients with severe pulmonary disease, hepatic congestion secondary to cor pulmonale must be considered in the differential diagnosis. The liver may also be palpated below the costal margin because of a flattened diaphragm. Therefore, the upper margin must always be delineated by percussion and the true size of the liver determined.

Hepatosplenomegaly

Hepatosplenomegaly may be the first indication of advanced hepatic disease. Because CF does not affect parenchymal cells directly, hepatic function may be well preserved, even in the face of longstanding portal hypertension. As a result, liver function tests have not proved to be very useful in detecting the presence or evaluating the progress of cirrhosis. Elevated fasting serum bile salt levels occur in up to 40 percent of patients with pancreatic insufficiency[87,88] and are correlated with hepatomegaly. Many of these cases probably have steatosis rather than cirrhosis. Bromsulphalein retention is abnormal[69] and may be useful as an indication of chronic liver disease. If abnormal liver function tests are present, other diagnoses such as chronic active hepatitis should be excluded. Hyperbilirubinemia and hypergammaglobulinemia are more likely to correlate with the level of pulmonary disease and emergence of cor pulmonale. Familial clustering has been reported, suggesting that genetic predisposing factors may condition the appearance of cirrhosis. Routine screening for an alpha$_1$-antitrypsin deficiency heterozygote state has been advocated, since several patients with CF and an abnormal Pi phenotype have been described.[86]

Portal hypertension in the absence of variceal bleeding requires no specific treatment, and further investigation is not necessary at this stage unless other diagnoses are suspected. A temptation to perform a liver biopsy often exists, but biopsy cannot distinguish focal biliary cirrhosis from multilobular cirrhosis and does not improve upon clinical judgment. Ultrasonography, since it is not invasive, is certainly worthwhile and may confirm portal venous obstruction.

Variceal Hemorrhage

The treatment of variceal hemorrhage is the same in patients with CF as in patients with portal hypertension due to other causes and is dealt with extensively elsewhere. An ongoing debate exists between proponents of prophylactic therapy and those who favor remedial therapy. Today the debate centers on injection sclerotherapy, which can be used prophylactically to obliterate varices or therapeutically to control acute bleeding episodes. Balloon tamponade, which was always a concern in patients with advanced pulmonary disease, is now rarely used, because sclerotherapy has proved to be more effective in treating acute episodes. The effectiveness of sclerotherapy has also reduced the pressure to intervene prophylactically. Definitive injection sclerotherapy after the first bleeding episode is generally considered desirable to lessen the risk of repeat hemorrhage in highly susceptible individuals. However, the treatment requires a number of endoscopic procedures, both initially, when three to five sessions may be necessary to produce complete obliteration, and later at 6-month intervals to obliterate new varices. In practice one's enthusiasm for obliterating varices in this manner varies inversely with the degree of respiratory embarrassment. Alternative, definitive approaches such as portosystemic shunting are of little use in patients with severe pulmonary failure. Shunting is associated with a significant risk to pulmonary function[89] and is now rarely employed.

Massive Splenic Enlargement

Occasionally a very large spleen becomes a source of discomfort or even respiratory embarrassment, and removal, coupled with a splenorenal shunt, may be indicated. Certainly the patient feels better, but one must balance the comfort against the risk at surgery, the susceptibility to pneumococcal infection, and the postsplenectomy hypercoagulable state. Hypersplenism is, in contrast, rarely if ever an indication for splenectomy in CF, no more than in other hepatic diseases.[90]

Decompensated Cirrhosis

Patients with cystic fibrosis rarely die of hepatic failure. As life expectancy increases, however, problems associated with advanced liver disease, such as intractable ascites, recurrent, refractory variceal bleeding, and portosystemic encephalopathy, will no doubt become more common. These patients may be aided by hepatic transplantation.[90]

Gallstones

Gallstones develop in one of every 10 patients with CF.[91] Gallbladder bile is lithogenic in untreated pancreatic insufficiency but responds to pancreatic enzymes.[92] Excessive loss of fecal bile acid[93] is the probable cause. Mucosal transport of conjugated bile salts by the ileum may be impaired and is possibly related to the genetic defect.[94,95] Steatorrhea may also contribute by solvation of bile salts in nonabsorbed fat, thus preventing access to ileal transport receptors. In six patients studied by Watkins et al,[96] pancreatic supplements sufficient to reduce fat excretion from a mean of 50 percent to 20 percent were associated with a doubling of the total bile acid pool. Weber and Roy[93] found a significant reduction in fecal bile acid excretion when steatorrhea was corrected. Effective control of steatorrhea may provide the additional dividend of reducing the future incidence of gallstones.

Cholestasis

The frequency of high fasting serum bile salt levels[87,88] suggests that a degree of impaired biliary secretion is common. Almost all patients with elevated serum bile salt levels have pancreatic insufficiency, suggesting that steatosis complicating malnutrition or possibly extrahepatic common duct compression by the pancreas[97] may be contributory. Elevated bile salt levels do not correlate well with the histologic severity of liver disease,[97,98] although most patients with normal hepatic morphology have normal bile salt levels. Patients with elevated fasting serum bile salt levels have reduced rates of bile acid secretion into the duodenum, as expected of cholestasis. Only about half of the patients with elevated levels[87] have hepatomegaly, and there is little correlation with other liver function tests. One is left with the impression that mild cholestasis without jaundice is common in CF but that its significance is currently unknown.

Extrahepatic Bile Duct Obstruction

Common duct strictures have been reported occasionally in CF, as well as other causes of chronic pancreatitis, owing to compression of the hepatic duct as it passes through the pancreas. Recent findings suggest that this complication may occur in patients with clinical liver disease more commonly than previously thought. It has even been suggested that multilobular cirrhosis may be a consequence of extrahepatic obstruction.[97]

Gaskin et al[97] found evidence of extrahepatic biliary tract obstruction on examination by hepatobiliary scintigraphy in all 45 patients with firm hepatomegaly or splenomegaly. In contrast to patients without clinical or biochemical evidence of liver disease, a high percentage of these patients had recurrent abdominal pain. The pain was usually in the right hypochondrium, precipitated by meals and improved by avoiding fatty foods. Strikingly, almost all of the 30 patients who ultimately had cholangiography had strictures of the distal common duct. Fourteen patients were operated on for abdominal pain, and all experienced complete relief of symptoms postoperatively. In eight of nine cases with preoperative evidence of cholestasis, fasting levels of serum bile acids and conjugated bilirubins returned to normal within 2 months of the operation. The incidence of hepatomegaly in Sydney is apparently 40 percent, much higher than in Toronto. It remains to be seen, therefore, whether the association of common duct strictures and firm hepatomegaly is a feature unique to Australia. Patients with hepatomegaly, splenomegaly, and disabling abdominal pain should nevertheless have a hepatobiliary scintiscan to look for evidence of biliary tract obstruction and, if the scan is suggestive, percutaneous cholangiography to define the duct. At present it seems reasonable to restrict corrective surgery to the relief of pain.

NUTRITIONAL DISTURBANCES IN CYSTIC FIBROSIS

Pathogenesis

Maldigestion and Malabsorption

Barely 2 percent of the total pancreatic capacity for secreting lipase is required to prevent steatorrhea. In those who exhibit steatorrhea very good correlations exist between pancreatic residual function and fat malabsorption up to a daily fat excretion of approximately 30 percent of intake.[45] Patients within this range may therefore have varying degrees of pancreatic function, however small, and their response to therapeutic agents may vary. These observations partially explain why some patients with pancreatic insufficiency appear to do much better than others when given pancreatic supplements. Many patients with CF, particularly infants, have steatorrhea in excess of 30 percent of intake. In these patients a variety of other factors may conspire to make the steatorrhea worse. Gastric acid entering the duodenum presents the small intestine with a relatively large challenge and, in the absence of pancreatic bicarbonate secretion, may not be neutralized by biliary and intestinal buffers until well into the jejunum. Lipase is less active at low pH, and the pK of bile acids is such that they are precipitated in an acid milieu.[49] As a result, the bile salt concentration may fall below the critical micellar concentration, exacerbating the degree of steatorrhea. Precipitated bile salts also appear to be lost from the enterohepatic circulation in greater quantities, and the loss contributes to the restriction in the total bile salt pool.[96] This tendency is exacerbated by the binding of bile salts to protein or neutral lipid droplets in extreme steatorrhea and perhaps by ileal transport abnormalities. It is also likely that the thickness of the intestinal unstirred layer is increased because of the excess mucus in the intestine, and this may lead to limited fat absorption.

Protein assimilation has not been studied well in CF. Stool nitrogen output seems to be increased to two or two and one half times the normal level,[44] but this may be more a reflection of rapid colonic transit and antibiotic usage than an indication of the degree of protein digestion that normally takes place.

As might be expected, in the presence of pancreatic insufficiency, fat-soluble vitamins are poorly absorbed. Absorption and utilization of water-soluble vitamins are normal, with the exception of vitamin B_{12}.

Increased Energy Expenditure

In addition to fecal losses, pulmonary infections and respiratory insufficiency increase the energy requirements of patients with CF. In 71 patients studied with open-circuit indirect calorimetry, free of acute lung infections, resting energy expenditures ranged from 85 to 153 percent of predicted values for age, sex, and weight. Energy expenditures were negatively correlated with pulmonary function and nutritional status.[99] Loss of body fat was associated quite strongly with increased energy expenditure as well as poor pulmonary function. Thin patients with poor pulmonary function are frequently unable to gain weight despite various attempts to supplement the diet. When they suffer pulmonary complications, energy expenditures increase further. Weight loss may be severe and recovery prolonged. Selective beta-adrenergic agonists, employed for long-term bronchodilator therapy, may also increase energy requirements.[100]

Underweight individuals with less extensive pulmonary disease, when free of acute pulmonary symptoms, appear to gain weight normally while consuming diets of 120 percent of the recommended dietary allowance (RDA).[101] Because normal growth may be achieved in the presence of extra energy loss due to steatorrhea, the inference is that their energy requirements are not very different from those of the general population. Some evidence suggests that energy requirements could also be marginally greater than normal owing to unexplained metabolic wastage.[102]

Inadequate Caloric Intake

Patients with CF are particularly prone to complications that limit appetite and oral intake. Esophagitis is commonly associated with advanced pulmonary disease and is frequently associated with anorexia and vomiting initiated by bouts of coughing. DIOS causes recurrent crampy abdominal pain, and patients often find that symptoms are exacerbated by eating. Pancreatitis, extrahepatic biliary obstruction, cholangitis, severe constipation, and cirrhosis are all associated with decreased dietary intake.

In addition, patients with CF are still treated unnecessarily with unpalatable diets in an effort to supplement caloric intake or normalize the appearance of the stools. In the past, a low-fat diet was particularly favored, because the number of stools was reduced and clinicians believed that steatorrhea interfered with the absorption of other nutrients. Too often the net effect of restrictive diets is to present young patients with tasteless choices and to deprive them of many of the energy-rich foods that are part of the normal peer's diet. Reduced caloric intake is an unfortunate and iatrogenic byproduct.

Acute respiratory exacerbations are the most common causes of restricted oral intake. Decreased appetite and weight loss are often the first signs of acute pulmonary infection. Early in the course of the disease appetite returns promptly on treatment, with rapid catch-up in weight following improvement of symptoms, but in the terminal stages chronic unremitting anorexia is a feature. Apathy, fatigue, and a disordered sense of smell and body image all seem to play a role.

Figure 8 summarizes many factors that contribute to energy deficit in the CF patient. As lung disease worsens, most commonly in older adolescents and young adults, there may be an increase in frequency and severity of pulmonary infections, which in turn induce anorexia. Chest infections often give rise to vomiting, which may further reduce intake. These factors, in combination with additional energy needs from increased work of breathing, may induce an energy deficit. Weight loss will result, initially producing a significant loss of adipose tissue, but over time there is a marked loss of lean tissue, with muscle wasting. Respiratory muscle wasting adversely affects respiratory motion and coughing, resulting in further deterioration of lung function. Malnutrition also adversely affects lung elasticity and a variety of aspects of immune function. All these factors contribute to progressive deterioration of lung function. In essence, a vicious circle is established, leading inevitably to end-stage pulmonary failure and death.

Clinical Features of Malnutrition

The common signs of malnutrition change as patients mature, but are all related to the protein-calorie deficit or malabsorption of essential nutrients (Table 4).

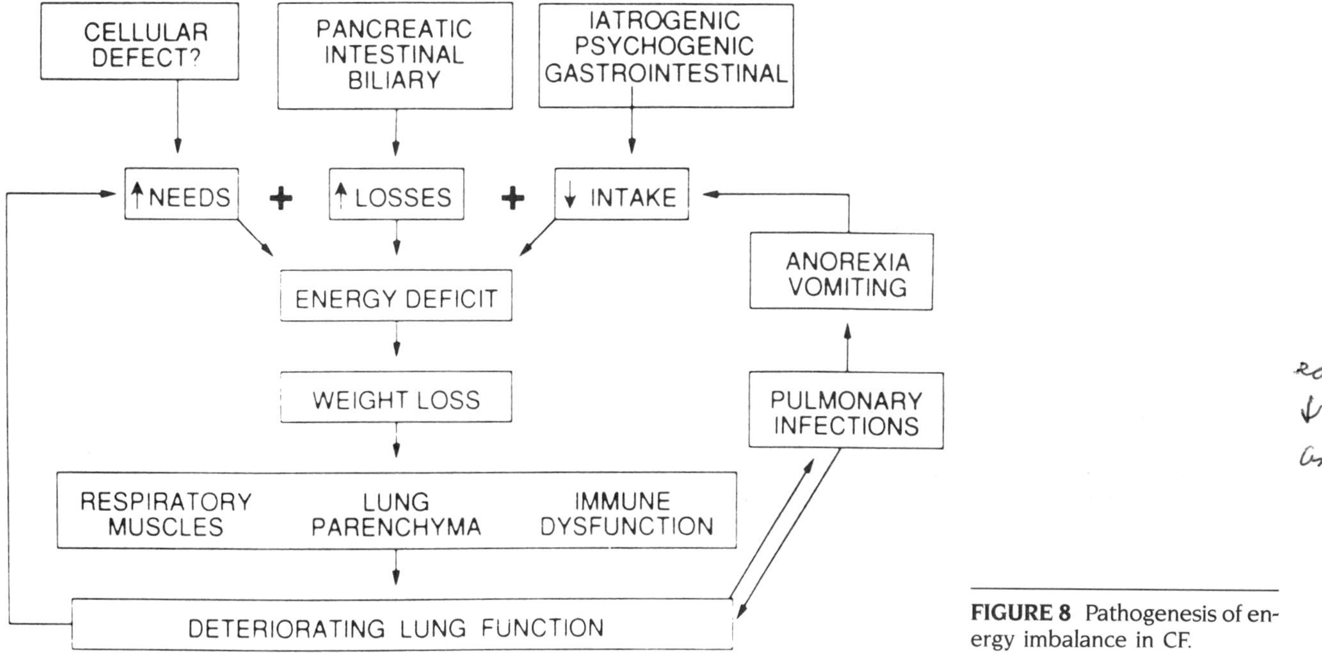

FIGURE 8 Pathogenesis of energy imbalance in CF.

edema
↓ alb
anemia

Protein-Calorie Deficit

Infants. CF infants have slightly low birth weights, amounting to an average reduction of 100 to 200 g. The majority of patients diagnosed in infancy present with some manifestation of maldigestion and are often malnourished. The abdomen is distended and muscles are wasted, particularly in the buttocks and thighs. The infant may appear listless, weak, and floppy. Growth failure is an early sign. Soon after the onset of symptoms, weight gain may cease or there may be actual weight loss. The appearance of edema, hypoalbuminemia, and anemia heralds severe protein-calorie malnutrition and, as noted above, usually occurs in infants under the age of 6 months.[28] An enlarged liver is a frequent finding in malnourished patients and is usually due to fat accumulation. Liver function tests are rarely deranged. If the infant is not treated and several months pass without weight gain, linear growth may halt as well, possibly leading to a permanent reduction in stature.

TABLE 4
Clinical Signs of Malnutrition in Cystic Fibrosis

In infancy and childhood
Growth retardation
Delayed bone age
Weight deficit
Muscle wasting
Pot belly
Rectal prolapse
Hypoalbuminemia
Edema
Anemia
Bruising
Bleeding
Skin rash
Hepatomegaly
Developmental delay
In late childhood and adolescence
Growth retardation
Weight deficit
Muscle wasting
Delayed puberty
Hepatomegaly
Hypoalbuminemia
Osteopenia
Ataxia
Ophthalmoplegia

Developmental delay may be evident in severely malnourished infants and may persist for the first 5 years of life. Beyond this age, with adequate nutritional and socioeconomic support, there appears to be no permanent effect on intellectual development.

Children and Adolescents. Growth retardation is a variable feature during childhood. In 1964 Sproul and Huang found significant evidence of bone, weight, and height age (6 to 14 months behind chronologic age) retardation in children of all ages, but they noted that growth retardation was most pronounced in preadolescents and adolescents.[103] Even then, however, growth rate was normal in 89 percent of the patients until the age of 9 years. Today, short children under age 9 years are less common because of earlier diagnosis, prompt treatment of chest infections in infancy, and improved nutritional support at the onset of the disease, all of which help to maintain linear growth when the child is most vulnerable. Thin, wasted children usually have severe chest disease; when they do not, other causes such as esophagitis-induced anorexia or an inadequate diet should be explored.

The onset of puberty and the pubertal growth spurt are delayed in the majority of children with CF.[104] In females, the onset of menarche is closely related to the severity of pulmonary disease and malnutrition, although most females eventually reach full sexual maturation.[105] No convincing studies have suggested any unusual endocrine abnormalities in CF and, in general, delayed sexual maturation appears related to the severity of malnutrition. Andersen noted that height growth often continued later than in normal children so that eventual mature height of patients with CF is usually within normal limits.[106] Reduced weight as a percentage of height is relatively common following adolescence, particularly in females, and is correlated with a greater severity of pulmonary disease and diminished overall survival.[107]

Terminally Ill Patients. Coincident with progressive deterioration in pulmonary function, there is a progressive loss of body tissue, initially as adipose tissue but eventually as loss of lean body mass. Patients with significantly diminished lung function are unable to increase their caloric intake to meet their increased energy requirements. Significant weight loss occurs in proportion to height, with severe generalized muscle wasting, electrolyte abnormalities, hypoalbuminemia, and edema.

Deficits of Essential Nutrients

Fat-Soluble Vitamin Deficiencies. All patients with pancreatic insufficiency malabsorb fat-soluble vitamins and are at risk of developing clinical signs and symptoms of deficiency.

Clinical signs of vitamin A deficiency are rarely seen. Increased intracranial pressure, probably secondary to vitamin A deficiency, has been reported.[108] Undiagnosed patients, or patients who for some reason fail to take pancreatic supplement, more often lack clinical signs but have biochemical evidence of diminished carotene and vitamin A stores. Supplemented patients commonly have diminished vitamin A levels, despite evidence of liver concentrations up to fivefold greater than in unsupplemented controls.[109] Low levels of retinol-binding protein resulting from diminished protein anabolism and zinc deficiency may inhibit mobilization and transport of these stores.

Ataxia, absence of deep tendon reflexes, peripheral nerve conduction defects, absence of vibration and position sense, ophthalmoplegia, and muscle weakness suggest vitamin E deficiency. Most reported cases have occurred in late adolescence and adulthood. Clinical symptoms are relatively rare, appearing in approximately 10 percent of patients with low serum vitamin E levels.[110]

Recurrent back pains and postural abnormalities are not uncommon in older patients with CF, and there is a high incidence of vertebral wedging secondary to osteopenia.[111] Diminished bone mineralization is common in older patients with CF and is probably due to a combination of prolonged malnutrition and chronic vitamin D deficiency. Hanly et al[34] found that 15 of 20 adolescent and adult patients with CF in Ireland had serum 25-hydroxyvitamin D values that were below normal when studied in the winter. Twelve had an elevated serum alkaline phosphatase. Nine had diminished bone mineral content measured by photon beam absorptiometry. Many of these patients had not received vitamin D supplements for at least 6 months prior to the study, whereas others were taking less than 800 IU daily. Patients were also somewhat thin and on a low-fat diet, suggesting that protein-calorie malnutrition might be a factor. Frank osteomalacia has been reported in a black man with CF and cirrhosis.[112] No doubt skin pigment and cirrhosis contributed to vitamin D malnutrition. Season and sunlight are important determinants.[113] Vitamin D supplements should receive particular attention in countries with long, cloudy winters.

Overt hemorrhagic manifestations of vitamin K deficiency may be seen in untreated individuals with CF.[30] In the newborn period or in infancy, they may present with unexplained purpura, intestinal blood loss, and bleeding from an injection site or from a minor surgical procedure such as circumcision. Catastrophic, sometimes fatal, intracranial hemorrhage can occur. Older children, particularly those on antibiotics or with advanced liver disease, are susceptible to coagulation abnormalities even when they receive supplementation with vitamin K.

Metal Ion Deficiencies. Although zinc deficiency has been reported in patients with CF, plasma zinc appears to be low only in those with moderate to severe malnutrition and correlates directly with plasma retinol-binding protein, vitamin A, and serum protein status. There is no obvious defect of zinc absorption or metabolism. Plasma levels of copper and ceruloplasmin may be elevated in patients with CF, but usually in proportion to the severity of pulmonary disease, and possibly because ceruloplasmin is an acute-phase reactant. Selenium deficiency appears to be of little clinical significance in CF.[114]

Iron deficiency anemia with low serum ferritin is seen frequently, even in the stable patient.[115] The mechanism has not been elucidated. In patients with advanced pulmonary insufficiency, polycythemia seems to occur less commonly than in other pulmonary disorders of comparable severity, suggesting that these individuals may have a relative anemia, even though their hemoglobin levels are within the normal range.

Symptomatic hypomagnesemia may develop in those receiving aminoglycosides. Green et al[116] reported 12 patients presenting with brisk reflexes, a positive Trousseau sign, weakness, tremulousness, and muscle cramps who required repeated doses of magnesium sulfate to raise serum magnesium levels. Patients with CF are prone to a number of problems that increase the risk of hypomagnesemia, such as malabsorption, hyperaldosteronism, and glycosemia.

Essential Fatty Acids. In infancy, particularly before diagnosis, clinical essential fatty acid deficiency, with desquamating skin lesions, increased susceptibility to infection, poor wound healing, thrombocytopenia, and growth retardation may rarely occur.[117] In older patients clinical essential fatty acid deficiency is extremely rare. Most patients with pancreatic insufficiency nevertheless have abnormal blood and tissue lipids.[118,119] Changes include decreased linoleic and increased palmitoleic, oleic, and eicosatrienoic acids. In a survey of 32 patients from our clinic we found that low essential fatty acid levels were confined to patients with less than 5 percent of pancreatic function. Occasional reports of patients with low levels and normal fat absorption presumably depend on the fact that some patients with 2 to 5 percent of pancreatic function do not have steatorrhea. Linoleic acid is absorbed as well as other fatty acids in the presence of pancreatic supplements. The low plasma and tissue levels may be due to increased metabolic usage in relatively undernourished patients. Long-term linoleic acid supplementation has often failed to normalize lipid profiles, whereas supplemental calories and an increase in ideal body weight may do so even when daily linoleic acid intake stays the same.[120]

CLINICAL EVALUATION

At diagnosis, height, weight (percentiles), and anthropometry (skinfolds, midarm circumference) should be careful measured. During routine clinic visits careful monitoring of growth rates should be instituted, preferably every 3 to 6 months. When patients receive an adequate diet, normal growth can be expected until advanced respiratory disease supervenes. Individuals failing to achieve normal growth velocity, particularly younger children without advanced pulmonary disease, deserve careful re-evaluation (Table 5). This may include assessment of caloric intake at home, evaluation of compliance with recommendations for pancreatic enzyme supplements, and assessment of the adequacy of absorption by a fecal fat collection while the patient is on pancreatic enzyme supplements. Patients with acute respiratory exacerbation invariably lose weight due to anorexia, but appropriate antibiotic therapy should produce rapid catch-up growth. Individuals suffering from recurrent abdominal pain due to distal intestinal obstruction syndrome often reduce their caloric intake to control symptoms, and aggressive treatment may be necessary. Similarly, signs of gastroesophageal reflux and esophagitis must be sought because severe symptoms reduce caloric intake. Generally, patients with hepatic disease continue to grow normally unless hepatic decompensation supervenes.

TABLE 5
Nutritional Assessment in Cystic Fibrosis

Initial examination

- Growth
  - Height/weight/skeletal age
- Protein anabolism
  - Lean body mass (anthropometry)
  - Serum albumin/serum zinc
  - Serum retinol-binding protein
- Diet
  - Caloric intake (by observation)
- Digestion/absorption
  - Fecal fat excretion (percent of intake)
  - Pancreatic stimulation test (if absorption normal)
  - Plasma vitamin E/hemogram, PT/PTT*
  - Plasma EFA*

Return visits

- Growth
  - Height/weight/anthropometry
- Diet
  - Caloric intake (24-hour recall)
- Digestion/absorption
  - Stool fat examination
  - Serum carotene
- Special problems
- Repeat initial measurements as indicated.
- Consider plasma vitamin A; 25-hydroxyvitamin D; serum B_{12}; serum iron; serum ferritin; radiographs of abdomen, upright and supine; barium studies of esophagus, small intestine, and colon; esophageal manometry, pH studies.

PT/PTT = prothrombin time/partial thromboplastin time; EFA = essential fatty acids.

Biochemical Evaluation

The initial examination should include a careful assessment of pancreatic function. Quantitative determination of fecal fat losses on adequate and known fat intake is still the recommended approach for documenting steatorrhea. Poor substitutes include documentation of fat on stool microscopy, stool chymotryptic activity, serum carotene, and vitamin A and E levels. These tests may be useful to monitor treatment on return visits.

As an index of nutritional state, the use of serum protein or albumin may be misleading. However, in the newly diagnosed infant hypoproteinemia and hypoalbuminemia are a true reflection of the malnourished state, and levels usually revert to normal with nutritional rehabilitation. With advancing age, particularly in those with severe disease, albumin levels may be depressed, although an elevated gamma globulin content may produce an increase in overall protein concentration. The increase in gamma globulin has been attributed to recurrent pulmonary infections.[121] The decreased albumin level is incompletely understood. Pittman et al[122] and Strober et al [123] found normal albumin turnover rates and expanded plasma volume in patients with cor pulmonale, suggesting that hemodilution is important. Low albumin concentrations are correlated with poor pulmonary function.[87]

Radiologic Evaluation

Skeletal films may be useful to assess bone age, the potential for sustained linear growth at puberty, and mineralization. Intestinal causes of anorexia and weight loss, particularly in the adolescent or adult, may require radiologic evaluation. Intestinal impaction and obstruction are the most common causes of recurrent abdominal pain. Signs of bowel obstruction or a palpable right lower quadrant mass may be present. A plain roentgenogram of the abdomen characteristically shows the distal small bowel and colon packed with highly viscid, bubbly fecal material. Dilated loops of small intestine with air-fluid levels may be recognized. A fecal mass within the cecum or ascending colon may be identified by barium enema examination. Gastroesophageal reflux may be demonstrated in patients with symptoms of esophagitis, with or without hiatal hernia. Esophageal stricture may be a secondary complication.

Plain roentgenograms, computed tomography (CT), ultrasonography, and cholangiopancreatography are useful to assess the exocrine pancreas and biliary tract and to detect gallstones. Patients with pancreatic insufficiency have a shrunken, fibrotic pancreas on ultrasonographic or CT examination. Calcification and macroscopic cyst formation are relatively rare but may be seen in patients with recurrent pancreatitis.

TREATMENT

Diet

The diet must be calorically adequate. Because fat is the most economical and appetizing energy source, it should not be restricted but encouraged. The diet should be as normal for

TABLE 6
Nutritional Recommendations in Cystic Fibrosis

Energy	RDA* × 1.3
Protein	RDA
Essential fatty acids	3–5% of total calories
Vitamins	
A	5,000–10,000 IU/day emulsified vitamin A alcohol
D	400–800 IU/day
E	100–200 IU/day, α-tocopherol acetate
K	5 mg twice weekly, vitamin K_1
B	RDA × 2
C	RDA × 2
Trace metals	
Zinc	15 mg daily
Iron	RDA
Pancreatic replacement	
Children and adults	
Regular capsules	48,000 units of lipase per meal ± adjunct
pH-sensitive microspheres	24,000 units of lipase per meal
Infants	8,000 units of lipase per 120 cc formula

RDA = recommended daily dietary allowances.

the age and peer group as possible. However, children should be encouraged to eat larger portions than their brothers and sisters or parents, to clean their plates with each feeding, to add fat in the form of cream or butter or untrimmed meat whenever possible, and to have high-calorie snacks between meals and before bed. Under these circumstances a growing child with CF has normal or slightly higher than normal caloric intake despite his or her illness. When a group of adolescents with CF who had followed this routine for years were investigated in Ontario,[124] we were surprised to learn that the average daily intake of calories and protein was in the same range as the diet normally eaten by Ontario school children. Perhaps the most significant finding was that the diets of the CF subjects were not lower in calories and protein, since a number of these patients had severe pulmonary disease.

Table 6 contains dietary supplement recommendations for individuals with CF. Fat-soluble vitamins should be given in large daily doses in water-miscible form. We normally give twice the daily minimum requirements of B vitamins, although the necessity for this has not been established.

Amino acid hydrolysate, medium-chain triglycerides (MCT), and polysaccharide supplements are rarely indicated. Patients who cannot maintain their weight with the high-calorie, constantly reinforced routine described above rarely do better when asked to take MCT or polysaccharide supplements unless the supplements are delivered by an unusual route such as parenteral alimentation or nasogastric, gastrostomy, or jejunostomy feeding. The exception occurs in infants with severe pulmonary problems in their first year of life because it is sometimes useful to begin feeding with MCT and hydrolysate formula when it is difficult to ensure adequate delivery of pancreatic enzymes. MCT mixtures should contain adequate essential fatty acids (or be supplemented with corn oil), and an attempt should always be made to provide some pancreatic supplementation, because digestion of MCT is thereby improved.[125]

Pancreatic Supplement

All patients with steatorrhea should receive regular supplementation with pancreatic enzymes. The pancreatic supplements should be taken at regular intervals throughout the meal. Infants can usually handle supplements if mixed in a small quantity of solids. Microspheres may not be swallowed well in the first year of life and may cause oral microulcers when they lodge in the mouth.

Nonspecific Measures

Dietary intake is closely related to an individual's sense of self-esteem and general well-being. It is therefore essential to ensure that patients who are having nutritional difficulties receive psychological support. Exercise programs aimed at improving physical capacity are also important. They may lead to a sense of accomplishment as muscle mass improves and stimulate genuine interest in providing nutritional support for physical goals. In addition, careful nutritional support must be individualized for those patients with diabetes, using standard guidelines.

Specific Approaches for Certain Complications

Hypoalbuminemia, Edema, and Anemia of Infancy

Patients may be profoundly anorexic and indifferent to food. A short course of total enteral nutrition may be the only way to ensure adequate nutrition in the first 5 to 10 days of care. Albumin infusions may be indicated to reduce edema. Vitamin E levels are invariably low, but all fat-soluble vitamins should be supplemented. When oral feeding is possible, patients improve rapidly with adequate caloric intake and pancreatic supplementation.

Neurologic complications of vitamin E deficiency are not easily reversed. Prolonged intramuscular administration of 200 to 400 IU per week has met with limited success.[33] Oral desiccated ox bile improves absorption, but for symptomatic cases it is prudent to supply the vitamin by injection. Progress may be followed by serial measurements of plasma or serum vitamin E level and periodic assessment of nerve conduction.

Anorexia and Weight Loss in Patients with Advanced Pulmonary Disease

These patients are particularly difficult to treat. Weight loss is often the first sign of a respiratory infection, and prompt treatment of pulmonary problems may improve appetite and restore weight. A major effort must be made to maintain caloric intake well in excess of RDA (Table 6). Adolescent dietary habits can never be altered by edict, but gentle and persistent persuasion can succeed. Low-calorie high-volume ingredients, such as carbonated beverages, tea, and coffee should be replaced with milk, cream, and milkshakes whenever possible. Commercial high-calorie supplements can often be worked into recipes for milkshakes, ice cream or puddings. The upper energy limit from the point of view of palatability and long-term tolerance is probably 1.5 kcal per milliliter, but if the patient can be induced to supplement the diet three times daily, it is often possible to add 400 to 600 kcal per day.

Unfortunately, as the disease progresses, intakes often fall to less than 1,200 kcal per day in spite of continued exhortation. Patients who fail to respond to intensive dietary counseling become candidates for alternative forms of alimentation. Long-term feeding by nasogastric intubation may be tried. Elemental preparations can be given via this route to ensure maximum absorption and utilization, and intakes of 3,000 to 4,000 kcal per day can be attained by gradually increasing the infusion volume over several weeks. Unfortunately, the caloric intake is limited by the volume that can be infused over time. Practical limits are about 1,000 kcal per 8-hour period. If the patient is to be fully ambulatory during the day, intubation is limited to overnight supplementation. Nasogastric tubes are not well tolerated by patients with acute respiratory symptoms or advanced chronic lung disease, and tubes are often dislodged by coughing. As a result, supplementation by this route tends to be intermittent and suboptimal. We have had more success recently with gastrostomy supplementation at night. Jejunostomy feeding and parenteral alimentation in hospital or at home have also been used. All these approaches are limited to adjunctive use in the ambulatory patient, and their value in slowing the progression of the disease or improving the quality of life must still be evaluated. It is doubtful whether any form of nutritional therapy has any impact on the outcome during the terminal stages, when the patient is frequently hospitalized and, in a practical sense, bedridden. Unfortunately, this is often the time when requests for a nutritional miracle become most intense. Perhaps the most important role of the nutritionist during this period is to discourage central lines, feeding tubes, and other examples of our technical versatility, which only add to the discomfort and pathos of the last days.

REFERENCES

1. Fanconi G, Uehlinger E, Knaucer C. Das Coelioksyndrom bei angeborener zystisher Pankreas Fibromatose and Bronchicktasis. Wein Med Wochensch 1936; 86:753–756.
2. Anderson D. Cystic fibrosis of the pancreas and its relation to celiac disease. Am Dis Child 1938; 56:344–399.
3. di Sant'Agnese P, Darling R, Perera G, Shea E. Abnormal electrolyte composition of sweat in cystic fibrosis of the pancreas. Pediatrics 1953; 12:549–563.
4. Gibbs GE, Bostick WL, Smith PM. Incomplete pancreatic deficiency in cystic fibrosis of the pancreas. J Pediatr 1950; 37:320–325.
5. Quinton PM. Chloride impermeability in cystic fibrosis. Nature 1983; 301:421–422.
6. Knowles MR, Gatzy JT, Boucher RC. Relative ion permeability of normal and cystic fibrosis nasal epithelium. J Clin Invest 1983; 71: 1410–1417.
7. Sato K, Sato F. Defective beta adrenergic response of cystic fibrosis sweat glands in vivo and in vitro. J Clin Invest 1984; 73:1763–1771.
8. Boucher RC, Stutts MJ, Knowles MR, Cantley L, Gatzy JT. Na^+ transport in cystic fibrosis respiratory epithelia. J Clin Invest 1986; 78:1245–1252.
9. Widdicombe JH, Welsh MH, Finkbeiner WE. Cystic fibrosis decreases the apical membrane chloride permeability of monolayers cultured from cells of tracheal epithelium. Proc Natl Acad Sci 1985; 82:6167–6171.
10. Li M, McCann CM, Liedtke C, Nairn A, Greengard P, Welsh M. Cyclic AMP dependent protein kinase opens chloride channels in wound but not cystic fibrosis airway epithelium. Nature 1988; 331: 358–360.
11. Frizzell RA. Cystic fibrosis: a disease of ion channels? Trends Neurosci 1987; 10:190–193.
12. Case RM, Scratcherd T. The actions of dibutyral cyclic adenosine 3′5′-monophosphate and methyl xanthines on pancreatic exocrine secretion. J Physiol 1972; 210:1–15.
13. Argent BE, Gray MA, Greenwell JR. Secretin regulated anion channel on the apical membrane of rat pancreatic duct cells in vitro. J Physiol 1987; 39:333
14. Kopelman H, Corey M, Gaskin K, Durie P, Weizman Z, Forstner G. Impaired chloride secretion as well as bicarbonate secretion underlies the fluid secretory defect in the cystic fibrosis pancreas. Gastroenterology 1988; 95:349–355.
15. Berschneider HM, Knowles MR, Azizkhan RG, Boucher RC, Tobey NA, Orlando RC, Powell DW. Altered intestinal chloride transport in cystic fibrosis. FASEB J 1988; 2:2625–2629.
16. Hopfer U. Pathophysiological considerations relevant to intestinal obstruction in cystic fibrosis. In: Quinton PM, Martinez JR, Hopfer K, eds. Fluid and electrolyte abnormalities in exocrine glands in cystic fibrosis. San Francisco, San Francisco Press, 1982: 241.
17. Kopelman H, Durie P, Gaskin K, Weizman Z, Forstner G. Pancreatic fluid secretion and protein hyperconcentration in cystic fibrosis. N Eng J Med 1985; 312:329–334.
18. Imrie J, Fagan D, Sturgess J. Quantitative evaluation of the development of the exocrine pancreas in CF and control infants. Am J Pathol 1979; 95:697–707.
19. Schutt W, Isles T. Protein in meconium ileus. Arch Dis Child 1968; 43:178–181.
20. Oppenheimer E, Esterly J. Cystic fibrosis of the pancreas. Arch Pathol 1973; 96:149–154.
21. Baxter PS, Goldhill J, Hardcastle J, Hardcastle PT, Taylor CJ. Accounting for cystic fibrosis. Nature 1988; 335:211.
22. Wainwright BJ, Scambler PJ, Schmidtke J, Watson E, Law H, Farrall M, Cooke H, Eiberg H, Williamson R. Localization of cystic fibrosis locus to human chromosome 7 cen-q22. Nature 1985; 318:384–385.
23. Knowlton RG, Cohen-Haguenauer O, Nguyen VC, Frezal J, Brown V, Barker D, Braman I, Schumm I, Tsui L, Buchwald M, Donis-Keleer H. A polymorphic DNA marker linked to cystic fibrosis is located in chromosome 7. Nature 1985; 318:380–381.
24. Kerem B, Buchanan JA, Durie P, Corey ML, Levison H, Rommens IM, Buchwald M, Tsue LC. DNA marker haplotype association with pancreatic sufficiency in cystic fibrosis; in press.
25. Gaskin K, Gurwitz D, Durie PR, et al. Improved respiratory prognosis in patients with cystic fibrosis with normal fat absorption. J Pediatr 1982; 100:857–862.
26. Kopito L, Shwachman H, Vawter G, Edlow J. The pancreas in cystic fibrosis: chemical composition and comparative morphology. Pediatr Res 1976; 10:742–749.
27. Liu P, Daneman A, Stringer D, Durie PR. Pancreatic cysts and calcification in cystic fibrosis. J Can Assoc Radiol 1986; 37:279–281.
28. Lee P, Roloff D, Howat W. Hypoproteinemia and anemia in infants with cystic fibrosis. JAMA 1974; 228:585–588.
29. Stern R, Izant RJ, Boat TF, Wood RE, Matthews LW, Doershuk CF. Treatment and prognosis of rectal prolapse in cystic fibrosis. Gastroenterology 1986; 82:707–710.
30. Torstenson O, Humphrey G, Edson J, Warwick W. Cystic fibrosis presenting with severe hemorrhage due to vitamin K malabsorption. A report of 3 cases. Pediatrics 1970; 45:857–860.
31. Farrell PM, Bieri JG, Frantantoni JF, Wood RE, di Sant'Agnese P. The occurrence and effects of human vitamin E deficiency: a study in patients with cystic fibrosis. J Clin Invest 1977; 60:233–241.
32. Elias E, Muller DP, Scott J. Association of spinocerebellar disorders with cystic fibrosis or chronic childhood cholestasis and very low vitamin E. Lancet 1981; ii:1319–1321.
33. Sitrin MD, Lieberman F, Jensen WE, Avertano N, Millurn C, Ad-

dington W. Vitamin E deficiency and neurologic disease in adults with cystic fibrosis. Ann Intern Med 1987; 107:51–54.
34. Hanly JG, McKenna M, Quigley C, Freaney R, Muldowney F, Fitzgerald M. Hypovitaminosis D and response to supplementation in older patients with cystic fibrosis. Q J Med 1985; 219:377–385.
35. Lindemans J, Neijens HJ, Kerrebijn KF, Abels F. Vitamin B_{12} absorption in cystic fibrosis. Acta Paediatr Scand 1984; 73:537–540.
36. Lindemans J, Abels F, Neijens J,Kerrebijn KF. Elevated serum vitamin B_{12} in cystic fibrosis. Acta Paediatr Scand 1984; 73:768–771.
37. Rosan R, Shwachman H, Kulczycki L. Diabetes mellitus and cystic fibrosis of pancreas. Am J Dis Child 1962; 104:625–634.
38. Wilmshurst E, Soeldner J, Holsclaw D, Kaufmann R, Shwachman H, Aoki TJ, Gleason R. Endogenous and exogenous insulin responses in patients with cystic fibrosis. Pediatrics 1975; 55:75–82.
39. Geffner ME, Lippe BM, Kaplan SA, Itami RM, Gillard BK, Levin S, Taylor IL. Carbohydrate tolerance in cystic fibrosis is closely linked to pancreatic exocrine function. Pediatr Res 1984; 18:1107–1111.
40. MacLean W, Tripp R. Cystic fibrosis with edema and falsely negative sweat test. J Pediatr 1973; 83:85–90.
41. Bonin A, Roy C, LaSalle R, Weber A, Morin S. Fecal chymotrypsin: a reliable index of exocrine pancreatic function in children. J Pediatr 1973; 83:594–600.
42. Cleghorn G, Benjamin L, Corey M, Forstner G, Dati F, Durie P. Age-related alterations in immunoreactive pancreatic lipase and cationic trypsinogen in young children with cystic fibrosis. J Pediatr 1985; 107:377–381.
43. Weizman Z, Forstner G, Gaskin KJ, Kopelman H, Wong S, Durie PR. Bentiromide test for assessing pancreatic dysfunction using analysis of para-aminobenzoic acid in plasma and urine. Gastroenterology 1985; 89:596–604.
44. Forstner G, Gall G, Corey M, Durie P, Hill R, Gaskin K. Digestion and absorption of nutrients in cystic fibrosis. In: Sturgess J, ed. Perspectives in cystic fibrosis. Proceedings of the 8th International Congress on Cystic Fibrosis. Mississauga, Canada: Imperial Press, 1980:137.
45. Gaskin KJ, Durie PR, Lee L, Hill R, Forstner GG. Colipase and lipase secretion in childhood onset pancreatic insufficiency. Delineation of patients with steatorrhea secondary to relative colipase deficiency. Gastroenterology 1984; 86:1–7.
46. Crossley JR, Smith PA, Edgar BW, Gluckman PD, Elliott RB. Neonatal screening for cystic fibrosis, using immunoreactive trypsin assay in dried blood spots. Clin Chim Acta 1981; 113:111–121.
47. Waters D, Dorney S, Gruca M, Brown J, Gaskin K. Pancreatic sufficiency in CF infants from a neonatal screening programme. Proceedings of the 10th International Congress on Cystic Fibrosis. Sydney, Australia, 1988. Excerpta Medica. Asia Pacific Congress Series 74, p 162.
48. Wilcken B. An evaluation of screening for cystic fibrosis in genetics and epithelial cell dysfunction. In: Riordan JR, Buchwald, M, eds. Cystic fibrosis. New York: Alan R. Liss, 1987: 201.
49. Zentler-Munro PL, Fine DR, Batten JC, Northfield TC. Effect of cimetidine on enzyme inactivation, bile acid precipitation and lipid solubilisation in pancreatic steatorrhea due to cystic fibrosis. Gut 1985; 26:892–901.
50. Durie PR, Bell L, Linton W, et al. Effect of cimetidine and sodium bicarbonate on pancreatic replacement therapy in cystic fibrosis. Gut 1980; 21:778–786.
51. Gow R, Bradbear R, Francis P, Shepherd R. Comparative study of varying regimens to improve steatorrhea and creatorrhea in cystic fibrosis. Lancet 1981; ii:1071–1074.
52. Stead RJ, Skypala I, Hodson ME, Batten JC. Enteric coated microspheres of pancreatin in the treatment of cystic fibrosis. Thorax 1987; 42:533–537.
53. Dressman JB, Shtohryn LV, Diokno D. Effects of product formation on in vitro activity of pancreatic enzymes. Am J Hosp Pharm 1985; 42:2502–2506.
54. Belli DC, Levy L, Darling P, Leroy C, Lepage G, Giguere R, Roy C. Taurine improves the absorption of a fat meal in patients with cystic fibrosis. Pediatrics 1987; 80:517–523.
55. Abrams CK, Hamosh M, Hubbard VS, Dutta SK, Hamosh P. Lingual lipase in cystic fibrosis. J Clin Invest 1984; 173:374–382.
56. di Sant'Agnese P. Fibrocystic disease of the pancreas with normal or partial pancreatic function. Pediatrics 1955; 15:683–695.
57. Schwachman H, Lebenthal E, Khaw K. Recurrent acute pancreatitis in patients with cystic fibrosis with normal pancreatic enzymes. Pediatrics 1975; 55:86–94.
58. Corey M, Gaskin K, Durie P, Levison H, Forstner G. Improved prognosis in CF patients with normal fat absorption. J Pediatr Gastroenterol Nutr 1984; 3 (suppl):S99–S105.
59. Tsui LC, Buetow K, Buchwald M. Genetic analysis of cystic fibrosis using linked DNA markers. Am J Hum Genet 1986; 39:720–728.
60. Lands L, Zinman P, Wise M, Kopelman H. Pancreatic function testing or meconium ileus in cystic fibrosis: two case reports. J Pediatr Gastroenterol Nutr 1988; 7:276–279.
61. Hurwitt E, Arnheim E. Meconium ileus associated with stenosis of the pancreatic ducts. Am J Dis Child 1942; 64:443–454.
62. Auburn R, Feldman S, Gadacz T, Rowe M. Meconium ileus secondary to partial aplasia of the pancreas: report of a case. Surgery 1969; 65:689–693.
63. Dolan T, Touloukian R. Familial meconium ileus not associated with cystic fibrosis. J Pediatr Surg 1974; 9:821–824.
64. Noblett H. Meconium ileus. In: Ravitch M, Welsh K, Benson C, et al, eds. Pediatric surgery. Chicago: Year Book Medical Publishers, 1979:943.
65. Wagget H, Bishop H, Koop E. Experience with Gastrografin enema in the treatment of meconium ilueus. J Pediatr Surg 1970; 5:649–654.
66. Kulczycki LL, Shwachman H. Studies in cystic fibrosis of the pancreas: occurrence of rectal prolapse. N Engl J Med 1958; 259:409–412.
67. Matseshe J, Go V, Di Magno E. Meconium ileus equivalent complicating cystic fibrosis in postneonatal children and young adults. Gastroenterology 1977; 72:732–736.
68. Davidson AC, Harrison K, Steinfort CL, Geddes DM. Distal intestinal obstruction syndrome in cystic fibrosis treated by oral intestinal lavage, and a case of recurrent obstruction despite normal pancreatic function. Thorax 1987; 42:538–541.
69. Park RW, Grand RJ. Gastrointestinal manifestations of cystic fibrosis. Gastroenterology 1981; 81:1143–1161.
70. Holsclaw D, Rocmans C, Shwachman H. Intussusception in patients with cystic fibrosis. Pediatrics 1971; 48:51–58.
71. Rosenstein BJ, Longbaum TS. Incidence of distal intestinal obstruction syndrome in cystic fibrosis. J Pediatr Gastroenterol Nutr 1983; 2:299–301.
72. Cleghorn GJ, Forstner GG, Stringer DA, Durie PR. Treatment of distal intestinal obstruction syndrome in cystic fibrosis with a balanced intestinal lavage solution. Lancet 1986; i:8–11.
73. Rubinstein S, Moss R, Lewiston N. Constipation and meconium ileus equivalent in patients with cystic fibrosis. Pediatrics 1986; 78:473–479.
74. Hernanz-Schulman M, Kirkpatrick J, Shwachman H, Herman T, Schulman G, Vawter G. Pneumatosis intestinales in cystic fibrosis. Radiology 1986; 160:497–499.
75. Bendig DW, Seilheimer DK, Wagner ML, et al. Complications of gastroesophageal reflux in patients with cystic fibrosis. J Pediatr 1982; 100:536–540.
76. Scott RB, O'Laughlin EV, Gall DG. Gastroesophageal reflux in patients with cystic fibrosis. J Pediatr 1985; 106:223–227.
77. Feigelson J, Girault F, Pecau Y. Gastroesophageal reflux and esophagitis in cystic fibrosis. Acta Paediatr Scand 1987; 76:989–990.
78. Kopel F. Gastrointestinal manifestations of cystic fibrosis. Gastroenterology 1972; 62:483–491.
79. Stern P, Stevens D, Boat T, Doershuk C, Izant R, Matthews L. Symptomatic hepatic disease in cystic fibrosis. Gastroenterology 1976; 70:645–649.
80. Oppenheimer E, Esterly J. Hepatic changes in young infants with cystic fibrosis. Possible relation to focal biliary cirrhosis. J Pediatr 1975; 80:683–689.
81. Hulterantz R, Mengarelli J, Strandvik B. Morphological findings in the liver of children with cystic fibrosis: a light and electron microscopic study. Hepatology 1986; 6:881–889.
82. Esterly J, Oppenheimer E. Observations in cystic fibrosis of the pancreas. 1. The gallbladder. Bull Johns Hopkins Hosp 1962; 110:247–254.
83. Talamo RC, Hendren WH. Prolonged obstructive jaundice: report of a case in a neonate with meconium ileus and jejunal atresia. Am J Dis Child 1968; 115:74–79.
84. Valman HB, France NE, Wallis PG. Prolonged neonatal jaundice in cystic fibrosis. Arch Dis Child 1971; 46:805–809.

85. Taylor WF, Qaqundah B. Neonatal jaundice associated with cystic fibrosis. Am J Dis Child 1972; 123:161-122.
86. Tanner MS. Current clinical management of hepatic problems in cystic fibrosis. J R Soc Med 1986; (suppl 12):38-43.
87. Davidson GP, Corey M, Hassel FM, Sondheimer JM, Crozier D, Forstner GG. Immunoassay of serum conjugates of cholic acid in cystic fibrosis. J Clin Pathol 1980; 35:390-394.
88. Robb TA, Davidson GP, Kirubakaran C. Conjugated bile acids in serum and secretions—response to cholecystokinin/secretin stimulation in children with cystic fibrosis. Gut 1985; 26:1246-1256.
89. Schuster S, Shwachman H, Toyama W. The management of portal hypertension in cystic fibrosis. J Pediatr Surg 1977; 12:201-206.
90. Mieles LA, Orenstein D, Teperman L, Podesta L, Koneru B, Starzl TE. Liver transplantation in cystic fibrosis. Lancet 1989; i:1073.
91. L'Heureux P, Isenberg J, Sharp H, Warwick W. Gallbladder disease in cystic fibrosis. AJR 1977; 128:953-956.
92. Roy C, Weber A, Morin C, Conbes JC, Nussle D, Megevand A, La Salle R. Abnormal biliary lipid composition in cystic fibrosis. N Engl J Med 1977; 297:1301-1305.
93. Weber A, Roy C, Morin C, La Salle R. Malabsorption of bile acids in children with cystic fibrosis. N Engl J Med 1973; 289:1001-1005.
94. Fondacaro JD, Heubi JE, Kellogg FW. Intestinal bile acid malabsorption in cystic fibrosis: a primary mucosal cell defect. Pediatr Res 1982; 16:494-498.
95. Colombo C, Roda A, Roda E, Sereni LP, Brega A, Fugazzo R, Giunta A. Bile acid malabsorption in cystic fibrosis with and without pancreatic insufficiency. J Pediatr Gastroenterol Nutr 1984; 3:556-562.
96. Watkins J, Tercyac A, Szczepanik P, Klein P. Bile salt kinetics in cystic fibrosis: influence of pancreatic enzyme replacement. Gastroenterology 1977; 73:1023-1028.
97. Gaskin KJ, Waters DLM, Howman-Giles R, de Silva M, Earl JW, Martin HCO, Kan AE, Brown JM, Dorney SFA. Liver disease and common-bile-duct stenosis in cystic fibrosis. N Engl J Med 1988; 318:340-346.
98. Strandvik B, Samuelson K. Fasting serum bile acid levels in relation to liver histopathology in cystic fibrosis. Scand J Gastroenterol 1985; 20:381-384.
99. Vaisman N, Pencharz P, Corey M, Canny G, Hahn E. Energy expenditure of patients with cystic fibrosis. J Pediatr 1987; 111:496-500.
100. Vaisman N, Levy L, Pencharz P, Tan Y, Soldin S, Canny G, Hahn E. Effect of solbutamol on resting energy expenditure in patients with cystic fibrosis. J Pediatr 1987; 111:137-139.
101. Shepherd R, Cooksley WGE, Domville-Cooke WD. Improved growth and clinical, nutritional and respiratory changes in response to nutritional therapy in cystic fibrosis. J Pediatr 1980; 97:351-357.
102. Buchdahl RM, Cox M, Fulleylove C, Marchant JL, Tomkins AM, Brenton MJ, Warner JO. Increased energy expenditure in cystic fibrosis. J Appl Physiol 1988; 64:1810-1816.
103. Sproul A, Huang N. Growth patterns in children with cystic fibrosis. J Pediatr 1964; 65:664-676.
104. Mitchell-Heggs P, Mearns M, Batten JC. Cystic fibrosis in adolescents and adults. Q J Med 1976; 45:479-504.
105. Moshang R, Holsclaw DS. Menarchal determinants in cystic fibrosis. Am J Dis Child 1980; 134:1139-1142.
106. Andersen DH. Cystic fibrosis of the pancreas. J Chron Dis 1958; 7:58-65.
107. Corey ML. Longitudinal studies in cystic fibrosis. In: Sturgess J, ed. Perspectives in cystic fibrosis. Proceedings of the 8th International Congress on Cystic Fibrosis. Mississauga, Canada: Imperial Press, 1980: 246.
108. Keating J, Feigin R. Increased intracranial pressure associated with probable vitamin A deficiency in cystic fibrosis. Pediatrics 1970; 46:41-46.
109. Underwood BA, Denning CR. Blood and liver concentrations of vitamin A and E in children with cystic fibrosis of the pancreas. Pediatr Res 1972; 6:26-31.
110. Willison HJ, Muller DPR, Matthews S, Jones S, Kriss A, Stead RJ, Hodson ME, Harding AE. A study of the relationship between neurological function and serum vitamin E concentrations in patients with cystic fibrosis. J Neurol Neurosurg Psychol 1985; 48:1097-1102.
111. Rose J, Gamble J, Schultz A, Lewiston N. Back pain and spinal deformity in cystic fibrosis. Am J Dis Child 1987; 141:1313-1316.
112. Friedman HZ. Langman CB, Favus MJ. Vitamin D metabolism and osteomalacia in cystic fibrosis. Gastroenterology 1985; 88:808-813.
113. Reiter EO, Brugman SM, Pike I, Pitt M, Dokoh S, Haussler M, Gerstle R, Taussig LM. Vitamin D metabolites in adolescents and young adults with cystic fibrosis: effects of sun and season. J Pediatr 1985; 106:21-26.
114. Castillo R, Landon C, Eckhardt K, Morris V, Levander O, Lewiston N. Selenium and vitamin E status in cystic fibrosis. J Pediatr 1981; 99:583-587.
115. Ater JL, Herbst JJ, Landaw SA, O'Brien RT. Relative anemia and iron deficiency in cystic fibrosis. Pediatrics 1983; 71:810-814.
116. Green CG, Doershuk CF, Stern RC. Symptomatic hypomagnesemia in cystic fibrosis. J Pediatr 1985; 107:425-428.
117. Chase HP, Long MA, Lavin MH. Cystic fibrosis and malnutrition. J Pediatr 1979; 95:337-347.
118. Hubbard VS, Dunn GD, di Santi'Agnese PA. Abnormal fatty acid composition of plasma lipids in cystic fibrosis. Lancet 1977; ii:1302-1304.
119. Lloyd-Still JD, Johnson SB, Holman RT. Essential fatty acid status in cystic fibrosis and the effects of safflower oil supplementation. Am J Clin Nutr 1981; 34:1-7.
120. Parsons HG, O'Loughlin EV, Forbes D, Cooper D, Gall DG. Supplemental calories improve essential fatty acid deficiency in cystic fibrosis patients. Pediatr Res 1988; 24:353-356.
121. Solomons NW, Wagonfeld JB, Rieger C, Jacob RA, Bolt M, Vander Horst J, Rothberg R, Sandstead H. Some biochemical indices of nutrition in treated cystic fibrosis patients. Am J Clin Nutr 1981; 34:462-474.
122. Pittman FE, Denning CR, Barker HG. Albumin metabolism in cystic fibrosis. Am J Dis Child 1964; 108:360-365.
123. Strober W, Peter G, Schwartz RH. Albumin metabolism in cystic fibrosis. Pediatrics 1969; 43:416-426.
124. Bell L, Linton WL, Corey ML, Durie PR, Forstner G. Nutrient intakes of adolescents with cystic fibrosis. J Can Diet Assoc 1981; 42:1-10.
125. Durie PR, Newth CJ, Forstner GG, Gall G. Malabsorption of medium-chain triglycerides in infants with cystic fibrosis: correction with pancreatic enzyme supplements. J Pediatr 1980; 96:862-864.

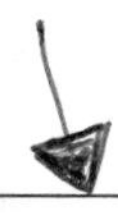

PART 3

Hereditary Disorders of the Pancreas

Kevin John Gaskin, M.B., B.S., F.R.A.C.P., FRCPC

A variety of other hereditary disorders of the exocrine pancreas have been described (Table 1). The incidence of these disorders is essentially unknown, although Shwachman's syndrome is at least five times less prevalent than cystic fibrosis (discussed elsewhere in this chapter). There have only been isolated reports of the remaining disorders.

SHWACHMAN'S SYNDROME

Shwachman's syndrome is characterized by short stature, exocrine pancreatic hypoplasia, a normal sweat chloride, and the variable features of neutropenia and radiologic skeletal changes. Following the original description of these anomalies by Bodian et al[1] and Shwachman et al,[2] other features have been documented (Table 2), and it is now clearly a multi-system disease. A recent report[3] estimated an incidence of one case per 10,000 live births; next to cystic fibrosis, it is the most common congenital abnormality of the exocrine pancreas. The etiology is unknown, although an unusual surface distribution of concanavalin A on neutrophils has been reported,[4] which may reflect a cellular cytoskeletal defect. Previously, analysis of sibship segregation ratios and family pedigrees supported an autosomal recessive mode of inheritance. However, one family with a child with pancreatic hypoplasia and neutropenia and the father with neutropenia has been documented,[5] and the author has seen two families each with a parent and child with pancreatic hypoplasia, and both children with documented neutropenia and metaphyseal dysplasia. An autosomal dominant pattern of inheritance with variable expressivity may thus prevail in some families.

TABLE 1
Other Hereditary Disorders of the Exocrine Pancreas

Shwachman's syndrome
Johanson-Blizzard syndrome
Exocrine pancreatic dysfunction with refractory sideroblastic anemia
Pancreatic agenesis
Congenital rubella
Isolated enzyme deficiencies
Lipase
Lipase/co-lipase
Co-lipase
Trypsin
Amylase

Clinical and Laboratory Manifestations

Short Stature

The most constant clinical feature of Shwachman's syndrome is short stature. The patients are below the third percentile for height but maintain a normal linear growth velocity. Of a total of 35 patients in two recently published series,[6,7] 22 were below the third percentile for height and 30 were below the tenth percentile. A delayed pubertal growth spurt was reported.[6] Although most adults described have short stature, at least two patients have reached the twenty-fifth percentile.[7]

TABLE 2
Features of Shwachman's Syndrome

Exocrine pancreatic hypoplasia
Short stature
with normal linear growth velocity
Skeletal changes
Clinical
Thoracic dystrophy
Clinodactyly
Genu and cubitus valgus
Radiologic
Metaphyseal dysplasia
Delayed bone age
Long bone tubulation
Short or flared ribs
Bone marrow
Hypoplasia
Neutropenia
Thrombocytopenia
Elevated fetal hemoglobin
Myelolymphoproliferative disorders
Recurrent infections
Neutropenia
Decreased neutrophil mobility
Immunoglobulin deficiency
Miscellaneous
Psychomotor retardation
Renal tubular dysfunction
Diabetes mellitus
Dental abnormalities
Ichthyosis
Hepatic dysfunction
Hirschsprung's disease

Pancreatic Hypoplasia

The invariable feature of this disease is pancreatic hypoplasia. Pathologically, there is extensive fatty replacement of pancreatic acinar tissue and normal ductular architecture.[1,2,6] These findings are consistent with pancreatic function studies[7-9] using intravenous secretin and cholecystokinin, demonstrating marked impairment of enzyme secretion, but only minimal impairment of bicarbonate secretion and water flow.

Clinically, patients present either with or without fat malabsorption.[7,8] The majority who have steatorrhea at their initial presentation in the infancy or toddler period show improvement in absorption to within the normal range at a later age. Quantitative pancreatic stimulation tests have demonstrated that those with steatorrhea have less than 1 percent of normal co-lipase and less than 2 percent of normal lipase secretion.[7,8] In contrast, patients with normal absorption have demonstrated co-lipase and lipase secretion up to 10 and 14 percent of normal, respectively.[7,8] Normal fat absorption does not, therefore, exclude a diagnosis of Shwachman's syndrome, and one should rely on the demonstration of exocrine pancreatic dysfunction using a quantitative pancreatic stimulation technique. However, as it is not a widely available investigation, noninvasive tests, including computed tomography and ultrasonography of the pancreas for lipomatosis[10] or serum trypsinogen[11] may assume increasing importance for diagnosis.

Bone Marrow Dysfunction

Bone marrow dysfunction is manifested principally as neutropenia, red cell hypoplasia, and thrombocytopenia.[6,7] Lymphoproliferative and myeloproliferative malignancies have also been reported.[3] Of the 35 patients in the two major series,[6,7] 30 manifested intermittent neutropenia, three persistent neutropenia, and two, on two and three counts respectively, normal neutrophil counts. Burke et al[5] had recommended that as the neutropenia (less than 1,500 neutrophils per cubic millimeter) was usually intermittent, twice-weekly counts over a three-week period should be performed during an interval when the patient is free of infections. Using these criteria, the presence of neutropenia is variable, occurring in 7 to 93 percent of counts in any individual patient.[6] Thrombocytopenia is also intermittent but less frequent than neutropenia. Bone marrow examinations have revealed varying degrees of marrow hypoplasia, fat infiltration, and myeloid maturation arrest.[6]

The clinical manifestations of neutropenia have included otitis media, bronchopneumonia, osteomyelitis, septicemia, and recurrent skin infections, and some patients have died of overwhelming sepsis early in life.[6] The frequency of infections appears to decline with age. Infections have occurred in the absence of neutropenia, and in this regard, reports of immunoglobulin deficiency[6] and neutrophil mobility defects may account for this phenomenon.[6]

Skeletal Abnormalities

The skeletal abnormalities are variable (see Table 2). They are manifested clinically in a small proportion of cases as thoracic dystrophy and in approximately 50 percent of cases as clinodactyly. One report[6] documented metaphyseal dysplasia in 60 percent, short flared ribs in 60 percent, long bone tubulation in 33 percent, and delayed bone maturation in at least 75 percent. Examples of the rib and metaphyseal changes are shown in Figures 1 and 2, respectively. It is important to note that although rib changes, with or without

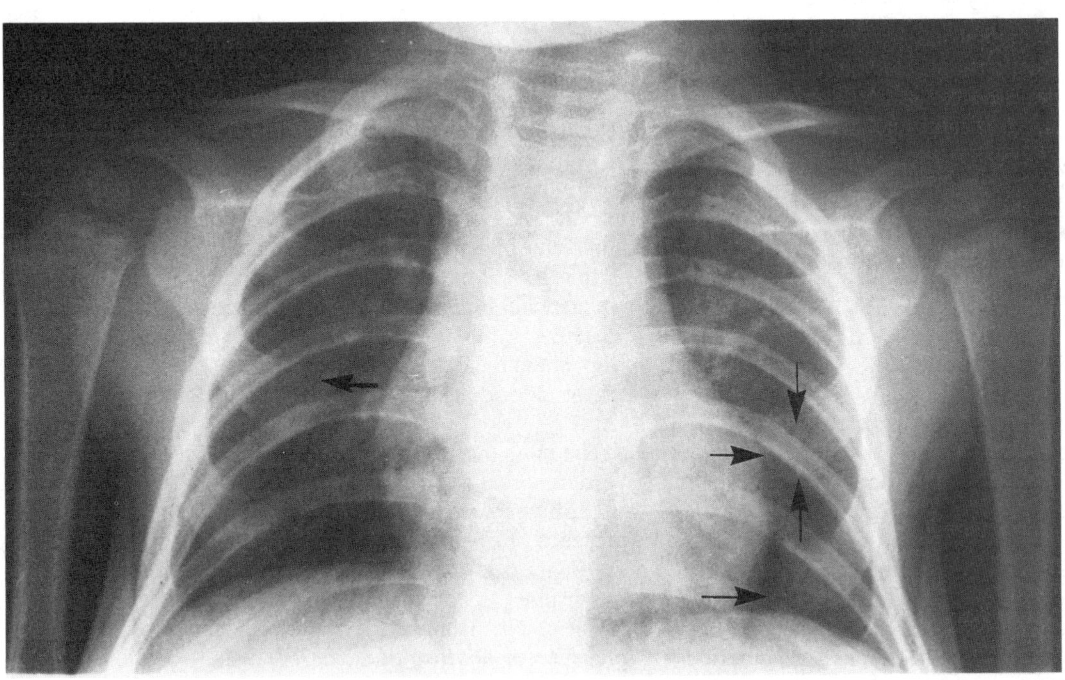

FIGURE 1 A chest radiograph from a 3-month-old male demonstrating short flared ribs (*arrows*).

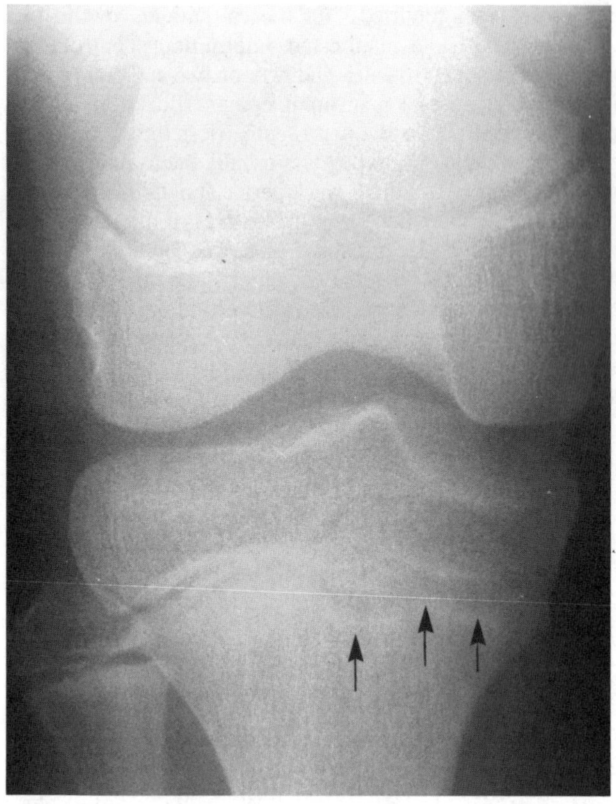

FIGURE 2 A radiograph of the right knee of a 13-year-old male demonstrating metaphyseal dysplasia (*arrows*).

thoracic dystrophy, have been noted early in life, metaphyseal dysplasia affecting long bones is not normally present until after 12 months of age. The metaphyseal changes also resolve during puberty, and so this feature is not usually recognizable in adults. The etiology of the metaphyseal changes is obscure, but poor vascularization of the columnar cartilage and a defect of endochondrial ossification have been noted. These lesions may produce the short stature that is clearly not related to pancreatic malabsorption, as correction of the latter produces no improvement in linear growth velocity in the vast majority of cases. The long-term sequelae of the bony changes are unknown, but in general they are mild and do not require intervention.

Treatment

Treatment of this disorder is symptomatic and supportive. Pancreatic enzyme replacement therapy is required for those with pancreatic insufficiency (fat malabsorption), but usually the dose required to achieve optimal absorption, i.e., greater than 90 percent of fat intake, is one-third to one-half the dose required by patients with cystic fibrosis. Supplemental therapy with fat-soluble vitamins may be necessary in a few cases with severe maldigestion. The management of neutropenia is symptomatic. On most occasions during periods of neutropenia the patient is asymptomatic and requires no therapy. The presentations with recurrent fevers or toxemia demand investigation to locate the focus of infection and the provision of appropriate antibiotic cover until the infection resolves.

JOHANSON-BLIZZARD SYNDROME

Another recognized cause of pancreatic lipomatosis during childhood is the syndrome described by Johanson-Blizzard,[12] manifested as anal imperforation, agenesis of the nasal cartilage, hair anomalies, mental retardation, deafness, and hypothyroidism associated with pancreatic insufficiency. The clinical hallmarks of the syndrome, namely imperforate anus and agenesis of the nasal cartilage, make detection of this syndrome reasonably obvious. The absence of bone marrow and skeletal changes differentiates it from Shwachman's syndrome. No quantitative pancreatic function data are available in this group of patients, but one would suspect from the pathologic appearances, which are similar to those of Shwachman's syndrome, that there would be impaired acinar function but reasonably normal ductal function.

EXOCRINE PANCREATIC DYSFUNCTION WITH REFRACTORY SIDEROBLASTIC ANEMIA

This syndrome, which is manifested as a refractory sideroblastic anemia with vacuolization of marrow precursors and exocrine pancreatic dysfunction, has been described in four unrelated children.[13] In infancy, these patients had a macrocytic anemia with variable degrees of neutropenia and thrombocytopenia. Their bone marrow aspirates were characterized by vacuolization of both the erythroid and myeloid precursors, a severe degree of hemosiderosis, and the presence of ringed sideroblasts. Family histories and hematologic examinations of parents were within normal limits. During infancy all four children failed to thrive and required regular transfusions to maintain a satisfactory hemoglobin level. Pancreatic stimulation tests using a nonquantitative technique revealed depressed acinar function with impaired enzyme secretion into the duodenum but also impaired water and bicarbonate secretion. Two of the infants died of sepsis in the first 2 years of life. The other two infants showed a spontaneous improvement with decreasing transfusion requirements, but moderate thrombocytopenia in one and neutropenia in the other infant persisted beyond 3 years of age. Sweat chloride estimates were normal for three of the patients.

The bone marrow changes were distinctly different from those reported in Shwachman's syndrome. The most distinctive differences were those of cell vacuolization and a marked presence of ringed sideroblasts. At postmortem examination the pancreatic changes were not those of lipomatosis but rather that of pancreatic acinar cell atrophy associated with fibrosis. No data were provided in the survivors of the presence or absence of steatorrhea; thus, at this stage the long-term requirements for persistent pancreatic enzyme replacement therapy are unknown.

CONGENITAL RUBELLA

A case of congenital rubella with chronic pancreatic insufficiency has been reported.[14] The infant presented at 12 weeks with gross emaciation. Subsequent investigation revealed steatorrhea but a normal sweat chloride and jejunal biopsy. Unstimulated duodenal juice contained amylase, but lipase and trypsin were absent. Over the next 7 years he was treated with pancreatic enzyme replacement therapy with improvement in absorption and growth and was finally weaned from the medication at 87 months. Pancreatic stimulation tests were performed at 35 and 87 months. However, both these results and the initial assays on unstimulated duodenal juice are difficult to interpret, as the tests were nonquantitative and during the stimulation tests only secretin was used.

PANCREATIC AGENESIS

This disorder usually presents with neonatal-onset diabetes mellitus without ketosis. The pancreatic insufficiency is seemingly a secondary clinical feature. In the one case studied in depth,[15] a quantitative pancreatic stimulation test demonstrated absent lipase and trypsin secretion, but no comment was made on H_2O and HCO_3^- secretion. There were no features of either cystic fibrosis or Shwachman's syndrome. To date, no follow-up report has been provided.

ISOLATED ENZYME DEFICIENCIES

A variety of selective deficiencies of lipase, trypsin, and amylase, or some combination thereof, have been reported. All are extremely rare anomalies, but they have provided some insight into the physiologic role of these specific enzymes and the sequelae resulting from their deficiency. It is important to note that most of these reports were made prior to the advent of pancreatic stimulation tests capable of quantitating pancreatic secretions via a marker perfusion technique during maximal stimulation of the pancreas with intravenous secretin and pancreozymin. Just as importantly, enzyme assays used were often insensitive and assays of unstimulated pancreatic secretions contaminated by gastric contents may have interfered with the results. These factors may account for some of the variability of the results.

Lipase Deficiency

Since Sheldon's original description in 1964 of isolated lipase deficiency,[16] seven subsequent cases have confirmed this entity. Sheldon described four patients who presented with characteristically oily bowel movements, with the oil separating easily from the rest of the stool. The patients had oil seepage and soiling of their underclothes, and the bowel movements were variably described as containing melted butter, bacon fat, or liquid oil. Despite their malabsorption of between 30 and 39 percent of fat intake, they thrived well and their absorption was documented to improve with pancreatic enzyme replacement therapy.

Analysis of unstimulated duodenal juice demonstrated absent or low lipase activity, and, in addition, in three cases either low amylase or trypsin activity. Cystic fibrosis was excluded in three children, but the fourth was noted to have a borderline sweat chloride result of 57 mEq per liter. Although none had neutrophil counts, three were of normal stature, thus seemingly excluding Shwachman's syndrome. Subsequently, Figarella et al[17] demonstrated a case of lipase deficiency, during pancreatic stimulation with intravenous pancreozymin and secretin. They could not detect lipase by immunologic double diffusion experiments but were able to demonstrate that co-lipase was present, although they did not quantitate the latter. Hildebrand et al[18] later reported two brothers of Assyrian origin with isolated co-lipase deficiency but seemingly normal lipase secretion. Recently Ghishan et al[19] demonstrated a patient with combined lipase and co-lipase deficiency.

These disorders appear relatively benign and most patients thrive well. Fat malabsorption is well controlled with oral enzyme replacement therapy and may improve spontaneously during later childhood years.

Trypsin Deficiency

Townes et al[20] reported two dysmorphic children with growth failure, hypoproteinemia, and edema. Proteolytic enzyme activity was absent in the duodenal juice but normalized on the addition of exogenous trypsin. Cystic fibrosis was excluded by the presence of a normal sweat test, but Shwachman's syndrome was not specifically excluded. As there were no quantitative pancreatic stimulation test data provided, it is difficult to assess the precise defect. The difference between this entity and enterokinase deficiency also remains unclear.

Amylase Deficiency

Lowe and May[21] reported one case of a selective absence of amylase and markedly reduced trypsin secretion. No follow-up data have been provided and no subsequent cases reported.

Enterokinase Deficiency

Congenital enterokinase deficiency was reported by Hadorn et al,[22] and its occurrence in siblings supports an autosomal recessive mode of inheritance. Patients have presented who were similar to the two patients with trypsin deficiency, manifesting malabsorption, hypoproteinemia, edema, and severe growth retardation. It was noted that amylase and lipase concentrations in unstimulated duodenal fluid were normal, but fat malabsorption was present, a factor that may be related to failure of activation of pro–co-lipase to co-lipase. The specific diagnosis of enterokinase deficiency rests on the addition of exogenous enterokinase to the duodenal juice with generation of normal tryptic activity. Pancreatic enzyme supplementation in these children generates normal proteolytic activity in the duodenum, and their clinical problems appear to resolve.

REFERENCES

1. Bodian M, Sheldon W, Lightwood R. Congenital hypoplasia of the exocrine pancreas. Acta Paediatr Scand 1964; 53:282–293.
2. Shwachman H, Diamond LK, Oski FA, Khaw KT. The syndrome of pancreatic insufficiency and bone marrow dysfunction. J Pediatr 1964; 65:645–663.
3. Woods WG, Roloff JS, Lukens JN, Krivit W. The occurrence of leukemia in patients with the Shwachman syndrome. J Pediatr 1981; 99:425–428.
4. Rothbaum RJ, Williams DA, Daugherty CC. Unusual surface distribution of concanavalin A reflects a cytoskeletal defect in neutrophils in Shwachman's syndrome. Lancet 1982; ii:800–801.
5. Burke V, Colebatch JH, Anderson CM, Simons MJ. Association of pancreatic insufficiency and chronic neutropenia in childhood. Arch Dis Child 1967; 42:147–157.
6. Aggett PJ, Cavanagh NPC, Mathew DJ, Pincott JR, Sutcliffe J, Harries JT. Shwachman's syndrome. Arch Dis Child 1980; 55:331–347.
7. Hill RE, Durie PR, Gaskin KJ, Davidson GP, Forstner GG. Steatorrhoea and pancreatic insufficiency in Shwachman's syndrome. Gastroenterology 1982; 83:22–27.
8. Gaskin KJ, Durie PR, Hill RE, Lee L, Forstner GG. Colipase and lipase secretion in childhood onset pancreatic insufficiency. Gastroenterology 1984; 86:1–7.
9. Gaskin KJ, Durie PR, Corey M, Wei P, Forstner GG. Evidence for a primary defect in pancreatic HCO_3^- secretion in cystic fibrosis. Pediatr Res 1982; 16:554–557.
10. Robberecht E, Nachtegaele P, Van Rattinghe R, Afschrift M, Kunnen M, Verharren R. Pancreatic lipomatosis in the Shwachman-Diamond syndrome. Pediatr Radiol 1985; 15:348–349.
11. Moore D, Forstner GG, Largman C, Cleghorn CJ, Wong SS, Durie PR. Serum immunoreactive cationic trypsinogen: a useful indicator of pancreatic exocrine function in the pediatric patient without cystic fibrosis. Gut 1986; 27:1362–1368.
12. Johanson A, Blizzard R. A syndrome of congenital aplasia of the alae nasi, deafness, hypothyroidism, dwarfism, absent permanent teeth, and malabsorption. J Pediatr 1971; 79:982.
13. Pearson HA, Lobel JS, Kocoshis SA, Naiman JL, Windmiller J, Lammi AT, Hoffman R, Marsh JC. A new syndrome of refractory anemia with vacuolization of marrow precursors and exocrine pancreatic dysfunction. J Pediatr 1979; 95:976–984.
14. Donowitz M, Gryboski JD. Pancreatic insufficiency and the congenital rubella syndrome. J Pediatr 1975; 87:241–243.
15. Howard CP, Go VLW, Infante AJ, Perrault J, Gerich JE, Haymond MW. Long-term survival in a case of functional pancreatic agenesis. J Pediatr 1980; 97:786–789.
16. Sheldon W. Congenital pancreatic lipase deficiency. Arch Dis Child 1964; 39:268–271.
17. Figarella C, Negri GA, Sarles H. Presence of colipase in a congenital pancreatic lipase deficiency. Biochim Biophys Acta 1972; 280:205–210.
18. Hildebrand H, Borgstrom B, Bekassy A, Eranson-Albertson C, Helin I. Isolated colipase deficiency in two brothers. Gut 1982; 23:243–246.
19. Ghishan FK, Moran JR, Durie PR, Greene HL. Isolated congenital lipase-colipase deficiency. Gastroenterology 1984; 86:1580–1582.
20. Townes PL, Bryson MF, Miller G. Further observations on trypsinogen deficiency disease: report of a second case. J Pediatr 1967; 71:220–224.
21. Lowe CU, May CD. Selective pancreatic deficiency. Am J Dis Child 1951; 82:459–464.
22. Hadorn B, Tarlow MJ, Lloyd JK, Wolff OH. Intestinal enterokinase deficiency. Lancet 1969; i:812–813.

PART 4

Acquired Disorders of the Pancreas

Kevin John Gaskin, M.B., B.S., F.R.A.C.P., FRCPC

Acquired disorders of the exocrine pancreas secondary to malnutrition, surgical resection, and enteropathies are well described in children. Both acute and chronic pancreatitis are described elsewhere in this chapter.

MALNUTRITION

There is now a cumulative body of pathologic data indicating that the exocrine pancreas is affected by protein-energy malnutrition.[1,2] At postmortem examination of children dying with kwashiorkor, profound pancreatic atrophy may be found.[3,4] Early in malnutrition, loss of zymogen granules from acinar cells and acinar cell atrophy are prominent findings, but diffuse pancreatic fibrosis is relatively uncommon and seemingly observed only in individuals with prolonged malnutrition.[5]

In severely malnourished children, duodenal aspiration has revealed low concentrations of lipase, trypsin, chymotrypsin, and amylase.[6,7] Semiquantitative pancreatic stimulation tests have demonstrated marked impairment of enzyme secretion but normal volume flow and the ability to raise the duodenal pH, suggestive of adequate bicarbonate secretion.[8] There was also prompt return of nearly normal enzyme secretion in response to dietary therapy, except in two patients who demonstrated persistently low enzyme secretion despite nutritional rehabilitation. The clinical manifestations of exocrine pancreatic dysfunction and malnutrition have been less well documented, although studies have suggested that there is sufficient enzyme secretion to produce normal digestion and absorption.[8-10]

Biochemically, acute malnutrition in children has been associated with elevated cationic trypsinogen levels, which are directly correlated with the severity of the malnutrition.[11]

Others have demonstrated persistently low immunoreactive trypsin levels in more chronically malnourished children.[12] These studies might well suggest, in the acute phase, that there is abnormal pancreatic cell membrane function with leakage of zymogen into the circulation, but more chronic malnutrition has been associated with extensive pancreatic acinar cell atrophy and diffuse fibrosis, thus producing the low trypsinogen levels. Juvenile tropical pancreatitis syndrome, which is frequently seen in developing countries, and its relationship to malnutrition are discussed elsewhere in this chapter.

SURGICAL RESECTION

The specific diseases requiring surgical resection, i.e., pancreatitis and nesidioblastosis, are covered elsewhere in this book. Exocrine pancreatic function following surgical resection has rarely been studied in children, but personal experience has suggested that even with 95 percent pancreatic resection for nesidioblastosis, few if any children develop malabsorption. Considering that recent studies of pancreatic lipase and co-lipase secretion in children[13] have demonstrated that malabsorption occurs only when values fall below 2 percent and 1 percent of mean normal values, respectively, it is not surprising that large pancreatic resections can be safely performed without inducing malabsorption. Massive pancreatectomy in infants and children, however, does require measurement of fat absorption to assess the necessity for pancreatic enzyme replacement therapy.

ENTEROPATHIES

Exocrine pancreatic dysfunction has been recognized in both children[14] and adults[15,16] with celiac disease. Although in most the pancreatic dysfunction is mild, in some it is profound, as evidenced by increased fecal neutral fat excretion and even rectal seepage of oil.[17] The etiology of the pancreatic dysfunction and/or fat maldigestion is unclear. Some studies[15,17,18] have indicated primary pancreatic dysfunction, as evidenced by impaired release of pancreatic bicarbonate and enzymes into the duodenum in response to exogenous stimulation with intravenous cholecystokinin and secretin. However, other patients have demonstrated intact pancreatic function in response to exogenous stimulation but an impaired response to stimulation with liquid test meals.[19,20] This finding is consistent with impaired release of endogenous cholecystokinin and secretin, a concept supported by the demonstration of low serum secretin levels in response to duodenal perfusion of citric acid in untreated celiac disease patients and normal levels following recovery of the intestinal lesion.[21] Impaired secretagogue release in untreated patients probably also explains the poor postprandial gallbladder emptying and diminished duodenal bile acid concentrations that, together with the impaired pancreatic enzyme release, contribute to the presence of fat maldigestion.

Profound irreversible pancreatic insufficiency with acinar atrophy and fibrosis has occurred rarely in celiac disease. This entity has been reported in adults with longstanding untreated celiac disease.[15,20,22,23] Recently, there has also been a report of a 17-year-old with a normal sweat test with biopsy-proven celiac disease and pancreatic insufficiency that appeared irreversible, as it did not improve with a gluten-free diet.[24] The etiology of this severe pancreatic lesion and its long-term reversibility are unknown. The lesion may be related to chronic understimulation of the pancreas due to impaired endogenous secretagogue release and subsequent induction of pancreatic cell atrophy, possibly aggravated by malnutrition.

In cases with seemingly irreversible pancreatic insufficiency and celiac disease, it is worthwhile considering the co-existence of celiac disease and cystic fibrosis.[25-27] However, such patients require careful follow-up with repeat sweat chloride examinations, as the latter may be falsely elevated in the presence of malnutrition.

REFERENCES

1. Pitchumoni CS. Special problems of tropical pancreatitis. Clin Gastroenterol 1984; 13:941–960.
2. Pitchumoni CS. Pancreas in primary malnutrition disorders. Am J Clin Nutr 1973; 26:374–373.
3. Davies JNP. The essential pathology of kwashiorkor. Lancet 1948; i:317–320.
4. Blackburn WR, Vinijchaikul K. The pancreas in kwashiorkor. An electron microscopic study. Lab Invest 1969; 20:305–318.
5. Veghelyi PV, Kemeny TT, Pozsonyi J, Sos J. Dietary lesions of the pancreas. Am J Dis Child 1950; 79:658–665.
6. Thompson MD, Trowell HC. Pancreatic enzyme activity in duodenal contents of children with a type of kwashiorkor. Lancet 1952; i:1031–1035.
7. Gomez R, Galvan RR, Cravioti J, French S. Enzymatic activity of the duodenal contents in children affected with third degree malnutrition. Pediatrics 1954; 13:544–552.
8. Barbezat GO, Hansen JDL. The exocrine pancreas and protein-calorie malnutrition. Pediatrics 1968; 42:77–92.
9. Hansen JDL, Schendel HE, Wilkins JA, Brock JF. Nitrogen metabolism in children with kwashiorkor receiving milk and vegetable diets. Pediatrics 1960; 25:258–282.
10. Gomez F, Galvan R, Cravioti J, French S, de la Pena R, Moreno ME, Villa ME. Influence of L-lysine supplements on the absorption and retention of nitrogen from milk by children with protein malnutrition. J Pediatr 1957; 51:262–266.
11. Durie PR, Forstner GG, Gaskin KJ, Weizman Z, Kopelman HR, Ellis L, Largman C. Elevated serum immunoreactive pancreatic cationic trypsinogen in acute malnutrition: evidence of pancreatic damage. J Pediatr 1985; 106:233–238.
12. Fedail SS, Karar ZA, Harvey RF, Read AE. Serum trypsin as measure of pancreatic function in children with protein-calorie malnutrition. Lancet 1980; ii:374.
13. Gaskin KJ, Durie PR, Hill RE, Lee L, Forstner GG. Colipase and lipase secretion in childhood onset pancreatic insufficiency: delineation of patients. Gastroenterology 1984; 86:1–7.
14. Peyrot M, Desjeux JF, Dumontier AM, Lestradet H. La sécrétion de lipase dans la maladie coeliaque de l'enfant. Gastroenterol Clin Biol 1981; 5:275–281.
15. Bustos Fernanez L, De Paula A, Prizont R, Tiscornia OM, Bragwinsky J, Carreras A, Hojman D. Exocrine pancreas insufficiency secondary to gluten enteropathy. Am J Gastroenterol 1970; 53:564–569.
16. Novis BH, Banks S, Marks IN. Exocrine pancreatic function in intestinal malabsorption and small bowel disease. Am J Dig Dis 1972; 17:489–494.
17. Weinstein LD, Herskovic T. Rectal seepage of oil in a patient with coeliac disease and secondary pancreatic insufficiency. Am J Dig Dis 1968; 13:762–765.
18. Dreiling DA. The pancreatic secretion in the malabsorption syndrome and related malnutrition states. J Mt Sinai Hosp NY 1957; 24:243–250.

19. Di Magno EP, Go VLW, Summerskill WHJ. Impaired cholecystokinin-pancreozymin secretion, intraluminal digestion, and maldigestion of fat in sprue. Gastroenterology 1972; 63:25–32.
20. Regan PT, Di Magno EP. Exocrine pancreatic function in coeliac sprue: a cause of treatment failure. Gastroenterology 1980; 78:484–487.
21. Besterman HS, Sarson DL, Johnston DI, Stewart JS, Guerin S, Bloom SR, Blackburn AM, Patel HR, Modigliani R, Mallinson CN. Gut hormone profile in coeliac disease. Lancet 1978; i:785–788.
22. Benson GD, Kowlessar OD, Sleisengar MH. Adult coeliac disease with emphasis upon response to a gluten free diet. Medicine (Baltimore) 1964; 43:1–40.
23. Fitzgerald O, Fitzgerald P, Fennelly J, McMullin JP, Boland SJ. A clinical study of chronic pancreatitis. Gut 1963; 4:193–216.
24. Weizman Z, Hamilton JR, Kopelman HR, Cleghorn G, Durie PR. Treatment failure in celiac disease due to coexistent exocrine pancreatic insufficiency. Pediatrics 1987; 80:924–926.
25. Hide DW, Burman D. An infant with both cystic fibrosis and coeliac disease. Arch Dis Child 1969; 41:533–535.
26. Goodchild MC, Nelson R, Anderson CM. Cystic fibrosis and coeliac disease: co-existence in two children. Arch Dis Child 1973; 48:684–691.
27. Taylor B, Sokol G. Cystic fibrosis and coeliac disease. Report of two cases. Arch Dis Child 1973; 48:692–696.

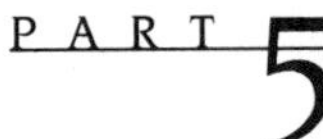

PART 5

Tumors of the Pancreas

Hinda Kopelman, M.D., FRCPC

Tumors of the pancreas are uncommon in children, and their classification has been confusing and controversial (Table 1). Pancreatic malignancy, largely carcinoma, may arise from duct cell, acinar cell, or islet cell or may be of uncertain origin. The most common of these is duct cell carcinoma. It carries the poorest prognosis. A tumor peculiar to pediatrics and termed *pancreatoblastoma*, or *infantile pancreatic carcinoma*, deserves special discussion. Rarely, pancreatic malignancy may arise in connective tissue elements.

When tumors arise in islet cells or from undifferentiated precursor cells, they often present because of the effects of the hormones they secrete in excessive amounts into the circulation. Such secretory or endocrine tumors may produce hormones normally secreted from functioning islet cells but in excessive amounts, or they may produce substances not normally secreted from the endocrine pancreas. They may be malignant with variable metastatic potential or, more frequently, may represent benign neoplastic growth as discrete adenomas or tissue hyperplasia.

This discussion covers tumors of the exocrine pancreas, which are largely malignant carcinomas, separately from endocrine pancreatic neoplasia, benign or malignant.

TUMORS OF THE EXOCRINE PANCREAS

Carcinoma of the Exocrine Pancreas

In adults, carcinoma of the pancreas is described as "an insidious, progressive and nearly universally fatal malignancy."[1] More than 90 percent are of pancreatic ductal origin and histologically are well-differentiated duct cell adenocar-

TABLE 1
Classification of Pancreatic Tumors

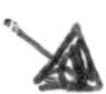

Location	Benign	Malignant
Exocrine pancreas	Duct adenoma Serous cystadenoma Mucinous cystadenoma Intraductal papilloma Papillary-cystic tumor	Duct cell adenocarcinoma Pancreatoblastoma Acinar cell carcinoma
Connective tissue	Hemangioendothelioma Lymphangioma Histiocytoma Neurilemoma	Sarcoma Lymphoma Leiomyosarcoma Histiocytoma Neurilemoma
Secretory/endocrine	Gastrinoma (40%) VIPoma Insulinoma (90%) Islet cell hyperplasia Islet cell adenoma	Gastrinoma (60%) Insulinoma (10%)

cinoma.[2] Under the best circumstances of treatment, published survival rates range between 1 and 6 percent at 3 to 5 years,[3-5] with an average survival of only 4 to 6 months following diagnosis.[6]

The experience with pancreatic carcinoma in childhood is somewhat different. Of the approximately 60 reported pediatric cases,[7-12] less than 50 percent were pancreatic ductal carcinoma, although this was still the single most common type. The remaining cases, including islet cell tumors (to be discussed later), acinar cell carcinoma, and pancreatoblastoma are known to be inherently less aggressive and more amenable to therapy. The proportional increase in these cases of carcinoma in the pediatric population probably accounts for the far less dismal survival rates in pancreatic carcinoma in children.[13,14]

Pathogenesis

The etiology of pancreatic carcinoma is unknown but is probably multifactorial.[15] The increasing incidence in the adult population suggests that environmental agents may play an important role in the rate of neoplastic transformation. Factors implicated include habitual wine-drinking, cigarette smoking, increased consumption of animal fat (cholesterol) and protein, ingestion of chemically decaffeinated coffee, and exposure to chemical carcinogens.[15] A history of chronic pancreatitis or diabetes mellitus has not been substantiated as an important risk factor by all investigators. Some of these environmental factors may have relevance in the discussion of pediatric carcinoma if exposure to them in utero, via breast milk, or in the household occurs, but this has not been investigated. One child, however, was reported to have adenocarcinoma occurring in a field of orthotopic irradiation.

The role of genetic predisposition in a multifactorial model for pancreatic carcinoma has been pointed out by reports of its familial occurrence.[16,17] Genetic predisposition may play a relatively significant role in the occurrence of pediatric pancreatic carcinoma. One child with Beckwith-Wiedemann syndrome, which has a high predisposition to malignancy, was reported to have developed a pancreatoblastoma at 19 days of age.[18] One child with tuberous sclerosis developed pancreatic adenocarcinoma.[7]

Clinical Presentation

Pancreatic carcinoma in the pediatric age group is not confined to adolescence. The age distribution is equal throughout childhood and adolescence. Almost half of the patients reported in two literature reviews[8,9] totaling 40 patients were less than 6 years of age. Of these 40 patients, the most frequent presentation was abdominal mass, and the most frequent complaint was abdominal pain. In adult patients, the typical description of pain is epigastric, dull, and aching, with radiation to the back. Nausea, vomiting, anorexia, weight loss, and a metallic taste are accompanying symptoms. Although obstruction of the common bile duct occurs frequently in the late presentation of adult carcinoma, causing jaundice in more than 50 percent of patients, pale stools, dark urine, pruritus, and a distended palpable gallbladder (Courvoisier's sign), this constellation is less common in children. Jaundice occurred in only one-quarter of pediatric patients, and Courvoisier's sign was rarely reported.

Nonspecific laboratory data may reveal anemia, elevated serum amylase, alkaline phosphatase, direct bilirubin, hepatocellular enzymes, and serum glucose, with depressed serum albumin.

Diagnosis

No tumor markers to date can specifically identify or exclude the diagnosis of pancreatic exocrine carcinoma. Some patients do have elevated carcinoembryonic antigen, alphafetoprotein, and human chorionic gonadotropin, but these are nonspecific and not consistently present. Widening and distortion of the duodenum with displacement of the stomach on upper gastrointestinal (GI) series in large tumors involving the head of the pancreas can often be appreciated, but this remains a poor diagnostic screening test.

Diagnosis of pancreatic carcinoma depends largely on the use of abdominal ultrasonography and computed tomography to visualize a pancreatic mass. Loss of tissue fat planes between the pancreas and retroperitoneum, dilated biliary and/or pancreatic ducts, and metastatic lesions may also be detected. The sensitivity and specificity of these investigations exceed 80 percent. Their limitation in detecting tumor is restricted to small foci of malignancy (less than 2 cm). Endoscopic retrograde cholangiopancreatography, allowing visualization of the pancreatic ductal system, may be sensitive enough to detect even small mass lesions, since they often occlude or distort the ductal system. Needle biopsy or aspiration of mass lesions for diagnostic cytology has not been widely used in pediatrics. Often, definitive diagnosis may await histologic examination of specimens obtained at laparotomy.

Treatment

Despite the dismal 5-year survival rate for adults, aggressive surgical resection is the only form of treatment that has resulted in long-term survival. In adults, pancreatoduodenectomy increased average survival from 3.6 months for patients who only had a biopsy performed to 20.3 months when histopathologic confirmation of surgical clearance of tumor was achieved.[6]

In children, the more limited experience has tended to agree with a radical surgical approach to pancreatic carcinoma. In one review of 28 cases,[8] average survival time from onset of symptoms was 4 months in nonresected patients and 12 years for those resected for whom follow-up was available. Unfortunately, these cases included patients with exocrine tumors such as pancreatoblastoma, thought to have a better prognosis. Palliative surgery, chemotherapy, and radiotherapy have not been particularly helpful. However, radiotherapy followed by a "second look" procedure aimed at radical resection is an alternative in some cases.

Two major alternatives exist for radical resection. The classic Whipple procedure consists of en bloc resection of the head of the pancreas, duodenum, common bile duct, gallbladder, and distal stomach. Three anastomoses are then required: a pancreaticojejunostomy, a gastrojejunostomy, and a choledochojejunostomy. Pancreatoduodenectomy has been accomplished even in infants[10] and is, perhaps, better tolerated than in adults. Because dilated bile ducts are less common in children and their size is small, the choledochojejunostomy may need to be replaced by a hepatojejunostomy. Removal of 60 to 70 percent of the gastric antrum and/or vagotomy minimizes the risk of peptic ulceration at the site of the gastrojejunostomy.

The alternative radical surgical approach, total pancreatectomy with en bloc resection of the duodenum, spleen, and greater omentum, subtotal gastrectomy, and lymphadenectomy, may not be superior to the Whipple procedure except if multiple tumor foci are present or if tumor is found in the body or tail of the pancreas as well.

Palliative biliary bypass by percutaneous transhepatic shunting of the common bile duct for decompression can be performed in children[19] when resection is considered impossible.

Pancreatoblastoma

Special discussion of this tumor is warranted. Pancreatoblastoma, or infantile carcinoma of the pancreas, has been reported not infrequently in children with pancreatic tumor.[11,12] Although it is generally classified as a carcinoma, the prognosis is much more favorable than that associated with classic ductal adenocarcinoma.[13,14]

Pathologically, this form of malignancy is contained within a dense fibrous capsule and consists of cords or nodules of squamous cells with elongated nuclei surrounding tubular structures of columnar epithelial cells and masses of poorly differentiated cells. It may contain islet cell features and/or acinar cells with zymogen granules. The histogenesis of this tumor remains uncertain: Some believe it to be of duct cell origin on the basis of ultrastructural findings[20]; others consider it primarily acinar.[21]

The clinical behavior of this tumor is different from that of either acinar, ductal, or islet cell tumors seen in adults, and it probably represents a unique childhood tumor of pluripotential nature and a substantially more favorable prognosis than adult pancreatic adenocarcinoma. Of 10 cases reported, all but two had substantially better survival after surgery, and the results with this tumor may be in part responsible for the generally better prognosis afforded to patients with childhood carcinoma of the pancreas.

Tumors of Connective Tissue Origin

Rare among pancreatic tumors, malignant neoplasia may occasionally arise from connective tissue elements of the pancreas and present as sarcoma, lymphoma, or even neuroblastoma. In addition, benign hamartomas and hemangioendotheliomas[19] have occasionally been reported.

ENDOCRINE PANCREATIC NEOPLASIA

Neoplasia of the endocrine pancreas represents a heterogeneous and fascinating group of lesions that have encouraged research into possible common embryologic origins of neuroendocrine cells and have provided valuable insight into some of the functions of the gastroenteropancreatic peptides. Endocrine pancreatic neoplasia includes both benign and malignant lesions, which themselves may be either secretory or nonsecretory.

Islet cell tumors in children represent a larger proportion of all pancreatic carcinoma than in adults. Although this entity accounts for 5 percent of adult pancreatic carcinoma,[1] it occurred in 20 percent of the 60 pediatric pancreatic malignancies reported.[7-12] Islet cell carcinoma carries a better prognosis[22] than pancreatic ductal carcinoma, as it is slower-growing and generally less aggressively metastatic. Its presentation is that of abdominal pain and mass as described under pancreatic exocrine carcinoma, and its treatment is similar. It will not be discussed further. The remainder of this discussion concerns secretory neoplastic lesions in children, both benign and malignant.

Secretory endocrine neoplasia in children is most often a diffuse or localized adenomatous growth, secreting a variety of hormones, peptides, amines, and prostaglandins. Clinical presentation is characteristic for identifiable syndromes resulting from the particular or dominant humoral substance being elaborated by the tumor. In children, the most common syndrome is hyperinsulinism[23] associated with beta-cell adenoma[15,24] or hyperplasia.[26] Insulin-secreting carcinoma is uncommon in adults and rarer in children. Zollinger-Ellison syndrome due to gastrinoma,[19,27] watery diarrhea/hypokalemia/achlorhydria (WDHA) syndrome due to VIPoma,[30] and multiple endocrine neoplasia I syndrome (MEN I)[31,32] have all been described in children and will be briefly considered. No findings of solitary glucagonoma or somatostatinoma have been reported in children, and these will not be discussed.

Pathogenesis

Although pancreatic secretory tumors are frequently called islet cell tumors, they are probably of ductular and not islet cell origin.[33] Current understanding of the normal cytodifferentiation of islet cells from pluripotent stem cells in the duct epithelium of the fetus suggests that it is these stem cells that give rise to neoplastic growth with the capacity to produce one or several hormones. It is of some interest, then, that pancreatic secretory tumors are able to elaborate hormones, such as gastrin, not normally produced by the well-differentiated pancreas.

One attempt to explain this finding and the relationship of pancreatic secretory tumors to other endocrine neoplasia was the amine precursor uptake and decarboxylation (APUD) cell theory.[34,35] It suggested that a family of gastroenteropancreatic peptide-containing cells have a common embryologic origin derived from the neural crest and may maintain the potential, under certain conditions, for secreting similar hormonal substances. This theory has now been modified by the proposal that both neural crest and alimentary endocrine cell precursors are derived from an earlier common cell origin,[36] and the term *neuroendocrine system* is favored over *APUD cell system*.

Clinical Syndromes

Zollinger-Ellison Syndrome: Gastrinoma

In 1955, Zollinger and Ellison described a syndrome of markedly increased gastric acid secretion, severe and intractable peptic ulcer disease, and non-beta islet cell tumors of the pancreas.[37] We now know that these tumors are usually but not always found in the pancreas, are often multifocal, and frequently are malignant. They contain and secrete gastrin. Although gastrinomas have been associated with neoplasms in other endocrine organs, in a review of 15 children with Zollinger-Ellison syndrome none had a second tumor type.[27]

Symptoms in Zollinger-Ellison syndrome[38] are due to the high circulating serum gastrin levels, which cause expansion of the gastric parietal cell mass and stimulation of excessive gastric acid secretion. The typical clinical features are thus those of peptic ulcer disease of persistent, progressive, and poorly responsive nature.

Symptoms in addition to those of ulcer disease may include diarrhea in more than one-third of patients due to the large quantity of concentrated gastric acid entering the duodenum, probably causing direct intestinal mucosal injury and the inhibitory effects of circulating gastrin on intestinal absorption; steatorrhea due to both lipase and bile salt inactivation by excessive duodenal acid; and B_{12} intrinsic factor complex malabsorption, also thought to be secondary to excess intestinal acid.

Gastrinoma should be suspected in patients with multiple ulcers, in those with ulcers distal to the first portion of the duodenum, when medical therapy is ineffective, or with recurrence of peptic ulcer disease following surgery. The most specific and reliable means of confirming the clinical diagnosis of Zollinger-Ellison syndrome or gastrinoma is the measurement of serum gastrin by radioimmunoassay. Markedly increased fasting serum gastrin levels in the absence of renal failure, massive small intestinal resection, and pernicious anemia with gastric achlorhydria are virtually diagnostic. However, increases in circulating gastrin can occur with chronic gastritis, gastric achlorhydria, peptic ulcer disease, and G cell (gastrin cell) hyperfunction.[39] Several provocative tests may then be useful as aids to the diagnosis. Basal and pentagastrin-stimulated gastric acid secretion is often markedly elevated in patients with gastrinoma and shows a smaller increase between basal and stimulated levels. This test by itself cannot establish or exclude the diagnosis of Zollinger-Ellison syndrome because of the overlap in values with normal and peptic ulcer patients. Bolus secretin infusion of 1 to 2 units per kilogram usually causes an increase in serum gastrin of more than 100 to 200 pg per milliliter in patients with gastrinoma but has little effect on patients with peptic ulcer disease, G cell hyperfunction, or achlorhydria. Intravenous calcium infusion of 5 mg per kilogram per hour causes increases in serum gastrin of more than 400 pg per milliliter in Zollinger-Ellison syndrome but is less specific and more hazardous than the secretin provocation. Serum gastrin values show very mild increases in response to feeding of a standard meal in patients with Zollinger-Ellison syndrome but increase by more than 200 percent in individuals with gastrin cell hyperfunction, making this a useful test for the diagnosis of the latter.

Treatment of Zollinger-Ellison syndrome involves control of the effects of hypergastrinemia, in particular acid-peptic disease, as well as treatment of a tumor that is frequently malignant and therefore progressive with metastatic potential. Medical management with potent H_2 antagonists at greater doses than are used in common peptic ulcer disease is usually effective in controlling acid-peptic disease and its complications and has offered an excellent alternative, often obviating gastrectomy with its significant morbidity and long-term complications.[40–42] Proximal gastric vagotomy has been introduced to facilitate treatment with H_2 antagonists because of the failure to control acid secretion with medical therapy alone in some patients.[43,44]

Medical therapy must be continued long-term and is not a solution to the progressive growth and spread of this tumor. Clearly, complete resection of tumor mass should be performed whenever possible, as it is associated with cure and obviates therapy directed at controlling the effects of hypergastrinemia. Complete tumor removal is most likely to occur with solitary extrapancreatic tumors, which may need to be identified at exploratory laparotomy. Pancreatic gastrinomas are far less frequently completely resectable. Chemotherapy, usually involving streptozotocin and 5-fluorouracil, has been successful in decreasing metastatic tumor mass but not in reducing the effects of acid secretion.

Watery Diarrhea/Hypokalemia/Achlorhydria Syndrome: VIPoma

In 1958, Verner and Morrison described a syndrome of profuse watery diarrhea, severe hypokalemia, and non–beta cell pancreatic islet adenomas.[45] Although its role may be controversial, vasoactive intestinal peptide (VIP) has been specifically associated with these tumors, and they are often referred to as VIPomas.

VIP has a variety of biologic properties that are related by its ability to stimulate the adenyl cyclase system. Stimulation of intestinal mucosal cells results in massive secretion of fluid and electrolytes and stimulation of intestinal motility; it is a potent vasodilator; it may inhibit gastric acid secretion, cause hyperglycemia and impaired glucose tolerance, release pancreatic insulin, cause hypercalcemia, and stimulate pancreatic fluid secretion.

Clinically, the severe secretory diarrhea may be intermittent or constant and is associated with abdominal cramps, flushing, and severe dehydration. In adults, about one-third of tumors are malignant.[46] The remainder are due to pancreatic adenomas, hyperplasia, or nonpancreatic ganglioneuromas. In children under 10 reported with WDHA syndrome, the lesion was virtually always a ganglioneuroma and not a pancreatic tumor.[47] However, occasional cases of a VIPoma of pancreatic origin have been reported in adolescents.[30]

Diagnosis of VIPomas depends on the measurement of plasma VIP levels by radioimmunoassay of greater than 60 pmol per liter and rules out most other causes of secretory diarrhea.

Management of this syndrome depends first on correction of the associated dehydration and electrolyte imbalances. Control of the diarrhea may be achieved medically using steroids, prostaglandin inhibitors, or somatostatin. This allows time to try to localize the secretory tumor. Surgical resection is mandatory if possible, and identification of the tumor site may require laparotomy. If at laparotomy no tumor is identified, recommendations in the past have been for a subtotal pancreatectomy. If malignant lesions are inoperable, response has been obtained with the combination of streptozotocin and 5-fluorouracil.

Multiple Endocrine Neoplasia Type I

MEN I is a complex of tumors or hyperplasia that may be found in at least two endocrine organs in the same individual. It is inherited in an autosomal dominant manner with a high degree of penetrance and is usually manifest in an affected individual before the age of 20 years.[31,32]

In MEN I, the associated endocrine organs include the pituitary, parathyroid, adrenal cortex, thyroid, and pancreas. Obviously, the clinical manifestations depend entirely on the endocrine organ involved and the functional nature of the secretory tumor. Pancreatic involvement is almost always multifocal, and each tumor may secrete several different products. The clinical picture is often determined, therefore, by the predominant circulating peptide.

Once an endocrine tumor is identified in an individual in the presence or absence of a positive family history, a thorough review for the possibility of other endocrinopathies is warranted. Approximately one-quarter of all gastrinoma patients, 4 percent of adults with insulinomas, and occasional patients with WDHA syndrome have MEN I.[48]

Presentation and management of the individual pancreatic entities have been discussed. Management should include genetic counseling and surveillance of family members, both affected and unaffected.

Insulinoma/Islet Cell Hyperplasia/Dysplasia

This is by far the most common pancreatic secretory neoplasia in children. It may manifest at birth or any time thereafter and presents clinically with symptoms due to hyperinsulinemic hypoglycemia. Characteristically, these patients experience hypoglycemia that is chronic, severe, and medically intractable.

Clinical symptoms are similar regardless of the presence of a discrete insulin-producing adenoma or diffuse involvement of the endocrine pancreas. In infants, diffuse adenomatosis or nesidioblastosis is frequently the cause of hyperinsulinemia.[26] In older patients, beyond the neonatal period, discrete insulinomas are more often found.[24] These are only occasionally malignant tumors.

Diagnosis depends on the demonstration of hyperinsulinemia or insulin levels inappropriate for the level of blood glucose. Furthermore, hypoglycemia in the absence of urinary ketones and the absence of elevated serum free fatty acids, glycerol, and beta-hydroxybutyrate levels (nonketotic hypoglycemia) are consistent with this diagnosis. It is often impossible to identify a discrete adenoma before surgery. Even at the time of laparotomy, the adenoma may be too small to be identified by palpation. Therefore, diagnosis is often dependent on histologic examination of resected material.

Medical treatment of hyperinsulinemic hypoglycemia[23] consists of the provision of continuous intravenous glucose and/or frequent feedings to prevent hypoglycemia and the use of diazoxide to inhibit insulin release. Glucagon may be of some value, but long-term use is not usually successful and may have paradoxical effects.

Definitive treatment of hyperinsulinemia requires surgical excision of the insulin-secreting tissue. Since it is often difficult to identify discrete adenomata, when this is not possible, recommendations are for resection of at least 85 percent and preferably 95 percent of pancreatic cell mass, leaving a residual rim of tissue along the duodenal loop. The generally aggressive surgical approach to this disorder in infants has been justified by its ability to control hypoglycemia in cases that have failed medical management and thus prevent the disastrous consequences of hypoglycemia on the brain.[23] In infants treated with 95 percent pancreatectomy early after failure of medical management, results have been remarkably good. Glucose homeostasis is almost always restored, although occasionally reoperation for further removal of tissue is needed. The residual rim of exocrine tissue appears sufficient to maintain normal digestion of nutrients and may have the potential for regeneration of exocrine pancreatic function with time.[49] Long-term effects on glucose homeostasis with the eventual need for insulin replacement are still unknown.

REFERENCES

1. Cello JP. Carcinoma of the pancreas. In: Sleisenger MH, Fordtran JS, eds. Gastrointestinal disease. Philadelphia: WB Saunders, 1983: 1514.
2. Kissane JM. Carcinoma of the exocrine pancreas: pathologic aspects. J Surg Oncol 1975; 7:167.
3. Shapiro TM. Adenocarcinoma of the pancreas: a statistical analysis of biliary by-pass vs Whipple resection in good risk patients. Ann Surg 1975; 182:715.
4. Forrest JF, Longmire WP. Carcinoma of the pancreas and perampillary region. Ann Surg 1979; 189:128–138.
5. Lerut JP, Gianello PR, Otte JB, Kestens PJ. Pancreaticoduodenal resection: surgical experience and evaluation of risk factors in 103 patients. Ann Surg 1984; 199:432–437.
6. Longmire WP, Traverso LW. The Whipple procedure and other standard operative approaches to pancreatic cancer. Cancer 1981; 47:1706–1711.
7. Lack EE, Cassady JB, Levey R, Vawter GF. Tumours of the exocrine pancreas in children and adolescents: a clinical and pathologic study of eight cases. Am J Surg Pathol 1983; 7:319–327.
8. Camprodon R, Quintanilla E. Successful longterm results with resection of pancreatic carcinoma in children: favorable prognosis for an uncommon neoplasm. Surgery 1984; 95:420–426.
9. Tersigni R, Arena L, Alessandroni L, Bufalni G, Bochicchio O, Gallo P, Stipa S. Pancreatic carcinoma in childhood: case report of long survival and review of the literature. Surgery 1984; 96:560–566.
10. Rich H, Weber JL, Shandling B. Adenocarcinoma of the pancreas in a neonate managed by pancreatoduodenectomy. J Pediatr Surg 1986; 21:806–808.
11. Horie A, Yano Y, Kotoo Y, Miwa A. Morphogenesis of pancreatoblastoma, infantile carcinoma of the pancreas. Report of two cases. Cancer 1977; 39:247–254.
12. Buchino JJ, Castello FM, Nagaraj HS. Pancreatoblastoma: a histochemical and ultrastructural analysis. Cancer 1984; 53:963–969.
13. Nagaraj H, Polk HC. Pancreatic carcinoma in children. (Editorial) Surgery 1984; 95:505.

14. Wetzel WJ. Re: Successful long-term results with resection of pancreatic carcinoma in children. (Letter) Surgery 1984; 96:946–947.
15. Lin RS, Kessler II. A multifactorial model for pancreatic cancer in man. Epidemiologic evidence. JAMA 1981; 245:147–152.
16. MacDermott RP, Kramer P. Adenocarcinoma of the pancreas in four siblings. Gastroenterology 1973: 65:137–139.
17. Danes BS, Lynch HT. A familial aggregation of pancreatic cancer: an in vitro study. JAMA 1982; 247:2798–2802.
18. Koh THHG, Cooper JE, Newman CL, Walker TM, Kiely EM, Hoffman EB. Pancreatoblastoma in a neonate with Wiedeman-Beckwith syndrome. Eur J Pediatr 1986; 145:435–438.
19. Sauer L, Harrison MR, Boud SJ, Flake AW, Heyman MB, Ring EJ. Longterm percutaneous biliary drainage in an infant with hemangioendothelioma. J Pediatr Surg 1987; 22:606–608.
20. Frable WJ, Still WJS, Kay S. Carcinoma of the pancreas, infantile type. Cancer 1971; 27:667–673.
21. Taxy JB. Adenocarcinoma of the pancreas in childhood. Cancer 1976; 37:1508–1518.
22. Brougham TA, Leslie JD, Soto JM, Hermann RE. Pancreatic islet cell tumours. Surgery 1986; 99:671–678.
23. Stanley CA, Baker L. Hyperinsulinism in infants and children: diagnosis and therapy. Adv Pediatr 1976; 23:315–355.
24. Mann JR, Rayner PHW, Gourevitch A. Insulinemia in childhood. Arch Dis Child 1969; 44:435.
25. Kitson HF, McCrossin RB, Jimenez M, Middleton A, Siliuk M. Somatostatin treatment of insulin excess due to beta cell adenoma in a neonate. J Pediatr 1980; 96:145–151.
26. Gould VE, Memoli VA, Daoli LE, Gould NS. Nesidiodysplasia and nesidioblastosis in infants. Scand J Gastroenterol 1981; (suppl 70):129–142.
27. Wilson SD, Schulte WJ, Meade RC. Longevity studies following total gastrectomy in children with the Zollinger Ellison syndrome. Arch Surg 1971; 103:108–115.
28. Buchta RM, Kaplan JM. Zollinger Ellison syndrome in a nine year old child: a case report and review of this entity in childhood. Pediatrics 1971; 47:594–598.
29. Drake DP, MacIver AG, Atwell JD. Zollinger Ellison syndrome in a child: medical treatment with cimetidine. Arch Dis Child 1980; 55:226–228.
30. Brenner RW, Sank LI, Kerner MB, Schrager GO, Elguezabal A, Roth J. Resection of a VIPoma of the pancreas in a 15 year old girl. J Pediatr Surg 1986; 21:983–985.
31. Werner P. Genetic aspects of adenomatosis of endocrine glands. Am J Med 1954; 16:363.
32. Ballard HS, Frame B, Hartsock RJ. Familial multiple endocrine adenoma–peptic ulcer complex. Medicine 1964; 43:481.
33. Larsson LI. Endocrine pancreatic tumours. Hum Pathol 1978; 9:401.
34. Pearse AGE. Common cytochemical and ultrastructural characteristics of cells producing polypeptide hormones (the APUD series) and their relevance to thyroid and ultimobranchial C cells and calcitonin. Proc R Soc Lond 1968; 107:71.
35. Pearse AGE. The cytochemistry and ultrastructure of polypeptide hormone–producing cells of the APUD series and the embryologic physiology and pathologic implications of the concept. J Histochem Cytochem 1969; 17:303.
36. Pearse AG, Tabot TT. Neuroendocrine embryology and the APUD concept. Clin Endocrinol 1976; (suppl 5):2295.
37. Zollinger RM, Ellison EH. Primary peptic ulcerations of the jejunum associated with islet cell tumours of the pancreas. Ann Surg 1955; 142:709.
38. Jensen RT, Gardner JD, Raufman JP, Pandol SJ, Doppman JL, Collen MJ. Zollinger Ellison syndrome: current concepts and management. Ann Intern Med 1983; 98:59–75.
39. Spindel E, Harty RF, Leibach JR, McGuigan JE. Decision analysis in evaluation of hypergastrinemia. Am J Med 1986; 80:11–17.
40. Deveney CW, Stein S, Way LW. Cimetidine in the treatment of Zollinger Ellison Syndrome. Am J Surg 1983; 146:116–123.
41. Bonfils S, Lander JH, Mignon M, Hervoir P. Results of surgical management in 92 consecutive patients with Zollinger Ellison syndrome. Ann Surg 1981; 194:692–697.
42. Thompson JC, Lewis BG, Wiener I, Townsend CM. The role of surgery in the Zollinger Ellison syndrome. Ann Surg 1983; 197:594–607.
43. Richardson CT, Peters MN, Feldman M, McClelland RN, Walsh JH, Cooper KA, Willeford G, Dickerman RM, Fordtran JS. Treatment of Zollinger Ellison syndrome with exploratory laparotomy, proximal gastric vagotomy, and H_2-receptor antagonists: a prospective study. Gastroenterology 1985; 89:357–367.
44. Maton PN, Fricht H, Vinayek R, Wonk SA, Gardner JP, Jensen RT. Medical management of patients with Zollinger Ellison syndrome who have had previous gastric surgery: a prospective study. Gastroenterology 1988; 94:294–299.
45. Verner JV, Morrison AB. Islet cell tumour and a syndrome of refractory watery diarrhea and hypokalemia. Am J Med 1958; 25:374.
46. Verner JV, Morrison AB. Endocrine pancreatic islet disease with diarrhea: report of a case due to diffuse hyperplasia of non-beta islet tissue with a review of 54 additional cases. Arch Intern Med 1974; 133:492.
47. Long RG, Mitchell SJ, Bryant MG, Polak JM. Bloom SR. Clinicopathological study of pancreatic and neural VIPomas. Gut 1979; 20:A934.
48. Yamada T. Secretory tumours of the pancreas. In: Sleisenger MH, Fordtran JS, eds. Gastrointestinal disease: pathophysiology, diagnosis, management. 3rd ed. Philadelphia: WB Saunders, 1983: 1527.
49. Kopelman H, Gaskin KJ, Durie PR, Sherwood G, Filler RM, Wesson DE, Forstner GG. Pancreatic exocrine function in islet cell dysplasia after 95 percent resection. Pediatr Res 1984; 18:203A.

PART 6

Pancreatitis

Peter R. Durie, B.Sc., M.D., FRCPC

Pancreatitis is considered to be a rare cause of abdominal pain in childhood, but it is probably more common than previously believed. It is less frequent in children than adults, but disease prevalence is largely undetermined. Alcohol abuse and biliary tract disease, the major causes of pancreatic inflammation in adulthood,[1,2] are rarely implicated in childhood-onset pancreatitis. Our own retrospective evaluation of childhood causes of pancreatitis,[3] which is corroborated by other clinical reports,[4–11] suggests that the predisposing factors are multiple and diverse. Single, self-limited attacks or recurrent attacks of acute pancreatitis are by far the most frequent feature of this disease in childhood.[3] Acute pancreatitis only rarely progresses to chronic pancreatitis. With the exception of two fascinating conditions of childhood, hereditary pancreatitis[12] and the juvenile tropical pancreatitis syndrome,[13] chronic pancreatitis is quite rare in the young patient. Hereditary pancreatitis is recognized only in defined kindreds, whereas juvenile tropical pancreatitis syndrome, which is described in detail in a companion chapter, is seen in certain developing countries abutting the equator.

CLASSIFICATION OF PANCREATITIS

The original clinical classification of pancreatic inflammation, established at the Marseilles symposium in 1963, was redefined at a second international symposium (Marseilles, 1984).[14,15] The revised classification, based largely upon experience in adults, is generally applicable to younger patients. The following is excerpted from the conference proceedings:

Pancreatitis should be classified only as *acute pancreatitis* or *chronic pancreatitis*. The terms "acute relapsing" pancreatitis and "chronic relapsing" pancreatitis have been dropped. Etiologic factors are not considered because pancreatitis is not a specific disease, and in many instances it is not possible to attribute a distinct clinical or morphologic entity to a distinct etiology.

Acute Pancreatitis

Clinically acute pancreatitis is characterized by acute abdominal pain accompanied by increased pancreatic enzymes in blood and/or urine. Although it usually runs a benign course, severe attacks may lead to shock, with renal and pulmonary insufficiency that may prove fatal. Acute pancreatitis may present with a single episode or it may recur.

Morphologically there is a gradation of lesions in acute pancreatitis. In the mild form, there are peripancreatic fat necrosis and interstitial edema, but as a rule pancreatic necrosis is absent. The mild form may develop into a severe form with extensive peri- and intrapancreatic fat necrosis, parenchymal necrosis, and hemorrhage. The lesions may be either localized or diffuse. Both exocrine and endocrine functions of the pancreas are impaired to a variable extent and for a variable duration.

If the primary cause and complications such as pseudocysts are eliminated, clinical, morphologic, and functional return to normal occurs. In some cases scarring and pseudocysts persist. Only rarely does acute pancreatitis lead to chronic pancreatitis.

Chronic Pancreatitis

Clinically chronic pancreatitis is characterized by recurrent or persisting abdominal pain, although in some cases chronic pancreatitis may be present without pain. Evidence of pancreatic insufficiency—for example, steatorrhea or diabetes—may be present.

Morphologically chronic pancreatitis is characterized by an irregular sclerosis with destruction and permanent loss of exocrine parenchyma that may be either focal, segmental, or diffuse. These changes may be associated with varying degrees of dilatation of segments of the ductal system. Thus, dilatation of the duct of Wirsung and of its smaller ducts may occur together or independently. No obvious cause of duct dilatation may be found, but most often it is associated with stricture of the ducts or intraductal protein plugs and calculi (calcification). All types of inflammatory cells may be present in varying degrees as well as edema and focal necrosis. Cysts and/or pseudocysts are not uncommon. Compared with the degree of acinar destruction, the islets of Langerhans are relatively well preserved.

The following terms can be used to describe chronic pancreatitis:

1. Chronic pancreatitis with focal necrosis
2. Chronic pancreatitis with segmental or diffuse fibrosis
3. Chronic pancreatitis with or without calculi

Obstructive chronic pancreatitis is a distinct morphologic form of chronic pancreatitis. It is characterized by dilatation of the ductal system proximal to the occlusion of all the major ducts (e.g., tumor or scars), diffuse acinar atrophy, and uniform fibrosis. Calculi are uncommon.

In chronic pancreatitis (except for obstructive chronic pancreatitis), the irreversible morphologic changes in the pancreas may lead to a progressive or permanent loss of exocrine and endocrine pancreatic function. In obstructive chronic pancreatitis, both structural and functional changes tend to improve when the obstruction is removed.

Hemochromatosis and cystic fibrosis were not classified as chronic pancreatitis. The question of whether chronic pancreatitis always progresses or may regress after removal of the primary cause or causes remains unanswered.

ACUTE PANCREATITIS

Typically, acute pancreatitis presents with severe abdominal pain, often with symptoms suggestive of ileus. No single, definitive diagnostic test exists, and the criteria for establishing a diagnosis rest upon (1) typical clinical manifestations, (2) increased serum concentrations of pancreatic enzymes (optimally two enzymes should be three to four times above the upper limits of normal), and (3) sonographic or radiologic evidence of pancreatic inflammation. The clinical course varies considerably from a mild, self-limited, uncomplicated attack to a severe complicated course that may be fatal. In general, the histologic severity of the pancreatitis correlates with the clinical course. With clinical recovery, there may be functional and morphologic derangement of both exocrine and endocrine pancreatic elements, but these usually recover fully after a variable period of time.[15] When the underlying cause remains, acute pancreatitis may recur, but if the precipitating factor is removed, sequelae are unlikely.

Pathogenesis of Acute Pancreatitis

It is generally agreed that acute pancreatitis is caused by autodigestion of the pancreas as a result of inappropriate activation of pancreatic zymogens to active enzymes within the pancreatic parenchyma (Fig. 1).[1,15–18] The pathologic changes within the pancreatic parenchyma support this concept and

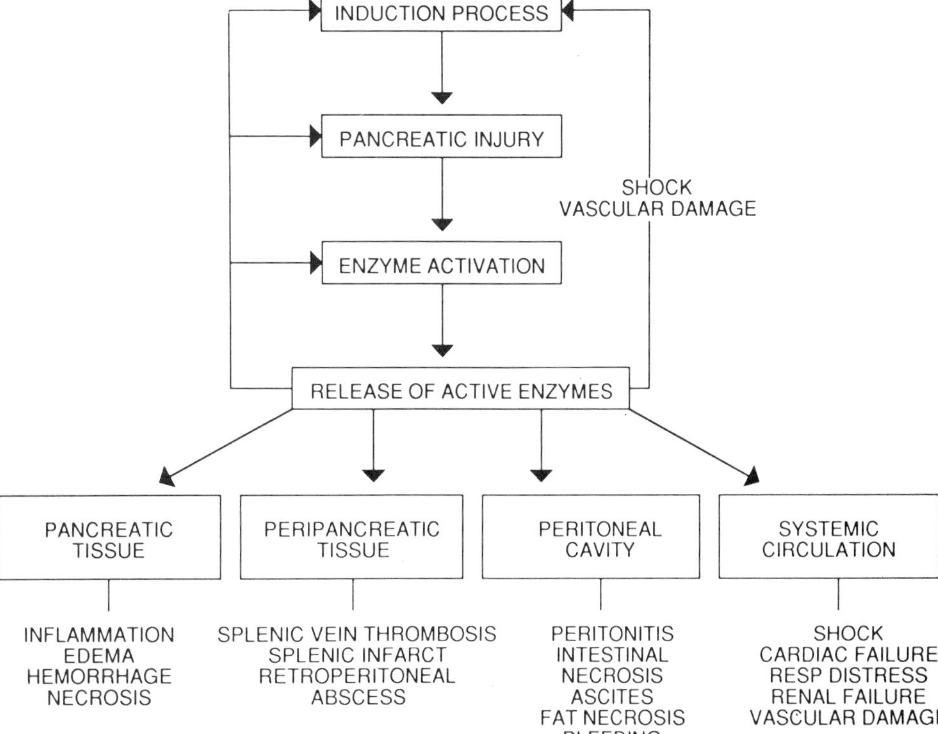

FIGURE 1 Pathogenetic mechanisms of acute pancreatitis. An unknown process induces pancreatic injury. Enzymes within the pancreatic parenchyma are activated and released into adjoining pancreatic tissue, peripancreatic tissue, the peritoneum, and the system circulation. Active enzymes are probably responsible for many of the local and systemic complications of acute pancreatitis.

so do animal models of pancreatic inflammation that induce similar morphologic and clinical effects.[15-21] The conditions whereby pancreatic enzymes are activated or the sequence of events required to trigger these events remains uncertain.[18] A wide spectrum of factors is known to predispose to acute pancreatitis (Table 1); therefore, a number of inductive mechanisms are likely responsible. Various experimental approaches have been devised to induce acute pancreatitis, but few if any provide useful insight into the triggering mechanisms of human disease.[19-21] Experimental studies do, however, permit evaluation of the secondary features and complications of pancreatic inflammation.

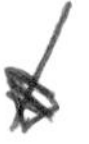

TABLE 1
Factors Causing Predisposition to Acute Pancreatitis

Mechanical/structural
Bile reflux
Outflow obstruction (congenital or acquired)
Duodenopancreatic reflux (congenital or acquired)
Trauma
Metabolic/toxic
Hyperlipidemia
Hypercalcemia
Cystic fibrosis
Malnutrition (refeeding pancreatitis)
Drugs/toxins
Renal disease
Hypothermia
Diabetes mellitus
Systemic diseases
Infections (bacterial, parasitic, viral)
Multisystem inflammatory disorders
Shock/hypoxemia
Unknown
Hereditary
Idiopathic

In normal circumstances, several protective mechanisms are in place to prevent pancreatic enzyme activation.[16,17,22,23] The proteolytic enzymes (trypsin, chymotrypsin, carboxypeptidases, elastase) and also phospholipase A are synthesized and stored as inactive zymogens, whereas the pancreatic enzymes amylase and lipase are synthesized and stored in the active form. Secondly, pancreatic enzymes are stored in membrane-bound zymogen granules, isolating them from other intracellular elements. The pancreatic tissue, pancreatic juice, and serum all contain potent protease inhibitors that can inactivate prematurely activated enzymes.

Under laboratory conditions, protease activation involves a cascade process (Fig. 2).[24] Trypsinogen is first activated either by enterokinase, a brush border intestinal peptidase, or by slow autoactivation under alkaline conditions. Small amounts of trypsin are capable of rapidly activating other proenzymes, including chymotrypsinogen, proelastase, procarboxypeptidase, and prophospholipase as well as nonpancreatic peptides (e.g., kallikrein, complement). Animal experiments have been used to study the local effects of active enzymes on the pancreas. Trypsin and chymotrypsin cause edema and in large quantities necrosis and hemorrhage. Elastase damages the walls of blood vessels, resulting in hemorrhage. Phospholipase A, which is enzymatically active in the presence of bile salts, destroys cellular phospholipid membranes, releasing lysolecithin, which in turn has strong cytotoxic properties. Lipase causes fat necrosis in the presence of its pancreatic co-factor co-lipase and bile acids.

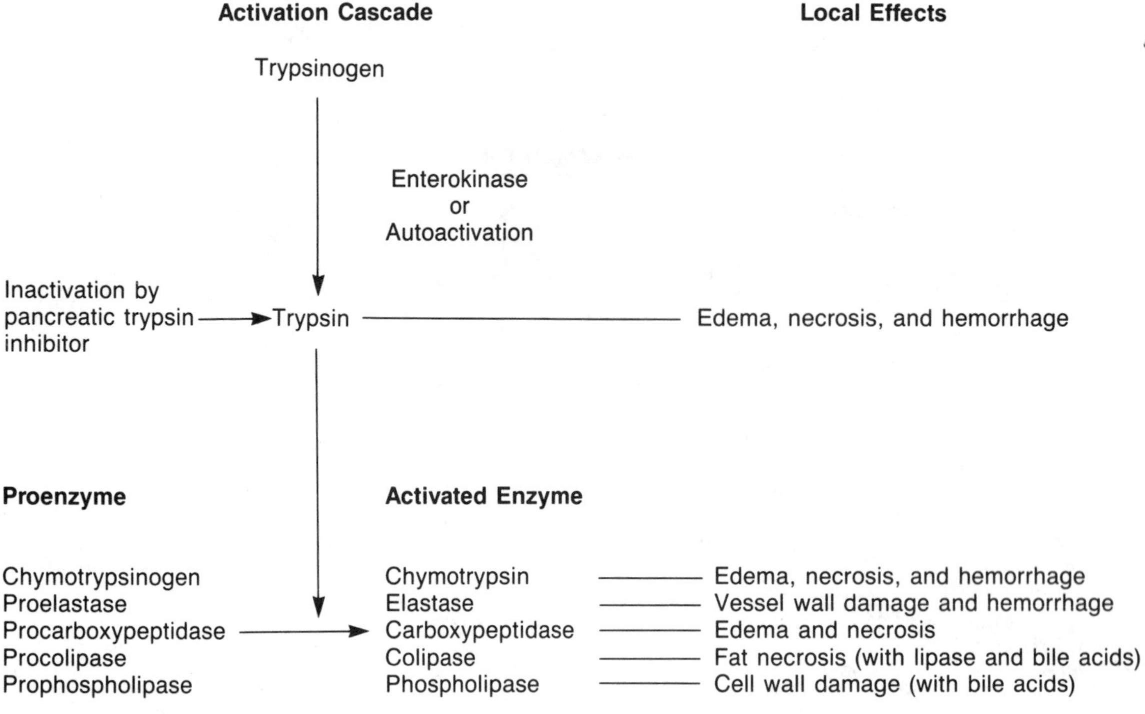

FIGURE 2 Activation of pancreatic enzymes.

Pathogenesis of Systemic Complications

Regardless of the method of induction, pancreatic enzyme activation remains the key process in the pathogenesis of disease and probably acounts for many well-recognized local and systemic complications. Until recently, remarkably little definitive biochemical evidence existed to confirm the presence of active pancreatic proteases in the bloodstream.[25] This was largely due to inadequate laboratory methodology to determine the activity and molecular forms of circulating pancreatic proteases. Since amylase and lipase are synthesized and secreted in the active form, their presence and activity in plasma bear no relationship to disease severity or to the degree of activation of pancreatic proteases.

In earlier studies, relatively crude, nonspecific biochemical tests of enzymatic activity showed increased levels of trypsin-like activity in sera of patients with acute pancreatitis, but because a number of proteases of nonpancreatic origin are normally present in sera, enzymatic activity could not be assigned specifically to pancreatic trypsin. To circumvent this problem, several laboratories have since developed immunologic methods to detect specific immunoreactive forms of circulating pancreatic proteases, including trypsin, chymotrypsin, carboxypeptidase, and elastase.[25-28] These methods cannot distinguish between proenzymes and active enzymes such as trypsinogen, trypsin, or trypsin-inhibitor complexes in unfractionated sera. Therefore, sera from patients with pancreatic inflammation were chromatographed under conditions that resolve trypsinogen from active trypsin bound to the major circulating protease inhibitors, alpha$_1$-protease inhibitor (alpha$_1$-antitrypsin) and alpha$_2$-macroglobulin.[25-31] In this regard, plasma from normal patients appears to contain only trypsinogen.[26] In most patients with acute pancreatitis, the major portion of the immunoreactive material also eluted in a position corresponds to free trypsinogen, but in patients with severe hemorrhagic pancreatitis, a minor fraction of immunoreactive trypsin was detected, bound to alpha$_1$-protease inhibitor, and following acid treatment the alpha$_2$-macroglobulin peak also yielded immunoreactive trypsin.[29,30]

We have employed similar techniques to define the longitudinal alterations in the molecular forms of circulating trypsin in children with acute pancreatitis.[31] Early in the course of the disease, predominantly trypsinogen was released into the circulation, but in considerably greater quantities than in normal individuals. In patients with severe hemorrhagic pancreatitis, confirmed by postmortem examination, serial samples showed increasing concentrations of active trypsin complexed to the two protease inhibitors, alpha$_2$-macroglobulin and alpha$_1$-protease inhibitor (Fig. 3). In patients with mild interstitial pancreatitis, plasma contained predominantly trypsinogen at all times. Although few patients were studied, a correlation appeared to exist between the histologic severity of acute pancreatitis and the amount of active trypsin complexed to circulating protease inhibitors. Subsequent studies involving analysis of active carboxypeptidase-B and its inactive proenzyme, which can be detected immunologically without the need for chromatography, suggest a generalized activation of all pancreatic enzymes in patients with severe pancreatitis.[32]

Laboratory techniques have been employed to evaluate temporal changes of the forms of circulating enzymes in animal models of acute pancreatitis. Studies in a canine model of bile-induced pancreatitis demonstrated that early samples con-

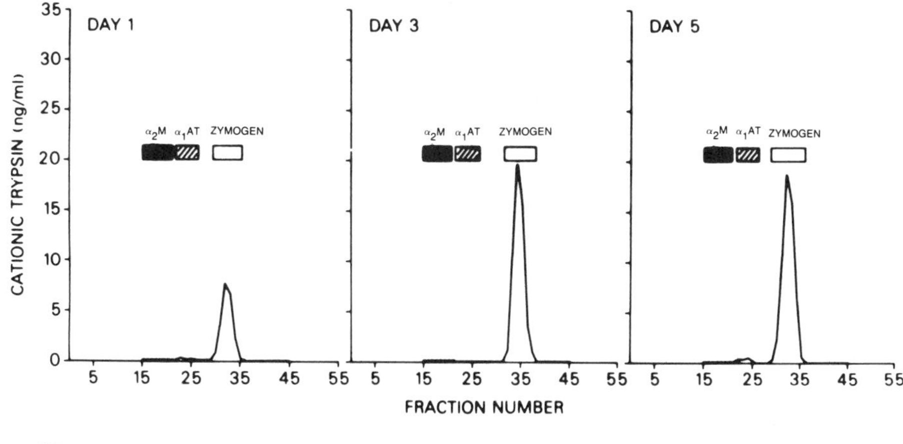

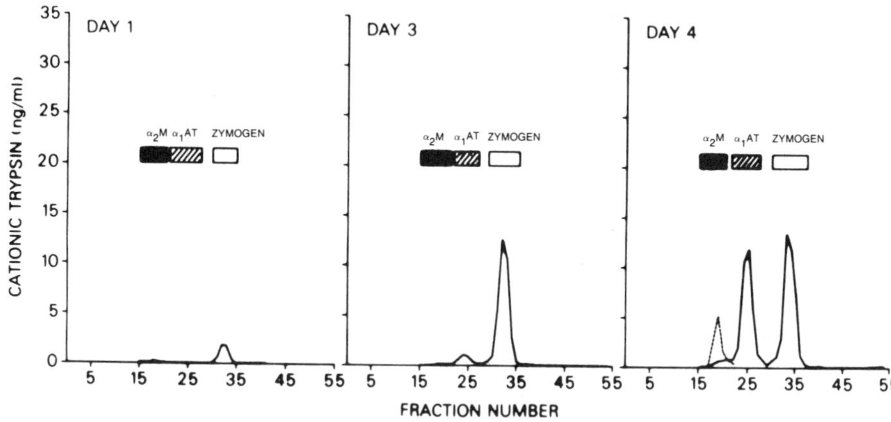

FIGURE 3 Molecular forms of immunoreactive cationic trypsin in serial fractionated plasma samples from two patients with acute pancreatitis. Superimposed bars show elution profiles of trypsin-α_2-macroglobulin complexes (α_2-M), trypsin-α_1-antitrypsin complexes (α_1-AT), and free trypsinogen (zymogen). *Top,* A patient with hemolytic uremic syndrome who had mild interstitial pancreatitis at postmortem. Only free trypsinogen is detected. *Bottom,* A patient with Reye's syndrome with severe hemorrhagic pancreatitis at postmortem. Increasing quantities of active trypsin complexed to protease inhibitors are detected.

tained predominantly free trypsinogen, but later in the disease process, plasma and ascites samples contained increasing quantities of active trypsin complexed to the major protease inhibitors.[33] In rats subjected to taurocholate-induced pancreatitis, the levels of active trypsin in the bloodstream correlated directly with mortality.[34] Other studies of experimental pancreatitis have shown a good correlation between mortality and the degree of depletion of circulating protease inhibitors, which are normally cleared by the reticuloendothelial system.[35] Similarly, experimental blockade of the reticuloendothelial system appears to increase mortality.[36] Although little is known about the effects of acute pancreatitis on reticuloendothelial system function, indirect evidence suggests that function may be compromised, which has the potential effect of retarding clearance of enzyme-inhibitor complexes.

Active enzymes complexed to protease inhibitors in the circulation and in the peritoneal cavity could be directly or indirectly responsible for a variety of systemic complications of pancreatitis; these complications include cardiovascular lesions, shock, hypotension, coma, adult respiratory distress syndrome, coagulation abnormalities, hypocalcemia, and acute renal failure. Since circulating active enzymes appear to be complexed primarily to various protease inhibitors, rather than in the free form, enzyme–protease inhibitor complexes must account for disease complications. In this regard, several vitally important biologically active peptides such as proinsulin, parathormone, and clotting enzymes are known to be degraded in vitro by plasma obtained from patients with severe acute pancreatitis.[37-39]

In addition, alpha$_2$-macroglobulin–bound active trypsin rapidly degrades low and medium molecular weight polypeptide hormones such as angiotensin, vasopressin, proinsulin, parathormone, complement, and porcine cholecystokinin.[37-41] Other biologically active peptides may also be activated—for example, kallikrein, which liberates bradykinin and kallidin, causing pain; these substances contribute to local edema formation, increased vascular permeability, and invasion by leukocytes. Thus, many of the well-recognized secondary systemic effects of acute pancreatitis, such as hyperglycemia, hypocalcemia, hypotension, complement activation, and coagulation abnormalities may be a direct result of degradation of vitally important biologically active peptides.

Predisposing Factors

Because we lack precise knowledge of the mechanisms of induction of acute pancreatitis, heavy reliance has been placed upon clinical and epidemiologic observations to determine disease etiologies.[1,3-11,16] Conditions are assumed to be associated if affected patients develop pancreatitis with a higher frequency than expected in the general population. Using this approach, acute pancreatitis has been associated with a broad spectrum of underlying conditions, but convincing proof of cause-effect relationships or the mechanisms involved frequently remains elusive.

In large prospective studies of adults, two major factors, biliary tract disease (gallstones) and alcohol abuse, appear to be associated in up to 80 percent of all cases; the prevalence and proportion of each vary considerably depending on the ethnic backgrounds and environmental conditions of the communities examined.[1,2,16,24] Both conditions are exceedingly rare in childhood, although biliary tract disease, from congenital anomalies and also from acquired disorders of the pancreaticobiliary system, can be implicated in a small number of patients.[3] In contrast to its close association with chronic pancreatitis in adults, ethanol abuse is virtually unheard of as a cause of acute or chronic pancreatitis in childhood. In a normal gland, acute pancreatitis rarely occurs following a single episode of ethanol intake and is probably a direct toxic effect of this drug.

In childhood-onset acute pancreatitis, four major predisposing factors (Table 1) appear to account for the majority of cases: (1) mechanical and structural factors, (2) toxic and metabolic disorders, (3) systemic disease, and (4) no known cause (hereditary or idiopathic).

Mechanical and Structural Factors

Bile Reflux. The "common duct" theory holds that acute pancreatitis may result from obstruction of the common biliary channel, which allows bile to flow via a common channel into the pancreatic duct.[42] It is postulated that reflux of bile into the pancreas causes local damage and inflammation. High-pressure injection of bile is commonly used to induce experimental pancreatitis in animal models.[33] Gallstone disease with distal obstruction is considered to be the most common predisposing factor in adults living in developed countries.[1,43] In autopsy series of adults, a close correlation has been shown between acute pancreatitis and biliary tract disease, but alcoholism was common in the populations examined.

A strong argument in favor of an association with gallstone disease is that pancreatitis rarely recurs following operative removal of gallstones, whereas recurring attacks of acute pancreatitis are commonly seen in patients in whom stones remain in the biliary tree.[43] Against this argument, clinical evidence of duct obstruction by stones is rare, occurring in less than 4 percent of patients during an acute episode. Other authors have suggested that inflammation within the gallbladder might spread to the pancreas via lymphatic pathways, but this argument eludes scientific logic. It is conceivable, nonetheless, that the common duct theory has some validity, since patients are often evaluated clinically some 24 to 48 hours or longer following the onset of clinical symptoms, by which time the obstructing stone may have passed.

Outflow Obstruction. It is proposed that obstruction to pancreatic flow might induce acute pancreatitis, but its true role is debated, since animal studies have shown that obstruction in the pancreatic duct produces atrophy without pancreatitis. Suggested clinical causes of outflow obstruction include sphincter of Oddi dysfunction, a variety of congenital anomalies of the pancreas and/or biliary tree (e.g., pancreas divisum, choledochal cyst, annular pancreas), and primary or secondary pancreatic tumors.

The muscular sphincter of Oddi is believed to induce increased resistance to outflow of pancreaticobiliary secretions and therefore may be responsible for acute pancreatitis. Dysfunction of the sphincter of Oddi could result from stenosis of the duct due to fibrosis and/or inflammation or functional abnormalities (dyskinesia). In adults manometric evaluation of sphincter of Oddi function is now becoming a standard technique in many specialized centers.[44,45] A perfusion catheter is used to cannulate the ampulla of Vater, and pressure recordings are made in the pancreatic duct and in the sphincter both before and after various drugs (cholecystokinin and smooth muscle relaxants) are administered to induce secretion or changes in sphincter contractility. In up to 20 percent of adult patients with idiopathic pancreatitis, abnormal tracings are seen; some of these patients appear to benefit from sphincteroplasty. Whether these observations represent a primary abnormality of sphincter function or are secondary effects of pancreatitis is debatable. This evaluation has not been routinely used in children, but a limited number of patients have been evaluated.[46]

Pancreas divisum, the embryologic failure of fusion of the ventral and dorsal pancreatic ducts, is also considered to be a frequent cause of outflow obstruction–induced acute pancreatitis in childhood. However, the true role of this common anomaly as a cause of pancreatitis is hotly debated.[46–51] The reader is referred elsewhere in this book for a detailed discussion of this interesting anomaly, which is recognized in close to 10 percent of the population, and in 2 percent of these patients the ventral duct is absent. Protagonists argue that the small orifice of the dorsal duct causes outflow obstruction, whereas detractors have indicated no difference in the frequency of pancreas divisum among patients with and without pancreatitis. Thus, demonstration of pancreas divisum creates a difficult dilemma—whether or not to proceed with surgical or endoscopic decompression.

Duodenopancreatic Reflux. Reflux of the duodenal contents through the papilla, for example following the passage of a stone or duodenal obstruction, might be a factor in triggering acute pancreatitis. Duodenal contents contain enterokinase and active pancreatic proteases, and these would be capable of activating proenzymes within the pancreas, triggering an autoactivation cascade. To some extent, the presence of protease inhibitors in the pancreas might be expected to limit this process.

A variety of clinical conditions have been implicated. Pancreatitis is known to occur as a complication of duodenal Crohn's disease, particularly in patients with obstruction from duodenal stricture. In addition, patients with duodenal diverticula and proximal blind-loop syndrome appear to have an increased susceptibility to acute pancreatitis.[52] Invasion of the pancreatic duct by worms has also been implicated as a cause of pancreatitis in childhood.[53] Instrumentation of the pancreas during endoscopic retrograde cholangiopancreatography (ERCP) invariably causes a transient rise in serum enzymes without symptoms of acute pancreatitis, but 1 to 7 percent of adult patients develop overt signs of acute pancreatitis.[54] This complication may be the direct result of injection of contrast material, but reflux of duodenal contents could follow duct cannulation. ERCP is now more commonly used in children; although no reliable data exist, a similar complication rate is anticipated.[46–50]

Trauma. There appears to be a true causal relationship between pancreatic trauma and acute pancreatitis.[1,3–11] Blunt abdominal trauma, child abuse, and penetrating wounds are frequent causes of pancreatic inflammation.[55] Pancreatitis is most likely to occur after disruption of the pancreatic ducts, impairment of the vascular supply, or severe compression injury of the pancreatic parenchyma. Extravasated pancreatic proenzymes in contact with catalytic agents, such as blood or intestinal contents, would provide the conditions for protease activation. Another cause of pancreatic inflammation, postoperative pancreatitis, is reported to have a high mortality rate in adults.[56] In the majority of reported cases, operations were performed on or near the pancreas. The true incidence and complication rate of postoperative pancreatitis in childhood are unknown.

Metabolic and Toxic Factors

A variety of toxic and metabolic disorders have been causally associated with acute pancreatitis (Fig. 2). In some of these examples the primary process may not be directly responsible, and acute pancreatic inflammation could result from a secondary metabolic derangement. Regardless of the process involved, it is believed that a variety of toxic and metabolic disturbances can induce acute pancreatitis by intrapancreatic enzyme activation. Animal models of acute pancreatitis provide some support for this contention. A choline-deficient, ethionine-supplemented diet consistently induces acute pancreatitis in mice.[20] Similarly, supramaximal doses of intravenous hormones known to stimulate the pancreas (cerulein or cholecystokinin) are capable of inducing acute pancreatitis in rodents.[21]

Hyperlipidemia. Reports on the association between hyperlipidemic conditions and acute pancreatitis are conflicting. Braunsteiner[57] reported a 25 percent incidence of acute pancreatitis in hyperlipidemic adults. Types I, IV, and V hyperlipoproteinemias are commonly associated with acute pancreatitis,[58] and in some of these patients chronic pancreatitis develops. However, it has been suggested that hyperlipidemia is a primary complication of alcoholism and in itself is not causative. Similarly, plasma lipids are frequently elevated during acute pancreatic inflammation, and most reports provide poor documentation of a pre-existing primary hyperlipidemia. In a retrospective review of childhood causes of acute pancreatitis, we observed three patients with acute pancreatitis who had primary hyperlipidemic disorders (types I and V).[3] Thus, although the data are suggestive, the true importance of hyperlipidemic states in the etiology of acute pancreatitis remains unresolved.[58]

Hypercalcemia. The causal relationship between hypercalcemia and acute pancreatitis is stronger, but the inductive mechanisms are unknown. In adult patients in hyperparathyroid crisis, overt pancreatic inflammation appears to be 10 to 20 times more frequent than in the general population.[59] Similarly, acute pancreatitis is frequently seen in adult patients with hypercalcemia from a variety of secondary conditions, including acute vitamin D intoxication, calcium intoxication, and metastatic carcinoma of the breast.[60,61] We have observed acute pancreatitis in a child following accidental infusion of excess calcium in an intravenous nutrition preparation.[3]

Cystic Fibrosis. Acute pancreatitis is an uncommon complication in patients with cystic fibrosis (CF).[62] The pathogenetic mechanisms are likely related to deficient fluid secretion within ducts, which appears to be a primary abnormality of all CF epithelial tissue, and inability to maintain hydration of pancreatic secretions leads to protein hyperconcentration, resulting in protein precipitation and pancreatic duct obstruction.[63] The pancreas rapidly atrophies and fails in the majority of CF patients, producing maldigestive symptoms from pancreatic insufficiency. However, approximately 15 percent of patients with CF retain sufficient residual pancreatic function for normal digestion, and this subgroup of "pancreatic-sufficient" patients appear susceptible to recurring attacks of acute pancreatitis.[64] Presumably duct obstruction damages proximal functional acinar epithelium, producing an inflammatory response. Rarely, patients with CF develop chronic pancreatitis, with formation of multiple cysts, scarring, and calcification.[65]

Malnutrition. In severely malnourished children, pancreatic enzyme synthesis and secretion are compromised.[66] The acini become markedly deranged and atrophied with profound changes of the intracellular organelles. Raised levels of pancreatic enzymes (serum trypsinogen), which correlate with the severity of malnutrition, appear to reflect pancreatic damage.[67] Recovery of pancreatic function can occur following refeeding, but vigorous, early feeding has been reported to induce acute pancreatitis.[68] There have also been occasional case reports of acute pancreatitis following forced refeeding in patients with anorexia nervosa.[69] The precise mechanisms of induction of acute pancreatitis following malnutrition are poorly understood, but the deranged acinar cells may be susceptible to injury following hormonal stimuli induced by feeding.

Drugs and Toxins. A vast pharmacopoeia of therapeutic agents, illicit drugs, and environmental toxins has been implicated in the pathogenesis of acute pancreatitis.[70,71] With some of these agents there is considerable doubt regarding a true cause-effect relationship, and in those in which there appears to be a true etiologic association, the pathogenetic mechanisms are often unknown or based on flimsy evidence. Frequently cited drugs and toxins are listed in Table 2, which provides an estimate of the probability of each agent's association with pancreatic inflammation. In some instances, there may be an indirect cause; for example, drugs known to induce an allergic vasculitis may affect the vascular supply of a number of organs, including the pancreas. Other drugs may induce a metabolic derangement that triggers pancreatic inflammation as a secondary phenomenon. Many drugs are used in the treatment of patients with a primary condition that itself is known to cause predisposition to acute pancreatic inflammation. Frequently, several drugs are used, for example in the treatment of malignancies, and consequently precise identification of the offending agent is often difficult.

In cases of accidental or suicidal drug intoxication, serum concentrations of pancreatic enzymes are frequently elevated, usually in the absence of symptoms of pancreatitis. Overt pancreatitis has been reported in a child after acetaminophen intoxication.[3] Agents commonly used by drug addicts may cause a necrotizing angiitis that sometimes induces pancreatitis; methamphetamines have been commonly implicated. There is convincing evidence to support an association between acute pancreatitis and poison from the scorpion *Tityus trinitatis*.[72] The pathogenetic mechanisms appear to be due to increased acetylcholine release from cholinergic neurons.

Renal Disease. Reports in adults have associated acute pan-

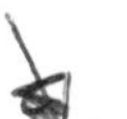

TABLE 2
Drugs and Toxic Agents Associated with Acute Pancreatitis

Therapeutic Agents
Definite
Chlorthiazides
Furosemide
Tetracyclines
Sulfonamides
Estrogens
6-Mercaptopurine
L-Asparaginase
Valproic acid
Possible
Corticosteroids
Nonsteroidal anti-inflammatory agents
Methyldopa
Phenformin
Nitrofurantoin
Azathioprine
Metronidazole
Nontherapeutic (Poisons, Drug Abuse, or Overdose)
Ethyl alcohol
Methyl alcohol
Heroin
Amphetamines
Organophosphate insecticides
Acetaminophen overdose
Iatrogenic hypercalcemia

creatitis with renal insufficiency.[73] However, pancreatic enzymes are often elevated in patients with impaired renal function due to reduced clearance.[74] Severe, acute pancreatitis appears to occur following renal transplantation, but the exact incidence and the etiologic factors are uncertain.[75] Acute attacks usually occur more than 6 months postoperatively, and some patients progress to chronic pancreatitis. Therapy with immunosuppressive agents may well be a contributing factor.

Hypothermia. Adult patients with hypothermia from exposure have developed acute pancreatitis.[76] There remains a possibility, in some cases, that hypothermia was a consequence of a severe illness that also contributed to acute pancreatitis. In our clinical experience, acute pancreatitis is not a common feature of children who are deliberately maintained under hypothermic conditions following near-drowning accidents.

Diabetes Mellitus. Children in ketoacidosis from diabetes mellitus frequently complain of abdominal pain. Serum amylase values are frequently raised, but analysis of the isoforms reveals increased salivary amylase. On occasion, however, acute pancreatitis has been reported in patients with diabetes mellitus, particularly during bouts of severe ketoacidosis.[77]

Systemic Diseases

Infections. A variety of systemic infectious agents have been implicated in the etiology of acute pancreatitis (Table 3). In most instances, supportive evidence is indirect—either an epidemiologic association or a concomitant rise in antibody titers.

TABLE 3
Infectious Agents Associated with Acute Pancreatitis

Bacteria
Typhoid fever
Verocytotoxin-producing *Escherichia coli**
Mycoplasma
Leptospirosis
Viruses
Mumps
Coxsackie B
Echovirus
Influenza A
Influenza B†
Varicella†
Epstein-Barr
Rubeola
Hepatitis A
Hepatitis B
Rubella
Parasites
Malaria
Ascariasis (duct obstruction)
Clonorchis sinensis (duct obstruction)

*Associated with the hemolytic-uremic syndrome.
†Associated with Reye's syndrome.

Acute pancreatitis has been rarely reported following severe bacterial infections. Several cases of pancreatitis following typhoid fever are reported. Acute pancreatitis has also been reported in association with *Mycoplasma pneumoniae* infections, but only on the basis of a concomitant rise in antibody titers.[78] Others have suggested that certain bacterial toxins may cause acute pancreatitis. In this regard, acute pancreatitis in childhood is a recognized complication of the hemolytic-uremic syndrome,[3] a multisystem disorder strongly associated with verocytotoxin-producing *Escherichia coli*.[79]

A number of viral agents have been implicated in the etiology of acute pancreatitis. Mumps is cited as the most frequent cause of acute pancreatitis inflammation in younger patients.[4–7] Although there is little doubt that the mumps may, on occasion, cause pancreatic damage,[80] the true incidence of acute pancreatitis with this viral agent is likely extremely low.[3,6] Hyperamylasemia due to the involvement of the parotid glands is common, and for this reason alternative evidence of pancreatic inflammation is imperative before a definite diagnosis can be established. Children with mumps parotitis frequently complain of mild abdominal pain, usually not severe enough to implicate acute pancreatitis. Other viral agents associated with acute pancreatitis include enterovirus strains (coxsackie B and strains of echovirus), Epstein-Barr, rubeola, hepatitis A, and in adults hepatitis B.[1,3,24] Interstitial pancreatitis has also been described in the rubella syndrome. Reye's syndrome is closely associated with epidemics of influenza B or endemic varicella, but, in addition, it has been linked with concomitant ingestion of acetylsalicylic acid. Severe, acute hemorrhagic pancreatitis is a frequent complication of this potentially fatal disease and occurs in up to 50 percent of cases with marked neurologic symptoms.[3,81] Pathologic evidence of acute pancreatitis was provided in Reye's original report.[82] Signs and symptoms of pancreatic inflammation may not be obvious clinically, because they may be masked by treatment protocols or the neurologic symptoms. In our experience acute pancreatitis can be severe enough to cause significant complications, to adversely affect the prognosis, and even to cause death.

Inflammatory Disorders. Acute pancreatitis has been reported in association with a variety of collagen-vascular diseases, such as systemic lupus erythematosus, rheumatoid arthritis, polyarteritis nodosa, and Behçet's syndrome. Antibodies against an antigen directed against the microsomal fraction of human pancreatic tissue have been isolated, but a recent report argues against immunologic mechanisms being a mediator of pancreatic inflammation.[83] Autoimmune mechanisms, however, remain a possibility in some cases. Interstitial pancreatitis has also been noted at postmortem examination in a considerable number of patients with inflammatory bowel disease. Clinical reports in both children and adults provide corroborative evidence. A recent case study in a 12-year-old patient with ulcerative colitis, for example, appears to provide a direct association unrelated to localized small bowel disease or drug ingestion.[84] Nevertheless, patients with collagen-vascular disorders or inflammatory bowel disease are frequently receiving medications considered to be precipitants of acute pancreatitis, making it difficult to establish a clear clinical or epidemiologic association with the primary disease process.

Shock. Any situation producing reduced oxygenation or impaired blood supply to the pancreas may precipitate acute pancreatitis. In our experience, pancreatitis can occur following systemic hypotension from severe blood loss or prolonged cardiopulmonary bypass during cardiac surgery.[3] Circulatory failure from septic shock is also implicated.

Unknown Causes

No precipitating factor is identified in up to 25 percent of children with acute pancreatitis.[3] Recurring attacks of acute pancreatitis are a consistent finding in these patients. Since childhood-onset acute pancreatitis is associated with a wide array of predisposing conditions, idiopathic pancreatitis should be considered only when all other inherited, congenital, and acquired causes have been carefully excluded. With further knowledge of the factors that contribute to acute pancreatic inflammation, identifiable causes are likely to be found in a considerable number of these patients.

Hereditary pancreatitis has been described in more than 40 kindreds. Inheritance patterns suggest autosomal dominant transmission, but the pathophysiologic mechanisms remain unknown.[12] Symptoms usually begin in childhood, often with an acute attack, but the clinical course resembles chronic pancreatitis with a high incidence of pancreatic calcifications, diabetes mellitus, and steatorrhea. A detailed description of this inherited condition is provided in the subsequent discussion of chronic pancreatitis.

TABLE 4
Clinical Features of Acute Pancreatitis

Symptoms
Abdominal pain
Anorexia
Nausea
Vomiting
Coma (rare)
Dyspnea (rare)
Signs
Localized epigastric tenderness
Abdominal wall rigidity
Rebound tenderness
Abdominal distention
Diminished or absent bowel sounds
Hypotension or shock
Low-grade fever
Pleural effusion
Ascites
Oliguria/anuria
Respiratory distress
Gray-Turner sign
Cullen's sign

Clinical Presentation in Childhood

Symptoms and Physical Findings

Acute pancreatitis can present with a wide spectrum of symptoms and complications[3–11]; the clinical course is frequently unpredictable. The diagnosis is difficult to establish unless a high index of suspicion is maintained. A combination of clinical signs and symptoms, in concert with supportive biochemical abnormalities and imaging techniques, is usually necessary to provide a certain diagnosis.

The important clinical features of acute pancreatitis are listed in Table 4. As is frequently the case in adults, abdominal pain is an outstanding symptom, but on rare occasions pain may be absent. Typically, pain is sudden in onset, increases gradually in severity, and reaches maximal intensity after a few hours. In a review of childhood cases from our center,[3] pain was most commonly located in the epigastrium; other sites included the right upper quadrant and the periumbilical area, and the occasional patient complained of diffuse pain over the entire abdomen. The quality of pain was difficult to determine. Radiation of the pain was noted in approximately one-third of cases, notably to the back, the middle, or lower part of the abdomen, to the right upper quadrant, and to the anterior aspect of the chest wall. In one-quarter of cases severe pain necessitated parenteral administration of narcotic analgesia (meperidine). Significant pain lasted from a few hours to 2 weeks, with an average duration of 4 days. Other frequent symptoms include anorexia, nausea, and persistent vomiting. Eating was found to be a common aggravating factor of pain and vomiting. Pain was associated with vomiting in 70 percent of the cases, and in 10 percent vomiting was bilious.

The most frequent physical finding was epigastric tenderness, and this finding was frequently seen with decreased or absent bowel sounds. Abdominal distention was observed in one-third of cases, particularly after 2 to 3 days of symptoms. Rebound tenderness and guarding were usually localized to the epigastrium or upper abdomen. Hypotension or circulatory shock was unusual, occasionally being seen in patients with severe pancreatitis later in the course of the disease. Fever was relatively infrequent and mild (usually less than 38.5°C), occurring in approximately one-third of cases.

In severe cases of hemorrhagic pancreatitis the Gray-Turner sign (bluish discoloration of the flanks) or the Cullen sign (bluish discoloration of the periumbilical area) may be seen. Both signs are due to ecchymosis with entrance of blood into the fascial planes and are not pathognomonic of acute pancreatitis. Other physical signs of patients with acute pancreatitis are infrequent and inconstant in occurrence and are generally nonspecific; these include coma, pleural effusion, respiratory distress, abdominal ascites, icterus, the presence of an abdominal mass, melena, and hematemesis.

Conditions Associated with Acute Pancreatitis in Childhood

There are surprisingly few comprehensive reports of acute pancreatitis in childhood. Many are of limited value, as they consist of individual case reports or are reviews of a limited number of patients. Thus, the true incidence of acute pancreatitis in childhood and the relative frequency of the many predisposing conditions have not been precisely determined. The condition is probably more frequent in children than was previously believed. Affected children can be any age, and the sexes appear to be equally affected. The most frequent causes of pancreatic inflammation in adulthood, namely alcohol abuse and gallstones, are rare in childhood. Table 5 provides a summary of the more common conditions associated with acute pancreatitis in children, which is based upon data from our own experience together with those from other clinical reports.[3-11]

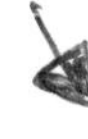

TABLE 5
Causes of Acute Pancreatitis in Childhood

	Approximate Frequency	Recurrence
Idiopathic	25%	Frequent
Mechanical/structural	25%	
Trauma		
Blunt injury		Rare
Child abuse		Rare
ERCP		Rare
Perforation		
Duodenal ulcer; other		Rare
Anomalies		
Pancreas divisum		Frequent
Choledochal cyst		Frequent
Stenosis		Frequent
Other anomalies		Frequent
Obstruction		
Stones		Variable
Parasites		Variable
Tumors		Frequent
Metabolic	10%	
Hyperlipidemia		Frequent
Hypercalcemia (primary or secondary)		Variable
Cystic fibrosis (pancreatic sufficiency)		Frequent
Diabetes mellitus (ketoacidosis)		Rare
Malnutrition (refeeding)		Rare
Drugs/toxins	3%*	Rare
Systemic/multisystem	35%	
Infections		Rare
Sepsis/peritonitis		Rare
Shock		Rare
Inflammatory bowel disease		Uncommon
Collagen-vascular diseases		Uncommon
Reye's syndrome		Rare
Henoch-Schönlein purpura		Rare
Hemolytic-uremic syndrome		Rare
Hereditary	2%†	Frequent

*Probably greatly underestimated.
†Incidence will vary according to kindred populations examined.
ERCP = endoscopic retrograde cholangiopancreatography.
Adapted from J Pediatr 1988; 113:24–29.

A severe multisystem disease appears to be the most common predisposing condition, and in our experience it accounts for approximately one-third of cases. This category encompasses patients with a wide variety of systemic conditions or disorders affecting multiple organs, such as sepsis, shock, systemic infections, collagen-vascular disease, inflammatory bowel disease, and Reye's syndrome. Structural or mechanical causes are also common. Traumatic pancreatitis, most frequently that following blunt abdominal injury, appears to account for approximately 10 to 15 percent of all childhood cases.[3,55] Similarly, anatomic obstruction from congenital or acquired anomalies of the pancreas or biliary tree is responsible for about 10 percent of cases. Metabolic disorders, such as hyperlipidemia, diabetic ketoacidosis, hypercalcemia, and CF, are also quite frequently associated with acute pancreatitis in childhood. Systematic investigation for a structural or metabolic cause is indicated when no obvious cause is found, since the predisposing factors may be amenable to therapy. In childhood, drugs or toxins have been infrequently implicated, but the true incidence may be considerably higher; this may be due to a low index of suspicion and lack of definite proof of an implicating agent. The incidence of hereditary pancreatitis varies considerably depending upon the kindreds in various communities. In our experience, in approximately 25 percent of cases, no predisposing factor is identified even when all other known predisposing factors have been carefully excluded.

Recurrent attacks of acute pancreatitis are more common in certain categories of disease; this is particularly true of cases in which the underlying cause perisists. Further attacks can be expected in patients with "idiopathic" pancreatitis, congenital anomalies of the pancreaticobiliary tree, primary metabolic abnormalities, and hereditary pancreatitis.[3] In contrast, it is unusual for patients with a self-limiting multisystem disorder, blunt trauma, or drug ingestion to experience further attacks unless the predisposing conditions persist or recur.

Diagnosis

General Approach

There is no single diagnostic test of acute pancreatitis, and histologic confirmation of pancreatic inflammation is rarely available. The clinical diagnosis rests on a gestalt of variable nonspecific clinical findings, supportive laboratory tests, and imaging techniques. Occasionally the diagnosis is made with certainty only at laparotomy or at autopsy. Evaluation of a patient suspected of acute pancreatitis requires a careful his-

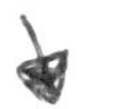

tory to determine the presence of any etiologic factors, such as a family history, associated inherited or acquired conditions, medications, and trauma. The patient and/or parents should also be questioned about previous unexplained episodes of abdominal pain. Although abdominal findings can be variable, the presence of epigastric tenderness, with or without guarding, possibly with abdominal distention and reduced or absent bowel sounds, suggests a significant organic disorder involving the abdominal organs. The differential diagnosis is determined by the history, symptoms, and clinical severity upon presentation. Mild disease may be confused with gastritis. On the other hand, severe disease may mimic a number of surgical emergencies, including small bowel obstruction or perforation. Thus, acute pancreatitis should be considered in any child with upper or diffuse abdominal pain or shock. A number of nonspecific and specific laboratory investigations and imaging procedures will provide supportive evidence of pancreatitis and may help to exclude alternative explanations. Severe pancreatitis should be recognized, since it requires close clinical monitoring and aggressive supportive therapy in the intensive care unit. Knowledge of the early and late complications of acute pancreatitis requires an adequate understanding of the disease process.

Laboratory Investigations

Nonspecific Laboratory Tests. A variety of laboratory abnormalities are described for adult-onset acute pancreatitis, but data in childhood are sparse.[1,3,24] Data in adults frequently show raised values for hemoglobin, hematocrit, leukocyte count, blood glucose, blood urea nitrogen, creatinine, bilirubin, serum lipids, alkaline phosphatase, transaminase, and lactic dehydrogenase. Serum calcium and magnesium and arterial oxygen tension may be reduced. Other nonspecific laboratory abnormalities include metabolic alkalosis, albuminuria, glycosuria, and coagulopathies.

Although not reported in children, in adults the observation of brown discoloration of the serum by methemalbumin is seen in association with necrotizing pancreatitis.[85] This phenomenon arises from the breakdown of hemoglobin in and around the pancreas and is caused by entry of heme into the plasma, where it combines with albumin. The diagnostic value of this test remains limited, however, since it occurs in any hemorrhagic or necrotizing intra-abdominal catastrophe.

Specific Laboratory Tests. The lack of a definitive diagnostic test for acute pancreatitis creates substantial problems in clinical practice, in the design and execution of appropriate clinical studies, and in the interpretation of published reports. Traditionally, considerable diagnostic importance has been attributed to the total serum amylase concentration,[86,87] but it is important to emphasize that patients can have severe pancreatitis with normal serum amylase levels. Conversely, hyperamylasemia is by no means specific for pancreatic disease (Table 6). The diagnostic usefulness of this test, together with a broader discussion of alternative biochemical tests, is given below.

Serum Amylase. This remains the most frequently utilized biochemical test of acute pancreatitis.[86] Alpha-amylase, which hydrolyzes the 1,4 linkages of starch, is synthesized in the active form by a number of organs but in significant amounts only by the pancreas and salivary glands. In normal individuals, small but measurable amounts of amylase enter the circulation directly by unknown mechanisms. Analysis of the major isoforms of the enzyme in normal serum shows that 33 to 45 percent of the amylase is of pancreatic origin, and the remainder is predominantly of salivary origin. Amylase is rapidly cleared from the bloodstream ($T_{1/2}$ 1 to 2 hours), and, unless large quantities of the enzyme continue to enter the bloodstream, serum concentrations equilibrate quickly. In animal studies, approximately 20 percent of infused amylase is recovered intact in the urine. The remainder is presumed to be catabolized, although the exact sites of catabolism are unknown. The renal tubules are important sites of catabolism, but in anephric subjects serum amylase levels are usually two- to threefold higher than normal, suggesting that alternative sites exist as well.[88]

TABLE 6
Causes of Hyperamylasemia

Pancreatic	Salivary	Mixed (Unknown)
Pancreatitis	Infection (mumps)	Cystic fibrosis
Pancreatic tumors	Trauma	Renal insufficiency
Pancreatic duct obstruction	Salivary duct obstruction	Pregnancy
Biliary obstruction	Lung carcinoma	Cerebral trauma
Pseudocysts	Ovarian tumors/cysts	Burns
Perforated ulcer	Prostate tumors	Macroamylasemia
Bowel obstruction	Diabetic ketoacidosis	
Acute appendicitis		
Mesenteric infarction/ischemia		
Endoscopic retrograde cholangiopancreatography		

Serum amylase values are elevated within hours of the onset of acute pancreatitis, and in uncomplicated cases they may remain elevated 3 to 5 days. A protracted elevation raises the suspicion of a local complication such as a pseudocyst or, alternatively, a pancreatic tumor or macroamylasemia. The degree of elevation of serum amylase and other pancreatic enzymes bears no relationship to the severity of pancreatic inflammation or to the clinical course. Although normalization of serum amylase usually indicates resolution of the inflammatory process, hemorrhagic or necrotizing pancreatitis can develop in the face of normal serum amylase.[89] In adults with acute pancreatitis, between 5 and 30 percent of patients have normal serum amylase, but a significant number of patients may have had chronic pancreatitis with advanced destruction of pancreatic acinar tissue. Similarly, children with clinical and sonographic evidence of pancreatitis frequently have normal serum amylase levels during the acute phase of the disease.[3,90]

Hyperamylasemia has numerous causes (Table 6). Symptoms and signs of other acute abdominal conditions are indistinguishable from those of acute pancreatitis. Raised amylase concentrations of pancreatic origin commonly occur with a variety of abdominal insults, including a perforated viscus, mesenteric ischemia, intestinal obstruction, acute cholecystitis, and renal failure. It is also common after uncomplicated endoscopic pancreatography. Obstruction to the pancreatic duct can yield high serum amylase levels, but acute pancreatic inflammation may be absent. Hyperamylasemia may occur as a result of elaboration of salivary amylase into the circulation from inflammation of the salivary gland, CF, calculi, and diabetic ketoacidosis.

Macroamylasemia develops when amylase forms a complex with normal serum proteins, but to our knowledge, it has been reported only in adults.[91] The serum amylase concentration depends upon the degree of protein binding, and levels range from slightly elevated to many times normal. Because the complex is not effectively cleared in the urine, macroamylasemia is associated with normal to low urinary amylase excretion. Macroamylase can be identified by gel filtration or electrophoretic techniques.

The sensitivity of amylase as a determinant of acute pancreatitis has been extensively evaluated. In studies of adults, it has been suggested than an amylase concentration more than threefold above the upper limits of normal strongly indicates pancreatic pathology when alternative salivary or intestinal pathology has been excluded. Application of this principle probably improves specificity but greatly reduces sensitivity. The sensitivity of amylase as a determinant of acute pancreatitis in childhood may be even less than in adults; in our experience and in that of others, up to 40 percent of cases can be missed by reliance solely on this test.[3,90] Thus, a normal serum amylase value does not exclude acute pancreatitis, and a raised value is quite nonspecific, particularly in the presence of a moderate elevation. Improved sensitivity might be expected if daily determinations were obtained, but our experience with a limited number of affected children provides no support for this contention.[3] Hypertriglyceridemia, which may be a primary event or secondary to acute pancreatitis, is known to produce false-negative amylase values.

Urinary Amylase–Creatinine Clearance Ratio. Levitt et al[92] were the first to report that patients with acute pancreatitis have an increased renal clearance of amylase in relation to creatinine. This is due to decreased renal tubular reabsorption (catabolism) of this small protein from the glomerular filtrate. The amylase-creatinine clearance ratio (ACCR), expressed in percent is calculated as follows:

$$\text{ACCR} = \frac{A_{\text{urine}} \times CR_{\text{serum}}}{A_{\text{serum}} \times CR_{\text{urine}}} \times 100$$

A and CR represent amylase and creatinine concentrations, respectively.

Previously, ACCR was advocated as a superior diagnostic test of acute pancreatitis. However, as one might expect, most conditions giving rise to elevated serum amylase also produce an elevated ACCR, and subsequent studies have failed to confirm its diagnostic superiority over a simple serum amylase determination.[93] Thus, ACCR is not more useful in the delayed diagnosis of acute pancreatitis and provides no additional diagnostic information when the serum amylase concentration is normal.

Serum Isoamylases. Various techniques are now available to measure the isoforms of amylase. These include electrophoresis, ion-exchange chromatography, plant-derived inhibitors of salivary amylase, and most recently immunoassay techniques using monoclonal antibodies directed against one or more of the isoforms.[94–96] Although most electrophoretic and chromatography techniques are labor-intensive, costly, and prolonged, the commercially available plant inhibitor assay can easily be performed in any routine clinical chemistry laboratory; despite technical limitations,[97] studies in adult patients have confirmed the superior sensitivity and specificity of the isoamylase method, providing data comparable to those of other assays of specific pancreatic enzymes.[95]

Lipase. Lipase assays are the next most commonly used tests in the routine laboratory diagnosis of acute pancreatitis. Lipase, a glycoprotein, hydrolyzes glycerol esters of long-chain triglycerides in the presence of micellar concentrations of bile salts and its pancreatic co-factor co-lipase.[98] There are two isoforms of this enzyme, which are immunologically identical. Lipases of nonpancreatic origin are found in salivary secretions, the stomach, and breast milk. Various nonpancreatic esterases have enzyme specificity to the same substrates commonly used in biochemical lipase assays,[99,100] but the contribution of nonpancreatic lipases to total activity is unclear. Current biochemical assays for serum lipase fall into two categories: those that use triglyceride substrates and those that use synthetic substrates.[98] Most triglyceride assays utilize photometric, nephelometric, or potentiometric techniques.[100] Difficulties in standardization, poor sensitivity, and lack of linearity are considerable, which together with their labor-intensive requirements have lessened their popularity. Other assays use exogenous co-lipase and bile salts to improve sensitivity and specificity for pancreatic lipase. A synthetic substrate, which is quite specific for pancreatic lipase, employs 2,3-dimercaptopropanol tributyrate, which is cleaved by lipase to release a compound that forms a color reaction. Short incubation time, ease of measurement, and the small amount of serum (20 μl) render this technique somewhat more advantageous than some of the conventional methods.

Considerable controversy exists regarding the superiority of lipase determination over the traditional amylase measurement.[95] Whether lipase values remain elevated longer than those of amylase is still debated, since most comparative studies are inconclusive because of different selection criteria and assay techniques. Commercial immunoassay techniques for the measurement of pancreatic lipase have now been developed; they provide superior test sensitivity and specificity beyond those seen with most biochemical approaches.[101]

Proteases. In the past, lack of substrate specificity of enzymatic techniques for measuring circulating pancreatic proteases greatly limited their clinical utility. However, with the development of highly sophisticated immunoassay techniques, a wide range of proteases can now be measured with a high degree of sensitivity and specificity.[25] These include immunoassays for anionic and cationic trypsin(ogen), elastase 1 and 2, chymotrypsin(ogen), and also carboxypeptidase A and B,[25–28] some of which are commercially available in kit form. The immunoassay for cationic trypsin(ogen), which has been extensively evaluated in both children and adults with acute pancreatitis,[3,29–31,95,102] appears to be a sensitive and specific diagnostic test. Steinberg et al[95] compared the sensitivity and specificity of various diagnostic assays including total amylase, pancreatic isoamylase (inhibitor assay), trypsin(ogen), and conventional lipase. The trypsin(ogen) assay had a higher degree of sensitivity than lipase and pancreatic isoamylase, without much difference in specificity. Our own data in childhood provide support for the superiority of the trypsin(ogen) assay over total serum amylase; when patient sera were studied in parallel, trypsinogen levels appeared to rise earlier in the disease process than did amylase levels and remained consistently elevated during the first 5 days in hospital.[3] The longer incubation time and increased cost of immunoassays limit their use as a first-line test of acute pancreatitis, but they should be utilized as a backup test. The trypsin(ogen) assay has the additional advantage of being able to detect active trypsin bound to plasma protease inhibitors following separation by chromatography.[29,31]

Trypsin(ogen) and other pancreatic proteases are excreted by the kidney, and some of the excreted material appears to be catabolized by the renal tubules. Elevated serum concentrations occur in nephrectomized patients and in those with chronic renal failure.[74] Plasma creatinine, a marker of glomerular filtration, is highly correlated with the serum concentration of cirulating trypsinogen in patients with renal disease, in which values range from 100 to 300 μg per liter.[74] In the majority of children with acute pancreatitis, however, serum trypsinogen levels are considerably higher.[31] Immunoassays toward other pancreatic proteases may be equally useful, but current clinical information is limited, particularly for children.

Ribonuclease. In humans, the concentration of circulating ribonuclease is low in both the serum and pancreatic juice. Pancreatic ribonucleases appear to differ in catalytic and immunologic properties from those obtained from the liver and the spleen. Warshaw and Lee[103] have suggested that raised pancreatic ribonuclease concentrations in the serum are indicative of pancreatic necrosis, but this interesting observation requires independent confirmation.

Imaging Techniques

The various radiologic modalities for evaluating pancreatitis are discussed in greater detail in pertinent parts of the chapter devoted to imaging techniques.

Conventional Radiology. Conventional radiology is of limited value in the diagnosis of acute pancreatitis.[104] Plain films of the abdomen, however, should be obtained in every child with acute abdominal pain to exclude other abdominal catastrophes such as a perforated viscus or appendicolith. In acute pancreatitis, they may show a "sentinel loop" (distention of a small intestinal loop near the pancreas), paralytic ileus involving the entire small intestine, "cut off" sign of the colon (absent colonic gas distal to the transverse colon), or diffuse haziness indicative of ascites. None of these findings is common, nor are they specific for acute pancreatitis, but they are indicative of an acute intra-abdominal or retroperitoneal event. Pancreatic calcification, which is rarely seen in childhood, is diagnostic of chronic pancreatitis and usually reflects a chronic pathologic process within the gland (Fig. 4).

A routine chest radiograph should be obtained in all suspected cases to identify diaphagmatic involvement or pulmonary complications of acute pancreatitis. Interstitial infiltrates within the pulmonary parenchyma are characteristic of pulmonary edema due to the adult respiratory distress syndrome. Similarly, accumulation of fluid within the pleural space may be visible on a chest radiograph, a complication indicative of severe pancreatic disease. Since high concentrations of amylase are generally present within pleural collections, this measurement can be helpful in confirming the diagnosis in difficult cases.

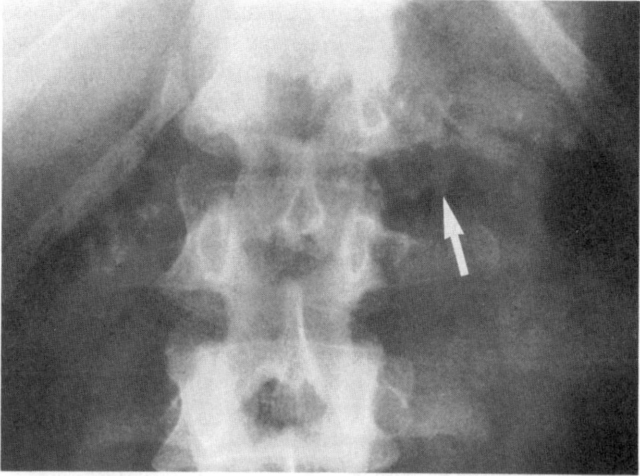

FIGURE 4 Chronic calcific pancreatitis. Speckled pancreatic calcification (*arrow*) is visible on the plain film. (Courtesy of Dr. D.A. Stringer.)

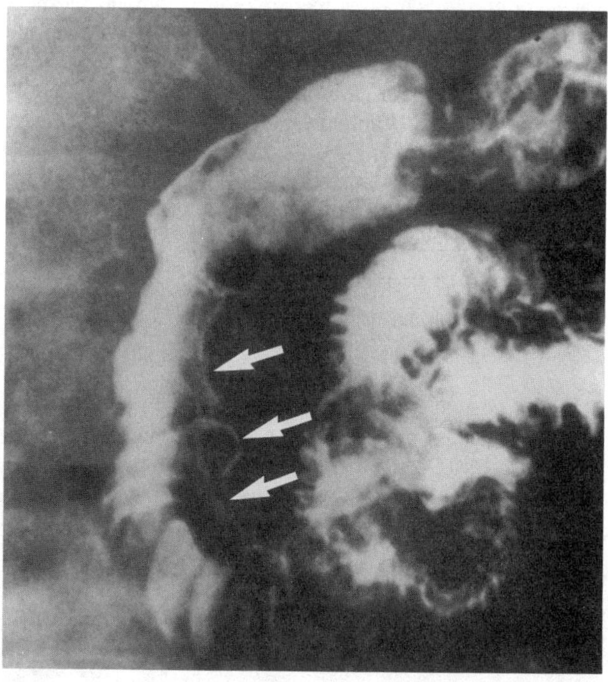

FIGURE 5 Acute pancreatitis. A barium meal study shows distortion of the medial aspect of the second part of the duodenum with a fixed deformity at the site of the pancreatic duct (*middle arrow*), giving the appearance of an inverted 3 to the medial aspect of the duodenum (*top and bottom arrows*). (Courtesy of Dr. D.A. Stringer.)

Contrast studies of the upper GI tract rarely provide useful information and have been largely superseded by alternative imaging techniques and by ERCP. Frequently, indirect evidence of pancreatic enlargement and peripancreatic inflammation may be present. The duodenal loop may appear widened and the mucosal folds effaced. Rarely, the swelling may give an inverted "3" appearance (Frostberg sign), with the middle apex of the "3" being the origin of the duct and the curves of the "3" indicating swelling of the pancreatic head (Fig. 5). The stomach may be displaced forward or medially by retroperitoneal swelling or a pseudocyst. Barium enema examination may show extrinsic compression and/or displacement of the midtransverse colon.

Sonography. Sonography enables direct visualization of the pancreas without subjecting the patient to ionizing radiation or the complications of invasive angiography.[104] Pancreatic size and contour, tissue echogenicity, calcification, and pseudocysts can be detected. Sonography is now the most frequently utilized technique in the preliminary evaluation of children with abdominal pain. There are considerable data to support its routine use in acute pancreatitis, not only as a diagnostic tool but also for identifying and monitoring patients for the development of local complications.[90,104–106] This relatively inexpensive imaging modality can be performed easily, even at the beside. Overlying gas may present technical difficulties, but this is rarely a problem in children. Water can always be given to fill the stomach and act as an acoustic window.

Considerable data have been accumulated in children in support of the argument that sonography is the method of choice in the diagnostic evaluation of any patient suspected of acute or chronic pancreatitis. Abdominal computed tomography (CT) should be reserved for difficult cases and situations in which sonography yields unclear information.[104] Dilatation of the pancreatic or biliary ducts can be readily identified by both techniques. Figure 6 shows a large choledochal cyst detected by sonography in a patient presenting with acute pancreatitis. In normal children and adults, the echodensity of the pancreas is equal to or slightly more than the left lobe of the liver. Pancreatic inflammation causes edema within the pancreatic parenchyma, producing a larger organ with reduced echodensity (Fig. 7). Cox et al[90] confirmed the usefulness of sonographic imaging in the diagnosis of acute pancreatic inflammation in childhood. They reported a poor correlation between pancreatic edema and serum amylase in cases of confirmed pancreatitis. In childhood, sonography may have a positive predictive value of 0.93 in comparison with a predictive value of 0.78 in the presence of a negative sonogram.[105] Normal size limits for the pancreas have been established for the pediatric age group, but many sonographers do not believe that measurement increases the accuracy of evaluation for pancreatic inflammation.

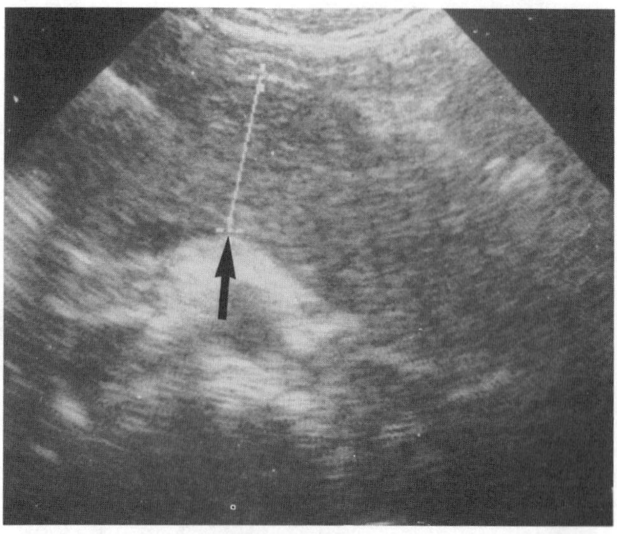

FIGURE 7 Acute pancreatitis. Transverse oblique sonogram shows a markedly enlarged body of the pancreas (*arrow*—between cursors). (Courtesy of Dr. D.A. Stringer.)

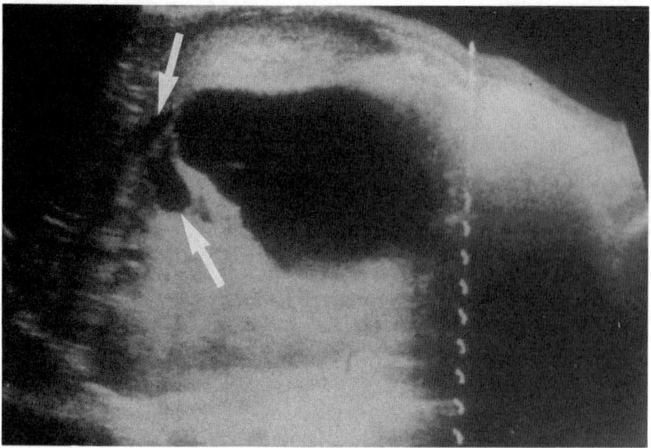

FIGURE 6 Large type I choledochal cyst. Longitudinal sonogram shows a large cyst extending into the porta hepatis separating the portions of the liver, with dilatation of the adjacent intrahepatic ducts (*arrows*).

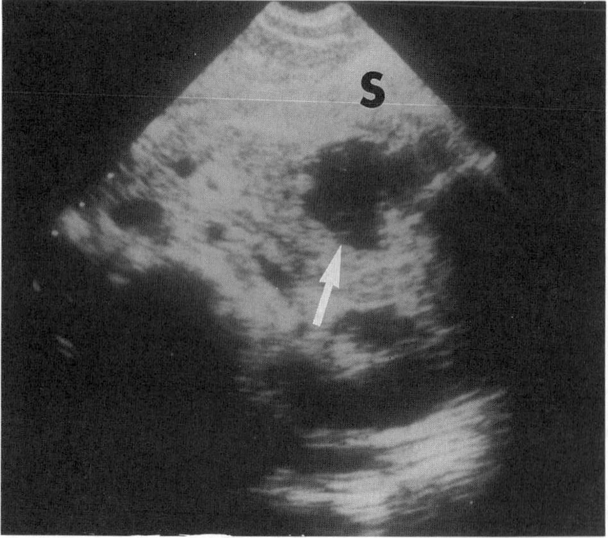

FIGURE 8 Pancreatic pseudocyst. Transverse sonogram shows a mainly cystic mass lying anterior to the tail of the pancreas (*arrow*) behind the stomach (S). (Courtesy of Dr. D.A. Stringer.)

Pancreatic pseudocysts can be readily demonstrated by sonography (Fig. 8). Percutaneous aspiration using sonographic (or CT) guidance is now considered a routine method of draining uncomplicated pseudocysts, and in our institution this approach is now used in preference to surgery.[55,104] Infected pseudocysts can also be drained by this approach.

Computed Tomography. Abdominal CT should be reserved for situations in which sonography is technically unsatisfactory or better anatomic definition is required. CT is particularly useful in the evaluation of abdominal trauma, because multiple organs can be visualized.[104] CT is also useful for identifying complications of pancreatitis such as pseudocysts (Fig. 9), pancreatic abscess, and duct enlargement. Nuclear magnetic resonance techniques show promise as an alterntive method of imaging the pancreas, but experience in childhood remains somewhat limited.[104]

Endoscopic Retrograde Cholangiopancreatography. ERCP is an invaluable diagnostic tool for the investigation of adults with pancreatic disease.[45,54] Increasing experience with this technique in children shows it to be a relatively safe and valuable diagnostic and therapeutic procedure in patients with pancreatic and biliary tract disease.[3,45–50] With the development of a smaller pediatric side-viewing endoscope, ERCP examination can be successfully performed in small children, and in the years ahead it is anticipated that ERCP will find increasing use in the pediatric patient. Since a large percentage of children with recurrent, acute pancreatitis are expected to have a congenital or acquired structural lesion of the pancreaticobiliary tree (Fig. 10), many of which are correctible, ERCP evaluation is strongly indicated in specific situations.[3,8,46] In our institution, ERCP is performed in patients with chronic pancreatitis and in those with recurrent acute pancreatitis following two or more attacks, provided that alternative causes have been eliminated.[3] General anesthesia may be necessary in small patients, but adolescents are usually studied under conscious sedation. Although relatively few pediatric cases have been reported, the risks appear to be the same as in adults. In adults, the principal morbidity is mild, self-limiting pancreatitis, which is estimated to occur in 1 to 3 percent of cases.[54] Mortality associated with the procedure ranges from 0.5 to 1.2 percent. In the largest series reported in children, mild pancreatitis occurred in 4 of 34 patients, but in all cases symptoms resolved with supportive therapy.[46] Therapeutic procedures such a sphincterotomy, stent placement, or balloon dilatation increase the risk of complications. Relative contraindications include unresolved acute pancreatitis, pancreatic pseudocysts, and abscess formation.

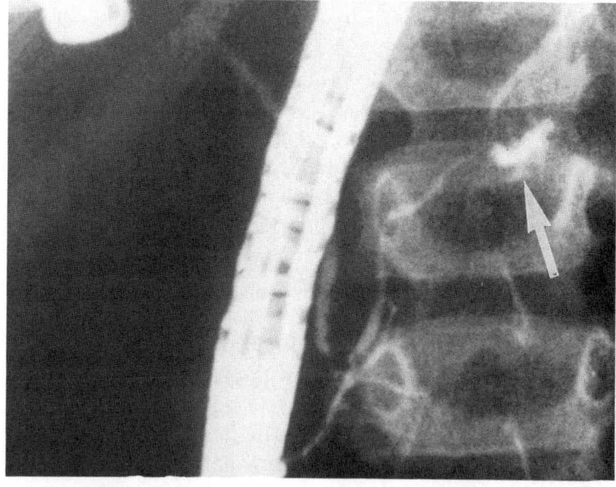

FIGURE 10 Pancreatic duct leak and pseudocyst. A 12-year-old patient developed traumatic pancreatitis. ERCP shows an attenuated, ruptured pancreatic duct and a leak of contrast overlying the L1-L2 disc space (*arrow*). The patient had the ERCP examination because a pancreatic cyst was persistent despite drainage procedures. (Courtesy of Dr. D.A. Stringer.)

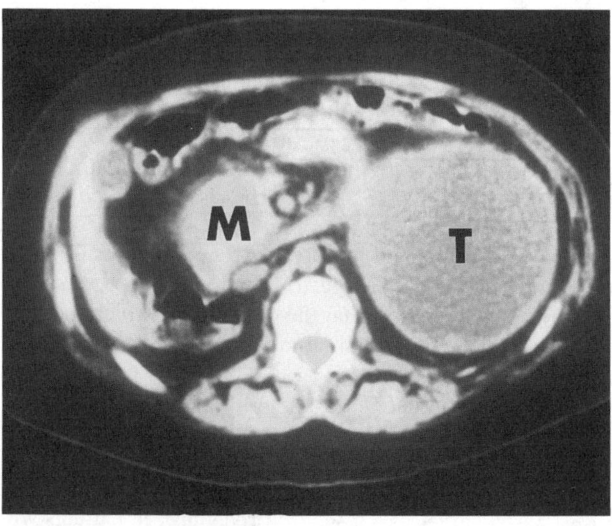

FIGURE 9 Pancreatic pseudocyst. CT scan demonstrates a mass (T) of low attenuation in the tail of the pancreas and a smaller low attenuation mass (M) in the head of the pancreas. The rest of the pancreas was seen on higher CT cuts. A large quantity of fat is present within the abdomen in this teenage girl who was receiving high-dose steroids for an extended period of time for her renal transplants. The fat obscured the pancreas on sonography. (Courtesy of Dr. D.A. Stringer.)

Clinical Course and Complications

There is considerable variation in the clinical course of acute pancreatitis.[1,3–11] The patient may have a mild illness, appearing only moderately ill with transient abdominal discomfort, or the course may be fulminating and rapidly progressive with the patient developing severe pain, renal failure, circulatory collapse, and a fatal outcome within hours or days. The histologic severity of pancreatic inflammation appears to correlate with the clinical course. Mild disease is usually seen in patients with interstitial edema of the pancreas, whereas patients with hemorrhagic and/or necrotic pancreatitis experience a fulminant, complicated, often fatal course. No accurate data exist regarding mortality in children. In adults, the overall mortality rate per attack is estimated to be approximately 9 percent, but in severe hemorrhagic pancreatitis the mortality is higher, ranging from 15 to 50 percent in large case reports.[1,24] Mortality is clearly influenced by the underlying cause of pancreatitis; whether the principal cause of death is a consequence of the underlying disorder or the result of local or systemic complications of pancreatitis is frequently difficult to determine. In our series, for example, 13 of 61 (21 percent) children with acute pancreatitis experienced a fatal outcome.[3] All fatalities occurred in patients with a severe multisystem disorder, but because each condition is associated with significant mortality in the absence of pancreatitis, it was often difficult to determine the precise cause of death. Reye's syndrome accounted for the majority of deaths, but fatalities were also seen in patients with hemolytic-uremic syndrome, sepsis, hypovolemic shock, and acetaminophen toxicity. In studies of adult patients, the predisposing condition or disease also appears to influence mortality. Patients with pancreatitis from biliary tract disease and alcoholism have a relatively low mortality rate (7 to 10 percent), whereas a higher mortality rate of 20 to 40 percent is seen in those with postoperative and traumatic pancreatitis.[1,24] Other factors influence prognosis. In adult patients, virtually all deaths occur during the first or second acute attack.[107] Clinical symptoms associated with a poor prognosis include the presence of shock, renal failure, and severe hypocalcemia; these secondary complications almost certainly occur as a result of severe hemorrhagic pancreatitis. Similarly, late complications, including hemorrhage or rupture of a pancreatic pseudocyst or development of pancreatic abscess, carry a high mortality rate.

Attempts have been made to develop clinically useful prognostic scores of disease severity in adults with acute pancreatitis by statistically analyzing early clinical features and biochemical measurements. Ranson performed multivariate analysis of 43 early objective measurements in patients with acute pancreatitis and identified 11 factors that provided important prognostic information.[108] Other investigators have developed modified systems, which appear to have some clinical utility.[109] A prognostic scoring system has not been developed for children, and most of those established for adults cannot be applied to the younger patient. For example, in the system developed by Ranson, prognostic features such as age (over 55 years) and volume of fluid sequestration are not applicable to children.[108] Because large numbers of patients are required for multivariate analysis of prognostic criteria, a useful scoring system is difficult to establish in the younger age group. However, certain clinical features of pancreatitis are clear indicators of severe disease, being frequent in patients with pancreatic hemorrhage or necrosis. These include disorders of body homeostasis, such as coma, hypotension, renal failure, pulmonary edema, shock, and hemorrhage. Similarly, laboratory indicators of severe disease include hyperglycemia, hypocalcemia, hypoxemia, hypoproteinemia, raised blood urea nitrogen, leukocytosis, and a drop in hematocrit. In adult studies, there appears to be a relationship between disease severity and the volume and color of peritoneal fluid obtained at early paracentesis; however, the potential hazards of paracentesis must be carefully considered before embarking on this approach.

Treatment

A variety of specific and nonspecific therapeutic approaches have been advocated for acute pancreatitis; some are based on considerations of the pathophysiology of pancreatitis, but most treat disease symptoms and complications.[110,111] In reality, most specific therapeutic interventions are of questionable or unproven benefit.[110] Based on current studies, no specific form of intervention has been proven to be efficacious in reducing the complication rate or improving mortality. One or more of these forms of therapy may prove to be beneficial, but existing studies have been inadequately designed or have failed to control for the multiple clinical variables of disease severity. The following specific and nonspecific treatment strategies have been proposed:

1. Removal of the initiating process
2. Halting the progression of the autodigestive process within the pancreas
3. Inhibition and/or removal of digestive enzymes and other toxic substances within the peritoneal cavity and/or circulation
4. Surgery
5. Treatment of local and systemic complications

Removal of the Initiating Process

Even if the initiating process is recognized or known, it may not be possible to modify or eliminate it. Frequently the autodigestive and inflammatory response within the pancreas is well advanced by the time the patient is seen. If the underlying cause is recognized, medical judgment will determine whether its elimination is possible. For example, if a primary metabolic cause such as hypercalcemia is present, immediate correction is mandatory.

Interruption of Autodigestion

Various nonspecific and specific clinical measures have been proposed to achieve this objective, but the therapeutic benefit of most conventional and unconventional strategies is either unproven or has been difficult to validate in clinical trials (Table 7). Current management of acute pancreatitis is based upon the concept that "putting the pancreas to rest" is beneficial,[110,111] because, in theory, it prevents or reduces pancreatic secretions, reduces the intensity of inflammation, decreases symptoms, and lowers the risk of complications. To achieve the goal of minimizing pancreatic secretions, patients are maintained in a fasting state, and gastric secretions are removed via nasogastric suction. This prevents acid and nutrients from reaching the duodenum, which theoretically minimizes hormonal stimulation of pancreatic secretions. A controlled trial to test the efficiency of nasogastric decompression in patients with mild to moderate alcoholic pancreatitis showed no therapeutic advantage, but no attempt was made to classify patients according to disease severity. At present, clinicians generally continue to fast patients and insert gastric tubes as a standard procedure; in patients with vomiting or paralytic ileus, little argument can be made against gastric decompression.

A variety of pharmacologic approaches designed to reduce pancreatic secretions have also been evaluated (Table 7). Unfortunately, most clinical studies have been inadequately designed and in almost every instance have failed to use strict criteria of disease severity to assess efficacy. None of the existing therapies is of proven benefit; some may even be harm-

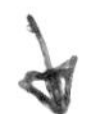

TABLE 7
Proposed Methods of Interrupting Autodigestion

Objective	Treatment(s)	Efficacy
Putting pancreas to rest	Nil per os	Questionable
	Nasogastric suction	Questionable
	Antacids	Questionable
	Histamine antagonists	Questionable
Inhibition/reduction of secretions	Anticholinergics	None
	Glucagon	None
	Somatostatin	None
	Vasopressin	None
	Hypothermia	None
	Calcitonin	None
Cell wall stabilizers	Prostaglandins	Questionable
Inhibition of proteases	Aprotinin	None
	Epsilon-aminocaproic acid	None
	Leupeptin	Animal studies only

ful. Nonspecific measures designed to reduce duodenal acidification (antacids or histamine antagonists) may be useful for the treatment or prevention of stress ulceration, particularly if GI bleeding is present. Other measures designed to reduce secretion of acid or reduce pancreatic flow, which include anticholinergics, glucagon, and vasopressin, are of unproven benefit. Similarly, drugs that in theory reduce cellular metabolism (propylthiouracil, 5-fluorouracil, or somatostatin) or those that stabilize cell membranes (prostaglandins) cannot be recommended on the basis of current knowledge of clinical efficacy.[1,24,110–112]

Inhibition or Removal of Pancreatic Enzymes

A variety of exogenous antiproteases have been tested experimentally in animal and human studies in an attempt to inhibit active pancreatic proteases within the circulation and in the peritoneal cavity. Aprotinin (Trasylol), a beef lung extract known to be a potent inhibitor of various proteases in vitro (trypsin, chymotrypsin, kallikrein, plasmin, and thrombin), has received considerable interest. Early animal studies of acute pancreatitis provided encouraging but conflicting reports of efficacy. Similarly, preliminary clinical studies created controversy regarding the effectiveness of aprotinin in reducing mortality or the complications of the acute phase of pancreatitis.[113] Subsequently, more carefully performed clinical trials demonstrated that aprotinin is of no value in the treatment of patients with acute pancreatitis.[114,115] Aprotinin inhibits alpha$_2$-macroglobulin–bound trypsin relatively slowly even at concentrations in excess of 100 M. In effect, the major form of circulating and peritoneal trypsin in acute pancreatitis, trypsin complexed to alpha$_2$-macroglobulin, is protected from aprotinin by the presence of alpha$_2$-macroglobulin.[31] In addition, aprotinin is unable to suppress the activity of other potentially destructive pancreatic proteases such as carboxypeptidase and elastase.

Other small molecular weight antiproteases have been evaluated in experimental and clinical studies. Epsilon-aminocaproic acid, which was used in earlier animal studies and clinical trials, has been abandoned because no obvious clinical benefit was observed.[110] Low molecular weight peptide-aldehyde inhibitors of bacterial origin (antipain, leupeptin) with a strong affinity for the active sites of a broad spectrum of pancreatic proteases rapidly inhibit the enzymatic activity of alpha$_2$-macroglobulin–bound trypsin in vitro and prolonged survival in rats with hemorrhagic pancreatitis.[116] Similarly, in a preliminary study, we were able to demonstrate that specific antiproteases (chloromethyl-ketone inhibitors) are capable of inhibiting circulating pancreatic enzyme–inhibitor complexes in a canine model of bile-induced pancreatitis.[33] FOY (gabexate mesilate), another low molecular weight protease inhibitor, capable of inhibiting enzyme-inhibitor complexes, has been quite extensively evaluated in clinical trials.[117] Preliminary studies show promising results, although double-blind trials and independent assessment of disease severity remain to be completed.

A number of investigators have suggested that peritoneal lavage might decrease morbidity and mortality in patients with severe pancreatitis.[11] In theory, patients would benefit by removal of proteolytic enzymes and other toxic agents released into the peritoneal cavity from the pancreas and surrounding tissues. Animal studies of peritoneal lavage suggest a positive effect on survival,[110] but none utilized delayed treatment after induction of acute pancreatitis. Clinical trials have, in general, been disappointing; many are uninterpretable, whereas others are unable to show a significant improvement in mortality or complication rate.

Surgery

Proposed indications for surgery in patients with acute pancreatitis include (1) uncertainty of the diagnosis of acute pancreatitis, (2) decompression of obstruction in the main pancreatic ducts or distal common bile duct (congenital or acquired), (3) correction of abdominal complications (e.g., cysts, abscesses), and (4) surgical measures to ameliorate the acute phase of the disease.

With the advent of improved imaging techniques in the diagnosis of acute abdominal conditions and its complications, the need for diagnostic laparotomy is waning. On occasion in children, however, the diagnosis of pancreatitis is still made at laparotomy, but in these cases the preoperative diagnosis is uncertain. In any event, diagnostic laparotomy is now hardly ever justified unless a treatable abdominal condition is strongly suspected.

Anatomic or structural lesions of the pancreas or hepatobiliary tree are sometimes anemable to surgical correction, but in the majority of instances surgery is performed electively once the precise cause has been identified and acute symptoms of pancreatitis have subsided. Emergency surgery

TABLE 8
Complications of Acute Pancreatitis

Complication	Mechanism(s)	Therapy
Systemic complications		
Hypocalcemia	↓Parathormone (degradation) Saponification	Intravenous calcium (magnesium)
Hyperglycemia	↓Insulin (degradation) Insulin resistance ↑Glucagon	Insulin Restrict glucose
Hyperlipidemia	Fat necrosis (lipase) Metabolic	Restrict intralipid and dietary fat Exclude primary cause
Acidosis	Cardiorespiratory failure Shock Renal failure	Fluids Cardiorespiratory support Intravenous bicarbonate Dialysis
Hyperkalemia	Acidosis Renal failure	Restrict potassium Glucose, insulin Correct acidosis Dialysis
Organ System Complications		
Circulatory failure	Fluid loss/sequestration Bleeding Pericarditis	Intravenous fluids Plasma expanders/blood Pressor agents
Renal failure	Hypovolemia/shock Vascular thrombosis DIC	Prevention of shock Dialysis
Respiratory failure	Diaphragmatic elevation Aspiration Pleural effusion DIC Adult respiratory distress	Nasogastric tube Oxygen Physiotherapy Drainage of effusion Mechanical ventilation
Gastrointestinal	Paralytic ileus Stress ulcers Hemorrhage	Nasogastric tube Histamine antagonists Blood transfusion
Hematologic	DIC Hemolysis Sepsis	Antibiotics Transfusions
Neurologic (psychosis or coma)	Metabolic Respiratory failure Shock Analgesics DIC	Controlled ventilation Correct metabolic derangement(s) Withdraw analgesics
Hepatobiliary	Bile duct obstruction Bile duct compression Primary liver disease Hepatic/portal vein thrombosis	Correct or relieve obstruction Treat varices Treat liver disease

DIC = disseminated intravascular coagulation.

may be required, however, such as operative removal of an impacted gallstone or for early (bowel perforation or hemorrhage) or late (abscess, infected pseudocyst) complications of acute pancreatitis.

Although experience is limited in childhood,[118] surgeons in adult practice have advocated the use of "therapeutic" surgery for severe necrotizing pancreatitis. The primary objective of surgical intervention is the early removal of necrotic tissue within and around the pancreas, which is intended to reduce complications and mortality by ameliorating the inflammatory process. Because of inadequate clinical or biochemical criteria for selecting patients at risk, there is considerable subjective opinion regarding the indications for surgical intervention. Advocates of this approach recommend early surgery when patients experience a fulminant course indicative of severe hemorrhagic pancreatitis. At present, however, the therapeutic advantages of surgery during an attack of acute pancreatitis remain uncertain. It should be emphasized, nevertheless, that proponents of this approach do not recommend surgery to treat patients with mild, uncomplicated pancreatitis.

Treatment of Local and Systemic Complications

In view of the apparent lack of efficacy of most specific forms of therapy of acute pancreatitis, current management consists of supportive care, together with anticipation and treatment of systemic and local complications as they arise (Table 8). Identification of the underlying cause, with a view to controlling the cause of inflammation and preventing recurring episodes, must remain a central treatment objective.

Supportive care of patients with acute pancreatitis comprises bed rest, close monitoring of vital signs, and adequate analgesia, together with restoration and maintenance of eletrolytes, acid-base balance, and intravascular volume. Chest radiographs, plain films of the abdomen, and an abdominal sonogram should be obtained when the patient is first assessed; abdominal sonography should be repeated every 3 to 4 days. In mild edematous pancreatitis, narcotic analgesia may be used if indicated, preferably meperidine given intravenously or intramuscularly every 3 to 4 hours. Meperidine induces less contraction of the sphincter of Oddi than does morphine. The fluid deficit must be assessed regularly by monitoring vital signs, urine output, skin turgor, hematocrit, and biochemical indices of renal function. A considerable proportion of the circulating plasma volume may become sequestered as peripancreatic exudate and abdominal ascites; additional fluid losses are likely from vomiting and nasogastric aspiration. Fluid losses must be adequately replaced, and abnormalities of acid-base balance and electrolytes should be corrected. With marked fluid losses, plasma expanders may be required. Continuous hemodynamic and arterial blood gas monitoring is not usually required in mild pancreatitis.

A severe attack of pancreatitis requires close monitoring in the intensive care unit, particularly when the patient is hypotensive, in shock, in renal failure, or showing neurologic impairment. Continuous monitoring of vascular hemodynamics and blood gases is usually necessary. If hypotension persists following adequate volume replacement (with plasma expanders), vascular pressor agents (dopamine or isoproterenol) may be required. In crucial situations, peritoneal lavage may be attempted despite uncertainty of efficacy. In our opinion, surgical intervention in an attempt to remove necrotic tissue or perform subtotal pancreatectomy carries considerable risk. Surgery should be reserved for patients with treatable primary causes or secondary complications of pancreatitis.

Additional supportive measures may be required to combat other secondary systemic and organ system complications (Table 8). Intravenous calcium replacement may be required to correct severe hypocalcemia; many of these patients have magnesium deficiency as well. Small doses of insulin are necessary for hyperglycemia. In adult patients with severe pancreatitis, respiratory insufficiency is quite common, although in our experience this complication is relatively infrequent in childhood. In the occasional patient it may be necessary to use anesthesia, endotracheal intubation, and controlled ventilation to maintain adequate respiratory control. Renal failure, considered to be a serious complication, usually presents with acute tubular necrosis due to hypovolemia and shock. Renal vein thrombosis occasionally occurs as a complication. In the presence of renal failure, fluid volume and electrolyte intake should be restricted, and acid-base and electrolyte balance requires careful monitoring and appropriate correction. Peritoneal dialysis or hemodialysis may be necessary. Encephalopathy or psychosis may occur in patients with severe hemorrhagic pancreatitis. Neurologic complication may be due to drugs, shock, hypoxemia, disseminated intravascular coagulation, or metabolic imbalance; in some cases cerebral edema has been noted.

In patients with a prolonged, complicated course, oral feeding may not be possible. Because nutritional deficits develop rapidly, particularly in the small child, total parenteral nutrition (with a central venous catheter) should be instituted early and should be continued until sufficient nutrient intake is possible via the oral route.

CHRONIC PANCREATITIS

Chronic pancreatitis is defined clinically as a condition characterized by recurring or persisting abdominal pain, with development of pancreatic exocrine or endocrine insufficiency in some patients.[2,15] Morphologically, the pancreas shows irregular sclerosis and focal, segmental, or diffuse destruction of exocrine tissue; frequently there are deformities of the pancreatic ducts as well as intraductal plugs containing protein and/or calculi (Fig. 11). These changes are considered to be irreversible and progressive, with the exception of "obstructive chronic pancreatitis," in which there may be partial or complete restitution if the obstruction is removed. Owing to the large reserve capacity of the exocrine pancreas, considerable deterioration of exocrine and endocrine pancreatic function is required before symptoms develop.[119] Therefore, loss of exocrine or endocrine function may be subclinical, and sensitive tests are needed to demonstrate dysfunction. Although recurring or unremitting pain is considered to be a hallmark of chronic pancreatitis, some patients experience no pain and may present clinically for the first time with symptoms of pancreatic failure and/or diabetes mellitus.

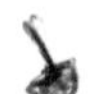

TABLE 9
Proposed Etiologies of Chronic Pancreatitis in Childhood

Calcific	Obstructive (Noncalcific)
Juvenile tropical pancreatitis	Trauma
Hereditary pancreatitis	Congenital anomalies
Hypercalcemia	Sphincter of Oddi dysfunction
Hyperlipidemia	Renal disease
Cystic fibrosis (pancreatic sufficiency)	Sclerosing cholangitis
Idiopathic	Idiopathic fibrosing pancreatitis

Etiology and Pathology

The precise causes of chronic pancreatic disease are frequently unknown.[2,120] Some well-recognized hereditary, congenital, and environmental factors are known to be causal, but as is the case in acute pancreatitis, the inducing mechanisms and the pathophysiologic causes of pancreatic damage are incompletely understood. Patients with acute and chronic pancreatitis frequently differ in etiology and in the pathogenetic mechanisms of pancreatic disease.

The two major morphologic forms of chronic pancreatitis, calcific and obstructive pancreatitis, are clearly different lesions,[15] and the known etiologies are often distinct (Fig. 11). Obstructive chronic pancreatitis, which is rare in childhood, occurs following occlusion of the main pancreatic duct or one of its major branches by a congenital anomaly, fibrosis, or a tumor. The ductal epithelium is relatively well preserved; protein precipitates are rare, and pancreatic calculi are not normally found. The pancreatic parenchyma is characterized by diffuse or focal infiltration and replacement by fibrous tissue. There have been isolated case reports of children who develop chronic fibrosing pancreatitis, and frequently these patients present with obstructive jaundice.[8,121,122] These patients appear to have chronic obstructive pancreatitis with pancreatic and biliary obstruction, presumably due to fibrotic narrowing at the head of the pancreas. Acute self-limiting pancreatitis usually follows pancreatic trauma, but on rare occasions healing may not be complete, producing focal chronic changes because of severe injury to the parenchyma, permanent disruption of a main pancreatic duct, obstruction from ductal strictures, or compression by pseudocysts. Congenital anomalies of the pancreaticobiliary tree are also believed to produce obstructive pancreatitis.

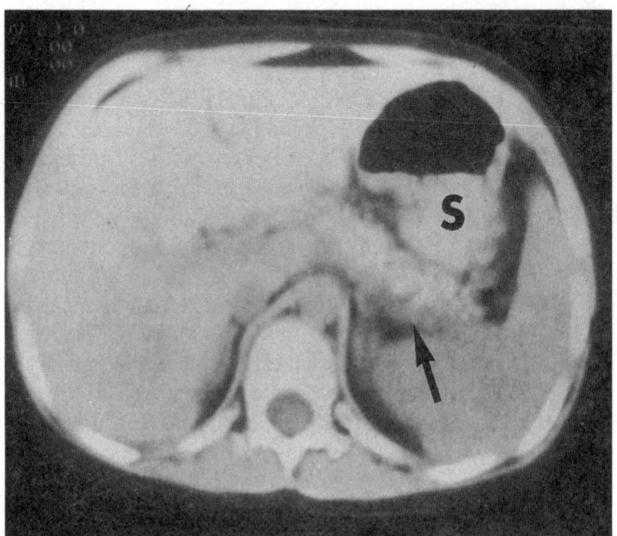

FIGURE 11 Pancreatic calcification. CT scan shows the tail of the pancreas behind the stomach (S) and anterior to the unopacifed splenic vein, which is full of high-attenuating calcium deposits (*arrow*). (Courtesy of Dr. D.A. Stringer.)

Calcific pancreatitis is also rare in childhood, but it is the most frequent form of chronic pancreatitis in adults, with an estimated frequency of 95 percent of adult cases. In calcific chronic pancreatitis, the pathologic lesions are similar and bear no relation to the apparent etiology. The distribution is generally patchy, with some pancreatic lobules showing complete destruction, whereas others appear completely normal. The duct lesions are often severe, with epithelial atrophy, scar formation, strictures, and retention cysts. The ducts contain protein plugs that evolve for years and later calcify.

In developed countries, adult-onset calcific pancreatitis is usually associated with chronic, excessive alcohol consumption,[2,120] whereas in developing countries, particularly those in tropical climates, the juvenile tropical pancreatitis syndrome is the most common cause of calcific pancreatitis.[13] In a small proportion of childhood cases of chronic calcific pancreatitis, other causes are implicated (Fig. 11). Metabolic disorders (hypercalcemia and hyperlipidemia), previously discussed as causes of acute pancreatitis, may also cause chronic pancreatitis. Also, pancreatic-sufficient CF patients on occasion show evidence of calcific pancreatitis.[62,65] Similarly, hereditary pancreatitis has been recognized as an important cause of chronic calcific pancreatitis in children and young adults.[12] In a considerable percentage of children with calcific pancreatitis, however, no cause is identified.

Pathogenesis

Sarles and co-investigators have pioneered many of the studies designed to evaluate the pathogenesis of the calcific lesions in chronic calcific pancreatitis.[123] They have suggested that the duct lesions arise as a result of protein- and calcium-containing plugs that form within the ducts and acini. Morphologic studies suggest that calculi originate after formation of protein plugs by the deposition of calcium bicarbonate in a network of protein fibrils. A low molecular weight phosphoprotein, pancreatic stone protein (PSP), purified and isolated in Sarles' laboratory, appears to be of central importance in the formation of the duct lesions.[124] PSP is abundant in zymogen granules and is secreted in large quantities in pancreatic secretions. Another protein, pancreatic thread protein (PTP), isolated by Gross et al,[125] was initially believed to be dissimilar to PSP in regard to physicochemical characteristics and amino acid composition, but subsequent studies suggest that the two proteins are identical.[126] In most calculi, calcium salts predominate, constituting 95 percent of total weight, but, in addition, there are small quantities of PSP/PTP.[123] The biochemical composition of these calculi appears to be the same in alcoholic pancreatitis, juvenile tropical pancreatitis, and "idiopathic" chronic pancreatitis. It has been suggested that PSP/PTP functions as a stabilizer of pancreatic juice by preventing calcium precipitation, since calcium is always present in saturated concentrations in pancreatic secretions. In vitro studies have shown that small quantities of PSP prevent precipitation of a supersaturated calcium chloride solution.[123] Similarly, PSP/PTP blocks crystallization after calcium precipitation commences by blocking the growth of crystals.

In chronic calcific pancreatitis, the initiating event could be reduced PSP/PTP secretion as a result of acinar damage, and once the concentration of PSP/PTP becomes sufficiently reduced, calcium calculi could form. However, this does not explain the observation of precipitated protein without calculus formation in many patients with chronic pancreatitis. Biochemical studies have shown that protein plugs within the pancreatic ducts contain high concentrations of PSP/PTP. Our studies of the precipitability of proteins in pancreatic secretions suggest that PSP/PTP is sparingly soluble in comparison with other pancreatic proteins.[126] We evaluated the relative precipitability of proteins in duodenal secretions from CF and non-CF subjects obtained during pancreatic stimulation with cholecystokinin and secretin, by concentrating them in stages by ultrafiltration. The only protein band regularly enriched in precipitates of CF and non-CF samples had a molecular weight similar to both PSP and PTP. Monoclonal antibodies directed against PSP and PTP reacted with this protein. Thus, our studies suggest that precipitability of PSP/PTP is clearly affected by concentration at neutral pH, and any abnormality of pancreatic function producing reduced fluid secretion or impaired ductal alkalinization may increase precipitation.[126] Loss through precipitation may provide an explanation for low concentration of PSP in pancreaticobiliary secretions of patients with chronic pancreatitis in comparison to those without pancreatic disease. In this regard, PSP/PTP may prove to be extremely important as a final common pathway in the pathogenesis of a wide variety of chronic calcific lesions of the pancreas, including alcoholic pancreatitis, juvenile tropical pancreatitis syndrome, CF, and hereditary pancreatitis.

Specific Entities Associated with Chronic Pancreatitis in Childhood

In one of the earliest descriptions of chronic pancreatitis in adults, Comfort and co-workers first recognized the association between excessive ethanol intake and chronic pancreatitis.[127] Subsequently, numerous epidemiologic studies have provided convincing evidence of the dominant role of alcohol intake in the pathogenesis of chronic calcific pancreatitis in adulthood.[2,120,123] In developed countries, there is a male predominance of affected individuals, and estimates of annual incidence range from 2 to 5 per 100,000 population. Several authoritative reviews are available on the subject.[2,120] Because alcohol abuse is not a factor in the etiology of childhood-onset chronic pancreatitis, it will not be discussed further in this text. Some of the more prevalent causes of chronic pancreatitis in childhood are discussed.

Hereditary Pancreatitis

Hereditary pancreatitis was first described by Comfort and Steinberg in 1952.[12] Since then, more than 200 patients have been described from a number of pedigrees in North America, Europe, and Japan.[8,12,128-135] Early studies raised doubts about the mode of inheritance, but subsequent reports have confirmed Comfort's original proposal—an autosomal dominant pattern of inheritance. The degree of penetrance appears to vary according to the pedigree studied. Despite accurate knowledge of inheritance, the pathophysiologic mechanisms of induction of pancreatic damage remain obscure, although precipitation of pancreatic proteins (PSP/PTP) within ducts or a primary defect of ductal fluid secretion may be responsible for the pancreatic pathology. Increased urinary excretion of certain amino acids (cysteine, lysine, arginine, and ornithine) has been reported in some kindreds.[134] Differentiation from other forms of chronic pancreatitis is usually not difficult owing to the early onset of symptoms, and the presence of multiple affected relatives.

Pathology. Most pathologic examinations have been carried out in patients with longstanding pancreatitis, and nonspecific changes of chronic calcific pancreatitis are seen that do not differ from other forms of chronic pancreatitis. Gross examination of autopsy specimens reveals a shrunken, fibrotic pancreas, frequently with small proteinaceous plugs and calculi within the pancreatic ducts. Light microscopy reveals extensive interstitial fibrosis, with nearly total acinar atrophy but relative preservation of normally appearing islets. The pathologic features of this disease are considered to resemble those seen in CF.

Clinical Features. Males and females appear to be affected equally. Symptoms usually begin at 10 to 12 years of age, and by 20 years of age up to 75 percent of patients are symptomatic. Symptoms can, however, begin in adulthood. Severe pain due to attacks of acute pancreatitis is the most common first symptom. Pain is frequently initiated by a large meal, alcohol, or stress. The character of the pain is no different from pancreatic pain of any other cause and is usually accompanied by nausea and vomiting. Spontaneous resolution of acute symptoms generally occurs over a period of 4 to 8 days. Severe hemorrhagic pancreatitis is rare, but if it occurs it is more likely during the first or second acute attack. Between episodes, patients are well but usually experience recurrent episodes of pain; symptoms of pain are variable in frequency and severity, ranging from weeks to years.

The physical findings during early attacks are typical of acute pancreatitis. As the disease progresses, symptoms and signs resemble those of chronic pancreatitis and laboratory tests are often normal. Sonography or CT may reveal a shrunken fibrosed pancreas; in patients with advanced disease calculi are common and the main pancreatic duct may be dilated. ERCP examination cannot differentiate hereditary pancreatitis from other forms of chronic pancreatitis. The main duct and its branches are dilated and deformed, and calculi are frequently observed. If surgery is contemplated, ERCP can provide useful information regarding the pancreatic ducts.

Treatment and Complications. Treatment of an acute attack is no different from treatment of other forms of acute pancreatic inflammation. As the disorder progresses, the pancreas is destroyed and the frequency and severity of attacks of abdominal pain are expected to decrease. Endoscopic sphincterotomy has been used in an attempt to relieve distal obstruction. A large percentage of patients undergo surgery in an effort to ameliorate pain. A variety of surgical procedures have been tried; choice of operation has depended upon the findings at ERCP. In the presence of dilated ducts a drainage procedure is usually attempted,[128] but subtotal pancreatectomy is performed when the ducts are small. Unfortunately, surgical intervention has not been particularly helpful for the relief of pain.

Diabetes mellitus is common, affecting 10 to 25 percent of patients with chronic pancreatitis. A high percentage of asymptomatic patients have an abnormal glucose tolerance test. Malabsorption due to exocrine pancreatic failure has been reported in 5 to 50 percent of patients; owing to the large functional reserve of the exocrine pancreas, pancreatic failure is a late complication that follows progressive destruction of the pancreas. Direct pancreatic function testing has been performed infrequently,[131] and in the patients studied, compromised ductular and acinar function was observed in symptomatic patients as well as in unaffected family members. Portal and splenic vein thromboses are infrequent secondary complications.[135]

One of the more significant associations of this hereditary condition has been the development of intra-abdominal carcinoma.[134] Among deceased patients of 21 kindreds, 18 percent had pancreatic adenocarcinoma, whereas other abdominal malignancies were present in 9 percent. Family members without chronic pancreatitis also have a higher incidence of pancreatic adenocarcinoma.

Metabolic Conditions

Some of the metabolic conditions previously discussed in association with acute pancreatitis can progress to chronic pancreatitis. These include CF (patients with pancreatic sufficiency), hypercalcemia, and certain hyperlipidemic conditions. Hyperlipidemic conditions appear to be more commonly associated with recurrent, acute pancreatitis, but chronic pancreatitis has been reported in type I and type V conditions.[57,58] Although CF was excluded from the Marseilles classification of pancreatitis, some patients clearly develop chronic calcific pancreatitis, with typical clinical symptoms and pathologic characteristics of intraductal plugging, calculi, and chronic inflammation.[62–65] However, the majority of patients with CF do not develop chronic pancreatitis, since they have pancreatic insufficiency at a very early age, owing to gland atrophy and fibrosis commencing in utero.[64] A single case of chronic pancreatitis in a patient with alpha$_1$-antitrypsin deficiency has been described, but the significance of this association remains unclear.[136]

Idiopathic Fibrosing Pancreatitis

Idiopathic fibrosis of the pancreas is a rare condition affecting both children and adults.[8,121,122] Only 16 cases have been reported in the literature. Extrinsic compression of the distal common bile duct by pancreatic fibrosis appears to be a consistent finding; many patients present with recurrent abdominal pain and biliary obstruction. Painless chronic pancreatitis has been described in adult patients and in a 3-year-old asymptomatic child with obstructive jaundice.[122] Percutaneous transhepatic cholangiography or ERCP shows extrinsic obstruction of the distal common bile duct, apparently due to fibrosis within the head of the pancreas. This observation is similar to that seen in some patients with CF.[137] Relief of common bile duct obstruction can be achieved surgically by choledochojejunostomy or endoscopic insertion of a biliary stent.

Other Causes of Chronic Pancreatitis

Sclerosing Cholangitis. Patients with sclerosing cholangitis (with or without inflammatory bowel disease) can present with concomitant chronic pancreatitis.[138] Most case reports are in adults, but this complication has been reported in children. The pathogenesis of chronic pancreatitis is unclear but may be due to obstruction in the common pancreaticobiliary channel.

Congenital Anomalies. The possible association between acute, recurrent pancreatitis and pancreas divisum has been discussed previously. Some surgical specimens with this common congenital anomaly show histologic changes consistent with chronic obstructive pancreatitis in the portion of the pancreas drained by the dorsal papilla. Chronic pancreatitis has also been reported as a complication of other congenital anomalies, including choledochal cyst, pancreatic ductal duplications, and sphincter of Oddi dysfunction.[2,8,118]

Trauma. Abdominal trauma usually causes self-limiting acute pancreatitis. Rarely, following severe damage to the pancreas, particularly with disruption of a major duct or compression from a pseudocyst, chronic pancreatitis may occur. Severe traumatic injury produces a focal fibrotic lesion in the damaged area, leaving the remainder of the gland entirely normal. Surgical correction may be necessary, with removal of the affected portion of the pancreas, but spontaneous resolution is likely in the majority of cases.

Renal Disease. In adults, the occasional patient with chronic renal failure has developed chronic pancreatitis.[73] Similarly, chronic pancreatitis has been observed following renal transplantation.[75] This complication may be secondary to a metabolic derangement of renal failure or to one of the drugs used for immunosuppression.

Idiopathic Chronic Pancreatitis. All known causes of chronic pancreatitis should be carefully excluded before a patient is relegated to the "idiopathic" category. In adults, idiopathic chronic pancreatitis is said to occur in 10 to 50 percent of patients, but high alcohol intake is common in the populations examined.[2,120] There are no precise data in childhood, although we estimate that idiopathic chronic pancreatitis accounts for approximately one-third of all cases.

Clinical Course

The clinical course of patients with chronic pancreatitis is much the same, regardless of etiology. Frequently, patients first present dramatically with episodes of acute pancreatitis. In adults, it is estimated that 50 percent present with symptoms of acute pancreatic inflammation,[2] but the exact incidence of children presenting with acute pancreatitis is not well defined. In other patients, acute episodes are absent, and pancreatic disease is characterized by an insidious, relentless form of pain which is continuous, intermittent, or variable in intensity. Since pain is either absent or negligible in a small percentage of patients, the diagnosis of chronic pancreatitis should always be considered in those who present with diabetes mellitus, malabsorption, or obstructive jaundice of undetermined cause. The age of onset, rate of disease progression, morbidity, and mortality vary according to the etiology and severity of the underlying pancreatic process.

Adult patients commonly demand narcotics for pain relief, particularly those with chronic pancreatitis secondary to ethanol abuse.[2] Narcotics in turn frequently aggravate the patients' difficulties because of addiction. In our experience, children with chronic pancreatitis not infrequently require narcotic analgesia for pain relief, and the risks of narcotic addiction must be carefully considered. Food intake may be limited, because eating frequently aggravates symptoms of pain. In most cases, the severity and frequency of pain improve with duration of the disease. In calcific pancreatitis, resolution of abdominal pain appears to correlate with the development of intrapancreatic calcification and exocrine-endocrine pancreatic failure, suggesting that symptomatic improvement coincides with end-stage "burn-out" of the gland.[2,120] Nevertheless, the time course is extremely variable, and some cases may take 10 to 20 years to progress to this point.

Patients with exocrine pancreatic failure have excessive appetites, since they compensate for maldigestive losses by eating more. It must be remembered that because of the large reserve capacity of the exocrine pancreas, symptoms of nutrient maldigestion do not become clinically manifest until 97 to 98 percent of the reserve capacity of the exocrine pancreas is lost.[119] Patients with malabsorption frequently experience abdominal discomfort and bulky, malodorous, greasy stools. Biochemical or clinical evidence of fat-soluble vitamin deficiencies and deficits of essential fatty acids may be apparent. Although carbohydrate malabsorption almost certainly occurs in severe pancreatic failure, clinical symptoms are uncommon, since salivary amylase secretion and intestinal brush border hydrolase activity are unimpaired. Malabsorption of ingested protein and fat is generally more severe. In the presence of pancreatic steatorrhea, there are increased fecal losses of bile salts, which reduces the total bile salt pool and increases bile lithogenicity. Patients with pancreatic failure usually have biochemical evidence of vitamin B_{12} malabsorption, but overt vitamin B_{12} deficiency hardly ever occurs. Reduced degradation of the cobalamin–R protein complexes by pancreatic proteases prevents cobalamin binding by intrinsic factor.

Early in the clinical course of chronic pancreatitis, insulin release is impaired following ingestion of carbohydrate, but the plasma glucose response is normal.[2] Eventually, with progressive pancreatic destruction, overt diabetes mellitus develops in a large percentage of patients. Severe diabetic ketoacidosis is uncommon. In adult-onset chronic pancreatitis, the systemic complications of diabetes mellitus, particularly the peripheral neuropathies and nephropathy, occur with a frequency similar to that in patients with other causes of diabetes mellitus.

Diagnosis

Chronic pancreatitis is relatively easy to diagnose when patients first present with florid symptoms of acute pancreatitis; this is usually followed by recurring attacks of pain. Those with painless disease and patients with milder symptoms, however, are more difficult to diagnose. Patients with pancreatic failure and untreated maldigestion exhibit growth failure, commonly having a weight deficit in relation to height. Some patients exhibit varying degrees of generalized malnutrition. Physical findings are usually nonspecific. Some localized tenderness may occur in the epigastrium, and very occasionally a vague epigastric mass may be palpable, suggestive of a pancreatic pseudocyst. Physical signs of fat-soluble vitamin deficiencies are usually absent, although night blindness may be apparent from longstanding vitamin A deficiency.

Laboratory Studies

Routine Tests. Routine urine and blood tests are usually normal unless the patient has diabetes mellitus.[1,120] There may be deficits of serum levels of carotene, fat-soluble vitamins, and essential fatty acids in patients with pancreatic failure. Clotting studies are usually normal. Liver function tests, particularly serum bilirubin, alkaline phosphatase, and other liver enzymes, may be elevated in the presence of concomitant liver disease; a persistent elevation in alkaline phosphatase with or without hyperbilirubinemia may suggest bile duct obstruction due to stenosis of the distal common duct or extrinsic fibrotic scarring of the head of the pancreas.

Serum Pancreatic Enzymes. Serum amylase, lipase, and protease concentrations are frequently normal even during attacks of chronic pain.[2,120] Patients experiencing attacks of acute pancreatitis and those with pancreatic pseudocysts or pancreatic ascites commonly show elevations of serum pancreatic enzymes. Patients with pancreatic insufficiency frequently have reduced serum concentrations of pancreatic enzymes (trypsinogen, lipase, and pancreatic isoamylase), and, in the absence of an alternative cause of pancreatic failure, these simple blood tests are useful tools for the diagnosis of severe pancreatic dysfunction due to chronic pancreatitis.[139] It must be emphasized, however, that serum enzyme concentrations are of no value in the detection of early or moderate chronic pancreatitis, since values are either normal or elevated.

Tests of Exocrine Pancreatic Dysfunction. The various direct and indirect pancreatic function tests are discussed in detail in the chapter devoted to pancreatic function testing. The choice of test will be determined by availability and the severity of pancreatic disease. For example, in the presence of radiologic evidence of pancreatic calcification and documented evidence of maldigestion, highly sophisticated, invasive tests of exocrine pancreatic function are seldom necessary. Alternatively, in a patient presenting with suspected chronic pancreatitis but no clinical evidence of pancreatic failure, indirect tests of exocrine pancreatic function frequently yield normal results. In these circumstances, a "direct" pancreatic function test involving duodenal intubation and aspiration of pancreatic secretions while stimulating of pancreatic flow would be invaluable.[119]

Imaging Techniques

For a detailed description of the imaging techniques (sonography and CT) currently used in the diagnosis, assessment, and treatment of patients with acute and chronic pancreatitis, the reader is referred to the preceding portion of this chapter on acute pancreatitis and also to the chapter devoted to gastrointestinal radiology.

Plain Films. Plain radiographs of the abdomen may reveal diffuse or focal pancreatic calcification. The presence of pancreatic calcification confirms the diagnosis of chronic pancreatitis with certainty, even in the absence of clinically apparent pancreatic disease (see Fig. 4). Bony abnormalities, such as medullary infarcts, and aseptic necrosis of the long bones of the arms and legs have been reported in a small percentage of adult patients with chronic pancreatitis. These lesions have been attributed to medullary fat necrosis following episodes of pancreatitis.

Barium Contrast Studies. These insensitive, nonspecific studies are no longer used for routine evaluation of chronic pancreatic disease. If they are performed, findings may suggest the possibility of chronic pancreatic disease, but confirmation will require more specific diagnostic imaging. On barium swallow, abnormalities include displacement of the stomach anteriorly by a pseudocyst, effacement and rigidity of the duodenum, and in some cases compression of the medial aspect of the duodenum by a cyst within the head of the pancreas. Barium enema examinations may show extrinsic narrowing and/or displacement of the midtransverse colon.

Angiography. With the advent of less invasive imaging techniques, angiography of the pancreas is rarely indicated in the routine evaluation and diagnosis of patients with suspected chronic pancreatitis. This is particularly true in childhood owing to the low incidence of malignancies of the pancreas.

Endoscopic Retrograde Cholangiopancreatography. ERCP has been extensively used in the diagnosis and management of adult patients with chronic pancreatic disease.[54] In recent years, following increasing use of this modality in younger patients, the relative indications for performing this procedure are better defined.[45-50] Alternative techniques, such as percutaneous transhepatic cholangiography, may provide superior information in cases with distal common duct obstruction.[121]

ERCP should be considered for (1) confirmation of the diagnosis of chronic pancreatitis, (2) identification of congenital or acquired anomalies of the pancreas or biliary tree, (3) preoperative assessment of surgically correctable lesions (strictures/cysts), and (4) sphincterotomy, stent placement, or stone removal.

In patients with early chronic calcific pancreatitis and occasionally in those with advanced disease, ductal changes may be minimal. With advanced calcific disease, however, the main pancreatic duct appears beaded, with areas of obstruction due to narrowing and intervening areas of dilatation. Ductal cysts, proteinaceous plugging calculi, or strictures may also be visualized. In a satisfactory examination, both the pancreatic and biliary channels should be visualized.

Local Complications

Pseudocysts

Pseudocysts usually arise within the pancreas and frequently communicate with the pancreatic duct; some extend well beyond the boundaries of the gland.[2] These collections of fluid are not encapsulated within epithelium-lined walls and contain a high concentration of pancreatic enzymes. True epithelium-lined pancreatic cysts are rare. Pancreatic pseudo cysts occur shortly after a severe attack of acute pancreatitis or develop insidiously with chronic pancreatitis. On occasion a pseudocyst is clinically palpable, but the majority require detection by sonography or CT. Pseudocysts occasionally produce pain, with localized abdominal tenderness in the upper abdomen or radiation to the back. A sensation of abdominal fullness may be present. Compression of the common bile duct by an adjoining pseudocyst may produce cholestasis. Subdiaphragmatic pseudocysts may cause local inflammation and fluid exudation into the pleural spaces or the mediastinal cavity. Rarely, a pseudocyst perforates through the diaphragm.

Serum pancreatric enzyme concentrations may be chronically elevated in patients with pancreatic pseudocysts, but the diagnosis can be reliably made only with the use of sonography or CT.[104-106] CT is useful for distinguishing pseudocysts from a pancreatic phlegmon. Distinction between pseudocysts and an abscess is frequently difficult, but patients with a pancreatic abscess usually exhibit signs and symptoms of sepsis.

Pancreatic pseudocysts frequently resolve with no management.[55] Those that remain for longer than 6 weeks are unlikely to resolve, and in most centers drainage is performed by either surgery or sonographic guidance. Studies in adults suggest that persistent pseudocysts are more likely to develop complications from rupture, hemorrhage, or infection.[2] No data for children support or negate this contention. Perforation of a pseudocyst into the free peritoneal cavity produces severe pain and abdominal rigidity owing to intense chemical peritonitis, which is often fatal. Emergency laparotomy should be performed with irrigation of the peritoneal cavity and drainage of the cyst. On occasion, pseudocysts erode and drain into an adjacent viscus, particularly into the colon or the stomach; few complications result and spontaneous resolution usually occurs. Erosion of small vessels lining a cyst may cause intracystic bleeding. Intracystic hemorrhage should be suspected with rapid enlargement of a previously diagnosed cyst; GI hemorrhage may result because cysts frequently drain into the duodenum via the pancreatic duct. Rarely, pseudocysts bleed directly into the peritoneum, the stomach, or the duodenum; the patient exsanguinates rapidly and emergency surgery is often required.

Infection of a pseudocyst is rare and to our knowledge has not been reported in childhood. Clinical presentation is striking, comprising shaking chills, high spiking fevers, severe pain, and a leukocytosis. The source of the organism may be the GI tract or contrast material injected during ERCP. Blood cultures may be positive, and on occasion sonography or CT of the abdomen may show pancreatic gas. Diagnostic fine needle aspiration of the cyst is recommended; large catheter drainage of infected cysts has been recommended, but surgical drainage remains the procedure of choice.

Distal Common Bile Duct Obstruction

In patients with chronic pancreatitis and cholestasis, the possibility of extrahepatic bile duct obstruction must be considered.[120,122] Following liver biopsy typical histologic findings of extrahepatic obstruction may also suggest this diagnosis. In childhood, diagnostic considerations include sclerosing cholangitis, idiopathic fibrosis of the pancreas, hereditary pancreatitis, and CF. A persistent obstruction should be relieved to prevent progressive hepatic damage, either by surgical means or by insertion of a biliary stent using ERCP or transhepatic approach. Biliary stents have been used in adult patients with considerable success, but experience in childhood remains limited.

Treatment

Treatment of uncomplicated chronic pancreatitis is usually medical. If a predisposing factor is identified, it may be modified or eliminated by medical or surgical intervention. Attacks of pancreatitis are usually more severe initially, but with disease duration symptoms become milder. Treatment should be conservative, with bowel rest and restriction of food and fluids by mouth. In the case of severe acute exacerbations, treatment should be directed as outlined in the discussion of acute pancreatitis.

Chronic Pain

Recurring, severe pain is the primary clinical manifestation of chronic pancreatitis. Pain may result in decreased food intake, weight loss, and, in children, growth failure. Nonnarcotic analgesics should be first attempted, but if they fail judicious use of narcotics should be contemplated; the risk of narcotic addiction is a major concern, and in the presence of severe pain, alternative medical or surgical treatments should be considered.

Medical measures such as a low-fat diet and abstinence from alcohol are frequently recommended, but there are no data to support their usefulness in relieving pain. A low-fat diet usually has the effect of restricting calories owing to its unpalatable nature and in children may result in growth failure. Recent reports suggest that regular administration of oral pancreatic enzyme supplements with meals helps to reduce the frequency and severity of pain in adults with chronic pancreatitis.[140] In animal studies, infusion of pancreatic proteases into the duodenum inhibits pancreatic secretions by preventing the release of cholecystokinin from the duodenum. Evidence of feedback inhibition of pancreatic secretions has also been observed in humans. In patients with chronic pancreatitis due to alcohol abuse, a significant reduction in the frequency and severity of pain with enzyme replacement therapy has been observed,[140] but other studies have been less convincing. A therapeutic trial of enzyme supplementation seems reasonable, however, before a surgical solution to alleviate the pain of chronic pancreatitis is considered. In the future, potent cholecystokinin receptor antagonists may prove beneficial.

Surgical intervention for the management of chronic pain is usually attempted in adult patients who fail medical management.[2,120] Because pain frequently remits spontaneously over a number of years, the decision to operate may be postponed, particularly when it is recognized that the outcome from surgery may not be beneficial. Prior knowledge of the pancreatic ductal anatomy by ERCP and/or CT is helpful in determining the choice of surgery. Various drainage procedures (Puestow, Du Val) are recommended if the intrapancreatic ducts are dilated. The Puestow technique is the most commonly used; the main pancreatic duct is opened longitudinally, and a longitudinally opened, defunctioned segment of jejunum is oversewn along the pancreatic duct, permitting drainage of pancreatic juice directly into the intestinal lumen. Experience in children is limited, but this technique is reported to afford relief of pain in 60 to 80 percent of adults with chronic pancreatitis. Sphincteroplasty is of value only in patients with localized obstruction within the spincter of Oddi. In the absence of intraductal dilatation, particularly when pancreatic resection may not relieve pain, and it may be necessary to remove up to 95 percent of the pancreas. Removal of a large portion of the pancreas carries the risk of diabetes mellitus and exocrine pancreatic failure. The Whipple procedure (pancreatoduodenectomy) is performed when obstruction in the head of the pancreas cannot be relieved. If pancreatic pathology is restricted to the tail of the pancreas, which generally occurs following traumatic duct rupture, resection of the affected portion produces excellent results.

Malabsorption

Impaired digestion of nutrients from pancreatic failure requires medical treatment. Before instituting therapy it is important to document the presence of pancreatic steatorrhea. Enzyme substitution with orally administered porcine pancreatic extracts helps to improve maldigestion, but complete correction of maldigestion is not readily achieved. The principles of enzyme replacement therapy and the attendant problems are discussed in the therapy section of the text.

Nutritional Support

Patients with pain from chronic pancreatitis often develop malnutrition and growth failure, since they frequently decrease nutrient intake because of abdominal pain. Patients who have pancreatic failure may be free of pain and frequently increase caloric intake in an attempt to compensate for fecal losses. In general, a high-energy diet, adequately supplemented with fat, is recommended to achieve normal growth. However, voluntary intake of nutrients may be inadequate for normal (or catch-up) growth, and nutritional supplements with an intact or partially digested commercial supplement may be needed. Total parenteral nutrition or enteral feeding (nasogastric or gastrostomy tube) may be used to nutritionally rehabilitate severely malnourished children with chronic pancreatitis. Additional fat-soluble vitamins are usually required.

Diabetes Mellitus

Patients who develop diabetes mellitus due to chronic pancreatitis usually have pancreatic exocrine failure as well. Control of the symptoms of diabetes is not easily achieved with dietary manipulations alone, and invariably growth failure results owing to reduced nutrient intake and increased fecal loss. In our experience, oral hypoglycemic agents are not effective. Most patients require daily injections of insulin, but insulin requirements are often low. Side effects, particularly the tendency toward hypoglycemia, are frequent because of deficient glucagon secretion. Severe diabetic ketoacidosis is a relatively uncommon complication in patients with diabetes mellitus due to chronic pancreatitis.

REFERENCES

1. Soergel KH. Acute pancreatitis. In: Sleisenger MH, Fordtran JS, eds. Gastrointestinal disease. 4th ed. Philadelphia: WB Saunders, 1989: 1814.
2. Grendell JH, Cello JP. Chronic pancreatitis. In: Sleisenger MH, Fordtran JS, eds. Gastrointestinal disease. 4th ed. Philadelphia: WB Saunders, 1989: 1842.
3. Weizman Z, Durie PR. Acute pancreatitis in childhood. J Pediatr 1988; 113:24–29.
4. Hendren WH, Greep JM, Patton AS. Pancreatitis in childhood: experience with 15 cases. Arch Dis Child 1965; 40:132–145.
5. Sibert JR. Pancreatitis in children: a study in the north of England. Arch Dis Child 1975; 50:443–448.
6. Jordan SC, Ament ME. Pancreatitis in children and adolescents. J Pediatr 1977; 91:211–216.
7. Buntain WL, Wood JB, Woolley MM. Pancreatitis in childhood. J Pediatr Surg 1978; 13:143–149.
8. Ghishan FH, Greene HL, Avant G, et al. Chronic relapsing pancreatitis in childhood. J Pediatr 1983; 102:514–518.
9. Tam PKH, Saing H, Irving IM, Lister J. Acute pancreatitis in children. J Pediatr Surg 1985; 20:58–60.
10. Ziegler DW, Long JA, Philippart AI, Klein MD. Pancreatitis in childhood. Experience with 49 patients. Ann Surg 1988; 207:257–261.
11. Nguyen T, Abramowsky C, Ashenburg C, Rothstein F. Clinicopathologic studies in childhood pancreatitis. Hum Pathol 1988; 19:343–349.
12. Comfort MW, Steinberg AG. Pedigree of a family with hereditary chronic relapsing pancreatitis. Gastroenterology 1952; 21:54–63.
13. Pitchumoni CS. Special problems in tropical pancreatitis. Clin Gastroenterol 1984; 13:941–959.
14. Sarles H, ed. "Pancreatitis" Symposium, Marseille, 1963. Basel: S Karger, 1965.
15. Gyr KE, Singer MV, Sarles H, eds. Pancreatitis. Concepts and classification. Amsterdam: Excerpta Medica, 1984.
16. Geokas MC. Acute pancreatitis. Ann Intern Med 1985; 103:86–100.
17. Rinderknecht H. Activation of pancreatic zymogens. Normal activation, premature activation, protective mechanisms against inappropriate activation. Dig Dis Sci 1986; 31:314–321.
18. Steer ML. Search for the trigger mechanism of pancreatitis. Gastroenterology 1984; 86:764–766.
19. Schiller WR, Suriyapa C, Anderson MC. A review of experimental pancreatitis. J Surg Res 1974; 16:69–90.
20. Lombardi B, Estes LW, Longnecker DS. Acute hemorrhagic pancreatitis with fat necrosis induced in mice by dl-ethionine fed with a choline deficient diet. Am J Pathol 1975; 79:465–476.
21. Lampel M, Kern HF. Acute interstitial pancreatitis in the rat induced by excessive doses of a secretagogue. Virchows Arch [A] 1977; 373:97–117.
22. Feinstein G, Hofstein G, Koifman J, Sokolovsky M. Human pancreatic proteolytic enzymes and protease inhibitors. Am J Biochem 1974; 84:574–583.
23. Lasson A, Ohlsson H. Protease inhibitors in human pancreatitis. Correlation between biochemical changes and clinical course. Scand J Gastroenterol 1984; 19:202–215.
24. Durr HK. Acute pancreatitis. In: Howat HT, Sarles H, eds. The exocrine pancreas. London: WB Saunders, 1969: 352.
25. Largman C, Brodrick JW, Geokas MC. Radioimmunoassay determination of circulating pancreatic endopeptidases. Methods Enzymol 1981; 74:272–290.
26. Geokas MC, Largman C, Brodrick JW, Johnson JH. Determination of pancreatic cationic trypsin in serum by radioimmunoassay. Am J Physiol 1979; 236:E77–83.
27. Geokas MC, Wollessen S, Rinderknecht H. Radioimmunoassay for pancreatic carboxypeptidase B in human serum. J Lab Clin Med 1974; 84:574–583.
28. Largman C, Brodrick JW, Geokas MC. Purification and characterization of two human pancreatic elastases. Biochemistry 1976; 15:2491–2500.
29. Brodrick JW, Geokas MC, Largman C, et al. Molecular forms of immunoreactive pancreatic cationic trypsin in pancreatitis patient sera. Am J Physiol 1979; 237:E474–480.
30. Borgstrom A, Ohlsson K. Immunoreactive trypsin in serum and peritoneal fluid in acute pancreatitis. Hoppe Seylers Z Physiol Chem 1978; 359:677–681.
31. Durie PR, Gaskin KJ, Ogilvie JE, Smith CR, Forstner GG, Largman C. Serial alterations in the forms of immunoreactive pancreatic cationic trypsin in plasma from patients with acute pancreatitis. J Pediatr Gastroenterol Nutr 1985; 4:199–207.
32. Delk AS, Durie P, Fletcher TS, Largman C. Radioimmunoassay of active pancreatic enzymes in sera from patients with acute pancreatitis. Detection of active carboxypeptidase B. Clin Chem 1985; 31:1294–1300.
33. Geokas MC, Largman C, Durie P, Brodrick JW, Ray SB. Immunoreactive forms of cationic trypsin in plasma and ascites of dogs following experimental pancreatitis. Am J Pathol 1981; 105:31–39.
34. Largman C, Reidelberger RD, Tsukamoto H. Correlation of trypsin-plasma inhibitor complexes with mortality in experimental pancreatitis in rats. Dig Dis Sci 1986; 31:961–969.
35. McMahon MJ, Bowen M, Mayer AD, Cooper EH. Relationship of α_2-macroglobulin and other antiproteases to the clinical features of acute pancreatitis. Am J Surg 1984; 147:164–169.
36. Adham NF, Song MK, Haberfelde GC. Relationship between the functional status of the reticuloendothelial system and the outcome of experimentally induced pancreatitis in young mice. Gastroenterology 1983; 84:461–469.
37. Largman C, Johnson JH, Brodrick JW, Geokas MC. Proinsulin conversion to desalanyl insulin by α_2-macroglobulin bound trypsin. Nature 1977; 269:168–170.
38. Brodrick JW, Largman C, Geokas MC, Ray SB. Proteolysis of parathyroid hormone in vitro by sera from acute pancreatitis patients. Proc Soc Exp Biol Med 1981; 167:588–594.
39. Harpel PC, Mosesson MW. Degradation of human fibrinogen by plasma α_2-macroglobulin-enzyme complexes. J Clin Invest 1973; 52:2175–2184.
40. Hermon-Taylor J, Magee AI, Grant DAW, et al. Cleavage of peptide hormones by α_2-macroglobulin-trypsin complex and its relation to the pathogenesis and chemotherapy of acute pancreatitis. Clin Chim Acta 1981; 109:203–209.
41. Lasson A, Ohlsson K. An in vitro study of the influence of plasma protease inhibitors and protein in trypsin-induced C3 cleavage in human serum. Biochim Biophys Acta 1982; 709:227–233.
42. Anderson MC, Mehn WH, Methad HL. An evaluation of the common channel as a factor in pancreatic or biliary disease. Ann Surg 1960; 151:379–392.
43. Howard MJ. Gallstone pancreatitis. In: Howard JM, Jordan GL, Reber HA, eds. Surgical diseases of the pancreas. Philadelphia: Lea & Febiger, 1987: 269.
44. Geenen JE, Hogan WJ, Dodds WJ, Stewart ET, Andorffer RC. Intraluminal pressure recording from the human sphincter of Oddi. Gastroenterology 1980; 78:317–324.

45. Venu RP, Geenen JE, Hogan WJ, Stewart ET, Dodds WJ, Johnson GK. Idiopathic recurrent pancreatitis: diagnostic role of ERCP and sphincter of Oddi manometry. Gastrointest Endosc 1985; 31:141–152.
46. Allendorph M, Werlin SL, Geenen JE, Hogan WJ, Venu RP, Stewart ET, Blank EL. Endoscopic retrograde cholangiography in children. J Pediatr 1987; 110:206–211.
47. Blustein PK, Gaskin K, Filler R, Ho C, Connon J. Endoscopic retrograde cholangiopancreatography in pancreatitis in children and adolescents. Pediatrics 1981; 68:387–393.
48. Cotton PB, Laage NJ. ERCP in children. Arch Dis Child 1982; 57:131–136.
49. Yedlin ST, Dubois RS, Philippart AI. Pancreas divisum: a cause of pancreatitis in childhood. J Pediatr Surg 1984; 19:793–794.
50. Forbes A, Leung JWC, Cotton PB. Relapsing acute and chronic pancreatitis. Arch Dis Child 1984; 59;927–934.
51. Cotton PB. Pancreas divisum—curiosity or culprit. (Editorial) Gastroenterology 1985; 89:1431–1433.
52. Lotveit T, Aune S, Johnsrud NK, Osnes M. The clinical significance of juxta-papillary duodenal diverticulae. Scand J Gastroenterol 1975; 10(suppl 34):22–26.
53. Das S. Pancreatitis in children associated with round worms. Indian Pediatr 1977; 14:81–83.
54. Cotton PB. Progress report ERCP. Gut 1977; 18:316–341.
55. Gorenstein A, O'Halpin D, Wesson DE, Daneman A, Filler RM. Blunt injury to the pancreas in children. Selective management based on ultrasound. J Pediatr Surg 1987; 22:1110–1116.
56. Corfield AP, Cooper MJ, Williamson RCN. Acute pancreatitis: a lethal disease of increasing incidence. Gut 1985; 26:724–729.
57. Braunsteiner H. Akute pankreatitis und hyperlipamie. Dtsch Med Wochenschr 1968; 93:492–493.
58. Cameron JL, Capuzzi DM, Zuidema GD, Margolis S. Acute pancreatitis with hyperlipemia. Evidence of a persistent defect in lipid metabolism. Am J Med 1974; 56:482–489.
59. Bess MA, Edis AJ, Van Heerden HA. Hyperparathyroidism and pancreatitis. Chance or causal association? JAMA 1980; 243:246–254.
60. Gafter U, Mandel EM, Har-Zahav L, Weiss S. Acute pancreatitis secondary to hypercalcemia. Occurrence in a patient with breast carcinoma. JAMA 1976; 235:2004–2005.
61. Hochgelernt EL, David DS. Acute pancreatitis secondary to calcium infusion in a dialysis patient. Arch Surg 1974; 108:218–220.
62. Shwachman H, Lebenthal E, Khaw K-T. Recurrent acute pancreatitis in patients with cystic fibrosis with normal pancreatic enzymes. Pediatrics 1975; 55:86–95.
63. Kopelman H, Durie P, Gaskin K, Weizman Z, Forstner G. Pancreatic fluid secretion and protein hyperconcentration in cystic fibrosis. N Engl J Med 1985; 312:329–334.
64. Durie PR, Forstner GG. Pathophysiology of the exocrine pancreas in cystic fibrosis. J R Soc Med 1989; 18(suppl 16):2–10.
65. Liu P, Daneman A, Stringer DA, Durie P. Large pancreatic cysts and pancreatic calcification in cystic fibrosis. J Can Assoc Radiol 1986; 37:279–282.
66. Pitchumoni CS. Pancreas in primary malnutrition disorders. Am J Clin Nutr 1973; 26:374–383.
67. Durie PR, Forstner GG, Gaskin KJ, Weizman Z, Kopelman HR, Ellis E, Largman C. Elevated serum immunoreactive cationic trypsinogen in acute malnutrition: evidence of pancreatic damage. J Pediatr 1985; 106:233–238.
68. Gryboski J, Hillemeier C, Kocoskis S, Anyan W, Seashore JS. Refeeding pancreatitis in malnourished children. J Pediatr 1980; 97:441–443.
69. Rampling D. Acute pancreatitis in anorexia nervosa. Med J Aust 1982; 2:194–195.
70. Nakashima Y, Howard JM. Drug-induced pancreatitis. Surg Gynecol Obstet 1977; 144:71–76.
71. Mallory A, Kern F. Drug-induced pancreatitis: a critical review. Gastroenterology 1980; 78:813–821.
72. Bartholomew C. Acute scorpion pancreatitis in Trinidad. Br Med J 1970; 1:666–667.
73. Robinson DO, Alp MH, Kerr-Grant A, Lawrence JR. Pancreatitis and renal disease. Scand J Gastroenterol 1977; 12:17–20.
74. Geokas MC, Reidelberger R, O'Rourke M, et al. The role of the kidney in plasma clearance of pancreatic trypsinogens. Am J Physiol 1982; 242:G177–182.
75. Corrodi P, Knoblauch M, Binswanger U, Scholzel E, Largiader F. Pancreatitis after renal transplantation. Gut 1975; 285:16–19.
76. Imrie CW, Whyte AS. A prospective study of acute pancreatitis. Br J Surg 1975; 62:490–494.
77. Schindler AM, Kowlessaar M. Prolonged abdominal pain in a diabetic child. Hosp Pract 1988; 134–136.
78. Mardh P-A, Ursing B. The occurrence of acute pancreatitis in *Mycoplasma pneumoniae* infection. Scand J Infect Dis 1974; 6:67–171.
79. Karmali MA, Petric M, Lim C, Fleming PC, Arbus GS, Lior H. The association between idiopathic hemolytic uremic syndrome and infection by verotoxin producing *Escherichia coli*. J Infect Dis 1985; 151:775–782.
80. Naficy K, Nategh R, Ghadimi H. Mumps pancreatitis without parotitis. Br Med J 1973; 1:529–530.
81. Ellis GH, Mirkin LD, Mills MC. Pancreatitis and Reye's syndrome. Am J Dis Child 1979; 113:1014–1016.
82. Reye RDK, Morgan G, Baral J. Encephalopathy and fatty degeneration of the viscera: a disease entity of childhood. Lancet 1963; ii:749–752.
83. Rumessen JJ, Marner B, Thorsgaard N, Permin H. Autoantibodies in chronic pancreatitis. Scand J Gastroenterol 1985; 20:966–970.
84. Forbes D, Scott RB, Trevenen C, Hershfield N, Gall DG. Chronic pancreatitis associated with ulcerative colitis. Clin Invest Med 1987; 10:321–324.
85. Geokas MC, Rinderknecht H, Walberg C, Weissman R. Methemalbumin in the diagnosis of acute hemorrhagic pancreatitis. Ann Intern Med 1974; 81:483–486.
86. Moosa AR. Diagnostic tests and procedures in acute pancreatitis. N Engl J Med 1984; 311:639–643.
87. Salt WB, Schenker A. Amylase—its clinical significance: a review of the literature. Medicine 1976; 55:269–289.
88. Johnson SG, Ellis CJ, Levitt MD. Mechanisms of increased renal clearance of amylase: creatinine in acute pancreatitis. N Engl J Med 1976; 295:1214–1217.
89. Spechler SJ, Dalton JW, Robbins AH, et al. Prevalence of normal serum amylase levels in patients with acute alcoholic pancreatitis. Dig Dis Sci 1983; 28:865–869.
90. Cox KL, Ament ME, Sample WF, et al. The ultrasonic and biochemical diagnosis of acute pancreatitis. J Pediatr 1980; 96:407–411.
91. Barrows D, Berk EJ, Fridhandler L. Macroamylasemia—survey of prevalence in mixed populations. N Engl J Med 1972; 286:1352–1353.
92. Levitt MD, Rapoport M, Cooperbrand SR. The renal clearance of amylase in renal insufficiency, acute pancreatitis and macroamylasemia. Ann Intern Med 1969; 71:919–925.
93. Levin RJ, Galuser FL, Berk JE. Enhancement of the amylase: creatinine clearance ratio in disorders other than acute pancreatitis. N Engl J Med 1975; 292:329–332.
94. Massey RM. Efficiency in the diagnosis of acute pancreatitis by improved electrophoresis of amylase isoenzyme P_3 on cellulose acetate. Clin Chem 1985; 31:70–75.
95. Steinberg WM, Goldstein SS, Davis ND, Shamma'a J, Anderson K. Diagnostic assays of acute pancreatitis. Ann Intern Med 1985; 102:576–580.
96. Rosenblum JL. Direct, rapid assay of pancreatic isoamylase activity by use of monoclonal antibodies with low affinity for macroamylase complexes. Clin Chem 1988; 34:2463–2468.
97. Gerstein M, Bank S, Lendrai S. Failure of inhibitor assay to determine isoamylase distribution. Dig Dis Sci 1983; 28:990–992.
98. Brockerhoff H, Jensen RG, eds. Lipolytic enzymes. New York: Academic Press, 1974.
99. Jensen RG, Dejong FA, Clark RM. Determination of lipase specificity. Lipids 1983; 18:239–252.
100. Desnuelle P, Figarella C. Biochemistry. In: Howart HT, Sarles H, eds. The exocrine pancreas. Philadelphia: WB Saunders, 1979: 86.
101. Grenner G, Deutsch G, Schmidtberger R, et al. A highly sensitive enzyme immunoassay for the determination of pancreatic lipase. J Clin Chem Clin Biochem 1982; 20:515–519.
102. Elias E, Redshaw M, Wood T. Diagnostic importance of changes in circulating concentrations of immunoreactive trypsin. Lancet 1977; ii:66–68.
103. Warshaw AL, Lee KH. Serum ribonuclease elevations and pancreatic necrosis in acute pancreatitis. Surgery 1979; 86:227–234.
104. Stringer DA. Pediatric gastrointestinal radiology. Toronto: BC Decker, 1989.
105. Fleischer AC, Parker P, Kirchner SG, James AF. Sonographic findings of pancreatitis in children. Radiology 1983; 146:151–155.
106. Coleman BG, Arger P, Rosenberg HK, Muthern CB, Ortega W, Stauffer D. Gray-scale sonographic assessment of pancreatitis in children. Radi-

ology 1983; 146:145-150.
107. Bank S, Wise L, Gersten J. Risk factors in acute pancreatitis. Am J Gastroenterol 1983; 78:637-642.
108. Ranson JHS, Pasternak BS. Statistical methods for quantifying the severity of acute pancreatitis. J Surg Res 1977; 22:79-91.
109. McMahon MJ, Playforth MJ, Pickford JR. A comparative study of methods for prediction of the severity of attacks of acute pancreatitis. Br J Surg 1980; 67:22-25.
110. Steinberg WH, Schlesselman SE. Treatment of acute pancreatitis. Comparison of animal and human studies. Gastroenterology 1987; 93:1420-1427.
111. Lasson A. Acute pancreatitis in man—a clinical and biochemical study of pathophysiology and treatment. Scand J Gastroenterol 1984; 19(suppl 99).
112. Standfield NJ, Kakkar VV. Prostaglandins and acute pancreatitis—experimental and clinical studies. Br J Surg 1983; 70:573-576.
113. Skyring A, Singer A, Tornya P. Treatment of acute pancreatitis with Trasylol: report of a controlled therapeutic trial. Br Med J 1967; 2:627-629.
114. Imrie CW, Benjamin IS, Ferguson JC, et al. A single centre double blind trial of Trasylol therapy in primary acute pancreatitis. Br J Surg 1978; 65:337-341.
115. MRC Multicentre Trial. Morbidity of acute pancreatitis: the effect of aprotinin and glucagon. Gut 1980; 21:334-339.
116. Jones PA, Hermon-Taylor J, Grant DAW. Antiproteinase chemotherapy of acute experimental pancreatitis using the low molecular weight aldehyde leupeptin. Gut 1982; 23:939-943.
117. Tanaka K, Tsuchiya R, Ishii I. Comparative clinical study of FOY and Trasylol in acute pancreatitis. In: Fujii S, Moriya H, Suzaki T, eds. Kinins II. New York: Plenum, 1979: 367.
118. Synn AY, Mulvihill SJ, Fonkalsrud EW. Surgical management of pancreatitis in childhood. J Pediatr Surg 1987; 22:628-632.
119. Gaskin KJ, Durie P, Lee L, Hill R, Forstner GG. Colipase and lipase secretion in childhood onset pancreatic insufficiency. Gastroenterology 1984; 86:1-7.
120. Sarles H, Sahel J, Staub JL, Bourry J, Laugier R. Chronic pancreatitis. In: Howart HT, Sarles H, eds. The exocrine pancreas. London: WB Saunders, 1969: 402.
121. Meneely RL, O'Neill J, Ghishan F. Fibrosing pancreatitis—an obscure cause of painless obstructive jaundice: a case report and review of the literature. Pediatrics 1981; 67:136-139.
122. Atkinson GO, Wyly JB, Gay BB, Ball TI, Winn KJ. Idiopathic fibrosing pancreatitis: a cause of obstructive jaundice in childhood. Pediatr Radiol 1988; 18:28-31.
123. Sarles H, Bernard JP. Pathogenesis of chronic pancreatitis. Can J Gastroenterol 1989; 3:15-20.
124. Multigner L, De Caro A, Lombardo D, Campese D, Sarles H. Pancreatic stone protein. A phosphoprotein which inhibits calcium carbonate precipitation from human pancreatic juice. Biochem Biophys Res Commun 1983; 110:69-74.
125. Gross J, Carlson RI, Brauer AW, Margolies MN, Warshaw AL, Wands JR. Isolation, characterization and distribution of an unusual pancreatic human secretory protein. J Clin Invest 1985; 76:2115-2126.
126. Forstner GG, Vesely SM, Durie PR. Selective precipitation of 14 kDa stone/thread proteins by concentration of pancreaticobiliary secretions: relevance to pancreatic ductal obstruction, pancreatic failure and CF. J Pediatr Gastroenterol Nutr 1989; 8:313-320.
127. Comfort MS, Gambill EE, Baggenstoss AH. Chronic relapsing pancreatitis: a study of 29 cases without associated disease of the biliary or gastrointestinal tract. Gastroenterology 1946; 6:239-285.
128. Perrault J, Gross JB, King JE. Endoscopic retrograde cholangiopancreatography in familial pancreatitis. Gastroenterology 1976; 71:138-144.
129. Appel MF. Hereditary pancreatitis. Arch Surg 1974; 108:63-65.
130. Lilja P, Evander A, Ihse I. Hereditary pancreatitis—a report of two kindreds. Acta Chir Scand 1978; 144:144-150.
131. Kattwinkel J, Lapey A, di Sant'Agnese PA, Edwards WA, Hufty MP. Hereditary pancreatitis: three new kindreds and a critical review of the literature. Pediatrics 1973; 51:55-69.
132. Fried AM, Selke AC. Pseudocyst formation in the hereditary pancreatitis. J Pediatr 1978; 93:950-953.
133. Rothstein FC, Wylie R, Gauderer MEL. Hereditary pancreatitis and recurrent abdominal pain of childhood. J Pediatr Surg 1985; 20:535-537.
134. Ricardi VM, Shih VE, Holmes LB, Nardi GL. Hereditary pancreatitis. Non-specificity of aminoaciduria and diagnosis of occult disease. Arch Intern Med 1975; 135:822-825.
135. McElroy R, Christiansen PA. Hereditary pancreatitis in a kinship associated with portal vein thrombosis. Am J Med 1972; 52:228-241.
136. Mihas AA, Hirschowitz BI. Alpha-l-antitrypsin and chronic pancreatitis. Lancet 1976; ii:1032-1033.
137. Gaskin KJ, Waters DLM, Howman-Giles R, deSilva M, Earl JW, Martin HCO, Kan AE, Brown JM, Dorney SFA. Liver disease and common bile duct obstruction in cystic fibrosis. N Engl J Med 1988; 318:340-346.
138. Borkje B, Vetrik K, Odegaard S, Schrumpf E, Larssen TB, Kolmannskog F. Chronic pancreatitis in patients with sclerosing cholangitis and ulcerative colitis. Scand J Gastroenterol 1985; 20:539-542.
139. Moore DJ, Forstner GG, Cleghorn GJ, Wong SS, Largman C, Durie P. Serum cationic trypsinogen—a useful indicator of pancreatic dysfunction in the pediatric patient without cystic fibrosis. Gut 1986; 27:1362-1368.
140. Slaff J, Jacobson D, Tillman CR, Curington C, Toskes P. Protease-specific suppression of pancreatic exocrine secretion. Gastroenterology 1984; 87:44-52.

PART 7

Juvenile Tropical Pancreatitis

C.S. Pitchumoni, M.D., M.P.H., FRCPC, FACP

Until recently, chronic pancreatitis has been considered mostly a disease of adults as a result of 10 to 15 years of heavy alcoholism. In children, the relatively rare form of hereditary chronic pancreatitis used to be referred to as the major type of chronic pancreatitis.[1] This perception has changed, largely as a result of innumerable reports from many Afro-Asian countries on hundreds of cases of a nonalcoholic juvenile chronic calcific pancreatitis syndrome, practically indistinguishable from the alcoholic variety.[2-15] Nutritional pancreatitis, tropical pancreatitis, juvenile trop-

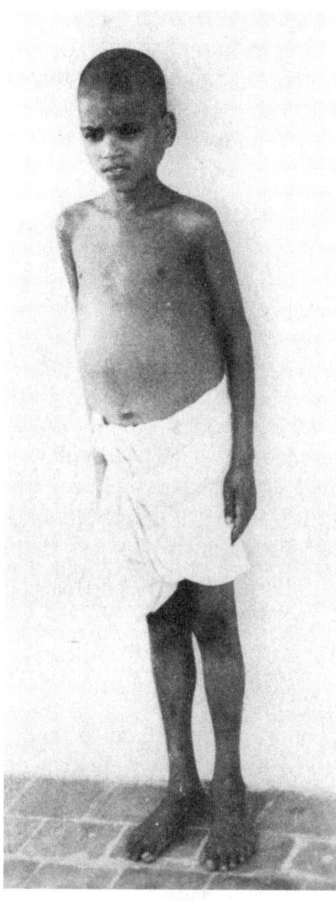

FIGURE 1 A 13-year-old boy with juvenile tropical pancreatitis. Note the emaciation and distended abdomen.

ical pancreatitis syndrome, Afro-Asian pancreatitis, and fibrocalculous pancreatic diabetes (FCPD) are the terms used in the literature to describe this entity.

DEFINITION

Juvenile tropical pancreatitis is a form of chronic pancreatitis characterized by recurrent abdominal pain, pancreatic calculi, and diabetes mellitus occurring in children and young adults of many developing nations (Figs. 1 to 3). The disease occurs almost exclusively among the children and teenagers of the impoverished sectors of developing nations and is accompanied by some characteristic signs of malnutrition such as emaciation, bilateral parotid gland enlargement, and hair and skin changes. The notable absence of other known causes of pancreatitis and experimental and clinical evidence that the pancreas is vulnerable to malnutrition implicate malnutrition as the most likely etiologic factor of this enigmatic disease.

EPIDEMIOLOGY

The first clear description of this syndrome was by Zuidema from Indonesia in 1955.[2] This classic paper described seven malnourished Indonesian patients with pancreatic lithiasis. The youngest, a 15-year-old girl, was markedly undernourished, weighing only 33.5 kg. Her main meal at home was rice, cassava (manihot esculenta), and vegetables and rarely included fish and never meat or eggs. The oldest in the group was 28 years of age. None had a history of alcohol consumption. In six patients diabetes mellitus dominated the clinical picture. Some of them had marked swelling of both parotid glands and changes in scalp hair resembling

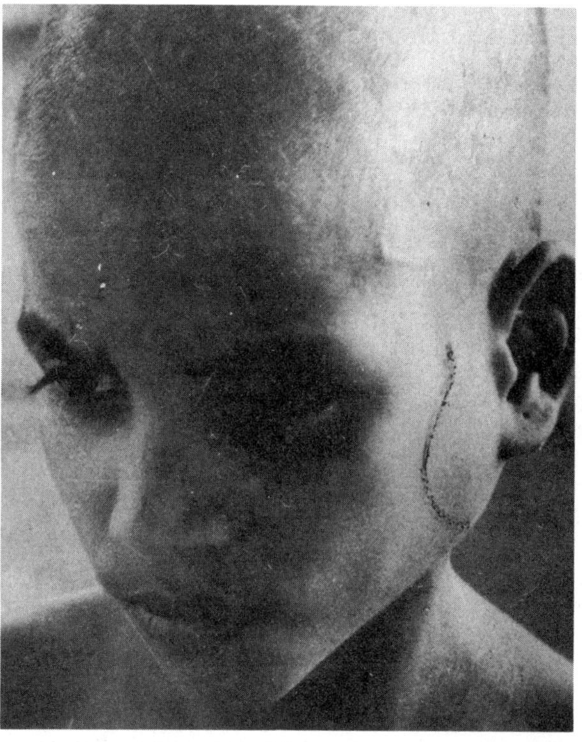

FIGURE 2 Parotid gland enlargement in the boy shown in Figure 1.

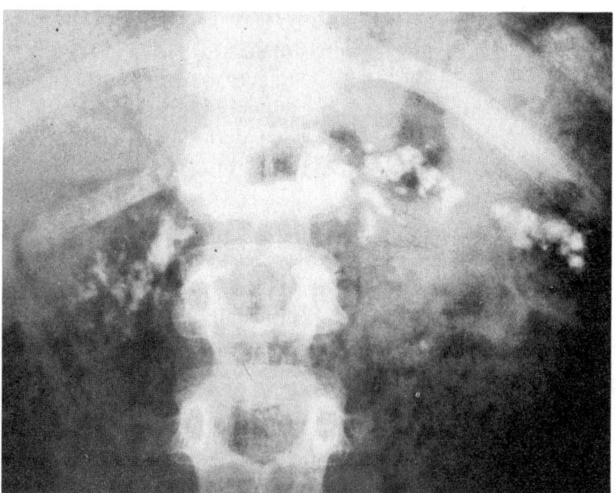

FIGURE 3 Flat plate of the pancreas in a case of juvenile topical pancreatitis. The entire main pancreatic duct and even some ductules are packed with calculi. A ductogram is seen.

that found in kwashiorkor. In one case autopsy showed firosis of the pancreas, destruction of the parenchyma, and pancreatic lithiasis. Zuidema subsequently (1959) reported on 45 patients from 12 to 45 years of age with the same clinicopathologic features.[3] The diabetes of the poor in Indonesia, Zuidema concluded, was a result of severe malnutrition.

Shaper in Uganda in 1960 observed a similar syndrome in the indigenous population around Kampala, whose diet was rich in carbohydrate but low in protein and fat.[4] The youngest patient was 10 years old. Most patients had a history of moderate to severe recurrent abdominal pain, suggestive of pancreatitis. Shaper felt that the high carbohydrate diet consumed under the circumstances of severe protein deficiency led to increased demands for pancreatic enzymes, potentiating the effect of protein depletion in the diet.

The syndrome of chronic pancreatitis with pancreatic calculi and diabetes has subsequently been reported by different observers from many countries such as Uganda, Nigeria, Congo, Malawi, Zambia, Ghana, Ivory Coast, and Madagascar in the African continent; Sri Lanka, Malayasia, Thailand, India, and Bangladesh in Asia; and Brazil in South America.[5-25] In support of the term *tropical pancreatitis*, the prevalence of nutritional pancreatitis is almost restricted to latitude 30 degrees north and south of the equator.

The largest series of cases of juvenile tropical pancreatitis to date is from the southwestern state of Kerala in India. GeeVarghese et al, in a series of reports, have presented data on this syndrome, which occurred in endemic proportions.[5,13,16-18,24,26] In India after 1962 a number of similar cases have been observed in the northeastern state of Orissa.[19] Recent epidemiologic data indicate that although less common, the disease is prevalent in many other parts of India.[27] This may be the result of an increased awareness and routine screening of young diabetics for pancreatic calculi with radiographic studies of the abdomen. Approximately 2,000 cases of this disease have been reported in the literature, more than 1,700 cases by GeeVarghese alone from the state of Kerala in India.[24]

The true prevalence of the disease is not well established, since the epidemiologic data are based exclusively on cases seen in major teaching hospitals of Afro-Asian countries and do not include cases seen outside these institutions. The hospital data often give an erroneously high prevalence, as most of the patients from villages tend to accumulate in the major teaching hospitals for treatment. In many countries men seek medical attention earlier and women are reluctant to go to hospitals except in life-threatening situations.

Calculation of the true prevalence of the disease is further complicated by a recent observation by the World Health Organization (1980) that a form of malnutrition-related diabetes mellitus (MRDM) seen in many developing nations is a variant of this syndrome.[28] Many cases of juvenile diabetes in the tropics, some of them previously described as "J" diabetes by Hugh-Jones in 1955, are at this time considered to be secondary to malnutrition.[29,30] (Note, however, that the most common type of diabetes in the tropics is not induced by malnutrition but is early-onset type II diabetes.) The abrupt onset of diabetes in an underweight teenager or young adult (with a body mass index below 18 kg per square meter), requirement of large doses of insulin (more than 2 units per kilogram body weight), and the absence of ketosis on withdrawal from insulin characterize MRDM.[30] In 1985 the WHO committee on diabetes in its third report included MRDM and FCPD as closely related entities but different from type I or II diabetes.[31] In support of the view that MRDM may be a variant of chronic pancreatitis is the experience of some observers in Afro-Asian countries who on routine screening of young diabetics could diagnose pancreatic calculi.[7,11]

PATHOLOGY

The pathologic changes in the pancreas and other organs in tropical pancreatitis have been well studied in material obtained postmortem or at surgery.[24,32] The histologic changes in the pancreas are almost identical to those seen in other forms of chronic pancreatitis.

The size of the pancreas varies inversely with the duration and severity of the disease. In advanced stages of the disease the pancreatic gland is as small as the little finger or the adrenal gland, and the surface is irregular and nodular. Uneven shrinkage and fibrous adhesions cause displacement of the pancreas from its normal location. The parenchyma may be replaced by fat and can become indistinguishable from surrounding adipose tissue. The pancreas is firm, fibrous, and gritty to touch. The consistency of the organ varies in different regions of the pancreas depending on the presence of fibrous tissue, cysts, or stones. Radiologic examination of the dissected pancreatic gland reveals multiple calculi, often not noted in recent antemortem radiologic studies (Fig. 4).

Homogeneous areas, early fibrosis, advanced fibrosis, cystic dilatation of the gland, and pancreatic calculi of different shapes and sizes distributed throughout the duct system characterize the cut-section appearance. The major pancreatic duct may be eccentrically placed as a result of uneven destruction of the glandular tissue. Areas of stenosis and dilatation of the ducts can be seen in the same gland. Incomplete pancreatic obstruction at the ampulla of Vater is noted in a large majority of carefully dissected cases, corresponding to the location of a solitary calculus ("sentinel stone") and/or larger stones.[24]

Pancreatic calculi vary in color, size, and shape. The larger stones are nearer the head, and they progressively diminish in size toward the tail. The stones may range in size from

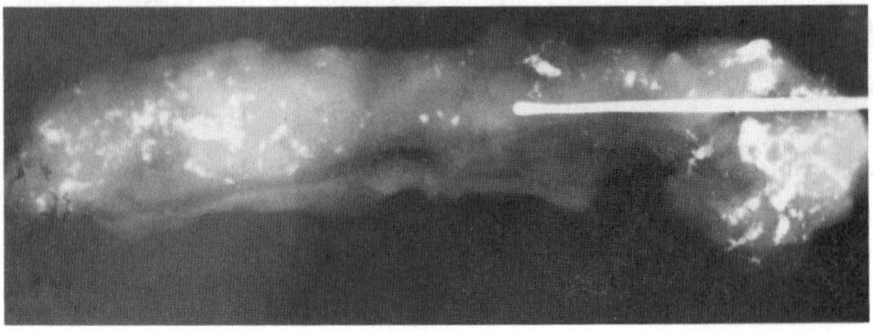

FIGURE 4 Radiologic study of the isolated postmortem pancreas. Note the numerous small radiodense areas, which are intraductal calculi. The probe is passed into the main duct to show the dilatation in relation to the shrunken pancreas.

FIGURE 5

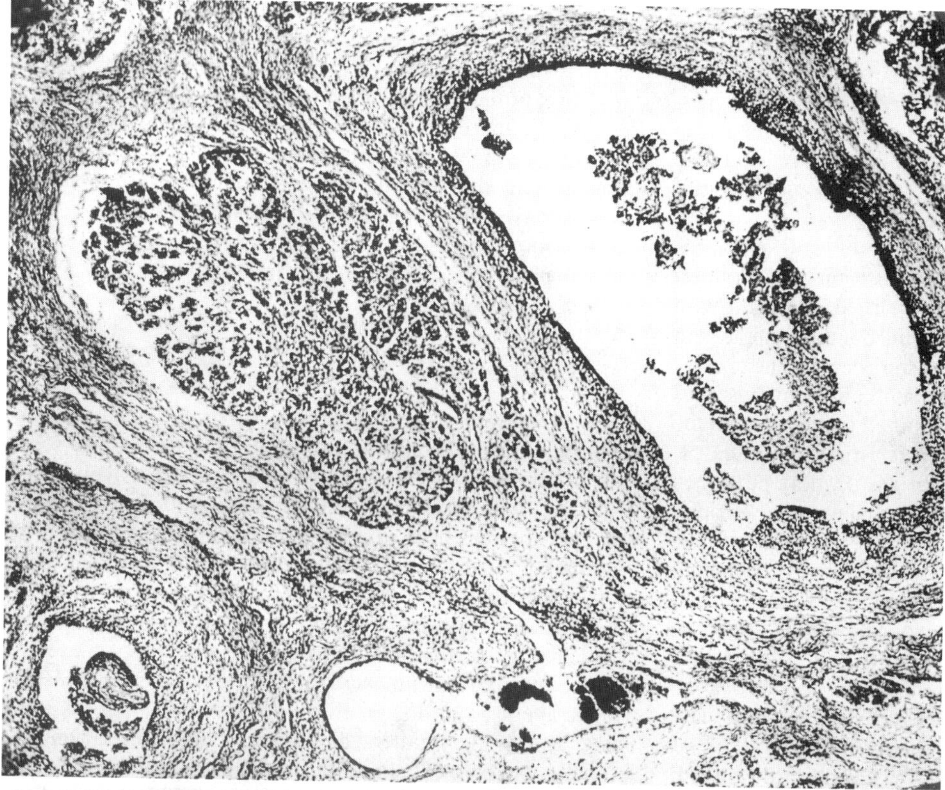

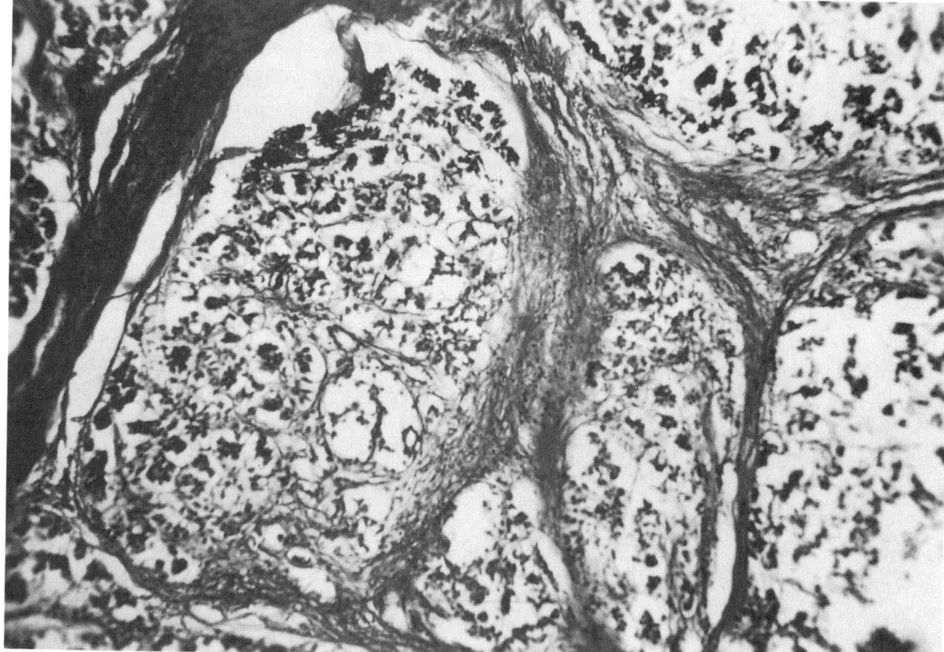

FIGURE 6

FIGURES 5 and 6 The pancreas shows extensive fibrosis, ductular dilatation, and intraductular calcium deposits. The intra- and interacinar fibrosis of the exocrine parenchyma produces the appearance of cirrhosis of the pancreas.

small sand particles to calculi 4.5 cm long, weighing up to 20 g. The shape of the stone is influenced by its location and may be smooth, rounded, or staghorn-like and may be incarcerated in the main pancreatic duct and major branches. Noncalcified protein plugs and caseous material may form soft stones. Sections of calcified stones have shown epithelial debris, fibrin, and mucinous material.

Pancreatic calculi are composed of 95.5 percent calcium carbonate and a small amount of calcium phosphate. Traces of magnesium, urate, and oxalate have been identified in some stones. X-ray diffraction studies of calculi have determined that calcium carbonate is predominantly in the form of calcite and rarely of vaterite.[33] Scanning electron microscopic studies and spectroscopic methods of analysis have shown that the calculi have an amorphous nidus and a cryptocrystalline periphery. The nidus is rich in iron, chromium, and nickel, and the periphery contains a number of trace elements and a preponderance of calcium.[34] These calculi are structurally and biochemically similar to stones obtained in other types of chronic pancreatitis. A nonenzymatic protein has been identified recently by some observers in the core of calculi. This protein, termed *pancreatic stone protein* (PSP), has been implicated in the pathogenesis of the disease and calculus formation.[35] The absence or decrease of PSP has been thought to promote nucleation of calcium carbonate and crystallization.

Microscopically, the characteristic feature is diffuse fibrosis of the pancreas (Figs. 5 and 6). The main duct, collecting ducts, and small ductules show marked dilatation with periductular fibrosis. Denudation of the ductular epithelium and squamous metaplasia are seen in some areas. The characteristic cellular infiltration of the pancreas is composed of lymphocytes and plasma cells, distributed mainly around the ducts. Interlobular fibrosis is characteristic of early cases, and focal, segmental, or diffuse fibrosis of more advanced cases. The acinar tissue shows varying degrees of atrophy and parenchymal destruction. Replacement by fibrous tissue is seen adjacent to relatively normal-looking parenchyma.

The islets of Langerhans appear relatively well preserved despite extensive destruction of exocrine parenchyma. In some instances, the islets appear even hypertrophied, and, as in other forms of pancreatic atrophy, a true nesidioblastosis is observed (Fig. 7). Limited histochemical studies have identified those hyperplastic islets as B-cell nesidioblasts.[36] As the disease advances, the islets become atrophic and get isolated and surrounded by dense fibrous tissue.[24] Vacuolation, ballooning, and glycogen infiltration of the islets characteristic of juvenile diabetes are seldom noted.

Pseudocysts of the pancreas are common in surgical and postmortem cases.[24] Pancreatic carcinoma has been noted in some surgically obtained tissues, indicating that tropical pancreatitis is a premalignant disease similar to hereditary pancreatitis and alcoholic calcific pancreatitis.[14]

Other organs such as the liver and parotid glands show changes indicative of uncontrolled diabetes mellitus and/or malnutrition. The liver in early stages shows glycogen infiltration of the cytoplasm and nuclei and fatty changes and cirrhosis in more advanced cases. Parotid glands show hypertrophied acini, with varying degrees of round cell infiltration around the intralobular and interlobular ducts. The pathogenesis of parotid enlargement is probably a functional or compensatory hypertrophy as an adaptative mechanism to pancreatic exocrine insufficiency.[37]

ETIOLOGY AND PATHOGENESIS

The etiology of tropical pancreatitis has not been well established. Data from different countries in the past 30 years stress the occurrence of the disease almost exclusively in association with poverty and childhood malnutrition. Protein malnutrition has been implicated as an important cause. The biologic plausibility of this association is an important factor in accepting the hypothesis. The turnover of protein in the pancreas is among the highest of any organ. The clinical evidence for protein malnutrition is that some of these patients have extreme emaciation, muscle wasting, and loss of subcutaneous fat. Pancreatic exocrine functional changes have been well documented in primary and secondary nutritional disorders. Glucose tolerance and insulin reserves are markedly affected in malnutrition.[38] Fasting insulin and insulin responses are markedly reduced. Pathologic changes that have been observed in the pancreas in autopsy studies of kwashiorkor include shrinkage and fibrosis.[39] Extreme atrophy of the exocrine cells, disorganization or loss of the acinar pattern, marked reduction in the amount of zymogen granules, vacuolization, occasional epithelial metaplasia, cystic dilatation of the ducts, and definite increase in fibrous

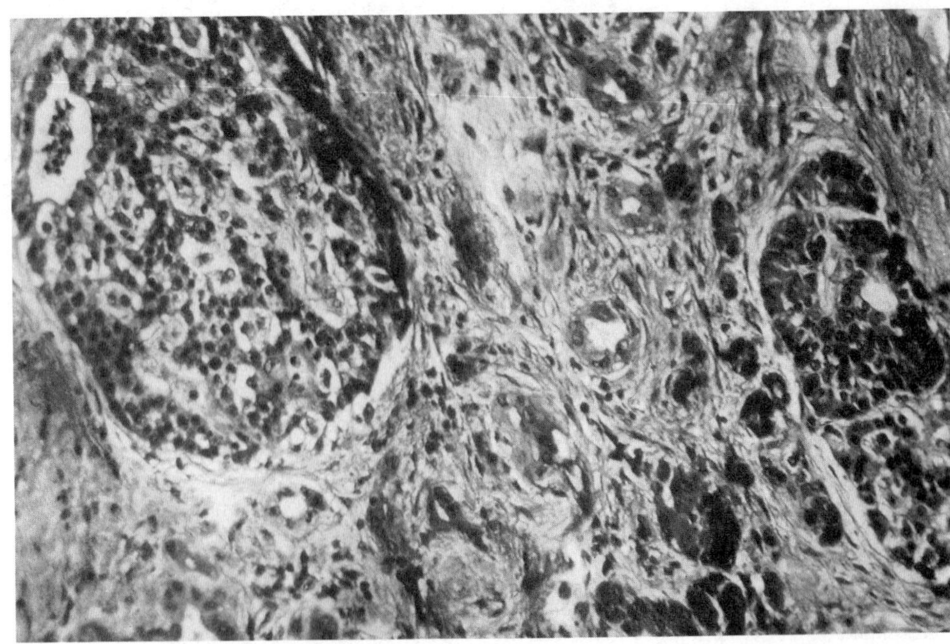

FIGURE 7 The islets show varying degrees of hypertrophy in the presence of fibrosis of the organ.

tissue are seen. A marked decrease in rough endoplasmic reticulum and mitochondria are the ultrastructural changes. Maternal malnutrition has also been a proposed, although not proven, cause of juvenile pancreatic injury.

There are many arguments against protein malnutrition being the sole factor in the initiation of the disease. In India and Africa the prevalence of the disease does not correlate well with the prevalence of kwashiorkor.[18,26] The pancreas in kwashiorkor does not develop pancreatic calculi, and calculous pancreatic disease does not exactly mimic the syndrome of kwashiorkor. Many patients with tropical pancreatitis have normal serum albumin. There have been a handful of cases reported recently in which there is no evidence at all of malnutrition.

However, one must realize that in all diseases of known causation accessory or secondary factors affect susceptibility. Our knowledge concerning the accessory factors in tropical pancreatitis is meager at this time. It is well known that human malnutrition is not a pure form of protein deficiency but is a combination of multiple deficiencies, exposure to toxins, immunologic disturbances, and viral, bacterial, and parasitic infections. There is experimental evidence that trace element deficiencies can cause pancreatic fibrosis. Deficiencies of selenium, zinc, and copper cause acinar cell injury and pancreatic fibrosis in experimental animals.[40] The role of micronutrient deficiencies in tropical pancreatitis has not been studied.

In many areas where tropical pancreatitis is endemic, such as Indonesia, parts of Nigeria, Uganda, the state of Kerala in India, and Thailand, a staple source of carbohydrate is the cassava root (manioc, manihot esculenta). Cassava is consumed as peeled, boiled, cut pieces of the root, sun dried chips, and fermented forms under different local names (gari in Nigeria, farinha in Brazil, cassarino in the Philippines, fufu in Zaire, tapioca in India and Sri Lanka).[24] The consumption of cassava is higher in northern Nigeria where nutritional pancreatitis is prevalent.[23] In the state of Kerala in India, the prevalence of the disease is highest in cassava-consuming areas.[24] The disease is rare in areas where malnutrition is prevalent, where rice is the staple food. The edible portion has a central core. The sap contains toxic cyanogenic glycosides, linamarin and lotaustralin, that liberate hydrocyanic acid on acid hydrolysis in the stomach, which may be responsible for this syndrome. The argument against this theory is that in some countries where cassava is consumed, pancreatitis is rare. The content of cyanogenic glycosides in the meal varies depending on the soil, season, method of storing, and cooking, affecting the exposure to cyanogens. There are important diseases well connected with chronic cassava toxicity, which include tropical ataxic neuropathy and endemic goiter. In an experimental study in which cyanide was administered in drinking water, rats developed diabetes, indicating its toxic effect on the islets.[41] On a cassava-based diet for 18 months, rats developed pancreatic changes suggestive of pancreatitis.[24] The detoxification of cyanides depends on the ready availability of methionine and/or vitamin B_{12}, notoriously deficient in the malnourished individual. It has also been hypothesized that cyanogens in their metabolism induce deficiency of cellular enzymes, including superoxide dismutase, which is required to scavenge oxygen-free radicals that are injurious to acinar cells.[42] Cyanide also binds and inactivates a multimeric enzyme complex vital for mitochondrial respiration.[42]

A third hypothesis is that a carbohydrate-rich diet is inadequate to stimulate pancreatic secretion and thus leads to protein plugs.[4,23] Cassava is 87.5 percent carbohydrate, but its protein content is only 0.7 percent and it is very low in essential amino acids, particularly methionine. Malnutrition, in association with infections and recurrent dehydration in children, was postulated to precipitate or enhance an environment conducive to protein plug formation inside the pancreatic ductules. Protein plug formation as a result of an increased viscosity of pancreatic secretion has been proposed as a mechanism for alcoholic pancreatitis.[23]

Ductal obstruction, noted at the ampullary region in many patients, is suspected as an initiating factor for pancreatitis, although it is not clear whether it is the cause or the result of pancreatitis.[24] Current data do not implicate infection as a cause, although recently, high titers of antibodies against cytomegalovirus, mumps, and coxsackie B have been noted in pancreatitis patients compared with hospital controls.[43] *Ascaris lumbricoides* (round worm) in the pancreatic duct has been shown in cases of acute pancreatitis in the tropics, but it is not an etiologic factor in chronic pancreatitis. Although a cluster of tropical pancreatitis patients is seen in many families, a hereditary factor is not discernible.[26]

In conclusion, the etiopathogenesis of this syndrome is controversial and remains largely in the realm of speculation owing to inadequate epidemiologic and experimental data. Malnutrition with some other unidentified factors appears to be the major accompaniment and carries the best strength of association among all postulated etiologic factors.

CLINICAL FEATURES

The cardinal manifestations of juvenile tropical pancreatitis are recurrent abdominal pain in childhood, followed by diabetes mellitus and pancreatic calculi by puberty and death in the prime of life.[24] Improvement in the management of diabetes has resulted in a longer life span not noted in earlier observations.

Pancreatalgia is a problem in young children with tropical pancreatitis, whereas pancreatic diabetes is noted in adolescence. The onset of the disease is insidious in early childhood with recurrent attacks of upper abdominal or periumbilical pain before the thirteenth year (Table 1). The history is often elicited from the patient's mother, who attests to the number of school days lost. About 5 percent of the juvenile diabetics with pancreatic calculi do not have abdominal pain. The patient usually keeps his palm on the abdomen to indicate a wide area of pain, as opposed to the finger tip as in duodenal ulcer. The pain radiates to the lower end of the sternum, the left costal margin and along the left side, or posteriorly to the lumbar spine. Radiation of pain to the right side is uncommon. The episodes of pain last for days, not minutes or hours. The pain is usually aggravated by small amounts of food, so that the patients refuse all food by mouth. In the early stages the bouts of pain are severe and are associated with vomiting. As years pass, painful attacks become less intense but more prolonged. In an attempt to obtain relief patients sit up, bend forward or walk, curl up in the

TABLE 1
Age of Onset of Pancreatic Pain in 100 Cases

Age (years)	Number of Cases
5–11	26
12–18	35
19–25	14
26–30	5
31–35	1
36–40	2
41–50	2
	85
No pain	6
Undetermined	9
TOTAL	100

Data from GeeVarghese et al.[5]

lateral decubitus position, clutch the skin of the abdomen, or apply hot water bottles to the area.

An interval of several years may pass between the cessation of painful attacks and the onset of diabetes mellitus. Pancreatic pain totally disappears in a large number of patients either before or some years after diabetes develops. It is uncommon for diabetes to precede abdominal pain.

Patients are often repeatedly treated with anthelminthics and antacids with the mistaken notion of parasitic disease or peptic ulcer. Persistent abdominal pain in childhood of undetermined etiology has often led to diagnostic laparotomy. In the absence of demonstrable pancreatic calculi, there is no easily available test to establish the diagnosis of chronic pancreatitis at this stage of illness.

Diabetes Mellitus

Most patients initially seek medical attention for diabetes mellitus, which becomes clinically manifest a few years after the onset of pancreatalgia. A pain-free period of 1 or 2 years and an apparent transient improvement in the clinical picture prior to the onset of diabetes are not unusual. The age of onset of diabetes in our series from India is presented in Table 2.

TABLE 2
Age of Onset of Pancreatic Diabetes in 100 Cases

Age (years)	Number of Cases
Below 13	2
14–15	3
16–20	19
21–25	10
26–30	9
31–35	7
36–40	4
41–50	2
Undetermined	44

Data from GeeVarghese and Pitchumoni.[16]

Diabetes associated with chronic pancreatitis (or that following total pancreatectomy) is termed *pancreatic diabetes* to differentiate it from type I (insulin-dependent juvenile type) and type II (the non–insulin-dependent maturity-onset type) diabetes. The fasting blood sugar range is between 200 and 400 mg per deciliter, although blood glucose levels greater than 1,000 mg per deciliter are not rare. Pancreatic diabetes is characteristically brittle, with marked fluctuations of blood glucose values with or without insulin therapy. Episodes of hypoglycemia are characteristic and may complicate the administration of even small doses of insulin. This may be a reflection of depleted glycogen reserves in the liver or decreased glucagon release from the pancreas. Spontaneous hypoglycemic episodes have been recorded without insulin therapy. True insulin resistance, defined as a daily requirement of over 200 units of insulin in the absence of infection or ketosis, occurs. This is surprising, since the insulin requirement after total pancreatectomy is only about 40 units, but the presence of a fibrosed pancreas increases insulin requirements. The nature of insulin resistance in pancreatic diabetes is poorly studied but is attributed to insulin antibodies. Metabolic acidosis is uncommon, but ketosis may be seen in 20 percent of cases.

The fasting serum insulin may be normal or in some cases higher than normal. However, as the disease progresses, there is a decline in amino acid–stimulated insulin release, indicating gradual beta cell failure.[44]

It was once believed that pancreatic diabetes seldom caused vascular complications. Recent studies indicate that vascular complications are related to the duration of uncontrolled diabetes or hyperglycemia. Fundic microaneurysms, exudates, and hemorrhages occur in varying frequency depending on the duration of illness. Almost 50 percent of patients develop sensory neuropathy, 10 percent develop combined sensory and motor neuropathy, 6 percent develop autonomic neuropathy, and about 2 percent develop mononeuritis. Other complications of pancreatic diabetes include recurrent urinary tract infections, intercapillary glomerulosclerosis, and pyelonephritis. The liver is palpably enlarged in 40 percent of diabetics, although the only liver function abnormality may be elevation of alkaline phosphatase, indicating fatty liver. Clinical and biochemical evidence of obstructive jaundice is a well-recognized complication secondary to stenosis and compression of the common bile duct which is tunnelled in the head of the pancreas. Pancreatic pseudocysts are not uncommon.

Exocrine Pancreatic Insufficiency

Overt exocrine pancreatic insufficiency characterized by steatorrhea is the least striking clinical feature. This may be attributable to the very low consumption of fat in the diet. However, pancreatic function tests have shown severe pancreatic exocrine insufficiency.[45] On a 100-g fat diet, more than 70 percent of patients develop biochemical steatorrhea.

DIAGNOSIS

The diagnosis of chronic pancreatic injury in early stages of the disease in young children is seldom made. Abdominal pain in childhood is often ignored or attributed to psychogenic causes or, in the tropics, to parasitic infestations. It is not clear whether endoscopic retrograde cholangiopancreatography (ERCP) or computed tomography (CT) will be of use. The cost and technical expertise needed prohibit the use of these techniques in developing nations. Sensitive, noninvasive blood and urine tests used for diagnosing pancreatitis are not available. Even in developed nations of the world, the diagnosis of chronic pancreatitis is often made very late.

On the other hand, the picture of a well-established case of tropical pancreatitis is so characteristic that one can make a diagnosis based on clinical features alone. The presenting complaints are those characteristic of diabetes mellitus, polyuria, polyphagia, and polydypsia with present or past history of recurrent abdominal pain suggestive of chronic pancreatitis. A family history of the disease may be seen. Extreme emaciation, peculiar cyanotic hue of the lips, bilateral parotid gland enlargement, and a distended upper abdomen are seen in most of the patients.

The diagnosis is established by demonstration of pancreatic calculi on a flat plate radiograph of the abdomen. Proper preparation of the patient for a satisfactory radiologic study of the abdomen and skillful radiologic technique are required in order to avoid missing small calculi. A lateral view of the abdomen, in addition to the standard anteroposterior view, is needed to differentiate renal stones and gallstones. The most common site of pancreatic calculi on the abdominal flat plate is to the right of the first and second lumbar vertebrae. The lateral extension is up to 2 to 5 cm to the right of these vertebrae. Calculi are most numerous in the head of the pancreas. In 30 percent of cases the calculi form a cast of the main duct. In the lateral film the stones are located anterior to the vertebral body but posterior to the gallbladder area.

The diagnosis of tropical pancreatitis does not depend on demonstration of pancreatic exocrine functional abnormality. Serum amylase determination is not highly useful in the diagnosis of chronic pancreatitis except in acute exacerbations. The amylase is below normal in a large number of cases. Steatorrhea is manifest only on a high-fat diet. Secretin cholecystokinin stimulation tests are academic but have shown a marked decrease in volume and enzyme output. Bicarbonate secretion is normal in some studies but markedly reduced in others. The newer diagnostic tests—bentiromide test, pancreolauryl test, and trypsin-like immunoreactivity assays in serum—have not been evaluated.

ERCP has shown ductal abnormalities similar to those observed in alcoholic pancreatitis.[43] However, ERCP cannot be routinely used in the early diagnosis of the disease in children with abdominal pain. Based on experience with other types of chronic pancreatitis, CT of the abdomen may be useful in identifying calculi in the pancreas, long before they can be identified by routine radiologic studies. The cost and limited availability, however, make it impractical.

MANAGEMENT

The management of tropical pancreatitis consists of treatment of diabetes, prevention of complications, alleviation of abdominal pain, and correction of nutritional problems.

The treatment of acute episodes of painful attacks is similar to the treatment of any other bout of pancreatitis. The measures to "put the pancreas to rest" include nasogastric suction, no feeding by mouth, and intravenous fluids and electrolytes. Nasogastric suction may be needed only in severe cases. Treatment of pain may require repeated injections of meperidine, but the fear of producing narcotic addiction is a real one.

Insulin therapy is the basis of treatment of diabetes in tropical pancreatitis. If the diabetes is mild, it is better to avoid insulin in order to prevent hypoglycemia. Oral hypoglycemic agents are used with moderate success in many patients with mild diabetes. In severe cases, insulin therapy is warranted. Although insulin requirement may exceed 60 units per day, it is advisable to avoid long-acting insulin and to use regular insulin in small doses at frequent intervals, preferably after meals.

The dietary treatment of diabetes in pancreatitis is complicated. The associated malnutrition, malabsorption, and tendency toward hypoglycemia deserve consideration in prescribing a suitable diet. A nutritious diet supplemented with vitamins and minerals is needed. It is not advisable to restrict the carbohydrate content of the diet below 300 g. The diet may have to be supplemented with pancreatic enzyme preparations in order to correct malabsorption. Temporary improvement in nutritional status can be achieved with dietary supplements of medium-chain triglycerides.

Although pain is an indication for surgical treatment, operative treatment of pancreatitis is often unrewarding. The best procedure is exploration of the pancreatic duct, removal of stones, and longitudinal anastomosis of the split surface of the pancreas to the jejunum as suggested by Puestow and Gillesby. The relief of pain may be temporary, even with surgery.[24]

In summary, juvenile tropical pancreatitis is a type of chronic pancreatitis that occurs in the setting of malnutrition in children and young adults in many developing nations. From a global point of view, the most common cause of pancreatitis in children is malnutrition. Although the etiology is not clear, malnutrition is an important association. Experimental and clinical observations provide conclusive evidence for the vulnerability of the pancreas to protein deprivation. Other proposed etiologic factors include dietary toxins, pancreatic ductal abnormalities, and trace element deficiencies. The role of cyanogens in the diet in inducing pancreatic injury in the presence of malnutrition is an attractive hypothesis but is not confirmed in epidemiologic or experimental studies. The occurrence of abdominal pain in childhood followed by onset of diabetes in an emaciated teenager is the clinical picture, and the radiologic demonstration of calculi in the pancreatic duct is the hallmark of the disease. Patient management in nutritional pancreatitis involves control of brittle diabetes with small frequent doses of insulin. Painful attacks of pancreatitis require the use of analgesics and other routine measures to provide rest for the pancreas. Nutritional management should include a diabetic diet with adequate complex carbohydrate, frequent small meals, and supplementation with oral pancreatic enzymes. Tropical pancreatitis is an enigmatic disease that requires further studies to explain its etiopathogenesis. It may be one of the preventable forms of diabetes in children in the tropics.

REFERENCES

1. Ghishan FK, Green HL, Avant G, O'Neill J. Chronic relapsing pancreatitis in childhood. J Pediatr 1983; 102:514–518.
2. Zuidema PJ. Calcification and cirrhosis of the pancreas in patients with deficient nutrition. Doc Med Geogr Trop 1955; 7:229–251.
3. Zuidema PJ. Cirrhosis and disseminated calcification of the pancreas in patients with malnutrition. Trop Geogr Med 1959; 11:70–74.
4. Shaper AG. Chronic pancreatic disease and protein malnutrition. Lancet 1960; i:1223–1224.
5. GeeVarghese PJ, Pillai VK, Joseph MP, Pitchumoni CS. The diagnosis of pancreatogenous diabetes mellitus. J Assoc Phys India 1962; 10:173–178.
6. Bourgoignie J, Sonnet J, Dechef G. Clinical study of diabetes mellitus in the Bantu region of Leopoldville. Ann Soc Belg Med Trop 1962; 3:261–294.
7. Kinnear TWG. Patterns of diabetes mellitus in a Nigerian teaching hospital. West Afr Med J 1963; 60:228–233.
8. Goodall JWD, Pilbeam STH. Diabetes in Nyasaland (Malawi). Trans R Soc Trop Med Hyg 1964; 58:575–578.
9. Sonnet J, Brisbois P, Bastin JP. Chronic pancreatitis with calcifications in Congolese Bantus. Trop Geogr Med 1966; 18:97–113.
10. Olurin EO, Olurin O. Pancreatic calcification: a report of 45 cases. Br Med J 1969; 4:534–539.
11. Nagaratnam N, Gunawardene KRW. Aetiological factors in pancreatic calcification in Ceylon. Digestion 1972; 5:9–16.
12. Osuntokun BO, Skinkugbe FM, Francis TI, Reddy S, Osuntokun O, Taylor GOL. Diabetes mellitus in Nigerians. A study of 832 patients. West Afr Med J 1971; 20:295–312.
13. Pitchumoni CS. Pancreas in primary malnutrition disorders. Am J Clin Nutr 1973; 26:374–379.
14. Narendranathan M. Chronic calcific pancreatitis of the tropics. Trop Gastroenterol 1981; 2:40–45.
15. Vannasaeng S, Vichayanrat A, Nitiyanant W, Tandhanand S. Diabetes mellitus in the tropics: a case with pancreatic calcification and chronic cassava toxicity. J Med Ass Thailand 1982; 65:330–332.
16. GeeVarghese PJ, Pitchumoni CS. Pancreatic diabetes in Kerala. In: Patel JC, Talwalker NG, eds. Diabetes in the tropics. Bombay: Diabetes Association of India, 1966: 223.
17. GeeVarghese PJ. Pancreatic diabetes. Bombay: Popular Prakashan, 1968.
18. Pitchumoni CS. "Tropical" or "nutritional pancreatitis"—an update. In: Gyr KE, Singer MV, Sarles H, eds. Pancreatitis—concepts and classification. Amsterdam: Elsevier Science Publishers, 1984: 359.
19. Kar BC, Tripathy BB. Clinical observations on a group of young diabetics. J Assoc Phys India 1967; 15:9–15.
20. Chandraprasert S, Samranvej P, Arthaschinta S, Isarsena S. Diabetes mellitus and tropical form of chronic calcific pancreatitis in Thailand. Aust N Z J Med 1976; 6:316–320.
21. Balasegaran M. Pancreatitis in the tropics. In: Howard JM, Jordan GL, Reber H, eds. Surgical diseases of the pancreas. Philadelphia: Lea & Febiger, 1987: 257.
22. Dani R, Nogueira CED. Chronische kalzifzierende pankreatitris in Brasilien. Eine analysse von 92 fallen. Leber Magen Darm 1976; 6:272–275.
23. Nwokolo C, Oli J. Pathogenesis of juvenile tropical pancreatitis syndrome. Lancet 1980; i:456–458.
24. GeeVarghese PJ. Calcific pancreatitis. Trivandrum: St. Joseph's Press, 1986.
25. Khan A. A brief statement on the problem of MRDM in Bangladesh. In: Tropical Diabetes Workshop. Position Papers. June 30–July 2, 1988. Wellcome Tropical Institute, London, UK.
26. Pitchumoni CS. Special problems in tropical pancreatitis. Clin Gastroenterol 1984; 3:941–959.
27. Mohan V, Ramachandran A, Viswanathan M. Tropical pancreatic diabetes. Diabetologia 1985; 29:128–138.
28. WHO expert committee on diabetes mellitus. Second report 1980. WHO Tech Rep Sec 1980; 646:23–24.
29. Hugh-Jones. Diabetes in Jamaica. Lancet 1955; ii:891.
30. Ahuja MMS. Profile of young Indian diabetics— biochemical studies. J Assoc Phys India 1073; 21:87–99.
31. WHO study group report on diabetes mellitus. WHO Tech Rep Ser No. 727. Geneva: WHO, 1985.
32. Nagalotimath SJ. Pancreatic pathology in pancreatic calcification with diabetes. In: Podolsky S, Viswanathan M, eds. Secondary diabetes: the spectrum of the diabetic syndromes. New York: Raven Press, 1980: 117.
33. Schultz AC, Moore PB, Pitchumoni CS. X-ray diffraction studies of pancreatic calculi associated with nutritional pancreatitis. Dig Dis Sci 1986; 31:476.
34. Pitchumoni CS, Viswanathan KV, GeeVarghese PJ, Banks PA. Ultrastructure and elemental composition of human pancreatic calculi. Pancreas 1987; 2:152–158.
35. DeCaro A, Multigner L, Lafont H, et al. Pancreatic stone protein: a phosphoprotein which inhibits calcium carbonate precipitation from human pancreatic juice. Gastroenterology 1983; 84:1120–1124.
36. Nair B, Latha P. The pancreas in chronic calcific pancreatitis. In: Balakrishnan V, ed. Chronic pancreatitis in India. Trivandrum: St. Joseph's Press 1987: 115.
37. Alapat JL, Ananthachari MD. A preliminary study of the structure and function of enlarged parotid glands in chronic relapsing pancreatitis by sialography and biopsy methods. Gut 1975; 64:13–22.
38. Rao H. The role of undernutrition in the pathogenesis of diabetes mellitus. Diabetes Care 1984; 7:595–600.
39. Blackburn WR, Vinijchaikul K. The pancreas in kwashiorkor in electron microscopic study. Lab Invest 1969; 20:305–331.
40. Pitchumoni CS, Scheele G, Lee PC, Lebenthal E. Effects of nutrition on the exocrine pancreas. In: Go VLW, et al, eds. The exocrine pancreas: biology, pathobiology and diseases. 1986: 387.
41. McMillan D, GeeVarghese PJ. Dietary cyanide and tropical malnutrition diabetes. In: Podolsky S, Viswanathan M, eds. Secondary diabetes: the spectrum of the diabetic syndromes. New York: Raven Press, 1980: 239.
42. Pitchumoni CS, Jain NK, Lowenfels A, DiMagno EP. Chronic cyanide poisonings: unifying concept for alcoholic and tropical pancreatitis. Pancreas 1988; 3:220–222.
43. Balakrishnan V. Tropical pancreatitis. Epidemiology, pathogenesis and etiology. In: Balakrishnan V, ed. Chronic pancreatitis in India. Trivandrum: St. Joseph's Press, 1987: 81.
44. Ahuja MMS, Sharma GP. Serum C-peptide content in nutritional diabetes. Horm Metab Res 1985; 17:267–268.
45. George PK, Banks PA, Pai KN. Exocrine pancreatic function in calcific pancreatitis in India. Gastroenterology 1971; 60:858–863.

SECTION V

Diagnosis of Gastrointestinal Disease in Children

CHAPTER 30

Endoscopy

PART 1

Fiberoptic Upper Intestinal Endoscopy

Marvin E. Ament, M.D.
Jorge Vargas, M.D.

During the last decade and a half, upper intestinal endoscopy has become one of the most frequently used tools in pediatric gastroenterology for the diagnosis and treatment of a variety of upper intestinal tract diseases. Until fiberoptic instruments were developed for children, more than half of all the complaints of hematemesis, melena, and abdominal pain went undiagnosed. The development of the instruments to evaluate the esophagus, stomach, duodenum, and hepatobiliary tract in infants and children has dramatically improved our understanding of the diseases that affect this part of the gastrointestinal (GI) tract.[1–8] It has led to an improvement in our approach to treatment.

Pediatricians have rapidly accepted the development of these tools and the indications used for upper and lower intestinal endoscopic examination and no longer fear these procedures. The practitioner has learned that, in the hands of a skilled pediatric endoscopist, these studies not only enhance diagnostic accuracy but can be performed safely.[1–8] They have learned that the decision to perform a procedure should be made on the basis of potential benefit versus risk in relation to other diagnostic tools and therapeutic maneuvers. In addition, some endoscopic therapeutic procedures widely used in adults have been safely adapted to children.[7–18]

INDICATIONS FOR UPPER INTESTINAL ENDOSCOPY

There are more than a dozen indications for performing an upper intestinal endoscopic examination in infants and children (Table 1). Most of the indications are diagnostic, but an increasing number of therapeutic measures can be done through the endoscope. Some of the therapeutic procedures have only rarely been reported in children, in part because of the infrequency with which they are indicated and because the therapeutic tools have not been available for small infants and children. Some techniques, such as photo- and thermocoagulation, have rarely been reported in children, whereas others, such as sclerotherapy, have been increasingly accepted in pediatric patients with variceal bleeding as a substitute for shunt procedures.[12–17] Endoscopic retrograde cholangiopancreatography (ERCP) is not commonly used because of the limited indications in the pediatric population for this diagnostic tool. However, recent developments in miniaturization of the instruments used for ERCP in children have increased the frequency with which this procedure is being done.[7,8] The endoscopic placement of gastrostomy and jejunostomy feeding tubes percutaneously has resulted in a nonoperative means of establishing feeding in compromised patients. Bleeding ulcers and angiomas may now be treated nonoperatively using heater probes and/or laser therapy.[10–12]

TABLE 1
Indications for Upper Gastrointestinal Tract Endoscopy in Children

1. Bleeding
   a. Hematemesis
   b. Melena
   c. Occult blood loss
2. Recurrent abdominal pain
   a. Localized to right upper quadrant midepigastric area
   b. Associated nausea, vomiting, diarrhea
   c. Weight loss
3. Indeterminate radiographic studies
4. Identification of mass lesions seen on radiographic studies
5. Vomiting
6. Caustic ingestion
7. Foreign body ingestion
8. Esophageal strictures
9. Sclerotherapy
10. Placement of gastrostomy tubes
11. Electro- or photocoagulation of bleeding gastric or duodenal ulcers
12. Electrocautery of antral webs

FREQUENCY OF INDICATIONS FOR UPPER GASTROINTESTINAL ENDOSCOPY

Table 2 shows the frequency of indications for upper intestinal fiberoptic endoscopy in 365 children.

Recurrent Abdominal Pain

Recurrent abdominal pain in the pediatric patient is the most common cause for which this procedure is done.[1-5,19,20] It is recognized that more than 90 percent of school-age children who have pain as their only symptom have no organic cause for it.[21] However, upper intestinal endoscopy should be considered a diagnostic test in children who consistently localize their pain to the epigastric region or right upper quadrant and have one or more of the following associated symptoms and signs: nausea, vomiting, diarrhea, weight loss, occult blood in the stool, and persistence or increasing severity of pain. A careful upper GI series should be done before endoscopy is considered. Should the study be nondiagnostic, the physician must then determine whether to proceed with endoscopy to remove any doubt about the normalcy of the esophageal, gastric, or duodenal mucosa. In most instances it should not be done. The willingness of parents to accept a functional diagnosis may influence the decision to perform endoscopy on a youngster, since some parents have doubts about the diagnosis unless they are given the definitive proof that endoscopy and biopsy give.

The endoscopist must be careful not to overinterpret observations. The observations to be made include presence or absence of ulcers, spontaneous friability, and induced friability and edema.[22-24]

Dysphagia and Odynophagia

Dysphagia and odynophagia are two other types of pain for which an endoscopic examination is indicated. Patients may have esophagitis (see Color Plate I*A*) and either spasm or stricture that may not be detected in an upper GI series. At least 10 percent of early strictures may be detected only by endoscopy.[3] Therefore, patients with these symptoms and a nondiagnostic radiographic examination of the esophagus should be examined endoscopically.

Patients with gastroesophageal reflux (GER) need to undergo endoscopy if they have hematemesis and/or occult blood-positive stools or associated dysphagia or odynophagia.

TABLE 2
Frequency of Indications for Upper Intestinal Fiberoptic Endoscopy in 365 Children

Abdominal pain	136
Hematemesis and melena	119
Dysphagia and vomiting, retrosternal pain, pyrosis	54
Abnormal but nondiagnostic radiographs	31
Portal hypertension	14
Foreign body removal	9
Caustic ingestion	2

Patients with reflux symptoms who have difficulty swallowing solid food should be considered prime candidates for endoscopic examination, since it is likely that they have esophagitis with or without associated stricture formation. Findings in such patients may vary from loss of vascular pattern in the distal esophageal mucosa to frank spontaneous friability or ulceration with or without stricture and/or spasm.[24] Chronic reflux with stricture formation is likely to be associated with Barrett's esophagus.

Patients need not have associated vomiting and pyrosis to have sufficient reason for endoscopic examination.

Indeterminate Gastrointestinal Series

Patients with indeterminate diagnosis on their upper GI series such as "pylorospasm," "duodenitis," "antral spasm," "delayed gastric emptying," and "gastritis" should be endoscoped to confirm or refute the radiologic findings.[2,3,5,19] Similarly, mass lesions seen on radiographic studies should be defined by endoscopic examination. Patients diagnosed as having ulcers in whom the radiologic signs cannot be seen in three or more views should undergo endoscopy to confirm the diagnosis.

Achalasia

Patients with achalasia may present with dysphagia for solids and recognize that doing a Valsalva maneuver helps to empty the esophagus. Although achalasia is usually diagnosed by typical features on esophagram and esophageal motility studies, rare cases may require endoscopy (see Color Plate I*B* and *C*) to differentiate the lesion from stricture formation or carcinoma at the gastroesophageal junction.

Hematemesis and Melena

Hematemesis and melena are probably the second most common reason why an endoscopic examination should be performed on an infant or child. They account for one of three indications for endoscopic examination.[1-5,19] Endoscopy clearly is superior to contrast studies to identify the cause of upper intestinal bleeding. This is especially true if the hematemesis is sufficient to cause a decrease in hemoglobin and hematocrit and the gastric aspirate is positive for blood. Upper GI series in children with hematemesis and melena will give greater than 50 percent false negatives compared with endoscopic examination. Endoscopy may not identify the site of bleeding in 10 to 20 percent of the cases.[1-5,19,20] This may occur because the blood loss was from the nasopharynx or was insignificant in amount.

Before an upper intestinal endoscopy is performed in a patient with hematemesis, a careful examination of the anterior nares and oropharynx should be done to look for signs of epistaxis. If it is found, measures should be directed at treating the epistaxis. The other problem encountered is delay between the episode of hematemesis and performance of the endoscopic procedure. The longer the delay beyond 24 hours, the less is the chance of finding the source of the bleed-

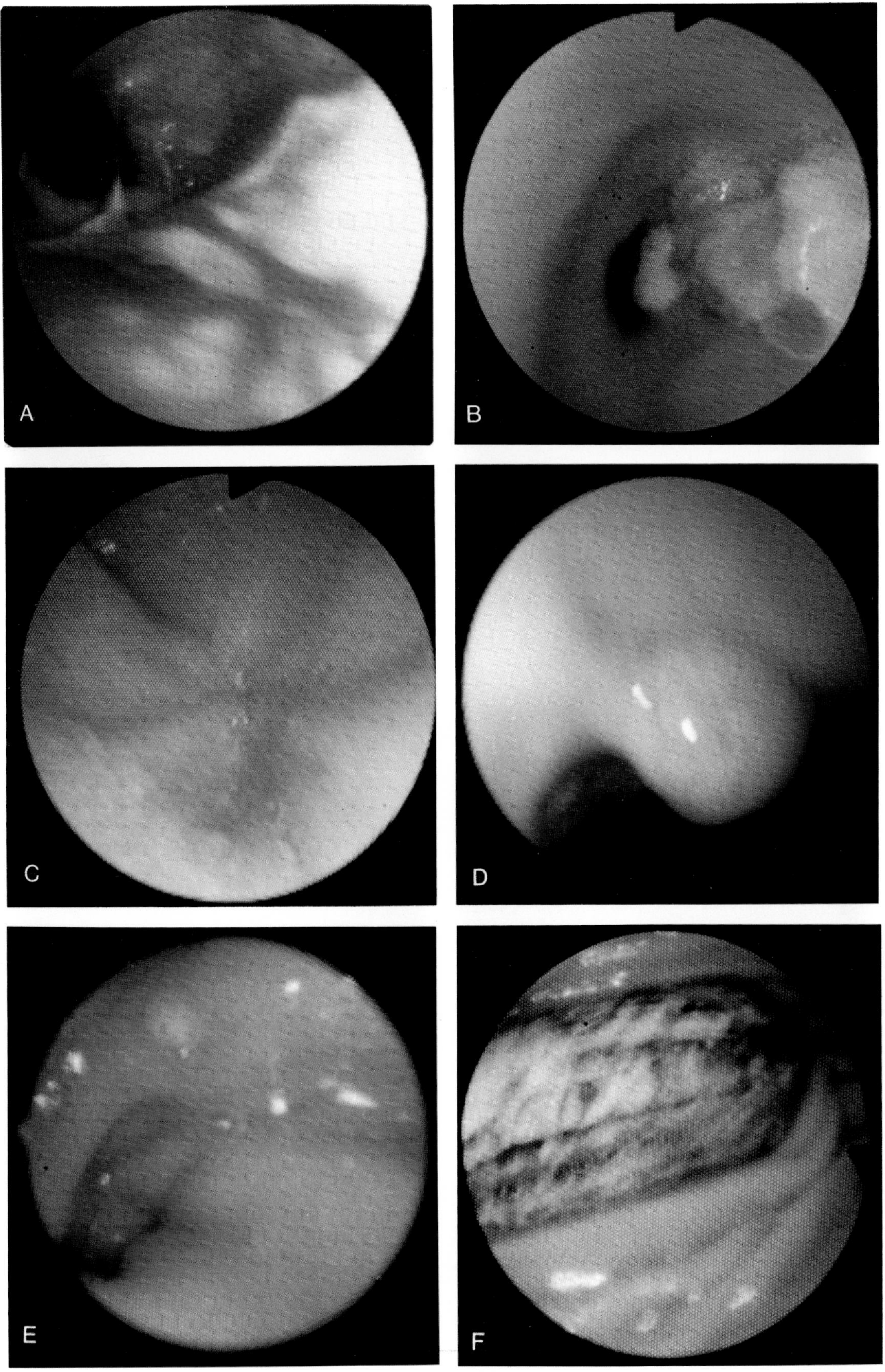

PLATE I *A*, Hemorrhagic esophagitis. *B*, Achalasia: typical finding of undigested food in the esophagus. *C*, Achalasia: tight lower esophageal sphincter that does not relax. Characteristic endoscopic finding of numerous radiating folds is demonstrated. *D*, Gastric polyp. *E*, Gastric ulcer in antrum. *F*, Battery ingestion with object in the stomach. (*A* to *F*, Courtesy of Harland S. Winter, M.D.)

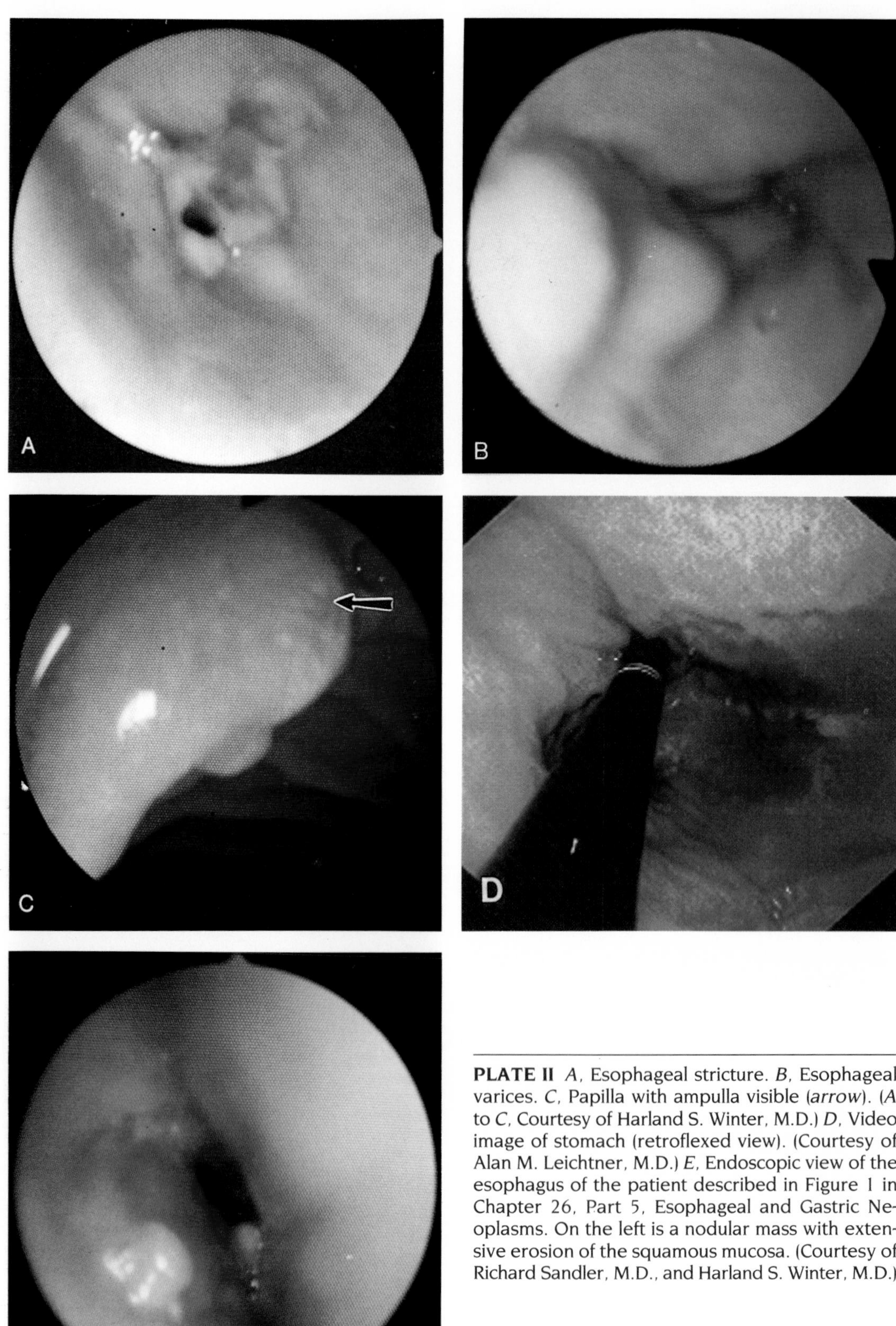

PLATE II *A*, Esophageal stricture. *B*, Esophageal varices. *C*, Papilla with ampulla visible (*arrow*). (*A* to *C*, Courtesy of Harland S. Winter, M.D.) *D*, Video image of stomach (retroflexed view). (Courtesy of Alan M. Leichtner, M.D.) *E*, Endoscopic view of the esophagus of the patient described in Figure 1 in Chapter 26, Part 5, Esophageal and Gastric Neoplasms. On the left is a nodular mass with extensive erosion of the squamous mucosa. (Courtesy of Richard Sandler, M.D., and Harland S. Winter, M.D.)

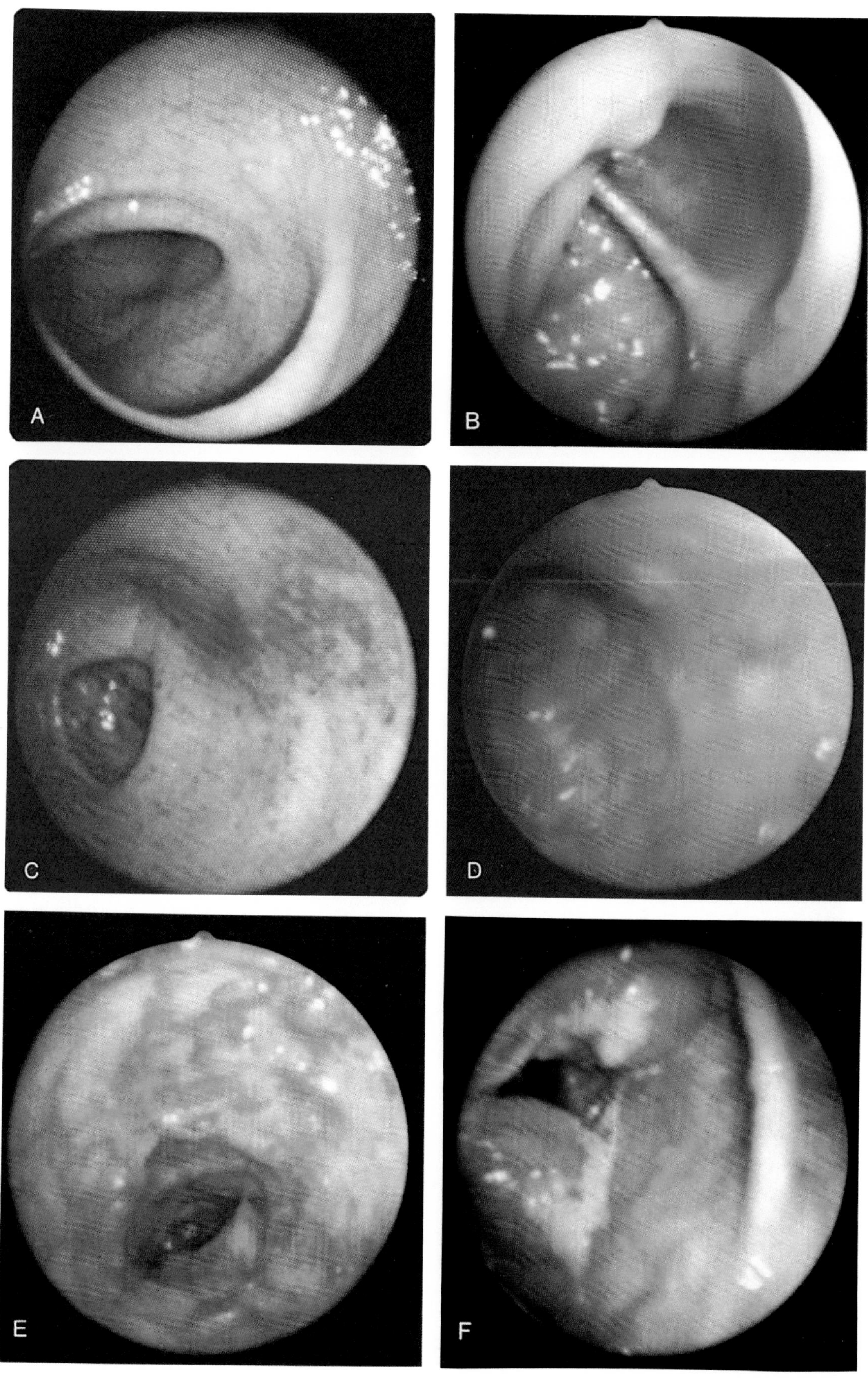

PLATE III *A*, Normal rectum. *B*, Normal splenic flexure. *C* and *D*, Ulcerative colitis. *E* and *F*, Crohn's colitis.

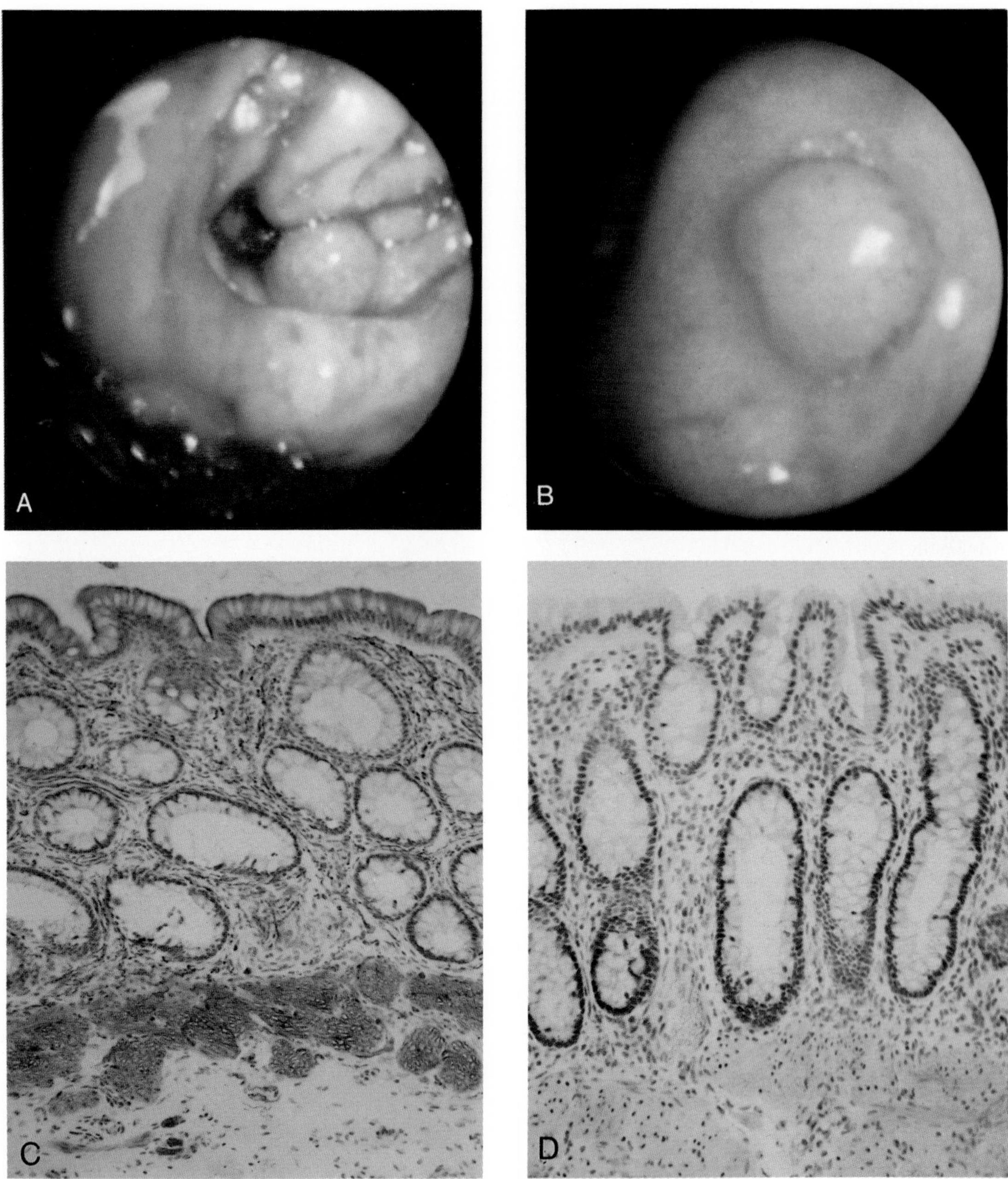

PLATE IV *A*, Juvenile polyp. *B*, Gardner's polyp. *C* and *D*, Histochemical reaction for acetylcholinesterase activity in Cryostat sections of rectal mucosal suction biopsies (original magnification, ×225). *C*, Aganglionic segment of rectum from a patient with Hirschsprung's disease. Note typical coarse cholinesterase-positive axons (brown stain) in lamina propria and intense cholinesterase activity in muscularis mucosae. *D*, Normally enervated rectal biopsy showing cholinesterase activity confined mainly to submucosal nerve plexus (Courtesy of Robert L. Wollmann, M.D.)

ing. Patients who present with hematemesis and/or melena and are considered candidates for endoscopic examination should have the procedure done as soon as they are stabilized in order to have the greatest yield with the diagnostic procedure.

Emergency endoscopy for hematemesis rarely is indicated at any age. Once the history of hematemesis is verified, the most important thing to do is to stabilize the patient. Establishing adequate venous access should be done first. It is extremely important that the physician establish a venous access that allows for rapid replacement of blood volume. Volume replacement should be done rapidly with normal saline in 5 percent albumin or saline alone until blood is available. Volume depletion is established by orthostatic changes in blood pressure and tachycardia. Fluids should be infused as rapidly as possible to normalize blood pressure. Once this has been achieved, the rate of infusion should be decreased to maintenance rates until blood becomes available for transfusion or until the patient rebleeds. The stomach should then be lavaged until the returned fluid is clear or until bleeding has slowed to a minimum. Most bleeding is stopped using these conservative measures, which then allow examination under controlled conditions with adequate support personnel.

If bleeding appears to be uncontrolled, requiring replacement of the patient's blood volume in less than 1 hour to an entire day, and surgery is contemplated, endoscopy truly is emergent. In situations such as this, it may not be possible to visualize the specific site of bleeding. If it is visualized, it can help direct the surgeon to the source.

Gastritis

In the past, hemorrhagic gastritis and both gastric and duodenal ulcers secondary to the use of acetylsalicylic acid for fever and pain were commonly diagnosed endoscopically. However, because pediatricians recognize the association between bleeding and use of salicylates, this medication is rarely recommended for fever control at this time. Parents have been educated not to use it; however, some still do and are unaware that many over-the-counter "cold medications" contain salicylates. This has significantly reduced the frequency of hemorrhagic gastritis and ulcers related to aspirin over the past decade.

Furthermore, because pediatricians have become aware that stress gastritis and ulcers develop in patients with increased intracranial pressure or sepsis or following cardiac, transplantation, and multiple trauma surgery, antacids and H_2 blockers are routinely used beginning in the first 24 hours after the procedure. This has reduced the number of patients who present with bleeding. However, in tertiary pediatric centers, these still are a frequent cause of upper GI bleeding. Rarely in immunocompetent but frequently in immunocompromised patients, infectious agents may be the cause of antral and/or fundal gastritis.

Among the currently used drugs, nonsteroidal anti-inflammatory agents are the more commonly recognized medications to cause gastritis and ulcers. Recent evidence has shown that simultaneous administration of prostaglandin analogues or sucralfate may prevent development of these lesions.[25,26] Gastritis may be generalized or confined to either the antrum or body of the stomach. Stress ulcers may be single or multiple and may be seen in the stomach and duodenum.

Idiopathic Peptic Ulcers

Patients with idiopathic peptic ulcers may present with a variety of GI symptoms.[27] These include abdominal pain, vomiting, and bleeding. Abdominal pain in children with peptic ulcers may be confusing. Preschool-age children with peptic ulcers may have no recognizable pain pattern. This is in part because the physician has to rely on the parents for the history. School-age children have pain patterns associated with ulcers that are more akin to those in adults. It is not uncommon for a child who has a peptic ulcer to present with hematemesis or melena. The preschool child is more likely to present with a complication of the condition than is a school-age child. Unfortunately, children who present with hematemesis or melena and who have ulcers typically have recurrence in the same fashion. If a child presents with melena or occult blood loss, he or she should have an endoscopy done first if the nasogastric aspiration is positive. Ten to 20 percent of upper GI hemorrhages from ulcers are Hemoccult-negative.[3] If the aspirate is negative, then the physician should consider doing radionuclide studies to exclude Meckel's diverticulum of the ileum or other bleeding sites in the small bowel distal to the ligament of Treitz or the colon. Polyps (see Color Plate *ID* and *E*), Crohn's disease, and hemangiomas are among the lesions seen in the area between the ligament of Treitz and the ileocecal valve. Idiopathic gastric ulcers (see Color Plate I*E*) should always be visualized and biopsied in pediatric patients because malignant ulcers have been described in teenagers.

Caustic Ingestion

Caustic ingestions have dramatically decreased in frequency since the development of safety caps on medications and household products. Despite this they occur, but fortunately with decreased frequency. Endoscopy is useful to determine whether any of the ingested substance actually has been swallowed, to assess the extent of the lesions, and to determine whether treatment needs to be started. Hospitalization may be avoided by early endoscopy and likewise treatment initiated rapidly in those established to have caustic burns in the esophagus and stomach. As a rule, patients free of burns on the lips, buccal mucosa, or pharynx rarely have a significant burn in the esophageal or gastric mucosa.[3] Endoscopic examination of the patient with caustic ingestion should proceed only as far as the instrument passes without resistance to reduce the risk of perforation. Typical lesions consist of a white or gray eschar where the caustic agent has made contact with mucosa. Edema is an early sign of caustic ingestion and stricture a late one.

Foreign Body Ingestion

Foreign body ingestion occurs commonly in infants and children. Fortunately, 90 percent of these reach the stomach and pass through it and out the body by allowing intestinal motility to remove them. Endoscopic removal is indicated emergently if the patient experiences symptoms of obstruction or if the object fails to progress through the stomach and GI tract.[3,28] If an object remains in the stomach for 14 to 28 days, it is unlikely to pass. Objects that become embedded in the mucosa usually become bound down by fibrous adhesions (see Color Plate I*F*). Smooth or round objects are unlikely to erode through the mucosa and perforate the stomach. There is a greater risk of perforation with sharp pins, broken glass, and bones. However, we have seen even these objects pass. As long as the patient is asymptomatic we have usually allowed 24 hours before we have removed objects such as these.

Objects obstructing the esophagus must be removed immediately. They usually impact in the upper third of the esophagus.

Esophageal Strictures

Peptic esophageal strictures (see Color Plate II*A*) are becoming increasingly rare in children because during the past decade, our ability to diagnose and treat clinically significant GER has dramatically improved. This has resulted in earlier diagnosis and treatment with fewer cases with late sequelae. We have seen only two new cases of stricture secondary to undiagnosed reflux in the past 5 years. In pediatric patients, most strictures are peptic in origin, with only an occasional one secondary to caustic ingestion or chronic infection with moniliasis. Patients with tracheoesophageal fistulas or esophageal atresia without a fistula have increased risk of developing esophageal strictures. This is because of their increased incidence of reflux. Strictures in these patients are most likely to occur in the lower esophagus or at the region of the anastomosis.

Barrett's esophagus in pediatric patients has a strong association with esophageal strictures. Virtually all cases of esophageal stricture that we have encountered have been associated with Barrett's esophagus.[29] The malignant potential of a Barrett's esophagus in the pediatric patient is real. We have seen one teenager who developed esophageal carcinoma 15 years after the recognition of her stricture and Barrett's esophagus.

Carcinoma of the esophagus is extremely rare; we have seen only one youngster who, in the late teens, developed a malignancy at the gastroesophageal junction.

Endoscopy serves as a guide for initiating the dilation of strictures. It allows for direct visualization and passage of balloon-type dilators in those patients with tight strictures in whom the blind passage of dilators would risk perforation.

Congenital strictures secondary to tracheobronchial remnants are rare, but endoscopy can help in the diagnosis by ruling out the presence of esophagitis.[30]

SCLEROTHERAPY

Injection sclerotherapy has increasingly been used in pediatric patients with portal hypertension and documented variceal bleeding as a means to reduce the frequency of recurrent bleeds (see Color Plate II*B*). Its advantages over shunting procedures are the rapidity with which it can be done, its decreased morbidity, and the lesser incidence of post-sclerotherapy hepatoencephalopathy. Sclerotherapy is not without its own complications: esophageal ulcers, stricture, perforation, mediastinitis, and recurrent bleeding can occur if the endoscopist is not careful with regard to the volume of sclerosant used.

Shunt procedures in children under 10 years of age are associated with an increased risk of post-shunt thrombosis in most surgeons' experience. The younger and smaller the child, the greater the chance that a shunt will become thrombosed. Sclerotherapy should be considered as a first level of therapy in patients with recurrent bleeding from varices.[12–18] It works best in those with extrahepatic portal hypertension. Sclerotherapy can function as a holding procedure until potential spontaneous shunt pathways develop or until a child's vessels are of sufficient size that an adequate surgical shunt can be created.

The number of sessions it takes to obliterate varices varies from as little as one to as many as eight.[12–17] Complications can occur if an excessive amount of sclerosing agent is injected. These complications are similar to those seen in adults. In series in which individuals have used excessive amounts of sclerosant, almost 50 percent of the patients have developed complications; ulceration has occurred in nearly half and hemorrhage in an equivalent number. Strictures have been recorded in 10 to 15 percent of pediatric patients following sclerotherapy. The role of sclerotherapy for children with liver disease is not well defined. Patients with liver disease with clotting disorders may not receive significant benefit from sclerotherapy, although we have shown a decreased requirement for blood transfusions. Sclerotherapy may be done either under general anesthesia with protection of the airway or with the use of sedation.[13,18] Either rigid or flexible instruments can be used. In almost all instances we have been able to do this procedure without the need for an operating room and an anesthesiologist. Our results indicate that the risk of complications is reduced if the volume of sclerosant does not exceed 4 to 5 ml per session. Sclerotherapy is extremely useful for the patient with extrahepatic portal hypertension, and in most of these instances it has stopped the bleeding. It is less useful for individuals bleeding from varices that have developed secondary to intrahepatic disease.

ENDOSCOPIC RETROGRADE CHOLANGIOPANCREATOGRAPHY

The indications for ERCP are recurrent, unexplained attacks of pancreatitis, unexplained obstructive jaundice, and the need to clarify pancreatic ductal anatomy prior to operation. Because relatively few children meet the indication for the procedure, experience with ERCP is limited.[7,8,31,32] In adults, alcohol abuse and choledocholithiasis are the primary causes of pancreatitis. In children the four leading causes are medications, trauma, infections, and pancreatic ductal abnormalities. In one recent series, nearly one-third of pediatric patients who underwent ERCP were found to have normal examinations.[8] More careful screening of this group of patients might have prevented the unnecessary procedures. Patients with abdominal pain with associated abnormalities in amylase, lipase, alkaline phosphatase, and liver function tests should be considered for ERCP. Patients with recurrent attacks of abdominal pain, in which liver and pancreatic blood tests are normal, are not likely candidates.

ERCP has been reported by one group as a means of differentiating biliary atresia from neonatal hepatitis.[7] Success of the procedure occurred in more than 85 percent of cases. Unfortunately, this study did not compare the results of diagnosis with those obtained by more conventional studies. Morbidity occurred in 10 to 15 percent of the patients secondary to overdose with sedation or compression of the trachea by the endoscope.[7]

A side-viewing pediatric duodenoscope for cannulation of the ampulla (see Color Plate II*C*) is an expensive piece of equipment and would not be as valuable if it were used only for an occasional infant. Only centers that see large numbers of infants with unexplained cholestatic liver disease should consider this modality of diagnosis, because diagnosis may be made rapidly with the use of radionuclide scan, sonography, and liver biopsy. Since diagnosis of biliary atresia by ERCP depends on failure to visualize the common duct and the ability to visualize the pancreatic duct, this diagnosis may be fraught with technical difficulties. Because biliary atresia is a condition in which 80 percent of the cases may be diagnosed by history, physical examination, and presence of acholic stools, relatively few patients truly require ERCP to diagnose it.[33] Although investigators have reported success in performing the procedure using intravenous sedation, some indicate that general anesthesia works more satisfactorily because breathing may be controlled.

Complications from this procedure are cholangitis and pancreatitis and occur in fewer than 3 percent of adults. Complication rates in children are based on small numbers of patients, but in the one large series of infants, respiratory depression, probably due to oversedation and tracheal compression, was the most common complication.[7]

PERCUTANEOUS ENDOSCOPIC GASTROSTOMY

An increasing number of pediatric patients are undergoing percutaneous endoscopic gastrostomy (PEG). Two different techniques are now widely used: the classic "pull," in which the "bumpered" gastrostomy tube is introduced through the mouth and pulled out through the abdominal wall site, and the "introducer," using "peel-away" type catheters, in which a balloon catheter is introduced directly through the abdominal incision.[34] Seven basic steps are necessary to place a percutaneous gastrostomy:

1. The patients must be sedated adequately and not become agitated when the stomach is distended.
2. Following sedation, the patient is placed in the supine, not in the left lateral decubitus, position; the endoscope is then advanced into the hypopharynx and down the esophagus to just below the cardioesophageal junction.
3. The stomach is then insufflated with air and the tip of the endoscope advanced to the position on the abdominal wall where the light of the endoscope shines through most brightly.
4. The assistant palpates the area so that the endoscopist can recognize the finger's imprint in an area on the anterior wall of the stomach where the body joins the gastric antrum and marks this spot with indelible ink.
5. The skin is then aseptically scrubbed, and a local anesthetic agent is infiltrated, using 1 percent lidocaine down through the subcutaneous tissue.
6. A ¼-inch stab wound is made at this site with a surgical blade.
7. The stomach is then insufflated and the Venocath (14 to 16 gauge) is thrust through the incision into the stomach.

At this point, the subsequent steps vary according to the available kit and technique chosen.

Pull Technique

1. The endoscopist passes a snare through the endoscope and opens its end as the assistant threads the soft tip of a guide wire through the catheter.
2. The endoscopist then snares the tip of the wire and withdraws the endoscope, with the snare in place, under visual control.
3. The guide wire is now recovered through the patient's mouth and advanced so that there is sufficient length to mount the entire gastrostomy tube into the wire, tapered (proximal) end first.
4. The gastrostomy tube is then lubricated and passed back through the pharynx into the esophagus and stomach and pulled out the abdominal wall opening. The "bumper" on the distal end of the gastrostomy tube keeps it from being dislodged and against the gastric mucosa. The guide wire is withdrawn.
5. The endoscope is passed into the stomach, and the position of the catheter and its "bumper" is documented.

In the second technique, a short guide wire is passed through the catheter, which is withdrawn, and several dilators of increasing diameter are passed through the tract until the desired size of the tube is reached. The endoscopist makes sure that the dilators penetrate the gastric lumen and that the wire remains in place. The gastrostomy tube is then passed and the "peel-away" introducer is withdrawn. The balloon of the catheter is then inflated and the gastrostomy tube secured.

There are no studies comparing the two techniques in children; in our experience, this latter procedure is more difficult in small infants. The potential for complications is higher owing to the use of dilators to increase the tract site of the introducer, the pressure and forceful manipulation on the abdominal wall, and the increased number of steps required prior to the passage of the tube, which add to the possibilities of leakage into the peritoneal cavity or even damage to adjacent structures.

The indications and goals should be clear: (1) to feed patients who are unable to swallow until they can resume oral feedings; (2) to improve or maintain nutritional status in neurologically impaired children; and (3) to reduce hospitalization in acute care centers and facilitate management either at home or in secondary care institutions in patients who are poor surgical risks, or when the need of antireflux procedure concomitant with the feeding gastrostomy is not apparent.

The indication for long-term feeding gastrostomy does not necessarily implicate the need for an antireflux procedure.[35-37] Even in neurologically impaired children with a history suggestive of, or respiratory complications from, GER, the placement of an endoscopic percutaneous gastrostomy may be done, and the risk of aspiration decreased by placing the actual feeding tube beyond the pylorus and distal to the angle of Treitz.

A gastric lumen or separate port may be used for drainage of gastric contents, if necessary; however, we believe that, in individuals with significant reflux, a surgically placed gastrostomy tube plus an antireflux procedure may be the best option.

The sedation required does not differ from that used in routine diagnostic endoscopy, but a trained assistant besides the endoscopy nurse is needed to carry out the various steps. The patient's anterior abdominal wall should be prepared surgically, and he or she should receive antibiotics perioperatively.

Complications (Table 3) are minimized when all the steps are followed for identifying the ideal site on the abdominal wall and in the stomach with the use of the endoscope's light and the indentation of the anterior wall for both the endoscopist and assistant. The intensity of the light in the videoendoscopes may not be great enough to be identifiable through the abdominal wall, but both the endoscopist and the assistant can simultaneously identify the ideal site on the screen with palpation.

Either of the techniques requires verification of hemostasis and the proper position of the tube. We find it useful to use surgical glue instead of sutures to secure the gastrostomy tube to the outer skin, because it seems more comfortable for the patients. Excessive pressure on the balloon or the "bumper" against the abdominal wall may cause necrosis of the different layers involved and should be avoided.

The most frequent complication of PEG is site infection; its incidence can be reduced by strict aseptic technique, perioperative antibiotics, and daily cleaning and changing of the dressing.[38-42]

A variety of complications and deaths have been reported in both children and adults with PEG placement. Most of them are from infections of the abdominal wall or peritoneum, fistulous tracts between the stomach and colon, puncture of adjacent organs or structures within the abdomen or the chest, and complications inherent to improper feeding techniques or tube migration.

In our experience, previous abdominal surgeries do not constitute a formal contraindication to the procedure, but the endoscopist should always consider the potential anatomic variations and the presence of adhesions as possible causes of complications.

The materials used to manufacture the tubes in the different commercially available kits are usually Silastic or polyurethane, ensuring prolonged tube life. However, the need for changing and replacing the tubes still exists. We have found that those tubes that cannot be pulled out because of the "bumper" may be cut at the skin level and the tube allowed to pass in the stool by gastric and intestinal transit. The recommendation from the manufacturer, however, is to remove them endoscopically.

CONTRAINDICATIONS TO ENDOSCOPY

There are few absolute contraindications to upper GI endoscopy in infants and children. They include shock, perforated hollow viscus, and cervical spine injury. Coma is not a contraindication unless the patient is combative. Most patients in coma may undergo endoscopy without the use of any sedation or anesthetics. If the patient is on a ventilator and is combative, small amounts of intravenous sedation may be used. Severe coagulopathy is not a contraindication to endoscopy, although it is to biopsy. The patient must be sedated to the point of not struggling to reduce the risk of traumatic injury by the endoscope and to reduce the risk of intracerebral hemorrhage. Correction of the coagulation defect should be considered prior to endoscopy if indicated.

Upper intestinal endoscopy should not be performed in an uncooperative patient. The most common reason for inadequate examination is incomplete sedation. Lack of experience in sedating infants and children is the most common reason for incomplete sedation. Sedation, if done carefully, may take 15 to 30 minutes. Patients who are receiving one or more medications that affect hepatic metabolism of drugs often require larger doses of medication.

TABLE 3
Complications in Upper Intestinal Fiberoptic Endoscopy in Children

	Patients Examined	Procedures	Complications	Phlebitis	Stridor
Gleason	25	27	0	0	0
Ament	142	163	3	2	0
Liebman	1	1	0	0	0
Graham	52	52	2	0	2
Akasaka	25	25	0	0	0
Kohli	63	63	0	0	0
Prolla	47	47	0	0	0
TOTAL	355	378	5	2	2

Endoscopy is not contraindicated in infants and children with congenital heart disease or with prosthetic devices such as central venous catheters, heart valves, and shunt for hydrocephalus. The risk of bacteremia is low. Only one study has been done in children, and it showed a 2 percent incidence of bacteremia. Data are not available on the routine use of prophylactic antibiotics. The most conservative approach would be to use prophylactic antibiotics as recommended by the American Heart Association to prevent infective endocarditis. This regimen could be used for others with prosthetic devices.

INSTRUMENTS AND TECHNIQUES FOR PERFORMING UPPER INTESTINAL ENDOSCOPY

Currently available instruments make an upper intestinal endoscopy possible in newborn infants. Infants between 1,500 and 2,500 g may undergo endoscopy effectively if instruments such as the Olympus OESGIF-XP10 or the Fujinon UGI-RU are used. The physical characteristics of these endoscopes for examination of the upper GI tract are listed in Table 4. Instruments that have an outer diameter of less than 10 mm can be passed without difficulty in all infants less than 2 years of age. Adequate examination of the esophagus, stomach, and duodenum can be done with any of these instruments. Obviously, the larger the patient, the larger is the diameter of the instrument that can be used. It is seldom necessary for pediatricians to use instruments with a diameter greater than 9.8 mm. The larger the instrument that is used, the greater the chance of tracheal compression. In children older than 10 years of age, any instrument 9 mm and larger would be satisfactory. Obviously a larger instrument will improve the visualization because of the increased number of fiber bundles carrying light. Therefore, it is uncommon to use anything smaller than 9.8 mm in this group. Virtually all of the procedures can be done with intravenous sedation. In the neonate, endoscopic examination can often be performed without the use of any sedation. This is often the most effective way to do procedures in the neonate. If intravenous sedation is used, the dosage must be slowly and carefully titrated to avoid respiratory depression. Tracheal compression should not be a problem in the hands of most experienced endoscopists, if the infant is sedated and restrained properly and the endoscopist is careful in the proper choice and manipulation of the instrument. It is preferable to examine the neonate with an endoscope of less than 9 mm in diameter. Endoscopy in the neonate and the young infant requires careful nursing assistance to bundle and fix the position of the infant and to help with monitoring and suction. All infants and children should have pulse oximeters attached during and after the procedures. This instrument helps the endoscopist monitor the effects of sedation before the procedure and the effects of the passage of the endoscope during the procedure. We believe the pulse oximeter should be placed before the procedure is begun. Once it is in place, sedation should be given following the placement of a secure line for intravenous medication. Initially we provide 0.15 mg per kilogram of midazolam (Versed) and repeat the dose 2 minutes after the first has been infused. Following the second dose of midazolam, 1 mg per kilogram of meperidine is infused. Two minutes after its infusion and if the patient's vital signs have remained stable, a second dose may be given, provided that the patient shows no signs of desaturation or abnormally low respiratory rate. Each dose of sedative is followed 2 minutes later by measurement of the patient's vital signs. As long as the

TABLE 4
Physical Characteristic of Upper Intestinal Endoscopes

Instrument (Manufacturer)	Length (cm)	Diameter (mm)	Field of View (Degrees)	Biopsy Channel Diameter (mm)
UGI-RU (Fujinon)	110.0	6.40	105	2.7
OES, GIF-XP10 (Olympus)	103.0	7.90	100	2.0
UGI-RB (Fujinon)	110.0	7.90	105	2.7
OES, GIF-P10 (Olympus)	103.0	9.00	100	2.0
UGI-FP2 (Fujinon)	110.0	9.50	105	2.7
FG-28B (Pentax)	110.0	9.50	93	2.5
OES, GIF-XQ10 (Olympus)	103.0	9.80	100	2.8
AG-RF (ACMI)	108.0	9.80	90	2.5
OES, GIF-Q10 (Olympus)	103.0	11.00	120	2.8
UGI-F2 (Fujinon)	110.0	11.00	105	2.8
FG-34JA (Pentax)	110.0	11.50	105	3.5
OES, GIF-IT10 (Olympus)	103.0	12.60	100	3.7

patient's saturation remains above 90 percent, further doses of medication are given if necessary. Once the patient is asleep and does not respond adversely to testing with the examiner's finger in the oral pharynx, the procedure is begun. The patient is turned on his or her side and wrapped or restrained.

Many endoscopists darken the endoscopy suite to improve visualization. We believe this is a poor practice, because the skin color of the infant or child should be carefully monitored. Some endoscopists feel more comfortable examining children under 2 years of age under general anesthesia. It then becomes the responsibility of the anesthesiologist to monitor the patient. Obviously, the use of an anesthesiologist and his or her equipment may greatly increase the cost of the procedure and does not necessarily lower the risk of complications.

Before any endoscopic procedure and, of course, depending on the age of the youngster, we try to explain in simple terms what type of test he or she is going to have. When school-age children are brought to the endoscopy suite, we show them the equipment and let them look through the endoscopes before we proceed with their sedation. We typically let the parents in the endoscopy suite while sedating their children, because it frequently alleviates the children's anxiety.

Infants less than 6 months of age should be fasted for a minimum of 4 hours before the procedure is done. After 6 months of age at least 6 to 8 hours of fasting should be done. If there is a question as to when the patient last ate or drank, a nasogastric tube should be passed into the stomach and the contents aspirated. The endoscopist should inquire about teeth and examine the oral cavity before beginning the procedure to check for loose teeth. If they are discovered, they may be removed before the procedure. This is an uncommon occurrence in the pediatric patient, and we have found only a handful of children whose teeth have become dislodged by the procedure. Some pediatric and adult endoscopists routinely anesthetize the throats of children to be examined with a topical agent. We normally do not do this because it has not improved our endoscopy success rate. Most children become rather agitated when they have lost their ability to swallow.

If the patient is not fully sedated, promethazine is given at a dose of 0.5 mg per kilogram to a maximum of 50 mg. We wait 5 minutes after the administration of the last medication before beginning the procedure. The patient is then placed in the left lateral decubitus position, and a bite block is placed in the mouth if the patient has teeth. This is to protect the instrument from the patient's teeth. If the patient is agitated with the passage of the instrument and tracheal compression is not present, further sedation may be given by administering another 0.5 to 1 mg of meperidine. Agitation may be a sign of hypoxia or gastric distention. The physician doing the procedure must assess this at all times. The use of the pulse oximeter has facilitated such assessment. Naloxone, with attached needle and syringe, should always be available in the endoscopy suite within reach of the endoscopist in case respiratory depression develops. Other forms of sedation have been used, including ketamine hydrochloride, 2 to 3 mg per kilogram intravenously, but this is considered an anesthetic agent and is administered by either an intensive care specialist or an anesthesiologist.

TECHNIQUE OF PASSING AN ENDOSCOPE

The endoscope may be passed down the pharynx in one of two ways: (1) with the mouthpiece in place and using the index finger as a guide or (2) under direct vision with the instrument being advanced while the endoscopist visualizes the oropharynx, glottis, and cricopharyngeal sphincter for the esophageal lumen through the endoscope. In either method, the endoscope must be kept in the midline and out of the pyriform sinuses. An instrument should never be advanced using force. Resistance to passage of the instrument and presence of light in the lateral neck warrant withdrawal and attempted repassage of the instrument. Once the tip of the endoscope has passed the upper esophageal sphincter, it should be advanced only under direct vision and only with enough air and insufflation to permit visualization. Once the tip is in the stomach, any fluid found should be aspirated. Folds should then be flattened and the fundus and antrum carefully inspected by forward viewing. The endoscope should then be advanced through the antrum to the pylorus. The pyloric channel and duodenal bulb should be viewed first from the outside. The instrument should be passed into the bulb and the tip turned down and to the right or clockwise into the second part of the duodenum. It is best to try to visualize the duodenal bulb while inserting as well as while withdrawing the instrument because trauma may alter its structure. Visualization of the duodenum may be accomplished with slow withdrawal of the scope, rotating its tip and torquing the shaft from side to side. The stomach should be evaluated on both entry and exit by slow withdrawal and rotation of the tip. Careful inspection of the cardia is done by retroflexing the instrument on itself and rotating it. Before the endoscope is removed, excessive air and fluid are suctioned from the stomach. Description of the findings should be objective and succinct.

Endoscopic findings should be confirmed histologically. The gross mucosal appearance may be a poor predictor of histologic change in the esophagus, stomach, or duodenum.[21] Erythema, paleness, and a lack of vascular pattern in the mucosa do not necessarily mean that inflammatory changes will be seen when biopsies are taken. Tissue that looks completely normal may have microscopic changes; therefore, in patients in whom esophagitis, gastritis, or duodenitis is suspected, biopsies should be performed. All gastric ulcers should be biopsied if there is no explanation for them, because carcinoma can occur in teenage children. Biopsy specimens from these ulcers should be obtained from the four quadrants of the ulcer and from the mucosa adjacent to the crater. Gastric biopsies should be taken if one is going to interpret the findings seen endoscopically. In the duodenum, ulcers need not be biopsied because they are not malignant. As in the stomach, duodenal erosion and so-called duodenitis should be biopsied to confirm the presence of inflammatory change. In the immunocompromised patient, opportunistic infections can produce ulcerous erosions. Patients with unexplained gastritis in biopsies of the antral mucosa should have a culture for *Campylobacter pylori*. Small intestinal biopsies taken under direct vision endoscopically can replace those taken by peroral small intestinal biopsy instruments. Biopsies taken through endoscopes are of sufficient size to be used diagnostically.[44,45] Their advantage is that they do not require radiation exposure. During the past 3 years, we have virtually stopped peroral small intestinal biopsies both because of parental concern about the risk of radiation and in order to stop our own exposure. Furthermore, we are almost 100 percent sure of obtaining biopsies endoscopically. Interpretation of such biopsies is not difficult if they are appropriately mounted and serially sectioned.

As a general rule, foreign bodies should be removed under general anesthesia. This reduces the risk of tracheal aspiration during withdrawal of the instrument. Whenever possible, the endoscopist should try to obtain an object similar to the foreign body and rehearse the maneuver to choose the most appropriate instrument and evaluate potential risks. Once the foreign body has been secured in a retrieval instrument, it is drawn up tightly to the end of the endoscope. The endoscope and object are then slowly withdrawn. Continued visualization of the object through the endoscope ensures that the object does not come loose. Care must be taken not to tear the esophagus if sharp objects are being removed. An overtube or rubber membrane attached to the endoscope may help prevent any laceration of the esophageal mucosa on retrieval. Large objects should either be broken up or removed surgically. No object should be forced up through the esophagus.

COMPLICATIONS

Upper intestinal endoscopy in children is a safe procedure. The complication rate is at most less than 2 percent.[1-5,18,19,44-50] Although the complication rate is higher than that reported in adults, most of the reported complications are minor and have been due to phlebitis from intravenous sedation. Probably this complication will all but disappear with the change from diazepam to midazolam. Transient respiratory arrest due to oversedation is perhaps the most common complication experienced. This, however, should be avoidable in most situations by careful monitoring and should be easily reversible with the use of naloxone. Bronchial spasm occurs in rare cases secondary to general anesthetics and from the use of any of the sedative agents. Complications secondary to the procedures themselves are extremely rare. Perforation, transient bleeding from an aspiration site, aspiration, retropharyngeal hematoma, and loosened or broken teeth have rarely been reported in children but have been seen in adults. Perforations have been recorded in fewer than 0.1 percent of adults and virtually a similar percentage of children. Bleeding secondary to biopsies or dislodged clot material is also seen in fewer than 1 percent of patients. Recognized aspiration occurs in fewer than 0.1 percent of patients. The risk of endoscopic procedures is comparatively low. Complications occur only when patients are inadequately sedated or oversedated and respond poorly to general anesthesia.[50] The potential for gathering information almost always outweighs the risks when doing endoscopic procedures in children.

VIDEO-ENDOSCOPY

The greatest advance in endoscopy in recent years has been the development of video-endoscopy (see Color Plate II*D*). The three essential components of an electronic video-endoscopy system are the endoscope with its charged couple device, the video processor, and a television monitor. Many components can be coupled to the basic system, including a keyboard to provide written information at the margin of the video display, a videotape deck, and a floppy disc system or an optical disc for storing images.

Video-endoscopy systems offer the ability to freeze frames for instant photographs; their quality is always superior. Whereas endoscopic television systems for use with fiberscopes represent an expense over and above that of the basic endoscope and light source, television and endoscopy are combined in video-endoscopy. Although television cameras for use with fiberscopes provide high-quality images, these do not approach the excellence of video-endoscopic images.

There are limitations of video-endoscopes. The light spectrum for good imaging has to be well adjusted. Distortions occur in mucosal appearance if illumination is too bright or too low. The focal range of the video-endoscope is not as good as that with a fiberoptic scope. The ability to distinguish small detail with a video-endoscope is slightly less than with fiberoptic instruments.

Video-endoscopy equipment is more cumbersome than fiberoptic systems and is not as portable because of its size. This makes it less easy to move to critical care areas and radiology suites. However, video-endoscopy is far superior to fiberoptic endoscopy for storage and retrieval of endoscopic data as well as for teaching purposes.[51]

REFERENCES

1. Cremer M, Peeters JP, Emonts P, Rodesch P, Cadranel S. Fiberendoscopy of the gastrointestinal tract in children. Experience with newly designed fiberscopes. Endoscopy 1974; 6:186–189.
2. Gleason WA, Tedesco FJ, Keating JP, Goldstein PD. Fiberoptic gastrointestinal endoscopy in infants and children. J Pediatr 1974; 85:810–813.
3. Ament ME, Christie DL. Upper gastrointestinal fiberoptic endoscopy in pediatric patients. Gastroenterology 1977; 72:1244–1248.
4. Liebman WM, Thaler MM, Bujanover Y. Endoscopic evaluation of upper gastrointestinal bleeding in the newborn. Am J Gastroenterol 1978; 69:697–698.
5. Graham DY, Klish WJ, Ferry GD, Sabel JS. Value of fiberoptic gastrointestinal endoscopy of infants and children. South Med J 1978; 71: 558–560.
6. Graham DY, Klish WJ, Ferry GD, Holcome BB. Endoscopy under gnotobiotic conditions. Gastrointest Endosc 1978; 24:298–299.
7. Guelrud M, Jaen D, Torres P, Jufica C, Mendoza S, Rivero E, Romer H, Avila B, Viera L. Endoscopic cholangiopancreatography in the infant: evaluation of a new prototype pediatric duodenoscope. Gastrointest Endosc 1987; 33:48.
8. Allendorph M, Werlin SL, Geenen JE, Hogan WJ, Venu RP, Stewart ET, Blank EL. Endoscopic retrograde cholangiopancreatography in children. J Pediatr 1987; 110:206–211.
9. Schwartz SE, Rowden DR, Dudgeon DL. Antral mucosal diaphragm. Gastrointest Endosc 1977; 24:33–34.
10. Fleisher D. Endoscopic therapy of upper gastrointestinal tract bleeding. Gastroenterology 1986; 90:217–224.
11. Tedesco FJ. Endoscopic therapy for vascular lesions: new challenges. J Pediatr Gastroenterol Nutr 1988; 7:321–322.

12. Noronha PA, Leist MH. Endoscopic laser therapy for gastrointestinal bleeding from congenital vascular lesions. J Pediatr Gastroenterol Nutr 1988; 7:375–378.
13. Dall'Oglio L, Bagolan P, Ferro F, Ponticelli A, Cadranel S, Rivosecchi M. Endoscopic injection sclerosis of oesophageal varices in children—indications and techniques. Endoscopy 1984; 16:98–100.
14. Hassall E, Ament ME, Berquist WE. Endoscopic sclerotherapy of esophageal varices in childhood. Gastrointest Endosc 1985; 31:130(21A).
15. Howard ER, Stamatokis JD. Management of oesophageal varices in children by injection. In: Westaby D, MacDougall RRD, Williams R, eds. Variceal bleeding. London: Pitman Books, 1982: 165.
16. Paquet KJ. Endoscopic paravasal injection of sclerosing agents in children with bleeding oesophageal varices. In: Westaby D, MacDougall BRD, Williams R, eds. Variceal bleeding. London: Pitman Books, 1982: 173.
17. Donovan TJ, Ward M, Shepherd RW. Evaluation of endoscopic sclerotherapy of esophageal varices in children. J Pediatr Gastroenterol Nutr 1986; 5:696–700.
18. Stamatakis JD, Howard ER, Psaharopoulos HT. Injection sclerotherapy for esophageal varices in children. Br J Surg 1982; 69:74–75.
19. Kohli Y, Fuse Y, Kodawa T, et al. Upper gastrointestinal endoscopy in pediatric patients. Gastroenterol Endosc 1981; 23:1294–1301.
20. Prolla JC, Diehl AS, Benvenuti GA, Loguercio SV, Magalhaes DS, Silveira TR. Upper gastrointestinal fiberoptic endoscopy in pediatric patients. Gastrointest Endosc 1983; 29:279–281.
21. Apley J. The child with abdominal pains. 2nd ed. Oxford: Blackwell Scientific Publications, 1975.
22. Oderda G, Forni M, Farina L, Dell'Olio D, Ansaldi N. Duodenitis in children: clinical endoscopic and pathological aspects. Gastrointest Endosc 1987; 33:366–369.
23. Black DD, Haggitt RC, Whitington PF. Gastroduodenal endoscopic-histologic correlation in pediatric patients. J Pediatr Gastroenterol Nutr 1988; 7:353–358.
24. Biller JA, Winter HS, Grand RJ, et al. Are endoscopic changes predictive of histologic changes in children? J Pediatr 1983; 103:215–218
25. Lanza FL. A double blind study of prophylactic effect of misoprostol on lesions of gastric and duodenal mucosa induced by oral administration of tolmetin in healthy subjects. Dig Dis Sci 1986; 31:131S.
26. Sucralfate for peptic ulcer—a reappraisal. Med Let Drugs Therap 1984; 26:43–45.
27. Murphy MS, Eastham EJ. Peptic ulcer disease in childhood. Long-term prognosis. J Pediatr Gastroenterol Nutr 1987; 6:721–724.
28. Christie DL, Ament ME. Removal of foreign bodies from the esophagus and stomach with flexible fiberoptic panendoscopes. Pediatrics 1976; 57:931–934.
29. Hassall E, Weinstein W, Ament ME. Barrett's esophagus in childhood. Gastroenterology 1985; 89:1331–1337.
30. Shoshany G, Bar Maor JA. Congenital stenosis of the esophagus due to tracheo-bronchial remnants: a missed diagnosis. J Pediatr Gastroenterol Nutr 1986; 5:977–979.
31. Waye JD. Endoscopic retrograde cholangiopancreatography in the infant. Am J Gastroenterol 1976; 65:461–463.
32. Blustein PK, Gaskin K, Filler R, et al. Endoscopic retrograde cholangiopancreatography in pancreatitis in children and adolescents. Pediatrics 1981; 68:387–393.
33. Ament ME. Is endoscopic cholangioprancreatography needed for the jaundiced infant? (Editorial) Gastrointest Endosc 1987; 33:49–50.
34. Deitel M, et al. Percutaneous endoscopic gastrostomy by the "pull" and "introducer" methods. Can J Surg 1988; 31:102–109.
35. Towkin RB, et al. Percutaneous gastrostomy and percutaneous gastrojejunostomy in children: antegrade approach. Radiology 1988; 168: 473–476.
36. Larson DE, et al. Percutaneous endoscopic gastrostomy: indications, success, complications and mortality in 314 consecutive patients. Gastroenterology 1987; 93:48–52.
37. Hashiba K. Endoscopic gastrostomy. Endoscopy 1987; 1(suppl):23–24.
38. Chobanian SJ. Persistent pneumoperitoneum following percutaneous endoscopic gastrostomy. (Letter to Editor) Gastrointest Endosc 1987; 33:462–463.
39. Fernandez ET, et al. Late presentation of gastrocolic fistula after percutaneous gastrostomy. (Letter to Editor) Gastrointest Endosc 1988; 34:308–309.
40. Korula J, et al. Necrotizing fascitis and percutaneous endoscopic gastrostomy. Gastrointest Endosc 1987; 33:335–336.
41. Shaldman RW, et al. Percutaneous endoscopic gastrostomy feeding tube migration and impaction in the abdominal wall. (Letter to Editor) Gastrointest Endosc 1988; 34:367–368.
42. Cappell NJ. Esophageal bleeding after percutaneous endoscopic gastrostomy. J Clin Gastroenterol 1988; 10:383–385.
43. Mago H, Chen Chao-Long, Wesson DE, Filler RM. Incisionless gastrostomy for nutritional support. J Pediatr Gastroenterol Nutr 1986; 5:66–69.
44. Graham MF, Wood R, Halpin TC. Endoscopic small bowel biopsy in children with a modified multipurpose biopsy tube. Gastrointest Endosc 1980; 26:36–37.
45. Hart MH, Vanderhoof JA, Antonson DL. Failure of blind small bowel biopsy in the diagnosis of intestinal lymphangiectasia. J Pediatr Gastroenterol Nutr 1987; 6:803–805.
46. Ament ME. Prospective study of risks of complication in 6,424 procedures in pediatric gastroenterology. Pediatr Res 1981; 15:524.
47. Tolia V, Fleming S. Spectrum of upper endoscopy findings in pediatric population. Gastrointest Endosc 1986; 32:150.
48. Akasaka Y, Misaka F, Miyaoka T, Nakajima M, Kawai K. Endoscopy in pediatric patients with upper gastrointestinal bleeding. Gastrointest Endosc 1977; 23:199–200.
49. Essenfeld-Sekler E, Paez CV, Toledano A, Congedo E, Guelrud M, Roa E. Bleeding lymphoid hyperplasia of the small bowel in an adolescent diagnosed by intraoperative endoscopy. Gastrointest Endosc 1979; 25:21–22.
50. Figueroa-Colon R, Gruen JE. Randomized study of premedication for esophagogastroduodenoscopy in children and adolescents. J Pediatr Gastroenterol Nutr 1988; 7:359–366.
51. Sivak MV. Videoendoscopy. In: Cotton PB, Tytgat GNJ, Williams CB, eds. Annual of gastrointestinal endoscopy. London: Gower Academy Journal; 1988: 115.

PART 2

Lower Endoscopy

Julie E. Bines, M.B.B.S.
Harland S. Winter, M.D.

Until the last decade diagnostic evaluation of the colon in childhood was limited to information obtained via rigid proctosigmoidoscopy and barium enema.[1] With improved technical expertise and experience, flexible fiberoptic colonoscopy can be performed safely and effectively using intravenous sedation in almost all infants and children.[2–6] Colonoscopy offers the advantage of allowing direct visualization of the colonic mucosa combined with the ability to obtain tissue for histologic assessment. It also enables therapeutic interventions such as polypectomy and electrocautery of vascular lesions.

INDICATIONS

Rectal bleeding is the most common indication for colonoscopy in infants and children[2] (Table 1). Polyps of the large bowel are the major cause.[2,3] Most polyps in children are juvenile polyps, which frequently spontaneously autoamputate, resulting in brisk, self-limited bleeding.[7,8] Based on studies using sigmoidoscopy and barium enema, 90 percent of juvenile polyps were thought to be solitary[8–10]; however, with the improved diagnostic yield of colonoscopy, 58 percent of children are found to have more than one juvenile polyp.[11] Although juvenile polyps do not undergo malignant transformation, adenomatous polyps have been reported in children.[2,11] A familial polyposis syndrome should be considered in patients with more than five colonic polyps and can be confirmed by histologic assessment of the polyps.[12] Therefore, for diagnostic, management, and prognostic reasons, histology should be obtained from all colonic lesions either by grasp biopsy or polypectomy.[2,11]

TABLE 1
Indications for Colonoscopy

1. Unexplained gastrointestinal bleeding
   a. Rectal bleeding
   b. Melena of unknown origin
   c. Fecal occult blood
2. Chronic inflammatory bowel disease
   a. Diagnosis
   b. Management
      1) Extent and severity
      2) Preoperative assessment
   c. Surveillance for colorectal cancer
3. Chronic diarrhea of uncertain etiology
4. Unexplained severe abdominal pain
5. Evaluation of an abnormality seen on barium enema
6. Family history of a familial polyposis syndrome
7. Cancer surveillance
   a. Ulcerative colitis
   b. Polyposis syndrome
   c. Adenomatous or mixed polyp
8. Intraoperative localization of a lesion that cannot be detected on external inspection or palpation
   a. Bleeding site
   b. Polypectomy site
9. Therapeutic
   a. Colonoscopic polypectomy
   b. Treatment of bleeding—angiodysplasia, polypectomy site
   c. Removal of foreign body
   d. Decompression of acute toxic megacolon or colonic volvulus
   e. Balloon dilation of stenotic lesions

Another potential cause of rectal bleeding in children is nodular lymphoid hyperplasia. Patients are usually not chronically ill, are not anemic, and have normal sedimentation rates. Nodular lymphoid hyperplasia has been observed in over 50 percent of children investigated with air-contrast barium enema and colonoscopy.[13] It is the only abnormality noted in one-third of the infants investigated for hematochezia.[14] Reports of direct observation of bleeding from lymphoid nodules adds strength to an underlying impression that these lesions can cause rectal bleeding in some infants.[15]

Vascular lesions, common in older adults, are rare in children. Nevertheless, colonoscopy remains a sensitive method of detecting vascular malformations of the colon.[16] Syndromes associated with vascular malformations of the gastrointestinal tract and rectal bleeding include Rendu-Osler-Weber syndrome, blue rubber bleb syndrome, dyschondroplasia (Maffucci's syndrome), sclerodactyly and telangiectasia (CRST) syndrome, Turner's syndrome, and pseudoxanthoma elasticum.[17–19] Bleeding angiodysplastic lesions can be electrocauterized at colonoscopy, providing significant therapeutic benefit.[16,20]

The sequence of investigation in patients presenting with rectal bleeding depends on the clinical pattern, nature, and activity of blood loss. In infants and young children an upper gastrointestinal source of bleeding is a common cause of rectal bleeding. It should always be considered prior to diagnostic testing directed at the colon. The main value of colonoscopy in the pediatric population is to differentiate an inflammatory process (e.g., infectious or idiopathic colitis or vasculitis) from a focal lesion (e.g., polyps, hemorrhage). For this reason, colonoscopy may be the initial procedure of choice for the diagnosis of acute or recurrent mild to moderate rectal bleeding. In patients with active moderate to severe bleeding, radionuclide scanning using ^{99m}Tc sulfur colloid or autologous labeled red blood cells may detect blood loss when the rate is greater than 0.1 ml per minute.[21] Since the interpretation of these scans may be difficult owing to reactive hyperemia following colonoscopy or obscured by barium, they should be considered as an initial investigation in patients with significant active bleeding.[5] At the same time the bowel can be prepared for colonoscopy using an oral lavage solution (Golytely: Braintree Laboratories, Braintree, MA). If no cause can be found on radionuclide scanning, air contrast enema, or colonoscopy, and the patient continues to have significant rectal bleeding, intraoperative enterocolonoscopy may be required.

Occult gastrointestinal blood loss with iron deficiency anemia can be caused from a slow, persistent, or intermittent ooze from a site anywhere in the upper or lower gastrointestinal tract. Possible colonic lesions include polyps, vascular malformations, nodular lymphoid hyperplasia, chronic inflammatory bowel disease, or even adenocarcinoma in a patient with a familial polyposis syndrome or ulcerative colitis. A third of children with symptomatic juvenile polyps have a microcytic hypochromic anemia.[11] Colonoscopy identified significant pathologic lesions in 30 percent of adults with anemia and melena who have no cause found on upper and lower barium studies and gastroduodenoscopy.[22]

Because most familial polyposis syndromes are inherited as an autosomal dominant trait, a high index of suspicion must exist for the offspring of affected parents.[12] Early diagnosis may avoid gastrointestinal blood loss, intussusception, and carcinoma.[12] Extracolonic manifestations such as osteomas, skin lesions, and retinal changes may suggest Gardner's syndrome; however, colonoscopy with biopsy is essential.[12] Once the diagnosis is established, surveillance colonoscopy should be routinely performed in those patients with syndromes associated with adenomatous polyps, such as familial polyposis coli and Gardner's syndrome.

In patients with inflammatory bowel disease, colonoscopy with biopsy can not only establish the diagnosis, but it also can help define the extent and severity of colitis and aid in the assessment of complications of the disease. Biopsies greatly enhance the diagnostic yield of colonoscopy by identifying areas of microscopic disease, detecting noncaseating granulomas, and defining the extension of inflammation into the submucosa.[2,5,23] The increased risk of adenocarcinoma of the colon in patients with ulcerative colitis is well recognized and correlates with the extent and the duration of disease.[24] Adenocarcinoma has, however, been reported in 3 percent of patients with a history of ulcerative colitis for less than 10 years.[24] To detect dysplasia or early carcinomatous change, routine surveillance colonoscopy with biopsy is recommended every 1 to 2 years in patients with pancolitis of more than 7 years duration or left-sided colitis of over 15 years duration.[25] Unfortunately, colonic carcinoma has been demonstrated in specimens that lack any histologic features of dysplasia, implying that even with regular colonoscopy some cancer will go undetected.[26]

Before undergoing diagnostic colonoscopy for rectal bleeding, children should have stool bacterial culture, parasite examination, and *Clostridium difficile* toxin assay performed to exclude a possible infectious etiology. Polymorphonuclear leukocytes in the stool make an inflammatory process more likely than a polyp. Even in the presence of negative microbiology studies, infectious pathogens may still exist. Colitis due to microorganisms such as *Salmonella*, *Shigella*, *Yersinia*, *Campylobacter*, *Aeromonas*, enteroinvasive *Escherichia coli*, and *Entamoeba hystolytica* can mimic the clinical and radiologic features of inflammatory bowel disease.[5,27,28] Because the majority of patients with infectious colitis have spontaneous resolution of symptoms, failure of clinical improvement is an indication for colonoscopy to exclude chronic inflammatory bowel disease. A patient with rectal bleeding following a course of antibiotics should be investigated for possible antibiotic-induced pseudomembranous colitis. The diagnosis is suggested by a positive *C. difficile* toxin assay and confirmed by colonoscopy with biopsy in which "volcano-type" lesions are found.[29] Although the distal colon is most commonly involved, the rectum may be spared and lesions may be localized to the right colon.[29,30]

Tuberculosis is an important cause of morbidity and mortality worldwide and is seen with increasing frequency in refugees and immigrants.[5] Gastrointestinal tuberculosis is most commonly localized in the ileocecal region. Caseating granulomas and acid-fast bacilli identified on endoscopic biopsies will help distinguish tuberculosis from Crohn's disease.[5]

In the immunocompromised host a wide spectrum of possible infectious pathogens can produce chronic diarrhea and colitis. *Candida* species, atypical mycobacteria, cryptosporidia, cytomegalovirus, and adenovirus infections have been seen in patients with acquired immunodeficiency syndrome and other immunodeficient states.[31,32] Colonoscopy and biopsy are the most efficient and accurate methods of detecting opportunistic infection in these patients when routine cultures are negative. After organ transplantation, the colitis of graft-versus-host disease can be distinguished by characteristic changes on biopsy.[33]

Allergic colitis is the most common cause of noninfectious colitis in infants under 1 year of age.[34] The diagnosis is suggested when rectal bleeding accompanied by watery stools with mucous, blood, and leukocytes symptoms resolves after elimination of the offending antigen.[35] Cow's milk proteins, soy protein, and proteins transmitted in breast milk have all been implicated as causes of allergic colitis of infancy.[34-37] Diagnosis by repeat antigen challenge following the guidelines established by Goldman and colleagues in 1963 has met with poor clinical acceptance due to the time and potential risk with each challenge.[35,38] The patchy, superficial mucosal features of allergic colitis can be missed on barium enema and sigmoidoscopy.[34,39] Colonoscopy with biopsy may identify the colitis, but only a biopsy can distinguish allergic colitis from other causes.[34,39,40]

Chronic abdominal pain in children is often an elusive clinical problem in which colonoscopy rarely plays a diagnostic role. If thorough clinical, laboratory, and radiologic investigations fail to identify an etiology and an organic cause is still suspected, colonoscopy with biopsy may be helpful to exclude chronic inflammatory bowel disease. Chronic colonic intussusception and appendiceal intussusception have been diagnosed on colonoscopy in two children with recurrent abdominal pain.[41,42] However, the benefit is low in patients who have no other clinical or radiologic abnormalities.[2,3]

CONTRAINDICATIONS

Colonoscopy is a safe procedure in the hands of an experienced endoscopist. However, respect must be given to colonic and extracolonic factors that can markedly increase the risks of this procedure. Most of these factors represent relative contraindications, and the examination may still be performed with particular attention given to the limit and technique of the procedure (Table 2). Clinical or radiologic features suggestive of bowel perforation represent an absolute contraindication to proceeding with colonoscopy.[2,25,44] Toxic megacolon and perforation may occur following barium enema or colonoscopy in patients with acute severe colitis.[2] However, a limited examination may be well tolerated by some patients.

Colonoscopy should be aborted if there is clear evidence of inadequate bowel preparation. Not only is the diagnostic yield compromised, but the risk of mucosal injury and perforation is increased if adequate visualization cannot be maintained throughout the procedure. Similarly in acute massive gastrointestinal bleeding, visibility of the bowel may be inadequate to enable a safe and diagnostically helpful examination. Advancement of the colonoscope along the bowel lumen may cause blunt trauma to adjacent organs.

The inherent risk of performing colonoscopy in patients with severe underlying medical illness needs to be weighed against the potential benefits of the procedure. In patients with a known coagulopathy, correction of the defect should be attempted prior to the procedure. In these patients, gentle technique and limited biopsies may also reduce the risk of bleeding.

PROCEDURE

Preparation

The potential for successful colonoscopy is greatly enhanced by the patient's cooperation. Without adequate bowel preparation and compliance with the preprocedure routine, even the most expert endoscopist will experience difficulties that may undermine the value and safety of the procedure. The thought of colonoscopy is often frightening for children and an introduction to the unit prior to the procedure may decrease anxiety. At this time a step-by-step account of the events before, during, and after the procedure should be offered, and both parent and child should be afforded an opportunity to ask questions.

Adequate bowel preparation is essential for colonoscopy. Particular attention should be paid to preparing the bowel in patients in whom polypectomy is anticipated. Limited visualization due to retained stool increases the risk of damage to the adjacent bowel wall during electrocautery. Bowel explosion has occurred during electrocautery resulting from the ignition of flammable gases produced from stool or by fermentation of carbohydrates used in bowel preparations such as mannitol.[45–47] There is no single ideal regimen, because age, underlying disease, and individual patient preference may make a particular regimen successful in one patient and ineffective or undesirable in another (Table 3). In infants on formula or breast feedings, adequate preparation is usually obtained by substituting clear liquids for 12 to 24 hours prior to the procedure. In children a soft or solid diet, and in adolescents a clear liquid diet for 48 to 72 hours combined with a laxative on each of the two evenings prior to the examination is generally effective. The choice of laxative is subject to individual experience. Bisacodyl (Dulcolax) (5 mg if less than 4 years, 10 mg if 4 to 10 years, 20 mg if more than 10 years) provides a suitable adjunct to bowel preparation without significant complaints of abdominal cramping. Alternatives include senna (Senokot) or magnesium citrate. A saline enema on the morning of the procedure may also be helpful.

Colonic lavage solutions containing the macromolecule polyethylene glycol are not absorbed from the small intestine and act as osmotic agents, inducing diarrhea (Table 4).[48] They are safe and effective methods of bowel preparation in children and adolescents and avoid dietary restriction, laxatives, or enemas.[49] Owing to the limited transmural flux of sodium and water with polyethylene glycol preparations, the risk of dehydration is minimal, even in younger children.[48,49] Their safe use in infants and children under the age of 5 years has not yet been confirmed. A major advantage is the rapid onset of action, making it particularly useful in the preparation of patients with acute rectal bleeding.[50] To achieve maximal effectiveness, a large volume of solution must be ingested over a short period of time.[48–51] In adults the recommended dose is 240 cc every 10 minutes until a total volume of 4 to 5 L is consumed or clear diarrhea commences. For pediatric patients, dosage varies with weight (see Table 3). In addition to the large volume required, the solution is also unpalatable and improves only minimally with refrigeration. Flavoring does not significantly improve the taste and is not recommended, as it may alter the osmolality of the solution.[49] Fermentation of sugars in flavoring may also increase hydrogen production, increasing the risk with electrocautery.[49] In children unable to drink the volume within the allotted time, instillation of the solution via a nasogastric tube may be a suitable alternative. Nausea, vomiting, and abdominal distention and cramps occur in some patients and may be avoided by a single dose of metoclopramide at the beginning of the therapy.[49]

Bowel preparation often needs to be tailored to the individual patient and disease presentation. In patients with a history of constipation, a more extensive purgative protocol may be considered. On the other hand, patients with diarrhea may require only minimal preparation. Enemas or suppositories

TABLE 2
Contraindications to Colonoscopy

1. Disorders of bowel integrity
   a.* Possible bowel perforation
   b.* Peritonitis or marked abdominal tenderness
   c. Acute severe colitis
   d. Intestinal obstruction
   e. Recent surgical anastomosis
2. Inadequate visualization
   a. Inadequate bowel preparation
   b. Acute massive gastrointestinal bleeding
3. Abnormalities of adjacent organs
   a. Aneurysms of iliac vessels or aorta
   b. Recent surgery
4. Underlying patient factors
   a. Coagulopathy
   b. Severe underlying medical illness

*Absolute contraindications. (Remaining factors are relative contraindications only.)

TABLE 3
Bowel Preparation

Children and Adolescents
1. a. Clear liquids for 48 to 72 hours
   b. Dulcolax 5 mg <4 years, 10 mg 4–10 years, 20 mg >10 years on the two evenings prior to the procedure
   or
   Magnesium citrate (1 oz per year up to 10 oz) 24 hours prior to the procedure
   or
   Senna—Senokot liquid (2½ oz) on the evening prior to the procedure
   c. NPO 8 hours prior to the procedure
   d. Saline enema on the morning of the procedure

2. a. Golytely, orally or via nasogastric tube:
   <10 kg, give 80 ml every 10 minutes, or total dose of 1100 ml
   10–20 kg, give 100 ml every 10 minutes, or total dose of 1600 ml
   20–30 kg, give 140 ml every 10 minutes, or total dose of 2200 ml
   30–40 kg, give 180 ml every 10 minutes, or total dose of 2900 ml
   40–50 kg, give 200 ml every 10 minutes, or total dose of 3200 ml
   >50 kg, give 240 ml every 10 minutes, or total dose of 4000 ml
   b. NPO 8 hours prior to the procedure

Infants
   a. Clear liquids (Pedialyte) 12–24 hours prior to the procedure
   b. NPO 6 hours prior to the procedure

can cause hyperemia, edema, petechiae, mucous depletion, and nonspecific inflammatory changes and should be avoided, if possible, in patients with suspected or known colitis.[1] Relapse of chronic inflammatory bowel disease has occurred after vigorous bowel preparation.[52]

Sedation

Colonoscopy can be performed safely and effectively under intravenous sedation in almost all infants and children.[2–5] Some patients will tolerate limited procedures without any sedation. General anesthesia is not only unnecessary in most children, but it also adds the inherent risks of anesthesia and ablates important warning signs of overdistention of the bowel. Therefore, general anesthesia should be reserved for the patient in whom the previous examination was inadequate or who has other medical problems requiring specialized monitoring.[2,5] On arrival in the endoscopy suite, the patient and parent should again have the procedure explained in detail and a formal consent obtained. The patient's weight and baseline vital signs are then obtained. In some centers, a premedication such as chlorpromazine is given an hour prior to the procedure,[3] but greater control of sedation is achieved in children by giving all medications intravenously. An intravenous cannula is inserted for initial sedation; one should try to avoid taping down a favorite sucking finger. The dose of intravenous meperidine (Demerol or Pethidine) ranges from 1.5 to 4.5 mg per kilogram (maximum 100 mg) with many children requiring 1 to 2 mg per kilogram.[2,5] This combined with midazolam (Versed) 0.15 to 0.30 mg per kilogram or diazepam (Valium) 0.30 mg per kilogram provides safe and effective sedation, amnesia, and analgesia.[2,3,5] The doses should be infused slowly and titrated against the individual's response. Compared with adults, the dose of these medications per kilogram of bodyweight is often large; in fact the sedative dose per kilogram required by children less than 10 years of age is usually twice that required by children older than 10 years.[2] The aims of sedation are to provide comfort and amnesia during the procedure, to allow maintenance of normal oxygenation, and to enable the patient to express discomfort. If additional medication is required during the examination, meperidine is preferred as this can be reversed by naloxone if necessary. Throughout the procedure, all children are followed with a continuous cardiorespiratory monitor, oxygen saturation monitor, and with intermittent blood pressure recordings.[53,54] Continuous monitoring of arterial oxygen saturation and heart rate via a pulse oximeter gives an early warning of hypoxemia and tachycardia related to cardiorespiratory dysfunction.[54] Facilities for suction and oxygen should be available at the bed head, and there should be easy access to pediatric resuscitation equipment.

TABLE 4
Composition of Golytely Solution

Sodium	125 mmol/L
Potassium	10 mmol/L
Chloride	35 mmol/L
Sulfate	40 mmol/L
Bicarbonate	20 mmol/L
Polyethylene glycol 3,350	17.6 mmol/L
Osmolality	280 mOsm/kg

Special Considerations

Transient bacteremia and endotoxemia have been reported following colonoscopy.[55–62] Despite this, the risk of bacterial endocarditis after colonoscopy is minimal, except in patients who have a predisposing factor such as congenital or acquired cardiac disease, prosthetic heart valves, surgically constructed systemic-pulmonary shunts, or a past history of bacterial endocarditis (Table 5).[56,63] In these patients routine antibiotic prophylaxis is recommended.[63,64] Patients with Harrington rods, ventriculoperitoneal shunts, indwelling central venous catheters, or immunodeficiency states should also be considered for antibiotic prophylaxis.[5] The current recommendation from the American Heart Association is for ampicillin 50 mg per kilogram per dose (not to exceed 2 g) and gentamicin 2 mg per kilogram per dose (not to exceed 80 mg) given intramuscularly or intravenously 30 minutes prior to the procedure with a follow-up dose 8 hours later.[63] In penicillin allergic patients, vancomycin 20 mg per kilogram per dose can be given with gentamicin.

TABLE 5
Cardiac Disease for Which Endocarditis Prophylaxis Is Recommended

1. Congenital cardiac malformations except:
   a. Isolated secundum atrial septal defect
   b. Secundum atrial septal defect repaired without a patch 6 or more months earlier
   c. Patent ductus anteriosus ligated and divided 6 months or more earlier
2. Rheumatic and other acquired valvular dysfunction
3. Idiopathic hypertrophic subaortic stenosis
4. Mitral valve prolapse with insufficiency
5. Surgically constructed systemic-pulmonary shunts
6. Prosthetic valves
7. Past history of bacterial endocarditis

Adapted from Shulman et al.[63]

Postprocedure

After the colonoscopy, the patient should be monitored for at least 1 hour to ensure complete recovery with no evidence of sedation or procedure-related complications. Clear liquids should be tolerated before the patient is discharged from the recovery room. Driving is not recommended after sedation, and a family member or friend should be available to escort the patient home. Outpatient follow-up for explanation of biopsy results and discussion of further patient management should be confirmed prior to patient discharge.

EQUIPMENT

Colonoscope

The flexible fiberoptic colonoscope consists of a hand held control unit with an eye piece and a flexible shaft with maneuverable scope tip (Fig. 1). The key to the flexibility and fiberoptics of the instrument are the thousands of fine glass fibers, each approximately 10 μm in diameter, organized into discrete fiber bundles.[52] As light hits each individual fiber, it is transmitted via internal reflection through the fiber, down the shaft of the scope to the eye piece. To prevent diffusion of light and subsequent distortion of the image, each fiber is coated with glass of a lower optical density. The difference between the internal and external character of each individual fiber gives the meshlike appearance that is sometimes seen superimposed on the final image as it is viewed through the eye piece.

Illumination is provided by cold light transmitted from an external light source. The shaft also contains a channel for air sufflation, water for irrigation, suction, and a biopsy channel through which a biopsy forceps, cytology brush, snare, or grasper can be introduced. The tip of the scope is adapted for maneuverability and can be directed up and down or right and left by wheels on the control unit. Retroflexion of the

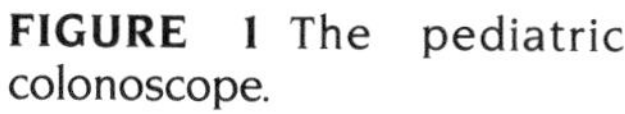

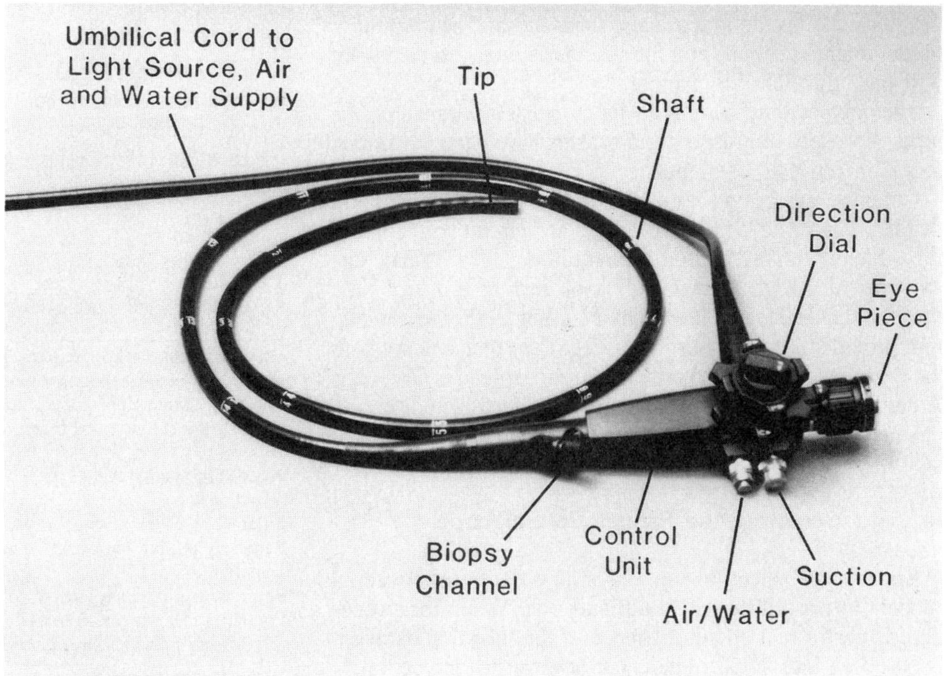

FIGURE 1 The pediatric colonoscope.

tip to greater than 180 degrees is possible with most newer colonoscopes. Additional rotation can be provided by gentle torquing of the scope shaft. This combination of features makes the fiberoptic colonoscope an extremely flexible system that can negotiate the tight curves and configurations of the bowel while still transmitting a clear and accurate image.

The control unit is constructed in a T configuration with the fiberoptic shaft and eye piece in linear continuity at the top of the T. At the base of the T the control unit is connected via an umbilical cord to the light source and air and water supply. The central portion of the unit contains the biopsy channel, air and water button, suction button, and the two dials for left and right, up and down tip control. Suction tubing is attached either to the control unit or to the umbilical cord. The control unit is held in the left hand with the thumb supporting the shaft to the eyepiece. The index and middle fingers are used to operate the suction and air/water buttons while the ring and fifth fingers support the shaft. This technique leaves the right hand free for manipulation of the tip dials and/or the shaft of the scope.

The new generation of video colonoscopes has enhanced the visual capabilities of the normal colonoscope. These scopes have a compact optical unit at the tip of the scope through which the image is received and transmitted up the shaft via wires to reproduce the image on a television screen. This system has the advantage of producing a larger, accurate image that all assistants can view simultaneously. The endoscopist is able to move more freely and subsequently can manipulate the scope with greater comfort.

Additional Equipment

A major advantage of colonoscopy over other diagnostic techniques is its capability of obtaining tissue biopsies for histologic examination. Biopsy forceps have a flexible wire cable with two opposing cups at one end. By squeezing a handle, the cups close, incising a small piece of tissue that usually includes the mucosa and submucosa. The amount of tissue obtained depends on the size of the biopsy forceps that will pass through the channel.

The polypectomy snare is a wire loop that is within a plastic tube. A variety of graspers and baskets have been developed to aid in retrieval of amputated polyps or foreign bodies.

Colonoscopic polypectomy requires an electrosurgical unit that has a separate "cut" and "coagulate" circuit with an ability to blend both these circuits if required. The coagulate circuit provides high voltage pulses of current that can pass through the desiccated layer. On the other hand, the cut current provides a continuous low voltage flow that will not pass the desiccated layer and therefore does not spread heat widely. A cutting action is produced by the more localized direction of current and the higher power of the cut circuit.[52]

Selecting the Proper Colonoscope

Appropriate selection can make the difference between a successful procedure and a difficult one. When the procedure is performed on adults, much of the selection decision is based on individual preference; however, in the pediatric group the size of the scope is a primary consideration. Most adolescents and older children can easily tolerate the adult size colonoscope with a diameter of 1.5 cm. Specific pediatric colonoscopes with a shaft diameter of 1.1 cm are ideal for younger children but are still too large for neonates and small infants. Smaller diameter scopes are currently being developed, but until they become widely available, many units use a small gastroduodenoscope with a 0.9-cm diameter.[2,3] Although the gastroduodenoscope is of a suitable diameter, it is intrinsically less flexible, making the procedure more difficult in infants. Also, the instrument is prone to fiber damage during excessive deflection and torquing. The length of the colonoscope is important if a complete examination is to be achieved in the adolescent or older child. An instrument length of approximately 140 cm in this age group is generally adequate.

FUNDAMENTALS OF COLONOSCOPY

To understand the techniques of good colonoscopic examination, knowledge of the intrinsic nature of the colon and its attachments is necessary. Viewed simply, the colon is a flexible, compliant tube connecting the anus to the terminal ileum. It is normally fixed at the rectum, descending colon, and ascending colon. The sigmoid and transverse colons are attached by a mesenteric sling, and are more freely mobile. If these features are ignored during colonoscopy, the colon can become long and tortuous, developing loops and sharp bends that add to the difficulty and discomfort of the examination (Table 6).

The Technique

Insertion of the Scope

The endoscopist and procedure assistants should wear protective clothing and gloves and should consider wearing protective glasses. The patient is placed in the left lateral position with knees bent (Fig. 2). All colonoscopies should be preceded by a careful examination of the perianal area. A digital rectal examination should be performed to assess the adequacy of the bowel preparation and sedation, to examine the rectal vault, and to relax the anus minimally to permit smooth

TABLE 6
Key Factors for Successful Colonoscopy

Ensuring adequate bowel preparation
Ensuring "good" sedation and careful patient monitoring
Checking colonoscope for all functions before introduction
Keeping the colonoscope direct and straight and keeping the lumen in view
Proceeding gently
Avoiding loops
Inflating as little air as possible
Regularly pulling back and "telescoping" the bowel onto the scope shaft
Being aware of scope location
Protecting the patient, yourself and staff from possible infection by following universal precautions

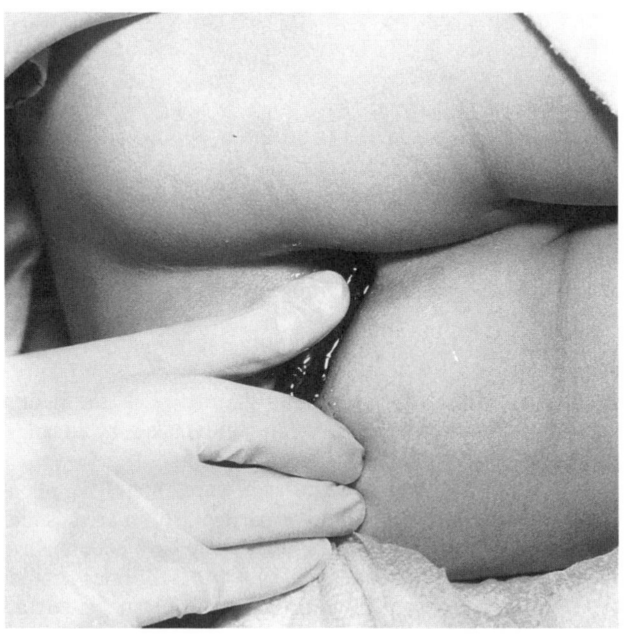

FIGURE 2 Insertion technique.

entry of the scope tip. Lubrication with xylocaine jelly during the digital examination may provide additional comfort for the patient with proctitis or perianal disease.

The tip of the scope should be generously lubricated. With the index finger adjacent to the scope tip, the anus is depressed from the side. As the anal sphincter relaxes, the scope tip is gently guided through the anus into the distal rectum (Fig. 2). The scope is steadied at this point, and with a small puff of air, the lumen of the rectum is found. If mucosa obscures the view, pulling the scope back slightly allows the lumen to appear. By directing the left-right and up-down dials, the tip can be directed and advanced toward the lumen. Rotating the shaft with the right hand can also help the execution of this maneuver. Even if a small amount of stool is present within the rectum and sigmoid the remainder of the colon may be clean, allowing adequate examination. A combination of washing and suction can aid in the removal of residual stool.

Scope Advancement

The rectosigmoid junction marks the first in a series of bends through the mobile sigmoid colon. As a bend is approached, the direction of the lumen may be indicated by the appearance of darker shadowing beneath a fold of mucosa. The mucosal blood vessels also tend to head in the direction of the lumen. Depending on the clues at the site of the bend, a plan should be followed, such as proceeding up and to the left. Once the lumen is viewed and the instrument progresses easily, the scope should be continued to be advanced. If the lumen is only partially seen or not seen, the tip should be pulled back, and the direction of the tip altered before continuing. If the bend still cannot be negotiated, an alteration in patient position may aid in changing the position of the bend, making it easier to advance. Occasionally these manuevers fail and a gentle blind sliding technique is attempted. Judging on the basis of previous attempts, the tip is pointed in the direction most likely to be in the direction of the lumen and pushed gently. The tip should slide over the mucosa with the vascular pattern passing across the view. If the tip continues to pass easily and the vascular pattern is sliding past, then the bend should be negotiated, and the lumen soon visualized. However, this procedure must be stopped if resistance is felt, mucosal blood vessels blanch, or the patient is in pain. These are all indications of excessive pressure on the bowel wall or mesentery. In this case the scope should be retracted, the lumen visualized, and the position reassessed. Anatomic variations, postsurgical and inflammatory changes can make the sigmoid colon difficult and even impossible to negotiate by endoscopy.

While advancing through the sigmoid colon the endoscopist should be establishing position for the remainder of the procedure. The inexperienced colonoscopist who simply "follows" the lumen often stretches the bowel over the scope, forming loops that add to the difficulty of the procedure. By using minimal amounts of air and withdrawing the scope regularly, a more direct scope course is likely.

Much has been said about loops, but how does an endoscopist know he or she has a loop, and are all loops disadvantageous? Under fluoroscopy, the configuration of the colonoscope is obvious. Fluoroscopy is rarely used in pediatric colonoscopy, however, owing to the risks of radiation and improving endoscopic techniques. A loop can be suspected whenever the one-to-one ratio of pushing with observed tip advancement is lost. When this is first noted, the scope should be withdrawn, straightened, and then readvanced. If the one-to-one ratio is still impaired, attempts at torquing the scope, aspirating air, or applying pressure to the abdominal wall may be helpful.[52]

A common loop formed in the sigmoid colon is the N loop (Fig. 3*A*). An N loop is formed when the sigmoid is stretched over the advancing scope, making the sigmoid-descending colon junction an acute and difficult bend. If this junction can be negotiated without excessive patient discomfort, the scope should then be straightened and the loop removed before proceeding further. When the sigmoid colon is stretched, it can twist on its mesentery to form an "alpha" loop (Fig. 3*B*). Although this loop can cause some patient discomfort, it does allow easy passage of the scope from the sigmoid to the descending colon. Most colonoscopists attempt to straighten this loop once in the descending colon or after the proximal transverse colon has been safely entered. The alpha loop can be straightened by a combination of withdrawal of the scope to reduce the size of the loop and clockwise rotation of the scope shaft to remove the twist in the mesentery, "telescoping" the sigmoid onto the shaft. This maneuver may be aided by the downward pressure of an assistant's hand on the lower abdomen. The more difficult N loop can be converted intentionally to an alpha loop to allow easier entry into the descending colon by the method called the alpha maneuver. Using this technique, the scope is withdrawn to just beyond the rectosigmoid junction and the tip angled firmly counterclockwise 180 degrees to form the twist in the mesentery. The scope is then advanced along the sigmoid colon to the sigmoid colon–descending colon junction.[52,65] Attempts at reducing sigmoid loops should be discontinued if patient dis-

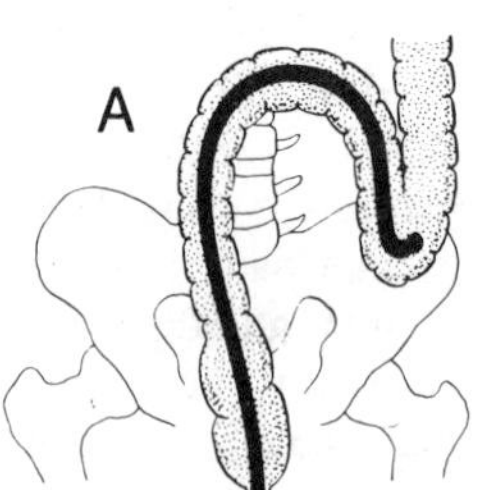

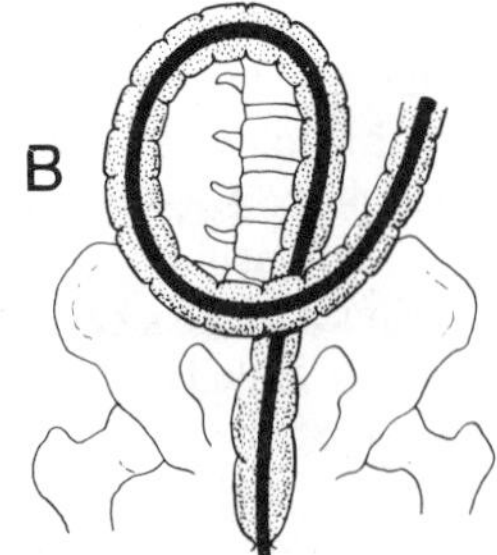

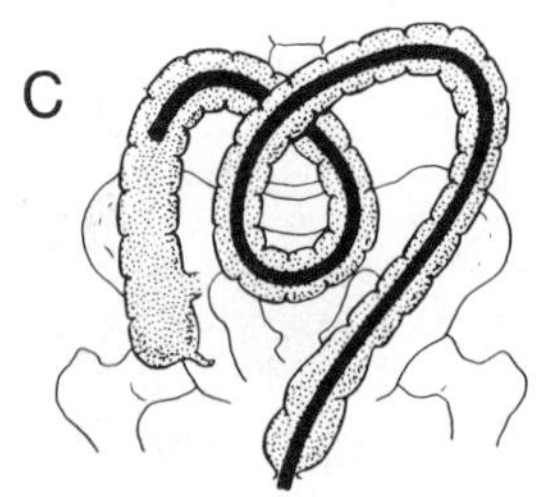

FIGURE 3 Colonoscopic "loops."

comfort is experienced. Adhesions and abnormal colonic attachments may not permit resolutions of the loops.

Once the scope is straightened, the tip will advance up the descending colon to the splenic flexure. The splenic flexure forms an acute angle that is most effectively passed if the tip is not too tightly deflected. In the transverse colon there is a risk of reforming an N loop in the sigmoid colon. This is again indicated by a disruption in the one-to-one movement ratio. By rotating the shaft in a clockwise direction in association with downward pressure on the lower abdomen, the scope can be straightened and the tip advanced. A reversed splenic flexure occurs when the attachment of the descending colon is mobile, and the descending colon approaches the splenic flexure medially rather than laterally. This is seen in over 5 percent of children undergoing colonoscopy.[52] In order to negotiate this flexure, a deep transverse colon loop is formed, making advancement to the cecum extremely difficult. Progress through the distal transverse colon can be aided by hooking the tip up and withdrawing the scope. This acts to straighten the transverse colon and often results in paradoxical advancement of the tip. In patients with a redundant transverse colon, a "gamma" loop may form (Fig. 3*C*). This can be straightened once the scope reaches the cecum by simply withdrawing the colonoscope.

The hepatic flexure is a very acute angle heralded by the bluish coloration of liver seen through the colonic mucosa. The flexure should first be approached and the likely direction of the lumen assessed. Then a combination of actions is performed. Firstly, air is aspirated, bringing the flexure toward the scope tip; then the scope is carefully withdrawn and rotated clockwise in the predetermined direction around the arc of the flexure. Once the lumen is visualized, short intermittent suction will cause the hepatic flexure and ascending colon to collapse back, and the tip will advance toward the cecum. Pushing the scope at this point may act to reform the transverse colon loop.

The cecum is characterized by obvious interhaustral markings and can be confirmed by identifying the appendiceal orifice and ileocecal valve or by localization by transillumination deep in the right iliac fossa. The ileocecal valve is located on the medial aspect of the cecum approximately 5 cm proximal to the pole in adults. Initially the scope should be advanced toward the appendiceal orifice then slowly withdrawn while the endoscopist watches closely for a slight irregularity in the medial aspect of the first prominent circular interhaustral fold. This represents the upper tip of the valve and characteristically lacks an overlying vascular pattern. Bile-stained fluid may be seen to exit through the valve. The tip is then maneuvered toward the valve, aiming to hook up on the lip and thereby falling into the orifice. If the ileum cannot be cannulated, biopsies can still be taken by advancing the forceps through the ileocecal valve.

As the scope is slowly withdrawn, care should be taken to examine the mucosa carefully, particularly in areas such as the major flexures where the views may have been inadequate during the initial passage of the scope. Biopsies should be taken of macroscopically normal and abnormal tissue at regular intervals.[2,3,23,66] The location of abnormalities and biopsies should be documented.

Localization of the Scope Tip

During colonoscopy, it is often important to know the correct localization of the scope tip. Due to the elasticity of the colon and its ability to stretch to form loops or to telescope along the scope, a polyp seen at 50 cm during insertion of the scope may be identified at 25 cm when the scope is being withdrawn. Therefore, the length of inserted scope is not an ideal way to localize colonic findings. In a dark room, the abdominal wall can be transilluminated by the light at the scope tip. If the tip is in the cecum, the light may be seen deep in the right iliac fossa. If the tip is at the hepatic and splenic flexures, the light will be seen posteriorly at the lower ribs. However, confusion can occur if the colonoscope stretches the sigmoid or transverse colon sufficiently so that the light appears in a position outside the normal anatomic configuration. In obese patients, transillumination may be difficult or even impossible.

The appearance of the mucosa and internal anatomy of the colon can also provide useful information regarding tip localization (see Normal Colonoscopic Appearance). The sigmoid and descending colon have interhaustral folds arranged in concentric rings that are usually easily distinguished from the triangular folds of the transverse colon. At the hepatic and splenic flexure, a sharp bend is approached. The organs may give a blue-grey tinge to the colonic mucosa due to the close physical proximity. The identification of the appendiceal orifice or ileocecal valve can document the position in the cecum.

Colonoscopic Polypectomy

Before proceeding with colonoscopic polypectomy, some additional factors need to be considered. Is the polyp of a type suitable for polypectomy? Is the bowel adequately prepared to minimize the risk of bowel wall heat damage due to poor visualization? Does the amount of retained stool or the type of bowel preparation, i.e., Mannitol, put the patient at risk for bowel explosion due to ignition of flammable gases by electrocautery? Is the bleeding status of the patient known? Polypectomy requires additional equipment including an electrosurgical unit with a cut and coagulation circuit, a plastic sheathed polypectomy snare, grabbers, or a basket to retrieve the polyp, and a return plate to ground the patient. Patients with a demand pacemaker should be monitored with an electrocardiography throughout the procedure, with the pacemaker on a fixed rate mode and the grounding plate situated distally on the thigh.[67]

When the patient's preparation is completed and the equipment is checked, polypectomy is ready to proceed. The snare is a loop of relatively thick wire covered by a thin plastic tube with a handle. The snare is advanced down through the biopsy channel of the colonoscope until the plastic tubing is seen exiting from the scope tip. As the assistant slowly opens the handle, the wire loop advances from the plastic covering. By maneuvering the scope tip, the polyp stalk can be lassoed at a point midway along its length. The plastic sheath should be pushed snugly against the stalk and the loop slowly closed. By gently moving the snare in and out, the placement of the loop can be assessed, noting if the loop contains any part of the polyp head. If it is positioned too basally or too high on the stalk, or if it contains any adjacent colonic mucosa, it must be repositioned. If any of these questions cannot be adequately answered because of poor visualization, then the snare should be opened and manipulated. Once satisfactory position of the loop is established, a puff of air is instilled and the polyp maneuvered into the center of the lumen so that there is minimal if any contact with the adjacent colonic wall. Current is then passed through the snare, initially with the coagulation circuit at a low setting (15 to 25 watts) for approximately 5 seconds. Successful coagulation is seen as whitening of the stalk with steam as a result of tissue desiccation. The snare is gently moved back and forth to disperse any heat injury to the adjacent colonic mucosa. An additional burst of current can be used if the polyp has not yet been amputated. Owing to the risks of heat dissipation with a prolonged coagulation current, it may be preferable to increase the power of the current if the polyp still remains attached. If no visible signs of coagulation can be seen, one should check the electrical source, connections, snare, and position of the loop.

Once amputated, the polyp can be removed with the snare loop, grasper, or basket designed for this purpose. Occasionally the polyp will escape efforts to secure it. If the amputated polyp is in the distal sigmoid or rectum, it can often be suctioned against the scope tip and removed along with the scope. If the polyp travels away from the scope and cannot be located, it may be helpful to instill some water and follow the path of the stream looking for the polyp. Once the polyp is retrieved, the scope should be reinserted, and the site of the polypectomy assessed for adequacy of polyp removal, bleeding, or damage to the adjacent colonic mucosa.

Although the polyp is easily visualized, it may be difficult to grasp with the polypectomy snare. Problems can arise when good scope tip position is not established before advancement of the snare or if the loop is tightened with the plastic sheath away from the polyp stalk, allowing the loop to slip over the head of the polyp. If the loop is closed too tightly in an inappropriate position, it may become imbedded in the polyp tissue and may be difficult to remove.

Variations in technique may need to be considered in the management of particular polyp types. Sessile polyps can often be snared and pulled up to form an adequate stalk. If the adjacent mucosa moves with the snare but the bowel wall does not, the risk of full-thickness injury to the bowel is minimal. Thick-stalked polyps usually require high-power settings, and transmission of heat to adjacent mucosa is often unavoidable because of the floppy polyp head. Small polyps such as those found in familial polyposis syndromes may be biopsied and removed at the same time using a biopsy forcep encased in a plastic sheath through which an electrical current can be passed. Although uncommon, malignant changes have been described in polyps removed from children.[2,11] This emphasizes the importance of accurate localization of polyps and formal histology on all polyps removed at colonoscopy.

COMPLICATIONS

Complications of colonoscopy in the pediatric age group can be divided into those related to bowel preparation and sedation and those directly related to colonoscopy (Table 7). All bowel preparation regimens have a potential for causing abdominal cramping, nausea, or vomiting. Fluid and electrolyte instability can be caused by aggressive or prolonged fasting or preparations using large volume lavage solutions (with the possible exception of Golytely). Fortunately, neonates and most infants can be adequately examined with minimal (if any) bowel preparation (see Preparation). The use of an intravenous line carries a small but potential risk. Dilution and slow infusion of intravenous medications such as diazepam and midazolam can reduce the incidence of chemical thrombophlebitis.

TABLE 7
Complications of Colonoscopy and Polypectomy in Infants and Children

1. Preparation-related
   a. Fluid and electrolyte imbalance
   b. Nausea and vomiting
   c. Abdominal cramping
2. Sedation-related
   a. Nausea and vomiting
   b. Thrombophlebitis
   c. Tachycardia
   d. Transient hypoxemia
   e. Apnea and bradycardia
   f. Hypotension
3. Procedure-related
   a. Hemorrhage
   b. Perforation
      1) Complete
      2) Incomplete
      3) Postpolypectomy coagulation syndrome
   c. Bowel explosion
   d. Bacteremia/Endotoxemia
   e. Cardiac arrhythmia
   f. Hypotension
   g. Abdominal distension

Adapted from Hassall et al.[2]

Respiratory depression with apnea and bradycardia are well-known complications of intravenous sedation. Forty-one percent of adult patients undergoing colonoscopy had desaturation to a Po_2 equivalent of less than 60 mm Hg.[53] Hypotension can result from intravenous sedation, vagal effects, or mechanical effects due to overdistention of the colonic viscera or simply from instrumentation in a sensitive patient. Arrhythmias and electrocardiograph changes in adults have been observed during colonoscopy.[68-70] With careful monitoring by an experienced assistant using a continuous heart rate monitor and pulse oximeter, early changes in the patient's condition can be detected and appropriately managed.

A small amount of rectal bleeding following colonoscopy is common. This is usually secondary to superficial mucosal trauma or ooze from biopsy sites. The risk of significant hemorrhage from endoscopic biopsy is minimal, and it occurred in only one patient in a series of 5,000 diagnostic biopsies.[44] Severe intra-abdominal bleeding can result from overly aggressive technique, causing trauma to mesenteric attachments, serosal tears, or even hepatic or splenic rupture.[71-74] The risk of hemorrhage following polypectomy is about 42 to 60 times greater than that occurring after routine diagnostic colonoscopy.[74] Bleeding is usually apparent soon after the procedure and will usually spontaneously resolve within 24 to 72 hours.[2,5] It is more frequent after removal of a thick stalk, large polyp, or if inappropriate coagulation is used.[74] If immediate hemorrhage is seen following polyp section, the stalk should be resnared and held for 10 to 15 minutes without further application of electrical current.[52,74] If the stalk cannot be resnared, electrical coagulation at a low voltage may be successful in stopping bleeding, or epinephrine 1:10,000, 5 ml diluted in 50 ml of iced water can be sprayed over the site of bleeding in an attempt at local vasoconstriction.[52,74] Severe hemorrhage requiring blood transfusion is rare, but necessary surgical exploration may be required to obtain adequate hemostasis. Secondary hemorrhage occurring 5 to 14 days after polypectomy is usually self-limited but may occasionally require repeat colonoscopy with local coagulation or surgery.[44]

The most common patient complaint during colonoscopy is abdominal discomfort and distention. This can be minimized with careful technique, using limited air sufflation and by avoiding the formation of bowel loops. Significant or persistent pain during or after colonoscopy demands a thorough clinical examination, radiologic studies, and close monitoring for features of perforation. Perforation of the colon is rare after routine colonoscopy with no reports in 508 pediatric diagnostic examinations.[5] The risk is highest in patients with active colitis, strictures, or adhesions.[74] The incidence of perforation in adults doubles with therapeutic procedures such as polypectomy and electrocautery, and in children the incidence of perforation with polypectomy has been reported to be between 0 and 5 percent.[2,3,9,74] With increasing expertise, a more accurate assessment of the risks of colonoscopic polypectomy in children should soon be available. Pain during polypectomy should alert the endoscopist to a possible transmural burn with a risk of immediate or delayed perforation.[74] Silent perforation has also been described.[75] In the event of clinical and radiologic evidence of perforation, immediate surgical intervention is warranted.[76] Incomplete perforation due to serosal rupture without mucosal tearing can result in intramural gas, pneumoperitoneum, pneumomediastinum, and/or cervical emphysema.[77,78] A nonperforating full-thickness burn to the colonic wall may present within 12 to 24 hours as localized abdominal pain, fever, and leukocytosis in the absence of free air in the peritoneum on abdominal x-ray film. This is sometimes called the postpolypectomy coagulation syndrome. Both these clinical sequelae can be conservatively managed with bowel rest, intravenous antibiotics, and close observation.[74]

Bacteremia is reported after colonoscopy in adults and children. The incidence following colonoscopy is not increased in the presence of inflammation or after therapeutic procedures such as multiple biopsies or polypectomy.[60,61] Although this bacteremia appears to be transient and not clinically significant for the normal host, there is a potential for bacterial endocarditis in patients who are immunocompromised, have cardiac disease, or have surgical prostheses.[58,63,64] Hence, prophylactic antibiotics should be considered in this group of patients (Table 5). Endotoxemia has been reported in 9 percent of adult patients following colonoscopy with no reported clinical sequelae.[59]

Therefore, colonoscopy is a procedure not without potential for serious complication. Careful patient preparation, sedation, and good scope technique can significantly minimize this risk, and the advantages of the procedure can be fully realized.

COLONOSCOPIC OBSERVATIONS

Interpretation of the endoscopic features of the colon requires consideration of the character of the mucosa and the internal anatomy of the colon. Both these features may alter dramatically during disease.

Normal Colonoscopic Appearance

When viewed through the colonoscope, the normal mucosa has a yellow to pink hue depending on the degree of illumination provided by the light source. The mucosal surface is moist and shiny because of the thin mucous layer overlying the epithelial surface. The normal mucosa is transparent, so the submucosal blood vessels can be identified. These are 1 to 2 mm in diameter and progressively branch until they finally form tiny capillaries. The prominence of the mucosal vascular pattern varies throughout the colon. It is easily seen in the rectum and transverse colon but is less obvious in the sigmoid and descending colon. Interhaustral folds or valves greatly increase the surface area, distensibility, and flexibility of the colon. These are mucosal folds with a sharp terminal border of less than 5 mm in diameter (see Color Plate III *A*). They are of variable height and intervals in different segments of the colon.

When the colonoscope first enters the rectum, the pink mucosa is seen with a prominent but fine branching network of mucosal blood vessels. Three semicircular folds of mucosa form the semilunar valves of Houston. Until reaching the rectosigmoid junction, there are no other bends or folds in the rectum.

The first obvious feature on entering the sigmoid colon is the circular interhaustral folds. These folds are generally less than 5 mm in height yet are separated only by millimeters. The mucosal vascular pattern is often barely visible. Progress through the sigmoid may be hampered by mobility of the colon on its mesenteric attachment, forming loops and sharp bends. The descending colon can be recognized by the relative lack of valvulae and greater distensibility. The mucosal pattern is normally difficult to appreciate. On approaching the splenic flexure, the descending colon expands. The flexure is recognized by a sharp angle usually heading to the left. The spleen may be visible as a bluish tinge seen through the colonic mucosa adjacent to the flexure (see Color Plate III *B*).

After one passes around the sharp bend of the splenic flexure, the characteristic triangular folds of the transverse colon can be recognized. These folds may extend to 1.5 cm in height with a sharp terminal border and are formed by the three longitudinal muscles or taeniae coli. The mucosa between these folds forms sacs or haustra. The mucosal vascular pattern is once again prominent, although the blood vessels are larger than the fine network identified in the rectum. The triangular folds disappear as the transverse colon enters the hepatic flexure. The liver is frequently recognized as a blue discoloration on the anterior aspect of the antimesenteric border of the transverse colon.

After progressing past the hepatic flexure, the ascending colon is entered. Here the interhaustral folds are taller, approximately 2 cm in height, but they still maintain their sharp terminal margin. They are separated by 2 to 3 cm of mucosa that form large saclike haustra. The cecum is recognized as a readily distensible, blind-ending area. The interhaustral folds are 3 to 5 cm long, 5 to 10 mm high, and converge onto a central point at the base of the cecum. The small indentation of the appendiceal orifice is located at the point of this confluence. After appendectomy, the appendiceal stump may appear as a small polypoid mass. On withdrawing the endoscope from the base of the cecum, the ileocecal valve can be identified as a slight irregularity on the medial aspect of the first interhaustral fold. The appearance of the normal ileocecal valve is thought to reflect the movement of the terminal ileum and may be described as three main types. The labial form appears as lips with a linear opening and is generally observed if the terminal ileum is empty and hypokinetic.[79] The papillary form is raised with the opening at its peak. Stool can be seen to emit through this valve. The intermediate form occurs as a transition between the two other valve types. The normal ileocecal valve can be observed to alter in shape from labial to papillary forms with the normal movement of the ileum and acts to regulate the flow of ileal contents into the colon.[79]

The terminal ileum is examined in up to half of children undergoing colonoscopy.[3] It is recognized endoscopically by the lack of circular interhaustral folds and intervening haustral sacs and the redder mucosal appearance. The mucosal surface is usually flat, although it may become undulating and granular as a result of prominent lymphoid follicles or Peyer's patches.

Inflammatory Bowel Disease

Colonoscopy has made a significant contribution to the diagnosis and management of patients with inflammatory bowel disease.

Ulcerative colitis is primarily a disorder of the colonic mucosa that extends proximally from the rectum in a continuous pattern. The mucosal changes observed in chronic, quiescent colitis may be subtle. They include blunting or loss of the normal mucosal vascular pattern and a coarse, granular appearance of the mucosa. Biopsies show histologic features of surface epithelial injury, crypt abscesses, mucin depletion, and crypt regeneration. The presence or loss of vascular patterns or spontaneous friability usually indicates acute disease activity (see Color Plate III*C*). Minimal scope trauma or biopsy may cause obvious mucosal hemorrhage known as induced friability.

In ulcerative colitis of moderate activity, single or multiple ulcers can be seen in association with a yellow mucopurulent exudate. These ulcers are pleomorphic in size and shape and may join to form confluent areas of ulceration (see Color Plate III*D*). Separating the ulcers, the mucosa is erythematous and friable, and in the presence of marked inflammation may form nodules or inflammatory polyps. The distinguishing feature between the cobblestoning effect seen in ulcerative colitis and Crohn's disease lies in the character of the intervening mucosa. In ulcerative colitis the mucosa is abnormal with evidence of acute inflammation, while in Crohn's disease the intervening mucosa is either normal or only slightly involved. In acute, severe colitis, ulcerations are larger (greater than 5 mm) and occur more frequently (more than 10 per 10 cm) so that the areas of intervening mucosa are minimal. This remaining mucosa is erythematous, edematous, and spontaneously bleeds. In patients with extensive colitis, the ileocecal valve may become effaced and patulous, allowing easy intubation of the terminal ileum. In these patients, the terminal ileum may be affected with absent mucosal folds, terminal narrowing, and areas of patchy erythema.[65,80]

Structural changes in the normal colonic anatomy may be seen endoscopically in acute ulcerative colitis. Edema secondary to acute inflammation may cause the valvulae to become thickened and blunt so that the sharp appearance of normal interhaustral folds is lost. Hypertrophy of the muscularis mucosae occurs in response to mucosal inflammation. As a result the normal haustral pattern disappears, and the lumen becomes narrowed and tubular. Occasionally during healing, areas of mucosa may form interconnections or bridges over intervening ulcers.[65] In areas of more focal inflammation, strictures may develop. These are short, generally less than 2 cm long, and are formed by focal muscular hypertrophy.[81] Colonoscopy in patients with ulcerative colitis, particularly those with a history of longstanding and extensive disease, should include examination for changes suggestive of malignant transformation. While most colonic cancers appear as ulcerated exophytic masses, carcinomas in ulcerative colitis tend to be infiltrating tumors.[65,82] They appear as a focal, slightly raised flat mass or plaque, a malignant stricture, or a single or multiple polypoid mass. Biopsies are essential to confirm the diagnosis.

Crohn's disease may involve the colon as ileocolonic disease in approximately 52 percent of children or the colon alone in 9 percent.[83] The rectum may be spared and segmental involvement with intervening areas of normal mucosa is characteristic.[65,84–86] Chronic, quiescent Crohn's colitis may appear endoscopically identical to ulcerative colitis with an abnormal vascular pattern and mucosal granularity. Aphthous ulceration occurring in moderately active Crohn's disease is the earliest endoscopic feature specific for Crohn's disease. These ulcers are flat, approximately 1 to 3 mm in diameter, are surrounded by a small rim of erythema with the adjacent mucosa being normal. Colonoscopic biopsies taken from these ulcers are more likely to contain granulomas and microgranulomas, characteristic histologic features of Crohn's disease.[87] In severe Crohn's colitis, these ulcers become large (greater than 5 mm) and deep, and they occur more frequently (more than five per 10-cm segment). Adjacent to ulcerations, the mucosa becomes edematous and hyperplastic, forming a cobblestone appearance or even inflammatory polyps (see Color Plate III*E* and *F*). Although this intervening mucosa may be more prominent than in ulcerative colitis, it lacks evidence of acute inflammation, ulceration, or friability.

Structural changes of the internal anatomy of the colon can also occur in patients with Crohn's disease. The interhaustral folds become thickened and blunted, the haustral pattern is lost, and the lumen becomes narrowed in response to acute submucosal inflammation. Strictures due to inflammation and fibrosis are common and tend to be longer than those found in ulcerative colitis.[65] Patients with Crohn's disease limited to the colon may also develop colonic fistulae.[85] The presence of a fistula can be confirmed by injecting methylene blue through the fistula orifice and watching for passage of the dye onto the skin surface or into the urine. Alternatively, meglumine diatrizoate (Gastrografin) followed by x-ray studies may localize the progression of the dye through the fistula. Although the incidence of colorectal cancer is greater in patients with Crohn's disease than in the normal population, these tumors do not usually present until the fourth or fifth decade.[88-90]

Allergic Colitis

The characteristic macroscopic and histologic appearance of allergic colitis differentiates it from other forms of colitis found in infants.[39,40] Colonoscopic findings include superficial aphthous ulcerations surrounded by a rim of erythema.[39] The intervening mucosa may be normal or have mild nonspecific features of colitis. The rectosigmoid colon is affected in the majority of infants, although involvement of the descending colon with rectal sparing occurs in about 14 percent of infants.[39] The transverse and ascending colon was involved in most infants undergoing complete colonoscopy.[39] Histologically, there is a diffuse increase in eosinophils in the lamina propria of greater than 60 per 10 high-power fields associated with a focal cryptitis.[40,91] Allergic proctitis has also been described in adults, although the pathogenesis of this entity is unknown.[92]

Polyps

Polyps are a common cause of rectal bleeding in childhood.[2,3,5,93,94] They can be differentiated endoscopically on the basis of their macroscopic appearance, number, and histologic characteristics.[11,12] The majority of colorectal polyps in children are juvenile polyps and are located in the sigmoid colon (55 percent) or rectum (37 percent).[95] These are pedunculated polyps ranging in size from 3 mm to 20 mm (see Color Plate IV*A*).[96] Histologically, juvenile polyps are composed of dilated, mucus-filled glands with edema and inflammation of the lamina propria.[8,10,96] The cells lining the glands have basally oriented nuclei, and there is no nuclear atypia or stacking of nuclei. The characteristic "swiss cheese" appearance due to the dilated mucous glands may be appreciated on sectioning the polyp after removal. The dense vascular supply to these polyps accounts for their major complication—rectal bleeding.

Inflammatory polyps may be found in any region of the colon undergoing active regeneration.[96] These are often large and may be single or multiple. The overlying mucosa may initially consist of inflammatory and granulation tissue but may later be indistinguishable from the normal colonic mucosa. Inflammatory polyps are common in inflammatory bowel disease but may also occur with bacterial or parasitic infections including amebiasis or schistosomiasis.[96] Neither juvenile nor inflammatory polyps have malignant potential. However, since inflammatory polyps are found in conditions such as ulcerative colitis, which is associated with an increased risk of carcinoma, biopsies should always be obtained. Adenomatous polyps may be pedunculated or sessile, or single or multiple. They result from abnormal proliferation of the colonic glandular epithelium and have been associated with malignant transformation in some patients.[96] Adenomatous polyps are a common observation in adult colonoscopic practice but are only occasionally found in children.[11] Factors associated with an increased risk of malignant transformation include large polyp size, histologic type, and the degree of dysplasia.[96] Mixed juvenile and adenomatous polyps have been described.[11]

The presence of multiple adenomatosis polyps is suggestive of a familial adenomatous polyposis syndrome. Familial polyposis coli is inherited as an autosomal dominant trait and is characterized by hundreds to thousands of individual polyps.[12] These polyps may appear endoscopically as a mass of tiny polyps totally covering the normal colonic mucosa, larger polyps with normal intervening mucosa, or a mixture of small and large polyps.[65] Although the average age of onset of these polyps is 24 years, familial polyposis coli can present as early as 4 years of age.[97] In Gardner's syndrome, the adenomatous polyps are multiple and widespread but generally fewer in number than those found in familial polyposis coli (see Color Plate IV*B*).[12] Gardner's syndrome frequently presents in childhood and may progress to carcinoma before the second decade.[98] Adenomas may also develop in the stomach and duodenum, particularly in the region of the ampulla of Vater.[12] Peutz-Jegher syndrome is an inherited hamartomatous polyposis syndrome involving the gastrointestinal tract in association with melanotic spots of the lips and buccal mucosa.[12] The colonic polyps in this syndrome may be sessile or pedunculated and are usually less than 2 cm in diameter.[65] They occur infrequently along the colon, only occasionally numbering over 20. In Cowden's disease, the tiny (1 to 3 mm) sessile polyps are often difficult to distinguish from the normal colonic mucosa. They are most frequently observed in the rectosigmoid colon.[12,65] Rarely an abnormality in the submucosa may expand to form a polypoid lesion. Lipomas, leiomyomas, leiomyosarcomas, lymphoid hyperplasia, neurofibromas, or carcinoid tumors rarely present in this way.[65] To sample the submucosa at colonoscopy multiple bites over the site may be required.

Vascular Abnormalities

Although uncommon, angiodysplasia of the colon is an important cause of acute and chronic blood loss in childhood. These lesions may be flat, 2- to 5-mm red spots or slightly raised, larger red areas. The irregular margins with radiating tiny capillary projections help distinguish angiodysplastic lesions from instrument induced trauma. If multiple lesions occur, they are usually small and may form clusters often linked by tiny capillaries. Although the proximal colon is most frequently involved, over 10 percent of adults had a second area of involvement in the transverse or descending colon.[99]

The colon may be involved as part of a systemic vasculitis.[100-102] In Henoch-Schönlein purpura the appearance of the colonic mucosa can mirror that occurring on the skin. Multiple petechiae and small ecchymoses ranging from 3 to 5 mm in diameter are noted in the colon of patients with moderate to severe disease. These lesions may have a segmental distribution and must be examined with care owing to the risk of intussusception, infarction, and perforation.[102] Uncommon causes of rectal bleeding in children detected at colonoscopy include colonic varices, hereditary telangiectasia, and cavernous hemangiomas.[65]

Pneumatosis Coli

Pneumatosis cystoides intestinalis is characterized by multiple gas-distended cysts in the submucosa of the colon and small intestine.[103] It is found predominantly in patients with pyloroduodenal obstruction, recent intestinal surgery, and chronic obstructive lung disease.[104-107] While in premature infants and neonates this usually indicates acute necrotizing enterocolitis, the significance in older children, adolescents, and adults is more benign.[107] At colonoscopy these cysts appear as multiple discrete polypoid masses with an intact overlying mucosa. They are usually soft, and with biopsy may collapse with a "popping" sound.

SUMMARY

The development of pediatric colonoscopy has added significantly to the diagnosis and management of pediatric colonic disease. It can be performed effectively and safely under intravenous sedation in most infants and children. By allowing direct visualization of the mucosa and internal anatomy of the colon and by providing the ability to obtain histologic specimens, colonoscopy has a marked advantage over other diagnostic modalities. The realm of therapeutic colonoscopy is still in its infancy but offers significant benefits in the management of many common pediatric diseases.

Acknowledgment

We wish to thank Stacia Langenbahn for her editorial and technical assistance.

REFERENCES

1. Vanderhoof JA, Ament ME. Proctosigmoidoscopy and rectal biopsy in infants and children. J Pediatr 1976; 89:911–915.
2. Hassall E, Barclay GN, Ament ME. Colonoscopy in childhood. Pediatrics 1984; 73:594–599.
3. Williams CB, Laage NJ, Campbell CA, et al. Total colonoscopy in children. Arch Dis Child 1982, 57:49–53.
4. Hassall E, Ament M. Total colonoscopy in children. (Letter) Arch Dis Child 1983; 58:76–77.
5. Rossi T. Endoscopic examination of the colon in infancy and childhood. Pediatr Clin North Am 1988; 35:331–356.
6. Howdle PD, Littlewood JM, Firth J, Losowsky MS. Routine colonoscopy service. Arch Dis Child 1984; 59:790–793.
7. Silverberg SG. Juvenile retention polyps of the colon and rectum. Dig Dis Sci 1970; 15:617–619.
8. Harris JW. Polyps of the colon and rectum in children. Dis Colon Rectum 1967; 10:267–272.
9. Liebman WM. Fiberoptic endoscopy of the gastrointestinal tract in infants and children. Am J Gastroenterol 1977; 68:452–455.
10. Toccalino H, Guastavino E, DePinni F, et al. Juvenile polyps of the rectum and colon. Acta Paediatr Scand 1973; 62:337–340.
11. Cynamon HA, Milov DE, Andres JM. Diagnosis and management of colonic polyps in children. J Pediatr 1989; 114:593–596.
12. Haggitt RC, Reid BJ. Hereditary gastrointestinal polyposis syndromes. Am J Surg Pathol 1986; 10:871–887.
13. Riddesberger MM, Lebenthal E. Nodular colonic mucosa of childhood: normal or pathologic? Gastroenterology 1980; 79:265–270.
14. Kaplan B, Benson J, Rothstein F, et al. Lymphonodular hyperplasia of the colon as a pathologic finding in children with lower gastrointestinal bleeding. J Pediatr Gastroenterol Nutr 1984; 3:704–708.
15. Berezin S, Newman LJ. Lower gastrointestinal bleeding in infants owing to lymphonodular hyperplasia of the colon. Pediatr Emerg Care 1987; 3:164–165.
16. Trudel JL, Fazio VW, Sivak MV. Colonoscopic diagnosis and treatment of arteriovenous malformations in chronic lower gastrointestinal bleeding. Dis Colon Rectum 1988; 31:107–110.
17. Morris SJ, Kaplan SR, Ballan K, Tedesco FJ. Blue rubber-bleb nevus syndrome. JAMA 1978; 239:1887.
18. Haddad HM, Wilkins L. Congenital anomalies associated with gonadal aplasia: review of 55 cases. Pediatrics 1959; 23:885–902.
19. Goodman RM, Smith EW, Paton D, et al. Pseudoelasticum: a clinical and histiopathological study. Medicine 1963; 42:297–334.
20. Lanthier PH, D'Harveng B, Vanheuverzwyn R, et al. Colonic angiodysplasia: follow-up of patients after endoscopic treatment for bleeding lesions. Dis Colon Rectum 1989; 32:296–298.
21. Winzelberg GG, Froelich JW, McKusick KA, Strauss HW. Scintigraphic detection of gastrointestinal bleeding: a review of current methods. Am J Gastroenterol 1983; 78:324–327.
22. Tedesco FJ, Pickens CA, Griffin JW, et al. Role of colonoscopy in patients with unexplained melena: analysis of 53 patients. Gastrointest Endosc 1981; 27:221–223.
23. Sanderson IR, Boyle S, Williams CB, Walker-Smith JA. Histological abnormalities in biopsies from macroscopically normal colonoscopies. Arch Dis Child 1986; 61:274–277.
24. Devroede GJ, Taylor WF, Sauer WG, et al. Cancer risk and life expectancy of children with ulcerative colitis. N Engl J Med 1971; 285:17-21.

25. Maloney WT, et al. Appropriate use of gastrointestinal endoscopy: a consensus statement from the American Society for Gastrointestinal Endoscopy. May 1989.
26. Ransohoff DF, Riddell RH, Levin B. Ulcerative colitis and colonic cancer: problems in assessing the diagnostic usefulness of mucosal dysplasia. Dis Colon Rectum 1985; 28:383–388.
27. Kirschner BS. Inflammatory bowel disease in children. Pediatr Clin North Am 1988; 35:189–208.
28. Doman DB, Golding MI, Goldberg HJ, Doyle RB. Aeromonas hydrophilia colitis presenting as medically refractory inflammatory bowel disease. Am J Gastroenterol 1989; 84:83–85.
29. Bartlett JG. The pseudomembranous enterocolitides. In: Sleisenger MH, Fortran JS, eds. Gastrointestinal diseases: pathophysiology, diagnosis, management. Philadelphia: WB Saunders, 1989: 1307.
30. Tedesco FJ, Corless JK, Brownstein RE. Rectal sparing in antibiotic-associated pseudomembranous colitis: a prospective study. Gastroenterology 1982; 83:1259–1260.
31. Cello JP. Gastrointestinal manifestations of HIV infection. Infect Dis Clin North Am 1988; 2:387–396.
32. Meyers JD. Infections in marrow transplant recipients. In: Mandell GL, Douglas RG, Bennett JE, eds. Principles and practice of infectious diseases. New York: Churchill Livingstone, 1990: 2291.
33. Sale GE, McDonald GB, Shulman HM, Thomas ED. Gastrointestinal graft-versus-host disease in man: a clinicopathologic study of the rectal biopsy. Am J Surg Pathol 1979; 3:291–299.
34. Jenkins HR, Pincott JR, Soothill JF, et al. Food allergy: the major cause of infantile colitis. Arch Dis Child 1984; 59:326–329.
35. Powell GK. Milk- and soy-induced enterocolitis of infancy. J Pediatr 1978; 93:553–560.
36. Chong SKF, Blackshaw AJ, Morson BC, et al. Prospective study of colitis in infancy and early childhood. J Pediatr Gastroenterol Nutr 1986; 5:352–358.
37. Lake AM, Whitington PF, Hamilton SR. Dietary protein-induced colitis in breast-fed infants. J Pediatr 1982; 101:906–910.
38. Goldman AS, Anderson DW, Sellers WA, et al. Milk allergy: I. Oral challenge with milk and isolated milk proteins in allergic children. Pediatrics 1963; 32:425–443.
39. Berezin S, Schwarz SM, Glassman M, et al. Gastrointestinal milk intolerance of infancy. Am J Dis Child 1989; 143:361–362.
40. Goldman H, Proujansky R. Allergic proctitis and gastroenteritis in children: clinical and mucosal biopsy features in 53 cases. Am J Surg Pathol 1986; 10:75–86.
41. Maurer G, Kratochvil P, Brandstatter G. The value of colonoscopy and ultrasonography in the diagnosis of chronic intussusception in childhood. Endoscopy 1986; 18:29–30.
42. Bailey DJ, Courington KR, Andres JM, et al. Cecal polyp and appendiceal intussusception in a child with recurrent abdominal pain: diagnosis by colonoscopy. J Pediatr Gastroenterol Nutr 1987; 6:818–820.
43. Duncan BR, Dohner VA, Priest JH. The Gardner syndrome: need for early diagnosis. J Pediatr 1968; 72:497–505.
44. Macrae FA, Tan KG, Williams CB. Towards safer colonoscopy: a report on the complications of 5000 diagnostic or therapeutic colonoscopies. Gut 1983; 24:376–383.
45. Bond JH, Levy M, Levitt MD. Explosion of hydrogen gas in the colon during proctosigmoidoscopy. Gastrointest Endosc 1976; 23:41–42.
46. Bigard MA, Gaucher P, Lassalle C. Fatal colonic explosion during colonoscopic polypectomy. Gastroenterology 1979; 77:1307–1310.
47. LaBrooy SJ, Avgerinos A, Fendick CL, et al. Potentially explosive colonic concentrations of hydrogen after bowel preparation with Mannitol. Lancet 1981; i:634–636.
48. Davis GR, Santa Ana CA, Morawski SG, Fordtran JS. Development of a lavage solution associated with minimal water and electrolyte absorption or secretion. Gastroenterology 1980; 78:991–995.
49. Tolia V, Fleming S, Dubois RS. Use of Golytely® in children and adolescents. J Pediatr Gastroenterol Nutr 1984; 3:468–470.
50. Caos A, Benner KG, Manier J, et al. Colonoscopy after Golytely preparation in acute rectal bleeding. J Clin Gastroenterol 1986; 8:46–49.
51. Thomas G, Brozinsky S, Isenberg JI. Patient acceptance and effectiveness of a balanced lavage solution (Golytely®) versus the standard preparation for colonoscopy. Gastroenterology 1982; 82:435–437.
52. Cotton PB, Williams CB. Practical gastrointestinal endoscopy. Oxford: Blackwell Scientific Publishers, 1985: 99.
53. Hayward SR, Sugawa C, Wilson RF. Changes in oxygenation and pulse rate during endoscopy. Am Surgeon 1989; 55:198–202.
54. Taylor MB, Whitwam JG. The current status of pulse oximetry. Anaesthesia 1986; 41:943–949.
55. Kelley CJ, Ingoldby CJH, Blenkharn JI, Wood CB. Colonoscopy related endotoxemia. Surg Gynecol Obstet 1985; 161:332–334.
56. Shorvon PJ, Eykyn SJ, Cotton PB. Gastrointestinal instrumentation, bacteremia, and endocarditis. Gut 1983; 24:1078–1093.
57. Norfleet RG, Mitchell PD, Mulholland DD, Philo J. Does bacteriemia follow colonoscopy? Gastrointest Endosc 1976; 23:31–32.
58. Pelican G, Hentges D, Butt J, et al. Bacteremia during colonoscopy. Gastrointest Endosc 1976; 23:33–35.
59. Kiss A, Ferenci P, Graninger W, et al. Endotoxemia following colonoscopy. Endoscopy 1983; 15:24–26.
60. Byrne WJ, Euler AR, Campbell M, Eisenach KD. Bacteremia in children following upper gastrointestinal endoscopy or colonoscopy. J Pediatr Gastroenterol Nutr 1982; 1:551–553.
61. Norfleet RG, Mulholland DD, Mitchell PD, et al. Does bacteriemia follow colonoscopy? Gastroenterology 1976; 70:20–21.
62. Dickman MD, Farrell R, Higgs RH, et al. Colonoscopy associated bacteremia. Surg Gynecol Obstet 1976; 142:173–176.
63. Shulman ST, Amren DP, Bisno AL, et al. Prevention of bacterial endocarditis. (Abstract) Circulation 1984; 70:1123–1127.
64. Simmons NA, Gawson RA, Clarke C, et al. The antibiotic prophylaxis of infective endocarditis: report of a working party of the British Society for Antimicrobial Chemotherapy. Lancet 1982; ii:1323–1326.
65. Blackstone MO. Endoscopic interpretation: normal and pathologic appearances of the gastrointestinal tract. New York: Raven Press, 1984: 401.
66. Prior A, Lessells AM, Whorwell PJ. Is biopsy necessary if colonoscopy is normal? Dig Dis Sci 1987; 32:673–676.
67. Rogers BHG. Complications and hazards of colonoscopy. In: Hunt RH, Wayne JD, eds. Colonoscopy, techniques, clinical practice and colour atlas. London: Chapman and Hall, 1981: 237.
68. Vawter M, Ruiz R, Alaama A, et al. Electrocardiographic monitoring during colonoscopy. Am J Gastroenterol 1975; 63:155–157.
69. Davison ET, Levine M, Meyerowitz R. Ventricular fibrillation during colonoscopy: case report and review of the literature. Am J Gastroenterol 1985; 80:690–693.
70. Alam M, Schuman BM, Duvernoy WFC, Madrazo AC. Continuous electrocardiographic monitoring during colonoscopy. Gastrointest Endosc 1976; 22:203–205.
71. Livstone EM, Kerstein MD. Serosal tears following colonoscopy. Arch Surg 1976; 111:88.
72. Ellis RW, Harrison JM, Williams RS. Rupture of spleen at colonoscopy. Br Med J 1979; i:307–308.
73. Telmos AJ, Mittal VK. Splenic rupture following colonoscopy. (Letter) JAMA 1977; 237:2718.
74. Hunt R. Towards safer colonoscopy. Gut 1983; 24:371–375.
75. Overholt BF, Hargrove RL, Farris RK, Wilson BM. Colonoscopic polypectomy: silent perforation. Gastroenterology 1976; 70:112–113.
76. Prorok JJ, Stahler EJ, Hartzell GW, Sugerman HJ. Surgical management of colonoscopic perforation. (Abstract) Gastrointest Endosc 1977; 23:238.
77. Foley B, Fielding JF. Cervical emphysema, pneumomediastinum and retroperitoneal gas after sigmoidoscopy. J Clin Gastroenterol 1982; 4:141–143.
78. Glouberman S, Craner GE, Ogburn RM, Burdick GE. Radiographic survey for extraluminal air following gastrointestinal tract fiberendoscopy. Gastrointest Endosc 1976; 22:165–167.
79. Nagasako N, Takemoto T. Endoscopy of the ileocecal area. Gastroenterology 1973; 65:403–411.
80. Newman SL. Ileoscopy, colonoscopy and backwash ileitis in children with inflammatory bowel disease: quid pro quo? J Pediatr Gastroenterol Nutr 1987; 6:325–327.
81. Goulston SJM, McGovern VJ. The nature of benign stricture in ulcerative colitis. N Engl J Med 1969; 281:290–295.
82. Cook MG, Goligher JC. Carcinoma and epithelial dysplasia complicating ulcerative colitis. Gastroenterology 1975; 68:1127–1136.
83. Gryboski JD, Spiro HM. Prognosis in children with Crohn's disease. Gastroenterology 1978; 74:807–817.
84. Pera A, Bellando P, Caldera D, et al. Colonoscopy in inflammatory bowel disease. Gastroenterology 1987; 92:181–185.
85. Mekhjian HS, Switz DM, Melnyk CS, et al. Clinical features and natural history of Crohn's disease. Gastroenterology 1979; 77:898–906.
86. Lennard-Jones JE, Lockhart-Mummery HE, Chir M, Morson BC.

Clinical and pathological differentiation of Crohn's disease and proctocolitis. Gastroenterology 1968; 54:1162–1170.
87. Potzi R, Walgram M, Lochs H, et al. Diagnostic significance of endoscopic biopsy in Crohn's disease. Endoscopy 1989; 21:60–62.
88. Traube J, Simpson S, Riddell RH, et al. Crohn's disease and adenocarcinoma of the bowel. Dig Dis Sci 1980; 25:939–944.
89. Gyde SN, Prior P, Macartney JC, et al. Malignancy in Crohn's disease. Gut 1980; 21:1024–1029.
90. Hamilton SR. Colorectal carcinoma in patients with Crohn's disease. Gastroenterology 1985; 89:398–407.
91. Antonioli DA, Marcial MA, Goldman H, Fukagawa NK, Winter HS. Utility of rectal biopsy in allergic proctitis. (Abstract) Lab Invest 1985; 52:3.
92. Rosekrans PCM, Meijer CJLM, Van der wal AM, Lindeman J. Allergic proctitis, a clinical and immunopathological entity. Gut 1980; 21:1017–1023.
93. Cucchiara S, Guandalini S, Staiano A, et al. Sigmoidoscopy, colonoscopy and radiology in the evaluation of children with rectal bleeding. J Pediatr Gastroenterol Nutr 1983; 2:667–671.
94. Daum F, Zucker P, Boley SJ, Bernstein LH. Colonoscopic polypectomy in children. Am J Dis Child 1977; 131:566–567.
95. Bartnik W, Butruk E, Ryzko J, et al. Short- and long-term results of colonoscopic polypectomy in children. Gastrointest Endosc 1986; 32:389–392.
96. Boland CR, Itzkowitz SH, Kim YS. Colonic polyps and the gastrointestinal polyposis syndromes. In: Sleisenger MH, Fordtran JS, eds. Gastrointestinal disease: pathophysiology, diagnosis, management. Philadelphia: WB Saunders, 1989: 1483.
97. Bussey HJR, Veale AMO, Morson BC. Genetics of gastrointestinal polyposis. Gastroenterology 1978; 74:1325–1330.
98. Naylor EW, Lebenthal E. Early detection of adenomatous polyposis coli in Gardner's syndrome. Pediatrics 1979; 63:222–227.
99. Tedesco FJ, Griffin JW, Khan AQ. Vascular ectasia of the colon: clinical, colonoscopic and radiographic features. J Clin Gastroenterol 1980; 2:233–238.
100. Burt RW, Berenson MM, Samuelson CO, Cathey WJ. Rheumatoid vasculitis of the colon presenting as pancolitis. Dig Dis Sci 1983; 28:183–188.
101. Reza MJ, Roth BE, Pops MA, Goldberg LS. Intestinal vasculitis in essential, mixed cryoglobulinemia. Ann Intern Med 1974; 81:632–634.
102. Martinez-Frontanilla LA, Haase GM, Ernster JA, Bailey WC. Surgical complications in Henoch-Schonlein purpura. J Pediatr Surg 1984; 19:434–436.
103. Koss LG. Abdominal gas cysts (pneumatosis cystoides intestinorum hominis). Arch Pathol 1952; 53:523–549.
104. Goodall RJR. Pneumatosis coli: report of two cases. Dis Colon Rectum 1978; 21:61–65.
105. Feinberg SB, Schwartz MZ, Clifford S, et al. Significance of pneumotosis cystoides intestinalis after jejunoileal bypass. Am J Surg 1977; 133:149–152.
106. Gruenberg JC, Grodsinsky C, Ponka JL. Pneumatosis intestinalis: a clinical classification. Dis Colon Rectum 1979; 22:5–9.
107. Earnest DL, Schneiderman DJ. Other diseases of the colon and rectum. In: Sleisenger MH, Fordtran JS, eds. Gastrointestinal diseases: pathophysiology, diagnosis, management. Philadelphia: WB Saunders, 1989: 1592.

CHAPTER 31

Liver Biopsy Interpretation

Antonio R. Perez-Atayde, M.D.

A vast number of diseases of the liver affect children and particularly manifest during infancy. Liver biopsy is of paramount importance in the diagnosis of these various and often complex disorders. In infants and children needle liver biopsy is easily accomplished under sedation and local anesthesia through a percutaneous transcostal or transdiaphragmatic approach.[1,2] It has become an invaluable, safe, and simple method of diagnosis of liver disease even in infants as young as 1 week of age. It is remarkably accurate in the diagnosis of diffuse parenchymal disorders that affect the liver evenly, such as extrahepatic biliary obstruction, hepatitis, cirrhosis, metabolic errors, and drug reactions. Liver biopsy also has a high diagnostic yield in disorders that affect the liver focally but extensively, such as immune cell-mediated rejection, graft-versus-host disease, granulomas, and neoplastic disorders. With the use of computed tomography (CT) scan and ultrasound-guided percutaneous liver biopsies using thin needles, it has become possible to diagnose isolated lesions of the liver.[2,3] This technique is increasingly gaining acceptance, especially for cytologic and bacteriologic diagnosis. Thin-needle biopsies, however, are usually inadequate for assessment of liver architecture.

The most frequent indications for needle liver biopsy are the following: hepatomegaly of uncertain origin, unexplained persistent conjugated hyperbilirubinemia, persistent elevations of hepatic enzymes, fever of unknown origin, systemic or infiltrative diseases such as sarcoidosis and miliary tuberculosis, primary or metastatic liver tumors, immune rejection in liver transplantation, and occasionally in bone marrow transplantation when graft-versus-host disease needs to be differentiated from hepatitis or drug toxicity. In addition, liver biopsy is often needed to assess the prognosis of an already-diagnosed hepatic disease by grading its severity, progression, or response to therapy and to monitor hepatotoxic drugs.

The light microscopic observation of hematoxylin and eosin (H & E)–stained sections of the liver biopsy can give extremely important and accurate information when properly processed and interpreted. However, the range of histopathologic reactions of the liver to various injuries is limited, so that frequently similar microscopic findings are observed as a result of etiologically unrelated disorders. Detailed clinical data should always be combined with the morphologic features in liver biopsy interpretation. Special stains such as periodic acid-Schiff (PAS), PAS after diastase digestion, reticulin, trichrome, and iron are part of the routine evaluation because they broaden the spectrum of hepatic reactions to injury by bringing out certain histologic or cytologic features not visible on H & E stains.

Tissue obtained by percutaneous liver biopsy can be used for enzyme analysis to detect inborn errors of metabolism, for biochemical analysis of stored material such as iron, copper, or specific metabolites, and for electron microscopy. The electron microscope has contributed greatly to the understanding of the subcellular pathogenetic mechanisms of disease.[4] It has become an essential tool in the diagnosis of various diseases of the liver, particularly in children. Such diseases include some inborn errors of metabolism, viral infections, drug toxicity, and certain intrahepatic diseases of unknown etiology.

Recently, immunoperoxidase techniques utilizing an ever-expanding list of polyclonal and monoclonal antibodies have been incorporated in the study of liver biopsies. They may render a specific diagnosis in some infectious, neoplastic, or metabolic disorders. In situ DNA hybridization has been used in the diagnosis of Epstein-Barr virus, hepatitis viruses, human immunodeficiency virus, adenovirus, and cytomegalovirus infection.[5-8] It is a technique that promises wider future applications along with the availability of new specific DNA probes.

DISORDERS OF BILIRUBIN METABOLISM

Most heritable disorders of bilirubin metabolism are associated with unconjugated hyperbilirubinemia and cause only nonspecific ultrastructural alterations in the liver. The Dubin-Johnson syndrome is an exception, since it produces conjugated hyperbilirubinemia and a distinctive hepatic histopathology without cholestasis. The centrilobular hepatocytes gradually accumulate within their lysosomes a melanin-like pigment that imparts to the liver a dark, almost black gross appearance.[9-11] Ultrastructural studies reveal characteristic pleomorphic pigment-containing lysosomes in the pericanalicular region.[4] Pathologic changes in Rotor's syndrome, a related disorder, are demonstrable only at the ultrastructural level with primitive, poorly developed canaliculi and nonspecific changes in cytoplasmic organelles.[4]

EXTRAHEPATIC BILIARY ATRESIA

In the newborn infant conjugated hyperbilirubinemia has a multitude of causes and generally is a challenging diagnostic puzzle for the physician. In only about 20 percent of children can a specific infectious or metabolic etiology be found.[12-17] Even less frequently, infants with conjugated

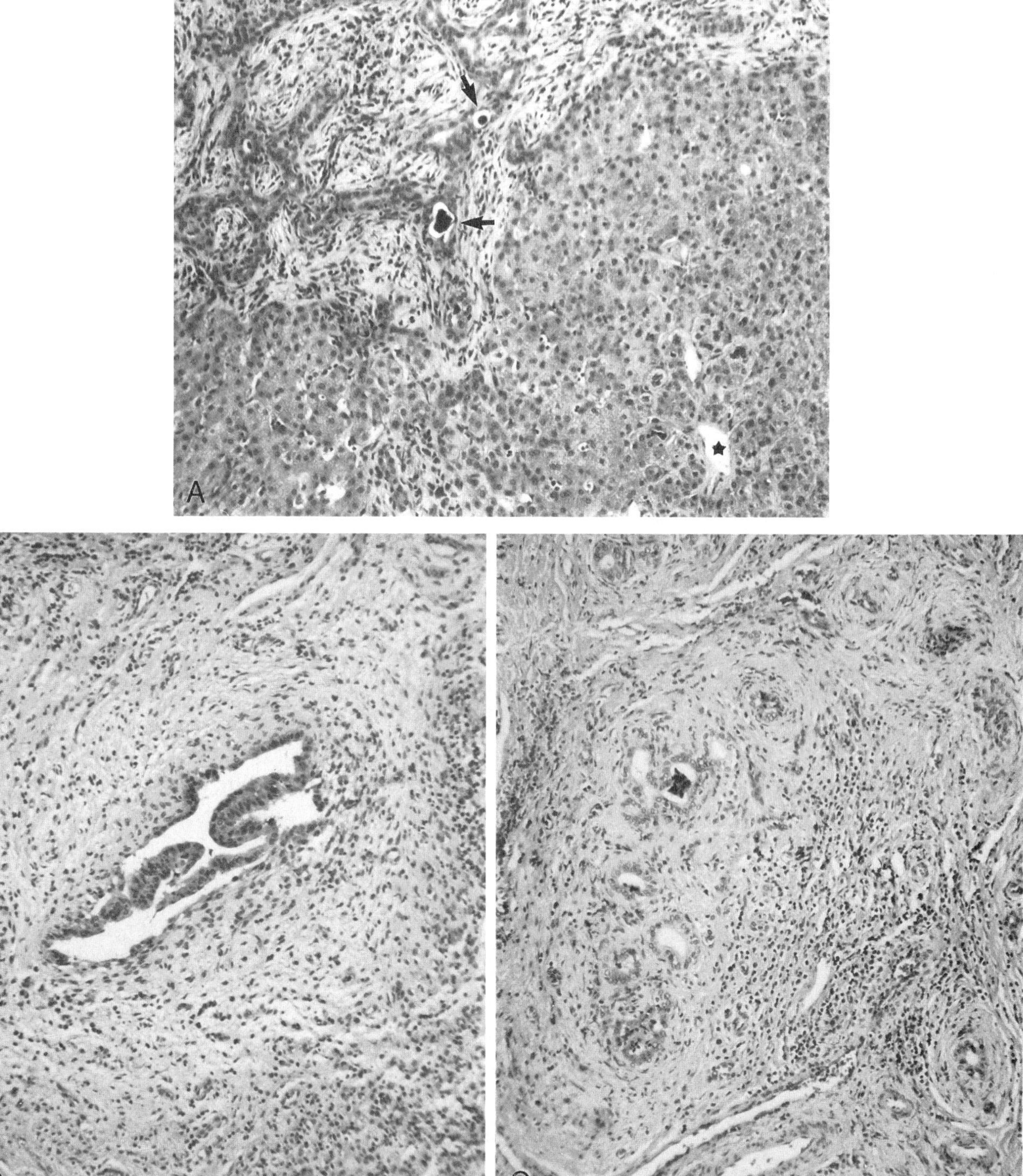

FIGURE 1 Extrahepatic biliary atresia. *A*, There is expansion of the portal tract (*left upper corner*) by fibrosis, bile duct proliferation, and mixed inflammatory infiltrate. Proliferating bile ducts are tortuous and contain bile plugs (*arrows*). The hepatic lobular architecture is maintained. Star indicates central vein. *B*, Porta hepatis showing a chronic fibrosing cholangitis. The bile duct is infiltrated by numerous lymphocytes and fibroblasts and is lined by a damaged epithelium with focal necrosis. *C*, Porta hepatis showing chronic inflammation and nodular scarring containing small bile ductules lined by cuboidal epithelium. (*A* to *C*, hematoxylin and eosin.)

hyperbilirubinemia have chronic intrahepatic cholestatic syndromes, a group of increasingly better recognized disorders of uncertain etiology, with variable nonspecific histopathologic findings and occasional familial incidence.[17-29] In these syndromes hypoplasia of the intrahepatic bile ducts is frequently but not always found. The majority of patients with obstructive-type jaundice fall into the category of idiopathic neonatal hepatitis and extrahepatic biliary atresia, the latter two to three times less frequent than the former.[29]

Extrahepatic biliary atresia is a rare syndrome, the incidence varying from 1 in 8,000 to 1 in 20,000 live births.[17,30] Despite its low incidence, it is the most common cause of extrahepatic cholestasis in infants. In extrahepatic biliary atresia there is interruption of bile flow from the liver to the duodenum because of a segmental anatomic discontinuity somewhere along the extrahepatic biliary tree (see Chapter 28, Parts 1 and 27).

In the diagnosis of extrahepatic biliary atresia the liver biopsy is of paramount importance. The histologic changes are not pathognomonic, but they are sufficiently characteristic to reach the correct diagnosis in 80 to 90 percent of the cases.[31-35] The consequences of extrahepatic biliary atresia observed on the histology of the liver are similar to those observed with other causes of chronic extrahepatic biliary obstruction such as choledochal cyst, inspissated bile plug syndrome, cholelithiasis, or extrinsic biliary compression. The portal tracts expand by edema, bile ductular proliferation, fibrosis, and a mixed inflammatory infiltrate of neutrophils and lymphocytes (Fig. 1*A*). Proliferating portal bile ductules are tortuous, are usually located along the limiting plate, and often reveal a mild nonspecific cholangitis. Intracellular and canalicular cholestasis is always observed early in the disease and is usually centrilobular, but in later stages it is present within hepatocytes and canaliculi and occasionally within the lumina of interlobular bile ducts. The rare interstitial bile leakage ("bile lakes") is seen only in advanced disease. The lobular hepatic architecture is generally well preserved until late stages of the disease. Giant cell transformation and ballooning of the hepatocytes occur, but they are usually inconspicuous and limited to the periportal hepatocytes. Fibrosis is always limited to portal tracts and the periphery of hepatic lobules, and its severity correlates with the state of the disease. The presence of intralobular and perisinusoidal fibrosis is not a feature of extrahepatic biliary obstruction.

The most important differential diagnosis of extrahepatic biliary obstruction is neonatal hepatitis, and generally the above-described features are sufficient to suggest one of the two diagnoses. There is, however, considerable overlap between the histologic findings, and on occasion accurate distinction of the two entities cannot be accomplished.[17,29,32] The most valuable histopathologic findings that favor the diagnosis of extrahepatic biliary obstruction over neonatal hepatitis are bile ductular proliferation, intraductal bile stasis, conspicuous portal fibrosis, partial preservation of the general lobular architecture, and absence of intralobular (particularly perisinusoidal) fibrosis (Table 1).

In patients suspected to have extrahepatic biliary atresia on the basis of clinical, radiologic, laboratory, and histologic features, exploratory laparotomy with operative cholangiography to document the presence and site of the atresia is indicated. It gives a definitive diagnosis and directs the surgical treatment.[29,35]

The anatomy of the abnormal extrahepatic bile ducts is markedly variable. Two main categories, however, can be distinguished. The most common type is the surgically "uncorrectable" atresia that occurs in 75 to 85 percent of the cases. In this type, the discontinuity occurs at or above the porta hepatis bile ducts. The "correctable" type of atresia occurs less frequently and is characterized by distal discontinuity of the biliary tree with a proximal permeable segment up to the porta hepatis and liver.[29,30]

The early differential diagnosis between intrahepatic and extrahepatic cholestasis is essential, since the latter requires surgical treatment before irreversible damage to the liver has occurred, usually at 2 to 3 months of age.[12,29,30,36,37] The consequences of extrahepatic biliary atresia left untreated are dismal, and the outcome is always lethal. Affected children suffer increasingly severe cholestasis and pruritus and die before reaching 2 years of age from chronic liver damage and the complications of cirrhosis. Until recently, only the "correctable" type of atresia was surgically treated with a Roux-en-Y choledochojejunostomy or direct anastomosis of the proximal permeable common bile duct to a jejunal loop. In 1959 Kasai and Suzuki demonstrated that hepatic portoenterostomy was an indicated surgical procedure for the until-then uncorrectable type of extrahepatic biliary atresia. In this operation a complete resection of the fibrous scar at the porta hepatis containing the atretic bile ducts is performed, with

TABLE 1
Histologic Features of Neonatal Hepatitis and Biliary Atresia

	Hepatitis	Atresia
Giant cells	Throughout the lobule; centrilobular (early)	Occasional and usually periportal
Portal bile ducts	No evidence of proliferation	Proliferation
Inflammation	Lymphocytic	Mixed portal
Nonspecific cholangitis	No	Yes
Cholestasis	Intracellular, intracanalicular	Intracellular, intracanalicular, intra-bile ducts
Fibrosis	No if uncomplicated Yes (portal, perisinusoidal)	Yes (portal)

anastomosis of a loop of small intestine to the hepatic hilus. Other authors have also subsequently achieved satisfactory results with this operation when they performed it early in the life of the infant. Restoration of the bile flow can be obtained in 60 to 90 percent of patients who are operated on before 2 months of age.[30]

Histologic examination of the resected porta hepatis during the Kasai operation (hepatic portoenterostomy) shows a chronic fibrosing destructive cholangitis, suggesting an inflammatory process acquired late in fetal or early postnatal life (Fig. 1*B*). Several studies have found a correlation of the severity of the extrahepatic biliary atresia with the success of the Kasai operation.[38,39] If the residual ducts on the porta hepatis scar have a luminal diameter of more than 100 μ, restoration of the bile flow occurs in 80 to 90 percent of the cases (Fig. 1*B*). If the porta hepatis scar is devoid of ductular remnants, the outcome of the operation is almost always poor. For this reason intraoperative evaluation of the porta hepatis by frozen sections is usually performed. If the sections lack bile ducts, the surgeon is compelled to remove further scar tissue higher at the porta hepatis. The presence of ductules lined by cuboidal epithelium conveys a less favorable outcome than the presence of ductules lined by columnar cells. Ductules lined by cuboidal epithelium probably represent periductal glands in no direct continuity with the intrahepatic biliary tree (Fig. 1*C*).

Patients with successful hepatic portoenterostomy have clearance of jaundice, normal growth, and slower progression of their hepatic damage. Most patients, however, eventually develop recurrent cholangitis, cirrhosis, and portal hypertension.[36,37,40–43] Therefore, patients with extrahepatic biliary atresia currently form the major group of children undergoing liver transplantation.

The etiology of extrahepatic biliary atresia is unknown. The term *infantile obstructive cholangiopathy* has been offered to include idiopathic neonatal hepatitis, extrahepatic biliary atresia, intrahepatic atresia, and choledochal cyst as different expressions of the same clinicopathologic process, with possible similar etiology and pathogenesis.[17,29,32] This is substantiated by the occurrence of different components of this group of disorders in members of the same family and by the overlapping histopathologic features.

Although extrahepatic biliary atresia is rarely recognized at birth, it has been described in siblings and in association with congenital malformations, including hypoplasia of the spleen, polysplenia syndrome, trisomy 17 or 18, and bronchobiliary fistula.[17,29,44] In the past it was considered a developmental anomaly acquired in utero; however, the presence of an active inflammatory process at the site of atresia suggests an infectious etiology. This is supported by the occasional association of extrahepatic biliary atresia with cytomegalovirus and Epstein-Barr virus infection. More recently reovirus type 3 has been implicated as a causative agent, since a high proportion of children with biliary atresia have antibody levels to this virus in their sera, and particles consistent with reovirus have been observed by electron microscopic studies of the atretic bile ducts.[45–48] Other studies, however, have challenged an etiologic role of reovirus type 3.[49]

In a series of 128 patients with extrahepatic biliary atresia, immunoglobulin deposits were found in the remnants of bile ducts of 44 cases. Deposits were observed by immunoperoxidase along the basement membranes of glandular structures.[50] Other studies have demonstrated circulating IgG antibiliary epithelial cell antibodies in children with extrahepatic biliary atresia by immunofluorescence studies on frozen sections of the porta hepatis obtained during hepatoportoenterostomy.[51] Positive immunofluorescence was observed only when the tissue was preincubated with the patients' sera. These studies support the notion that extrahepatic biliary atresia is an acquired, progressively destructive inflammatory process.

NEONATAL HEPATITIS

Neonatal hepatitis, also known as giant cell neonatal hepatitis, is a morphologic alteration of the infant's liver that occurs as a nonspecific reaction to different kinds of insults, of which infectious (20 percent) and metabolic derangements (15 percent) are the most commonly identified. A familial occurrence of neonatal hepatitis is observed in 10 percent of the cases. Drug-related neonatal hepatitis is rare. Unfortunately, in the largest group of infants with neonatal hepatitis a cause cannot be identified (55 percent).[12,17,29] This idiopathic form of neonatal hepatitis is a frequent frustrating challenge for the pediatric hepatologist and urgently needs a scientific breakthrough.

Regardless of the etiology, the general histologic changes observed in giant cell neonatal hepatitis are similar. These changes are characterized by a preservation of the zonal hepatic distribution of portal tracts and central veins and a diffuse loss of the lobular architecture. Most hepatocytes show ballooning degeneration and fusion of their membranes with extensive transformation into multinucleated giant cells (Fig. 2*A* and *B*). Inflammation is variable and usually difficult to discern from the abundant extramedullary hematopoiesis. Intracanalicular and intrahepatocytic cholestasis is usually marked. Hepatocyte necrosis and swelling produce distortion and condensation of the reticulin framework. Histopathologically, the main differential diagnosis of neonatal hepatitis is to suggest a metabolic cause and to exclude extrahepatic biliary obstruction. The latter has already been discussed. In general the presence of steatosis, pseudoacinar transformation, persinusoidal fibrosis, various cytoplasmic inclusions or storage, and a positive family history frequently indicate a metabolic etiology (see Chapter 28, Part 1).

The viruses most frequently implicated in the etiology of giant cell neonatal hepatitis are rubella, coxsackie, cytomegalovirus, hepatitis B, and parainfluenza.[52] The light microscopic alterations in the liver are indistinguishable, and clinical or laboratory data or culture of the virus is necessary to reach an etiologic diagnosis (see Chapter 28, Part 2).

Cytomegalovirus may, however, induce distinct cytopathic changes with cytomegalia and characteristic nuclear and cytoplasmic inclusions with or without multinucleated giant cell transformation.[9,29,52] A discrete neutrophilic infiltrate around the damaged hepatocyte is occasionally present (Fig. 3*A*). Often, however, the only pathologic changes observed are occasional single heptocytes with characteristic cytopathic changes with minimal or no inflammatory reaction. Similar cytomegalovirus inclusions may be observed in bile duct epithelial cells.[9] The ultrastructural characteristics of

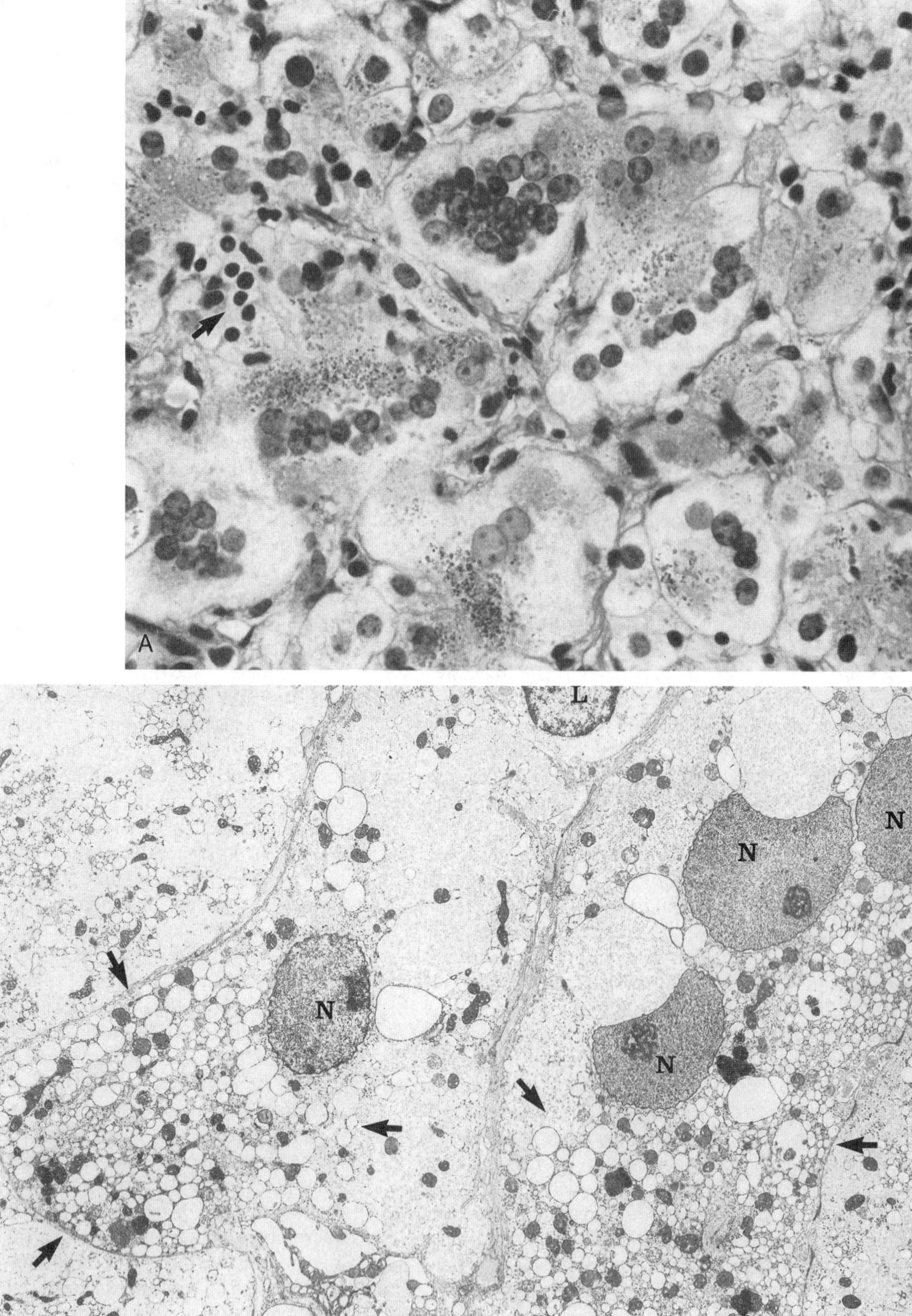

FIGURE 2 Giant cell neonatal hepatitis. *A*, There is loss of the lobular organization with ballooning and diffuse transformation of hepatocytes into multinucleated giant cells. Occasional lymphocytes and erythroblasts are scattered throughout (*arrow*) (hematoxylin and eosin). *B*, Electron micrograph showing multinucleated hepatocytes with cytoplasmic distention and vesicular transformation of endoplasmic reticulum (*between arrows*). N = nuclei; L = lymphocyte (uranyl acetate and lead citrate, ×2,500).

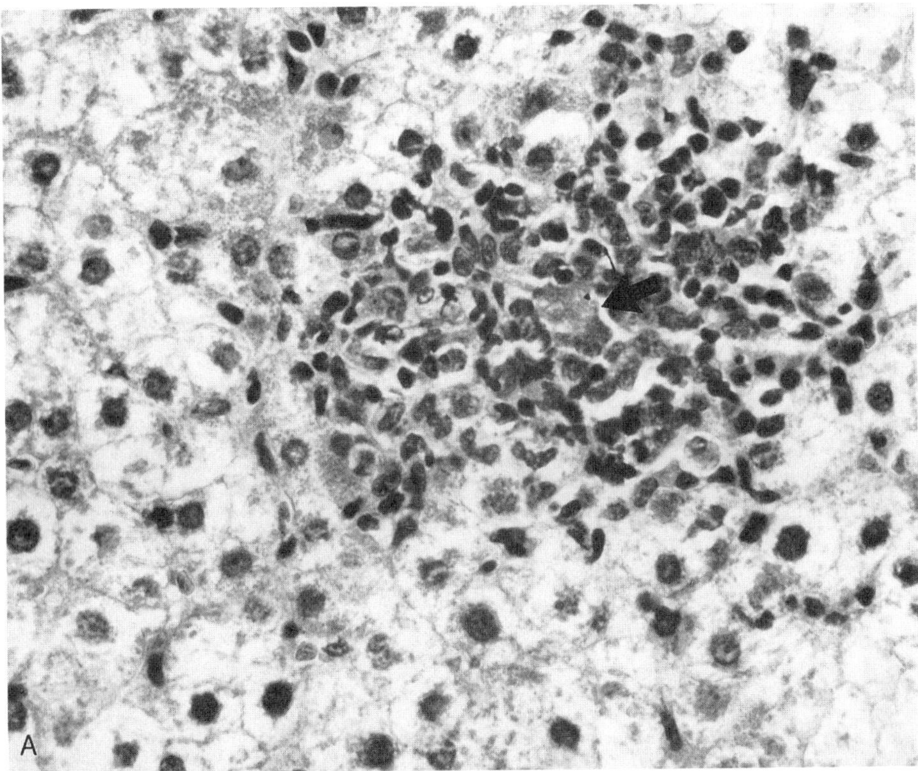

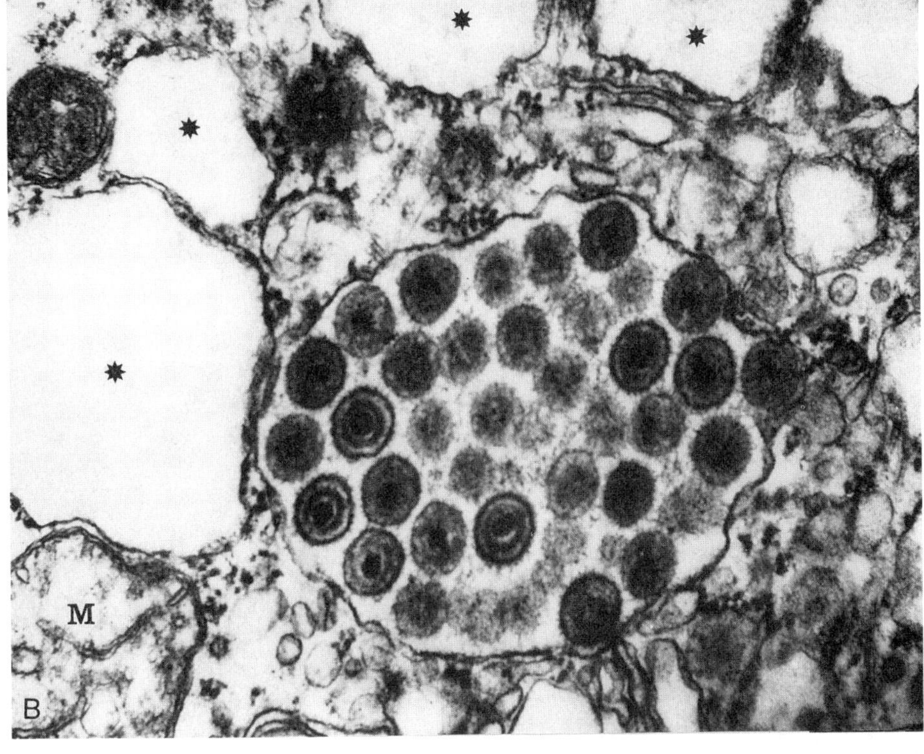

FIGURE 3 Cytomegalovirus hepatitis. *A*, Discrete cluster of mixed inflammatory cells, mainly neutrophils, surrounding a degenerating, transformed hepatocyte with nuclear and cytoplasmic basophilic granular inclusions (*arrow*). Adjacent hepatic parenchyma is unremarkable (hematoxylin and eosin). *B*, Ultrastructure of cytoplasmic inclusion showing a cisterna of endoplasmic reticulum containing numerous complete viral particles. Complete viruses are composed of nucleoid, capsid, and envelope. Vacuolar change of endoplasmic reticulum is also seen (*asterisk*). M = mitochondria (uranyl acetate and lead citrate, ×60,000).

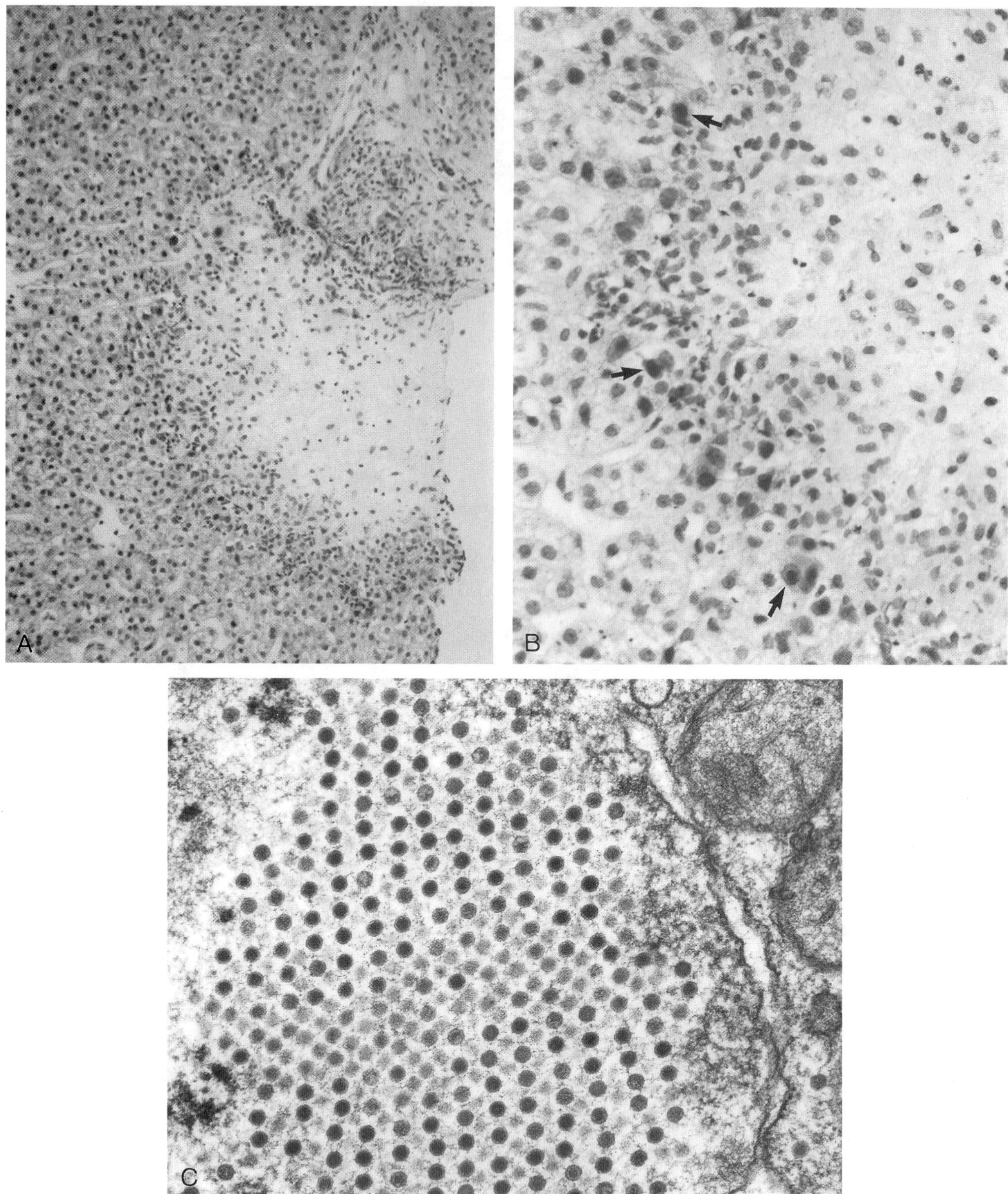

FIGURE 4 Adenovirus hepatitis. *A*, Well-circumscribed, pale, round area of necrosis containing cellular debris, occasional mononuclear inflammatory cells, and amorphous granular material. The surrounding hepatocytes are transformed, contain viral inclusions, and are undergoing degeneration and necrosis. Adjacent hepatic tissue shows normal appearance. *B*, A rim of transformed hepatocytes reveals large purple nuclei with viral inclusions (*arrows*). The cytoplasm is basophilic and retracted. (*A* and *B*, hematoxylin and eosin). *C*, Ultrastructural appearance of intranuclear adenovirus with the characteristic geometric arrangement of icosahedral nucleocapsids (uranyl acetate and lead citrate, ×100,000).

cytomegalovirus are those seen in the herpes family virus[4] (Fig. 3*B*). This kind of cytomegalovirus hepatitis without multinucleated giant cell transformation and preservation of the lobular architecture is usually observed in older children with congenital or acquired immunodeficiency. Rare associations of cytomegalovirus infections include paucity or proliferation of intrahepatic bile ducts, confluent necrosis, and sinusoidal fibrosis with noncirrhotic portal hypertension.[53,54]

Epstein-Barr virus and cytomegalovirus may cause the mononucleosis syndrome. The histopathology of the liver shows a conspicuous accumulation of large atypical lymphocytes within sinusoids and portal tracts and phlebitis of portal and central veins.[55]

Discrete round areas of confluent necrosis with peripheral inconspicuous inflammatory infiltrate are characteristic of herpes simplex and adenovirus hepatitis,[9,29,52] the intervening hepatic parenchyma remaining intact (Fig. 4*A*). Viral cytopathic changes typical for each virus are observed in transformed hepatocytes surrounding the necrotic foci (Fig. 4*B*). The ultrastructural features are distinctive for each type of virus[4] (Figs. 4*C* and 5). Echovirus 11 is an established cause of massive hemorrhagic necrosis of the liver in the newborn infant.[52,56]

INHERITED AND METABOLIC DISEASES

Various inherited disorders present in infancy with progressive cholestatic liver disease and variable histopathologic changes in the liver.[10,11] Some of these disorders are well defined because they occur in association with characteristic congenital anomalies or with singular metabolic defects. Variable, often nonspecific histologic changes occur in the liver of these patients. Most of these features are not constant for any specific disorder and usually change within the course of the disease.

In *arteriohepatic dysplasia (syndromatic paucity of intrahepatic bile ducts, Alagille's syndrome)*,[20-23,25,57] the most characteristic histopathologic findings are paucity of intrahepatic bile ducts, mild intrahepatic cholestasis, and sparse portal lymphocytic infiltrate without significant fibrosis (Fig. 6). The hepatocellular damage is usually mild. Some infants, however, present with a giant cell neonatal hepatitis or with bile duct proliferation that later progresses to the more typical picture of intrahepatic bile duct paucity. More rarely, some infants develop extrahepatic biliary atresia. The histologic diagnosis of paucity of intrahepatic bile ducts requires serial liver biopsies or bilateral wedge liver biopsies for quantification of portal tracts and bile ducts. The number of portal tracts devoid of bile ducts varies from 30 to 100 percent. The absolute concentration of portal tracts is also decreased.

Ultrastructurally, bile retention at the convex side of the Golgi complex has been described and is considered to be characteristic of the disorder.[58] Arteriohepatic dysplasia remains, however, a clinicopathologic diagnosis associated with multiple manifestations. These include characteristic facies, butterfly vertebrae, peripheral pulmonary artery stenosis, embryotoxon, hypogonadism, and growth and mental retardation.

When the hepatic findings occur in isolation (*nonsyndromatic paucity of intrahepatic bile ducts*),[17,18] the disease can have a variable course but is usually more severe with progressive portal fibrosis. This type of intrahepatic bile duct pau-

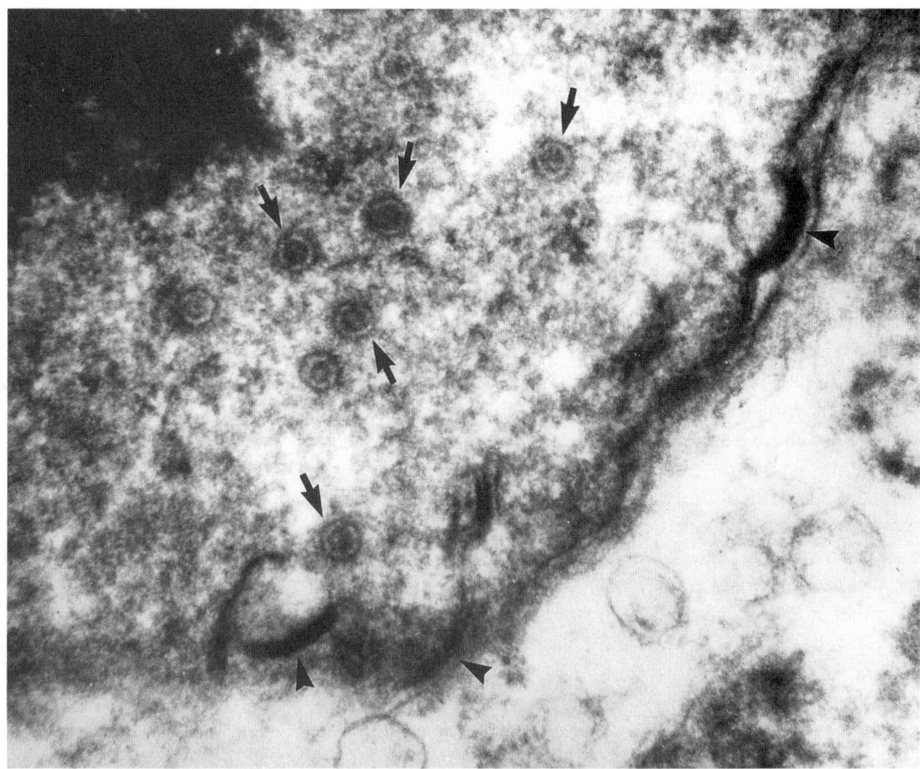

FIGURE 5 Ultrastructure of herpes virus hepatitis. Nucleus of hepatocyte contains numerous viral nucleocapsids (*arrows*). Fragments of the nuclear envelope (*arrowheads*) are acquired by the virus prior to its release into the cytoplasm as a complete viral particle (uranyl acetate and lead citrate, ×58,000).

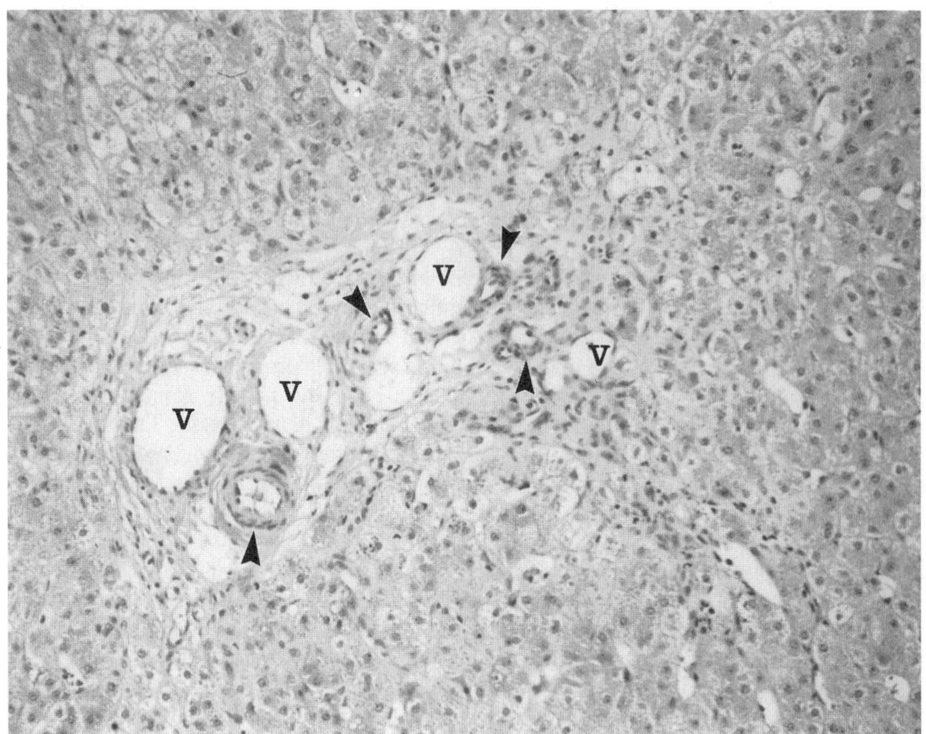

FIGURE 6 Syndromatic intrahepatic paucity of bile ducts (Alagille's syndrome). Portal tract is devoid of bile ducts. Portal vein (V), hepatic artery (*arrowheads*). Note absence of inflammation and preserved parenchymal architecture (hematoxylin and eosin).

city is usually idiopathic; however, it occurs as well in a variety of better-defined disorders (see below).

The *cerebrohepatorenal (Zellweger's) syndrome*[26–28,59–62] is an autosomal recessive disorder causing progressive cholestatic liver disease in infancy. Infants afflicted by this syndrome may have various of the following features: characteristic facies, hypotonia, renal cortical cysts, punctate calcifications of bones, and severe neurologic deficits. Eye abnormalities may also occur. The histologic changes in the liver are variable, but the most frequently encountered is diffuse hepatocellular damage with pseudoacinar transformation of hepatocytes, cholestasis, and perisinusoidal fibrosis. Steatosis may also be present. The fibrosis is usually progressive, leading to micronodular cirrhosis in the first few months of life. Hepatocellular and phagocyte-mononuclear iron deposits may be abundant. Paucity of intrahepatic bile ducts may be present early in the course. Absence or decreased number of peroxisomes and abnormal mitochondria are the ultrastructural hallmarks of the disease. The characteristic abnormalities in the metabolism of lysine, bile acids, very long chain fatty acids, and glycero-ether lipids all appear to be secondary to the peroxisomal deficiency.

Diffuse hepatocellular damage with pseudoacinar transformation, intracanalicular and cellular cholestasis, perisinusoidal fibrosis, and excessive hepatocellular iron occurs in *neonatal idiopathic hemochromatosis*.[62–67] Multinucleated giant hepatocytes may also be present. Iron accumulation occurs in other organs as well and characteristically spares the phagocyte-mononuclear system. The very existence of neonatal hemochromatosis as a clinicopathologic entity has recently been challenged.[67] In this report, iron contents in various organs were semiquantitated in autopsies of infants who died with severe subacute or chronic liver disease of undetermined cause and were compared with the iron contents in 14 children who died of severe subacute or chronic liver disease of known etiology and with those of nine who died with massive hepatic necrosis. Fourteen of 15 infants with liver disease of unknown cause showed heavy iron accumulation in parenchymal cells of more than one organ, in contrast to only one of 23 in the other two groups. The authors raise the possibility that neonatal hemochromatosis may represent a single disease entity or alternatively may be the result of severe in utero liver injury. The conclusion in this report, however, is hindered by the use of age-unmatched controls. The well-defined *familial hemochromatosis*[68] due to a defect in the regulation of intestinal iron absorption manifests rarely in childhood. Hemolytic anemias and blood transfusions are the leading causes of *secondary hemochromatosis*.[68]

Diffuse hepatocellular damage with the triad of pseudoacinar transformation, canalicular and cellular cholestasis, and conspicuous macro-microvesicular steatosis typically occurs in three metabolic disorders—*hereditary fructose intolerance, galactosemia due to transferase deficiency*, and *neonatal tyrosinemia* (Fig. 7) (see Chapter 28, Parts 9 and 10).[10,11] Nonspecific portal inflammatory changes, hematopoiesis, and occasional giant cell transformation of hepatocytes may be observed. Intralobular (perisinusoidal) fibrosis occurs in severe or advanced disease leading to micronodular cirrhosis. There are no specific changes that distinguish one disorder from another, and the same findings can be seen in unclassifiable cases. A combination of clinical, biochemical, and pathologic data is necessary to reach a diagnosis. Liver disease in fructose intolerance occurs only when fructose is part

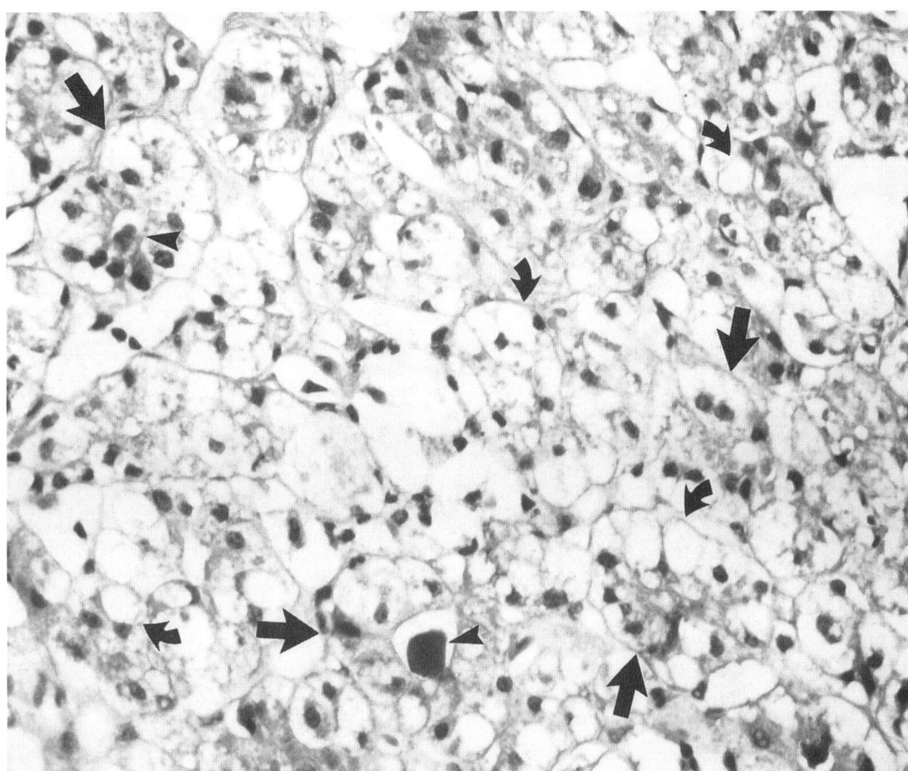

FIGURE 7 Hereditary fructose intolerance. There is diffuse hepatocellular damage with disarray of the lobular architecture, pseudoacinar transformation of hepatocytes (*arrows*), steatosis (*curved arrows*), and cholestasis (*arrowheads*) (hematoxylin and eosin).

of the diet. An ultrastructural lesion, the "fructose hole," has been claimed as distinctive of the disorder.[4] In neonatal tyrosinemia, the defective enzyme is fumarylacetoacetic acid hydrolase leading to an impaired conversion of fumarylacetoacetate to the Krebs cycle intermediate, fumerate, and the ketone body acetoacetate. There is excess iron in hepatocytes and nodular regeneration; adenomas and hepatocellular carcinoma occur frequently in the chronic form. Dietary restrictions may stop or reverse the hepatic damage in fructose intolerance and galactosemia. In tyrosinemia, however, dietary manipulations had been unsuccessful, and liver transplantation is the only alternative for cure.

Most children with *alpha$_1$-antitrypsin deficiency* and hepatic disease present during infancy with a cholestatic syndrome that usually resolves promptly.[10,11,69–78] The histologic changes in the liver are diverse and include giant cell neonatal hepatitis, portal fibrosis with bile duct proliferation, chronic active hepatitis, and intrahepatic paucity of bile ducts. The most frequently encountered early pathology includes mild hepatocellular damage with ballooning, mild neutral fat deposition, and occasional giant cell transformation; mild portal fibrosis with bile duct proliferation; hepatocellular and canalicular cholestasis; and the distinctive alpha$_1$-antitrypsin inclusions in periportal hepatocytes (Fig. 8*A*). These inclusions represent alpha$_1$-antitrypsin and stain positively with PAS even after diastase digestion and specifically with antibodies against alpha$_1$-antitrypsin (Fig. 8*B*). They are usually present regardless of the pathologic picture and can appear as early as the first week of life. However, they are inconspicuous before 10 to 12 weeks and increase in number with age. Ultrastructurally, they appear as proteinaceous amorphous material located in dilated cisternae of endoplasmic reticulum (Fig. 8*C*). After a variable asymptomatic period of months or years, the hepatic lesion can progress to cirrhosis in severe cases. Pi typing is required to confirm the diagnosis (see Chapter 28, Part 13).

The *familial progressive intrahepatic cholestatic syndromes* include a group of rare, ill-defined disorders that manifest in infancy and have variable clinical course.[17,19,29,79–84] Histologically, they are characterized by diffuse hepatocellular damage with lobular disarray, pseudoacinar transformation, canalicular and hepatocellular cholestasis, and absence of steatosis (Fig. 9). In some of these disorders a giant cell neonatal hepatitis may be the earliest manifestation. Intrahepatic paucity of bile ducts and/or progressive fibrosis may occur. A defect in bile acid metabolism[80] and abnormal canalicular microfilaments[79] have been identified in some of these disorders.

Pure cholestasis, mainly intracanalicular, and no other morphologic changes in the liver are observed in *benign recurrent cholestasis*[85] and generalized *sepsis* among others.

Indian childhood cirrhosis is a usually fatal familial disorders that affects primarily Indian children during the first decade of life.[86–88] It is associated with high levels of hepatic copper and marked deposits of copper-binding protein in hepatocytes. The histopathology resembles alcoholic liver disease with marked ballooning of hepatocytes, intracytoplasmic Mallory hyaline, and neutrophilic inflammation. Progressive fibrosis of terminal hepatic veins and Disse spaces leads to cirrhosis. The disease has been described in India, Pakistan, Sri Lanka, Burma, and recently in the United States and Great Britain.

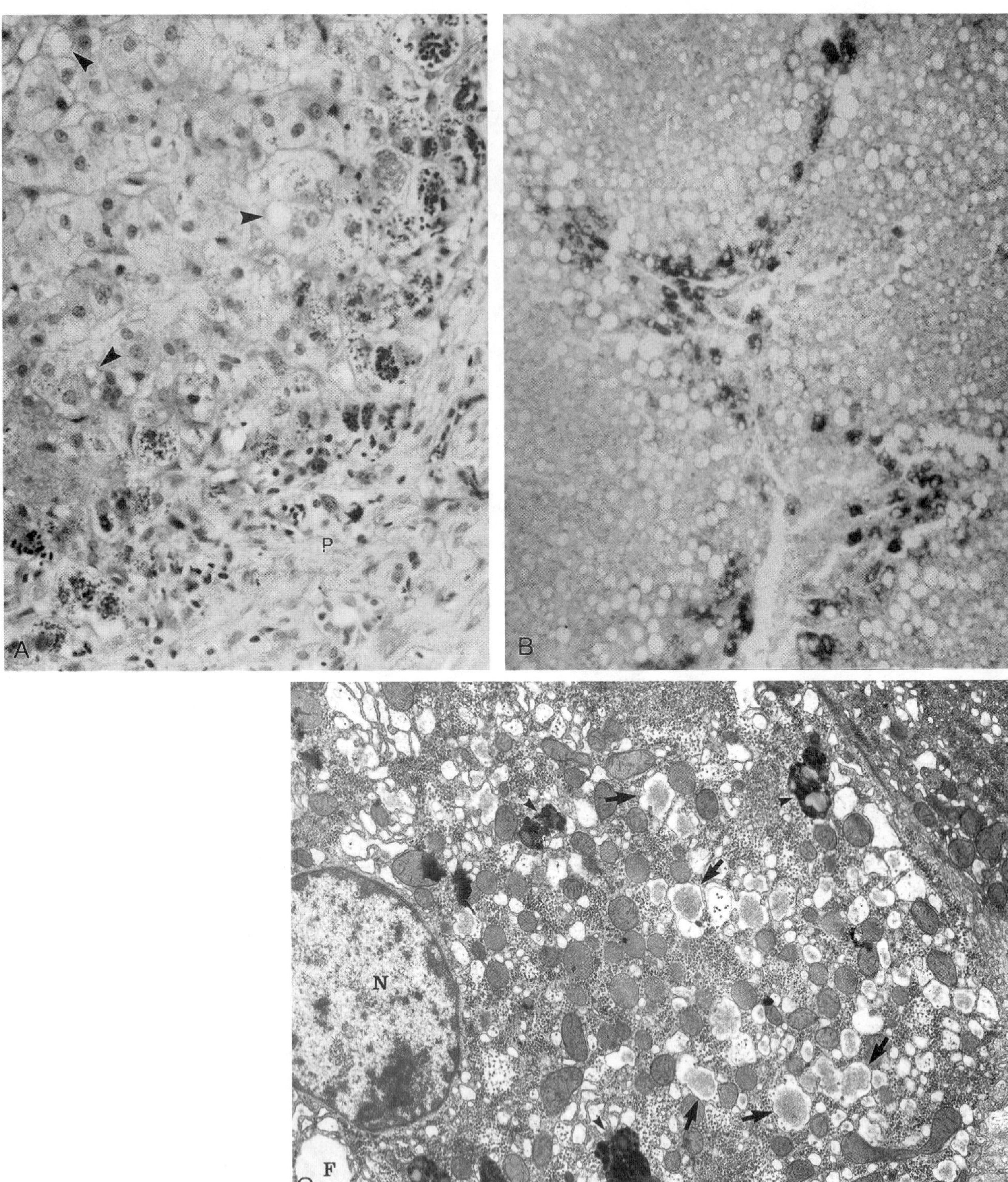

FIGURE 8 Alpha$_1$-antitrypsin deficiency. *A*, There is diffuse hepatocellular damage with ballooning, steatosis (*arrowheads*), pseudoacinar transformation, and cholestasis. The periportal hepatocytes contain numerous intracytoplasmic PAS-positive, diastase-resistant globules characteristic of the disease. The portal tract (P) is expanded with fibrosis, bile duct proliferation, and mild chronic inflammatory infiltrate (PAS stain after diastase digestion). *B*, Specific immunohistochemical staining of periportal alpha$_1$-antitrypsin droplets (dark brown staining cells). Note the moderate neutral fat deposition in hepatocytes (avidin-biotin complex with hematoxylin counterstain). *C*, Ultrastructure of hepatocyte showing dilated cisternae of endoplasmic reticulum containing amorphous proteinaceous material that represents alpha$_1$-antitrypsin (*arrows*). N = nucleus; arrowheads = lipofuscin granules; F = neutral fat (uranyl acetate and lead citrate, ×8,500).

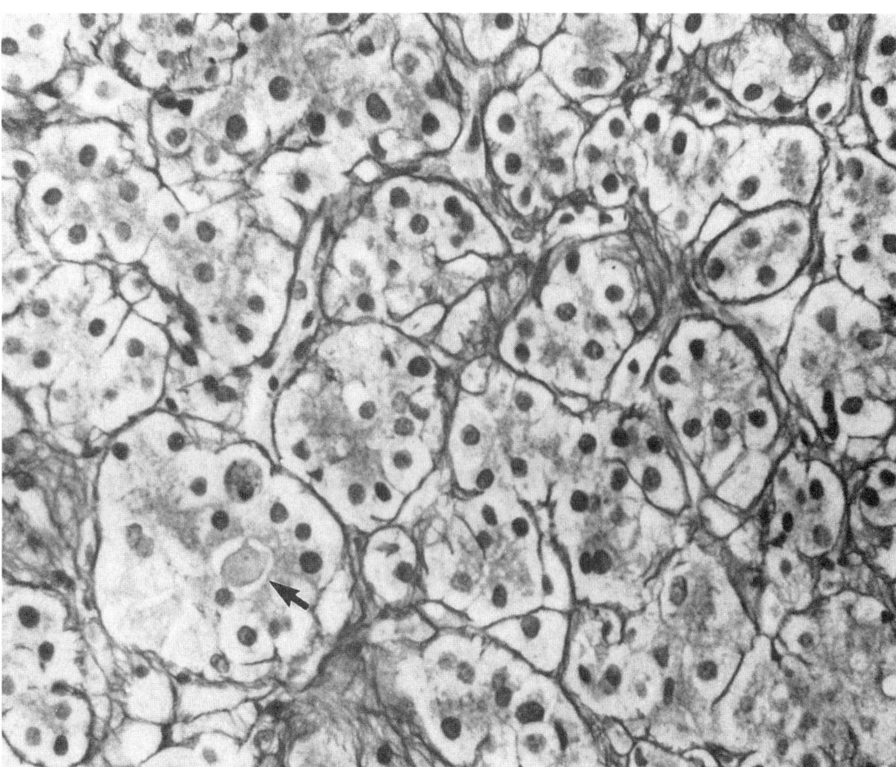

FIGURE 9 Familial progressive intrahepatic cholestasis. There are diffuse pseudoglandular transformation of hepatocytes, cholestasis (*arrow*), and pericellular fibrosis (reticulin stain).

Wilson's disease (hepatolenticular degeneration) is a rare, autosomal recessive inherited disorder that occurs predominantly in young people and is characterized by toxic accumulations of copper in the liver, brain, cornea (Kayser-Fleischer rings), and other organs. Clinical manifestations of copper excess are rare before 6 years of age, and 50 percent of untreated patients remain asymptomatic through adolescence. Increased liver copper precedes the development of histologic changes. The presence of copper storage can be suspected in H & E sections of liver biopsies when periportal hepatocytes contain unusually large and pleomorphic lipofuscin granules.[10,11] Specific staining for lysosomal copper and copper-binding protein can be accomplished with rhodamine and orcein stains, respectively.[9–11,89] These stains are important for the diagnosis of Wilson's disease; however, the absence of stainable copper does not exclude the diagnosis. In early stages of Wilson's disease copper accumulates in periportal hepatocytes. When it localizes diffusely in the cytosol of hepatocytes, histochemical reaction can be negative despite a high concentration of copper in the tissue. On the other hand a positive reaction for copper is not pathognomonic for Wilson's disease, since copper deposition can also be seen in chronic cholestatic syndromes, alpha$_1$-antitrypsin deficiency, Indian childhood cirrhosis, and normal neonatal liver. In the cirrhotic stages of Wilson's disease the stainable copper has a variable distribution; it may be present in some nodules and absent in others (Fig. 10*A*). When present, it may have a periportal or a diffuse distribution throughout the nodule. Measurement of copper content per gram of dry liver weight is the most accurate way to assess copper storage (see Chapter 28, Part 15).

The histologic changes in the liver range from nonspecific inflammation and steatosis to acute, chronic active, and fulminant hepatitis and cirrhosis. Patients with acute or fulminant hepatitis are rarely biopsied. Cirrhosis is by far the most frequent diagnosis. The constellation of histologic changes seen in early and late stages of the disease may be sufficient to suggest the diagnosis of Wilson's disease (Fig. 10*A*). There are ballooning of hepatocytes with occasional cytoplasmic Mallory hyaline, single cell necrosis, and variable fatty degeneration with occasional mild lymphocytic and/or neutrophilic infiltrate. Some hepatocytes characteristically have densely eosinophilic cytoplasm. Zone 1 hepatocytes contain atypically coarse lipofuscin granules with copper storage. In addition, portal inflammation with piecemeal necrosis and variable fibrosis is observed in chronic active hepatitis. The hepatic ultrastructural findings in Wilson's disease are very characteristic, especially those involving the mitochondria[4] (Fig. 10*B*). Pleomorphic mitochondria with dilated cristae and dense matrices containing a different kind of inclusions are frequently seen. Typical lysosomes containing copper are prominent in zone 1 hepatocytes.

The main histologic changes observed in *cystic fibrosis*[11] are secondary to segmental obstruction of bile flow by intraductal inspissated mucous secretions. The involved portal tracts reveal bile duct proliferation, intraductal cholestasis, fibrosis, chronic inflammation, and occasionally characteristic eosinophilic mucous plugs in bile ducts (Fig. 11). The hepatic lobular architecture is usually spared with the exception of cholestasis. Acute ascending cholangitis may be associated. The fibrosis usually progresses in an uneven manner, involving more the subcapsular zone, and leads to

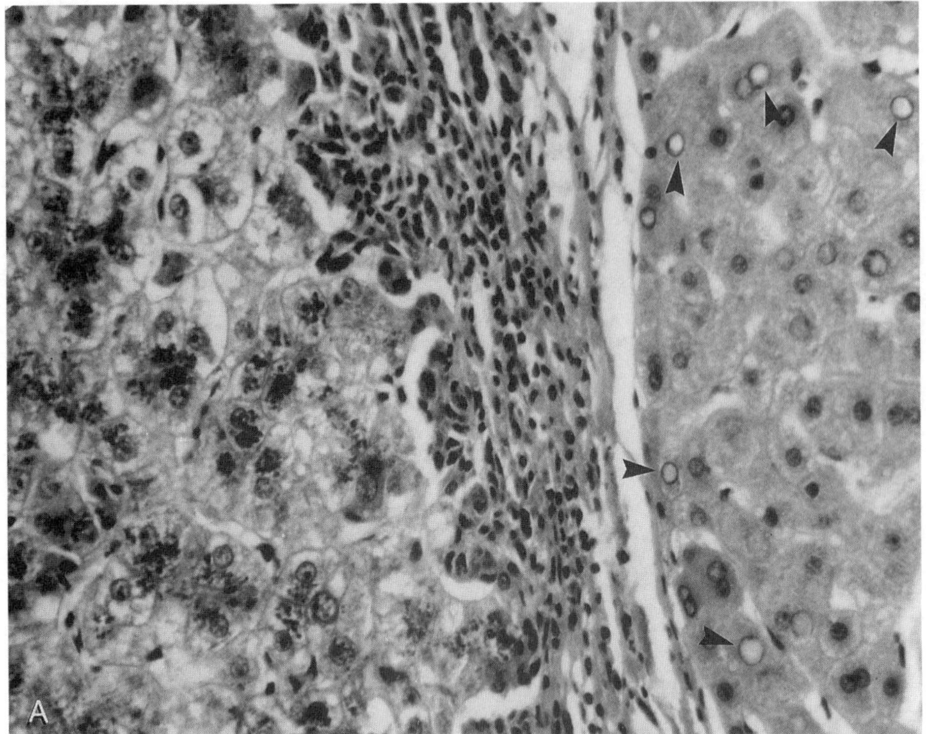

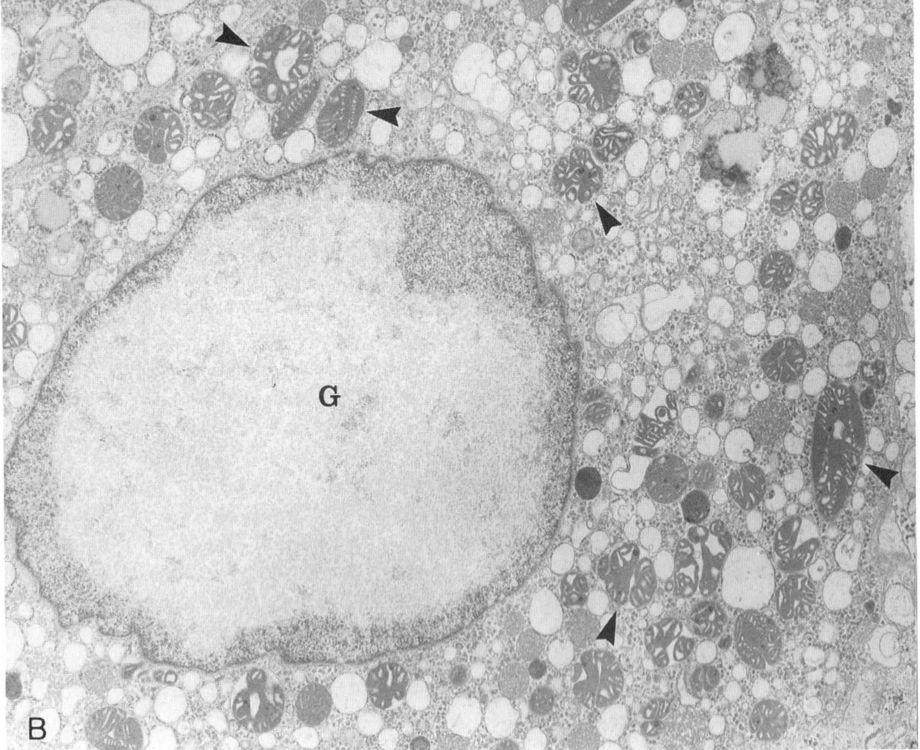

FIGURE 10 Wilson's disease. *A*, Two cirrhotic nodules, separated by a narrow fibrous septum, have different appearance. On the left, hepatocytes are swollen and contain neutral fat and numerous copper granules in the pericanalicular pole. On the right, hepatocytes have "glycogenated" nuclei (*arrowheads*) and normal appearance of the cytoplasm. The fibrous septum contains mixed inflammatory cells (hematoxylin and eosin). *B*, Ultrastructure of hepatocyte showing a large "glycogenated" nucleus (G) with margination of the chromatin and abundant free glycogen. The cytoplasm reveals enlarged mitochondria (*arrowheads*) with dense matrix, dilated cristae with angulated profiles, prominent intramatrical granules, and paracrystalline inclusions. The endoplasmic reticulum shows a vesicular change (uranyl acetate and lead citrate, ×11,000).

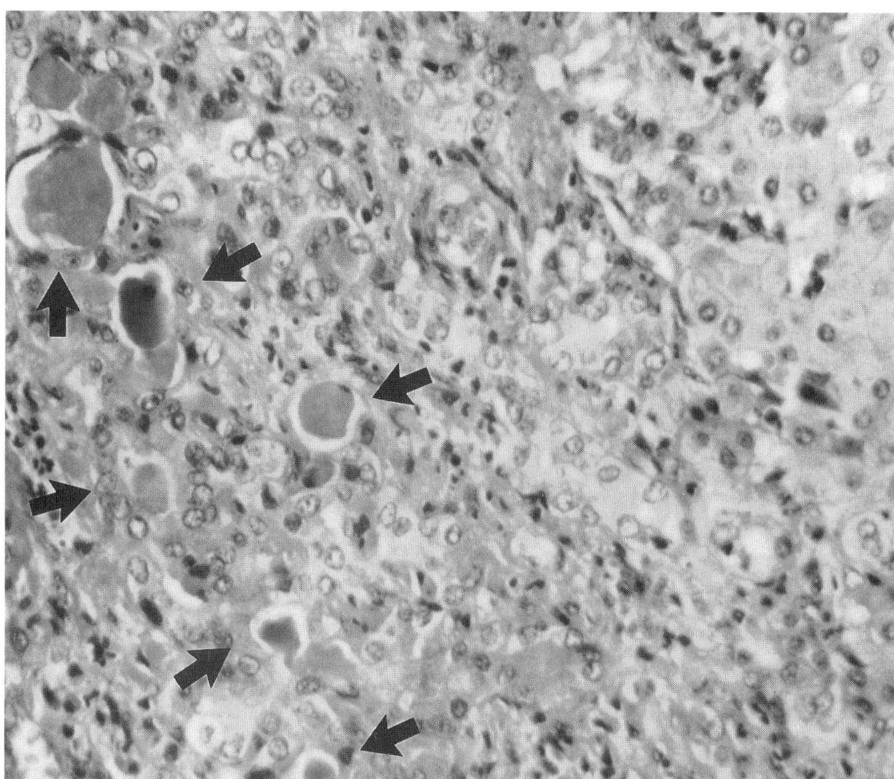

FIGURE 11 Cystic fibrosis. Broad fibrous septum with mixed inflammatory infiltrate and proliferating bile ducts. Inspissated eosinophilic material is seen within the lumina of bile ducts (*arrows*) (hematoxylin and eosin).

the characteristic focal biliary cirrhosis. Massive steatosis frequently observed in the past was probably related to inadequate nutrition. Amyloidosis has been described in older patients.[29,90]

ACUTE AND CHRONIC VIRAL HEPATITIS

Children may develop hepatitis due to A, B, non-A and non-B (NANB), and delta viruses, with histologic alterations in the liver similar to those of adults. Regardless of the etiologic agent, *acute viral hepatitis*[9,91–96] is characterized by generalized panacinar disarray with swelling or ballooning degeneration of hepatocytes, regenerative activity, single cell necrosis, and lymphoplasmacytic infiltrate. These changes are more pronounced in perivenular regions. A variable degree of cholestasis is usually present. Hepatocytes undergoing necrosis acquire densely eosinophilic retracted cytoplasm and pyknotic nuclei, leading to the formation of acidophilic bodies. Acidophilic bodies are round eosinophilic masses with or without pyknotic nuclei which represent apoptotic hepatocytes. Although nonspecific, they are particularly numerous in acute hepatitis. Extrusion of necrotic hepatocytes leads to cellular dropout with focal reticulin collapse. The lymphocytic and plasmacytic infiltrate has a portal and focally lobular distribution. In areas, lymphocytes are in close contact with degenerating and necrotic hepatocytes. There is diffuse hyperplasia of the phagocyte-mononuclear system, with Kupffer cells containing abundant PAS-positive diastase-resistant cytoplasmic granules (heterophagolysosomes). In severe cases of acute hepatitis there may be bridging hepatic necrosis with formation of loose connective tissue bands devoid of elastic fibers, connecting portal tracts to central veins. This bridging hepatic necrosis, although reversible, is associated with a poor course. Prominence of eosinophilic hepatocytes and steatosis occurs more commonly in hepatitis as the result of delta and NANB virus.[91,92,94] In NANB hepatitis, circulating sinusoidal lymphocytes, portal lymphoid follicles, and bile duct damage, although not always present, appear to be particularly characteristic.[91,96]

Acute viral hepatitis usually resolves with complete recovery and hepatic repair. A fatal outcome occurs, however, in a minority of patients who develop *massive hepatic necrosis* with fulminant hepatic failure. Histologically, there is panacinar confluent necrosis of hepatocytes with sparing of portal tracts and adjacent hepatocytes. The hepatic parenchyma is collapsed with approximation of portal tracts (Fig. 12*A* and *B*). Other causes of massive hepatic necrosis are diverse and include Wilson's disease, drugs, toxins, metabolic errors, and other viral infections.

Acute viral hepatitis may become chronic when inflammation of the liver persists for more than 6 months. Two types of *chronic hepatitis*[9,97–103] are distinguishable histopathologically by the presence or absence of piecemeal necrosis: *chronic active* and *chronic persistent hepatitis*, respectively. In both types there is portal lymphocytic inflammation. In chronic persistent hepatitis the inflammation is confined to portal tracts, and the lobular interface with the portal tract connective tissue, the limiting plate, is intact. Mild fibrosis and occasional foci of single cell necrosis may occur. However, in chronic active hepatitis, lymphocytes obscure the limiting plate and infiltrate the lobular periphery surround-

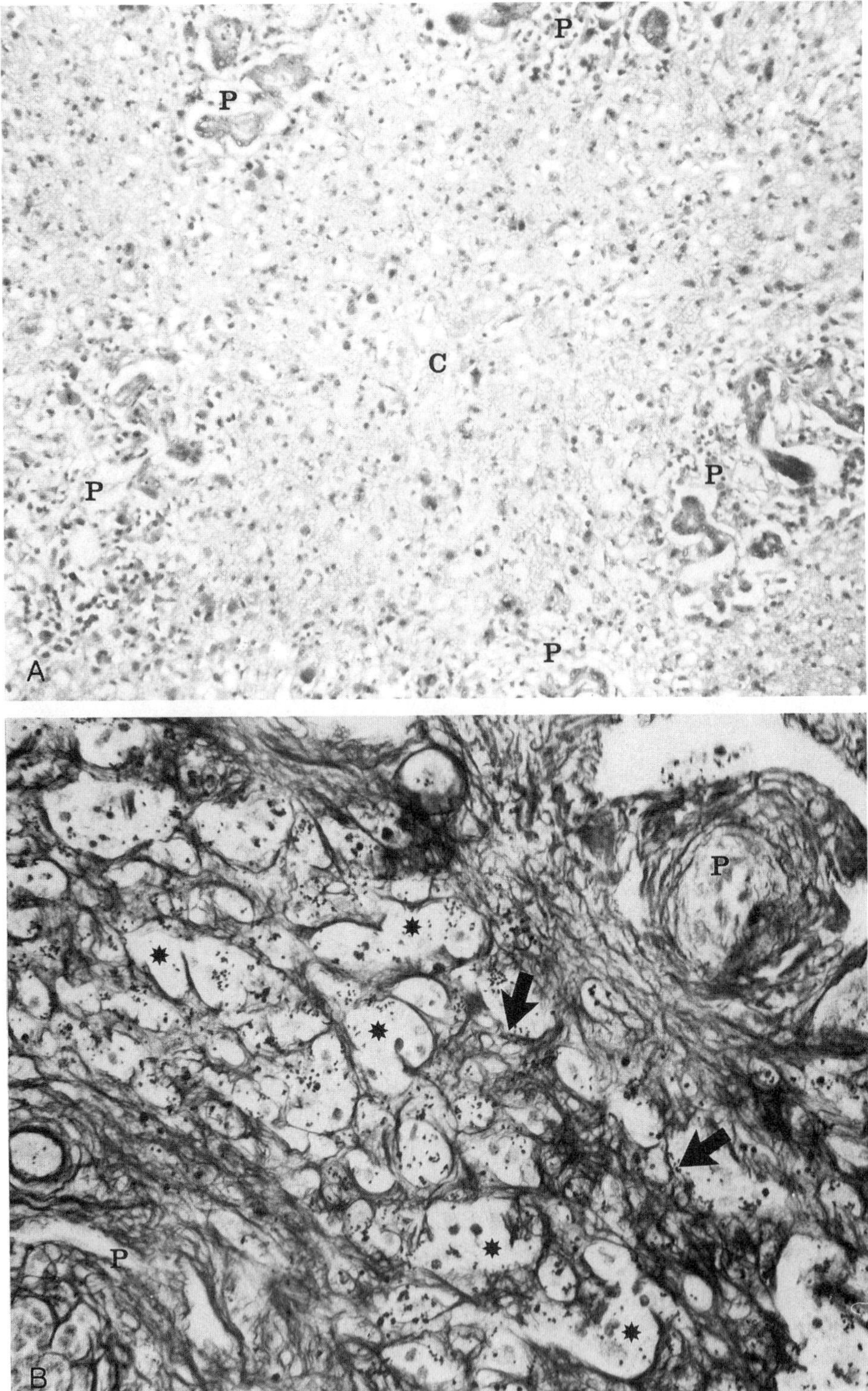

FIGURE 12 Massive hepatic necrosis. *A*, There is extreme collapse of the parenchyma due to extensive necrosis of hepatocytes. Hepatic lobule is replaced by blood, endothelial cells, and macrophages. Portal tracts (P) are preserved and in close proximity to each other. Necrotic central vein (C) (hematoxylin and eosin). *B*, Massive collapse of the reticulin framework (*arrows*). P = portal tracts; asterisks = sinusoids (reticulin stain).

ing single hepatocytes (piecemeal necrosis) (Fig. 13*A* and *B*). There may be bridging necrosis with distortion of the general acinar architecture and loss of portal and central vein relationships (Fig. 13*C*). Pathologic assessment of the degree of inflammatory activity, severity of portal fibrosis, and lobular collapse are essential for evaluation of prognosis and potential treatment (see Chapter 28, Part 3).

Chronic lobular hepatitis has recently been added as a rare type of chronic hepatitis and is characterized histologically by persistent lobular activity and inconspicuous portal and

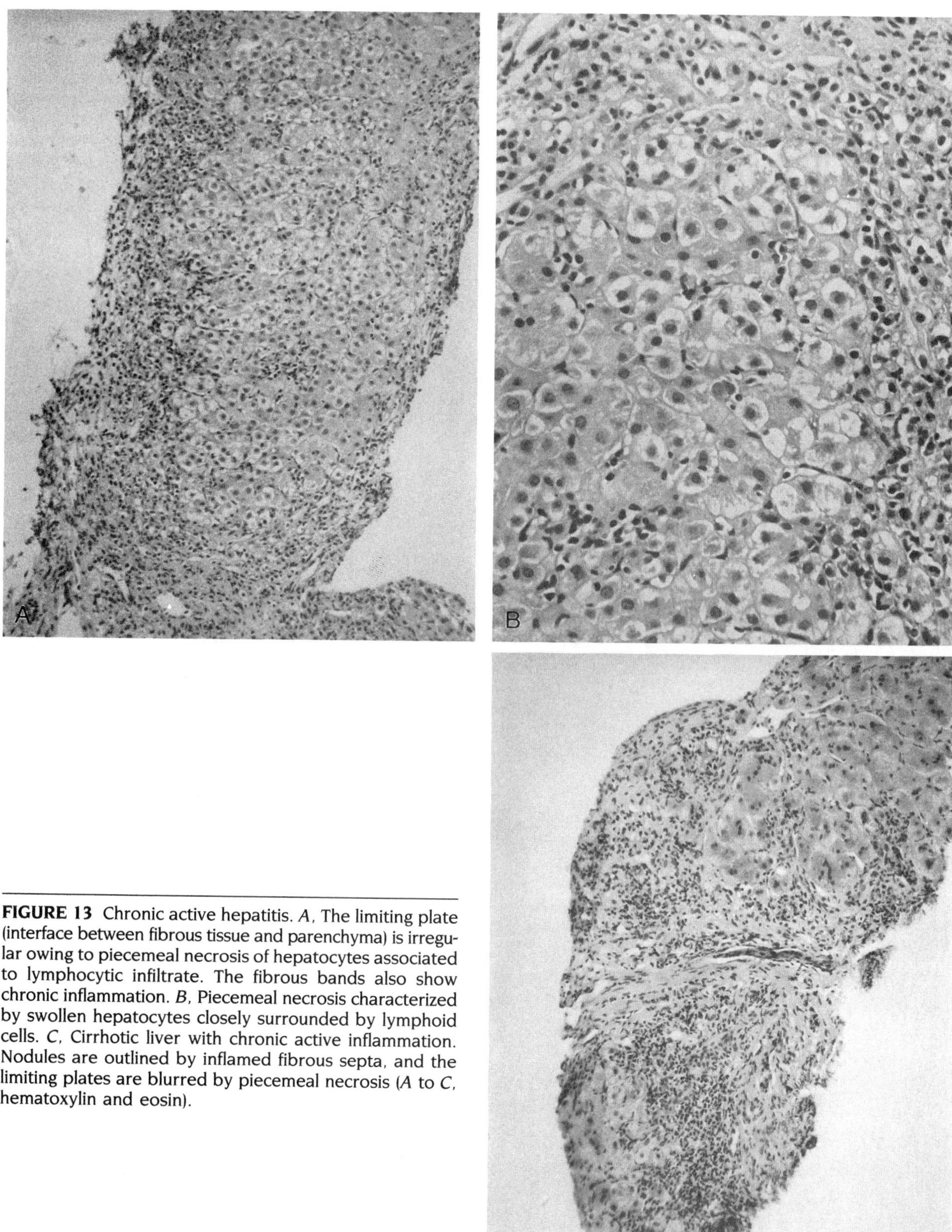

FIGURE 13 Chronic active hepatitis. *A*, The limiting plate (interface between fibrous tissue and parenchyma) is irregular owing to piecemeal necrosis of hepatocytes associated to lymphocytic infiltrate. The fibrous bands also show chronic inflammation. *B*, Piecemeal necrosis characterized by swollen hepatocytes closely surrounded by lymphoid cells. *C*, Cirrhotic liver with chronic active inflammation. Nodules are outlined by inflamed fibrous septa, and the limiting plates are blurred by piecemeal necrosis (*A* to *C*, hematoxylin and eosin).

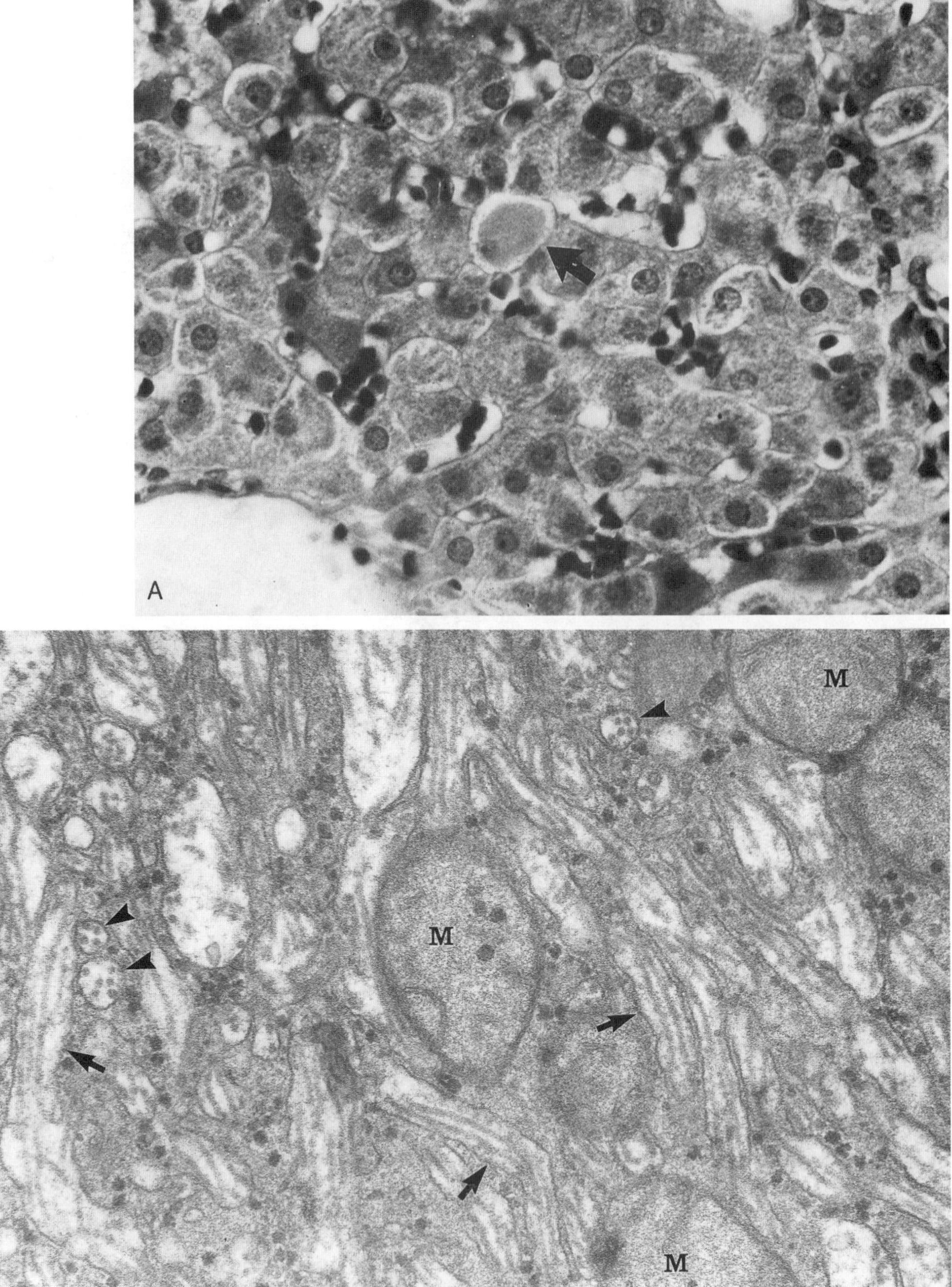

FIGURE 14 Chronic type B hepatitis. *A*, Characteristic ground-glass hepatocyte (*arrow*). The granular, slightly eosinophilic cytoplasm is separated from the cell membrane by a clear halo (hematoxylin and eosin). *B*, Ultrastructure of ground-glass hepatocyte. Numerous cisternae of smooth endoplasmic reticulum (*arrows*) are filled with tubular profiles of hepatitis B surface antigen, which can be observed on longitudinal and cross section (*arrowheads*). Mitochondria (M) (uranyl acetate and lead citrate, ×44,000).

TABLE 2
Causes of Chronic Active Hepatitis

Hepatitis B virus and delta agent
Hepatitis non-A, non-B viruses
Human immunodeficiency virus
Wilson's disease
Alpha$_1$-antitrypsin deficiency
Drugs
Autoimmune (lupoid hepatitis)
Unknown

periportal inflammation.[103,104] The lobular hepatocellular necrosis and spotty lymphocytic infiltrate histologically resemble acute hepatitis, but the clinical course is protracted with relapsing episodes. Chronic lobular hepatitis occurs more often in Taiwan in carriers of hepatitis B virus.

In contrast to chronic active hepatitis, which is a leading cause of cirrhosis, chronic persistent and chronic lobular forms of hepatitis have a good prognosis and rarely progress to cirrhosis.

The causes of chronic hepatitis are multiple[9,103,105] (Table 2), and the histologic appearance is usually not sufficiently specific to suggest an etiology. In chronic hepatitis B, however, the presence of ground-glass hepatocytes is characteristic. These display eosinophilic cytoplasmic inclusions with a marginal halo (Fig. 14*A*). These inclusions stain specifically with orcein and aldehyde fuscin stains as well as with immunoperoxidase techniques using antibodies to membrane-associated hepatitis B surface antigen (HBsAg). Ultrastructurally, the inclusions are composed of proliferated endoplasmic reticulum cisternae containing HBsAg tubular particles[4,106] (Fig. 14*B*). The presence of nuclear and cytoplasmic hepatitis B core antigen (HBcAg) and nuclear hepatitis B delta antigen (HBDAg) can be demonstrated immunohistochemically using specific antibodies. In situ hybridization techniques can detect the presence of HBV DNA in tissue sections. Ultrastructurally, HBcAg is characterized by intranuclear spherical particles measuring 27 nm in diameter. Target-like Dane particles may be observed within endoplasmic reticulum cisternae in association with HBsAg tubules. Tubuloreticular and cylindric (test tube–like) inclusions are described ultrastructurally in NANB hepatitis and in the acquired immunodeficiency syndrome.[4,107] In the liver, tubuloreticular inclusions are usually present in the cytoplasm of endothelial cells and less frequently in Kupffer and bile duct epithelial cells. Cylindric inclusions are usually present within the cytoplasm of hepatocytes. In addition, complex cytoplasmic structures of probable viral origin are frequently present in the cytoplasm of hepatocytes in NANB hepatitis.[4] They are composed of filamentous strands, vesicles, and membranous fragments arranged in various configurations (see Chapter 28, Part 23).

In *autoimmune lupoid chronic hepatitis* (Table 2)[9,101,103] liver biopsy usually reveals a florid chronic active hepatitis with marked piecemeal necrosis, conspicuous plasma cell infiltrate, and pseudoacinar transformation of hepatocytes.

CIRRHOSIS

Cirrhosis is defined as diffuse fibrosis of the liver associated with parenchymal regenerative nodules and generalized distortion of the acinar architecture (Fig. 15).[9] Three morphologic types can be distinguished regarding the size of the

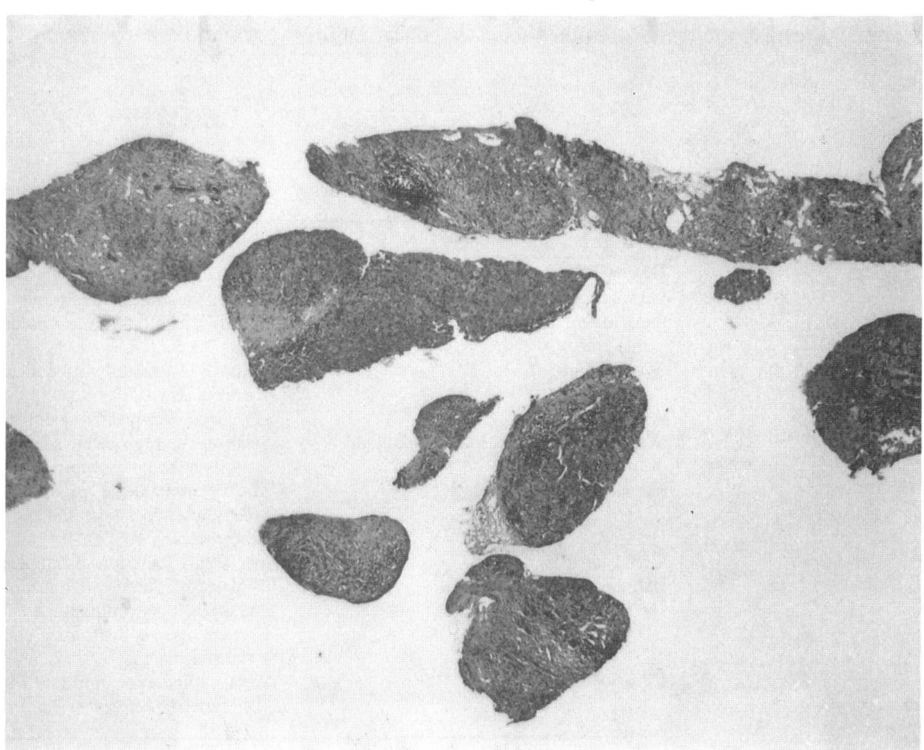

FIGURE 15 Macronodular cirrhosis. There is fragmentation of the needle biopsy core. Fragments of tissue have round edges and are partially covered by thick fibrous septa (hematoxylin and eosin).

TABLE 3
Histopathologic Features of Cirrhosis

Fragmentation of the biopsy tissue core
Active hepatocyte regeneration with adjacent hepatocytes showing different growth rates and different nuclear and cytoplasmic appearances
Abnormal orientation of reticulin fibers
Fibrosis at the edge of or through tissue fragments
Excessive number of terminal hepatic venules
Approximation of terminal hepatic venules and portal tracts
Nodules devoid of terminal hepatic veins
Poorly formed and unusually small portal tracts
Elastic tissue–rich septa linking terminal hepatic venules to portal tracts
Hepatic cords made up of two or more rows of hepatocytes
Pleomorphism of hepatocyte nuclei (nuclear dysplasia)

From Scheuer.[9]

regenerative nodules: micronodular cirrhosis when the nodules are uniform and measure less than 3 mm in diameter, macronodular when the nodules are larger, and mixed. The diagnosis of macronodular cirrhosis can be difficult by needle liver biopsy alone, since the fibrous septa may not be present in the biopsy. Important histopathologic features in the diagnosis of cirrhosis and diseases associated with it are listed in Tables 3 and 4. The pathologic assessment of the inflammatory activity based primarily in the degree of piecemeal necrosis (co-existence with chronic acitve hepatitis) is important for treatment considerations (see Fig. 13*C* and Chapter 28, Part 24).

BACTERIAL INFECTIONS AND SEPSIS

Multiple factors contribute to the pathogenesis of liver disease in sepsis and often occur in combination. Direct invasion of bacteria to the liver, toxemia, shock, and dehydration are probably the most important.[9,52,108–110] Direct invasion of the liver by bacteria may cause acute ascending cholangitis, phlebitis of the portal veins (pylephlebitis), hepatic abscesses, or granulomatous hepatitis. Acute ascending cholangitis is characterized by neutrophilic infiltration of the wall and lumina of portal bile ducts and focal bile duct epithelial cell necrosis (Fig. 16). Microabscesses may form adjacent to the wall of the ducts (cholangitis abscesses). Hepatic abscesses vary in size from microscopic clusters of a few neutrophils to large collections of pus. Multiple microabscesses occur in terminal stages of sepsis and are rarely seen in liver biopsies. Chronic bacterial infections of the liver are rare, and the pathologic findings are usually nonspecific, with portal lymphocytic infiltrate, hyperplasia of the phagocyte-mononuclear system, and occasionally cholestasis.[109] The terms *cholangitis lenta* and *bacterial hepatitis* have been used to describe these chronic lesions. Bacterial cultures are essential for the diagnosis (see Chapter 28, Part 5).

Liver disease may occur without direct bacterial invasion. Jaundice is a common clinical finding in children with gram-negative bacterial sepsis.[111,112] Histologically the liver often reveals canalicular cholestasis without hepatocellular necrosis and occasionally nonbacterial cholangitis. The pathogenesis of these lesions has been attributed to bacterial endotoxins.

GRANULOMATOUS HEPATITIS

The basic definition of granuloma is that of an aggregate of epithelioid histiocytes. In the liver, as in other organs or tissues, granulomas vary in their morphology from discrete clusters of epithelioid histiocytes to better-developed granulomas containing other inflammatory cells and multinucleated giant cells, often of Langhans' type (Fig. 17).

It has been estimated that only 5 to 7 percent of cases of granulomatous hepatitis occur in children.[29] The causes of

TABLE 4
Diseases Associated with Cirrhosis in Children

Disease	Distinguishing Features
Glycogenosis type I	Plantlike hepatocytes
Glycogenosis type IV	Large ground-glass inclusions
Galactosemia and hereditary fructose intolerance	Steatosis, cholestasis, and pseudoglands
Tyrosinemia	Steatosis, cholestasis, pseudoglands, and adenomas
$Alpha_1$-antitrypsin deficiency	Periportal PAS-positive globules
Wilson's disease and Indian childhood cirrhosis	Steatosis, empty nuclei, neutrophils, Mallory bodies, copper storage
Neonatal hemochromatosis	Marked iron storage in liver and ductal cells, pseudoglands, and perisinusoidal fibrosis
Cystic fibrosis	Inspissated secretion in bile ducts
Extrahepatic biliary atresia	Cholestasis, portal inflammation, fibrosis, and bile duct proliferation
Neonatal hepatitis	Lobular disarray with giant cell transformation
Chronic active hepatitis	Portal lymphocytic infiltrate with piecemeal necrosis

From Ishak and Sharp[10] and Ishak.[11]

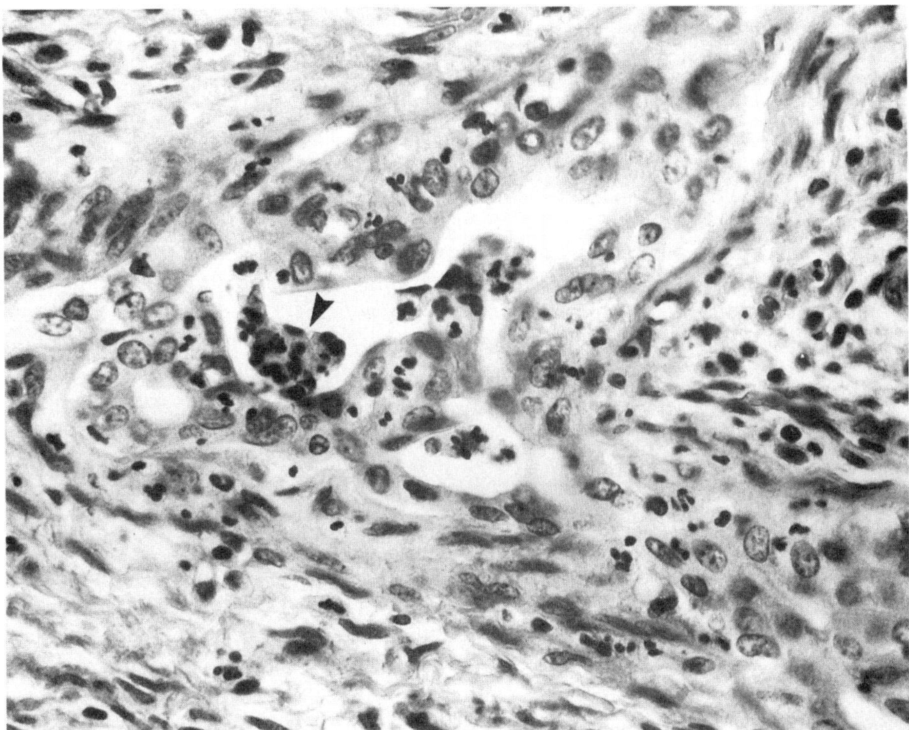

FIGURE 16 Acute ascending cholangitis. Portal bile duct reveals numerous polymorphonuclear leukocytes around and within the wall and lumen. The bile duct epithelium is poorly oriented and has irregular nuclei. *Arrowhead* indicates a cluster of intraluminal neutrophils (hematoxylin and eosin).

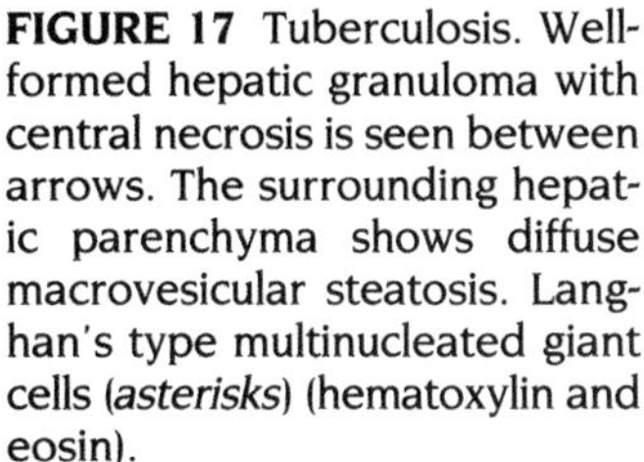

FIGURE 17 Tuberculosis. Well-formed hepatic granuloma with central necrosis is seen between arrows. The surrounding hepatic parenchyma shows diffuse macrovesicular steatosis. Langhan's type multinucleated giant cells (*asterisks*) (hematoxylin and eosin).

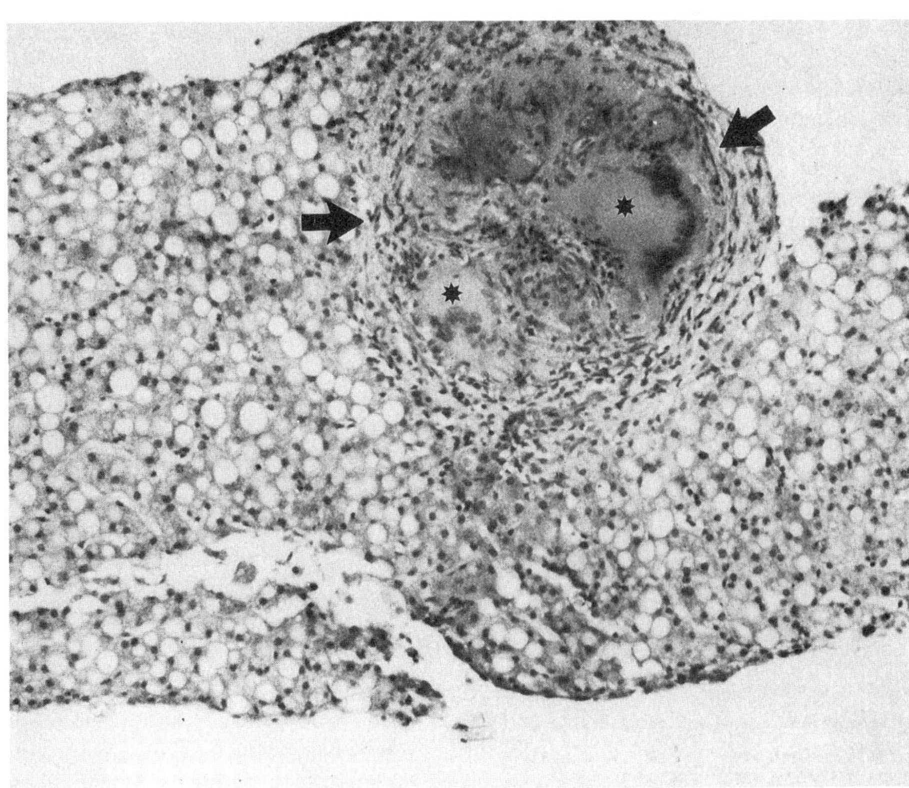

granulomatous hepatitis are diverse and vary from one geographic area to another. An etiologic diagnosis is usually not possible by morphology alone, and special stains often fail to reveal an etiologic agent. When granulomas are suspected a fragment of the liver should be sent for bacterial cultures, and the entire biopsy should be serially sectioned when granulomas are not observed in the initial sections.

Tuberculosis including typical and atypical forms is the most frequent etiology in our institution. Tuberculous granulomas are usually well developed, and central acellular (caseous) necrosis often occurs. However, the absence of necrosis does not exclude the diagnosis. In a small proportion of cases, acid-fast bacilli can be demonstrated by special stains. Granulomas in atypical tuberculosis are usually larger and stellate in appearance and have a higher tendency to coalesce and form large, irregular masses.

Sarcoidosis rarely affects children; when it does it is usually during adolescence. Sarcoid granulomas are usually small and noncoalescent with each other. They reveal little or no necrosis, and the multinucleated giant cells on rare occasions contain asteroid or Schaumann bodies. Sarcoid granulomas have a prominent reticulin framework and a tendency to undergo fibrosis.[9] Some cases of sarcoidosis are associated with diffuse fibrosis of the liver.

Infective granulomas of various etiologies may occur in association with immunodeficiency states. Often, however, T-cell immunodeficiencies including acquired immunodeficiency syndrome (AIDS) are associated with poorly formed or well-developed sarcoid granulomas of no demonstrable infectious origin.[29,113-115] Similar sarcoid granulomas occur also in association with Hodgkin's disease.[29]

Chronic granulomatous disease of childhood due to a defect of bacterial killing by phagocytes is often associated with infective hepatic granulomas of various etiologies.[10] They are usually large, coalesce with each other, display abundant necrosis, and are frequently purulent. In chronic granulomatous disease periportal macrophages and Kupffer cells usually contain ceroid pigment. Similar pigmented macrophages are present in other organs and tissues.

TOTAL PARENTERAL NUTRITION SYNDROME

The hepatic changes associated with total parenteral nutrition may resemble a genetic metabolic disorder. The classic triad of mild to moderate micro- and macrovesicular steatosis, canalicular and cellular cholestasis, and nonspecific mild neutrophilic cholangitis is characteristic.[9,29] Cholestasis is the most constant finding. In severe and prolonged cases, hepatocellular damage with ballooning, pseudoacinar transformation, and occasional giant multinucleated hepatocytes often progresses to portal and lobular fibrosis and rarely even cirrhosis (see Chapter 28, Part 20).

FATTY LIVER, REYE'S SYNDROME, AND REYE'S-LIKE DISORDERS

Chronic (longstanding) fatty change of the liver may be clinically silent or may manifest with asymptomatic hepatomegaly. Histologically, there is macrovesicular cytoplasmic accumulation of neutral lipid. The hepatocytes appear enlarged and contain large round punched-out vacuoles on routine sections stained with H & E. The neutral fat produces flattening and displacement of the nucleus to the cytoplasmic periphery. In severe cases of longstanding steatosis, macrovesicular fat accumulates diffusely throughout the hepatic lobule. Hepatocytes may rupture, leading to coalescence of fat vacuoles and the formation of microcysts. In subacute steatosis perivenular hepatocytes may display a microvesicular pattern, whereas larger vacuoles occur in periportal zones. Chronic debilitating diseases such as tuberculosis and malignant tumors, malnutrition, diabetes mellitus, morbid obesity, and drugs (e.g., methotrexate, prednisone, asparaginase) are the most frequent causes of macrovesicular steatosis in children (Fig. 17).

Acute accumulation of significant amounts of fat may manifest clinically with hepatic failure. Histologically, the hepatocytic cytoplasm is distended by numerous small droplets of neutral fat which do not displace the nucleus. The fat droplets might be so small that special stains such as oil red O are needed to demonstrate their presence. Diffuse panacinar steatosis of this type, with no evidence of necrosis, inflammation, or cholestasis, occurs in Reye's syndrome (Fig. 18*A* and *B*).[116] Ischemic centrilobular necrosis, however, may be observed at autopsy in patients who die in shock. Ultrastructurally, there are characteristic mitochondrial changes with swelling and enlargement, cristolysis, ameboid deformation, and dissolution of intramatrical granules (Fig. 18*C*).[4] Biochemical analysis of hepatic tissue typically reveals depletion of multiple mitochondrial enzymes. Histologic, biochemical, and ultrastructural changes in Reye's syndrome are short-lived, and the biopsy should be done in the acute stage of the disease during the first 4 days.

In children, similar microvesicular steatosis occurs with salicylates and sodium valproate toxicity[29,117,118] and in several syndromes that clinically are characterized by recurrent symptoms resembling Reye's syndrome.[119-126] These metabolic errors include urea cycle enzyme deficiencies; the syndrome of hyperammonemia, hyperornithinemia, and homocitrullinuria; systemic carnitine deficiency; carnitine palmitoyl transferase deficiency; and medium- and long-chain acyl CoA dehydrogenase deficiencies. In urea cycle enzyme disorders and in the syndrome of hyperammonemia, hyperornithinemia, and homocitrullinuria, the steatosis is usually milder, and discrete islands of swollen hepatocytes with clear cytoplasm and collapse of adjacent sinusoids may characteristically but rarely occur. These hepatocytes have the appearance of vegetable cells reminiscent of glycogenosis. The ultrastructural findings of all these metabolic errors are also characterized by abnormal mitochondria.[4] The changes, however, differ from those observed in Reye's syndrome. Mitochondria are mildly pleomorphic with elongated shape, preservation of matrical granules, and without ameboid deformation (Fig. 19). They may contain matrical paracrystalline inclusions (see Chapter 28, Part 18).

STORAGE DISEASES

Numerous inborn errors of metabolism are characterized by deposition and storage of particular substances in tissues[10,11] (Table 5). Many of these storage disorders involve the liver,

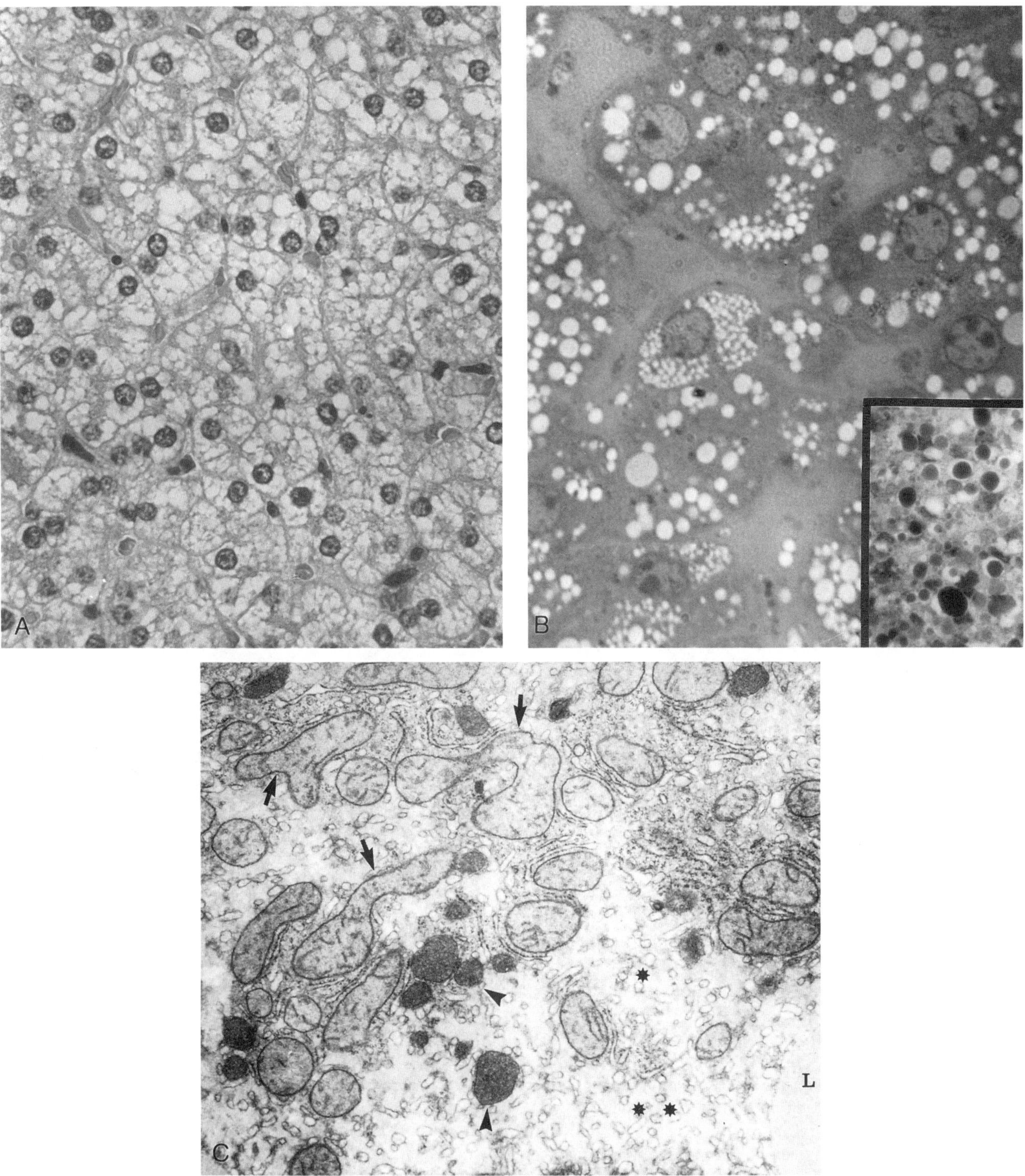

FIGURE 18 Reye's syndrome. *A*, Diffuse microvesicular steatosis. The cytoplasms are distended by numerous round vacuoles without evidence of nuclear displacement (hematoxylin and eosin). *B*, One micron thick section of Epon-embedded tissue showing the fine vesicular steatosis. On occasion, owing to the small size of the vesicles, the steatosis can be overlooked on routine sections (toluidine blue stain). The inset shows numerous neutral fat droplets brightly stained by oil red O. *C*, Ultrastructure of hepatocyte showing characteristic deformed mitochondria (*arrows*) with ameboid configuration, matrical expansion, cristolysis, and loss of intramatrical granules. Cluster of microbodies (*arrowheads*), fat droplets (L), vesiculated smooth endoplasmic reticulum (*asterisks*) (uranyl acetate and lead citrate, ×11,000).

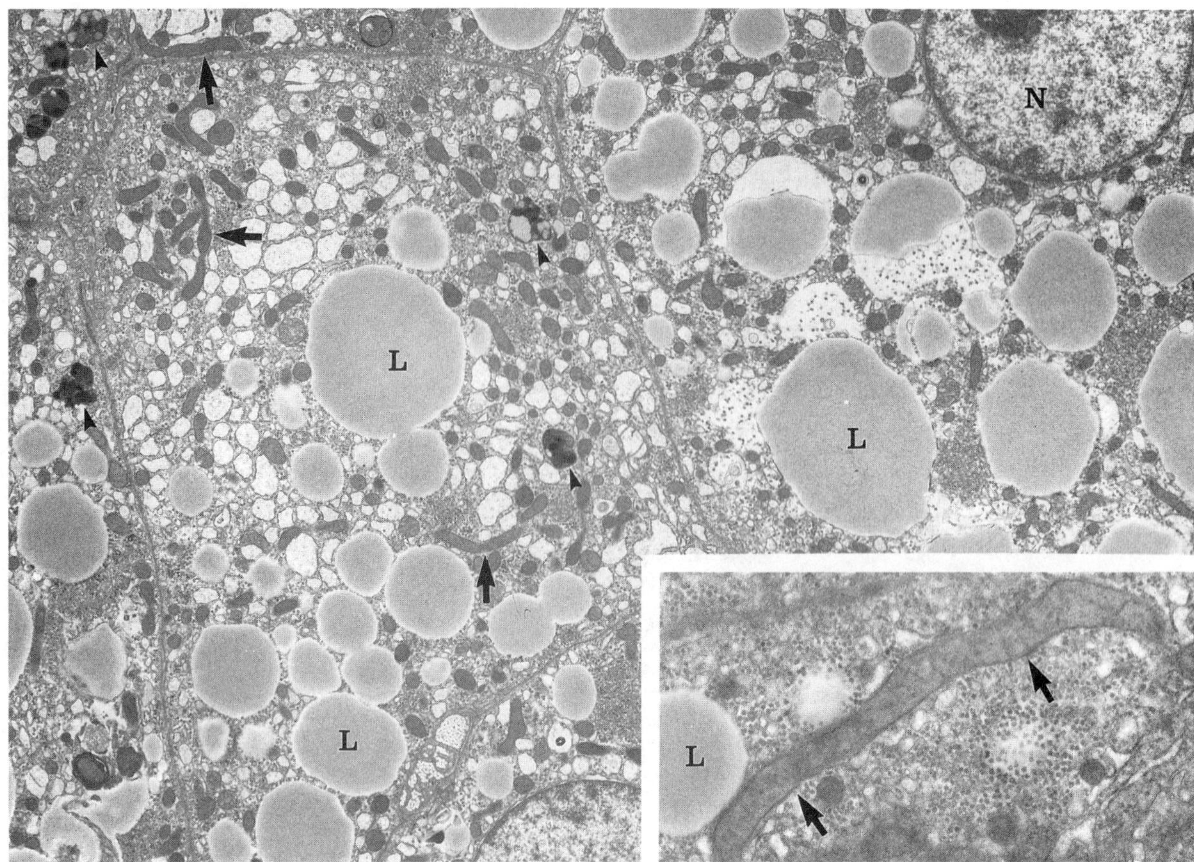

FIGURE 19 Medium-chain acyl CoA dehydrogenase deficiency. There is microvesicular fatty change (L) and vesicular dilation of endoplasmic reticulum. Mitochondria are elongated and slightly tortuous (*arrows*). Nucleus (N), lipofuscin (*arrowheads*) (uranyl acetate and lead citrate, ×4,000). Inset shows elongated mitochondrium (*arrows*) (uranyl acetate and lead citrate, ×12,000).

so that liver biopsy is often an important tool for the diagnosis. In the liver, the storaged metabolite may accumulate in hepatocytes (e.g., glycogenosis), in the phagocyte-mononuclear system (e.g., Gaucher's disease), or in both (e.g., Niemann-Pick disease). Light and electron microscopy and biochemical analysis are essential for a precise diagnosis. *Glycogen storage diseases (glycogenoses)*[10,11] often involve the liver (Table 5). The light microscopic appearance of the liver in these disorders denotes abundant accumulation of cytoplasmic glycogen and mild microvesicular steatosis of hepatocytes. Hepatocytes are markedly enlarged with clear cytoplasm, central nuclei, and compression of adjacent sinusoids, giving a mosaic appearance reminiscent of vegetable cells (Fig. 20*A*). Glycogenated nuclei are usually numerous in acinar zone 1. There are no specific histologic changes that distinguish different types of glycogenosis, so that biochemical detection of the missing enzyme is necessary for the diagnosis. Three types of glycogenosis have more or less distinguishing features. In type III glycogenosis, portal fibrosis, which may progress to cirrhosis, is frequently found. Neutral fat is less conspicuous. In type II the glycogen accumulation is primarily lysosomal. Hepatocytes contain round cytoplasmic vacuoles that represent glycogen-rich lysosomes. In type IV glycogenosis (amylopectinosis) large, irregular cytoplasmic PAS-positive diastase-resistant inclusions are present in enlarged hepatocytes with displaced nuclei (Fig. 20*B*). Fibrosis may also be present.

Electron microscopic findings in glycogenosis are characteristic, with cytoplasmic accumulation of free glycogen particles displacing organelles to the perinuclear zone and cytoplasmic periphery (Fig. 20*C*).[4] In type II glycogenosis, glycogen is predominantly single membrane bound within lysosomes, and in type IV characteristic filamentous inclusions of amylopectin displace nucleus and organelles.

In *Gaucher's disease* (glycosyl ceramide lipidosis), the storage metabolite glycocerebroside accumulates throughout the phagocyte-mononuclear system. In the liver, storage histiocytes (Gaucher cells) are distributed throughout the parenchyma within sinusoids. They are large and slightly eosinophilic with characteristic striated cytoplasm (wrinkled paper appearance) (Fig. 21*A*).[10,11] Gaucher cells are PAS-positive and diastase-resistant and contain a small amount of iron. Ultrastructurally, Gaucher cells contain cytoplasmic single membrane saccules containing twisted tubular structures arranged in rods (Fig. 21*B*).[4] Hepatocytes do not contain storage material but may appear compressed and atrophic.

TABLE 5
Hepatic Pathology of Some Storage Diseases

	Light Microscopy	Electron Microscopy
Hepatic glycogenosis		
Type I (von Gierke's disease)	Mosaic pattern (plant-like hepatocytes) Mild steatosis Glycogenated nuclei	Cytoplasmic free glycogen storage with displacement of organelles Abnormal mitochondria Glycogenated nuclei
Type II (Pompe's disease)	Cytoplasmic glycogen-rich vacuoles Glycogenated nuclei	Intralysosomal glycogen storage
Type III (Forbes/Cori's disease)	Similar to type I with less steatosis Fibrosis	Similar to type I Fibrosis
Type IV (Andersen's disease, amylopectinosis)	PAS-positive, diastase-resistant large cytoplasmic inclusions Fibrosis	Free cytoplasmic fibrillar and granular inclusions of amylopectin
Other (types VI, VIII, IX)	Similar to type I	Similar to type I
Mucopolysaccharidosis, mucolipidosis II (I-cell disease), and mucolipidosis III	Swollen vacuolated and clear hepatocytes and Kupffer cells Fibrosis and cirrhosis may occur.	Single membrane-bound vacuoles containing electrolucent and finely granular material in hepatocytes and Kupffer cells
Oligosaccharidosis (sialidosis, mannosidosis, fucosidosis)	Swollen vacuolated (foamy) hepatocytes and Kupffer cells	Single membrane-bound vacuoles containing granular, membranous, and filamentous material
Gangliosidosis	Foamy histiocytes and faintly vacuolated hepatocytes	Large single membrane-bound vacuoles containing granular and fibrillar material Concentric lamellar membrane Zebra bodies
Fabry's disease	Vacuolated Kupffer cells and portal histiocytes	Concentric and geometric lamellar inclusions in Kupffer cells, hepatocytes, and endothelial cells
Gaucher's disease	Sinusoidal clusters of Gaucher cells	Single membrane-bound inclusions containing twisted tubules
Niemann-Pick disease	Foamy histiocytes and vacuolated hepatocytes	Concentrically arranged round lamellar inclusions
Wolman's disease and cholesteryl ester storage disease	Vacuolated hepatocytes and Kupffer cells Fibrosis	Neutral fat droplets and cholesterol crystals in hepatocytes, Kupffer cells, and endothelial cells

From Ishak and Sharp[10] and Ishak.[11]

In *Niemann-Pick disease* (sphingomyelin lipidosis) sphingomyelin accumulates in hepatocytes and the phagocyte-mononuclear system. Storage cells have a vacuolated cytoplasm with a foamy appearance (Fig. 22*A*).[10,11] Special stains for lipids are positive. Ultrastructurally characteristic cytoplasmic myelin figures and concentrically arranged phospholipid membranes are present (Fig. 22*B*).[4]

PRIMARY SCLEROSING CHOLANGITIS

Primary sclerosing cholangitis is a syndrome of unknown etiology, which occurs rarely in children and is characterized by chronic fibrosing inflammation of intra- and extrahepatic bile ducts.[127-129] The hepatic lesion slowly progresses to characteristic lamellar (onion skin) fibrosis with obliteration of intrahepatic bile ducts and to biliary cirrhosis. The diagnosis is usually based on cholangiographic changes. The liver biopsy is only occasionally diagnostic; more frequently it reveals nonspecific chronic cholangitis. Primary sclerosing cholangitis is often associated with chronic inflammatory bowel disease, particularly ulcerative colitis, and less frequently with Langerhans cell histiocytosis, immune disorders, and chronic active hepatitis.

CONGENITAL BILIARY ECTASIA AND NONCIRRHOTIC HEPATIC FIBROSIS

The autosomal recessive condition *congenital hepatic fibrosis* usually presents in childhood and occasionally in adulthood with abdominal enlargement, hepatosplenomegaly, or hematemesis.[1,17] The morphology of the liver is characteristic.[9,17] The general hepatic architecture is maintained with normal vascular relationships. The portal tracts are markedly expanded by broad fibrous bands that transect the periphery of hepatic lobules, giving a cirrhotic appearance. Unlike cirrhosis, however, the hepatocytes show no evidence of regeneration, necrosis, or inflammation. In addition, the bands of fibrous tissue in congenital hepatic fibrosis typically contain numerous large, malformed, often cystically dilated bile ducts with occasional bile plugging (Fig. 23). This

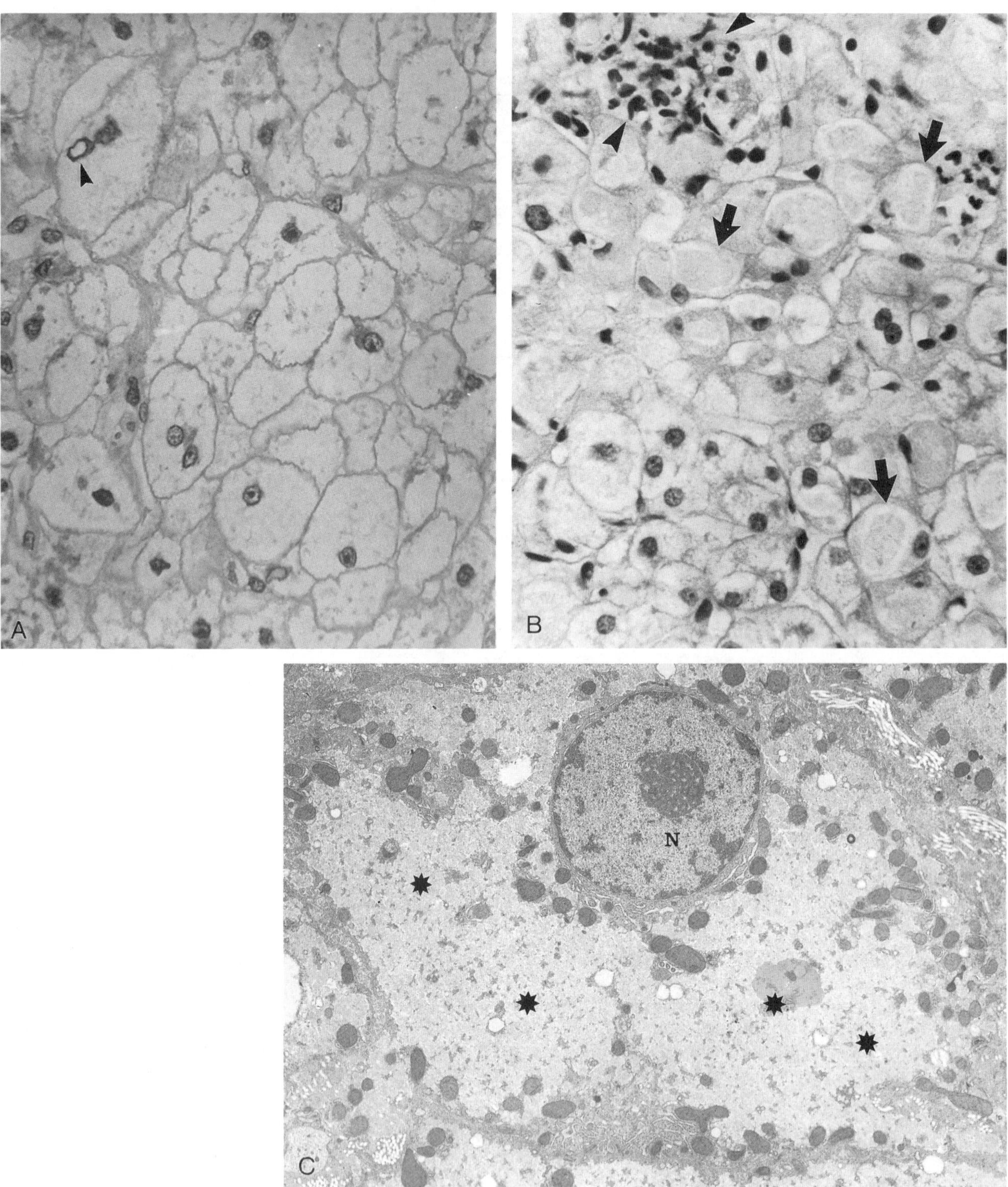

FIGURE 20 Glycogen storage disease. *A*, Type I glycogenosis showing diffuse expansion of hepatocytic cytoplasms and compression of sinusoids, giving the appearance of plant cells. "Glycogenated" nucleus (*arrowhead*) *B*, Type IV glycogenosis. Hepatocytes have cytoplasmic distention with polygonal contours. Large cytoplasmic slightly eosinophilic inclusions surrounded by a clear halo are indicated by arrows. Foci of single cell necrosis with inflammatory cells are rarely a feature (*arrowheads*) (*A* and *B*, hematoxylin and eosin). *C*, Ultrastructure of hepatocyte in type I glycogenosis showing accumulation of free glycogen particles (*asterisks*) with distention of the cytoplasm and displacement of organelles to the periphery of the cell and perinuclear zone. Nucleus (N) (uranyl acetate and lead citrate, ×5,000).

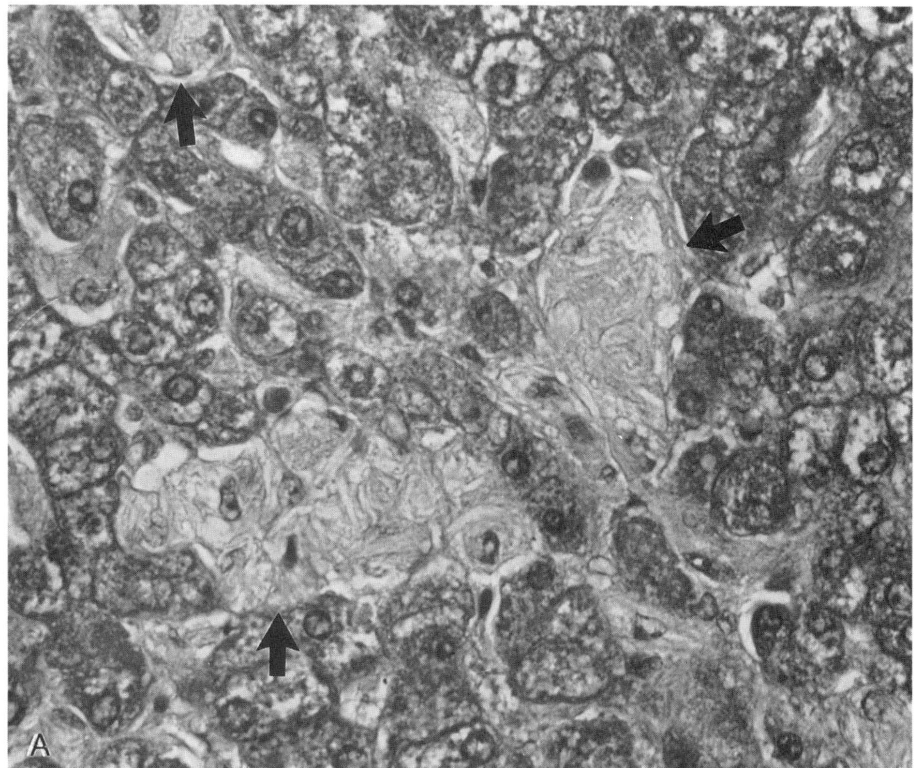

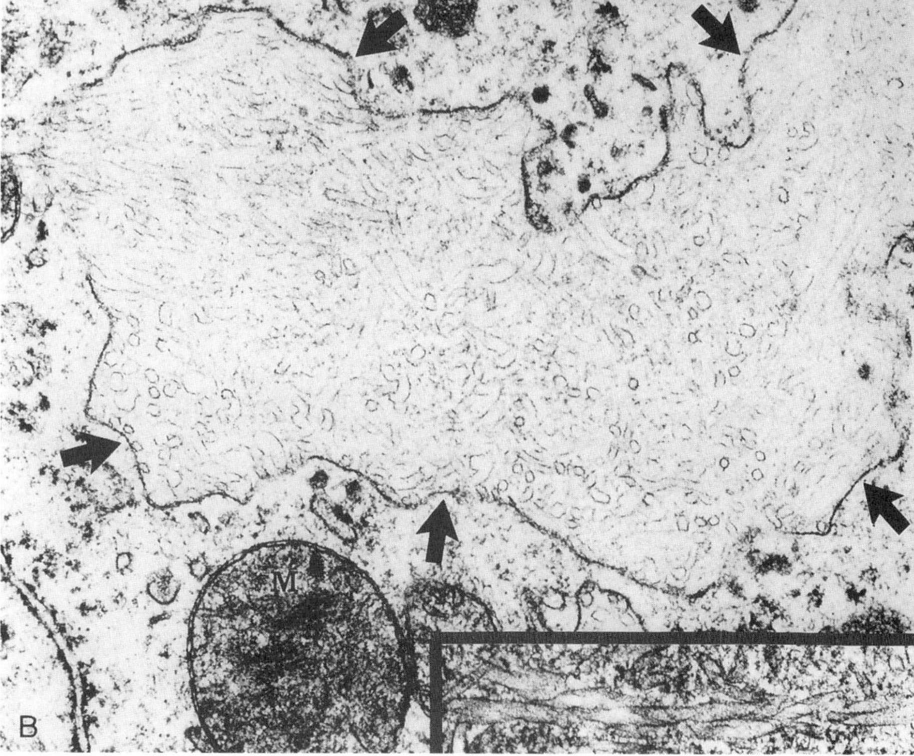

FIGURE 21 Gaucher's disease. *A*, Cluster of histiocytes (Gaucher cells) with striated cytoplasm contains storage material (*arrows*). Adjacent hepatocytes (dark staining cells) show compression atrophy (trichrome stain). *B*, Ultrastructure of cytoplasmic storage in Gaucher cell. A large group of elongated tubular structures are bound by a single membrane between arrows (intralysosomal storage). Mitochondria (M) (uranyl acetate and lead citrate, ×40,000). Inset shows a close-up of tubules with the characteristic twisted appearance (uranyl acetate and lead citrate, ×60,000).

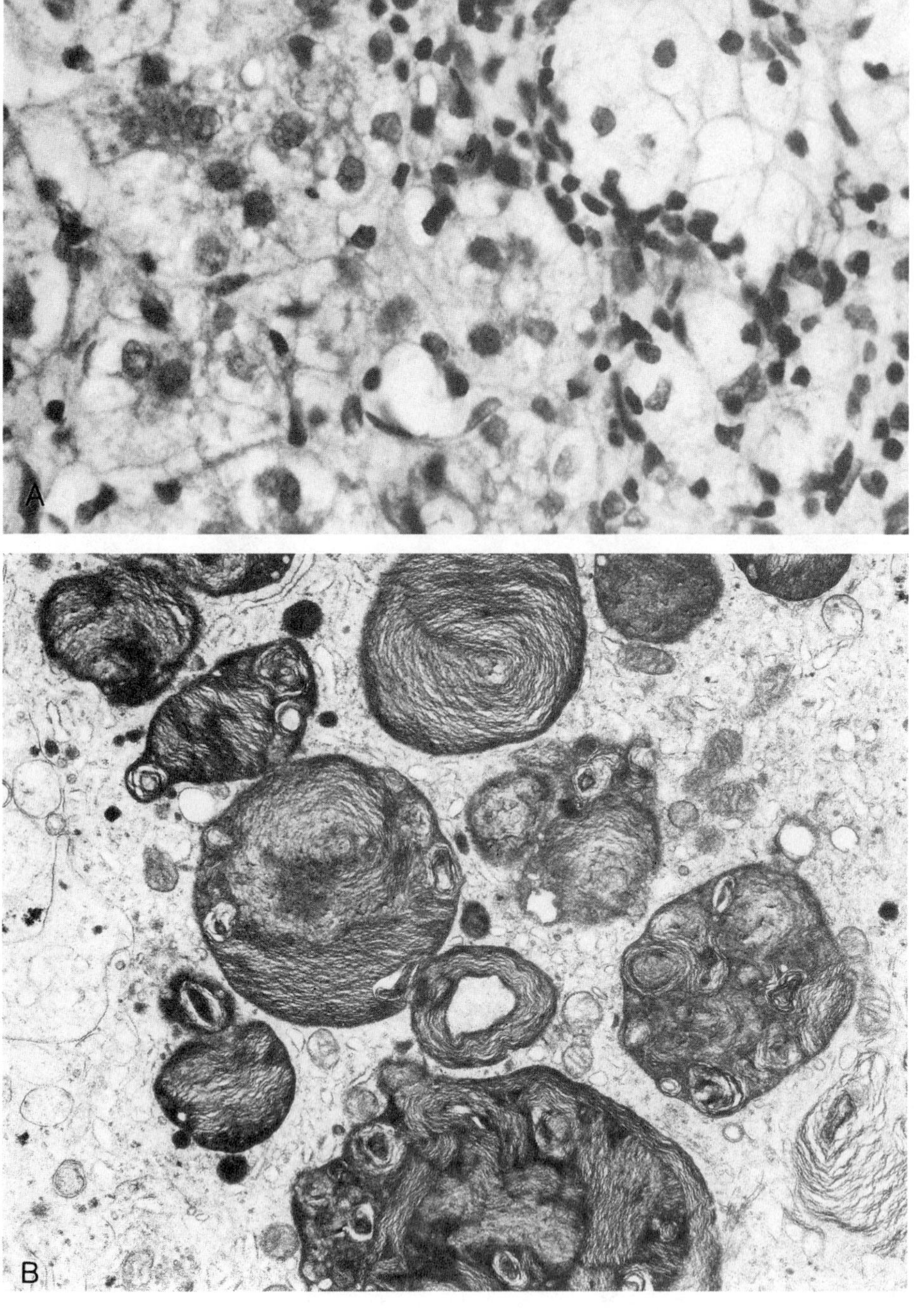

FIGURE 22 Niemann-Pick disease. *A*, On the left, there are lipid-containing hepatocytes with ballooning degeneration and vacuolization of the cytoplasm; to the right, clusters of foamy histiocytes and Kupffer cells with lipid storage (hematoxylin and eosin). *B*, Ultrastructure of hepatocyte showing large intracytoplasmic whorls of sphingomyelin membranes within lysosomes. The inclusions vary in size and consist of concentrically arranged lamellar membranes (uranyl acetate and lead citrate, ×9,000).

condition is thought to represent a defect in the development of the lobular ductal plate. Portal vein branches may be hypoplastic and narrowed.

A related condition that may co-exist with congenital hepatic fibrosis is the *congenital dilation of the intrahepatic bile ducts*, also known as *Caroli's disease*.[9,17,130] This grossly visible multiple cystic malformation usually involves the entire liver, and the cysts communicate with the rest of the biliary tree. The condition occasionally is segmental or lobar. Recurrent cholangitis is frequently associated.

Hepatic solitary cysts and *polycystic liver disease* occur rarely in children.[9,17,29] The proliferated cystic ducts in polycystic liver disease are lined by a single layer of columnar epithelium with intraluminal papillary projections.[17] All

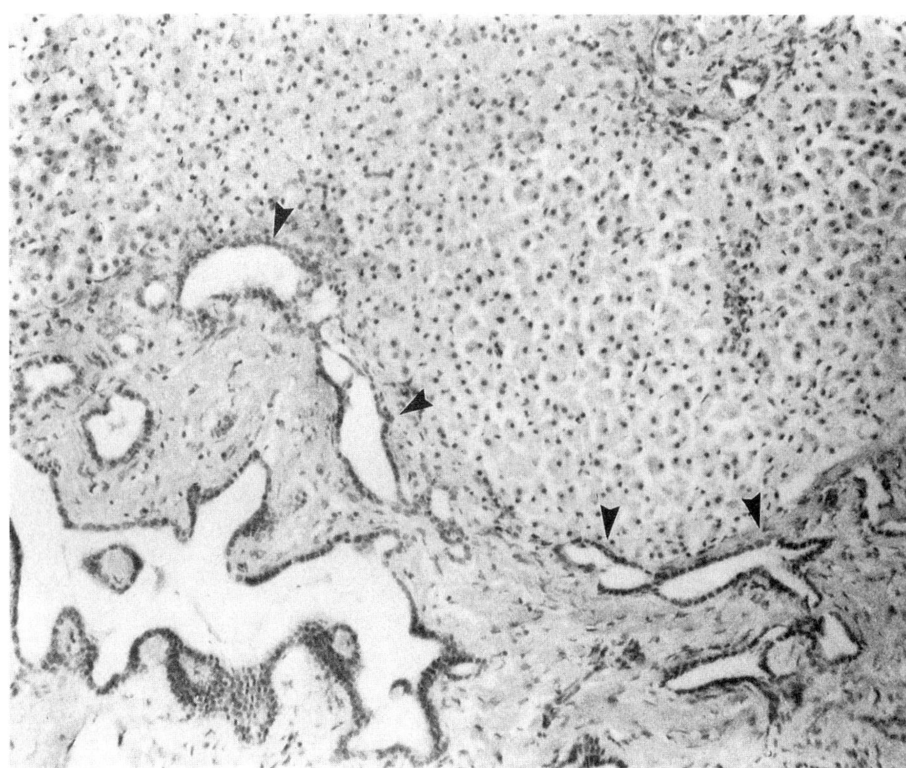

FIGURE 23 Congenital hepatic fibrosis. A broad fibrous septum with cystically dilated tortuous bile ducts is seen below. The persistent and dilated ductal plate is indicated by arrowheads. Above, hepatocytes show normal size and orientation. Note the absence of inflammation (hematoxylin and eosin).

those conditions have reportedly been associated with various cystic diseases of the kidneys and pancreas.[131-133]

Most of the hepatic disorders described in this chapter may induce hepatic fibrosis and subsequent cirrhosis. There are, however, patients with *idiopathic noncirrhotic portal fibrosis*[29] who present with asymptomatic hepatomegaly and minimal alteration of serum hepatic enzymes. Histologically, the portal fibrosis may produce bridging and completely encircle hepatic lobules in the absence of nodular regeneration. Inflammation and cholestasis are absent. A thorough clinicopathologic correlation is important to exclude known causes of portal fibrosis such as chronic hepatitis, chemotherapy, radiation, chronic cholangitis, and infiltrating malignant tumors such as neuroblastoma and leukemia.

VASCULAR DISORDERS[9,134]

Hepatic infarcts, represented by confluent areas of coagulative necrosis, usually occur as a result of occlusion, usually thrombosis, of the *hepatic arterial* flow. Periarteritis nodosa and hepatic transplantation are the most common predisposing conditions. The arterial lesion in both disorders involves usually medium-sized vessels, which are usually not included as part of needle liver biopsies. Periarteritis nodosa is often associated to hepatitis B virus, and specific immune complexes can be detected in the affected vessels. Hepatic infarcts may be caused by disseminated intravascular coagulation and sickle cell disease. In the former, sinusoidal fibrin thrombi can be seen in the biopsy. In sickle cell disease intrasinusoidal sickling of red blood cells can be found. Infarction of the right lobe of the liver occurs in infancy and may be associated with hepatic artery hypoplasia.

Infarcts occur rarely as a result of occlusion of the *portal venous* flow. The effects of portal vein occlusion depend on the extent and location of the thrombosis. Focal, subcapsular parenchymal atrophy with congestion (Zahn's infarct) occurs with occlusion of a peripheral portal vein and segmental or lobar atrophy when thrombosis is extensive. In some cases portal vein obstruction may cause partial nodular transformation of the liver. Thrombosis of the main portal vein may result from infection or invasion of the veins by tumor (hepatoblastoma or hepatocellular carcinoma) or in association with cirrhosis. In pylephlebitis, septic thrombi may be observed in the intrahepatic portal veins. Cavernous transformation of the portal vein is probably the result of recanalized thrombosis rather than congenital malformation. The lumen of the main portal vein is replaced by a spongy mass. It may be secondary to neonatal umbilical infection. The histology of the liver is usually unremarkable. Congenital aplasia or strictures of the portal vein are difficult to recognize in liver biopsies.

Occlusion of the main *hepatic vein* or large hepatic veins, usually due to thrombosis, causes the Budd-Chiari syndrome.[134,135] In the acute form, there is marked sinusoidal congestion and dilatation with compression of hepatocytes and focal disruption of liver cell plates in acinar zones 2 and 3 (Fig. 24). Occlusion of the terminal hepatic veins characterizes veno-occlusive disease, a disease that can be familial and most frequently affects infants. In the acute stage, there is centrilobular sinusoidal congestion with hemorrhage and necrosis of adjacent hepatocytes. The central veins show luminal narrowing or occlusion by loose connective tissue and intimal edema with or without thrombosis (see Chapter 28, Part 21).

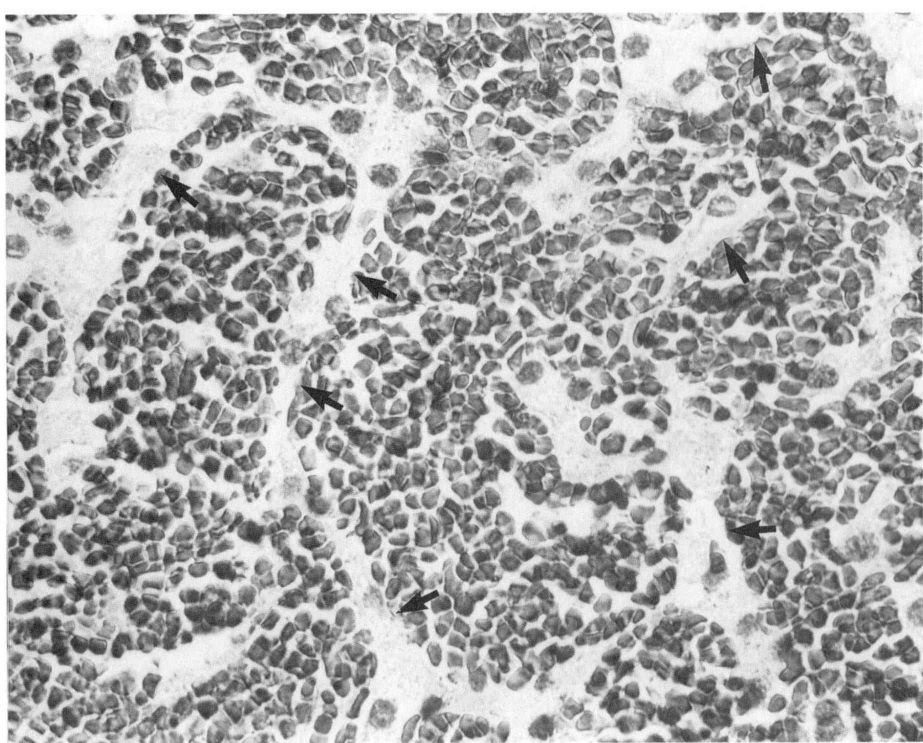

FIGURE 24 Budd-Chiari syndrome. Markedly dilated sinusoids are filled with blood. Light-stained, displaced hepatocytes show compression atrophy and elongation (*arrows*) (hematoxylin and eosin).

TABLE 6
Some Drugs Associated with Hepatic Injury in Children

Drug	Hepatic Findings
Acetaminophen (paracetamol)	Confluent necrosis of acinar zone 3
Salicylate	Hemorrhagic necrosis Microvesicular steatosis (Reye's-like)
Amethopterin (methrotexate)	Macrovesicular steatosis, hepatocellular swelling, and mixed inflammatory infiltrate (alcoholic liver disease–like) Portal fibrosis
Asparaginase	Diffuse macrovesicular steatosis
6-Mercaptopurine and azathioprine	Intracellular and canalicular cholestasis and single cell necrosis
Prednisone	Macrovesicular steatosis
Isoniazid	Hepatocellular damage resembling acute viral hepatitis Chronic active hepatitis Massive hepatic necrosis
Phenytoin	Massive hepatic necrosis Hepatocellular degeneration Cholestasis Granulomatous hepatitis
Sodium valproate	Diffuse hepatocellular damage Microvesicular steatosis (Reye's-like)
Hypervitaminosis A	Perisinusoidal fibrosis Increased number of Ito cells

From Dehner[29] and Zimmerman and Ishak.[137]

Severe hypoxemia or hypoperfusion of the liver produces a noninflammatory necrosis of the acinar zone 2 and 3 hepatocytes. There is usually associated congestion, hemorrhage, and sinusoidal dilatation. Acute heart failure and shock are the most common causes of ischemic centrilobular necrosis.

In the chronic form of Budd-Chiari syndrome, veno-occlusive disease, and congestive heart failure, perivenular and perisinusoidal fibrosis supervenes, leading to "reversal" of the lobular architecture and rarely to nodular regeneration and cirrhosis. Special connective tissue stains should be used to recognize the usually fibrotic and obscured central veins.

Sinusoidal dilatation may also be observed in association with neoplasia, granulomatous diseases, and the use of contraceptive or anabolic steroids. In peliosis hepatis, well-circumscribed, small, blood-filled cysts occur throughout the parenchyma. They are lined by a focally interrupted endothelium.[9,134,136]

TOXIC LIVER DISEASE[29,137]

Toxic liver disease is less common in children than in adults. In Table 6 are listed the most important drugs associated with hepatic injury in children. In clinical practice, antineoplastic, analgesic, and anticonvulsive drugs are the most frequently implicated (see Chapter 28, Part 6).

HEPATIC AND BONE MARROW TRANSPLANTATION

Hepatic transplantation is a well-established mode of therapy for progressive or terminal hepatic disorders. In children, the most frequent indication for liver transplantation is extrahepatic biliary atresia with advanced cirrhosis. Various metabolic disorders and massive hepatic necrosis follow in frequency.

Liver biopsy is the most reliable method to monitor the status of the graft.[138-142] Biopsies of the donor's liver before and 2 hours after implantation are important to exclude preexisting hepatic damage and serve as a baseline for comparison with subsequent biopsies. The causes of transplant failure are diverse and include extensive coagulative necrosis, extrahepatic biliary leakage and obstruction, acute ascending cholangitis, failure of vascular anastomosis, viral hepatitis, opportunistic infections, drug toxicity, and acute and chronic rejection. Recurrence of the primary disease is rare. In the differential diagnosis of these disorders, liver biopsy is essential.

The biopsies taken at the time of transplantation usually reveal diffuse hydropic degeneration of hepatocytes and occasional single cell necrosis. Clusters of polymorphonuclear leukocytes, commonly intrasinusoidal, might be numerous and are related to surgical manipulation. On occasion, the necrosis is confluent, especially in the subcapsular zone. With the use of new preservation fluids during procurement and transport of the graft, these histologic changes probably induced by cold ischemia, have become minimal.

Histologic changes associated to ischemia usually dominate the pathology during the first month following transplantation. The cause of this ischemia is probably multifactorial and includes poor organ preservation, vascular insufficiency, and poor condition of the recipient, who may have suffered hypovolemic or hypoxemic episodes. Mild cold ischemia may cause centrilobular ballooning of hepatocytes, cholestasis, and mild elevation of liver enzymes in the postoperative period. This nonspecific cholestasis usually reverses without treatment in well-vascularized grafts. A marked increase in serum hepatic enzymes, usually during the first 2 weeks, heralds a more severe ischemic process with confluent coagulative necrosis of hepatocytes. Well-perfused grafts might be able to regenerate. Biopsies of these organs usually show extensive regenerative activity characterized by ductular metaplasia of hepatocytes, cholestasis, and nonbacterial neutrophilic cholangitis. If coagulative necrosis is extensive or the ischemia persists, failure of the graft supervenes. The failed organ usually shows nearly complete infarction with bacterial overgrowth and focal dystrophic calcification of necrotic hepatocytes (see Chapter 28, Part 25).

The triad of portal inflammation, bile duct damage, and endothelialitis characterizes acute graft rejection (Fig. 25*A* and *B*). The portal inflammation is mixed and includes lymphocytes, plasma cells, neutrophils, and eosinophils. It is usually confined to the portal tracts, but on rare occasions there is transgression of the limiting plate and involvement of the lobular periphery. The portal bile duct damage is highly characteristic, with loss of nuclear polarity of epithelial cells, cytoplasmic degeneration and vacuolization, increased nuclear-to-cytoplasmic ratio, epithelial cell necrosis, and intramural and intraluminal mixed inflammation. In endothelialitis, there is attachment of lymphocytes to endothelial surfaces in central and portal veins and in sinusoids. When endothelialitis is severe, there is necrosis and sloughing of endothelial cells, and lymphocytes separate basal lamina from endothelium. Acute rejection may start as early as the first week and peaks during the second month following transplant.

Biopsies in successfully treated cases of acute rejection reveal a decrease in the number of inflammatory cells and absence of endothelialitis. The bile duct damage and cholestasis persist for a period of time until complete regeneration occurs. The sequelae of healed acute rejection are represented by minute scars in the portal tracts, often in the vicinity of bile ducts, and by eccentric scars of the central vein walls. Mild fibrosis of portal tracts may occur, but portal bridging or cirrhosis is rare.

By definition, chronic rejection occurs beyond day 100 following transplantation. Histopathologic features include those of acute rejection; however, endothelialitis is usually minimal. In addition, arterial changes are frequently encountered in chronic rejection. There is an arteritis of medium-sized arteries with transmural mixed inflammation, necrosis of the media with fibrous replacement of the smooth muscle coat, disruption of elastic membranes, and intimal infiltration by foamy macrophages (Fig. 25*C*). Vascular occlusion is common. Discrete foci of hepatocyte drop-out with preservation of sinusoidal outlines and no evidence of reticulin collapse are probably caused by vascular insufficiency.

Chronic bile duct damage may progress to extensive, often complete loss of portal bile ducts, the so-called vanishing bile

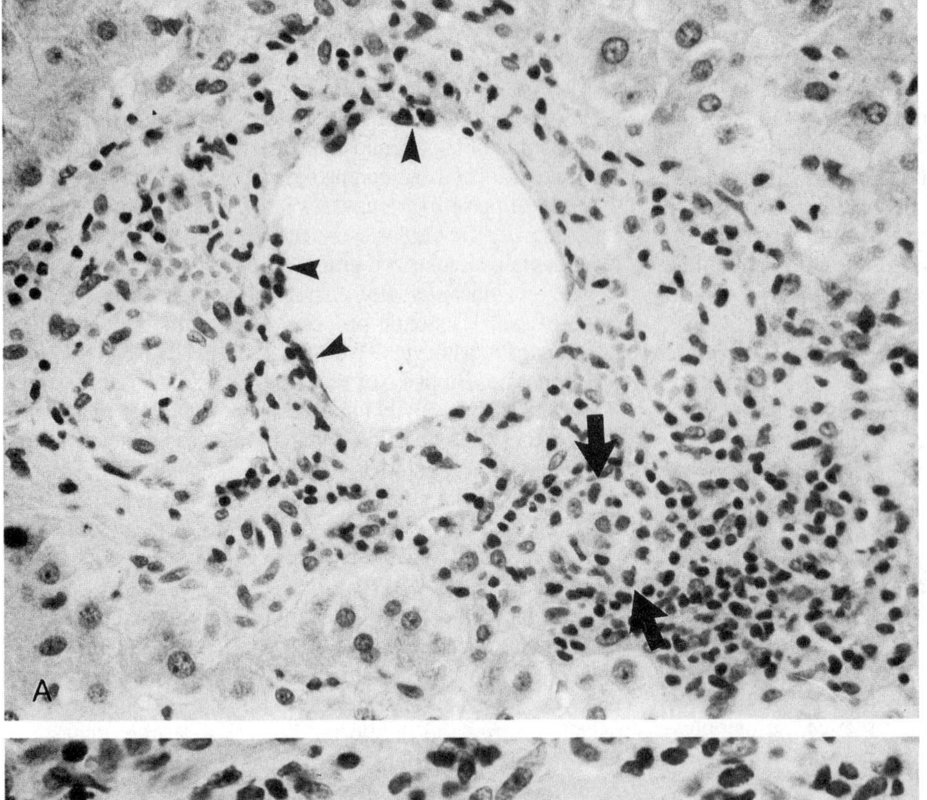

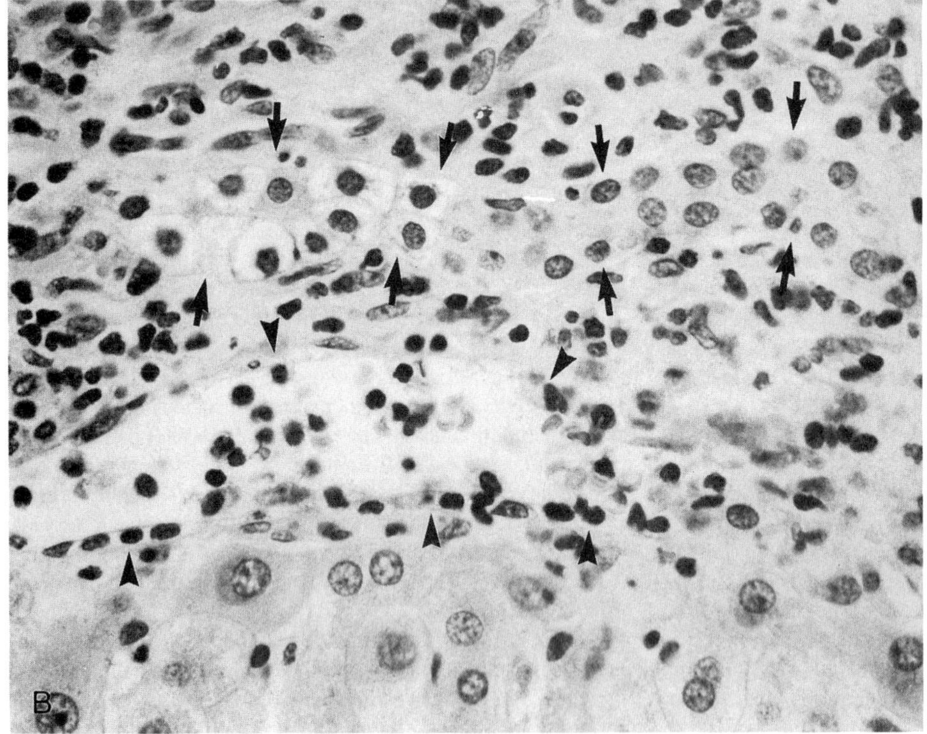

FIGURE 25 Hepatic graft rejection. *A*, Acute rejection. Portal tract reveals predominantly lymphocytic inflammation with infiltration around and within bile duct wall (*between arrows*) and endothelialitis of portal vein (*arrowheads*) (hematoxylin and eosin). *B*, Acute rejection. Close-up showing portal vein endothelialitis with disruption of endothelium associated with activated lymphocytes (*arrowheads*). Lymphoid cells are within the lumen, beneath detached endothelial cells, and on top of the endothelial surface. The bile duct (*between arrows*) shows lymphocytic infiltrate, loss of nuclear polarity, and focal cytoplasmic vacuolar degeneration.

duct syndrome. The biopsy reveals cholestasis, other features of chronic rejection, and replacement of bile ducts by scar tissue and lymphocyte aggregates (Fig. 25*D*).

Recipients of bone marrow grafts are subjected to *graft-versus-host disease* (GVHD), which is one of the most important complications of the procedure.[143,144] Acute GVHD closely resembles histologically acute rejection, with cholestasis and the triad of portal inflammation, bile duct damage, and endothelialitis. The bile duct inflammation is, however, predominantly lymphocytic and of a lesser degree. Endothelialitis is also less pronounced in GVHD and is often accompanied by hemosiderosis. Mild hepatocellular damage is usually present as well. As in chronic rejection, in chronic GVHD, there is progression of the ductal damage with even-

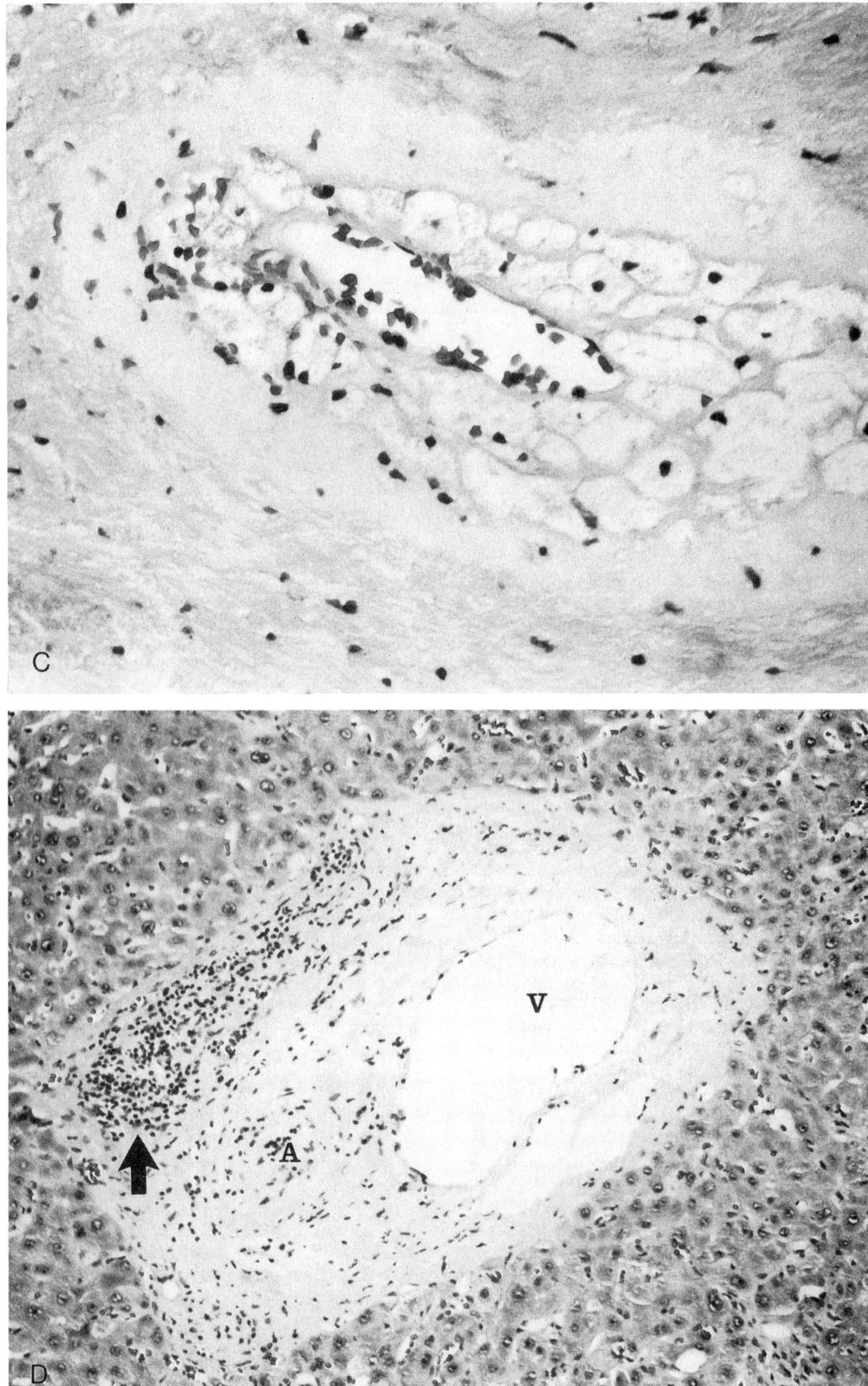

FIGURE 25 *Continued* *C*, Chronic rejection. Arteritis of medium-sized artery. The media is hyalinized and necrotic. The intima is thickened by numerous foamy histiocytes and occasional lymphocytes. The lumen is markedly reduced (hematoxylin and eosin). *D*, Chronic rejection. Vanishing bile duct syndrome. The portal tract shows a burned-out bile duct replaced by a cluster of lymphoid cells (*arrow*). A = hepatic artery; V = portal vein (hematoxylin and eosin).

tual loss of bile ducts, cholestasis, liver cell damage, and fibrosis. Biliary-type cirrhosis has been reported.[145] Veno-occlusive disease of the liver is another complication of bone marrow transplantation and is probably induced by chemotherapy or radiation or possibly is secondary to GVHD.

Acknowledgment

I am indebted to Dr. Gordon F. Vawter for his critical comments in the preparation of this manuscript.

REFERENCES

1. Sherlock S. Diseases of the liver and biliary system. 8th ed. Oxford: Blackwell Scientific Publications, 1989.
2. Schaffner F. Liver biopsy. In: Mac Sween RNM, Anthony PP, Scheuer PJ, eds. Pathology of the liver. 2nd ed. Edinburgh: Churchill Livingstone, 1987: 689.
3. Limberg B, Hopker WW, Kommerell B. Histologic differential diagnosis of focal liver lesions by ultrasonically guided fine needle biopsy. Gut 1987; 28:237–241.
4. Phillips MJ, Poucell S, Patterson J, Valencia P. The liver. An atlas and text of ultrastructural pathology. New York: Raven Press, 1987.
5. Tozuka S, Uchida T, Suzuki K, Esumi M, Shikata T. State of hepatitis B virus DNA in hepatocytes of patients with noncarcinomatous liver disease. Arch Pathol Lab Med 1989; 113:20–25.
6. Enns RK. DNA probes. An overview and comparison with current methods. Lab Med 1988; 19:295–300.
7. Grody WW, Cheng L, Lewin KJ. In situ viral DNA hybridization in diagnostic surgical pathology. Hum Pathol 1987; 18:535–543.
8. Masih AS, Linder J, Shaw BW Jr, Wood RP, Donovan JP, White R, Markin RS. Rapid identification of cytomegalovirus in liver allograft biopsies by in situ hybridization. Am J Surg Pathol 1988; 12:362–367.
9. Scheuer PJ. Liver biopsy interpretation. Philadelphia: WB Saunders, 1988.
10. Ishak KG, Sharp HL. Metabolic errors and liver disease. In: Mac Sween RNM, Anthony PP, Scheuer PJ, eds. Pathology of the liver. 2nd ed. Edinburgh: Churchill Livingstone, 1987: 99.
11. Ishak KG. Hepatic morphology in the inherited metabolic diseases. Semin Liver Dis 1986; 6:246–258.
12. Balistreri WF. Neonatal cholestasis. J Pediatr 1985; 106:171–184.
13. Brough AJ, Bernstein J. Conjugated hyperbilirubinemia in early infancy. A reassessment of liver biopsy. Hum Pathol 1974; 5:507–516.
14. Johnson JD. Neonatal nonhemolytic jaundice. N Engl J Med 1975; 292:194–197.
15. Popper H. Cholestasis: the future of a past and present riddle. Hepatology 1981; 1:187–191.
16. Heathcote J, Doedhar KP, Scheuer PJ, Sherlock S. Intrahepatic cholestasis in childhood. N Engl J Med 1976; 295:801–805.
17. Ishak KG, Sharp HL. Developmental abnormality in liver disease in childhood. In: Mac Sween RNM, Anthony PP, Scheuer PJ, eds. Pathology of the liver. 2nd ed. Edinburgh: Churchill Livingstone, 1987: 66.
18. Kahn E, Daum F, Markowitz J, Teichberg S, Duffy L, Harper R, Aiges H. Nonsyndromatic paucity of interlobular bile ducts: light and electron microscopic evaluation of sequential liver biopsies in early childhood. Hepatology 1986; 6:890–901.
19. Desmet VJ. Cholestasis: extrahepatic obstruction and secondary biliary cirrhosis. In: Mac Sween RNM, Anthony PP, Scheuer PJ, eds. Pathology of the liver. 2nd ed. Edinburgh: Churchill Livingstone, 1987: 364.
20. LaBrecque DR, Mitros FA, Nathan RJ, Romanchuk KG, Judisch GF, El-Khoury GH. Four generations of arterio-hepatic dysplasia. Hepatology 1982; 2:467–474.
21. Kahn EI, Daum F, Markowitz J, Aiges HW, Schneider KM, So HB, Altman P, Chandra R, Silverberg M. Arteriohepatic dysplasia. II. Hepatobiliary morphology. Hepatology 1983; 3:77–84.
22. Markowitz J, Daum F, Kahn EI, Schneider KM, So HB, Altman P, Aiges HW, Alperstein G, Silverberg M. Arteriohepatic dysplasia I. Pitfalls in diagnosis and management. Hepatology 1983; 3:74–76.
23. Dahms BB, Petrelli M, Wyllie R, Henoch MS, Halpin TC, Morrison S, Park MC, Tavill AS. Arteriohepatic dysplasia in infancy and childhood: a longitudinal study of six patients. Hepatology 1982; 2:350–358.
24. Odievre M, Gautier M, Hadchouel M, Alagille D. Severe familial intrahepatic cholestasis. Arch Dis Child 1973; 48:806–812.
25. Levin SE, Zarvos P, Milner S, Schmaman A. Arterio-hepatic dysplasia: association of liver disease with pulmonary arterial stenosis as well as facial and skeletal abnormalities. Pediatrics 1980; 66:876–883.
26. Dalta NS, Wilson GN, Hajra AK. Deficiency of enzymes catalyzing the biosynthesis of glycerol-ether lipids in Zellweger's syndrome. A new category of metabolic disease involving the absence of peroxisomes. N Engl J Med 1984; 311:1080–1083.
27. Monnens L, Bakkeren J, Parmentier G, Janssen G, van Haelst U, Trijbels F, Eyssen H. Disturbances in bile acid metabolism of infants with the Zellweger (cerebro-hepato-renal) syndrome. Eur J Pediatr 1980; 133:31–35.
28. Powers JM, Moser MW, Moser AB, Upshur JK, Bradford BF, Pai SG, Kohn PH, Frias J, Tiffany C. Fetal cerebrohepatorenal (Zellweger) syndrome. Dismorphic, radiologic, biochemical, and pathologic findings in four affected fetuses. Hum Pathol 1985; 16:610–620.
29. Dehner LP. Liver, gallbladder, and extrahepatic biliary tract. In: Dehner LP, ed. Pediatric surgical pathology. 2nd ed. Baltimore: Williams & Wilkins, 1987: 433.
30. Alagille D. Extrahepatic biliary atresia. Hepatology 1984; 4:7S–10S.
31. Mowat AP, Psacharopoulos HT, Williams R. Extrahepatic biliary atresia versus neonatal hepatitis. Review of 137 prospectively investigated infants. Arch Dis Child 1976; 51:763–770.
32. Ghishan FK, LaBrecque DR, Mitros FA, Younoszai MK. The evolving nature of "infantile obstructive cholangiopathy." J Pediatr 1980; 97:27–32.
33. Hirsing J, Rickham PP. Early differential diagnosis between neonatal hepatitis and biliary atresia. J Pediatr Surg 1980; 15:13–15.
34. Brough AJ, Bernstein J. Liver biopsy in the diagnosis of infantile obstructive jaundice. Pediatrics 1969; 43:519–526.
35. Hays DM, Wooley MM, Snyder WH, Reed GB, Gwinn JL, Landing BH. Diagnosis of biliary atresia: relative accuracy of percutaneous liver biopsy, open liver biopsy, and operative cholangiography. J Pediatr 1967; 71:598–607.
36. Dessanti A, Ohi R, Hanamatsu M, Mochizuchi I, Chiba T, Kasai M. Short term histological liver changes in extrahepatic biliary atresia with good postoperative bile drainage. Arch Dis Child 1985; 60:739–742.
37. Kobayashi A, Itabashi F, Ohbe Y. Long-term prognosis in biliary atresia after hepatic portoenterostomy: analysis of 35 patients who survived beyond 5 years of age. J Pediatr 1984; 105:243–246.
38. Gautier M, Jehan P, Odievre M, Hugon RN. Histologic study of biliary fibrous remnants in 48 cases of extrahepatic biliary atresia: correlation with postoperative bile flow restoration. J Pediatr 1976; 89:704–709.
39. Chandra RS, Altman RP. Ductal remnants in extrahepatic biliary atresia: a histopathologic study with clinical correlation. J Pediatr 1978; 93:196–200.
40. Dick MC, Mowat AP. Hepatitis syndrome in infancy—an epidemiological survey with 10 year follow up. Arch Dis Child 1985; 60:512–516.
41. Deutsch J, Smith AL, Danks DM, Campbell PE. Long term prognosis for babies with neonatal liver disease. Arch Dis Child 1985; 6:447–451.
42. Ecoffey C, Rothman E, Bernard O, Hadchouel M, Valayer J, Alagille D. Bacterial cholangitis after surgery for biliary atresia. J Pediatr 1987; 111:824–829.
43. Houwen RHJ, Zwierstra RP, Severignen RSVM, Bouquet J, Madern G, Vos A, Bax NMA, Heymans HSA, Bijleveld CMA. Prognosis of extrahepatic biliary atresia. Arch Dis Child 1989; 64:214–218.
44. Marksem JA. Polysplenia syndrome and splenic hypoplasia associated with extrahepatic biliary atresia. Arch Pathol Lab Med 1980; 104:212–214.
45. Morecki R, Glaser JH, Johnson AB, Kress Y. Detection of reovirus type 3 in the porta hepatis of an infant with extrahepatic biliary atresia: ultrastructural and immunocytochemical study. Hepatology 1984; 4:1137–1142.
46. Glasser JH, Balistreri WF, Morecki R. Role of reovirus type 3 in persistent infantile cholestasis. J Pediatr 1984; 105:912–915.
47. Morecki R, Glaser JH, Cho S, Balistreri WF, Horwitz MS. Biliary atresia and reovirus type 3 infection. N Engl J Med 1982; 307:481–484.
48. Morecki R, Glasser JH, Cho S, Balistreri WF, Horwitz MS. Biliary atresia and reovirus type 3 infection. N Engl J Med 1984; 310:1610.
49. Dussaix E, Hadchouel M, Tardieu M, Alagille D. Biliary atresia and reovirus type 3 infection. N Engl J Med 1984; 310:658.
50. Hadchouel M, Hugon RN, Odievre M. Immunoglobulin deposits in the biliary remnants of extrahepatic biliary atresia: a study by immunoperoxidase staining in 128 infants. Histopathology 1981; 5:217–221.
51. Vacanti JP, Perez-Atayde AR, Tewksbury J, Morse MA, Leung DYM. Presence of antibiliary epithelial cell antibodies to biliary epithelium in children with biliary atresia. Gastroenterology. Submitted for publication.
52. Simson IW, Gear JHS. Other viral and infectious diseases. In: Mac Sween RNM, Anthony PP, Scheuer PJ, eds. Pathology of the liver. 2nd ed. Edinburgh: Churchill Livingstone, 1987: 224.
53. Finegold MJ, Carpenter RJ. Obliterative cholangitis due to cytomegalovirus: a possible precursor of paucity of intrahepatic bile ducts. Hum Pathol 1982; 13:662–665.

54. Ghishan FK, Greene HL, Halter S, Barnard JA, Moray JR. Noncirrhotic portal hypertension in congenital cytomegalovirus infection. Hepatology 1984; 4:684–686.
55. Snover DC, Horwitz CA. Liver disease in cytomegalovirus mononucleosis: a light and immunoperoxidase study of six cases. Hepatology 1984; 4:408–412.
56. Mostoufizadeh M, Lack EE, Gang DL, Perez-Atayde AR, Driscoll SG. Postmortem manifestations of echovirus 11 sepsis in five newborn infants. Hum Pathol 1983; 14:818–823.
57. Kocoshis SA, Cottrill CM, O'Connor WN, Haugh R, Jonnson GL, Noonan JA. Congenital heart disease, butterfly vertebrae, and extrahepatic biliary atresia: a variant of arteriohepatic dysplasia? J Pediatr 1981; 99:436–439.
58. Valencia-Mayoral P, Weber J, Cutz E, Edwards VD, Phillips MJ. Possible defect in the bile secretory apparatus in arteriohepatic dysplasia (Alagille's syndrome): a review with observations on the ultrastructure of liver. Hepatology 1984; 4:691–698.
59. Pfeifer U, Sandhage K. Licht- und elektronenmikroskopische leberbefunde beim cerebro-hepato-renalen syndrom nach Zellweger (Peroxisomen-Defizienz). Virchows Arch [A] 1979; 384:269–284.
60. Moser AE, Singh I, Brown FR, Solish GI, Kelley RI, Benke PJ, Moser HW. The cerebrohepatorenal (Zellweger) syndrome. Increased levels and impaired degradation of very-long-chain fatty acids and their use in prenatal diagnosis. N Engl J Med 1984; 310:1141–1146.
61. Mathis RK, Watkins JB, Szczepanik-Van Leeuween P, Loft IT. Liver in the cerebro-hepato-renal syndrome: defective bile acid synthesis and abnormal mitochondria. Gastroenterology 1980; 79:1311–1317.
62. Heymans HSA, Schutgens RBH, Tan R, van den Bosch H, Borst P. Severe plasmalogen deficiency in tissues of infants without peroxisomes (Zellweger syndrome). Nature 1983; 306:69–70.
63. Knisely AS, Magid MS, Dische MR, Cutz E. Neonatal hemochromatosis. Birth Defects 1987; 23:75–102.
64. Goldfischer S, Grotsky HW, Chang C-H, Berman EL, Richert RR, Karmarkar SD, Roskamp JO, Morecki R. Idiopathic neonatal iron storage involving the liver, pancreas, heart and endocrine and exocrine glands. Hepatology 1981; 1:58–64.
65. Silver MM, Beverley DW, Valberg LS, Cutz E, Phillips MJ, Shaheed WA. Perinatal hemochromatosis. Clinical, morphologic, and quantitative iron studies. Am J Pathol 1987; 128:538–553.
66. Escobar GJ, Heyman MB, Smith WB, Thaler MM. Primary hemochromatosis in childhood. Pediatrics 1987; 80:549–554.
67. Witzleben CL, Uri A. Perinatal hemochromatosis: entity or end result? Hum Pathol 1989; 20:335–340.
68. Searle JW, Kerr JFR, Halliday JW, Powell LW. Iron storage disease. In: Mac Sween RNM, Anthony PP, Scheuer PJ, eds. Pathology of the liver. 2nd ed. Edinburgh: Churchill Livingstone, 1987: 181.
69. Alagille D. Alpha-l-antitrypsin deficiency. Hepatology 1984; 4:11S–14S.
70. Ghishan FK, Greene HL. Liver disease in children with PiZZ alpha$_1$-antitrypsin deficiency. Hepatology 1988; 8:307–310.
71. Nemeth A, Strandvik B. Natural history of children with alpha-l-antitrypsin deficiency and neonatal cholestasis. Acta Paediatr Scand 1982; 71:993–999.
72. Nemeth A, Strandvik B. Liver disease in children with alpha-l-antitrypsin deficiency without neonatal cholestasis. Acta Paediatr Scand 1982; 71:1001–1005.
73. Psacharopoulos HT, Mowat AP, Cook PJL, et al. Outcome of liver disease associated with alpha-l-antitrypsin deficiency (PiZ). Arch Dis Child 1983; 58:882–887.
74. Nemeth A, Samuelsson K, Strandvik B. Serum bile acids as markers of juvenile liver disease in alpha-l-antitrypsin deficiency. J Pediatr Gastroenterol Nutr 1982; 1:479–483.
75. Nebbia G, et al. Early assessment of evolution of liver disease associated with alpha-l-antitrypsin deficiency in childhood. J Pediatr 1983; 102:661–665.
76. Sveger T. Prospective study of children with alpha-l-antitrypsin deficiency: eight-year-old follow-up. J Pediatr 1984; 104:91–94.
77. Hodges JR, et al. Heterozygous MZ alpha-l-antitrypsin deficiency in adults with chronic active hepatitis and cryptogenic cirrhosis. N Engl J Med 1981; 304:557–560.
78. Hultcrantz R, Mengarelli S. Ultrastructural liver pathology in patients with minimal liver disease and alpha-l-antitrypsin deficiency: a comparison between heterozygous and homozygous patients. Hepatology 1984; 4:937–945.
79. Weber AM, Tuchweber B, Yousef I, Brochu P, Turgeon C, Gabbiani G, Morin CL, Roy CC. Severe familial cholestasis in North American Indian children: a clinical model of microfilament dysfunction? Gastroenterology 1981; 81:653–662.
80. Williams CN, Kaye R, Baker L, Hurwitz R, Senior JR. Progressive familial cholestatic cirrhosis and bile acid metabolism. J Pediatr 1972; 81:493–500.
81. Sharp HL, Krivit W. Hereditary lymphedema and obstructive jaundice. J Pediatr 1971; 78:491–496.
82. Ballow M, Margolis CZ, Schachtel B, Hsia YE. Progressive familial intrahepatic cholestasis. Pediatrics 1973; 51:998–1007.
83. Greco MA, Finegold MJ. Familial giant cell hepatitis. Report of two cases and review of the literature. Arch Pathol 1973; 95:240–244.
84. Linarelli LG, Williams CN, Phillips MJ. Byler's disease: fatal intrahepatic cholestasis. J Pediatr 1972; 81:484–492.
85. De Pagter AGF, Van Berge Henegouwen GP, Ten Bokkel Huinink JA, Brandt K-H. Familial benign recurrent intrahepatic cholestasis. Interrelation with intrahepatic cholestasis of pregnancy and from oral contraceptives? Gastroenterology 1976; 71:202–207.
86. Nayak NC. Indian childhood cirrhosis. In: Mac Sween RNM, Anthony PP, Scheuer PJ, eds. Pathology of the liver. 2nd ed. Edinburgh: Churchill Livingstone, 1987: 358.
87. Klass HJ, Kelly JK, Warnes TW. Indian childhood cirrhosis in the United Kingdom. Gut 1980; 21:244–350.
88. Lefkowitch JH, Honig CL, King ME, Hagstrom JWC. Hepatic copper overload and features of Indian childhood cirrhosis in an American sibship. N Engl J Med 1982; 307:271–277.
89. Goldfischer S, Popper H, Sternlieb I. The significance of variations in the distribution of copper in liver disease. Am J Pathol 1980; 99:715–730.
90. Travis WD, Castile R, Vawter G, Shwachman H, Warwick W, Burke BA, Skinner M. Secondary (AA) amyloidosis in cystic fibrosis. Am J Clin Pathol 1986; 85:419–424.
91. Dienes HP, Popper H, Arnold W, Lobeck H. Histologic observations in human hepatitis non-A, non-B. Hepatology 1982; 2:562–571.
92. Buitrago B, Popper H, Hadler SC, Thung SN, Gerber MA, Purcell RH, Maynard JE. Specific histologic features of Santa Marta hepatitis: a severe form of hepatitis delta-virus infection in northern South America. Hepatology 1986; 6:1285–1291.
93. Lefkowitch JH, Goldstein H, Yatto R, Gerber MA. Cytopathic liver injury in acute delta virus hepatitis. Gastroenterology 1987; 92:1262–1266.
94. Verme G, Amoroso P, Lettier G, Pierri P, David E, Sessa F, Rizzi R, Bonino F, Recchia S, Rizzetto M. A histological study of hepatitis delta virus liver disease. Hepatology 1986; 6:1303–1307.
95. Govindarajan S, Cock KM, Peters RL. Morphologic and immunohistochemical features of fulminant delta hepatitis. Hum Pathol 1985; 12:262–267.
96. Wands JR. Non-A, non-B hepatitis. Hepatology 1983; 3:764–766.
97. Rakela J, Redeker AG. Chronic liver disease after acute non-A,non-B viral hepatitis. Gastroenterology 1979; 77:1200–1202.
98. Chang M-H, Hwang L-Y, Hsu H-C, Lee C-Y, Beasley RP. Prospective study of asymptomatic HBsAg carrier children infected in the perinatal period: clinical and liver histologic studies. Hepatology 1988; 8:374–377.
99. Maggiore G, DeGiacomo C, Marzani D, Sessa F, Scotta MS. Chronic viral hepatitis B in infancy. J Pediatr 1983; 103:749–752.
100. Hsu H-C, Lin Y-H, Chang M-H, Su I-J, Chen D-S. Pathology of chronic hepatitis B virus infection in children: with special reference to the intrahepatic expression of hepatitis B virus antigens. Hepatology 1988; 8:378–382.
101. Sherlock S. Chronic hepatitis and cirrhosis. Hepatology 1984; 4:25S–28S.
102. Popper H. Changing concepts of the evolution of chronic hepatitis and the role of piecemeal necrosis. Hepatology 1983; 3:758–762.
103. Bianchi L, Spichtin HP, Gudat F. Chronic hepatitis. In: Mac Sween RNM, Anthony PP, Scheuer PJ, eds. Pathology of the liver. 2nd ed. Edinburgh: Churchill Livingstone, 1987: 310.
104. Liaw Y-F, Chu C-M, Chen T-J, Lin D-Y, Chang-Chien C-S, Wu C-S. Chronic lobular hepatitis: a clinicopathological and prognostic study. Hepatology 1982; 2:258–262.
105. Duffy LF, Daum F, Kahn E, Teichberg S, Pahwa R, Fagin J, Kenigsberg K, Kaplan M, Fisher SE, Pahwa S. Hepatitis in children with

acquired immune deficiency syndrome. Histopathologic and immunocytologic features. Gastroenterology 1986; 90:173–181.

106. Kamimura T, Ponzetto A, Bonino F, Feinstone SM, Gerin JL, Purcell RH. Cytoplasmic tubular structures in liver of HBsAg carrier chimpanzees infected with delta agent and comparison with cytoplasmic structures in non A, non B hepatitis. Hepatology 1983; 3:631–637.
107. Marciano-Cabral F, Rublee KL, Carithers RL, Galen EA, Sobieski TJ, Cabral GA. Chronic non-A, non-B hepatitis: ultrastructural and serologic studies. Hepatology 1981; 1:575–582.
108. Zimmerman HJ, Fang M, Utili R, Seeff LB, Hoofnagle J. Jaundice due to bacterial infection. Gastroenterology 1979; 77:362–374.
109. Lefkowitch JH. Bile ductular cholestasis: an ominous histopathologic sign related to sepsis and "cholangitis lenta." Hum Pathol 1982; 13:19–24.
110. Weinstein L. Bacterial hepatitis: a case report on an unrecognized cause of fever of unknown origin. N Engl J Med 1978; 299:1052–1054.
111. Banks JG, Foulis AK, Ledingham IMcA, Mac Sween RNM. Liver function in septic shock. J Clin Pathol 1982; 35:1249–1252.
112. Ishak KG, Rogers WA. Cryptogenic acute cholangitis—association with toxic shock syndrome. Am J Clin Pathol 1981; 76:619–626.
113. Lebovics E, Thung SN, Schaffner F, Radensky PW. The liver in the acquired immunodeficiency syndrome: a clinical and histologic study. Hepatology 1985; 5:293–298.
114. Gordon SC, Reddy KR, Gould EE, McFadden R, O'Brien C, De-Medina M, Jeffers J, Schiff ER. The spectrum of liver disease in the acquired immunodeficiency syndrome. J Hepatology 1986; 2:475–484.
115. Schneiderman DJ, Arenson DM, Cello JP, Margaretten W, Weber TE. Hepatic disease in patients with the acquired immune deficiency syndrome (AIDS). Hepatology 1987; 7:925–930.
116. Heubi JE, Partin JC, Partin JS, Schubert WK. Reye's syndrome: current concepts. Hepatology 1987; 7:155–164.
117. Partin JS, Daugherty CC, McAdams AJ, Partin JC, Schubert WK. A comparison of liver ultrastructure in salicylate intoxication and Reye's syndrome. Hepatology 1984; 4:687–690.
118. Starko KM, Mullick FG. Hepatic and cerebral pathology findings in children with fatal salicylate intoxication; further evidence for a causal relation between salicylate and Reye's syndrome. Lancet 1983; i:326–329.
119. Treem WR, Witzleben CA, Piccoli DA, Stanley CA, Hale DE, Coates PM, Watkins JB. Medium-chain and long-chain acyl Co A dehydrogenase deficiency: clinical, pathologic and ultrastructural differentiation from Reye's syndrome. Hepatology 1986; 6:1270–1278.
120. Latham PS, LaBrecque DR, McReynolds JW, Klatskin G. Liver ultrastructure in mitochondrial urea cycle enzyme deficiencies and comparison with Reye's syndrome. Hepatology 1984; 4:404–407.
121. Chapoy PR, Angelini C, Brown WJ, Stiff JE, Shug AL, Cederbaum SD. Systemic carnitine deficiency—a treatable inherited lipid-storage disease presenting as Reye's syndrome. N Engl J Med 1980; 303:1389–1394.
122. Glasgow AM, Eng G, Engel AG. Systemic carnitine deficiency simulating recurrent Reye's syndrome. J Pediatr 1980; 96:889–891.
123. Treem WR, Stanley CA, Finegold DN, Hale DE, Coates PM. Primary carnitine deficiency due to a failure of carnitine transport in kidney, muscles and fibroblasts. N Engl J Med 1988; 319:1331–1336.
124. Nyhan WL. Abnormalities of fatty acid oxidation. N Engl J Med 1988; 319:1344–1346.
125. Rinaldo P, O'Shea JJ, Coates PM, Hale DE, Stanley CA, Tanaka K. Medium-chain acyl-CoA dehydrogenase deficiency. Diagnosis by stable-isotope dilution measurement of urinary *N*-hexanoylglycine and 3-phenylpropionylglycine. N Engl J Med 1988; 319:1308–1313.
126. Winter HS, Perez-Atayde AR, Levy HL, Shih VE. Unique hepatic ultrastructural changes in a patient with hyperammonemia (HAM), hyperornithinemia (HOR), and homocitrullinuria (HC). Pediatr Res 1980; 14:583.
127. LaRusso NF, Wiesner RH, Ludwig J, MacCarty RL. Primary sclerosing cholangitis. N Engl J Med 1984; 310:899–903.
128. Sisto A, Feldman P, Garel L, Seidman E, Brochu P, Morin CL, Weber AM, Roy CC. Primary sclerosing cholangitis in children: study of five cases and review of the literature. Pediatrics 1987; 80:918–923.
129. El-Shabrawi M, Wilkinson ML, Portmann B, Mieli-Vergani G, Chong SKF, Williams R, Mowat AP. Primary sclerosing cholangitis in childhood. Gastroenterology 1987; 92:1226–1235.
130. Nakanuma Y, Terada T, Ohta G, Kurachi M, Matsubara F. Caroli's disease in congenital hepatic fibrosis and infantile polycystic disease. Liver 1982; 2:346–354.
131. Tazelaar HD, Payne JA, Patel NS. Congenital hepatic fibrosis and asymptomatic familial adult-type polycystic kidney disease in a 19-year old woman. Gastroenterology 1984; 86:747–760.
132. Kudo M, Tamura K, Fuse Y. Cystic dysplastic kidneys associated with Dandy-Walker malformation and congenital hepatic fibrosis. Report of two cases. Am J Clin Pathol 1985; 84:459–463.
133. Witzleben CL, Sharp AR. "Nephronophthisis-congenital hepatic fibrosis": an additional hepatorenal disorder. Hum Pathol 1982; 13:728–733.
134. Bras G, Brandt KH. Vascular disorders. In: Mac Sween RNM, Anthony PP, Scheuer PJ, eds. Pathology of the liver. 2nd ed. Edinburgh: Churchill Livingstone, 1987:478.
135. Carlson RA, Arya S, Gilbert EF. Budd-Chiari syndrome presenting as sudden infant death. Arch Pathol Lab Med 1985; 109:379–380.
136. Usatin MS. Peliosis hepatis in a child. Arch Pathol Lab Med 1976; 100:419–421.
137. Zimmerman HJ, Ishak KG. Hepatic injury due to drugs and toxins. In: Mac Sween RNM, Anthony PP, Scheuer PJ, eds. Pathology of the liver. 2nd ed. Edinburgh: Churchill Livingstone, 1987: 503.
138. Snover DC, Sibley RK, Freese DK, Sharp HL, Bloomer JR, Najarian JS, Ascher NL. Orthotopic liver transplantation: a pathological study of 63 serial liver biopsies from 17 patients with special reference to the diagnostic features and natural history of rejection. Hepatology 1984; 4:1212–1222.
139. Fennel RH. Ductular damage in liver transplant rejection. Its similarity to that of primary biliary cirrhosis and graft-versus-host disease. Pathol Ann (Part 2) 1981; 16:289–294.
140. Demetris AJ, Lasky S, Van Thiel DH, Starzl TE, Dekker A. Pathology of hepatic transplantation. A review of 62 adult allograft recipients immunosuppressed with a cyclosporine/steroid regimen. Am J Pathol 1985; 118:151–161.
141. Vierling JM, Fennell RH. Histopathology of early and late human hepatic allograft rejection: evidence of progressive destruction of interlobular bile ducts. Hepatology 1985; 5:1076–1082.
142. Fennel RH, Vierling JM. Electron microscopy of rejected human liver allografts. Hepatology 1985; 5:1083–1087.
143. Shulman HM, Sharma P, Amos D, Fenster LF. McDonald GB. A coded histologic study of hepatic graft-versus-host disease after human bone marrow transplantation. Hepatology 1988; 8:463–470.
144. Snover DC, Weisdorf SA, Ramsay NK, McGlave P, Kersey JH. Hepatic graft versus host disease: a study of the predictive value of liver biopsy in diagnosis. Hepatology 1984; 4:123–130.
145. Knapp AB, Crawford JM, Rappeport JM, Gollan JL. Cirrhosis as a consequence of graft-versus-host disease. Gastroenterology 1987; 92:513–519.

CHAPTER 32

Intestinal Biopsy

John A. Walker-Smith, M.D.(Syd.), F.R.C.P.(Lon., Edin.), F.R.A.C.P.
Alan D. Phillips, B.A.(Hon.)
Paul I. Richman, M.B.B.S., Ph.D., M.C.C.Path.

SMALL INTESTINAL BIOPSY

The introduction of the techniques of proximal small intestinal mucosal biopsy to pediatric practice by Shiner in 1957[1] was a major advance. It has led to a great increase in knowledge of small intestinal mucosal pathology in relation to disease states in children.

Crosby and Kugler[2] in the same year developed a capsule for small intestinal biopsy in adults which has come to be known as the Crosby capsule. In 1962,[3] a modification of this capsule was produced, and a pediatric version known as the Watson capsule is now widely used for small intestinal biopsy in children. An adaptation of the pediatric Crosby capsule with two adjacent portholes, which provide two smaller biopsies simultaneously, may be useful when the presence of a patchy lesion is suspected, e.g., cows' milk–sensitive enteropathy. The use of this further modification does *not* increase the risks of the procedure, and the capsule is recommended for routine use in children.[4]

The safety of a capsule in children is related to its porthole size, which in the Watson capsule is 2.5 to 3 mm, compared with 5 mm in the adult capsule.

It is dangerous to use the adult capsule in small children, as the size of the tissue biopsied may be too large and may occasionally lead to perforation. Use of the pediatric capsule, however, is safe in the experience of most observers, although there is still a small risk of complications.

During the experience of 704 biopsies by one of us (JW-S) in the 6-year period from 1966 to 1972 at the Royal Alexandra Hospital for children in Sydney, Australia, there was only one serious complication—an intraduodenal hematoma that settled spontaneously without any surgical intervention.[5] However, a further experience of 2,101 biopsies at Queen Elizabeth Hospital for Children in London from 1973 to 1987 has been without morbidity.

It is vitally important that a small intestinal biopsy in children be performed only in specialty centers where considerable experience and expertise both in the technique itself and in the interpretation of biopsy findings is available. In this way safety, minimal disturbance to the child, and reliable results will all be appropriately combined. The occasional small intestinal biopsy performed by inexperienced hands may lead to a disturbed child and often yields inconclusive results.

Technique of Small Intestinal Biopsy

The child should be fasted overnight, although small amounts of water may be given as required. Infants may have a 10 PM and sometimes a 2 AM feeding if necessary. On the morning of the biopsy the child is sedated. A useful regimen of oral sedation is that currently used at the Queen Elizabeth Hospital for Children, namely trimeprazine (Vallergan), chloral hydrate, and metoclopramide in appropriate dose for age. If the child becomes highly restless or distressed during the procedure intravenous diazepam (Valium) may be given at a maximum dose of 0.5 mg per kilogram. This should be done only when there is no risk to the child because of heavy sedation and resuscitation equipment is immediately available. Grossly enlarged tonsils or any compromise to the upper airways is clear contraindication to its use. Once the child is appropriately sedated, the capsule is passed. This is done in the small child by placing a tongue depressor in the mouth and placing the capsule at the back of the tongue. The depressor is withdrawn, the chin is held up, and the child swallows. The tubing is then gently advanced until the capsule is in the stomach. Resistance is often felt at the cardioesophageal junction. The child is then placed on his right side and the capsule further advanced. It should then fall toward the pylorus.

The next step depends upon whether a flexible tubing is being used or a more rigid tubing and whether there is to be fluoroscopic screening (the preferred technique) or if progress is to be assessed by plain radiograph of the abdomen. In addition, if a nonradiopaque tube is used, radiopaque material such as Urografin needs to be injected down the tubing before the position of the capsule can be checked radiologically. Using a flexible tubing and a plain radiograph of the abdomen is a time-consuming procedure, but it does have the virtue of providing an exact record, i.e., radiograph, of the exact site of the biopsy. The more rapid technique of using a radiopaque relatively rigid tube and positioning the capsule under fluoroscopic control is, however, to be preferred. Such a semirigid catheter is the metal braided angiocardiographic catheter, which successfully transmits torque. It is also helpful to inject some air into the stomach via the capsule. A practical advantage of this technique is its usual speed, which makes the procedure preferable from the child's point of view. Care should be taken to monitor the fluoroscopy time. This should not exceed 2 minutes and is usually far shorter.

Metoclopramide introduced into the tubing in the dose of 2.5 mg for infants under 2 years and 5 mg for those over 2 years usually speeds the passage of the capsule when there is hold-up at the pylorus. Using either procedure, once the capsule is positioned in the fourth part of the duodenum, the duodenojejunal flexure, or the first loop of the jejunum, it is "fired" by suction with a 20-ml syringe and then withdrawn. Ideally, biopsies should be taken from a constant standard site. A virtue of the screening technique is that it can be done easily and accurately. In order to ensure that the tube is not blocked (if Urografin or metoclopramide syrup has been injected down the tube), it is helpful to inject 2 ml of water followed by 2 ml of air before firing the capsule.

It is possible to fire the capsule under screening. This can allow the movement of the blade to be seen, confirming that the capsule has indeed fired. However, this involves extra screening time, is not completely reliable, and increases the time between taking the sample and processing it.

Ideally, some duodenal juice should be obtained either by free drainage before the capsule is fired or at the time of firing. The juice should be examined immediately by light microscopy, under phase-contrast or high-contrast conditions, for the presence of *Giardia lamblia* and should be sent for culture if bacterial overgrowth or enteroadherent enteropathogenic *Escherichia coli* infection is considered a diagnostic possibility.

Once the capsule has been withdrawn, the biopsy specimens should be rapidly removed from the capsule onto a gloved finger using a blunt seeker. The samples are opened out carefully so that the mucosal surface is facing downward (this can be checked using a dissecting microscope or hand lens if required). A piece of dry, black card is then applied gently to the serosal surface for a few seconds, resulting in the sample adhering to the card. The card and sample, with the mucosal surface now facing upward, are placed into cold (4°C) normal saline. The black card optimizes contrast of the specimen for study and photography. Under the dissecting microscope the appearance of the mucosa can be assessed, and samples can be taken for other studies for which fixation with formalin is to be avoided, e.g., electron microscopy, disaccharidase assay, and immunohistochemistry.

The specimens, still on the black card, are then placed in 10 percent phosphate-buffered formalin and processed for histology. Routinely, 10 to 20 serial sections are cut, mounted on a single glass slide, and stained with hematoxylin and eosin and with periodic acid–Schiff (PAS) stain.

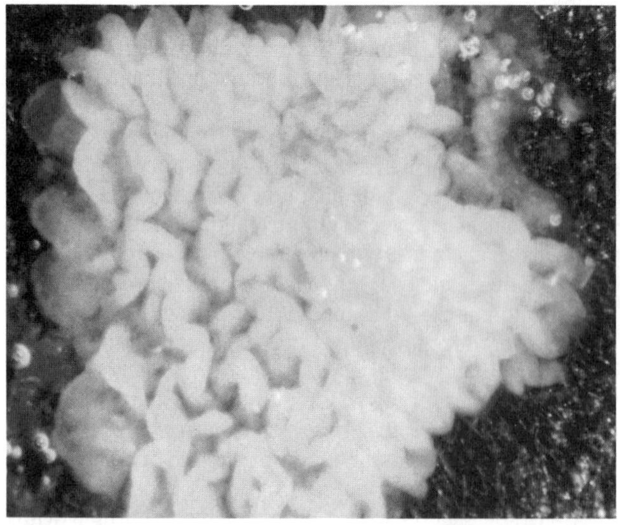

FIGURE 1 Dissecting microscopy. Patchy appearance showing ridgelike villi on the left side with low, closely packed ridges on the right (male, 13 months, postenteritis syndrome).

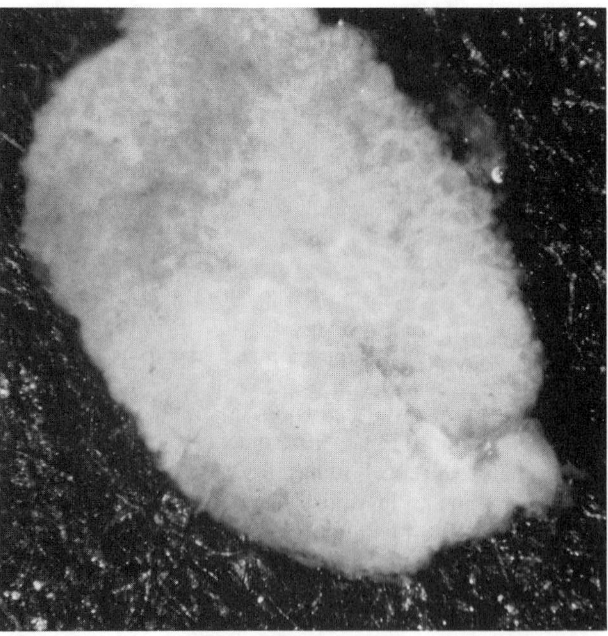

FIGURE 2 Dissecting microscopy. Flat mucosa showing visible crypt openings (female, 13 months, untreated celiac disease).

Hygiene Precautions

It is sensible practice, when handling the biopsy capsule following firing, to wear surgical gloves. The biopsy capsule should be cleaned thoroughly after use and disinfected for at least 10 minutes in 0.5 percent chlorhexidine gluconate (weight per volume) in 70 percent alcohol, followed by a minimum of 1 hour in Cidex (2 percent activated glutaraldehyde solution—Surgikos, Ltd.), rinsed in water, and allowed to dry.

Morphologic Observations of Small Intestinal Biopsy Specimens

Dissecting Microscopy

The value of initial examination of biopsy samples with the dissecting microscope has been confirmed by many workers, both in adult medicine and in pediatrics.[6,7] Many now consider examination of a small intestinal biopsy specimen without a dissecting microscopic assessment to be an inadequate examination. The value of this method includes the following:

1. It greatly facilitates orientation of biopsy specimens in readiness for sectioning.
2. It allows study to be made of the three-dimensional arrangements of mucosal architecture.
3. The entire biopsy specimen may be examined, which is particularly important in children, in whom patchy mucosal lesions often occur (Fig. 1).
4. It allows rapid diagnosis of the presence or absence of a flat mucosa.

5. It allows parents to see the mucosa themselves, e.g., a flat mucosa (Fig. 2), and therefore reinforces the need for a gluten-free diet, particularly in postgluten challenges when symptoms may not arise.

The drawbacks of the method are that if due care is not taken fixation may be postponed, giving rise to the possibility of autolytic changes, and the severity of an abnormality other than a flat mucosa can be underestimated.

Some authors[8] have considered that this method of examination adds little to histology and that its only value lies in the rapid recognition of a flat mucosa. They advocate, instead, serial sectioning for histology of the whole biopsy specimen. However, such an approach is idealistic, as it is not practical in most hospitals, whereas dissecting microscopy is simple and straightforward and can easily be performed routinely.

In normal, healthy adults the small intestinal mucosa is characterized principally by finger-like, with some leaflike, villi, but in children the villi tend to be broader. The term "tonguelike" is used to describe such villi, and when they are extremely wide the term "thin ridgelike villi" is used. The latter appearance is frequently seen in children in the first 5 years of life[9] (Fig. 3).

When the small intestine is studied at postmortem examination by means of a dissecting microscope, a remarkable variation of small intestinal mucosal morphology in relation to age can be demonstrated.[10] Throughout childhood up to the age of 10 years, finger-like villi occur uncommonly in the duodenum and broader villi are characteristic. This is true, but to a somewhat lesser extent, in the jejunum. In the ileum, finger-like villi are most often found in the neonate; this changes from 1 month to 4 years of age, when broader villi are found to be characteristic. Over the age of 4 years, finger-like villi are again the dominant finding in the ileum, as occurs in adult life.

Thus, the observation under the dissecting microscope of broad villi described as leaflike, tonguelike, or thin ridgelike villi on proximal small intestinal biopsy is accepted as a normal finding in children. Certainly Wright et al[11] found that in childhood controls the epithelial cell transit time in the crypts was 40 percent less than in adult controls. Also the corrected mitotic index was 20 percent greater. Thus, in early childhood the mucosal surface area is reduced and epithelial cell turnover is greater than in adults.

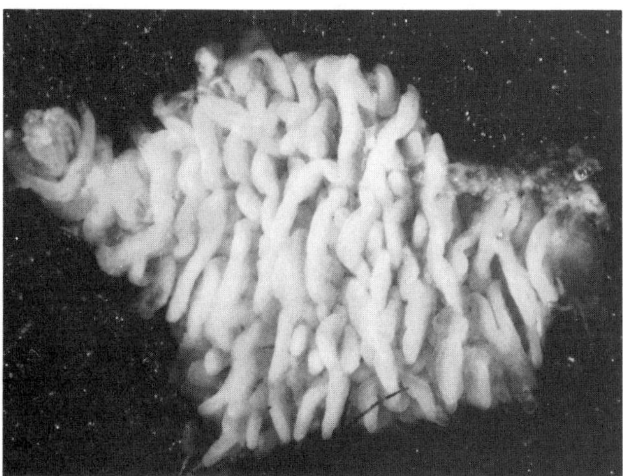

FIGURE 3 Dissecting microscopy. Normal appearance of tall, thin, ridgelike villi interspersed with leaflike villi (male, 5 months, intermittent diarrhea).

TABLE 1
Classification of Dissecting Microscope Appearances

Group I
Flat mucosa
Flat and barren
Flat mosaic
Group II
Thickened ridges
Short
Taller
Group III
Broad villi
Long, thick, ridgelike villi and tonguelike villi
Tongue- and leaflike villi with occasional finger-like villi
Leaflike and finger-like villi

The explanation for this observation of reduced surface area, i.e., broader forms of villi, is unknown. As it is found in infants of 26 or more weeks' gestation who have not been fed,[12] it cannot be due to ingestion of food and bacteria after birth. However, in utero ingestion of amniotic fluid or gastric acid secretions per se may play a role.

Abnormal appearances seen under the dissecting microscope are broadly grouped under two headings: a flat mucosa and a ridged or convoluted mucosa. In both types of mucosae the normal villous architecture is lost. Table 1 indicates a classification of the dissecting microscope appearances of small intestinal biopsy specimens.[13] Patchy changes in architecture can also be appreciated with the dissecting microscope.

It is important that a photographic record be kept of each biopsy examined in order to correlate appearances seen with those observed with the light microscope. The dissecting microscope also allows isolated lymphoid follicles to be seen. They may be frequently found in children around 1 to 2 years old but are not commonly seen in children over 6 years of age. Dilated lacteals may also be visible, but they are not indicative of lymphangiectasia in the absence of other clinical features.

Possible artifacts and misinterpretation to be aware of include the mounting of a specimen upside down on the card so that it appears flat and obtaining a gastric, rather than a proximal small intestinal, biopsy, which also appears flat. Both of these findings are apparent on histologic examination. Around 50 percent of samples show some hyperemia, an artifactual result of the suction technique. However, such artifacts are much less common than those found when endoscopy is used to take the samples. Endoscopic biopsies are not adequate for complete morphologic assessment.

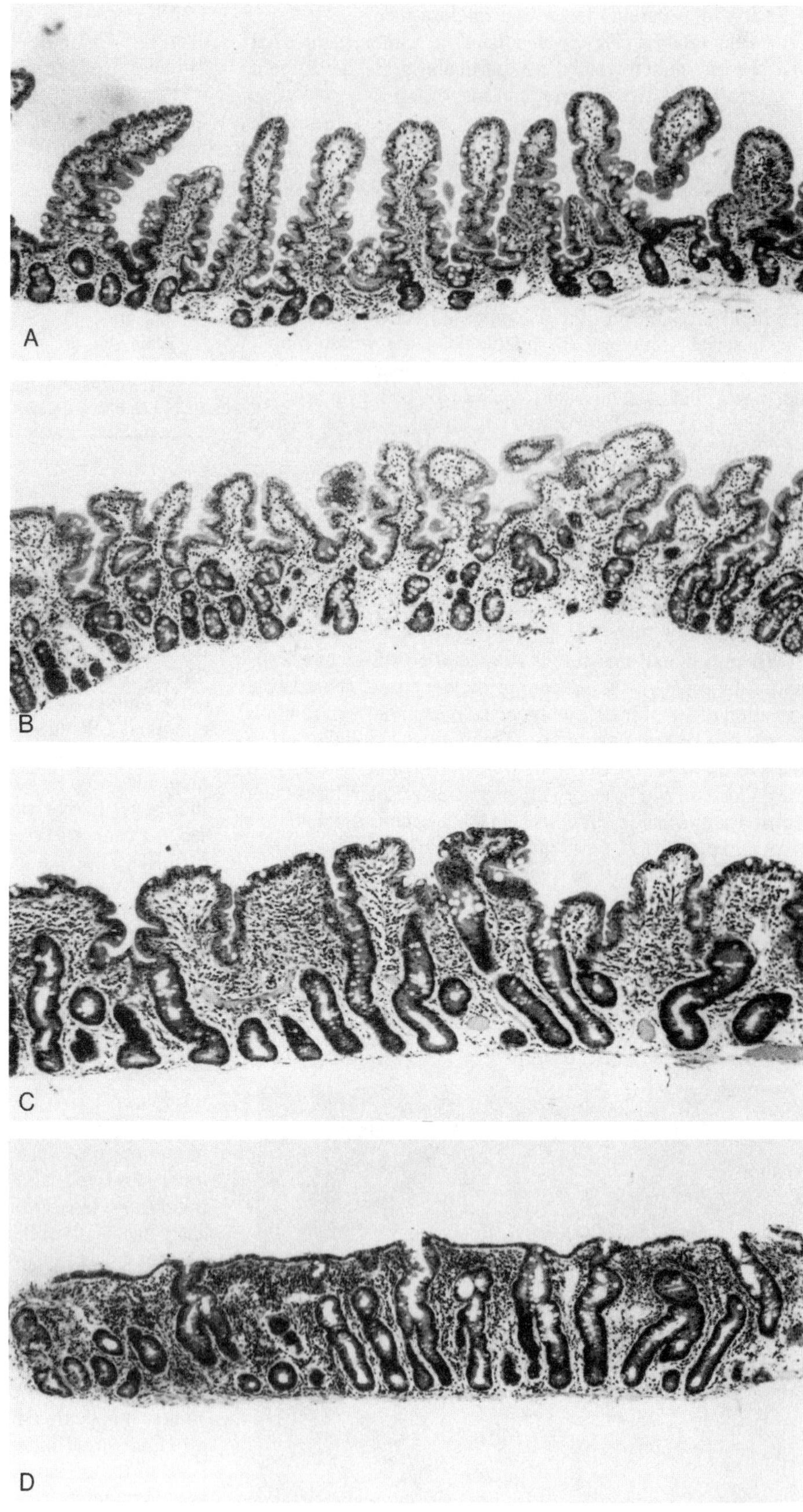

FIGURE 4 Light microscopy. *A*, Histologically normal small intestinal mucosa (female, 12 months, failure to thrive). *B*, Minor enteropathy (female, 5 months, chronic diarrhea with failure to thrive). *C*, Moderate enteropathy (male, 6 years 9 months, celiac disease—postgluten challenge). *D*, Severe enteropathy (female, 6 years 10 months, untreated celiac disease) (×75 for all).

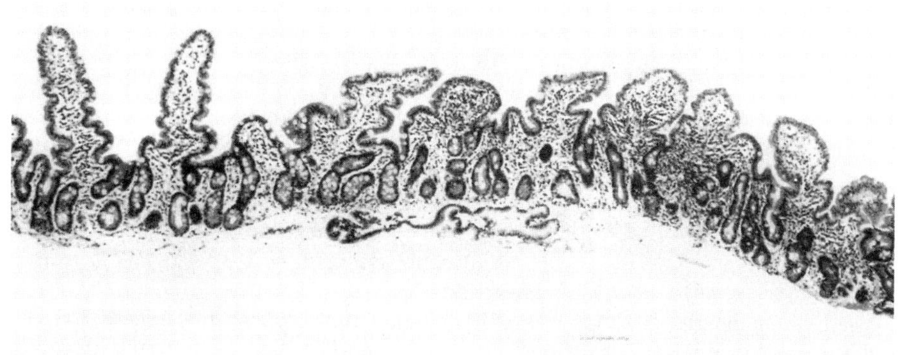

FIGURE 5 Light microscopy. Patchy enteropathy (female, 2 years 2 months, diarrhea postcolectomy) (×60).

Light Microscopy

Small intestinal biopsy sections are routinely examined with the light microscope after staining the sections with hematoxylin and eosin. At present an unsatisfactory situation exists in relation to histologic terminology. The earliest reports divided pathologic small intestinal mucosae into "subtotal" and "partial" villous atrophy. The former category was characterized by a flat mucosa with thickening of the glandular layer beneath an atrophic epithelium and the latter by a less abnormal mucosa. Some authors have further qualified "partial villous atrophy" with the terms "mild" and "severe." Others have used the term "total villous atrophy"

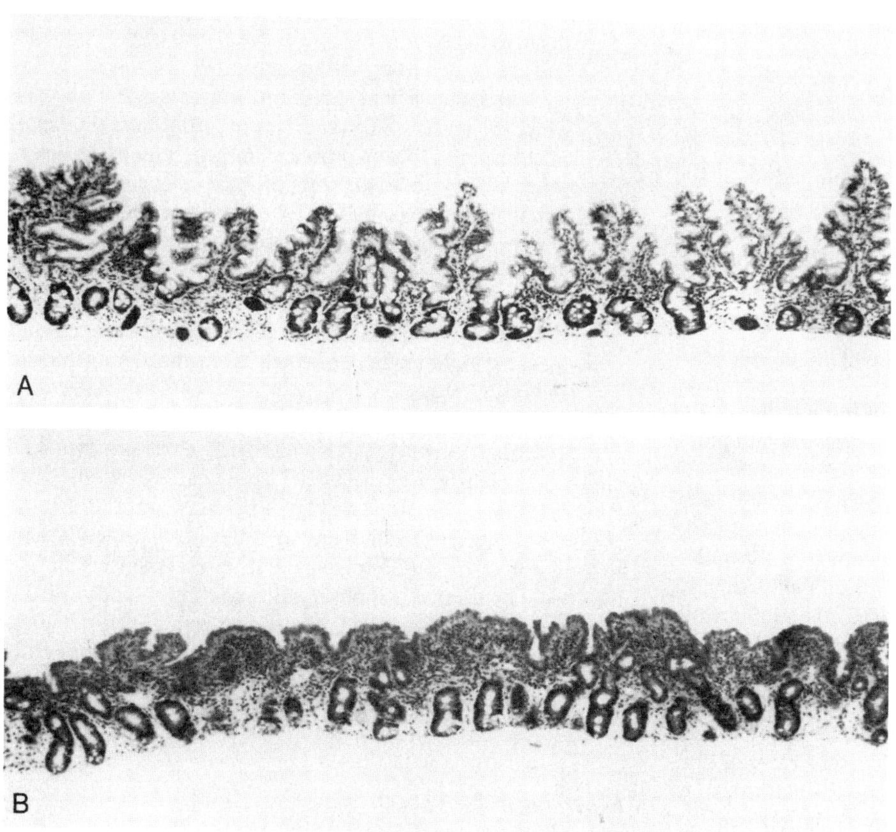

FIGURE 6 Light microscopy. Villous atrophy without marked crypt hyperplasia. *A*, Mild enteropathy (female, 1 year 7 months, cows' milk protein intolerance). *B*, Moderate enteropathy (male, 11 months, cows' milk protein intolerance) (×75 for both).

(the term used by some authors of this text) to describe a flat mucosa. In fact, the mucosa described as either "total" or "subtotal villous atrophy" is not a truly atrophic mucosa, i.e., not thinner than normal.

Many parameters of mucosal structure may be appreciated on light microscopy. However, classification of the appearance has, in the main, continued to center on villous height and crypt depth.

Currently, most pathologists avoid the terms referred to above and use the term "crypt hyperplastic villous atrophy" to describe lesions in which villi are shortened and crypts are lengthened. This is the most frequently observed abnormality of the small intestinal mucosa. When villous height and crypt depth are approximately equal, this is termed a mild or minor abnormality (Fig. 4B); a moderate abnormality involves crypt depth greater than villous height (Fig. 4C); and a flat mucosa (Fig. 4D) is a severe abnormality. Just as observed under the dissecting microscope, a patchy histologic abnormality may be seen, i.e., a patchy enteropathy (Fig. 5).

It should be recognized that it is possible to find villous atrophy without marked crypt hyperplasia. This may be referred to as crypt hypoplastic villous atrophy; however, crypt dimensions are normal. Thus, a more accurate description would be "crypt normoplastic villous atrophy." This produces a thin mucosa, and lesions of variable severity are seen (Fig. 6). It is also possible to see villous hyperplasia with crypt hyperplasia.[14]

It is important to study other aspects of the mucosa as well as villous height and crypt depth, as these can give specific diagnoses. These include the following:

1. Looking for the presence of luminal, surface-attached, and intramucosal organisms (e.g., *G. lamblia, Cryptosporidium*, and enteropathogenic *E. coli*).
2. Assessing the state of the epithelium, in particular the enterocyte, e.g., cell height and degree of vacuolation. The latter finding can indicate abeta- and hypobetalipoproteinemia if extensive vacuolation of villous epithelium is seen in an otherwise normal mucosa. But it should not be confused with the lesser degree of vacuolation seen in celiac disease and the postenteritis syndrome.
3. Noting the presence and number of intraepithelial and other epithelial cells, i.e., lymphocytes, eosinophils, neutrophils, mast cells, and goblet cells.

   Counting the number of lymphocytes within the small intestinal epithelium is of great value for routine diagnostic use.[15] It is used to make a count of the lymphocytes within the villous epithelium, i.e., measuring the intraepithelial lymphocyte count (IEL) per 100 villous epithelial cells. These lymphocytes are intercellular—i.e., they lie between the enterocytes—but are intraepithelial, since they occur within the surface epithelium. Phillips and his colleagues[16] found a mean of 23.4 IEL per 100 villous epithelial cells in a group of children on a normal diet who had normal small intestinal mucosae. There was no significant variation with age in the children studied, and the value is similar to the mean level of 21.1 described in 40 adults.[17] Marsh[18] has pointed out that different results are found when absolute lymphocyte numbers are counted. An IEL count in fact represents the density of the IELs within the epithelium.

   Significantly raised counts of IEL are characteristically found in the small intestinal mucosa of untreated celiac disease both in children and in adults and also in the mucosa of untreated dermatitis herpetiformis in adults. Increased levels have also been reported in tropical sprue, in some children with giardiasis, and in some with unexplained diarrhea and failure to thrive,[15] as well as in some children with cow's milk–sensitive enteropathy.[16]

   The IEL count falls to the normal range after introduction of a gluten-free diet in children with celiac disease. It has been shown that the increase found in the flat mucosa of celiac disease reflects reduction in surface area.[18] However, when IEL counts are related to surface area in children with a flat mucosa due to celiac disease but to other causes as well, it is clear that there is no consistent relationship between the reduction in surface area and the IEL count. Furthermore, there may be localized or patchy areas of increased IELs, which argues against the level merely reflecting reduced surface area per se.
4. Studying the lamina propria for degree and nature of the cellular infiltrate and the appearance of lacteals. Using monoclonal antibodies, it is possible to investigate the T-cell receptors on lymphocytes in the mucosa.
5. Performing a PAS stain to allow the preservation of the brush border to be visualized. The presence of PAS-positive material in the apical cytoplasm of the epithelial cells indicates microvillous atrophy[19]; PAS-positive inspissated mucus in crypt lumina suggests cystic fibrosis.
6. Mucosal mast cells in the lamina propria of the small intestine may be quantitated and their density determined. There are two sorts of mast cells: mucosal and connective tissue mast cells. The latter are present in the lamina propria and are best studied using Carnoy's solution as fixative[20,21] and chloroacetoesterase reaction for staining so that they can be clearly seen.[22] Using this technique, Sanderson et al have demonstrated that there is higher mast cell density in the ileum than in the colon.[23]

Histologic Normality. Knowledge of what is normal in children is clearly difficult to determine. It is obviously not ethical to biopsy healthy children, but observation of morphology of biopsies taken from (1) children suspected of having gastrointestinal (GI) disease but whose biopsies in fact turn out to be normal, (2) observation of control biopsies from children with celiac disease in remission on a gluten-free diet, and (3) postmortem studies of the small intestine from children dying without evidence of GI disease, does allow some knowledge of "normal" small intestinal mucosal morphology to be acquired (Fig. 4*A*).

Electron Microscopy

Transmission electron microscopy (TEM) and scanning electron microscopy (SEM) have been used to study the morphology of small intestinal biopsies taken from children as

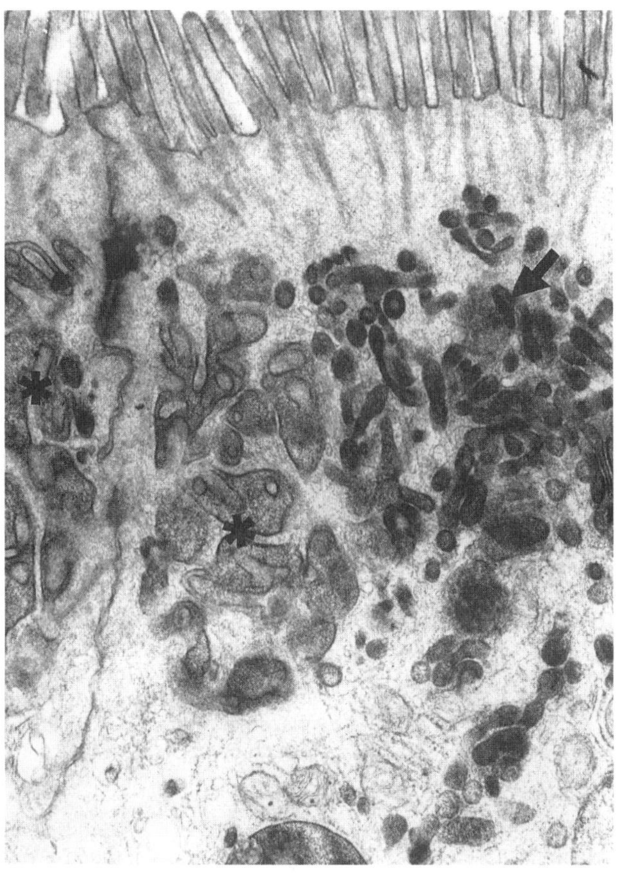

FIGURE 7 Electron microscopy. Microvillous atrophy (female, 14 months). Increased presence of secretory granules (*arrow*) with membranous inclusions containing microvillus-like projections (*asterisk*) (×40,000).

well as adults. Certain differences in morphology in children have been found.[24] Ultrastructural studies are now routine in cases of chronic diarrhea. Disorders such as microvillous atrophy[19] (Fig. 7), attaching and effacing *E. coli*[25] (Fig. 8), and cryptosporidiosis[26] (Fig. 9) are diagnostic possibilities. Small intestinal biopsies from patients with AIDS should also be studied by electron microscopy, as many infectious agents are beyond the resolution of the light microscope, e.g., microsporidiosis.

Biochemistry

A mucosal sample should be taken and frozen for biochemical studies in cases in which primary or secondary disaccharidase deficiencies are possible. Although it is possible to assess enzyme levels on histochemistry of frozen tissue sections or on duodenal juice, the usual practice is to analyze tissue homogenates.[27,28] Other techniques are possible and may be required to diagnose rare disorders such as glucose-galactose malabsorption and defective proton transport.

The Role of Small Intestinal Biopsy in Diagnosis

At present, a single small intestinal biopsy has two specific roles that are of value in making a diagnosis in clinical pediatrics. The first is to demonstrate the presence of a proximal small intestinal enteropathy. Enteropathy may be defined as an abnormality of the small intestinal mucosa which can be demonstrated with the light microscope. The second is to provide a piece of small intestinal mucosa for enzyme assay in order to diagnose a specific enzyme deficiency.

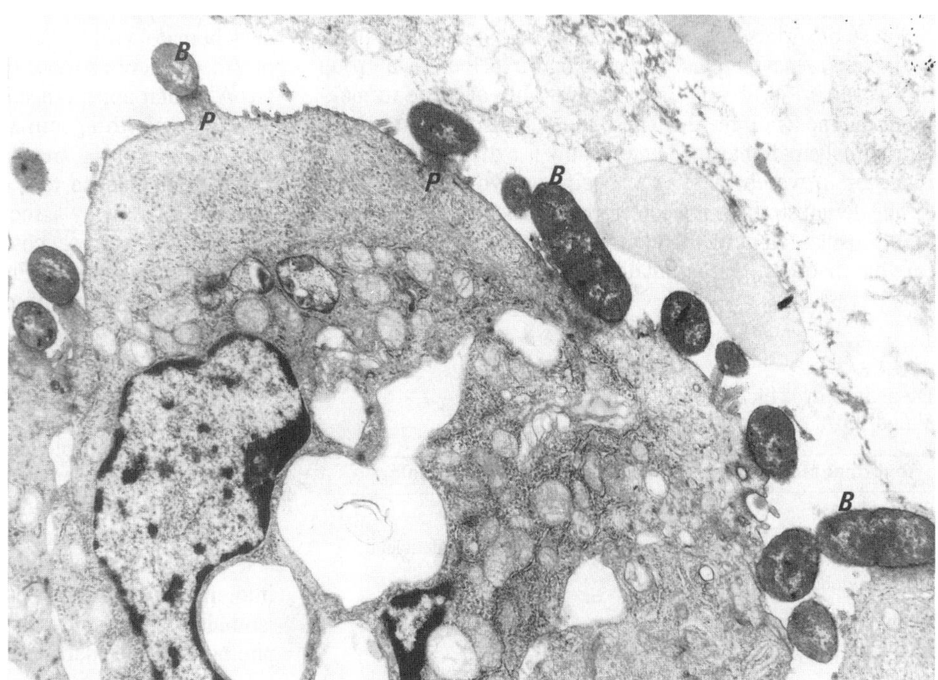

FIGURE 8 Electron microscopy. Enteropathogenic *Escherichia coli* enteritis (male, 8 months) *E. coli* 0128 (B) attached to apical surface of epithelium in association with microvillous effacement and pedestal formation (P) (×18,000).

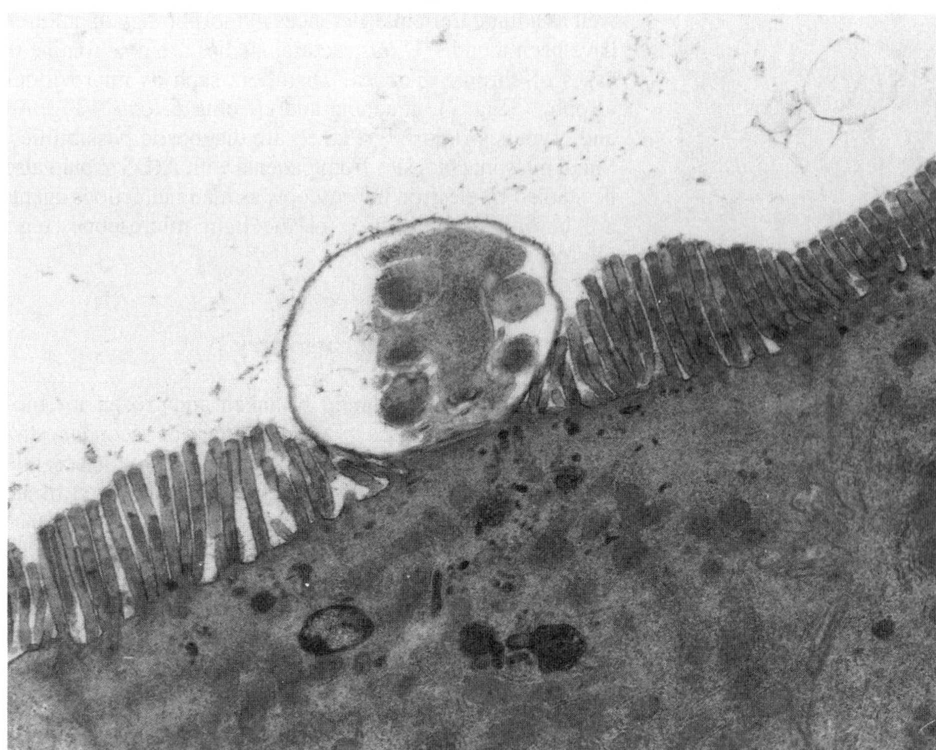

FIGURE 9 Electron microscopy. Cryptosporidiosis (male, 13 months). Cryptosporidial schizont adhering to the epithelial surface. Note displacement of microvilli at site of attachment (×18,000).

It is clear that two or more biopsies over a period of time, that is, serial small intestinal biopsies related to dietary change (i.e., elimination and challenge), are sometimes required before a final diagnosis can be made. Classic examples of this approach are provided by celiac disease and cow's milk–sensitive enteropathy. The use of serial biopsy in this way, initially a research procedure, has now become routine. It enables a specific diagnosis to be made that is not at present possible by any other means.

Those disorders in which small intestinal biopsy has a role in diagnosis may be placed in groups. First, there is a group of disorders for which biopsy is invariably of value in making a diagnosis (Table 2). These include disorders in which a proximal small intestinal enteropathy is a diagnostic prerequisite or in which there is a specific enzyme deficiency.

The demonstration of an enteropathy is an absolute requirement for the diagnosis of celiac disease, but it is not specific for this disorder. A flat small intestinal mucosa is characteristic of celiac disease, but there are other causes of a flat mucosa in childhood, and on occasion lesser degrees of mucosal abnormality may be found in children who do have celiac disease.

TABLE 2
Disorders in Which Biopsy Is Invariably Valuable

Abnormal Morphology	Normal Morphology
Celiac disease	Congenital alactasia
Abetalipoproteinemia	Sucrase-isomaltase deficiency
Agammaglobulinemia	
Autoimmune enteropathy	
Microvillous atrophy	

The enterocyte in abetalipoproteinemia cannot synthesize betalipoprotein and, as a result, chylomicron formation is impaired. Thus, absorbed dietary fat is not properly mobilized from the enterocyte. As a result the cytoplasm of those cells lining the upper half of the villi appears vacuolated in ordinary hematoxylin and eosin sections. By using special stains on frozen sections these cells can be shown to be filled with fat. A similar appearance is seen in hypobetalipoproteinemia.

Children with agammaglobulinemia lack plasma cells in the lamina propria, but the mucosal architecture may range from a flat mucosa to a completely normal one.

In the enteropathy associated with multisystem autoimmune disease and the presence of circulating autoantibodies (autoimmune enteropathy) (Fig. 10), the mucosa is severely abnormal at the time of diagnosis, sometimes with a flat mucosa. The demonstration of an enteropathy in the presence of circulating autoantibodies against the enterocyte in a child who has chronic diarrhea is essential for diagnosis of this syndrome.

Microvillous atrophy can be diagnosed only by the demonstration of the characteristic microvillous involutions and an increase in secretory granules on electron microscopy of a small or large intestinal mucosal biopsy.[19]

Children who have either of the two primary disaccharide intolerances, namely congenital alactasia and sucrase-isomaltase deficiency, have a normal small intestinal morphology, but the characteristic enzyme deficiencies are present on disaccharidase assay.

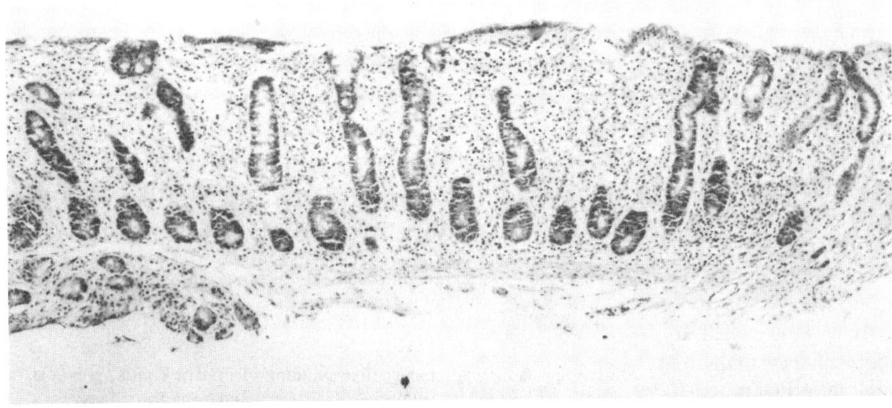

FIGURE 10 Light microscopy. Autoimmune enteropathy (male, 14 months), severe enteropathy (×120). (From Pediatr Gastroenterol Nutr 1982; 1:503–515.)

Second, when the lesion is nonuniform, i.e., patchy, or when there is penetration of the mucosa by a parasite, biopsy may provide a specific diagnosis, but in this group of disorders the absence of abnormality (i.e., a normal mucosa) does not exclude the diagnosis (Table 3). It is possible in parasitic and "attaching-effacing" *E. coli* infections that a more distal site of the intestine is affected, and the diagnosis is made on stool microbiology.

The trophozoite of *G. lamblia* is often found in the duodenal juice of children with giardiasis but may also be found on section of small intestinal biopsy specimens. Similarly, in children with strongyloidiasis, larvae of *Strongyloides stercoralis* may be found in juice and on section of the mucosal biopsy specimens. Cryptosporidial schizonts may just be visible by light microscopy, but the characteristic morphology is readily identifiable by electron microscopy. Similarly, electron microscopy is required to show the microvillous loss and pedestal formation typical of enteropathogenic *E. coli* infections[25] (see Fig. 8).

Small intestinal lymphangiectasia may be diagnosed by biopsy of the small intestinal mucosa, but as the lesion is often patchy it can be missed on a single biopsy and multiple biopsies may be indicated.

Rarely, small intestinal lymphoma may be diagnosed by biopsy if the lesion has invaded the mucosa.

Children with hypogammaglobulinemia may be found to have hyperplastic lymphoid follicles on small intestinal biopsy as well as a diminished number of plasma cells and variable morphologic abnormalities. *G. lamblia* is often found in the duodenal juice of such children.

TABLE 3
Disorders in Which Biopsy May or May Not Be of Specific Diagnostic Value

Giardiasis
Strongyloidiasis
Small intestinal lymphangiectasia
Small intestinal lymphoma
Hypogammaglobulinemia
Enteroadherent *Escherichia coli*

TABLE 4
Disorders in Which Biopsy May Be Abnormal but Abnormality Is Nonspecific

Postenteritis syndrome
Cows' milk protein intolerance
Transient gluten intolerance
Soy protein intolerance
Intractable diarrhea syndrome
Tropical sprue
Radiation enteritis
Drug-induced lesions, e.g., by methotrexate
Protein-energy malnutrition
AIDS

Third, in another group of disorders, in which the lesion may also be patchy, the demonstration of an enteropathy is nonspecific (Table 4). However, the finding of mucosal abnormality is diagnostically useful in such patients because it indicates the presence of pathology in the small intestine. Some disorders in this group, e.g., cows' milk–sensitive enteropathy, may be diagnosed by serial biopsy related to dietary protein withdrawal and challenge, although there is no specific

TABLE 5
Disorders in Which Biopsy Is Normal

Cirrhosis
Hepatitis
Exocrine pancreatic insufficiency
Toddler's diarrhea

pathology for this disorder. To the list of nonspecific abnormalities must now be added acquired immunodeficiency syndrome (AIDS).

Finally, for completeness, a group of disorders in which small intestinal biopsy is characteristically normal is listed in Table 5.

To conclude this section on the role of small intestinal biopsy in diagnosis, it is important briefly to review the diagnostic approach to a child suspected of having small intestinal disease. This is summarized in Table 6. The emphasis is not so much upon demonstrating malabsorption, e.g., steatorrhoea or xylose malabsorption, as formerly was the case, but upon pinpointing an anatomic abnormality of the small intestine, a structural abnormality of the small intestinal mucosa (i.e., an enteropathy), or a specific infectious etiologic agent. Thus barium studies, small intestinal biopsy, and stool examination are particularly important investigations. Hematologic investigations, such as a full blood count and serum folate, can provide important evidence of a deficiency state that may need to be treated immediately or followed up as a marker of response to treatment. Radiologic studies are particularly important for diagnosing Crohn's disease and congenital anatomic lesions of the small intestine.

LARGE INTESTINAL BIOPSY

From its introduction in the early 1960s, the value of fiberoptic colonoscopy as a diagnostic procedure in adult patients has become well established. It is now clear that this is a very useful technique in pediatric practice as well. In fact, the most useful aspect of fiberoptic colonoscopy is the provision of multiple colonic biopsies. It is also possible in the hands of an expert endoscopist to enter the ileum in a high percentage of cases. In one series,[29] the terminal ileum was entered in 75.3 percent of cases. This then affords an opportunity to study ileal histology as well as colonic histology. The availability of pediatric colonoscopy is restricted to pediatric gastroenterologic centers and is dependent upon the availability of endoscopy skills. When these are available, this approach has largely overtaken the need for barium enema examination in the investigation of rectal bleeding and suspected chronic inflammatory bowel disease.[30]

The role of colonoscopy when used in this way[29] has been evaluated. The findings at first colonoscopy in 412 children examined were as follows: 239 children (58.0 percent) had abnormal endoscopies. Crohn's disease was diagnosed and confirmed in 118 of the 412 patients (28.6 percent), ulcerative colitis in 62 (15.0 percent), indeterminate colitis in 21 (5.1 percent), polyps in 18 (4.4 percent), and other abnormalities in 20 (4.9 percent). Eighty-six of the 328 positive colonoscopies, i.e., 26.2 percent, revealed abnormalities that would have been beyond the range of flexible sigmoidoscopy. Most of these were patients with ileocecal Crohn's disease, although eight of the 18 (44 percent) patients with polyps would also have remained undiagnosed on limited examination, three (17 percent) of whom had other polyps more proximally. When colonoscopy is not available, rigid sigmoidoscopy must be used to obtain colonic and rectal biopsies.

The principal purpose of obtaining intestinal colonic biopsies in this context is for the diagnosis of chronic inflammatory bowel disease, and Crohn's disease in particular. However, there are other reasons, and Table 7 lists the indications for fiberoptic colonoscopy in children.

Large intestinal biopsy is also used for the diagnosis of Hirschsprung's disease. In recent years mucosal biopsy has replaced full-thickness biopsy. However, full-thickness biopsy still has its place in diagnosis.

TABLE 6
Diagnostic Approach to Child Suspected of Having Small Intestinal Disease

Initial assessment
- Detailed case history
- Physical examination
- Analysis of centile charts for height and weight

Initial investigations
- Full blood count and also erythrocyte sedimentation rate in older child (? Crohn's disease)
- Serum and red cell folate
- Stool culture for bacteria
- Stool electron microscopy for viruses
- Stool examination for *Giardia lamblia* and *Cryptosporidum*
- Stool-reducing substances

Next stage
- Small intestinal biopsy
- Duodenal juice examination for *Giardia lamblia*
- Bacterial culture for bacteria (anaerobic and aerobic [as indicated])
- Barium follow-through
- Gut antibodies
- Response to elimination diet

TABLE 7
Indications for Proceeding to Fiberoptic Colonoscopy in the Pediatric Patient

- Unexplained rectal bleeding
- Bloody diarrhea in the absence of stool pathogens (with or without abdominal pain)
- Abdominal pain associated with weight loss (with or without diarrhea)
- Other features suggesting a diagnosis of chronic inflammatory bowel disease (e.g., strictures, fistulae, disease activity extent as a guide to therapy)
- Surveillance for malignancy (longstanding ulcerative colitis, polyposis coli, Peutz-Jeghers syndrome, Gardner's syndrome)
- Polypectomy

Technique of Colonoscopy

Table 8 outlines the recommended regimen used to prepare the bowel prior to endoscopy. Children should be admitted to hospital 24 hours before the examination and placed

TABLE 8
Standard Bowel Preparation Prior to Colonoscopy

Admit to ward 24 hours prior to procedure—fluid diet only allowed
Senna syrup (Sennokot X-prep)—1ml/kg 18 hours before procedure
Picolax Under 1 year of age—not given Ages 1 to 4 years—¼ package in warm water Ages 4 to 6 years—½ package in warm water Over 6 years of age—1 whole package in warm water
2 doses of Picolax—one 15 hours and the other 3 hours prior to procedure
Phosphate enema given to all infants less than 1 year and if above preparation fails
If child presents with severe diarrhea, give rectal saline wash-outs only

on a diet limited to clear fluids. The standard bowel preparation consists of a single dose of senna syrup (1 ml per kilogram) during the afternoon of the day before colonoscopy, and two doses of a sodium picosulfate/magnesium citrate mixture (Picolax) approximately 15 hours and 3 hours prior to the procedure. Children are instructed to drink copiously to avoid dehydration. Picolax should not be given to infants under 12 months of age. Bowel preparation is considered successful if the patient has clear watery diarrhea by the morning of procedure. If this is not the case, a phosphate enema should be given. Patients with profuse diarrhea should have a modified bowel preparation, some receiving a smaller dose of Picolax and others being given a rectal washout with 0.9 percent saline 30 minutes before the endoscopy.

Endoscopy should be performed routinely under intravenous sedation without the need for general anesthesia. Most younger children may require a premedication of trimeprazine or chlorpromazine some 90 minutes before the procedure. Immediately prior to endoscopy intravenous sedation consisting of diazepam (0.2 mg per kilogram) in the lipid suspension form (Diazemuls, Kabi) and pethidine, 1 to 2 mg/per kilogram, is to be administered by an experienced pediatrician via butterfly needle into a peripheral vein. Further doses of pethidine may be given as required during difficult colonoscopies to provide adequate analgesia. Additional diazepam is not recommended. The dose of intravenous sedation should be titrated against individual patient's requirements. In general, sedation sufficient to allow early and easy insertion of the colonoscope should predict satisfactory tolerance during the remainder of the procedure. Naloxone, 0.01 mg per kilogram, is administered to some patients at the end of the procedure if there is excessive sedation induced by pethidine. Full resuscitation equipment should be available in cases of a respiratory emergency.

Colonoscopy should be performed to the left lateral position in most cases, except in a few young infants in whom supine performance may be easier. Change of position to right lateral may sometimes be useful for improving visualization of the descending colon or passage around the splenic flexure. A variety of fiberoptic colonoscopes may be used. The ones favored in the authors' experience are pediatric instruments—the Olympus PCF 10; in older children, standard adult endoscopes such as the Olympus CFBLB 3 or SCF 1 OL may be used.

Disorders Diagnosed by Large Intestinal Biopsy in Childhood

These disorders may be broadly grouped into inflammatory disorders and motility disorders. The principal features of biopsy diagnosis are outlined. The histologic diagnosis of chronic inflammatory bowel disease in children specifically has been reported by Chong et al.[31]

Inflammatory Disorders

Ulcerative Colitis. This is a chronic intermittent disease that affects the large bowel mucosa. It is possible to make a suggested histopathologic diagnosis from biopsies taken at the initial presentation. Confident biopsy diagnoses can certainly be made in established disease. Sequential biopsies form part of the diagnostic work-up. Ulcerative colitis usually commences in the rectum and may extend to involve the rest of the colon. Both the clinical picture and the histopathology may be considered in terms of three phases: (1) active, (2) resolving, and (3) in remission (quiescent).[32]

Active Phase. The most specific feature is loss of crypt architecture with crypt distortion and branching (Fig. 11). Polymorphonuclear neutrophils are present within the crypt epithelium, and there may be crypt abscesses (Fig. 12). The epithelium shows varying amounts of degeneration and regeneration. There is mucin depletion and increased mitotic activity. The lamina propria shows capillary congestion and edema; it contains a heavy mixed inflammatory cell infiltrate. This is diffuse throughout the lamina propria and is composed of plasma cells, lymphocytes, and neutrophils. Eosinophils are also found and when prominent have been associated with an improved prognosis.[33] Inflammatory cells may also be found in the submucosa; this may be associated with severe ulceration.

Resolving Phase. An important feature of ulcerative colitis is the fact that the biopsy appearances vary with time. In the resolving phase, the crypts remain distorted and branched; the surface may take on a villous appearance. Goblet cells reappear in the crypts but may be elongated. Inflammation in the lamina propria is reduced and may become focal; there is then a possibility of confusion with other disease such as Crohn's disease. There are few polymorphs at this stage.

Remission Phase. Here the crypts are atrophied and distorted. There is a gap between the muscularis mucosae and the crypt bases. Goblet cells are present, but there may be Paneth cell metaplasia and increased numbers of crypt endocrine cells.[34-36] There is no active inflammation; neutrophils are therefore absent.

Inflammatory Polyps (Pseudopolyps). These consist of granulation tissue, a mixture of glands and granulation tissue, or a tag of virtually normal mucosa. They are a frequent

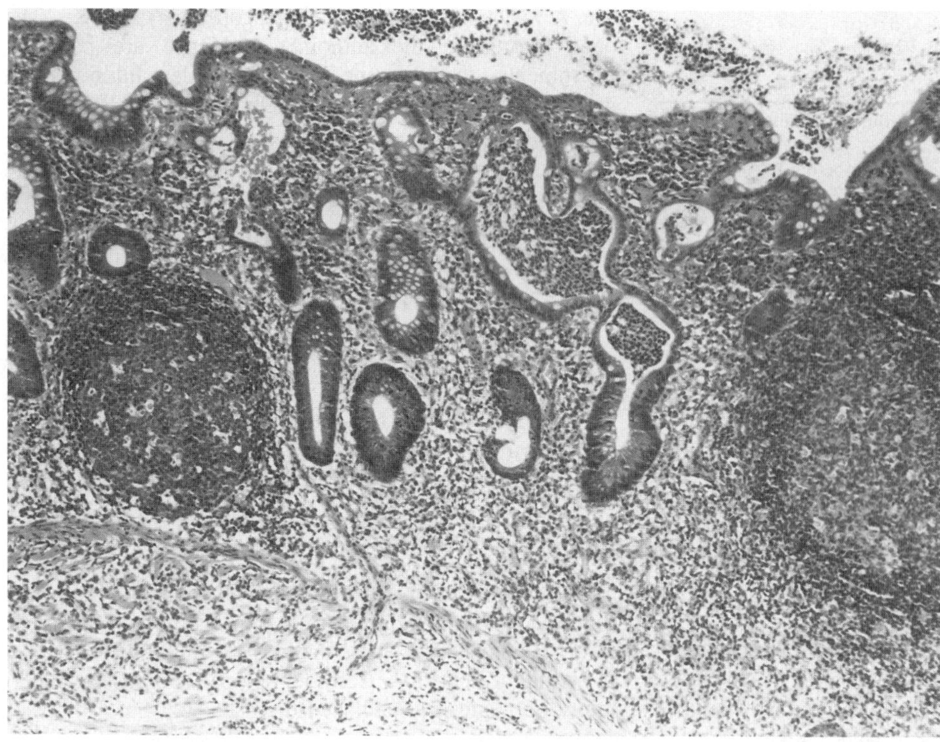

FIGURE 11 Chronic ulcerative colitis, active phase. Crypts are distorted and show mucus depletion; several contain neutrophils resulting in crypt abscesses. There is diffuse inflammation of the mucosa. Lymphoid follicles are also present (hematoxylin and eosin, ×100).

finding and indicate prior severe mucosal ulceration with irregular healing. Biopsy allows them to be distinguished from neoplastic polyps (adenomas).

Fulminant Acute Dilatation. This has been recorded in up to 13 percent of patients with ulcerative colitis.[37,38] The rectum is relatively spared, and the transverse colon is most severely affected. There are several misleading features in biopsies in this condition: Inflammation may be transmural and there may be fissuring ulceration, the crypt architecture is often intact, and inflammation may be mild.

Follicular Proctitis. Prominent lymphoid follicles are present, and there is an accompanying diffuse infiltrate of

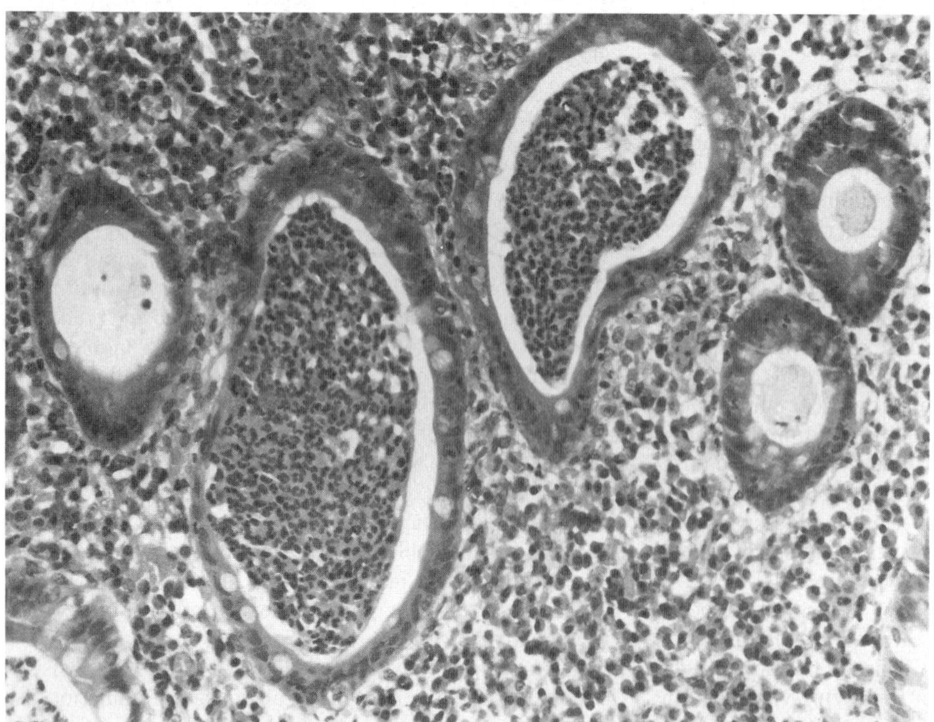

FIGURE 12 Chronic ulcerative colitis, active phase. High-power view showing crypt distortion, mucus depletion, and crypt abscesses. There is diffuse inflammation in the lamina propria (hematoxylin and eosin, ×250).

plasma cells and neutrophils. These features cause thickening of the mucosa. The crypt architecture is irregular. The differential diagnosis in this condition includes lymphoid polyps, malignant lymphoma, and lymphomatous polyposis.

Crohn's Disease

Crohn's disease may affect any part of the GI tract,[39,40] but most commonly it presents as regional ileitis,[41] ileocolitis, colitis, or perianal disease. It is characterized by its focal distribution and, unlike ulcerative colitis, it often involves the full thickness of the bowel wall. The endoscopic appearances form an important part of the diagnosis in Crohn's disease. The features include tiny aphthoid ulcers,[42] serpiginous ulceration, edema, linear ulceration ("cobblestoning"),[43,44] and inflammatory polyps. Areas of normal mucosa appear between abnormal areas, which are thus termed "skip lesions." Anal lesions consist of painless fissures, ulcers, fistulae, skin tags, and perianal abscesses.

The crypt architecture and goblet cell population are usually preserved despite considerable inflammation (Fig. 13).[45,46] However, there may be some crypt distortion close to areas of ulceration; such distortion may also occur in the early healing phase.[47] The inflammatory cell component consists of a mixture of lymphocytes, plasma cells, and polymorphs; their density varies across the biopsy.[48] Neutrophils are less conspicuous than in ulcerative colitis or infectious colitis, but crypt abscesses may be found.[49] Small aggregates of lymphocytes occur adjacent to crypt bases.[50] Granulomas are also found; these are composed of collections of epithelioid histocytes, Langerhans giant cells, and a cuff of lymphocytes (Fig. 14).

Granulomas occur throughout the bowel wall in Crohn's disease and may be seen both in inflamed mucosa and in endoscopically normal mucosa.[31,51] Microgranulomas consisting of clusters of histocytes and small numbers of inflammatory cells also occur.[51] Confluent granulomas with florid central necrosis suggest a diagnosis of tuberculosis; however, a small focus of central necrosis may be seen in granulomas in Crohn's disease.

The incidence of granulomas in biopsies is variable, and published figures in adults range from 0 to nearly 30 percent.[51-54] In a series of 104 endoscopic biopsies from children with Crohn's disease,[31] epithelioid granulomas were present in 21 (36 percent). This is clearly an underestimate and is a question of sampling, as in an analysis of 17 operative specimens from children with Crohn's disease 14 had noncaseating granulomas (82 percent) (Fig. 14).

Other features of biopsies in Crohn's disease include aphthoid ulcers; these are seen as small areas of ulceration immediately over a lymphoid follicle.[50] Fissuring ulcers also occur; they penetrate down through the submucosa and are characteristic of Crohn's disease.

Biopsies in Crohn's disease should include at least the superficial half of the submucosa: this will often show "disproportionate inflammation"[47] with a mixed inflammatory cell infiltrate. This reflects the transmural nature of the inflammatory process in the disease. Granulomas in the submucosa are helpful in the diagnosis. The following features are considered to be the most helpful in the diagnosis of Crohn's disease when granulomas are absent: the patchy na-

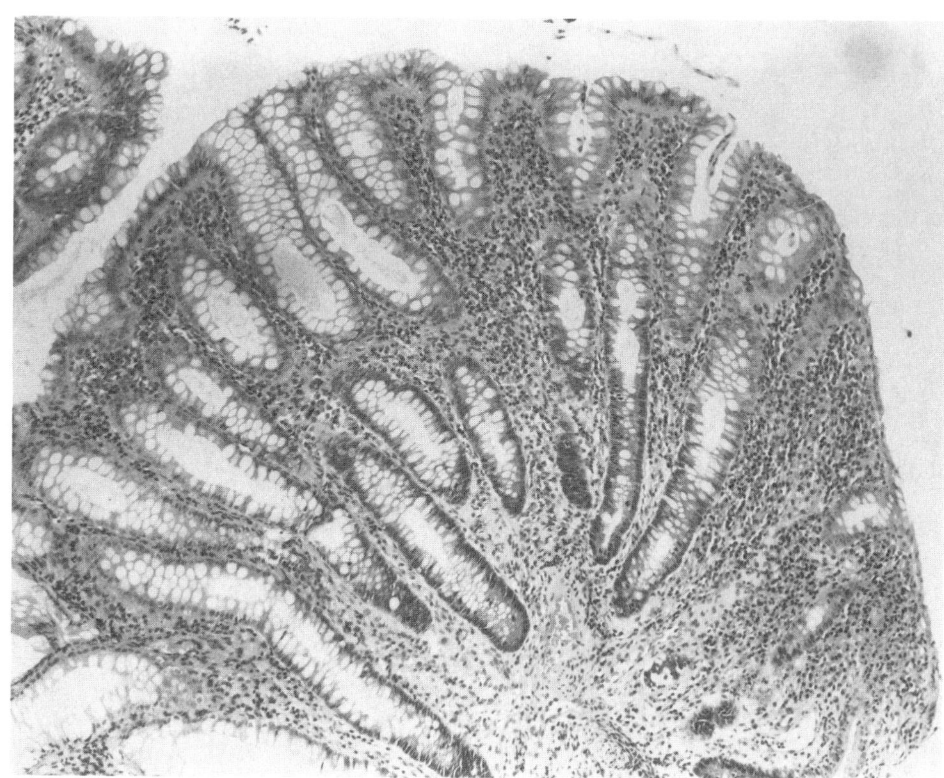

FIGURE 13 Rectal biopsy in Crohn's disease. There is chronic inflammation in the lamina propria, but crypt architecture is well preserved (hematoxylin and eosin, ×100).

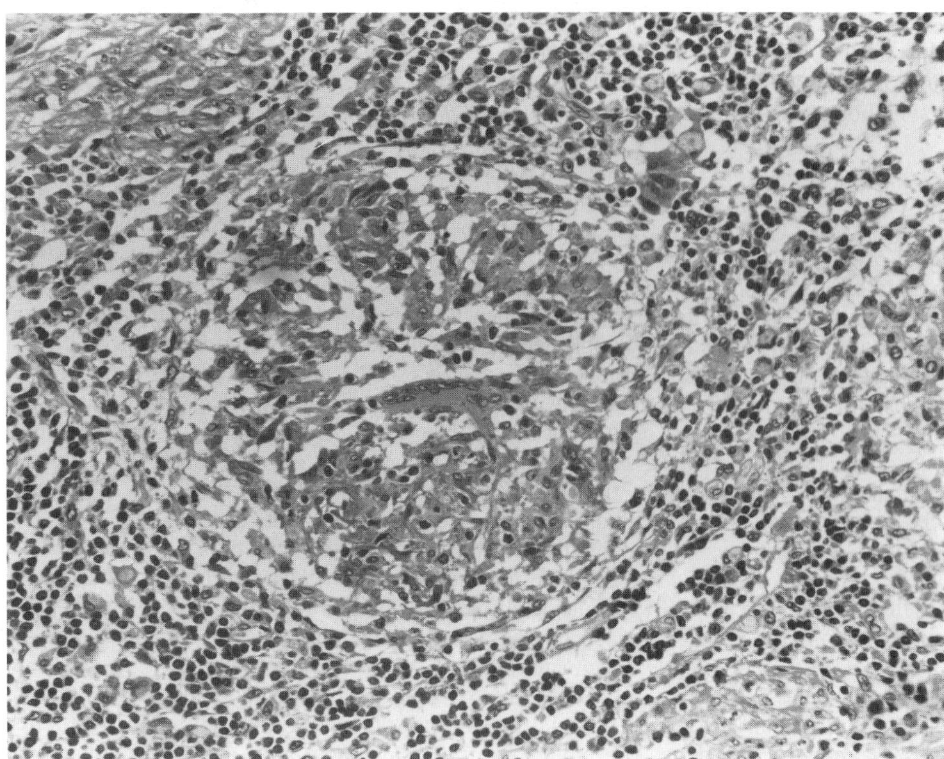

FIGURE 14 Crohn's disease. A noncaseating granuloma in the submucosa (hematoxylin and eosin, ×250).

ture of the inflammation; relatively little crypt distortion or goblet cell depletion; the presence of basal lymphoid aggregates. Unfortunately, aphthoid ulceration and fissure are rare in biopsies.

No studies have yet been able to correlate specific features with disease activity.[55] As already mentioned, granulomas may occur in normal-appearing mucosa. Fibrosis in the submucosa and splitting up of the muscularis mucosae indicate longstanding disease. Granulomas have been claimed to indicate a favorable prognosis,[56,57] but not all studies are in greement with this.[58,59] Ulceration and fissuring have been claimed to be indicative of a poor prognosis.[60] Overall, there appears to be no universally accepted prognostic microscopic feature.[47]

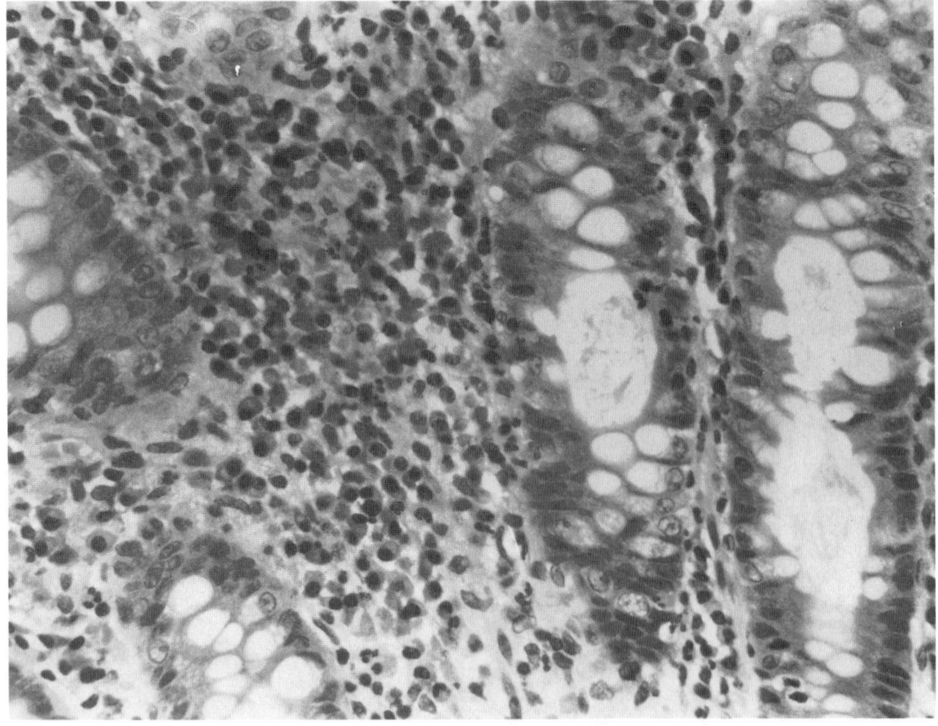

FIGURE 15 Infective colitis (*Campylobacter*). High-power view of a rectal biopsy showing patchy inflammation with neutrophil polymorphs in the lamina propria. One crypt is infiltrated by neutrophils (hematoxylin and eosin, ×400).

Infective Colitis

Infective colitis may be classified etiologically into bacterial, viral, protozoal, and fungal infections and infestations by helminths. The bacterial diarrheas cause the vast majority of diagnostic problems. *Salmonella* species, *Shigella* species, enteroinvasive *E. coli* and *Campylobacter* species may all produce similar histopathologic appearances, which have been termed "infective" biopsy pattern (Fig. 15). It is important to be familiar with these histologic features so that patients with infectious disease are not mislabeled as having ulcerative colitis or Crohn's disease.

It is not usually possible from a biopsy to distinguish among the main causes of bacterial colitis.

Examination of the biopsy specimen indicates that the mucosa is widened by edema. Clusters of polymorphs are present throughout the biopsy, often adjacent to dilated capillaries or next to crypts. Polymorphs may be present between the crypt epithelial cells, and, although crypt abscesses occur, they are less common than in active ulcerative colitis or Crohn's disease.[61] Clusters or polymorphs also infiltrate between the cells of the surface epithelium. Although plasma cells and lymphocytes may be increased, this is often masked by edema and polymorphonuclear neutrophils dominate the picture (Fig. 15).

The crypt pattern is regular, although the superficial crypt epithelium may show degenerative changes and there is dilatation of luminal parts of the crypt (crypt "withering").[62,63] Mucin depletion and flattening of epithelial cells are also seen. Crypt destruction may be marked by a multinucleate giant cell. Other, less specific, abnormalities include luminal pus, margination of polymorphs, and capillary microthrombi.[64]

The above description represents a characteristic pattern and is most common in biopsies taken at the onset of symptoms or within the first 7 days.[62]

The Differential Diagnosis of the Major Inflammatory Bowel Disease Entities

No single specific histologic feature is invariably present in one condition or absent from the others. The concept of a spectrum of histologic appearances in chronic inflammatory bowel disease in childhood is useful and convenient for practical assessment.[31] This is particularly true in the early histologic appearance of children with Crohn's disease when the definitive criteria may not be present. From the point of view of histologic assessment, particularly of mucosal biopsies, which are small in size, the histopathologist is faced with an apparent range of inflammatory changes falling within a continuous spectrum. This approach is not intended to imply that inflammatory bowel disease is genuinely a continuous spectrum of a single disease. It reflects only the difficulty of making a confident diagnosis by extrapolation from a very restricted sample of the organ in question.

Key features of the various disorders are the following:

Ulcerative Colitis. There is crypt distortion, villous surface, goblet cell depletion, prominent crypt abscesses, diffuse predominantly plasma cell infiltrate of the lamina propria.

Crohn's Disease. Granulomas (25 to 28 percent of biopsies) are present. Crypts remain well aligned with little mucin depletion despite a moderate inflammatory cell infiltrate. The infiltrate is often patchy. Basal lymphoid aggregates are helpful. Crypt abscesses and cryptitis are less constant than in ulcerative or infective colitis. There are microganulomas (focal collections of inflammatory cells including histocytes) and definite patchy inflammation.

Infective Colitis. Crypts remain aligned but show degeneration. Polymorphs are the most conspicuous inflammatory cells; they cluster in the lamina propria and migrate between crypt epithelial cells. Plasma cell infiltrate is light to moderate. Edema is prominent.

Nonspecific Minor Abnormalities

The most common abnormality under this heading is a cellular infiltrate in the lamina propria with regular crypt architecture and variable goblet cell depletion. In some biopsies, a focal polymorph infiltrate in the lamina propria may be seen. A mild increase in plasma cells and lymphocytes may be an accompanying feature. The changes can be interpreted only after consideration of the clinical data; e.g., Crohn's disease may be suggested if there is evidence of disease at another site.[47] Some specific features that can easily be overlooked include the following:

1. Microgranulomas in Crohn's disease.
2. Spirochetosis. This represents infection of colorectal epithelium by spirochetes that belong to the genus *Borrelia*. Histologically, this is seen as a basophilic fringe along the apical border of surface epithelial cells. It is not clear whether infection produces symptoms.
3. Amebae. *Entamoeba histolytica* may cause large intestinal infection, which may closely resemble chronic inflammatory bowel disease in childhood.[65] Ulcers occur which may result in perforation of the bowel wall. Amebae are found on or just beneath the surface of ulcers, but in severe cases they enter the inflamed bowel wall and may be seen within blood vessels. Diastase-PAS is a useful staining method for demonstrating them in histologic preparations.
4. Cytomegalovirus. This viral infection may occur in immunosuppressed children both in disease states such as AIDS and following renal transplantation. Inclusions occur in endothelial cells, fibroblasts, and macrophages. More rarely, they are found in epithelial cells.
5. Chronic granulomatous disease. This rare disorder is characterized by recurrent infections with catalase-positive organisms; the patients' neutrophils are unable to kill the organisms. GI involvement is well recognized; there may be narrowing of the gastric antrum due to local granulomas; perianal fistulae may occur; rectal biopsy may show granulomas and lipid-laden histiocytes. Clinically, the disease may mimic Crohn's disease or tuberculosis, especially when there is ileal involvement with intestinal obstruction.[66,67]
6. Indeterminate colitis. This diagnosis is made when endoscopy shows erythema and sometimes ulceration. However, the histologic picture shows features suggestive of both ulcerative colitis and Crohn's disease. This is regarded as a provisional diagnosis or "holding category." In a recent study of 104 children, 15 were labeled as having indeterminate colitis.[31] In a study of the outcome of 18 children in whom this diagnosis was

made with a follow-up of 0.6 to 10 years, six were well and apparently disease free, three had developed histologically proven Crohn's disease, one had chronic granulomatous disease, and seven still had evidence of active but indeterminate colitis.

Disorders of Motility

Three categories of abnormality are recognized under the term *neuronal dysplasia*.[68] Any of these may present with a Hirschsprung's-like syndrome: (1) aganglionosis (Hirschsprung's disease), (2) hypoganglionosis, and (3) hyperganglionosis.[69]

Normal Innervation

The submucosa and wall of the rectum are normally deficient in ganglia for a distance of up to 1 cm above the dentate line, the hypoganglionic zone.[70] In this zone there are reduced numbers of submucosal ganglia; a small mucosal biopsy often appears to be aganglionic. The myenteric plexus in this zone shows few ganglion cells but prominent nerve bundles.

Above this level, there are submucosal ganglia situated immediately beneath the muscularis mucosae and, more sparsely, immediately superficial to the circular muscle coat. Small, inconspicuous nerve bundles are scattered through the submucosa. Sparse, fine nerve fibers are present in the muscularis mucosae and lamina propria. They may be detected by acetylcholinesterase histochemical staining.

Full-thickness biopsies from above the hypoganglionic zone contain the myenteric plexus (Auerbach), which lies between the circular and longitudinal muscle layers. Acetylcholinesterase staining reveals fine nerve fibers passing between the muscle cells, vertically in the circular muscle coat and horizontally in the longitudinal muscle coat.

Technical Considerations

Hematoxylin and eosin staining can be used to detect the more obvious abnormalities. Acetylcholinesterase histochemistry is the most useful stain for diagnostic purposes.[70] Nonspecific esterase histochemistry is rapid and may be used for preoperative guidance for the surgeon in citing a colostomy. Immunohistochemical methods have been studied but are not widely used yet.

The diagnostic biopsy must be high enough to be clear of the hypoganglionic zone but low enough to avoid missing a short segment abnormality. The initial biopsy may be mucosal; it requires a special stain: acetylcholinesterase. Therefore the biopsy must be fresh when received in the laboratory. For operative biopsies, a rapid nonspecific esterase technique and toluidine blue staining can be used to identify nerves and ganglia. Full-thickness biopsies are required.

Neuronal Dysplasias

Aganglionosis. Ganglia are absent from both submucosal and myenteric plexuses in the affected bowel segment. Eighty percent of cases are confined to the rectum or rectum and sigmoid colon.

Coarse, irregular acetylcholinesterase-positive nerve fibers are seen in the muscularis mucosae and in the lamina propria. Irregular large submucosal nerve bundles are also present.[47] If there is doubt about a mucosal biopsy, full-thickness biopsies must be examined. Acetylcholinesterase staining reveals irregular, coarse nerve fibers in the circular muscle coat as well as between smooth muscle cells.

A zone of hypoganglionosis is found immediately above the affected segment. There is frequent hyperplasia of myenteric ganglia and nerves more proximally, and this may extend for a considerable distance along the colon. This must be distinguished from hyperganglionosis A, in which there is also an increase in numbers and thickness of acetycholinesterase-positive nerve fibers between muscle cells.

Hypoganglionosis. Ganglion cells may be reduced to one-tenth of their normal numbers. This may be the cause of constipation with overflow incontinence. The diagnosis is difficult using hematoxylin and eosin–stained mucosal biopsies; if hypoganglionosis is suspected, full-thickness biopsies should be performed to delineate the extent of the abnormality and also to avoid confusion with a zone of hypoganglionosis adjacent to an aganglionic segment.

Acetylcholinesterase histochemistry shows a few scattered myenteric ganglion cells and prominent nerve trunks. There is a reduction in the fine intramuscular nerve fibers in both the muscularis mucosae and muscularis propria.

Hyperganglionosis ("Neuronal Colonic Dysplasia").[70,71] This condition causes constipation and may present after the age of 6 months. Abnormally large and numerous ganglia and ganglioneuroma-like structures are present in the submucosal and myenteric plexus sites. Smooth muscle fibers may occur in the lamina propria of the mucosa. Full-thickness biopsies (multiple) should be examined.

REFERENCES

1. Sakula J, Shiner M. Coeliac disease with atrophy of the small intestine mucosa. Lancet 1957; ii:876.
2. Crosby WH, Kugler HW. Intraluminal biopsy of the small intestine; the intestinal biopsy capsule. Am J Dig Dis 1957; 2:236.
3. Read AE, Gough KR, Bones JA, McCarthy CF. An improvement to Crosby peroral intestinal capsule. Lancet 1962; i:894.
4. Kilby A. Paediatric small intestinal biopsy capsule with two ports. Gut 1976; 17:158.
5. Walker-Smith JA. Intramural jejunal haematoma complicating peroral mucosal biopsy. Arch Dis Child 1972; 47:676.
6. Holmes R, Hourhane DO, Booth CC. Dissecting microscope appearances of jejunal biopsy specimens from patients with idiopathic steatorrhoea. Lancet 1961; i:81.
7. Walker-Smith JA. Dissecting microscope appearance of small bowel mucosa in children. Arch Dis Child 1967; 42:626.
8. Rubin CE, Dobbins WO. Peroral biopsy of the small intestine. A review of its diagnostic usefulness. Gastroenterology 1965; 49:676.
9. Walker-Smith JA. Variation of small intestinal morphology with age. Arch Dis Child 1972; 47:80.
10. Walker-Smith JA. Uniformity of dissecting microscope appearances in proximal small intestine. Gut 1972; 13:17.
11. Wright NA, Watson AJ, Morley AR, Appleton DR, Marks JM. Cell kinetics in flat (avillous) mucosa of human small intestine. Gut 1972; 14:701–710.
12. Ferguson A, Maxwell JD, Carr KE. Progressive changes in the small intestinal villous pattern with increasing length of gestation. J Pathol 1969; 99:87.
13. Walker-Smith JA, Reye RDK. Small intestinal morphology in aboriginal children. Austral NZ J Med 1971; 4:477.

14. Lee FD, Toner PG. Biopsy pathology of the small intestine. London: Chapman and Hall, 1980: 53.
15. Ferguson A. Intraepithelial lymphocytes of the small intestine. Gut 1977; 18:921.
16. Phillips AD, Rice SJ, France NE, Walker-Smith JA. Small intestinal lymphocyte levels in cows; milk protein intolerance. Gut 1979; 20:509.
17. Ferguson A, Murray D. Quantitation of intraepithelial lymphocytes in human jejunum. Gut 1971; 12:988.
18. Marsh MN. Studies of intestinal lymphoid tissue: III-quantitative analysis of epithelial lymphocytes in the small intestine of control subjects and of patients with coeliac sprue. Gastroenterology 1980; 79:481–492.
19. Phillips AD, Jenkins P, Raafat F, Walker-Smith JA. Congenital microvillous atrophy specific diagnostic features. Arch Dis Child 1985; 60:730–735.
20. Enerbach L. Mast cell in rat gastrointestinal. Acta Pathol Microbiol Scand 1966; 66:289–302.
21. Strobel S, Miller HPR, Ferguson A. Human intestinal mast cells: evaluation of fixation and staining techniques. J Clin Pathol 1981; 34:851–858.
22. Heder LD. The chloracetoesterase reaction. A useful means of histological diagnosis of haematological disorders from paraffin sections of skin. Am J Dermatopathol 1979; 1:39–42.
23. Sanderson IR, Slavin G, Walker-Smith JA. Density of mucosal mast cells in the lamina propria of the colon and terminal ileum of children. J Clin Pathol 1985; 38:771–773.
24. Phillips AD, France NE, Walker-Smith JA. The structure of the enterocyte in relation to its position on the villus in childhood—an EM study. Histopathology 1979; 3:117–130.
25. Ulshen MH, Rollo JL. Pathogenesis of *Escherichia coli* gastroenteritis in man: another mechanism. N Engl J Med 1980; 302:99–101.
26. Phillips AD, Hunt G, Price E, et al. Cryptosporidium in the postenteritis syndrome. In: Walker-Smith JA, McNeish AS, eds. Diarrhoea and malnutrition in childhood, London: Butterworths, 1986: 82.
27. Dalqvist A. Assay of intestinal disaccharidases. Enzymol Biol Clin 1970; 11:52–56.
28. Phillips AD, Avigad S, Sacks SJ, France NE, Walker-Smith JA. Microvillous surface area in secondary disaccharidase deficiency. Gut 1980; 21:44–48.
29. Evans CM, Lipson AB, Sanderson IR, Walker-Smith JA, Williams CB. Fibreoptic colonoscopy in childhood, 1990: In preparation.
30. Chong SKF, Bartram C, Campbell GA. Chronic inflammatory bowel disease in childhood. Br Med J 1982; 284:1–3.
31. Chong SKF, Blackshaw AJ, Boyle S, Williams CB, Walker-Smith JA. Histological diagnosis of chronic inflammatory bowel disease in childhood. Gut 1985; 26:55–59.
32. Morson BC, Dawson IMP. Gastrointestinal pathology. 2nd ed. Oxford: Blackwell, 1979.
33. Heatly RV, James PD. Eosinophils in the rectal mucosa. A simple method of predicting the outcome of ulcerative proctitis. Gut 1978; 20:787–791.
34. Watson AJ, Roy AD. Paneth cells in the large intestine in ulcerative colitis. J Pathol Bacteriol 1960; 80:309–316.
35. Skinner JM, Whitehead R, Pins J. Argentaffin cells in ulcerative colitis. Gut 1971; 12:636–638.
36. Gledhill A, Enticott ME, Howe S. Variation in the argyrophil cell population of the rectum in ulcerative colitis and adenocarcinoma. J Pathol 1986; 149:287–291.
37. Edwards FC, Truelove SC. The course and prognosis of ulcerative colitis, Parts III and IV. Gut 1964; 5:1–22.
38. Jalan KN, Sinus W, Card WI, Falconer CWA, Bruce J, Crean GP, McManus JPA, Small WP, Smith WP. An experience of ulcerative colitis. 1. Toxic dilatation in 55 cases. Gastroenterology 1969; 57:68–82.
39. Basu MK, Asquith P, Thompson RA, Cooke WT. Oral manifestations of Crohn's disease. Gut 1975; 16:249–254.
40. Dunne WT, Cooke WT, Allan RN. Enzymatic and morphometric evidence for Crohn's disease as a diffuse lesion of the gastrointestinal tract. Gut 1977; 18:290–294.
41. Higgins BC, Allan RN. Crohn's disease of the distal ileum. Gut 1980; 21:933–940.
42. Morson BC. The early histological lesion of Crohn's disease. Proc R Soc Med 1972; 65:71–72.
43. Geboes M, Vantrappen G. The value of colonoscopy in the diagnosis of Crohn's disease. Gastrointest Endosc 1975; 22:18–23.
44. Waye JD. Endoscopy in inflammatory bowel disease. Clin Gastroenterol 1980; 9:297–306.
45. Cook MG, Dixon MF. An analysis of the reliability of detection and diagnostic value of various pathological features in Crohn's disease and ulcerative colitis. Gut 1973; 14:255–262.
46. Yardley JH, Donowitz M. 1977. Colorectal biopsy in inflammatory bowel disease. In: Yardley JH, Morson BC, Abell MR, eds. The gastrointestinal tract. International Academy of Pathology Monograph. Baltimore: Williams & Wilkins, 1977: 50.
47. Talbot IC, Price AB. Biopsy pathology in colerectal disease. London: Chapman and Hall, 1987.
48. Hamilton SR, Bassey HJR, Morson BC. En face histological technique to demonstrate mucosal inflammatory lesions in macroscopically uninvolved colon of Crohn's disease resection specimens. Lab Invest 1980; 42:121.
49. Morson BC. Rectal biopsy in inflammatory bowel disease. New King J Med 1972; 287:1337–1339.
50. McGovern VJ, Goulston SJM. Crohn's disease of the colon. Gut 1968; 9:164–179.
51. Rotterdam H, Korelitz BI, Sommers SC. Microganulomas in grossly normal rectal mucosa in Crohn's disease. Am J Clin Pathol 1977; 67:550–554.
52. Surawicz CM, Meisel JL, Ylvisaker T, Saunders DR, Rubin CE. Rectal biopsy in the diagnosis of Crohn's disease: value of multiple biopsies and serial sectioning. Gastroenterology 1981; 81:66–71.
53. Anderson FH, Bogoch A. Biopsies of the large bowel in regional enteritis. Can Med Assoc J 1968; 98:150–153.
54. Petri M, Poulsen SS, Christensen K, Jamum S. The incidence of granulomas in serial sections of rectal biopsies from patients with Crohn's disease. Acta Pathol Micro Immunol Scand A 1982; 90:145–147.
55. Gomes P, DuBoulay C, Smith CC, Holdstock G. Relationship between disease activity indices and colonoscopic findings in patients with colonic inflammatory disease. Gut 1968; 27:92–95.
56. Glass RG, Baker WNW. Role of the granuloma in recurrent Crohn's disease. Gut 1976; 17:75–77.
57. Chambers TJ, Morson BC. The granuloma in Crohn's disease. Gut 1979; 20:269–274.
58. Wilson JAP, Burkhardt RT, Kumar N, Appleman HD. Relationship of granulomas to clinical parameters in Crohn's disease. Gastroenterology 1980; 78:1292.
59. Wolfson DM, Sachar DB, Cohen A, Goldberg J, Stczynskir J, Greenstein AJ, Glerntim, Jenowitz HD. Granulomas do not affect postoperative recurrence rates in Crohn's disease. Gastroenterology 1982; 83:405–409.
60. Ward M, Webb JN. Rectal biopsy as a prognostic guide in Crohn's disease. J Clin Pathol 1977; 30:126–131.
61. Anand BS, Malhotra V, Bhattachanya SK, Patta P, Datta D, Sen D, Bhattachanja MK, Makherjee PP, Pal SC. Rectal histology in acute bacillary dysentery. Gastroenterology 1986; 90:654–660.
62. Kumar NB, Nostrant JJ, Appleman HD. The histopathologic spectrum of acute self-limited colitis (acute infectious-type colitis). Am J Surg Pathol 1982; 6:523–529.
63. Surawicz CM, Belic L. Rectal biopsy helps to distinguish acute self-limited colitis from idiopathic inflammatory bowel disease. Gastroenterology 1984; 86:104–113.
64. Mathan MM, Mathan VI: Local Schwartzman reaction in the rectal mucosa in acute diarrhoea. J Pathol 1985; 146:179–187.
65. Sanderson IR, Walker-Smith JA. Indigenous amoebiasis: an important differential diagnosis of chronic inflammatory bowel disease. Br Med J 1984; 289:823–824.
66. Issacs D, Wright VM. Shaw DG, Raafat F, Walker-Smith JA. Chronic granulomatous disease mimicking Crohn's disease. J Paediatr Gastroenterol Nutr 1985; 4:498–501.
67. Harris BH, Boles ET. Intestinal lesions in chronic granulomatous disease of childhood. J Pediatr Surg 1973; 8:955.
68. Garrett JR, Howard ER. Myenteric plexes of the hind-gut: developmental abnormalities in humans and experimental studies. In: Development of the autonomic nervous system. (Ciba Found. Symp. 83) London: Pitman Medical, 1981: 236.
69. Meier-Ruge W. Hirschsprung's disease: its aetiology, pathogenesis and differential diagnosis. In: Grundman E, Kirsten WH, eds. Current topics in pathology, Vol 59. Berlin: Springer-Verlag 1974:131.
70. Aldridge RT, Campbell PE. Ganglion cells distribution in the normal rectum and anal canal. A basis for the diagnosis of Hirschsprung's disease by a rectal biopsy. J Pediatr Surg 1968; 3:475–489.
71. Puri P, Lake BD, Nixon HH, Mishalang H, Claireaux AE. Neuronal colonic dysplasia: an unusual association of Hirschsprung's disease. J Pediatr Surg 1977; 12:681–685.

CHAPTER 33

Motility Studies

Brent Scott, M.D.C.M., FRCPC

Motility is a term that, when applied to the gastrointestinal (GI) tract, encompasses two distinct but interdependent phenomena: the movements of the wall of the GI tract and the propulsion of contents through the lumen. The study of GI fluid dynamics, how wall motions generate hydraulic forces and initiate intestinal fluid flow, unifies these concepts and is reviewed elsewhere.[1] The techniques that have been developed to study intestinal motility evaluate wall motion or luminal fluid flow, or in some cases a combination of the two.[2] This chapter reviews these techniques and then focuses on the methodology of infused catheter manometry.

TECHNIQUES FOR THE EVALUATION OF MOTILITY

Radiology

This remains the most widely available and most commonly utilized method of evaluating GI motor function. A variety of procedures, each with its own application, is available and utilizes radiopaque solid markers, radiopaque solutions, radioisotopes, and the nonradiographic imaging technique of ultrasonography. The ingestion of radiopaque solid markers, followed by serial plain films of the abdomen, has been used to assess the rate of gastric emptying of solids, colonic transit, and mouth-to-anus transit time.[3] The latter may be measured without patient radiation by taking plain films of serial collections of feces. Solid markers have certain disadvantages: they are not triturated and emptied from the stomach in the same way as solid ingested food, they are particularly difficult to localize in the small bowel, and documenting the location of markers reveals little about the mechanism of their luminal transit.

Barium sulfate or other radiopaque fluid media can be ingested orally or given by enema to permit radiographic visualization of the anatomy and the contour of the upper and lower GI tract, respectively. Plain films repeated at intervals give some indication about gastric emptying, the rate of intestinal transit, or the efficiency of colonic evacuation. Fluoroscopy, with or without cine or video recording, allows subjective assessment of the patterns of motor activity and the effectiveness of peristalsis. However, radiopaque fluid media are not physiologic, and their transit is not necessarily representative of the gastric emptying, intestinal transit, or colonic propulsion of ingested food. Radiation exposure limits the period of observation, and the technique does not permit quantification of contraction amplitude or sphincter pressure. Nonetheless, cineradiography is especially effective in the evaluation of pharyngeal swallowing disorders, making possible frame-by-frame analysis of the co-ordinated action of the tongue, palate, pharyngeal musculature, and upper esophageal sphincter.[4,5] Simple modifications of the standard barium swallow can increase its usefulness in the assessment of motor disorders. Gravity alone empties barium from the esophagus, and this effect can be eliminated by requiring that esophageal function be examined when the patient is supine. Bread or a marshmallow dipped in barium and swallowed permits radiologic tracking of a solid bolus in patients complaining of dysphagia. In the absence of mechanical obstruction, the arrest of the bolus at one or more sites in the esophagus or its aimless propagation to and fro within the esophagus is suggestive of a motor disorder.

Radionuclide scintigraphy is now routinely used in the evaluation of biliary,[6] esophageal,[7] gastric,[8] and colonic[9] motor function. Radionuclide is given intravenously so that it may be concentrated in bile and stored in the gallbladder, ingested so that esophageal or gastric emptying may be studied, or given as an enema so that colonic motility may be evaluated. The proportion of the total radioactivity that is present in an area of interest can be plotted against time to generate a measure of transit or emptying with a minimum of radiation exposure. At the present time, image resolution is such that motor patterns cannot be assessed. In the case of gastric emptying, radioisotopes have been incorporated into a variety of foods, and the use of multiple markers has permitted the evaluation of the different emptying rates of liquid and solid phases of a meal.

The imaging technique of sonography is used routinely for the assessment of gallbladder filling and emptying. Development of the technique and degree of resolution may some day expand its application.

Marker-Perfusion Studies

This is a well-validated method of studying intestinal absorption, secretion, and bolus propulsion.[10] It has been used to measure gastric emptying, biliary secretion, and intestinal transit. The principle is relatively simple. A test solution containing an inert marker (one that is not absorbed, degraded, or adsorbed during its transit through the gut and does not influence intestinal motility or digestion of the test substance) is infused at a constant rate, and intestinal contents are sampled continuously distal to the infusion site. Flow rate past the sampling site can be calculated accurately from the infusion rate and the difference in marker concentration between test solution and the aspirated sample. Solute transport is similarly calculated by the difference in the amount of solute (flow rate × concentration) entering and leaving the study segment. In gastric emptying studies, the technique can be modified so that multiple markers are utilized to label aqueous, lipid, and solid phases of a meal.[11] The technique requires gastric or intestinal intubation, and the possibility of secretion or absorption must be taken into account in the interpretation of results.

Breath Tests

Mouth-to-cecum transit time can be measured using the lactulose breath hydrogen tolerance test.[12] The technique is based on the observation that hydrogen is produced when carbohydrate is fermented by colonic bacteria, and the hydrogen produced results in an increase in breath hydrogen excretion.[13] The time between the ingestion of lactulose, a nonabsorbable carbohydrate, and a rise in breath hydrogen excretion represents the mouth-to-cecum transit time for the head of the carbohydrate load as it passes through the gut.[14] Accurate interpretation requires recognition of the false-negative results due to an inability (spontaneous or antibiotic-induced) of the colonic bacterial flora to ferment carbohydrate. Early elevation of breath hydrogen may occur in patients with upper small bowel bacterial overgrowth.

The ^{14}C-glycocholate breath test depends upon colonic bacterial metabolism of ^{14}C-labeled glycine and the release of $^{14}CO_2$ in the expired breath. ^{14}C-breath tests represent a small but finite radiation exposure and have been avoided in children.[12]

Manometry

Unlike the radiographic techniques, which image luminal contents and assess transit or marker perfusion, and breath tests, which assess only transit, manometry is a technique that monitors movements and quantitates the force of contraction of the muscular wall of the gut. Sensors at multiple locations permit description of muscular activity in terms of the amplitude, direction, duration, and velocity of propagation of contraction.

Air-filled balloon kymographs were used for the detection of movement within the GI tract over a century ago. With the advent of force transducers, they were replaced by the more efficient water-filled balloon connected by a fluid column to a sensor. The disadvantages of a balloon system are that it (1) is a tethered obstruction that can induce a motor response, (2) represents a relatively large sensor that integrates all pressure changes over an area several millimeters in length, and (3) is highly compliant, which diminishes the fidelity of the pressure recording.

The most widely available and a well-validated technique for accurately measuring intraluminal pressure is the infused, multiple-lumen manometry catheter with distal side-hole recording orifices.[15] Catheters are continuously infused with distilled water by a low-compliance pump. Compression of the distal side-hole of the catheter by a contraction causes an increase in pressure within the catheter lumen which is sensed by a pressure transducer located outside the body. At least two recording orifices spaced along a multilumen manometry catheter are required to determine the direction and velocity of propagation of a contraction. The system is appropriate for recording motility in a narrow lumen viscus, but in a larger organ such as the body of the stomach a localized contraction will not occlude the catheter lumen, and the only recorded response will be an attenuated simultaneous change in pressure recorded from all sensory sites within the cavity (a common cavity phenomenon). The advantages of the infused catheter manometry system are that it is relatively cheap, rugged, versatile, and easy to use. Multiple-lumen catheters are commercially available or individually constructed by bonding together polyvinyl chloride tubes, and the side-hole recording orifices can be cut at any desired location. The frequency response characteristics of an infused catheter manometry system are sufficient for esophageal or GI recording but insufficient for accurate recording of higher-frequency activity in the pharynx and upper esophageal sphincter.[15-17]

Similar recordings can be obtained with commercially available intraluminal strain-gauge force transducers mounted on catheter probes (Honeywell Biomedical and Millar Instruments). These assemblies eliminate the need for infusion and have frequency response characteristics that substantially exceed those necessary for accurate recording of pharyngeal, esophageal, or GI activity.[17] The disadvantages of these systems are that they are more expensive and fragile. The recording sites are fixed in position, and with increasing numbers of lumens they become more rigid and uncomfortable than a comparable manometry catheter.

Recently, radiopills—small capsules containing a pressure sensor, a coil transmitting a signal, and a battery—have been stationed at a fixed point in the gut lumen and tethered by a fine thread to provide information comparable to that obtained with the intubation systems described above.[18] Multiple pills are required to determine direction and velocity of propagation of a wave form. Presently, the system remains technically complex, expensive, and subject to intermittent signal loss. A reliable system would achieve a greater degree of patient mobility and comfort.

Electromyography

Intestinal smooth muscle is an electrically excitable tissue. Rapid high-amplitude oscillations of the smooth muscle membrane potential (action or spike potentials) have a one-to-one association with contraction. Thus, a recording of electrical spike activity at successive locations within the gut would provide information similar to that of manometric or intraluminal strain gauge probes. The recording of smooth muscle myoelectric activity (electromyography) in humans has been attempted in a variety of ways, none of which has as yet been shown to have wide clinical application. Catheter probes have been constructed with suction, ring, wick, or clip electrodes and in all cases the major difficulty has been to maintain continuous contract between the mucosa and the electrode, a condition necessary for uninterrupted recording of the electrical signal.[19] These systems all suffer from a very low signal-to-noise ratio, and the suction and the clip electrodes may cause mucosal damage or even perforation. A number of workers have implanted electrodes into gut muscle through the serosal surface at the time of operation.[20] They were secured with catgut sutures, which dissolved and allowed them to be removed together with a surgical drain up to 5 days postoperatively. The method is possible only after laparotomy and allows recording only during a time interval when the gut has not yet returned to a normal state.

Recent research in surface electromyography (body surface recording of GI myoelectrical activity analogous to electrocardiography) suggests that, with technical improvements, electrogastrography may one day prove useful.

METHODOLOGY OF INFUSED CATHETER MANOMETRY

Factors Affecting Fidelity of Performance

Proper performance of manometry and reporting of manometric data are essential in order that information be quantitatively accurate and reproducible. The factors affecting the fidelity of intraluminal infused manometric recording systems have been reviewed.[15,16] Recording fidelity is determined by the characteristics of the pressure phenomenon being recorded and the performance capabilities of the recording system.

Pressure Phenomenon Being Recorded. The accuracy with which a recording system is able to record a change in pressure is directly related to the duration of the change but inversely related to the amplitude, the rate of change, and the frequency of variation. The amplitude, frequency, and wave form of pressures induced by contractions within the GI tract vary with location along the gut. For example, the frequency of pharyngeal pressure variation is in the range of 1 to 3 Hz, the frequency of esophageal pressure events is just less than 1 Hz, gastric contractions occur at about three per minute, and duodenal contractions occur at about 12 per minute. Pharyngeal contractions have amplitudes in the range of 200 mm Hg, a duration of 0.2 second, and a rate of rise of 1,000 mm Hg per second. Within the esophagus peristaltic waves range from 20 to 200 mm Hg in amplitude, are 2 to 6 seconds in duration, and have rates of rise of 20 to 500 mm Hg per second. In the intestinal tract more distal to the esophagus, contractile events range from 20 to 200 mm Hg in amplitude and 2 to 5 seconds in duration and exhibit rates of rise considerably below those recorded in the esophagus.

Recording System Performance. The infused catheter manometry system comprises the following components: manometry catheter, infusion pump, external volume-displacement transducers, preamplifier-amplifier, and a pen chart recorder. Recording fidelity is directly related to the infusion rate and inversely related to the total compliance of the infused catheter systems.[15] Compliance is a measure of the ease with which the system accommodates a change in volume, i.e., the volume change resulting from the application of a unit pressure. Circularly oriented contractions of the gut lumen create forces that tend to seal the side-hole recording orifices of water-filled catheters. Recording accuracy is achieved only if the rate of infusion is high enough and the compliance of the system is low enough that a contraction does not seal the recording orifice. Catheter infusion rate can be regulated by varying the infusion pressure. When using multilumen infused catheters it is desirable to keep the rate of infusion as low as possible to minimize fluid loading of the patient and permit longer recording periods. With this restriction in mind, recording system fidelity is best achieved by minimizing the compliance of the volume-displacement transducers, the infusion system, and the manometric tube assembly. The performance characteristics of commercially available volume-displacement transducers and polygraph recorders greatly exceed those necessary to accurately record pressure wave forms in the pharynx, esophagus, stomach, and intestinal tract, and their compliance is negligible.[15] This may not be true for the infusion system and the manometry catheter.

Until recently, the most commonly utilized infusion apparatus consisted of water-filled syringes whose emptying was driven by a gear train and an electrical motor. During pressure loading the fluid delivered by such a system fell to as little as 15 percent of the baseline delivery rate,[21] owing to a high compliance or deformability of the pump, syringes, and gear train. While this compliance can be reduced by greasing the syringes and using a heavier duty pump, the pneumohydraulic capillary infusion pump is a superior mechanism that achieves minimal compliance and permits accurate recording at low infusion rates of 0.5 ml per minute.[16] Such a system is without syringes or moving parts (Fig. 1). A nitrogen gas source is connected through a step-down pressure regulator to a fluid reservoir containing demineralized water. Pressurized water exits the pressure chamber through an on/off valve. Microcapillary tubing connects the outlet valve to a pressure transducer and a manometry catheter in series. By substituting a manifold of valves at the outlet of the pressure reservoir, multiple capillaries can be connected in parallel to infuse as many pressure transducer and manometry catheter lumens as desired. The low compliance of this pneumohydraulic-capillary infusion system is based on the fact that fluid flow from the manometry catheter is proportional to the pressure difference across the capillary tubing. If reservoir pressure is high (1,000 mm Hg) relative to the catheter pressure generated by intestinal contractions (e.g., 100 mm Hg), the pressure gradient across the capillary tubing decreases only 10 percent (from 1,000 to 900 mm Hg) and there is only a small reduction in flow rate.

Compliance of the manometry catheter itself is inversely related to luminal diameter, wall thickness, and wall rigidity and directly related to length.[16] Catheter compliance can be decreased by using minimally elastic, thick-walled catheters of the shortest length and smallest internal diameter possible. Infusion catheters may be made from polyvinyl chloride or polyethylene. The advantages of the polyvinyl chloride catheters are that they are softer, more pliable, and more comfortable for the patient, and single catheters can be fused together in their longitudinal axis (with tetrahydrofuran) to form a multilumen manometric assembly. A lateral recording orifice is cut in each lumen at an appropriate location along the assembly and a plug of radiopaque material is used to obstruct the catheter lumen distal to the recording orifice. Although selection of a smaller diameter catheter decreases compliance and increases the number that may be incorporated into a multilumen bundle of acceptable size, the resistance to flow increases with decreased internal diameter.

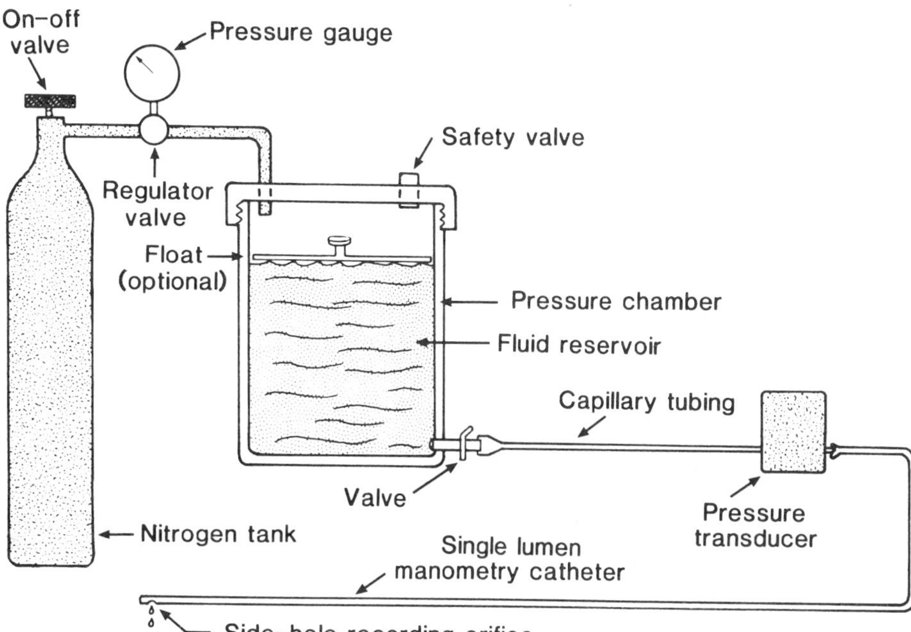

FIGURE 1 Pneumohydraulic capillary infusion system. (Redrawn from Arndorfer et al.[16])

A catheter lumen that is too small will result in an undesirable elevation of baseline pressure (the perfusion pressure) recorded at the pressure transducer. Polyvinyl chloride or polyethylene catheters with internal diameters of 0.7 to 0.8 mm seem to be an appropriate compromise and, when infused with bubble-free water at 0.5 ml per minute by a pneumohydraulic capillary infusion system, have been shown to have a low compliance and a high fidelity of recording at frequencies and pressures encountered within the GI tract.

Multilumen tubes of fused or extruded construction are available commercially in a variety of specifications. The total compliance of any infusion system (at a specific rate of infusion) can be measured as the rate of rise of pressure in millimeters of mercury per second after occlusion of the side-hole recording orifice on the manometry catheter. Accurate recording from the cervical esophagus requires a rise rate of 300 mm Hg or more and a rate of 150 mm Hg per second or more in the thoracic esophagus.[15] These rise rates are more than sufficient for recording from the more distal GI tract.

Recording Technique—A Regional Application

Patient Preparation. All oral intake should be stopped 4 hours before intubation. A variety of medications are known to affect intestinal motility (e.g., anticholinergics, prokinetic agents, antidiarrheals, laxatives, narcotics) and must be discontinued for an appropriate interval prior to study if a record of basal motor activity is desired. Satisfactory recordings can be obtained in infants less than 6 months of age without sedation; however, between the ages of 6 months and 6 years sedation with chloral hydrate, 50 to 75 mg per kilogram, may be necessary to obtain a good quality recording in the period immediately following intubation. In small infants the manometry catheter can be passed orally through a feeding nipple. In older patients a lubricated manometry tube is passed through the external nares and causes less gagging, obviates the risk of the patient biting and perforating the manometry catheter, and allows easy fixation by taping the catheter to the nose. The tube should be inserted into the nose perpendicular to the face until the tip reaches the oral pharynx. The catheter can be advanced into the esophagus during a wet or dry swallow when the larynx is closed. In the older patient, lidocaine gel on the catheter and topical Xylocaine spray to the pharynx minimize the discomfort of intubation. For esophageal manometry the catheter can be advanced until the most proximal recording orifice is in the stomach, a distance of about 40 cm from the external nares in adults and approximately 20 cm in infants. Once it is in the stomach, abdominal compression and inspiration both produce a rise in pressure. Upper intestinal intubation has been achieved using fluoroscopy and a manometry catheter stiffened with a flexible-tip Teflon-coated guide wire. Some centers have utilized endoscopy or steerable catheters to position a flexible-tip Teflon-coated guide wire, removed the steerable catheter or endoscope, and then fed the manometric assembly down over the guide wire until the position of the manometric ports as identified by radiopaque markers was appropriate at fluoroscopy.[22] For prolonged intubation the catheter should be firmly anchored to the patient's external nares, as peristaltic activity tends to advance it. Once proper location of the manometry catheter is established, the patient should be put in the supine position, and the catheters flushed with water and connected to their respective pressure transducers. A pressure artifact generated by the hydrostatic force of the column of water in the manometry catheter is minimized if the transducers are positioned at the same level as the intraluminal recording, i.e., at the midaxillary line of the supine patient. If sufficient channels are available respiration can be recorded using a belt pneumograph positioned around the thorax. Adults and older children may tolerate a belt pneumograph positioned around the neck to record laryngeal movement and provide a record of swallowing.

Prior to each use, the pneumohydraulic infusion system should be flushed clear of bubbles (which greatly increase compliance because of the compressability of air) and calibrated in millimeters of mercury. The calibration record, infusion rate, pressure response (rise rate in millimeters of mercury per second), paper speed during recording, and relevant patient information should be noted on the manometric tracing.

Esophageal Manometry. Manometric evaluation of the esophagus requires assessment of the functional characteristics of the lower esophageal sphincter (LES), esophageal body, and upper esophageal sphincter (UES); the sphincters are evaluated for the strength of their resting closure and their ability to relax with swallowing, while the body is assessed for the presence of peristaltic or nonperistaltic motor activity. Variation in instrumentation and recording technique among laboratories, recording assembly diameter (recorded pressure increases with larger assembly diameters because of muscle length-tension characteristics), scoring technique, and age introduce variability into recorded pressures.[15] Normal values in one laboratory cannot necessarily be used as reference values elsewhere.

The UES is a slit-shaped orifice with its long axis in the coronal plane and a narrow zone of high pressure in the sagittal plane.[23] The LES also exhibits radial asymmetry, with its zone of highest pressure in the levoposterior direction.[24] To minimize radial asymmetry as a source of recording error, the manometry catheter should have side-hole recording orifices oriented in different directions. Young infants are unable to comfortably accommodate manometry catheters with more than three lumens, and in this age group we use a three-lumen catheter with recording orifices 2 cm apart in the longitudinal direction and 120 degrees apart in their radial orientation. In the older patient a six-lumen catheter can be constructed with four recording orifices spaced 5 cm apart and two additional sites, one opening 1 cm above and another 1 cm below the most distal side-hole. The three distal sites should be 120 degrees apart in radial orientation. The upper and lower esophageal sphincters move proximally a distance of up to several centimeters during deglutition.[25] It is useful to be able to place the three closely spaced recording orifices in the sphincter zone to verify that a fall in pressure is due to sphincter relaxation and not an artifact related to axial movement of the sphincter away from the recording orifice. A modification (Dent sleeve) of the infused catheter system allows prolonged monitoring of sphincter pressure unaffected by axial displacement of the digestive tube with respect to the viscus.[26] In this system a side-hole recording orifice opens into the closed end of a 5.0-cm long Mylar sleeve, and infused water must drain out through the distal open end of the sleeve. A rise in pressure anywhere along the sleeve impedes the outflow of distilled water and causes a rise in pressure sensed by the transducer.

When a manometry catheter is positioned with the distal orifices in the stomach, and is withdrawn at increments of 0.5 to 1.0 cm at intervals of 20 seconds or so, a station pull-through pressure profile of LES, body of esophagus, and UES is obtained. Ideally the patient should be encouraged or induced to swallow at each interval during the station pull-through technique. As each recording orifice is withdrawn from the abdomen into the chest, the pressure deflection produced by inspiration changes from positive to negative—the pressure inversion point. Because respiratory artifact is superimposed upon LES pressure, LES pressure has been variously scored and reported as a peak inspiratory, end-expiratory, or average midrespiratory value. Recent experimental evidence suggests that the true LES pressure is the end-expiratory value.[27] An alternative method of measuring LES pressure is the rapid pull-through technique.[28] This measurement is performed by continuously withdrawing the pressure sensor at a rate of 0.5 to 1.0 cm per second across the LES while the patient suspends respiration for 10 to 15 seconds. The method is obviously not suitable for infants or the uncooperative child. Most laboratories report LES pressure as the mean of the measures obtained from at least three recording orifices with representative radial orientation using the station pull-through technique. LES pressure ranges between 10 and 35 mm Hg in normal adults.[15] In children LES pressure is age-dependent, with normal values being 43.3 $\pm$ 2.4 mm Hg below 1 year of age and 30.6 $\pm$ 2.3 mm Hg above 1 year of age.[29] The LES relaxes to gastric pressure after 95 percent of swallows in normal subjects.[15] Relaxation is initiated immediately with deglutition and lasts 6 to 12 seconds while a peristaltic contraction wave propagates from the pharynx through the body of the esophagus and the sphincter segment. LES relaxation is verified (1) if relaxation occurs simultaneously at three closely spaced recording sites, located within the sphincter zone, (2) if it occurs with each swallow during incremental withdrawal of a single recording orifice across the sphincter zone, or (3) if a Dent sleeve is employed and relaxation is documented.[15,26]

Within the body of the esophagus peristaltic pressure wave amplitude, duration, and velocity depend upon bolus volume, consistency, and temperature.[15] If swallows are elicited at each increment of catheter withdrawal, the entire length of the body of esophagus is evaluated with respect to the presence and nature of peristaltic activity. Wet swallows consistently elicit esophageal peristaltic waves that are of greater amplitude and slower velocity than those of dry swallows. After a swallow the velocity of contraction varies from 1 to 5 cm per second, with the contraction wave moving fastest in the proximal esophagus, slowing at the aortic arch, regaining speed in the midesophagus, and slowing once again in the distal esophagus. The amplitude varies between 25 and 150 mm Hg. The amplitude of a swallow wave decreases as it propagates toward the aortic arch and then increases as it propagates more distally to the LES. The duration of the swallow wave varies between about 2 and 6 seconds and is inversely related to wave speed. Abnormal responses to swallowing include aperistalsis, frequent failure of peristaltic waves to traverse the entire esophagus, frequent failure of deglutition to initiate a propagated swallow, and quantitative abnormalities of amplitude, velocity, and duration of wave form.

An evaluation of UES function and pressure is subject to the same concerns regarding axial movement of the sphincter with swallowing and radial asymmetry as have been discussed in relation to the LES. In addition, most patients choke as soon as perfused catheter orifices are withdrawn into the hypopharynx. In this situation the infusion to each recording orifice may be turned off as it enters the hypopharynx and the station pull-through recording continued. The normal UES pressure is 32 ± 10 mm Hg in adults[15] and 21.3 ± 7.4 mm Hg in children.[30]

Gastrointestinal Manometry. It is little more than a decade since manometry was first utilized as a tool in the clinical assessment of patients with symptoms suggestive of disordered GI motility.[31] Despite a paucity of normal data from healthy humans,[32-34] and marked intra- and interindividual variability of motility in the normal human, disturbances or abnormalities of gastric and intestinal motor patterns have been appreciated which appear to be pathogenetic and of diagnostic significance.[22,31-33] Although slower rates of infusion (0.1 ml per minute) and longer lengths of tubing (150 to 450 cm) are utilized and markedly diminish the rise rates recorded in response to catheter occlusion, manometry accurately records motility of the human distal small bowel and proximal colon.[32] There is no standardization for the arrangement of recording orifices in catheters for GI manometric recording, and most are constructed to meet specific requirements, e.g., an eight-lumen catheter with three proximal recording sites several centimeters apart that can be localized within the antrum and five more distal recording sites with orifices 5 to 10 cm apart for recording duodenal and jejunal contractile activity. Longer tubes are employed to assess ileal or ileocolonic activity.

Patients should be studied both in the fasting state to identify and define the characteristics of the migrating myoelectric complex (MMC) and after feeding to document the change to the fed motor pattern. Manometric abnormalities are found in about three-fourths of patients with unexplained nausea, vomiting, or abdominal pain,[33] and in patients with a wide variety of primary and secondary pseudo-obstructive disorders.[22] Most laboratories record for 3 to 6 hours during fasting, give a standard meal, and continue recording for 1 to 2 hours after feeding. Because of marked intra- and interindividual variability and the possible effects of stress, much longer periods of assessment would be desirable if they were practical or could be tolerated by the patient. For example, the average interval between MMCs in the normal individual is approximately 90 minutes, but the range is 15 minutes to more than 3 hours. If a period of observation less than 3 hours is utilized, the MMC may not be identified in normal patients.[32] It is inevitable that there will be increasing utilization of GI motility for diagnostic and prognostic purposes. We must be cautious not to make interpretations that exceed our understanding of what is normal or pathologic.

Colonic manometry remains an experimental procedure, with interpretation and clinical usage greatly hampered by the limited level of understanding of both normal and disordered colonic motor function.

Rectoanal Manometry. There is currently no standardized method for performing anorectal manometry, and there is considerable variability in the equipment, technique, and results described in the literature.[35,36] For recording anal sphincter pressures, and specifically the response of the internal anal sphincter to rectal distention, we employ a multilumen probe with a distal latex balloon. Three or more side-hole openings are spaced 0.5 cm apart in the catheter's longitudinal axis and are equally separated in radial orientation. The balloon can be filled or emptied with air through a distal catheter orifice. The size of the balloon and probe must be appropriately adjusted to accommodate premature and newborn infants, children, and adults.[36] The distal latex balloon and more proximal catheter orifices are inserted through the anus until they are all located within the rectum. The catheter is withdrawn by 0.5- to 1.0-cm increments at equal intervals until a station pull-through pressure profile of the internal and external anal sphincter is obtained. Cooperative children are asked to make voluntary contractions of the external anal sphincter at each station. Once the location of the sphincter zone is established, the catheter can be re-introduced until the side-hole recording orifices are optimally located within the sphincter zone. Then the latex balloon is inflated with incremental volumes of air until a sensory threshold for rectal distention and the threshold for rectoanal inhibitory reflex are established. The rectoanal inhibitory reflex was first described by Denny-Brown and Robertson.[37] Distention of the rectum by stool or artificially by a balloon causes relaxation of the internal anal sphincter and contraction of the external anal sphincter.[37,38] This response persists in patients with acquired functional or idiopathic constipation but is absent in those with Hirschsprung's disease. A rectal biopsy should be done for histologic confirmation of a manometric diagnosis of Hirschsprung's disease. A false-positive manometric diagnosis can be made if there has been insufficient rectal distention to produce the rectoanal inhibitory reflex, if the rectum has not been cleared of feces prior to assessment, if the rectal balloon has not been properly placed, or if crying and body movements cause axial displacement of the catheter with respect to the sphincter zone and produce artifact. To avoid this situation, patients should have a cleansing enema before the test to permit correct placement of the distending balloon in the rectum and to permit distention of the rectal wall by the inflated balloon. Anxious and uncooperative young children may be lightly sedated to facilitate an accurate recording.

Other clinical applications for rectoanal manometry include evaluation of anal sphincter function (1) in neuromuscular disease, (2) in rectoanal surgery, and (3) for behavioral modification of incontinent patients.

REFERENCES

1. Weems WA. Intestinal fluid flow: its production and control. In: Johnson LR, ed. Physiology of the gastrointestinal tract. 2nd ed. New York: Raven Press, 1987: 571.
2. Wingate DL. Methodology of motility. In: Christensen J, Wingate DL, eds. A guide to gastrointestinal motility. Boston: Wright PSG, 1983: 215.
3. Metcalf AM, Phillips SF, Zinsmeister AR, MacCarty RL, Beart RW, Wolff BG. Simplified assessment of segmental colonic transit. Gastroenterology 1987; 92:40–47.
4. Fisher SE, Painter M, Milmoe G. Swallowing disorders in infancy. Pediatr Clin North Am 1981; 28:845–853.
5. Bowen A'D, Ledesma-Medina J, Fujioka M, Oh KS, Young LW. Radiologic imaging in otolaryngology. Pediatr Clin North Am 1981; 28:905–939.
6. Shaffer EA, McOrmond P, Duggan H. Quantitative cholescintigraphy: assessment of gallbladder filling and emptying and duodenogastric reflex. Gastroenterology 1980; 79:899–906.
7. Russell CDH, Hill LD, Holmes ER, Hull DA, Gannon R, Pope CE. Radionuclide transit: a sensitive screening test for esophageal dysfunction. Gastroenterology 1981; 80:887–892.
8. Houghton LA, Read NW, Heddle R, Horowitz M, Collins PJ, Chatterton B, Dent J. Relationship of the motor activity of the antrum, pylorus, and duodenum to gastric emptying of a solid-liquid mixed meal. Gastroenterology 1988; 94:1285–1291.

9. Krevsky B, Malmud LS, D'Ercole F, Maurer AH, Fisher RS. Colonic transit scintigraphy. A physiologic approach to the quantitative measurement of colonic transit in humans. Gastroenterology 1986; 91:1102–1120.
10. Fordtran JS. Marker perfusion techniques for measuring intestinal absorption in man. Gastroenterology 1966; 51:1089–1093.
11. Cortot A, Phillips SF, Malagelada J-R. Gastric emptying of lipids after ingestion of a solid-liquid meal in humans. Gastroenterology 1981; 80:922–927.
12. Barr RG, Perman JA, Schoeller DA, Watkins JB. Breath tests in pediatric gastrointestinal disorders: new diagnostic opportunities. Pediatrics 1978; 62:393–401
13. Bond JH, Levitt MD. Investigations of small bowel transit time in man utilizing pulmonary hydrogen (H_2) measurements. J Lab Clin Med 1975; 85:546–555.
14. Read NW, Miles CA, Fisher D, Holgate AM, Kime ND, Mitchell MA, Reeve AM, Roche TB, Walker M. Transit of a meal through the stomach, small intestine, and colon in normal subjects, and its role in the pathogenesis of diarrhea. Gastroenterology 1980; 70:1276–1282.
15. Dodds WJ. Instrumentation and methods for intraluminal esophageal manometry. Arch Intern Med 1976; 136:515–523.
16. Arndorfer RC, Stef JJ, Dodds WJ, Linehan JH, Hogan WJ. Improved infusion systems for intraluminal esophageal manometry. Gastroenterology 1977; 73:23–27.
17. Dodds WJ, Hogan WJ, Lydon SB, Stewart ET, Stef JJ, Arndorfer RC. Quantitation of pharyngeal motor function in normal human subjects. J Appl Physiol 1975; 39:693–696.
18. Thompson DG, Wingate DL, Archer L, Benson MJ, Green WJ, Hardy RJ. Normal patterns of human upper small bowel motor activity recorded by prolonged radiotelemetry. Gut 1980; 21:500–506.
19. Fleckenstein P. A probe for intraluminal recording of myoelectrical activity from multiple sites in the human small intestine. Scand J Gastroenterol 1978; 13:767–770.
20. Catchpole BN, Duthie HL. Post-operative gastrointestinal complexes. In: Duthie H, ed. Gastrointestinal motility in health and disease. Lancaster: MTP Press, 1978: 29.
21. Stef JJ, Dodds WJ, Hogan WJ, Linehan JH, Stewart ET. Intraluminal esophageal manometry: an analysis of variables affecting recording fidelity of peristaltic pressures. Gastroenterology 1974; 67:221–230.
22. Malagelada J-R, Camilleri M, Staghellini V. Manometric diagnosis of motility disorders. New York: Thieme Inc, 1986.
23. Winans CS. The Pharyngoesophageal closure mechanism: a manometric study. Gastroenterology 1972; 63:768–777.
24. Kaye MD, Showalter JP. Manometric configuration of the lower esophageal sphincter in normal human subjects. Gastroenterology 1971; 61:213–223.
25. Dodds WJ, Stewart ET, Hogan WJ, Stef JJ, Arndorfer RC. Effect of esophageal movement on liminal esophageal pressure recording. Gastroenterology 1974; 67:592–600.
26. Dent J. A new technique for continuous sphincter pressure measurement. Gastroenterology 1976; 71:263–267.
27. Boyle JT, Altschuler SM, Nixon TE, Tuchman DN, Pack AI, Cohen S. Role of the diaphragm in the genesis of lower esophageal sphincter pressure in the cat. Gastroenterology 1985; 88:723–730.
28. Dodds WJ, Hogan WJ, Stef JJ, Miller WN, Lydon SB, Arndorfer RC. A rapid pull-through technique for measuring lower esophageal sphincter pressure. Gastroenterology 1975; 68:437–443.
29. Moroz S, Espinoza J, Cumming W, Diamant NE. Lower esophageal sphincter function in children with and without gastroesophageal reflux. Gastroenterology 1976; 71:236–241.
30. Sondheimer JM. Upper esophageal sphincter and pharyngoesophageal motor function in infants with and without gastroesophageal reflux. Gastroenterology 1983; 85:301–305.
31. Vantrappen G, Janssens J, Ghoos Y. The interdigestive motor complex of normal subjects and patients with bacterial overgrowth of the small intestine. J Clin Invest 1977; 59:1158–1160.
32. Kerlin P, Phillips S. Variability of motility of the ileum and jejunum in healthy humans. Gastroenterology 1982; 82:694–700.
33. Malagelada J-R, Stanghellini V. Manometric evaluation of functional upper gut symptoms. Gastroenterology 1985; 88:1223–1231.
34. Kellow JE, Borody TJ, Phillips SF, Tucker RL, Haddad AC. Human interdigestive motility: variations in patterns from esophagus to colon. Gastroenterology 1986; 91:386–395.
35. Coller JA. Clinical application of anorectal manometry. Gastroenterol Clin North Am 1987; 16:17–33.
36. Rosenberg AJ, Vela AR. A new simplified technique for anorectal manometry. Pediatrics 1983; 71:240–245
37. Denny-Brown D, Robertson EG. An investigation of the nervous control of defecation. Brain 1935; 58:256–310.
38. Schuster MM, Hendriz TR, Mendeloff AI. The internal anal sphincter response: manometric studies on its normal physiology, neural pathways, and alteration in bowel disorders. J Clin Invest 1963; 42:192–207.

CHAPTER 34

Esophageal pH Monitoring

Judith M. Sondheimer, M.D.

Monitoring pH in the distal esophagus is an accurate method of evaluating acid reflux events over time. Although this technique cannot measure the volume of gastric contents passing retrograde from stomach to esophagus, it does quantify the number of reflux events and their duration. The use of intraluminal pH recordings as a diagnostic test for gastroesophageal (GE) reflux was first proposed and tested in adults by Tuttle and Grossman in 1956 using a flexible, bipolar, glass electrode passed through the mouth.[1] The size of this electrode made it impractical for use in small children. Since the late 1970s, smaller, more flexible unipolar electrodes with external reference electrodes have been developed, which can be passed with relative ease via the nares. The miniaturized glass electrodes have relatively high impedance and are relatively fragile and unstable with prolonged use. The response times of glass electrodes are variable and sometimes quite long. Newer electrodes with sensing elements of monocrystalline antimony have lower impedance and require less shielding than glass electrodes, which allows for even finer caliber. The pH-dependent function of the antimony electrode is determined by an oxidative process, and thus the electrode properties will change as the element corrodes during use.[2,3] One recent study estimates the life expectancy of a fine antimony electrode as 800 hours of use before the effects of oxidation cause deterioration of function.[4]

When properly adjusted and standardized, both glass and antimony electrodes are adequate for 24-hour studies.[5] The electrodes are connected to an external pH meter whose output may be directly transcribed on a strip chart or sampled at intervals and stored for later print-out. Recording devices that transmit to a remote receiver allow for immediate evaluation of pH events in ambulatory patients.[6,7] Strip chart recorders give the most accurate second-by-second reflection of esophageal pH but, because of their size, limit the normal patient activity during testing. Miniaturized, battery-powered pH meters and recorders carried by the patient permit nearly normal activity during monitoring. Most portable recorders are capable of receiving other input signals, allowing the subject to key in events such as meals, pain, episodes of cough, and changes in body position. Some portable recording devices are equipped with position sensors, either attached to the patient or included in the recorder, which indicate whether the subject is upright or recumbent. Data from pH recordings can be analyzed either by visual inspection of records or by computer programs.[8] There is no uniformly accepted method of analyzing these records and no universally recognized criteria for the diagnosis of GE reflux based on pH recordings (see Interpretation of Results).

INDICATIONS AND CONTRAINDICATIONS FOR pH TESTING

In healthy young children with typical GE reflux characterized by repetitive postprandial emesis, the diagnosis of GE reflux can be made by a combination of typical history, careful physical examination, and an upper gastrointestinal (GI) series that shows no evidence of gastric outlet obstruction.[9] When symptoms are less characteristic or the consequences of delay in diagnosis greater, more sensitive and specific diagnostic tests are needed. The barium swallow is essential to rule out gastric outlet obstruction in patients who vomit but is less useful in confirming a diagnosis of GE reflux. False-positive diagnosis of GE reflux may be as high as 31.3 percent, and the false-negative rate may be as high as 14.0 percent.[10] Continuous monitoring of esophageal pH is especially useful in the child with atypical symptoms, not only to confirm the diagnosis but also to clarify the relationship between reflux episodes and nongastrointestinal symptoms such as apnea, colicky spells, dysphagia, cough, and wheezing. Evaluation of pH records may reveal relationships between reflux episodes and body position, type of feeding, and physical activity that cannot be obtained from radiographs. pH monitoring can also be used as a check on response to therapy, especially in situations in which nongastrointestinal symptoms are the primary complaint.[11]

Esophageal pH monitoring may be contraindicated if placement of the electrode in the nares causes respiratory compromise. Results will be misleading in infants and children who remain agitated after placement of pH electrodes or in children who gag or wretch uncontrollably, as increased abdominal pressure will produce reflux.[12] Prolonged monitoring should not be performed in infants or children if careful observation cannot be assured. Supervision by an informed adult greatly increases the information derived from this study and is necessary for the safety of the child.

TECHNICAL ASPECTS

Prior to insertion, the flexible electrode must be standardized with buffers bracketing the expected range of pH to be measured. Buffers should be at body temperature, and the patient should be connected to the buffer reservoir by a salt bridge. Reaction time of glass electrodes should be checked, as this tends to increase with repeated use. The reference electrode can be attached to a mucosal surface or, more conveniently, to an area of thoroughly cleaned skin using standard ECG electrodes. Electrodes should be sterilized between uses by gas sterilization. Gastric pH must be checked before study to ensure that reflux can be detected.

In adults, the tip of the pH electrode is usually placed 5 cm above the GE junction (13 percent of the standard adult esophageal length from teeth to lower esophageal sphincter). Despite the fact that the pH electrode in pediatric patients is usually passed through the nares, the tip of the electrode is customarily placed above the lower esophageal sphincter (LES), 13 percent of the nares-to-LES distance. The most accurate and reproducible method of electrode placement is obtained by manometrically determining the nares-to-LES distance. Fluoroscopic placement of probes in the distal third of the esophagus is probably sufficiently accurate for a single study in a subject with normal body habitus and esophageal anatomy. However, the presence of hiatus hernia, thoracic deformity, or previous esophageal or thoracic surgery makes this method of placement inaccurate. Esophageal length, from nares to the middle of the LES, can be estimated from the patient's height. The formula, which is derived from manometric measurements in 30 children ranging in age from 3 weeks to 235 months, estimates esophageal length to within 3.1 cm and assumes a normal body habitus and esophageal anatomy. Within these limitations, it provides a relatively reliable means of positioning intraesophageal electrodes. Esophageal length in centimeters from nares to LES is 5 + 0.252 (height in centimeters).[13] Estimating esophageal length by observing the location of a sudden drop in pH as the electrode tip is advanced beyond the LES is not recommended, as mucus clinging to the electrode can prevent a change in pH exactly at the GE junction and result in an overestimate of esophageal length. Accuracy in probe position may not be essential in an individual study, as pH records of the upper third of the esophagus in patients with reflux are abnormal when compared with the distal esophageal records of normal subjects.[14] However, if repeated studies in the same patient are performed, positioning is critical to ensure comparability.

Duration of monitoring depends upon the information desired. If pH monitoring is performed for diagnosis only, there may be no need for a 24-hour study. Several clinical studies have shown that pH monitoring for as short as 3 hours is as sensitive and specific as long-term monitoring.[15] Short-term monitoring is performed in the fasted state and in the recumbent position to avoid the frequent episodes of reflux that occur normally in the immediate postprandial period.[16,17] Monitoring after administration of an acid clear liquid increases test sensitivity and permits further shortening of the monitoring period (Tuttle test). The patient is given a standard acidified liquid meal (300 cc per 1.73 square meters), and esophageal pH is monitored for 30 to 60 minutes. Standards for interpretation vary. According to some authors, two episodes or reflux characterized by a sudden drop in pH to less than 4.0 or a single episode that lasts more than 30 percent of the monitored time is pathologic. The sensitivity of the Tuttle test is high, and there is a false-positive rate of about 30 percent when this test is compared with more prolonged monitoring.[18,19] Longer periods of monitoring have the diagnostic advantages of greater specificity and less sensitivity than the short-term studies. Stanciu and colleagues have shown that when the number of reflux episodes per hour and the average duration of reflux episodes are extracted from 15-hour pH records, the false-positive rate in asymptomatic controls is 0 percent and the false-negative rate in symptomatic subjects is 10 percent.[20]

Prolonged monitoring allows for detailed evaluation of the events surrounding reflux episodes. This may be important to therapy, to understanding the role of reflux in producing symptoms, and to an appreciation of reflux characteristics of normal individuals. Prolonged pH recordings in normal subjects have confirmed the fact that reflux episodes are common in the immediate postprandial period. Up to five episodes per hour in the first 2 postprandial hours may be seen.[16] Reflux is more likely to occur in the upright position in normal infants and children, whereas episodes of reflux during sleep are distinctly unusual.[21] It is also apparent that the reflux episodes occurring during sleep are different from awake and postprandial episodes. Whereas awake episodes occur with a sudden drop in esophageal pH and a stepwise return to normal, about 50 percent of episodes occurring during sleep are characterized by a gradual drift of pH to a level just below 4.0.[22] Whether this difference in pH pattern reflects a difference in volume or refluxed material or a different mechanism of awake and asleep reflux is not known.

A major problem with prolonged studies of esophageal pH is the lack of standard methods of performing the test. Controlling all variables of feeding, sleeping, activity, medication, and so on over a 24-hour period is impossible. However, the effect of some variables must be recognized and controlled to avoid erroneous interpretation of results. Body position, especially in the infant under 6 months, has a profound effect on the frequency of reflux. In the prone position, reflux episodes normally occur less frequently than in the supine position. In a recent study of normal infants, the time spent with a pH less than 4.0 increased sevenfold simply by moving the infant from prone to supine.[23] Feedings with an acid pH will cause an increase in the number of reflux episodes detected, as will reflux-promoting foods containing caffeine or alcohol. Liquid meals tend to reflux more often than solid meals. Feeding at short intervals or continuous feeding will buffer gastric contents and reduce measurable reflux. The pH of medications must be considered. In particular, antacids and histamine receptor antagonists decrease measurable reflux by raising gastric pH. Therapies such as tracheal suctioning, physical therapy, and inhalation treatments often produce reflux episodes.

Maintaining monitoring accuracy for a prolonged time requires durable equipment and some good luck. Electrodes may be inadvertently dislodged and inaccurately replaced. Electrical interference from other equipment in the area can cause inaccurate functioning of pH meter or recording equipment. Extremely hot or cold feedings can change the sensitivity of the pH electrode. Loose connection of the reference electrode to the skin causes artifact. Inadequate observation or inadequate diaries kept by ambulatory patients decrease the information gathered from this lengthy study.

INTERPRETATION OF RESULTS

Methods of interpretation of prolonged esophageal pH monitor recordings vary widely. Only a few published scoring systems have been developed with adequate controls, and few have taken into consideration such basic variables as age, body position, percent of monitored time spent in sleep, feeding frequency, and neurologic status.[24-28] It is generally agreed that an episode of reflux starts when the pH falls below 4.0 and ends when the pH is restored to a value above 4.0. Above pH 4.0 there is little activation of gastric peptic activity. However, some authors define reflux as any sudden drop in pH of one or more units. Some authors consider a drop in pH lasting 15 seconds as an episode, and some count only episodes lasting 60 seconds.

Computer-assisted scoring systems are based to a great extent upon the work of Johnson and Deemester.[27] This system, developed and validated in adults, depends upon six variables—percentage of total monitored time during which the esophageal pH is less than 4.0, percentage of total supine time spent with esophageal pH less than 4.0, percentage of total upright time spent with pH less than 4.0, number of reflux episodes per 24 hours, number of reflux episodes lasting more than 5 minutes per 24 hours, and duration in minutes of the longest episode of reflux. The number of standard deviations by which each patient variable differs from the normal population mean is calculated, and the sum is taken. A score above 12 (two standard deviations from the mean for each of six variables) is considered abnormal. A critical look at these six variables shows that five depend upon reflux episode duration and only one upon reflux episode frequency. This emphasis may be appropriate, since individuals with pathologic reflux are more likely to have delayed acid clearance than increased reflux episode frequency. Occasionally, an entire study may be scored as abnormal on the basis of a single variable (this is particularly true if the patient has one very long episode of reflux in an otherwise normal record). This scoring system may be inappropriate in infants who are fed at frequent intervals and spend most of their time recumbent. Slavish adherence to computer-generated scores without examination of the raw data generally leads to overdiagnosis of GE reflux. Some norms for adults and pediatric patients are shown in Table 1. It should be noted that the infant patients reported in Table 1 were fed frequently with a formula that may have buffered gastric contents, thus masking some reflux episodes.[29] Some scoring systems have attempted to take both the acidity of the reflux episodes and their duration into account under the assumption that peptic damage to the esophagus is a function both of acidity of refluxed material and duration of acid exposure. Computer programs that calculate the "area under the pH 4.0 curve" are available, but the scores derived do not seem to improve on the test's diagnostic accuracy or its correlation with symptoms.[30,31]

Studies of reproducibility have not been performed in pediatric patients. Repeated studies in normal adults indicate that although there may be some variability from test to test in

TABLE 1
Normal Values for 24-Hour Esophageal pH Records in Asymptomatic Infants, Children, and Adults

	Infants[31] (n = 92) (age < 15 days)	Children[14] (n = 11) (mean age—61.5 months)	Adults[27] (n = 15)	Adults[28] (n = 42)
Time pH < 4.0 (%)				
Overall	1.2 ± 9*	3.2 ± 1.9*	1.5 ± 1.3*	2.6 (0–45.2†)
Supine	—	2.9 ± 2.5	0.3 ± 0.5	0.5 (0–26.5)
Upright	—	5.2 ± 5.6	2.3 ± 2.0	3.8 (0–53.3)
Reflux episodes/hr				
Overall	0.3 ± 0.3	0.8 ± 0.4	0.9 ± 0.6	—
Supine	—	0.6 ± 0.4	—	0.1 (0–6.5)
Upright	—	1.7 ± 1.5	—	1.5 (0–10.3)
Reflux episodes > 5 min/24 hr				
Overall	0.6 ± 0.5	3.4 ± 2.6	0.6 ± 1.2	0 (0–21)
Supine	—	1.9 ± 2.1	—	0 (0–4)
Upright	—	4.6 ± 8.2	—	0 (0–17)
Acid clearance time				
Overall	—	2.3 ± 1.0	—	—
Supine	—	2.4 ± 1.1	—	0.5 (0–19.0)
Upright	—	2.0 ± 1.4	—	1.3 (0–4.9)
Duration of longest episode (min)				
Overall	3.8 ± 1.9	—	3.9 ± 2.7	4.5 (0–127.0)
Supine	—	—	—	0.3 (0–29.5)
Upright	—	—	—	4.5 (0–127.0)

*Mean values ±SD.
†Median values (range).
Data from Vandenplas and Sacre-Smits,[31] Sondheimer and Haase,[14] Johnson and Demeester,[27] and Schindlbeck et al.[28]

a single subject, results vary within the normal range.[32] Other extended pH studies in adult patients with reflux indicate that overall scores usually relate directly to symptoms but may not be accurate predictors of the presence of esophagitis.[33-35] Some studies in children have shown a correlation of esophagitis with increased total time of acid exposure (abnormal frequency and clearance of reflux) during sleep.[36] Most studies agree that extended pH monitoring is a more diagnostically accurate test for GE reflux than the upper GI series, esophageal scintiscan, endoscopy, manometry, or short-term pH testing in subjects with typical symptoms. It is assumed by extension that prolonged monitoring is equally accurate in patients without typical symptoms.

UTILITY OF EXTENDED pH MONITORING

When properly performed and carefully analyzed, extended pH recordings provide a wealth of information about the circumstances under which reflux occurs in both normal and abnormal individuals. Study of pH records has pointed out the stepwise return of esophageal pH to normal during clearance and has led to an appreciation of the role of swallowing in acid clearance, which has been confirmed by combined monitoring of esophageal pH and electromyography of the muscles of deglutition.[37] Monitoring of esophageal pH in patients with hiatus hernia has revealed retention of acid in the hernia sac, which may in part explain the tendency for these subjects to have pathologic reflux.[38] Monitoring of esophageal pH simultaneously in several sites has shown that the upper esophagus is also subjected to abnormal acid exposure during reflux, whereas episodes of reflux in normal individuals tend to be limited to the distal esophagus.[39] Prolonged monitoring of gastric pH has proved useful in assessing effectiveness of antacid medications.[40] It was hoped that a combination of esophageal pH monitoring with cardiac, respiratory, and EEG monitoring would quickly reveal the cause of infant apnea spells. Although there is some indication that infants with repetitive unexplained apneic spells have a higher incidence of pathologic pH studies, particularly during sleep, there is yet no convincing proof that GE reflux is the consistent cause of infant apnea spells.[41,42] Similarly, infants and children with asthma have been shown to have a higher incidence of pathologic reflux by 24-hour pH monitoring, but these studies have not proved that the pathologic reflux is a cause of bronchospasm.[43]

REFERENCES

1. Tuttle SG, Grossman MI. Detection of gastroesophageal reflux by simultaneous measurement of intraluminal pressure and pH. Proc Soc Biol Med 1958; 98:225–227.
2. Edwall G. Improved antimony-antimony (III) oxide pH electrodes. Med Biol Eng Comput 1978; 16:661–669.
3. Ask P, Edwall G, Tibbing L. Combined pH and pressure measurement device for oesophageal investigations. Med Biol Eng Comput 1981; 19:443–446.
4. Markdahl-Bjarme M, Edwall G. Modified conventional type of pCO_2 electrode with monocrystalline antimony as the pH sensing element. Med Biol Eng Comput 1981; 19:447–456.
5. Anderson J, Naesdal J, Strom M. Similar 24-hour intragastric pH profiles with antimony and glass electrodes compared with aspirated gastric juice. Gastroenterology 1988; 94:A7.
6. Falor WH, Chang B, White HA, Kraus JM, Taylor B, Hamsel JR, Kraus FC. Twenty-four hour esophageal pH monitoring by telemetry. Am J Surg 1981; 142:514–516.
7. Braniki FJ, Evans DF, Ogilvie AL. Ambulatory monitoring of oesophageal pH in reflux oesophagitis using a portable radiotelemetry system. Gut 1982; 23:992–998.
8. Troxell RB, Kohn SR, Gray JE, Welch RB, Harloe ED, Goyal RK. A computer assisted technique for 24 hour esophageal monitoring. Dig Dis Sci 1982; 27:1057–1062.
9. Herbst JJ. Gastroesophageal reflux. J Pediatr 1981; 98:859–870.
10. Meyers WF, Roberts CC, Johnson DG, Herbst JJ. Value of tests for evaluation of gastroesophageal reflux in children. J Pediatr Surg 1985; 20:515–520.
11. Strickland AD, Chang JHT. Results of treatment of gastroesophageal reflux with bethanechol. J Pediatr 1983; 103:311–315.
12. Werlin SL, Dodds WJ, Hogan WJ, Arndorfer RC. Mechanisms of gastroesophageal reflux in children. J Pediatr 1980; 97:244–249.
13. Strobel CT, Byrne WJ, Ament ME, Euler AR. Correlation of esophageal lengths in children with height: application of the Tuttle test without prior esophageal manometry. J Pediatr 1979; 94:81–86.
14. Sondheimer JM, Haase GA. Simultaneous pH recordings from multiple sites in children with and without distal gastroesophageal reflux. J Pediatr Gastroenterol Nutr 1988; 7:46–51.
15. Reyes HM, Ostrovsky E, Radhakrishnan J. Diagnostic accuracy of a 3-hour continuous intraluminal pH monitoring of the lower esophagus in the evaluation of gastro-esophageal reflux in infancy. J Pediatr Surg 1982; 17:626–631.
16. Jolley SG, Herbst JJ, Johnson DG, Book LS, Matlak ME, Condon VR. Patterns of post-cibal gastroesophageal reflux in symptomatic infants. Am J Surg 1979; 138:946–950.
17. Kaye MD. Post-prandial gastro-oesophageal reflux in healthy people. Gut 1977; 18:709–712.
18. Euler AR, Ament ME. Detection of gastroesophageal reflux in the pediatric age patient by esophageal intraluminal pH probe measurement (Tuttle test). Pediatrics 1977; 60:65–68.
19. Skinner DB, Booth DJ. Assessment of distal esophageal function in patients with hiatal hernia and/or gastroesophageal reflux. Am Surg 1970; 172:627–637.
20. Stanciu C, Hoare RC, Bennett JR. Correlation between manometric and pH tests for gastro-oesophageal reflux. Gut 1977; 18:536–540.
21. Sondheimer JM. Clearance of spontaneous gastroesophageal reflux in awake and sleeping infants: role of swallowing and esophageal peristalsis. Gastroenterology 1989; 97:821.
22. Sondheimer JM. Personal observation.
23. Vandenplas Y, Sacre-Smits L. Seventeen hour continuous esophageal pH monitoring in the newborn: evaluation of the influence of position in asymptomatic and symptomatic babies. J Pediatr Gastroenterol Nutr 1985; 4:356–361.
24. Sondheimer JM. Continuous monitoring of distal esophageal pH: a diagnostic test for gastroesophageal reflux in infants. J Pediatr 1980; 96:804–807.
25. Jolley SG, Johnson DG, Herbst JJ, Alberto-Pena R, Garnier R. An assessment of gastroesophageal reflux in children by extended pH monitoring of the distal esophagus. Surgery 1978; 84:16–24.
26. Euler AR, Byrne WJ. Twenty-four hour esophageal intraluminal pH probe testing: a comparative analysis. Gastroenterology 1981; 80:957–961.
27. Johnson LF, Demeester TR. Twenty-four hour pH monitoring of the distal esophagus, a quantitative measure of gastroesophageal reflux. Am J Gastroenterol 1974; 62:325–332.
28. Schindlbeck NE, Heinrich C, Konig A, Dendorfer A, Pace F. Müller-Lissner SA. Optimal thresholds, sensitivity and specificity of long-term pH-metry for the detection of gastroesophageal reflux disease. Gastroenterology 1987; 93:85–90.
29. Wallin L, Madsen T, Boesby T, Sorensen O. Gasto-oesophageal acid reflux and oesophageal peristalsis. Method for 12 hour simultaneous recording of pH and peristaltic activity in the esophagus. Scand J Gastroenterol 1979; 14:481–487.
30. Vandenplas Y, Franckx-Goosens A, Pipeleers-Marichal M, Darde MP, Sacre-Smits L. Area under pH 4: advantages of a new parameter in the interpretation of esophageal pH data infants. J Pediatr Gastroenterol Nutr 1989; 9:34–39.
31. Vandenplas Y, Sacre-Smits L. Continuous 24-hour esophageal pH monitoring in 285 asymptomatic infants 0-15 months old. J Pediatr Gastroenterol Nutr 1987; 6:220–224.

32. Boesby S. Continuous esophageal pH recording and acid clearing test: a study of reproducibility. Gut 1977; 12:245–247.
33. Schlesinger PK, Donahue PE, Schmid B, Layden TJ. Limitations of 24-hour intraesophageal pH monitoring in the hospital setting. Gastroenterology 1985; 89:797–804.
34. Irvin TT, Perez-Avila C. Diagnosis of symptomatic gastroesophageal reflux by prolonged monitoring of the lower esophageal pH. Scand J Gastroenterol 1977; 12:715–720.
35. Hyams JS, Ricci A, Leichtner AM. Clinical and laboratory correlates of esophagitis in young children. J Pediatr Gastroenterol Nutr 1988; 7:52–56.
36. Baer M, Maki M, Nurminen J, Turjanmaa V, Pukander J. Vesikari T. Esophagitis and findings of long term esophageal pH recording in children with repeated lower respiratory tract symptoms. J Pediatr Gastroenterol Nutr 1986; 5:187–190.
37. Helm JF, Dodds WF, Pelc LR, Palmer DW, Hogan WJ, Teeter BC. Effect of esophageal emptying and saliva on clearance of acid from the esophagus. N Engl J Med 1984; 310:284–288.
38. Mittal RK, Lange RC, McCallum RW. Identification and mechanism of delayed esophageal acid clearance in subjects with hiatus hernia. Gastroenterology 1987; 92:130–135.
39. Ferrarini F, Longanesi A, Angeloni M, Ragazzini M, Oletti-Montanari M, Barbara L. Extension of acid gastroesophageal reflux and its relation with symptoms: an assessment with double esophageal pH recording. Gastroenterology 1988; 94:A19.
40. Sutphen JL, Dillard VL, Pipan ME. Antacid and formula effects on gastric acidity in infants with gastroesophageal reflux. Pediatrics 1986; 78:55–57.
41. Ariagno RL, Guilleminault C, Baldwin R, Owen-Boeddiker M. Movement and gastroesophageal reflux in awake term infants with "near miss" SIDS unrelated to apnea. J Pediatr 1982; 100:894–897.
42. Walsh JK, Farrell MK, Keenan WJ, Lucas M, Kramer M. Gastroesophageal reflux in infants: relation to apnea. J Pediatr 1981; 99:197–201.
43. Orenstein SR, Orenstein DM. Gastroesophageal reflux and respiratory disease in children. J Pediatr 1988; 112:847–858.

CHAPTER 35

Gastric Function Tests

Paul E. Hyman, M.D.

GASTRIC ACID SECRETION

The relatively noninvasive methods required for the collection of gastric contents make gastric secretory testing a useful means of investigating the development of specific physiologic functions. The gastric mucosa secretes hydrochloric acid, bicarbonate, mucus, enzymes (pepsinogens and lipases), and a number of regulatory peptides and eicosanoids. The ease of measuring hydrogen ion concentration in the collected samples and the simplicity of interpreting the unidirectional outward flux of hydrogen ions have fostered enthusiasm for the study of gastric acid secretion in infants. The disadvantages to the study of in vivo human gastric acid secretion as a model of developmental change are the inability to control the variety of complex regulatory interactions of neural, hormonal, and paracrine origin and to differentiate primary from secondary effects.

Indications

Gastric secretory testing in infants and children is used most often for research purposes to assess normal developmental changes and perturbations of normal function, such as the effects of drugs or disease states on acid secretion.

Clinical utility for gastric secretory testing often relates to the assessment of children with conditions associated with gastric acid hypersecretion. Children whose ulcers fail to heal with treatment are candidates for acid secretory studies and fasting serum gastrin determinations. Gastric acid hypersecretion is associated with recurrent or intractable peptic ulcer disease or esophagitis.[1-3] In patients with giant gastric rugal hypertrophy, acid secretory testing is useful for defining the presence of hypersecretion or protein-losing gastropathy, as an adjunct in the diagnosis of the Zollinger-Ellison syndrome and Ménétrier's disease. After acid hypersecretion is identified in a child with recurrent or refractory peptic ulcer disease, effective medical treatment is determined by repeated acid secretory tests, titrating the dosage of antisecretory medication to achieve the desired suppression of acid secretion.

Methods

Neonates are fasted for at least one feeding before study of basal secretion.[4,5] Older infants and children fast overnight before gastric secretory studies. Medications that might affect secretion, such as histamine H_2-receptor antagonists and anticholinergics, are discontinued for at least 24 hours prior to study, but longer periods may be required depending on drug metabolism. Intravenous infusions of glucose and electrolyte solutions may be used to maintain a normal fluid balance. Solutions containing amino acids and calcium are discontinued because they may stimulate acid secretion.[6]

Continuous Aspiration of Gastric Contents

This method is employed for studies of acid, pepsin, and intrinsic factor secretion in the basal state and following drugs. It cannot be used for studies evaluating the effect of meals or gastric distention. A vented plastic tube with several orifices is best for collecting gastric secretions. Infant feeding tubes may be necessary for the study of very small infants, but unvented tubes are more likely than vented tubes to induce traumatic bleeding from the gastric mucosa. When using unvented tubes the attendant injects small volumes of air intermittently into the tube. Aspiration of the injected air serves to verify proper tube placement and patency. Neonates appear to be most comfortable when the tube is positioned through the oropharynx, but older infants and children favor nasogastric placement. Positioning the tube in the most dependent portion of the stomach is important for ensuring that the collection is accurate. Tube position may be verified by fluoroscopy or assumed to be correct after the immediate and complete recovery of a bolus of water instilled after the stomach is emptied of residual contents. Gastric secretions are collected continuously by hand aspiration or with a suction pump applying cycles of intermittent negative pressure. The stomach should be empty at the start of the test. Secretions are collected continuously and saved in 10- or 15-minute periods.

Basal Acid Output. Aliquots of aspirated gastric juice are collected for 1 hour. Normal values are proportional to weight and range from 10 to 70 μmol per kilogram per hour.[2] Basal acid output varies during the day, depending on the state of arousal and diurnal rhythms as well as other factors. Periods of no acid secretion occur in normal infants and children, but achlorhydria is rare except in very sick or very preterm infants.

Pentagastrin-Stimulated Acid Output. The synthetic, nonantigenic, carboxy-terminal pentapeptide of gastrin retains full biologic activity of the naturally occurring peptide gastrin. In adults pentagastrin stimulates maximal acid output. It is not clear that pentagastrin stimulates maximal acid output in neonates, because pentagastrin fails to stimulate acid secretion in healthy 1-day-old infants,[5] but gastric distention with sugar water or a complex liquid meal increases acid secretion twofold above basal.[7] In neonates it is appropriate to define acid secretion in the hour following pentagastrin as pentagastrin-stimulated acid output rather than maximal acid output. In toddlers and children this distinction is unnecessary. A subcutaneous injection of 2 mg per kilogram is equal in effect to a dose of 6 mg per kilogram.[2] The time course of effect appears to be similar to the time course in adults following subcutaneous injection, the peak in secretion occurring after 20 minutes and the effect waning after an hour.[7,8] Pentagastrin appears to be a safe drug, even in preterm infants. Side effects reported in adults include nausea, sweating, abdominal cramps, lightheadedness, and, rarely, hypotension. A mature response with increases to pentagastrin of fivefold or more over basal develops by 1 year of age. Normal values for pentagastrin-stimulated acid output range from 150 to 450 μmol per kilogram per hour.[2,7]

Histalog-Stimulated Acid Output.[4] Until pentagastrin became available, the stimulant favored for studies of acid secretion was Histalog (Eli Lilly and Co.). Pain at the injection site is common. Other side effects include dizziness, nausea, palpitations, abdominal cramps, headache, and flushing. Hypotension following a 2 mg per kilogram dose occurred in 2.5 percent of adults tested. The acid secretory responses to Histalog and pentagastrin are equivalent, but Histalog has a higher rate of side effects. Pentagastrin is preferred for clinical studies because of its safety profile.

Analysis of Acid Secretory Studies. The volume and pH of each sample are recorded. Using an autotitrator, 1.0-ml samples of gastric aspirate are titrated to pH 7.0 with 0.01 N NaOH to provide the number of equivalents of acid per milliliter. Multiplying the equivalents of acid per milliliter by the total volume of the aspirated sample gives the total acid output for that sample. Basal acid output consists of addition of samples from 1 hour of unstimulated collection. Maximal acid output consists of the acid in the samples from the hour following administration of pentagastrin. Peak acid output is an attempt to express the results as the highest rate of acid secretion attainable. Peak acid output is calculated by adding the two highest 10- or 15-minute periods following pentagastrin administration. This result is then multiplied by a factor of 2 or 3 so that results are expressed as equivalents per hour or equivalents per kilogram per hour. The ratio of basal to maximal acid output is useful in the differential diagnosis of Zollinger-Ellison syndrome. In Zollinger-Ellison syndrome basal acid hypersecretion co-exists with a basal to maximal acid output ratio greater than 0.6.

Marker Dilution Techniques

To measure secretion in response to meals, a nonabsorbable marker is added to the meal, so that gastric volume and secretion can be calculated from the changes in marker concentration. Phenol red is a commonly used marker with the advantage that visible light spectrophotometry can be used to determine marker concentration but the disadvantage that the meal must be transparent in order to avoid contributing to the measurement of optical density. Polyethylene glycol is used as a marker for studies of the effects of complex, opaque liquids such as infant formula.[9] The concentration of polyethylene glycol is determined by a turbidometric method.[10] Samples are titrated to determine gastric acid concentration. Subtracting the volume of secretions from the total intragastric volume, provides an estimate of the amount emptied from the stomach (see below). A mathematical correction in total acid secretion to include the volume emptied into the duodenum results in higher values for basal acid secretion using dye dilution than using aspiration.[11]

Extragastric Titration[7]

One of two ways to measure acid secretion in response to meals in children, extragastric titration was an adaptation of the intragastric titration method used to measure meal-stimulated acid secretion in adults.[12] Using a double-lumen tube with afferent and efferent channels, gastric contents are continuously circulated to and from an extragastric mixing chamber. NaOH is added in the mixing chamber to maintain pH 5.5, and the quantity of NaOH added corresponds to the acid secreted. Results are expressed as acid neutralized per unit of time.

Intrinsic Factor Secretion

Intrinsic factor is a glycoprotein that avidly binds cobalamin (vitamin B_{12}) in an acid environment. Intrinsic factor secretion from parietal cells is stimulated by the same agonists that stimulate acid secretion. This relationship is maintained in infants.[4] The Schilling test (part 1, without intrinsic factor) is an in vivo bioassay establishing the presence or absence of biologically active intrinsic factor. There are in vitro methods to quantitate intrinsic factor in gastric juice, utilizing either functional or immunologic approaches.

Pepsinogen Secretion

Pepsinogens are a group of at least seven different acid proteinases secreted by the gastric mucosa. Gastric chief cells secrete pepsinogens in response to the same agonists that simulate acid secretion. After adjusting for body weight, Histalog-stimulated pepsinogen secretion in infants is well below adult values but increases with postnatal age.[4] In studies using a marker dilution technique, a formula meal given to 3- to 4-week-old preterm infants stimulated pepsinogen secretion.[13] There are several assays for estimating total pepsinogen activity by quantitating the ability of gastric juice to release trichloroacetic acid–soluble peptides from a protein substrate. No proteolytic assay is specific for a single pepsinogen, and none provides optimal conditions for the determination of all molecular forms. Individual pepsinogens may be measured by specific radioimmunoassay. There is no known clinical utility to gastric pepsinogen determination in the pediatric patient.

INTRAGASTRIC pH MONITORING[14]

Microelectrodes positioned in the stomach record intragastric pH continuously. Results from intragastric pH monitoring are not good estimates of acid secretion except at neutral pH values, because during fasting intragastric pH is normally 1.0 to 2.0, and rates of acid secretion are related to the volume secreted, a parameter not assessed by pH monitoring. There may be clinical utility in intragastric pH monitoring for patients whose intragastric hydrogen ion concentration must be maintained above a specific pH, as in patients with stress-associated gastrointestinal bleeding in an intensive care setting. Titration of antisecretory drugs or antacids may be done with added accuracy using intragastric pH monitoring. Care must be taken to ensure that the electrode floats free in the gastric lumen and does not become wedged between gastric folds, causing a false recording.

SERUM GASTRIN

The most apparent effect of gastrin is stimulation of gastric acid secretion, although the peptide also has trophic effects on the gastric mucosa and effects on motility. Gastrin is synthesized by and secreted mainly from antral G cells. In the human fetus, gastrin is found in higher concentration in the duodenum than in the antrum.[15] Gastrin is measured routinely by highly sensitive and specific antisera.[16] Gastrin is released in response to meals and to activation of neural reflexes and by circulating catecholamines. Fasting serum gastrin concentrations in neonates are twice the adult values. Hypergastrinemia is found in children with gastrin-producing tumors and sometimes after massive bowel resection.

Clinical indications for measuring serum gastrin relate to the diagnosis of Zollinger-Ellison syndrome in children with recurrent or severe peptic ulcer disease. In the majority of patients with symptomatic gastrinomas, fasting serum gastrin concentrations are greater than 500 pg per milliliter, or more than twice the upper limit of normal in most laboratories. A few patients have values between normal and 500 pg per milliliter. Because antisecretory medications may result in achlorhydria, which in turn stimulates gastrin secretion, histamine H_2-receptor antagonists are discontinued prior to measuring serum gastrin. The hormone secretin is used as a provocative test when results of fasting gastrin determinations are equivocal. Secretin, which has no effect on serum gastrin in normal individuals, stimulates gastrin secretion in patients with gastrinomas.[17] An intravenous bolus of 2 IU per kilogram GIH secretin (Pharmacia, Inc.) is injected, and blood is drawn before the injection and at 2, 5, 10, 15, and 30 minutes following injection. Increases in serum gastrin concentration greater than 200 pg per milliliter above mean basal values are strong evidence for the presence of a gastrinoma.

GASTRIC EMPTYING TESTS

There are difficulties in standardizing gastric emptying tests for pediatric patients. There is no general agreement concerning a correct test meal volume or composition. Lack of patient co-operation is a serious problem for studies that require voluntary immobility. Do the stomachs of agitated toddlers empty at the same rate as the stomachs of sleeping toddlers? How is the study interpreted if a portion of the test meal is vomited? Each laboratory or testing center develops a set of normal values based on expectations and independent experience.

Indications. As with acid secretory testing, most published gastric emptying studies in infants and children were designed to investigate developmental changes or abnormalities related to specific pathologic conditions.

The major clinical indications for studies of gastric emptying in infants and children is to assess the contribution of delayed gastric emptying to symptomatic gastroesophageal reflux. Since gastric emptying is delayed in a substantial minority of patients with gastroesophageal reflux,[18] gastric emptying studies should be considered in pediatric patients deemed candidates for fundoplication. In patients with a prolonged delay in gastric emptying, fundoplication may result in difficulty in vomiting and, when added to gastroparesis, may be associated with symptoms including repeated retching, abdominal distention, and pain. Gastric emptying studies are indicated for patients with unexplained nausea or vomiting and in patients with suspected dumping syndrome. The effect of motility drugs to aid gastric emptying can be assessed by repeated studies.

Radiologic Methods.[19] Radiopaque meals of barium or iodinated contrast medium provide information concerning the anatomy of the stomach and the presence or absence of a physical obstruction but cannot be used for quantitative estimates of gastric emptying. Two-dimensional films poorly estimate intragastric volume.

Gastric Aspiration.[20] A tracer amount of nonabsorbable marker substance is mixed with the test meal. The volume of the meal V_M and the concentration of marker in the meal C_M are known. At a predetermined time following administration of the meal, a nasogastric tube is placed into the stomach and the gastric contents are completely aspirated. Gastric emptying is calculated from the concentration of marker in the gastric aspirate C_G and is reported as the volume of the meal remaining in the stomach V_G, according to the following formula:

$$V_G = V_M \, (C_M / C_G)$$

The test must be repeated with different times of aspiration on different days in order to obtain a complete time course of emptying. The nonabsorbable marker chosen for use depends on the meal: The pH indicator dye phenol red is used when test meals are clear liquids, and polyethylene glycol is used when test meals are opaque liquids. Gamma-emitting radionuclides are used infrequently in aspiration method studies because of the radiation dose to the patient and relative inconvenience to the investigators, but radionuclides may be utilized to mark any test meal,[21] including solids. The major disadvantage to serial testing is that it takes several days to complete a time course of emptying. The aspiration method does not estimate the contributions of swallowed saliva or gastric secretions to the intragastric volume.

Marker Dilution Method.[22] The marker dilution method utilizes repeated sampling of gastric contents to calculate the intragastric volume without the need to empty the stomach. Samples are taken before and after addition of a small volume V_2 of concentrated marker C_2 to the stomach. V_1, the volume in the stomach, can be calculated from the equation:

$$V_1C_1 + V_2C_2 = (V_1 + V_2)C_3$$

where C_1 is the concentration of marker from the gastric sample before addition of concentrated marker and C_3 is the concentration of marker from the gastric sample aspirated after addition of the concentrated marker. Solving for V_1:

$$V_1 = V_2(C_2 - C_3/C_3 - C_1)$$

This procedure is repeated at predetermined intervals. A number of assumptions are made concerning this method (and the aspiration method, above): (1) Markers are not absorbed, adsorbed, secreted, or digested in the stomach; (2) mixing of injected marker with the gastric contents is rapid and complete; (3) the rate of emptying of the marker is identical to the rate of emptying of the meal; (4) there is no emptying or secretion during the mixing and sampling periods. The final assumption creates a large error when the gastric volume is small or if secretions are large. Mathematical corrections for the error can be performed, providing an assessment of volume secretion.[11,23]

An advantage of marker-dilution methods over radionuclide scanning is that with marker-dilution testing the volume of secretions can be calculated from the data; moreover, when concentrations of a solute are determined in each sample, the amount of solute secretion can be calculated. Most commonly, hydrogen ion is the solute of interest, and rates of gastric acid secretion, volume secretion, and gastric emptying are assessed simultaneously.[11]

Marker dilution tests require considerable preparation before testing, precision and nearly constant attention from the operator during the procedure, followed by a laboratory analysis of two samples from each time point and computer analysis of the data. Because of the time and multidisciplinary expertise required for satisfactory execution, the marker dilution method is rarely used in routine clinical assessment.

Radionuclide Imaging. Radionuclide studies are used for the clinical evaluation of gastric emptying in pediatric patients in most medical centers. Patient acceptability is high, because intubation of the stomach is unnecessary. Physicians favor radionuclide studies over marker dilution techniques because of the availability of nuclear medicine facilities and the rapid access to results.

^{99m}Tc-sulfur colloid is mixed with the meal that is fed to the patient. The rate of gastric emptying is estimated from the emissions recorded by a gamma camera. The camera is focused over a specific "area of interest" that corresponds to the stomach. Upon entry into the camera, photons emitted by the radionuclide are filtered through a collimator, which directs them to a detector. A two-dimensional image of the radioactivity is created and transformed into an electrical signal, which is amplified by the photomultiplier. The electrical signal is proportional to the amount of radionuclide present in the area of interest. The signal is visualized as an image and recorded for quantitative analysis by computer. It is possible to study the emptying of solid food or the emptying of solids and liquids simultaneously (using two radionuclide markers), but in studies of pediatric patients liquid meals such as water,[24] apple juice,[25] or milk[26] have been typical.

Inaccuracy in this method may be related to lack of cooperation by the pediatric patient. It is important that the meal be completed quickly, so that the initial images of the stomach record the maximal number of counts present before gastric emptying has progressed. Infants and toddlers may not drink on command or finish quickly, and the use of nasogastric feeding for the radionuclide study is undesirable. Body movement in any direction changes the position of the camera relative to the stomach, creating inaccurate acquisition of counts, but most young children find it difficult to remain motionless for the 30-minute to 1-hour study period.

Another inaccuracy is due to the acquisition of counts in a two-dimensional image from a three-dimensional object. The amount of radioactivity that is measured varies with the depth and thickness of the tissue. The gastric fundus is more posterior and the antrum more anterior. To correct for this problem in adults, two cameras—one anterior and one posterior—are employed simultaneously. In children who cannot sit, the two-camera approach is not possible. There are no standards for meal content or volume. Each facility designs a protocol and develops normal values from experience.

Sonography. Sonography has the advantage of high patient acceptability because it requires neither gastric intubation nor radiation exposure. In studies of adults the total gastric volume is measured by rapidly moving the ultrasound probe along the longitudinal axis of the stomach. Measurements of the area of the stomach are acquired in successive planes, and these are used to reconstruct the appearance of the stomach and estimate intragastric volume. This procedure is repeated at predetermined times to provide a time course of gastric emptying. The contribution of secretion to gastric volume cannot be determined. Because gas reflects ultrasound in all directions, the stomach must be full of liquid at the time of study.

In infants it was possible to estimate gastric volume after a meal based on the assumption that the lateral and anteroposterior diameters of the gastric antrum were linearly related to the gastric volume.[27] The diameters immediately following the meal were maximal, and measurements repeated every 15 minutes were expressed as percent of maximal.

Analysis of Gastric Emptying Results. In most cases the gastric emptying of liquids is best described by the simple exponential curve: $f = ae^{-kt}$. In this equation f is the fraction of the meal in the stomach at time t, a is the fraction present at $t = 0$, e is the constant 2.718, and k is the rate of gastric emptying. For individual gastric emptying tests the gastric volumes at each time point are analyzed by nonlinear least squares regression to solve for k. One goal of analysis is to characterize individual curves so that one or two parameters can be used to describe the time course. One means of achieving this goal is to calculate $t_{1/2}$, the time required for half the meal to empty. Following the solution of the equation for k, f is set to 50 percent to find $t_{1/2}$. Another choice is to determine the percent of the meal remaining at predetermined times during and at the completion of the test. A final alternative is to determine the fractional emptying rate k for the period between each time point and express the data as the mean fractional emptying rate.

REFERENCES

1. Christie DL, Ament ME. Gastric acid secretion in children with duodenal ulcer. Gastroenterology 1976; 70:242–244.

2. Euler AR, Byrne WJ, Campbell MF. Basal and pentagastrin-stimulated gastric acid secretory rates in normal children and in those with peptic ulcer disease. J Pediatr 1983; 103:766–768.
3. Tam PHK, Saing H. Gastric acid secretion and emptying rates in children with duodenal ulcer. J Pediatr Surg 1986; 21:129–131.
4. Agunod M, Yamaguchi N, Lopez R, Luhby L, Glass GBJ. Correlative study of hydrochloric acid, pepsin, and intrinsic factor secretion in newborns and infants. Am J Dig Dis 1969; 14:400–414.
5. Euler AR, Byrne WJ, Meis PJ, Leake RD, Ament ME. Basal and pentagastrin-stimulated acid secretion in newborn infants. Pediatr Res 1979; 13:36–37.
6. Hyman PE, Everett SL, Harada T. Intravenous amino acids and stimulation of gastric acid secretion in infants. J Pediatr Gastroenterol Nutr 1986; 5:62–65.
7. Harada T, Hyman PE, Everett SL, Ament ME. Meal-stimulated gastric acid secretion in infants. J Pediatr 1984; 104:534–538.
8. Lari J, Lister J, Duthie HL. Response to gastrin pentapeptide in children. J Pediatr Surg 1968; 3:682–689.
9. Cavell B. Postprandial gastric acid secretion in infants. Acta Paediatr Scand 1983; 72:857–860.
10. Malawer SJ, Powell DW. An improved turbidometric analysis of polyethylene glycol utilizing an emulsifier. Gastroenterology 1967; 53:250–256.
11. Hyman PE, Abrams C, Dubois A. Effect of metoclopramide and bethanechol on gastric emptying in children. Pediatr Res 1985; 19:1029–1032.
12. Richardson CT, Walsh JH, Hicks MI, Fordtran JS. Studies on the mechanism of food-stimulated gastric acid secretion in normal human subjects. J Clin Invest 1976; 58:623–630.
13. Yahav J, Carrion V, Lee PC, Lebenthal E. Meal-stimulated pepsinogen secretion in premature infants. J Pediatr 1987; 110:949–951.
14. Sondheimer JM, Clark DA, Gervaise EP. Continuous gastric pH measurement in young and older preterm infants receiving formula and clear liquid feedings. J Pediatr Gastroenterol Nutr 1985; 4:352–355.
15. Larsson LI, Rehfeld JF, Goltermann N. Gastrin in the human fetus. Distribution and molecular forms of gastrin in the antro-pyloric gland area, duodenum and pancreas. Scand J Gastroenterol 1977; 12:869–872.
16. Rosenquist G, Walsh J. Radioimmunoassay of gastrin. In: Jerzy Glass GB, ed. Gastrointestinal hormones, Vol 33. New York: Raven Press, 1980: 769.
17. McGuigan JE, Wolfe MM. Secretin injection test in the diagnosis of gastrinoma. Gastroenterology 1980; 79:1324–1327.
18. Hillemeier AC, Lange R, McCallum R, Seashore J, Gryboski J. Delayed gastric emptying in infants with gastroesophageal reflux. J Pediatr 1981; 98:190–193.
19. Schell NB, Karelitz S. Epstein BS. Radiographic study of gastric emptying in premature infants. J Pediatr 1963; 66:342.
20. Husband J, Husband P. Gastric emptying of water and glucose solutions in the newborn. Lancet 1969; ii:409–411.
21. Sidebottom R, Curran JS, Williams PR, Kanarek KS, Bramson RT. Effects of long-chain vs medium-chain triglycerides on gastric emptying time in premature infants. J Pediatr 1983; 102:448–450.
22. George JD. New clinical method for measuring the rate of gastric emptying: the double sampling test meal. Gut 1968; 9:237–242.
23. Seigal M, Lebenethal E, Topper W, Krantz B, Li PK. Gastric emptying in prematures of isocaloric feedings with differing osmolalities. Pediatr Res 1982; 16:141–147.
24. Guillet J, Basse-Cathalinat B, Christophe E, Ducassou D, Blanquet P, Wynchank S. Routine studies of swallowed radionuclide transit in pediatrics: experience with 400 patients. Eur J Nucl Med 1984; 9:886–890.
25. Jolley SG, Leonard JC, Tunnell WP. Gastric emptying in children with gastroesophageal reflux. I. An estimate of effective gastric emptying. J Pediatr Surg 1987; 22:923–926.
26. Heyman S, Kirkpatrick JA, Winter HS, Treves S. An improved radionuclide method for the diagnosis of gastroesophageal reflux and aspiration in children (milk scan). Radiology 1979; 131:479–482.
27. Lambrecht L. Ultrasonic evaluation of gastric clearing and of hypertrophic pyloric stenosis in infants. Vern K Acad Geneska Belg 1978; 49:345–370.

CHAPTER 36

Pancreatic Function Tests

Richard Couper, M.B., Ch.B., F.R.A.C.P.,
Peter R. Durie, B.Sc., M.D., FRCPC

Exocrine pancreatic function is notoriously difficult to assess. In practical terms, the organ and its secretions are relatively inaccessible, and direct assessment requires duodenal intubation to collect pancreatic secretions. The other obstacle rendering assessment difficult is the enormous functional reserve capacity of the exocrine pancreas. Digestive enzymes are synthesized and secreted by the pancreatic acini in considerable excess. Considerable reduction of exocrine pancreatic function must occur before nutrients are malassimilated and the functional loss becomes a homeostatic threat. Di Magno et al[1] found in adult patients that steatorrhea and creatorrhea did not occur unless lipase and trypsin outputs, respectively, were less than 10 percent of normal control values. Similarly, in pediatric patients with cystic fibrosis and Shwachman's syndrome, Gaskin et al[2] found that lipase and co-lipase outputs had to be less than 2 percent and less than 1 percent of normal values, respectively, before steatorrhea was apparent. The corollary is that between 98 and 99 percent of pancreatic reserve for lipase and co-lipase must be lost before fat maldigestion is evident.

Steatorrhea is a useful indicator of pancreatic function. Patients are pancreatic-insufficient if steatorrhea is present, which is defined as a fecal fat output in excess of 7 percent of ingested fat. These patients, by definition, have lost more than 98 percent of pancreatic reserve for lipase and co-lipase. Patients are pancreatic-sufficient if steatorrhea is absent and may have pancreatic function in excess of 2 percent of normal. Pancreatic-insufficient subjects can be detected reliably by a variety of tests. The challenge has been to develop a test that evaluates the range of function in pancreatic-sufficient subjects.

TESTS OF EXOCRINE PANCREATIC FUNCTION

There are three categories of exocrine pancreatic function tests (Table 1):

Direct tests assess the secretory capacity of the exocrine pancreas. Pancreatic secretions are collected via small intestinal intubation, usually under stimulated conditions, and analyzed for the output of water, ions, and enzymes. Stimulation of the pancreas allows an accurate assessment of pancreatic functional reserve. Collection of unstimulated secretions from a rested organ provides little information.

Indirect tests detect abnormalities secondary to loss of pancreatic function such as the maldigestion and consequent malabsorption of fat and/or nitrogen. Alternatively, they

TABLE 1
Tests of Exocrine Pancreatic Function

Direct Tests
- Exogenous hormonal stimulants
  - Secretin
  - Cholecystokinin*
  - Cerulein*
  - Bombesin*
- Nutrient stimulants
  - Lundh test meal
  - Fatty acids
  - Amino acids
  - Hydrochloric acid
  - Bile salts
- Other tests
  - ^{75}Se-methionine incorporation and release
  - Pure pancreatic juice
  - Haptocorrin

Indirect Tests
- Stool
  - Microscopy—fat, meat fibers
  - Steatocrit
  - Fecal balance studies
  - Excretion of ^{131}I-triolein
  - Dual radiolabeled fat
  - Trypsin, chymotrypsin
- Breath tests
  - ^{14}C-lipids
  - ^{13}C-lipids
  - ^{14}C-cholesterol octanoate
  - Starch breath hydrogen tests
- Urinary/plasma markers
  - Bentiromide
  - Fluorescein dilaurate (pancreolauryl)
  - Oral tolerance tests (fat and vitamins)
  - Dual-label Schilling test
  - Urinary lactulose

Blood Tests
- Total amylase or lipase
- Isoamylase
- Cationic/anionic trypsinogen
- Pancreatic polypeptide

*Used in various dose combinations with or without secretin.

depend upon the ability of pancreatic enzymes to cleave specific synthetic substrates, generating absorbable, measurable end-products that are detectable in breath, in serum, or in urine. Additionally, pancreatic enzymes such as chymotrypsin are relatively nonbiodegradable and can be detected in the stool.

Blood tests depend upon the fact that a small but significant proportion of the enzymes and enteroendocrine hormones that are synthesized by the pancreas enter the systemic circulation. In certain circumstances, the serum concentration of specific pancreatic enzymes, such as immunoreactive trypsinogen, and specific hormones, such as pancreatic polypeptide, may reflect residual exocrine pancreatic function.

The criteria for an ideal pancreatic function test are listed in Table 2. All currently available tests of pancreatic function have at least one (in most cases several) major drawback. Direct pancreatic function tests are expensive, invasive, unsuitable for longitudinal evaluation, and poorly reproducible between laboratories, and pancreatic enzyme supplements interfere with the test. However, because they are specific for pancreatic disease, define the exact level of pancreatic function, and are the only tests capable of delineating the range of function in pancreatic-sufficient subjects, they are the yardstick against which other tests are measured. Because of the manifest disadvantages of the direct tests, considerable ingenuity has been applied to the development of indirect tests. Currently available indirect tests often fail to discriminate between pancreatic disease and other causes for nutrient malassimilation. They also often fail to evaluate the degree of functional impairment in pancreatic-sufficient patients, and because the pancreas is usually unstimulated they do not evaluate functional reserve.

DIRECT TESTS

The exocrine pancreas secretes fluid and ions in response to endogenous secretin and enzymes in response to endogenous cholecystokinin (CCK). Endogenous secretin and CCK are released from small intestinal mucosa exposed to nutrients or gastric acid. The pancreas is also stimulated by neural pathways. It is supplied by vagal efferents that act on muscarinic receptors. Intestinal nutrients provoke stimulation of enzyme secretion via this pathway as well as by CCK release. Stimulation of the exocrine pancreas is undertaken by utilizing one or both of these pathways by supplying either exogenous hormones or intestinal nutrients.

TABLE 2
Criteria for the Ideal Pancreatic Function Test

Inexpensive and easily performed
Noninvasive
Specific for pancreatic disease and able to exclude patients with other digestive disorders due to small bowel mucosal disease, inherited defects of fat transport, or cholestasis
Defines the exact level of pancreatic function in subjects with pancreatic sufficiency in whom partial impairment of exocrine function is present but nutrient assimilation is unaffected
Repeatable, reproducible between laboratories, and able to monitor exocrine function longitudinally
Lack of interference from exogenous pancreatic supplements

Successful quantitation of human pancreatic exocrine function is contingent on the following conditions:

1. The development of appropriate intravenously administered hormonal stimuli or appropriate intestinally administered nutrients
2. The ability to quantitatively measure pancreatic secretions
3. The ability to exclude gastric acid and pepsin

Exogenous Hormonal Stimulation

There is no standard method of hormonal stimulation. Consequently, techniques vary among centers, and each laboratory is required to establish its own range of normal values. The doses of hormones used, the mode of administration (intravenous bolus or intravenous infusion), the duration of infusion, and, in the case of a combined secretin-CCK infusion, the sequence of administration may differ. For further information regarding testing regimens and doses of secretin and CCK in adults, the reader is referred to Gowenlock,[3] Arvanitakis and Cooke,[4] and Regan et al.[5] Little information exists regarding optimal doses in children, especially for synthetic secretin and CCK, and in most cases doses have been extrapolated from adult data on a weight per kilogram basis. Current sources of supply of pancreatic secretagogues are listed in Table 3. Synthetic preparations of secretin and CCK are preferable to animal extracts in that they are not contaminated with other gut-derived peptides and are less allergenic. Combined stimulation is optimal, as there is evidence that CCK or similar hormones act synergistically with secretin.[6] Other investigators have used cerulein, a decapeptide from an amphibian source, or bombesin, a tetradecapeptide also from an amphibian source, since these peptides have effects on the exocrine pancreas similar to those of CCK. No published information exists regarding their use in children.

Quantification of secretions requires that precise volume data be obtained. Two approaches are used: either distal occlusion of the duodenum by a balloon[7] or continuous perfusion of a nonabsorbable marker,[8] allowing correction for distal losses. Balloon occlusion techniques are less physiologic in that they may cause luminal distention and possible stimulation by this means. Similarly, gastric acid and pepsin can be excluded either by continuous nasogastric suction or by a pyloric balloon.

The technique used at The Hospital for Sick Children employs practical solutions to the above conditions and is readily adaptable. The test is a quantitative technique modified from Go et al[9] and is represented diagrammatically in Figure 1. Subjects should be fasting and, in the case of patients on pancreatic enzyme supplements, these should be discontinued at least 48 hours prior to the test. Under fluoroscopic control, a double-lumen tube is inserted into the duodenum. The tube is constructed so that one lumen opens proximally at the ampulla of Vater and the other lumen, which has several distal ports, is positioned 5 to 12 cm distally at the ligament of Treitz. Through the proximal lumen, a non-

TABLE 3
Sources of Pancreatic Secretagogues

Secretagogue	Supplier
Secretin	
Natural porcine secretin Kabisecretin (GIH secretin)	Pharmacia (Stockholm, Sweden)
Synthetic porcine secretin Sekretolin	Hoechst Co. (Frankfurt/M, Federal Republic of Germany)
Synthetic human secretin	Peninsula Laboratories (Belmont, California)
Cholecystokinin	
Natural porcine cholecystokinin (CCK, GIH CCK)	Pharmacia (Stockholm, Sweden)
Synthetic CCK octapeptide Kinevac/Sincalide	E.R. Squibb & Sons Inc. (Princeton, New Jersey)
Cerulein	Farmitalia Research Laboratories (Milan, Italy)
Bombesin	Farmitalia Research Laboratories (Milan, Italy) Calbiochem (Behring, La Jolla, California)

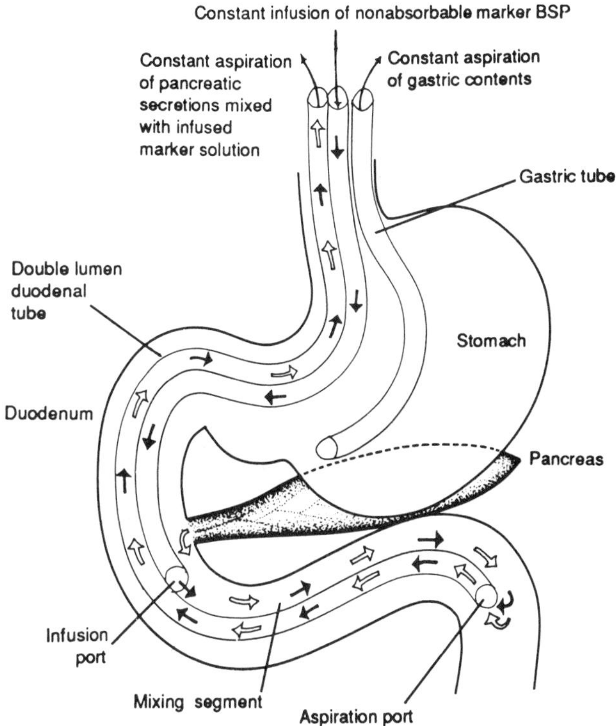

FIGURE 1 Gastric juice is removed via the nasogastric tube. Through the proximal lumen of the double-lumen intestinal tube, the nonabsorbable marker Bromsulphalein (BSP) is perfused at a constant rate. Pancreatic secretions mix with BSP in the mixing segment, and the mixture is aspirated via the distal port. Pancreatic secretions are collected over a specific time period (60 to 80 minutes) while maximally stimulating pancreatic secretion with intravenous hormones (CCK and/or secretin). (Adapted from Durie.[86])

absorbable marker solution sulfobromophthalein sodium ([Bromsulphalein] in 5 percent mannitol) is infused into the duodenum at a constant rate. Pancreatic juice mixed with infused marker solution is aspirated distally by intermittent low-pressure suction and collected over four 20-minute collection periods into flasks on ice. The first period allows equilibration of marker solution with pancreatic juice and also allows residual luminal pancreatic enzymes to be washed out. During the subsequent three periods, duodenal juice mixed with marker is collected while continuously and simultaneously infusing intravenous secretin and CCK at doses known to achieve maximal pancreatic stimulation. A separate nasogastric tube facilitates aspiration of gastric juice and minimizes contamination of duodenal contents with acid and pepsin.

This technique allows both the collection and quantification of pancreatic secretions. Although both the biliary tree and the duodenal mucosa contribute to fluid secretion, the vast bulk of the secretory response is generated by the action of secretin on the pancreatic ductular epithelium and acini and the effect of CCK on the acini. This fact, coupled with the use of a nonabsorbable marker, allows us to correct for distal losses of fluid and enzyme by assuming that once equilibration has been attained, the degree of distal loss of the marker is the same as the degree of enzyme and fluid loss. A simple volume correction factor can be calculated:

$$\frac{\text{BSP in mg per period infused}}{\text{BSP in mg per period recovered}}$$

The determination of fluid, electrolyte, and enzymatic output can be adjusted accordingly. Trypsin,[10] co-lipase, and total lipase[11] outputs are measured routinely by titrimetric techniques and bicarbonate output by a colorimetric technique.[12] Sodium, potassium, and chloride outputs are also measured. Other investigators have measured total protein, amylase, chymotrypsin, carboxypeptidase, elastase, cholesterol esterase, and deoxyribonuclease and viscosity.

The techniques employed for enzymatic determination, especially amylase and lipase, may differ. The substrates used for the colorimetric determination of amylase activity vary, and consequently the units used to express activity differ. In the case of lipase, the results vary depending on whether a short-chain triglyceride such as glycerol tributyrate or a long-chain triglyceride such as olive oil is used as the substrate.

The invasiveness of this test tends to discourage routine clinical use, particularly in pancreatic-sufficient patients, the group in which it is most helpful. It is worthwhile reiterating that this test has helped to delineate pancreatic function in both healthy and diseased individuals. For example, the fact that co-lipase is the rate-controlling factor for lipolysis became apparent with analysis of stimulated secretions from both normal individuals and patients with steatorrhea.[13] Additionally, in patients with cystic fibrosis, deficits in electrolyte secretion, particularly chloride[14] and bicarbonate secretion,[15] have been identified, which in turn may lead to reduced fluid secretion.[16] As a result, protein is hyperconcentrated in ductal secretions, leading to ductal obstruction and acinar atrophy.[16]

Nutrient Stimulation

Nutrient stimulation of the exocrine pancreas can be undertaken by directly adapting the methods used in the secretin-CCK stimulation test and substituting intraluminal nutrients for the intravenous secretagogues. This method is more physiologic in that the stimulus is provided by both release of endogenous secretin and CCK directly into the splanchnic circulation and by a vagal mechanism that can be inhibited by atropine.

The most-utilized test meal has been that devised by Lundh,[17] which consists of dry milk, vegetable oil, and dextrose for use in adult patients. The total volume is 300 ml, and the final composition is 6 percent fat, 5 percent protein, and 15 percent carbohydrate. The Lundh meal is composed of intact nutrients. The presence of intact fat, protein, and carbohydrate render the enzymatic determinations of lipase, protease, and amylase activity difficult. Although Lundh used a nonabsorbable marker to provide a reference for absorption of nutrients, the lack of continuous duodenal marker perfusion coupled with the presence of salivary and gastric secretions makes this test relatively qualitative. Although the test is more physiologic, these practical difficulties have led other investigators to develop more quantitative methods of nutrient stimulation.

Alternative nutrients have been used. The most potent nutrient stimuli are essential amino acids, particularly phenylalanine, but methionine, valine, and tryptophan have all been shown to stimulate the pancreas.[18] Amino acids are usually given as duodenal infusions. Amino acids do not interfere with enzymatic or electrolytic determinations. For physiologic purposes, amino acid solutions should have a pH approximating that of the duodenal lumen in that hydrogen ions neutralize bicarbonate, rendering assessment of secretin response difficult, and can also directly stimulate the pancreas through secretin release. The volume of the infusions should be low, because duodenogastric reflux of nutrients can stimulate the pancreas via gastrin release. With the exception of the Lundh meal, nutrient stimulation has not been used clinically in children.

In addition to nutrients, both dilute hydrochloric acid[19] and bile acids have been used in luminal perfusion mixtures as stimulants,[20] but owing to lingering doubts as to physiologic relevance, they have never been widely accepted.

OTHER DIRECT TESTS

A variety of alternative approaches has been used in adult patients. These include the use of radioisotopes to assess uptake, incorporation and release of amino acids, direct ductal sampling of secretions, and other methods employing microtechniques to assess protease activity. Pancreatic synthetic capacity is measured by the ability to incorporate ^{75}Se-labeled methionine. Subsequently, in response to a stimulus, ^{75}Se-labeled methionine is then released into pancreatic secretions as a constituent of enzymes and other proteins. Measurement of ^{75}Se activity serves as a guide to acinar function. Endoscopic collection of pure pancreatic juice allows the assessment of uncontaminated samples, but it is technically difficult.[22] The haptocorrin test measures total pancreatic protease activity, particularly trypsin and chymotrypsin, by measuring the degradation of a salivary glycoprotein.[23] These tests are unlikely to find a niche in pediatric practice.

INDIRECT EXOCRINE PANCREATIC FUNCTION TESTS

The actions of individual pancreatic enzymes are assessed indirectly by quantifying the malassimilation of specific nutrients in the feces—for example, fecal fat—or by measuring metabolic products in the blood, urine, or breath—for example, the bentiromide test and radiolabeled breath tests. Alternatively, the stool content of enzymes such as chymotrypsin may reflect residual pancreatic function. Most of these tests cannot reliably assess the level of function in pancreatic-sufficient subjects or exclude biliary or intestinal causes of malabsorption. However, because they are relatively noninvasive, some of the tests, such as fecal fat, can be used to evaluate the success of pancreatic enzyme supplementation in pancreatic-insufficient subjects.

Fecal Tests

Microscopic Examination

Microscopic examination of the stools may reveal meat fibers, neutral fat droplets, or free fatty acid crystals, suggesting partial fat hydrolysis. Sudan III is the preferred stain for neutral fat, although the fat droplets can be seen quite easily without staining. Free fatty crystals are birefringent and are best visualized by a microscope with a polarizing filter. They can also be visualized by lowering the pH of the Sudan III stain.[24] If stool is obtained by rectal examination, lubricants containing oil or petroleum jelly should be avoided.

Attempts have been made to quantify the degree of steatorrhea by counting the number and determining the size of fat globules in a high-power field.[25] If, on cursory examination, steatorrhea is present, it is sensible to quantify fecal fat losses using balance studies. Microscopic examination of the stool should be mandatory in all cases of suspected malabsorption. However, it should not be regarded as more than a highly useful, albeit crude, screening test for malabsorption.

Steatocrit

The steatocrit, a measurement of fat malabsorption, works on the principle that if homogenized feces are centrifuged, the lipid and liquid phases and stool residues separate with the lipid phase on top of the liquid and the stool residue phases.[26] The lipid phase can be measured in a hematocrit tube if the tube is centrifuged at 15,000 rpm for 15 minutes. This may prove to be a useful adjunct in laboratories with limited technical expertise and may also provide a crude method for monitoring the response of patients receiving pancreatic enzyme supplements.

Pooled Stool Collections for Fat, Nitrogen, and Carbohydrate

Because of the functional reserve of the exocrine pancreas, these tests detect only pancreatic-insufficient subjects. All three nutrient classes—fat, protein, and carbohydrate—have been measured in stool to assess pancreatic function. Fecal fat analysis is the most widely used and the most informative of these tests. Pooled stool collections detect malabsorption but do not discriminate between patients with pancreatic and nonpancreatic malabsorption. Despite these limitations, fecal fat analysis is useful longitudinally, especially for assessing the effectiveness of porcine pancreatic enzyme supplements in patients with cystic fibrosis. Because of the odious nature of the test for both patients and laboratory technicians, it has fallen into disfavor in some circles.[27] Alternative tests that rely on isotopic methods are more expensive, are almost as inconvenient, and still fail to differentiate among the various causes of malassimilation.

The method most commonly used for the measurement of fecal fat is the titrimetric van de Kamer method.[28] In adults, the test involves a diet containing 100 g of fat for 3 to 5 days.[29] Stools collected over 72 to 96 hours are collected, pooled, and refrigerated. Steatorrhea is defined as a fecal excretion of more than 7 g of fat per day (7 percent of dietary intake). The mechanics of collection can be improved by the use of a nonabsorbable marker at the start and the end of the diet. In children, the collection period is usually 3 days, although it is occasionally extended to 5 days. It is difficult to adhere to a strictly regimented diet; meticulous weighing of food and careful dietary records are required to allow the calculation of mean daily fat intake. Steatorrhea is present if more than 7 percent of ingested fat is excreted. Owing to physiologic immaturity of the pancreatic and biliary secretions, infants under 6 months of age can excrete up to 15 percent of dietary fat.[30] The van de Kamer method must be modified if the diet contains appreciable amounts of medium-chain triglycerides, as these are not detected by the standard method.[31] The potential for error is great, as collections may be incomplete, fat intake may be inaccurately quantitated, and the occasional patient may have delayed intestinal transit. Other methods of estimating fat in feces, such as nuclear magnetic resonance spectrometry[32] and near-infrared reflectance spectroscopy,[33] may make laboratory analysis easier and less odious.

Fecal nitrogen has been used as an index of exocrine pancreatic function but does not provide further diagnostic information, since it is unlikely that significant creatorrhea will occur if steatorrhea is absent.[1] The same criticism can be made of fecal carbohydrate measurements. The most commonly used assessment of carbohydrate relies on the measurement of reducing sugars and does not assess total carbohydrate. Recently, the anthrone method, which assesses all hexose carbohydrates, has provided better quantitation of carbohydrate losses.[34] Carbohydrate measurements are likely to be elevated with small intestinal mucosal disease, and additionally both nitrogen and carbohydrate are subject to variable colonic absorption and substrate utilization by fecal flora. For the above reasons, they are less accurate than neutral fat as a guide to pancreatic insufficiency.

Stool Isotopic Methods

Most of these methods are inappropriate for pediatric use because they use gamma-ray–emitting isotopes. Single isotopes (^{131}I, ^{125}I) bound to triglycerides are expensive, and the test necessitates a 3-day stool collection, but the need for strict dietary records is eliminated. Dual-isotope methods append markers to a nonabsorbable lipid such as glycerol triether and to an absorbable lipid such as glycerol trioleate. This technique allows fat malabsorption to be estimated from single stool samples. Although some of the dual labeling systems use beta-emitting isotopes,[35] none of these methods has been adapted for pediatric use.

Fecal Trypsin and Chymotrypsin

The capacity to measure both fecal trypsin and chymotrypsin has existed for 20 years.[36,37] The initial tests measured enzymatic activity by means of a laborious titrimetric estimation utilizing low molecular weight substrates. A number of problems existed with these tests. The enzymes are subject to proteolytic degradation by both pancreatic and bacterial proteases, and the interpretation varies with intestinal transit. Chymotrypsin is the favored measurement because it is more resistant to inactivation by colonic bacteria. However, a high proportion of chymotrypsin is strongly bound to insoluble stool residue,[38] and, until recently, this thwarted attempts to develop accurate and more convenient photometric methods. A new photometric method, the BMC test developed by Boehringer Mannheim Corporation, employs a detergent to solubilize chymotrypsin in stool[39] and is convenient, reproducible, and sensitive. The patients who receive pancreatic enzymes should discontinue them at least 5 days prior to measurement. Fecal chymotrypsin reliably differentiates between pancreatic-insufficient and pancreatic-sufficient patients. However, it does not reliably discriminate pancreatic-sufficient from normal subjects. Compliance with pancreatic enzyme supplements can be checked in pancreatic-insufficient subjects. Patients with pancreatic insufficiency can be differentiated from those with intestinal disease of biliary disease.[40] This method has been validated for pediatric use by showing a good correlation between 72-hour fecal output of chymotrypsin and CCK-secretin–stimulated duodenal output of chymotrypsin.[41] Other observers have shown good correlation between duodenal chymotrypsin output following CCK stimulation[42] and three random stool samples collected within 72 hours of pancreatic stimulation with CCK. Fecal chymotrypsin is relatively stable at 18°C for up to 72 hours and thus can be sent from peripheral centers to a reference laboratory. If random stool samples are used and a low value is obtained, repeating the test eliminates most false-negative results.

Breath Tests

Radiolabeled Breath Tests

The techniques and principles of breath testing are described in a separate chapter. Ingested lipids are predominantly hydrolyzed by pancreatic lipases in the small intestine, absorbed as free fatty acids and monoglycerides, and transported to the liver, where oxidative metabolism liberates CO_2. The radiolabeled breath tests take advantage of this fact by appending either ^{14}C or ^{13}C to triglycerides. The three triglycerides of different carbon chain lengths that have been commonly used are trioctanoin, tripalmitate, and triolein. All three substrates labeled with ^{14}C are sensitive in detecting fat malabsorption.[43,44] Triolein is more specific than either trioctanoin and tripalmitate for fat malabsorption; however, it does not differentiate between pancreatic and nonpancreatic causes of fat malabsorption. Normal release of CO_2 from triolein and tripalmitate requires adequate lipolysis, bile salt solubilization, and an adequate mucosal surface and transport capability. The release of CO_2 from trioctanoin is limited by lipolysis alone and can distinguish pancreatic insufficiency from bile salt deficiency and mucosal defects. Using these substrates in combination with one another, for example, testing with triolein and repeating the test with trioctanoin, improves specificity but not sensitivity. Other confounding variables are the action of lingual and gastric lipases on the substrate, varying individual lipid pool sizes and the variable respiratory excretion of CO_2 in chronic respiratory disease. The labeling with ^{14}C militates against using the tests in children.

The specificity of these tests may be improved by repeating them after administering pancreatic enzyme supplements. The same compounds have been labeled with ^{13}C, a stable isotope that is measurable by mass spectroscopy, and similar results have been obtained in children.[45] Recently, ^{14}C cholesteryl octanoate, which is hydrolyzed by the pancreatic-specific cholesterol esterase, has been utilized as a substrate.[46] Studies suggest that hydrolysis by cholesterol esterase is the rate-limiting step and that the test is adaptable to ^{13}C labeling.[46] Because stable isotopes and mass spectroscopy are expensive, these breath tests are unlikely to find a niche for routine pediatric use.

Hydrogen Breath Test

This test measures breath hydrogen excretion following starch ingestion. Starch is normally cleaved enzymatically into oligosaccharides by pancreatic isoamylase prior to further cleavage by brush border disaccharidases. When amylase secretion is impaired, undigested starch is digested by colonic bacteria, generating hydrogen, which is absorbed and excreted in the breath. A two-stage test with concomitant ingestion of oral pancreatic enzymes results in reduced breath hydrogen. This test is extremely nonspecific; false-positive results may occur in blind-loop syndromes and also when small intestinal transit time is reduced. False-negative results may occur when the colon is colonized with non–hydrogen-producing bacteria and in subjects who have recently received antibiotics. Currently there are no pediatric data.

Urinary/Plasma Markers

Bentiromide Test

Bentiromide is a nonabsorbable synthetic peptide (*N*-benzoyl-L-tyrosyl-*p*-aminobenzoic acid) that is specifically cleaved by pancreatic chymotrypsin in the upper small intestine, resulting in the release of *p*-aminobenzoic acid (PABA). PABA, which serves as a marker, is rapidly absorbed, conjugated in the liver, and excreted in the urine. The principles involved are illustrated diagrammatically in Figure 2. PABA can be measured in both blood and urine by a colorimetric assay, and its detection and quantification form the basis of the test. Falsely abnormal results have been demonstrated in subjects with bowel, liver, or renal disease due to defects in absorption, conjugation, or excretion of PABA. Additionally, both intestinal bacteria and the intestinal brush border may demonstrate chymotrypsin-like activity, reducing specificity.[47,48] Ingestion of a number of drugs and foods may result in elevated aromatic amines that may interfere with laboratory determinations of PABA.[49] Recently, high-pressure liquid chromatography techniques have been developed to sensitively detect PABA and its metabolites and may prove to be superior.

The bentiromide test was introduced in 1972 and the initial reports relied on a one-stage test with a urinary collection.[50] The methods used involved collections over varying time periods and varying doses of substrate. Consequently, reports of test specificity and sensitivity vary widely. In North America the recommended method for adults entails receiving a 500-mg dose of bentiromide (170 mg of PABA), ingesting sufficient fluid to maintain an adequate diuresis, and collecting urine for a period of 6 hours.[51] The urinary recovery of PABA is expressed as a percentage of the orally ingested PABA. Less than 50 percent PABA excretion purportedly reflects pancreatic insufficiency. In order to correct for potential defects of absorption, hepatic conjugation, or excretion, a two-stage test has been suggested with an equivalent dose of free PABA administered subsequently and the urine collected for an identical time period.[52] This allows the urinary recovery of PABA after bentiromide to be corrected for the urinary recovery of equimolar free PABA, and the results are expressed as a PABA excretion index (PEI):

$$\text{PEI} = \frac{\text{PABA recovered after bentiromide (\%)}}{\text{PABA recovered after free PABA (\%)}}$$

This maneuver improves sensitivity and specificity, but the test is cumbersome and time-consuming. Additionally, timed urine collections make the test awkward to perform in infants. In adults, this drawback has been circumvented by the simultaneous administration of ^{14}C-free PABA[53] or by the simultaneous administration of a free structural analogue of PABA, *p*-aminosalicylic acid (PAS).[54] The ^{14}C PABA method is impractical for pediatric use. The PAS method has been used in the pediatric age group and has improved the sensitivity of the test.[55]

The initial pediatric experience with the bentiromide test concentrated on timed urine collections.[56] However, the specificity and sensitivity of the test have been improved with the development of methods to measure plasma PABA,[57,58]

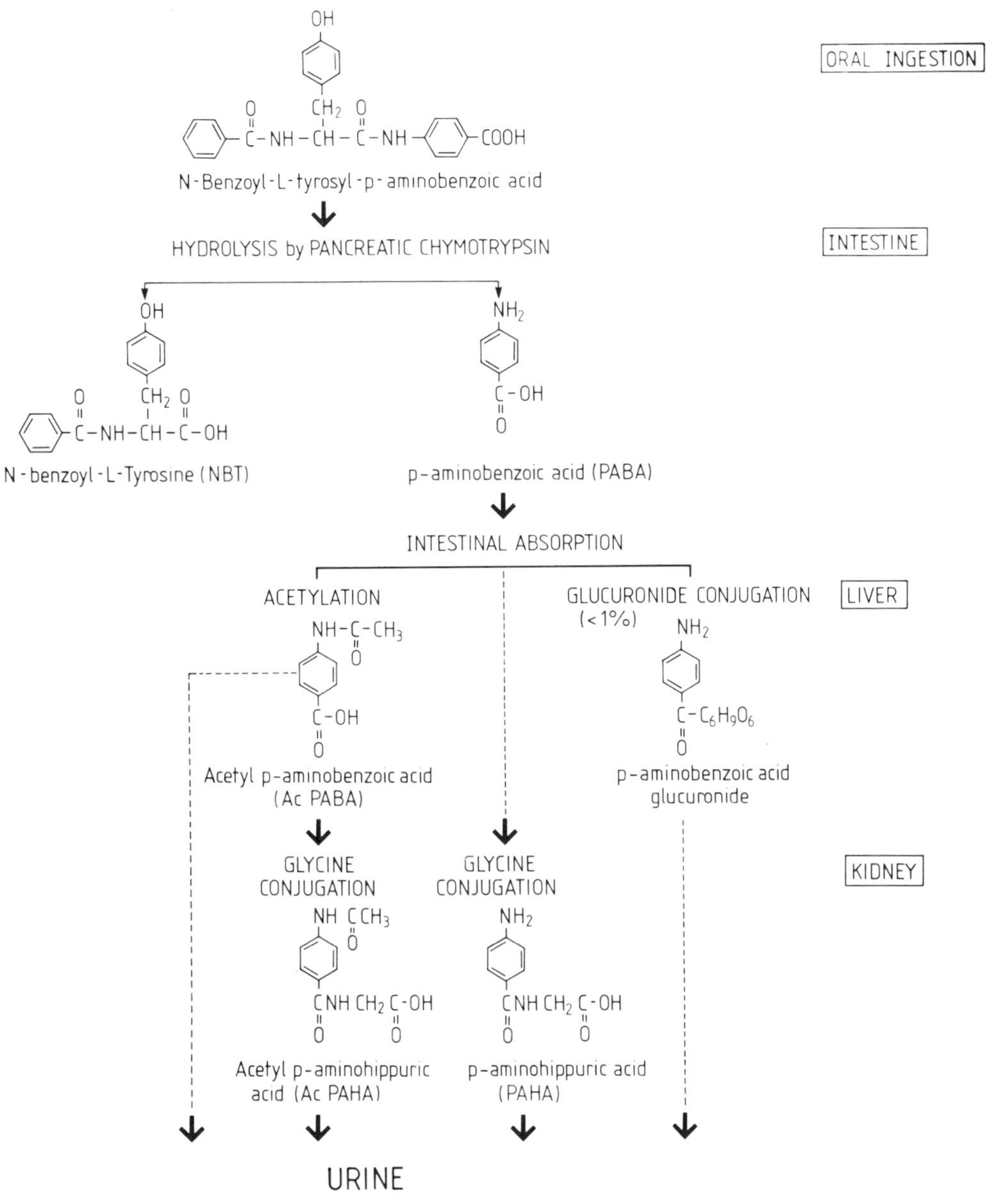

FIGURE 2 Scheme of the bentiromide test and the metabolism of *p*-aminobenzoic (PABA). (From Scharpé and Iliano.[62] Original illustration courtesy of Professor S. Scharpé.)

and the need for dual collections and urinary collections has been eliminated. The recommended pediatric dosage of bentiromide of 15 mg per kilogram has been used in older children and is based on extrapolation from adult data. For the first 3 hours following ingestion of the dose, plasma PABA concentrations rise, and optimal discrimination between normal adolescent controls and patients with pancreatic insufficiency is obtained at the 90- and 120-minute time points.[59] Reliable detection was not obtained in patients with cystic fibrosis and pancreatic sufficiency (between 5 and 10 percent of normal pancreatic chymotrypsin output as measured by the secretin-CCK test). In patients with Shwachman's syndrome, none of whom had malabsorption, the plasma test failed to detect pancreatic dysfunction in patients with enzyme output as low as 1 percent of normal. Bentiromide, 15 mg per kilogram, has not proved useful for assessment in infants if clear fluids are given with the dose. Test sensitivity may be improved by using a liquid meal and by increasing the dose to 30 mg per kilogram. Further refinement may improve the capability of this test to identify patients with lesser degrees of impairment of exocrine function. Thus, the bentiromide test may discriminate pancreatic steatorrhea from other causes of steatorrhea and could potentially provide a method of monitoring the effect of pancreatic enzyme supplementation.

4-*N* acetyl-L-tyrosyl aminobenzoic acid has been used as a substrate for chymotrypsin in both adults[60] and children,[61] and in comparison with the standard bentiromide test has been reported to allow better differentiation between controls and patients with chronic pancreatitis.[61] A modified Lundh meal was used in the pediatric study and extremely good separation was obtained between normal controls and patients with cystic fibrosis. However, no information exists on its usefulness in subjects who have pancreatic sufficiency but reduced functional reserve.

Fluorescein Dilaurate Test (Pancreolauryl)

This test is based on a principle similar to that of the bentiromide test. Orally administered fluorescein dilaurate is hydrolyzed by pancreatic cholesterol esterase, liberating lauric acid and free water-soluble fluorescein. Fluorescein is readily absorbed in the small intestine, partially conjugated in the liver, and excreted in the urine, predominantly as fluorescein diglucuronide. The steps involved in the metabolism of fluorescein dilaurate are illustrated in Figure 3. Fluorescein is nontoxic and can be easily measured in both serum and urine by spectrophotometric or fluorometric techniques.

The commercial version of this test in adult patients involves the ingestion of 0.5 mmol of fluorescein dilaurate with a standard meal. To enhance diuresis, 1 liter of unsweetened tea is consumed between the third and fifth hour of the test. All urine is collected over a 10-hour period. In order to correct for individual differences in intestinal absorption, conjugation, and urinary excretion, the test is repeated using equimolar free fluorescein after an interval of at least 24 hours. The results are expressed as a ratio of the fluorescein detected on the test and the control days. A ratio of greater than 30 percent is considered normal, a ratio of between 20 and 30 percent equivocal, and a ratio of less than 20 percent abnormal.[62] Equivocal results should be repeated. The dose can be modified for pediatric purposes.[63–65]

The serum test is more convenient because it is less time-consuming, and the need for urine collection is eliminated. Peak serum levels occur at approximately 210 minutes after absorption, and the best cut-off point for discriminating between pancreatic exocrine–insufficient patients and controls appears to be between 240 and 300 minutes.[66]

This test has some advantages over the bentiromide test but is not capable of detecting subtle impairment of function in pancreatic-sufficient subjects. Analysis is easier and there is less interference by exogenous compounds, although it is recommended that niacin and sulfasalazine be avoided prior to the test.[62] False-positive results can be found in patients with biliary tract and mucosal disorders. Cholesterol esterase is pancreatic-specific, and therefore the test is not subject to the influence of brush border enzymes. However, bacterial overgrowth can influence the results, as some bacteria, in particular streptococci, are able to hydrolyze fluorescein dilaurate.[62]

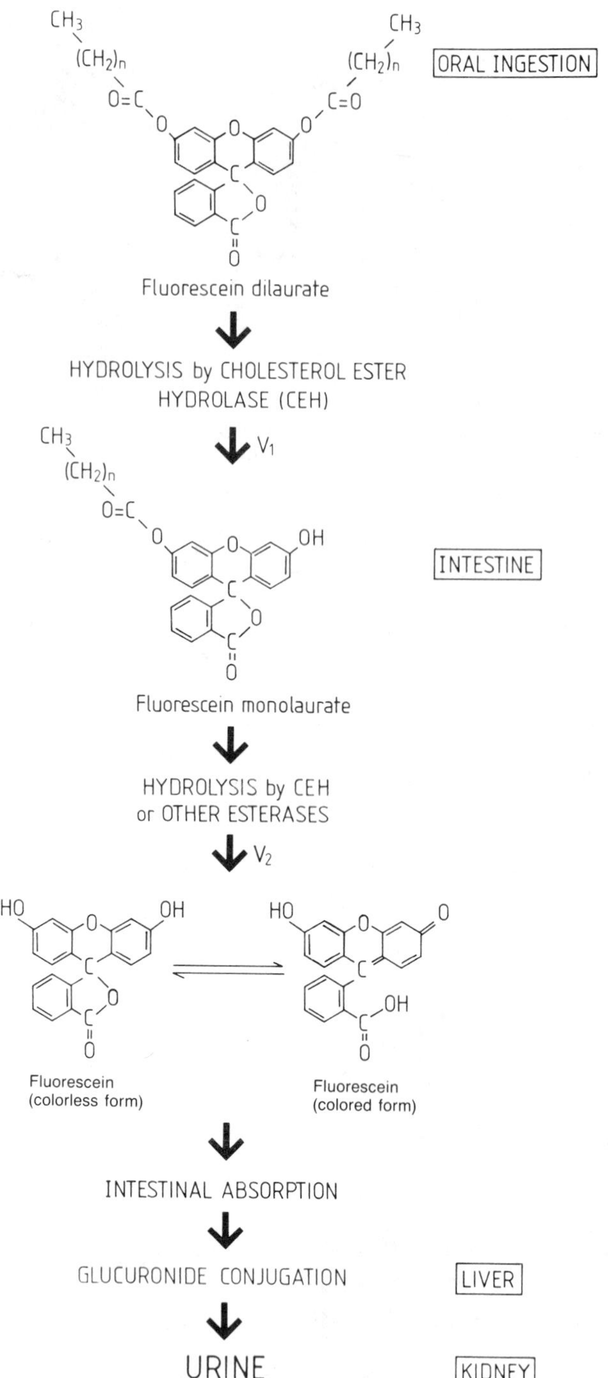

FIGURE 3 Scheme of the pancreolauryl test and the metabolism of fluorescein dilaurate. (From Scharpé and Illiano.[62] Original illustration courtesy of Professor S. Scharpé.)

Oral Tolerance Tests

Oral fat loading tests may provide useful information in patients from whom a reliable stool sample cannot be obtained. Serum triglycerides and chylomicron levels are measured at 2, 3, and 5 hours following the ingestion of a meal consisting of 50 g of fat, containing equal amounts of butter and margarine, emulsified in 70 ml of water. Serum triglycerides usually peak at 3 hours after ingestion. An abnormal result consists of a serum triglyceride rise of less than 1.13 mmol per liter, or less than 100 percent above the fasting level, and/or the appearance of less than 7 percent chylomicrons.[67] This test does not differentiate among patients with pancreatic disease, intestinal mucosal defects, and bile salt deficiency.

Attempts have been made to improve test specificity by using radiolabeled lipids. Initial tests in adults employed triolein labeled with ^{131}I, but subsequently a dual-label lipid system was evaluated, using tritium-labeled free fatty acid (oleic acid) and ^{14}C-labeled triglyceride (triolein). The substrates are administered simultaneously and the serum ratio $^{3}H:^{14}C$ is calculated.[67] Patients with pancreatic insufficiency have a higher ratio than normal patients or patients with mucosal disease. However, this test does not exclude patients with defects of bile salt delivery or synthesis. Labeling with radioisotopes precludes using this test in children.

Previously, tolerance tests such as the vitamin A tolerance test were used to evaluate the assimilation of fat-soluble nutrients. In patients with suspected pancreatic disease, the rise in serum profile of vitamin A following administration can be compared, with and without supplements.[68] This test is mentioned as a historical footnote and is currently out of vogue.

Dual-Label Schilling Test

Patients with exocrine pancreatic insufficiency often have an abnormal Schilling test. Pancreatic enzymes are responsible for the cleavage of intrinsic factor from the R protein–intrinsic factor complex secreted by the parietal cells. This step is required in order for intrinsic factor–cyanocobalamin binding to occur before renal absorption. A dual-label Schilling test has been developed utilizing this principle.[69] ^{57}[Co] cobalamin–intrinsic factor complex is administered with ^{58}[Co] cobalamin–hog R protein complex. Free human intrinsic factor and a cobalamin analogue are administered to prevent endogenous human R protein from stripping ^{57}[Co] cobalamin from intrinsic factor. The excretion of ^{58}Co and ^{57}Co is measured in the urine and expressed as a ratio. A low ratio is said to denote severe pancreatic insufficiency. This test is not suitable for pediatric use owing to the radiation dose.

Urinary Lactulose

Lactulose is a poorly absorbed and nonmetabolized disaccharide. Increased permeability to lactulose, reflected by increased urinary lactulose excretion, has been demonstrated in patients with pancreatic insufficiency due to chronic pancreatitis and cystic fibrosis. The mechanisms responsible for this finding are unknown, but the test could prove to be a useful screening test for pancreatic exocrine insufficiency. Unfortunately, it does not exclude mucosal defects such as celiac disease.

BLOOD TESTS

All pancreatic enzymes are detectable in small quantities (nanograms per millilter) in the sera of normal individuals. Some enzymes, such as lipase and amylase, are released as active enzymes, whereas others, such as trypsin, are released as the zymogen or proenzyme trypsinogen. Excessive quantities of circulating pancreatic enzymes are seen in three circumstances.

1. **Acute Pancreatitis.** Enzymes are released directly into the circulation as a consequence of inflammation. Enzymes that are normally detected only as proenzymes may be present in the zymogen or activated form. For example, both trypsin(ogen) and trypsin are present in severe pancreatitis. In mild pancreatitis only the zymogen is released.
2. **Ductal Obstruction.** Obstruction of pancreatic enzymatic outflow may result in elevated levels of pancreatic enzymes in sera in the absence of inflammation. The mechanism responsible is thought to be regurgitant release of enzymes from the acini or ducts. A good example of this mechanism is cystic fibrosis in which obstruction is thought to result from inspissated secretions, and in these circumstances serum enzyme concentrations may be elevated in the presence of impaired secretion.
3. **Impaired Renal Function.** Pancreatic enzymes are cleared from the circulation by the kidneys. Impaired renal function may result in significant elevations of pancreatic enzymes in the absence of pancreatic disease.

   Theoretically, in the absence of inflammation, ductal obstruction, or impaired renal function, the serum level of a particular enzyme should reflect the amount of functioning acinar tissue, and this consideration forms the rationale for enzyme determination in sera. However, until recently, two considerations have prevented this goal from being attained: lack of test specificity and variable maturation of pancreatic enzymes.

Lack of Test Specificity. Biochemical determinations of enzymes in sera, particularly total amylase, have been used for many years as a crude screening test for acute pancreatitis. The major limitation of enzymatic techniques has been the lack of substrate specificity. For example, the traditional starch and iodine method does not distinguish between salivary and pancreatic isoamylases. Similarly, trypsin substrates are subject to degradation by other circulating serine proteases. Recently, immunoassay techniques have been developed that sensitively detect and measure specific pancreatic enzymes. Because techniques vary, it is vital that each laboratory establish its own normative data.

Variable Maturation of Pancreatic Enzymes. Concentration of serum enzymes varies with age, especially in early infancy. In most instances serum enzyme levels increase with age and reflect the ongoing maturation of the exocrine pancreas and consequent pancreatic parenchymal enzyme levels. For example, at birth the pancreas synthesizes and secretes very little amylase and continues to produce very little during the first year of life. In contrast, however, trypsin(ogen) production is relatively mature, and comparatively larger amounts of trypsin are secreted.[70] Serum trypsinogen levels change relatively little during childhood, whereas serum amylase levels increase markedly. The different rates of maturation of pancreatic enzymes lead to varying degrees of usefulness of serum enzyme determinations for diagnosing pancreatic disease or determining function. An appreciation of the dynamics of enzyme maturation helps in the interpretation of serum enzyme data. These considerations are best addressed by detailed examination of the various tests.

Serum Amylase

Total amylase measurements are extremely nonspecific, as the enzymatic determination does not distinguish salivary and pancreatic isoenzymes. Refinement of amylase measurement has concentrated on distinguishing between pancreatic and salivary isoamylase. Biochemical methods include column chromatography, electrophoresis, isoelectric focusing, salivary isoenzyme inhibitors derived from wheat, and differential thermolability. In addition, highly specific monoclonal antibodies to the pancreatic isoenzyme have been raised, permitting the development of immunoassay techniques. The pancreatic isoenzyme peak on isoelectric focusing or electrophoresis appears to correlate with the level of function in older patients with cystic fibrosis and Shwachman's syndrome.[71] However, in patients with slight or moderate reduction of function, values are within the normal range. This test is therefore of little use in pancreatic-sufficient individuals. Additionally, levels of pancreatic isoenzyme are low in both normal neonates and neonates with cystic fibrosis, and they rise throughout childhood.[72] This finding limits the interpretability of the test in younger patients.

Serum Lipase

The enzymatic measurement of serum lipase relies on a titrimetric or turbidometric method in which lipase hydrolyzes a triglyceride substrate, producing free fatty acids and glycerol. These methods are not conducive to the assessment of large numbers of sample. A sensitive enzyme-linked immunosorbent assay (ELISA) is available commercially and allows rapid determination of lipase in sera from multiple patients.[73] Cross-sectional evaluation of the usefulness of serum lipase as a measure of pancreatic exocrine function was undertaken in a population with cystic fibrosis and compared with normal controls. The results were validated by fecal fat evaluation and/or secretin-CCK stimulation test in younger patients (less than 5 years of age) and in older patients (greater than 5 years) with cystic fibrosis.[74,75] The patterns seen in each group are distinctive. In all cystic fibrosis patients, serum lipase is much higher than control values during the first year of life. In pancreatic-insufficient patients, after the first year of life the levels decline, gradually reaching a nadir of 25 percent of control values after 5 years of age. In pancreatic-sufficient subjects, levels also decline during early childhood, but after 5 years of age they remain elevated approximately threefold above control levels. There is a wide scatter, however, and some pancreatic-sufficient patients have levels within the normal range. The elevated serum lipase in the first year of life has encouraged the adaptation of serum lipase as a screening test for cystic fibrosis.[76] However, the test has not attained the same popularity as cationic trypsinogen. It is less sensitive, with a detection rate of 76 percent in the first year of life as opposed to a 90 percent detection rate with cationic trypsinogen. After 5 years of age the test is reasonably sensitive and specific for the detection of pancreatic insufficiency (95 percent and 85 percent, respectively) but remains relatively imprecise for the detection of pancreatic-sufficient subjects. There is no information about the usefulness of serum lipase in delineating pancreatic insufficiency in other pancreatic diseases of childhood.

Serum Immunoreactive Trypsin(ogen)

Two forms of trypsin(ogen) (cationic and anionic trypsinogen) exist and are detectable in sera. Specific radioimmunoassays,[77,78] particularly for the cationic form, have permitted the population screening of pediatric groups at risk of pancreatic disease. Recently, an ELISA utilizing a monoclonal antibody specific for the zymogen trypsinogen has been developed.[79] This technique has the advantages of being quicker, easier to perform, and less labor-intensive. Neonatal screening for cystic fibrosis using dried blood spots is now routine in some parts of the world.[80,81]

Serum immunoreactive trypsinogen levels have been evaluated both cross-sectionally and longitudinally in pediatric patients with cystic fibrosis[82] and also in children with exocrine pancreatic functional impairment due to other causes.[83] The findings have been validated in comparison to normal controls. In cystic fibrosis, two patterns emerge. In all individuals with cystic fibrosis the serum immunoreactive trypsinogen level is grossly elevated during the first year of life. In pancreatic-insufficient patients a rapid decline is noted during the second year of life, with levels becoming subnormal by 6 years of age. In pancreatic-sufficient patients with cystic fibrosis no consistent pattern of decline is seen; indeed, many older patients continue to have elevated serum levels. However, there is a wide scatter, and in this group the test is of little predictive value of the degree of functional impairment. The control group provides a reasonably narrow normal range, with individual values being unrelated to age. Serum immunoreactive trypsinogen measurement in cystic fibrosis is useful in two circumstances. In infants less than 1 year of age, the test is a sensitive diagnostic screening test; the detection rate is 90 percent. In patients over 7 years of age, depressed serum levels are highly predictive of pancreatic insufficiency. In 199 cystic fibrosis patients over 7 years of age who had pancreatic insufficiency, only nine had normal values and three had elevated values, resulting in a predictive rate of 94 percent. Although this test does not delineate pancreatic-sufficient subjects from normal individuals, it is a sensitive, relatively noninvasive method of screening for pancreatic insufficiency in older subjects. Below 7 years of age, a fecal fat determination is recommended.

In patients with other pancreatic diseases of childhood, this test has proved useful in delineating pancreatic steatorrhea from nonpancreatic steatorrhea. At The Hospital for Sick Children (Toronto) this test provided absolute separation of 10 children with pancreatic steatorrhea from 22 children with other causes of steatorrhea (Fig. 4). The patients with the pancreatic steatorrhea include those with Shwachman's syndrome, insulin-dependent diabetes mellitus, idiopathic pancreatic insufficiency, and celiac disease with primary pancreatic insufficiency.

Serum Pancreatic Polypeptide

Pancreatic polypeptide, a 36-amino acid straight-chain peptide, is predominantly confined to the pancreatic islets of Langerhans and is also located between acinar cells. Pancreat-

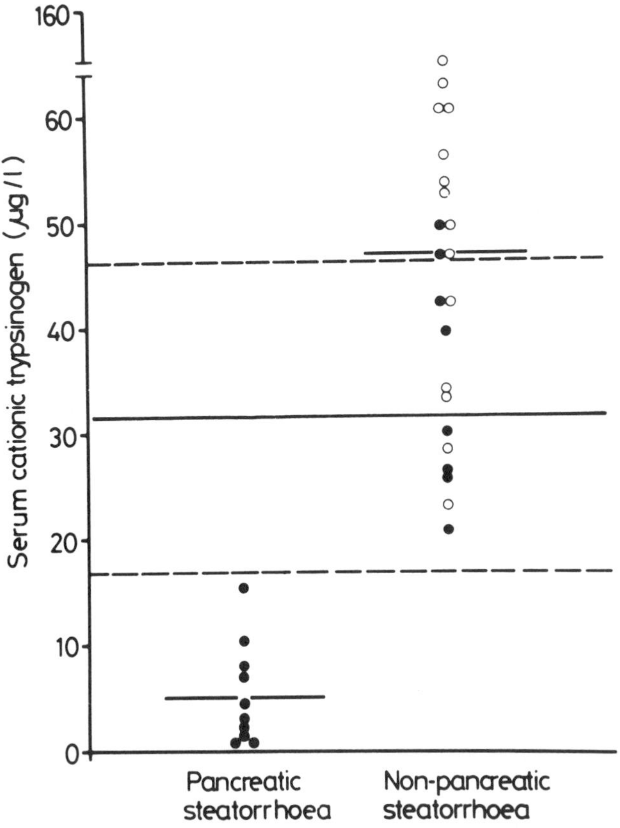

FIGURE 4 Serum cationic trypsinogen values in patients with pancreatic and nonpancreatic steatorrhea. The solid and interrupted horizontal lines indicate mean normal cationic trypsinogen of ±2 SD, respectively (31.4 ± 14.8 μg per liter). Closed circle = patients who underwent a pancreatic stimulation on test. Open circle = patients with nonpancreatic steatorrhea who did not have a pancreatic stimulation test. (From Moore et al.[83])

ic polypeptide is an inhibitor of pancreatic enzyme secretion and is released into the circulation in response to various stimuli, particularly protein meals and CCK.

A radioimmunoassay technique has been used to assess fasting pancreatic polypeptide levels or to assess serial responses of serum pancreatic polypeptide evoked by CCK infusions or in response to various nutrients.[84,85] In adult patients with chronic pancreatitis, fasting serum pancreatic polypeptide levels are low. Additionally, in response to CCK octapeptide, patients with chronic pancreatitis display either no rise in pancreatic polypeptide or a greatly limited rise compared with both normal controls and patients with other causes of steatorrhea. Thus the test is capable of differentiating between patients with pancreatic steatorrhea and those with nonpancreatic steatorrhea. However, the test fails to discriminate between pancreatic-sufficient and pancreatic-insufficient subjects with chronic pancreatitis and as such gives no indication of actual pancreatic function.[85] Serial responses evoked by a stimulus are difficult to control and are an inconvenience both to the patient and to the technical staff. This test has not been widely used in pediatric practice.

SUMMARY AND CONCLUSIONS

The ideal pancreatic stimulation test has yet to be developed to displace the pantheon of pretenders currently holding court. Direct pancreatic function testing provides the most information and when performed properly and with adequate normative data remains the only truly accurate test of pancreatic function. It is the only test capable of delineating pancreatic-sufficient patients with mild to moderate degrees of functional impairment. The invasive, complex nature of the direct stimulation test precludes its routine use and limits its value for serial monitoring purposes. Although none of the currently available indirect tests of pancreatic function is sensitive enough to reliably detect patients with impairment of function not severe enough to result in steatorrhea, they remain useful in specific circumstances. The bentiromide, pancreolauryl, radiolabeled breath tests, and fecal fat, chymotrypsin, and serum cationic trypsinogen measurements are useful in that they allow pancreatic insufficiency to be reliably detected. The pancreolauryl test, fecal chymotrypsin measurements, and serum cationic trypsinogen measurements are more specific for exocrine pancreatic disease and are less liable to be confounded by biliary tract and mucosal disease. The quantitative fecal fat is useful for serial assessment of function, particularly in patients who receive pancreatic enzyme supplements.

REFERENCES

1. Di Magno EP, Go VLW, Summerskill WJH. Relations between pancreatic enzyme outputs and malabsorption in severe pancreatic insufficiency. N Engl J Med 1973; 288:813–815.
2. Gaskin KJ, Durie PR, Lee L, Hill R, Forstner GG. Colipase and lipase secretion in childhood-onset pancreatic insufficiency. Gastroenterology 1984; 86:1–7.
3. Gowenlock AH. Tests of exocrine pancreatic function. Ann Clin Biochem 1977; 14:61–89.
4. Arvanitakis C, Cooke AR. Diagnostic tests of exocrine pancreatic function and disease. Gastroenterology 1978; 74:932–948.
5. Regan PT, Go VLW, Di Magno PE. Comparison of the effects of cholecystokinin and cholecystokinin octapeptide on pancreatic secretion, gallbladder contraction and plasma pancreatic polypeptide in man. J Lab Clin Med 1980; 96:743–748.
6. Meyer JH, Spingola LJ, Grossman MI. Endogenous cholecystokinin potentiates exogenous secretin on pancreas of dog. Am J Physiol 1971; 221:742–747.
7. Hadorn B, Zoppi G, Shmerling DH, Prader A, McIntyre I, Anderson CM. Quantitative assessment of exocrine pancreatic function in infants and children. J Pediatr 1968; 73:39–50.
8. Lagerloff HO, Schutz HB, Holmer S. A secretin test with high doses of secretin and correction for incomplete recovery of duodenal juice. Gastroenterology 1967; 52:67–82.
9. Go VLW, Hofmann AF, Summerskill WHJ. Simultaneous measurements of total pancreatic, biliary and gastric outputs in man using a perfusion technique. Gastroenterology 1970; 58:321–328.
10. Dyck WP. Titremetric measurements of fecal trypsin and chymotrypsin in cystic fibrosis with pancreatic exocrine insufficiency. Am J Dig Dis 1967; 12:310–317.
11. Gaskin KJ, Durie PR, Hill RE, Lee LM, Forstner GG. Colipase and maximally activated pancreatic lipase in normal subjects and patients with steatorrhea. J Clin Invest 1982; 69:427–434.
12. Skegg LT. An automatic method for the determination of carbon dioxide in blood plasma. Am J Clin Pathol 1960; 33:181–185.
13. Borgstrom B, Hildebrand H. Lipase and colipase activities of human small intestinal contents after a liquid test meal. Scand J Gastroenterol 1975; 10:585–591.

14. Kopelman H, Corey M, Gaskin K, Durie P, Weizman Z, Forstner G. Impaired chloride secretion, as well as bicarbonate secretion, underlies the fluid secretory defect in the cystic fibrosis pancreas. Gastroenterology 1988; 95:349–355.
15. Gaskin KJ, Durie PR, Corey M, Wei P, Forstner GG. Evidence for a primary defect of pancreatic HCO_3^- secretion in cystic fibrosis. Pediatr Res 1982; 16:554–557.
16. Kopelman H, Durie P, Gaskin K, Weizman Z, Forstner G. Pancreatic fluid secretion and protein hyperconcentration in cystic fibrosis. N Engl J Med 1985; 313:329–334.
17. Lundh G. Pancreatic exocrine function in neoplastic and inflammatory disease: a simple and reliable new test. Gastroenterology 1962; 42:275–280.
18. Go VLW, Hofmann AF, Summerskill WHJ. Pancreozymin bioassay in man based on pancreatic enzyme secretion: potency of specific amino acids and other digestive products. J Clin Invest 1970; 49:1558–1564.
19. Wormsley KG. The physiological implications of secretin. Scand J Gastroenterol 1980; 15:513–517.
20. Osnes M, Hanssen LE, Figten O, Myron J. Exocrine pancreatic secretion and immunoreactive secretin (IRS) release after intraduodenal instillation of bile in man. Gut 1978; 19:180–184.
21. Shichiri M, Etani N, Yoshida M, Haraon Y, Hoshi M, Shigeta Y, Abe H. Radioselenium pancreozymin-secretin test for pancreatic exocrine function. Am J Dig Dis 1975; 20:460–468.
22. Denyer ME, Cotton PB. Pure pancreatic juice studies in normal subjects and patients with chronic pancreatitis. Gut 1978; 20:89–97.
23. Gueant JL, Champgneulle B, Djalali M, Bigard MA, Gaucher P, Hassouni A, Nicolas JP. In-vitro test of haptocorrin degradation for biological diagnosis of exocrine pancreatic insufficiency using duodenal juice collected during endoscopy. Lancet 1986; ii:709–712.
24. Khouri MR, Huang G, Shiau YF. Sudan stain of fecal fat: new insight into an old test. Gastroenterology 1989; 96:421–427.
25. Drummey GD, Benson JA Jr, Jones CM. Microscopic examination of the stool for steatorrhea. N Engl J Med 1961; 264:85–87.
26. Columbo C, Maiavacca R, Ronchi M, Consalvo E, Amoretti M, Giunta A. The steatocrit: a simple method for monitoring fat malabsorption in patients with cystic fibrosis. J Pediatr Gastroenterol Nutr 1987; 6:926–930.
27. Holmes GKT, Hill PG. Do we still need to measure fecal fat? Br Med J 1988; 1961; 1552–1553.
28. van de Kamer JK, ten Bokkel Huinink H, Weyers HA. Rapid method for the determination of fat in feces. J Biol Chem 1949; 177:347–355.
29. Thompson JB, Su CK, Ringrose RE, Welsh JO. Fecal triglycerides. II. Digestive vs absorptive steatorrhea. J Lab Clin Med 1969; 73:521–530.
30. Fomon SJ, Ziegler ER, Thomas LN, Jensen RL, Filer LJ. Excretion of fat by normal full-term infants fed various milks and formulas. Am J Clin Nutr 1970; 23:1299–1313.
31. Jeejeebhoy KN, Ahmed S, Kozak G. Determination of fecal fats containing both medium and long chain triglycerides and fatty acids. Clin Biochem 1970, 3:157–163.
32. Schnieder MU, Demling L, Jones SA, Barker PJ, Domschke S, Heptner G, Domschke W. NMR spectrometry: a new method for total stool fat quantification in chronic pancreatitis. Dig Dis Sci 1987; 32:494–499.
33. Koumentakis G, Radcliff PJ. Estimating fat in feces by near infrared reflectance spectroscopy. Clin Chem 1987; 33:502–506.
34. Green VZ, Powel GK. A simple spectrophotometric method for quantitative fecal carbohydrate measurement. Clin Chim Acta 1985; 152:3–9.
35. Nelson LM, Mackenzie JF, Russell RI. Measurement of fat absorption using [^{3}H] glycerol triether and [^{14}C] glycerol trioleate in man. Clin Chim Acta 1980; 103:325–334.
36. Haverback BJ, Dyce VJ, Gutentag PJ, Montgomery DW. Measurement of trypsin and chymotrypsin in stool: a diagnostic test for pancreatic exocrine function. Gastroenterology 1963; 44:588–597.
37. Ammann RW, Tagwercher E, Kashiwagi H, Rosenmund H. Diagnostic value of fecal chymotrypsin and trypsin assessment for detection of pancreatic disease. Am J Dig Dis 1968; 13:123–126.
38. Goldberg DM, Campbell R, Roy AD. Fate of trypsin and chymotrypsin in the human small intestine. Gut 1969; 10:477–483.
39. Kaspar P, Möller G, Wahlefeld A. New photometric assay for chymotrypsin in stool. Clin Chem 1984; 30:1753–1757.
40. Durie PR, Goldberg DM. Biochemical tests of pancreatic function in infancy and childhood. Adv Clin Enzymol 1986; 4:77–92.
41. Bonin A, Roy CC, Lasalle R, Weber A, Morin CL. Fecal chymotrypsin: a reliable index of exocrine pancreatic function in children. J Pediatr 1973; 83:594–600.
42. Brown GA, Sule D, Williams J, Puntis JWL, Booth IW, McNeish AS. Faecal chymotrypsin: a reliable index of exocrine pancreatic function. Arch Dis Child 1988; 63:785–789.
43. Mills PR, Horton PW, Watkinson G. The value of the ^{14}C breath test in the assessment of fat absorption. Scand J Gastroenterol 1979; 14:913–921.
44. Newcomer AD, Hormann AF, DiMagno EP, Thomas PJ, Carlson GL. Triolein breath test: a sensitive and specific test for fat malabsorption. Gastroenterology 1979; 76:6–13.
45. Watkins JB, Klein PD, Schoeller DA, Kirschner BS, Park R, Perman JA. Diagnosis and differentiation of fat malabsorption in children using ^{13}C-labelled lipids: trioctanoin, triolein and palmitic acid breath tests. Gastroenterology 1982; 82:911–917.
46. Cole SG, Rossi S, Stern A, Hofmann AF. Cholesteryl octanoate breath test: preliminary studies on a new noninvasive test of human pancreatic exocrine function. Gastroenterology 1987; 93:1372–1380.
47. Sterchi EE, Green JR, Lentz MJ. Non pancreatic hydrolysis of *N*-benzoyl-L-tyrosyl-*p*-aminobenzoic acid (PABA-peptide) in the human small intestine. Clin Sci 1982; 62:557–560.
48. Gyr K. Felsenfeld O, Imondi AR. Chymotrypsin-like activity of some intestinal bacteria. Dig Dis Sci 1978; 23:413–416.
49. Heyman MB. The bentiromide test: how good is it? Gastroenterology 1985; 89:685–687.
50. Imondi AR, Stradley RP, Wolgemuth R. Synthetic peptides in the diagnosis of exocrine pancreatic insufficiency in animals. Gut 1972; 13:726–731.
51. Toskes PP. Bentiromide as a test of exocrine pancreatic function in adult patients with pancreatic exocrine insufficiency: determination of appropriate dose and urinary collection interval. Gastroenterology 1983; 85:565–569.
52. Mitchell CJ, Humphrey CS, Bullen AW, Kelleher H, Losowsky MS. Improved diagnostic accuracy of a modified oral pancreatic function test. Scand J Gastroenterol 1979; 14:737–741.
53. Mitchell CJ, Field HP, Simpson FG, Parkin A, Kelleher J, Losowsky MS. Preliminary evaluation of a single day tubeless test of pancreatic function. Br Med J 1981; 282:1751–1753.
54. Hoek FJ, van den Berg FAJTM, Klein Elhorst JT, Meyer JL, Timmer E, Tytgat GNJ. Improved specificity of the PABA test with *p*-aminosalicylic acid (PAS). Gut 1987; 28:468–473.
55. Puntis JWL, Berg JD, Buckley TM, Booth IW, McNeath AS. Simplified oral pancreatic function test. Arch Dis Child 1988; 63:780–784.
56. Sacher M, Kobsa A. Shmerling DH. PABA screening test for exocrine pancreatic function in infants and children. Arch Dis Child 1979; 53:639–641.
57. Dockter G, Nacu I, Kohlberger E. Determination of protease-cleaved *p*-aminobenzoic acid (PABA) in serum after oral administration of *N*-benzoyl-L-tyrosyl-*p*-aminobenzoic acid (PABA-peptide) in children. Eur J Pediatr 1981; 135:277–279.
58. Delchier J-C, Soule J-C. BT-PABA test with plasma PABA measurements: evaluation of sensitivity and specificity. Gut 1983; 24:318–325.
59. Weizman Z, Forstner GG, Gaskin KJ, Kopelman H, Wong S, Durie PR. Bentiromide test for assessing pancreatic dysfunction using analysis of para-aminobenzoic acid in plasma and urine: studies in cystic fibrosis and Shwachman's syndrome. Gastroenterology 1985; 89:596–604.
60. Mališ F, Frič P, Kasahrek E, Slabý J. Comparative study of the estimation of exocrine pancreatic function using *p*-(*N*--acetyl-L-tyrosyl) and *p*-(*N*-benzoyl-L-tyrosyl) aminobenzoic acid. Acta Hepatogastroenterol 1983; 30:99–101.
61. Mališ F, Frič P, Kasahrek E, Jodl J, Vavsová V, Slabý J. A paroral test of pancreatic insufficiency with 4-(*N*-acetyl-L-tyrosyl) aminobenzoic acid in children with cystic fibrosis. J Pediatr 1979; 94:942–944.
62. Scharpé S, Iliano L. Two indirect tests of exocrine pancreatic function evaluated. Clin Chem 1987; 33:5–12.
63. Lankisch PG, Brauneis J, Otto J, Göke B. Pancreolauryl and NBT-PABA tests: are serum tests a more practicable alternative to urine tests in the diagnosis of exocrine pancreatic insufficiency? Gastroenterology 1986; 90:350–354.
64. Schönberger W, Weitzel D. Diagnose per exorrinen pankrean-insuffizienz mit flurescein-dilawat bei patienten mit cysticher fibrose. Monatsschr Kinderheelkd 1980; 128:195–198.
65. Neis P, Zeub F, Uber die anwendbarkeit von fluoresceindilaurat zur exokrinen pankreasfunktionsprüfung bei kindern. Monatsschr Kinderheilkd 1981; 129:347–348.
66. Cumming JGR, Forsyth JS, Boyd EJS, Frost GJ, Cuschieri A. Diag-

nosis of exocrine insufficiency in cystic fibrosis by use of fluorescein dilaurate test. Arch Dis Child 1986; 61:573–575.

67. Goldstein R, Blondheim O, Levy E, Stankiewicz H, Freier S. The fatty meal test: an alternative to stool fat analysis. Am J Clin Nutr 1983; 38:763–768.
68. Shwachman H, Dooley RR. Tests of exocrine functions of the pancreas in childhood. Pediatr Clin North Am 1955; 2:201–271.
69. Brugge WR, Goff JS, Allen NC, Podell ER, Allen RH. Development of a dual label Schilling test for pancreatic exocrine function based on the differential absorption of cobalmin bound to intrinsic factor and R protein. Gastroenterology 1980; 78:937–949.
70. Lebenthal E, Lee PC. Development of functional response in human exocrine pancreas. Pediatrics 1980; 66:556–560.
71. Davidson GP, Koheil A, Forstner GG. Salivary amylase in cystic fibrosis: a marker of disordered autoimmune function. Pediatr Res 1978; 12:967–970.
72. O'Donnell MD, Miller NJ. Plasma pancreatic and salivary type amylase and immunoreactive trypsin concentrations: variations with age and reference ranges for children. Clin Chim Acta 1980; 104:265–273.
73. Grenner G, Deutsch G, Schmidtberger R, Dati F. A highly sensitive enzyme immunoassay for the determination of pancreatic lipase. J Clin Chem Clin Biochem 1982; 20:515–520.
74. Cleghorn G, Benjamin L, Corey M, Forstner G, Dati F, Durie P. Age-related alterations of immunoreactive pancreatic lipase and cationic trypsinogen in young children with cystic fibrosis. J Pediatr 1985; 107:377–381.
75. Cleghorn G, Benjamin L, Corey M, Forstner G, Dati F, Durie P. Serum immunoreactive pancreatic lipase and cationic trypsinogen for the assessment of exocrine pancreatic function in older patients with cystic fibrosis. Pediatrics 1986; 77:301–306.
76. Adriaenssens K, van Riel L. Serum pancreatic lipase as a screening test for cystic fibrosis. Arch Dis Child 1982; 57:553–555.
77. Borgström A, Ohlsson K. Radioimmunological determination and characterization of cathodal trypsin-like immunoreactivity in normal human plasma. Scand J Clin Lab Med 1976; 36:809–814.
78. Geokas MC, Largman C, Brodrick JW, Johnston DH. Determination of human pancreatic cationic trypsinogen in serum by radioimmunoassay. Am J Physiol 1979; 236:E77–E83.
79. Bowling FG, Watson ARA, Rylatt DB, Elliot JE, Bunch RJ, Bundesen PG. Monoclonal antibody-based enzyme immunoassay for trypsinogen in neonatal screening for cystic fibrosis. Lancet 1987; i:826–827.
80. Crossley JR, Smith PA, Edgar BW, Gluckman PD, Elliot RB. Neonatal screening for cystic fibrosis using immunoreactive trypsin assay in dried blood spots. Clin Chim Acta 1981; 113:111–121.
81. Wilcken B, Brown ARD, Urwin R, Brown DA. Cystic fibrosis screening by dried blood spot trypsin assay: results in 75,000 newborn infants. J Pediatr 1983; 102:383–387.
82. Durie PR, Forstner GG, Gaskin KJ, Moore DJ, Cleghorn GJ, Wong SS, Corey ML. Age-related alterations of immunoreactive pancreatic cationic trypsinogen in sera from cystic fibrosis patients with and without pancreatic insufficiency. Pediatr Res 1986; 20:209–213.
83. Moore DJ, Forstner GG, Largman C, Cleghorn GJ, Wong SS, Durie PR. Serum immunoreactive cationic trypsinogen: a useful indicator of severe exocrine dysfunction in the pediatric patient without cystic fibrosis. Gut 1986; 27:1362–1368.
84. Owyang C, Scarpello JH, Vinik AI. Correlation between pancreatic enzyme secretion and plasma concentration of human pancreatic polypeptide in health and in chronic pancreatitis. Gastroenterology 1982; 83:55–62.
85. Koch MB, Go VLW, Di Magno EP. Can plasma human pancreatic polypeptide be used to detect diseases of the exocrine pancreas? Mayo Clin Proc 1985; 60:259–265.
86. Durie PR. Pancreatic function tests. Med Clin North Am 1988; 20:3842–3845.

CHAPTER 37

Breath Analysis

Jay A. Perman, M.D.

Breath analysis for the purpose of assessing gastrointestinal (GI) function depends on metabolism of an orally administered substrate to a freely diffusible gas that is ultimately excreted by the lungs. The substrate is selected based on the digestive function being assessed. The detected gas may indicate either deficiency or intactness of a digestive process.

For example, measurement of hydrogen following administration of lactose assesses the completeness of lactose digestion and absorption. The presence of H_2 in breath indicates lactase activity insufficient to hydrolyze the lactose load, thus demonstrating deficiency. Conversely, evolution of labeled carbon dioxide in breath following tissue oxidation of an orally administered labeled lipid such as ^{14}C triolein indicates intactness of fat digestion.

Breath analysis offers readily apparent advantages for noninvasive investigation of digestive function in the child. Breath is sampled noninvasively, permitting frequently repeatable measurements. No separation steps are required prior to analysis of the sample, thus allowing rapid measurement. Alternatively, the potential for sample storage exists, and this facilitates testing at sites distant from the laboratory and analysis at a later time.

The two major gases in expired air pertinent to investigation of GI function are hydrogen and carbon dioxide. Breath tests dependent on the measurement of these gases are discussed in detail in this chapter. In addition, measurement of methane in breath has attracted recent interest.[1] Methane is excreted by approximately one-third of the general population.[2] An increased frequency of CH_4 excretion in patients with colonic cancer and in premalignant colonic disorders has been reported,[3] but these observations have not been uniformly confirmed.[4] Furthermore, a recently completed study utilizing an experimental model of colon cancer failed to show an influence of the presence of tumor on methane excretion.[5] The utility of breath CH_4 measurements for the investigation of GI function, therefore, remains to be elucidated. Expired air methane measurements are not further discussed in this chapter.

Similarly, ethane and pentane require further investigation regarding their significance in expired air and their utility as breath tests. The presence of these hydrocarbons in expired air originates from in vivo peroxidation of unsaturated fatty acids, especially those found in the lipid bilayers of various cell membranes. Thus, it appears possible to investigate factors that could affect lipid peroxidation in intact animals or humans by utilizing measurement of these gases in breath. For example, both vitamin E and selenium deficiencies have recently been studied using this methodology.[6]

BREATH HYDROGEN TESTS

Performance

Breath hydrogen tests are generally performed by obtaining samples of expired air before and at 30-minute intervals for 3 hours following administration of aqueous sugar solutions, which represent the test substrate.[7] Such a 3-hour monitoring period detects mono- or disaccharide malabsorption, with more than 90 percent of malabsorbers exhibiting hydrogen excretion curves consistent with a positive response by 2 hours following substrate ingestion. Detection of carbohydrate malabsorption following administration of a complex test meal, such as detection of lactose malabsorption after ingestion of milk or yogurt, requires a longer testing period to compensate for the slower gastric emptying induced by fat in the test meal.[8] Detection of starch malabsorption, especially in patients with cystic fibrosis, may require a monitoring period of 8 to 10 hours.[9]

Sampling

Original techniques for breath hydrogen measurements were not readily applicable to the child. These techniques required a closed continuous collection system in which the patient remained for hours. Using this method, total excretion of specific components of breath could be determined without concern for minute-to-minute variation in endogenous gas production. Because this methodology was complicated and unwieldy, interval sampling methods have been developed that are less precise than closed continuous collection systems but are certainly adequate for patient care and clinical research. A semiquantitative estimate of the total excretion of a gas component over time can be determined using interval sampling by assuming a constant output of respiratory gases. More specifically, the total amount of gas expired during a period of observation can be calculated, assuming a constant production per unit time of the specific components of breath being measured and taking the mean value of two sample points.[10] For most clinical applications, however, the concentration of the specific gas is sufficient, and calculation of the total quantity excreted is not required.

Application of breath tests in the pediatric population has required the development of well-tolerated collecting systems, which, in the case of infants and toddlers, do not require the child's active co-operation. Face masks are commonly used for collection techniques in infants and children.[11] Much of my work has utilized a simple nasal prong into which the patient breathes normally while the prong is held at the nose by either the patient or the examiner.[12] While watching the subject's breathing pattern, the examiner aspirates 3 to 5 cc during the latter half of expiration until a sample sufficient for analysis has been obtained. The nasal prong technique has been found to be well tolerated by patients of all ages, and satisfactory samples have been obtained (Fig. 1).

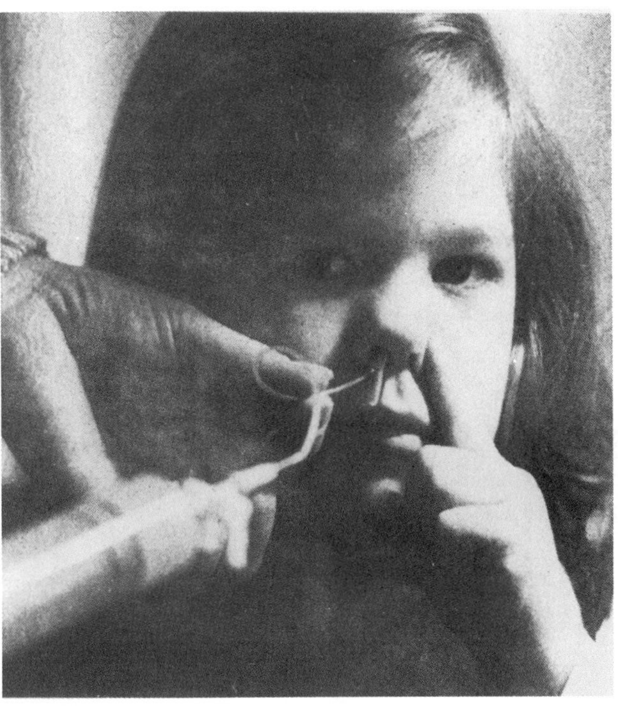

FIGURE 1 Demonstration of "nasal prong" device used for collection of expired air. (From Perman et al.[12])

Substrate Selection

Flexibility of substrate selection, substrate form, and dosage is characteristic of breath hydrogen testing. The only rigid requirement is that the substrate be appropriate to the function that one wishes to evaluate. Thus, detection of lactose malabsorption requires the administration of lactose as the test substrate. Conventionally, 2 g per kilogram of lactose in a 20 percent solution is the test dosage.[7] This dosage was adapted from the standard lactose tolerance test using blood glucose as the measured response. The osmolality of the solution may need to be modified in patients younger than 6 months of age. This investigator commonly uses a 10 percent solution in this age group. Should one wish to determine whether an individual malabsorbs a more physiologic dose, one could use lactose in a given serving of milk or yogurt as the test substrate.[8]

Sample Analysis

Hydrogen is usually measured by gas chromatography, and relatively inexpensive and dedicated instruments are available commercially for this purpose. Other methods of measuring breath hydrogen are available. These include electrochemical cells, helium ionization detectors, and reduction gas detectors.[13,14] Samples are conventionally collected in plastic syringes. It is not necessary to use glass syringes for this purpose. Alternatively, samples may be collected in specialized collection bags and transferred to syringes for application directly to the sample loop of the instrument. No intermediate separation steps are required prior to analyzing the sample.

Sample Storage

Breath hydrogen methodology has been applied to outpatient and field studies because of its ease and simplicity and because samples can be stored in a variety of systems. Samples stored in the collection syringes themselves over an 8-hour period demonstrated no change in hydrogen concentration, but deterioration does occur over a period of days.[15] Sealing methods and refrigeration of samples appear to retard the deterioration in the sample if stored in a syringe over time. Specialized nonsterile Vacutainers have been successfully used to store and ship samples, and these Vacutainers have been demonstrated to be stable for periods exceeding 30 days.[12] Mylar bags are also available for prolonged sample storage.

Interpretation of Data

Criteria for a Positive Response. Results are most commonly expressed as the concentration of hydrogen excreted in parts per million (ppm) above baseline. Hydrogen concentrations tend to decline during the fasting state, and the baseline value can therefore be defined as the lowest value of hydrogen obtained at any sampling time (Fig. 2).[7] Parts per million above baseline, or delta ppm, is then calculated by subtraction of this value from the subsequent hydrogen concentrations. An increase in breath hydrogen of greater than 10 ppm above baseline completely discriminates biopsy-proven isolated lactase-insufficient subjects from lactase-sufficient subjects. If this increase occurs later than 120 minutes after ingestion of substrate, more specifically at 180 minutes, the result may be consistent with either normal mucosal function or partial or secondary lactase deficiency due to mucosal injury.[7] In practice, most clinicians prefer to use a rise above baseline of 20 ppm or more, rather than 10 ppm, as the criterion for an unequivocal positive response, with rises of 10 to 20 ppm considered equivocal.

In addition, an early rise in H_2 concentration in the first 30 minutes following substrate ingestion may be consistent

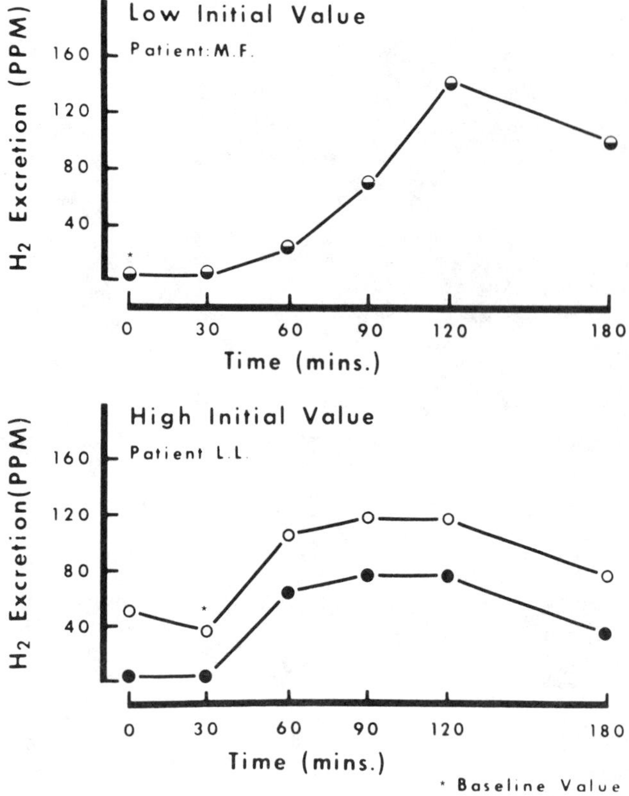

FIGURE 2 To determine parts per million above baseline (Δppm), baseline value is defined as the lowest value of H_2 excretion obtained at any sampling time. In patient M.F. with low initial value, actual H_2 excretion (*open circles*) and delta ppm (*solid circles*) are synonymous. In patient L.L., with high initial value, 30-minute sample is taken as baseline value, such that delta ppm (*solid circles*) is determined by subtraction of that value from subsequent H_2 responses. (From Barr et al.[7])

with small bowel bacterial overgrowth, especially if accompanied by a subsequent second peak in expired hydrogen.[16] The latter is thought to be consistent with the bolus of the substrate reaching the colon. Unfortunately, the second peak does not commonly occur in practice, and one must therefore rely on either the early rise in breath hydrogen or the elevation of the fasting H_2 (discussed below) as an indicator of bacterial overgrowth.

Normalization to an Alveolar Concentration. Hydrogen concentration in expired air may be normalized to an alveolar concentration using CO_2 as an internal standard.[17] This corrects for variations in the phase of expiration from which samples were obtained. Correction using CO_2 requires the assumption that ventilation is relatively constant over interval sampling times. If there are wide swings in minute ventilation, correction using CO_2 as the internal standard may actually exacerbate the error.[18] Some investigators use oxygen and nitrogen rather than CO_2 as an internal standard.[19] In actual practice, the use of an internal standard to correct hydrogen values is unnecessary when sampling is done by an experienced individual, since the shape and interpretation of the hydrogen curve are commonly unaltered by corrected values, especially in children older than 6 or 7 years in whom sampling generally occurs in the same phase of expiration.

Fasting Breath H_2. Criteria for interpretation of breath hydrogen tests in the detection of carbohydrate malabsorption may vary, but all are based on comparisons of hydrogen concentrations in interval samples with a pretest value obtained after an overnight fast. The diagnostic significance of the fasting breath hydrogen (FH_2) concentration itself has been examined. In our hands, values defined as greater than 42 ppm may indicate the presence of GI stasis and bacterial overgrowth (Table 1).[20] Since laboratories may vary, an elevated FH_2 can probably more generically be described as that which exceeds two standard deviations beyond the mean FH_2 for that laboratory. FH_2 is of use in this manner only if the pretest dinner meal has been standardized (Fig. 3).[20,21] A red meat and rice meal with no source of carbohydrate other than the rice should be ingested the night before a morning breath test if FH_2 is to be reliably used as a screening test for stasis and bacterial overgrowth.

DEVELOPMENTAL ASPECTS OF HYDROGEN PRODUCTION

Approximately 75 percent of infants excrete hydrogen by 1 week of age, and virtually all infants produce and excrete hydrogen by the end of the third week of life.[22] Hydrogen production in early infancy is dependent on colonization of the GI tract with hydrogen-producing bacteria. Colonization,

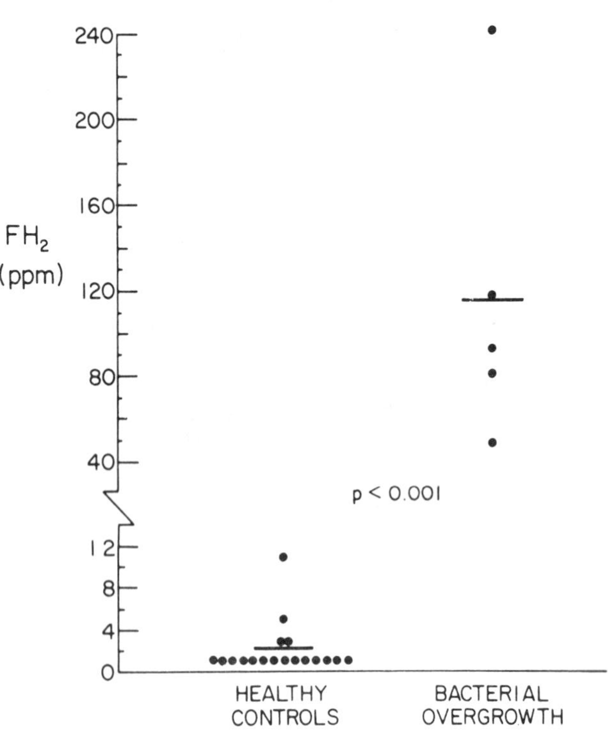

FIGURE 3 Fasting breath hydrogen after a standard dinner meal of meat and rice bread in 18 healthy subjects and five patients with intestinal pseudo-obstruction and bacterial overgrowth. The mean for each group is indicated by the line. The *P* value was calculated using Student's unpaired *t*-test. (From Perman et al.[20])

TABLE 1
Diagnosis and Clinical Features in Patients with Elevated Fasting Breath Hydrogen

Patient	Fasting Breath Hydrogen (ppm)	Diagnosis	Documentation
1	48	Chronic diarrhea	Positive culture*
2	224	Scleroderma	X-ray,† steatorrhea, abnormal glycocholate breath test, no culture done
3	101	Diabetes mellitus	X-ray, bacteria adherent to aspirated duodenal mucus
4	245 163	Intestinal pseudo-obstruction	Positive culture, x-ray
5	134 77	Colonic interposition	Positive culture; steatorrhea
6	105	Crohn's disease with multiple resections	Steatorrhea, no culture done
7	45	Post-Billroth II gastrectomy	X-ray, hypoalbuminemia, no culture done
8	54	Idiopathic steatorrhea	Abnormal Schilling test, abnormal glycocholate breath test, no culture done
9	73 112	Chronic diarrhea	Severe combined immunodeficiency syndrome
10	195 141	Intestinal pseudo-obstruction	Positive culture, x-ray
11	156 191	Intestinal pseudo-obstruction	Positive culture, x-ray
12	48	Intestinal pseudo-obstruction	Positive culture, x-ray
13	136 80	Intestinal pseudo-obstruction	Positive culture, x-ray
14	47	Recurrent abdominal pain	
15	43	Recurrent abdominal pain	

*Greater than 10^4 organisms per milliliter of duodenal fluid.
†Stasis.
From Perman et al.[20]

in turn, is dependent on the mode of delivery of the infant and the nature of the infant's feeding, breast versus bottle.[23] In addition to the flora, production of hydrogen requires the presence of fermentable substrate in the neonate's colon. Since the capacity to digest and absorb carbohydrate continues to evolve after birth, entrance of fermentable substrate into the colon appears to be a normal phenomenon over the first several months of life.

From the foregoing discussion, it can be seen that both colonization of the gut and the infant's capacity to absorb carbohydrates are evolving. The infant's capacity to produce and excrete hydrogen over the first several months of life is thus not in steady state. Studies by MacLean and Fink[22] and by Barr et al[24] support these observations. Excretion of hydrogen in concentrations associated with pathologic malabsorption in later life are common in the infant through the first 3 to 4 months of life. Accordingly, applications of breath hydrogen methodologies, which were developed and validated in the older infant and child, are not easily applicable in early infancy. Furthermore, breath hydrogen tests are generally performed after an overnight fast, and both baseline values and expected hydrogen response following ingestion of substrate are predicated on a previous overnight fast. Because overnight fasting cannot be carried out in early infancy except in infants who are receiving intravenous therapy, standard breath hydrogen testing in this age group becomes fraught with difficulty.

Breath hydrogen testing in early infancy has nevertheless been advocated in several conditions, including necrotizing enterocolitis (NEC)[25] and in intractable diarrheal states.[26] Early interest in application of breath hydrogen methods in the nursery centered on identification of NEC. It was reasoned that carbohydrate malabsorption is an early sign of NEC, and hydrogen is the principal component of the gases formed in the intramural blebs in this condition. Thus, it was hypothesized that hydrogen excretion would be elevated beyond what is normally seen in infants in those who were developing early NEC. This possibility has recently gained support in data published by Cheu et al using the ratio of H_2 to CO_2 in expired air samples.[27] It has been reported that ratios below 8 ppm per millimeter of mercury are inconsistent with NEC. These data require confirmation.

Shermeta et al[28] and Lifschitz[26] have described the utility of spot breath H_2 measurements, i.e., single measurements, in infants receiving continuous nutritional drips following intra-abdominal surgery or in those with intractable diarrhea. Their data support the use of spot measurements to guide advancement in nutritional therapy. This technique, however, has not gained widespread use, and further evaluation of the value of such applications is necessary. It should be emphasized that spot measurements in infants on continuous drip feedings do not carry the same implications as a FH_2 value in an older child. An elevated spot hydrogen in the continuously fed infant cannot be taken to imply bacterial overgrowth.

TABLE 2
Clinical Applications of H_2 Breath Tests

Clinical Question	Substrate	Dose	Interval/Duration	Reference
Lactose malabsorption	Lactose	2 g/kg; maximum 50 g in 20% solution 10% solution in infants less than 6 months old	Every 30 min for 3 hours	7
Sucrose malabsorption	Sucrose	Same	Every 30 min for 3 hours	12
Glucose malabsorption	Glucose	1 g/kg; maximum 50 g in 20% solution*	Every 30 min for 4 hours	—
Bacterial overgrowth	Glucose or lactulose	50 g* 10 g†	Every 30 min for 4 hours	41 16
Pancreatic insufficiency	Rice flour	100 g carbohydrate‡	Every 30 min–1 hour for 8 hours	9

*Dose of glucose and conduct of test in infants and small children not well established.

†Dose for patients under 30 kg body weight not well established. I conventionally use 0.3 g/kg; maximum 10 g in 20 percent solution.

‡Application in children not established. I use a serving of pancakes from rice flour and measure the amount eaten to determine quantity of starch ingested.

APPLICATION OF BREATH HYDROGEN TESTS

Specific applications of breath hydrogen methodology are listed in Table 2. Breath hydrogen testing is performed principally for the investigation of lactose malabsorption. Abundant data support its position as the most accurate indirect test of lactase insufficiency.[7,29-32] Similarly, sucrase deficiency can be accurately diagnosed by breath hydrogen testing.[12,33,34]

Breath hydrogen methodology has also been used to evaluate monosaccharide malabsorption. Glucose malabsorption can be evaluated in a manner analogous to that for lactose and sucrose malabsorption. Fructose malabsorption has been demonstrated utilizing breath hydrogen measurements,[35-37] and it has been demonstrated that children as well as adults may physiologically malabsorb fructose. Until the developmental aspects of fructose absorption are established, it will not be possible to apply a standard breath hydrogen test in investigating patients for fructose malabsorption. In other words, normality remains to be defined. Similarly, the breath hydrogen test has been used to demonstrate sorbitol malabsorption in children.[38] As with fructose, one cannot simply use the breath hydrogen test to demonstrate abnormality, since it appears that sorbitol is commonly malabsorbed in the healthy individual.

Starch absorption has been evaluated with breath hydrogen methodology in adults,[9] and this method may have some applicability in the evaluation of pancreatic insufficiency in childhood. The substrate for starch absorption tests is generally rice. As much as 100 g of carbohydrate as rice starch has been shown to be completely absorbed in normal adults.[39] Thus, rice becomes an appropriate substrate in the evaluation of starch absorption. Preliminary results by this author in the evaluation of pancreatic insufficiency among patients with cystic fibrosis suggest that this technique has promise.[40]

Several substrates have been utilized for breath hydrogen tests intended to identify patients with bacterial overgrowth. Initial interest was focused on the use of lactulose for this purpose.[16] Fermentation of lactulose by bacteria in the upper small bowel results in early release of hydrogen, generally within the first 30 minutes after administration of lactulose. This may be followed by a later peak when the balance of the lactulose bolus reaches the colon, resulting in a double-humped curve that is considered indicative of overgrowth. Such characteristic curves do not frequently occur. Alternatively, glucose has been demonstrated to be a particularly effective substrate in hydrogen breath tests for the identification of bacterial overgrowth.[41] Administration of glucose will be followed by a breath hydrogen peak within the first 2 hours after administration in patients with overgrowth. In addition, the fasting breath hydrogen itself is often elevated in bacterial overgrowth and can be utilized as an additional expired air marker of this disorder.

CARBON DIOXIDE BREATH TESTS

Dodds was the first to recognize the potential of breath CO_2 measurements as a means of evaluating intestinal function.[42,43] He demonstrated a rise in breath CO_2 concentration after meals and documented changes in postprandial CO_2 excretion in GI disorders, including pancreatic insufficiency and pernicious anemia. In contrast to hydrogen and methane, CO_2 is normally present in percent quantities in expired air, and breath tests dependent on changes in breath CO_2 concentration require labeled substrates. ^{14}C is used as this label. The nonradioactive stable isotope of carbon, ^{13}C, has been used in children and pregnant women.[44] Measurement of ^{13}C-containing compounds currently requires mass spectrophotometry, which is not readily available.

The labeled carbon is placed in a specific small molecular weight segment of the test substrate, which will be cleaved off by the enzymatic process being studied, yielding a moiety that is oxidized to CO_2 by mammalian enzymes or bacteria. Cleavage of the target bond is the rate-limiting step in the function being evaluated. Thus, the rate of labeled CO_2 excretion can be used as a measure of enzymatic activity. Substrates utilized include fatty acids, carbohydrates, and bile acids. As with hydrogen breath tests, the specific application dictates the substrate required. Following administration of the substrate, breath samples are collected at 30- to 60-minute intervals for a period of 4 to 6 hours. Techniques for performance of CO_2 breath tests and expression of data are reviewed elsewhere.[45] $^{13}CO_2$ collection and measurement methods have been described in detail by Schoeller et al.[44,46]

Safety

^{14}C is a beta emitter with a long half-life, but the dose generally used is 10 μCi, which results in little total body radiation. It is thought that the radiation delivered in a ^{14}C-glycocholate breath test represents approximately one-tenth of the radiation delivered to the gonads by a chest radiograph.[45] While the test appears to be safe for adults, even this small dose of radiation may be unacceptable for children or women of child-bearing age, establishing the rationale for development of the $^{13}CO_2$ breath tests.

APPLICATIONS

Applications of carbon dioxide breath tests have included evaluation of mucosal function,[47,48] lipid digestion and absorption, and bacterial overgrowth.

CO_2 Breath Tests for the Detection of Fat Malabsorption

Utilization of lipid breath tests in which the substrate is labeled with ^{14}C or ^{13}C for the demonstration of fat malabsorption depends on the assumption that intestinal absorption is the rate-limiting step in the interval from ingestion of a labeled fat to expiration of labeled CO_2. The tests utilize lipids labeled with either the radioactive isotope of carbon (^{14}C) or the stable isotope of carbon (^{13}C) in the carboxyl moiety and dissolved in a corn oil preparation for oral administration. Subsequent recovery of labeled CO_2 in breath in amounts within a range established in healthy individuals is assumed to indicate normal digestive and absorptive mechanisms for dietary fat.

Many factors independent of fat digestion and absorption, including gastric emptying, small bowel transit time, rate of tissue lipid deposition and oxidation, the size of the endogenous CO_2 pool, and pulmonary factors affecting CO_2 excretion, have been cited as influencing the abundance of labeled CO_2 in breath.[49] Despite these variables, the triglyceride breath tests are reproducible within individuals studied serially, and the magnitude of recovery of labeled CO_2 in breath following administration of labeled medium and long-chain triglycerides generally shows the required negative correlation with results of 3-day quantitative fecal fat determination (Fig. 4).[50-52] However, some investigators have reported a good correlation between breath and fecal fat results only in patients with steatorrhea secondary to pancreatic insufficiency.[53] If application of the lipid breath test is restricted to patients with lipolytic disorders, excellent separation from healthy controls is observed. Absorption of the medium-chain triglyceride trioctanoin is impaired when lipolysis is inadequate, and a mean eightfold reduction in labeled CO_2 recovery in patients versus controls has been reported.[51] Similar separation has been demonstrated using the long-chain triglyceride tripalmitin.[54]

Overlapping of results between controls and steatorrheic individuals occurs when the patient group includes individuals

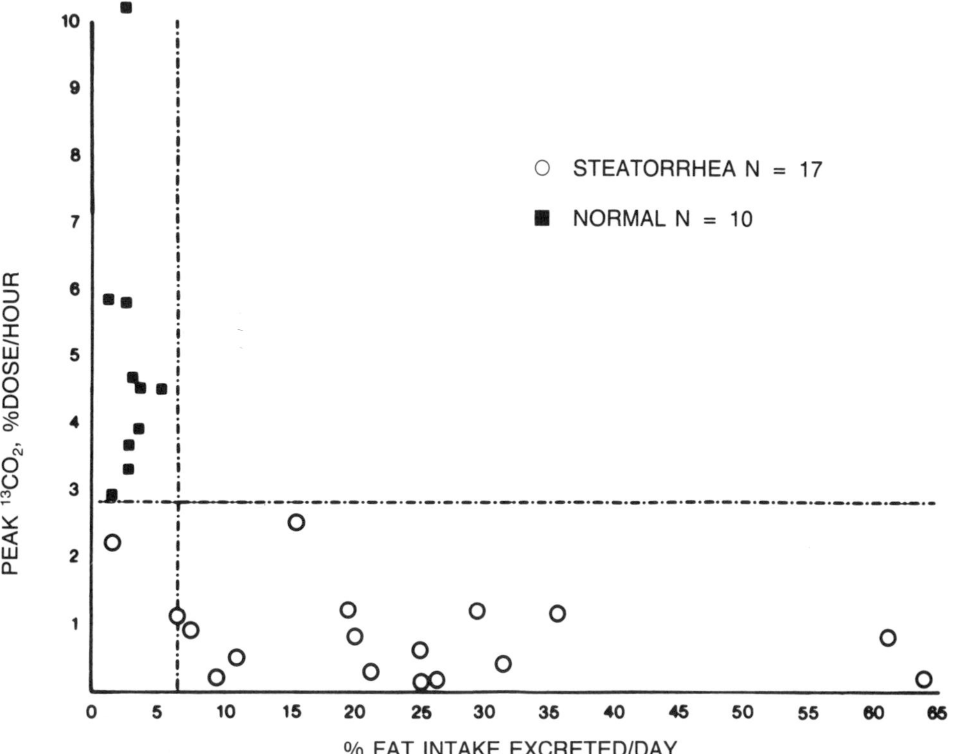

FIGURE 4 Peak breath excretion of $^{13}CO_2$ after ingestion of ^{13}C triolein. Vertical line depicts upper limit of normal fecal fat excretions for children (less than 7 percent of intake), and horizontal line depicts the lower limit of $^{13}CO_2$ excretion (greater than 2.73 percent dose per hour). (From Watkins et al.[52])

with fat malabsorption from a variety of causes. Newcomer et al[49] compared the trioctanoin and tripalmitin breath tests with triolein in a diverse group of patients with steatorrhea. In contrast to the relatively poor performance of trioctanoin (31 percent) and tripalmitin (42 percent), specificity was 96 percent utilizing triolein. Poor discrimination between normals and patients with mucosal disease is not surprising when triocanoin is utilized, since medium-chain triglycerides may be efficiently absorbed in the presence of mucosal damage.

To enhance the utility of lipid breath testing, various strategies have been devised to determine whether an abnormal result is attributable to inadequate lipolysis. One approach requires successive breath tests, administering a single triglyceride with and without pancreatic enzyme. Goff reported no overlap between patients with pancreatic insufficiency and those with other causes of malabsorption following repetition of a triolein breath test with pancreatic replacement enzymes.[55] Watkins et al[52] have demonstrated that the use of a series of breath tests to include triolein, palmitic acid, and trioctanoin not only indicates the presence of fat malabsorption in children but also provides direction as to the basis for the fat malabsorption. By utilizing a series of breath tests it is possible to discriminate steatorrhea attributable to pancreatic insufficiency from that attributable to mucosal disease, ileal dysfunction, or liver disease (Fig. 5).

Bile Acid Breath Tests for Bacterial Overgrowth and Ileal Dysfunction

The ^{14}C or ^{13}C cholylglycine or bile acid breath test utilizes, as a substrate, cholic acid conjugated to labeled glycine. In patients with bacterial overgrowth, the amide bond of cholylglycine is split by bacteria in the small intestine, releasing a free bile acid and the labeled glycine. Most of the cholic acid is absorbed from the small intestine, whereas the glycine[45] may enter the body glycine pool with eventual metabolism to labeled CO_2. Alternatively, the glycine may be metabolized by colonic bacteria with release of CO_2, which is absorbed and exhaled. The presence of abnormally high concentrations of labeled CO_2 in the breath therefore is an indication of bile salt deconjugation and provides indirect evidence of bacterial overgrowth.

Evolution of labeled CO_2 in breath following administration of cholylglycine may also occur in the presence of ileal dysfunction. Interruption of the enterohepatic circulation results in entrance of the orally administered cholylglycine into the colon, where the process described above will occur. Thus, a potential reason for a false-positive cholylglycine breath test when one seeks the presence of bacterial overgrowth is ileal dysfunction. In an attempt to differentiate bacterial overgrowth from ileal dysfunction, measurement of fecal labeled carbon has been advocated.[45] In comparison with luminal aspiration and culture of contents, the sensitivity of bile acid breath tests for the detection of bacterial overgrowth has been estimated to be 70 percent and the specificity 90 percent.[56]

Use of the ^{13}C glycocholate breath test has not been incorporated into clinical practice, and little use of this modality currently occurs. There has been insufficient experience in children to establish sensitivity and specificity.

^{14}C-D-Xylose Breath Test

King and Toskes[57] have reported use of ^{14}C-D-Xylose (10 μCi) administered in 1 g xylose for the detection of bacterial overgrowth. $^{14}CO_2$ results from intraluminal fermentation of the sugar by bacteria, and the rate of expired $^{14}CO_2$ accurately discriminates patients with overgrowth from healthy controls within 1 hour after administration of test substrate. Direct comparison of this test with the glycocholate breath test is not yet available, but the initial results are promising.

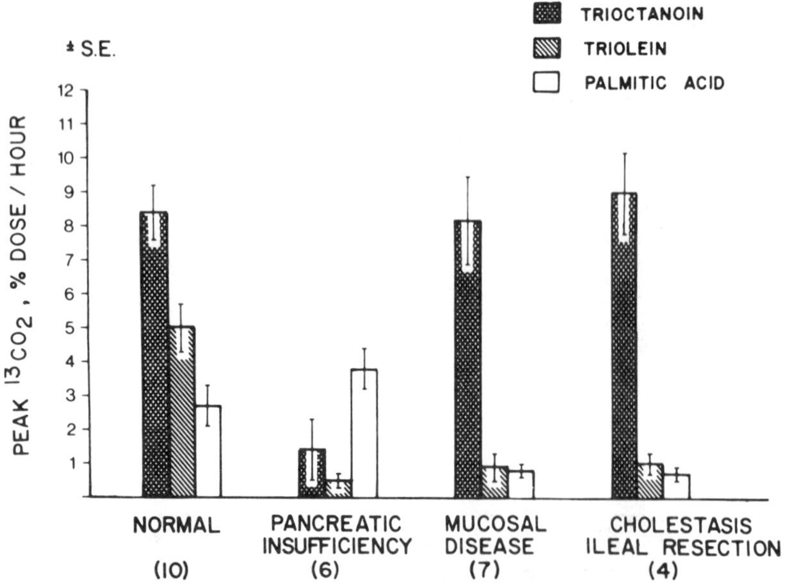

FIGURE 5 Peak excretion rate for each substrate in normals and patients with fat malabsorption, depicted according to substrate and diagnosis; n = number of patients in each group. (From Watkins et al.[52])

REFERENCES

1. Perman JA. Methane and colorectal cancer. Gastroenterology 1984; 87:728–730.
2. Bond JH, Engel RR, Levitt MD. Factors influencing pulmonary methane excretion in man. J Exp Med 1971; 133:572–588.
3. Piqué JM, Pallarés M, Cusó E, Vilar-Bonet J, Gassull MA. Methane production and colon cancer. Gastroenterology 1984; 87:601–605.
4. Karlin CA, Mastromarino AJ, Jones RD, Stroehlein JR, Lorentz O. Fecal skatole and indole and breath methane and hydrogen in patients with large bowel polyps or cancer. J Cancer Res Clin Oncol 1985; 109:135–141.
5. Flick JA, Perman JA. Nonabsorbed carbohydrate: Effect on fecal pH in methane-excreting and nonexcreting individuals. Am J Clin Nutr 1989; 49:1252–1257.
6. Lemoyne M, Van Gossuma A, Kurian R, Jeejeebhoy K. Plasma vitamin E and selenium and breath pentane in home parenteral nutrition patients. Am J Clin Nutr 1988; 48:1310–1315.
7. Barr RG, Watkins JB, Perman JA. Mucosal function and breath hydrogen excretion: comparative studies in the clinical evaluation of children with nonspecific abdominal complaints. Pediatrics 1981; 68:526–533.
8. Solomons NW, Garcia-Ibanez R, Viteri FE. Reduced rates of breath hydrogen (H_2) excretion with lactose tolerence tests in young children using whole milk. Am J Clin Nutr 1979; 32:783–786.
9. Kerlin P, Wong L, Harris B, Capra S. Rice flour, breath hydrogen and malabsorption. Gastroenterology 1984; 87:578–585.
10. Solomons NW, Viteri F, Rosenberg IH. Development of an interval sampling hydrogen (H_2) breath test for carbohydrate malabsorption in children; evidence for a circadian pattern of breath H_2 concentration. Pediatr Res 1978; 12:816–823.
11. Bujanover Y, Katz A, Peled Y, Gilat T. Lactose malabsorption in Israeli children. Isr J Med Sci 1985; 21:32–35.
12. Perman JA, Barr RB, Watkins JB. Sucrose malabsorption in children; non-invasive diagnosis by interval breath hydrogen determination. J Pediatr 1978; 93:17–22.
13. Bartlett K, Dobson JV, Eastham E. A new method for the detection of hydrogen in breath and its application to acquired and inborn sugar malabsorption. Clin Chim Acta 1980; 108:189–194.
14. Stevenson D, Cohen RS, Ostrander CR, Shahin SM, Kerner JA, Wetmore DL, Werner SB, Tomczyk M, Johnson JD. A sensitive analytical apparatus for measuring hydrogen production rates. II. Application to studies in human infants. J Pediatr Gastroenterol Nutr 1982; 1:233–237.
15. Ellis CJ, Kneid JM, Levitt MD. Storage of breath samples for hydrogen analysis. Gastroenterology 1988; 94:822–824.
16. Rhodes JM, Middleton P, Jewell DP. The lactulose hydrogen breath test as a diagnostic test for small-bowel bacterial overgrowth. Scand J Gastroenterol 1979; 14:333–336.
17. Niu H, Schoeller DA, Klein PD. Improved gas chromatographic quantitation of breath hydrogen by normalization to respiratory carbon dioxide. J Lab Clin Med 1979; 94:755–763.
18. Perman JA, Modler S, Engel RR, Heldt G. Effect of ventilation on breath hydrogen measurements. J Lab Clin Med 1985; 105:436–439.
19. Robb TA, Davidson GP. Advances in breath hydrogen quantitation in pediatrics: sample collection and normalization to constant oxygen and nitrogen levels. Clin Chim Acta 1981; 111:281–283.
20. Perman JA, Modler S, Barr RG, Rosenthal P. Fasting breath hydrogen concentration: normal values and clinical application. Gastroenterology 1984; 87:1358–1363.
21. Kotler DP, Holt PR, Rosensweig NS. Modification of the breath hydrogen test: increased sensitivity for the detection of carbohydrate malabsorption. J Lab Clin Med 1982; 100:798–805.
22. MacLean WC, Fink BB. Lactose malabsorption by premature infants: magnitude and clinical significance. J Pediatr 1980; 97:383–388.
23. Long SS, Swenson RN. Development of anaerobic fecal flora in healthy newborn infants. J Pediatr 1977; 91:298–301.
24. Barr RG, Hanley J, Patterson DK, Wooldridge J. Breath hydrogen excretion in normal newborn infants in response to usual feeding patterns: evidence for "functional lactase insufficiency" beyond the first month of life. J Pediatr 1984; 104:527–533.
25. Kirschner BS, Lahr C, Lahr D, et al. Detection of increased breath H_2 in infants with necrotizing enterocolitis, abstracted. Gastroenterology 1977; 72:1080.
26. Lifschitz CH. Breath hydrogen testing in infants with diarrhea. In: Lifshitz F, ed. Carbohydrate intolerance in infancy. New York: Marcel Dekker, 1982: 31.
27. Cheu HW, Brown DR, Rowe MI. Breath hydrogen excretion as a screening test for the early diagnosis of necrotizing enterocolitis. Am J Dis Child 1989; 143:156–159.
28. Shermeta DW, Ruaz E, Fink BB, MacLean WC Jr. Respiratory hydrogen secretion: a simple test of bowel adaptation in infants with short gut syndrome. J Pediatr Surg 1981; 16:271–274.
29. Newcomer AD, McGill DB, Thomas PJ, Hofmann AF. Prospective comparison of indirect methods for detecting lactase deficiency. N Engl J Med 1975; 293:1232–1236.
30. Metz G, Blendis LM, Jenkins DJA. H_2 breath test for lactase deficiency. N Engl J Med 1976; 294:730.
31. Douwes AC, Fernanades J, Degenhart HJ. Improved accuracy of lactose tolerance test in children, using expired H_2 measurement. Arch Dis Child 1978; 53:939–942.
32. Maffei HVL, Metz G, Bampoe V, Shiner M, Herman S, Brook CGD. Lactose intolerance, detected by the hydrogen breath test, in infants and children with chronic diarrhea. Arch Dis Child 1977; 52:766–771.
33. Metz G, Jenkins DJA, Newman A, Blendis LM. Breath hydrogen in hyposucrasia. Lancet 1976; i:119–120.
34. Douwes AC, Fernandes J, Jongbloed AA. Diagnostic value of sucrose tolerance test in children evaluated by breath hydrogen measurement. Acta Paediatr Scand 1980; 69:79–82.
35. Ravich WJ, Bayless TM, Thomas M. Fructose: incomplete intestinal absorption in humans. Gastroenterology 1983; 84:26–29.
36. Barnes G, McKellar W, Lawrence S. Detection of fructose malabsorption by breath hydrogen test in a child with diarrhea. J Pediatr 1983; 103:575–577.
37. Kneepkens CMF, Vonk RJ, Fernanades J. Incomplete intestinal absorption of fructose. Arch Dis Child 1984; 59:735–738.
38. Hyams JS. Sorbitol intolerance: an unappreciated cause of functional gastrointestinal complaints. J Pediatr 1983; 84:30–33.
39. Anderson IH, Levin AS, Levitt MD. Incomplete absorption of the carbohydrate in all-purpose wheat flour. N Engl J Med 1981; 304:891–892.
40. Perman JA, Rosenstein BJ. Carbohydrate digestion in cystic fibrosis (CF): application of breath H_2 measurements. Pediatr Res 1986; 20:246A.
41. Kerlin P, Wong L. Breath hydrogen testing in bacterial overgrowth of the small intestine. Gastroenterology 1988; 95:982–988.
42. Dodds EC. Variations in alveolar carbon dioxide pressure in relation to meals. J Physiol 1921; 54:342–348.
43. Dodds EC. A new method of investigating gastrointestinal secretion. Lancet 1921; ii:605–607.
44. Schoeller DA, Schneider JF, Solomons NW, et al. Clinical diagnosis using the stable isotope ^{13}C in CO_2 breath test: methodology and fundamental consideration. J Lab Clin Med 1977; 90:412–421.
45. Thaysen EH. Diagnostic value of the ^{14}C-cholylglycine breath test. Clin Gastroenterol 1977; 6:227–245.
46. Schoeller DA, Klein PD. A simplified technique for collecting breath CO_2 for isotope ratio mass spectrometry. Biomed Mass Spectrom 1978; 5:29–31.
47. Cozzetto FJ. Radiocarbon estimates of intestinal absorption. Am J Dis Child 1964; 107:605–611.
48. Barr RG, Perman JA, Schoeller DA, Watkins JB. Breath tests in pediatric gastrointestinal disorders: new diagnostic opportunities. Pediatrics 1978; 62:393–401.
49. Newcomer AD, Hofmann AF, DiMagno EP, Thomas PJ, Carlson GL. Triolein breath test–sensitive and specific test for fat malabsorption. Gastroenterology 1979; 76:6–13.
50. Kaihara S, Wagner HN Jr. Measurement of intestinal fat absorption with carbon-14 labeled tracers. J Clin Med 1968; 71:400–411.
51. Hepner GW, Vesell ES. Quantitative assessment of hepatic function by breath analysis after oral administration of [^{14}C] aminopyrine. Ann Intern Med 1975; 83:632–638.
52. Watkins JB, Klein PD, Schoeller DA, Kirschner BS, Park R, Perman JA. Diagnosis and differentiation of fat malabsorption in children using ^{13}C-labeled lipids: trioctanoin, triolein, and palmitic acid breath tests. Gastroenterology 1982; 82:911–917.
53. Levy-Gigi C, Mandelowitz N, Peled Y, Ayalon D, Gilat T. Is the fat breath test effective in the diagnosis of fat malabsorption and pancreatic disease? Digestion 1978; 18:77–85.
54. Burrows PJ, Fleming JS, Garnet ES, Ackery DM, Collin-Jones DG, Bamfort J. Clinical evaluation of the ^{14}C fat absorption test. Gut 1974; 15:147–150.

55. Goff JS. Two-stage triolein breath test differentiates pancreatic insufficiency from other causes of malabsorption. Gastroenterology 1982; 83:44–46.
56. Lauterburg BH, Newcomer AD, Hofmann AF. Clinical value of the bile acid breath test. Mayo Clin Proc 1978; 53:227.
57. King CE, Toskes PP. Comparison of the 1-gram [^{14}C] xylose, 10-gram lactulose-H_2 and 80-gram glucose-H_2 breath tests in patients with small intestine bacterial overgrowth. Gastroenterology 1986; 91:1447–1451.
58. Davidson GP, Robb TA, Kirubakaran CP. Bacterial contamination of the small intestine as an important cause of chronic diarrhea and abdominal pain: diagnosis by breath hydrogen test. Pediatrics 1984; 74:229–235.

CHAPTER 38

Laboratory Studies

PART 1

Biochemical Studies: Liver and Intestine

Patrick J. St. Louis, Ph.D., Dip.C.C.

The pediatric gastroenterologist should be critically aware of the diagnostic advantages and disadvantages of various laboratory tests, the complications of their performance, and the interpretation of the results. Optimum benefit to the patient can be achieved if there is a healthy dialogue between the laboratory staff and the clinician. This discussion deals in a general way with biochemical approaches to the investigation of the pediatric patient with presumed gastrointestinal disorders. Specific diseases and related tests will not be discussed. The reader is referred to appropriate sections elsewhere in the text.

GENERAL

Reference Ranges

Many analytes measured in the pediatric population exhibit age-related variation in their reference ranges, especially in the neonatal and in the pubertal periods (Table 1). In addition to age-related distributions, numerous analytes also show sex-related intervals and the number of intervals may vary from one analyte to another. The situation is further complicated in preterm infants where gestational age at birth might influence the definition of normal values. These facts must be remembered when interpreting test results relative to alterations expected in pathologic conditions.

In pediatric hospitals, laboratories usually indicate these age- or sex-related ranges in the laboratory handbook or data system. In a general hospital (adult) or in the case of external testing sites this may not be the case. Pediatric clinicians have to be aware of this and should rely on communication with the appropriate laboratory. Furthermore, for a variety of technical reasons, reference ranges frequently vary from laboratory to laboratory. The clinical correlates of these interlaboratory variations might not always be clear but should always be considered. An example of this is shown in Table 1, where the reference ranges for the enzyme gamma glutamyltransferase (GGT) are quoted from two different sources.

Specimens

Patient Preparation

The requirement for obtaining a fasting sample is problematic for some tests; examples include lipid analysis, lactose breath tests, and the xylose absorption test. Although

TABLE 1
Reference Values for Gamma Glutamyltransferase (GGT)

A*		B†	
Age	Enzyme Activity (IU/L)	Age	Enzyme Activity (IU/L)
<1 mo	<385	Newborn	<206
1-2 mo	<225	1-2 mo	<118
2-4 mo	<135	2-4 mo	<71
4-7 mo	<75	4-7 mo	<37
7 mo–15 yr	<45	7 mo–15 yr	1-22
>15 yr—male	<75	>15 yr—male	5-38
—female	<45	—female	5-27

*From Handbook of laboratory reference values; assay on the Kodak Ektachem clinical chemistry analyzer at 37 °C. The Hospital for Sick Children, Toronto, 1988.

†From Kincaid HL. Clinical enzymology in pediatrics. In: Hicks JM, Boeckx RL, eds. Pediatric clinical chemistry. Philadelphia: WB Saunders, 1984: 349.

adults are usually required to fast for at least 12 hours prior to some tests, in younger patients the time required for fasting is frequently reduced to 8 or 4 hours in infants. In the neonate, requirements for fasting are usually met by testing or sampling the patient immediately prior to the next feeding. However, instructions should be clear; frequently children and adolescents travel some distance to undergo a test and, having fasted overnight, unwittingly ingest juice or milk just before arriving at the test center.

Blood

Phlebotomy is frequently a problem for the clinician, the laboratory, and the young patient. There is the difficulty of finding a suitable access site, especially when frequent sampling is required. Sample volume is an evident problem in obtaining blood samples from children, especially neonates. Owing to an increasing number of tiny, often premature, infants being cared for in tertiary care units, there has been increasing use of capillary samples. These are frequently contaminated by body fluids and from sample hemolysis. Also, techniques for skin puncture, including the selection of optimum sites and the effects of depth and width of lancets, require constant evaluation.[1,2] The emphasis on skin puncture is partly attributable to the fact that accessible veins in the sick infant must be reserved for parenteral therapy; one report indicates that up to 57 percent of the inpatients in a pediatric hospital were receiving intravenous fluids.[2] Although the present generation of analyzers is capable of providing a wide range of tests on microliter volumes of blood, some specific tests still require larger sample volumes. When the patient has to be repeatedly tested, for example, when there is prolonged jaundice in the neonate, test ordering patterns may have to be adjusted in relation to sample volume requirements so that maximum information is obtained. All these considerations reinforce the need for critical evaluation of test results and consultation with laboratory staff.

Urine and Stool

The complete collection of urine and stool for timed or pooled samples presents special challenges in a pediatric setting, where even older children may not be cooperative. In infants and children who are not yet toilet-trained, urine samples are best obtained using urine bags and, depending on the test in question, may require special collecting tubes such as the U-Bag system (Hollister Inc.). Catheterization should be required only in difficult cases. Collection of specimens for timed clearance tests is more critical, and special attention must be paid to the separation of stool and urine. It may be necessary to catheterize the patient to avoid the fecal contamination of urine.

For stool collections from babies and infants, diapers lined with nonabsorbent material (e.g., Saran Wrap) may be used if the stools are formed. With looser stools as much as 30 percent may be lost by absorption and adherence to the diaper. For patients with diarrhea, it may be necessary to use a metabolic collection frame or a special bed (or walker) with restraints and a cutaway section under which a collecting vessel is placed. This arrangement, while restraining and unpleasant for the patient and difficult for the nursing staff, may be absolutely necessary to ensure complete collections.

THE LIVER

The algorithms applied to differential diagnoses of liver disease are somewhat similar in adult and in pediatric populations. The major exception in pediatric practice is the higher incidence of genetic metabolic disorders (e.g., glycogen storage disease, alpha$_1$-antitrypsin deficiency, tyrosinemia) as well as congenital disorders such as biliary atresia. These cases are seen with some frequency in a tertiary care referral center but are rare in a general practice setting. Since most cases of liver disease require specific diagnostic laboratory tests, early referral to an appropriate center is essential when the clinical indications warrant it and when standard diagnostic tests yield uncertain results. The reader is referred to appropriate sections elsewhere in this book for the discussion of specific diseases and related tests.

Impairment of liver function can be evaluated by (1) measurement of levels of liver-derived enzymes in blood; (2) determination of the bilirubin content of blood, urine, or stool; (3) tests of the integrity of liver function, generally referred to as "liver function tests"; (4) and quantitation and fractionation of bile salts in serum.

Enzymes

Serial changes in the serum levels of the various liver enzymes listed in Table 2 can be useful in evaluating liver disease. Increases in circulating levels can be due to (1) increased synthesis with spillover (for example the induction of GGT in patients on anticonvulsant therapy); (2) release caused by cellular destruction as in acute hepatocellular diseases; or (3) reflux caused by intrahepatic or extrahepatic obstruction. Disorders that affect primarily the hepatocyte cause alterations in the serum levels of transaminases, while the functional impairment of ductal cells within the hepatic canaliculi and biliary tree, including cholestasis, is reflected by changes in levels of alkaline phosphatase (ALP), GGT or 5′ nucleotidase (5′ NT).[3] Unfortunately, such a clear distinction is not always present.

Published reference ranges for various liver-derived enzymes usually relate to total catalytic activities. For most enzymes the assay system is straightforward, using specific substrates, but in some circumstances assay conditions may be less than optimal. For example, aspartate aminotransferase (AST; serum glutamate oxaloacetate transaminase) requires the presence of pyridoxal phosphate as enzymatic co-factor. Pyridoxal phosphate, the co-enzyme form of vitamin B_6, may be deficient in the serum of alcoholic and of uremic patients and, consequently, in the absence of added co-factor in the assay, results for catalytic activity would be less than optimum. Therefore, it has been recommended that assays for AST include added co-factor, although the validity of this approach remains a matter of debate.[4] The use of immunologic methods for the assay of enzymes and their isoforms is increasing. The advantage of immunoassays is their capability to quantify specific isoforms of each enzyme and, in some cases, catalytically inactive forms of the enzyme.[5] The major disadvantages lie in the varying degrees of cross-reactivity (even in the case of monoclonal antibody–derived assays), the longer time required for the assay, and the cost. Immunoassays generally measure the mass of the enzyme,

TABLE 2
Characteristics of Various Liver Enzymes

	Alkaline Phosphatase*	Aspartate Transaminase	Alanine Transaminase	Gamma Glutamyltransferase	5′-Nucleotidase
Source of serum enzyme	Isoforms from: Liver (L)† Bone (B) Intestine (I) Placenta/tumors (P)	Hepatocyte: Cytosol (c) Mitochondria (m) Muscle	Hepatocyte	Membranes of: liver canaliculi, kidney, pancreas Isoforms present	Cell membranes Biliary tree membranes
Causes of ↑ (other than liver disease)	Growth (age-related) Bone repair Vitamin D deficiency Malignancy Transient	Acute myocardial infarction Muscle disease		Age-related Induced by alcohol, drugs Malignancy Sarcoidosis	Slight ↑ in other diseases (renal, cardiovascular, etc.)
Analytic and technical concerns	Differential reactivity of isoforms Differential elevations of isoforms Wide choice of assay substrates Use of phosphate (product) acceptor to enhance the assay Avoid complexing anticoagulants in sample e.g., oxalate, EDTA Temperature dependence of catalytic activity of isoforms L and B isoforms not easily separated	Interference from hemoglobin ↑ Proteins (e.g., multiple myelomas) cause +ve bias relative to normals Requires pyridoxal phosphate as co-factor added in the assay Catalytic activity of mAST low compared with cAST	Interference with hemolysis Requires pyridoxal phosphate; co-factor added in some assays; low in some patients, e.g., in chronic renal disease	Use of specific substrate Temperature dependence of assay	Nonspecific hydrolysis of substrate (5′ AMP) No reference method available Interference with hemolysis Sample storage at room temp. Causes false ↑ in methods using NH_3 determinations

*See also table 5.
†Abbreviations for isoforms.
‡5′AMP = 5′ adenosine monophosphate.

which may not be equivalent to the catalytic activity. Furthermore, some antibodies, for example antialkaline phosphatase (anti-ALP), react with fragments of the target proteins, thus producing spuriously elevated results. At present, of the various hepatically derived enzymes measured by immunoassay, only isoenzyme fractionation of ALP is of some clinical use in cases in which the distinction needs to be made between elevations of total activity due to increases in the liver isoform and those due to increases in other isoforms. Alternatively, separation by gel electrophoresis with and without heat treatment provides a reliable and widely available method for qualitative and semiquantitative analysis.

Transaminases

Serum levels of AST and alanine aminotransferase (ALT, serum glutamate pyruvate transaminase) are sensitive indicators of hepatocellular damage.[3] The usefulness of a relative increase in the levels of the transaminases in the differential diagnosis of acute hepatocellular damage, chronic liver disease, and biliary disease is comparable in adult and in pediatric populations. Very high levels suggest acute hepatocellular disease, whereas in chronic hepatitis prolonged moderate enzyme elevations are apparent. Increased serum AST is not specific for liver disease. Moderate increases occur in cases with acute myocardial infarction (not generally a problem in pediatric patients), as well as in myocarditis and pericarditis. Inflammatory or destructive diseases of skeletal muscle, including myositis and muscular dystrophy, can cause 5- to 10-fold increases in serum AST. Thus ALT is more specific for liver disease, although AST is the more sensitive enzyme. Unfortunately hemolysis, which is a frequent problem in pediatric sampling, also increases AST results. The diagnostic application of the ratio AST:ALT is confined to the identification of alcoholic liver disease and thus is of limited use in pediatric populations.[6]

At levels within and close to the normal (reference) range for transaminases (0 to 50 units per liter for most groups), assay precision for most methods is in the range of 10 to 15 percent, while some are as high as 20 percent. For example, a reported result of 60 units per liter could represent a true value between 55 units per liter and 65 units per liter. Clinicians should thus determine the level of precision of their testing site and interpret changes in enzyme levels accordingly. In most laboratories, assay precision improves significantly at levels above 100 units per liter. In some diseases transaminase levels can be high, sometimes 100-fold or more above the upper limit of normal. Analytically, this may cause problems because of the rapid depletion of substrate and may result in the generation of falsely low results. Many of the present generation of analyzers can identify this problem and flag the operator. This prompts protocols designed to reassay, usually requiring dilution of the sample and reassay. However, if a high dilution is required, the matrix and properties of the sample could be far removed from those of the original specimen. Most laboratories compromise by using a fixed maximum dilution; this results in reports in the form of "greater than x units." Some clinicians might request a more specific test result, but this is both inappropriate and not diagnostically useful.

There are cytosolic and mitochondrial isoforms of liver-derived AST that can be distinguished by immunoassays; their kinetic and catalytic properties are similar. There appears to be no diagnostic advantage to separately quantitating these isoforms, although several papers address the issue in a research setting.

Alkaline Phosphatase

Levels of total ALP in serum vary with sex and age; normal values are high in the newborn and during periods of active growth, particularly puberty (Table 3).[7] The use of inappropriate reference ranges in the evaluation of assay results in children frequently leads to improper interpretations of test results. Of the four major isoforms of ALP (bone, liver, intestinal, and placental), the combination of bone and liver isoenzymes generally represent over 90 percent of the total enzyme activity. In individuals undergoing active growth the relative contribution of the bone isoenzyme to the total ALP pool is enhanced. Thus, in childhood and adolescence the bone isoenzyme represents about 80 percent of the total enzyme activity, although this value decreases to 30 percent in adults.[8]

Increases in the liver isoform of ALP are responsible for the increase in total serum activity commonly seen in hepatobiliary disease. Generally much higher increases are seen in cholestasis than in hepatocellular disease, but because of considerable overlap in the two situations, this distinction is not always diagnostically useful.

Because high serum levels of ALP can occur in several conditions other than liver disease (Table 4), care must be taken in their interpretation. When one must determine whether increased ALP directly reflects liver disease, one of two approaches may be followed. Direct fractionation for the ALP isoenzymes can be performed: electrophoretic methods are most frequently used for separating liver and bone isoenzymes, while differential heat or chemical inactivation is best applied to the identification of placental and P-type isoforms.[8,9] Although these methods are useful, they are difficult to perform, are at best semiquantitative, and do not provide rapid answers. Alternatively, the serum levels of other enzymes, such as GGT and 5′NT, can be measured (for a more detailed description see below). Assay methodology for these enzymes, especially for GGT, is comparatively simple and rapid. The latter approach is recommended if the question simply concerns whether or not the elevation of total ALP is due to a hepatic cause.

TABLE 3
Reference Values for Alkaline Phosphatase

Males		Females	
Age (yr)	Value (U/L)	Age (yr)	Value (U/L)
<1	175–600	<1	185–555
1–8	175–400	1–2	185–520
9–11	180–475	3–8	185–425
12–15	200–630	9–13	160–500
16–17	100–455	14–15	90–400
18–19	80–210	16–18	45–140
>19	60–150	>18	25–100

From Handbook of laboratory reference values: assay on the Kodak Ektachem clinical chemistry analyzer, p-npp at 37 °C. The Hospital for Sick Children, Toronto, 1988.

TABLE 4
Causes of Elevated Alkaline Phosphatase in Pediatric Patients

Disorders	Major Isoenzyme
Active growth	Bone
Healing fractures	Bone
Vitamin D deficiency (rickets and osteomalacia)	Bone
Hyperparathyroidism	Bone
Metastatic disease malignancy	Placental (P-type)
With osteoblastic activity	+ Bone
Of liver	+ Bone
Liver disease	Liver
Acute hepatocellular disease	
Cholestasis (intra- and extrahepatic)	
Cirrhosis	
Ascending cholangitis	
Infection, inflammation	?
Pregnancy	Placental
Transient hyperphosphatasemia	Bone and liver

Several isolated case reports have described the occurrence of very high levels of ALP in pediatric patients, in the absence of liver disease (when all other liver-derived enzymes are normal and there is no other identifiable underlying pathology). This observation has been referred to as transient hyperphosphatasemia.[10,11] It has been suggested that subclinical viral infection might be an underlying cause. One theory, based on isoenzyme analysis by liquid chromatography, holds that the elevation might be due to a viral-induced decrease in the hepatic clearance of enzyme fragments, many of which retain their catalytic properties.[10] In my experience with these cases, isoenzyme fractionation by conventional electrophoretic methods does not yield useful diagnostic information. In children with marked elevation of serum ALP, but no other laboratory or clinical evidence of hepatic disease, I recommend that the assay for ALP be repeated 5 to 7 days later before further investigations are considered.

Gamma Glutamyltransferase and 5′Nucleotidase

Since both of these enzymes are localized to cellular membranes of canalicular cells, serum levels are generally elevated in disorders affecting the biliary tree.[3] GGT is present in the plasma membranes and microsomal membranes of epithelial cells of the biliary tract and hepatic canaliculi; other sources include the proximal renal tubules and the pancreatic ducts.

The largest amount is present in the kidney, but in practical terms the serum enzyme is almost entirely derived from the liver.[12] Levels are increased in cholestatic liver disease; the highest increases occur in primary biliary cirrhosis and malignancies, while moderate increases are seen in chronic active hepatitis and extrahepatic obstruction. Thus, although serum elevations of GGT are specific for liver disease, the enzyme is not of proven value in the differential diagnosis of extrahepatic biliary obstruction. Various isoforms exist, but their identification does not provide a clear diagnostic benefit.

5′NT is present in surface membranes of tissues including liver, brain, and heart. In the liver the enzyme is localized to canalicular and sinusoidal membranes, and serum levels increase during cholestasis.[3] The enzyme is a specific indicator of hepatobiliary disease. However, since 5′NT may be normal in the presence of increased liver-derived ALP, it is not a sensitive indicator.

Since GGT and 5′NT in serum are derived from membranes of canalicular cells, then increases in the levels of these enzymes can be helpful in distinguishing biliary causes of elevations of ALP and transaminases from hepatocellular causes. GGT has the advantage over 5′NT, because essentially all the enzyme measured in serum is derived from the liver. Also, GGT is easier to assay; a highly specific substrate is available and its hydrolysis is readily measured. In contrast almost all of the available substrates for 5′NT are hydrolyzed by numerous other serum enzymes thereby reducing reaction specificity. Thus, in theory GGT is the measurement of choice, but unfortunately, for clinical reasons, it is not always chosen. GGT is an inducible enzyme, and levels increase when liver microsomal hydroxylation systems are stimulated. For example, the use of phenytoin for chronic anticonvulsant therapy can lead to elevations in serum GGT.[14] In these circumstances elevations in GGT levels should be interpreted with caution and the 5′NT assay, either alone or in conjunction with GGT, should be used for discriminating causes of transaminase elevation. Similarly, in adults and in some adolescents, where elevations of GGT may be due to chronic alcohol use, 5′NT should be the enzyme of choice.

In infants, early diagnostic differentiation of biliary atresia from neonatal hepatitis and other causes of jaundice continues to be a difficult clinical problem. The discriminant value of various liver enzymes has been suggested, most recently including GGT.[15] Presently, however, the data do not support any of these claims.

Bilirubin

In pediatric practice, hyperbilirubinemia during the neonatal period and in infants and older children can be considered to represent separate diagnostic problems. In the neonate it is often necessary to distinguish physiologic jaundice from other causes of prolonged hyperbilirubinemia, such as hemolytic disease, neonatal hepatitis, and hepatobiliary obstruction. Early diagnosis is important, since it is recognized, for example, that the early identification of biliary atresia can have important benefits with respect to long-term therapy and outcome. In older children causes of jaundice include hemolytic disorders, acute and chronic hepatitis, genetic-metabolic diseases, and biliary obstruction.

Considerable diagnostic value is attached to the determination, in serum, of total bilirubin as well as the quantitation of the unconjugated and conjugated bilirubin fractions. The different bilirubin species present in serum can be separated and quantitated using high-performance liquid chromatography (HPLC).[16,17] The method is not suitable for routine use in the chemistry laboratory but is recommended as a reference method. The classic diazonium reaction, with its various modifications, is still the most widely used procedure for measuring bilirubin. The determination of total and conjugated bilirubin requires two separate analyses: total bilirubin is determined in the presence of an "accelerator" added in the assay, allowing for the simultaneous measurement of both the unconjugated and the conjugated fractions; the conjugated fraction alone (Bc; direct bilirubin) is measured in the absence of the accelerator; the unconjugated fraction (Bu; indirect bilirubin) is mathematically derived (Bu = total − Bc).

The following are some technical problems related to the diazonium reaction.

1. Hemolysis is a significant cause of interference. This is of concern in pediatrics owing to the likelihood of hemolysis in capillary blood samples.
2. Assay precision is often poor (coefficient of variation up to 15 percent) at low to modest levels of bilirubin (up to approximately 4 mg per deciliter; 70 μmol per liter).
3. Most assays for direct bilirubin measure only 70 percent of the diconjugated bilirubin fraction.[16] At moderate levels of conjugated bilirubin this can result in spuriously high values for unconjugated bilirubin, leading to an inappropriate classification of mixed hyperbilirubinemia.
4. Pure stable standards, especially for conjugated bilirubin, are difficult to obtain and to prepare for analysis; nonphysiologic standards, for example synthetic ditaurine bilirubin, are therefore often used.[17,18] In the assay these compounds do not react in exactly the same way as normal bilirubin. Therefore, each laboratory should establish its own reference ranges. Apparent inaccuracies and differences in results obtained using different methods, both within and between laboratories, are often due to variations in standardization.

Bilirubin can also be quantitated by measuring absorbance at selected wavelengths. This method is particularly sensitive to interference from hemoglobin and from carotenoid pigments derived from dietary sources. In the healthy neonate bilirubin is virtually all unconjugated and the absence of significant carotenoid in the diet permits quantitation of serum bilirubin, using this simpler direct spectrophotometric method, with appropriate corrections for hemoglobin. Bilirubinometers are simple differential spectrophotometers dedicated to this purpose[17,18]; they require only microliter volumes (up to 200 μl) of blood. Standardization, which generally makes use of solutions of inorganic salts (e.g., methyl orange at pH 7.4), continues to be a problem; several studies have shown a lack of equivalence between direct spectrophotometry and colorimetric methods for bilirubin. The bilirubinometer, when properly maintained and used, is an adequate instrument for the rapid detection of trends in bilirubinemia in the neonate. However, a diminishing number of laboratories use bilirubinometers, since, with available technology, it is now possible to obtain a fast and accurate bilirubin measurement from a microvolume of blood by chemical analysis using the diazonium reaction.

The transcutaneous bilirubinometer, which is used solely for neonates, is a hand-held spectrophotometer capable of measuring light reflected from subcutaneous tissue when the instrument is placed against a test site, usually the forehead. Bilirubin is quantitated by measurement at selected wavelengths with appropriate correction for hemoglobin.[16] Transcutaneous bilirubinometry is attractive for at least two reasons: it is noninvasive (no need for blood sampling), and it is convenient in settings remote from a traditional chemistry analyzer. Accuracy and precision are not as good as for other methods, but performance, in the hands of trained nonlaboratory personnel, is sufficient to permit routine noninvasive monitoring of simple neonatal jaundice in a nursery setting.

It has been shown, using HPLC, that total bilirubin measured by the colorimetric diazo reaction includes unconjugated and conjugated bilirubin and a bilirubin species covalently bound to albumin.[16] This last fraction, which reacts in the diazonium reaction as a conjugated bilirubin, is called delta bilirubin. Delta bilirubin is not present in measurable amounts in the normal neonate, but in infants, older children, and adults the levels are markedly increased, especially in those with cholestatic disorders, in whom it may represent as much as 70 percent of the total bilirubin.[19,20] It appears to be formed as a result of a spontaneous chemical reaction between albumin and bilirubin glucuronides, particularly when conjugated bilirubin levels are very high. Since delta bilirubin reacts in the diazonium test as conjugated bilirubin, it contributes to the "direct" bilirubin fraction. At this time its measurement has no clear diagnostic use, but, because the specific fraction is not measured in most laboratories, its contribution to results for conjugated bilirubin could be misleading.

In the neonate as well as in older patients, the ability to distinguish direct from indirect hyperbilirubinemia is becoming increasingly important. However, this is not always technically convenient, since, as noted above, measurement of direct (conjugated) bilirubin by the chemical diazonium method requires a test separate from the assay for total bilirubin, which is not available in many laboratories. Regardless of the method used, its performance characteristics, including sensitivity, limits of linearity, and potential interferents, must be understood by both the laboratory staff and the clinician.

Stool Bilirubin

The examination of stool for bilirubin is a useful screening test, especially in the neonate and young infant, for distinguishing between neonatal hepatitis and extrahepatic biliary atresia (EHBA). In this situation the lack of deconjugating bacteria in the GI tract means that bilirubin is normally present in the stool. A positive stool bilirubin in the neonate tends to exclude biliary atresia, but its absence does not exclude hepatitis. Most laboratories use a modification of the Ictotest Tablet test (Ames Division of Miles Laboratories) for this analysis. This test is qualitative, devised primarily for the determination of bilirubin in urine, and yields a positive result at concentrations of approximately 1.0 μmol per liter (0.05 mg per deciliter). It is important that the test be done on a fresh specimen of stool not contaminated with urine. It can easily be performed by the clinician at the bedside.

Urine

Qualitative dipstick tests for bilirubin and urobilinogen are easy to perform and should be done on a fresh sample close to the bedside. The test for bilirubin has a sensitivity in the range of 7 to 14 μmol per liter (0.4 to 0.8 mg per deciliter; Ames Reagent Strips, Miles Laboratories). In comparison, the Ictotest tablet has a sensitivity in the range of 0.9 to 1.8 μmol per liter (0.05 to 0.1 mg per deciliter); this is the lowest level at which bilirubin in the urine is abnormal. If there is uncertainty about the diagnosis, particularly in the case of suspected porphyria, then screening for coproporphyrin and porphobilinogen can be performed, which, if necessary, can be followed by more detailed testing.

Liver Function Tests

The liver is the major site of synthesis, degradation, and detoxification of various molecules. It is also involved in the elimination of bilirubin via its uptake, conjugation, and secretion into bile. Tests for the functional capability of the liver would be useful especially in situations where there is minimal or no change in the usual biochemical indices of liver function such as serum enzyme levels. Several exogenous molecules have been advocated as probes useful in the evaluation of liver function. Since these molecules are metabolized, in various ways, by the liver (e.g., uptake and secretion; conjugation; hydroxylation), then quantitation of the recovery of selected metabolites of the particular probe can provide some information on liver function. Procedures using this approach are generally designated "liver function tests." Probe molecules used in these liver function tests include sulfobromophthalein sodium (Bromsulphalein, BSP), aminopyrine, and caffeine.

BSP is an anion that is handled like bilirubin; it undergoes uptake, conjugation with glutathione, and secretion into bile. The BSP test for liver function involves intravenous infusion of the dye with the determination of plasma levels at timed intervals. Alternatively, BSP can be administered as a bolus injection and a single sample determination taken after 45 minutes. Normally uptake and clearance are rapid; alteration at any step in uptake and clearance causes increased plasma retention of the dye. The BSP test is not specific and is rarely used. However, the bolus test has been proposed as a simple, sensitive test for the early detection of liver dysfunction and the prolonged test as an aid in distinguishing Rotor's syndrome from Dubin-Johnson syndrome.[21] Problems with this test include the need for continuous infusion and repeated blood sampling. In addition, the BSP test has fallen into disfavor because of concerns about side effects.

The aminopyrine breath test uses ^{14}C-labeled aminopyrine and measures $^{14}CO_2$ production as a result of hepatic demethylation of the substrate.[22,23] It is no more sensitive than other serum tests such as AST and bile acids and because it involves radioisotopes cannot be used in pediatric patients. Use of the stable isotope-labeled ^{13}C aminopyrine overcomes the latter objection but is not routinely used because both the ^{13}C probe and the instrumentation required for analysis are expensive. Finally, there remains some debate as to whether the aminopyrine test is simply a test of hepatic microsomal enzyme activity rather than a test of overall liver function.

Other tests of liver function include amino acid quantitation (either of total or specific amino acids) and the evaluation of caffeine metabolism following an oral load of caffeine.[23] These tests are still being evaluated in research laboratories, and most of the available data relate to adults. Amino acid quantitation is highly dependent on diet and might not be useful. In a pediatric setting the caffeine test could be advantageous since the test material is easy to administer. A recent report suggests that saliva can be used as the test fluid, making it a relatively noninvasive procedure.[24] It is not known, however, whether this test is better than the BSP test, which is not universally accepted. Furthermore, the caffeine test is probably simply a test of hepatic microsomal demethylation function, rather than of liver function.

Bile Acids

Quantitation of bile acids is useful in some clinical circumstances, such as in evaluating the cause of fat malabsorption in the absence of signs of cholestasis. It has been suggested that bile acid determinations are superior to conventional liver tests for the detection of severe chronic liver disease. However, the routine use of serum bile salt determinations in the diagnosis and management of liver disease is not justified.[25,26] The relative advantage of determining serum bile acids in the fasting state versus sampling postprandially (two- to sixfold increases occur after a meal) has been debated. However, because analytically sensitive assay methods are now available, there is no major advantage to using postprandial samples.[25-27]

The most common method of determining bile salts in blood (serum) is by radioimmunoassay (RIA) using a labeled cholylglycine tracer. This assay is based on the principle that the major bile salt is cholylglycine and that the relative proportions of bile acids in the sample will remain the same. However, in pathologic conditions these assumptions obviously cannot be made. There is also antibody crossreactivity with other bile salts, particularly deoxycholylglycine (concentrations in normal serum: cholylglycine (CG) = 0.2 to 0.9 mmol per liter; deoxycholyglycine = 0.08 to 0.7 mmol per liter). Serum bile acids may also be nonspecifically quantitated using available enzymatic-fluorometric procedures, but these have limited analytic sensitivity.[25-27] More specific and accurate analysis of bile salts in serum, in bile itself, and in duodenal aspirates and feces requires either HPLC or gas-liquid chromatographic methods that can separate, identify, and quantitate individual species.[23,25] These are available only in specialized research centers.

TABLE 5
Factors Affecting the Usefulness of Tests of Intestinal Permeability

Nature of probe (whether radiolabeled) and its availability
Cost of probe
Test dose (pediatric versus adult)
Specimen-type, timed collection, number required
Analytic method
Reference interval (pediatric versus adult)
Sensitivity and specifity

THE INTESTINAL TRACT

The description of various disease-specific tests of gastrointestinal disorders are discussed elsewhere in this text. This discussion is restricted to the description of tests of malabsorption and impaired mucosal permeability together with tests for evaluating intestinal protein loss.

Malabsorption and Permeability

The intestinal mucosa acts as a barrier to the unrestricted movement of molecules between the gastrointestinal lumen and the body. Some molecules undergo absorption by active or facilitated transport mechanisms while others simply penetrate (permeate) the mucosa, to a varying extent, by mechanisms that are often undefined. Although the processes of absorption and permeation are dissimilar, in many disorders with malabsorption there is also impairment of the integrity of the mucosa, which, in turn, is accompanied by abnormalities of permeation. Conversely, alterations of the integrity of the intestinal mucosa will adversely affect absorption. Biochemical tests of the intactness of the small bowel mucosa are based on alterations in the transmucosal passage of various probe molecules. These tests are noninvasive and permit screening of the integrity of the small bowel mucosa, and they are particularly useful in cases of minimal symptomatology. They may provide support for more extensive radiologic and/or endoscopic investigations. Following oral administration of a known dose of the probe, the passage of the probe across the small bowel mucosa is evaluated by measuring levels either in the blood, after a predetermined interval or in a timed urine collection. The probes to be discussed include xylose, other carbohydrates, polyethyleneglycol polymers, and ^{51}Cr EDTA.

Most tests of small bowel mucosal permeability assume that the probe molecule enters via the small bowel alone, but frequently this assumption cannot be made. For example, ^{51}Cr EDTA is readily absorbed in the colon.[28] The absorption characteristics of suggested probe molecules should therefore be carefully examined. Factors that can influence the usefulness of these tests are listed in Table 5. The specific tests will be discussed in terms of these factors where relevant.

The D-Xylose Test

D-Xylose is a monosaccharide absorbed in the proximal small bowel either by passive diffusion or by a weak carrier mechanism. It is partially metabolized, but a large fraction of the dose (approximately 50 percent) is excreted unmetabolized by the kidney. Following an oral dose of D-xylose, the amount of xylose excreted in a timed urine collection (usually 5 hours) is used as the index of absorptive function. Xylose excretion is influenced by renal function. There are also practical limitations of obtaining an accurate, timed urine collection, especially in pediatric practice. Thus, although more invasive, measurement of blood levels is preferred. In adults, serum xylose is determined 2 hours after administering the dose but in children a 1-hour sampling time has been recommended.[29,30]

There is controversy concerning the loading dose in pediatric patients. The usual dose in adults is 25 g. In pediatric patients there have been various recommendations. Christie[31] has used 5 g of xylose for all children, while others have recommended this dose for children up to 30 kg body weight (approximately 8 years of age).[32] Buts et al[29] have used dosage based on surface area (14.5 g per square meter^2 to a maximum of 25 g). Following a dose of 5 g, side effects are minimal but with this small dose the rate of absorption might not be optimal. Higher doses can lead to adverse patient reactions, including abdominal discomfort and intestinal hurry, even in adults and older children. Given the wide range in size of pediatric patients, I recommend the use of a dose based on surface area.

The routine methods of analysis involves the colorimetric measurement of xylose. This is a simple technique and provides a clear advantage for the xylose absorption test when compared with other tests for absorption or permeability. Low urinary excretion of xylose or low serum levels indicate malabsorption but do not suggest the underlying cause. The xylose absorption test has been promoted as a test for carbohydrate malabsorption and particularly as a screening test for celiac disease. In the case of celiac disease in children, test sensitivity of 70 percent and specificity of 95 percent has been reported.[32a] Some investigators use the test as an aid in the selection of patients for jejunal biopsy. A normal xylose test result is highly predictive of a normal biopsy with a predictive value of a negative result (i.e., sensitivity) as high as 96 percent.[30] However, other reports of a high incidence of false-positive (46 percent[31]) and particularly false-negative (25 percent[31]; 30 percent[32a]) results argue against its use as a screening test. It must be remembered that the disease entities included in any evaluation of test performance influence the sensitivity and specificity derived for that test; this is clearly the case with the xylose absorption test. In addition, false positives (low values) can result from various causes, including delayed gastric emptying, rapid transit time, and small bowel bacterial overgrowth. Reactions to xylose, particularly if intestinal transit is affected, can also invalidate the test result. Nevertheless, the test remains a somewhat useful screening test for malabsorption. However, it is not diagnostic for any one disease entity.

Other Carbohydrates

Nonabsorbed carbohydrates such as lactulose have been used as probes for the evaluation of intestinal permeability. Following oral administration, the urinary excretion of the probe is determined in a timed urine collection. Practical problems include the need for a complete urine collection, the effect of renal function on the clearance of the probe, and the analysis of lactulose in urine.

The dual sugar tests purportedly minimize the practical concerns of an accurate urine collection and the effect of renal function on clearance of the probe. This is achieved by determining the ratio of the urinary concentration of two coadministered probes. In this procedure a monosaccharide and a disaccharide, for example, lactulose and mannitol, lactulose and L-rhamnose, or cellobiose and mannitol, are coadministered. Interpretation is based on the relative concentration (ratio) of probe molecules excreted in a timed urine collection.[33-35] These tests are based on the observation that, in patients with small intestinal mucosal disease, the transmucosal passage of monosaccharides such as mannitol is decreased while the transfer of disaccharides is increased relative to controls. However, using lactulose and mannitol in control subjects, it has been shown that the ratio of probe recovery in urine is influenced by the period over which collection is made.[28] This implies that each probe can have different rates of intestinal transit and that the test results will be influenced by the time over which the test is performed.

Adverse reactions to the sugars can be a problem that is further complicated by the coadministration of an osmotic "filler" such as lactose or glucose. So far, no ideal combination of probe molecules has been identified, particularly if one considers difficulties of analysis. To some extent, this is because of the use of a combination of probes and the presence of the osmotic filler. Age-related control ratios have not been established in pediatric patients.

The probe molecules are difficult to measure, and specialized laboratories are usually necessary for analysis. Quantitation is usually performed using chromatographic separation (paper or thin layer) followed by scanning densitometry. The precision of these methods is frequently less than 10 percent. To circumvent this problem, more precise enzyme-linked spectrophotometric methods have been described,[34] but interference from endogenous molecules such as glucose and mannitol create considerable analytic and interpretative difficulties.

^{51}Cr EDTA Test

In this procedure a test dose of ^{51}Cr EDTA is administered orally and recovery of the radiolabeled probe is evaluated in a timed 24-hour urine collection; recovery is expressed as a percentage of the radioactivity of the administered dose. A clear distinction has been shown between controls and the higher values obtained in patients with impaired mucosal permeability; the test is abnormal in patients with enteropathies due to various causes including infectious and inflammatory lesions.[36,37] In addition to the problem of requiring a timed urine collection, the test involves exposure to radioactivity, which obviously should be avoided in children.

Polyethyleneglycol Test

The polyethyleneglycol (PEG) test uses a preparation of low molecular weight polymers of PEG (200 to 600) and the measurement of PEG excretion in a timed urine collection (up to 6 hours). The assay requires the separation and quantitation of different molecular weight polymers of PEG. Results are expressed as a score of the relative excretion of the various PEG polymers in the urine, usually the longer polymer units. Hence, accuracy of urine collection is not a critical factor. A PEG score below the reference value reflects decreased urinary recovery resulting from decreased permeation across the gastrointestinal mucosa.[33,38] Abnormal results are frequently seen in infants and children with celiac disease and may reflect a decrease in intestinal surface area available for permeation due to villous atrophy. Measurement of PEG polymers is done by gas chromatography, which is difficult and expensive to perform. The test has a high false-negative rate with a sensitivity of 78 percent.[39] Various drugs, particularly nonsteroidal anti-inflammatory drugs, also affect the test results.

Summary

Although the tests described above are sensitive to changes in mucosal integrity and permeability, they are not specific for particular disease entities. Abnormal results are obtained in a wide variety of gastrointestinal disorders including celiac disease, Crohn's disease, and acute gastroenteritis. These tests frequently do not provide sufficient discrimination to be of practical use in the individual patient. Nonetheless noninvasive screening tests for the impairment of the integrity of the small bowel mucosa clearly have a role to play in various clinical settings. Furthermore, the clinician should be aware that, except for the xylose test, the tests discussed here measure the permeability properties of the mucosa and not absorption. The dual sugar tests appear to be the most promising of these. However, they still suffer from drawbacks such as the lack of defined reference ranges, especially for pediatric groups, and the difficulty of analytic methods that continue to limit their wide application to clinical practice.

Intestinal Protein Loss

A variety of plasma proteins, representing 2.5 percent of the total plasma pool and including albumin, gamma globulins, and alpha$_1$-antitrypsin (alpha$_1$-AT), are normally lost through the gastrointestinal tract. In protein-losing enteropathies, due to a wide variety of causes such as inflammatory bowel disease, celiac disease, radiation enteritis, and obstruction to lymph flow, excessive plasma protein losses occur via the gastrointestinal tract. Methods presently available for the laboratory measurement of enteric protein loss include the ^{51}Cr albumin excretion test and the determination of the fecal loss of endogenous proteins such as alpha$_1$-AT.

Albumin

Excessive protein loss is often reflected by low serum levels of albumin due to its relative concentration in plasma (approximately 50 percent of total protein) and its relatively long half-life (21 days). On the other hand, considerable intestinal protein loss can occur without a detectable fall in serum albumin. Important causes of hypoalbuminemia, other than in protein losing enteropathies, include decreased production due to deficient protein intake (malnutrition) or to chronic liver disease and increased loss via the kidneys (nephrotic syndrome) or skin (burns). Most of these causes can be eliminated from consideration by appropriate clinical and laboratory evaluation.

Since albumin is subject to proteolytic degradation in the intestinal tract, its direct measurement in feces is problematic. The availability of methods for the labeling of albumin with radioactive tracers, especially ^{51}Cr, and for the measurement of the tracer in feces, led to the development of tests based on the measurement of these radiolabeled albumin molecules. For some time, the standard laboratory test for protein-losing enteropathies involved the intravenous administration of a dose of ^{51}Cr-labeled albumin, followed by the measurement of the amount of radiolabel excreted in the feces over a fixed time (3 to 5 days).[40] ^{51}Cr chloride has also been used as the probe molecule. Results are expressed as a percentage of the injected dose excreted in the stool (normal value: up to 1 percent of dose). Like many other tests involving the use of radioisotopes, this test is not recommended in pediatrics.

In any event, other problems associated with this test include:

1. the appropriate dose for children of different sizes;
2. the need for an accurate timed stool collection, free from urine contamination; and
3. the measurement of radioactivity in the stool; here considerations include the need for an appropriate counter and sample quenching and the efficiency of counting.

Alpha$_1$-Antitrypsin Test

The plasma protein alpha$_1$-AT, a protease inhibitor with a molecular weight similar to that of albumin, is present at concentrations of approximately 1 to 2 g per liter. In comparison with albumin, it is more resistant to proteolysis in the gastrointestinal tract and has a shorter half-life of 7 days. Since the first report of high fecal alpha$_1$-AT in patients with proven protein losing enteropathy (measured by ^{51}Cr chloride excretion) appeared a number of studies have confirmed that fecal losses of alpha$_1$-AT correlate well with the excretion of ^{51}Cr chloride in both normals and patients with protein-losing enteropathy.[41–43] With the ready availability of specific and sensitive immunoassays for the measurement of alpha$_1$-AT, it has seen increasing use as an endogenous probe for protein-losing enteropathies. However, there are also studies that suggest that the sensitivity of the test is poor and so it may not be a reliable measure of enteric protein loss.[44,45]

Fecal loss of alpha$_1$-AT can be expressed as a clearance:

$$\text{Clearance (in ml per day)} = (F \times W)/P$$

F = fecal concentration of alpha$_1$-AT
W = weight of stool in g per day
P = plasma concentration of alpha$_1$-AT

This approach requires a timed stool collection, usually 24 hours, and a concurrent serum sample. Loss of alpha$_1$-AT can also be expressed as excretion, given either as a rate based on timed collections (mg per day) or as concentration related to dry weight or to wet volume of stool. Defining fecal excretion in terms of concentration is advantageous because a random stool sample can be used and the problems associated with timed collections would be eliminated. This approach could permit a more rapid turnaround time for the test result, but further validation is necessary before it becomes widely accepted.

Gastric Protein Loss. In patients with gastric protein loss, the high acidity (pH less than 3.5) within the stomach can effect sufficient denaturation of alpha$_1$-AT to result in falsely low fecal values when measured by immunoassay. The administration of H_2-antagonists has been effectively used to neutralize gastric acidity and permit the accurate measurement of fecal alpha$_1$-AT.[48]

Laboratory Analysis

Sample Preparation. The fecal concentration of alpha$_1$-AT is commonly determined using aqueous extracts of lyophilized stool. This is advantageous since fecal concentrations of alpha$_1$-AT are usually low, necessitating concentration prior to analysis. Concentrations are further reduced with diarrhea, a common occurrence in patients with conditions giving rise to excessive intestinal protein loss. However, lyophilization requires time and special equipment. Heat-drying (37 °C for 24 hours) has been suggested as an alternative method[40]; results show a good correlation between the two methods, although the mean alpha$_1$-AT concentration after heat drying was slightly lower. Normal concentrations of alpha$_1$-AT in stool are low (about 4 mg per gram of dry weight or 1.3 g per liter of wet volume).[44]

Assay Methods. Radial immunodiffusion (RID) on plates is still used by many laboratories to quantitate alpha$_1$-AT. Results obtained using plates from different manufacturers can disagree by as much as 30 percent, but distinction between normals and abnormals remain.[46] Thus, between-laboratory performances cannot be readily compared, and attention must be given to the effects of changing suppliers and even between different batches of plates from the same supplier. RID assays may require several hours to set up and read, and the entire process can take 1 to 3 days to perform. Precision, especially at the low concentrations of alpha$_1$-AT in feces, is about 10 percent at best. Automated immunonephelometric methods unfortunately require expensive analyzers. However, they permit rapid analysis and excellent assay precision is achieved, usually better than 5 percent.

Homogeneity of Alpha$_1$-Antitrypsin. It is assumed that little or not degradation of alpha$_1$-AT occurs in the gastrointestinal tract and that the immunoassay measures all the fecal alpha$_1$-AT. Nevertheless, complexes of alpha$_1$-AT with proteases such as leukocyte elastase as well as denatured forms of alpha$_1$-AT have been found in the feces of both healthy subjects and patients with gastrointestinal disease.[47] The denaturation of alpha$_1$-AT in feces might be due to a variety of factors including the effects of bile salts or bacterial proteases. The potential thus exists for underestimating the amount of alpha$_1$-AT lost into the gastrointestinal tract due to altered reactivity in immunologic assays that could lead to spuriously low (false-negative) test results.

BIOCHEMICAL INDICES OF NUTRITIONAL STATUS

Failure to thrive and overt malnutrition are common complications of gastrointestinal disease in pediatrics. Many patients may be subclinically malnourished on presentation and, if they remain unrecognized, may suffer from increased morbidity and mortality. Also, since nutritional status correlates with growth and development in the young child, it is important to be assured of proper nutritional status. Anthropometric measurements, such as height and weight (percentiles) and skin fold thickness, are useful indices of nutritional sta-

TABLE 6
Nutritional Markers

Protein	Reference Range* (g/L)	Half-Life (Days)	Analytic Method	Causes of Change (Other than Poor Nutrition)
Albumin	32–48 (0–1 yr) 33–58 (>1 yr)	21	Colorimetric: dye-binding methods	↑ Acute-phase response ↓ Chronic liver disease, protein-losing enteropathy, renal disease, burns
Transferrin	2.5–4.3	8	Immunonephelometry (automated) RID, RIA, ELISA	↑ Iron deficiency, estrogen/pregnancy ↓ Acute phase response, chronic liver disease, protein-losing enteropathy, renal disease, burns
Prealbumin (transthyretin)	0.116–0.280 (up to 3 yr) 0.170–0.420 (adults)	2	Immunonephelometry (automated) RID	↑ Oral contraceptives, Hodgkin's disease, alcoholism, NSAIDs ↓ Liver disease, acute inflammation, nephrotic syndrome
Retinol-binding protein	0.030–0.065	0.5–1	Manual immunonephelometry RIA, RID, ELISA	↓ Oral contraceptives, glucocorticosteroids, nephrotic syndrome, hyperthyroidism
Fibronectin	0.178–0.380 0.250–0.400	1	ELISA, manual immunonephelometry	↑ Chronic active hepatitis ↓ Fulminant hepatic failure, hepatic cirrhosis, shock, burns, infection

*Unless otherwise stated, these values are adult ranges.
RID = radial immunodiffusion; RIA = radioimmunoassay; ELISA = enzyme-labeled immunosorbent assay; NSAIDs = nonsteroidal anti-inflammatory drugs.

tus but generally reflect long-term changes. Other indices of nutritional status that are capable of providing more timely information are obviously important. In this regard, the serum concentrations of several proteins reflect the balance between synthesis and loss and have been proposed as tests of nutritional status (Table 6). The liver is the predominant site of synthesis of these proteins and, in the absence of liver disease, the serum concentrations should, in theory, reflect the nutritional status of the individual.

A decreased serum albumin concentration is frequently used as a marker of nutritional status, but its value is questionable. Owing to its relatively long half-life (21 days) albumin is not a sensitive indicator of short-term nutritional deficits or of short-term nutritional response. Proteins with a shorter half-life may be more useful (see Table 6).[49,50] These include transferrin (8 days), prealbumin (48 hours), retinol-binding protein (12 to 24 hours), and fibronectin (24 hours). Although most of these proteins are present in significantly lower serum concentrations than albumin, they are more sensitive to acute changes in protein homeostasis. However, not all are useful indicators of nutritional status. For example, transferrin levels are greatly influenced by iron status; levels at birth correlate with gestational age and are affected by intrauterine growth retardation.[51] Transferrin is a negative acute-phase protein. Prealbumin has a higher concentration in serum than either retinol-binding protein or fibronectin but, in a study of adult males with mild malnutrition due to chronic intestinal disease, it failed to reflect the nutritional deficit.[49] Fibronectin may well be an acceptable marker of nutritional status, since serum levels respond more rapidly than other serum proteins and have been shown to reflect nutritional response in infants.[49,52]

There are several other problems regarding the use of the serum protein concentrations as laboratory indices of nutritional status. Excessive losses of these proteins can occur via the intestinal tract, the kidneys, and, in the case of burns, through the skin. In addition, the serum concentrations of some are affected by acute phase responses to a variety of diseases. It should also be noted that neonates, especially premature babies, have immature livers with poorly developed protein synthesizing ability. The normal analyte levels in the neonate are greatly influenced by factors such as gestational age, and for this reason reference ranges derived for adult populations are not applicable.[53]

Albumin, with a mean serum concentration of 45 g per liter, is easily measured by automated analysis using specific albumin-binding dyes. Transferrin (2.5 to 4.5 g per liter) is usually measured by automated immunonephelometry, a rapid, accurate, and relatively inexpensive procedure. Other serum proteins mentioned above are present at much lower concentrations, generally in the mg per liter or μg per liter range, and consequently more sensitive and precise analytic methods are required for their quantitation. Immunologic methods such as radioimmunoassay (RIA), RID, and enzyme-labeled immunosorbent assay (ELISA) have now been developed for their measurement. These methods are time-consuming, expensive, and only moderately precise. Fortunately, cross-reactivity has not been a problem. Automated immunoassays for prealbumin are now becoming available but methods for fibronectin determination remain a research tool. The type of sample used is important, since methods for protein quantitation generally require serum rather than plasma and most published reference ranges refer to serum. For example, the plasma concentration of prealbumin is, on the average, 7 percent greater than in serum.[53]

For the above-mentioned analytic reasons, serum albumin continues to be the most frequently used marker of nutritional status. However, with further technical advances it should be possible to develop rapid and inexpensive clinically useful methods for quantifying other serum proteins such as fibronectin. This would allow the laboratory to provide relevant, clinically useful information regarding nutritional deficits in the pediatric patient.

REFERENCES

1. Rutledge JC. Pediatric Specimen Collection for Chemical Analysis. Pediatr Clin North Am 1989; 36:37–45.
2. Meites S. Skin-puncture and blood-collecting technique for infants: update and problems. Clin Chem 1988; 34:1890–1894.
3. Reichling JJ, Kaplan MM. Clinical use of serum enzymes in liver disease. Dig Dis Sci 1988; 33:1601–1614.
4. Murray RL. Aspartate aminotransferase. In: Pesce AJ, Kaplan LA, eds. Methods in clinical chemistry. St. Louis: CV Mosby, 1987: 1093.
5. Ogawa M. Immunoassay of circulating enzymes: current status. Enzyme 1986; 36:254–260.
6. Williams AL, Hoofnagle JH. Ratio of serum aspartate to alanine aminotransferase in chronic hepatitis. Gastroenterology 1988; 95:734–739.
7. Kovar IZ, Mayne PD. Postnatal and gestational age and the interpretation of plasma alkaline phosphatase activity in preterm infants. Ann Clin Biochem 1989; 26:193–194.
8. Chapman JF, Woodard LL, Silverman LM. Alkaline phosphatase isoenzymes. In: Kaplan LA, Pesce AJ, eds. Clinical chemistry. 2nd ed. St. Louis: CV Mosby, 1989: 902.
9. Meyer-Sabellek W, Sinha P, Kottgen E. Alkaline phosphatase. Laboratory and clinical implications. J Chromatogr 1988; 429:429–444.
10. Schonau E, Herzog KH, Bohles HJ. Transient hyperphospatasaemia of infancy. Eur J Pediatr 1988; 148:264–266.
11. Lockitch G, Pudek MR, Halstead AC. Isolated elevation of serum alkaline phosphatase. Clinical and laboratory observations. J Pediatr 1984; 105:773–775.
12. Nemesanszky E, Lott JA. Gamma-glutamyltransferase and its isoenzymes: progress and problems. Clin Chem 1985; 31:797–803.
13. Ellis G. 5′-nucleotidase. In: Pesce AJ, Kaplan LA, eds. Methods in clinical chemistry, St. Louis: CV Mosby, 1987:1125.
14. Keeffe EB, Sunderland MC, Gabourel JD. Serum gamma-glutamyl transpeptidase activity in patients receiving chronic phenytoin therapy. Dig Dis Sci 1986; 31:1056–1061.
15. Fung KP, Lau SP. γ-Glutamyl transpeptidase activity and its serial measurement in differentiation between extrahepatic biliary atresia and neonatal hepatitis. J Pediatr Gastroenterol Nutr 1985; 4:208–213.
16. Rutledge JC, Ou CN. Bilirubin and the laboratory. Pediatr Clin N Am 1989; 36:189–198.
17. Sherwin JE, Obernolte R. Bilirubin. In: Pesce AJ, Kaplan LA, eds. Methods in clinical chemistry. St. Louis: CV Mosby, 1987: 1105.
18. Isherwood DM, Fletcher KA. Neonatal jaundice: investigation and monitoring. Ann Clin Biochem 1985; 22:109–128.
19. Weiss JS, Gautam A, Lauff JJ, Sundberg MW, Jatlow P, Boyer JL, Seligson D. The clinical importance of protein-bound fraction of serum bilirubin in patients with hyperbilirubinemia. N Engl J Med 1983; 309:147–150.
20. Ostrea EM Jr, Ongtengco EA, Tolia VA, Apostol E. The occurrence and significance of the bilirubin species, including delta bilirubin, in jaundiced infants. J Pediatr Gastroenterol Nutr 1988; 7:511–516.
21. Wolpert E, Pascasio FM, Wolkoff AW, Arias IM. Abnormal sulfobromophthalein metabolism in Rotor's syndrome and obligate heterozygotes N Engl J Med 1977; 296:1099–1101.
22. Bircher J. Quantitative assessment of deranged hepatic function: a missed opportunity? Semin Liver Dis 1983; 3:275–284.
23. Balistreri WF, Setchell KD. Newer liver function tests. Front Gastrointest Res 1989; 16:220–245.

24. Jost G, Wahllander A, von Mandach U, Preisig R. Overnight salivary caffeine clearance: a liver function test suitable for routine use. Hepatology 1987: 7:338–344.
25. Whiting MJ. Bile acids. Adv Clin Chem 1986; 25:169–231.
26. Cravetto C, Molino G, Biondi AM, Cavanna A, Avagnina P, Frediani S. Evaluation of the diagnostic value of serum bile acid in the detection and functional assessment of liver diseases. Ann Clin Biochem 1985; 22:596–605.
27. Mannes GA, Stellaard F, Paumgartner G. Diagnostic sensitivity of fasting and postprandial serum bile acids determined by different methods. Clin Chim Acta 1987; 162:147–154.
28. Elia M, Behrens R, Northrop C, Wraight P, Neale G. Evaluation of mannitol, lactulose and ^{51}Cr-labelled ethylenediaminetetra-acetate as markers of intestinal permeability in man. Clin Sci 1987; 73:197–204.
29. Buts J-P, Morin CL, Roy CC, Weber A, Bonin A. One-hour xylose test: a reliable index of small bowel function. J Pediatr 1978; 92:729–733.
30. McNeely MD. D-Xylose. In:Pesce AJ, Kaplan LA, eds. Methods in clinical chemistry. St. Louis: CV Mosby, 1987: 862.
31. Christie DL. Use of the one-hour blood xylose test as an indicator of small bowel mucosal disease. J Pediatr 1978; 92:725–728.
32. Rolles CJ, Kendall MJ, Nutter S, Anderson CM. One-hour blood-xylose screening-test for coeliac children. Lancet 1973; ii:1043–1045.
32a. Hill R, Cutz E, Cherian G, Gall DH, Hamilton JR. An evaluation of D-xylose absorption measurements in children suspected of having small intestinal disease. J Pediatr 1981; 99:245–247.
33. Walker-Smith JA. Evaluation of intestinal protein loss and intestinal permeability. Front Gastrointest Res 1989; 16:126–134.
34. Juby LD, Rothwell J, Axon ATR. Lactulose/mannitol test: an ideal screen for celiac disease. Gastroenterology 1989; 96:79–85.
35. Hamilton I, Hill A, Bose B, Bouchier AD, Forsyth JS. Small intestinal permeability in pediatric clinical practice. J Pediatr Gastroenterol Nutr 1987; 6:697–701.
36. Turck D, Ythier H, Maquet E, Deveaux M, Marchandise X, Farriaux JP, Fontaine G. Intestinal permeability to [^{51}Cr] EDTA in children with Crohn's disease and celiac disease. J Pediatr Gastroenterol Nutr 1987; 6:535–537.
37. Forget P, Sodoyez-Goffaux F, Zappitelli A. Permeability of the small intestine to [^{51}Cr] EDTA in children with acute gastroenteritis or eczema. J Pediatr Gastroenterol Nutr 1985; 4:393–396.
38. Lifschitz CH, Irving CS, Marks LM, Klein PD, Finegold MJ, Nichols BL. Polyethylene glycol polymers of low molecular weight as probes of intestinal permeability. II. Application to infants and children with intestinal disease. J Lab Clin Med 1986; 108:37–43.
39. Lifschitz CH, Shulman RJ, Langston C, Gopalakrishna GS. Comparison of the D-Xylose and polyethylene glycol absorption tests as indicators of mucosal damage in infants with chronic diarrhea. J Pediatr Gastroenterol Nutr 1989; 8:47–50.
40. Durie PR. Intestinal protein loss and fecal α-1-antitrypsin. J Pediatr Gastroenterol Nutr 1985; 4:345–347.
41. Hill RE, Hercz A, Corey ML, Gilday DL, Hamilton JR. Fecal clearance of α_1-antitrypsin: A reliable measure of enteric protein loss in children. J Pediatr 1981; 99:416–418.
42. Crossley JR, Elliott RB. Simple method for diagnosing protein-losing enteropathies. Br Med J 1977; 2:428–429.
43. Bernier JJ, Florent C, Desmazures C, Aumes C, L'Hirondel C. Diagnosis of protein-losing enteropathy by gastrointestinal clearance of alpha-1-antitrypsin. Lancet 1978; ii:763–764.
44. Quigley EM, Ross IN, Haeney MR, Holbrook IB, Marsh MN. Reassessment of faecal α-1-antitrypsin excretion for use as screening test for intestinal protein loss. J Clin Pathol 1987; 40:61–66.
45. Haeney MR, Carter RA, Fields J, Thompson RA, Asquith P. Faecal α_1-antitrypsin excretion a reliable screening test for protein-losing enteropathy. Lancet 1979; ii:1161–1162.
46. Wilson CM, McGilligan K, Thomas DW. Determination of fecal α_1-antitrypsin concentration by radial immunodiffusion: two systems compared. Clin Chem 1988; 34:372–376.
47. Mizon C, Becuwe C, Balduyck M, Columbel J-F, Cortot A, Mizon J. Qualitative study of fecal α_1-proteinase inhibitor in normal subjects and patients with Crohn's disease. Clin Chem 1988; 34:2268–2270.
48. Florent Ch., Vidon N, Flourie A, Carmantrand A, Zerbani A, Maurel M, Bernier JJ. Gastric clearance of alpha-1-antitrypsin under cimetidine perfusion new test to detect protein-losing gastropathy. Digest Dis Sci 1986; 31:12–15.
49. Haider M, Haider SQ. Assessment of protein-calorie malnutrition. Clin Chem 1984; 30:1286–1299.
50. Rassin DK. Evaluation of protein nutritional status. J Pediatr Gastroenterol Nutr 1987; 6:7–9.
51. Chockalingam U, Murphy E, Ophoven JC, Georgieff MK. The influence of gestational age, size for dates, and prenatal steroids on cord transferrin levels in newborn infants. J Pediatr Gastroenterol Nutr 1987; 6:276–280.
52. Yoder MC, Anderson DC, Gopalakrishna GS, Douglas SD, Polin RA. Comparison of serum fibronectin, prealbumin, and albumin concentrations during nutritional repletion in protein-calorie malnourished infants. J Pediatr Gastroenterol Nutr 1987; 6:84–88.
53. Sherry B, Jack RM, Weber A, Smith AL. Reference interval for prealbumin for children two to 36 months old. Clin Chem 1988; 34: 1878–1880.

PART 2

Hematologic Studies

Melvin H. Freedman, M.D., FRCPC

Hematologic abnormalities often accompany serious gastrointestinal (GI) and hepatic diseases of childhood and adolescence. This discussion describes the two major hematologic changes that occur in this setting, namely, anemia and disordered hemostasis. The important diagnostic tests that lead to a specific diagnosis in each category are emphasized.

IRON DEFICIENCY

Essentially, there are two causes of iron deficiency: inadequate iron availability and excessive iron loss. Inadequate iron availability can be caused by an absolute dietary deficiency from an iron-poor diet or malabsorption, or a relative dietary deficiency in the face of increased physiologic requirements such as rapid growth in infancy and adolescence. Excessive iron loss is seen with acute or chronic blood loss, especially a loss that is gastrointestinal in origin, and with hemosiderinuria in chronic intravascular hemolysis.

The transition from adequate iron balance to overt iron deficiency anemia occurs in a sequence of three stages. The first event is a depletion of storage iron in the liver, spleen, and bone marrow. This is followed by a decrease in circulating transport iron characterized by a declining concentration of serum iron and an increase in the iron-binding capacity of transferrin. The final stage develops when the supply of transport iron decreases sufficiently to produce a fall in hemoglobin below the age-related range of normal.

No single laboratory test or combination of tests reliably confirm iron deficiency in all clinical situations. In general, if the degree of iron deficiency is severe, laboratory studies usually are useful and diagnostic. In mild deficiency, laboratory studies do not always conform to our understanding of the three sequential stages in the development of iron deficiency anemia. Mild iron deficiency, especially when it evolves gradually, can be in a steady state, and laboratory studies may not be confirmatory. In this situation, a panel of tests is recommended because the sensitivity of laboratory diagnosis is enhanced if more than a single test is used.

Peripheral Blood and Bone Marrow

Iron deficiency anemia is classified morphologically as hypochromic and microcytic. These descriptive terms are substantiated by standard electronic cell counting, from which red cell indices can be derived. In chronic iron deficiency anemia, the mean cell volume (MCV), mean cell hemoglobin (MCH), and mean cell hemoglobin concentration (MCHC) are all reduced, although the MCV and MCH are far more sensitive than the MCHC for confirmation of iron deficiency.[1] It should be noted that the MCV and MCH normally change during development in the first two decades of life,[1,2] and therefore age-specific reference standards should be used in evaluating data.

The relative number of reticulocytes is often slightly increased, but when corrected for the degree of anemia, the reticulocyte count is usually in a normal range.

Changes in red cell morphology may be highly subtle in patients with mild iron deficiency. In severe deficiency all cells are deficient in hemoglobin, have a large central area of pallor, and sometimes appear as distorted, small rings (Fig. 1). Other findings include variation in cell size, microcytes, target cells, elliptocytes ("pencil" cells), and red cell fragments.

Currently the bone marrow aspirate is not a routine test in the investigation of iron deficiency in children. When the test is performed, however, stainable iron is always absent. The marrow morphology is characterized by mild to moderate erythroid hyperplasia. Individual nucleated red cells appear small and often have scanty cytoplasm with irregular, ragged borders.

The major diagnostic tests for evaluation of anemia caused by suspected iron deficiency are serum ferritin, serum iron and iron-binding capacity, and erythrocyte protoporphyrin (Table 1).

Serum Ferritin

The level of serum ferritin is proportional to that of storage iron[3] and hence is a useful test in determining a patient's iron status. The test has, for the most part, replaced the bone marrow aspirate as an index of iron stores. Age-related changes in serum ferritin levels occur that reflect normal variations in body iron with increasing age. However, serum con-

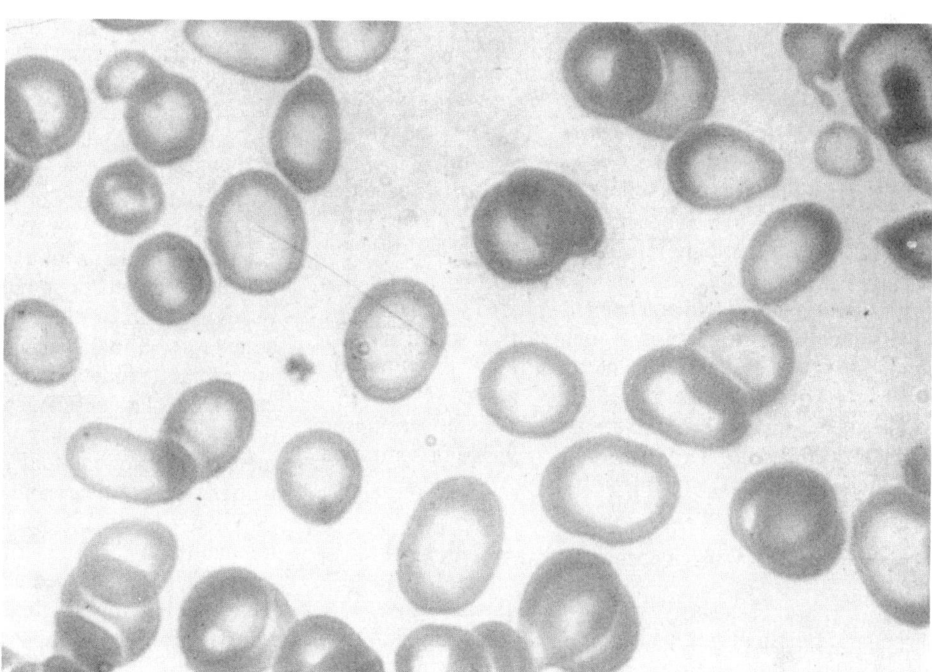

FIGURE 1 Hypochromic-microcytic red cells in iron deficiency anemia.

TABLE 1
Laboratory Tests for Iron Deficiency: Limits of Age-Related Normal Values

Age (years)	MCV* (fl or μ^3)	MCH* (pg)	Serum Ferritin* (μg/L)	Transferrin Saturation* (%)	Erythrocyte Protoporphyrin† (μg/g Hb)
0.5–4	72	24	10	7–16	2.3
5–10	75	25	10	7–16	2.0
11–14	78	26	10	16	2.0
>15	79	27	12	16	2.0

*Lower limits of normal.
†Upper limits of normal.
MCV = mean cell volume; MCH = mean cell hemoglobin.

centrations of less than 10 μg per liter in children or 12 μg per liter in adults are diagnostic of storage iron depletion.

Values for serum ferritin may be in the normal range, despite the presence of iron deficiency. This occurs in association with certain diseases such as mild or severe infection, acute or chronic inflammation, and metastatic malignancy, including leukemia. It is possible that enteritis and parasitic infestation may provoke sufficient inflammation to increase serum ferritin values as well. Liver disease, even mild forms, can result in major elevations of serum ferritin[4]; hence, its measurement is not useful in diagnosing iron deficiency in this group of patients.

The elevation of serum ferritin in all of the cited disorders can be explained by a shift of iron from the red cell mass to storage sites and by increased ferritin synthesis as a nonspecific response to inflammation.[5,6] Thus, ferritin is an acute-phase reactant.

Serum Iron and Iron-Binding Capacity

Almost all the iron in the serum is bound to the iron-binding transport protein, transferrin. By itself, a low serum iron value is of little diagnostic significance. It is subject to wide diurnal variation after 3 years of age, usually with high values in the morning and low values at night.[7] The serum iron also decreases abruptly with a variety of infections and inflammatory disorders.

The test for total iron-binding capacity (TIBC) measures the amount of iron that can be bound to transferrin. The TIBC is less subject to biologic variation than the serum iron and usually varies inversely with iron stores. However, a decline in circulating transferrin and hence a fall in TIBC can occur independently of iron stores in malnutrition states, inflammation, liver disease, protein enteropathy, and the nephrotic syndrome.[8]

Therefore, it is more useful to examine both the serum iron and TIBC in a ratio that yields the percentage of saturation of transferrin:

$$\frac{\text{serum iron}}{\text{TIBC}} \times 100 = \text{percentage transferrin saturation}$$

The transferrin saturation is more consistently helpful than either value alone because it reflects the biologic variability and laboratory errors of both measurements and also functionally assesses the adequacy of iron flow from blood to developing red cells in the bone marrow. In adults, a transferrin saturation below 16 percent is indicative of iron deficiency. The corresponding value for children is lower. Although a transferrin saturation less than 7 percent is highly suggestive of iron deficiency in children, values between 7 and 16 percent are supportive of the diagnosis only in conjunction with a low MCV or other evidence of a lack of iron.

Erythrocyte Protoporphyrin

Erythrocyte protoporphyrin (EP), formerly called FEP (free erythrocyte porphyrin), increases in red cells when insufficient iron is available to combine with protoporphyrin to produce heme. Values higher than 2.3 μg per gram of hemoglobin in patients up to 4 years of age and higher than 2.0 μg per gram of hemoglobin in older patients are considered abnormal. EP increases with progressive degrees of iron deficiency anemia and may be more sensitive in identifying infants with iron deficiency than either transferrin saturation or serum ferritin. The EP has the advantage of being less sensitive to abrupt changes in iron balance or recent iron medication than either transferrin saturation or serum ferritin, and the EP returns to normal only after 2 to 3 months of iron therapy. Moderate increases in EP (3 to 18 μg per gram of hemoglobin) occur in chronic inflammatory disorders and mild lead poisoning; values above 18 μg per gram of hemoglobin indicate moderate to severe lead intoxication.

FOLATE AND VITAMIN B_{12} DEFICIENCIES

Megaloblastic anemia is the end result of deficiencies of folate and vitamin B_{12}, either alone or in combination. The laboratory manifestations of both deficiency states are identical. In an experimental setting, the dietary folate deprivation in an otherwise healthy human evolves into full-blown megaloblastic anemia within only 18 to 20 weeks.[10] Because body stores of vitamin B_{12} are large, especially hepatic (normal liver contains 1 μg of vitamin B_{12} per gram of tissue) and postpubertal daily needs are small (about 1 μg per day), the development of megaloblastic anemia due to an acquired nutritional deficiency of vitamin B_{12} usually takes considerably longer than anemia due to folate deficiency.

Megaloblastic anemia in the pediatric age group is highly unusual. The most common cause is folate deficiency usually resulting from dietary lack, faulty absorption as part of a generalized malabsorption syndrome, or inhibition of dihydrofolate reductase by chemotherapeutic agents. Other causes of folate deficiency are congenital defects in absorption, congenital and acquired disorders of folate metabolism, increased folate requirements, and increased excretion accompanying severe heart and liver disease.

When vitamin B_{12} deficiency is the cause of megaloblastic anemia in children, it is usually due to defective absorption, either from congenital or acquired lack of intrinsic factor or from failure of intestinal absorption. Rarely, defects in vitamin B_{12} transport or disorders of metabolism can be identified.

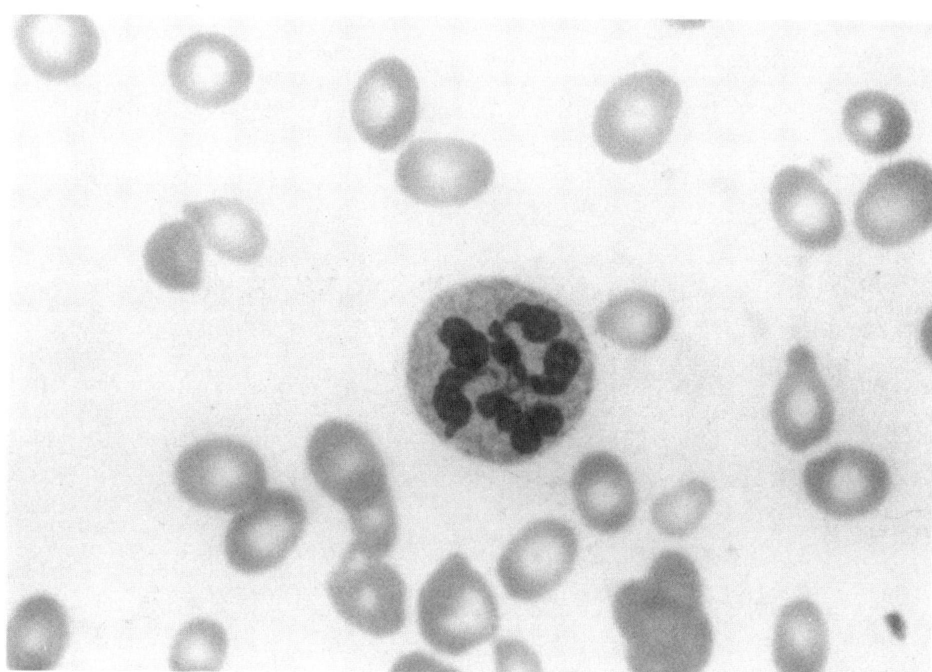

FIGURE 2 Hypersegmentation of neutrophils in either folate or vitamin B_{12} deficiency.

Peripheral Blood and Bone Marrow

In anemia due to a deficiency of either folate or vitamin B_{12}, red cell morphology is classified as normochromic and macrocytic. The increase in MCV is usually proportional to the degree of anemia. Compared with an upper normal pediatric MCV value of 94 fl (μ^3), MCV values of 95 to 110 fl are usual in mild to moderate anemia. In severe anemia, the MCV generally ranges between 110 and 130 fl, but it may be higher. The MCHC is always normal.

The total white cell count may be normal or decreased. When it is decreased, the leukopenia is usually the result of neutropenia and lymphopenia. Thrombocytopenia may also be present, occasionally with bizarre platelet forms including giant platelets.

The two cardinal morphologic findings on blood smear are hypersegmentation of granulocytes (Fig. 2) and macro-ovalocytosis of red cells (Fig. 3). The granulocyte changes are important because they appear very early in the evolution of the megaloblastic state and are often evident, even in mixed

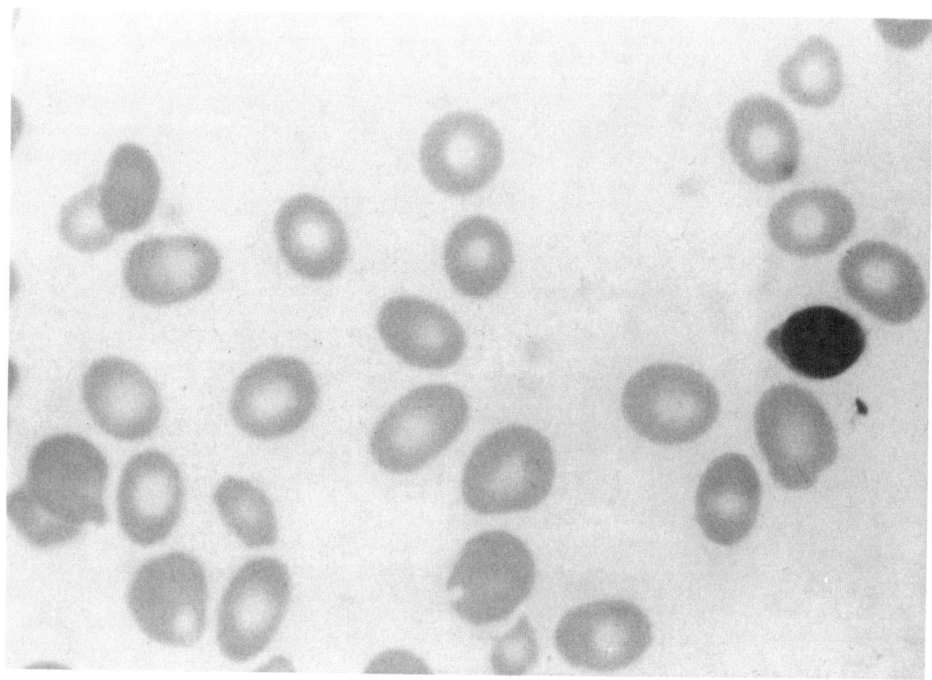

FIGURE 3 Macrocytic and ovalocytic red cells in either folate or vitamin B_{12} deficiency.

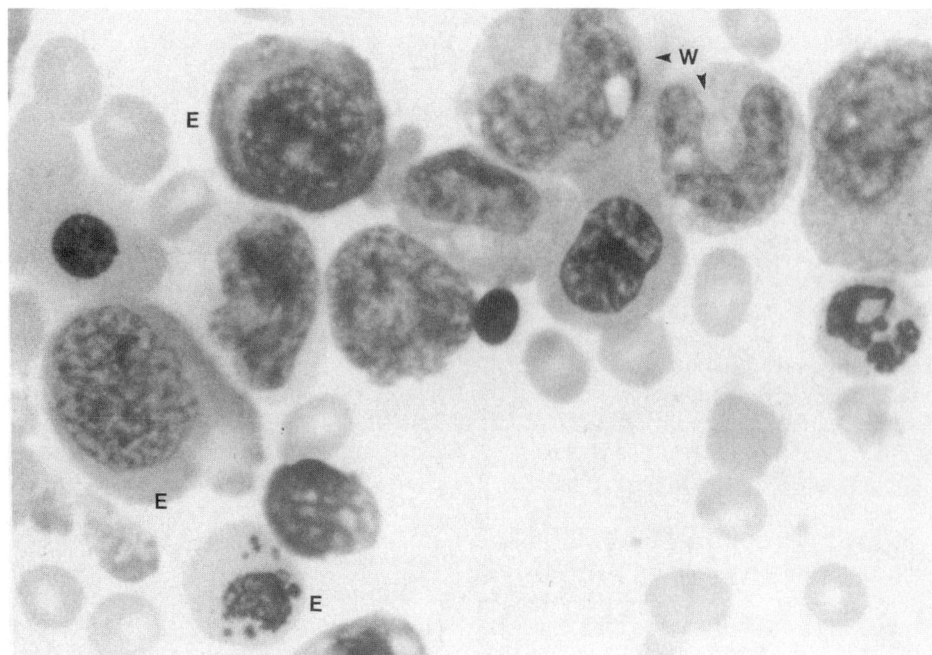

FIGURE 4 Megaloblastic changes in bone marrow red cell and white cell precursors in either folate or vitamin B_{12} deficiency. E = megaloblastic erythroid cells; W = megaloblastic white cells.

deficiency states involving iron and lack of protein. Usually nuclei of circulating neutrophils have less than five lobes, but in megaloblastic anemia segmentation is increased, and cells with six or more lobes are commonly seen. A formal lobe count can be performed, and an average of more than 3.42 lobes per cell in 100 neutrophils is considered abnormal.

The oval macrocytes, well-filled with hemoglobin, are also always evident. Additionally, red cell size and shape may vary considerably. In advanced anemia, a variety of red cell inclusions can be identified, including fine and coarse punctate basophilic stippling, Howell-Jolly bodies, acidophilic (Cabot's) rings, and nucleated erythrocytes.

Examination of bone marrow morphology in conjunction with peripheral blood makes possible the firm diagnosis of megaloblastic anemia. Megaloblastic erythroid cells at all stages of development are larger than corresponding cells of the normoblastic series and often have a higher-than-normal ratio of cytoplasmic area to nuclear area (Fig. 4). The

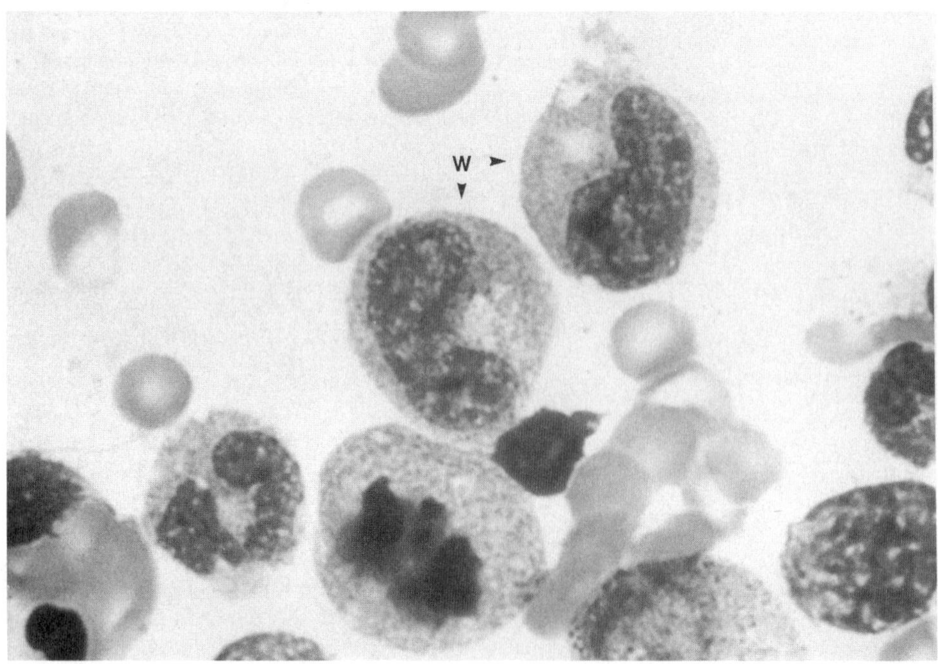

FIGURE 5 Giant metamyelocytes in bone marrow in either folate or vitamin B_{12} deficiency. W = megaloblastic white cells.

megaloblastic nuclei also have an open, stippled, or lacy appearance, and there are often bi- and tri-nucleated forms. In normoblastic maturation, the red cell nucleus and cytoplasm mature in parallel. In megaloblastosis, the nucleus matures more slowly than the cytoplasm, a feature termed *nuclear-cytoplasmic dissociation* or *asynchrony.* White cell changes are also evident, the most striking being the appearance of giant metamyelocyte forms that have a horseshoe-shaped nucleus (Figs. 4 and 5). Megakaryoctyes may also, but not always, show altered morphology.

Bone marrow erythropoiesis is considered to be ineffective and is associated with considerable intramedullary destruction of red cell precursors. Red cell survival is also shortened. The level of unconjugated bilirubin in the serum is usually increased. Ineffective erythropoiesis and myelopoiesis also result in raised levels of serum lactate dehydrogenase and muramidase. Plasma iron clearance and turnover are rapid, but iron incorporation into circulating erythrocytes is decreased. Marrow cytogenetics are abnormal, with elongated chromosomes, spreading of the centromere, and randomly distributed breaks.[12]

Serum Folate

Serum folate[13] is measured microbiologically with a mutant strain of *Lactobacillus casei*, which grows in the presence of 5-methyltetrahydrofolic acid, the predominant form of serum folate. This assay is accurate, reproducible, and available in most diagnostic laboratories; however, it may be invalidated by previous administration of folic acid or by antibiotics. Isotope dilution methods may also be employed for determining serum folate. The normal ranges for serum folate show a wide variation, but in most laboratories levels below 3.0 ng per milliliter are low, 3.0 to 5.0 are borderline, and above 5.0 to 6.0 are normal.

Serum folate levels are highly labile with respect to folate intake and become normal quickly when a folate-deficient patient is treated with folic acid or is placed on an adequate diet. Therefore, serum folate cannot be used to make a retrospective diagnosis of folate deficiency in a recently treated patient. However, the diagnosis can be confirmed by measuring red cell folate, because the folate in red blood cells changes little over the life span of the cell and remains low in a patient with recent folate deficiency, even if the serum folate level has returned to normal.

Red Cell Folate

Red cell folate[14] levels are also measured microbiologically with *Lactobacillus casei*. The isotope dilution methods are less dependable than the bioassay in measuring red cell folate. The normal levels are between 160 and 640 ng per milliliter, and the result is subnormal in patients with megaloblastic anemia caused by folate deficiency. However, it should be noted that the red cell folate level is also subnormal in about 60 per cent of patients with megaloblastic anemia caused by vitamin B_{12} deficiency. Also, if patients with severe folate deficiency have received transfusions prior to blood being taken for an assay, red cell folate levels may be normal, since the folate in mature, transfused red cells is not released until the cell dies.

Other Studies

Although no longer widely used in the routine investigation of folate deficiency, the deoxyuridine suppression ("dU suppression") test[15] and the formiminoglutamic acid (FIGLU) excretion test[16] may provide additional information. The dU suppression test has been used to diagnose the cause of megaloblastic anemia in cases in which serum levels of vitamin B_{12} or folate are equivocal. The test is based on the observation that incorporation of labeled thymidine into normal bone marrows cells or peripheral blood lymphocytes is decreased to less than 10 per cent after preincubation with an excess of deoxyuridine, whereas a smaller decrease in labeled thymidine incorporation is observed in marrow cells of lymphocytes from patients with megaloblastic anemia caused by folate or vitamin B_{12} deficiency.

FIGLU is a normal intermediate product of the metabolism of histidine and requires active tetrahydrofolic acid for further degradation to glutamic acid. In folate deficiency, FIGLU accumulates and its excretion in the urine serves as an indication of the deficiency state. Oral "loading" doses of L-histidine to folate-deficient patients can increase the sensitivity of the test for FIGLU excretion.

Serum Vitamin B_{12}

Serum vitamin B_{12} is measured microbiologically with organisms such as *Euglena gracilis*[17] and *Lactobacillus leishmanii,*[18] which grow in the presence of the nutrient. Currently, microbiologic measurements have been supplanted in most laboratories by isotope dilution techniques using protein-coated charcoal.[19]

Normal values for serum vitamin B_{12} range from 200 to 800 pg per milliliter, and overt deficiency is unlikely with levels greater than 100 pg per milliliter. For reasons that are not clear, one-third of patients with folate deficiency may have low or borderline serum B_{12} levels that return to normal levels within 1 to 3 weeks of starting treatment with folic acid. The presence of antibiotics in a patient's serum may affect the microbiologic assays for serum B_{12} but not the isotope dilution assays.

Vitamin B_{12} Absorption Studies

Vitamin B_{12} absorption tests are useful in diagnosing a defect in vitamin B_{12} absorption. After the oral administration of vitamin B_{12} labeled with radioactive cobalt, its appearance may be measured in the feces, urine, plasma, or liver, or its retention in the whole body may be determined directly by a whole-body counter.

The widely used Schilling test[20] measures the intestinal phase of vitamin B_{12} absorption as well as the availability of gastric-derived intrinsic factor. The test is performed by administering 0.5 to 2.0 μg of radioactive vitamin B_{12} orally.

This is followed in 2 hours by intramuscular injection of 1,000 μg of nonradioactive vitamin B_{12} to saturate the vitamin B_{12}-binding proteins and allow the subsequently absorbed oral radioactive vitamin B_{12} to be excreted in the urine. Urine is usually collected for 24 hours, and the radioactivity is determined. Normal subjects excrete 10 to 35 percent of the administered dose, and those with severe malabsorption of vitamin B_{12} because of lack of intrinsic factor or intestinal malabsorption excrete less than 3 percent.

The Schilling test is a sensitive test of ileal function and is abnormal in any type of vitamin B_{12} malabsorption. When abnormal, the test is repeated with commercial intrinsic factor administered with the oral radioactive vitamin B_{12}. In pernicious anemia due to congenital or acquired deficiency of intrinsic factor, the abnormality in vitamin B_{12} absorption is corrected in the repeat Schilling test with commercial intrinsic factor. Vitamin B_{12} malabsorption persists despite the addition of intrinsic factor if the cause is intestinal malabsorption. When bacterial competition is suspected, as in the "blind-loop syndrome," the test may be repeated after treatment with an appropriate antibiotic and results often revert to normal.

Other Studies

Deficiency of vitamin B_{12} impairs the activity of the enzyme methylmalonyl-CoA mutase. This results in the accumulation of L-methylmalonyl-CoA, which is excreted in the urine as methylmalonic acid. Hence, methylmalonic acid excretion in the urine is increased in vitamin B_{12} deficiency[21] but not in pure folate deficiency.

OTHER NUTRITIONAL ANEMIAS

Protein Deficiency Anemia

Protein deficiency is essentially a disease of underdeveloped countries, although it is also seen in North America, primarily in children of strict vegetarians and in those with chronic diseases such as cancer and GI disorders. A mild to moderate normochromic and normocytic anemia frequently results from the protein deficiency.[22]

The anemia is due primarily to decreased red cell production[23] and is characterized by decreased red cell and reticulocyte counts, with normal numbers of platelets and white cells. Serum and urinary erythropoietin levels are abnormally decreased relative to the low hemoglobin level. The bone marrow is normocellular to mildly hypocellular with a relative decrease in erythroid elements and frequently a variable maturation arrest of erythroid precursors.[24]

At diagnosis, low total serum protein and serum albumin concentrations are indicative of protein deficiency. Normochromic, normocytic red cells with decreased serum iron and decreased TIBC are compatible with this form of nutritional anemia.

Occult deficiencies of iron, folate, riboflavin, vitamin E, vitamin B_{12}, and copper may complicate protein deficiency, and the classic hematologic picture of protein deficiency anemia might be modified at presentation. Usually, however, these complicating nutritional deficiencies become evident only with treatment after partial correction of the protein deficiency.

Copper Deficiency Anemia

A hypochromic and microcytic anemia has been described in association with copper deficiency in malnourished children, exudative enteropathies, nephrosis, Menke's kinky hair syndrome, and prolonged intravenous alimentation.[23,25,26]

Copper is essential for the absorption and utilization of iron. In the form of ferroxidase, copper converts ferrous iron to ferric iron and maintains it in this state for transport by transferrin. Thus, the anemia of copper deficiency results primarily from the decreased transport of iron to the marrow erythroid progenitor cells.

Copper deficiency, therefore, can mimic iron deficiency anemia both morphologically and by the presence of low serum iron concentrations; however, the anemia is refractory to iron supplementation. Copper deficiency anemia can also be distinguished from iron deficiency anemia because copper deficiency is usually associated with neutropenia, leukopenia, and vacuolated erythroid precursors in the bone marrow, features generally not seen with iron deficiency. Copper deficiency can be confirmed by documentation of a low serum copper concentration (less than 70 μg per deciliter after the patient is 3 months of age).

Miscellaneous Anemias

Vitamin E, alpha-tocopherol, is a fat-soluble vitamin that serves as an antioxidant in humans but has no essential cofactor functions.[27] Nutritional vitamin E deficiency in humans is rare and seems to be limited to the neonatal period, to chronic cholestasis, and to fat malabsorption syndromes such as cystic fibrosis.[28] In these clinical settings, a hemolytic anemia due to vitamin E deficiency has been described.[27] The anemia appears to be the consequence of peroxidation of the lipid component of the red cell membrane initiated by the generation of free radicals.

Vitamin A deficiency can cause a hypochromic and microcytic anemia associated with a low serum iron concentration.[24] However, in contrast to iron deficiency anemia, body iron stores are increased, serum transferrin is normal or decreased, and the anemia does not respond to iron therapy. Treatment with vitamin A supplements corrects the anemia. The pathophysiology of this anemia may involve a defect in iron utilization caused by the vitamin A deficiency.[29]

About 80 percent of patients with scurvy have anemia, but it has not been shown that vitamin C deficiency itself is the cause of the anemia. Attempts to induce anemia in human volunteers by vitamin C restriction have been unsuccessful.

Isolated nutritional deficiencies of pyridoxine, riboflavin, pantothenic acid, or niacin are rare, and it is not clear whether these deficiencies per se can cause anemia. Nevertheless, malnourished patients with pyridoxine deficiency and hypochromic, microcytic anemia unresponsive to iron therapy have responded to the administration of pyridoxine. Moreover, patients with riboflavin deficiency and pure red cell aplasia have improved with the administration of riboflavin. Deficiencies of niacin and of pantothenic acid have been associated with anemias in certain animals, but no such relationships in humans have been demonstrated.

ANEMIA OF CHRONIC DISORDERS

The anemia of chronic disorders is associated with a wide variety of chronic infectious, inflammatory, and neoplastic diseases.[30] Since these diseases may produce anemia for a number of reasons, a diagnosis of anemia of chronic disorders cannot be made without considering other possible causes.

This form of anemia develops slowly and is usually mild. The hematocrit seldom falls below 30 percent in adults or below 20 percent in children. Morphologically, the anemia is usually classified as normochromic and normocytic with a low or normal reticulocyte count. Occasionally the red cells are hypochromic and normocytic and, less frequently, hypochromic and microcytic.

The anemia of chronic disorders is characterized by decreased serum iron levels, decreased TIBC, decreased saturation of transferrin, decreased numbers of iron-containing nucleated red cells in bone marrow (sideroblasts), normal or increased stores of reticuloendothelial iron, and an increase of EP. The serum ferritin is normal or raised, even in the presence of reduced serum iron levels. Serum copper levels are usually raised.

The pathophysiology of the anemia is complex. At least three factors play a role: shortened red cell survival, impaired marrow response to anemia, and defective transfer of iron from reticuloendothelial storage sites to the bone marrow.

The shortened red cell survival appears to be mild and is not a universal finding. When present, the mechanism is ill-defined, but the cause appears to be extracorpuscular. The bone marrow also fails to respond to the anemia with an effective increase in erythropoiesis. This may be due in part to defective production or release of erythropoietin. The impaired iron release from the reticuloendothelial system is an important factor in the anemia of chronic disorders and accounts for the iron-deficient type of erythropoiesis that is frequently observed. In iron kinetic studies, plasma iron clearance is normal, but incorporation into new, circulating red cells is markedly diminished, indicating a severe block in iron utilization that occurs in chronic disorders.

Iron absorption from the gut may be either normal or diminished in patients with this type of anemia. Diminished iron absorption appears to result from an inability to release intracellular iron from the intestinal cells rather than from defective uptake of iron into the cells. Reduced levels of transferrin and, hence, reduced TIBC are explained by either diminished production of transferrin or increased transferrin binding to iron-overloaded reticuloendothelial cells.

Anemia of Liver Disease

In addition to the anemia of chronic disorders that may be seen in a variety of chronic GI diseases, an anemia occurs commonly in otherwise "uncomplicated" acute and chronic liver disease and appears to be multifactorial in etiology.[31]

Shortened red cell survival is seen in some patients with liver disease but without evidence of blood loss. The explanation for the shortened survival is not clear, but patients with active hepatic disease have an increased tendency toward Heinz body formation following red cell incubation with oxidant chemicals, such as acetylphenylhydrazine. The increase in Heinz body formation is associated with increased instability of the red cell and altered hexose monophosphate shunt activity.[32]

The significance of the metabolic changes in the red cells is unclear, but they can be reproduced in normal erythrocytes by incubating the cells in plasma from patients with active liver disease. Metabolism in patients' red cells returns to normal within a few weeks after the resolution of hepatic disease.

The erythrocytes in patients with liver disease are often macrocytic, and MCV values range from 100 to 110 fl. Target cells, spur cells, and acanthocytes may also be seen, and, along with the macrocytic changes, they appear to be due to increases in red cell membrane phospholipid and cholesterol that occur with obstructive hepatic disease. The membrane lipid changes result in an increased red cell membrane area, which ultimately leads to target and spur cell formation.

DISORDERS OF HEMOSTASIS

Normal hemostasis depends on an interaction of blood vessels, platelets, and the coagulation system.

Hemostatic "Plug" Formation

The first event whereby bleeding is arrested at the level of the capillary and small vessel is the formation of a hemostatic "plug." Vascular injury exposes subendothelial collagen fibrils and provides a site for platelet adhesion. The process of adhesion requires an interaction of platelet membrane glycoprotein Ib, the von Willebrand component of the Factor VIII molecule, and the damaged vessel endothelium.

Aggregation of additional platelets is promoted by agonists such as adenosine diphosphate (ADP), collagen, thrombin, and epinephrine and is mediated through interaction with platelet membrane glycoproteins IIb-IIIa with fibrinogen. Upon aggregating, platelets release or secrete ADP, thromboxane A_2, and serotonin, which facilitate further clumping, termed *secondary platelet aggregation*. Platelet thromboxane A_2, a potent inducer of platelet secretion and aggregation, is synthesized within the cell via the arachidonic acid metabolic pathway as a direct result of stimulation of the platelet membrane during the aggregation process.

At the time of platelet aggregation, thromboplastic material called *tissue factor* is released as a result of vascular injury. Tissue factor and phospholipid released from platelets, termed *platelet factor 3*, promote thrombin formation in the coagulation system. Fibrin is subsequently formed and is pulled together with the clumped platelets as a tight "plug." The process is facilitated by a platelet contractile protein called thrombasthenin.

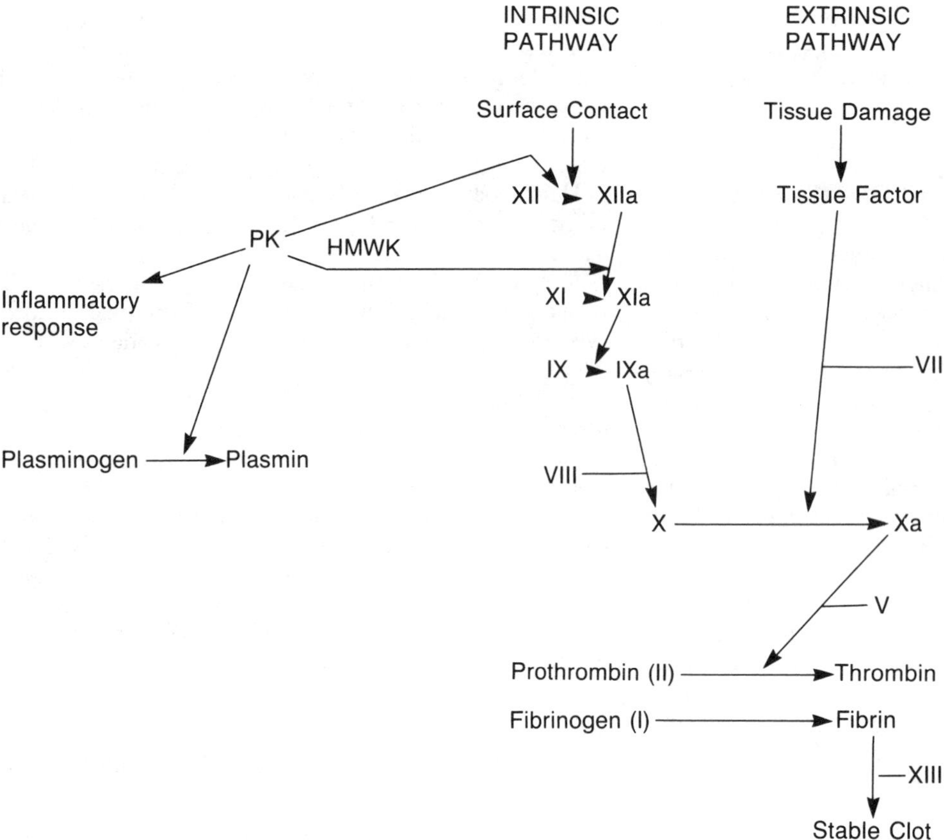

FIGURE 6 Pathways of blood coagulation. Table 2 shows the nomenclature of the coagulation factors. Activated factor with enzyme activity has a suffix "a". PK = prekallikrein; HMWK = high molecular weight kininogen.

Fibrin Clot Formation

Events in the coagulation system lead to a definitive fibrin clot. The system consists of a sequence of reactions by serine proteases or their specific substrates (Fig. 6). The nomenclature for the coagulation factors is shown in Table 2. Fibrin clot formation may be initiated by either of two pathways.

The first pathway, called the *intrinsic pathway*, is initiated by the surface activation of Factor XII. The process is accelerated by the presence of prekallikrein (Fletcher factor) and high molecular weight kininogen (Fitzgerald factor), which also link the coagulation system to the kinin system. The intrinsic pathway progresses through the stepwise acti-

TABLE 2
Nomenclature of Blood Coagulation Factors

Factor Number	Alternate Names
I	Fibrinogen
II	Prothrombin
III	Thromboplastin, tissue factor
IV	Calcium
V	Proaccelerin, accelerator globulin
VI	Number no longer used
VII	Proconvertin
VIII	Antihemophilic factor (AHF) *or* Antihemophilic globulin (AHG)
IX	Christmas factor *or* Plasma thromboplastin component (PTC)
X	Stuart-Prower factor
XI	Plasma thromboplastin antecedent (PTA)
XII	Hageman factor
XIII	Fibrin-stabilizing factor
No number	Prekallikrein (Fletcher factor)
No number	High molecular weight kininogen (Fitzgerald factor)
No numbers	Platelet factors: Platelet factor 3 (PF-3); phospholipoprotein Platelet factor 4 (PF-4); antiheparin

vation of Factors XI and IX. Activated Factor IX forms a complex with Factor VIII, phospholipid, and calcium to activate Factor X.

The second pathway, called the *extrinsic pathway*, is initiated by the release of tissue factor from injured parenchymal and vascular tissues. Tissue factor forms a complex with Factor VII and calcium, which in turn activates Factor X.

The last steps in coagulation are shared by the two pathways. The formation of thrombin is mediated by the action of activated Factor X, Factor V, and phospholipid. Thrombin then accelerates the polymerization of fibrinogen to fibrin through the intermediate formation of fibrin monomer. The fibrin clot that finally results is stabilized by a cross-linking enzyme, Factor XIII.

Fibrinolysis

The fibrinolytic system is a physiologic response that helps prevent excessive formation of clot at the site of injury. The system is activated by plasma and tissue plasminogen activators that convert the inert precursor, plasminogen, to the fibrinolytic enzyme, plasmin. When fibrin is degraded by plasmin, the resulting fibrin degradation products (FDP) inhibit further conversion of fibrinogen to fibrin. The FDP are removed from the blood by the liver over several hours.

Inhibitors of Coagulation

When the coagulation system is activated, protease inhibitors provide a controlling and regulating mechanism. The activated coagulation Factors XIIa, XIa, IXa, and Xa and thrombin, all of which are serine proteases, are inhibited by the protease inhibitor antithrombin III (AT-III). Activated Factors VIII and V are inhibited by another mechanism—degradation by the serine protease protein C and its co-factor protein S. Plasmin is neutralized by the action of alpha$_2$-antiplasmin and alpha$_2$-macroglobulin.

Diagnostic Approaches to Bleeding Disorders

In patients with suspected GI disease and bleeding, it is important to exclude a primary bleeding disorder as the cause. The history and physical findings are important in this regard.

A family history may identify the hereditary nature of the bleeding. The history may include, for example, X-linked recessive inheritance in Factors VIII and IX deficiency, an autosomal dominant pattern in von Willebrand's disease, and autosomal recessive inheritance in Factor XI deficiency. The past history and surgical records may also be helpful. Patients with Factor XIII deficiency characteristically have umbilical cord bleeding during the newborn period. Prolonged bleeding after dental extractions, or after tonsillectomy or adenoidectomy, is a useful clue to an abnormal bleeding disorder.

The type of bleeding observed on physical examination is also helpful. Thrombocytopenia, abnormalities of platelet function, and von Willebrand's disease are frequently manifested by bleeding from mucous membranes, for example, by epistaxis. "Deep" bleeding with hematomas and hemarthroses is characteristic of the hemophilias.

Screening Tests

A panel of laboratory screening tests can be performed to determine and identify the presence of a bleeding disorder (Table 3). These include a *platelet count* or an estimation of platelet numbers on the blood smear; a *bleeding time* by

TABLE 3
Results of Screening Tests for Various Bleeding Disorders

Disorder	Platelet Count	BT	PTT	PT	TT
Severe liver disease	N or low	N or Abn	Abn	Abn	N or Abn
Vitamin K lack (II, VII, IX, X deficiencies)	N	N	Abn	Abn	N
Disseminated intravascular coagulation	Low	Abn	Abn	Abn	Abn
Hemophilias (VIII, IX, XI, XII deficiencies)	N	N	Abn	N	N
von Willebrand's disease	N	Abn	Abn	N	N
Factor VII deficiency	N	N	N	Abn	N
Afibrinogenemia	N	Mild Abn	No clot	No clot	No clot
Platelet function defects	N or low	Abn	N	N	N

BT = bleeding time; PTT = partial thromboplastin time; PT = prothrombin time; TT = thrombin time; N = normal; Abn = abnormal.

a standardized method, which measures platelet-vessel interaction; a *partial thromboplastin time* (PTT), which measures thrombin generation in the intrinsic pathway and is a function of all the coagulation factors except Factor VII; a *prothrombin time* (PT), which measures thrombin generation in the extrinsic pathway and is a function of Factors II, V, VII, and X activity and of the fibrinogen level; and *thrombin time* (TT), which estimates the amount and function of fibrinogen and is particularly sensitive to the presence of fibrin degradation products or heparin.

Additional laboratory tests, such as fibrinogen level, clot retraction, specific coagulation factor assays, platelet function tests, alpha$_2$-antiplasmin, Factor XIII, and heparin assay, may be indicated to establish a diagnosis.

Bleeding Disorder Due to Vitamin K Deficiency

Deficiency of vitamin K results in the failure of the vitamin K–dependent coagulation Factors II, VII, IX, and X to develop calcium-binding sites essential to their function in the coagulation process. In the absence of vitamin K, the polypeptide chains of vitamin K–dependent factors are produced normally, but an essential carboxylation step does not take place. The acarboxy forms of the factors cannot bind calcium and thus cannot participate in the coagulation sequence.[33]

Beyond the newborn period, vitamin K is absorbed from the colon, and synthesis by bacterial flora provides a major source. Vitamin K is not absorbed from the colon in older children or adults but is absorbed from the ileum. The daily requirement of this fat-soluble vitamin is probably about 1 μg per kilogram of body weight, which is supplied readily in most normal diets, particularly those containing green, leafy vegetables. After absorption from the upper small intestine, vitamin K is stored in the liver.

Conditions associated with malabsorption of vitamin K that may result in a bleeding disorder include cystic fibrosis, biliary atresia, cholelithiasis, obstructive jaundice, and disorders leading to upper small intestine dysfunction. An additional cause of hemorrhagic problems due to vitamin K deficiency may be the excessive administration of the anticoagulant coumarin. In the absence of marked dietary deficiency of vitamin K, malabsorption due to alteration of GI bacterial flora by antibiotic therapy is rare.

Laboratory findings of vitamin K deficiency (Table 3) include a normal platelet count and bleeding time, a prolonged PTT and PT, and a normal TT. Assays of the individual coagulation factors can provide confirmation of the diagnosis.

Bleeding Disorder in Liver Disease

The liver synthesizes most coagulation factors: fibrinogen, prothrombin, prekallikrein, high molecular weight kininogen, and Factors V, VII, IX, X, XI, XII, and XIII. It also produces plasminogen, the three regulators of coagulation, AT-III, proteins C and S, and inhibitors of fibrinolysis—alpha$_2$-antiplasmin and alpha$_1$-antitrypsin. The liver is also involved in the clearance of activated coagulation factors and activators of fibrinolysis from the circulation.

As a consequence, severe hepatocellular damage is frequently associated with multiple hemostatic defects than can predispose to bleeding. Hepatic failure can also lead to disseminated intravascular coagulation (DIC) as the result of decreased synthesis of AT-III and decreased hepatic clearance of activated coagulation factors.

In general, screening tests for a bleeding disorder in liver disease give variable results (Table 3). In mild liver disease, screening tests for coagulation disturbances often fail to show that liver dysfunction exists. For example, most patients with acute viral or toxic hepatitis do not demonstrate marked abnormalities of coagulation. In contrast, in fulminant hepatitis hemostatic abnormalities are more pronounced, are often associated with hemorrhagic symptoms, and have prognostic significance.[34] In chronic liver disease, results of coagulation screening tests are unpredictable. Although most studies have failed to show close correlations between coagulation tests and cholesterol, transaminase, or gamma globulin levels, the prothrombin time still appears to be the most convenient coagulation test for monitoring liver function.

Specific assays may provide additional information in hepatic disorders. *Fibrinogen* levels are usually normal in liver disease because fibrinogen synthesis occurs in liver cells but is also produced in extrahepatic sites. An increased catabolic rate of labeled fibrinogen has been noted in acute and chronic active hepatitis, despite normal levels of plasma fibrinogen.[35] Altered rates of fibrinogen catabolism may be the result of primary fibrinolysis induced by liver disease or may be due to DIC. The low levels of fibrinogen occasionally observed in some cases of acute liver failure have been explained on the basis of DIC with depletion of some of the clotting factors.

High levels of fibrinogen are occasionally observed in liver disease, mainly because fibrinogen is an acute phase reactant. Elevated levels of fibrinogen have been observed in obstructive jaundice, biliary cirrhosis, and hepatoma.

An abnormal fibrin monomer aggregate, termed *dysfibrinogen*, has been described in a number of patients with liver dysfunction.[36] Coagulation abnormalities involving a prolongation of the thrombin time despite a normal fibrinogen concentration should suggest that dysfibrinogenemia is present.

The levels of *vitamin K–dependent factors*, Factors II, VII, IX, and X, are frequently reduced in patients with liver disease, even in the absence of vitamin K deficiency. This appears to result primarily from impaired hepatic synthesis. Of the factors that may reflect hepatocellular damage, Factor VII appears to be the most sensitive. Factor VII is synthesized almost exclusively in the liver and has the most rapid biologic half-life of all the liver-dependent factors (about 5 hours). In a study of patients with acute liver failure, it appeared that those with Factor VII activity exceeding 8 percent survived, whereas the others died,[34] suggesting that the assay can be used prognostically.

Factor V activity usually parallels the activity of Factors II and X in liver disease when the defect is due to decreased hepatic synthesis. If DIC occurs in association with liver disease, the Factor V level may be significantly depressed. Markedly elevated levels of Factor V may be seen in obstructive liver disease as an acute phase reactant phenomenon.

Factor VIII activity is generally normal or elevated in all forms of liver disease because extrahepatic production of Factor VIII is very extensive. *Factor XI and XII* activity is usually normal in hepatocellular disease but may be decreased. Both factors may be elevated when the primary problem is obstructive.

There are contradictory data concerning *Factor XIII* levels in liver disease. Reports of low activity have been based primarily on results of clot solubility tests; however, when immunologic or radioisotopic techniques are used, more variable results are seen.

Plasminogen levels are commonly decreased in liver disease. In one study, levels were depressed in 45 percent of patients who had liver disease but not hepatic failure, whereas all patients with hepatic failure demonstrated diminished plasminogen levels.[36]

Antithrombin III levels are frequently decreased in patients with acute and chronic liver disease, whereas elevations may be observed in those with obstructive disease.[37]

Disseminated Intravascular Coagulation in Liver Disease

Patients with liver disease commonly show a profile of coagulation abnormalities which is highly suggestive of DIC. The abnormalities include hypofibrinogenemia, increased fibrinogen catabolism, increased levels of fibrin degradation products, thrombocytopenia, and depressed levels of Factors V and VIII. This pattern of abnormalities is not specific for DIC and may simply reflect the severity of the hepatocellular disease process. For example, fibrinogen levels may be depressed owing to decreased production, although this is unusual. Increased catabolism of fibrinogen may reflect distribution in extravascular spaces such as in the formation of ascitic fluid; alternatively, proteolysis by enzymes other than thrombin can produce increased fibrinogen catabolism. Because fibrin degradation products are cleared by the liver, severe liver dysfunction itself may cause elevations of these products in the absence of DIC. Thrombocytopenia may occur for a variety of reasons such as hypersplenism. Changes in the levels of Factors V and VIII are widely variable and nonspecific. Thus, the hemostatic abnormalities in liver disease may be similar to those found in DIC, and differentiating the abnormalities due to liver disease from those due to DIC may be difficult.

REFERENCES

1. Dallman PR, Siimes MA, Stekel A. Iron deficiency in infancy and childhood. Am J Clin Nutr 1980; 33:86–118.
2. Yip R, Johnson C, Dallman PR. Age-related changes in laboratory values used in the diagnosis of anemia and iron deficiency. Am J Clin Nutr 1984; 39:427–436.
3. Worwood M. Ferritin in human tissue and serum. Clin Haematol 1982; 11:275–307.
4. Lipschitz DA, Cook JD, Finch CA. A clinical evaluation of serum ferritin as an index of iron stores. N Engl J Med 1974; 290:1213–1216.
5. Cartwright GE, Lee GR. The anaemia of chronic disorders. Br J Haematol 1971; 21:147–152.
6. Konijn AM, Hershko C. Ferritin synthesis in inflammation. I. Pathogenesis of impaired iron release. Br J Haematol 1977; 37:7–16.
7. Schwartz E, Baehner RL. Diurnal variation of serum iron in infants and children. Acta Paediatr Scand 1968; 57:433–435.
8. Brittenham GM, Danish EH, Harris JW. Assessment of bone marrow and body iron stores: old techniques and new technologies. Semin Hematol 1981; 18:194–221.
9. Koerper MA, Dallman PR. Serum iron concentration and transferrin saturation in the diagnosis of iron deficiency in children: normal developmental changes. J Pediatr 1977; 91:870–874.
10. Herbert V. Experimental nutritional folate deficiency in man. Trans Assoc Am Physicians 1962; 75:307–320.
11. Herbert V. Megaloblastic anemias—mechanisms and management. DM, pp 1-40, August, 1965.
12. Lawler SD, Roberts PD, Hoffbrand AV. Chromosome studies in megaloblastic anaemia before and after treatment. Scand J Haematol 1971; 8:309–320.
13. Hoffbrand AV, ed. Megaloblastic anaemia. Clin Haematol 1976; 5:547–618.
14. Hoffbrand AV, Newcombe FA, Mollin DL. Method of assay of red cell folate activity and the value of the assay as a test for folate deficiency. J Clin Pathol 1966; 19:17–28.
15. Herbert V, Tisman G, Go LT, Brenner L. The dU suppression test using 125 I-UdR to define biochemical megaloblastosis. Br J Haematol 1973; 24:713–723.
16. Spray GH, Witts LJ. Excretion of formiminoglutamic acid as an index of folic-acid deficiency. Lancet 1959; ii:702–704.
17. Anderson BB. Investigations into the Euglena method for the assay of vitamin B_{12} in serum. J Clin Pathol 1964; 17:14–26.
18. Skeggs HR. *Lactobacillus leishmannii* assay for vitamin B_{12}. In: Kavanaugh F, ed. Analytical microbiology. New York: Academic Press, 1963.
19. Lau KS, Gottlieb C, Wasserman LR, et al. Measurement of serum vitamin B_{12} level using radioisotope dilution and coated charcoal. Blood 1965; 26:202–214.
20. Schilling RF. Intrinsic factor studies. II. The effect of gastric juice on the urinary excretion of radioactivity after the oral administration of radioactive vitamin B_{12}. J Lab Clin Med 1953; 42:860–866.
21. Barness LA, Young D, Mellman WJ, Kahn SB. Methylmalonate excretion in a patient with pernicious anemia. N Engl J Med 1963; 268:144–146.
22. Reissmann KR. Protein metabolism and erythropoiesis. I. The anemia of protein deprivation. Blood 1964; 23:137–145.
23. Dallman PR. Iron deficiency and related nutritional anemias. In: Nathan DG, Oski FA, eds. Hematology of infancy and childhood. 3rd ed. Philadelphia: Saunders, 1987: 274.
24. Oski FA. Anemia related to nutritional deficiencies other than vitamin B_{12} and folic acid. In: Williams WJ, Beutler E, Erslev AJ, Lichtman MA, eds. Hematology. 3rd ed. New York: McGraw-Hill, 1983: 532.
25. Graham GG, Cordano A. Copper depletion and deficiency in the malnourished infant. Johns Hopkins Med J 1969; 124:139–150.
26. Joffe G, Etzioni A, Levy J, Benderly A. A patient with copper deficiency anemia while on prolonged intravenous feeding. Clin Pediatr 1981; 20:226–228.
27. Lubin B, Machlin LJ, eds. Vitamin E: biochemical, hematological, and clinical aspects. Ann NY Acad Sci 1982; 393:1–504.
28. Farrell PM, Bieri JG, Fratantoni JF, et al. The occurrence and effects of human vitamin E deficiency. A study in patients with cystic fibrosis. J Clin Invest 1977; 60:233–241.
29. Hodges RE, Sauberlich HE, Canham JE, et al. Hematopoietic studies in vitamin A deficiency. Am J Clin Nutr 1978; 31:876–885.
30. Hansen NE. The anaemia of chronic disorders. A bag of unsolved questions. Scand J Haematol 1983; 31:397–402.
31. Kimber C, Deller DJ, Ibbotson RN, et al. The mechanism of anaemia in chronic liver disease. Q J Med 1965; 34:33–64.
32. Smith JR, Kay NE, Gottlieb AJ, et al. Abnormal erythrocyte metabolism in hepatic disease. Blood 1975; 46:955–964.
33. Olson RE. Vitamin K. In: Colman RW, Hirsh J, Marder VJ, Salzman EW, eds. Hemostasis and thrombosis: basic principles and clinical practice. Philadelphia: JB Lippincott, 1982: 582.
34. Dymock IW, Tucker JS, Woolf IL, et al. Coagulation studies as a prognostic index in acute liver failure. Br J Haematol 1975; 29:385–395.
35. Clark RD, Gazzard BG, Lewis ML, et al. Fibrinogen metabolism in acute hepatitis and active chronic hepatitis. Br J Haematol 1975; 30:95–102.
36. Gallus AS, Lucas CR, Hirsh J. Coagulation studies in patients with acute infectious hepatitis. Br J Haematol 1972; 22:761–771.
37. Cederblad G, Korsan-Bengsten K, Olsson R. Observations of increased levels of blood coagulation factors and other plasma proteins in cholestatic liver disease. Scand J Gastroenterol 1976; 11:391–396.

PART 3

Microbiologic Tests

Susan E. Richardson, B.Sc., M.D., C.M.
Martin Petric, Ph.D.
Mohamed A. Karmali, M.B., Ch.B., FRCPC

Numerous gastrointestinal (GI) syndromes warrant the consideration of a wide variety of infectious agents. An accurate microbiologic diagnosis enables appropriate treatment to be instituted and rules out other conditions, the treatment of which could be harmful to the prompt resolution of an infectious process (e.g., steroid therapy for inflammatory bowel disease). Specific antimicrobial management is indicated for some GI infections, although many spontaneously resolve without treatment, e.g., most causes of acute infectious diarrhea. In some cases, therapy is *not* indicated, as in uncomplicated *Salmonella* enterocolitis,[1] in which the use of antimicrobials prolongs the fecal excretion of organisms and has no effect on clinical symptoms. Similarly, the use of antibiotics in verocytotoxin-producing *Escherichia coli* infections may be a factor in the progression of the disease to the hemolytic-uremic syndrome and should therefore be withheld.[2] These considerations underscore the need for consultation with the laboratory in the interpretation of microbiologic data. The following discussion is intended to be a guide to the capabilities of the routine microbiology laboratory in the diagnosis of GI infections, with mention of the more specialized tests that are obtainable at reference laboratories. Full details of these illnesses are discussed elsewhere in the text.

GASTROENTERITIS AND RELATED SYNDROMES

Although a detailed etiologic investigation of all known enteropathogens is not feasible in most laboratories, appropriate clinical and epidemiologic information can provide a valuable guide for the microbiologist in search of unusual pathogens. A history of diarrhea in contacts of an affected patient provides good evidence of an infectious etiology. The length of the incubation period can suggest a particular etiology in outbreaks. It is usually not possible to establish an accurate correlation between clinical features and microbial etiology because the spectrum of clinical manifestations of specific enteric infections is wide and variable. On the other hand, certain classic features can be suggestive of a particular etiology, for example, dysentery (shigellosis, enteroinvasive *E. coli*, amebiasis), bloody diarrhea (salmonellosis, shigellosis, campylobacteriosis, enteroinvasive *E. coli*), "rice-water" stools (cholera), significant vomiting and watery diarrhea in a young infant (rotavirus), hemorrhagic colitis (verocytotoxin [VT]-producing *E. coli*), subacute or chronic diarrhea with flatulence (giardiasis), and appendicular syndromes (yersiniosis). Histories of recent travel (especially to the tropics) and recent antibiotic usage are helpful.

Laboratory findings may be influenced by a number of factors, including the nature of the methods used for diagnosis, the spectrum of microbial agents tested for, the timing of collection of the specimen related to the onset of symptoms, the quality of the specimen obtained, and delays in transportation of the specimen to the laboratory.

Investigation of feces is the main approach to diagnosing enteric infection. Occasionally, other specimens, especially upper small bowel biopsies or aspirates, can be helpful in the investigation of chronic diarrhea for giardiasis, attaching and effacing *E. coli* infection, or bacterial overgrowth in the blind-loop syndrome.

Specimen Collection and Transport

A fresh stool sample submitted promptly to the laboratory in a clean container is the best specimen for the diagnosis of bacterial and viral diarrhea. The less satisfactory rectal swab may be unavoidable in some instances, but it eliminates viral diagnosis. If delay in transportation is anticipated, stools for bacterial culture should be placed in an appropriate transport medium such as Cary-Blair or buffered glycerol citrate, since this prevents changes in pH that may be detrimental to the survival of the pathogen.

For the diagnosis of parasitic enteric infection, microscopy of fresh stool promptly after collection may be rewarding in that characteristic motile trophozoites may be seen, if present. On the other hand, trophozoites tend to disintegrate rapidly after collection. Thus it is advisable to place all stools to be investigated for parasites in an appropriate fixative such as sodium acetate formalin (SAF), polyvinyl alcohol (PVA), or Schaudinn's fixative, which preserves the trophozoites and cysts of protozoa as well as eggs and larval forms.

Microscopic Examination of Stools

Whereas light microscopy is a standard procedure for the investigation of parasitic disease, it may also, in selected instances, be rewarding in the diagnosis of bacterial diarrhea.

Few to moderate numbers of inflammatory cells may be seen in stained fecal smears of patients with enterocolitis or bloody diarrhea. These may point to causes such as salmonel-

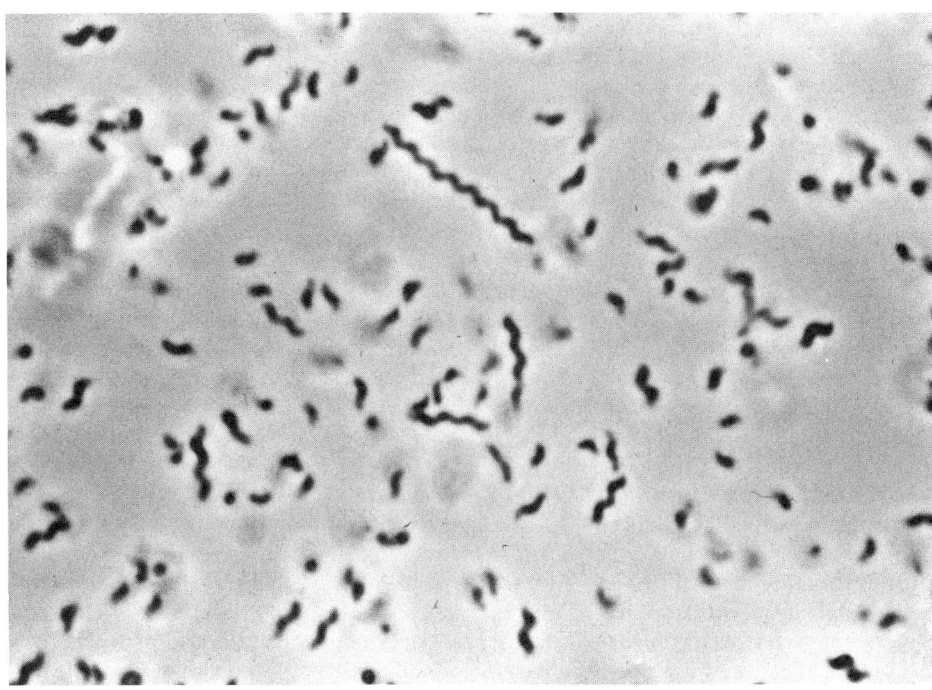

FIGURE 1 Phase contrast microscopy of a 24-hour culture of *Campylobacter jejuni* (×2,000).

losis, campylobacteriosis, and shigellosis. Frank bacillary dysentery (pus in the stools) is usually associated with sheets of polymorphonuclear leukocytes on the smear, a picture that is also seen in ulcerative colitis. In areas endemic for amebic dysentery, the type of cellular exudate may be helpful in distinguishing amebic dysentery (mononuclear cell exudate) from bacillary dysentery (polymorphonuclear cell exudate).

A rapid presumptive diagnosis of *Campylobacter* enterocolitis or cholera can be made by direct microscopy (preferably phase-contrast) by visualizing characteristic highly motile curved (Vibrio) or S-shaped/spiral (*Campylobacter*) bacteria (Fig. 1).

Bacterial Enteropathogens

The definitive laboratory diagnosis of bacterial diarrhea is based on the isolation, by culture, of a potential enteropathogenic bacterium or, in appropriate cases, the demonstration of a specific bacterial toxin in fecal filtrates. Further studies (e.g., biochemical or serologic tests of strain discrimination or virulence tests) may be necessary to distinguish pathogenic strains from nonpathogenic ones. Since the normal fecal flora in humans contains a large number of different bacterial species, the isolation of a specific bacterial pathogen requires the use of selective methods that enable the specific pathogen to grow while ensuring the suppression of normal fecal flora. Bacterial enteropathogens that are routinely screened for in many laboratories include *Salmonella* spp., *Campylobacter* spp., *Shigella* spp., *Yersinia enterocolitica*, *Clostridium difficile*, and, increasingly, verocytotoxin-producing *E. coli* serotype O157:H7. Vibrios are not screened for routinely in nonendemic regions. Enteropathogenic *E. coli* serotypes, enterotoxigenic and enteroinvasive *E. coli*, and the food-poisoning organisms (*Staphylococcus aureus*, *Clostridium perfringens*, and *Bacillus cereus*) are usually investigated only during outbreaks and by suitable reference laboratories. The status of *Aeromonas* spp. and *Plesiomonas* spp. in gastroenteritis is controversial, and the systematic detection of these organisms is confined to a limited number of laboratories.

Campylobacter. Culture requires incubation on special selective media at 43°C for up to 2 days under conditions of reduced oxygen tension. The most common enteropathogenic species is *C. jejuni*. Less frequently isolated species include *C. coli*, *C. laridis*, *C. upsaliensis*, and *C. hyointestinalis*.

***Salmonella* and *Shigella*.** Well-established selective methods are available for the routine isolation of these bacteria from stools. Preliminary identification of *Salmonella* involves biochemical and serologic tests to distinguish nontyphoidal salmonellae from *S. typhi* and other varieties generally associated with enteric fever. Nontyphoidal salmonellae can be subdivided into over 1,500 serovars, the most common of which is serovar Typhimurium.

Shigellae are subdivided into four species, *S. dysenteriae*, *S. flexneri*, *S. boydii*, and *S. sonnei*, and each species can be further subdivided into various bioserotypes.

Enteropathogenic *Escherichia coli* (EPEC) Serotypes. Certain serotypes of *E. coli*, referred to as enteropathogenic *E. coli* serotypes, have a longstanding historical association with outbreaks of diarrhea among infants, although such outbreaks are now rare in industrialized countries. The best-known EPEC serotypes include O26:H11, O26:H$^-$, O55:H$^-$, O55:H6, O55:H7, O86:H$^-$, O86:H34, O86:H2, O111:H$^-$, O111:H2, O111:H12, O111:H21, O114:H2, O119:H6, O125ac:H21, O126:H27, O127:H9, O127:H21, O127:H$^-$, O127:H6, O128ab:H2, O142:H6, and O158:H23. Identification of the strains is based on screening for these particular "O" (somatic) and "H" (flagellar) antigens in multiple colonies of *E. coli* from the suspect stool specimen. The association between EPEC serotypes and diarrhea is based on epidemiologic evidence consisting of isolating the same serotype from a number of individuals in the same outbreak. The serotype designation is thus only a marker for a particular enteropathogenic strain and does not necessarily imply that all strains of that serotype are pathogenic. The clinical significance of isolating an EPEC serotype from a sporadic case of diarrhea is difficult to interpret.

Some EPEC serotyped strains have been observed to show in vivo a specific type of "attaching and effacing" adherence to intestinal mucosal epithelial cells. The nature, mechanism, and genetic basis of this phenomenon are under intense study.[3] Future developments in this area should enable EPEC to be identified in routine laboratories using tests for a specific virulence factor.

Enterotoxigenic *Escherichia coli* (ETEC). The microbiologic diagnosis of ETEC infection is based on identifying ETEC in stool cultures and/or specifically demonstrating enterotoxin activity in fecal filtrates. At least five separate *E. coli* colonies from primary agar cultures are tested for the presence of the heat-labile toxin (LT) and the heat-stable toxin (ST) in broth culture filtrates. LT activity is conventionally detected in various cell lines (Y-1 adrenal, Chinese hamster ovary, or vero) in which it produces a characteristic reversible cytotonic effect, but immunologic methods such as the enzyme-linked immunosorbent assay (ELISA), receptor-binding ELISA, and latex agglutination are available in some centers. ST activity is detected by the infant mouse test, which involves the intragastric administration of culture filtrates to infant mice and the monitoring for weight increase in the gut that is associated with fluid accumulation. Genetic methods using DNA probes specific for LT and ST genes have been used successfully for detecting ETEC in individual bacterial colonies and in stools.

Enteroinvasive *Escherichia coli.* EIEC is associated with a bacillary dysentery–like syndrome and has been investigated mostly in the epidemic setting. They belong to certain characteristic O serogroups, including 28, 112, 136, 143, 144, 152, and 164. Typically if an epidemic strain belonging to one of these (or other rare) serogroups is identified, it is tested for invasiveness by laboratory tests such as the Serény test (production of keratoconjunctivitis in the guinea-pig eye) or for invasiveness in HeLa or HEp 2 cells. The genes determining "invasiveness" are encoded on plasmids. They have been cloned and shown to hybridize well with corresponding genes cloned from shigellae. DNA probes specific for these genes have been used successfully for detecting EIEC in feces and in primary cultures.

Verocytotoxin-Producing *Escherichia coli* (VTEC).[4] VTEC is associated with a spectrum of illnesses including nonspecific diarrhea, hemorrhagic colitis, and the hemolytic-uremic syndrome (HUS). About 50 different VTEC serotypes have been associated with human disease,the most common being O157:H7. Individual strains may elaborate one or both of at least two related, but immunologically distinct, VTs, VT 1 and VT 2, in broth culture filtrates. Because VTEC are often present in relatively low numbers and cannot (with the exception of serotype O157:H7) be differentiated from commensal *E. coli*, the most sensitive diagnostic approach for VTEC disease is to demonstrate free VT activity in fecal filtrates (Fig. 2). Serotype O157:H7 strains can be differen-

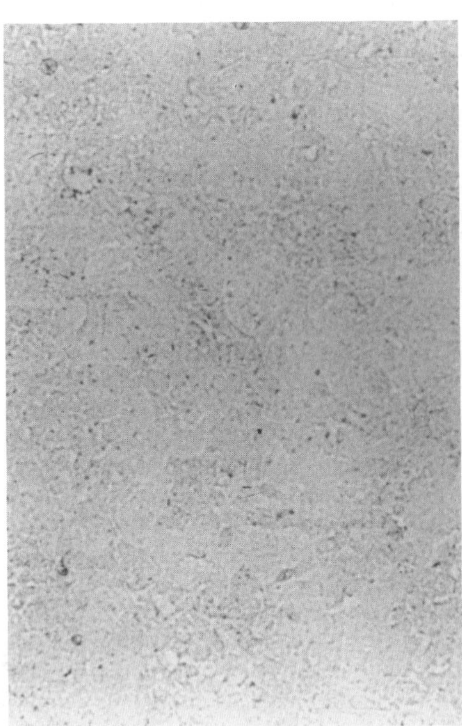

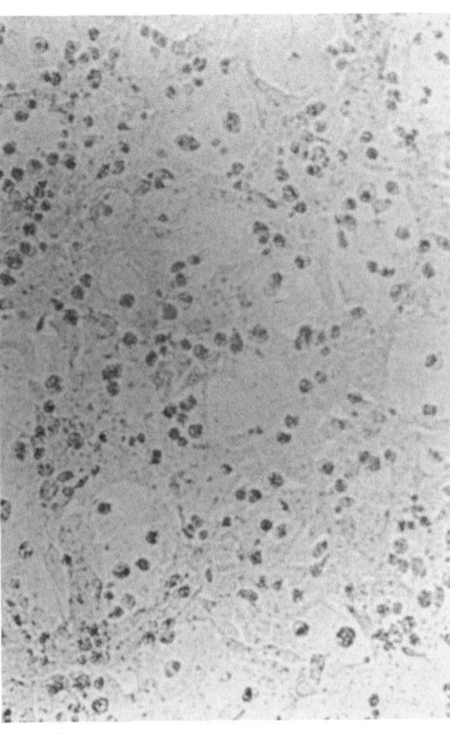

FIGURE 2 Cytotoxic effect of a culture filtrate of verocytotoxin-producing *Escherichia coli* on a vero cell monolayer after 36 hours of exposure. Control monolayer on left and affected monolayer on right.

tially isolated on sorbitol-containing media because, unlike most other *E. coli*, they fail to ferment sorbitol. DNA probes specific for VT 1 and VT 2 genes are used in some centers for diagnostic purposes.

Yersinia.[6] *Y. enterocolitica* is classically associated with diarrhea in young children, and with an appendicular syndrome and/or mesenteric adenitis in older children and adults. The laboratory diagnosis is made by the isolation of this organism from feces on selective culture media. Strains of *Y. enterocolitica* may be subdivided into over 50 different O serogroups, but not all of these are virulent. Serotypes commonly associated with virulence are O3 (North America, Europe, and Japan), O8 (mostly North America), and O9 (mostly Europe). Serologic tests based on the detection of O agglutinins may be of value in the diagnosis of postinfectious complications such as reactive arthritis and erythema nodosum.

Y. pseudotuberculosis infection typically presents with an appendicular syndrome in children. Diarrhea is usually absent. Stool cultures are often negative, but the organism may be recovered from affected mesenteric lymph nodes. Serologic tests are of value in diagnosing this infection in patients with an unexplained appendicular syndrome.

Vibrio. The optimal isolation of *V. cholerae* from stools requires the use of special selective media, not included in the routine media for stool culture and thereby requiring special consultation with a microbiologist. *V. cholerae* can be subdivided into over 50 different O serogroups, the cholera vibrio being serogroup O1. Other *V. cholerae* serogroups, whose clinical significance is uncertain, are referred to as noncholera vibrios (NCV) or nonagglutinable vibrios (NAG). Isolates of *V. cholerae* O1 should be referred to a reference laboratory for confirmation of biotype (classic or El Tor) and cholera toxin production.

V. parahaemolyticus is associated with food-borne outbreaks and sporadic cases of gastroenteritis, typically following the consumption of contaminated seafood. It may be detected in nonselective media by the alert microbiologist, but optimal isolation requires the use of selective media.

Aeromonas hydrophila* and *Plesiomonas shigelloides. *A. hydrophila* and *P. shigelloides* are taxonomically related to the vibrios. *A. hydrophila* has been associated with acute gastroenteritis, but the nature and etiologic significance of this association are still controversial. During acute infection, presumably when large numbers of organisms are present in the feces, the organism can be detected on nonselective blood agar media where it produces oxidase-positive beta-hemolytic colonies. Optimal isolation requires the use of an appropriate selective medium containing ampicillin to which the organism is resistant.

P. shigelloides has been associated with sporadic cases of diarrhea as well as outbreaks. When present in large numbers, it should be detectable on routine enteric media by most laboratories.

Enterotoxin-Producing Strains of *Clostridium perfringens, Staphylococcus aureus*, and *Bacillus cereus.* These organisms are commonly implicated in community outbreaks of food-borne disease. Food poisoning is diagnosed by isolating large numbers of the organisms (10^5 per gram or more) belonging to the same serotype (or phage type in the case of *S. aureus*) from epidemiologically related cases and from the suspect food; *C. perfringens* diarrhea can also be diagnosed by detecting specific enterotoxin in fecal filtrates. Preformed staphylococcal enterotoxin may also be detected in suspect food.

Clostridium difficile.[5] The most sensitive and reliable laboratory test for the diagnosis of pseudomembranous colitis (PMC) or antibiotic-associated diarrhea caused by *C. difficile* is the tissue culture assay for the detection of cytotoxic activity in fecal filtrates that is neutralized by antitoxin to *C. difficile* or *C. sordellii*. This test is highly sensitive, detecting 50 pg per milliliter of toxin B (cytotoxin). The enterotoxin, or toxin A, is responsible for the fluid response in the ileal loop model. Although it also has cytotoxic activity, it is much less potent than toxin B, and its effect is masked in the tissue culture assay. Although there is some evidence that toxin A plays a more important role in the pathogenesis of disease than toxin B, both toxins are co-produced in all isolates so characterized, thus supporting the validity of screening for either toxin. The isolation of *C. difficile* from the stool should be interpreted with caution because not all strains produce toxins. Proof of its ability to produce toxin, or concomitant fecal cytotoxin, would be required to provide evidence of a role in disease. It should be noted that children under the age of 2 years may carry large numbers of toxigenic *C. difficile* in their stool without any GI symptoms. Other tests are available for the identification of the toxin(s) or the organism, such as counterimmunoelectrophoresis, ELISA, or latex agglutination, but all suffer from problems in sensitivity or specificity, making them inappropriate for routine use at the present time.

Viral Enteropathogens

The viruses associated with gastroenteritis include the rotaviruses, fastidious enteric adenoviruses, a group of small round viruses (Norwalk, astrovirus), calicivirus, and possibly coronaviruses. These agents were originally discovered by electron microscopy (EM) of stool specimens, which remains the cornerstone of diagnosis. The viruses of gastroenteritis, in general, are difficult to isolate by conventional cell culture methods. Except for some immunoassays for rotavirus, the diagnosis of most of these agents still requires EM availability.

Rotaviruses. These agents are a major worldwide cause of gastroenteritis in infants and young children and the most common agent of nosocomial pediatric diarrhea. They are double-stranded RNA viruses, 75 nm in diameter, and have two concentric icosahedral shells resembling a wheel (rota) (Fig. 3). Laboratory diagnosis is usually made by EM examination of stools, although a wide variety of commercial immunoassays are now available. In addition, electropherotyping and nucleic acid probes can also be used effectively for epidemiologic studies on rotavirus.

Adenoviruses. Adenoviruses are nonenveloped, icosahedral, double-stranded DNA viruses with a diameter of about 80 nm (Fig. 4). Most adenoviruses (types 1 to 39) are considered pathogens of the respiratory tract. Their association with gastroenteritis is based on their consistent diagnosis by EM, in relatively high concentrations, in stools of symptomatic patients. In contrast, adenovirus types 40 and

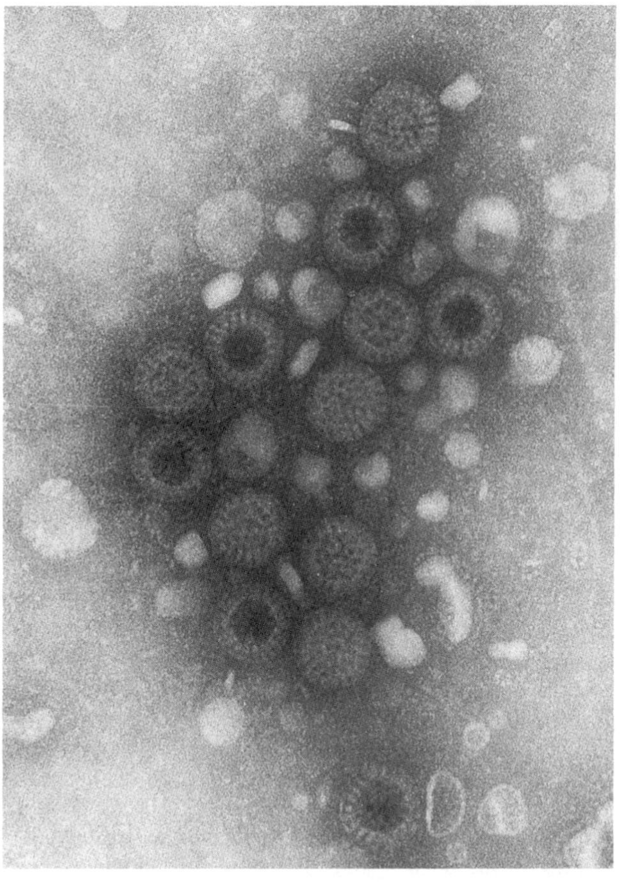

FIGURE 3 Electron micrograph of rotavirus in a stool specimen (×250,000).

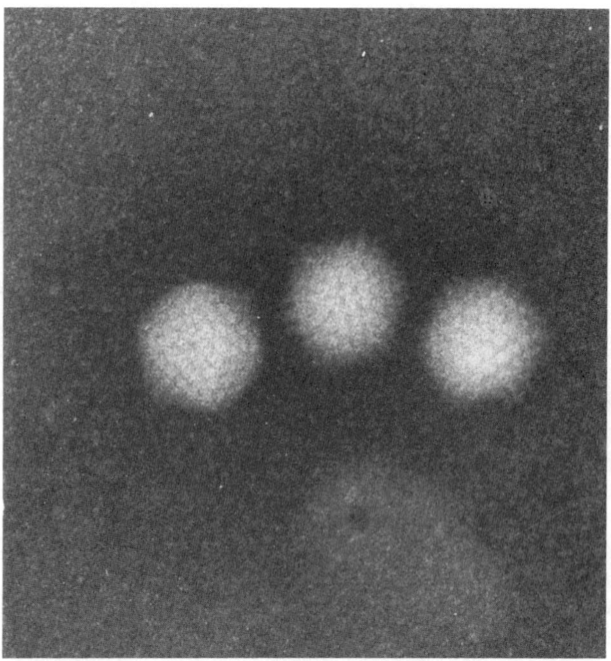

FIGURE 4 Electron micrograph of adenovirus (×275,000).

41 are associated only with gastroenteritis and are called fastidious enteric adenoviruses, since they can not be readily isolated from EM-positive stool specimens by conventional cell culture techniques. Adenoviruses account for approximately 15 percent of pediatric viral gastroenteritis, and half of this is due to adenovirus types 40 and 41. The latter agents can be identified by immunospecific assays or by the analysis of viral DNA after restriction endonuclease treatment.

Norwalk and Norwalk-like Viruses. This group of small (25 to 35 nm), round viruses having Picorna- or Parvovirus-like morphology causes vomiting and diarrhea in infants, older children, and adults and is a noted cause of institutional outbreaks of illness. The Norwalk virus is reported to have a single-stranded RNA genome but is as yet unclassified, since it cannot be grown in cell culture or collected in sufficient quantities from stools to be adequately analyzed. These agents are present in low quantities in stool specimens and their diagnosis by EM requires concentration by centrifugal or immunologic means. Diagnosis by serology is possible in epidemiologically related cases.

"Minireo" viruses have been associated with cases of gastroenteritis of infants and young children and are sometimes included in the Norwalk group of viruses by virtue of their small size (35 nm) and their spherical structure. However, their morphology is suggestive of a double-shell configuration seen with reoviruses. EM is the method of diagnosis.

Caliciviruses and Astroviruses. These small, round, single-stranded RNA viruses associated with gastroenteritis have distinct EM morphologic features (Fig. 5). The calicivirus (30 to 40 nm diameter) has large cup-shaped subunits that produce a scalloped outline. Astrovirus (25 to 30 nm diameter) has a subunit arrangement that appears as a five- or

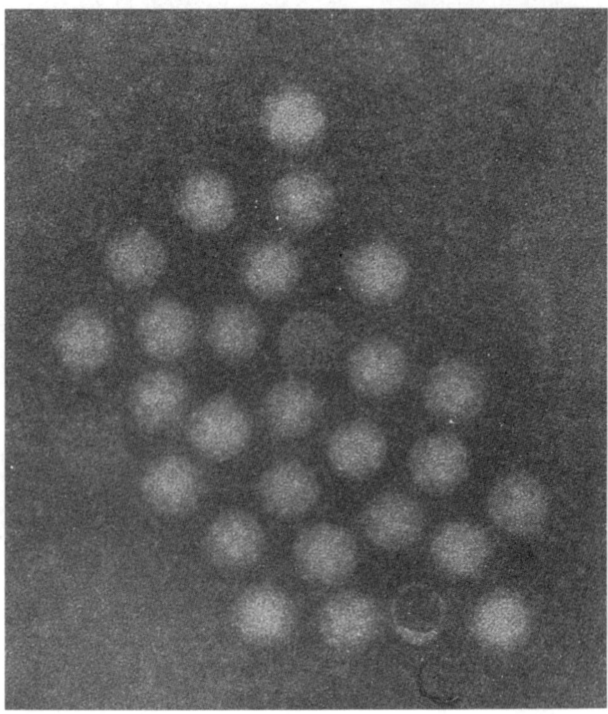

FIGURE 5 Electron micrograph of astrovirus (×300,000).

six-pointed star on the surface of at least 10 percent of the particles. The diagnosis is usually made by EM, but immunologic assays are available, mainly for use in outbreaks.

Other Viruses. Coronaviruses and bredaviruses are associated with significant gastroenteritis in young mammals. Their role in human disease is not yet firmly established.

Parasites

Intestinal parasites can be associated with a wide spectrum of GI symptoms, including acute, subacute, and chronic diarrhea, dysentery, malabsorption, steatorrhea, constipation, abdominal pain and colic, intestinal obstruction, melena, and anemia in association with nonspecific GI symptoms, and features of hepatobiliary disease.

Most parasitic diseases occur in the tropics and may be seen in nonendemic areas in returning travelers, visitors, and refugees from endemic areas. Parasitic diseases that are commonly seen in the temperate climes include giardiasis, cryptosporidiosis, and infection by *Dientamoeba fragilis*. A parasitic investigation of stools may reveal a variety of unexpected agents whose significance should be discussed with a microbiologist. In the laboratory, a concentration step (formalin-ether) and a permanent staining method (iron-hematoxylin, Gomori's trichrome stain) are performed on the preserved stool for optimal visualization of the internal structure of the parasites and reliable identification.

Although the investigation of feces is the mainstay of diagnosis for intestinal parasites, an examination of upper small bowel biopsy or aspirate may be helpful in the investigation of subacute or chronic diarrhea or malabsorption, particularly in association with giardiasis. Serologic tests are of value mainly in the diagnosis of extraintestinal parasitic diseases, some of which may originate from the bowel or may be associated with GI symptoms.

Intestinal Protozoans

Intestinal protozoa are identified by demonstrating living forms (e.g., trophozoites) and/or latent forms (e.g., cysts or oocysts) in feces or in duodenal aspirates.

Intestinal Amebae. The only ameba of clinical relevance is *Entamoeba histolytica*. A variety of others may be reported by the laboratory, including *E. hartmanni*, *E. coli*, *E. polecki*, *Iodamoeba buetschlii*, and *Endolimax nana*. None of the latter is a recognized pathogen and should not usually be interpreted as having clinical significance. The great majority of patients (85 to 95 percent) whose stools contain *E. histolytica* are asymptomatic. Most symptomatic patients have amebic dysentery or nondysenteric colitis, and a few may develop extraintestinal disease, e.g., hepatitis or liver abscess. Because only a minority of patients with intestinal amebiasis are symptomatic, it has long been suspected and has now been confirmed that there are pathogenic and nonpathogenic strains of *E. histolytica*, and these can be distinguished in appropriate research laboratories on the basis of isoenzyme patterns, although this finding is not directly applicable to therapy at the present time.

Laboratory diagnosis requires demonstration of *E. histolytica* trophozoites and cysts in stained smears. Serologic methods (e.g., indirect hemagglutination and enzyme immunoassay [EIA]) are also available for diagnosing amebiasis, but these are more likely to be positive in extraintestinal or invasive colonic disease.

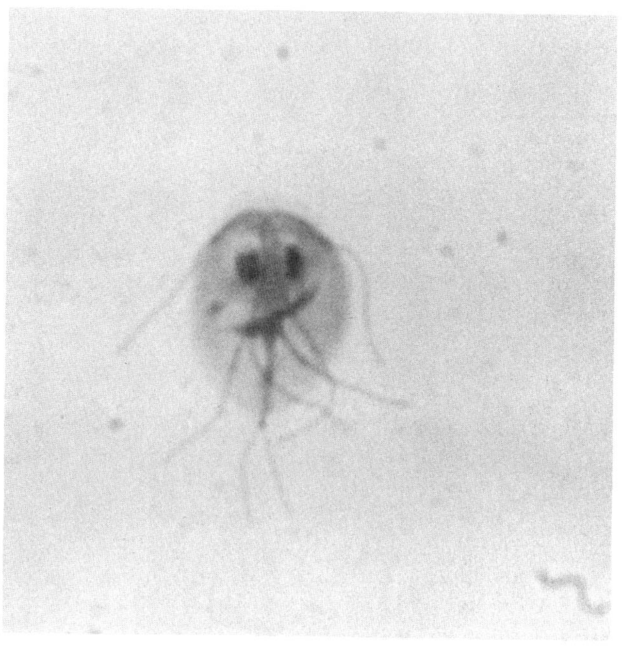

FIGURE 6 *Giardia lamblia* trophozoite (×2,200). (Courtesy of Dr. J. Yang.)

Intestinal Flagellates. Of the four common species of intestinal flagellates, *Giardia lamblia*, *Chilomastix mesnili*, *Trichomonas hominis*, and *D. fragilis*, only *G. lamblia* and *D. fragilis* are of clinical significance.

Giardia lamblia. Often found in completely asymptomatic individuals, *G. lamblia* has the potential to cause a wide range of enteric illness including mild to moderate acute, subacute, or chronic diarrhea, abdominal cramps, flatulence, anorexia, epigastric tenderness, steatorrhea, and a full-blown malabsorption syndrome.

The mean incubation period of giardiasis is about 8 days. During the acute phase of the illness the organisms may be detectable only in samples from the upper small bowel. The prepatent period in giardiasis, i.e., the period between the onset of symptoms and the detection of *Giardia* in the stools, may be as long as about a month. Because *Giardia* does not appear consistently in the stools of all patients, at least three stool samples should be examined at intervals of a few days for the presence of *G. lamblia* cysts or trophozoites. Diagnosis may also be made by demonstrating trophozoites (Fig. 6) in duodenal fluid obtained by intubation or string test, or by biopsy if clinical suspicion is high and the stool examination is negative. Antigen detection methods for detecting *Giardia* antigens in feces (e.g., ELISA or immunofluorescence) are available in some centers.

Dientamoeba fragilis. Long considered to be an ameba, this parasite is now known to be a flagellate. It is characteristically binucleate and lacks recognizable flagellae or cyst forms (Fig. 7). *D. fragilis* can be identified only in appropriately stained fecal smears, not in an unstained preparation.

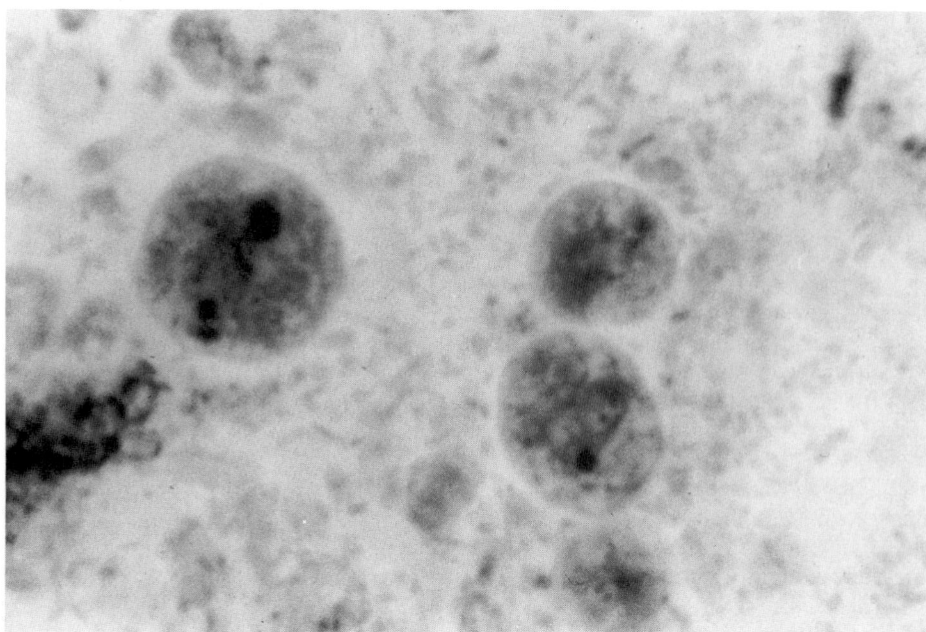

FIGURE 7 *Dientamoeba fragilis* trophozoites (×2,500). (Courtesy of Dr. J. Yang.)

The parasite has been found in asymptomatic cases as well as in those with a variety of symptoms, including diarrhea and abdominal pain. Interestingly, there is an impressive association between *D. fragilis* infection and pinworm (*Enterobius vermicularis*) infection.

Ciliates. The only ciliate of clinical significance, *Balantidium coli*, occurs mainly in the tropics and may be associated with a variety of GI symptoms including abdominal cramps and diarrhea that is watery, mucoid, or, rarely, bloody. It is a large protozoan that may be detected in fecal smears either in its cystic form or in an easily recognizable ciliated trophozoite form.

Coccidia. The two main coccidia of medical importance are *Isospora belli* and *Cryptosporidium*, which can cause acute diarrhea in normal hosts, particularly children in daycare centers, and acute or chronic diarrhea in immunosuppressed hosts, especially acquired immunodeficiency syndrome (AIDS) patients. The laboratory diagnosis is usually made by demonstrating characteristic oocysts in fresh or preserved fecal concentrates after staining them with a modified acid-fast procedure.

Trematodes (Flukes)

Intestinal Flukes. The most common intestinal flukes of medical importance are the giant fluke (*Fasciolopsis buski*), which is endemic in parts of Asia, and the heterophyids (*Heterophyes heterophyes* and *Metagonimus yokogawai*), which occur in Asia, the Middle East, and Southern Europe. The adult worms live in the intestine, and the laboratory diagnosis is made by the demonstration of characteristic eggs in feces. Worms may be seen following purgation after anthelminthic therapy. Heavy worm burdens may be associated with a wide range of symptoms, including diarrhea, abdominal pain, and features of duodenal ulcer. In heavy infestation, features of malabsorption, intestinal obstruction, and protein-losing enteropathy may result.

Liver Flukes. The medically important liver flukes, typically inhabitants of the biliary passages in humans, include *Clonorchis sinensis* (Chinese liver fluke), *Opisthorchis* (endemic in Asia and Eastern Europe), and *Fasciola hepatica* (sheep liver fluke endemic in Southern Europe, North Africa, and Latin America). These worms all produce hyperplastic changes in the epithelium and fibrosis of the bile ducts. Light infestations are generally asymptomatic, but heavier infestations may give rise to features of biliary obstruction, cholangitis, cholecystitis, and secondary liver abscess.

Laboratory diagnosis is by the recovery of the characteristic eggs from the feces or, occasionally, from duodenal aspirates.

Blood Flukes (Schistosomes). The three schistomes of major medical importance are *S. mansoni*, *S. japonicum*, and *S. haematobium*. The adult worms of *S. mansoni* and *S. japonicum* live in the mesenteric venules and produce eggs that are shed in the feces. *S. haematobium* resides in the bladder venules and sheds eggs into the urine. Clinically, schistosomiasis is a complex multisystem disease that has GI manifestations of hepatosplenomegaly with portal hypertension and granulomatous enteritis. The diagnosis is usually made by demonstrating characteristic eggs in feces. Occasionally the number of eggs may be very low, and in this situation rectal biopsy, serology, or, in some centers, culture is available for diagnosis.

Cestodes (Tapeworms)

Tapeworms are flattened worms that have a ribbon-like body made up of a chain of segments or proglottids and an attachment organ known as a scolex. Many different tapeworms are capable of infesting humans. These include *Diphyllobothrium latum* (fish tapeworm), *Taenia saginata* (beef tapeworm), *Taenia solium* (pork tapeworm), and *Echinococcus granulosus* and *E. multilocularis* (agents of hydatid disease).

In *Taenia* and fish tapeworm infection, the ingested larva matures in the gut into the adult worm, which then produces eggs. The diagnosis is made by the demonstration of eggs or proglottids in fecal smears. The presence of these worms in the gut is not associated with significant GI symptomatology, although the fish tapeworm may be associated with features of vitamin B_{12} deficiency.

In hydatid disease, ingested eggs hatch into larval forms in the host's intestinal tract. The larvae penetrate the circulation and localize primarily in the liver, where they give rise to the hydatid cyst. Serology is the main diagnostic method. The Casoni skin test is no longer recommended owing to its low sensitivity and specificity. Diagnostic cyst aspiration is contraindicated owing to the possibility of rupture and dissemination of cyst contents throughout the peritoneal cavity. If surgical removal of the intact cyst is performed as treatment, the cyst contents should be stained and examined microscopically for the presence of hooklets and brood cysts. Occasionally, the diagnosis can be made from the presence of hooks in the sputum, duodenal contents, feces, urine, and peritoneal or pleural fluid.

Intestinal Nematodes (Roundworms)

Nematodes are nonsegmented and generally cylindrical with tapered ends. Stages in the life cycle include the egg, one or more larval stages, and the adult worm. Diagnosis is usually made by the demonstration of characteristic eggs and, in some cases, of larval forms in fecal smears. Adult worms may occasionally be passed.

Intestinal nematodes of gastroenterologic interest include *Ascaris lumbricoides*, *Trichuris trichiura* (whipworm), the hookworms (*Ancylostoma duodenale* and *Necator americanus*), *Strongyloides stercoralis*, and *Anisakis* (fish nematodes). They are associated with a variety of GI presentations, and, in the case of *S. stercoralis*, with systemic infection due to the hyperinfection syndrome in the immunocompromised host. The presence of characteristic eggs in stained fecal smears is the main method of diagnosis for *Ascaris*, *Trichuris*, and hookworm infections. The larvae of *Strongyloides* may be seen in stained smears of feces or duodenal aspirates, whereas the diagnosis of anisakiasis is usually made by the demonstration of the worm in surgical specimens of the intestines or by upper GI radiology or endoscopy. Occasionally, culture of hookworm-like eggs is necessary to differentiate various species (*Strongyloides*, *Necator*, Ancylostoma). Systemic infection with the nonhuman ascarids, *Toxocara canis* and *Toxocara cati*, is associated with visceral larva migrans, which may present to a gastroenterologist as a case of hepatomegaly and chronic eosinophilia. Serology is used to diagnose these infections.

Acid Peptic Disease

Increasing evidence of an association between *C. pylori* infection and primary antral gastritis and/or duodenal ulcer warrants a microbiologic investigation in all patients suspected of having acid peptic disease. The definitive diagnosis of *C. pylori* infection is made by the isolation of the organism in culture. Indirect evidence of infection may be provided by direct visualization of bacteria morphologically resembling *C. pylori* in silver-stained sections of the antral mucosa (e.g., by the Warthin Starry method), or by tests for a potent urease enzyme that is produced by *C. pylori*. The best specimen for culture is antral biopsy, although the organism may also be recovered, less frequently, from antral brushings and gastric aspirates. *C. pylori* has been cultured only infrequently from the site of duodenal ulcers. In many patients with duodenal ulcer who have been investigated, the organism has been isolated from biopsies of concurrently inflamed antral mucosa.

Material for culture should be transported to the laboratory in a small quantity of normal saline or 20 percent glucose solution and processed promptly. The organism is irregularly distributed in biopsy material, and optimal culture results are obtained when the biopsy is ground prior to culture.[7] The material is cultured on appropriate selective and nonselective media, which are incubated for up to 5 days at 37° C under conditions of reduced oxygen tension. Most positive cultures are evident within 3 days of incubation.

C. pylori cultures produce a rapid positive urease reaction that has been exploited in several ways to provide a rapid presumptive diagnosis, including inoculation of biopsy material or gastric juice into urease broth, and a urea-derived $^{13}CO_2$ breath test.

Blind-Loop Syndrome

The normal upper small bowel is only sparsely populated with bacteria, with counts ranging from about 10 to 10^4 organisms per milliliter. Both aerobes and anaerobes may be present, but coliforms and *Bacteroides* spp. tend to be absent. The term *blind-loop syndrome* refers to the development of malabsorption in a patient with overgrowth of bacteria in the small bowel, which occurs secondary to a large number of surgical or medical conditions.[8]

The most direct evidence of bacterial overgrowth is achieved by quantitative bacterial counts of upper small bowel aspirates. These specimens should be obtained anaerobically, serially diluted, and cultured anaerobically using a calibrated loop. A total bacterial count exceeding 10^5 per milliliter is considered to be consistent with the overgrowth syndrome. A variety of indirect methods are commonly used for diagnosing this syndrome. They rely on the measurement of breath excretion of volatile metabolites produced by intraluminal bacteria (e.g., bile acid breath test, ^{14}C-xylose breath test, breath hydrogen test, $^{13}CO_2$ bile salt breath test). These tests have varying sensitivities and specificities and may need to be employed together or confirmed by microbiologic analysis.

Anoproctitis

Anoproctitis can occur in children in relation to inflammatory bowel disease, foreign bodies, or specific infections of the GI tract. Anal infections may occur alone or in conjunction with more proximal infection in the GI tract. Depending on the pathogen isolated, sexual abuse or other forms of sexual activity (especially homosexual) should be considered. Severe disease may be associated with immunosuppression, including infection with the human immunodeficiency virus. Microbes that should be considered in the diagnosis of infectious anoproctitis include *Neisseria gonorrhoeae*, *Campylobacter* spp., *Salmonella* spp., *Shigella* spp., *Treponema pallidum*, *Chlamydia trachomatis*, herpes simplex virus, and *E. histolytica*. Investigation of most of these agents from anorectal specimens is not conducted routinely and should be specially arranged with the microbiologist.

Hepatobiliary Disease

All classes of microbes may be associated with hepatobiliary disease. The laboratory aspects of viral and bacterial diseases of the liver are discussed below. Parasitic infections relating to hepatobiliary disease have been discussed above.

Viral Hepatitis

The most common primary agents of viral hepatitis are hepatitis A (enterovirus 72), hepatitis B, hepatitis non-A, non-B, and the hepatitis delta virus.

Hepatitis may also be an occasional feature of clinical syndromes associated with other viruses such as the herpes viruses (Epstein-Barr virus [EBV], cytomegalovirus [CMV]) and the viruses of hemorrhagic fevers (yellow fever, Marburg, Ebola, Lassa, Rift Valley fever, and the Crimean-Congo hemorrhagic fever virus). Hepatitis is a major feature of disseminated viral infections that overwhelm neonates (herpes simplex virus [HSV], varicella zoster virus [VZV], CMV, and congenital rubella) or immunocompromised patients (HSV, VZV, and CMV).

Laboratory Diagnosis. *Hepatitis A Virus.* Virus is detectable in the feces during the week prior to the appearance of the cardinal clinical signs of hepatitis, and it disappears when serum transaminase levels reach their peak. The presence of anti-HAV IgM, detected by either EIA or radioimmunoassay (RIA), is diagnostic of hepatitis A. This antibody is demonstrable in the serum from the time signs and symptoms appear until about 4 to 6 months later.

Hepatitis B Virus. Serology forms the basis of diagnosing hepatitis B virus infection and of differentiating the various clinical forms of hepatitis B. The serologic markers used include hepatitis B surface antigen (HBsAg), hepatitis B e antigen (HBeAg), viral DNA polymerase, antibody to hepatitis B core antigen (anti-HBc), and antibody to HBsAg (anti-HBs).

In *acute hepatitis B*, HBsAg appears in the blood during the last month of the incubation period, rises to a peak shortly after onset of symptoms, and disappears with convalescence, paralleling the fall in transaminase levels. HBeAg and viral DNA polymerase appear at about the same time as HBsAg but disappear abruptly when symptoms and liver enzyme levels peak. Anti-HBc is detectable shortly before the onset of symptoms and persists indefinitely. Anti-HBs, on the other hand, becomes detectable only when HBsAg has disappeared and recovery is complete, usually around 5 to 6 months following infection. Anti-HBc is the single most consistent marker of past or present HBV infection. Anti-HBs is the major protective antibody, and its presence indicates recovery and immunity to reinfection.

Chronic hepatitis B infection is characterized by persistence of HBsAg for prolonged periods (HBsAg carrier state). There is no anti-HBs, but anti-HBc is present in high titer and persists for life. the HBsAg carrier state may be asymptomatic or associated with progressive liver damage (chronic active hepatitis). The persistence of HBeAg, DNA polymerase, and Dane particles (hepatitis B virions detected by EM) implies active viral multiplication, progressive liver damage, and a poor prognosis.

Hepatitis Delta Virus (Delta Agent). The delta agent is a defective virus that depends upon hepatitis B virus for its replication. It may produce a co-primary infection with HBV or a superinfection in an HBsAg-positive individual. Superinfection of an asymptomatic HBsAg-positive individual may cause a severe and often fulminating hepatitis. Delta virus infection may be an important determinant of a fulminant course or progression to chronic disease in acute HBV infection. A diagnosis is made by demonstrating the presence of HDAg (delta antigen) in blood early during acute infection or the presence of anti-delta IgM at later stages.

Herpes Virus Group. Liver involvement in HSV infection occurs in disseminated disease, usually in the neonate. It is diagnosed by EM of cutaneous lesions, if present, or by the isolation of the virus from skin, respiratory secretions, or organs. Disseminated VZV infections may cause extensive liver damage in the immunocompromised patient and neonate. The laboratory diagnosis is made by EM of cutaneous vesicles, by viral isolation from these lesions, or by serology. Isolation of VZV may take up to a week, whereas HSV cultures are usually positive within 3 days, and sometimes as early as 1 day when the virus inoculum is high. CMV infection may involve the liver to varying degrees in the immunocompetent and immunosuppressed hosts. CMV is diagnosed by isolation of the virus from peripheral blood leukocytes, respiratory secretions, and urine. Although immunospecific assays and nucleic acid probes have proved effective in the diagnosis of CMV in tissues, current isolation technology enables the infection to be diagnosed within 24 to 48 hours. Serologic diagnosis is also available and may be positive prior to detectable viruria.

Infectious mononucleosis is frequently accompanied by transient abnormalities in liver function tests, but overt clinical hepatitis is rare. The diagnosis of EBV infection can usually be made by the detection of high levels of heterophile agglutinins in the blood (Paul-Bunnell test, Monospot test) or by the presence of the more reliable EBV-specific antibody tests (anti–viral capsid antigen [anti-VCA] IgM and IgG antibodies and anti–early antigen [anti-EA] antibody). The anti-EA and anti-VCA IgM develop to a high titer early in the illness and decline rapidly within about 3 months, whereas the anti-VCA IgG remains high as a marker of past illness.

Congenital Rubella. Rubella virus can be isolated from the throat, urine, CSF, or (at autopsy) virtually any organ of an infant with the congenital rubella syndrome. Diagnosis may also be made by demonstrating rubella IgM in cord blood or serum.

Viral Hemorrhagic Fevers. The laboratory diagnosis (particularly virus isolation) of the viral hemorrhagic fevers is a highly specialized investigation that is generally confined to specialized laboratories working under high levels of containment. Serologic tests, particularly IgM serology, are generally used for making the diagnosis.

Pyogenic Liver Abscess

Liver abscesses may be associated with septicemia, septic emboli in the portal venous system arising from pelvic or intra-abdominal sepsis, umbilical vein sepsis (in neonates), suppurative cholangitis related to abnormalities in the biliary system, infection from adjacent organs, and penetrating injury.[9] In many cases, the explanation is not apparent.

Systemic bacteremia with hematogenous spread of bacteria to the liver is probably the most common source of liver abscess in children. Major causes of liver abscess in children are *S. aureus* and fecal bacteria (coliforms and anaerobes); polymicrobial infection is common. Less common causes include *Candida albicans* (particularly in immunocompromised patients who have received hyperalimentation) and *Actinomyces* spp.

The specific microbial etiology may be obtained by blood culture in more than 50 percent of cases or by diagnostic or therapeutic aspiration of the abscess cavity. Care should be taken in transporting the pus to the laboratory under anaerobic conditions (capped syringe or a special anaerobic transport system) to facilitate the recovery of anaerobes.

Other bacteria that may be involved in liver disease, and for which special diagnostic methods are required, include *Mycobacterium tuberculosis*, *Leptospira* spp., *Brucella* spp., *Rickettsia*, and *Chlamydia*.

Note: For further discussion in major texts on these subjects, see references 10 through 14.

REFERENCES

1. Hook EH. *Salmonella* species (including typhoid fever). In: Mandell GM, Gordon RG, Bennett JE, eds. Principles and practices of infectious diseases. 2nd ed. New York: John Wiley & Sons, 1985: 1256.
2. Carter AO, Borczyk AA, Carlson JAK, Harvey B, Hockin JC, Karmali MA, Krishnan C, Korn DA, Lior H. A severe outbreak of *Escherichia coli* 0157:H7–associated hemorrhagic colitis in a nursing home. N Engl J Med 1987; 317:1496–1500.
3. Levine MM. *Escherichia coli* that cause diarrhea: enterotoxigenic, enteropathogenic, enteroinvasive, enterohemorrhagic, and enteroadherent. J Infect Dis 1987; 155:377–389.
4. Karmali MA. Infection by verocytotoxin-producing *Escherichia coli*. Clin Microbiol Rev 1989; 2:15–38.
5. Lyerly DM, Krivan HC, Wilkins TD. *Clostridium difficile*: its disease and toxins. Clin Microbiol Rev 1988; 1:1–18.
6. Weinstein L. Yersiniosis. In: Feigin RD, Cherry JD, eds. Textbook of pediatric infectious disease. 2nd ed. Philadelphia: WB Saunders, 1987: 689.
7. Goodwin CS, Blincow ED, Warren JR, Waters TE, Sanderson CR, Easton L. Evaluation of cultural techniques for isolating *Campylobacter pyloridis* from endoscopic biopsies of gastric mucosa. J Clin Pathol 1985; 38:1127–1131.
8. Toskes PP, Donaldson RM. The blind loop syndrome. In: Sleisenger MH, Fordtran JS, eds. Gastrointestinal disease. 3rd ed. Philadelphia: WB Saunders, 1983: 1023.
9. Kaplan SL. Pyogenic liver abscess. In: Feigin RD, Cherry JD, eds. Textbook of pediatric infectious disease. 2nd ed. Philadelphia: WB Saunders, 1987: 746.
10. Lifshitz F, Ribeiro H, Silverberg M. Childhood infectious diarrhea. In: Silverberg M, Daum F, eds. Textbook of pediatric gastroenterology. 2nd ed. Chicago: Year Book Medical Publishers, 1988: 284.
11. Markell EK, Voge M, John DT. Medical parasitology. 6th ed. Philadelphia: WB Saunders, 1986.
12. White DO, Fenner FJ. Medical virology. 3rd ed. New York: Academic Press, 1986.
13. Finegold SM, Sutter VL, Mathison GE. Normal indigenous intestinal flora. In: Hentges DJ, ed. Human intestinal microflora in health and disease. New York: Academic Press, 1983.
14. Pickering LK, Cleary TG. Gastrointestinal infections. In: Feigin RD, Cherry JD, eds. Textbook of pediatric infectious disease. 2nd ed. Philadelphia: WB Saunders, 1987: 622.

CHAPTER 39

Imaging

PART 1

Overview

David A. Stringer, B.Sc., M.B.B.S., F.R.C.R., FRCPC

Indications for the examination of the gastrointestinal (GI) tract in children, particularly in infants, and the techniques of these examinations are often very different from those of adults. Significant morbidity and, indeed, mortality can result from a careless or improperly performed technical procedure.

Patient co-operation is essential to the success of radiologic procedures. In infants and young children, sedation may be necessary for invasive procedures, but it is rarely if ever indicated for noninvasive techniques because children usually co-operate if the examiner treats them with consideration and attempts to inspire their confidence. Hence, great care must be taken to inform the child of the exact nature of each procedure in an appropriate, friendly, and reassuring manner.

The success of the investigation of a child also depends on the clinical findings. A careful history and physical examination play an essential role here, as does a good rapport between the referring physician and radiologist. These factors are crucial to the expeditious and safe completion of radiologic tests with a minimum of distress or harm to the patient.

Sonography, because it does not require radiation, is the preferred initial modality for the investigation of many pediatric abdominal conditions. However, because bowel gas reduces the usefulness of sonography in the GI tract, contrast studies are often used initially. Ionizing radiation is, however, potentially harmful. It can cause chromosomal anomalies, especially to cells undergoing mitosis. In addition, the risk of neoplasia is of particular concern in children because of their long life expectancy. The aim in pediatric radiology is to keep the radiation dosage to a minimum yet still obtain the required diagnostic information.

The techniques used in subsequent investigations depend on these findings and those of the clinical assessment. This discussion provides an overview of the value and indications for each modality that are considered in more detail in subsequent chapters.

SONOGRAPHY

The use of sonography should be considered first in the radiologic investigation of any child because it requires no radiation and little patient preparation and because it allows the radiologist to view many organs simultaneously. As far as we know, sonography, when used at diagnostic levels, is completely safe. It is generally easier to perform and more reliable in children because of their lack of fat planes and smaller size than it is in adults.[1]

At The Hospital for Sick Children (HSC), Toronto, we have found that sonography is a more useful investigative tool than computed tomography (CT) or magnetic resonance imaging (MRI) for evaluating cystic or other benign lesions in children because they have less intra-abdominal fat to degrade the sonogram and not enough to enhance the CT image. However, in many other instances, sonography and CT are complementary and together give a high diagnostic accuracy.[2] Generally, sonography is the first cross-sectional imaging modality used, with CT and MRI reserved for situations in which sonography fails to provide enough information for a diagnosis or in which more complete information is required.[3]

The value of spectral Doppler or color Doppler sonography is still being assessed, but early findings indicate that these modalities can be used to demonstrate accurately the presence and direction of flow and flow profiles in the major abdominal vessels. We have found it to be most helpful in evaluating portal hypertension because it shows abnormal or absent portal vein flow and the presence of any collateral circulation.[4] It is also useful in the management of the liver transplant patient, especially since the procedure can be performed in the intensive care unit at the bedside of these extremely ill children.[4] This modality has also proved itself most valuable in the evaluation of major vessel thrombosis in the neonate.[5]

PLAIN FILM RADIOGRAPHY

The major value of plain films is their ability to reveal bowel gas patterns and to exclude obstruction or perforation in the GI tract. Calcification, appendicoliths, and mass lesions may also be detected.

CONTRAST EXAMINATIONS

Contrast examinations are the radiologic mainstay of investigations of suspected bowel abnormalities. In children, the type of examination performed depends on the clinical circumstances to a larger degree than it does in adults. There is more risk involved in the procedures, particularly in the neonatal period when the fluid-electrolyte balance is fragile and perforations of the gut caused by improperly performed examinations can occur easily. A number of fatalities have been reported. In view of this risk, contrast examinations should not be performed on infants or young children by radiologists who are inexperienced in pediatric examinations.

The indications for and techniques of radiologic examinations for children are quite different from those for adults because of the different disease entities and because of the greater susceptibility of children to radiation, especially with their longer life expectancy. Because of this, it is no accident that most low radiation dose techniques were first perfected in pediatric institutions.

When making a decision about which contrast examination should be performed, the radiologist and the referring physician must have a close rapport to minimize conflicts and to maximize the co-operation and the well-being of the patient. Although ultimately the radiologist, who performs any necessary radiologic studies, determines which contrast medium and procedure will be used, the referring gastroenterologist or other attending physician should make the initial assessment. This initial assessment should include the possibility of endoscopy. The different choices are therefore briefly considered here and covered further in the discussion on contrast studies.

Endoscopy or Radiology

Endoscopy has had a most significant impact on the radiologic techniques for investigating the GI tract. It has enabled close clinical-pathologic-radiologic correlation and has stimulated advances in double-contrast techniques. Unfortunately, too often endoscopy and double-contrast studies are viewed as antagonistic techniques when in fact they are complementary.[6] In some situations, one may be more sensitive in any given patient. It is very clear, however, that single-contrast as compared with double-contrast techniques are extremely poor for the detection of mucosal disease. In addition, even compared with double-contrast techniques, endoscopy has a better detection rate for many mucosal diseases. The radiologic techniques, however, are less invasive and require no sedation, a most important feature in pediatrics. Again, in the choice of technique, the rapport between radiologist and physician becomes vital to promote the best interests of the patient.

Choice of Contrast Media

A variety of contrast media are now available. These may be divided into three main groups: barium sulfate, water-soluble contrast, and air. The choice of contrast medium depends on the diagnostic problem and the procedure.

Barium sulfate is the most commonly used contrast medium unless there is a contraindication, such as a suspected perforation, aspiration, or impaction. Barium in the retroperitoneum or mediastinum can result in granuloma formation and fibrotic scarring.

Water-soluble contrast media include conventional hyperosmolar contrast media and new low-osmolar contrast media. The new iso-osmolar water-soluble contrast media are safer but more expensive. Because Gastrografin, one of the conventional hyperosmolar water-soluble media with a very high osmolality, has many side effects on the small and large bowel, it is never used at HSC. None of the conventional hyperosmolar contrast media should ever be used in the upper GI tract because of the risk of lung toxicity and pulmonary edema, which could lead to death if aspirated.[7,8]

The new low-osmolar water-soluble contrast media include the nonionic iopamidol (Niopam in Europe or Isovue in North America) and iohexol (Omnipaque) or the ionic ioxaglate (Hexabrix) and fulfill the criteria for the ideal medium except for their high cost. As far as we know, they have no effect on the lungs or peritoneum and are not absorbed by the bowel. They are being used with increasing regularity to evaluate the GI tract in pediatric patients.

The advantages of these media are many. So little contrast medium is absorbed that the gut can be clearly visualized for prolonged periods of time, an advantage when delayed films are required, as is the case in the diagnosis of Hirschsprung's disease. Indeed, nonionic media (iopamidol and iohexol) are probably not absorbed from the pediatric gut at all,[9] and thus the discovery of a pyelogram indicates a perforation even if the leak itself is not visible. Table 1 summarizes the indications for the expanding uses of the new low-osmolar water-soluble contrast media in the gut.[9]

TABLE 1
Criteria For Use of Low-Osmolality Contrast Media in the Pediatric Gut

Risk of lung aspiration
Laryngopharyngeal dyskinesia
H-type fistula
Vomiting or refluxing child
Risk of bowel leak
Recent surgery on bowel
Demonstration of site of leak
Demonstration of fistula(e)
Risk of barium inspissated in
Cystic fibrosis
Blind loop of bowel
Hirschsprung's disease
Neonatal obstruction/meconium ileus
Endoscopic deep biopsy immediately following examination

Air is rarely regarded as a contrast medium, but in pediatrics it can be extremely safe and useful in specific situations. Air is an excellent, safe contrast medium for the diagnosis of esophageal, duodenal, jejunal, or large bowel atresia. Diagnosis is generally possible from plain films, but the injection of air into the large or small bowel may facilitate the delineation of any obstruction.

Although not universally accepted, air enemas have been used in the diagnosis and treatment of intussusception and are now the contrast medium and technique of choice at HSC.

Single- or Double-Contrast Barium Examinations

If a barium study is indicated, a single-contrast or double-contrast examination can be performed. A single-contrast study uses only barium, often of low density, whereas a double-contrast study uses a smaller amount of high-density barium and a relatively large amount of gas, usually air.

The choice between single- and double-contrast examinations is dependent on the suspected diagnosis and age of the patient. Single-contrast examinations best delineate gross anatomy and function. Double-contrast studies are reserved for the examination of the mucosa to diagnose such problems as inflammatory bowel disease, polyps, other mass lesions, and peptic ulceration. Of these, the most common suspected diagnosis requiring double-contrast examinations at HSC is inflammatory bowel disease.

Double-contrast examinations are more difficult to perform in children than in adults. The radiation dosage is higher than that for a single-contrast examination because there is more fluoroscopy performed and more images taken.

Choice of Type of Study

Because there are many varieties of studies that can be performed, the choices can be confusing. Table 2 defines the various GI studies used at HSC and briefly reviews the information they provide. However, the vast majority of examinations performed are barium meals and large bowel enemas, which are therefore considered here in more detail.

TABLE 2
Types of Gastrointestinal Studies Performed at The Hospital for Sick Children, Toronto

Study	Use
Speech study	Study used to assess the soft palate and pharyngeal structures for evaluation of velopharyngeal insufficiency.
Feeding study	Study used to evaluate the bolus formation in the mouth and to assess the best method of feeding a child with neuromuscular dysfunction.
Barium swallow (esophagus)	Contrast study used to assess esophageal abnormalities. The esophagus is assessed at least from the level of the oropharynx down to the gastroesophageal junction.
Swallowing study	Study similar to the barium swallow, except that it concentrates on oropharyngeal kinesia and is recorded by videofluoroscopy.
Upper GI study (stomach and duodenum)	Contrast study used for the evaluation of the stomach and duodenum, including the position of the duodenojejunal flexure. This study is usually performed in conjunction with a barium swallow, although occasionally it may be performed through a nasogastric or gastrostomy tube.
Small bowel follow-through	Study used for the assessment of small bowel abnormalities, usually performed in conjunction with an upper GI study. The small bowel is assessed from the duodenojejunal flexure all the way down to the ileocecal valve.
Peroral pneumocolon (POP)	Double-contrast study to assess specifically the ileocecal region, performed at the end of a conventional small bowel follow-through by insufflation of air through the rectum.
Small bowel enema (enteroclysis)	Special barium study of the small bowel requiring nasojejunal intubation with a long wide-bore feeding tube. Barium is introduced through this tube to fully distend the small bowel.
Colon study	Contrast study used for the evaluation of the colon. The contrast agents may be barium, water-soluble contrast media, or air.
Defecogram	Barium study specifically used to assess the functional abnormalities of the rectum and anal canal during defecation.

Barium Meal

The clinical problems of infants and young children differ from those of adults. These problems are often related to congenital anomalies such as malrotation and duodenal web, to conditions peculiar to childhood such as hypertrophic pyloric stenosis, or to functional problems such as achalasia and infantile chalasia. Because ulcers, tumors, and other mucosal lesions are rare in children, single-contrast examinations are usually more than adequate for infants and for many older children.

Single-contrast studies may be necessary in an older child to exclude obstruction, varices, or gastroesophageal reflux, or they may be performed as part of a small-bowel follow-through examination.

Double-contrast barium meal examinations are generally reserved for children over 7 years of age, when esophagitis, erosions, ulcers, or mass lesions are suspected. Under 5 years of age, it is exceedingly rare for a child to be co-operative enough for a satisfactory examination that would include the use of an effervescent agent and high-density barium. Endoscopy and double-contrast barium meal studies are complementary techniques in children, although one may prove more sensitive than the other in any one patient.[10]

Water-soluble contrast examinations of the upper GI tract in children are rarely necessary. If there is a perforation, water-soluble contrast media are indicated, but care must be taken to prevent aspiration; consequently, hyperosmolar contrast media should never be used.

TABLE 3
Progression of Investigative Techniques for the Small Bowel

Conventional small bowel follow-through
⬇
If the terminal ileum is poorly seen, a peroral pneumocolon is performed.
⬇
If the terminal ileum is still poorly seen and if a double-contrast barium enema is being performed for other reasons, reflux may occur into terminal ileum and aid in visualization of the terminal ileum.
⬇
If terminal ileum is still poorly seen or if there is still a diagnostic dilemma, a small-bowel enema is performed.

The major indications for the newer, more expensive low-osmolar contrast media (see Table 1) include patients at risk for lung aspiration, suspected malrotation, bowel perforation, barium inspissation, and neonatal obstruction, especially meconium ileus. It is also used for contrast examinations prior to endoscopic biopsy.[9]

Small Bowel Follow-Through, Peroral Pneumocolon, and Small-Bowel Enema

There are many types of studies that can be performed to examine the small bowel, such as the small bowel follow-through, peroral pneumocolon, and small bowel enema. The choice is best made in consultation with the radiologist. At HSC, the most common order of studies is shown in Table 3.

The small bowel follow-through examination is generally considered the most appropriate initial technique for examining the small bowel.[11] The examination is best performed after a single-contrast barium meal study because the gas and high-density barium used in double-contrast examinations degrade the delineation of the small bowel. The small bowel follow-through examination can be combined with a peroral pneumocolon (see Table 2) when the terminal ileum is difficult to visualize or when the evidence for fistulae is equivocal.[12-16]

In children, visualization of the terminal ileum is important, primarily to diagnose or exclude Crohn's disease or to evaluate the extent of the disease preoperatively. Since Crohn's disease is extremely rare under the age of 8 years, peroral pneumocolon is rarely necessary in younger children. The peroral pneumocolon is well tolerated in children, requires no patient preparation, and requires little additional radiation.[12]

Occasionally, when the peroral pneumocolon is not helpful, the terminal ileum may later be delineated by the reflux of air and barium that occurs in a double-contrast barium enema study performed to evaluate the large bowel.

The small bowel enema (see Table 2) is a more invasive technique and is, therefore, reserved for those very few patients in whom the small bowel follow-through and peroral pneumocolon examinations have failed to resolve a diagnostic dilemma.[11] This occurs most commonly in the terminal ileum but may also occur if there is a mass effect from possible Crohn's disease or lymphoma, if small mass lesions are suspected, or if fine detail is required.[11]

The major indication for the small bowel enema at HSC is a failure of the small bowel follow-through to solve a diagnostic problem.[11] In particular, the small bowel enema can be helpful in the examination of mass lesions and a poorly delineated terminal ileum, as well as in the differentiation between a normal and abnormal small bowel when this distinction is unclear from the small bowel follow-through.

Large Bowel Enema

As in the upper GI tract, the clinical problems in the large bowel in infants and young children differ from those in adults. They are often related to congenital anomalies such as malrotation, to conditions peculiar to childhood such as meconium ileus and meconium plug syndrome (functional immaturity of the large bowel or the hypoplastic left hemicolon syndrome), or to functional problems such as constipation or Hirschsprung's disease. Because polyps, tumors, ulcers, and other mucosal lesions are rare in children, single-contrast examinations are usually more than adequate for infants and for many older children. For infants, I prefer to use walter-soluble contrast media, since inspissation or perforation causes fewer complications with these media. In many instances, such as in meconium ileus and the meconium plug syndrome, water-soluble media also have a therapeutic effect. In older infants and children, water-soluble contrast media are rarely used; they are reserved for the few patients in whom perforation is suspected.

For older children, single-contrast examinations are usually indicated to exclude malrotation and to investigate problems of bowel habits such as Hirschsprung's disease or functional constipation.

Double-contrast examinations are reserved for children with rectal bleeding and other symptoms that suggest inflammatory bowel disease, polyps, or other mucosal diseases. When a high-density, low-viscosity barium sulfate suspension is used, there is excellent correlation with colonoscopic and histologic findings.[6]

Colonoscopy and double-contrast barium enema are complementary techniques used in children. Different patients are often more sensitive to one study than the other.[6] Colonoscopy provides direct vision and facilitates biopsies and polypectomies. However, a colonoscopy is a more invasive procedure than a double-contrast barium enema: It often requires significant sedation in children and has been associated with a small incidence of serious complications such as bleeding, perforation, or even bowel gas explosion when a polypectomy is performed.[17-20] A double-contrast barium enema is less invasive, does not require sedation, permits easy and rapid visualization of the entire large bowel and often of the terminal ileum as well, and has negligible complications in a viable large bowel.

Both radiologic and endoscopic studies have limitations. The extent of colitis may be underestimated by either procedure.[6] Infrequently, both double-contrast barium enema and colonoscopy fail to detect small polyps in adults and children.[6,14,21,22] Colonoscopy may fail to detect polyps if they are hidden by a haustral fold or a valve of Houston or if they are located in a region of sharp angulation.[15] Occasionally, histology detects an unsuspected abnormality not revealed during a colonoscopy or a double-contrast barium enema—the so-called *microscopic colitis*—although the existence of this entity is controversial.[6,23] But the most common disparity between double-contrast barium enema and colonoscopy is the failure of double-contrast barium enema to detect early mild distal colitis and proctitis when the only colonoscopic findings are the loss of the normal vascular mucosal pattern caused by edema.[6]

NONANGIOGRAPHIC BODY INTERVENTIONAL AND INVASIVE STUDIES

Pediatric body interventional procedures in radiology are mostly composed of the techniques of abscess drainage and biopsy. Many different types of collections, such as pancreatic pseudocysts, can be successfully drained. Percutaneous gastrostomy obviates the need for endoscopy or surgery[24,25] and may be suitable for some pediatric patients. Blunt foreign bodies such as coins may be removed with a Foley catheter.[26,27] This technique has been used regularly with excellent results in some centers; however, the safety of the procedure has been seriously questioned because of the risk of aspiration.[28] Great caution is therefore advised. The technique should be attempted only by the experienced.

Gastrojejunal tubes, nasojejunal tubes, small bowel biopsy capsules, and pancreatic enzyme aspiration tubes often require fluoroscopy for accurate placement. However, if the radiologist allows ample time for the tubes to pass into the small bowel without screening, fluoroscopy can be kept to an absolute minimum.

Percutaneous transhepatic cholangiography (PTC), an invasive procedure with some risks, often requires heavy sedation or a general anesthetic when performed on children. It also requires radiation from fluoroscopy and spot films; moreover, fluoroscopy may be prolonged, especially if a drainage procedure is performed. Consequently, careful consultation between clinicians is necessary before the patient is examined. Percutaneous cholecystography with a sonographically guided puncture of the gallbladder is an alternative technique for delineating the biliary tree.[29-31]

When other, less invasive investigative methods have failed, PTC is usually indicated to demonstrate biliary anatomy and drainage in a patient with obstructive jaundice or a dilated biliary tree that has been revealed by sonography.[32] Occasionally, depending on such findings as those of a bile duct stricture or cholangitis, a percutaneous drainage procedure or biliary duct dilatation may be performed.[33]

If the bile ducts are not dilated, PTC is still possible, as has been shown in the preoperative evaluation of biliary atresia patients.[34] PTC has also been used in the follow-up examination of patients with biliary atresia who have undergone a Kasai operation[34] and in the assessment of drainage from bile lakes that may be associated with the recurrence of jaundice and cholangitis, a not uncommon sequela of the Kasai operation. Initial results suggest that irrigation and drainage of the bile-filled cysts can result in reopening the cysts into the hepatoportoenterostomy, with the eventual disappearance of the cyst.[35] PTC can also be a valuable technique in the investigation of complications following liver transplantation.

COMPUTED TOMOGRAPHY

CT is a most useful modality for visualizing structures in the pediatric abdomen,[36] particularly in malignant disease and complex lesions, especially in older children. However, CT is an invasive procedure because oral and/or intravenous contrast media are usually required, and rectal or intravaginal contrast may sometimes be necessary. The invasiveness and cost of the procedure, along with the added disadvantage of sedation of younger children, mean that we reserve CT for problems that cannot be adequately solved by other safer and less invasive modalities, such as sonography.

CT is particularly useful in blunt abdominal trauma,[37] since multiple organs, such as the liver, spleen, pancreas, and adjacent bones, are quickly and accurately visualized. It is now the procedure of choice in the investigation of significant trauma at HSC. Intra-abdominal abscesses can be well defined[38] if sonography has failed to delineate them satisfactorily. CT has also been used to investigate the retroperitoneum.[37]

CT can help solve diagnostic difficulties. It can image thickened bowel walls such as may occur in diagnostically problematic patients with possible abscess formation because of Crohn's disease. It is also useful in the identification of tumors of the gut, although these are not commonly found in children.

Abdominal masses in children can be investigated with CT.[39] However, this method should be reserved for those patients in whom sonography has failed to demonstrate the anatomy sufficiently, especially in those with malignant primary tumors of the liver or retroperitoneum. Metastases are also well delineated. Benign masses of the liver can be well visualized but may be difficult to differentiate from malignant lesions because these may have similar patterns of enhancement unless they are cystic or have a vascular etiology, such as hemangiomas or aneurysms.

CT can accurately show calcification in the biliary tree or pancreas. CT may also be used to investigate hepatic parenchymal disease because it demonstrates enhancing nodules in cirrhosis, dilated intrahepatic ducts, and fat or iron deposition. Fat, which is characteristically found in the pancreas in older patients with cystic fibrosis, is well delineated with CT.

ANGIOGRAPHY

The advent of high-quality sonography, CT, nuclear scintigraphy, and now MRI has led to a continuing reassessment of the role of angiography. Angiography is now used mostly to assess solid hepatic mass lesions and bleeding in the pediatric GI tract. Arterial chemotherapy infusion may require angiographic techniques; arterial occlusion with embolization is possible in benign and malignant tumors, especially hemangioendotheliomas.

NUCLEAR MEDICINE

There are many conditions of the GI tract that can be investigated by nuclear scintigraphy. A variety of techniques are used with or without sedation. The primary value of nuclear scintigraphy in the GI tract lies in the detection of ectopic gastric mucosa and the evaluation of biliary, liver, and splenic function. Inflammatory or neoplastic lesions can also be detected. Less common uses include the evaluation of gastroesophageal reflux, abnormalities of gastric emptying, and salivary gland assessment.

MAGNETIC RESONANCE IMAGING

MRI is a relatively new body-section imaging modality that does not use ionizing radiation. It has no significant complications and causes no discomfort to the child. However, as with CT examinations, sedation is usually necessary in children aged 1 to 4 years. MRI has certain other advantages over CT and sonography: It can image in different planes, better delineate soft tissues, and does not produce artifacts from bone or nonferromagnetic implanted metal. Moreover, in the future, tissue characterization may be possible by spectroscopic analysis, although initial results are less promising than anticipated.[40]

There are, however, relative disadvantages of MRI. These include the cost of the equipment and the length of the examination (30 to 90 minutes). The time of examination is long because the signals detected are weak, and any movement, such as that caused by respiration and peristalsis, degrades the image. Although respiratory gating (synchronizing the acquisition of images with the phases of respiration) can overcome one of these problems, it further lengthens the examination.[41] In addition, calcium and bone are not directly visualized with MRI, so calcium deposition and subtle bone destruction may be missed.[42,43] Sick infants and children often need close monitoring, and electrical equipment that uses ferromagnetic material may malfunction because of the magnetic field.[44] These problems can be alleviated if the radiologist uses nonferrous electrodes and monitors respiration with a pneumonic tube taped to the abdomen, as well as blood pressure and heart rate with Doppler probes.[44]

When MRI has been chosen, the radiologist fully explains and demonstrates the equipment to the child to allay any fears. The child is then asked to evacuate the bladder (and if necessary the bowels) prior to being positioned comfortably on the table. A parent is encouraged to remain to reassure the child. Neither should be in possession of any magnetic material.

For the evaluation of the GI tract in children, the full indications for MRI are still being evaluated. Unfortunately, in the abdomen, peristalsis interferes with intestinal imaging. Bowel loops are also difficult to distinguish from the pancreas, which is further obscured by respiratory movement. In the gut, however, inflammatory disorders, tumors such as lymphoma, and bowel wall hematomas from trauma or Henoch-Schönlein purpura can be seen.[40,45]

Abdominal abscesses may be visualized, but these are best detected if they are adjacent to the liver, where they should also be visible sonographically.[40,46] Elsewhere in the abdomen, abscesses are difficult to distinguish from bowel loops. However, CT may also have this difficulty.[46]

MRI is sensitive enough to detect liver lesions, but it is often not specific enough to distinguish between tumors and infection, since both can give similar images on both T1- and T2-weighted slices. However, cavernous hemangiomas often appear different from malignant liver tumors with MRI.[47]

Blood vessels in the liver are visible with MRI,[40] but the bile ducts are usually not appreciated. The gallbladder is seen if it is present. Gallstones are not detectable because they produce a very weak signal and hence are appreciated only as negative defects if the bile is sufficiently concentrated to be visible.[48]

Diffuse hepatic fatty infiltration is difficult to detect because it is less sensitive to MRI than to CT,[49] but focal fat, diffuse hepatitis, or iron deposition[50] can be more easily differentiated with MRI.

In the spleen and pancreas, abscesses, cysts, and tumors can all be identified with MRI, but this represents no improvement, since other modalities perform similar functions more inexpensively.

As the technology improves, MRI will likely become as important as sonography in the investigation of childhood disorders—a most promising and exciting prospect for the future of radiologic studies.

Note: For further reading on this topic, references 51 and 52 are suggested.

REFERENCES

1. Cremin BJ. Real time ultrasonic evaluation of the paediatric abdomen: technique and anatomical variations: a personal view. Br J Radiol 1985; 58:859–868.
2. Brasch RC, Abols IB, Gooding CA, Filly RA. Abdominal disease in children: a comparison of computed tomography and ultrasound. AJR 1980; 134:153–158.
3. Holm HH, Smith EH, Bartrum RJ Jr. The relationship of computed tomography and ultrasonography in diagnosis of abdominal disease. J Clin Ultrasound 1977; 5:230–237.
4. Stringer DA, Daneman A, St. Onge O. Doppler assessment of abdominal and peripheral vessels in children. Presented at the 71st meeting of the Radiological Society of North America. Chicago, Illinois, November 18, 1985.
5. Stringer DA, Manson D, Krysl J, Babiak C, Liu P, Daneman A. The value of Doppler sonography in the detection of major vascular thrombosis in the neonatal abdomen. Presented at the 32nd Annual Meeting of the Society of Pediatric Radiology. San Antonio, Texas, April 5–9, 1989.
6. Stringer DA, Sherman PM, Jakowenko N. Correlation of double-contrast high-density barium enema, colonscopy and histology in children with special attention to disparities. Pediatr Radiol 1989; 16:298–301.
7. Chiu CL, Gambach RR. Hypaque pulmonary edema—a case report. Radiology 1974; 111:91–92.
8. Reich SB. Production of pulmonary edema by aspiration of water-soluble nonabsorbable contrast media. Radiology 1969; 92:367–370.
9. Ratcliffe JF. Low osomolality water soluble (LOWS) contrast media and the paediatric gastro-intestinal tract. Radiol Now 1985; 8:8–11.

10. Drumm B, Rhoads JM, Stringer DA, Sherman PM, Ellis LE, Durie PR. Peptic ulcer disease in children: etiology, clinical findings, and clinical course. Pediatr 1988; 82:410–414.
11. Stringer DA, Cloutier S, Daneman A, Durie P. The value of the small bowel enema in children. J Can Assoc Radiol 1986; 37:13–16.
12. Stringer DA, Sherman PM, Liu P, Daneman A. Value of the peroral pneumocolon in children. AJR 1986; 146:763–766.
13. Kelvin FM, Gedgaudas RK, Thompson WM, Rice RP. The peroral pneumocolon: its role in evaluating the terminal ileum. AJR 1982; 139:115–121.
14. Kellett MJ, Zboralske FF, Margulis AR. Per oral pneumocolon examination of the ileocecal region. Gastrointest Radiol 1977; 1:361–365.
15. Laufer I. Upper gastrointestinal tract: technical aspects. In: Laufer I: Double-contrast gastrointestinal radiology with endoscopic correlation. Philadelphia: WB Saunders, 1979: 59.
16. Kressel HY, Evers KA, Glick SN, Laufer I, Herlinger H. The peroral pneumocolon examination. Radiology 1982; 144:414–416.
17. Geenen JE, Schmitt MG Jr, Wu WC, Hogan WJ. Major complications of colonoscopy: bleeding and perforation. Am J Dig Dis 1975; 20:231–235.
18. Burdelski M. Endoscopy in pediatric gastroenterology. Eur J Pediatr 1978; 128:33–39.
19. Bigard M-A, Gaucher P, Lassalle C. Fatal colonic explosion during colonoscopic polypectomy. Gastroenterology 1979; 77:1307–1310.
20. Kozarek RA, Earnest DL, Silverstein ME, Smith RG. Air-pressure-induced colon injury during diagnostic colonoscopy. Gastroenterology 1980; 78:7–14.
21. Gans SL, Ament M, Christie DL, Liebman WM. Pediatric endoscopy with flexible fiberscopes. J Pediatr Surg 1975; 10:375–380.
22. Williams CB, Hunt RH, Loose H, Riddell RH, Sakai Y, Swarbrick ET. Colonoscopy in the management of colon polyps. Br J Surg 1974; 61:673–682.
23. Bo-Linn GW, Vendrell DD, Lee E, Fordtran JS. An evaluation of the significance of microscopic colitis in patients with chronic diarrhea. J Clin Invest 1985; 75:1559–1569.
24. Ho C-S. Percutaneous gastrostomy for jejunal feeding. Radiology 1983; 149:595–596.
25. Ho C-S, Gray RR, Goldfinger M, Rosen IE, McPherson R. Percutaneous gastrostomy for enteral feeding. Radiology 1985; 156:349–351.
26. Shackelford GD, McAlister WH, Robertson CL. The use of a Foley catheter for removal of blunt esophageal foreign bodies from children. Radiology 1972; 105:455–456.
27. Carlson DH. Removal of coins in the esophagus using a Foley catheter. Pediatrics 1972; 50:475–476.
28. Berdon WE. Editorial comment. Pediatr Radiol 1983; 13:119.
29. Franken EA. Examination techniques and gastrointestinal symptoms in infants and children. In: Franken EA, Smith WL, eds. Gastroentestinal imaging in pediatrics. 2nd ed. Philadelphia: Harper & Row, 1982: 1.
30. Carty H. Percutaneous transhepatic fine needle cholangiography in jaundiced infants. Ann Radiol 1978; 21:149–154.
31. Brunelle F, Amedee-Manesme O, Bernard O, Madchouel M, Alagille D, Chaumont P. Sclerosing cholangitis in infancy. Presented at the 29th Annual Meeting of the Society for Pediatric Radiology. Boston, Massachusetts, April 19, 1985.
32. Brunelle F, Riou JY, Douillet P, Chaumont P. Percutaneous transhepatic cholangiography in biliary duct dilatation in children. Ann Radiol 1981; 24:131–139.
33. Stringer DA. Gruntzig angioplasty balloon catheters in the treatment of bile duct stenosis. Ann Radiol 1984; 27:125–129.
34. Chaumont P, Martin N, Riou JY, Brunelle F. Percutaneous transhepatic cholangiography in extrahepatic biliary duct atresia in children. Ann Radiol 1982; 25:94–100.
35. Brunelle F, Amedee-Manesme O, Bernard O, Armangaud D, Alagille D, Chaumont P. Percutaneous drainage of biliary cysts in biliary atresia in children. Presented at the 29th Annual Meeting of the Society for Pediatric Radiology. Boston, April 19, 1985.
36. Daneman A. Pediatric body CT. London: Springer-Verlag, 1987: 85.
37. Kuhns LR. Computed tomography of the retroperitoneum in children. Radiol Clin North Am 1981; 19:495–501.
38. Afshani E. Computer tomography in abdominal abscesses in children. Radiol Clin North Am 1981; 19:515–526.
39. Kirks DR, Merten DF, Grossman H, Bowie JD. Diagnostic imaging of pediatric abdominal masses: an overview. Radiol Clin North Am 1981; 19:527–545.
40. Cohen MD. Pediatric magnetic resonance imaging. Philadelphia: WB Saunders, 1986: 17.
41. Johnston DL, Liu P, Wismer GL, et al. Magnetic resonance imaging: present and future applications. Can Med Assoc J 1985; 132:765–767.
42. Bydder GM, Steiner RE, Young IR, et al. Clinical NMR imaging of the brain: 140 cases. AJR 1982; 139:215–236.
43. Brant-Zawadzki M, Badami JP, Mills CM, Norman D, Newton TH. Primary intracranial tumor imaging: a comparison of magnetic resonance and CT. Radiology 1984; 150:435–440.
44. Roth JL, Nugent M, Gray JE, et al. Patient monitoring during magnetic resonance imaging. Anesthesiology 1985; 62:80–83.
45. Hahn PF, Stark DD, Vici L-G, Ferrucci JT Jr. Duodenal hematoma: the ring sign in MR imaging. Radiology 1986; 159:379–382.
46. Wall SD, Fisher MR, Amparo EG, Hricak H, Higgins CB. Magnetic resonance imaging in the evaluation of abscesses. AJR 1985; 144:1217–1221.
47. Ohtomo K, Itai Y, Furui S, Yashiro N, Yoshikawa K, Iio M. Hepatic tumors: differentiation by transverse relaxation time (T2) of magnetic resonance imaging. Radiology 1985; 155:421–423.
48. Moon KL, Hricak H, Margulis AR, Bernhoft R, Way LW, Filly RA, Crooks LE. Nuclear magnetic resonance imaging characteristics of gallstones in vitro. Radiology 1983; 148:753–756.
49. Buonocore E, Borkowski GP, Pavlicek W, Ngo F. NMR imaging of the abdomen: technical considerations. AJR 1983; 141:1171–1178.
50. Brasch RC, Wesbey GE, Gooding CA, Koerper MA. Magnetic resonance imaging of transfusional hemosiderosis complicating thalassaemia major. Radiology 1984; 150:767–771.
51. Stringer DA. Pediatric gastrointestinal imaging. Philadelphia: BC Decker, 1989.
52. Dobranowski J, Stringer DA, Somers S, Stevenson GW. Procedures in gastrointestinal radiology. New York: Springer Verlag, 1990.

PART 2

Radiography: Plain Film

Paul Babyn, M.D.C.M.
David A. Stringer, B.Sc., M.B.B.S., F.R.C.R., FRCPC

The conventional plain film of the abdomen remains one of the most commonly obtained films in everyday practice, despite the upsurge of newer imaging modalities. Plain films are indicated in the evaluation of abdominal pain, abdominal distention, and suspected intestinal obstruction, and they are used as a prelude to contrast studies of the urinary tract. The findings of initial plain films or scout radiographs often help direct the radiologist to the appropriate radiologic study, and thereby help avoid unnecessary examinations and preparatory procedures.

The following discussion of the plain radiographic evaluation of the abdomen, primarily of the gastrointestinal (GI) tract, is subdivided into two main sections. The first deals with the radiographic approach to the plain film, normal anatomy, and normal variants. The second examines commonly encountered radiographic abnormalities, illustrated by several of the most important pediatric abdominal conditions in which plain radiography plays an important diagnostic role.[1–9]

NORMAL RADIOGRAPHIC APPEARANCE

The standard radiographic examination of the abdomen is a frontal film of the entire abdomen and pelvis from the domes of the diaphragm down to the symphysis pubis, taken when the patient is supine. Additional films obtained with the patient in the erect, prone, or lateral decubitus position are often indicated, especially if pneumoperitoneum or bowel obstruction is suspected. The erect or lateral decubitus position enhances visualization by aiding the movement of free intraperitoneal air to the most superior aspect of the abdomen, either under the diaphragm or adjacent to the liver margins. Here, smaller amounts of air can be more readily distinguished than on the supine film. Similarly, the air-fluid levels of bowel obstructions are more easily noted in the erect position. For infants, particularly in critically ill premature infants in whom the absolute minimum of handling is desired, the horizontal cross-table lateral film replaces the erect film. Here the film cassette is placed perpendicular to the floor, adjacent to the lateral abdominal wall, with the x-ray beam directed horizontally across the supine infant.

TABLE 1
A Systematic Approach to the Abdominal Film

Area	Features and Abnormalities
Abdominal contour	Position of hemidiaphragms, abdominal wall, and properitoneal flank stripes
Extra-abdominal structures	Visualized skeleton
	Retroperitoneum: psoas margins, renal outlines
	Lung bases
	Pelvic organs: bladder, uterus
Intra-abdominal organs	Liver abnormalities—position, size, contour, density
	Spleen abnormalities—position, size, contour, density
Bowel gas pattern	Distribution of air
	Bowel distention
	Mucosal outline
Abnormal densities	Calcification
	Foreign bodies
	Soft tissue masses, including organomegaly
	Ascitic fluid
	Extraluminal gas

Radiographic evaluation of the pediatric abdomen requires a thorough knowledge not only of normal anatomy and radiologic techniques but also of the normal development of the neonate from infancy to adolescence and of the normal variants that may simulate disease. The radiologist must combine this knowledge with a systematic approach to the film to search diligently for subtle abnormalities, such as those of density and of bowel gas patterns, as well as to look for normal features (Table 1). Because basilar pneumonia can often cause abdominal pain, careful attention must be paid to the lung bases. In addition, abdominal disease, such as pancreatitis, may cause pleural effusions.

The normal radiographic anatomy for the older child or adolescent outlined in Figure 1 shows the soft tissue densities of the liver and spleen, with smooth tapering in density superiorly, overlying the posterior lung bases. The abdominal wall, with the properitoneal flank stripes and psoas muscle margins, is well defined. The bowel gas pattern is similar to that observed in a normal adult: air is present predominantly in the stomach and colon, and minimally in the small bowel. This contrasts with the normal radiographic anatomy of an infant's abdomen in Figure 2, which shows the bulging flanks and the relatively larger size of the liver. With the paucity of fat in this age group, the psoas margins may not be clearly seen and may be asymmetrically visualized. The presence of relatively more gaseous distention of the stomach and/or more gas in the small bowel is a common and normal finding. Several normal air-fluid levels may also be noted in the small and large bowel.[10] Clinical correlation is mandatory if the significance of any one finding is to be interpreted accurately.

In infancy, the normal bowel mucosa may not be visible on plain radiography, nor can the large and small bowel be reliably distinguished with plain films. Cross-table lateral

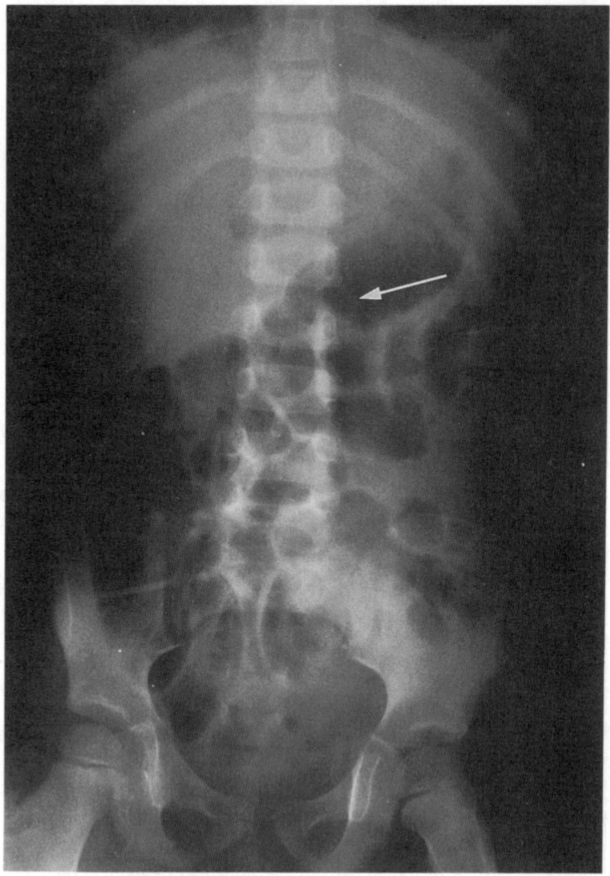

FIGURE 1 Normal abdominal plain film in an 8-year-old. The stomach is small and part of the outline of the psoas muscle is visible (*arrow*) (compare with Fig. 2).

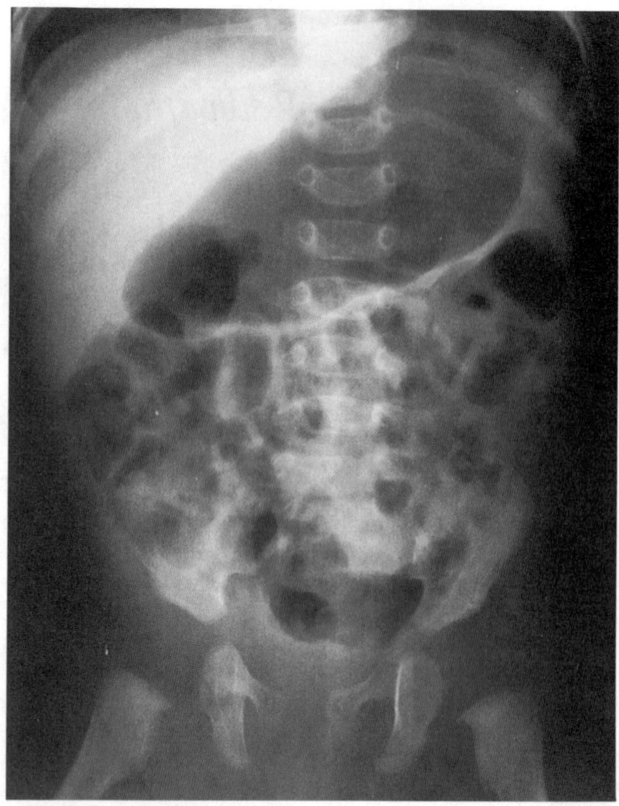

FIGURE 2 Normal abdominal plain film in an infant. The stomach is large and the psoas outline is not visible (compare with Fig. 1). In addition the flanks bulge slightly and the femoral heads are not ossified.

films may help show the posterior location of the ascending and descending colons. The mucosal pattern becomes more obvious with increasing age and is more prominent in the proximal small bowel, less so in the distal ileum.[11] In older children, the colonic haustral pattern does not extend across the entire bowel lumen as it does in infants, thus allowing a presumptive differentiation of the large from the small bowel.

The normal bowel gas pattern is established within 24 hours of birth. With normal swallowing, air progresses through the stomach and duodenum into the small bowel. This generally occurs very rapidly, often within the first 5 minutes. Distal colonic air (i.e., that of the distal transverse and descending colon) is typically seen at 12 hours.[1,2,6] Identifiable rectal air may not be seen because of its intermittent emptying.

In normal children and adults, feces are readily identifiable within the colon, most commonly in the ascending colon. The radiographic fecal pattern typically appears foamy or bubbly because the feces are intermixed with air. This normal fecal pattern is rarely present in newborns and is usually established by 2 weeks of age.[12] Its presence in the immediate postnatal period, however, suggests a distal bowel disease such as Hirschsprung's disease, meconium ileus, or early development of pneumatosis intestinalis in necrotizing enterocolitis.[12]

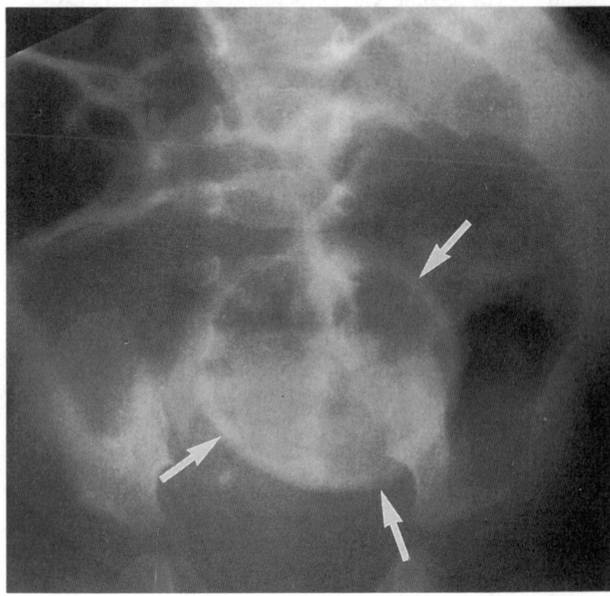

FIGURE 3 Umbilical protrusion. An apparent air-filled mass lesion (*arrows*) represents an umbilical protrusion. It is rarely a problem and nearly always disappears spontaneously by 6 months of age, though some persist until the age of 5 years. (From Stringer.[1])

Normal variants include skin folds or overlying dressings that can cause inhomogeneity of the abdomen, particularly of hepatic or splenic densities. Other extra-abdominal soft tissue masses, such as a myelomeningocele or the umbilical stump, can also cause confusing densities (Fig. 3). Pneumoperitoneum may be simulated by colonic interposition anterior to the liver (Chilaiditi's syndrome), the Mach effect (a radiolucent line seen adjacent to a thoracic rib, which is a visual artifact), or the superimposition of several air-filled loops of bowel creating a misleading appearance of free intraperitoneal air outside the bowel wall. Abscesses and other masses might be suspected in patients with colonic interposition or fluid-filled loops of bowel. Reidel's lobe, an inferior projection of the right lobe most commonly found as a normal variant in girls, may suggest a right lower quadrant mass or hepatomegaly.[13-15]

ABNORMAL PLAIN FILM OF ABDOMEN AND GASTROINTESTINAL TRACT

Abnormalities apparent from the plain film examination of the abdomen and gastrointestinal tract can be somewhat simplistically divided into three main categories: abnormal bowel gas patterns, abnormal densities, and abnormal abdominal contours. Although considered separately here, there is usually considerable overlap in presentation, with multiple abnormalities often occurring together. Only occasionally are the plain film findings specific enough, when correlated with the clinical examination, to permit an exact diagnosis. Most often, further diagnostic evaluation with contrast studies or another imaging modality such as sonography is necessary.

Abnormal Bowel Gas Patterns

Many abnormal bowel gas patterns have been described, each with a fairly specific gamut of diagnoses ranging from the airless abdomen to diffuse dilatation of the bowel. These are discussed below.[1-9] Recognition of an abnormal bowel gas pattern depends primarily on the determination of the presence of one or more of the following three features: abnormal distribution of alimentary tract air, abnormal bowel caliber, or mucosal abnormalities. The differential diagnosis will depend not only on the age of the patient, but also on the associated clinical features.

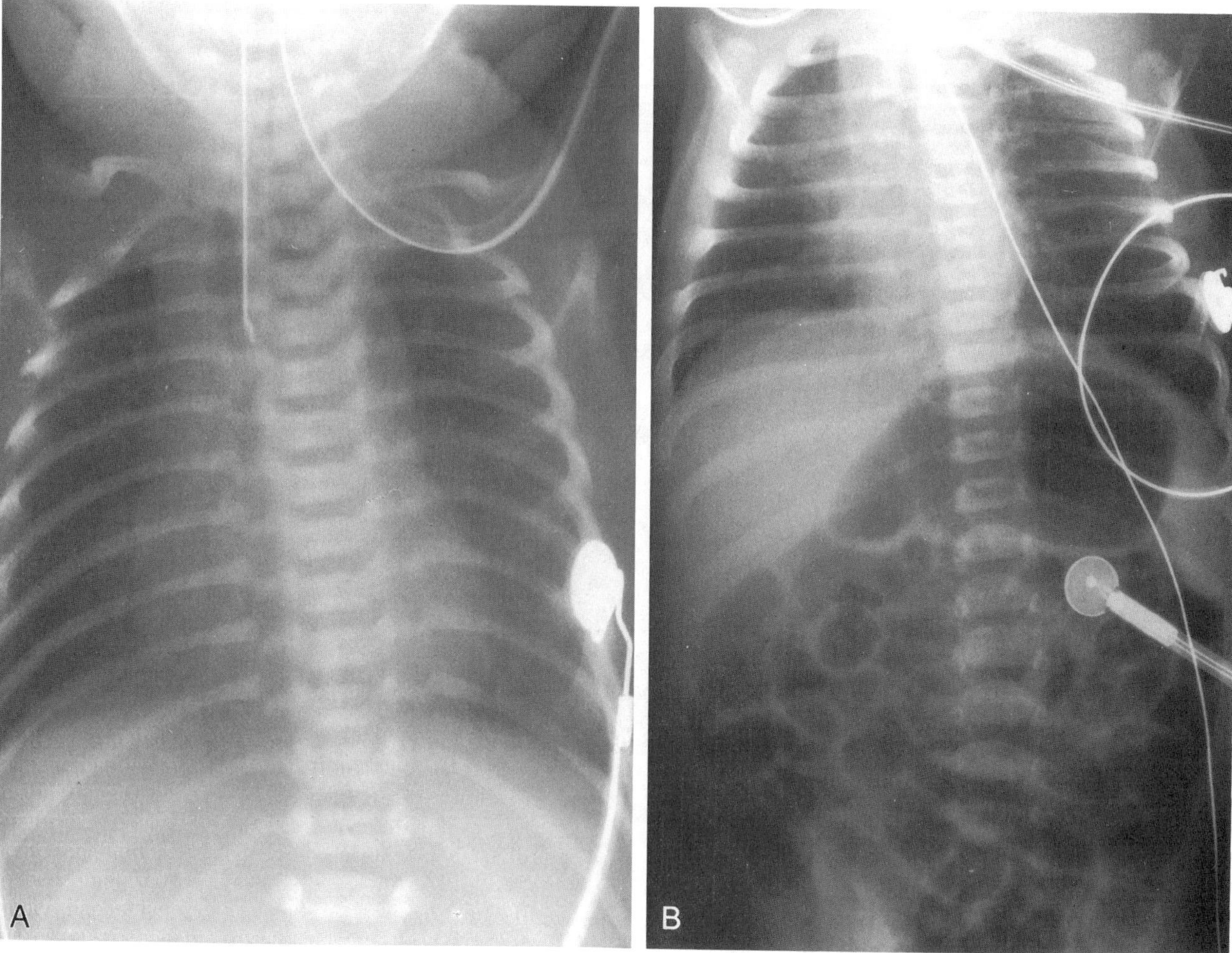

FIGURE 4 Esophageal atresia. *A*, Without a fistula, the plain films show absence of upper abdominal bowel gas. *B*, There is extensive bowel gas caused by a distal fistula. A nasogastric tube shows the limit of the proximal pouch in both *A* and *B*.

Abnormal Distribution of Alimentary Tract Air

Airless Abdomen. A complete absence of air within the abdomen may be seen when the normal progression of air from hypopharynx to stomach cannot occur. This condition is seen in neonates who have pure esophageal atresia without tracheobronchial fistula (Fig. 4). Infants with depressed cerebral or respiratory functions often have diminished swallowing functions and consequently diminished abdominal air. It is also uncommon in infants with adrenogenital syndrome or Addison's disease. In older children, the airless abdomen is most often seen in patients who have gastroenteritis or appendicitis, when vomiting and diarrhea empty the gastrointestinal tract.[1,14]

Intestinal Obstruction. In patients with bowel obstruction, the bowel proximal to the level of the obstruction is distended with air and/or fluid, coupled with decreased or absent bowel contents distally.[16] In infants, congenital obstructions are by far the most common causes; acquired causes assume increasing importance in later life.

Congenital Obstruction. In neonates, the lack of normal progression of gastrointestinal-tract air through the bowel is associated with focal bowel dilatation and is almost always attributable to a congenital obstructing anomaly, whether caused by canalization, duplication, rotation, or innervation.[1–9] As almost all these lesions require surgery, close cooperation between the radiologist and surgeon is needed to ensure prompt therapy and to avoid unnecessary investigations.

The clinical and radiographic appearance of these congenital obstructions varies with the level, severity, chronicity, and underlying etiology of the obstruction. Naturally, atresias and severe stenoses present quite soon after birth; milder narrowings often present late and may be discovered only in adulthood. Complete obstructions show no air distal to the level of blockage. Because stenosis allows passage of air distally, a contrast study is often necessary to ascertain the exact level of the obstruction; generally, the more proximal the obstruction, the fewer are the visible distended loops of bowel.

Gastric obstruction, whether the result of gastric atresia, antral webs, or other causes, gives rise to the so-called *single-bubble* sign of a large distended viscus with or without an associated solitary air-fluid level (Fig. 5). Duodenal obstructions may show two air collections, one in the stomach and the second in the distended duodenum (Fig. 6). Although the surgeon can best differentiate among the various lesions causing duodenal obstruction, several features help differentiate midgut volvulus from duodenal atresias, duodenal stenosis, or rarer causes such as mesenteric bands.[1–9] Duodenal atresias occur early in fetal life, causing greater bowel distention. Midgut volvulus typically obstructs the third portion

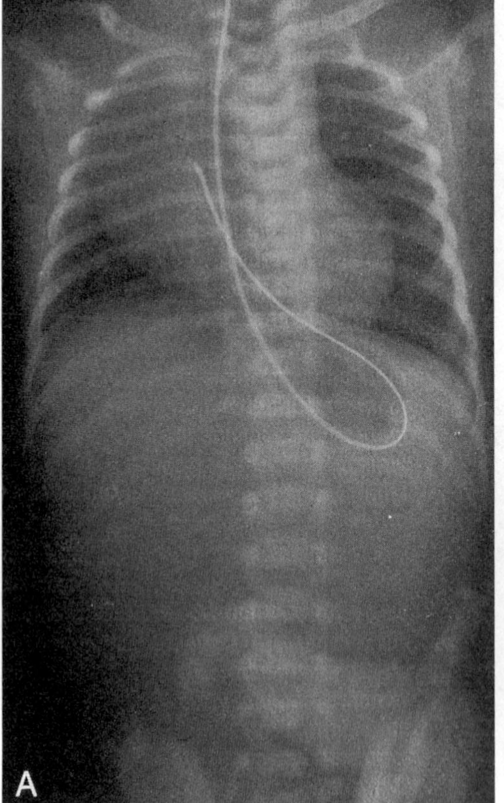

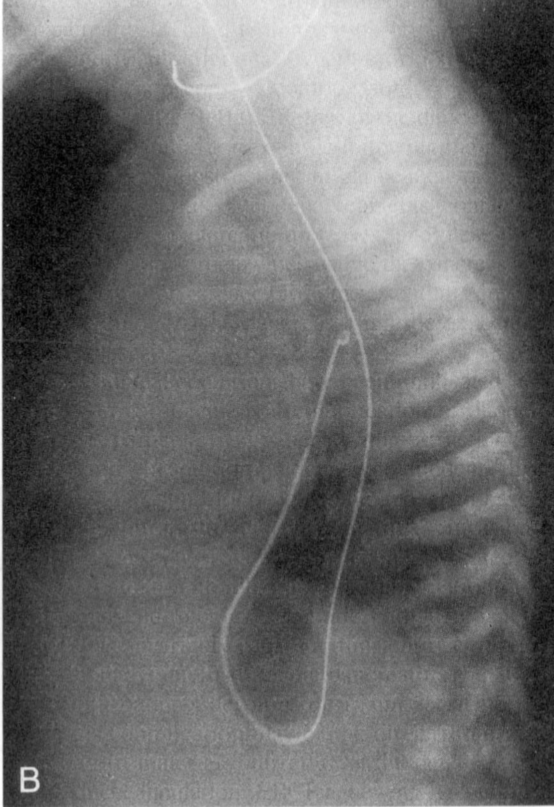

FIGURE 5 Agastria (absent stomach) with atresia. *A*, On anteroposterior plain films, and *B*, lateral plain films, a nasogastric tube curled back into the esophagus from below the hemidiaphragm. Injected barium confirmed the complete obstruction, and a ^{99m}Tc scan showed no functioning gastric mucosa. No stomach was found on surgery, and there was a dilated distal esophagus in which the nasogastric tube was curled. This example represents the most extreme form of gastric atresia. (From Stringer.[1])

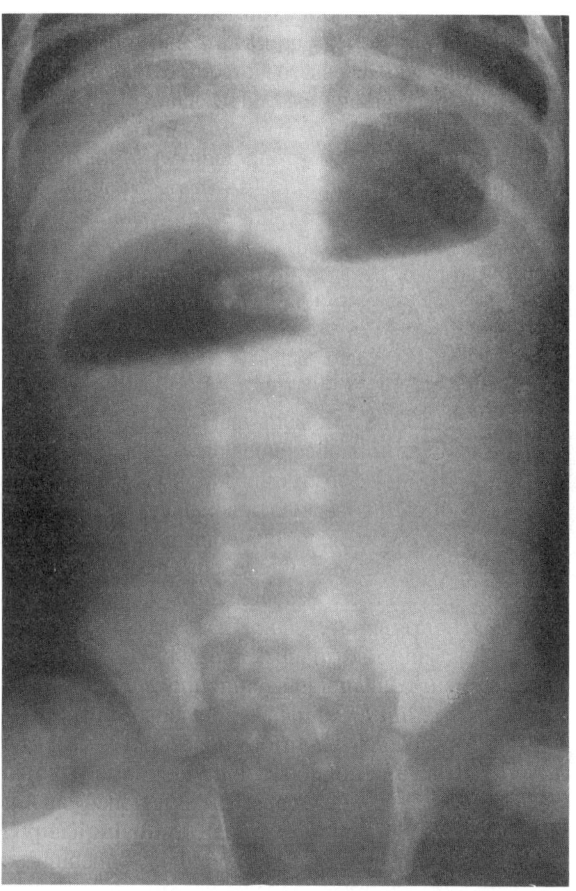

FIGURE 6 Duodenal atresia. On an erect film, prominent gas-fluid levels are present in the stomach and duodenum, the double-bubble appearance. (From Stringer.[1])

of the duodenum, whereas most other congenital obstructions involve the descending duodenum. However, the degree of distention and apparent level of obstruction are not reliable enough to distinguish duodenal atresia from midgut volvulus. Malrotation must be excluded by further radiographic evaluation if surgery is not being performed immediately. To facilitate correct surgical management, it is important to remember the strong association of duodenal atresias with other abnormalities such as Down's syndrome, rib and vertebral anomalies, and other atresias of the bowel, particularly esophageal and imperforate anus.

Plain films of jejunal obstructions, typically caused by atresias and stenoses, show several gas-filled loops of bowel, predominantly in the left upper quadrant (Fig. 7). Multiple sites of involvement are not uncommonly seen in small bowel atresias and are often associated with intraluminal calcifications. With a more distal obstruction such as ileal atresia, an increasing number of dilated bowel loops are seen (Fig. 8). Along with the increased bowel caliber, the small bowel loses its normal polygonal outline, assuming a more circular cross-sectional appearance. The bowel loops may appear stacked and displaced laterally, filling the entire abdomen.[10] Often distal small bowel and large bowel obstructions cannot be differentiated on plain films. In such cases, contrast enemas should be performed.

In addition to ileal atresia, meconium ileus, total colonic aganglionosis, necrotizing enterocolitis, and duplication cysts (Fig. 9) occur frequently and must be considered in the diagnosis.[14] Meconium ileus, the earliest presentation of cystic fibrosis, presents with abnormally thick meconium obstructing the terminal ileum. A paucity of air-fluid levels, along with the increased density and mottled appearance of meconium, may be seen in the right lower quadrant (Fig. 10). Meconium ileus may be associated with small bowel atresias, volvulus,meconium peritonitis, and pseudocyst formation. Meconium peritonitis represents a chemical inflammation of the peritoneum secondary to a spillage of meconium from a bowel perforation, usually occurring in utero. Plain films typically show an intestinal obstruction, frequently associated with calcification or pneumoperitoneum or both. A localized mass or pseudocyst may form from the extravasated meconium.[17]

Colonic distention in the neonate also often indicates obstruction. Anorectal anomalies are common and readily recognized clinically. Differentiation of the level of the imperforate anus (either above or below the level of the levator ani) may require more extensive radiologic investigation, including voiding cystourethrograms, contrast enemas following colostomy, computed tomography (CT), and more recently, magnetic resonance imaging (MRI). Hirschsprung's disease and functional immaturity of the small bowel (meco-

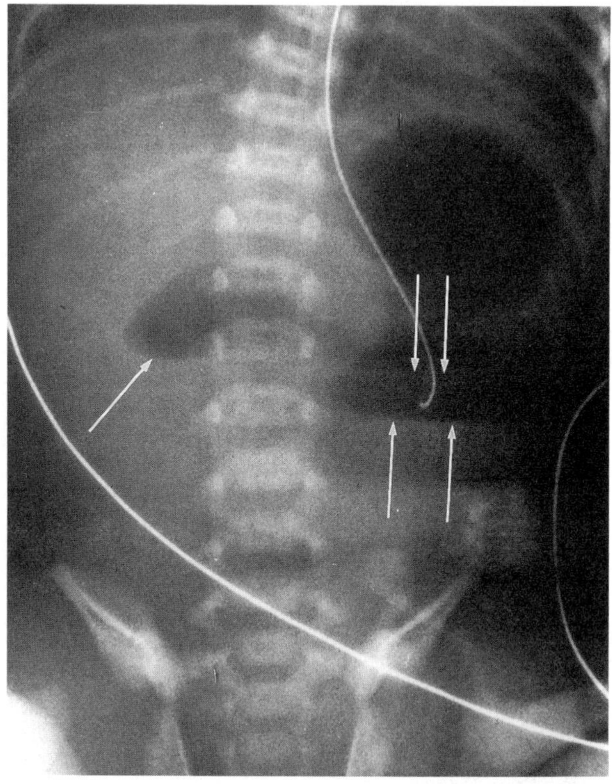

FIGURE 7 Jejunal atresia. Gas-filled levels in the stomach (*arrow aimed inferiorly*), duodenum (*oblique arrow*), and proximal jejunum (*arrow aimed superiorly*) indicate high jejunal atresia and produce the triple-bubble appearance. (From Stringer.[1])

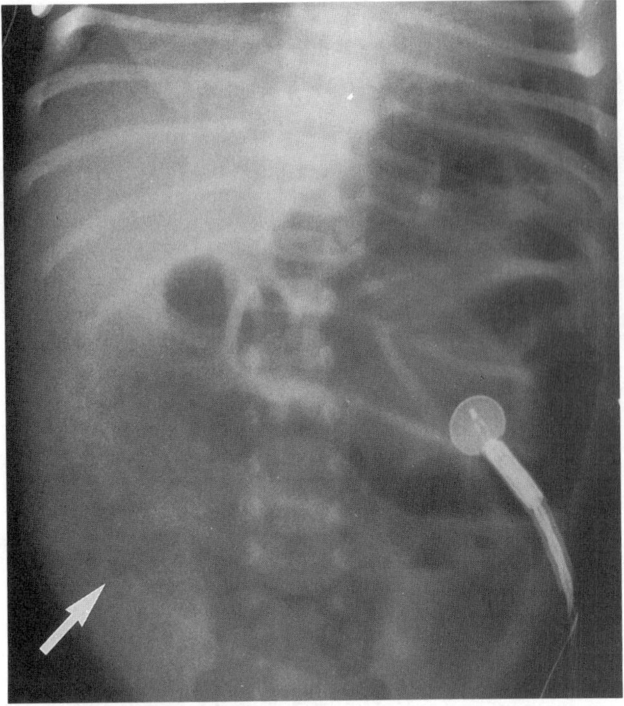

FIGURE 8 Ileal atresia. A bubbly pattern in the right iliac fossa (*arrow*) suggests meconium ileus, but this patient had an atresia and the dilated distal small bowel proximal to the atresia was filled with meconium (see Figs. 10 and 25). (From Stringer.[1])

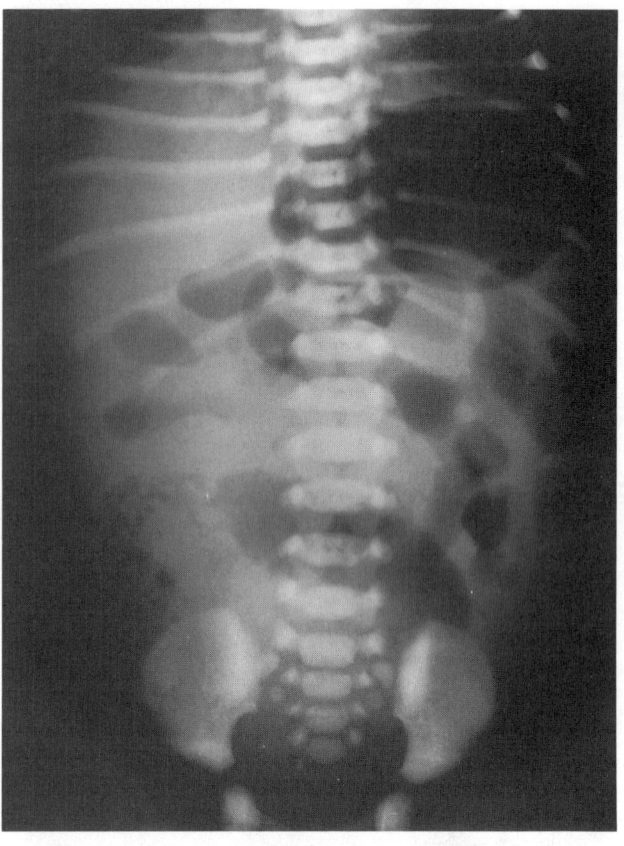

FIGURE 10 Meconium ileus. A typical granular pattern is noted in the right iliac fossa, and the small bowel is dilated (see Figs. 8 and 25).

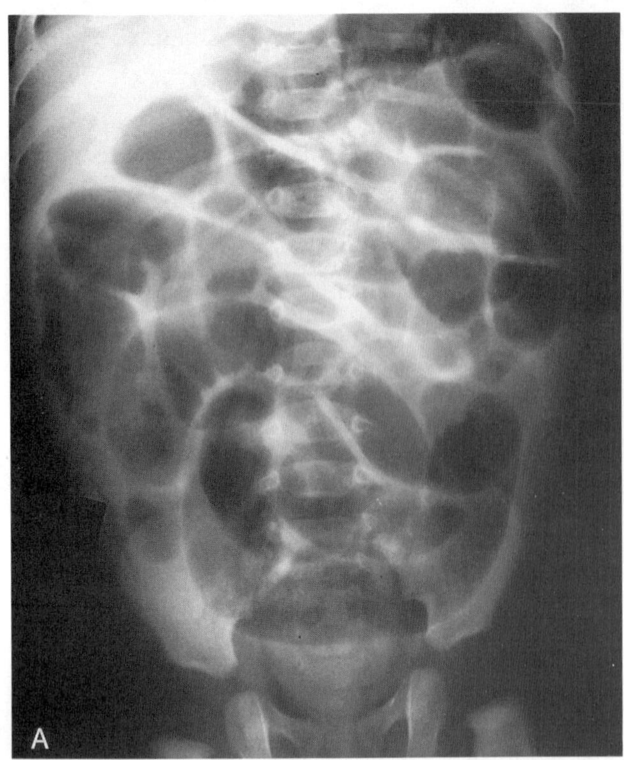

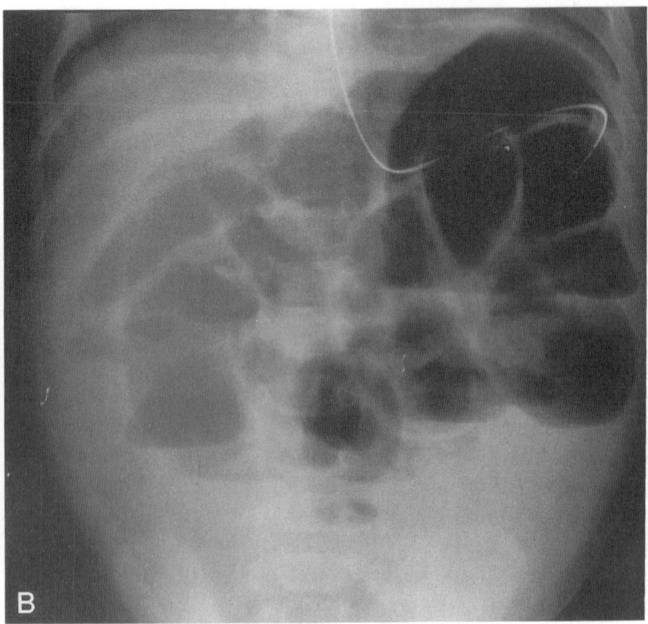

FIGURE 9 Duplication of the terminal ileum. *A*, Plain supine radiograph shows dilated loops of small bowel with multiple air-fluid levels on erect film. *B*, Indicating distal small bowel obstruction.

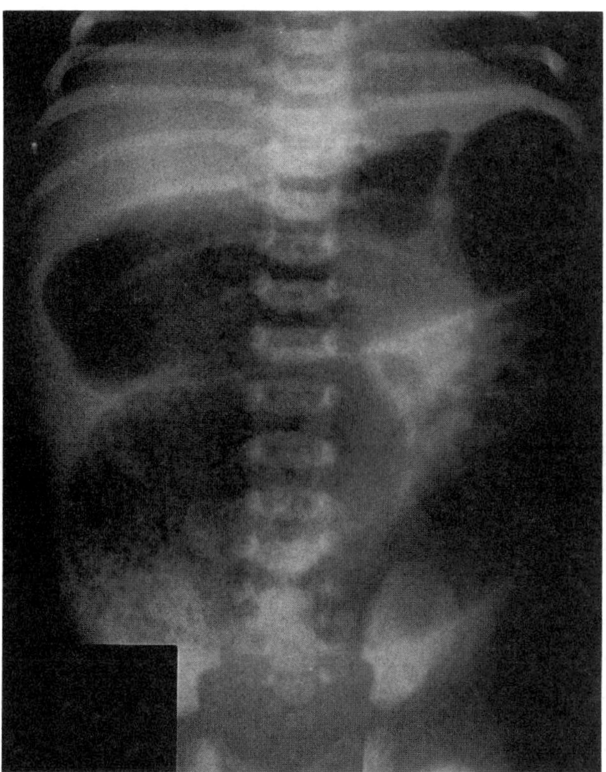

FIGURE 11 Colonic atresia. Supine film shows speckled meconium in a dilated loop of bowel in the right iliac fossa. The other very dilated loops of bowel are in the location of the transverse and descending colon, suggesting distal large bowel obstruction. (From Stringer.[1])

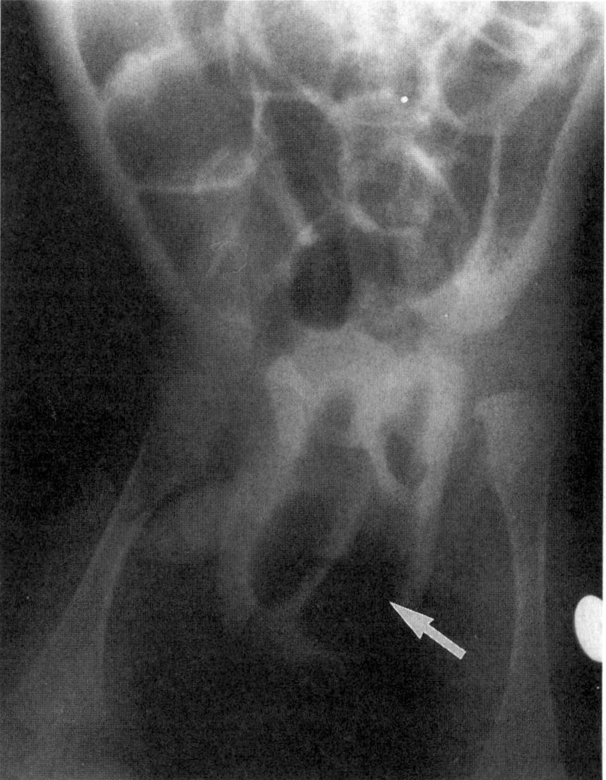

FIGURE 12 Left inguinal hernia. A gas-filled loop of bowel (*arrow*) is present in a left inguinal hernia.

nium plug or hypoplastic left-hemicolon syndrome) are relatively common causes. Colonic atresia is uncommon (Fig. 11) and rarely may be associated with Hirschsprung's disease.[18,19] Contrast enemas can usually distinguish among all these lesions.[1-9]

Acquired Obstruction. Beyond the neonatal period, acquired causes of bowel obstruction become more common. Gastric distention from pylorospasm or hypertrophic pyloric stenosis is best differentiated by sonography. Traumatic hematomas of the duodenum can cause obstruction, usually of the third portion of the duodenum. Small-bowel obstructions are commonly due to appendicitis, intussusception, incarcerated hernias, and postoperative adhesions. Specific features of appendicitis and intussusception are discussed later. Incarceration of inguinal and umbilical hernias may appear mottled because of the presence of air within the hernia or more commonly may just show fullness of the soft tissues in these regions (Fig. 12).

Abnormal Bowel Caliber

Distention of bowel loops, either focal or diffuse, is the most commonly encountered abnormal bowel gas pattern. Although occasionally a subjective determination (complicated by the extremes in size, from premature infants to adult-sized teenagers, with which pediatric radiology must deal), bowel distention is an important radiologic feature that may indicate an underlying bowel obstruction (as already discussed), localized inflammation, or a more generalized disorder.[1-9]

Dilatation of the esophagus may be seen in cardiospasm, achalasia, and during gastroesophageal reflux. An absent gastric air-fluid level may also be seen in achalasia.[1] Gastric distention is often a normal finding in infants when the distal bowel-gas pattern appears normal. Isolated gastric distention, however, may herald sepsis such as that caused by necrotizing enterocolitis or gastroenteritis.[20] Following abdominal trauma, there may be marked gastric dilatation that can cause respiratory difficulty if not relieved by a nasogastric tube.[1]

Isolated fixed focal dilatation of a loop of either the large or the small bowel, termed a *sentinel loop*, is most commonly caused by an inflammatory disease of the bowel itself or an adjacent organ. Sentinel loops may also be seen in ischemia, trauma, or early bowel obstruction.[14] Associated mucosal thickening or irregularity can be noted. The location of the sentinel loop often provides a helpful clue to the underlying inflammatory process. In patients with pancreatitis, plain films may delineate not only the fixed distention of the duodenum (Fig. 13), but also the colon cut-off sign where the transverse colon is dilated. Appendicitis can involve the adjacent bowel in the right lower quadrant, namely, the cecum and terminal ileum. Serial films are useful in distinguishing normal transient focal bowel dilatation from sentinel loops.[1,2,4]

Diffuse dilatation of the large and the small bowel, a normal finding in infants and children who have been crying for prolonged periods, may normally be seen because of aeropha-

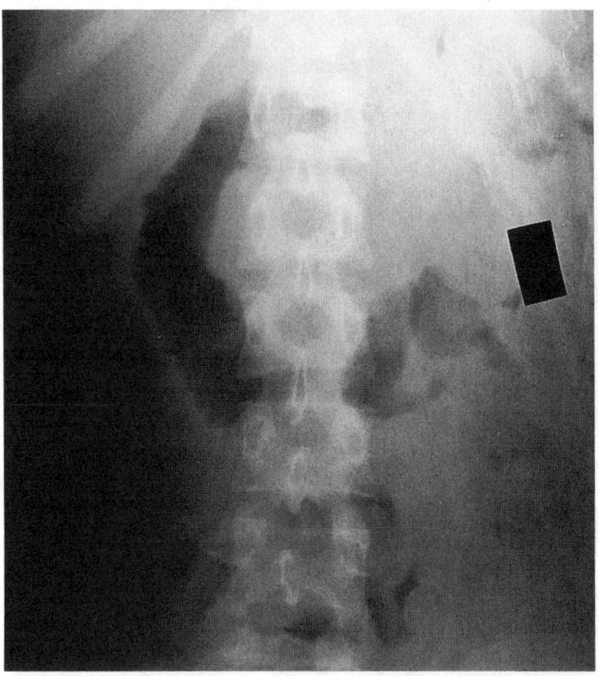

FIGURE 13 Acute pancreatitis. There is gas in a dilated duodenal loop because ileus occurs secondary to pancreatitis. (From Stringer.[1])

gy or meteorism. Paralytic ileus, a nonobstructive bowel dilatation of large and small bowel, may be seen in the postoperative period or reflect a wide variety of disorders, including metabolic disease, vasculitis, and response to drugs, as well as gastroenteritis (Fig. 14).[1,7,10,14,16]

Focal narrowing of the bowel usually occurs with abnormalities of the mucosa or submucosa, such as intramural hemorrhage, edema, inflammation, or neoplasm.

Abnormal Mucosa

Occasionally, abnormalities of the bowel mucosa can be appreciated on plain radiographs. Most often this condition represents abnormal mucosal thickening. Not uncommonly, however, loss of mucosal detail may also be demonstrated, particularly when obstruction causes marked dilatation of the small bowel. Mucosal enlargement may be due to the infiltration of the mucosa or submucosa by edema, pus, blood, or tumor. Generalized diffuse regular fold thickening is most often seen in cases of hypoproteinemia. Irregular fold thickening may be seen in Henoch-Schönlein purpura and Kawasaki's disease, as well as other vasculitides in which segmental bowel wall involvement (caused by hemorrhage and edema) is often associated with bowel dilatation suggestive of obstruction.[21] Thumbprinting refers to the enlargement of the mucosal folds, generally of the colon, perceived as thumb-sized marginal indentations along the colonic wall. Inflammatory bowel disease—ulcerative colitis, Crohn's colitis, or infectious colitis— is probably the most common cause in the pediatric population (Figs. 15 and 16).[14] Loss of the nor-

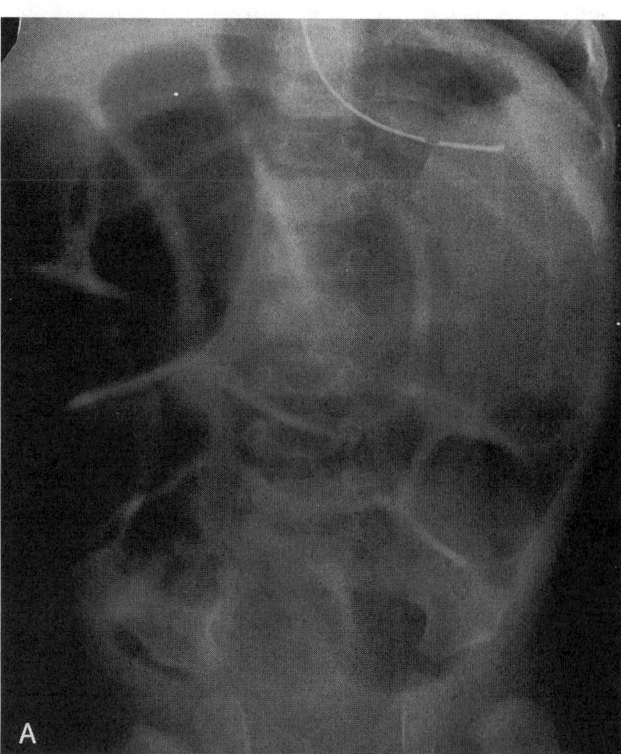

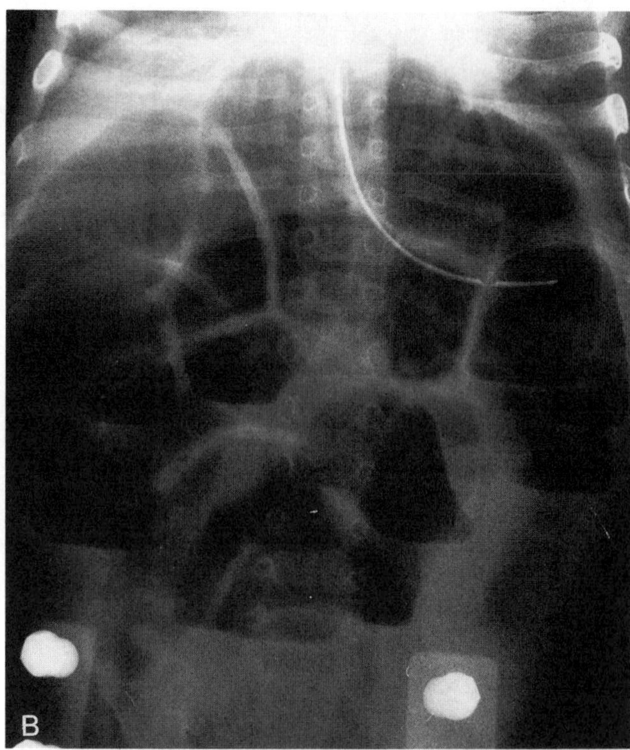

FIGURE 14 Gastroenteritis. *A*, Supine radiograph shows gas-filled loops of bowel, mimicking intestinal obstruction, and multiple air-fluid levels on erect film (*B*).

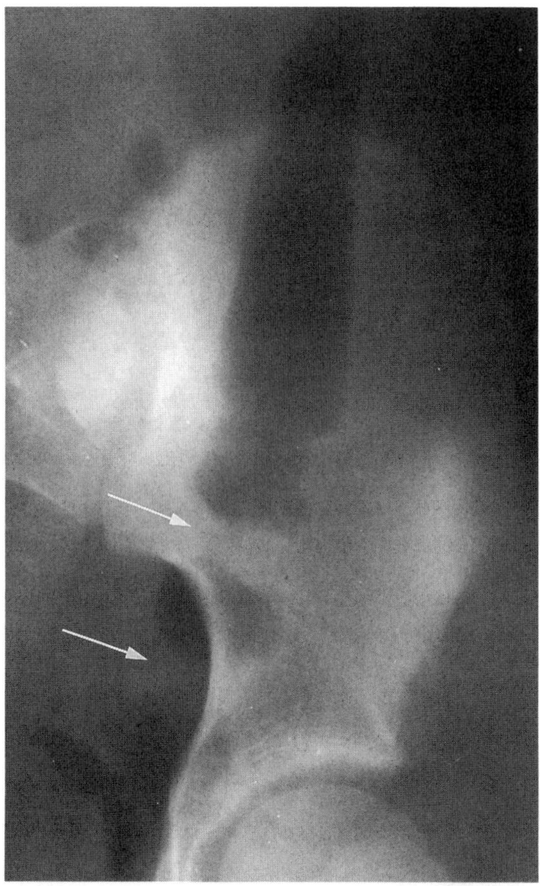

FIGURE 15 Ulcerative colitis. The plain film shows haustral thickening (*arrows*) in the descending colon and proximal sigmoid colon. (From Stringer.[42])

mal mucosa may be associated with shortening of the colon in longstanding ulcerative colitis. These changes are better assessed with contrast studies of the small or large bowel, if they are clinically warranted.[42]

Toxic megacolon may present acutely in children, but fortunately it is rare in the pediatric population. It is important that the radiologist recognize this condition from the plain films to avoid the potential hazard of perforation with contrast enemas. In films of patients with toxic megacolon, the normal haustral pattern is lost. It is replaced by nodular inflammatory soft tissue masses that project into the bowel lumen. Marked dilatation of the transverse colon is also usually evident,[22-24] but pneumatosis intestinalis or frank ulceration is rare.[14] The enterocolitis associated with Hirschsprung's disease can present similarly.

Abnormalities in Abdominal Density

Plain film evaluation of the abdomen may reveal abnormal densities that are caused by a wide variety of lesions that focally increase or decrease abdominal density, including abnormal organ densities, abdominal calcifications, foreign bodies, soft tissue masses, ascites, and extraluminal air.[14]

Abdominal Organ Density

The liver and spleen normally show a soft tissue density similar to that of the surrounding abdominal wall musculature. In patients with hemochromatosis, increases in liver density can occasionally be appreciated on plain films, but iron deposition is most reliably evaluated with CT or MRI. Similarly, a fatty liver, often seen in patients with chronic malnutrition, cystic fibrosis, or chemotherapy, may be recognized by a relative decrease in hepatic density, compared with that of the spleen or abdominal musculature.[25]

Abdominal Calcification and Foreign Bodies

Calcification within the abdomen of the pediatric patient is usually easily detected by the presence of a focal increase in radiographic density on plain films. Almost always abnormal, it is a common finding among all age groups in the pediatric population, from newborns to adolescents. Most abdominal calcifications arise from either the genitourinary tract (including adrenal glands) or the gastrointestinal tract. Table 2 lists the more common causes of abdominal calcifications.

The outline of hepatic calcification on plain films most often appears focal and irregular. The calcification may occur after infarction or the formation of an abscess, especially when

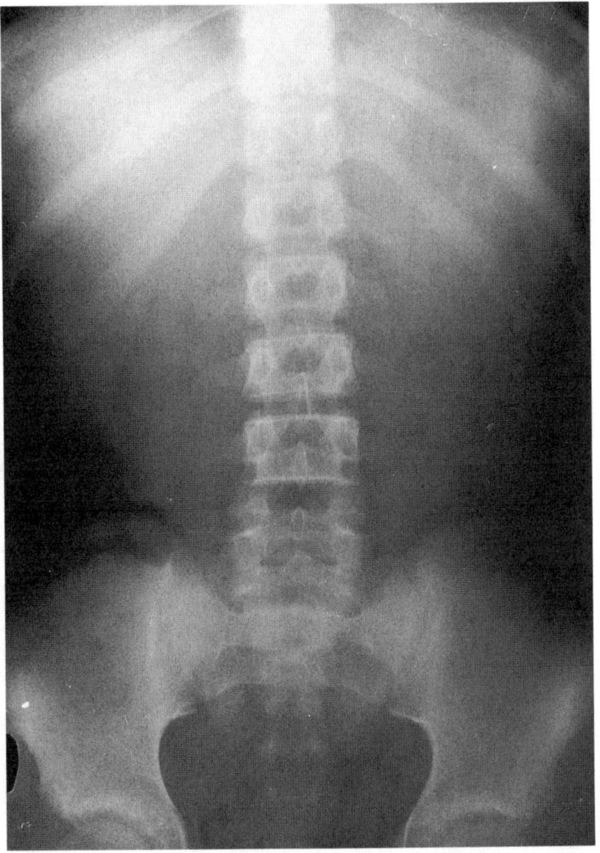

FIGURE 16 Crohn's colitis. The plain abdominal film shows no fecal material, which in a patient with acute bloody diarrhea suggests a pancolitis.

TABLE 2
Common Causes of Abdominal Calcifications

Location	Cause
Genitourinary	
Kidney	Nephrolithiasis
	Nephrocalcinosis (e.g., renal tubular acidosis)
	Renal infarction
	Wilms' tumor
Adrenal Glands	Posthemorrhagic
	Postinflammatory
	Neuroblastoma
Gastrointestinal	
Bowel	Intraluminal: foreign bodies, enteroliths, appendix, and Meckel's diverticulum
	Other: necrotic bowel, meconium peritonitis
Liver and Spleen	Postinfarction
	Postabscess
	Inferior vena caval and portal vein thrombus
	Neoplasm (e.g., hepatoblastoma)
Gallbladder	Gallstones
Pancreas	Pancreatic calcifications

associated with granuloma formation such as occurs in chronic granulomatous disease of childhood. Associated splenic calcifications may also be seen. Other infectious causes include echinococcal cysts, TORCH infections (congenital infections due to Toxoplasmosis, Rubella, Cytomegalovirus, Herpes), and visceral larva migrans. Neoplasms such as hepatocellular carcinoma, hepatoblastoma, neuroblastoma, and hemangioma may have more extensive calcifications or be associated with a soft tissue mass or hepatomegaly. Linear densities, often caused by umbilical catheterization, may represent calcifications within the vascular system, particularly in the inferior vena cava or portal venous system.[1,14]

Cholelithiasis and other biliary tract calcifications are much less common in childhood than in adulthood (Fig. 17). If these calcifications are multiple, the diagnosis is straightforward; however, if they are single, they may easily be confused with right renal calculi or hepatic calcification. Further localization by means of sonography is recommended for most upper abdominal calcifications.

Pancreatolithiasis may occasionally be recognized by its anatomic distribution (Fig. 18). It most often occurs in heredi-

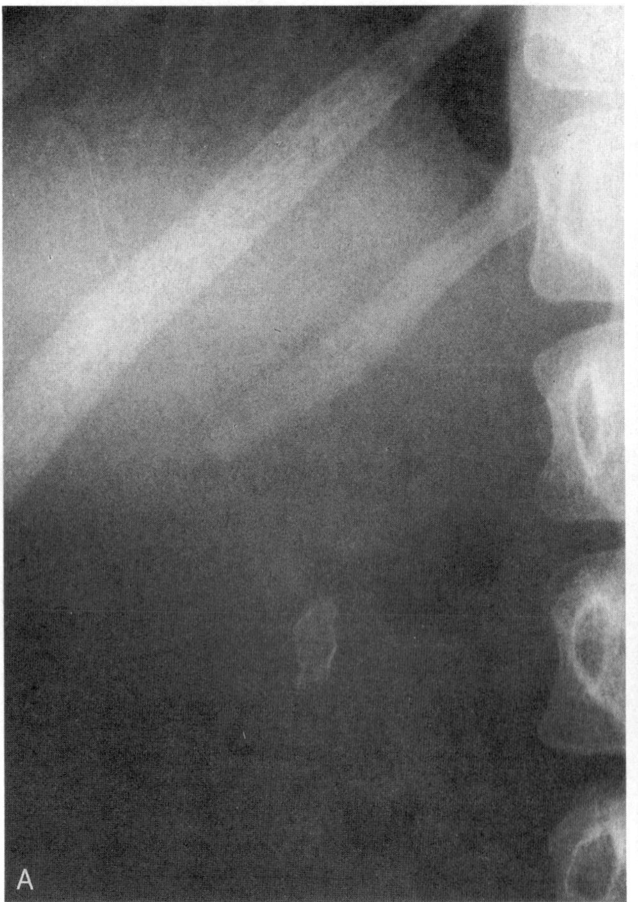

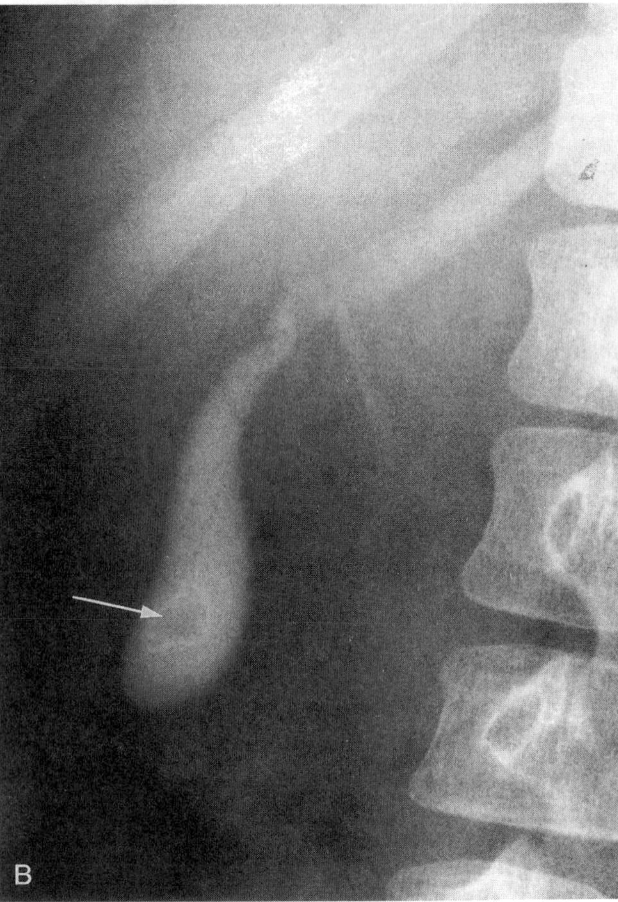

FIGURE 17 Gallstone in a 9-year-old girl with tetralogy of Fallot. *A*, Plain film shows a calcified right upper quadrant opacity with a well-demarcated calcific margin. *B*, Oral cholecystography partially obscures the gallstone, which appears as a faint lucency (*arrow*). (From Stringer.[1])

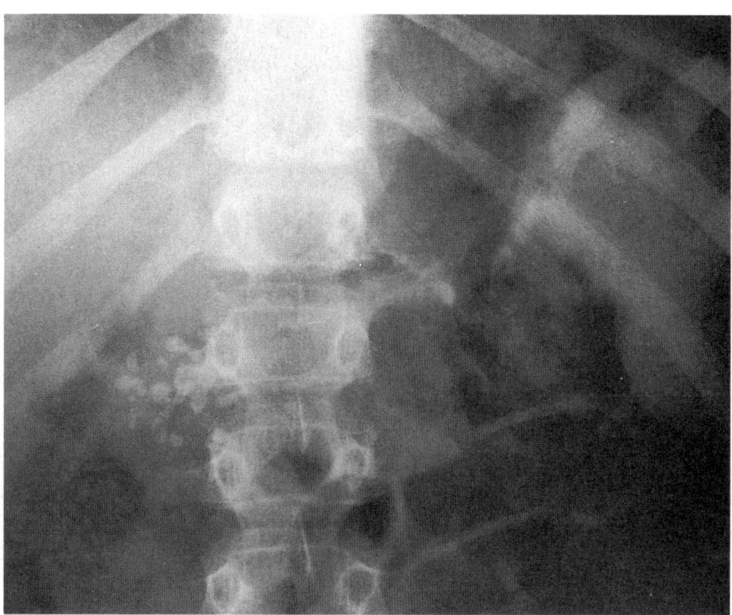

FIGURE 18 Chronic relapsing pancreatitis. Pancreatic calcification is visible on the plain film of a 14-year-old boy. (From Stringer.[1])

tary chronic pancreatitis, but it may also be seen in individuals with cystic fibrosis. It rarely occurs in individuals with pancreatic tumors.[26]

Although only found in the minority of cases, the appendicolith is one of the most important signs of appendicitis. A teardrop shape may provide the clue to its diagnosis, particularly when it occurs in the right lower quadrant.[27] The rare Meckel's diverticulum enterolith can be confused with an appendicolith.

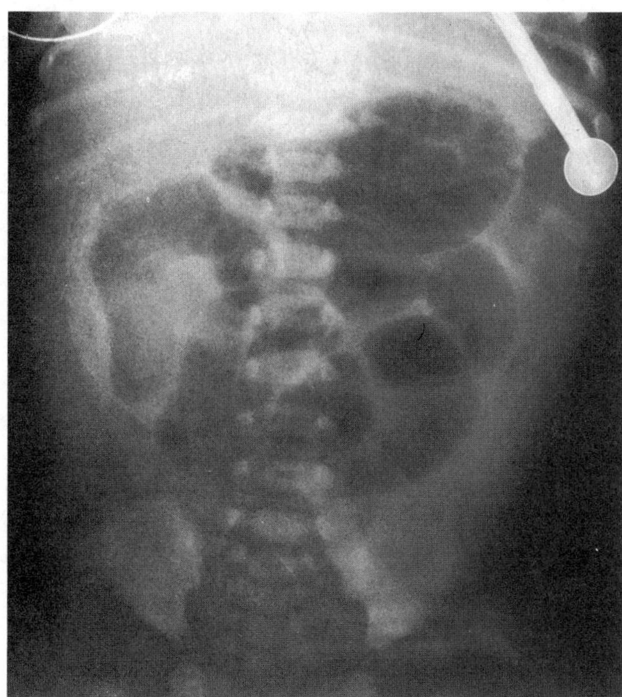

FIGURE 19 Meconium peritonitis. Faint intraperitoneal calcification is present because of meconium peritonitis, secondary to intrauterine perforation. (From Stringer.[1])

In neonates, other causes of bowel-related calcification are more numerous. In meconium peritonitis, focal or generalized calcification may outline a portion of the peritoneal cavity or pseudocyst wall, or extend down into the scrotum through a patent processus vaginalis (Fig. 19). Meconium calcification with mucosal tears may remain confined to the bowel wall or even be intraluminal, particularly in cases of multiple small bowel atresias. Associated features of ascites and bowel obstruction are usually present.

Soft Tissue Masses

Plain film demonstration of a soft tissue mass is dependent upon the visualization of the displacement of either gas-filled portions of the GI tract, abdominal organs, organomegaly, abnormal density, or, infrequently, skeletal changes.

Plain film assessment of an abdominal mass includes its localization within the abdomen, its contour, and its density (Fig. 20). Localization of the mass in the various abdominal quadrants and contour provide only a rough guide to the origin and nature of the lesion. Similarly, most abdominal masses show a nonspecific soft tissue density. A specific diagnosis can rarely be suggested by the relative lucency of fatty tumors. The presence, type, and distribution of calcification may also be a helpful diagnostic feature. It is important to be aware of gastrointestinal intraluminal soft tissue masses or intussusception so that diagnostic and therapeutic enemas can be administered (Fig. 21).

Sonography and CT are better radiologic diagnostic tools for the evaluation of palpable soft tissue masses. Plain radiography is of little additional benefit.

It is important to remember that abdominal pseudomasses such as a distended urinary bladder, fluid-filled stomach, or fluid-filled loops of bowel often mimic soft tissue masses. Gastric contents such as feces may appear bubbly on the plain films and thus may simulate a mass lesion, especially an abscess. Sonography can help in these cases, particularly in the postoperative period.

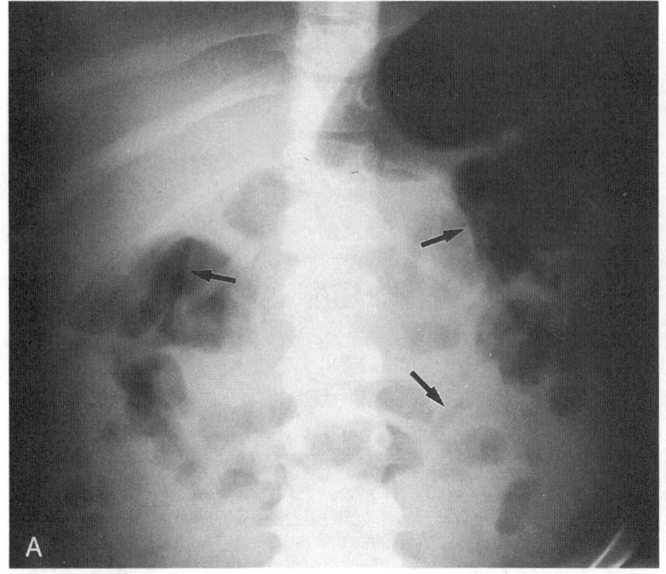

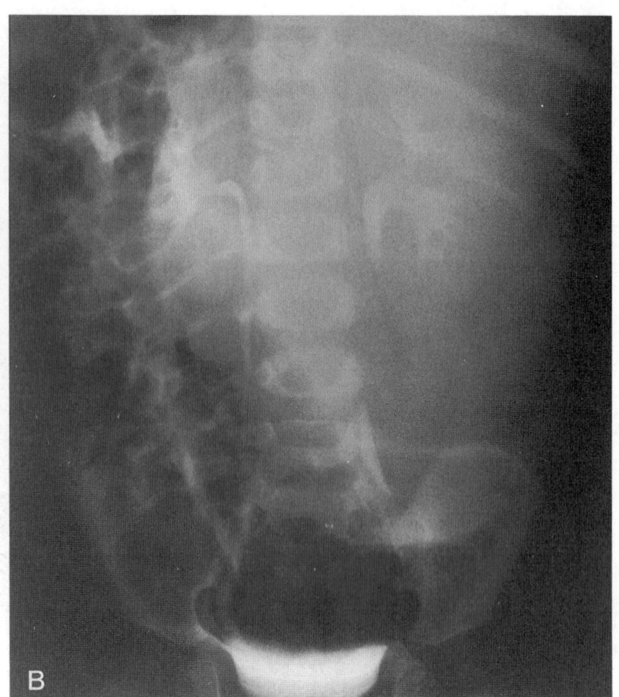

FIGURE 20 Pancreatic pseudocyst. *A*, The central soft tissue mass of a pseudocyst (*arrows*) indents and displaces contiguous loops of bowel. *B*, A large pseudocyst in the left side of the abdomen displaces bowel loops, giving a gasless appearance. There is slight compression of the left kidney seen on urography. (From Stringer.[1])

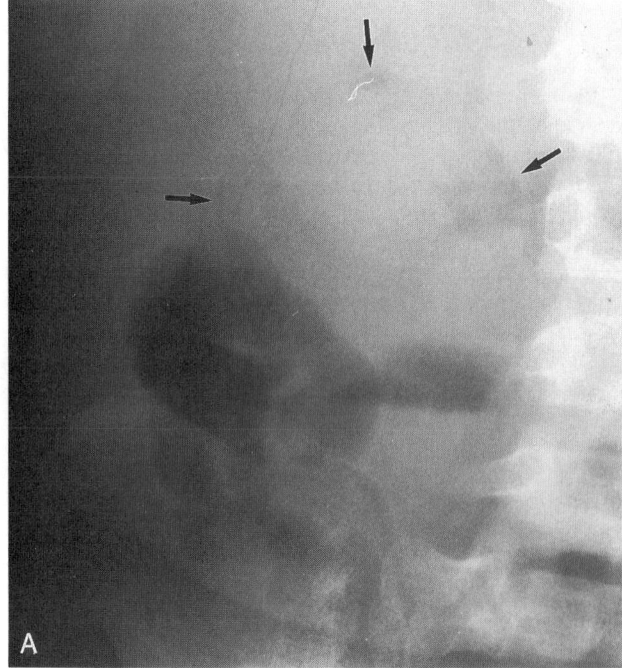

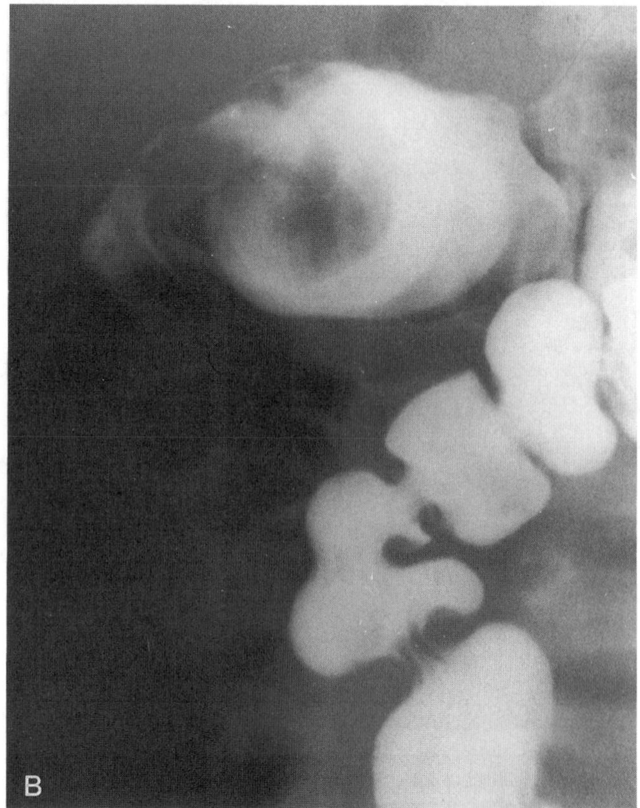

FIGURE 21 Ileocolic intussusception. *A*, Intussusception produces a right upper quadrant mass with a faint curvilinear rim of bowel gas (*arrows*). *B*, Intussusception is confirmed on barium enema; the gas lucencies around the intussusceptum fill with barium. (From Stringer.[1])

TABLE 3
Signs of Pneumoperitoneum

Abnormal air collections
Football sign: oval radiolucent shadow in the midabdomen, representing a massive pneumoperitoneum
Air in lesser peritoneal sac or Morrison's pouch
Air in scrotum or groin through patent processus vaginalis
Triangle sign: air accumulation between adjacent bowel loops
Visualization of structures not normally seen
Falciform ligament
Urachus
Umbilical arterial folds
Rigler's sign: both inner mucosal and outer serosal walls of bowel outlined by air
Lateral margin of liver or spleen on decubitus views

Ascites

The presence of intraperitoneal fluid, whether blood, chyle, pus, or serous fluid, is best evaluated by sonography. However, certain signs on plain film are suggestive of ascites. These include the displacement of the colon away from the properitoneal flank stripe, a centrally located floating small bowel, the separation of bowel loops, the presence of pelvic fluid causing the increased density above the bladder (commonly termed *dogears*), and the presence of fluid lateral to the liver and spleen. On occasion, chyloperitoneum may look less dense than other forms of ascites, but it cannot always be reliably distinguished from hemoperitoneum or other causes of fluid collections on plain films.[29,30]

Extraluminal Air (Pneumoperitoneum)

Extraluminal air can occur anywhere within the abdomen but is most commonly free within the peritoneal cavity. Pneumoperitoneum may be due to a wide variety of causes, including bowel perforation, inferior extension of pneumomediastinum, trauma, and postoperative air. In neonates, pneumoperitoneum is almost always caused by a gastrointestinal perforation of the stomach, small bowel, or colon (Fig. 22). Although pneumoperitoneum is best evaluated radiographically with erect films to assess the presence of free air under the diaphragm, this is not clinically possible in every case. A multitude of signs on supine, prone, lateral decubitus, or cross-table lateral films help identify pneumoperitoneum (Table 3 and Fig. 22). Delineation of air-fluid levels in the peritoneal cavity almost always represents a bowel perforation. Postoperative pneumoperitoneum usually disappears quickly, but occasionally it can last for 1 to 2 weeks, or even longer.[31,32]

Extraluminal air also includes air within the intestinal wall, liver, and other organs; loculated peritoneal collections such as abscesses (Fig. 23); and air within the retroperitoneum. Hepatic air can be found within the biliary or portal venous systems. Biliary air is often caused by biliary-enteric fistu-

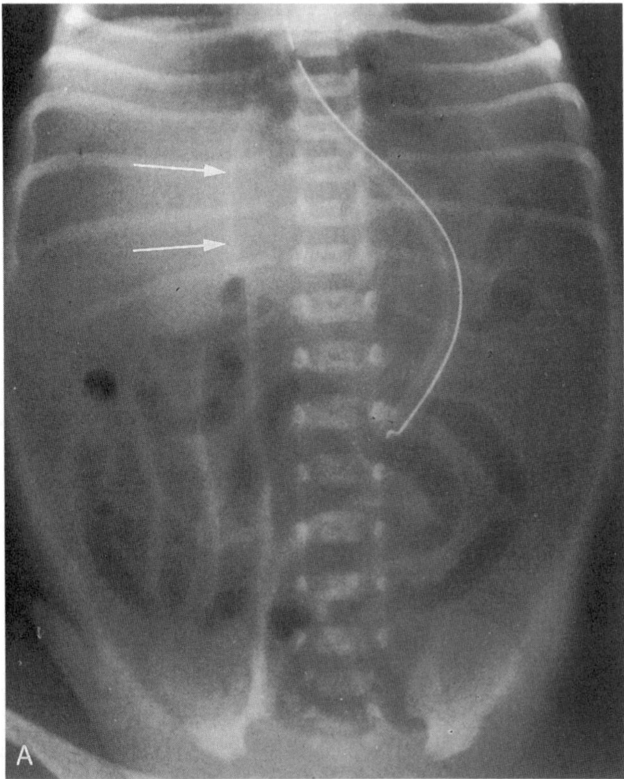

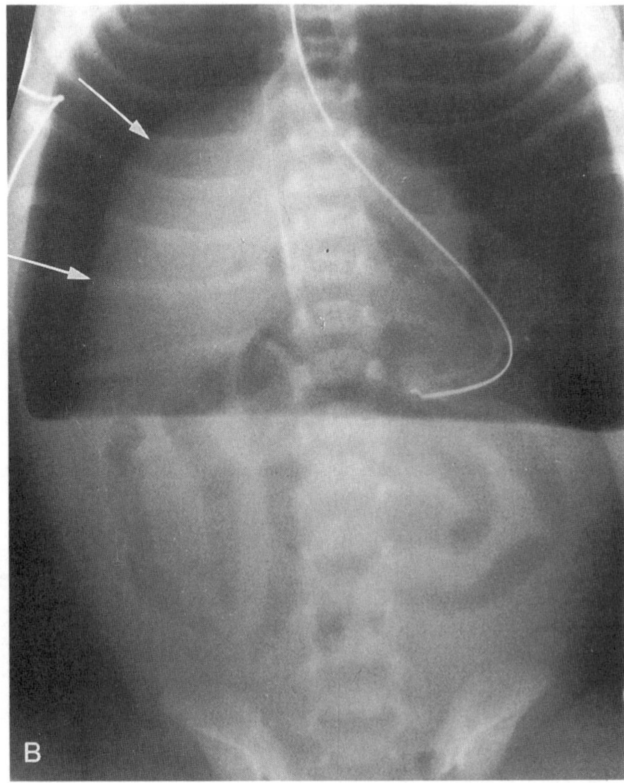

FIGURE 22 Neonatal gastric rupture. Massive hydropneumoperitoneum is present. *A*, The stomach is devoid of gas on the supine film, and *B*, there is no gastric gas-fluid level on the erect film. The falciform ligament (*A, arrows*) and liver (*B, arrows*) are outlined by free intraperitoneal gas. (From Stringer.[1])

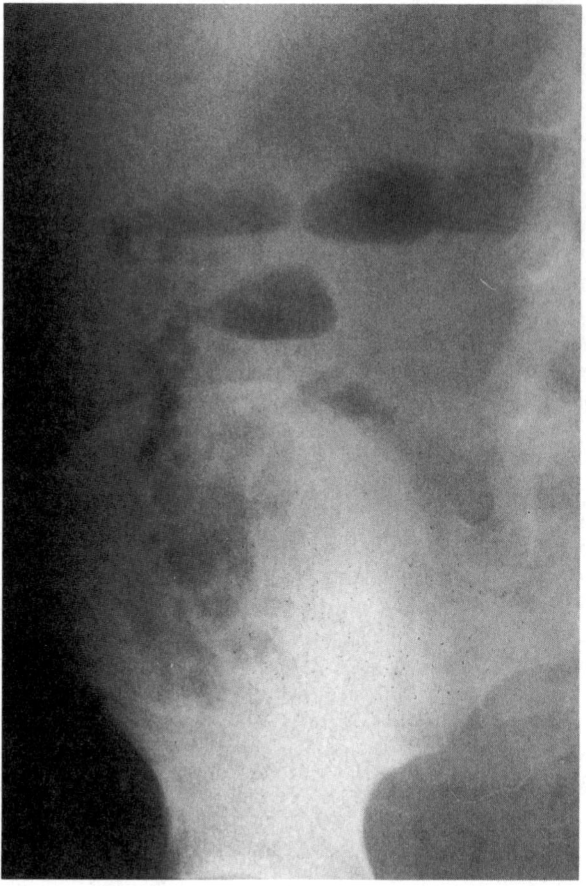

FIGURE 23 Typhlitis (neutropenic colitis) in a child with leukemia. The gas pattern is highly abnormal, with a speckled appearance in the cecum caused by gas in an abscess that developed following perforation of a severely affected cecum.

las. It tends to conglomerate centrally, whereas portal air flows more peripherally. Trauma and abscess formation can also cause loculated air collections within the liver and other abdominal viscera, or within the peritoneal cavity. A rare cause of hepatic air is bronchobiliary fistulas. Retroperitoneal air may represent the inferior extension of pneumomediastinum, or it may be secondary to duodenal or colonic trauma. Retroperitoneal air appears as abnormal lucencies adjacent to the psoas muscles or kidneys on plain film.

Abnormal Abdominal Contours

The normal contours or borders of the abdomen are formed superiorly by the diaphragm, and anteriorly and laterally by the abdominal wall, with the bony support (i.e., the spine, ribs, and pelvis) forming the posterior and inferior aspects of the abdomen, respectively. Most abnormalities in abdominal configuration represent congenital defects in the formation of the diaphragm and anterior abdominal wall. The abdominal contents can thus protrude into the thoracic cavity or anteriorly outside the normal confines of the abdomen.[1]

Diaphragmatic defects represent a spectrum of lesions ranging in severity from complete absence of the diaphragm to pathologic (Bochdalek and Morgagni hernias) and physiologic orifices (hiatal hernias) through which abdominal viscera protrude. Bochdalek hernias, the most common defects in the neonatal period, are posterolateral defects in the diaphragm. In the great majority of patients, they occur on the left side; commonly, they include a variable amount of small bowel but may also include stomach, spleen, kidney, and colon. Larger defects include a greater proportion of the small bowel, causing a scaphoid abdomen. Massive diaphragmatic defects are associated with a shift of the heart and mediastinum to the opposite sides and severe respiratory distress. Initially, the hemithorax after birth appears opaque, but with increasing small bowel gas, multiple cystlike lucencies will be identified. Within the abdomen proper, decreased small bowel gas may be noted. Placement of a nasogastric tube may demonstrate herniation of the stomach up into the hemithorax (Fig. 24). If the stomach is not herniated, it may lie low and central within the abdomen. Evidence of associated anomalies may be noted in the cardiovascular system or central nervous system. Morgagni hernias are much less common and occur in the parasternal region, most typically on the right, but they may also be bilateral. The liver is the most often herniated viscus. Eventration, a focal area of muscular thinning, occurs with elevation of the involved portion of the diaphragm. Other diaphragmatic defects include hiatal and paraesophageal hernias. On plain films, abnormal retrocardiac soft tissue and gas collections may be noted.

Anterior abdominal wall defects are readily apparent clinically after birth and include gastroschisis, omphalocele, and caudal fold defects such as bladder exstrophy. Plain radiography plays little role in their assessment. Prenatal sonography is gaining increasing importance in the assessment of these lesions and is particularly useful because it enables physicians to plan the management of the condition and parental counseling.

Miscellaneous Abdominal Abnormalities

Necrotizing Enterocolitis

Despite improvements in neonatal management over the last several years, necrotizing enterocolitis (NEC) remains a common serious disease found in every neonatal intensive care unit. Plain film radiography plays a vital role, in both the diagnosis and the subsequent management of the affected infants.[33-35] The radiologist must maintain a high index of suspicion because radiologic evidence of NEC may precede the clinical findings by several hours. The classic radiographic manifestations are nonspecific and include dilated bowel, intramural gas, and portal venous gas (Figs. 25 to 27). The small and large bowel may be involved, with dilatation of the small bowel alone being most commonly involved.[33] With colonic involvement, pneumatosis is commonly seen. The degree and extent of bowel dilatation are generally related to the clinical severity of the disease. The small bowel dilatation may resemble small bowel obstruction; therefore, correlation of radiographic findings with clinical ones is important (Fig. 25).[33] Intramural gas or pneumatosis has been considered a

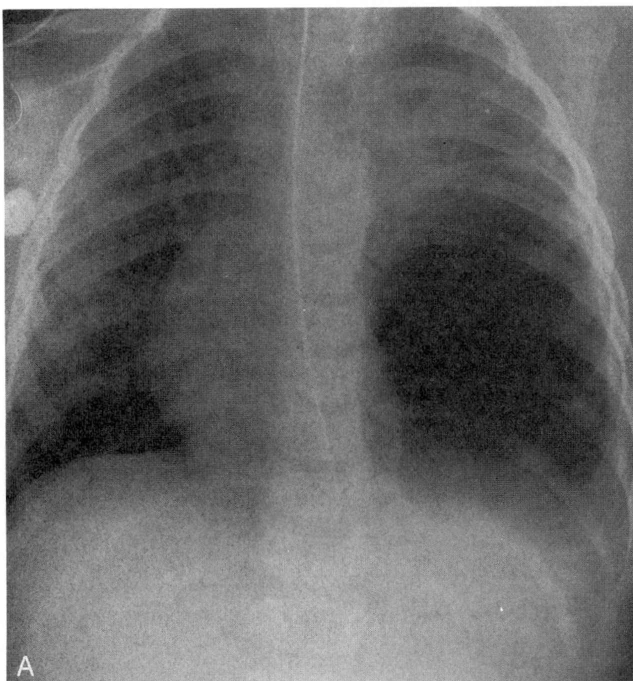

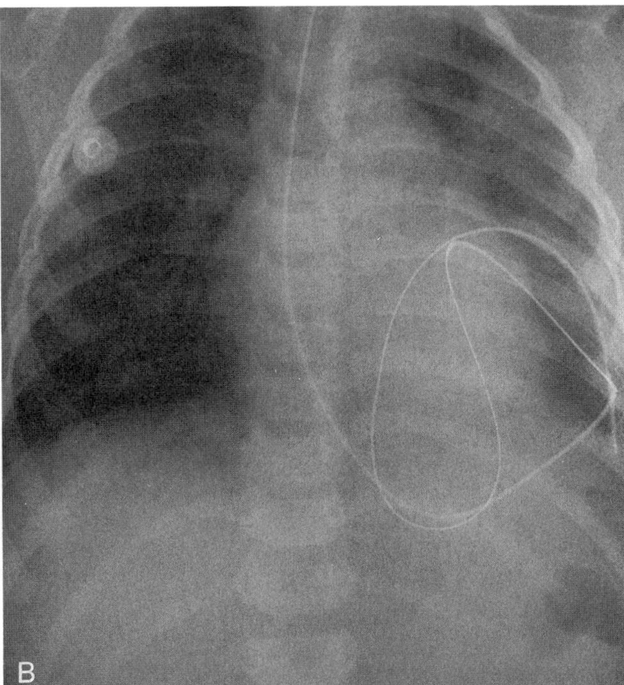

FIGURE 24 Left-sided Bochdalek (pleuroperitoneal) hernia. *A*, Gas in the intrathoracic stomach displaces the heart to the right, exacerbating the respiratory distress. The tip of the nasogastric tube lies at the esophagogastric junction, and the stomach has twisted up into the chest. *B*, If the situation is acute, aspiration of gas through a nasogastric tube can decompress the stomach and can be life-saving. (From Stringer.[1])

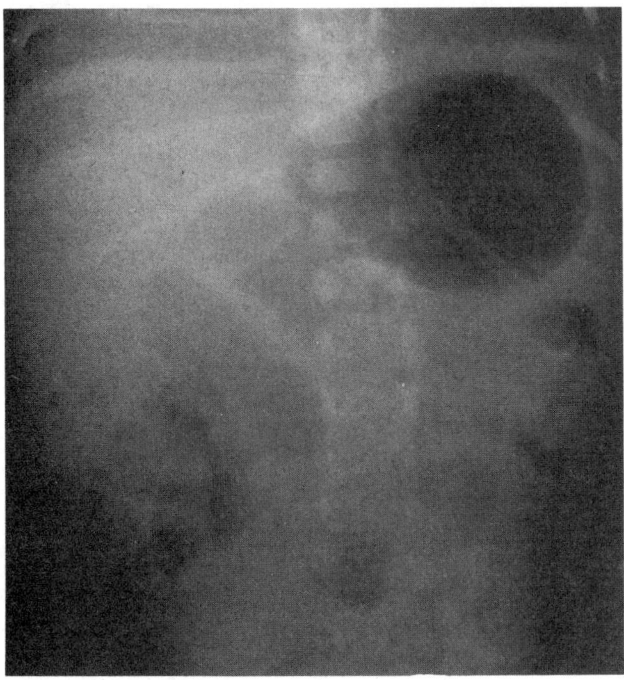

FIGURE 25 Necrotizing enterocolitis. Some dilated loops of small bowel superficially mimic obstruction; however, careful inspection shows an abnormal bowel gas pattern in the left midabdomen and a foamy pattern of intramural air in the right lower abdomen. Note similarity to Figures 8 and 10.

pathognomonic sign of NEC in the appropriate clinical situation. However, its absence does not exclude NEC. Pneumatosis typically occurs early in the clinical course and may be seen throughout the stomach and small or large bowel, most commonly in the terminal ileum. The ileal involvement may simulate the bubbly appearance of meconium ileus. Its disappearance, however, is not always related to clinical improvement. On radiographs, it appears to consist of localized cystic collections or diffuse linear strips of air density that parallel the bowel wall (Fig. 26). Pneumatosis also has been found with gastric distention, small bowel or colonic obstruction, or infection with gas-forming organisms; it has been found following ingestion of corrosives or after bone marrow transplantation.[36]

Portal venous gas, like intramural gas, may appear and disappear rapidly (Fig. 27). It is generally seen in the more severe cases, but again, its disappearance does not necessarily reflect improvement. Portal venous gas is typically located in the periphery of the liver, unlike biliary air, which is central and less commonly seen in the neonatal period.

Radiologic signs of deterioration that reflect perforation or bowel necrosis with impending perforation that may require surgery include evidence of pneumoperitoneum (Fig. 28), ascites, diminished bowel gas with asymmetric dilated loops, and persistently dilated bowel loops. Other indications for operation include fistulas, abscess formation, and adhesions.[33,34]

Late complications include stricture formations in the large and small bowel (Fig. 29). Routine contrast examination is

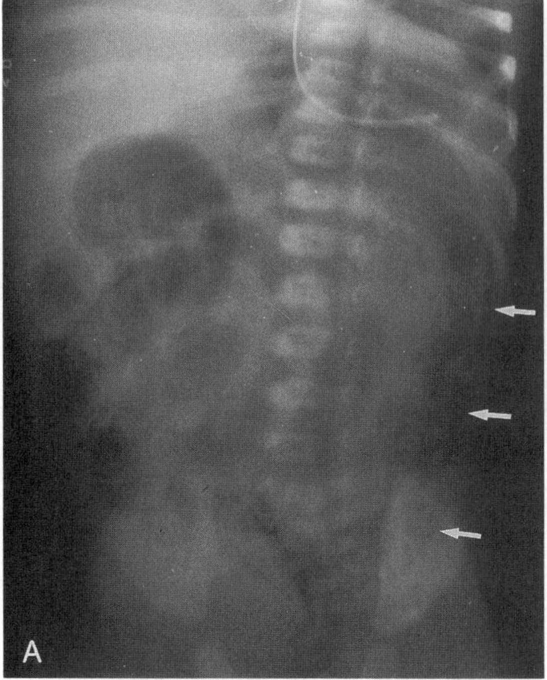

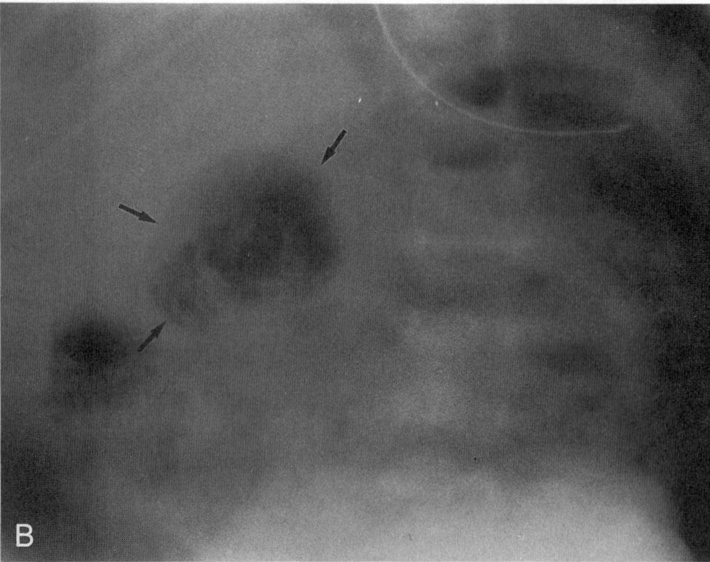

FIGURE 26 Extensive necrotizing enterocolitis. *A*, A supine plain film shows linear lucencies (*arrows*), especially surrounding the left hemicolon. *B*, A spot film of the upper abdomen shows curvilinear gas (*arrows*) affecting the hepatic flexure. In addition, in *A* and *B* there is a bubbly pattern of intramural gas throughout the large bowel.

recommended because no relationship between the formation of the stricture and the clinical severity of disease has been found. Enterocysts may be seen in cases of multiple strictures.

Intussusception

Intussusception is a frequent cause of abdominal pain in late infancy and early childhood. Plain film radiologic evaluation, usually with supine, erect, or lateral decubitus films, often precedes a diagnostic enema in clinically suspected cases. Cross-table lateral films with horizontal beam have recently been proved valuable for demonstrating the level of obstruction. Positive radiographic findings include the demonstration of an intraluminal mass (see Fig. 21), sparse feces within the large bowel, small bowel obstruction (Fig. 30), and decrease in overall bowel gas, particularly in the right lower quadrant. However, none of these signs need be evident on plain films, and a normal plain film appearance does not exclude intussusception. Similarly, intussusception may not always be reliably diagnosed by plain film evaluation.[35,38]

Appendicitis

Appendicitis represents one of the most common causes of abdominal pain in childhood and the most frequent reason for abdominal surgery. The large majority of patients are diagnosed clinically without need for any radiologic imaging. However, when the clinical presentation is not straightforward, as is often the case in the very young infant, radiologic evaluation becomes more important.[36,39] Initial evaluation with plain films can help confirm the diagnosis by demonstrating an appendicolith or exclude appendicitis if another cause for the pain, such as intussusception, is found. If not, further evaluation with sonography or contrast study may then be helpful.

The numerous radiologic features of acute appendicitis and its complications, such as perforation, appendiceal abscess, and peritonitis, have been well described in the literature.[39-41] Most are nonspecific and can be seen in asymptomatic children with lesser frequency. Therefore, it is important to correlate the clinical findings with those of the film. Plain film findings roughly correspond to the degree of inflammation and the stage of disease in the appendix. Early on, the plain film may be completely normal or show decreased overall bowel gas caused by associated nausea and vomiting. Later on, but still before perforation occurs, localized sentinel loops in the right lower quadrant, scoliosis convex to the left, and obscuration of the right psoas margin may all be noted because of the underlying inflammatory response (Fig. 31).

If the inflammatory process is allowed to continue to perforation, with subsequent development of peritonitis, the obliteration of the properitoneal fat line and a positive flank-stripe sign (increased soft tissue distance between the abdominal wall and air-filled colon) are evident. Bowel changes include air-fluid levels in the right lower quadrant in the cecum or terminal ileum, cecal wall edema, distended bowel with functional small bowel obstruction from reflex paralytic ileus, and compression from the inflammatory exudate. With the formation of an abscess, the increased soft tissue density in the right lower quadrant, pelvic cul-de-sac, or subhepatic space may be noted with or without air-fluid levels. Free air is not commonly seen and is not usually massive when present. Gas in the appendix may reflect infection caused by a gas-forming organism. Appendicoliths or calcific coproliths, which are typically found in only 15 percent

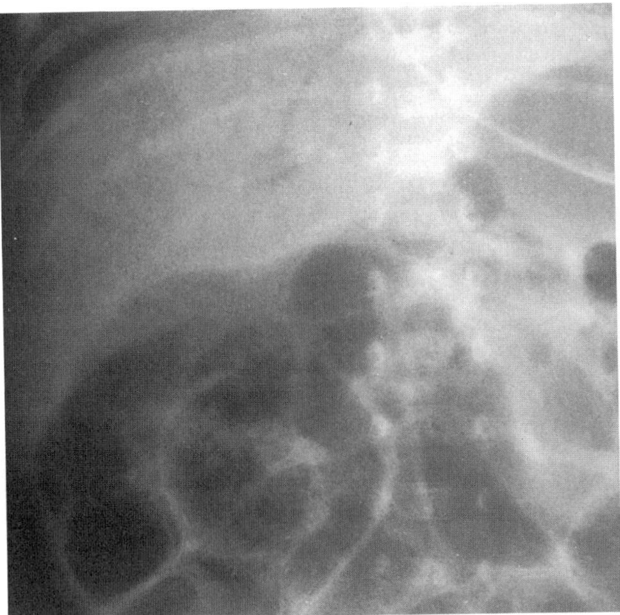

FIGURE 27 Severe necrotizing enterocolitis with portal vein gas. Branching lucencies within the liver parenchyma represent gas in the portal venous system. Unlike gas in the biliary tree, the lucencies extend to the periphery of the liver. Except after biliary tract surgery, gas is rarely present in the biliary tree of infants.

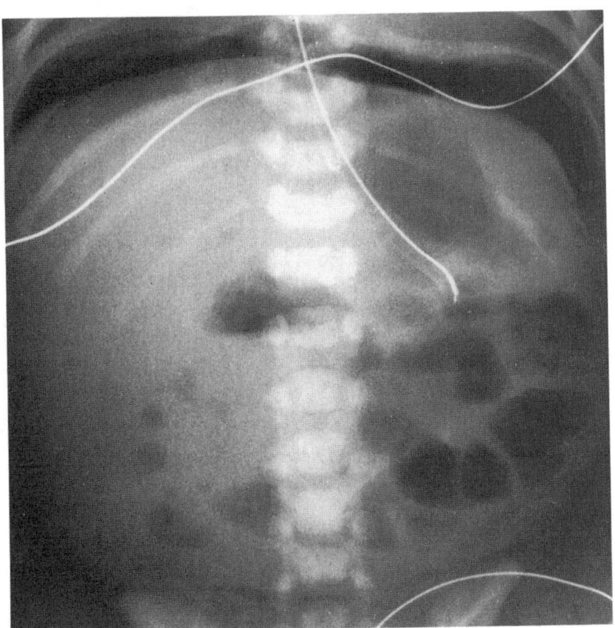

FIGURE 28 Perforation resulting from necrotizing enterocolitis. The presence of large lucencies under both hemidiaphragms indicate gross intraperitoneal free air.

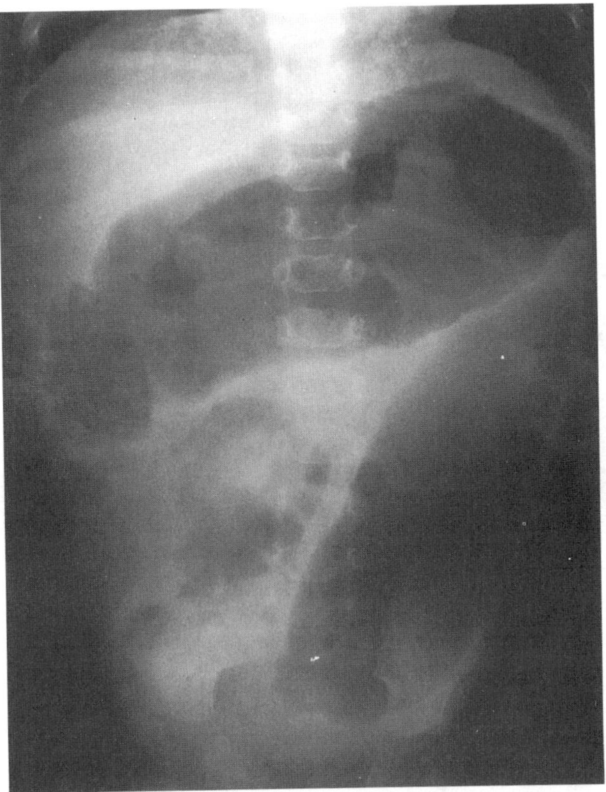

FIGURE 29 Strictures resulting from necrotizing entercolitis. A stricture in the distal colon has resulted in gross dilatation of the more proximal large bowel.

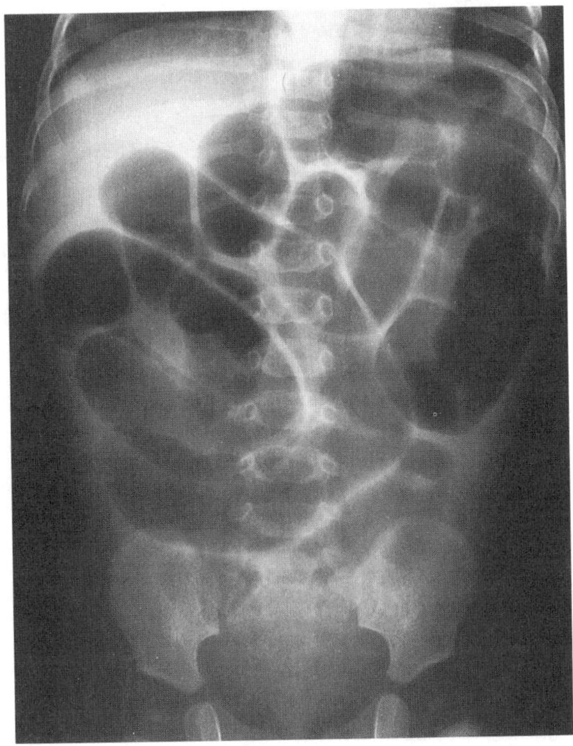

FIGURE 30 Ileocolic intussusception. The presence of dilated loops of small bowel indicate distal small bowel obstruction.

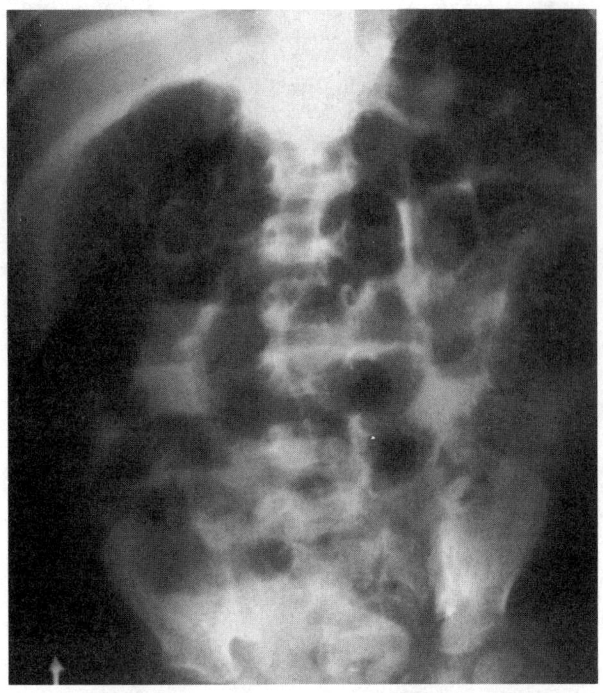

FIGURE 31 Acute appendicitis. There are multiple right iliac fossa air-fluid levels caused by local inflammation, producing localized ileus. (From Stringer.[1])

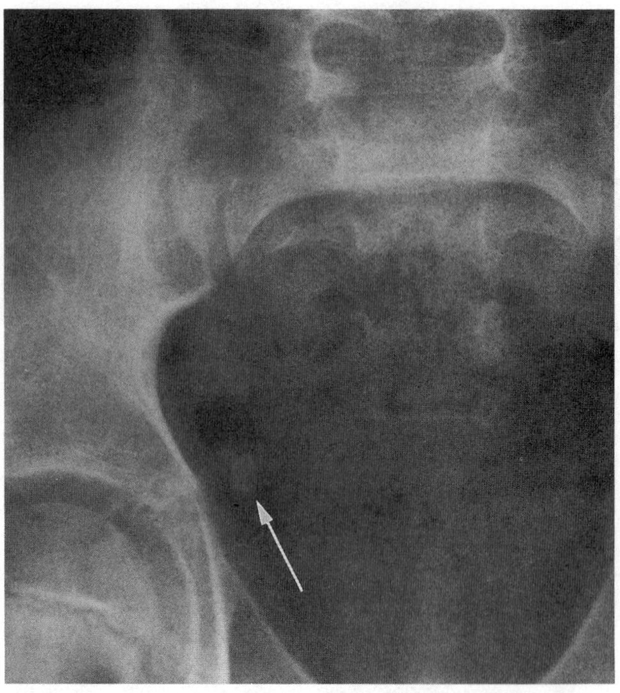

FIGURE 32 Appendicolith in an appendiceal abscess. The plain film shows an easily visualized appendicolith (*arrow*). (From Stringer.[1])

of patients with appendicitis, indicate a higher risk of perforation (Fig. 32). They can occur singly or be multiple and are often laminated.

The type and number of radiologic findings are influenced by the position of the appendix and age of the patient. Those with atypical appendiceal position and younger patients often demonstrate a multiplicity of findings because of the delay in diagnosis.[39–41] Sonography has been used increasingly, not only to demonstrate appendiceal abscesses but also to differentiate the inflamed appendix from the normal one.

REFERENCES

1. Stringer DA. Pediatric gastrointestinal imaging. Philadelphia: BC Decker, 1989.
2. Franken JR. Gastrointestinal imaging in pediatrics. 2nd ed. Philadelphia: Harper & Row, 1982.
3. Kirks DR. Practical pediatric imaging: Diagnostic radiology of infants and children. Boston: Little, Brown, 1984: 536.
4. Girdany BR. The abdomen and gastrointestinal tract. In: Silverman FN, ed. Caffey's pediatric x-ray diagnosis: an integrated imaging approach. 8th ed. Chicago: Year Book Medical Publishers, 1985: 1353.
5. Eisenberg RL. Gastrointestinal radiology: a pattern approach. Philadelphia: JB Lippincott, 1983.
6. Swischuk LE. Radiology of the newborn and young infant. 2nd ed. Baltimore: Williams & Wilkins, 1980: 322.
7. Swischuk LE. Emergency radiology of the acutely ill or injured child. 2nd ed. Baltimore: Williams & Wilkins, 1986: 154.
8. Singleton EB. Gastrointestinal tract. In: Margulis AR, Burhenne HJ, eds. Alimentary tract radiology. 3rd ed. St. Louis: CV Mosby, 1983: 1961.
9. Rabinowitz JG. Pediatric radiology. Philadelphia: JB Lippincott, 1978: 49.
10. Singleton EB, Wagner ML. The acute abdomen in the pediatric age group. Semin Roentgenol 1973, 8:339–356.
11. Maglinte DDT. The small bowel: Anatomy and examination techniques. In: Taveras JM, Ferrucci JT, eds. Radiology—diagnosis—imaging—intervention. Vol 4. Philadelphia: JB Lippincott, 1989.
12. Patriquin HB, Fisch C, Bureau M, Black R. Radiologically visible fecal gas patterns in "normal" newborns and young infants. Pediatr Radiol 1984; 14:87–90.
13. Rice RP. The plain film of the abdomen. In: Taveras JM, Ferrucci JT, eds. Radiology—diagnosis—imaging—intervention. Vol 4. Philadelphia: JB Lippincott, 1989: 1.
14. Swischuk LE. Differential diagnosis in pediatric radiology. Baltimore: Williams & Wilkins, 1984: 129.
15. Keats TE. Atlas of normal roentgen variants that may simulate disease. 4th ed. Chicago: Year Book Medical Publishers, 1984: 753.
16. Schwartz SS. The differential diagnosis of intestinal obstruction. Semin Roentgenol 1973; 8:323–338.
17. Pan EY, Chen LY, Yang JZ, Lee Z, Wang ZZ. Radiographic diagnosis of meconium peritonitis. A report of 200 cases including six fetal cases. Pediatr Radiol 1983; 13:199–205.
18. Johnson JF, Dean BL. Hirschsprung's disease coexisting with colonic atresia. Pediatr Radiol 1981; 11:97–98.
19. Hiller HG, McDonald P. Neonatal Hirschsprung's disease. In: Kaufman HJ, ed. Progress in pediatric radiology. Vol 2. Chicago: Year Book Medical Publishers 1969: 340.
20. Odita JC, Omene JA, Okolo AA. Gastric distension in neonatal necrotising entercolitis. Pediatr Radiol 1987; 17:202–205.
21. Miyake T, Kawamori J, Yoshida T, Nakano H, Kohno S, Ohba S. Small bowel pseudo-obstruction in Kawasaki disease. Pediatr Radiol 1987; 17:383–386.
22. Taylor GA, Nancarrow PA, Hernanz-Schulman M, Teele RL. Plain abdominal radiographs in children with inflammatory bowel disease. Pediatr Radiol 1986; 16:206–209.
23. Eklöf O. Abdominal plain film diagnosis in infants and children. In: Kaufman HJ, ed. Progress in pediatric radiology. Vol 2. Chicago: Year Book Medical Publishers, 1969: 3.
24. Eklöf O. Roentgenological aspects of ulcerative colitis. In: Kaufman HJ, ed. Progress in pediatric radiology. Vol 2. Chicago: Year Book Medical Publishers, 1969: 374.
25. Griscom NT, Capitanio MA, Wagoner NL, Culham G, Morris L. The

visibly fatty liver. Radiology 1975; 117:385–389.
26. Ring EJ, Eaton SB Jr, Ferrucci JT, Short WF. Differential diagnosis of pancreatic calcification. AJR 1973; 117:446–452.
27. Miller WT Jr, Greenan TJ, Miller WT. The solitary teardrop: Sign of an appendicolith. AJR 1988; 151:1252.
28. Alexander WJ, Kadish JA, Dunbar JS. Ingested foreign bodies in children. In: Kaufman HJ, ed. Progress in pediatric radiology. Vol 2. Chicago: Year Book Medical Publishers, 1969: 256.
29. Franken EA Jr. Ascites in infants and children: roentgen diagnosis. Radiology 1972; 102:393–398.
30. Griscom NT, Colodny AH, Rosenberg HK, Fliegel CP, Hardy BE. Diagnostic aspects of neonatal ascites: Report of 27 cases. AJR 1977; 128:961–970.
31. Wiot JF, Benton C, McAlister WH. Postoperative pneumoperitoneum in children. Radiology 1967; 89:285–288.
32. Svartholm F, Zwetnow N. Resorption of postoperative pneumoperitoneum in children. Acta Radiol (Diagn) 1969; 8:514–518.
33. Daneman A, Woodward S, de Silva M. The radiology of neonatal necrotizing enterocolitis (NEC): A review of 47 cases and the literature. Pediatr Radiol 1978; 7:70–77.
34. Virjee J, Somers S, DeSa D, Stevenson G. Changing patterns of neonatal necrotizing enterocolitis. Gastrointest Radiol 1979; 4:169–175.
35. LeVine M, Schwartz S, Katz I, Burko H, Rabinowitz J. Plain film findings in intussusception. Br J Radiol 1964; 37:678–681.
36. Yeager AM, Kanof ME, Kramer SS, et al. Pneumatosis intestinalis in children after allogeneic bone marrow transplantation. Pediatr Radiol 1987; 17:18–22.
37. Frey EE, Smith W, Franken EA Jr, Wintermezer KA. Analysis of bowel perforation in necrotizing enterocolitis. Pediatr Radiol 1987; 17:380–382.
38. Eklöf O, Hartelius H. Reliability of the abdominal plain film diagnosis in pediatric patients with suspected intussusception. Pediatr Radiol 1980; 9:199–206.
39. Soter CS. The contribution of the radiologist to the diagnosis of acute appendicitis. Semin Roentgenol 1973; 8:375–388.
40. Olutola PS. Plain film, radiographic diagnosis of acute appendicitis: An evaluation of the signs. J Can Assoc Radiol 1988; 39:254–256.
41. Franken EA Jr. The child with abdominal pain. In: Saskia von Waldenburg Hilton, Edwards DK, Hilton JW, eds. Practical pediatric radiology. Philadelphia: WB Saunders, 1984: 199.
42. Stringer DA. Imaging inflammatory bowel disease in the pediatric patient. Radiol Clin North Am 1987; 25:93–113.

PART 3

Radiography: Contrast Studies

Peter Liu, M.D.
David A. Stringer, B.Sc., M.B.B.S., F.R.C.R., FRCPC

Despite the proliferation of new imaging modalities, such as sonography, computed tomography (CT), magnetic resonance imaging (MRI), and radionuclide studies, contrast studies still play a major role in the investigation of the pediatric gastrointestinal (GI) tract because of their ability to assess luminal and bowel wall abnormalities. The newer modalities, on the other hand, evaluate primarily extraluminal abnormalities and masses. Conventional contrast studies and newer imaging modalities are thus complementary.

CONTRAST AGENTS

Barium sulfate and iodinated water-soluble compounds are the two basic types of contrast agents for the study of the GI tract. For most investigations of the GI tract, barium is preferred because it has ideal radiographic contrast properties and does not usually flocculate even in the presence of fluid and mucus. It is not hypertonic and thus does not lead to electrolyte imbalance or to dehydration, unlike some of the hypertonic water-soluble contrast agents.[1] In cases of aspiration, barium is also less harmful to the lungs than the conventional hypertonic water-soluble agents, which may induce pneumonitis and pulmonary edema.[2] In infants with suspected Hirschsprung's disease or meconium ileus, some researchers[3,4] also advocate the use of barium because hypertonic contrast agents may cause irritation of the bowel, which can stimulate bowel evacuation and mask the signs of Hirschsprung's disease.

Iodinated water-soluble contrast agents are preferred when perforation is suspected. The leakage of barium and its suspending agents may result in severe inflammation of the mediastinal or peritoneal compartments, eventually leading to adhesions and fibrosis. Because of their greater safety, water-soluble agents are also preferred for neonates and infants under 6 months of age.

Both the conventional hyperosmolar water-soluble contrast and the new iso-osmolar water-soluble contrast media can clearly delineate the anatomy of the upper and lower GI tracts of infants; however, these same agents are often unsatisfactory for the radiographic visualization of those of older children with larger body sizes. Gastrografin and other hyperosmolar media can be dangerous because of their osmolality.

For neonates and infants under 6 months of age, radiologists prefer the newer generation of iso-osmolar water-soluble contrast agents.[5,6] If aspirated into the lungs, they are less toxic than barium or the conventional hyperosmolar water-soluble contrast.[5,6] The new low-osmolar water-soluble contrast agents (ioxaglate, iohexol, iopamidol) are also preferred for colon studies in infants because they are available in almost iso-osmolar concentrations and therefore do not cause dehydration and electrolyte imbalances, unlike conventional hyperosmolar water-soluble agents (e.g., Hypaque, Conray, Gastrografin). In addition, the new agents cause less peritoneal irritation if perforation occurs. The colon of the neonate is more fragile than that of the older child. We have found that microcolon is common in our neonatal patient population. Also, a small bowel atresia may rarely be associated with a bowel wall defect.[7] Hence, the added safety of the new agents is reassuring if perforation cannot be avoided. Gastrografin is never used at The Hospital for Sick Children (HSC), Toronto, because of its high osmolality.

The choice of water-soluble contrast material for colonic examinations of neonates and infants is controversial. We have used a variety of conventional and newer iso-osmolar contrast agents over the last few years, all with equally good results. If meconium ileus is the primary diagnosis, we have often added *N*-acetylcysteine (Mucomyst) to the water-soluble contrast agents because its lytic effect is supposed to hasten the passage of the meconium.[8] There is also some debate about the actual usefulness of the *N*-acetylcysteine: Some believe that the primary stimulus for colonic evacuation is probably caused by the distention of the colon by the enema rather than by the *N*-acetylcysteine itself.

Currently, we use a low-osmolar contrast on all colonic studies in neonates and infants under 4 months of age, since most cases of Hirschsprung's disease can be detected with a water-soluble contrast without the risk of compounding an obstruction with barium. In addition, because other conditions may mimic Hirschsprung's disease in the neonate, a water-soluble contrast medium is a safer choice than barium. Unfortunately, the one major disadvantage of the newer low-osmolar water-soluble contrast is its high cost.

In older children, barium is the preferred contrast medium for most colonic studies. If, however, intussusception is the only concern, then air alone may be used as the contrast medium. Most institutions in North America still use barium as the contrast agent for the diagnosis and reduction of intussusception; however, we and other centers have begun to use air only and have achieved a higher success rate than we had with hydrostatic reduction.

SINGLE- VERSUS DOUBLE-CONTRAST STUDIES

A single-contrast examination of the GI tract is based on careful fluoroscopy with graded compression of the area of interest as necessary to demonstrate the abnormalities of bowel contour and motility usually associated with disease.[9] A double-contrast examination of the GI tract relies on multiple spot films of the various areas of GI tract to demonstrate the fine mucosal details to detect early ulceration and tumor.[9]

Because the spectrum of the pathology of the pediatric GI tract is different from that of an adult, in pediatric radiology most studies of the upper and lower GI tracts are performed with a single-contrast technique. There are numerous reasons for this. Double-contrast studies can be performed on children of any age, including newborns, but they do require unpleasant and time-consuming techniques, such as the injection of contrast by nasogastric tube. Moreover, the bowel preparation required for a double-contrast study causes the patient more discomfort because loops of bowel must be distended with gas. The amount of radiation is also significantly greater because of the multiple film exposures required. Children under the age of 6 years are unlikely to co-operate for such a study. Generally, the most co-operative children are over the age of 9 years. Hence, requests for a double-contrast study in children under the age of 6 years should be carefully screened; the single-contrast study is more likely to solve the clinical problem. If, however, a mucosal disease is suspected, then a double-contrast is essential because it complements and correlates well with endoscopy.[10]

RADIOGRAPHIC EXAMINATIONS OF THE PHARYNX

Speech Study

Speech study, which is always performed in consultation with a speech pathologist,[11] is used to evaluate velopharyngeal insufficiency in speech disorders.[12,13] High-density barium is used to coat the nasopharyngeal outline and palatal contour, and the movement of the velopharyngeal structures is then assessed by fluoroscopy in a variety of projections while the patient repeats various sentences selected to accentuate the velopharyngeal abnormalities.[12,13] The results obtained help the radiologist and speech pathologist formulate the course of therapy and may also aid in planning any necessary surgery (such as the pharyngeal flap) to improve the speech.

Feeding Study

A feeding study is designed to provide information about the best method of feeding a child with a major neuromuscular dysfunction such as cerebral palsy. It is a time-consuming study that is not used as a routine test for the investigation of swallowing disorders. The procedure is performed with the patient in an erect sitting position, in the presence of an occupational therapist and the parents or guardians, if possible. Bolus formation in the mouth is assessed by fluoroscopy. A variety of prostheses, nipples, spoons, and nasogastric tubes may be used to feed the patient. Different textures of barium including pablum, and low- and high-density mixtures may be given.

Swallowing Study of the Oropharynx

A swallowing study, which is often combined with an upper GI examination, evaluates suspected oropharyngeal abnormalities in children. A single-contrast medium, usually a barium sulfate solution, is used to examine the swallowing action of the pharynx of a patient who is either sitting erect or lying prone. The oropharynx is viewed so that the lateral projection includes the soft palate, the upper trachea, and the cricopharyngeal region.

Deglutition consists of two parts: sucking and bolus formation caused by mandibular and tongue movements and swallowing caused by pharyngeal movement. This mechanism of sucking and swallowing is complex and rapid. Because it takes less than a second for a mouthful of fluid to reach the upper esophagus, the radiologic evaluation has to be dynamic; static images are rarely helpful.

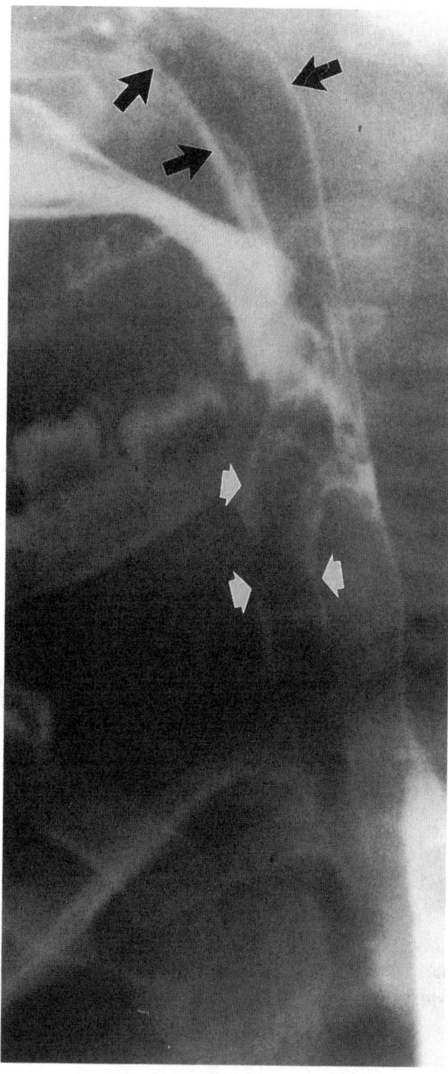

FIGURE 1 Nasal escape and aspiration. Cerebral palsy patient with pharyngeal inco-ordination, showing nasal escape (*black arrows*) and aspiration into the trachea (*white arrows*). (From Stringer.[14])

Videofluoroscopy is the best method for the radiologic assessment because it results in significantly less radiation than cineradiography. A videofluoroscopic barium study is used to assess the adequacy of bolus formation and to detect any pharyngeal inco-ordination, such as nasal escape and aspiration into the trachea (Fig. 1).[14]

Nasal escape may occur in the first few days after the birth of a normal-term infant, but it is more common in those with swallowing disorders. If it persists after the first week of life in a full-term infant, it is almost always abnormal.

Aspiration is the most serious of the findings associated with swallowing disorders. In crying or struggling infants and children, intermittent slight aspiration during the study may occur, often because of the patient's lack of co-operation. This slight aspiration is usually accompanied by coughing and prompt clearing of the barium. If no cough follows the aspiration, the child is more likely to have respiratory problems related to aspiration. Fatigue aspiration, accompanied by a decreased cough reflex, may develop toward the end of feeding during the examination of premature babies.[15] Repeated spontaneous aspiration from the beginning of the procedure is highly significant and usually results in the termination of the examination.

Abnormalities in swallowing can be caused by abnormal anatomy, neuromuscular dysfunction, or a combination of the two. Anatomic abnormalities include cleft palate, macroglossia, and micrognathia, as well as tumors and diverticula. The more common neuromuscular disorders affecting swallowing include cerebral palsy, myelomeningocele with Arnold-Chiari malformation, and cricopharyngeal dysfunction.

UPPER GASTROINTESTINAL TRACT EXAMINATIONS

The areas assessed in a routine upper GI study, whether single- or double-contrast, include the esophagus, the stomach, and the duodenal bulb and loop, including the position of the duodenojejunal flexure. The presence of nasopharyngeal inco-ordination and of gastroesophageal reflux is also routinely assessed in this study.[9]

The stomach should be empty for this study: Infants should fast for 3 to 4 hours prior to the study; children between 1 and 2 years, for 6 hours; and those older than 2 years of age, for 8 hours. For most children, a single-contrast study is performed. In an older co-operative patient, especially when inflammatory bowel disease or ulcer is suspected, a double-contrast study is usually carried out.

Single-Contrast Study

A single-contrast study of the upper GI tract, which requires the patient to drink thin diluted barium, permits complete distention of the esophagus, stomach, and duodenum. It reveals any alteration of the contour by either extrinsic masses (such as vascular rings) or intrinsic abnormalities (tumors, inflammation). Motility and gastroesophageal reflux can also be assessed.

Although the examination is usually terminated when aspiration into the trachea occurs, if further assessment of the GI tract is needed, barium can be introduced into the stomach through the nasogastric tube. The examiner must, however, be watchful for the signs of gastroesophageal reflux during the remainder of the study.

Vascular Rings

When clinical signs suggest the presence of vascular rings, the diagnosis is usually confirmed radiologically by a combination of plain films, barium swallow, and angiography. Careful study of the plain chest radiograph generally shows an abnormal position of the trachea and aorta.[16]

For practical purposes, the lateral view of the esophagus during the barium swallow can predict the type of vascular abnormality in a great majority of cases. The frontal view of the esophagus is also routinely obtained, whereas the oblique views do not yield additional significant information.[17,18] For a definite diagnosis, angiography, CT scanning, and/or MRI would be required.

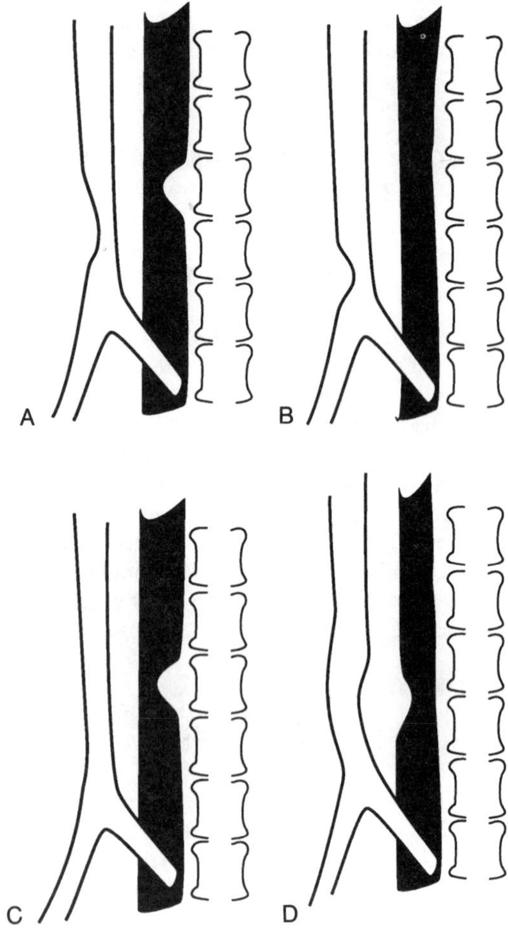

FIGURE 2 The four lateral esophagram patterns. *A*, Posterior esophageal and anterior tracheal impression. *B*, Anterior tracheal impression and normal esophagus. *C*, Posterior esophageal impression and normal trachea. *D*, Anterior esophageal and posterior tracheal impression. (From Stringer.[14])

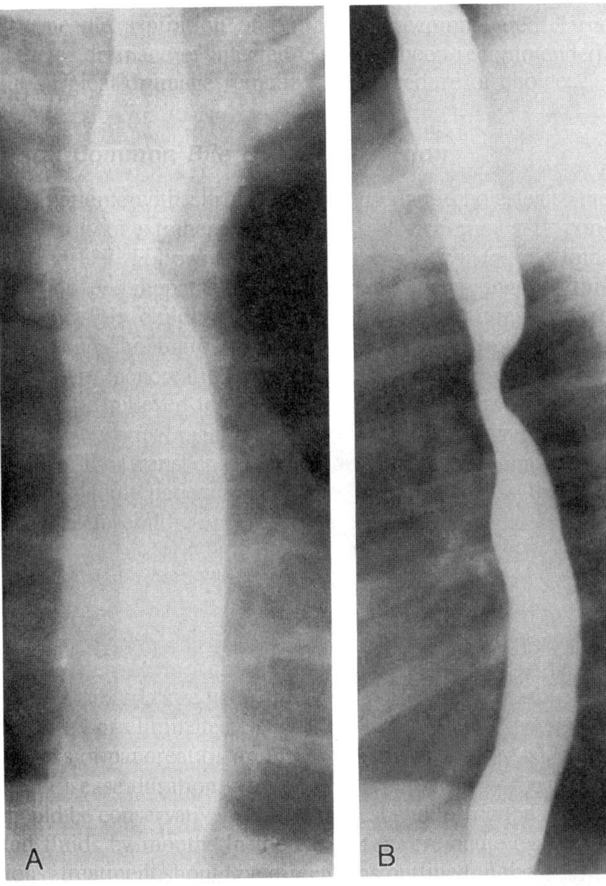

FIGURE 3 Double aortic arch. *A*, On the anteroposterior view, the esophagus is compressed on both sides at the level of the aortic arch. *B*, The posterior impression on the esophagus and anterior compression of the trachea on the lateral esophagram suggest the diagnosis for an 11-month-old infant. (From Stringer.[14])

On the lateral view of the esophagus, four patterns of extrinsic compression may be seen (Fig. 2)[17,18]: (1) posterior esophageal impression and anterior tracheal compression, (2) anterior tracheal compression and normal esophagus, (3) posterior esophageal impression and normal trachea, (4) anterior esophageal impression and posterior tracheal compression.

For the first pattern, the two most common vascular causes are the double aortic arch (Fig. 3) and the complex of right aortic arch associated with a left ductus arteriosus and aberrant left subclavian artery. Although the exact distinction between these two conditions is not possible from the esophagram alone, the double aortic arch appears to be more common.

For the second pattern, the major cause is compression by the innominate artery. The management of this condition, however, is controversial. Many centers suggest that surgery is neither indicated nor curative.

The third pattern is usually caused by an aberrant right subclavian artery with a normal left aortic arch (Fig. 4), the most common true vascular anomaly of the aortic arch, found in 0.5 percent of the general population. The frontal view of the esophagus shows its oblique course, which almost never causes any respiratory symptoms or dysphagia. The vast majority of patients remain asymptomatic throughout life, and no further investigation is usually required. Very rarely, an aberrant left subclavian artery with a right aortic arch may mimic this pattern.

The only vascular cause of the fourth pattern is a pulmonary sling, a condition in which the left pulmonary artery arises from the right pulmonary artery and then loops posteriorly around the trachea before passing to the left. In infancy it may cause respiratory distress, but it has also been found in asymptomatic adults. During a barium swallow study, a soft tissue mass is seen between the trachea and esophagus at the level of the carina (Fig. 5). The mass is indistinguishable from a bronchogenic cyst. Hence, additional imaging studies are needed. The condition may be associated with the tracheostenosis secondary to complete cartilage rings. If the complete cartilage ring–pulmonary sling complex is present, the prognosis is poor, even with surgery.[19,20]

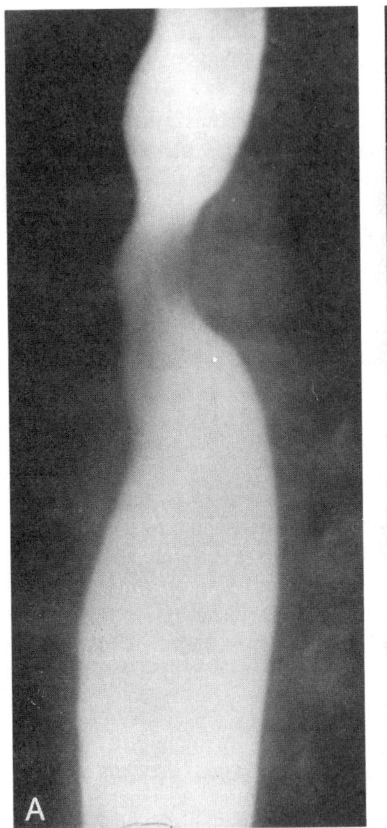

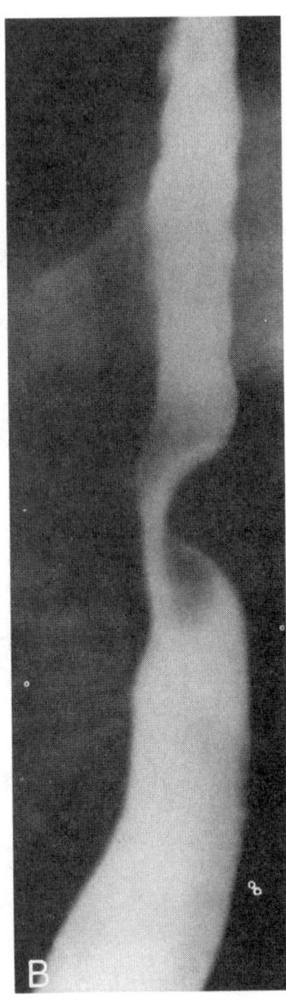

FIGURE 4 *A* and *B*, Aberrant right subclavian artery with left-sided aortic arch in a 5-month-old infant. Esophagram shows a posterior indentation on the lateral view, which is slightly more triangular than the indentation caused by an aberrant left subclavian artery because the course of the vessel is more oblique. This finding is usually asymptomatic.

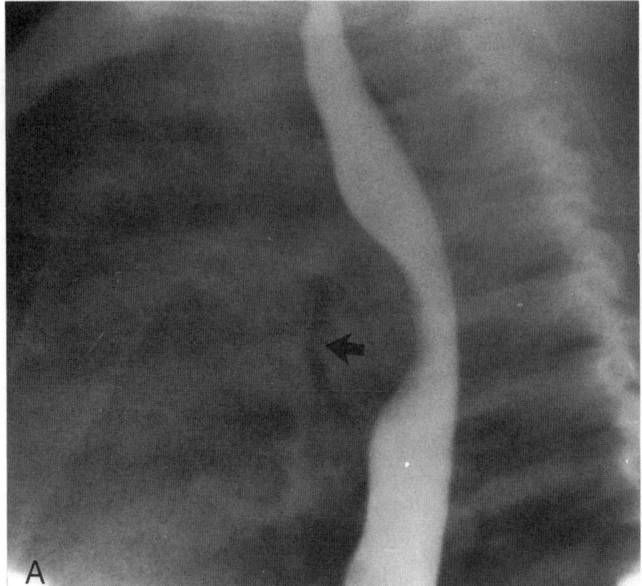

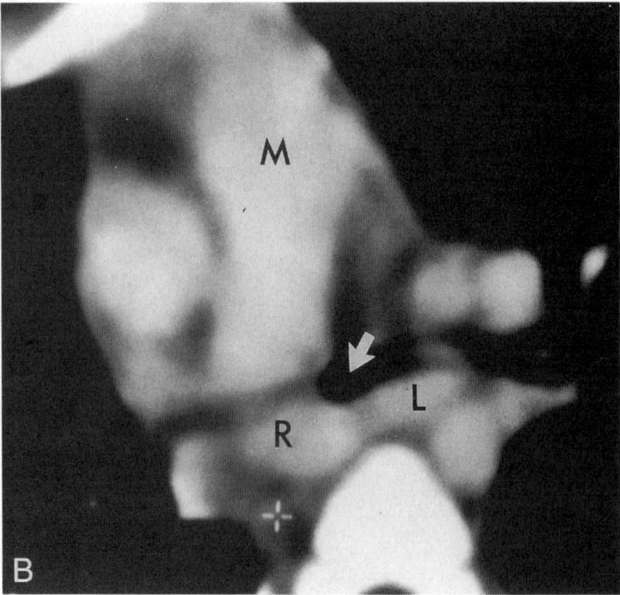

FIGURE 5 Aberrant left pulmonary artery. *A*, A faint soft tissue mass indents the posterior part of the trachea (*arrow*) and the anterior aspect of the esophagus. *B*, Contrast-enhanced CT confirms the presence of the pulmonary sling. M = main pulmonary artery; R = right pulmonary artery; L = left pulmonary artery; white arrow = trachea; cursor = esophagus.

Achalasia

Achalasia is a neuromuscular disorder of the esophagus, usually caused by the absence of myenteric plexus in the lower esophagus.[21] As a result, the esophagram shows disordered motility and an unrelaxed lower esophageal sphincter. The lack of relaxation of the distal esophagus leads to a rat-tail appearance, with minimal periodic passage of barium (Fig. 6). With longstanding achalasia, the esophagus becomes dilated and elongated and fills with fluid and food debris. In advanced cases, these findings may be apparent from plain chest radiographs.

Esophageal Varices

Esophageal varices are best shown in the collapsed or resting stage of the barium swallow when the varices are serpiginous with the multiple round or oval filling defects (Fig. 7).[9] These filling defects are much less obvious with full distention of the esophagus and may be completely obscured by the full distention of the barium column. Most varices secondary to portal hypertension are confined to the lower third of the esophagus.

Hiatal Hernia and Gastroesophageal Reflux

The subject of the significance and role of hiatal hernia and its relationship to gastroesophageal reflux (GER) is still controversial.[22,23] A barium study is the simplest method to assess the gastroesophageal junction and to check for the presence of a hiatal hernia.[24,25] This study also seems to detect most of the clinically significant GER.[26]

The earliest manifestation of hiatal hernia is a tenting or beaking of the gastroesophageal junction (Fig. 8*A*). As the

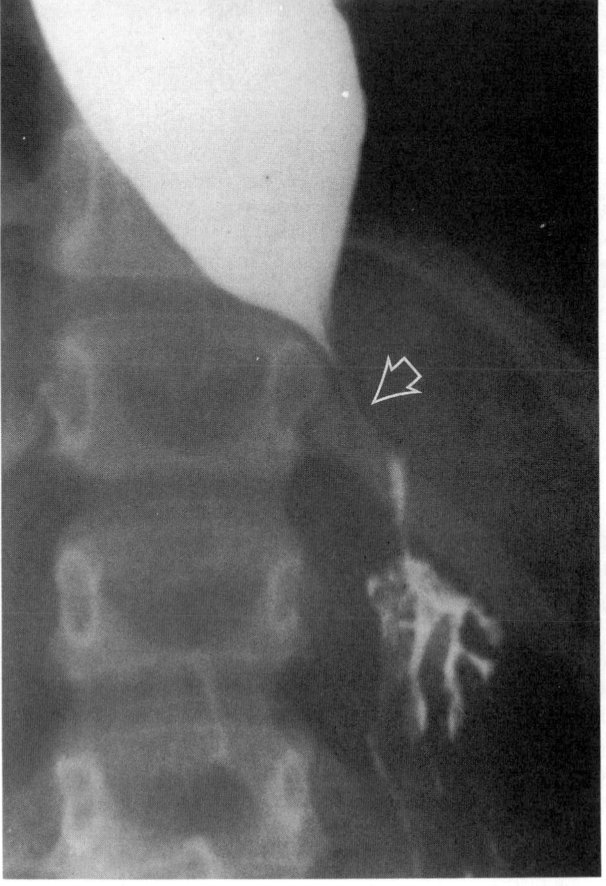

FIGURE 6 Achalasia. The dilated barium-filled esophagus shows characteristic tapering and obstruction at the gastroesophageal junction (*open arrow*). Note that the lower esophagus is the same caliber as the vertebral column.

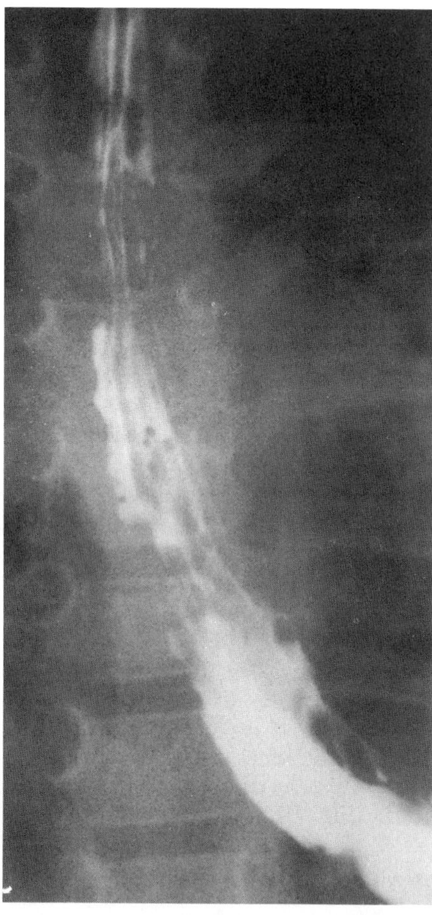

FIGURE 7 Esophageal varices. Serpiginous filling defects in the lower esophagus indicate varices.

hiatal hernia becomes larger, gastric mucosal folds may converge superiorly above the hiatus (Fig. 8*B*).

There is no consensus about the best method of testing for GER with a barium swallow study. The significance of the reflux observed to the patient's symptoms is also not always clear.

A minor degree of lower esophageal reflux is common under 1 year of age, probably because of the immaturity of the lower esophageal sphincter. Reflux is most significant if it occurs spontaneously, if it is extensive, and if it reaches a level above the clavicles in a quiet infant lying supine after having been burped.[26] If spontaneous reflux is not seen, it may be elicited by gently rocking the supine infant or child from the left to right posterior oblique position. Palpating the abdomen and placing the patient in a head-down position, which are nonphysiologic maneuvers, elicit reflux of uncertain significance.

The presence of esophagitis or stricture obviously makes the reflux highly significant (Fig. 9). If reflux or hiatal hernia is detected during the study, particular attention is also paid to the gastric outlet because of the increased likelihood of obstruction such as hypertrophic pyloric stenosis.

Gastric Outlet Obstruction

The causes of gastric outlet obstruction can be divided into three subgroups—decreased peristalsis, abnormal function or anatomy of the pylorus, and other anatomic causes such as atresia, webs, ulcers, or extrinsic mass lesions.[14] Radiology is used to determine whether or not a surgically correctable lesion is present.

Decreased peristalsis of the stomach, which has multiple causes, is often evident from clinical symptoms. If the clinical findings are not definite, then an upper GI study may be

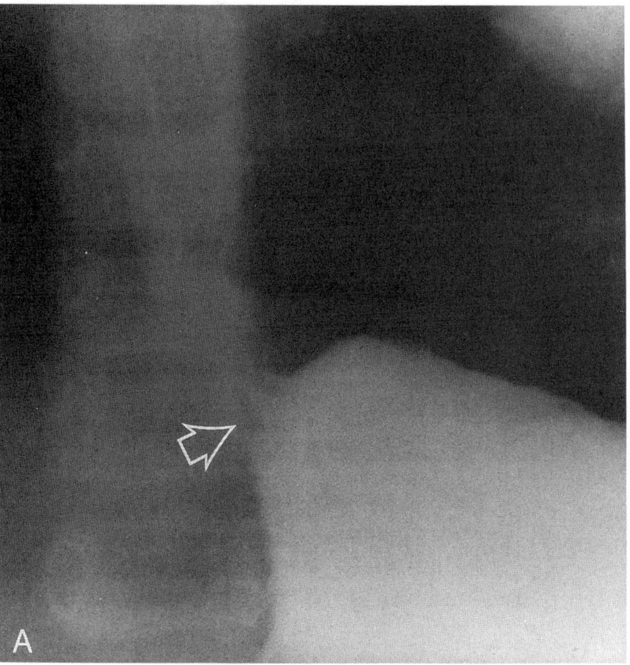

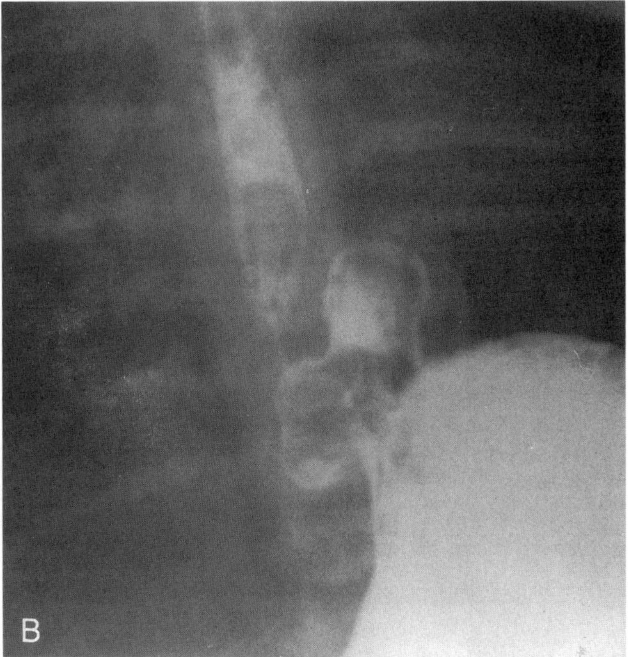

FIGURE 8 Small hiatal hernia. *A*, The esophagogastric junction is tented with converging gastric folds entering the hiatus (*arrow*), the earliest sign of hiatal hernia. *B*, A small part of the stomach has herniated superior to the diaphragm in a different patient.

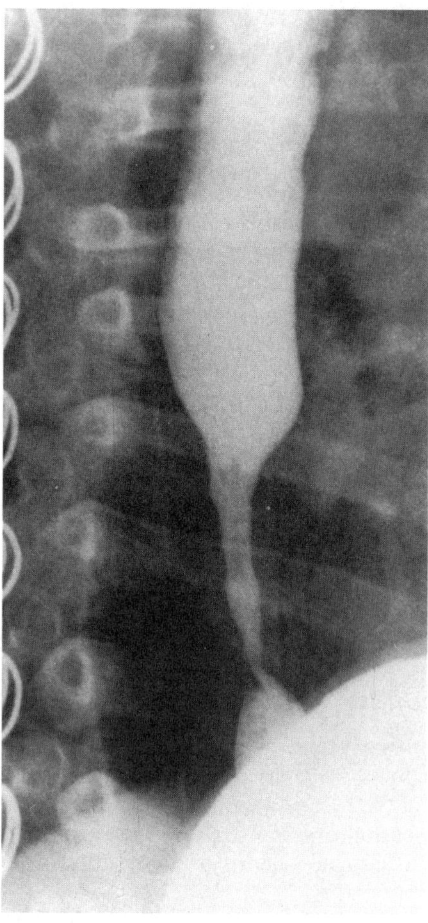

FIGURE 9 Reflux esophagitis stricture. A long stricture is present with gradual tapering at either end and some mucosal irregularity in a child with cerebral palsy and gross gastroesophageal reflux.

performed to rule out any organic lesions. The plain films usually show a greatly distended stomach, often with an air-fluid level, whereas an upper GI study should reveal decreased peristalsis and prolonged gastric emptying. At the end of the study, the barium is aspirated from the stomach to prevent GER and subsequent aspiration into the tracheobronchial tree.

Pylorospasm, which is a poorly defined and self-limiting entity, may present with symptoms of gastric outlet obstruction and should not be confused with hypertrophic pyloric stenosis. A single-contrast study is sufficient for the diagnosis because it shows the delay in gastric emptying as secondary to the pyloric spasm. The narrowed pyloric channel may resemble hypertrophic pyloric stenosis, but as the study progresses, it reveals pyloric opening to a variable degree. If there is still clinical uncertainty, a repeat examination may be done after a few days of medical management.

Because most patients with hypertrophic pyloric stenosis have a clear clinical presentation, the patient may proceed directly to surgery after the clinical assessment. In a small percentage of patients with an atypical presentation, diagnostic imaging can play a role in determining if surgery is needed. Because sonography can clearly show the hypertrophied pyloric muscles and a narrowed pyloric channel, this technique is now the preferred imaging modality used to confirm the diagnosis.[27,28] It has completely replaced the upper GI study in most major centers.

The radiologic and sonographic appearances of hypertrophic pyloric stenosis are similar (Fig. 10). The pyloric channel never distends well and has a constant elongated appearance (the string sign), with a gentle curve that is concave superiorly.[29,30] The pyloric channel often has a double track of barium because of the folding of the compressed mucosa. The hypertrophied pyloric muscle bulges into the distal antrum and the base of the duodenal cap, producing an appearance that resembles a shoulder.[29,30] A pyloric tit deformity may be seen on the lesser curve adjacent to the pyloric mass.[29] Complete obstruction results in a beak sign at the expected entrance of the pyloric channel. The rate of gastric emptying is quite variable but is decreased in all cases.

There are numerous other causes of gastric outlet obstruction. Antral membranes are usually evident in the upper GI examination, but membranes in the prepyloric region may be difficult to identify.[31] Gastric duplication located in the region of the gastric outlet may mimic hypertrophic pyloric stenosis. Sonography is useful in assessing the abdominal masses. The presence of a submucosal nodule with a central niche is suggestive of an ectopic pancreas, a very rare cause of obstruction (Fig. 11).

Duodenal Obstruction

Duodenal obstruction may be caused by duodenal atresia, stenosis, and web; annular pancreas; duodenal bands and malrotation; preduodenal portal vein; and traumatic duodenal hematoma.

Duodenal atresia usually shows a characteristic double-bubble appearance on plain films, but very occasionally a small amount of gas is evident distally in the jejunum or ileum because of gas bypassing the atresia through the pancreatic ducts.[32] Such cases may require a barium examination to show the obstruction. To prevent reflux and aspiration, a nasogastric tube should be used to instill only a small amount of barium, which should then be promptly aspirated at the end of the procedure.

With a duodenal stenosis and an incomplete web, an upper GI study is often required. The findings depend on the degree of obstruction. A web may appear as a linear lucency in the barium column and may balloon distally in the lumen of the duodenum to give the appearance of a wind sock (Fig. 12).

An annular pancreas often produces an appearance identical to that of duodenal stenosis during the barium study but may be detected with sonography or CT.[33] Preduodenal portal vein is difficult to diagnose with barium studies but may cause an indentation on the anterior aspect of the duodenum between its first and second portions. It is usually associated with other anomalies of the GI tract, especially malrotation.

An obstruction may also be caused by peritoneal (Ladd) bands, which probably result from the attempt by the peritoneum to fix a malpositioned bowel. The bands, therefore, are usually associated with malrotation; co-existing midgut vol-

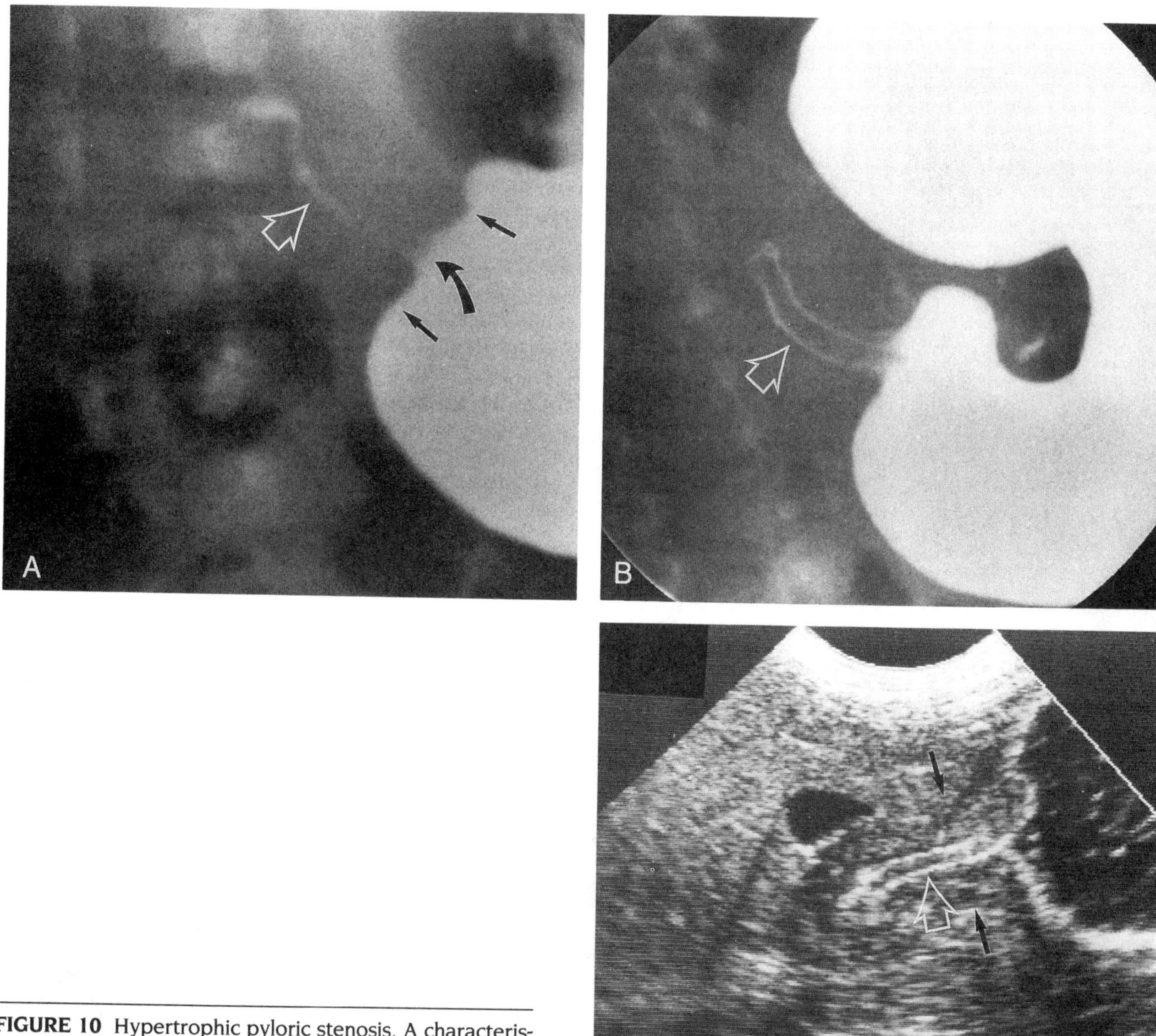

FIGURE 10 Hypertrophic pyloric stenosis. A characteristic single track (*A*) or double track (*B*) (*open arrows*) of barium connects the antrum to the duodenal cap. Other signs include shouldering (*black arrows*) and beaking (*curved arrow*) in the gastric antrum and gastric hyperperistalsis. *C*, Oblique longitudinal sonography shows findings similar to those of the barium examination. In addition, sonography directly shows the markedly thickened pyloric muscle (*black arrows*). Open arrow = pyloric channel.

vulus may also be present. These bands cross and partially compress the duodenum, resulting in the obstruction symptoms. They often arise from the peritoneum of the posterior abdominal wall adjacent to the liver, extend to a loosely attached right colon, and pass anterior to the duodenum. The exact cause of the duodenal obstruction may not be apparent on the barium studies. Surgery is required in most symptomatic patients.

Malrotation and Volvulus

The choice between barium enema and upper GI study for the assessment of the malrotation is controversial. In North America, the barium enema study is preferred, whereas in Europe, an upper GI study is more often used initially. Many North American surgeons prefer the barium enema because they have more confidence in the images, but there may be

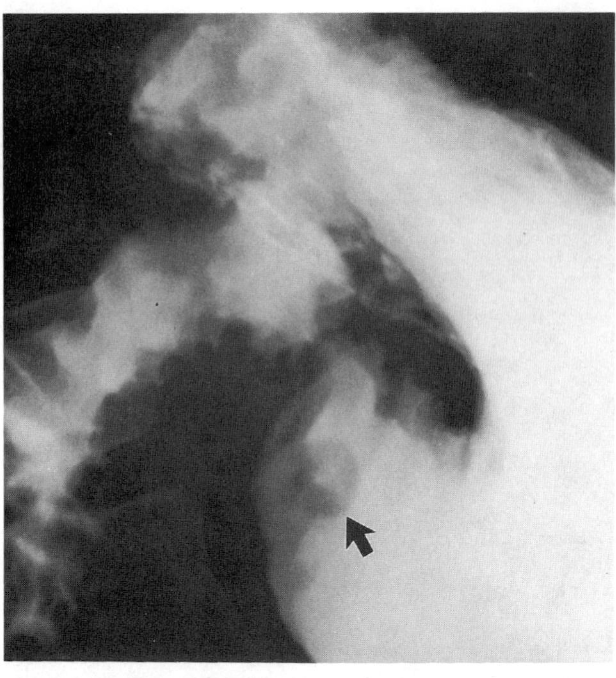

FIGURE 11 Ectopic pancreas. A smooth dome-shaped umbilicated mass (*arrow*) projects into the lumen of the antrum on the greater curvature. The central niche represents a rudimentary duct system.

diagnostic problems that are better clarified by the upper GI study.[34,35] The cecum is mobile in 16 percent of all age groups (Fig. 13), and it can be higher than usual in neonates, especially if it is displaced by dilated bowel loops. The duodenojejunal junction is, therefore, a more reliable indicator of the point of fixation than the cecum.[36] In addition, the large bowel may be normal with an isolated incomplete rotation of the duodenum[37] (Table 1). Hence, the upper GI study plays an important role in the investigation of these patients.

Because there are multiple causes of bowel obstruction, we first use a contrast enema to investigate this problem in infants. If, however, plain films indicate proximal disease, then an upper GI study is performed first.

Problems with the Interpretation of Contrast Studies. The major complication of malrotation is a volvulus of the small bowel around the superior mesenteric artery. This can be life-threatening because of the complications of vascular compromise and infarction of the entire small bowel. The risk of volvulus depends on the fixation of the mesentery. Unfortunately, contrast examinations reveal only the position of the gut. But because the positions of the bowel and the root of the mesentery are independent, the radiologist can make only an educated guess about the location of the root (i.e., the fixation) of the mesentery. Fortunately, in a large majority of patients, the bowel tends to follow certain patterns for each different form of malrotation, thus offering a reasonable chance for success (Table 1).

If either the contrast enema or upper GI study fails to give a clear-cut answer, both examinations should be performed, because some patients appear abnormal on only one of them.

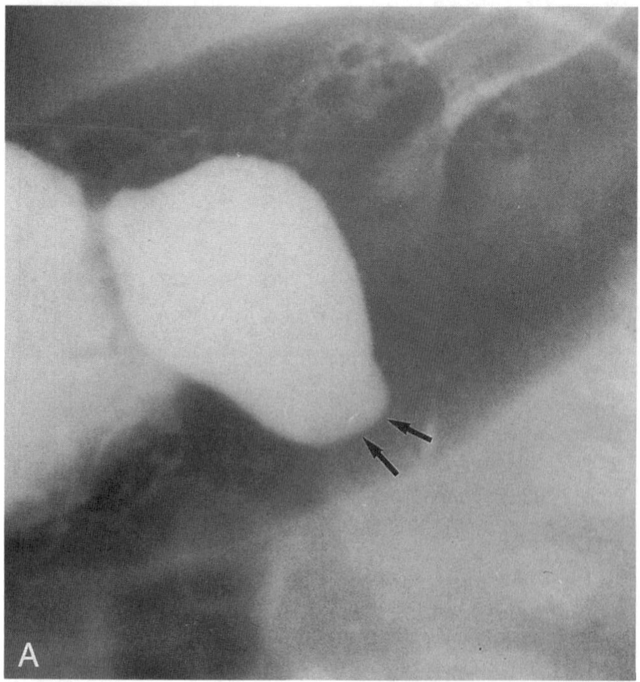

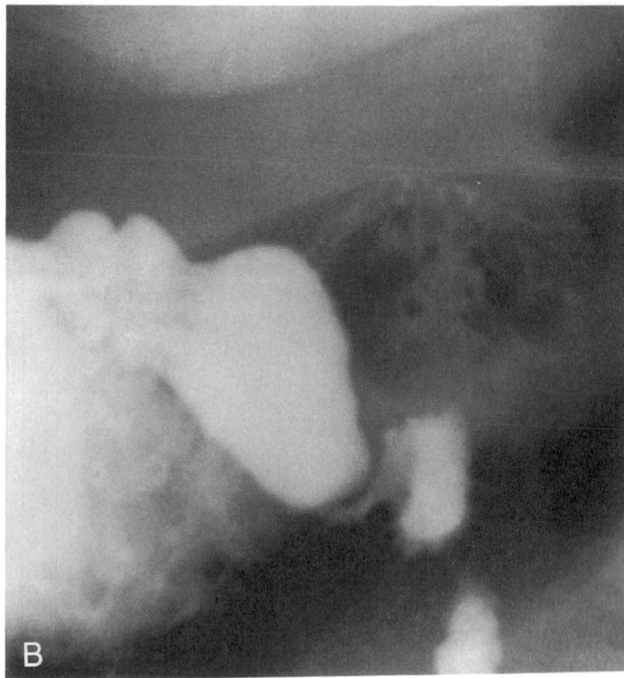

FIGURE 12 Duodenal web. A very dilated duodenum shaped like a wind sock, seen on early barium meal films (*A*), lies proximal to a linear lucency (*arrows*), which represents a duodenal web seen on a delayed film (*B*). A jet of barium passed through the defect in the web.

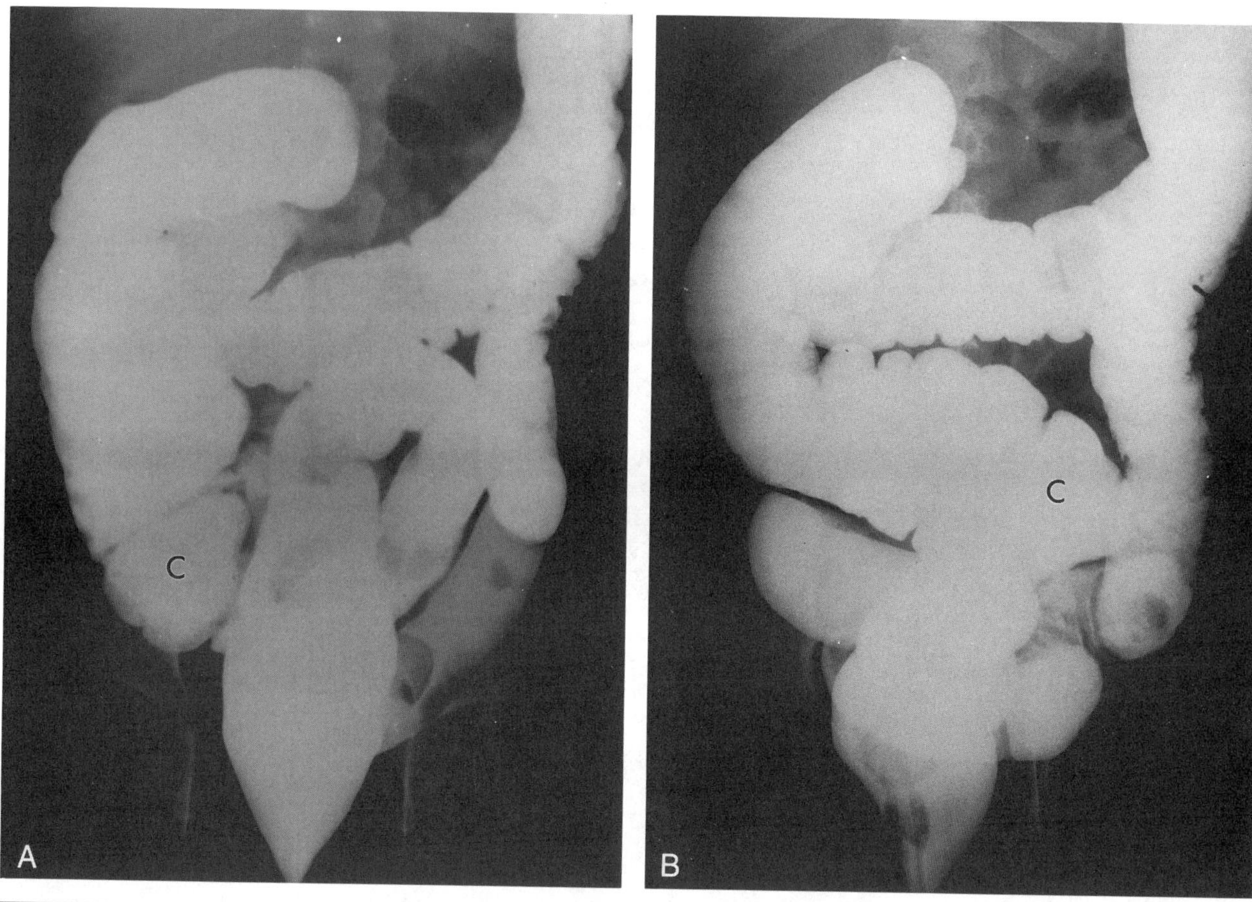

FIGURE 13 Mobile cecum. The position of the cecum (C) moved from normal (*A*) to a high position (*B*). (From Stringer.[14])

If both examinations are inconclusive and there is any clinical concern, a laparotomy is advisable, because a missed malrotation can undergo acute catastrophic volvulus even with minimal preceding symptoms. It is essential that malfixation be actively excluded on every contrast study performed on any child.

Upper Gastrointestinal Study for Malrotation. If the plain films show a complete proximal obstruction in the neonate, then surgery rather than investigation is indicated. However, if obstruction appears incomplete, the upper GI study has some advantages.[14] It quickly and easily reveals the extent of duodenal obstruction as well as the position of

TABLE 1
Radiologic Findings of Major Types of Malrotation

Embryologic Classification	Position of Duodenojejunal Flexure (DJ)	Position of Large Bowel and Cecum
I (nonrotation)	The DJ and proximal jejunum lie on the right side of the abdomen.	The large bowel lies on the left side of the abdomen with the cecum overlying the left iliac crest.
Type IIA (duodenal malrotation)	The DJ lies to the right of the lumbar spine.	The cecum is in the normal position overlying the right iliac crest.
Type IIIA	The DJ lies in the midline, to the right of the left lumbar spine pedicle.	The transverse colon crosses the midline, then doubles back so that the cecum is in the midline.
Type IIIC (mobile cecum)	The DJ is in normal position, just to the left of the lumbar spine pedicle.	The mobile cecum can move from the right iliac crest to the midline of the abdomen.

Adapted from Stringer.[17]

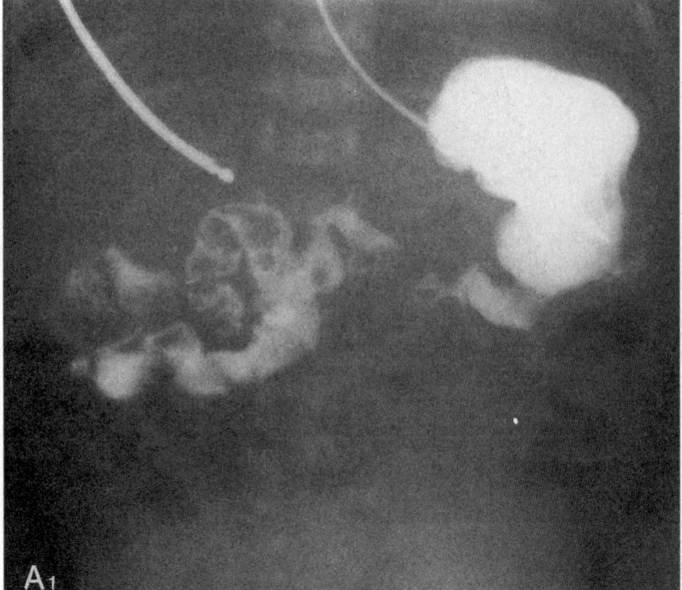

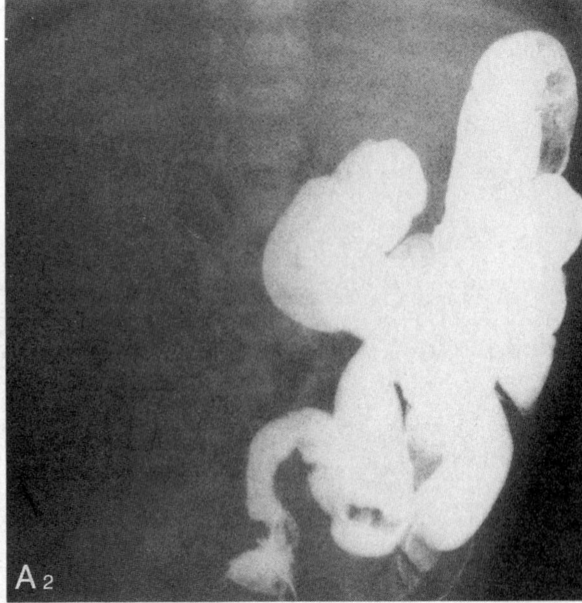

FIGURE 14 Types of significant malrotation. *A*, Type I malrotation or nonrotation: Upper GI study (*A*1) shows the duodenojejunal junction and proximal jejunum lying on the right side of the abdomen. *B*, Barium enema (*A*2) shows all the large bowel lying on the left. (From Stringer.[14])

the duodenojejunal junction (Fig. 14*A*1,*B*1,*C*1). The risk of aspiration is minimal with the use of modern fluoroscopic units and careful technique. Contrast media can and should be aspirated through a nasogastric tube at the end of the procedure.

An upper GI study demonstrates any intrinsic duodenal obstruction, like a web, which is found in 10 percent of the cases of malrotation. Barium should be followed beyond any duodenal obstruction, if possible, since in cases of malrotation and volvulus it is rare for the obstruction to be complete, and the proximal jejunum may be found lying on the right. When volvulus is present, a twisted-ribbon or corkscrew appearance of the duodenum and jejunum may occur, as well as thickened jejunal folds indicating mucosal edema (Fig. 15). If the obstruction is complete in a volvulus, a beak appearance may be found at the site of duodenal obstruction (Fig. 16). Occasionally, the site of obstruction is not beaked but smooth and round, indistinguishable from a duodenal atresia.

Unfortunately, the signs of malrotation in the upper GI study may be subtle and can be missed unless great care is taken. Therefore, if malrotation is still suspected, it is advisable to perform a contrast enema as well.

Double-Contrast Study

Because of the different spectrum of pediatric disease, double-contrast studies are usually less advantageous in children than in adults and are not performed routinely. Double-contrast studies are most often performed in older, more co-operative children if mucosal disease is suspected.[38,39] The patient must drink a high-density viscous barium to coat the mucosal surface of the upper GI tract and ingest effervescent tablets that release gas on contact with the stomach contents to distend the esophagus, stomach, and duodenum.

Esophagitis

Many children with esophagitis do not tolerate gas granules or tablets, so a single-contrast study must be performed. In these patients, the earliest signs of esophagitis are decreased motility, irregular contractions, and spasm.[14] Although a single-contrast study is less sensitive to the early superficial changes, it can show the moderate to advanced changes of esophagitis very well. These later changes include spasm, mucosal thickening and irregularity, shaggy esophageal outline, and deep erosions and ulcers.

In more co-operative older patients, a double-contrast examination, a study more sensitive to early mucosal changes,[14] is performed. Signs of esophagitis include superficial erosions and ulcerations and nodular lesions and plaques, especially the latter if the cause is candidiasis (Fig. 17).[14]

The cause of esophagitis cannot be determined from the radiologic appearances in most cases, although it may be obvious in the clinical setting. However, in the early stages, the presence of discrete ulcers on an otherwise normal mucosa suggests herpetic involvement. Infection is the second most common cause of esophagitis; the most common cause in pediatrics is GER.

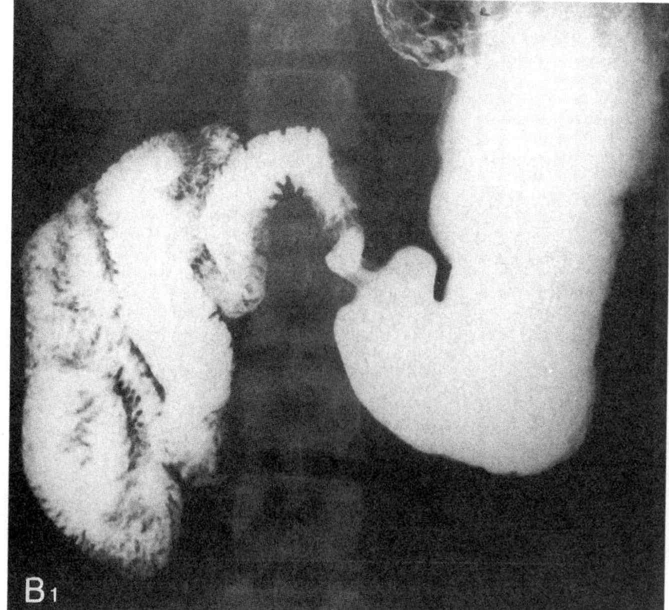

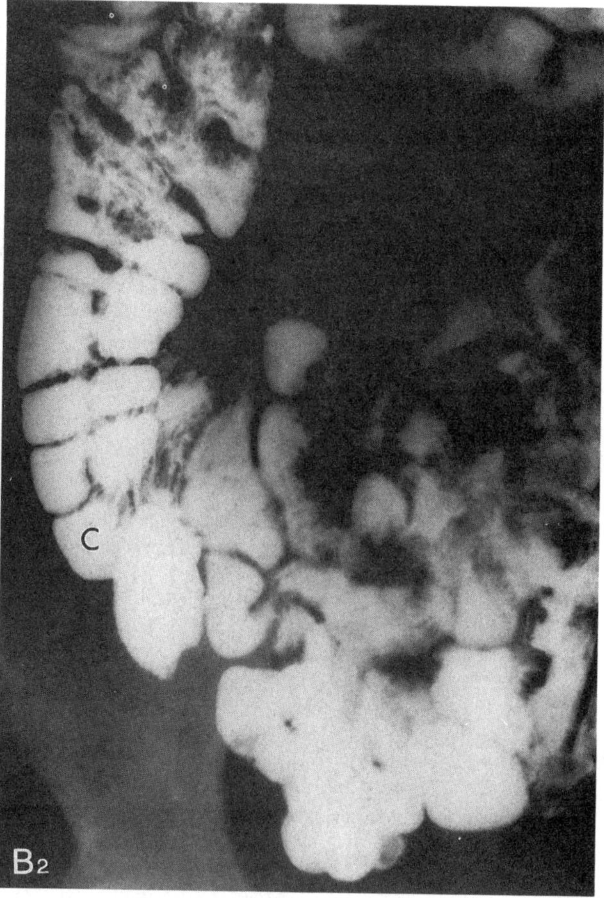

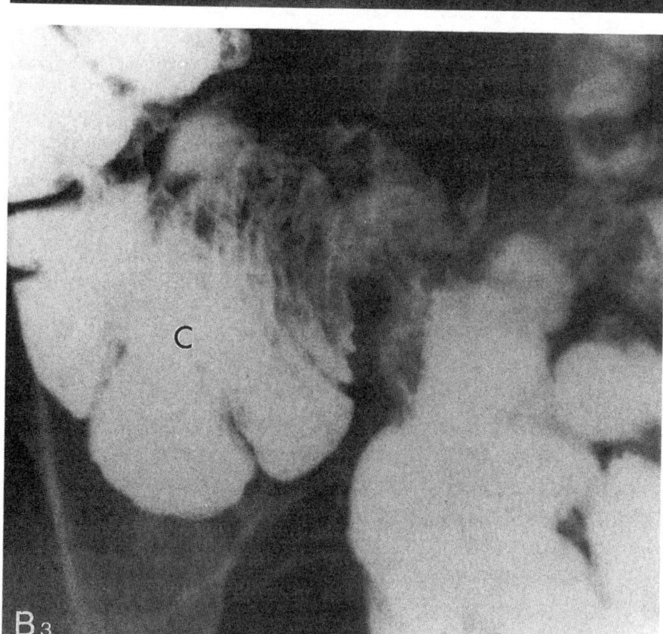

FIGURE 14 *Continued. B,* Type IIA malrotation or duodenal malrotation: (*B*1) On upper GI study, the position of the duodenojejunal junction is to the right of the spine, but the cecum (C) lies in the right iliac fossa as seen on a barium follow-through (*B*2) and spot films (*B*3). At operation, the position of the bowel was confirmed; a volvulus was found in this 13-year-old girl who had only minor symptoms. (From Stringer.[14])

Peptic Ulceration of the Stomach and Duodenum

Although peptic ulcers are uncommon in children,[38,40,41] if gastritis or a gastric ulcer is suspected, then a double-contrast study is recommended; a single-contrast study does not detect these abnormalities well.[41] The radiologic appearance of a peptic ulcer in children is similar to that in adults: The ulcer is most commonly found near the pylorus. In a single-contrast study, the ulcer may appear as an outpouching from the lesser curve of the stomach. In double-contrast examinations, large ulcer craters may fill with a pool of barium (Fig. 18).[14] More subtle findings of these studies include mucosal folds radiating from the central ulcer niche.

The radiologic findings of duodenal ulcer in children are also identical to those in adults; an ulcer crater is diagnostic (Fig. 19).[14] Most patients with duodenal ulcers also have mucosal edema and inflammation of the duodenal bulb. Marked spasm and delay in gastric emptying are often seen in association with the duodenal ulcer.[14]

Longstanding ulceration may result in deformity of the duodenum, especially in the bulb where the majority of the duodenal ulcers occur. However, longstanding ulceration is

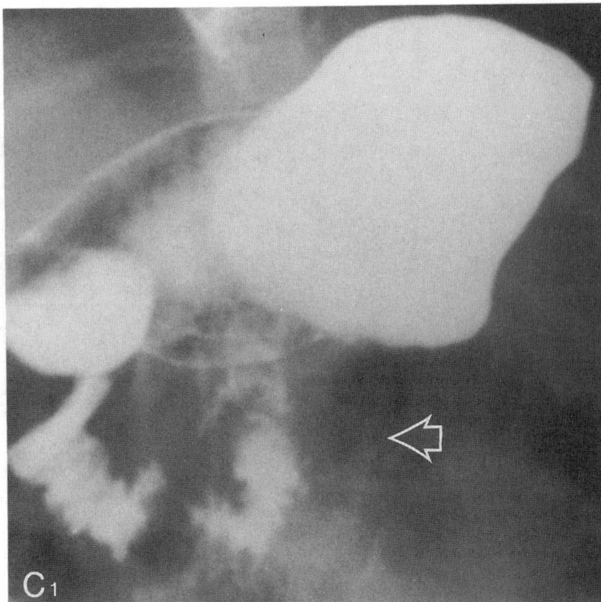

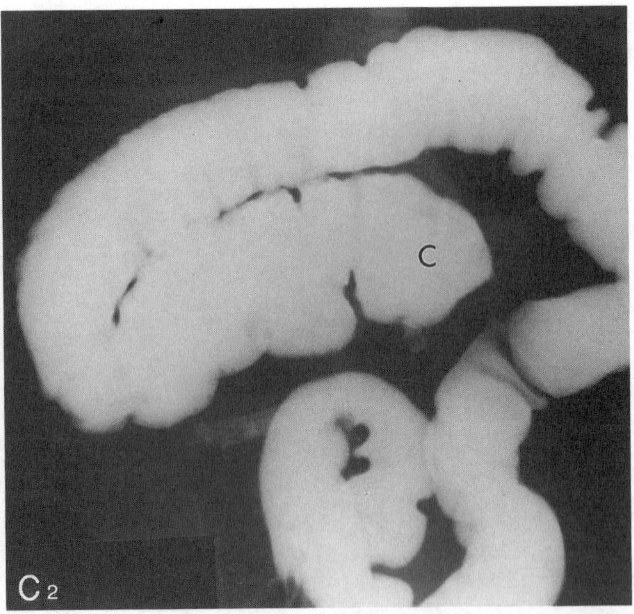

FIGURE 14 *Continued. C,* Type IIIA malrotation with volvulus: On upper GI study (*C1*), the supine film shows the duodenojejunal junction lying in the midline to the right of the left lumbar spine pedicle (*arrow*). This view is the most important one for making the diagnosis of malrotation. Normally the duodenojejunal junction lies to the left of the left lumbar spine pedicles as well as almost as high as the duodenal cap. The barium enema (*C2*) shows the transverse colon crossing the midline but then doubling back so that the cecum lies in the midline. (From Stringer.[14])

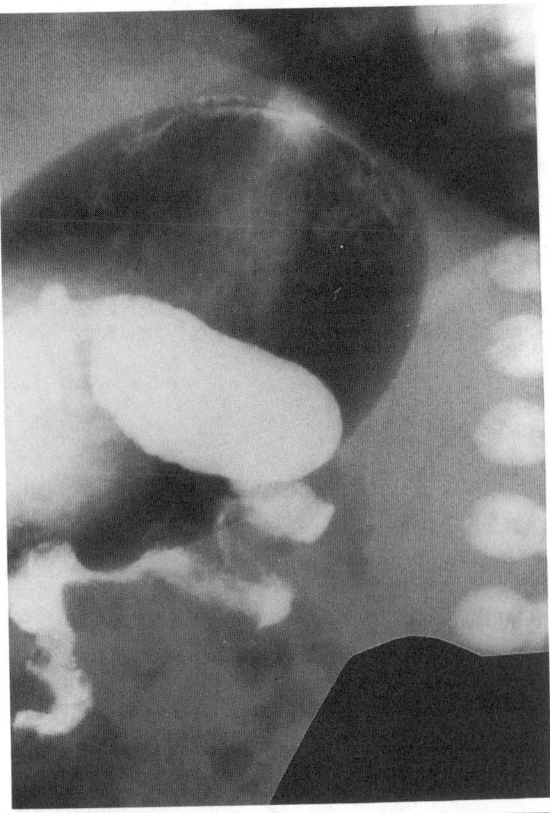

FIGURE 15 Malrotation with midgut volvulus. The duodenum has the appearance of a twisted ribbon or corkscrew. (From Stringer.[14])

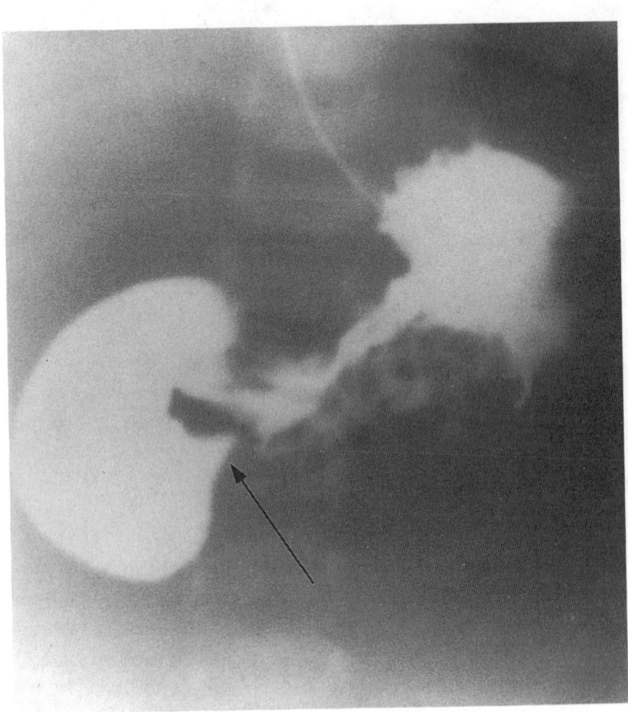

FIGURE 16 Malrotation with volvulus and complete obstruction. The barium has a beaked appearance at the site of obstruction (*arrow*), indicating probable volvulus. (From Stringer.[14])

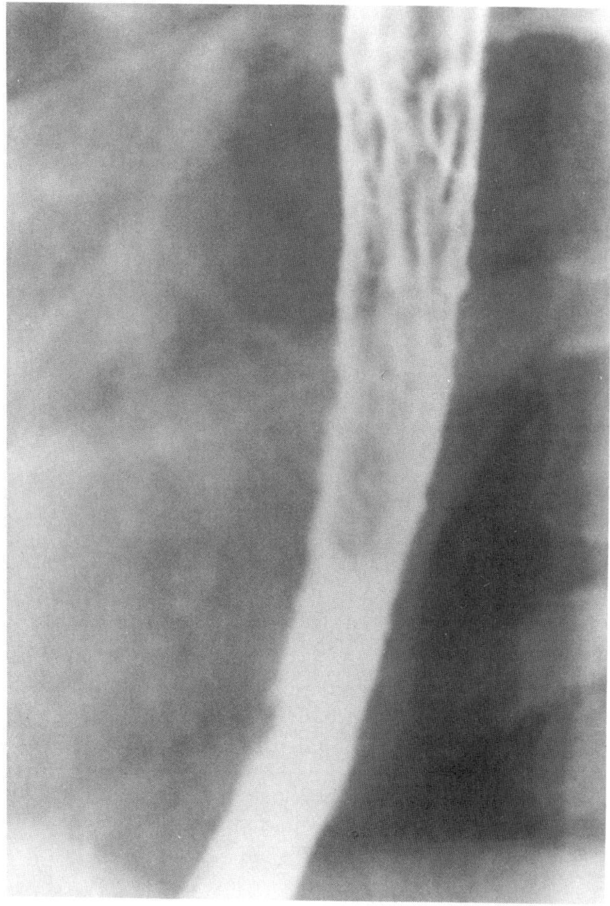

FIGURE 17 Monilial esophagitis. There are raised nodules representing monilial plaques and mucosal irregularity.

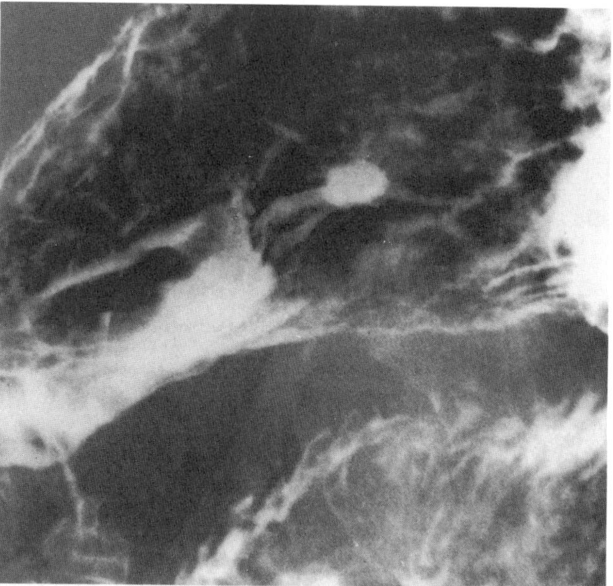

FIGURE 18 Gastric ulcer. A large posterior ulcer crater is filled with a pool of barium on double-contrast examination and shows radiating folds.

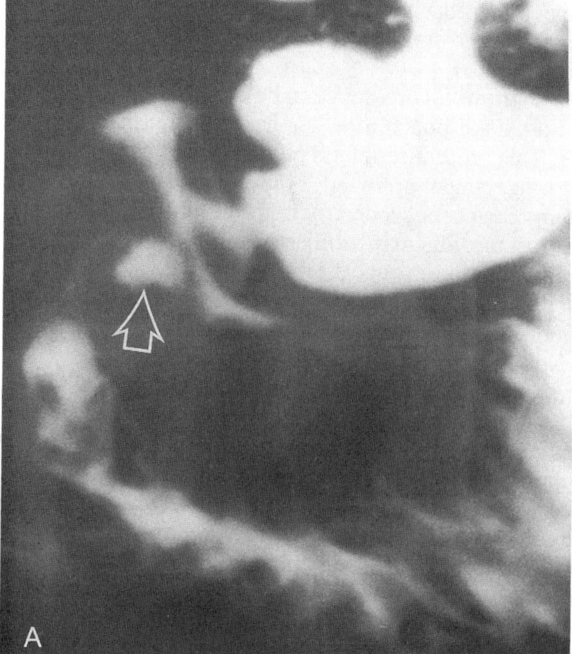

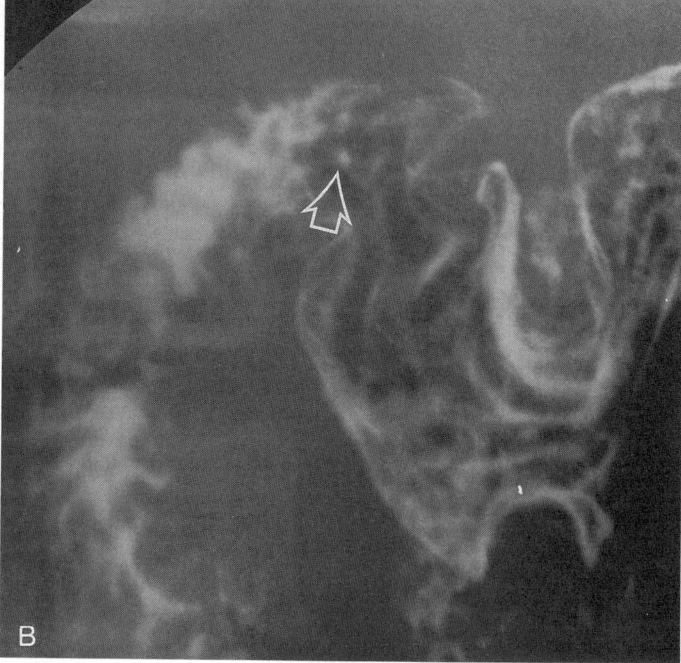

FIGURE 19 Duodenal ulcer. *A*, On single-contrast barium meal there is a large ulcer crater (*arrow*) in a very deformed duodenal cap, indicating a chronic duodenal ulcer. *B*, On double-contrast barium meal, in another patient, there is a small constant collection of barium (*arrow*) lying in a posterior ulcer crater, indicating an acute duodenal ulcer. This acute duodenal ulcer was confirmed endoscopically.

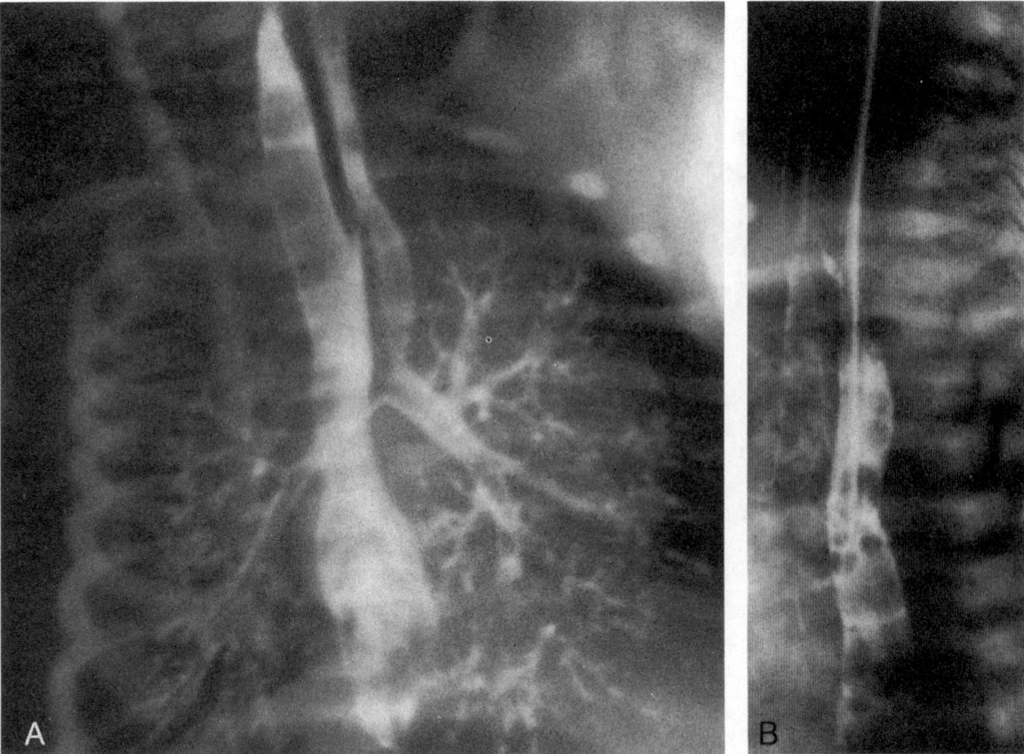

FIGURE 20 H-type tracheoesophageal fistula. *A*, A large fistula passes obliquely and superiorly from the esophagus to the trachea. More of the tracheobronchial tree is filled with barium than is desirable. *B*, A tube esophagram was necessary to fill this smaller fistula in another patient.

unusual in childhood. Perforation of the duodenal ulcer can result in free peritoneal air, which is best detected on the upright or right lateral decubitus plain film.

Special Technique for Tracheoesophageal Fistula

All patients with esophageal atresia present on the first day of life with coughing and choking during the first feeding, a condition that may be associated with cyanosis.[42] A diagnosis of esophageal atresia should be considered if a catheter cannot be passed into the stomach. H-type tracheoesophageal fistula, which usually presents later and may even be found in adulthood, usually presents with chronic or intermittent respiratory symptoms and can be difficult to diagnose if the fistula is small.

After birth, plain films are usually sufficient to make the diagnosis of the more common types of esophageal atresia and tracheoesophageal fistula. After a nasogastric tube is positioned, frontal and lateral radiographs of the chest and upper abdomen show the extent of the proximal pouch and the presence of a distal fistula. A lack of gas in a scaphoid abdomen indicates lack of a distal fistula. If a proximal fistula is suspected, a pouchogram may be performed; if an H-type fistula is likely, a prone video esophagram may be performed (Fig. 20).[43,44]

Pouchogram. Fluoroscopy can be used to delineate the size of the proximal pouch after air has been injected into the pouch. This procedure should be carried out with heart rate monitoring, since profound bradycardia and respiratory problems can occur secondary to the esophageal distention.

Contrast medium may be injected into the proximal pouch through the nasoesophageal tube to eliminate a diagnosis of proximal fistula. After the pouch is filled, the barium should be removed through the nasoesophageal tube by prompt suction. However, we have not found that this technique is generally necessary. The rare proximal fistula in the chest will be found intraoperatively. Fluoroscopy is necessary to prevent the patient from aspirating the barium. Water-soluble bronchographic media may also be used, but barium or the new low-osmolar contrast media are preferable.

Prone Video Esophagram. When a routine barium swallow fails to demonstrate the communication, a prone esophagram with barium injected through a tube may be performed to assess specifically for the presence of a tracheoesophageal fistula (Fig. 21).[43,44] The patient remains in a prone position for this special test.[9,14,44] A nasogastric tube is placed in the esophagus, and barium is injected through this tube to achieve maximal distention of the esophagus.

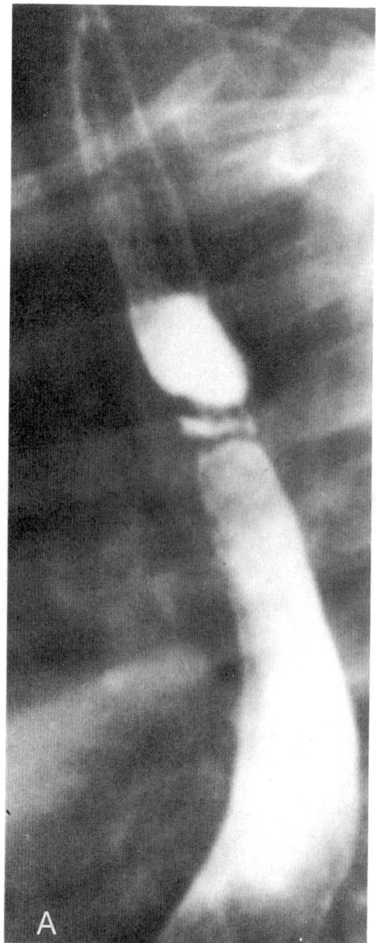

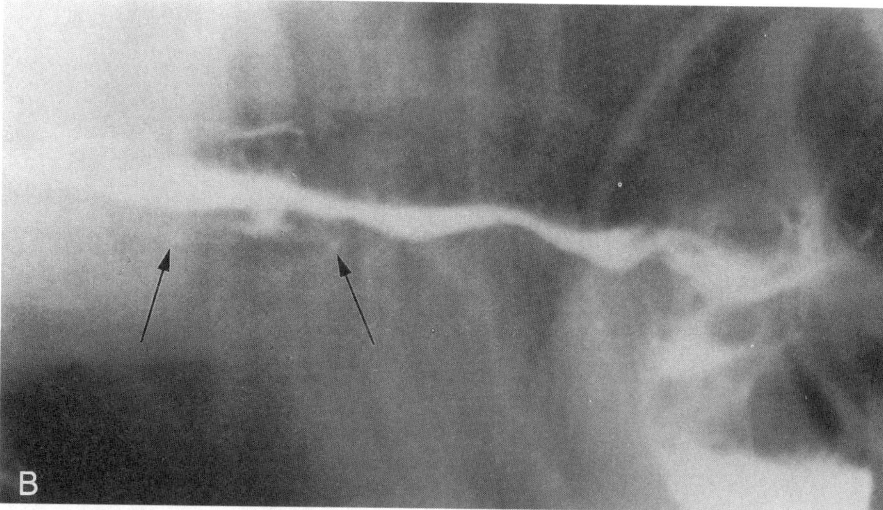

FIGURE 21 Recurrent tracheoesophageal fistula. *A*, A barium swallow shows a beak at the site of the repair of an esophageal atresia and tracheoesophageal fistula, but no fistula was seen. *B*, A subsequent prone video esophagram shows a recurrent fistula that could not be demonstrated by other techniques. Faint traces of barium are evident in the trachea (*arrows*).

SMALL BOWEL EXAMINATION (JEJUNUM AND ILEUM)

The small bowel can be examined by a follow-through examination or by a small bowel enema (enteroclysis).[45,46] Small bowel follow-through findings can be supplemented by a peroral pneumocolon[45,46] or a subsequent double-contrast barium enema.

Small Bowel Follow-Through Technique

The small bowel follow-through examination may be performed as the only examination of the GI tract if the small bowel is the only area of clinical concern. But this study is usually performed immediately after a single-contrast upper GI study. It should not follow a double-contrast study, since the high-density barium and gas degrade the images of the small bowel. The patient is asked to drink a large quantity of barium (at least two 16-oz cups if the patient is older than 10 years) so that all the small bowel loops can be filled with a single-contrast column of barium. Overhead radiographs are taken about every 30 minutes until the barium has reached the right side of the colon. Spot films of the terminal ileum and the ileocecal valve are obtained routinely under fluoroscopic control. If any area appears abnormal on the overhead films, further spot films of these areas are also obtained.

Of all the small bowel examinations, the conventional small bowel follow-through most closely approximates the natural peristalsis and morphology of the small bowel. The small bowel caliber may be best assessed with this study because it is not distorted by the barium pressure as it is in the small bowel enema. Partial mechanical obstruction may be more evident from the small bowel follow-through study.

The disadvantage of this technique is that the entire small bowel may not be distended adequately, causing problems with the interpretation of the results. For instance, an area of limited distensibility of the small bowel may be normal; the apparent narrowing may simply be caused by peristalsis. However, spasm and actual narrowing of this area are other possibilities. Usually the series of films obtained with a small bowel follow-through and additional spot films of the area of concern help to clarify any uncertainties.

The appearance of the small bowel pattern is much more variable in children than in adults. Hence malabsorption may be difficult to assess on the basis of a small bowel follow-

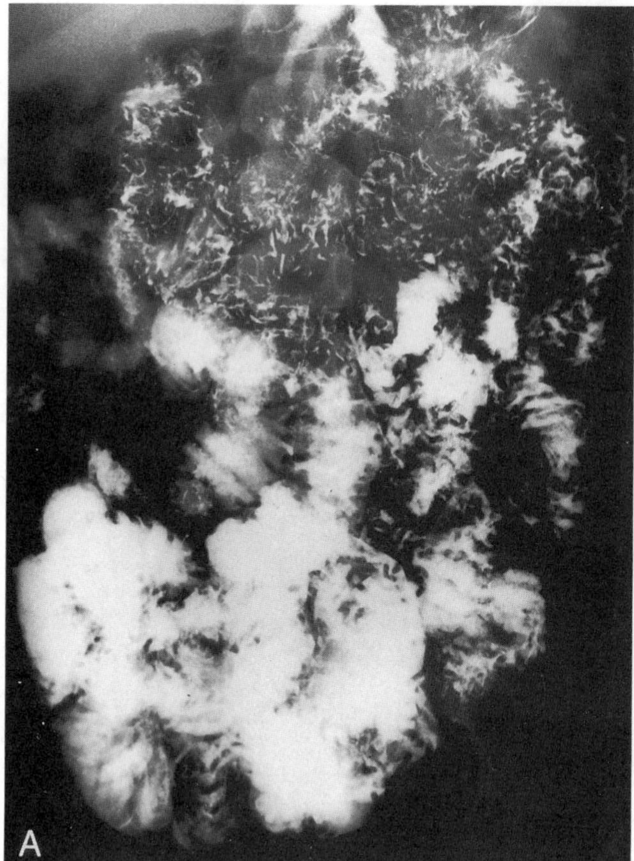

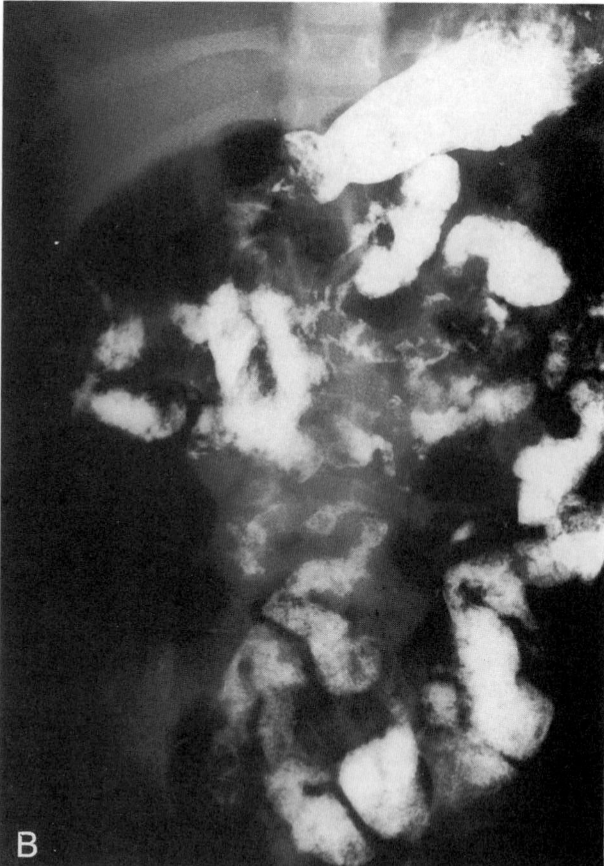

FIGURE 22 Malabsorption pattern. Both patients have segmentation, flocculation, and mild bowel dilatation, a nonspecific malabsorption pattern. *A*, Celiac disease. The mucosal biopsy was abnormal, and biochemically proven malabsorption was present with a high fecal fat excretion. *B*, Failure to thrive due to poor intake. Small bowel biopsy was normal, and there was no biochemical evidence of malabsorption. The patient thrived when given an adequate diet. (From Stringer.[14])

through alone (Fig. 22).[47] Small bowel biopsy is still the preferred study for the assessment of malabsorption in children.

In most cases of inflammatory bowel disease, small bowel follow-through provides sufficient information for diagnosis and clinical management without the need for a more invasive study such as small bowel enema.[45,46] The overhead films and additional spot films usually clearly show the abnormal segments of small bowel. For moderate-sized tumors and polyps, the small bowel follow-through should also be able to detect these abnormalities.

Peroral Pneumocolon

A peroral pneumocolon (POP) is usually performed at the end of the conventional small bowel follow-through to more accurately assess the terminal ileum and ileocecal valve.[45] As the single-contrast barium column reaches the ileocecal valve area, air is insufflated rectally through a tube in an attempt to reflux air into the terminal ileum.[45] This procedure gives a double-contrast view of the ileocecal valve and terminal ileum, providing fine mucosal details and improving the assessment of the distensibility of the terminal ileum (Fig. 23).[45] For example, an area of narrowing in the terminal ileum may distend with air insufflation, thus demonstrating that it is not fibrotic but possibly merely spastic.[45] Questionable areas of abnormality may also be more clearly shown with air insufflation.[45]

In the assessment of inflammatory bowel disease, a well-planned and executed small bowel follow-through, together with a peroral pneumocolon, should answer most clinical questions (Fig. 24).[45]

Small Bowel Enema (Enteroclysis)

Although small bowel enema is the most sensitive test for subtle small bowel disease, it should be reserved only for patients in whom the small bowel follow-through fails to provide a satisfactory study.[46] This test is invasive, requiring intubation of the patient orally or nasally. The positioning

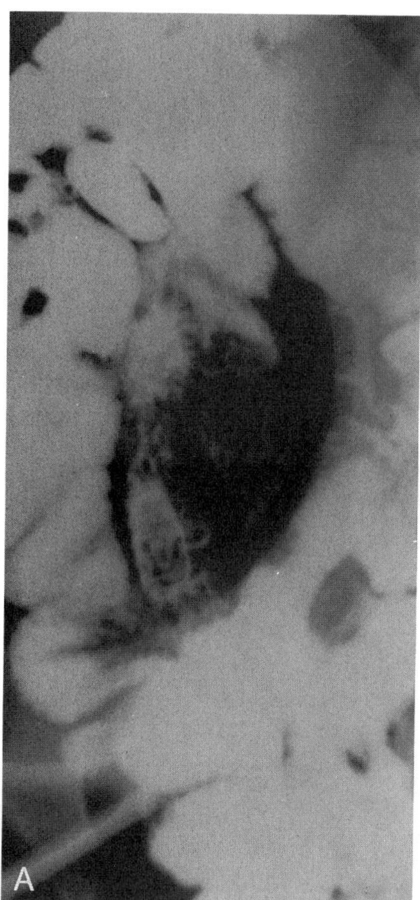

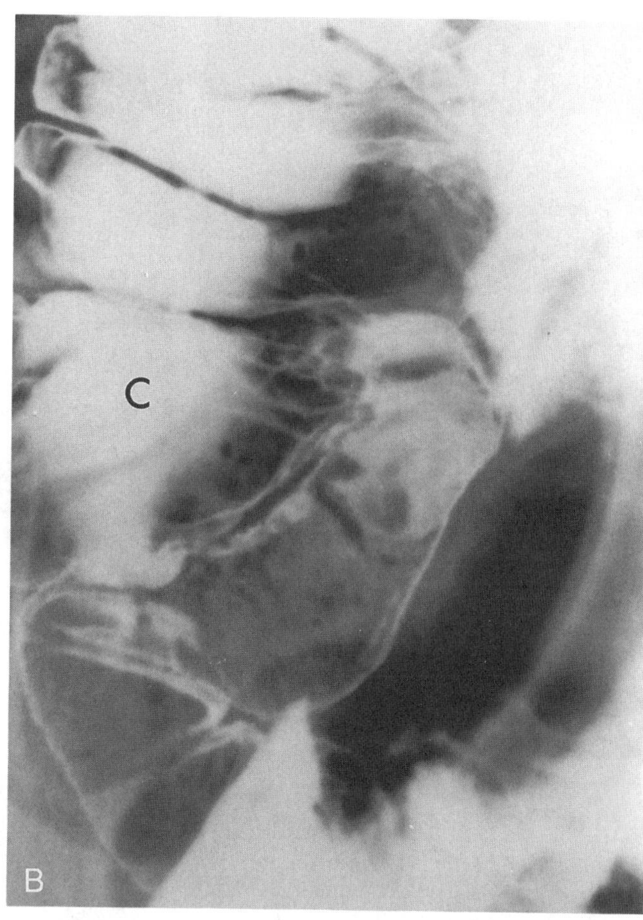

FIGURE 23 Normal terminal ileum on peroral pneumocolon. *A*, The terminal ileum is poorly seen during a conventional small bowel follow-through examination, despite compression. *B*, A peroral pneumocolon performed within minutes of *A* demonstrates a normal terminal ileum. C = cecum. (From Stringer et al[45]; © 1986 by the Am Roentgen Ray Soc.)

of the tip of a long feeding tube in the proximal jejunum to minimize reflux into the stomach[9] is relatively smooth in many cases, but it can be difficult, often requiring extra fluoroscopic time and, in other instances, giving considerable distress to the patient. It is important, therefore, that the child be co-operative for the intubation.

After the jejunal tube placement, barium is injected through the tube to fill the small bowel, followed by an injection of water and/or methylcellulose solution to give a double-contrast effect.[9] Good distention of the small bowel is obtained when the barium is introduced into the jejunum under some pressure. Depending on the size of the patient, the transit time of barium is about 15 to 30 minutes.[9] Multiple spot films and overhead radiographs of the various segments of the small bowel are obtained, including the ileocecal valve.

A small bowel enema is able to show the smaller polyps, smaller mass lesions, and subtle mucosal involvement of inflammatory bowel disease more clearly than the conventional small bowel follow-through; however, it is unlikely to provide significant additional information for the patient's management. If exquisite details are essential and the child is co-operative, then the small bowel enema may be considered after an unsatisfactory small bowel follow-through has been obtained (Fig. 25).

In summary, for most common abnormalities of the small bowel, the small bowel follow-through, especially if combined with a peroral pneumocolon, should be able to answer clinical questions and supply information adequate for the patient's management.[45,46] The small bowel follow-through should, therefore, be the initial screening study.[45,46]

Selected Abnormalities Revealed in Small Bowel Studies

Hemorrhage and Trauma to the Small Bowel

Hematoma in the small bowel wall may be the result of trauma or spontaneous causes such as Henoch-Schönlein purpura and bleeding disorders. The duodenum, which is the most immobile part of the small bowel, is the part most at risk from trauma.[48] Usually a water-soluble contrast medi-

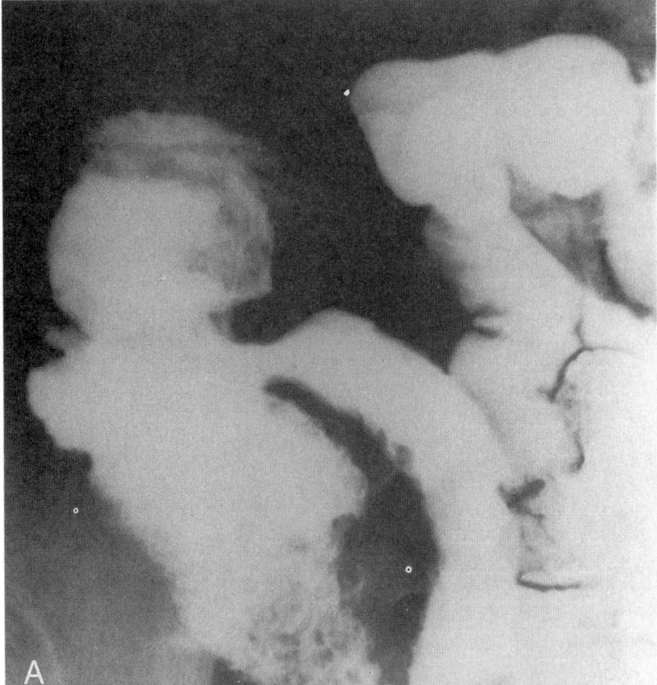

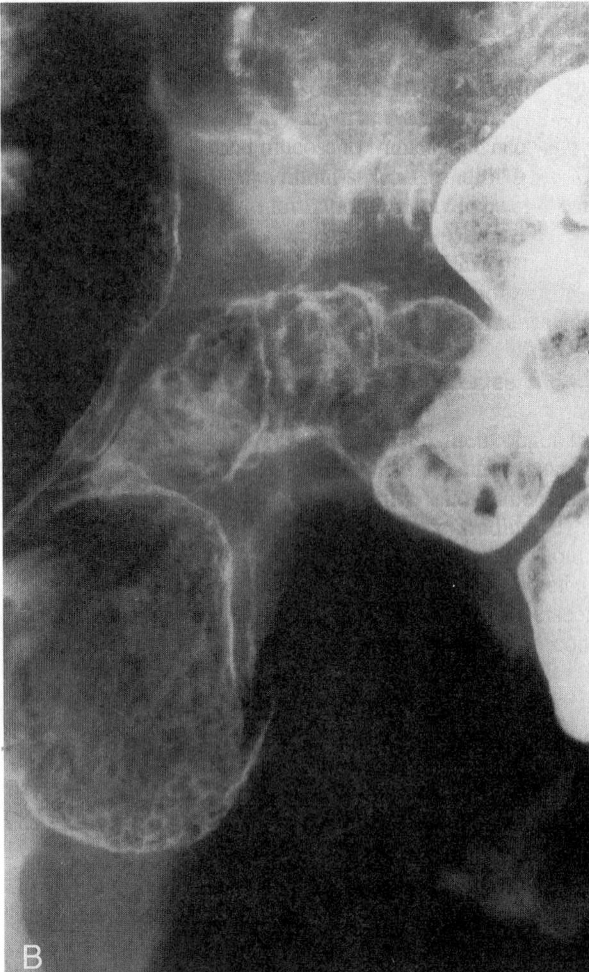

FIGURE 24 Crohn's disease of the terminal ileum. The terminal ileum appeared more rigid than usual on a conventional small bowel follow-through (*A*), and a peroral pneumocolon performed immediately demonstrated extensive and relatively unsuspected ulceration (*B*). (From Stringer et al[45]; © 1986 by the Am Roentgen Ray Soc.)

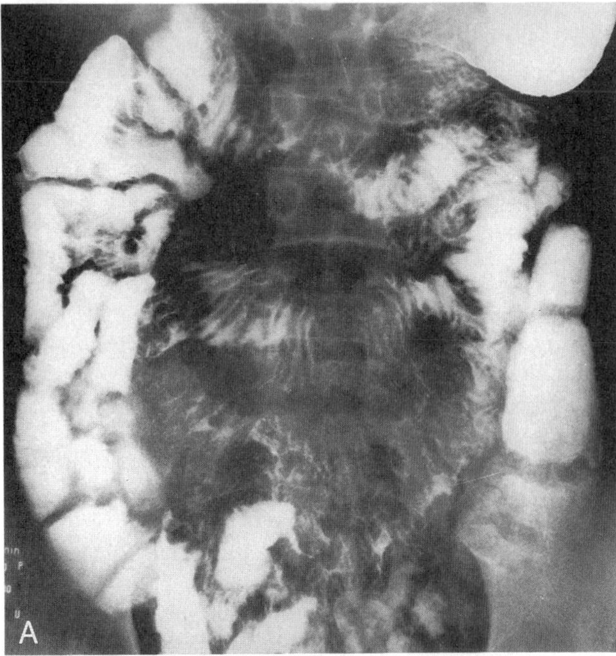

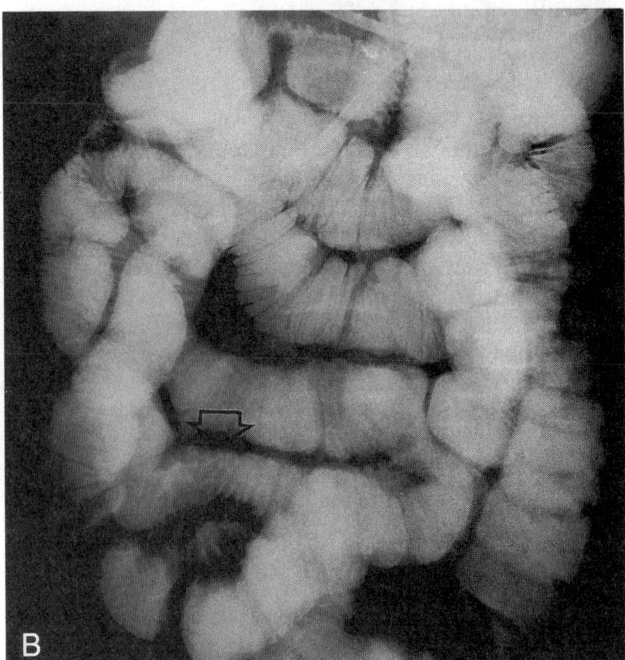

FIGURE 25 Crohn's disease of the mid small bowel. *A*, Barium follow-through gives poor detail of the mid small bowel. *B*, Subsequent small bowel enema shows that the mid small bowel has an area of limited distensibility and irregular bowel wall thickening.

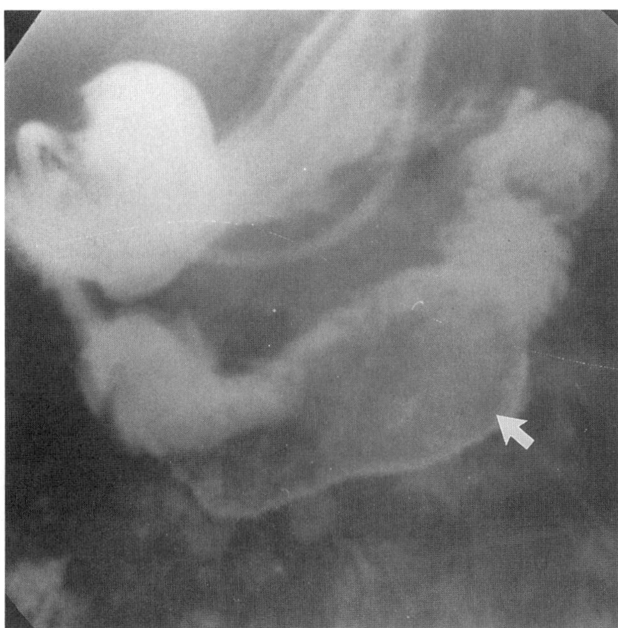

FIGURE 26 Duodenal hematoma. A smooth mass (*arrow*) projects into the duodenal lumen and almost obstructs the duodenal lumen.

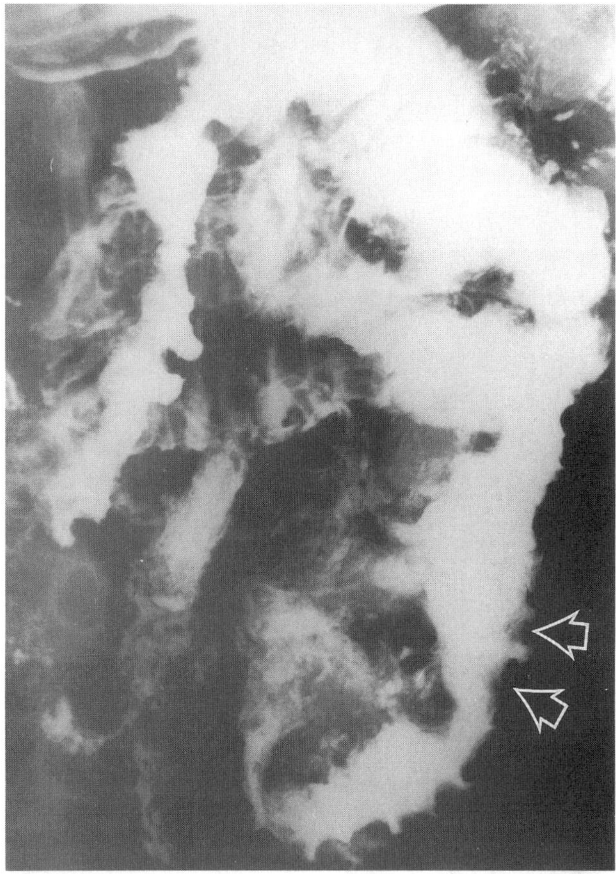

FIGURE 27 Henoch-Schönlein purpura. The small bowel follow-through shows gross thickening of mucosal folds, thumbprinting (*arrows*), and separation of bowel loops.

um is used to assess any traumatic injury to the duodenum because of the risk of perforation. It shows the hematoma as a smooth intramural mass (Fig. 26) and also reveals the thickening and crowding of the valvulae conniventes in a picket-fence pattern.

Hematoma in the jejunum or ileum is more likely the result of other causes such as Henoch-Schönlein purpura. Hemorrhage and edema into the small bowel wall cause a thickening of the valvulae conniventes, making them look like stacked coins or a picket fence in the affected region. In cases of more severe bleeding, gross thickening of the mucosal folds, thumbprinting, and separation of the bowel loops appear on the films (Fig. 27). Occasionally, a small hematoma may act as a lead point of an intussusception.

Malabsorption

Many diseases can result in malabsorption. They can be grouped into two major categories: those associated with pancreatic enzyme deficiency, such as cystic fibrosis, and those associated with mucosal diseases of the small bowel, such as celiac disease. Regardless of the cause, a small bowel follow-through does not reveal any specific signs of these diseases.[47]

Cystic Fibrosis

The first striking feature of cystic fibrosis is the lack of barium abnormality in the ravenously hungry child who fails to put on weight because of malabsorption. Nonspecific signs sometimes appear, and the small bowel may be irregularly dilated with thick mucosal folds.[49] The intestinal wall may be thickened, and the transit time of barium can be prolonged. Flocculation, fragmentation, and segmentation of the barium are nonspecific findings, more often found in the past when malnutrition was common in cystic fibrosis patients and when barium preparations were less resistant to precipitating out of suspension. Marginal filling defects in the small bowel have also been found. These may be caused by adherent mucus from the hyperplastic goblet cells.[50] The duodenum is especially distorted with very thick folds (Fig. 28) that may be distorted further by a dilated colon filled with stool. Smudging of the prominent duodenal folds may extend into the jejunum and ileum. The cause of the mucosal pattern of the small bowel is uncertain.

Large bowel complications include intussusception, fecaloma, pneumatosis coli, and constipation.[51] Although the distal intestinal obstruction syndrome affects the distal ileum, it is the large bowel that is examined radiologically.

Celiac Disease

The small bowel pattern in a follow-through examination has been used to detect celiac disease, but it appears normal in 5 percent of proven cases. In celiac disease, the barium follow-through examination may show small bowel dilatation

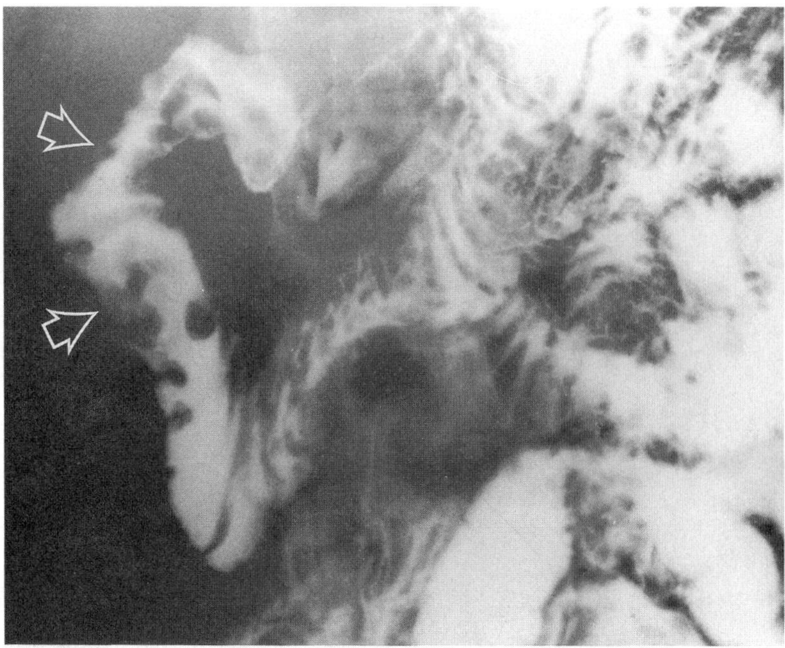

FIGURE 28 Cystic fibrosis. The duodenal mucosal folds are prominent (*arrows*). (From Stringer.[14])

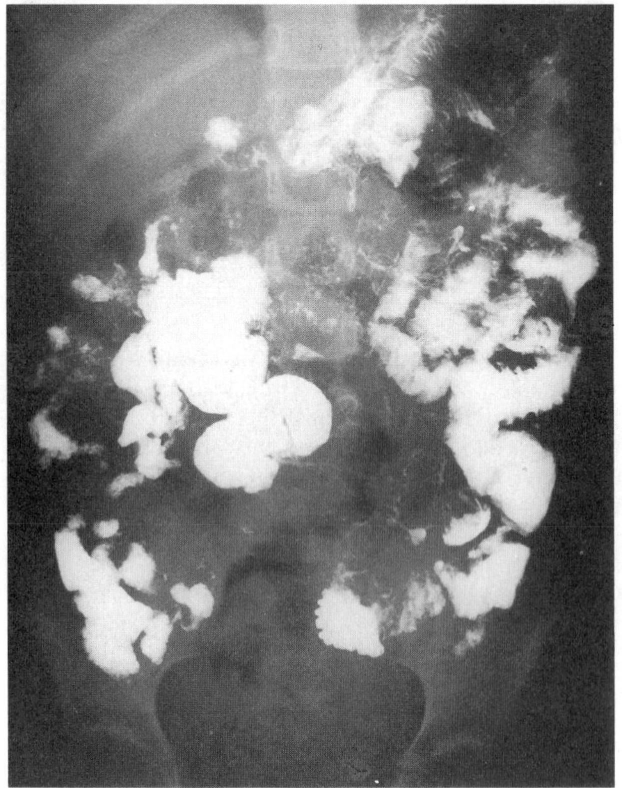

FIGURE 29 Malabsorption pattern in celiac disease. There are segmentation, flocculation, and mild bowel dilatation, a nonspecific malabsorption pattern (see also Fig. 22). (From Stringer.[14])

with thickened transverse mucosal folds, flocculation, segmentation, and delay in the transit of barium. However, with the use of new barium preparations, flocculation and segmentation occur in less than 20 percent of patients; with mild small bowel dilatation, in 70 percent (Fig. 29). Duodenal abnormalities, such as erosion or thickened mucosal folds, occur in up to 80 percent of patients. Other radiologic signs include a reversal of the normal jejunal-ileal fold pattern with a featureless jejunum and transverse folds in the ileum. An abnormal barium pattern, however, is nonspecific and is not diagnostic of either celiac disease or malabsorption (see Fig. 22).[47]

Small bowel intussusception, a well-recognized complication of celiac disease, is transient and may be found in up to 20 percent of patients. Celiac disease is also associated with an increased incidence of GI lymphoma and carcinoma.

Infections

Most infections of the small bowel result in a nonspecific small bowel pattern on the barium study. They include spasm, mucosal thickening, and irregularity. However, the distribution of the abnormality may suggest a possible infectious agent in the clinical setting. Giardiasis tends to involve the proximal small bowel, whereas tuberculosis and *Yersinia* tend to involve the ileocecal region. A more specific diagnosis can be made only with certain parasitic infections such as ascariasis, in which the barium examination may sometimes clearly outline single or multiple worms in the small bowel lumen and may fill their threadlike intestine (Fig. 30).

Meckel's Diverticulum

Meckel's diverticula lie on the antimesenteric border of the ileum within 40 to 50 cm of ileocecal valve. They are found in 2 percent of the general population. Ectopic gastric mucosa

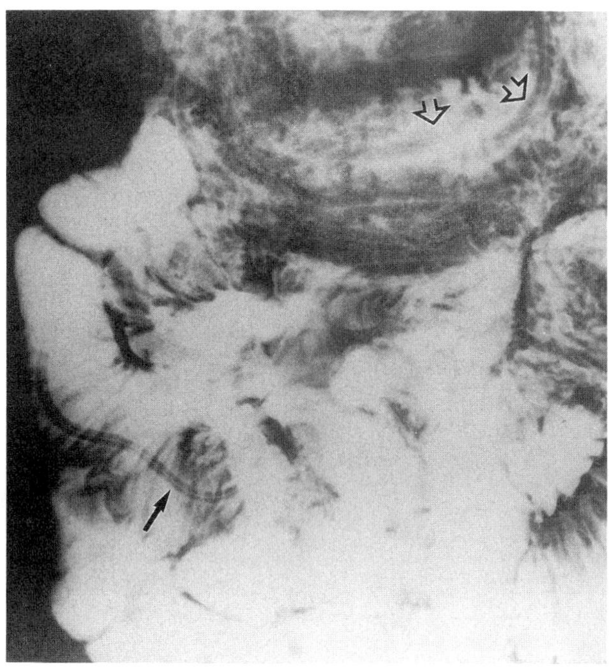

FIGURE 30 Ascariasis. Multiple worms (*open arrows*) are seen in the proximal bowel. A solitary worm, whose alimentary tract is outlined by barium, is seen more distally (*black arrow*). (From Stringer.[14])

is found in 15 percent of all patients with Meckel's diverticula and in over 50 percent of those who are symptomatic. Therefore, a ^{99m}Tc-pertechnetate radionuclide scan is the preferred screening modality because this radionuclide is taken up by the gastric mucosa.[52]

A small bowel follow-through examination may occasionally reveal a soft tissue mass in the midabdomen or right lower quadrant, but the diverticulum is not usually filled (Fig. 31*A*). A small bowel enema may sometimes fill the diverticulum and show spasm and ulceration in the adjacent bowel loop (Fig. 31*B*).[53] Barium studies can also show the complications of a Meckel's diverticulum, including obstruction, intussusception, volvulus, and local inflammation and ulceration. If a Meckel's diverticulum acts as a lead point of an intussusception, then this type of intussusception is usually impossible to reduce by barium enema and will be found during surgery.

Duplication Cyst and Other Abdominal Masses

For an investigation of abdominal masses, sonography is the initial modality of choice. The amount of detail revealed in a barium study of duplication cysts varies according to the size, shape, and location of the mass. Most duplication cysts have a spherical shape and do not communicate with the GI tract. Barium studies simply show the mass effect of these lesions with a displacement of the bowel loops around the

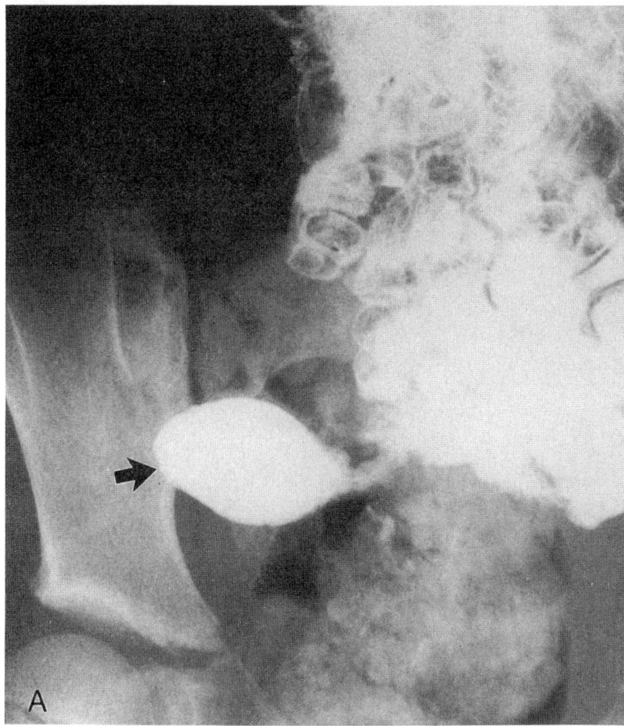

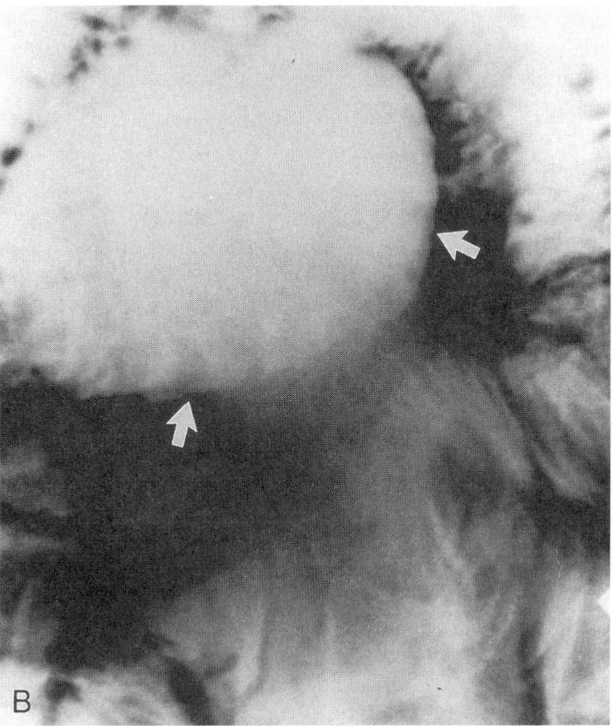

FIGURE 31 Meckel's diverticulum. A large Meckel's diverticulum (*arrow*) has filled with barium during a small bowel follow-through examination (*A*). More commonly, a small bowel enema is needed to fill the Meckel's diverticulum (*arrows*) (*B*). (From Stringer.[14])

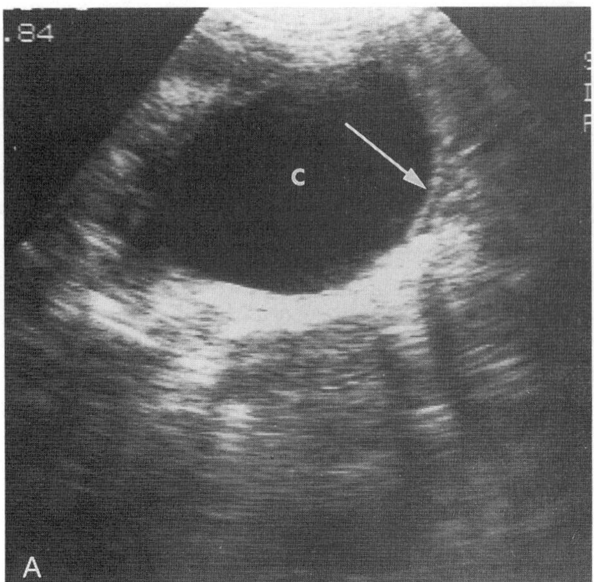

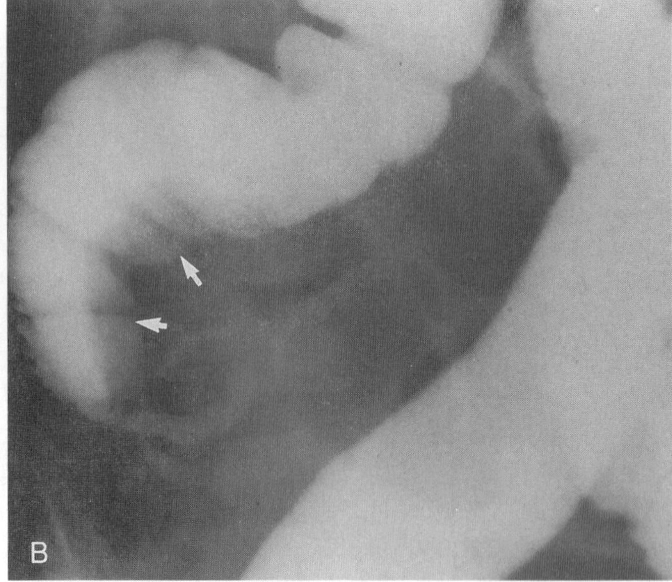

FIGURE 32 Duplication cyst. *A*, Longitudinal sonography shows a large cyst (c) on the right side of the abdomen. The wall of the cyst is bowel, as it has an echogenic line (the mucosa) (*arrow*), surrounded by a hypoechoic line (the muscle). *B*, A barium enema shows a filling defect (*arrows*) caused by extrinsic compression from a duplication cyst. The sonogram is the more helpful examination. (From Stringer.[14])

mass and the possible bowel obstruction (Fig. 32). Occasionally, the rarer tubular duplications may communicate with the bowel lumen. These may sometimes fill with barium but more often do not. Barium studies generally show only the mass effect but may show localized inflammation and ulceration in the adjacent bowel loop when the duplication cysts contain gastric mucosa (as they do in about 15 percent of cases).

Crohn's Disease

Since Crohn's disease can affect any part of the GI tract from the mouth to the anus, specific radiologic investigation should be aimed at the part of the gut in which disease is clinically suspected. In children, the ileocecal region is affected most often; thus, contrast examination of both the large and small bowel is often required.[9,14,54] If small bowel disease is suspected, a small bowel follow-through is the best routine examination in children,[46] whereas an air-contrast barium enema is the most useful study for the assessment of colonic involvement.

The air-contrast upper GI study can be reserved for the few patients with esophageal, gastric, or duodenal involvement, since in our experience inflammatory bowel disease rarely (in only 1 percent of cases) affects the upper GI tract in children and is then associated with suggestive symptoms. If an air-contrast upper GI examination is required, it is best to perform this on a separate occasion from the small bowel examination, since the high-density barium and gas degrade the follow-through images.[9,14,54]

In small bowel disease, the terminal ileum is most commonly affected, but in children, a normal terminal ileum is found in up to 20 percent of cases of small bowel disease

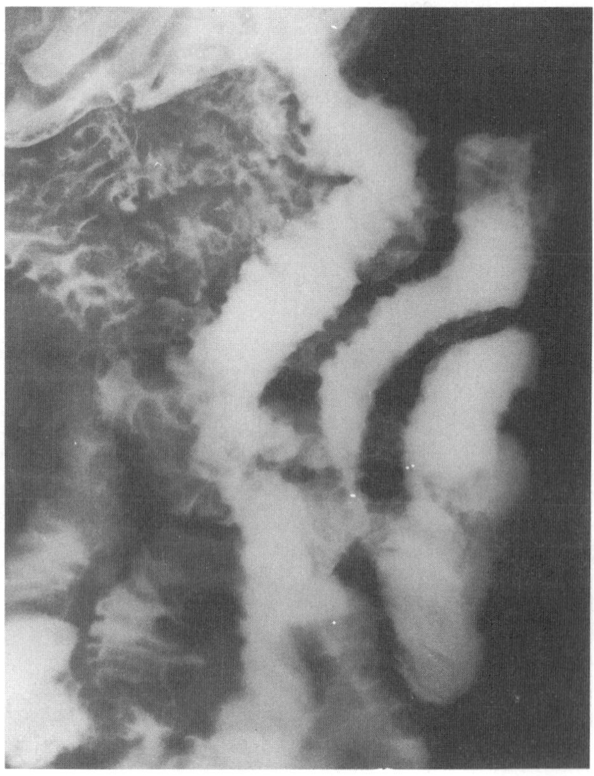

FIGURE 33 Crohn's disease of the jejunum. A large portion of proximal jejunum shows marked nodularity with bowel wall thickening, resulting in separation of bowel loops. The terminal ileum was normal on other views.

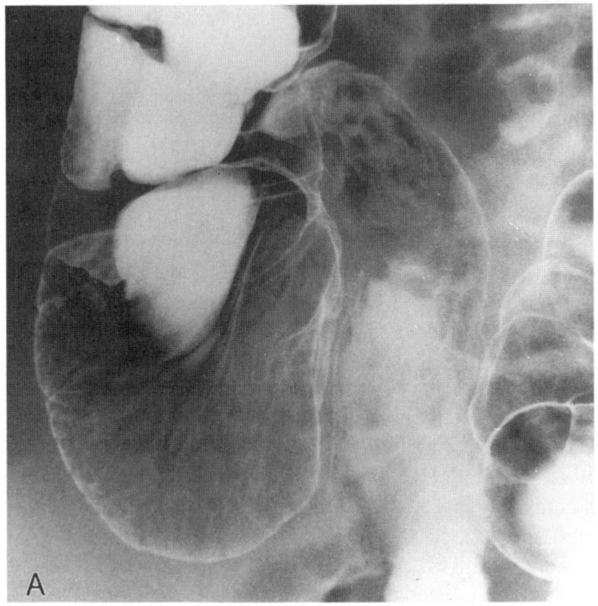

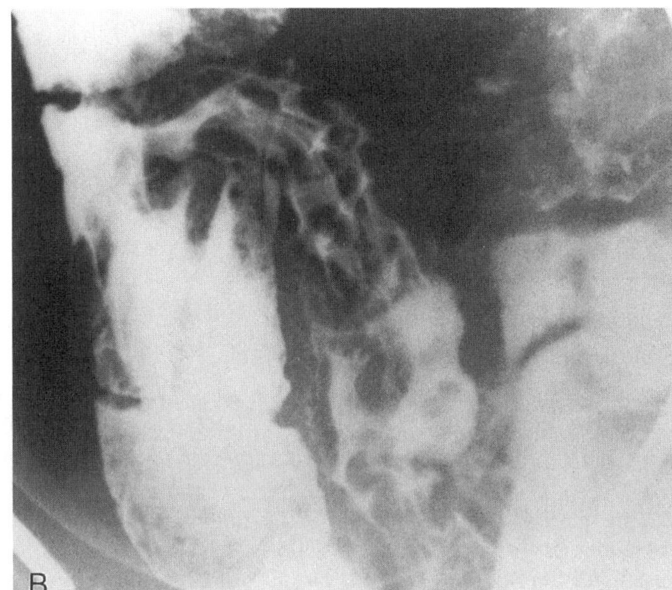

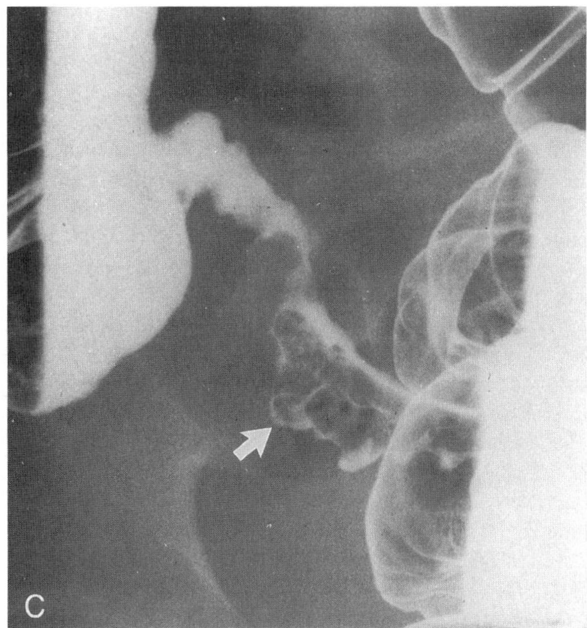

FIGURE 34 Crohn's disease of the terminal ileum. *A*, Early disease with the terminal ileum showing irregularity and fine nodules, which become more prominent as the disease progresses (*B*). An aphthous or umbilicated appearance is seen on some of the nodules. (From Stringer.[54]) *C*, Eccentric pseudodiverticula (*arrow*) and strictures form as a result of fibrosis.

(Fig. 33). Skip lesions may also be present. The terminal ileum is the most difficult portion of the bowel to visualize. If it is seen incompletely on the small bowel follow-through or if there are equivocal fistulae, a peroral pneumocolon may be performed.[9,14,45,54] If an air-contrast examination of the terminal ileum is performed, either by reflux in a double-contrast barium enema or by a peroral pneumocolon, subtle ulceration can be revealed, likely the earliest detectable sign of Crohn's disease.[45]

More commonly, as in adults, the terminal ileum shows more florid irregularity and nodules, some of which can appear aphthous (Fig. 34).[14,54] Linear ulcers or a spiculated outline may be seen, and a variable narrowing and mass effect are present because of inflammation, associated spasm, and fibrosis.[14,54]

Stenosis may be found, but it occurs less frequently than in adults and usually affects only the terminal ileum.[14,54] When the stenosis is tight, the proximal small bowel may be dilated. Since fibrosis usually occurs eccentrically, pseudodiverticula may be seen (Fig. 34), and progressive narrowing results in a small bowel obstruction.[14,54]

When a large mass effect suggests the possibility of a lymphoma, small bowel enema, which can overcome spasm, may demonstrate sufficient detail to obviate laparotomy in the correct clinical setting (see Fig. 25).[46] If an area of narrowing stays constant, it may not be possible to decide radiologically if it is caused by fibrosis or by a superimposed complication such as a malignancy. Because small bowel enema is an invasive and unpleasant procedure in children and usually requires more radiation,[9,14,46,54] it is reserved for the few cases in which the conventional small bowel follow-through, peroral pneumocolon, and double-contrast barium enema (if performed) have failed to give adequate information.[9,14,46,54]

LARGE BOWEL EXAMINATIONS

The large bowel can be examined easily from anus to cecum by contrast enema. In addition, filling the appendix and terminal ileum is common and provides additional information. In children, and especially infants, a single-contrast study is usually performed. This enables evaluation of rotational anomalies (malrotation) and obstruction. The causes of obstruction in children are varied, but all can be adequately evaluated by contrast enema. The double-contrast study is reserved for older children with suspected mucosal disorders such as inflammatory bowel disease or polyps; infants under the age of 1 year rarely suffer from these.[55]

Single-Contrast Enema in Neonates

A distal small bowel or large bowel obstruction, a relatively common occurrence in the first week of life, requires an enema examination. The differential diagnosis includes a wide list of disparate diagnoses such as malrotation, bowel atresia, meconium ileus, functional immaturity of the colon (meconium plug syndrome), and Hirschsprung's disease.[56]

Because of the risk of perforating the bowel in these infants, we always perform these studies with an iso-osmolar water-soluble contrast medium.[7,9] A soft catheter such as a Foley catheter is inserted just inside the rectum and the buttocks of the child are taped together. With the patient prone, contrast medium is injected into the rectum manually through a syringe attached to the catheter, and fluoroscopy is performed intermittently. Spot films of the lateral rectum, cecum, and encountered abnormalities are obtained. If meconium is encountered, the contrast medium is slowly and gently injected so that it passes around the plugs and hence facilitates the passage of this material.

Single-Contrast Enema in Older Children

In older children, a single-contrast enema is usually performed to diagnose malrotation and differentiate Hirschsprung's disease from functional constipation caused by other factors.[9]

In a single-contrast study, the bowel is not prepared. Barium is introduced through the rectal tube and colonic motility, distensibility, and contour are studied by fluoroscopy. Spot films of the rectum in a lateral position and of the cecum on a frontal view are obtained routinely. The former is used for assessment of possible Hirschsprung's disease in all patients with constipation, and the latter is used to assess for possible malrotation in patients with abdominal pain. An overhead film of the abdomen is obtained at the conclusion of the study. A postevacuation film of the abdomen is also obtained to assess colonic emptying.

Selected Abnormalities Observed in a Single-Contrast Enema

Malrotation

The most significant finding in the contrast enema of a malrotation is a transverse colon that crosses the midline but doubles back so that the cecum lies near the midline in the upper abdomen (type III A) (see Fig. 14; Table 1) instead of overlying the right iliac crest.[34–37] This is a dangerous form of malrotation because the root of the mesentery is very short and volvulus easily occurs.[34–37] An unusual but characteristic appearance of volvulus in an enema examination is a beak sign at the head of the contrast column either in the region of the ileocecal valve or in the distal ileum, which has filled by retrograde flow.[57]

In older children and adults, a large bowel that is confined to the left side of the abdomen may be discovered by chance; the cecum is in the left iliac fossa and the duodenojejunal junction on the right side of the abdomen (type I) (see Fig. 14; Table 1).[34–37] This situation is commonly called nonrotation, although a rotation of up to 90 degrees has occurred. The duodenum and large bowel lie lateral to the superior mesenteric artery, but on the opposite sides.[34–37] This form of malrotation rarely undergoes volvulus because malfixation is highly uncommon.[34–37]

A mobile cecum, which occurs in 14 percent of infants and children, is caused by the incomplete attachment of the cecum and the mesocolon; it has been included in the embryologic classification of malrotation as type III C (see Fig. 13).[34–37] However, in the absence of other anomalies, this finding is rarely clinically significant.

Conversely, a normally positioned cecum does not always exclude malrotation and volvulus.[34–37] The tip of the cecum observed in an enema examination may be considerable distance lateral to the root of the mesocolon and is a less precise marker for the root of mesocolon than is the position of the duodenojejunal junction (see Fig. 13).[36] In some cases, the duodenum may be the only abnormally rotated bowel (see Fig. 14*B*; Table 1). Therefore, in any child with symptoms suggestive of malrotation, an upper GI study should be performed if the enema examination appears normal.

Small Bowel (Jejunal or Ileal) Atresia

The level of obstruction of the small bowel can often be determined by plain abdominal films,[56] although the large bowel and a dilated small bowel may have a similar appearance in the neonate, since the haustral pattern is not well developed. A contrast enema is the most useful examination for excluding large bowel causes of obstruction, for demonstrating meconium ileus, or for preoperatively delineating its anatomy for the surgeon.

Water-soluble contrast media are preferable to barium for the enema examination because an atresia may rarely com-

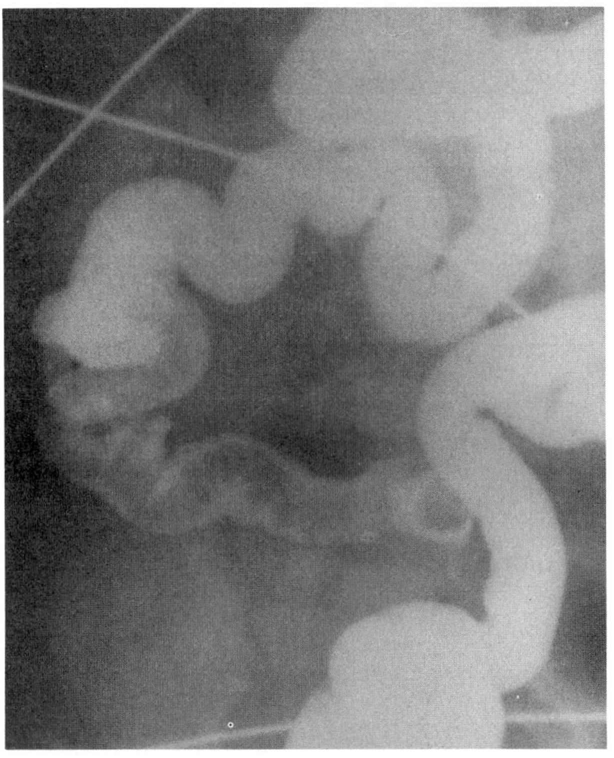

FIGURE 35 Meconium ileus. A water-soluble contrast enema demonstrates a microcolon, and reflux into the terminal ileum outlines many meconium plugs.

municate freely with the peritoneum and because the bowel adjacent to the atresia may be necrotic and at risk of perforation.[7,9]

A microcolon is usually seen in low ileal atresia with or without meconium ileus. The colon is usually of a more normal size in jejunal or proximal ileal atresia. The size of the large bowel is dependent on the amount of succus entericus that is present, since this distends the large bowel from its embryologic size to that found in a normal neonate.[56] However, these generalizations are not infallible.

Meconium Ileus

A contrast enema shows a microcolon and inspissated meconium in the ileum (Fig. 35). Previously, barium was invariably used for outlining the mass of meconium in a meconium ileus. The great advantage of diatrizoate meglumine and diatrizoate sodium solutions with polysorbate (Gastrografin), which were first introduced in 1969, is that the relief of the obstruction may occur during or following the procedure, thus obviating the need for surgery.[58] However, Gastrografin is hypertonic and when administered at full strength can be particularly dangerous because it draws fluid into the bowel lumen.[1] In animals, the osmotic effect of Gastrografin increases the hematocrit and decreases the pulse rate and cardiac output. These effects have been implicated in fatal complications.

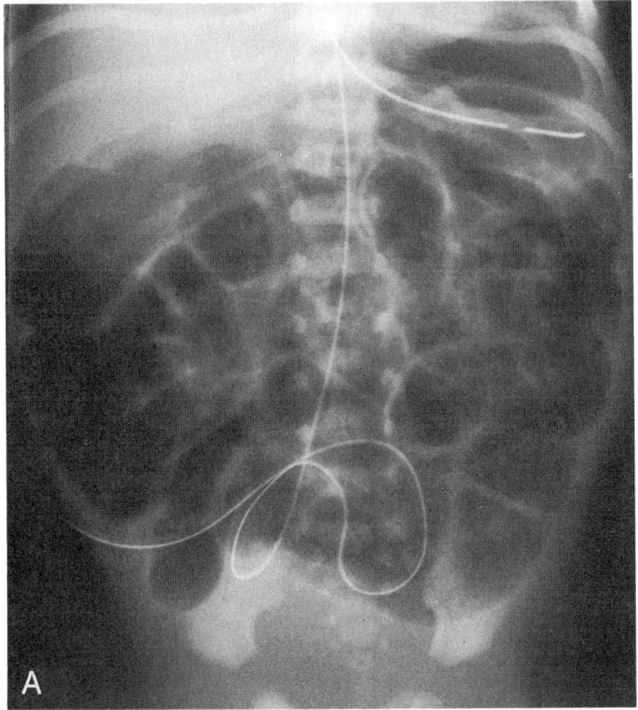

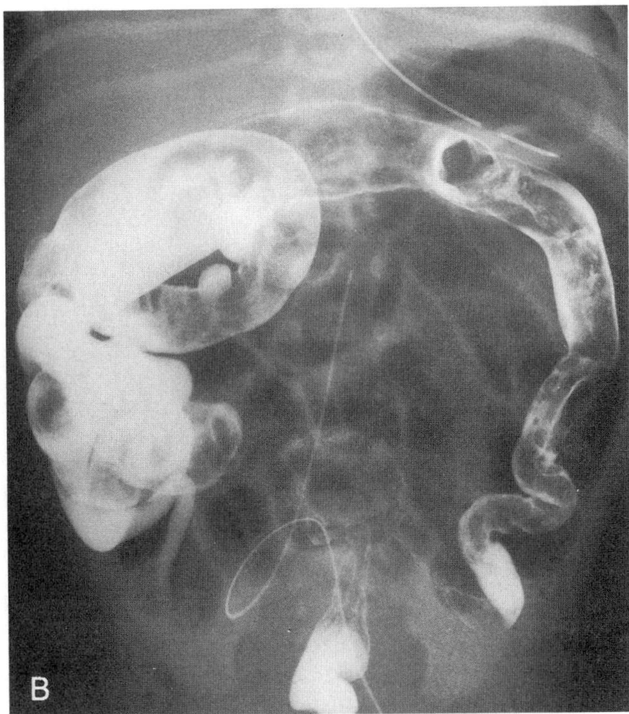

FIGURE 36 Neonatal functional immaturity of the large bowel (meconium plug syndrome). *A*, Plain film in a 2-day-old boy indicates distal obstruction with many dilated loops of bowel and no rectal gas. *B*, Water-soluble contrast enema shows a distal microcolon that gently tapers proximally to the normal-sized colon. The entire colon contains many plugs of meconium. The water-soluble contrast enema aided passage of the meconium; no further treatment was necessary. The major differential diagnosis is Hirschsprung's disease. (From Stringer.[14])

Many other preparations have been successfully used in the enema treatment of meconium ileus, including polysorbate 80 (Tween 80), *N*-acetylcysteine, diatrizoate sodium (Hypaque), and iothalamate meglumine (Conray). These other contrast media are also associated with the side effects, such as necrotizing enterocolitis following a diatrizoate meglumine and diatrizoate sodium (Renografin-76) enema. Consequently, there has been much debate regarding the correct contrast medium to use.[1,3,59–61] We do not use Gastrografin.

The new low- or iso-osmolar contrast media are ideal because they are safe and not absorbed; therefore, delayed films may be taken. However, they are expensive for routine use.[9]

In view of the many different media available, caution is urged in the investigation of any neonate with intestinal obstruction. Since there is little difference in the efficacy of the various water-soluble preparations, we use an iso- or hypo-osmolar contrast medium mixed with *N*-acetylcysteine.[9,64] We do not use barium sulfate because it may inspissate. Barium also causes peritoneal inflammation and adhesions if peritoneal spill occurs. In our experience, approximately one-third of neonates with meconium ileus can be treated successfully with this contrast-enema technique. The rest are unsuccessful, but half of these require surgery for other intra-abdominal pathology. Included in the unsuccessful enemas are approximately 20 percent who have sustained a perforation during the procedure.[63] Despite this risk, the technique is worth performing because the successfully treated patients require no further intervention, and those who perforate suffer no postoperative sequelae.

Functional Immaturity of the Colon (Meconium Plug Syndrome, Small Left Hemicolon Syndrome)

Contrast-enema examinations of a functionally immature colon show a narrowed descending colon with the marked change of caliber, which usually occurs at the splenic flexure (Fig. 36), but is occasionally located more proximally.[66] Meconium plugs are often present. Water-soluble contrast media are useful in the treatment of neonatal functioning immaturity of the colon because they often facilitate decompression.[9,14]

Functional immaturity of the colon must be differentiated from Hirschsprung's disease. Hirschsprung's disease seldom affects the splenic flexure or more proximal large bowel. Moreover, it is more often associated with an aganglionic bowel of a normal rather than small size; the aganglionic section appears relatively small, however, when compared with the proximal dilated ganglionic bowel. Patients with functional immaturity of the colon tend to improve within 48 hours of the enema, whereas patients with Hirschsprung's disease

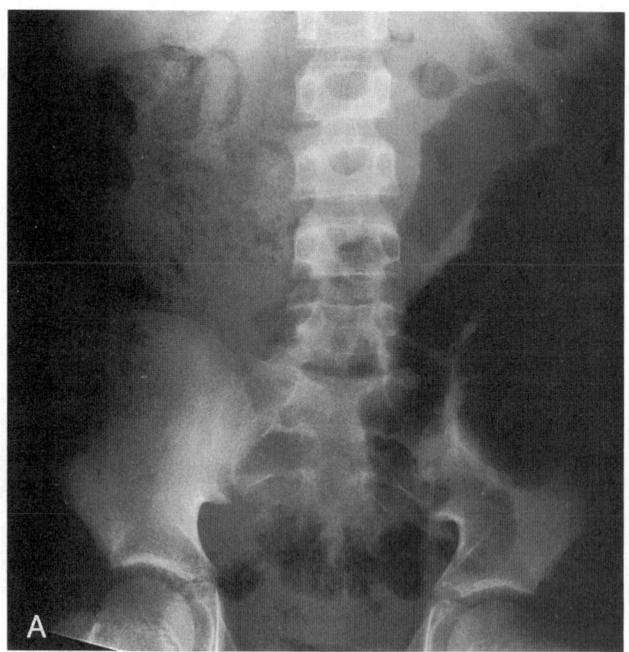

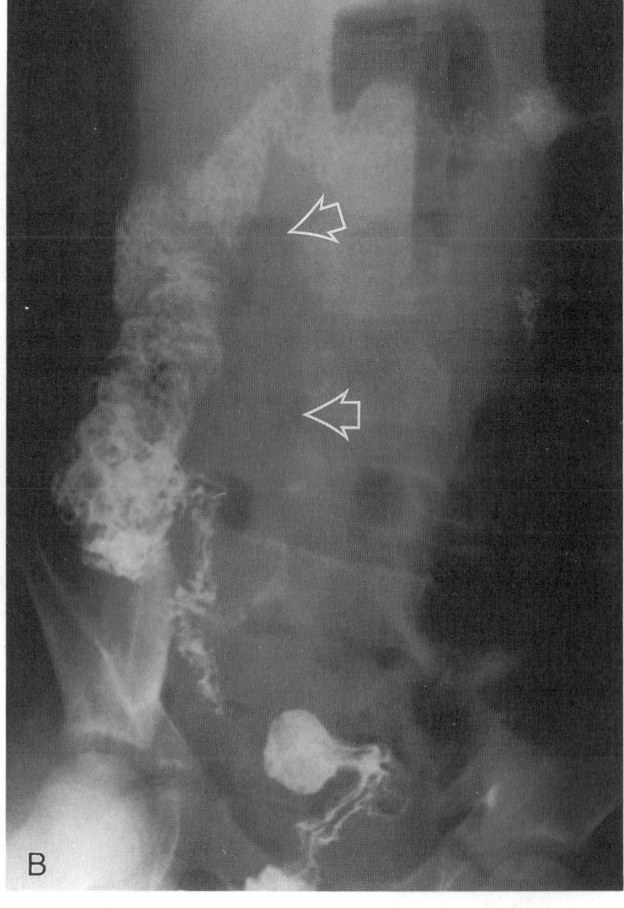

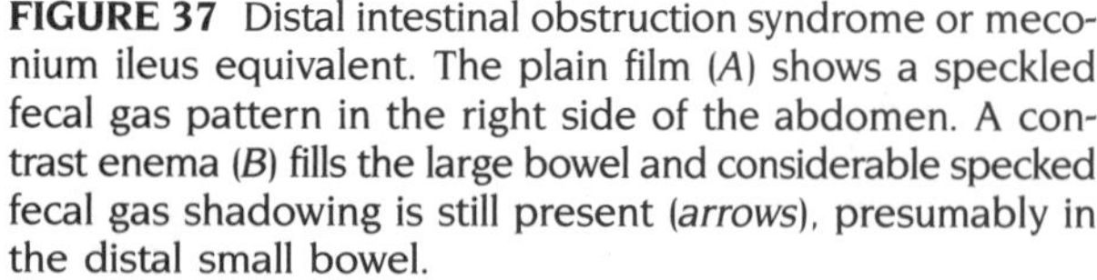

FIGURE 37 Distal intestinal obstruction syndrome or meconium ileus equivalent. The plain film (*A*) shows a speckled fecal gas pattern in the right side of the abdomen. A contrast enema (*B*) fills the large bowel and considerable specked fecal gas shadowing is still present (*arrows*), presumably in the distal small bowel.

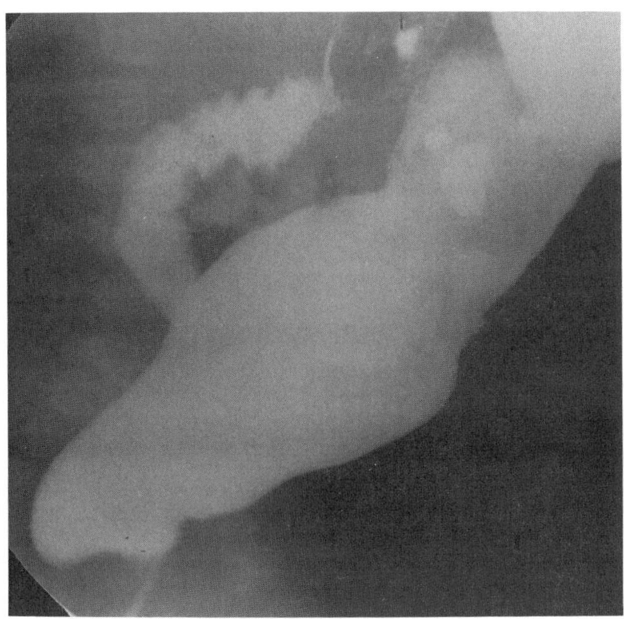

FIGURE 38 Hirschsprung's disease. A gradual transitional zone is seen from ganglionic proximal bowel that is dilated to an aganglionic distal bowel that has a normal caliber.

invariably return with further symptoms. Doubt concerning the diagnosis may remain in a number of cases; if so, a definite biopsy may be necessary.

Distal Intestinal Obstruction Syndrome

The distal intestinal obstruction syndrome (or meconium ileus equivalent), found in patients with cystic fibrosis and pancreatic insufficiency, may result in sticky bowel contents and may cause an ileocecal obstruction (Fig. 37). Gastrografin or other water-soluble contrast media have been advocated in the treatment of this condition, but we have found that oral GoLytely (a balanced electrolyte solution) yields better results and is more readily tolerated by the patient.[65,66]

Hirschsprung's Disease

A high index of suspicion is required if Hirschsprung's disease is to be detected. In the neonate, other causes of obstruction, such as neonatal functional immaturity of the colon (meconium plug syndrome), can mimic Hirschsprung's disease both clinically and on plain films.

In all suspected cases of Hirschsprung's disease, the child should not undergo bowel preparation prior to an enema. A rectal examination should also be avoided, although there is some evidence that it does not affect the diagnostic accuracy.

The most reliable indicator of Hirschsprung's disease is a transitional zone, typically found in the distal sigmoid colon. It most often appears in a contrast enema as a disparity in size between the distal bowel, which has a small or normal caliber, and the proximal bowel, which is dilated. This zone can be abrupt or gradual (Figs. 38 and 39*A*).[67]

Not all patients have transitional zones. They are more fully defined in older children than in infants. A recognizable transitional zone may be particularly difficult to see in the first weeks of life.[67] Diagnosis becomes more difficult in the absence of a transitional zone. An inflated balloon catheter or a previous vigorous digital examination may obscure the transitional zone by dilating the narrow caliber of the distal bowel. Usually the transitional zone marks the junction of ganglionic and aganglionic bowel, but passive dilatation of the proximal portion of the aganglionic segment may occur so that some

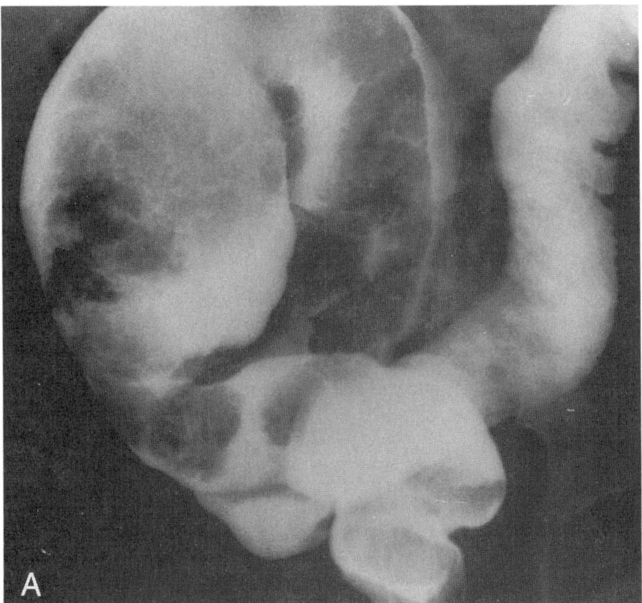

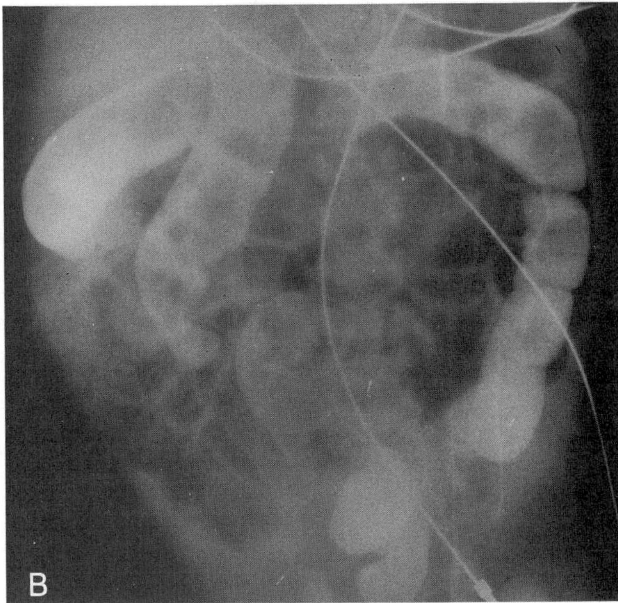

FIGURE 39 Hirschsprung's disease. *A*, The zone of abrupt transition from a grossly dilated ganglionic large bowel proximally to an aganglionic large bowel distally is easily assessed on the frontal view in this 10-month-old child with classic rectosigmoid Hirschsprung's disease. *B*, The colon is normal in this other child with total colonic aganglionosis.

of the dilated proximal bowel is aganglionic. Occasionally, this transitional zone is most clearly delineated on delayed films.

Occasionally, neonatal functional immaturity of the large bowel may mimic Hirschsprung's disease by appearing to have a zone of transition, usually in the region of the splenic flexure. This is best distinguished on clinical grounds. The patients are generally premature babies, often with diabetic mothers; moreover, the symptoms spontaneously resolve within 24 hours of the contrast enema—all of which is highly atypical for Hirschsprung's disease. In rare cases of total colonic ganglionosis, a transitional zone does not exist.

There is some controversy concerning which contrast medium should be used in infants thought to have Hirschsprung's disease. Barium is used in many places because it conveniently allows delayed films to be taken. Because excess barium can become impacted, only an amount sufficient to demonstrate the transitional zone should be instilled unless isoosmolar water-soluble contrast media are used.

In our opinion, dilute water-soluble contrast medium is the preferred contrast medium because in most cases it reveals the presence of Hirschsprung's disease without running the risk of compounding the obstruction with barium. If, however, barium is used and neonatal functional immaturity of the colon is detected during the examination, a change to a water-soluble contrast medium is possible. When doubt about the diagnosis still remains, a follow-up enema examination or biopsy is necessary.

The rectosigmoid index has been used to indicate the presence of a zone of transition, but some believe that it is not useful because it is sensitive only to the presence of an obvious transitional zone.[68,69] This index is calculated from the division of the maximum diameter of the rectum by the maximum width of the sigmoid colon. Normally the rectum is larger than the sigmoid at their widest points, making the index equal more than 1.0. When the rectum is smaller, as in Hirschsprung's disease, the index is less than 1.0 and usually less than 0.9. The value of this index has been disputed because an abnormal index may indicate only an obvious zone of transition and a normal index can be misleading, as is often the case for long-segment Hirschsprung's disease. However, in doubtful cases, finding sigmoid loops larger than the rectum facilitates making the diagnosis when the zone of transition has not been adequately demonstrated on the available images.

Irregular, bizarre, saw-tooth contractions seen in the aganglionic segment of the large bowel may help in making the diagnosis when no transitional zone is present.[14,67] Fine marginal serrations may be present in ganglionic and aganglionic segments, but they may be seen in normal large bowel and are attributable to circular muscle contraction. Mucosal irregularity and prominent thickened folds are seen in enterocolitis, a serious complication.

Some barium retention may occur normally following enema examination, but the barium tends to collect in the more distal portions of the large bowel. With aganglionosis, barium may remain in the bowel proximal to the transitional zone for an extended period of time, often for as long as 24 hours. Occasionally, complete evacuation of barium may occur despite a distal segment of aganglionosis; therefore, complete evacuation does not exclude Hirschsprung's disease.[70] Barium retention is nonspecific and does not necessarily indicate the presence of Hirschsprung's disease. Conversely, it may be the only indication of the presence of Hirschsprung's disease. We use bisacodyl USP (Dulcolax) in the enema to expedite evacuation and allow an early postevacuation film.

Total Colonic Aganglionosis. The radiologic findings are often not diagnostic for total colonic aganglionosis.[71,72] On plain films, total colonic aganglionosis usually presents evidence of distal small bowel obstruction; however, other causes of distal small bowel obstruction also have to be considered. A contrast-enema examination may show a microcolon (23 percent) or a normal colon (77 percent) (Fig. 39*B*). A short colon with loss of the normal redundancy of the splenic and hepatic flexures and of the sigmoid colon appears in 23 percent of patients. Meconium plugs are commonly seen but are nonspecific, since they are found in the meconium plug syndrome, meconium ileus, short-segment Hirschsprung's disease, and even some normal patients. Occasionally, a pseudotransition zone may be present, mimicking the more common forms of Hirschsprung's disease. This finding reinforces the need for a full-contrast examination and biopsy confirmation during surgery. Colonic wall irregularity, probably caused by spasm, may be seen in up to 46 percent of patients. There may be delayed evacuation, or the examination may be completely normal. The terminal ileum may be relatively more dilated than the large bowel. Significant reflux to the terminal ileum occurs in 33 percent of patients, and complete reflux of barium through the small bowel has also been found in patients with total colonic aganglionosis.

Ultrashort Segment Hirschsprung's Disease. The importance or even existence of ultrashort segment Hirschsprung's disease is a subject of controversy. This diagnosis is rarely suspected in infants. In older children, the appearance of the colon in a barium-enema study is identical to that of functional constipation. The rectum is dilated and filled with feces down to the anus. The diagnosis can be made only on manometric studies followed by biopsy. Ganglia are normally absent in the anal region, so great care is required to ensure that the correct diagnosis is made. Biopsies must, therefore, be taken just proximal to the anus.

Zonal Colonic Aganglionosis. Exceptionally rarely, a segment of the large bowel may be aganglionic with normal ganglia found more proximally and distally.[73] These segments of aganglionic large bowel are usually single, but occasionally a second segment is present. A relatively narrow portion of the large bowel may be seen radiologically. Overdiagnosis must be avoided, since this condition is extremely rare and there is some controversy over its true nature. Careful diagnosis is important, particularly because finding aganglionosis proximally (e.g., in the appendix) does not necessarily mean that there is total aganglionosis distally, and further biopsies should be taken.

Intussusception

If an intussusception is suspected, a colon study is the preferred imaging modality because it quickly confirms or disproves the diagnosis. If an intussusception is encountered, it can also be immediately reduced during the same study in the fluoroscopic suite without moving the sick child to another part of the hospital.

Plain films are not reliable for a definite diagnosis, and in any case, reduction of the intussusception is still required. Sonography and CT may also show the intussusception, but the simplest and most reliable method for both the patient and the physician is the colon study, since it permits both quick diagnosis and reduction of the intussusception.

In most North American and European centers, barium enema is the preferred method for the investigation and treatment of intussusception.[9,14,74] A water-soluble contrast enema has been advised by some radiologists, especially if there is a high risk of perforation. However, if conventional water-soluble contrast media are being used when a perforation occurs, there is a risk of serious electrolyte disturbance because the contrast media are absorbed from the peritoneum. Using the new low-osmolar contrast media would avoid this problem, but they are expensive.

In China and other parts of the world, air, instead of barium, is used as the contrast medium. Over the past 25 years, the successful use of air in the reduction of intussusception has been reported in several large series.[75] This method is not really new. In the nineteenth century, air given by hand bellows was used for the reduction of intussusception. Since 1985, we have also used this technique. Our results have been so positive that air is now the contrast medium of choice in the diagnosis and reduction of intussusception.[75] However, this air-enema technique has not yet been widely accepted.

Liquid Contrast Enema (Barium or Water-Soluble Contrast). If there is no evidence of peritonitis barium-enema reduction of intussusception can be performed. The standard method of reduction is to place a reservoir of barium 1 meter above the patient so that a constant hydrostatic pressure is generated. However, there is little if any scientific evidence to support this arbitrary height of 1 meter. With experience, and depending on the clinical status of the child, a more vigorous reduction can be undertaken.

We place no time limit on the examination, and we may raise the height of the barium column to the ceiling if difficulty in reduction occurs.[9,14] Reduction is complete only when a good portion of the distal ileum is filled with barium, thus excluding ileoileal intussusception. Radiographs are kept to a minimum. Our standard series consists of a spot film when the intussusception is first encountered and an abdominal film when the reduction is complete.[9] We have not found the postevacuation film advocated by some[76] to be useful; hence, we save the child from this extra dose of radiation.

In a typical ileocolic intussusception, the barium column is met as an intraluminal filling defect (the intussusceptum) that is the caliber of the normal colon (Fig. 40). The intussusceptum can be found in any part of the large bowel, including the rectum. Occasionally, some barium may coat the outer surface of the intussusceptum and the inner surface of the intussuscipiens, resulting in a coiled-spring pattern.

Ileoileocolic intussusception may be more difficult to reduce because the barium often percolates along the loops of small bowel in the colon, dissipating the effective pressure of the enema. During the study, the cecum and ascending colon may be filled with obvious loops of bowel (Fig. 41). On reflux of the barium through the ileocecal valve, an intussusceptum may be seen in the terminal ileum. These ileoileocolic intussusceptions may be reducible and do not necessarily recur.

A postreduction filling defect in the cecum is not uncommonly seen, probably the result of residual edema in the il-

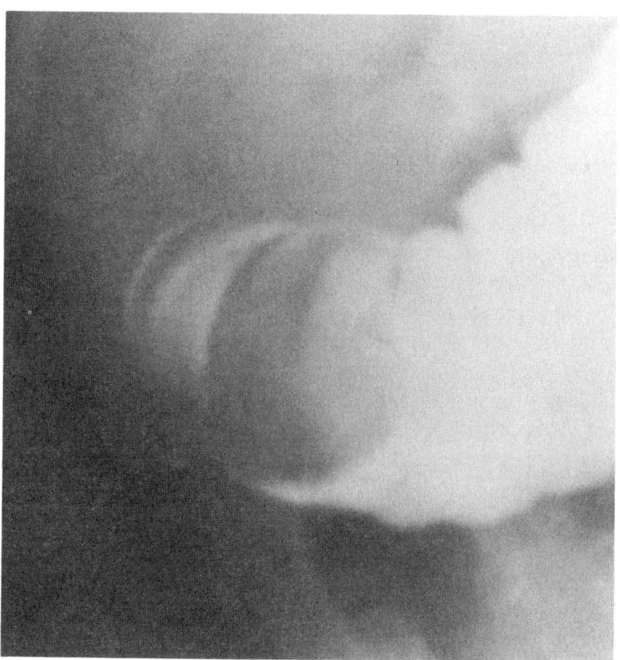

FIGURE 40 Ileocolic intussusception. Barium shows the intussusceptum as an intraluminal filling defect occluding the bowel lumen. The intussusception was reduced easily.

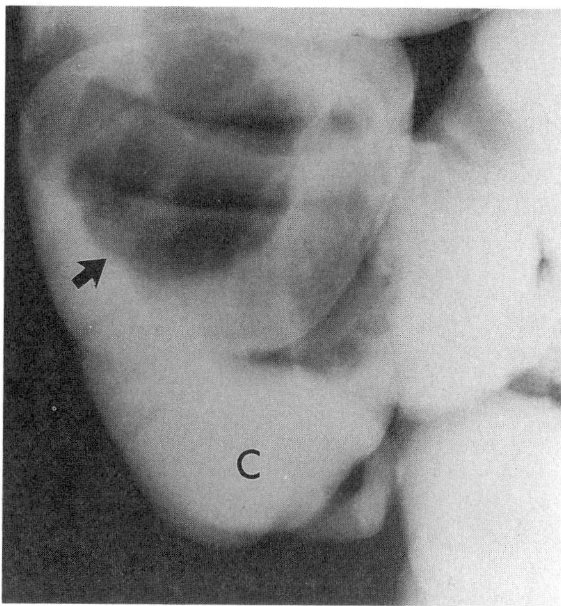

FIGURE 41 Ileoileocolic intussusception. Barium outlines loops of small bowel (*arrow*) coiled within the ascending colon. C = cecum.

eocecal valve. Follow-up barium enemas are useful to exclude a small mass lesion as a cause of the intussusception.

Air Enema. We have been the first in North America to use the air-enema technique. We have found that it is effective and convenient, allowing for easy and quick reduction of the intussusception in the majority of cases.[75] The fluoroscopic time and the time of reduction are reduced to less than half, compared with that of our previous experience with barium.

The technique is simple. A Foley catheter is inserted into the rectum. Fluoroscopy is used to assess the presence of bowel gas in the abdomen. Then air is instilled, initially by hand pump, until the diagnosis is made[9,14] (Fig. 42) and the intussusceptum is pushed gently back. If the intussusceptum stops moving despite the use of the hand pump, an electric pump is connected. Both these pumps must have a pressure-release system, so that the pressure remains between 80 and 120 mm Hg.[9,14] The initial 80 mm Hg corresponds to the hydrostatic pressure generated by a 1-meter column of barium sulfate suspension, whereas 120 mm Hg corresponds to about a 1.5-meter column of barium. If a perforation occurs during the procedure, the abdomen can very rapidly fill with gas, and an 18-gauge needle should be rapidly passed through the anterior abdominal wall to deflate the distention, thus preventing respiratory or cardiovascular compromise.[9,14]

The use of air is advantageous because of the ease of intussusception reduction, the reduced radiation and cost, and the relatively harmless nature of air in the peritoneal cavity compared with that of other contrast media.[9,14] Carbon dioxide can also be used and has the added advantage of being absorbed rapidly from the gut, causing less discomfort, and being less dangerous than air, which could potentially cause an air embolism. However, air embolisms have never been reported with this air-enema technique.

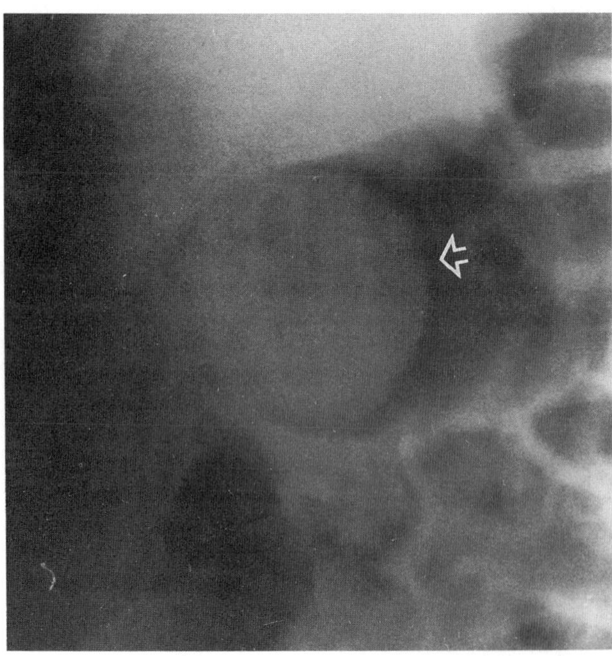

FIGURE 42 Ileocolic intussusception. Air shows the intussusceptum (*arrow*) as an intraluminal filling defect occluding the bowel lumen. Note the coiled-spring appearance. The right iliac fossa is relatively gasless. After easy reduction, the right iliac fossa is full of large and small bowel gas.

Complications. *Perforation.* The most serious complication of attempted reduction is colonic perforation with barium entering the peritoneal cavity. This perforation may occur distal to the intussusception but most commonly occurs where the intussusception is first shown by the barium,[77] although it has also been reported more proximally.[78]

Perforation most commonly occurs in infants under 6 months of age, especially if there is evidence of small bowel obstruction. Although there is no increase in mortality if perforation occurs, these patients require a more cautious and gentle approach. Some authors have advised against trying to reduce any intussusception in infants under 3 months because they have had poor success in this age group. This has not been the experience at our institution or other hospitals.[14] To reduce the risk of perforation, it is our policy to have a pediatric surgeon examine all patients before the procedure. In this way the most seriously ill infants are prevented from undergoing a possibly hazardous enema, especially if there is evidence of peritonitis.

Recurrent Intussusception and Lead Points. After reduction by barium enema, recurrent intussusception occurs in about 5 percent of cases.[79] At present, data are insufficient to show the recurrence rate after an air enema, although our initial results show a slightly lower recurrence rate than that after a barium enema.

Adequate filling of the ileum with barium or air ensures complete reduction of an ileoileal intussusception and likely helps to prevent recurrence of the problem. Repeated barium- or air-enema reductions are both possible and safe. Reduction of an intussusception with barium is more likely to fail in children over the age of 5 years or under the age of 1 year; lead points are more often found in these age groups.[79]

With experience with barium enema, the risk of missing a surgically significant lesion acting as a lead point is negligible. However, occasionally an ileocolic intussusception may be caused by a significant lead point, such as a lymphoma, and yet be totally reducible by barium enema.[80] Over a 9-year period and 300 intussusceptions, we have had five children whose intussusceptions were caused by a lead point and yet were completely reduced. Some of these children could not be separated on age or clinical grounds from the usual child with intussusception but were detected because of relatively subtle defects in the ileocecal region.[80]

Benign and malignant lesions cannot be distinguished by radiologic examination alone. An ileocecal valve can appear large because of edema following an intussusception reduction. Hence, a follow-up study is indicated if there is concern over the appearance of this area. If a defect, however subtle, is present on a repeat examination, then laparotomy is indicated.[80]

Failed Reduction of Intussusception. Our success rate with the reduction of intussusception with barium is 75 percent and with air enema about 85 percent. The usual range reported in the literature is 45 to 65 percent.[75] The patients with failed reductions all require surgical reduction. Intravenous or intramuscular glucagon has been advocated as a means of decreasing the number of failed barium-enema reductions, but this technique is not in widespread use. The value of glucagon in the hydrostatic reduction of intussusception is uncertain; we have not found glucagon to be useful.

Double-Contrast Enema

A double-contrast enema is an excellent technique for the visualization of fine mucosal details; it is, therefore, the preferred technique for the detection of inflammatory bowel disease and polyps. Inflammatory bowel disease is usually not a major concern in the younger age groups and is rare in children less than 6 years of age.[9,14]

For a double-contrast study, more vigorous bowel preparation is required than for a single-contrast study. For children over 2 years of age, clear fluids are given for 36 hours prior to the examination. A dose of castor oil or magnesium citrate or other purgative, 1 ml per kilogram of body weight, is given the afternoon prior to the examination if not clinically contraindicated; the dose is reduced for smaller children.[9,14] A saline or Fleet enema is given the evening before and the morning of the examination.[9,14] For children under 2 years of age, we find that it is safest to prepare the patient in the department.[9,14]

The double-contrast colon study requires the use of high-density barium mixture to coat the mucosal surface of the entire colon, followed by rectal insufflation or air.[10] The presence of lymphoid follicles is a normal feature in the large bowel of infants and can be used as an indicator of the adequacy of the examination.[81] After a good air-contrast effect has been achieved, multiple large overhead films of the colon (at least six) are then obtained so that all areas of the colon can be visualized in an air-contrast phase. Spot films may also be obtained as needed to more completely document any observed pathology. In young children, spot films may suffice.

Ulcerative Colitis

Most clinicians[10,39] believe that the double-contrast barium enema still plays an important role in the diagnosis of ulcerative colitis, although some believe colonoscopy with biopsy is the only diagnostic test necessary.[10] Using high-density barium and an average of only 30 seconds of fluoroscopy, and taking only six films (supine, prone, both decubitus, and spot films of the cecum and lateral rectum), we achieve results comparable to those of colonoscopy. The small disparity occurs primarily in our failure to detect early proctitis (8 percent).[10] This is hardly surprising, since the earliest endoscopic finding in early ulcerative colitis is a blurring of the normal superficial rectal blood vessel pattern because of edema, a feature unlikely to be detected by a double-contrast barium enema.[10] Hence, the more invasive colonoscopy technique can be limited primarily to the examination of the distal large bowel. Colonoscopy and biopsy are necessary if the specific diagnosis remains in doubt.

Plain film evidence of toxic megacolon is an absolute contraindication to the contrast study of the colon.[54] The radiologic appearances are similar to those in adults. Mild colitis shows as a subtle granularity of the mucosa extending uniformly from the rectum for a variable distance proximally.[54] Circumferential superficial involvement is a characteristic feature that helps to distinguish ulcerative colitis from Crohn's colitis (see Fig. 7).[54] Minor haustral thickening secondary to edema is common in the early stages, and this can become quite marked (Fig. 43).[54]

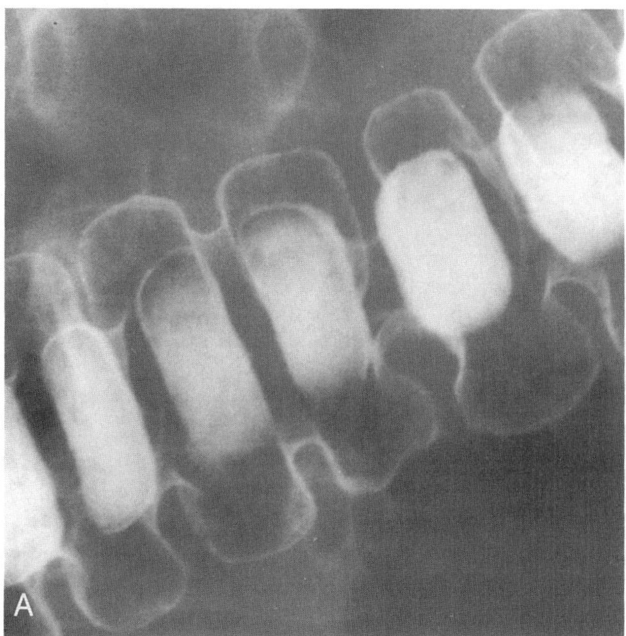

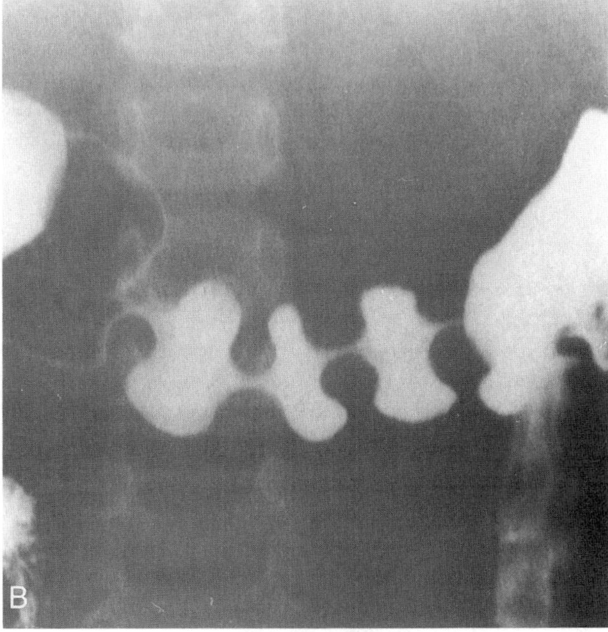

FIGURE 43 Ulcerative colitis. *A*, There is minor subtle haustral fold thickening of the transverse colon secondary to edema seen in the early stages of ulcerative colitis. *B*, There is marked haustral fold thickening of the transverse colon as shown on a barium enema in a different patient. (From Stringer.[14])

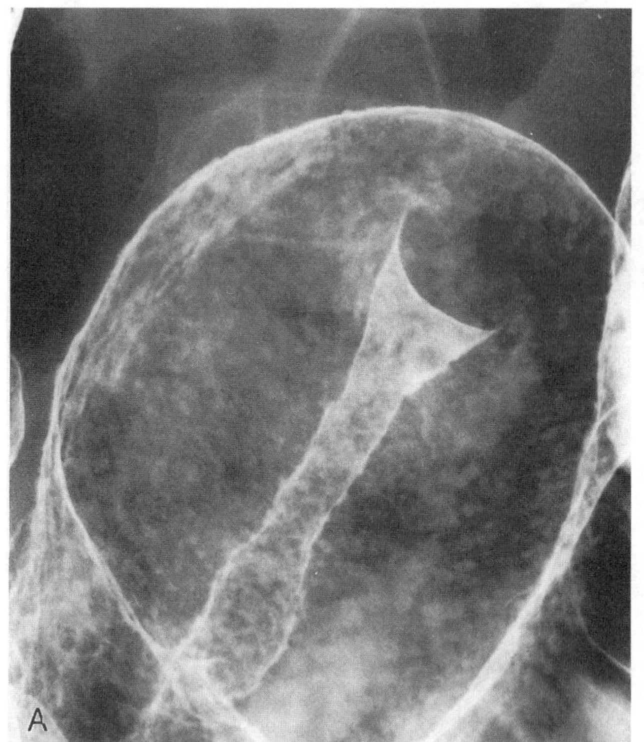

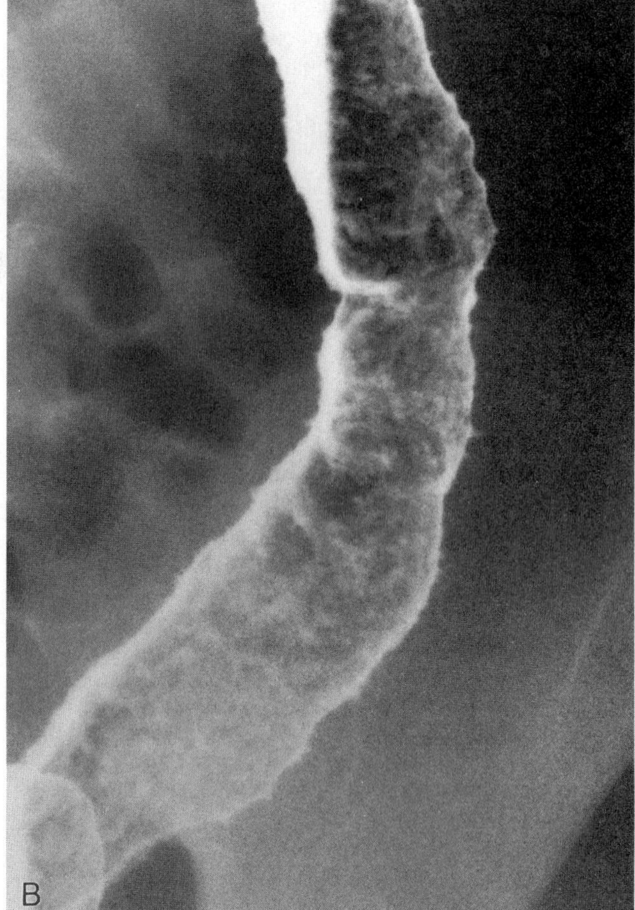

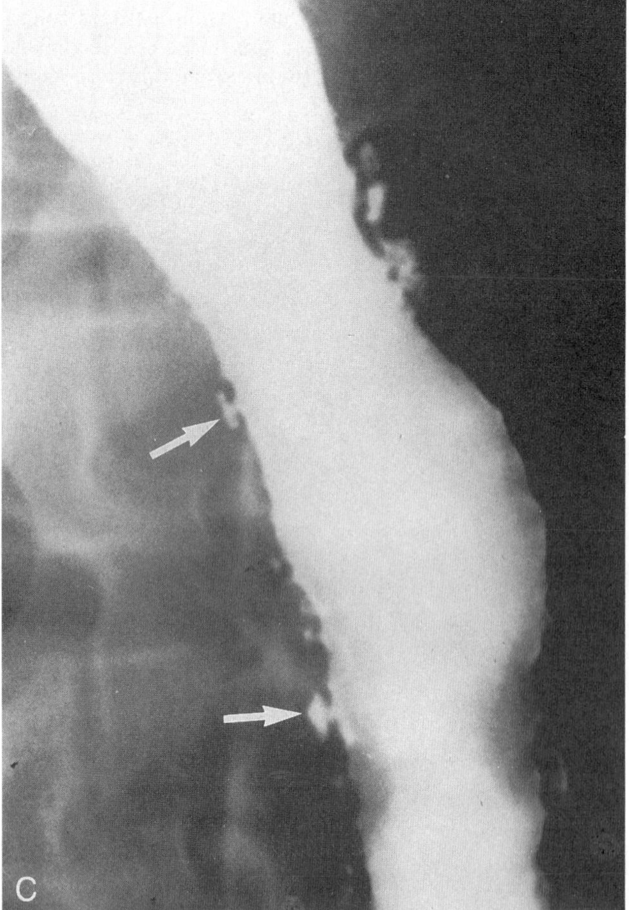

FIGURE 44 Ulcerative colitis. *A*, There are moderate mucosal irregularity and punctate ulceration seen on double-contrast barium enema. *B*, In another patient, there is more severe disease with deep ulceration, and as the disease progresses (*C*), there is a submucosal tracking with formation of collar-button ulcers (*arrows*). (From Stringer.[54])

As the disease progresses, more severe mucosal irregularity and punctate ulceration are seen (Fig. 44). When submucosal tracking occurs, an ulcer the shape of a collar button is formed, and pseudopolyps of the remaining islands of mucosa or granulation tissue may result.[54] In the healing phase, filiform (postinflammatory) polyps may form and often have a characteristic branching or wormlike appearance (Fig. 45).[54] In the late stages of the disease, the entire large bowel may be short and tubular, with a widening of the postrectal space and the loss of the valves of Houston.[54] The ileocecal valve becomes patulous, and reflux ileitis may occur.[54]

Crohn's Colitis

Because the ileocecal region is the most commonly affected by Crohn's disease, it is common to require both large and small bowel studies. The double-contrast high-density barium enema is the preferred imaging modality for the evaluation of the fine detail of the bowel mucosa.[9,14,54] If the child is too sick for a double-contrast examination, a single-contrast study helps show the distribution of a gross colitis but is not sensitive enough to detect early mucosal disease. As in adults, plain film evidence of a toxic megacolon contraindicates a contrast examination.

In the colon, the earliest evidence of Crohn's disease is ulceration, which occurs at the apices of enlarged lymphoid follicles, the ulcers being commonly designated aphthae.[14,54] (*Aphthae* is the Greek term for ulcers and is preferable to *aphthous* or *aphthoid* ulcer, which after all means "ulcer-like ulcer.") These aphthae have a characteristic appearance with smooth, raised edges (Fig. 46). As the disease progresses, the aphthae enlarge and coalesce and can penetrate to deeper tissues (Fig. 46). Extension of the ulceration can occur along the wall of the bowel, resulting in linear ulcers (Fig. 46) or penetration of the bowel wall, forming sinus or fistulous tracks.[14,54] Associated inflammation gives a nodular appearance with progressive thickening of the bowel wall.[14,54]

In contrast to ulcerative colitis, Crohn's disease characteristically involves areas asymmetrically, causing discrete ulceration separated by normal mucosa (Fig. 46).[14,54] It tends to affect the right hemicolon and less commonly the rectum. When the rectum is involved, it is often localized in a small area and the ulceration is more severe than it is in ulcerative colitis. However, occasionally Crohn's disease affects the entire colon with minimal colitis indistinguishable from ulcerative colitis.[14,54]

In longstanding disease, fibrosis can lead to strictures that may result in bowel obstruction (Fig. 47). Fibrosis may also

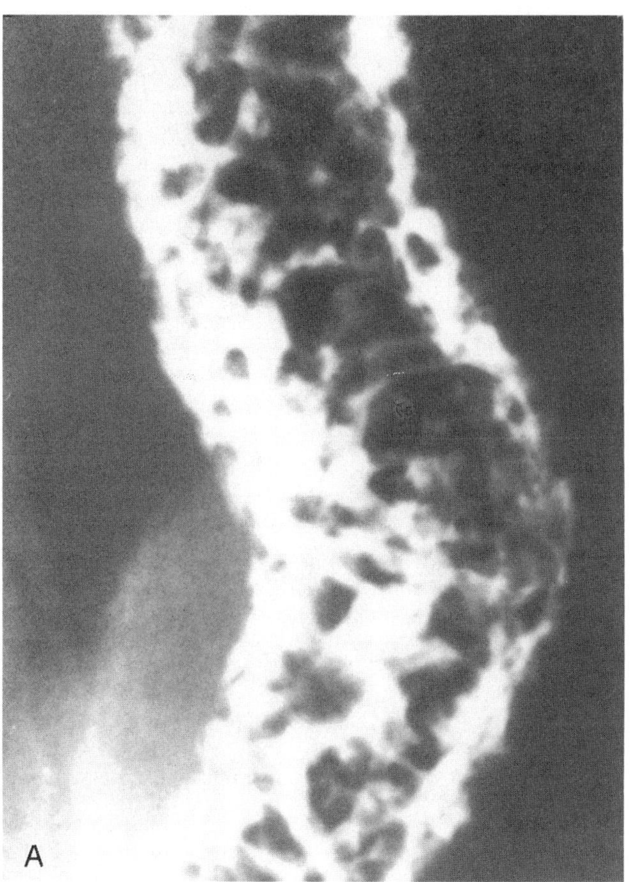

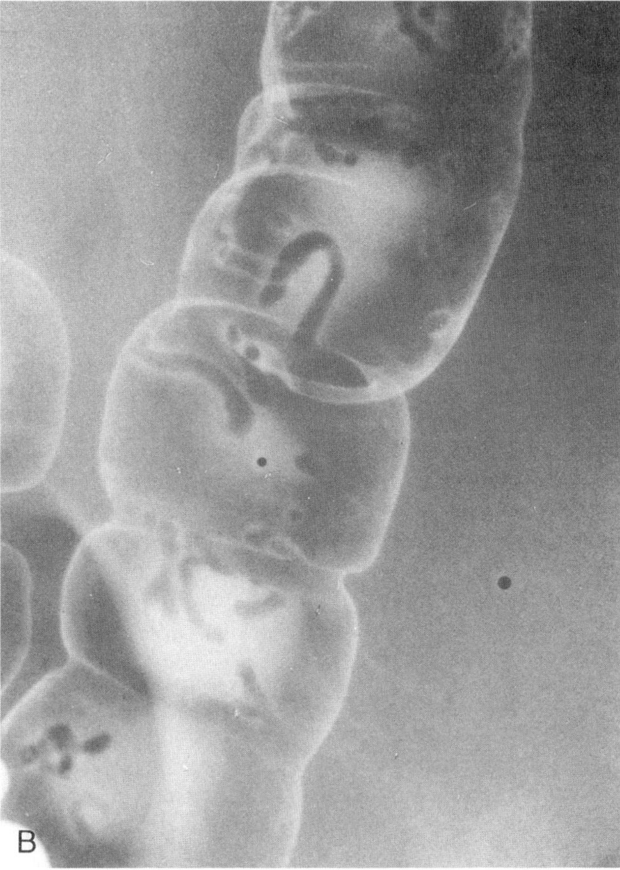

FIGURE 45 Filiform (postinflammatory) polyps in ulcerative colitis. *A*, There is gross colitis, as indicated by mucosal irregularity and nodularity seen on single-contrast barium enema. *B*, Four years later, a double-contrast study shows branching or wormlike polyps.

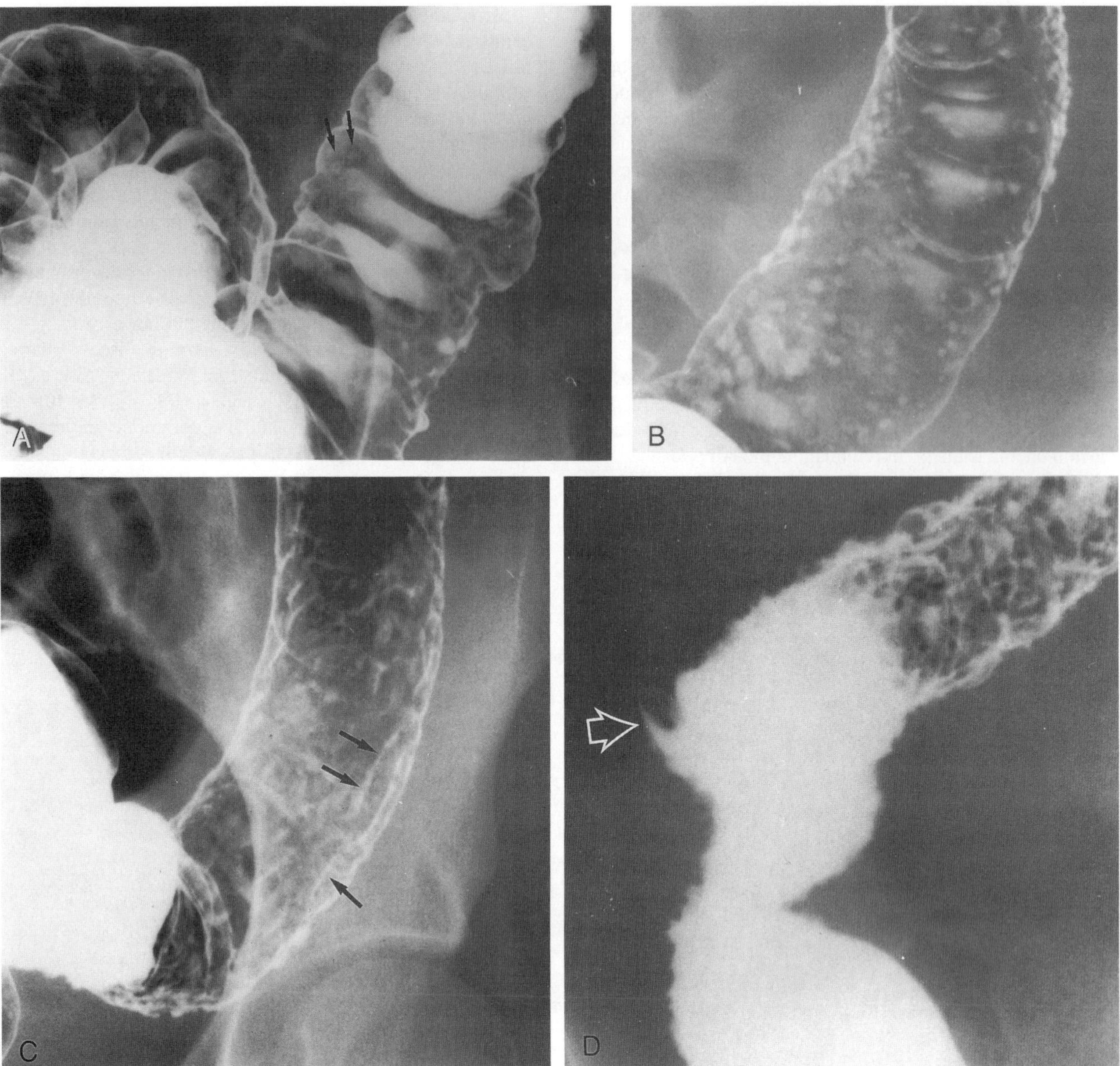

FIGURE 46 Crohn's colitis. *A*, In mild disease double-contrast barium enema shows asymmetric disease and multiple aphthae, which have a characteristic appearance of smooth, raised edges and a central umbilication (*arrows*). More severe disease shows *B*, deeper punctate ulceration, or *C*, linear ulceration (*arrows*). *D*, Severe disease gives extensive mucosal ulceration with marked irregularity of the mucosa and a deep ulcer (*arrow*) resembling a rose thorn. (From Stringer.[14])

lead to the formation of pseudodiverticula.[14,54] In children, Crohn's disease rarely causes filiform polyposis.[14,54]

Occasionally reflux of barium into the terminal ileum during the barium enema, a common occurrence in children, can be most helpful in excluding terminal ileal disease; however, usually a dedicated small bowel study with or without a peroral pneumocolon is required. We have found that the appearance of the terminal ileum in a barium enema study alone may underestimate the extent of terminal ileal involvement.[14,54]

The colon study may also show such complications of Crohn's disease as abscess of fistula formation, as well as the development of malignancy in longstanding cases.

Polyps

For the investigation of possible polyps and polyposis syndromes, a double-contrast study is preferred.[9,14] The appearance of the polyps of the various polyposis syndromes is indistinguishable, but the distribution of the polyps in the GI

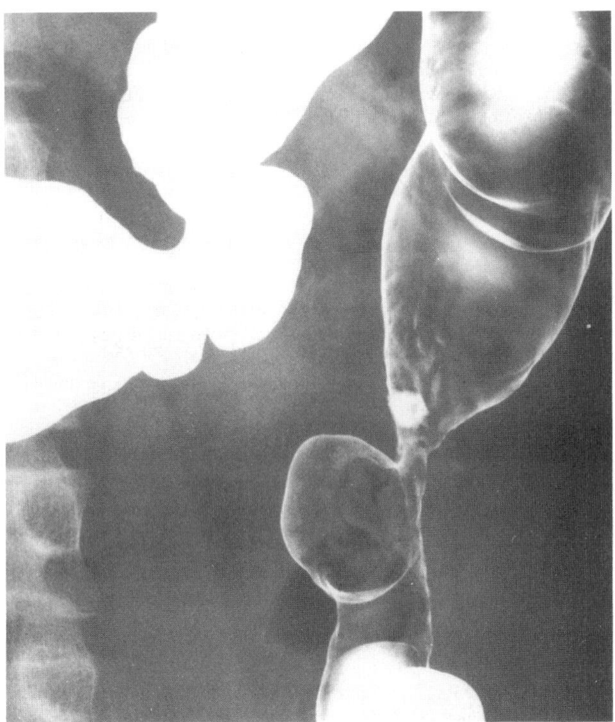

FIGURE 47 Crohn's disease stricture. There is an irregular narrowed area in the descending colon shown on double-contrast barium enema. Within and adjacent to this stricture, the mucosa is ulcerated, but elsewhere the mucosa is normal.

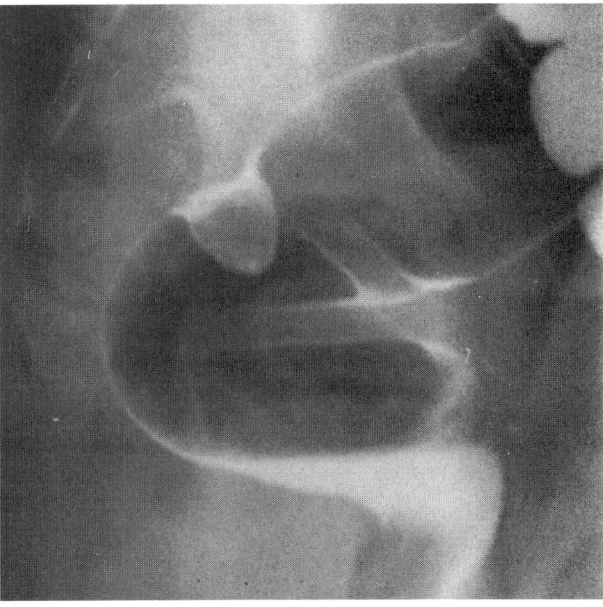

FIGURE 48 Sessile juvenile polyp. A smooth polyp arises from the posterosuperior wall of the rectum on a double-contrast barium enema.

tract together with the clinical features may suggest a more specific diagnosis.[82] For example, patients with Peutz-Jeghers syndrome may have polyps in the stomach, small bowel, and colon.[82] Juvenile polyps are the most common polyps in children and are not premalignant (Fig. 48). The incidence of malignancy increases with polyps larger than 1 cm. Biopsy may be needed for assessment of these larger polyps.

Unusual Large Bowel Techniques

Loopogram

A loopogram is a gentle enema, usually performed through an ostomy with water-soluble contrast material, to delineate an isolated loop of bowel before or after surgery. The anatomy and presence of any leaks or obstruction can thus be assessed.

Defecogram

Although a defecogram is occasionally helpful in the assessment of constipation in adults, its value in similar assessments in children is less clear.[83,84] It is used to assess patients with rectal prolapse, pain, blockage, or incontinence. The passage of barium from the rectum though the anal canal is assessed during defecation, during which the patient should be in a sitting or squatting position to simulate normal defecation.

SUMMARY

Contrast studies remain the primary means of assessment of the pediatric GI tract. The radiologist should be consulted so that the appropriate contrast study is performed to assess the clinical problem.

In selected diseases and for the assessment of abdominal masses, sonography is now playing a larger role as the screening modality. The newer imaging modalities complement the traditional contrast studies, which are still the most effective way to assess luminal and bowel wall abnormalities.

REFERENCES

1. Harris PD, Neuhauser EBD, Gerth R. The osmotic effect of water soluble contrast media on circulating plasma volume. AJR 1964; 91:694–698.
2. Chiu CL, Gambach RR. Hypaque pulmonary edema. A case report. Radiology 1974; 111:91–92.
3. Leonidas JC, Burry VF, Fellows RA, Beatty EC. Possible adverse effect of methylglucamine diatrizoate compounds on the bowel of newborn infants with meconium ileus. Radiology 1976; 121:693–696.
4. Grantmyre EB, Butler GJ, Gillis DA. Necrotizing enterocolitis after renografin-76 treatment of meconium ileus. AJR 1981; 136:990–991.
5. Ratcliffe JF. Low osmolality water soluble (LOWS) contrast media and the pediatric gastrointestinal tract. Radiology Now 1985; 8:8–11.
6. Ratcliffe JF. The use of ioxaglate in the paediatric gastrointestinal tract: a report of 25 cases. Clin Radiol 1983; 34:579–583.
7. Wolfson JJ, Williams H. A hazard of barium enema studies in infants with small bowel atresia. Radiology 1970; 95:341–343.

8. Shaw A. Safety of *N*-acetylcysteine in treatment of meconium obstruction of the newborn. J Pediatr Surg 1969; 4:119–125.
9. Dobranowski J, Stringer DA, Sommers S, Stevenson G. Manual of procedures in gastrointestinal radiology. New York: Springer-Verlag, 1990.
10. Stringer DA, Sherman PM, Jakowenko N. Correlation of double-contrast high-density barium enema, colonoscopy and histology in children with special attention to disparities. Pediatr Radiol 1986; 16:298–301.
11. Skolnick ML. A plea of an interdisciplinary approach to the radiological study of the velopharyngeal portal. Cleft Palate J 1977; 14:329–330.
12. Stringer DA, Witzel MA. Waters projection for evaluation of lateral pharyngeal wall movement in speech disorders. AJR 1985; 145:409–410.
13. Stringer DA, Witzel MA. Velopharyngeal insufficiency on videofluoroscopy: comparison of projections. AJR 1986; 146:15–19.
14. Stringer DA. Pediatric gastrointestinal imaging. Philadelphia: BC Decker, 1989.
15. Cumming WA, Reilly BJ. Fatigue aspiration. Radiology 1972; 105:387–390.
16. Wolf EL, Berdon WE, Baker DH. Improved plain-film diagnosis of right aortic arch anomalies with high kilovoltage-selective filtration-magnification technique. Pediatr Radiol 1978; 7:141–146.
17. Berdon WE, Baker DH. Vascular anomalies and the infant lung: rings, slings, and other things. Semin Roentgenol 1972; 7:39–64.
18. Klinkhamer AC. Esophagography in anomalies of the aortic arch system. Baltimore: Williams & Wilkins, 1969: 1.
19. Williams RG, Jaffe RB, Condon VR, Nixon GW. Unusual features of pulmonary sling. AJR 1979; 133:1065–1069.
20. Berson WE, Baker DH, Wung J-T, et al. Complete cartilage-ring tracheal stenosis associated with anomalous left pulmonary artery: the ring-sling complex. Radiology 1984; 152:57–64.
21. Moersch HJ. Cardiospasm in infancy and in childhood. Am J Dis Child 1929; 38:294–298.
22. Steiner GM. Review article: gastro-oesophageal reflux, hiatus hernia and the radiologist, with special reference to children. Br J Radiol 1977; 50:164–174.
23. Astley R, Carre IJ, Langmead-Smith R. A 20-year prospective follow-up of childhood hiatal hernia. Br J Radiol 1977; 50:400–403.
24. McCauley RGK, Darling DB, Leonidas JC, Schwartz AM. Gastroesophageal reflux in infants and children: a useful classification and reliable physiologic technique for its demonstration. AJR 1978; 130:47–50.
25. Leonidas JC. Gastroesophageal reflux in infants: role of the upper gastrointestinal series. AJR 1984; 143:1350–1351.
26. Darling DB, McCauley RGK, Leonidas JC, Schwartz AM. Gastroesophageal reflux in infants and children: correlation of radiological severity and pulmonary pathology. Radiology 1978; 127:735–740.
27. Stunden RJ, LeQuesne GW, Little KET. The improved ultrasound diagnosis of hypertrophic pyloric stenosis. Pediatr Radiol 1986; 16:200–205.
28. Pilling DW. Infantile hypertrophic pyloric stenosis: a fresh approach to the diagnosis. Clin Radiol 1983; 34:51–53.
29. Shopfner CE. The pyloric tit in hypertrophic pyloric stenosis. AJR 1964; 91:674–679.
30. Shopfner CE, Kalmon EH, Coin CG. The diagnosis of hypertrophic pyloric stenosis. AJR 1964; 91:796–800.
31. Cremin BJ. Congenital pyloric antral membranes in infancy. Radiology 1969; 92:509–512.
32. Kassner EG, Sutton AL, De Groot TJ. Bile duct anomalies associated with duodenal atresia; paradoxical presence of small bowel gas. AJR 1972; 116:577–583.
33. Inamoto K, Ishikawa Y, Itoh N. CT demonstration of annular pancreas: case report. Gastrointest Radiol 1983; 8:143–144.
34. Bill AH. Malrotation of the intestine. In: Ravitch MM, Welch KJ, Benson CD, et al, eds. Pediatric surgery. 3rd ed. Chicago: Year Book, 1979: 921.
35. Snyder WH, Chaffin L. Embryology and pathology of the intestinal tract: presentation of 40 cases of malrotation. Ann Surg 1954; 140:368–380.
36. Steiner GM. The misplaced caecum and the root of the mesentery. Br J Radiol 1978; 51:406–413.
37. Firor HV, Harris VJ. Rotational abnormalities of the gut: re-emphasis of a neglected facet, isolated incomplete rotation of the duodenum. AJR 1974; 120:315–321.
38. Drumm B, Rhoads M, Stringer DA, et al. Etiology, presentation and clinical course of endoscopically diagnosed peptic ulcer disease in children. Pediatrics; 1988; 82:410–414.
39. Winthrop JD, Balfe DM, Shackelford GD, et al. Ulcerative and granulomatous colitis in children. Comparison of double- and single-contrast studies. Radiology 1985; 154:657–660.
40. Seagram CGF, Stephens CA, Cumming WA. Peptic ulceration at the Hospital for Sick Children, Toronto, during the 20-year period 1949-1969. J Pediatr Surg 1973; 8:407–413.
41. Drumm B, Rhoads JM, Stringer DA, et al. Peptic ulcer disease in children: etiology, clinical findings, and clinical course. Pediatrics 1988; 82:410–414.
42. Ein SH, Friedberg J. Esophageal atresia and tracheoesophageal fistula: review and update. Otolaryngol Clin North Am 1981; 14:219–249.
43. Ein SH, Stringer DA, Stephens CA, et al. Recurrent tracheoesophageal fistulas: seventeen-year review. J Pediatr Surg 1983; 18:436–441.
44. Stringer DA, Ein SH. Recurrent tracheo-esophageal fistula: a protocol for investigation. Radiology 1984; 151:637–641.
45. Stringer DA, Sherman P, Liu P, Daneman A. Value of the peroral pneumocolon in children. AJR 1986; 146:763–766.
46. Stringer DA, Cloutier S, Daneman A, Durie P. The value of the small bowel enema in children. J Can Assoc Radiol 1986; 37:13–16.
47. Weizman Z, Stringer DA, Durie PR. Radiologic manifestations of malabsorption: a nonspecific finding. Pediatrics 1984; 74:530–533.
48. Kleinman PK, Brill PW, Winchester P. Resolving duodenal-jejunal hematoma in abused children. Radiology 1986; 160:747–750.
49. Djurhuus MJ, Lykkegaard E, Pock-Steen OC. Gastrointestinal radiological findings in cystic fibrosis. Pediatr Radiol 1973; 1:113–118.
50. Jones B, Bayless TM, Hamilton SR, Yardley JH. "Bubbly" duodenal bulb in celiac disease: radiologic-pathologic correlation. AJR 1984; 142:119–122.
51. Berk RN, Lee FA. The late gastrointestinal manifestations of cystic fibrosis of the pancreas. Radiology 1973; 106:337–381.
52. Rosenthall L, Henry JN, Murphy DA, Freeman LM. Radiopertechnetate imaging of the Meckel diverticulum. Radiology 1972; 105:371–373.
53. Maglinte DDT, Elmore MF, Isenberg M, Dolan PA. Meckel diverticulum: radiologic demonstration by enteroclysis. AJR 1980; 134:925–932.
54. Stringer DA. Imaging inflammatory bowel disease in the pediatric patient. Radiol Clin North Am 1987; 25:93–113.
55. Spencer R. Gastrointestinal hemorrhage in infancy and childhood: 476 cases. Surgery 1964; 55:718–734.
56. Berdon WE, Baker DH, Santulli TV, Amoury RA, Blanc WA. Microcolon in newborn infants with intestinal obstruction. Its correlation with the level and time of onset of obstruction. Radiology 1968; 90:878–885.
57. Siegel MJ, Shackelford GD, McAlister WH. Small bowel volvulus in children: its appearance on the barium enema examination. Pediatr Radiol 1980; 10:91–93.
58. Noblett HR. Treatment of uncomplicated meconium ileus by gastrografin enema: a preliminary report. J Pediatr Surg 1969; 4:190–197.
59. Lutzger LG, Factor SM. Effects of some water-soluble contrast media on the colonic mucosa. Radiology 1976; 118:545–548.
60. Seltzer SE, Jones B. Cecal perforation associated with gastrografin enema. AJR 1978; 130:997–998.
61. Wood BP, Katzberg RW, Ryan DH, Karch FE. Diatrizoate enemas: facts and fallacies of colonic toxicity. Radiology 1978; 126:441–444.
62. Shaw A. Safety of *N*-acetylcysteine in the treatment of meconium obstruction of the newborn. J Pediatr Surg 1969; 4:119–125.
63. Ein SH, Shandling B, Reilly BJ, Stephens CA. Bowel perforation with nonoperative treatment of meconium ileus. J Pediatr Surg 1987; 22:146–147.
64. Le Quesne GW, Reilly BJ. Functional immaturity of the large bowel in the newborn infant. Radiol Clin North Am 1975; 13:331–342.
65. Cleghorn GJ, Stringer DA, Forstner GG, Durie PR. Treatment of distal intestinal obstruction syndrome in cystic fibrosis with a balanced intestinal lavage solution. Lancet 1986; i:8–11.
66. Koletzko S, Stringer DA, Cleghorn GJ, Durie PR. Lavage treatment of distal intestinal obstruction syndrome in cystic fibrosis; accepted by Pediatrics, 1989; 83:727–733.
67. Cremin BJ. The early diagnosis of Hirschsprung disease. Pediatr Radiol 1974; 2:23–28.
68. Pochaczevsky R, Leonidas JC. The "recto-sigmoid index". A measurement for the early diagnosis of Hirschsprung disease. AJR 1975; 123:770–777.
69. Siegel MJ, Shackelford GD, McAlister WH. The rectosigmoid index. Radiology 1981; 139:497–499.
70. Johnson JF, McMurdo KK. Spontaneous complete evacuation of barium in a baby with Hirschsprung [sic] disease. AJR 1982; 139:594–595.

71. Cremin BJ, Golding RL. Congenital aganglionosis of the entire colon in neonates. Br J Radiol 1976; 49:27–33.
72. De Campo JF, Mayne V, Boldt DW, De Campo M. Radiological findings in total aganglionosis coli. Pediatr Radiol 1984; 14:205–209.
73. Haney PJ, Hill JL, Sun CCJ. Zonal colonic aganglionosis. Pediatr Radiol 1982; 12:258–261.
74. Ein SH, Stephens CA. Intussusception: 354 cases in 10 years. J Pediatr Surg 1971; 6:16–27.
75. Gu L, Alton DJ, Daneman A, et al. Intussusception reduction in children by rectal insufflation of air. AJR 1988; 150:1345–1348.
76. Eklöf O, Hugosson C. [Post-evacuation findings in barium-enema treated intussusceptions.] Ann Radiol 1976; 19:133–139.
77. Humphry A, Ein SH, Mok PM. Perforation of the intussuscepted colon. AJR 1981; 137:1135–1138.
78. Armstrong EA, Dunbar JS, Graviss ER, Martin L, Rosenkrantz J. Intussusception complicated by distal perforation of the colon. Radiology 1980; 136:77–81.
79. Ein SH. Leading points in childhood intussusception. J Pediatr Surg 1976; 11:209–211.
80. Ein SH, Shandling B, Reilly BJ, Stringer DA. Hydrostatic reduction of intussusceptions caused by lead points. J Pediatr Surg 1986; 21:883–886.
81. Miller M, Stringer DA, Chiu-Mei T, Daneman A, Juodis E. Lymphoid follicular pattern in the colon: an indicator of barium coating. J Can Assoc Radiol 1987; 38:256–258.
82. Dodds WJ. Clinical and roentgen features of the intestinal polyposis syndromes. Gastrointest Radiol 1976; 1:127–142.
83. Ekberg O, Nylander G, Fork FT. Defecography. Radiology 1985; 155:45–48.
84. Brown BSJ. Defecography or anorectal studies in children including cinefluorographic observations. J Can Assoc Radiol 1965; 16:66–76.

PART 4

Sonography

Paul Babyn, M.D.
David A. Stringer, B.Sc., M.B.B.S., F.R.C.R., FRCPC

In the last 15 years, pediatric radiology has witnessed an explosive increase in use of sonography. Sonography has become the primary imaging modality for the evaluation of any suspected problem associated with the abdominal viscera. This discussion provides an introduction to some general principles as well as an overview of the value of sonography in the evaluation of the pediatric gastrointestinal tract.

The main advantages of sonography include its noninvasiveness (particularly its lack of ionizing radiation), real-time imaging, and Doppler flow analysis. Sonography is applicable across the entire pediatric age spectrum, from the early embryo to the adolescent. In addition, sonographic visualization of the intra-abdominal contents is easier in children than in adults, because of their smaller size and relative lack of fat. When these advantages are coupled with the wide availability and portability of ultrasound it is easy to see why sonography has become an indispensable tool in pediatric radiology. However, sonography is not without limitations. Its primary disadvantages include the fact that it is operator-dependent, has limited section analysis, and requires direct access to the skin. These can be overcome to a large degree with adequate training and experience.[1,2,3]

GENERAL PRINCIPLES OF SONOGRAPHY

Diagnostic sonography depends upon the transmission of ultrasound in the frequency range of 3 to 10 MHz generated by a piezoelectric crystal located in the transducer. On returning to the transducer, the reflected signals are then analyzed, allowing identification and differentiation of underlying structures within the tissue examined. It is important to have a basic understanding of the nomenclature of sonography. *Echogenicity* refers to the brightness of the returning echos and is related to the percentage of the sound being reflected back from a tissue interface. *Attenuation* is the decrease in intensity of the ultrasound beam as it passes through a defined tissue. For example, calcification is more attenuating than most soft tissue, which gives rise to the decreased distal acoustic signal (also known as distal acoustic shadowing) (see Fig. 13). Calcification is also more echogenic, appearing quite bright on sonographic images because of the high proportion of reflected sound. Sonography is commonly utilized to differentiate cysts from solid masses. Typical cysts appear anechoic (that is, without internal echoes) with a clearly defined deep wall that demonstrates enhanced through transmission (a relative increased echogenicity at and beyond this deep wall compared with the background) (see Fig. 18). The terms *hypo-* and *hyperechogenicity* refer to internal echogenicity, typically the echogenicity of a lesion within an abnormal organ or one tissue relative to another. Similarly, echogenicity may be variable over time. Hematomas, for example, generally are hyperechoic initially, becoming more hypoechoic as they liquefy (see Fig. 29). Not all pathologic conditions will demonstrate similar echogenicity. Abscesses, for example, may be hypo- or hyperechoic, depending upon internal characteristics (see Figs. 8, 9, and 31). Solid masses are echogenic lesions that may be irregular or poorly defined without increased through transmission (see Figs. 5, 6, and 7). Bowel gas is also echogenic and can cause acoustic shadowing because of its high attenuation. This limits visualization of underlying structures and may be responsible for a technically unsatisfactory scan.[4]

The early B-mode static scanners have been long surpassed by present day machines featuring real-time imaging, computerized processing, spectral Doppler imaging (see Figs. 11 and 12), and color flow imaging. These have improved gray scale imaging and permit dynamic evaluations of blood flow. Doppler signals result from the interaction of the transmitted sound beam and a moving medium, generally red blood cells within a vessel. Reflected signals are thereby generated and can be used to determine not only the presence and direction of blood flow but the velocity wave form of the sampled vessel.[5] Over the last 5 years an increased range of applications for Doppler sonography within the abdomen have been found. Primary indications include evaluation of suspected portal hypertension, liver transplantation, and assessment of shunt patency. These are discussed further in the hepatobiliary section.

TECHNIQUE OF EXAMINATION

The normal scan protocol depends upon the area to be examined and the nature of the clinical problem. Generally there is no need, at any age, for sedation prior to examination. In preparation for examination of the gallbladder fasting for approximately 4 hours is recommended. A multitude of transducers can be utilized. In neonates we usually use 5-MHz transducers, whereas in older children we use either 3- or 5-MHz depending on patient size. We scan the entire abdomen including the pelvis, since sonography provides a useful screening examination and organ-specific scans are too limiting diagnostically. Initial survey views of the upper abdomen and pelvis are obtained along with more focused views of any pathology. Although the normal sonographic anatomy does not change with the age of the patient, the sonographic appearance of the viscera may vary with age, both in relative size and echogenicity of organs. The sonologist should have a precise understanding of the normal variations at each age and know the potential sonographic artifacts.

PRENATAL SONOGRAPHY

The application of prenatal sonography in gastrointestinal tract imaging has grown rapidly over the last decade.[1] The normal development and appearance of the upper abdomen viscera, gastrointestinal tract, and abdominal wall are now well established.[6,7] Prenatal sonography, however, requires considerable operator expertise, excellent equipment, and also knowledge of the gestational development and growth of the fetus. Certain findings at one gestational age may be normal and abnormal later on.[8] For example, before the normal bowel migrates from the extraembryonic coelom back into the abdomen, differentiation from omphaloceles is almost impossible. Naturally more detail will be visible during the latter stages of gestation than earlier when the embryo is only 1 to 2 cm in length, although vaginal sonography gives excellent delineation early in gestation.

The assessment of the abdominal wall is an important area of interest in prenatal sonography. Many anomalies of the abdominal wall can be imaged including omphaloceles and gastroschisis. Normal embryologic development of the anterior abdominal wall depends upon fusion of four endomesodermic folds, the cephalic and caudal folds, and the two lateral folds. Omphaloceles are ventral wall defects that are characterized by herniations of the intra-abdominal contents into the base of the umbilical cord and are covered by amnioperitoneal membrane. Gastroschisis is a lateral defect, usually on the right, with herniation of the bowel without a surrounding membrane. In every fetal examination, the entrance of the umbilical cord into the fetus should be scanned to screen for the presence of omphalocele and caudal fold defects.[1] On sonography, omphaloceles are generally midline masses adjacent to the anterior abdominal wall often associated with polyhydramnios (Fig. 1).[6] With careful scanning, gastroschisis can be seen separate from the umbilical cord insertion.[6] Omphaloceles may be associated with the Beckwith-Wiedemann syndrome or the complex of ectopia cordis and sternal and diaphragmatic defects as in the pentalogy of Cantrell.[6] In gastroschisis the abdominal wall defect is thought to result from vascular compromise of either the umbilical vein or an inflamed mesenteric artery. There is also a strong association between jejunal atresia, gastroschisis, and bowel malrotation.[6]

Abnormalities of the diaphragm are common and include Bochdalek and Morgagni hernias as well as eventration; these may be identified by prenatal sonography. In the fetus, the normal diaphragm is seen as a hypoechoic line separating lungs and liver and is completely formed by 8 weeks of gestation. Severe defects of the diaphragm are associated with lung hypoplasia as well as bowel malrotation. On sonography one may appreciate fluid-filled cystic structures with peristalsis in the thoracic cavity at the level of the heart. There is often associated cardiac displacement and polyhydramnios.[6]

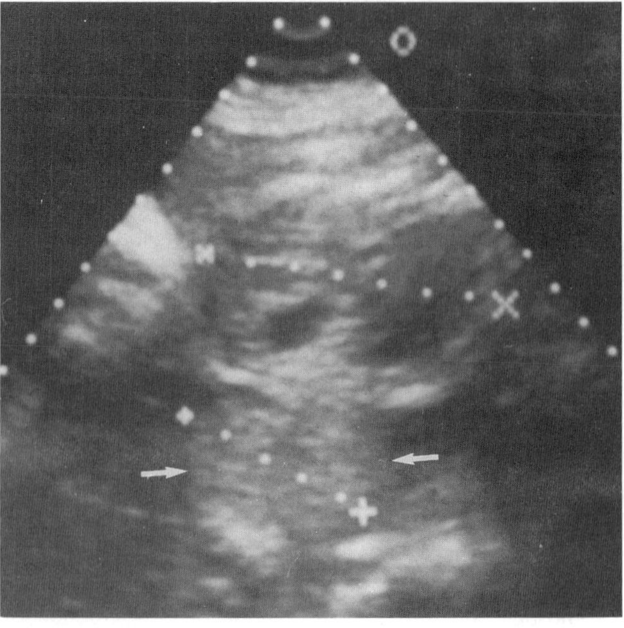

FIGURE 1 Omphalocele. Prenatal sonography shows an anterior abdominal wall sac (*between arrows*). (From Stringer.[3])

Prenatal sonography is helpful in evaluating suspected bowel obstruction. By 9 weeks of gestation the stomach can be routinely visualized. Small and large bowel can usually be distinguished by sonography, and normal measurements have been determined.[7] Small bowel is centrally located and changes with peristalsis; only short segments can be imaged at one time. The large bowel appears tubular around the periphery of the abdomen without peristalsis. Haustral clefts can be seen by 31 weeks.[7] When meconium appears, it is hypoechoic compared with the abdominal wall. Obstruction is suggested if the small bowel is larger than 7 mm in diameter or the colon exceeds 18 mm.[7,9] Polyhydramnios is often associated with bowel obstruction, particularly in cases of upper intestinal atresia. In the presence of polyhydramnios, esophageal atresia without tracheoesophageal fistula should be suspected, if there is no fluid-filled stomach. In duodenal atresia, the most common type of congenital small bowel obstruction, one can image distention of both the stomach and duodenum, a sonographic double bubble.[7] Multiple distended fluid-filled loops of small bowel suggest more distal obstruction that may represent meconium ileus.[10] However, not all bowel distention represents intestinal obstruction, as it has rarely been seen in association with chronic chloride-losing diarrhea.[7]

Meconium peritonitis may be diagnosed when there is intra-abdominal hyperechogenicity with shadowing compatible with calcification; often it is associated with fetal ascites and polyhydramnios. A loculated fluid collection representing a meconium cyst may be seen. Soon after birth, echogenic ascites termed a *snowstorm* pattern has been found in meconium peritonitis. A variety of miscellaneous abnormalities of the gastrointestinal tract can be detected prenatally. These include visceromegaly of the liver or spleen, congenital hepatic tumors (congenital hepatoblastoma, hemangioendothelioma), and hepatic cysts. Choledochal cysts and other cysts of the peritoneal cavity (mesenteric and retroperitoneal cysts) have also been noted.[6]

LIVER AND BILIARY SYSTEM

The liver is readily accessible in its entirety with real-time sonography from the dome of the hemidiaphragm down to its inferior margin. Sonography is the initial modality of choice for investigation of suspected congenital anomalies, focal masses, and diffuse disease. The hepatic artery and veins, including the portal venous system, form the vascular scaffolding that helps define the lobar anatomy of the liver. The hepatic vasculature is readily subdivided by vessel origin, characteristic course, branching pattern, and vessel wall echogenicity. [11,12] Caudal hepatic veins may be seen in 10 percent of the population and are of no clinical concern.[13] The normal hepatic parenchyma is homogeneous in echogenicity, displaying relatively increased echogenicity compared with the renal cortex, and echotexture similar to that of the spleen. Occasionally the main right and left hepatic ducts can be visualized anterior to the portal vein bifurcation, but the smaller branches are not normally seen. Infrequently, during transverse sonography, the falciform ligament and ligamentum venosum can appear as hyperechoic structures simulating pseudotumors, which are usually easily defined by longitudinal scanning. Assessment of hepatic size is usually evaluated subjectively by the experienced sonographer, but standardized age-related tables are available.[14] A rounded inferior margin and extension of the liver beyond the inferior aspect of the right kidney are helpful features suggestive of enlargement.

Congenital and Developmental Anomalies

Congenital lobar anomalies of the liver, such as agenesis and lobar hypoplasia, are rare. Other congenital and developmental anomalies that more commonly involve the biliary tract include choledochal cysts, biliary atresia, and Alagille's syndrome. Choledochal cysts are commonly divided into four main types, the two most common being fusiform dilatation of the common bile duct (Fig. 2) and saccular diverticula extending off the common bile ducts.[11,12] Choledochoceles or Caroli's disease is seen much less commonly (Fig. 3). Large choledochal cysts are easily appreciated with sonography as fluid-filled structures in the region of the porta hepatis. Associated intrahepatic biliary tract dilatation, choledocholithiasis, or internal debris may be noted. Fortunately, minimal degrees of choledochal dilation are rare, but these may require further investigation with endoscopic retrograde cholangicopancreatography or percutaneous transhepatic cholangiography to differentiate from other causes of a dilated biliary tree. Choledochoceles are not usually seen by sonography. In Caroli's disease there is often marked nonobstructive segmental dilatation of the intrahepatic biliary system (Fig. 3).[11,12,15,16]

Cystic lesions in the right upper quadrant also encompass a wide variety of other cystic lesions besides choledochal

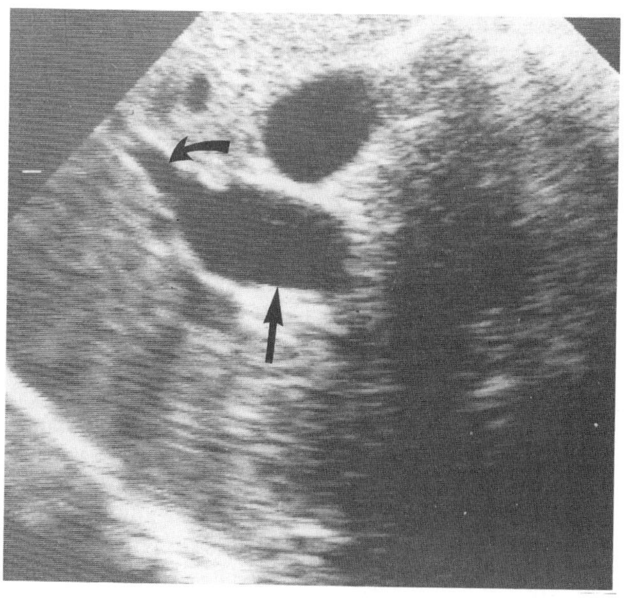

FIGURE 2 Type I choledochal cyst. Oblique sonography shows fusiform dilatation of the common bile (*straight arrow*) and hepatic ducts (*curved arrow*) extending into the porta hepatis separating the portions of the liver with intrahepatic extension.

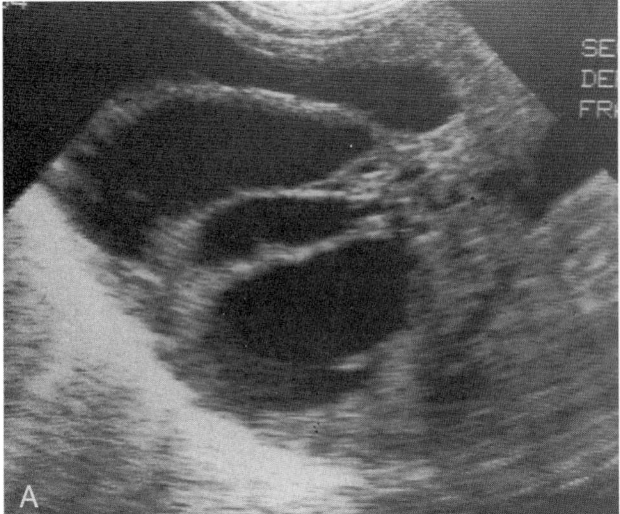
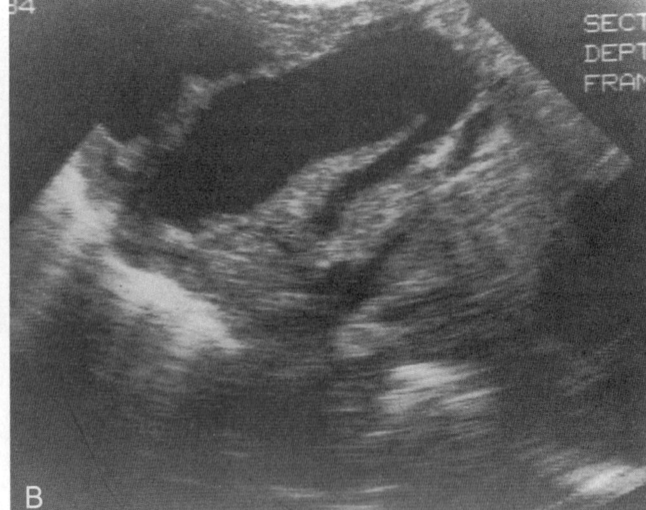
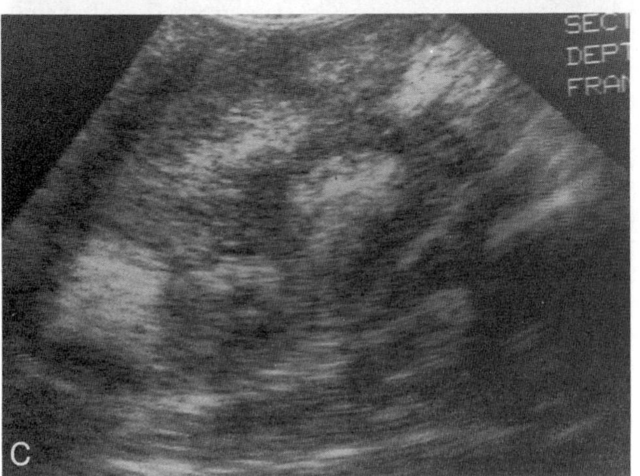

FIGURE 3 Type IV choledochal cyst or Caroli's disease. *A*, Longitudinal sonography shows multiple cystic structures enlarging the liver. *B*, Some of the cystic structures appear to communicate. *C*, Longitudinal sonography through both kidneys showed marked increased echogenicity of the renal pyramids in grossly enlarged kidneys. A postmortem specimen showed gross dilatation of the biliary tree with congenital hepatic fibrosis and multiple tiny cysts in the kidney. (From Stringer.[3])

cysts, such as duplication cysts and ovarian cysts. Usually no further imaging is necessary prior to surgery.[11]

Biliary atresia is an important cause of infantile cholestatic jaundice, necessitating prompt diagnosis and therapy with a Kasai portoenterostomy and/or liver transplantation. Sonography is utilized primarily to exclude other surgical causes of obstructive infantile cholestasis. In a minority of cases sonography can differentiate biliary atresia from neonatal hepatitis by documenting the presence of ductal dilatation and increased periportal echogenicity in biliary atresia.[11] Infrequently, biliary atresia is associated with polysplenia and/or choledochal cysts. In the past, documentation of the presence of a normal gallbladder was thought sufficient to exclude biliary atresia; however, a normal-size gallbladder may occasionally be found in biliary atresia. Similarly, sonographic absence of the gallbladder may be seen in neonatal hepatitis. Following a Kasai procedure, progressive intrahepatic ductal dilation and bile lake formation are frequently noted and sonography is useful in monitoring these (Fig. 4).[11,12]

In Alagille's syndrome, a congenital form of biliary hypoplasia, a general increase in hepatic echogenicity may be noted. Another congenital cause of increased echogenicity is congenital hepatic fibrosis. This disorder, inherited as autosomal dominant or recessive, is almost invariably associated with polycystic renal disease. Congenital hepatic fibrosis may be recognized and diagnosed by the associated marked abnormal enlargement and echogenicity of the kidneys. Occasionally, liver cysts may be noted in autosomal dominant polycystic disease, appearing as anechoic fluid-filled structures similar to any cyst seen sonographically. Isolated hepatic cysts are rare, but they can occur, particularly in the right lobe of the liver.[11,12]

Focal Hepatic Masses

Sonography is preferred as the initial modality for the radiologic assessment of any known or suspected abdominal mass, particularly of the upper abdominal viscera, largely owing to its inherent advantages, particularly its ready availability and the lack of exposure to radiation. For lesions that are clearly benign (e.g., a simple hepatic cyst), no further imaging is required before instituting therapy. Computed tomography (CT) is reserved for cases requiring more extensive investigation, either for clearer anatomic delineation or definition of malignant spread. Liver masses include neoplasms, abscesses, cysts, and hematomas. Considerable overlap in sonographic appearance exists among the various etiologies of focal masses, for example, between abscesses and tumors. Therefore, one must carefully integrate the clinical and labora-

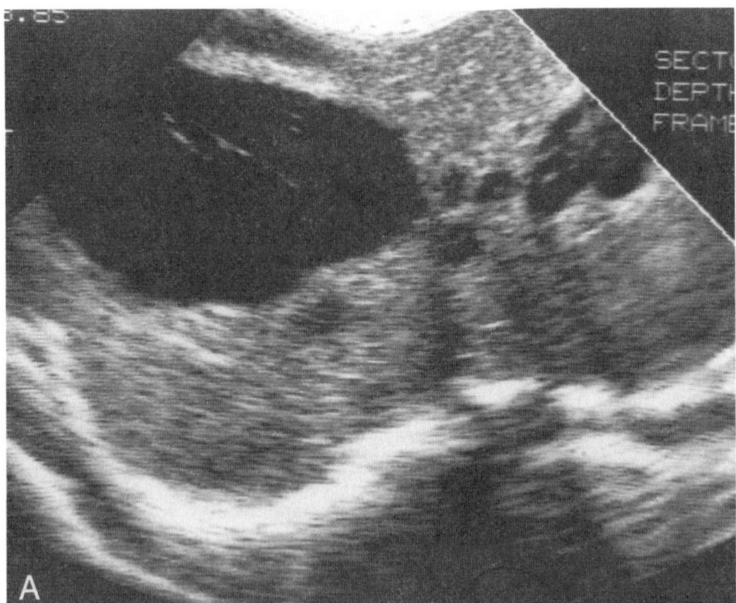

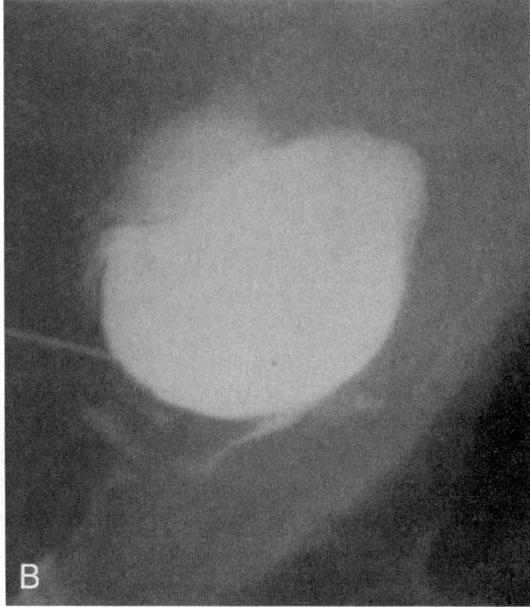

FIGURE 4 Bile lakes in biliary atresia after the Kasai procedure. *A*, There is a large intrahepatic cystic slightly trabeculated structure on transverse sonography. *B*, A percutaneous cholangiogram demonstrated a large bile lake. Drainage of the lake did not improve hepatic status in this patient. (From Stringer.[3])

tory information with the radiographic results to most accurately define the lesion.[11,12,17,18]

Hepatic Tumors

Benign hepatic tumors can be classified into two main groups according to their cellular origin as either mesenchymal or epithelial. Mesenchymal tumors include vascular tumors (infantile hemangioendotheliomas) and mesenchymal hamartomas. Epithelial tumors include congenital hepatic cysts, which were discussed previously, together with focal nodular hyperplasia and hepatic adenomas.

Hemangioendothelioma is the most common benign hepatic tumor of infancy, which presents with liver enlargement, an abdominal mass, or congestive heart failure. Associated cutaneous hemangiomas are found in slightly less than half the cases. Sonographically these lesions are of variable echogenicity: hyperechoic, isoechoic, or hypoechoic (Fig. 5). They may be diffuse, multifocal, or localized to one hepatic lobe. Enlargement of feeding vessels (aorta, hepatic artery) and draining hepatic veins may occur with or without arteriovenous shunting.[19-21] Sonography can monitor the resolution of these tumors, which generally occurs with focal development of calcifications over 6 months to 1 year.

Mesenchymal hamartomas are not true neoplasms but more likely represent a developmental anomaly of the bile ducts and mesenchymal tissue. The majority arise from the right lobe of the liver, and they usually present with abdominal distention or a palpable abdominal mass. Sonographically, they are rounded, anechoic, predominantly cystic lesions of variable size and contain thin intervening septa (Fig. 6). Infrequently, solid echogenic components may be found.[22,23]

Hepatic adenomas are uncommon benign hepatic tumors of childhood and are often associated with glycogen storage disease or other metabolic disorders. Typically, the lesions are rounded, but they vary in size and echogenicity. In glycogen storage disease, sonography and routine alpha-fetoprotein measurement have been recommended to monitor for malignant transformation of hepatic adenomas.[24]

Focal nodular hyperplasia are tumor-like lesions of the liver that are uncommon during childhood. Sonographically these lesions are solitary, large, rounded masses of variable echogenicity (either hyperechoic, isoechoic, hypoechoic, or complex). Occasionally they have a characteristic central echogenic stranding that corresponds to the central stellate fibrosis that is seen pathologically. ^{99m}Tc–sulfur colloid scans often show normal uptake that strongly supports the diagnosis.[25]

Metastases to the liver occur more commonly than primary malignant tumors of the liver. Neuroblastoma and Wilms' tumor, as well as lymphoma are among the metastatic tumors that more commonly spread to the liver. Most metastates show as hypoechoic, solitary, or multiple masses located anywhere within the hepatic parenchyma. Hyperechoic or complex masses may also be seen. In neuroblastoma or leukemia, liver metastases may be so extensive that discrete nodules may not be detectable, and the enlarged liver may show diffuse coarse echogenicity.[11,12]

Hepatoblastomas and hepatocellular carcinomas are the most common primary hepatic malignancies of childhood that typically present with hepatomegaly and/or abdominal distention. Hepatoblastomas almost always occur in children under 5 years of age, whereas hepatocellular carcinomas are found in older children. Both are similar sonographically. Typically they are large, usually solitary, hyperechoic but

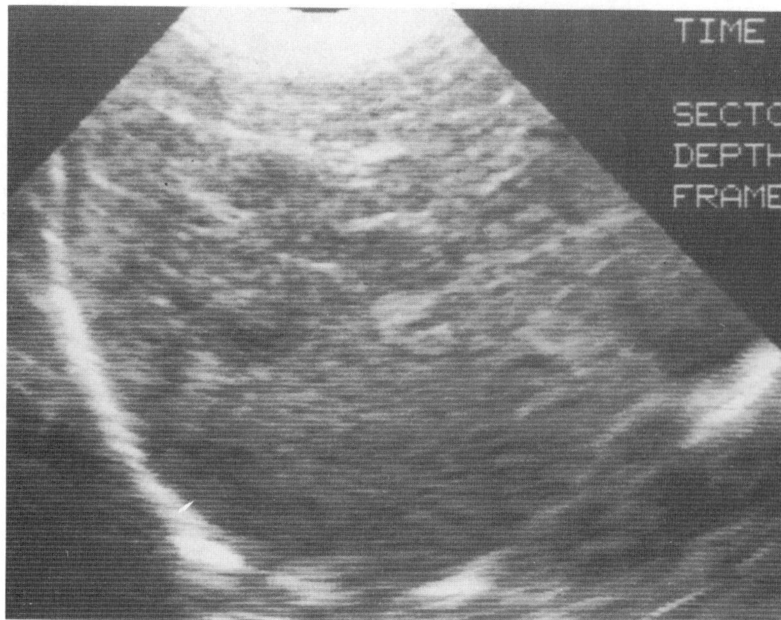

FIGURE 5 Hepatic hemangioendothelioma. Longitudinal sonography shows an irregular area of mixed hyper- and hypoechoic signals in the anterior portion of the liver. (From Stringer.[3])

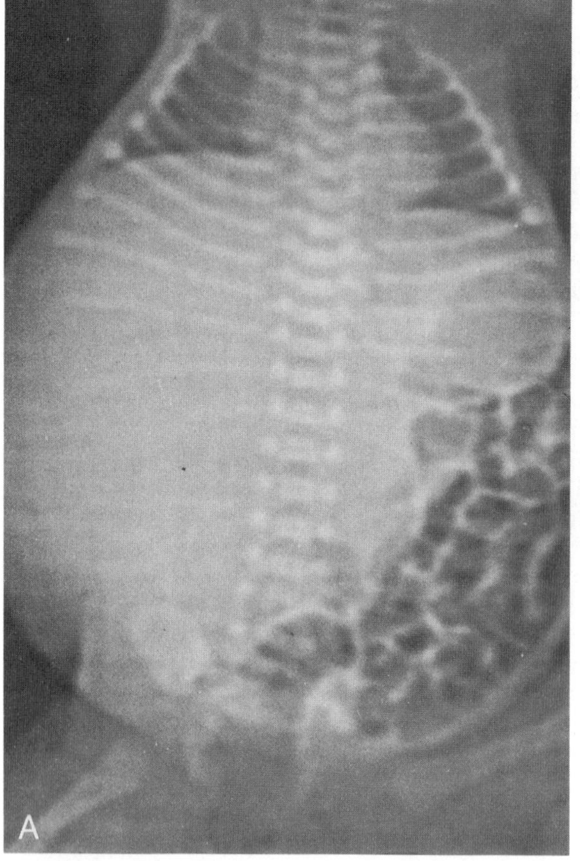

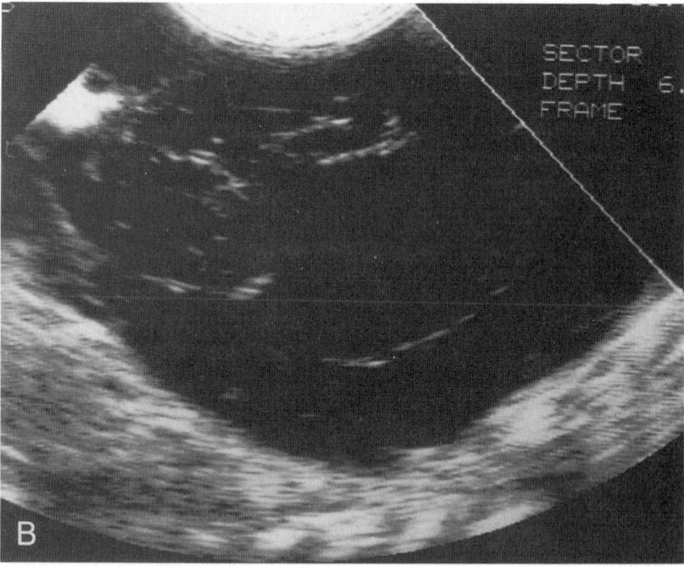

FIGURE 6 Hepatic hamartoma. *A*, The plain film shows a large soft tissue mass in the right side of the abdomen. *B*, Longitudinal sonography shows a cystic mass containing a few thin echogenic septa. (From Stringer.[3])

sometimes hypoechoic (Fig. 7) masses of variable homogeneity, most often arising from the right lobe of the liver.[11,12] A multifocal or diffuse pattern is slightly more common with hepatocellular carcinoma.[12] Brunelle and Chaumont have emphasized the importance of careful examination of the portal-venous system.[26] Malignant tumors characteristically invade and amputate the portal veins, which is not seen in benign tumors. This can be demonstrated with angiography or sonography. A variant of hepatocellular carcinoma is fibrolamellar hepatocellular carcinoma, which usually occurs in adolescence and is more found in the left lobe of the liver. They may have a central echogenic stellate scar similar to that seen in focal nodular hyperplasia.[17]

Hepatic Abscesses

Hepatic abscesses, whether pyogenic, fungal, or due to other infections, are uncommon lesions in infancy and childhood. Abscesses show a wide spectrum of sonographic appearances dependent upon age of the abscess, the inflammatory response, and the underlying organism.[27-30] Sonography confirms the presence and number of lesions and provides a rough guide to etiology while providing internal characteristics and anatomic localization of potential use for aspiration and drainage. Pyogenic abscesses are uncommon in children, being found mainly in immunocompromised or malnourished patients. They are usually solitary, round or ovoid lesions that are most often located in the periphery of either lobe of the liver. The abscess wall may be irregular and poorly or well defined. A hypoechoic halo is infrequently seen. Centrally the abscess is usually hypoechoic, but may be anechoic due to liquefactive necrosis (Fig. 8). Echogenic debris or gas may be seen. Distal acoustic enhancement is often present, suggesting a cystic origin.[27,28] Small staphylococcal abscesses can occasionally stimulate a target sign with central echogenic areas surrounded by an hypoechoic periphery. This appearance is more commonly seen in hepatic candidiasis (Fig. 9).[29]

Parenchymal Liver Disease and Vascular Abnormalities

Parenchymal liver disease may occur as a result of a spectrum of disease processes including hepatitis, metabolic disease, and drug toxicity. None of these disorders has a characteristic sonographic appearance.[31] Diagnosis is usually established by associated clinical and laboratory findings and pathologic examination from a biopsy. When abnormal, the liver is usually enlarged with a coarse increased parenchymal echogenicity, often associated with decreased visualization of the hepatic vasculature and decreased through transmission (Fig. 10). This bright liver pattern is most frequently seen in diffuse hepatic injury and fatty infiltration. A centrilobular pattern of increased periportal echogenicity may be seen with hepatitis,[32] but is less frequent in childhood than in adulthood.

Progressive hepatic injury can lead to cirrhosis. In cirrhosis, variable sonographic findings can be present. In early stages, the liver may appear entirely normal, but with advanced disease, the liver becomes small, often irregular in outline, and there is diffusely increased echogenicity probably from fibrosis. Associated findings include the development of portal hypertension, splenomegaly, and ascites.[12] Concomitant with the onset of portal hypertension, the portosystemic collaterals develop, which can be seen sonographically. Gastroesophageal varices, a paraumbilical vein, an enlarged coronary vein, and perirenal retroperitoneal varices may be visualized. The lesser omentum may be thickened. Doppler examination can demonstrate venous flow in the varices, and document direction of portal venous flow. Por-

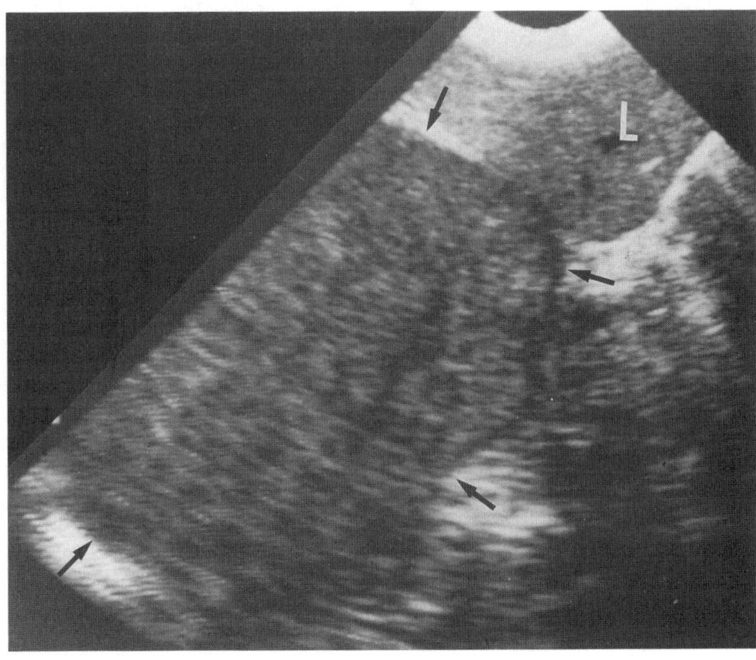

FIGURE 7 Hepatoblastoma. A large mass (*arrows*) posterior to normal liver tissue (L) on longitudinal sonography has an irregular hypoechoic pattern that more nearly resembles liver than is usual for hepatoblastomas.

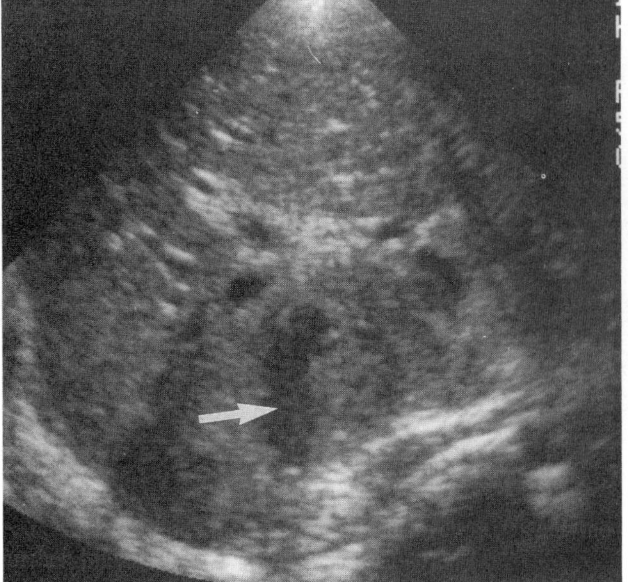

FIGURE 8 Pyogenic hepatic abscess. Transverse sonography shows one of many echo-poor lesions (*arrow*) seen within the liver of a 4-year-old boy who had chronic granulomatous disease of childhood.

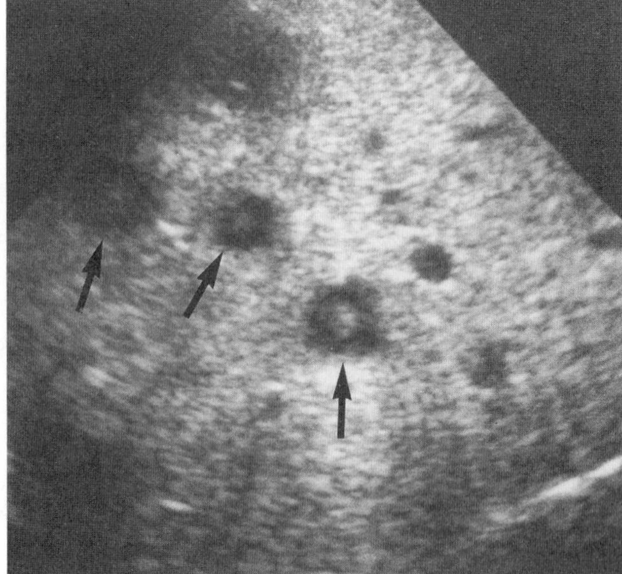

FIGURE 9 Hepatic candidiasis. Transverse sonography shows multiple relatively well-defined hypoechoic areas in the liver, some of which have an echogenic center (*arrows*), the so-called target lesion.

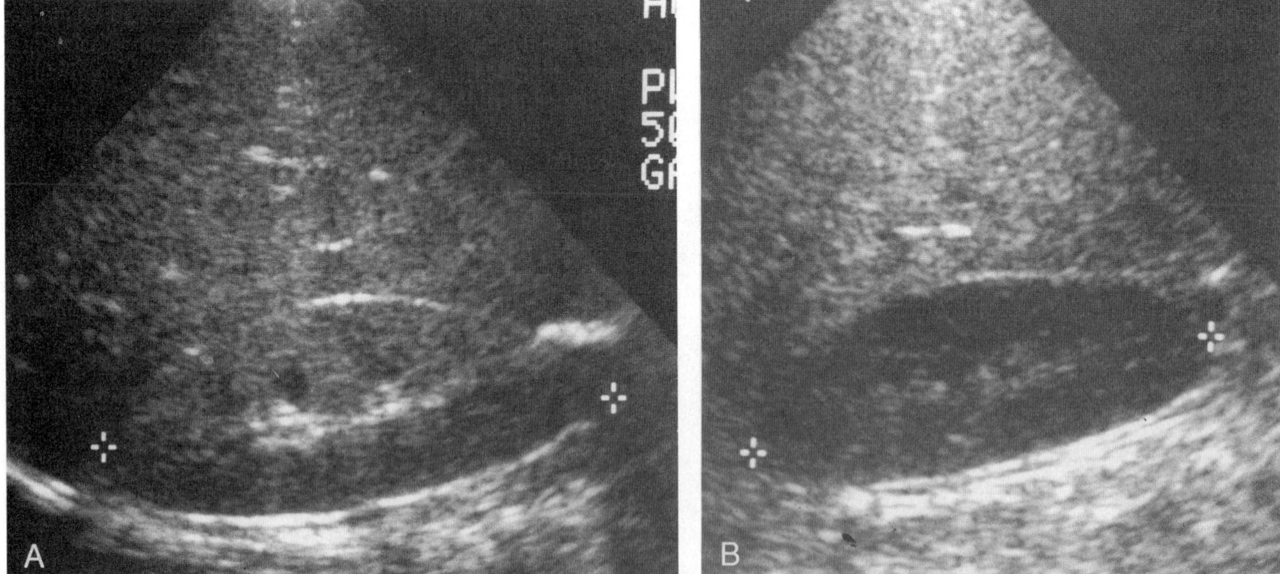

FIGURE 10 Fatty infiltration of the liver. *A*, Soon after starting cytotoxic therapy, longitudinal sonography showed the liver and right kidney to have approximately the same echogenicity. *B*, After continued cytotoxic therapy the liver became increasingly echogenic with respect to the kidney owing to fat deposition in the liver. The kidney remained normal but appeared hypoechoic on this image because the gain was at a very low level to aid visualization of the liver. (From Stringer.[3])

tal hypertension may be accompanied by a loss or diminution of the normal respiratory variation of portal flow (Fig. 11).[5] In childhood, portal hypertension more commonly develops from thrombosis of the portal vein, which may occur early in perinatal life. The normal portal vein is no longer seen sonographically. Instead it is replaced by a tangle of enlarged venous collaterals termed *cavernous transformation of the portal vein* (Fig. 12). Rarely one can see septic or neoplastic thrombus in the portal vein.[12] Doppler has also been beneficial in confirming patency or obstruction of the inferior vena cava[33] or, in Budd-Chiari syndrome, of the hepatic veins.[12]

Liver Transplantation

The number of children undergoing hepatic transplantation continues to grow each year. Potential candidates for transplantation must be carefully assessed for the presence of malignancy, extent of hepatic disease, vascular anomalies, and presence of other disorders that may complicate or contraindicate surgery.[34] For example, biliary atresia may be associated with polysplenia. Sonography can identify the vascular anomalies of the inferior vena cava (IVC) such as interruption of the IVC with azygous continuation. The portal vein should be assessed for size and patency. If sonography is nondiagnostic, further evaluation with angiography may be indicated.

Postoperatively, sonography is helpful in evaluation for major surgical complications, including vascular thrombosis, biliary obstruction or leakage, bleeding, graft rejection, or infarction.[35] Sonography is the initial investigation of choice because it is portable and may be performed at the bedside. We routinely scan the patient within the first 24 hours and when clinically indicated thereafter.

Vascular compromise may be detected with Doppler evaluation of either the hepatic artery or portal vein. A mild degree of turbulence may be noted at the site of vascular anastomosis, but increasing turbulence or absence of signal suggests severe stenosis and occlusion. In cases of infarction or severe ischemia, abnormal focal or diffuse hepatic echogenicity can develop. In rejection there may be a nonspecific decrease in diastolic flow (presumably from increased hepatic resistance) or periportal echogenicity. Periportal echogenic-

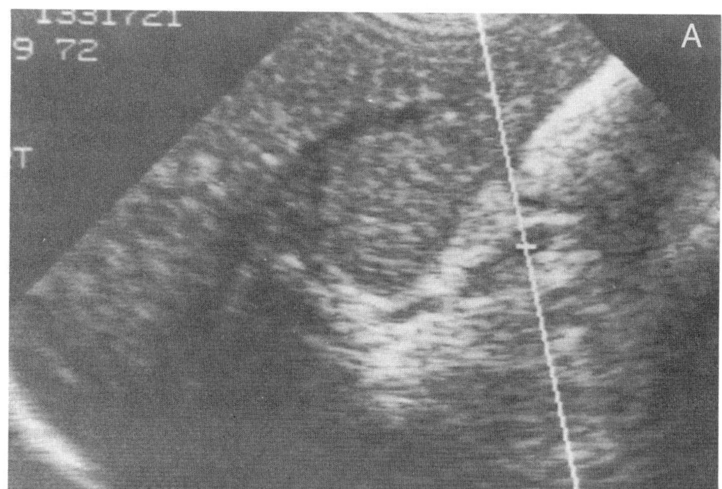

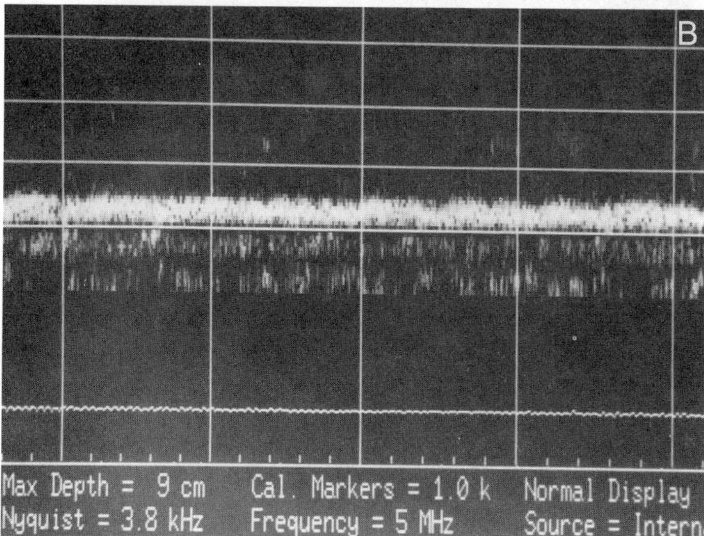

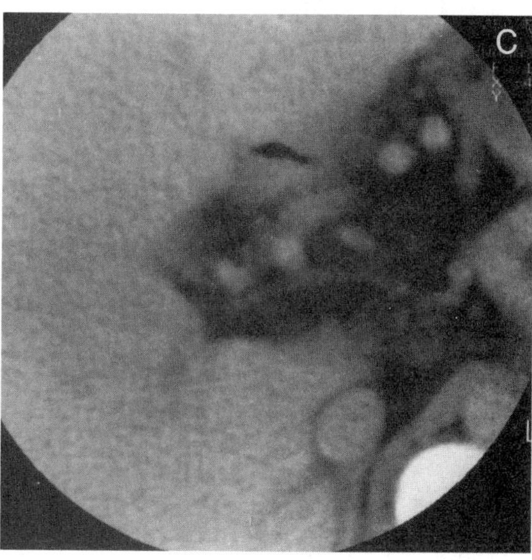

FIGURE 11 Portal hypertension. *A*, An abnormal collateral vessel was interrogated (see cursor line) by duplex range gated Doppler sonography and flow was seen in the direction of the porta hepatis. Blood could also be detected flowing into the liver from the porta. *B*, Doppler sonography showed loss of the respiratory pulsation suggestive of portal hypertension. A portal cavernoma with small sonographically invisible collaterals was suspected. *C*, Dynamic contrast-enhanced CT scan shows a loss of normal vascular structure with sinuous enhanced pathways around the outside of the porta. Compare with Figure 12. (From Stringer.[3])

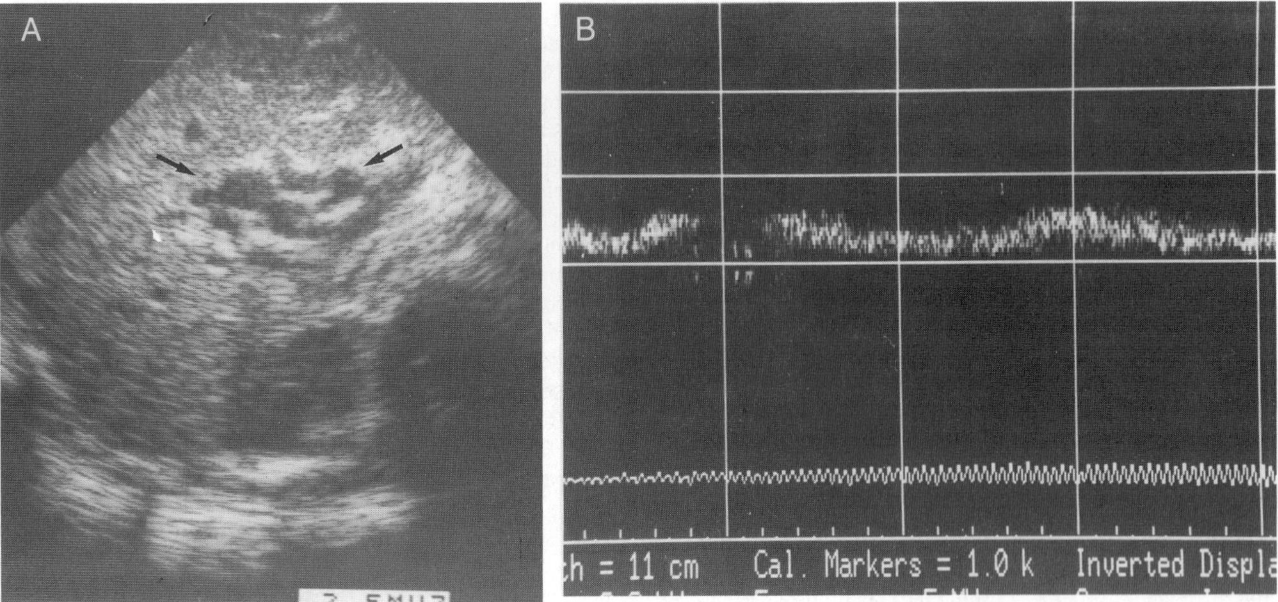

FIGURE 12 Portal cavernoma in extrahepatic portal vein obstruction. *A*, Tortuous vessels (*between arrows*) are seen in the porta hepatis on this oblique sonogram. *B*, Duplex range gated Doppler sonography shows good flow with respiratory pulsations indicating good compensation in a child who had little if any evidence of portal hypertension. Compare with Figure 11. (From Stringer.[3])

ity is not specific for rejection and may result from lymphedema. In our experience allograft rejection is not reliably diagnosed with sonography or CT.

Biliary dilatation may result from bile duct strictures and often reflects underlying hepatic artery thrombosis. Bile lakes can form in focal areas of infarction and may require aspiration or drainage. Extrahepatic surgical complications including hematomas, abscesses, other fluid collections, adrenal hemorrhage, and pancreatitis may also be detected by sonography.[11]

Hepatic Trauma

The liver is the most frequently injured organ in blunt abdominal trauma. We find CT to be the most useful and cost-efficient imaging modality for evaluating the extent of injury following blunt trauma. However, sonography is adequate for follow-up of any lesion previously demonstrated on CT or for documentation of post-traumatic complications. Frequently a hematoma is first hyperechoic and ill defined within the hepatic parenchyma, but with time and progressive liquefaction, the lesion becomes anechoic and diminishes in size.[12] Biliary complications of hepatic trauma include hematobilia and biloma formation. Echogenic debris in the gallbladder suggests intraluminal hemorrhage.[11,12] Bilomas or bile lakes can occur and may simulate a liquefied hematoma on follow-up scans.

Biliary Disease

Biliary ductal dilation may result from congenital anomalies, stones, strictures, or neoplasms. Intrahepatic ductal enlargement is recognized sonographically by visualization of tubular canals, either anterior or posterior to the portal veins. The obstructed common bile duct may dilate to more than 4 mm. Not infrequently, however, the cause of the obstruction is not apparent and further evaluation with endoscopic retrograde cholangiopancreatography (ERCP) or percutaneous transhepatic cholangiography is necessary.

Cholelithiasis may be noted from birth through adolescence as a result of multiple causes. Sonographically, gallstones may be multiple or single and are seen as mobile, echogenic areas within the gallbladder. Distal acoustic shadowing is almost always seen. In infants, so-called gallstones are common but probably result from aggregations of sludge (Fig. 13). Sludge does not usually cause shadowing, although progression to stones does occur. Subsequent spontaneous resolution has been noted (Fig. 13).[11]

Calculous cholecystitis is less common in children than adults. Gallbladder wall thickening, which is common in adults (Fig. 14), is not usually seen in pediatric cholecystitis, but more frequently occurs in other disorders such as hypoalbuminemia.[37] Radionuclide scanning may be more helpful for the diagnosis of cholecystitis than sonography. Acalculous cholecystitis is reported to be more common than calculous cholecystitis, but many of these cases probably represent hydrops of the gallbladder (Fig. 15).[11] Hydrops is characterized by marked distention of the gallbladder occurring in the absence of frank cholecystitis, but may be associated with a mild inflammatory reaction. In most cases it is self-limiting.

PANCREAS

Sonography is the modality of choice in evaluating children suspected of having pancreatic disease.[40] The pancreas is

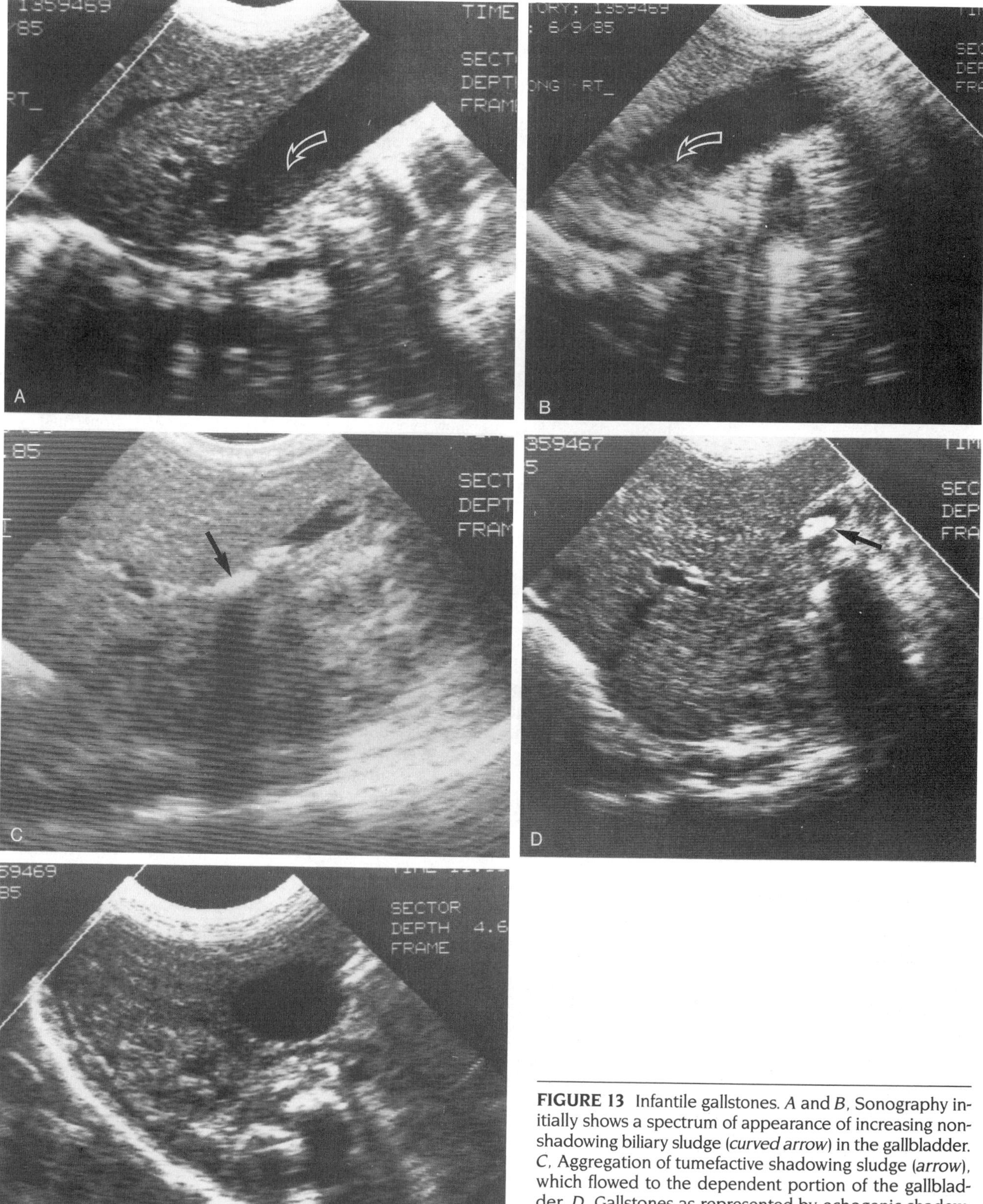

FIGURE 13 Infantile gallstones. *A* and *B*, Sonography initially shows a spectrum of appearance of increasing nonshadowing biliary sludge (*curved arrow*) in the gallbladder. *C*, Aggregation of tumefactive shadowing sludge (*arrow*), which flowed to the dependent portion of the gallbladder. *D*, Gallstones as represented by echogenic shadowing opacities (*arrow*), which moved as distinct stones to the dependent portion of the gallbladder. *E*, These gallstones disappeared with time and caused no symptoms in this neonate. (From Stringer.[3])

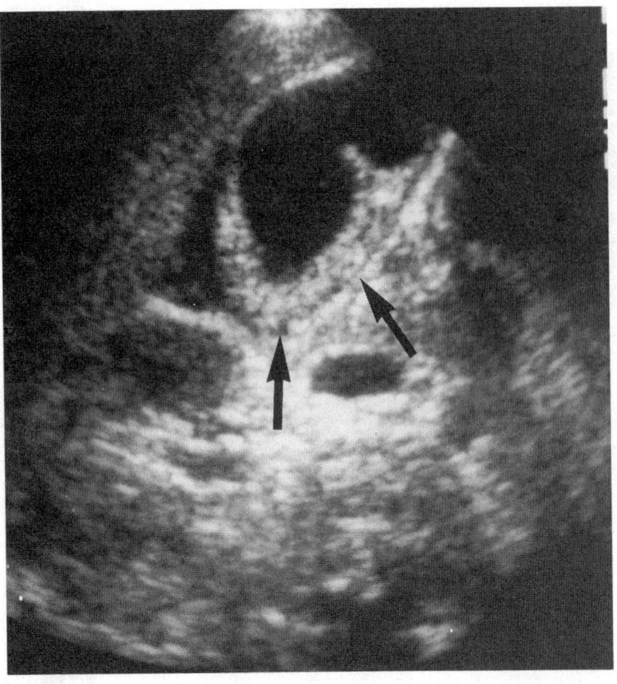

FIGURE 14 Thick-walled gallbladder. Sonography shows a very thick-walled gallbladder (*arrows*) in a patient with hypoalbuminemia. (From Stringer.[3])

almost always easily defined during routine scanning in children. Lying obliquely or transversely within the retroperitoneum, the posterior vasculature—particularly the splenic and superior mesenteric veins—helps define the normal pancreatic anatomy, including the pancreatic head, body, and tail (Fig. 16). The normal pancreas is of uniform echogenicity, usually similar to that of the liver, but occasionally it may be more hyperechoic or even hypoechoic.[38-40] Not uncommonly the normal pancreatic duct may be visualized as a thin tubular structure less than 2 mm in diameter that courses through the pancreatic body and tail. Within the pancreatic head, one may note the common bile duct and occasionally one or two gastroduodenal arteries. The normal age-related range of pancreatic size has been established and may be particularly useful for borderline enlargement of the pancreas in acute pancreatitis.[38,39] The pancreatic head and tail are normally similar in size with a thinner intervening body.[38]

Congenital Anomalies

Congenital anomalies of the pancreas most commonly involve the ductal system. Visualization of ductal anomalies by sonography has not been reliably achieved. In patients with annular pancreas, sonography is usually normal but occasionally can detect a parenchymal extension from the pancreatic head surrounding the duodenum.[40] Rarely sonography may show hypoplasia or agenesis of the pancreas. Congenital cysts may be encountered, either isolated or in association with polycystic disease of the kidneys and liver.[40]

Pancreatitis

Causes of pancreatitis in children include multisystem disease, structural anomalies, trauma, infection, and drug toxicity.[41] Other less common etiologies include hereditary pancreatitis and metabolic diseases such as cystic fibrosis. Trauma represents one of the most common causes of pancreatitis in childhood. Blunt trauma to the upper abdomen may produce the entire spectrum of pancreatic injury ranging from mild focal pancreatitis, to pancreatic transection. Sonography is helpful in the initial evaluation and follow-up, both for the diagnosis of acute pancreatitis and for identification of complications such as pseudocysts.[38-43] The most common finding in acute pancreatitis is focal or diffuse pan-

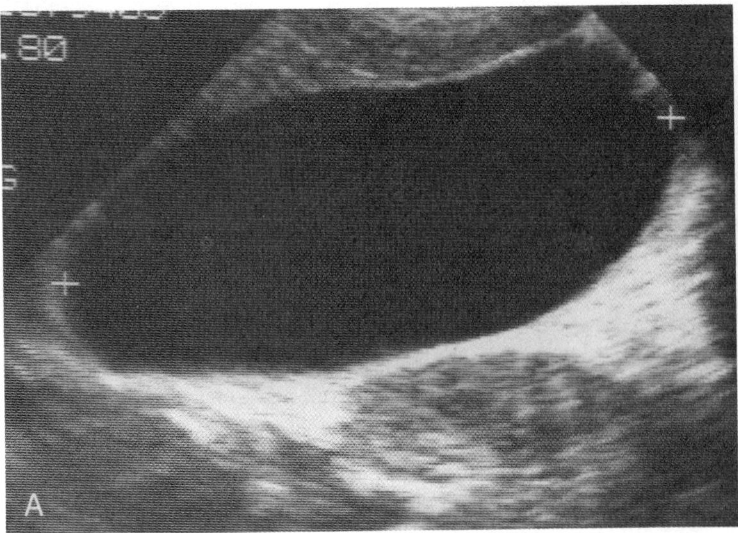

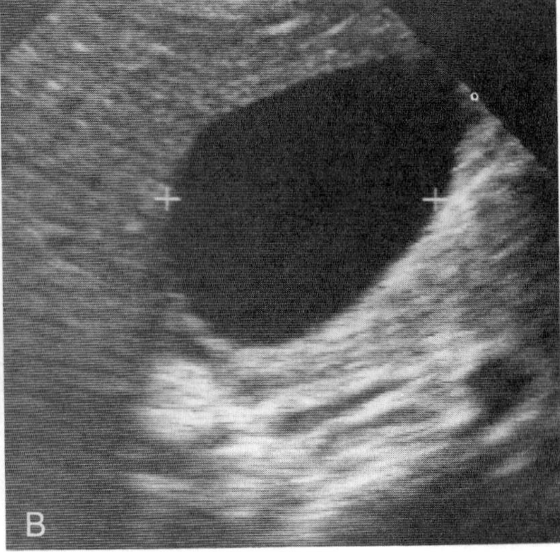

FIGURE 15 Hydrops of the gallbladder in Kawasaki's syndrome. *A*, Longitudinal sonogram and *B*, transverse sonogram, show a markedly distended spherical gallbladder with normal intrahepatic ducts.

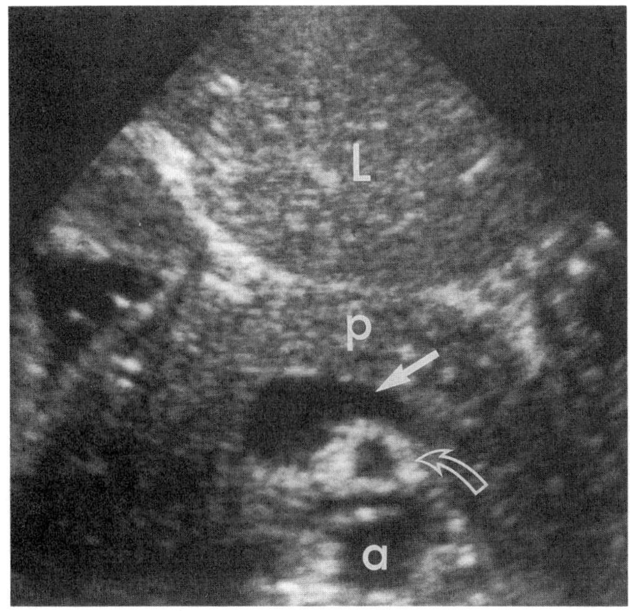

FIGURE 16 Normal pancreas. Sonography shows the body and tail of the pancreas (p) lying posterior to the left lobe of the liver (L), anterior to the splenic vein (*white arrow*), superior mesenteric artery (*curved arrow*), and aorta (a). The left renal vein lies between the superior mesenteric artery and aorta.

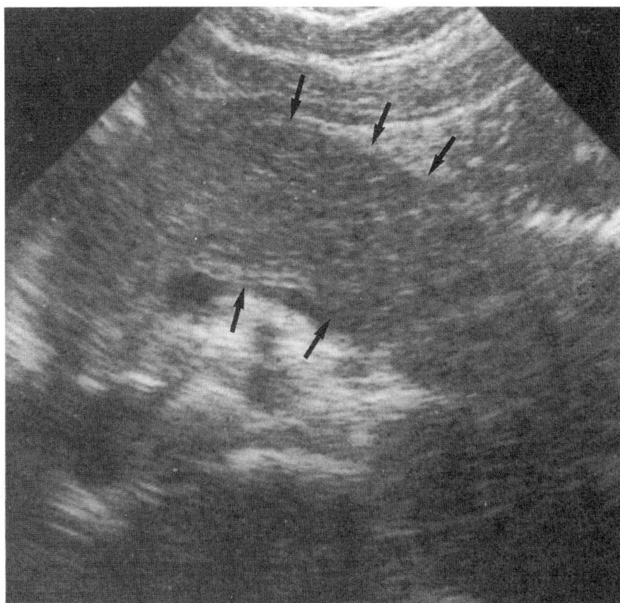

FIGURE 17 Acute pancreatitis. Transverse oblique sonography shows a diffusely enlarged pancreas (*between arrows*). (From Stringer.[3])

creatic enlargement (Fig. 17). However, the normal variability of the size of the pancreatic gland may occasionally make determination of pancreatic enlargement problematic. Other findings include ductal enlargement, decreased echogenicity, inhomogeneous echogenicity, or hyperechogenicity of the pancreas. Pararenal space hyperechogenicity has also been reported in children, but this is more often seen in adults owing to a relative decrease in the amount of retroperitoneal fat in children.[42,43]

Collections of peripancreatic fluid, a known complication of acute pancreatitis, may be loculated or free in the intraperitoneal space. Pseudocysts may be seen most commonly in the lesser sac within 1 to 2 days following pancreatic injury (Fig. 18.) Sonography is very helpful in monitoring the size of the pseudocysts over time and in evaluating their internal characteristics. Most fluid collections resolve within 1 month. The presence of echogenicity within the pseudocyst may reflect hemorrhage, infection, or increased tissue (Fig. 18). Occasionally, fluid-fluid levels may be noted as a result of hemorrhage. Echogenic foci with distal acoustic shadowing suggests the possibility of air within the lesion, and immediate drainage is recommended because of the possibility of a pancreatic pseudocyst abscess. Other complications of pancreatitis that may be recognized by sonography include ascites, pleural effusions, phlegmons, fistula formation, and persistent pseudocysts.[42-44] The assessment of the size of the duct is important, for if ductal dilatation is associated with pseudocyst formation, surgery may be indicated.[45] Rarely, splenic vein thrombosis and secondary splenomegaly may be found.[43] Sonography is usually adequate in the evaluation of these complications and CT should be reserved for the few complicated cases in which further information is needed. If pseudocyst drainage is required, sonography may be used for guidance.

Features of chronic pancreatitis, which in childhood is rare, include ductal dilatation, irregularity, pancreatic calcification, and pseudocyst formation.[40,43] In cystic fibrosis changes consistent with acute or chronic pancreatitis may be seen but neither is common. More commonly, in cystic fibrosis, pancreatic echogenicity is increased due to glandular atrophy, fibrosis, and fat deposition (Fig. 19); gland size is frequently small.[46] Fatty replacement may also be noted in Shwachman's syndrome.[43] True cyst formation has rarely been noted in cystic fibrosis. Numerous microcysts are seen histologically, but it is rare to see these sonographically, although rare cases of macrocysts have been reported. Infrequently, pancreatic calcification may also be noted.[46]

Pancreatic Tumors

Most children with pancreatic tumors present clinically with a palpable mass, abdominal enlargement, or a variety of secondary endocrine abnormalities.[40,43] Benign islet cell tumors, which are rare, include insulinoma, gastrinoma, and VIPoma. These tumors are usually small on presentation and are difficult to visualize, despite application of multiple imaging modalities. Intraoperative sonography may be helpful for locating small lesions.[47] Other uncommon benign tumors of the pancreas include lymphangiomas, hemangiomas, and dermoids.

Malignant tumors of the pancreas are extremely rare in children; they may or may not secrete hormones. Nonfunctioning tumors such as adenocarcinoma or pancreatoblastomas

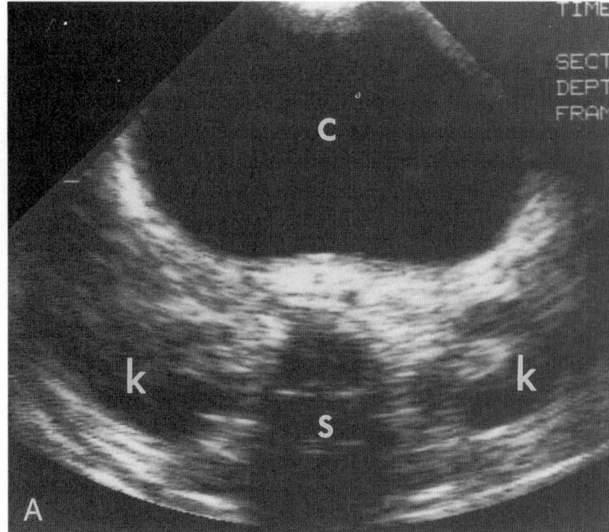

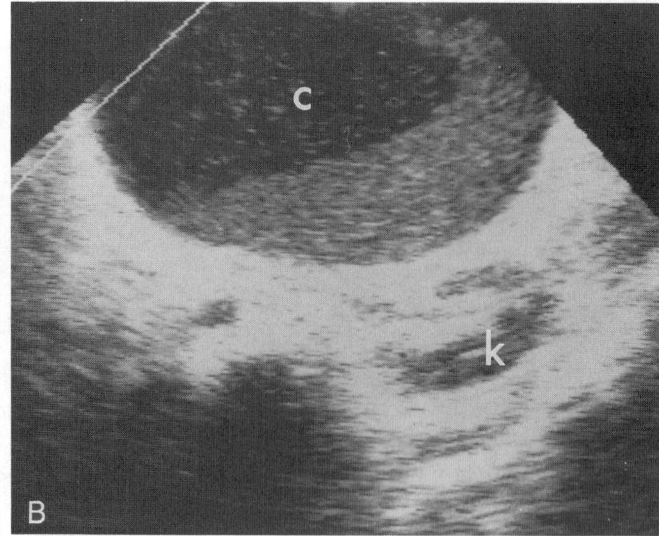

FIGURE 18 Acute pancreatic pseudocyst formation. *A*, Transverse sonography shows massive unilocular cystic mass (c) filling the upper abdomen anterior to both kidneys (k) and spine (s). *B*, Transverse sonography in another patient shows a large amount of echogenic debris within a large pseudocyst (c) anterior to the left kidney (k). The debris may be desquamated cells, blood clot, or pus.

have been found at all ages from infancy through adolescence.[48] Sonography will show an echogenic tumor mass, and metastases may be present. The echogenicity of these lesions can be variable owing to areas of tumor necrosis or hemorrhage intermixed with more solid homogeneous tumor tissue (Fig. 20).[43,48] Cystic neoplasms of the pancreas are uncommon in children. Other malignant tumors of the retroperitoneum, such as neuroblastoma, can invade the pancreas directly or by hematogenous spread. Abdominal lymphoma can extend into the pancreas. We have found CT evaluation superior to sonography, since neoplastic masses in the lung parenchyma and upper abdomen can be performed simultaneously, permitting more extensive evaluation of tumor characteristics, location, and spread.

SPLEEN

Sonography is almost always satisfactory in evaluating splenic anatomy and pathology. The normal spleen shows a homogeneous echogenicity similar to the liver and normally lies adjacent to the left hemidiaphragm and stomach.[49] The size of the normal spleen will vary depending on the patient's age and body habitus. An appreciation of splenic enlarge-

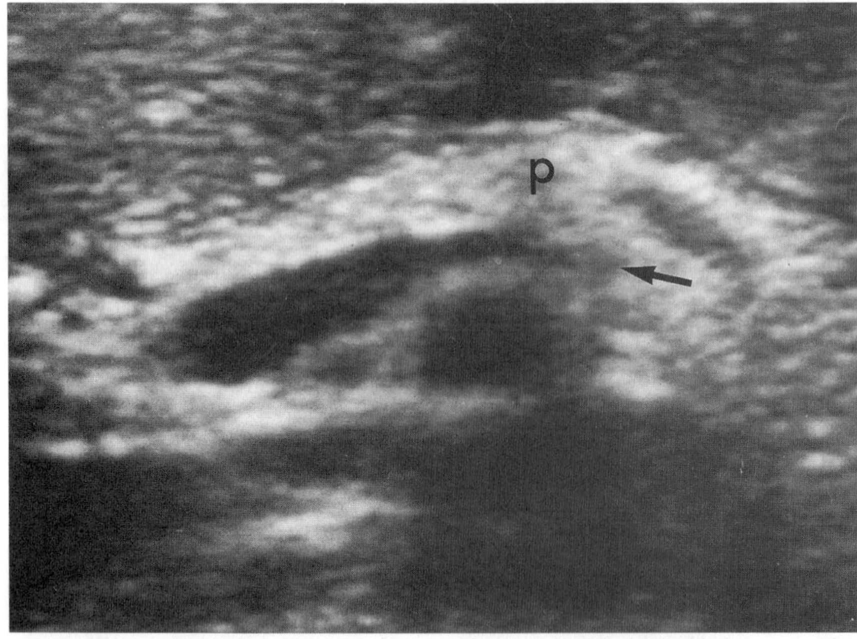

FIGURE 19 Pancreatitis in cystic fibrosis. Transverse sonography shows a small echo-dense pancreas (p) just anterior to the splenic vein (*arrow*). The pancreatic duct is dilated.

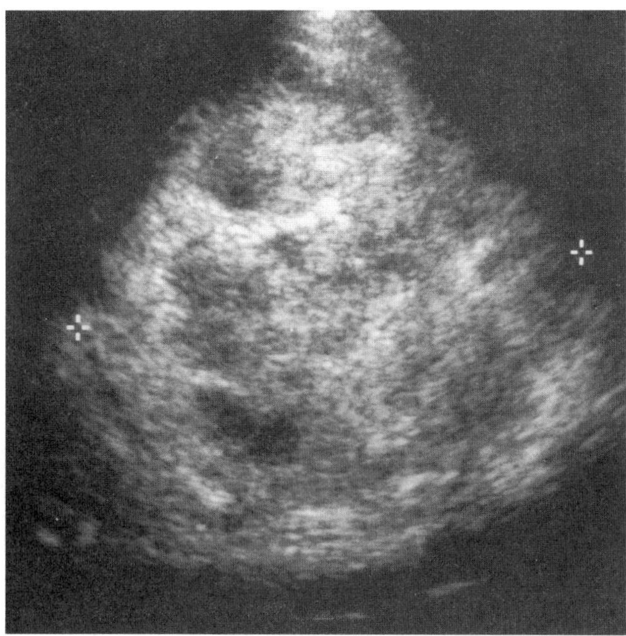

FIGURE 20 Solid and papillary epithelial tumor of the pancreas. Longitudinal sonography shows a poorly defined mass of mixed echogenicity between cursors.

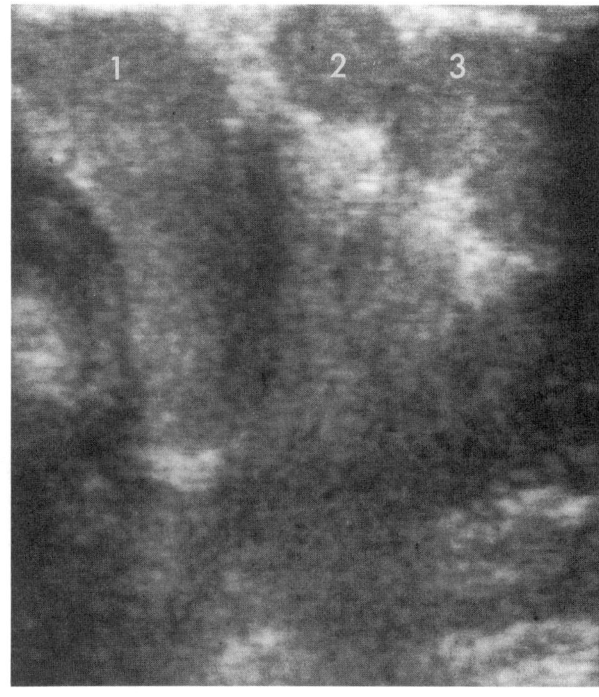

FIGURE 21 Polysplenia. Oblique sonography demonstrates at least three spleens (*1* to *3*) on the left side of the abdomen.

ment can be achieved with sonography using established biometric tables, but their use is cumbersome.[14] In actual practice most estimates of splenic size are subjective and based upon personal experience. The splenic hilum is directed medially, and both the splenic artery and vein can be identified. Within the splenic hilum, note may be made of small rounded densities with similar echogenicity to the spleen representing accessory spleens. Accessory spleens may be located in other areas of the left upper quadrant and may hypertrophy following splenectomy.

Congenital Anomalies

Congenital anomalies of the spleen include abnormalities of situs: asplenia and polysplenia. Although polysplenia (Fig. 21) rarely occurs in isolation, more often it is associated with cardiovascular and gastrointestinal anomalies. Absence of the spleen is almost always associated with cardiovascular anomalies. Since the left lobe of the centrally positioned liver may simulate splenic tissue, it may be difficult with sonography to diagnose asplenia. In difficult cases, correlation and radionuclide scanning is suggested. Associated anomalies of liver, biliary system (absent or hypoplastic gallbladder, biliary atresia), and gastrointestinal tract (imperforate anus, duodenal atresia) may be evident.[49,50] Occasionally the spleen is not located in its normal position, which is abutting the left hemidiaphragm, and instead is ectopic, because of either congenital absence or secondary absence of the normal splenic attachments. Sonography can show the abnormal location and mobility of the spleen. Torsion of the spleen may be associated with a wandering spleen.[49,50]

Inflammation and Tumors

Focal lesions of the spleen may be due to abscesses, cysts, hematomas, or infarcts. Abscesses most often appear as irregular poorly defined hypoechoic masses (Fig. 22), either as multiple small lesions or as a large single lesion.[49–53] Splenic cysts may be congenital in origin or secondary to prior hemorrhage or infection.[49,50] Congenital cysts and secondary cysts are usually well-defined anechoic fluid-filled masses (Fig. 23). Internal echogenicity may represent evidence of resolving hemorrhage or infection. Homogeneous echogenicity may be seen with cholesterol crystals within congenital cysts (Fig. 24). Focal echogenicity within the wall of these lesions may reflect calcification, and correlation of the sonograms with plain films may be helpful in this regard.[49,50] Lymphangiomas can on occasion also present as a multilocular cystic lesion. Other benign tumors of the spleen include hemangiomas and hamartomas. These are rare in childhood and are usually seen as complex masses within the splenic parenchyma.[49,50]

The most common malignancies affecting the spleen are lymphoma and leukemia (Fig. 25). There is considerable variability in the appearance of the spleen in these diseases.[49,50] Splenomegaly with normal echogenicity may be noted. In rare cases this may reflect diffuse infiltration of the spleen by neoplastic tissue, but in a large percentage of patients it may simply represent splenic reaction. Focal areas

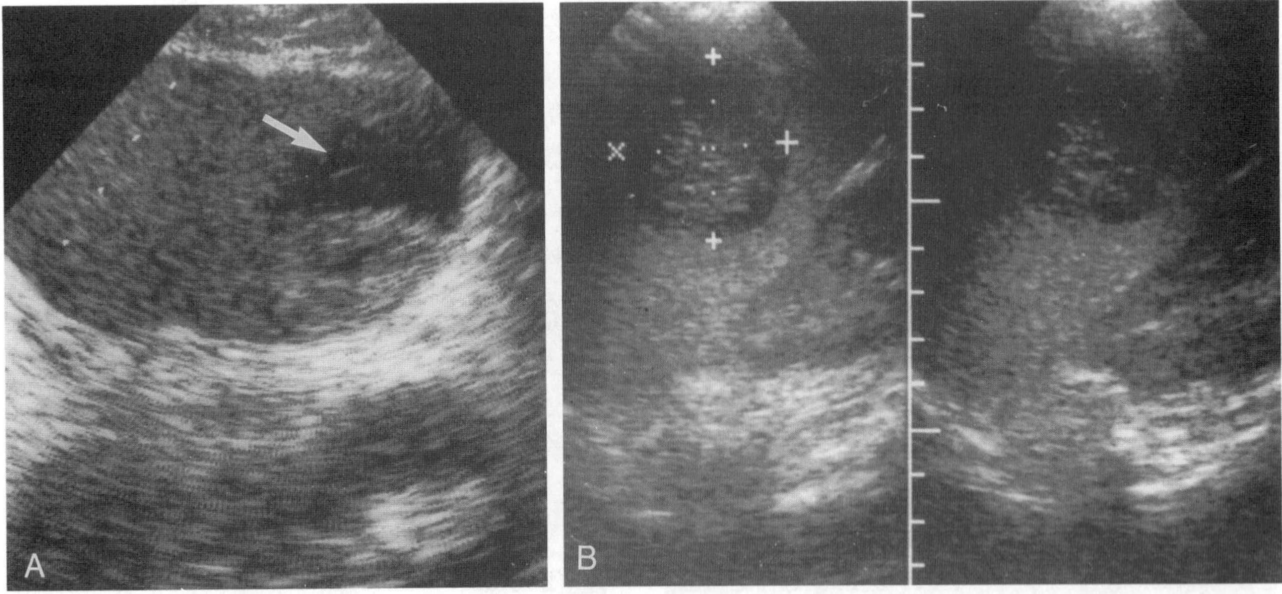

FIGURE 22 Splenic abscess. *A*, Oblique sonography demonstrates a small ill-defined hypoechoic area in the spleen (*arrow*). *B*, In another child with an abscess of longer duration, two longitudinal sonographic images show a well-defined hypoechoic area (between cursors on left-hand image) that contains some hyperechoic debris.

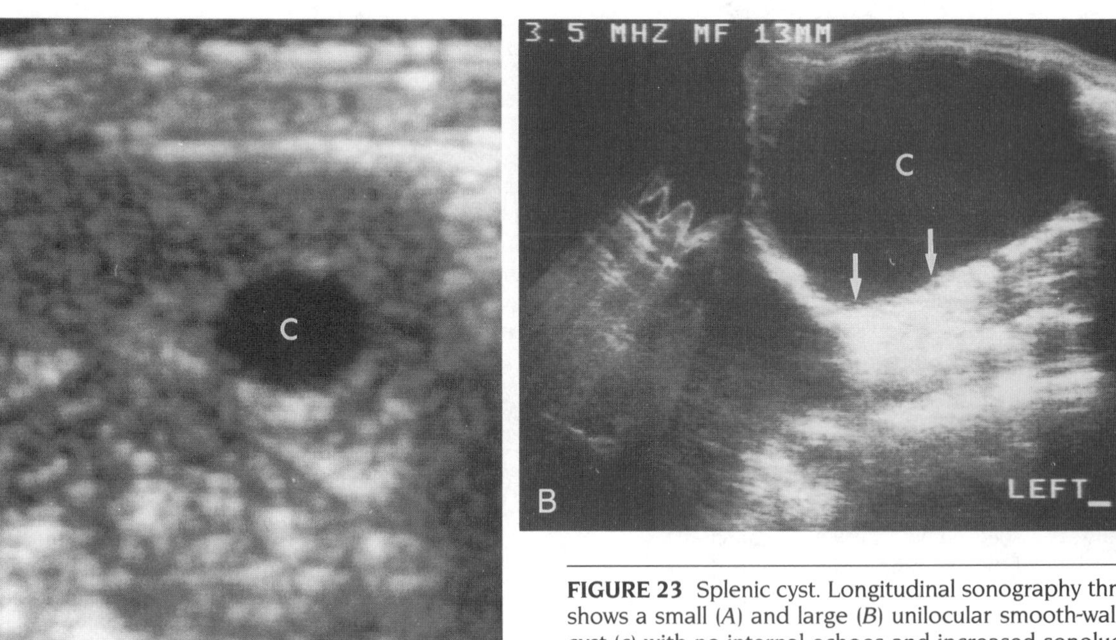

FIGURE 23 Splenic cyst. Longitudinal sonography through the spleen shows a small (*A*) and large (*B*) unilocular smooth-walled well-defined cyst (c) with no internal echoes and increased sonolucency as indicated by increased through transmission (posterior hyperechogenic area—*arrows*).

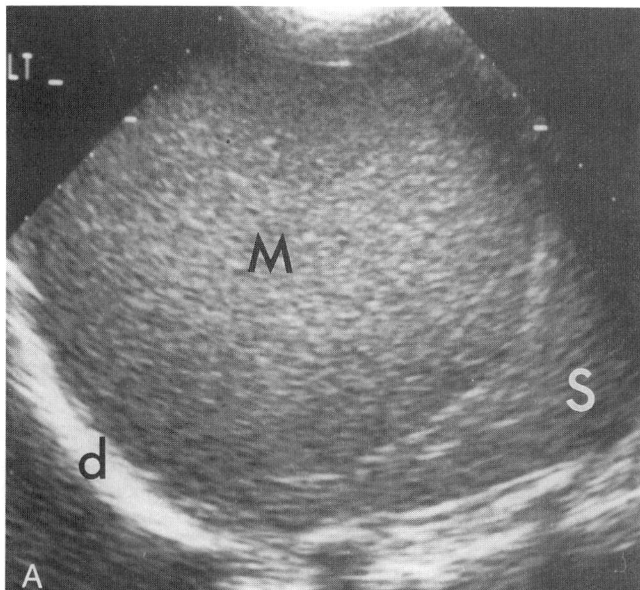

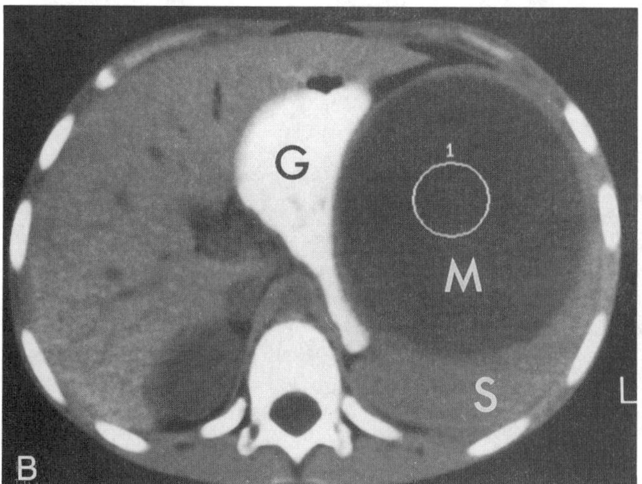

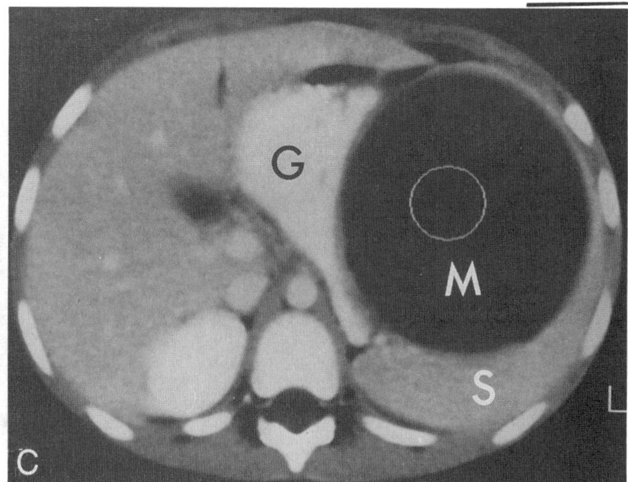

FIGURE 24 Splenic cyst. *A*, Longitudinal sonography through a left upper quadrant abdominal mass shows an echogenic lesion with fine echoes throughout the mass (M) almost but not quite as echogenic as the more normal position of spleen (S) seen inferiorly. The diaphragm (d) is shown superior to the mass. The echoes were found pathologically to the cholesterol crystals. *B*, Unenhanced CT shows the mass (M) to be a cystic lesion in the spleen (S), lateral to the stomach (G), which failed to enhance with intravenous contrast injection (*C*). (From Stringer.[3])

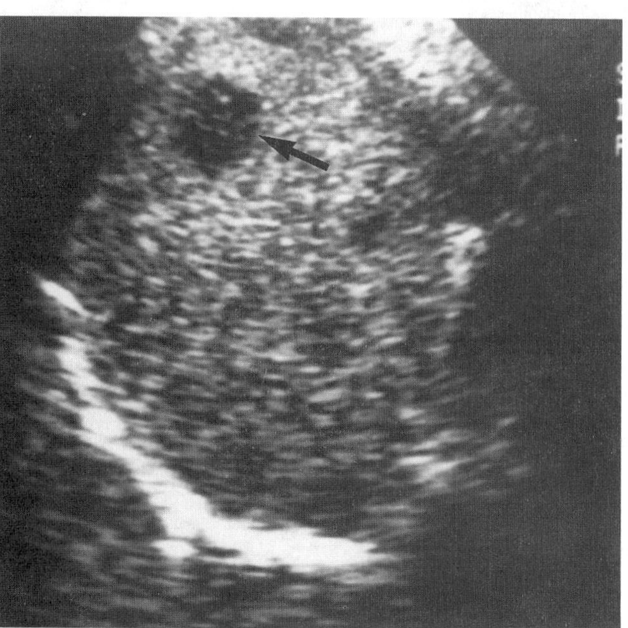

FIGURE 25 Splenic lymphoma. Sonography shows highly inhomogeneous echogenicity of the spleen, which contains a relatively well-defined hypoechoic mass (*arrow*).

of abnormal echogenicity that are usually hypoechoic are more likely to represent actual malignant infiltration of the spleen (Fig. 25).

Trauma

In patients with abdominal trauma, initial evaluation of the spleen is best performed by using CT.[54,55] Sonography, however, may be of use in the initial investigation if the degree of trauma is not severe. This modality is of unquestioned value for follow-up examination. Sonographic signs of splenic injury include splenic enlargement, irregular contour, and its association with subcapsular fluid collections and free intraperitoneal fluid (Fig. 26). Intraparenchymal hemorrhage following parenchymal laceration or contusion may initially show a hyperechogenic area, but it subsequently becomes hypoechoic. However, early hematomas may be isoechoic with normal splenic parenchyma, making visualization difficult.[54]

Splenomegaly

Splenomegaly is the most common manifestation of diffuse parenchymal disease and the spleen may be enlarged owing to neoplastic infiltration (histiocytosis X, leukemia, or lymphoma), infection, hematologic disorders, or portal hypertension (Fig. 27).

Sonographic findings are often nonspecific with regard to changes in splenic parenchymal echogenicity. In Gaucher's disease, multiple hypo- or hyperechoic areas may be found within the spleen, representing infiltration by Gaucher cells, fibrosis, or infarction. In hereditary spherocystosis, focal hyperechoic areas may be noted within the spleen as a result of intrasplenic hematopoiesis. Infarction of the spleen is often

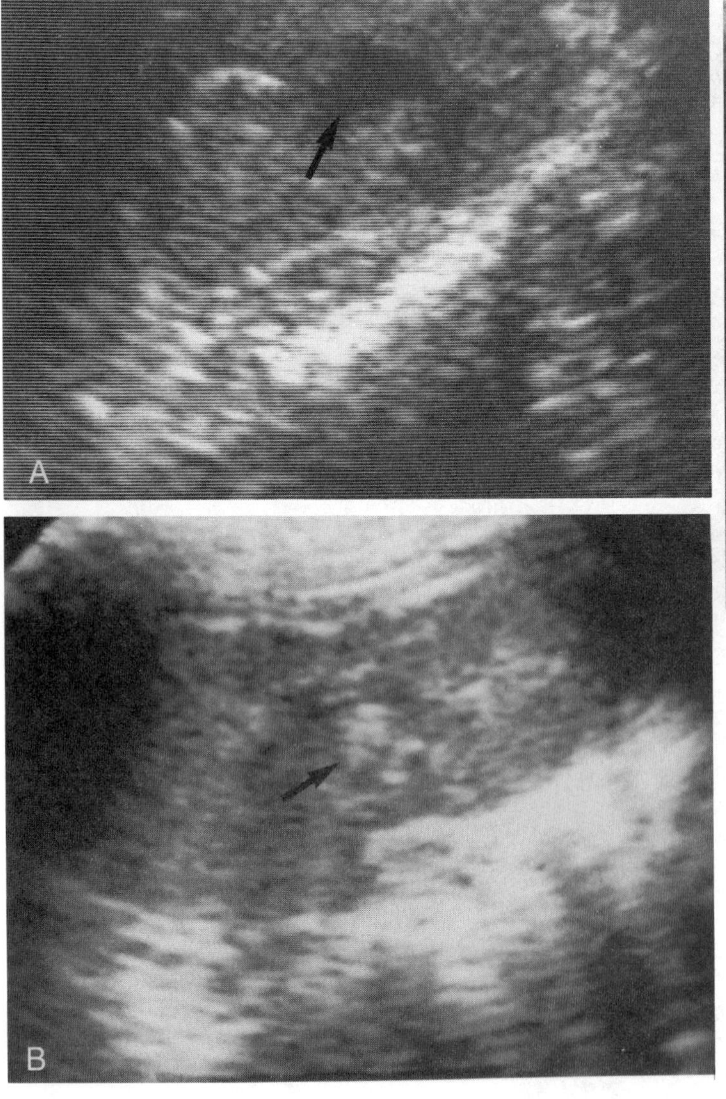

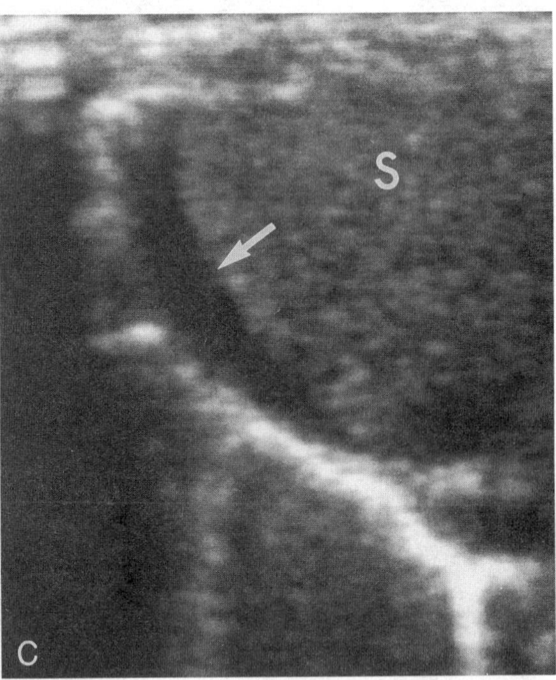

FIGURE 26 Ruptured spleen due to trauma. *A*, On admission, longitudinal sonography shows a hypoechoic inferior tip to the spleen, which contains a small anechoic area (*arrow*). *B*, Eight weeks later, a repeat study showed filling in of the anechoic area with hyperechoic material (*arrow*). Over the next 6 months the appearance returned to normal. *C*, In another patient, longitudinal sonography shows a hypoechoic linear collection (*arrow*) between the left hemidiaphragm and spleen (s) representing a subcapsular hematoma. (*B*, From Stringer.[3])

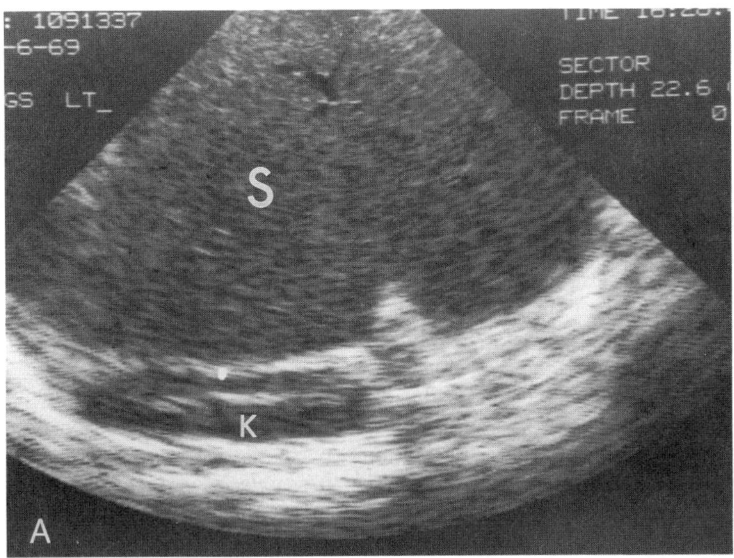

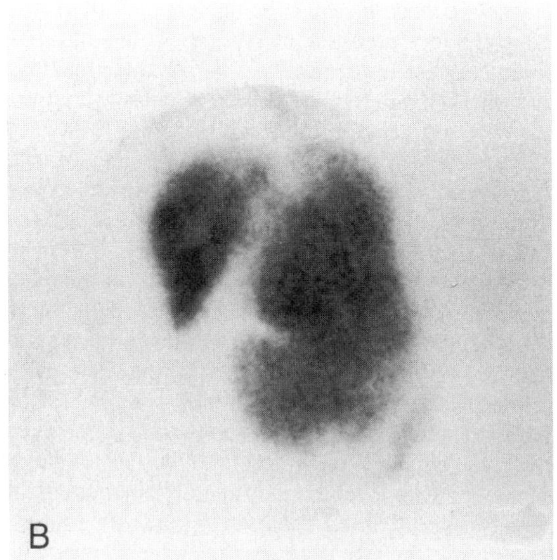

FIGURE 27 Splenomegaly in a 15-year-old boy with cystic fibrosis secondary to portal hypertension. *A*, Longitudinal sonography shows a very large spleen (S) that is isoechoic relative to the compressed left kidney (K). *B*, ^{99m}Tc–sulfur colloid liver spleen scan shows a very enlarged spleen on the right and smaller liver on the left showing patchy activity due to the cirrhosis that has resulted in hypersplenism. (From Stringer.[3])

hypoechoic and is commonly seen in sickle cell disease and hereditary spherocytosis together with a number of other causes.[49,50]

THE GASTROINTESTINAL TRACT

General Considerations

The advent of real-time scanning has caused sonography to rapidly assume both a primary role and a screening role in the evaluation of a variety of lesions of the pediatric gastrointestinal tract.[56,57] Sonography can be used to evaluate a wide spectrum of intestinal diseases, from observing the swallowing and sucking movements of the tongue in newborns[58] to assessing pelvic inflammatory bowel disease in adolescents. Sonography has added a new dimension to imaging of the gastrointestinal tract beyond that provided by contrast studies, since it enables direct observation not only of the intraluminal contents but also of the bowel wall and extraluminal extension.[56-62]

The normal sonographic appearance of bowel consists of an outer hypoechoic bowel wall musculature and an inner ring of more echogenic bowel mucosa with variable intraluminal contents. On transverse views this has been described as a target sign, doughnut, or bull's eye and is normally seen in the undistended gastric antrum or gastroesophageal junction[59-61] (the same terms are used for pathologic thickening). Small bowel can usually be distinguished from large bowel by the presence of peristalsis and pliability. The valvulae conniventes of the small bowel may be sonographically detected, whereas haustra, increased lumen size, and peripheral location are seen in the large bowel.[57,59-62] The stomach is readily identifiable throughout its length from the gastroesophageal junction through the pyloric canal and into the duodenum. The intraluminal bowel contents normally consist of a variable admixture of fluid, feces, and gas. Gas is highly echogenic, often displaying distal acoustic shadowing, which may interfere with imaging. Fortunately, simple changes in positioning the patient or in administering water (either orally or through a nasogastric tube) can usually displace the gas allowing satisfactory imaging. Feces may simulate pelvic masses clinically and sonographically. Scanning following water enemas is usually sufficient to document these masses as pseudotumors.

Types of Abnormalities Detected

Sonography can be useful for defining a variety of pathologic abnormalities of the gastrointestinal tract, including thickened bowel wall musculature and/or mucosa, bowel dilatation, or motility disturbances, regardless of whether they are associated with extraluminal masses, fluid collections, or abnormal vasculature such as varices.

Thickened Bowel Wall

Thickening of the bowel wall may arise from muscular hypertrophy or infiltration by blood, pus, edema, or tumor.[57] The normal bowel wall is usually less than 2 to 3 mm thick, particularly when distended with fluid. Pathologic thickening may be concentric or eccentric and should be suspected if the wall is greater than 4 to 5 mm.[59,61,62] The thickened bowel wall may show an exaggerated ring of sonolucency if the thickening is due to muscular hypertrophy and/or infiltration. Mucosal thickening is often nodular and centrally echogenic. Most benign conditions, such as hypertrophic pyloric stenosis, inflammation, and intussusception, cause concentric thickening.[59,62] Eccentric masses, such as intestinal lymphomas, are usually neoplastic but may also occur with abdominal trauma and Henoch-Schönlein purpura.

Muscular Hypertrophy. Hypertrophic pyloric stenosis is a common cause of gastrointestinal obstruction in early infancy. If the typical pyloric tumor is not palpable, sonography is the imaging modality of choice for investigating suspected pyloric stenosis. Hypertrophy of the pyloric musculature is often associated with hypertrophy of the prepyloric antral region. There is usually delayed gastric emptying, and gastroesophageal reflux may be present. The pyloric musculature is best assessed with sonography in both transverse and longitudinal planes. Transversely, the hypertrophied muscle gives rise to a target sign.[56,57,63,64] On longitudinal cuts one sees the hypoechoic musculature surrounding the echogenic, usually curved mucosa (Fig. 28). A double mucosal tract may be seen. In our experience, the most reliable criterion is the length of the pyloric canal on longitudinal scan. A normal term infant has a pyloric canal less than 12 mm in length. A firm diagnosis of hypertrophic pyloric stenosis can be established in those with canal lengths exceeding 17 mm, whereas those with canal lengths between 12 and 17 mm are considered to be borderline cases.[63,64] It is important to assess the rate of gastric emptying as well, and the administration of fluid, either orally or via a nasogastric tube. Placing the patient in the right lateral decubitus position is usually helpful.[56,57,63,64] In some children with borderline measurements, good gastric emptying makes the diagnosis of hypertrophic pyloric stenosis an unlikely one. In premature infants, absolute canal length is not reliable and subjective interpretation must be made.[56]

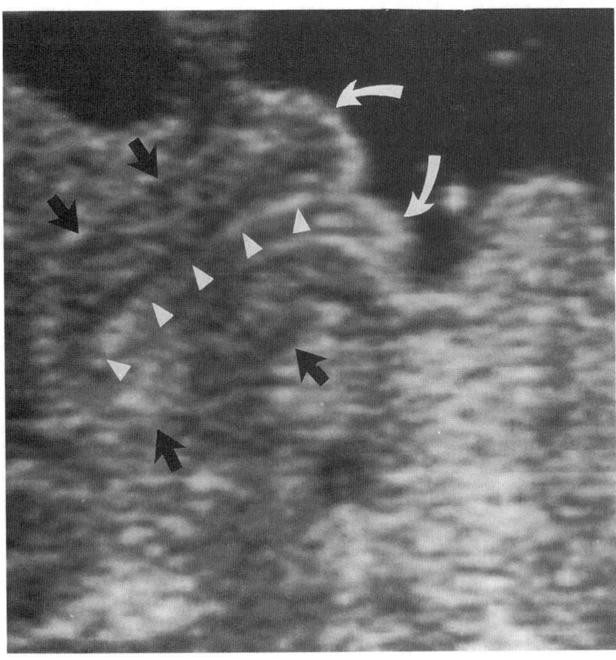

FIGURE 28 Hypertrophic pyloric stenosis. The continuity of the thickened muscle with the stomach wall can be seen on oblique sonographic cuts along the long axis of the pylorus. The pyloric canal appears as an echogenic curved line (*arrowheads*) in the middle of the hypertrophied muscle (*arrows*). Other signs seen include shouldering and beaking in the gastric antrum (*white curved arrows*) and gastric hyperperistalsis. (From Stringer.[3])

The indirect signs of pyloric hypertrophy seen on barium studies can also be observed with sonography. These include the impression by the hypertrophied muscle on the gastric antrum (shoulder sign); gastric fluid extending into the pyloric canal (beak sign), and angulation in the gastric wall at the level of the pyloric canal (tit sign). Sonography may occasionally miss pyloric stenosis and, if clinical concern persists, a barium meal is recommended for further assessment. After surgery, the pylorus decreases in size, usually assuming a normal configuration by 6 weeks postoperatively.[57]

Trauma. Trauma to the gastrointestinal tract most often involves the duodenum or proximal jejunum. Although not recommended for initial imaging in severe trauma, sonography may demonstrate intramural hematomas of the duodenum (Fig. 29). Initially, they appear as eccentric complex solid masses, often abutting the pancreas. As time passes, these hematomas liquefy and become more cystic in appearance. Sonographic monitoring will show a progressive decrease in size. Sonography is of value for detecting intramural hematomas resulting from other conditions such as hemophilia or Henoch-Schönlein purpura.[56,57]

Inflammatory Disease. Sonography can be helpful for evaluating inflammatory disease of the stomach, particularly for follow-up of a known lesion. On occasion it has been useful in demonstrating unsuspected gastric pathology. In gastritis there may be eccentric bowel wall thickening or mucosal edema, and rarely sonography may actually demonstrate ulceration. In chronic granulomatous disease marked thickening of the antrum may be apparent, which on barium images reveals antral deformity.[65] Crohn's disease involving the stomach may be sonographically visible with wall thickening. In Crohn's disease, sonography of the small bowel not only can demonstrate the extent of disease involvement of the bowel wall (Fig. 30) but can show evidence of extraluminal complications such as abscesses (Fig. 31), fistula formation, phlegmons, and associated fluid collections.[59,60,66] Abscesses may need surgical or percutaneous drainage. Typically they are hypoechoic, rounded irregular collections adjacent to abnormal inflamed bowel. On occasion, however, it may be difficult to differentiate an abscess from phlegmon sonographically, as both may appear either hypoechoic or hyperechoic. In this situation, CT may be of benefit.[68] Sonography can help differentiate confusing cases of Crohn's disease and other causes of terminal ileocolitis that may mimic the acute presentation of appendicitis. In Crohn's disease there may be abundant enlarged mesenteric nodes and bowel wall thickening of the terminal ileum and/or cecum without visualization of an inflamed appendix.[66]

Appendicitis is the most common abdominal inflammatory process requiring surgery. In straightforward cases imaging studies are unnecessary. Unfortunately, in up to 30 percent of cases, the clinical presentation may be atypical, which may delay the diagnosis and increase the risk of perforation. This is particularly true for infants. Other pathologic entities such

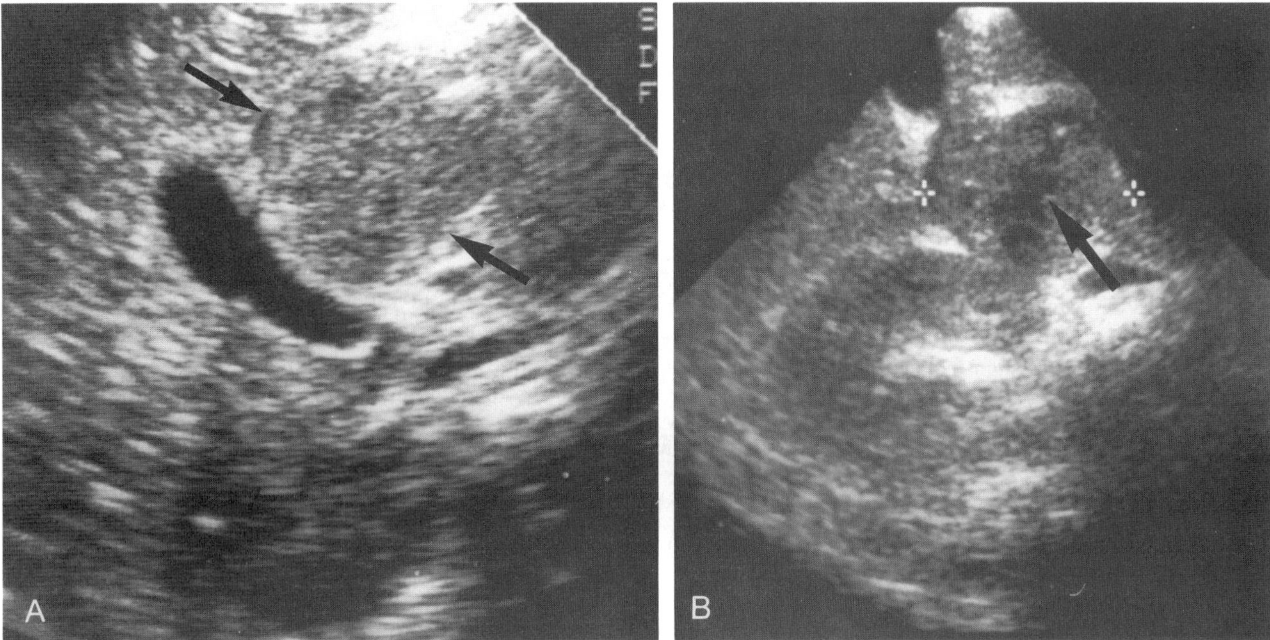

FIGURE 29 Duodenal hematoma. *A*, Oblique sonography shows an echogenic mass (*between arrows*), anterior to the right kidney adjacent to the gallbladder. *B*, Follow-up examination 3 weeks later shows some liquefaction as indicated by hypoechoic areas (*arrow*) in the hematoma (*between cursors*).

as mesenteric adenitis and acute terminal ileitis may mimic acute appendicitis.[67] In approximately 20 percent of cases laparotomy is negative.

Sonography has long been employed to investigate suspected appendiceal complications, but only recently is it being recommended as a diagnostic tool in the assessment of the inflamed appendix.[68–74] The right lower quadrant is carefully examined utilizing the graded compressive technique as described by Puylaert.[73] Graded compression is well tolerated even in those with peritoneal signs. It allows bowel gas

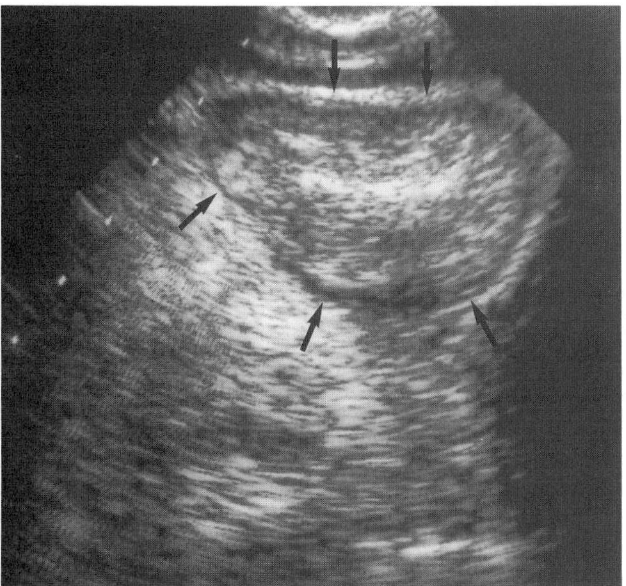

FIGURE 30 Crohn's disease without abscess formation. Longitudinal sonography shows a constant mass with a hyperechoic center and a hypoechoic border (*arrows*), indicating an intact muscular layer. (From Stringer.[3])

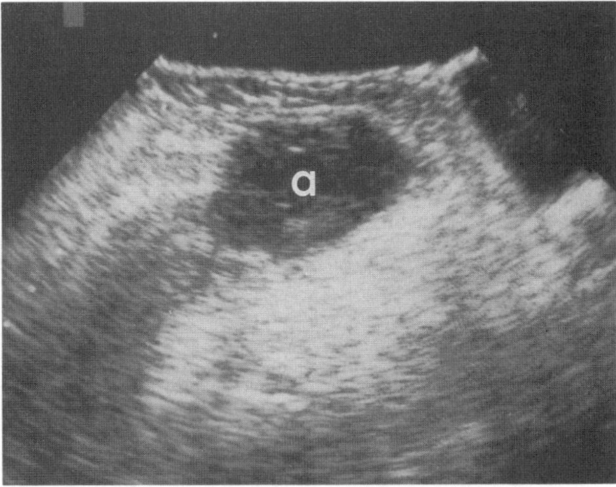

FIGURE 31 Crohn's disease with abscess formation. *A*, Longitudinal sonography shows a constant mass (a) of mixed echogenicity in the right lower quadrant.

and mobile small bowel loops to be displaced away from the area of interest. The normal appendix is rarely imaged by sonography. It is thin-walled (less than 6 mm in diameter) and nontender on examination. The inflamed appendix is enlarged, usually greater than 6 mm in diameter, and a typical target sign is seen on transverse images. It is noncompressible and often tender on examination.[70,71,74] In early appendicitis one can see thickening of the appendiceal wall musculature, submucosa, and serosa (Fig. 32). With increasing suppuration there is progressive distention of the appendiceal lumen with even more thickening of the appendiceal wall. Eventually, there are perforation and abscess formation. Perforation is suggested by asymmetric wall thickening, localized fluid collections, or free intraperitoneal fluid and lack of tenderness over the appendix. Appendicoliths may be noted in approximately one-quarter of cases as highly echogenic focus with distal acoustic shadowing. Although sonography is quite accurate in the diagnosis of acute appendicitis, false-positive and false-negative examinations have been reported.[70,71] False-positive examinations may be due to visualization of a normal thick-walled appendix or to cases of appendicitis that have resolved spontaneously. Most cases of false-negative examinations arise from technically unsatisfactory studies. In patients in whom an appendix is not identified, the entire abdomen and pelvis should be scanned to exclude other pathology. Rare complications of appendicitis include pyelophlebitis and liver abscess. Sonography may be useful for percutaneous aspiration and drainage of appendiceal abscesses and for monitoring postappendectomy fluid collections.[75]

Typhlitis is a necrotizing inflammatory disease of the cecum that is most often found in acute leukemia patients undergoing chemotherapy. The cecum is often secondarily infected. Sonography reveals thickening of the bowel wall with an unusual distinctive appearance of the mucosa. The mucosa is highly echogenic, thickened, irregular, and often polypoid in configuration (Fig. 33). Ascites and fat necrosis may be seen. These changes may resolve rapidly after antibiotic therapy is instituted.[76]

In other inflammatory diseases of the colon, such as ulcerative colitis and Crohn's disease, thickening of the bowel wall may be visualized. Crohn's disease tends to show more marked transmural thickening than ulcerative colitis, where mild to moderate thickening of only a portion of bowel wall is common.[66]

Sonographic examination of premature infants occasionally reveals bowel wall thickening. Although this finding is nonspecific it should raise the possibility of necrotizing enterocolitis, as other causes in the premature infant, such as intussusception, are rare. The differentiation of necrotic gangrenous bowel from inflamed viable bowel cannot reliably be performed. Other features may be present, however, such as ascites or localized collections, and these would suggest perforation. Sonography may also confirm necrotizing enterocolitis by detecting portal-venous gas, perhaps with a degree of sensitivity greater than plain films. Mobile, small, very echogenic bubbles are noted within the portal venous system flowing to the nondependent areas of the liver. It is important to emphasize that other causes of portal venous gas, such as recent umbilical vein catheterization, should be

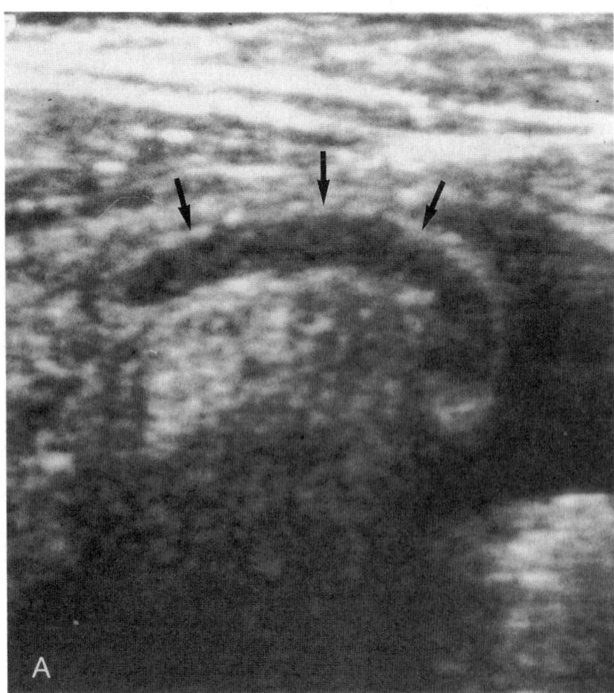

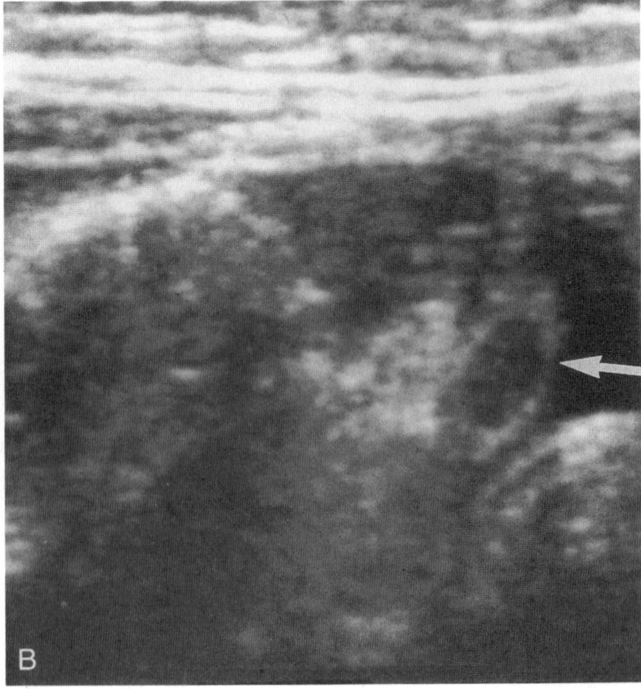

FIGURE 32 Acute appendicitis. *A*, Longitudinal graded compression sonography shows a noncompressible tubular structure, the appendix (*arrows*), with a small adjacent collection fluid. No enlarged mesenteric lymph nodes can be seen. *B*, On transverse sonography the appendix appears round (*arrow*). (From Stringer.[3])

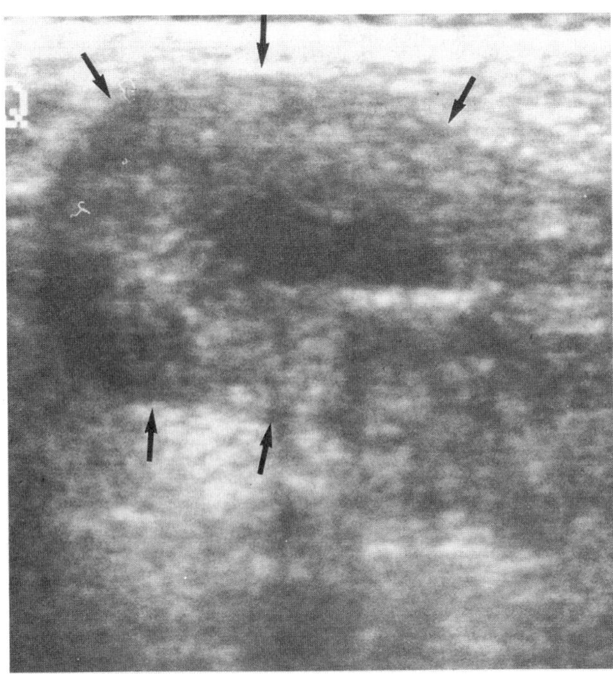

FIGURE 33 Typhlitis (neutropenic colitis) in a leukemic child. Sonography shows thickening of the bowel wall (*arrows*) of the cecum, which contains a small amount of fluid. (From Stringer.[3])

excluded. Pneumatosis intestinalis can occasionally be detected sonographically by echogenic foci within abnormal bowel wall[56,58,77,78] before the plain film diagnosis is established.

Intussusception. Intussusception, a common cause of intestinal obstruction in children, arises when one portion of the bowel invaginates into another. Most often it is ileocolic but may also be ileoileocolic, colocolic, or ileoileal. Sonography has been found helpful not only in the diagnosis of intussusception but also in monitoring the effects of hydrostatic reduction.[79-81] We utilize sonography primarily for evaluation of patients with atypical clinical presentations in whom the diagnosis is not suspected. We do not scan children in whom intussusception is suspected, because sonography is more time-consuming and unlike contrast enema is not therapeutic.

The typical appearance of intussusception has again been likened to a doughnut or bull's eye on transverse images. The edematous intussusceptum or invaginated bowel displays a hypoechoic appearance surrounding the more echogenic central invaginated loop mucosa. Longitudinal images have been termed *pseudokidney* because of the similarity with the normal sonographic appearance of the kidney with an echogenic center and echolucent periphery. The sonographic findings are not pathognomonic of intussusception, since similar images are seen in other lesions including necrotizing enterocolitis, sigmoid volvulus, and midgut volvulus. Swischuk et al[80] have described a rough correlation between the sonographic appearance and reducibility. If multiple sonographic layers are imaged, which probably reflects lesser degrees of edema, successful hydrostatic reduction appears to be more likely.[80]

Bowel Dilatation

Dilatation of the bowel, usually due to paralytic ileus or intestinal obstruction, can be assessed sonographically, especially when distended with intraluminal fluid. The presence of intraluminal fluid allows visualization of the valvulae conniventes or haustra, which helps localize the lesion; more importantly, it may permit sonographic diagnosis of bowel obstruction in cases in which the plain films are nondiagnostic because of the lack of bowel gas.[82] Adynamic ileus may show distended loops of bowel, and bowel peristalsis may be normal, increased, or reduced. Usually the bowel loops remain somewhat compliant.[59] With bowel obstruction and increasing degrees of distention, there is usually less compliance of the individual loops.[59] Congenital causes of obstruction may be recognized, including meconium ileus, duplication cysts and midgut volvulus, and atresias.[56,57,83]

Duplication cysts are usually well-defined, ovoid or tubular cystic masses adjacent to the bowel. They often cause underlying bowel obstruction but can be seen as an incidental finding. Typically they are anechoic with a double layered wall similar to normal bowel—the central layer is echogenic from bowel mucosa, the peripheral sonolucent layer from surrounding musculature (Fig. 34). This finding for the cyst wall is specific but is not always seen. Internal cyst hemorrhage or air may be present, giving rise to increased echogenicity within the cyst.[56,57]

In midgut volvulus, an obstructive pattern of bowel distention may be noted. Occasionally one can appreciate an underlying rotational anomaly by the unusual position of the superior mesenteric vein, which may be to the left or directly in front of the superior mesenteric artery.[84]

Sonography is a useful aid in the diagnosis of intestinal atresia by excluding extrinsic lesion to the bowel such as duplication cysts. In addition, if sonography reveals that the level of obstruction is similar to that defined by contrast enema, multiple atresias would be excluded.[83] Sonography is not recommended for simple cases of proximal atresia where plain films are satisfactory. In meconium ileus, sonography can reveal the distended small bowel loops filled with homogeneous hypoechoic meconium.

Motility Disorders

Peristalsis and fluid movement within the bowel can be observed by sonography. The flow of intraluminal contents can be observed.[59,85] It is important to assess gastric emptying as discussed in pyloric stenosis and normal peristalsis. Abnormal peristalsis can be found in adynamic ileus and bowel obstruction as discussed above. By scanning the region of the gastroesophageal junction, it is possible to observe fluid entering the stomach and also reflux of gastric contents into the distal esophagus. Comparative studies of barium meals and sonography have shown similar results for documenting gastroesophageal reflux.[85] Sonography can continuously

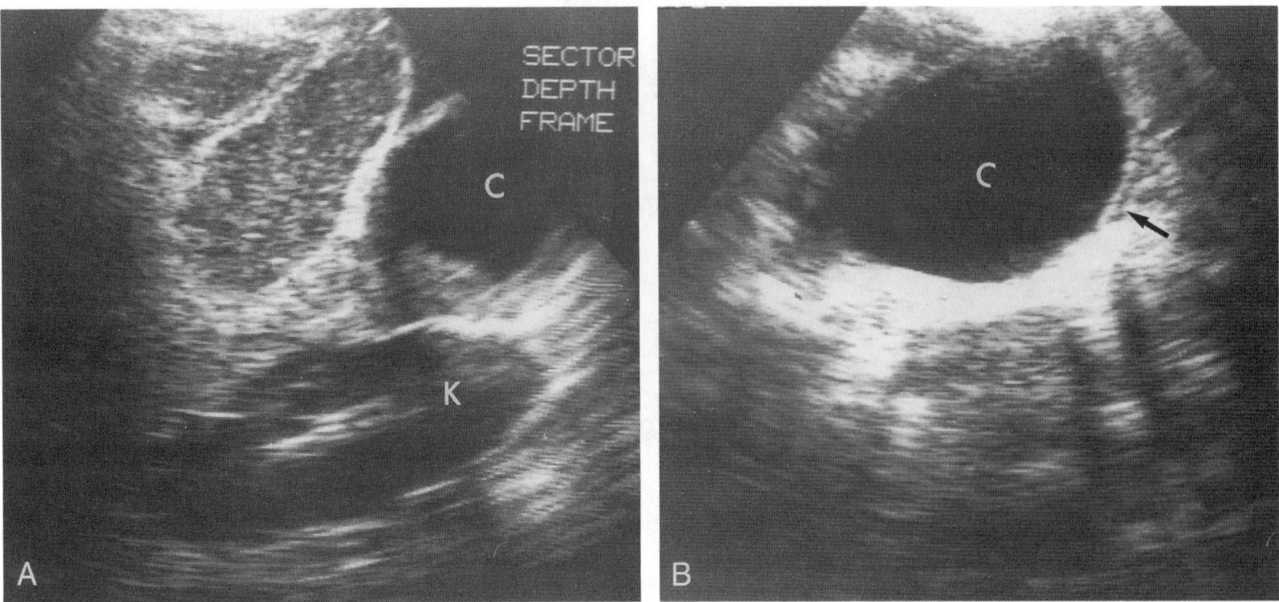

FIGURE 34 Duplication of the terminal ileum. *A*, Longitudinal sonography shows a cystic mass (C) anterior to the right kidney (K) with adjacent dilated loops of hyperperistalsing small bowel. *B*, Further sonographic views show the cyst (C) and its echogenic inner rim of gastrointestinal mucosa and hypoechoic muscular layer (*arrow*). (From Stringer.[3])

monitor the gastroesophageal junction for reflux without the risk of exposure to radiation, but patient co-operation is required, and it does not allow one to assess the height of reflux.

Ascites

Free intraperitoneal fluid (ascites) may arise from a multiplicity of causes ranging from obstructive uropathy, meconium peritonitis, birth trauma, and infection in the neonate, to portal hypertension, trauma, and neoplasms in the older child. Sonography is one of the most sensitive means of detecting the presence of free or loculated fluid within the peritoneal cavity.[86] Depending upon the amount of fluid present, it will typically appear as an anechoic area within the pelvis, paracolic gutters, or Morrison's pouch, or as outlining the margins of the liver and spleen. The smallest

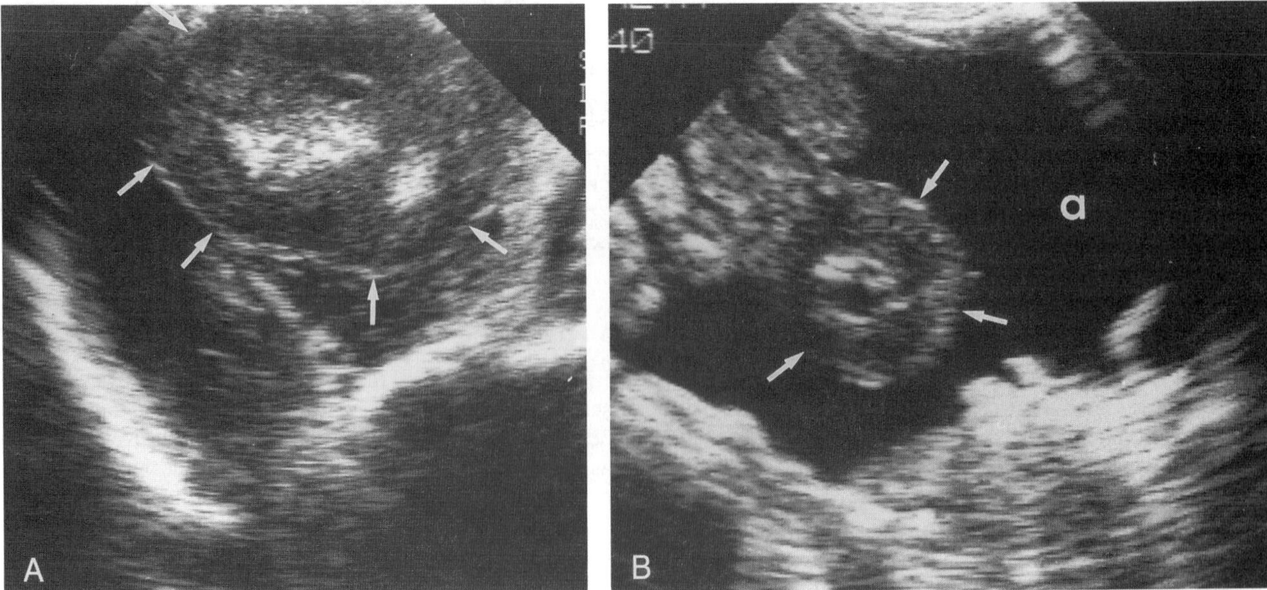

FIGURE 35 Non-Hodgkin's lymphoma. *A*, A loop of bowel has a thick wall (*arrows*) and an echogenic center with some adjacent ascitic fluid. *B*, Another bowel loop has a thick and irregular wall (*arrows*) outlined by surrounding ascitic fluid (a). (From Stringer.[3])

volumes of fluid are best noted within the pelvis adjacent to the bladder when the pelvis is the most dependent portion of the peritoneal cavity. Transudates or hemoperitoneum without clotted blood is usually anechoic. Echoes within the fluid suggest exudates, hemoperitoneum with clotted blood, meconium peritonitis, or malignancy. The sonographic appearance is almost invariably nonspecific, and causes for the fluid should be actively sought (Fig. 35). Loculated collections remain in the same site as the position of the patient changes.[86]

Acknowledgment

We appreciate the dedicated secretarial assistance provided by Ms. Carolyn MacDonald.

REFERENCES

1. Sherman NH, Boyle GK, Rosenberg HK. Sonography in the neonate. Ultrasound Q 1988; 6:91–149.
2. Cooperberg PL, Allen Rowley V. Abdominal sonographic examination technique. In: Taveras JM, Ferrucci JT, eds. Radiology diagnosis—imaging—intervention. vol 4. Philadelphia: JB Lippincott, 1989: 1.
3. Stringer DA. Pediatric gastrointestinal tract imaging. Philadelphia: BC Decker, 1989.
4. Sample WF, Erikson K. Basic principles of diagnostic ultrasound. In: Sarti DA, Sample WF, eds. Diagnostic ultrasound: text and cases. Boston: GK Hall Medical, 1980: 3.
5. Taylor KJW. Gastrointestinal Doppler ultrasound. In: Taylor KJW, Burns PN, Wells PNT, eds. Clinical applications of Doppler ultrasound. New York: Raven Press, 1988: 162.
6. Romero R, Pilu G, Jecintfy P, Ghidini A, Hobbins JC. Prenatal diagnosis of congenital anomalies. Norwalk, CT: Appleton and Lange, 1988: 209.
7. Nyberg DA, Mack LA, Patten RM, Cyr DR. Fetal bowel: normal sonographic findings. J Ultrasound Med 1987; 6:3–6.
8. Gray DL, Martin CM, Crane JP. Differential diagnosis of first trimester ventral wall defect. J Ultrasound Med 1989; 8:255–258.
9. Nyberg DA, Hastrup W, Watts H, Mack LA. Dilated fetal bowel: a sonographic sign of cystic fibrosis. J Ultrasound Med 1987; 6:257–260.
10. Lawrence PW, Chrispin A. Sonographic appearance in two neonates with generalized meconium peritonitis: the snowstorm sign. Br J Radiol 1984; 57:340–342.
11. Stringer DA. Pediatric gastrointestinal tract imaging. Philadelphia: BC Decker, 1989: 471–583.
12. Hayden CK, Swischuk LE. Pediatric ultrasonography. Baltimore: Williams & Wilkins, 1987: 169.
13. Hausdorf G. Sonography of caudal hepatic veins in children. Incidence, importance and relation to cranial hepatic veins. Pediatr Radiol 1984; 14:376–379.
14. Dittrich M, Milde S, Dinkel E, Baumann W, Weitzel D. Sonographic biometry of liver and spleen size in childhood. Pediatr Radiol 1983; 13:206–211.
15. Papanicolaou N, Abramson SJ, Teele RL, Treves S. Specific preoperative diagnosis of choledochal cysts by combined sonography and hepatobiliary scintigraphy. Ann Radiol 1985; 28:276–282.
16. Carty H, Pilling DW. Jaundice in children: A spectrum of causes. Ann Radiol 1985; 28:267–275.
17. Friedman AC, Fishman EK, Radecki PD, Scatarige JC, Sherman JL, Farmlett EJ, Markle BM, Dachman AH, Pakter RL. Focal diseases. In: Friedman AC, ed. Radiology of the liver, biliary tract, pancreas and spleen. Baltimore: Williams & Wilkins, 1987: 151.
18. Miller JH, Greenspan BS. Integrated imaging of hepatic tumors in childhood. I. Malignant lesions (primary and metastatic). Radiology 1985; 154:91–100.
19. Abramson SJ, Lack EE, Teele RL. Benign vascular tumors of the liver in infants: sonographic appearance. AJR 1982; 138:629–632.
20. de Campo M, de Campo JF. Ultrasound of primary hepatic tumors in childhood. Pediatr Radiol 1988; 19:19–24.
21. Dachman AH, Lichtenstein JE, Friedman AC, Hartman DS. Infantile hemangioendothelioma of the liver: a radiologic—pathologic—clinical correlation. AJR 1983; 140:1091–1096.
22. Stanley P, Hall TR, Woolley MM, Diament MJ, Gilsang V, Miller JH. Mesenchymal hamartomas of the liver in childhood: sonographic and CT findings. AJR 1986; 147:1035–1039.
23. Ros PR, Goodman ZD, Ishak KG, Dachman AH, Olmsted WW, Hartman DS, Lichtenstein JE. Mesenchymal hamartoma of the liver: radiologic—pathologic correlation. Radiology 1986; 158:619–624.
24. Brunelle F, Tamman S, Odievre M, Chaumont P. Liver adenomas in glycogen storage disease in children. Pediatr Radiol 1984; 14:94–101.
25. Welch TJ, Sheedy PF, Johnson CM, Stephens DH, Charboneau JW, Brown ML, May GR, Adson MA, McGill DB. Focal nodular hyperplasia and hepatic adenoma: Comparison of angiography, CT, US, and scintigraphy. Radiology 1985; 156:593–595.
26. Brunelle F, Chaumont P. Hepatic tumors in children: ultrasonic differentiation of malignant from benign lesions. Radiology 1984; 150:695–699.
27. Oleszczuk-Raszke K, Cremin BJ, Fisher RM, Moore SW, Millar AJ. Ultrasonic features of pyogenic and amebic hepatic abscesses. Pediatr Radiol 1988; 19:230–233.
28. Ralls PW, Barnes PF, Radin DR, Colletti P, Halls J. Sonographic features of amebic and pyogenic liver abscesses: a blinded comparison. AJR 1987; 149:499–501.
29. Pastakia B, Shawker TH, Thaler M, O'Leary T, Pizzo PA. Hepatosplenic candidiasis: wheels within wheels. Radiology 1988; 166:417–421.
30. Merten DF, Kirks DR. Amebic liver abscess in children: the role of diagnostic imaging. AJR 1984; 143:1325–1329.
31. Henschke CI, Goldman H, Teele RL. Hyperechogenic liver in children: Cause and sonographic appearance. AJR 1982; 138:841–846.
32. Needleman L, Kurtz AB, Rifkin MD, Cooper HS, Pasto ME, Goldberg BB. Sonography of diffuse benign liver disease: accuracy of pattern recognition and grading. AJR 1986; 146:1011.
33. Slovis TL, Clapp SK, Farooki ZQ. Non-invasive evaluation of the inferior vena cava: The value of sonography. Am J Dis Child 1984; 38:277–280.
34. Ledesma-Medina J, Dominguez R, Bowen A, Young LW, Bron KM. Pediatric liver transplantation: I. Standardization of preoperative diagnostic imaging. Radiology 185; 157:335–338.
35. Dominguez R, Young LW, Ledesma-Medina J, Cienfuegos J, Gartner JC, Bron KM, Starzl TE. Pediatric liver transplantation: II. Diagnostic imaging in postoperative management. Radiology 1985; 157:339–344.
36. Callahan J, Haller JO, Cacciarelli AA, Slovis TL, Freedman AP. Cholelithiasis in infants: association with total parenteral nutrition and furosemide. Radiology 1982; 143:437–439.
37. Patriquin HB, DiPietro M, Barber FE, Teele RL. Sonography of thickened gallbladder wall: causes in children. AJR 1983; 141:57–60.
38. Siegel MJ, Martin KW, Worthington JL. Normal and abnormal pancreas in children: US studies. Radiology 1987; 165:15–18.
39. Coleman BG, Arger PH, Rosenberg HK, Mulhern CB, Ortega W, Stauffer D. Gray-scale sonographic assessment of pancreatitis in children. Radiology 1983; 146:145–150.
40. Stringer DA. Pediatric gastrointestinal imaging. Philadelphia: BC Decker, 1989: 585.
41. Weizman Z, Durie PR. Acute pancreatitis in childhood. J Pediatr 1988; 113:24–29.
42. Fishman EK, Siegelman SS. Pancreatitis and its complications. In: Taveras JM, Ferrucci JT, eds. Vol. 4. Philadelphia: JB Lippincott, 1988: 1.
43. Hayden CK Jr, Swischuk LE. Pediatric ultrasonography. Baltimore: Williams & Wilkins, 1987: 231.
44. DeVanna T, Dunne MG, Haney PJ. Fistulous communication of pseudocyst to the common bile duct: a complication of pancreatitis. Pediatr Radiol 1983; 13:344–345.
45. Garel L, Brunelle F, Lallemand D, Sauvegrain J. Pseudocysts of the pancreas in children: which cases require surgery? Pediatr Radiol 1983; 13:120–124.
46. Liu P, Daneman A, Stringer DA, et al. Pancreatic cysts and calcification in cystic fibrosis. J Can Assoc Radiol 1986; 37:279.
47. Rueckert KF, Klotter HJ, Kiimmerle F. Intraoperative ultrasonic localization of endocrine tumors of the pancreas. Surgery 1984; 96:1045–1047.
48. Robey G, Daneman A, Martin DJ. Pancreatic carcinoma in a neonate. Pediatr Radiol 1983; 13:284–286.
49. Stringer DA. Pediatric gastrointestinal imaging. Philadelphia: BC Decker, 1989: 611.

50. Hayden CK, Swischuk LE. Pediatric ultrasonography. Baltimore: Williams & Wilkins, 1987: 225.
51. Goske Rudick M, Wood BP, Lerner RM. Splenic abscess diagnosed by ultrasound in the pediatric patient: Report of three cases. Pediatr Radiol 1983; 13:269–271.
52. Laurin S, Kaude JV. Diagnosis of liver and spleen abscesses in children with emphasis on ultrasound for the initial and follow-up examinations. Pediatr Radiol 1984; 14:198–204.
53. Mittelstaedt CA, Partain CL. Ultrasonic-pathologic classification of splenic abnormalities: gray-scale patterns. Radiology 1980; 134:679–705.
54. Booth AJ, Bruce DI, Steiner GM. US diagnosis of spleen injuries in children and the importance of free peritoneal fluid. Clin Radiol 1987; 38:395.
55. Brick SH, Taylor GA, Potter BM. Hepatic and spleen injury: role of CT in the decision for laparotomy. Radiology 1987; 165:643.
56. Stringer DA. Pediatric gastrointestinal imaging. Philadelphia: BC Decker, 1989.
57. Hayden CK, Swischuk LE. Pediatric ultrasonography. Baltimore: Williams & Wilkins, 1987: 101.
58. Smith WL, Erenberg A, Nowak A, Franken EA Jr. Physiology of sucking in the normal term infant using real-time US. Radiology 1985; 156:379–381.
59. Miller JH, Kemberling CR. Ultrasound scanning of the gastrointestinal tract in children: subject review. Radiology 1984; 152:671–677.
60. Miller JH, Kemberling CR. Ultrasound of the pediatric gastrointestinal tract. Semin US CT MR 1987; 8:349.
61. Teele R. A dozen pediatric ultrasonic doughnuts. Mt Sinai J Med 1984; 51:528–534.
62. Fleischer AC, Muhletaler CA, James AE Jr. Sonographic patterns arising from normal and abnormal bowel. Radiol Clin North Am 1980; 18:145–159.
63. Haller JO, Cohen HL. Hypertrophic pyloric stenosis: diagnosis using US. Radiology 1986; 161:335–339.
64. Graif M, Itzchak Y, Avigad I, Strauss S, Ben-Ami T. The pylorus in infancy: overall sonographic assessment. Pediatr Radiol 1984; 14:14–17.
65. Kopen PA, McAlister WH. Upper gastrointestinal and ultrasound examinations of gastric antral involvement in chronic granulomatous disease. Pediatr Radiol 1984; 14:91–93.
66. Limberg B. Diagnosis of inflammatory and neoplastic large bowel disease by conventional abdominal and colonic sonography. Ultrasound Q 1988; 6:151–166.
67. Puylaert JBCM. Mesenteric adenitis and acute terminal ileitis: US evaluation using graded compression. Radiology 1986; 161:691–695.
68. Jeffrey RB. Management of the periappendiceal inflammatory mass. Semin Ultrasound CT MR 1989; 10:341–347.
69. Parulekar SG. Ultrasonographic findings in diseases of the appendix. J Ultrasound Med 1983; 2:59–64.
70. Jeffrey RB, Laing FC, Townsend RR. Acute appendicitis: sonographic criteria based on 250 cases. Radiology 1988; 167:327–329.
71. Abu-Yousef MM, Franken EA. An overview of graded compression sonography in the diagnosis of acute appendicitis. Semin Ultrasound CT MR 1989; 10:352–363.
72. See CC, Glassman M, Berezin S, Inamdar S, Newman LJ. Emergency ultrasound in the evaluation of acute onset abdominal pain in children. Pediatr Emerg Care 1988; 4:169–171.
73. Puylaert JBCM. Acute appendicitis: US evaluation using graded compression. Radiology 1986; 158:335–360.
74. Jeffrey RB, Laing FC, Lewis FR. Acute appendicitis: high-resolution real-time US findings. Radiology 1987; 163:11–14.
75. Baker DE, Silver TM, Coran AG, McMillin KI. Postappendectomy fluid collections in children: incidence, nature, and evolution evaluation using US. Radiology 1986; 161:341–344.
76. Alexander JE, Williamson SL, Seibert JJ, Golladay ES, Jimenez JF. The ultrasonographic diagnosis of typhlitis (neutropenic colitis). Pediatr Radiol 1988; 18:200–204.
77. Griffiths DM, Gough MH. Gas in the hepatic portal veins. Br J Surg 1986; 73:173–176.
78. Kodruff MB, Hartenberg MA, Goldschmidt RA. Ultrasonographic diagnosis of gangrenous bowel in neonatal necrotizing enterocolitis. Pediatr Radiol 1984; 14:168–170.
79. Bisset GS, Kirks DR. Intussusception in infants and children: diagnosis and therapy. Radiology 1988; 168:141–145.
80. Swischuk LE, Hayden CK, Boulden T. Intussusception: indications for ultrasonography and an explanation of the doughnut and pseudokidney signs. Pediatr Radiol 1985; 15:388–391.
81. Bolia AA. Case report: Diagnosis and hydrostatic reduction of an intussusception under ultrasound guidance. Clin Radiol 1985; 36:655–657.
82. Fleischer A, Dowling A, Weinstein M. Sonographic patterns of distended, fluid-filled small and large bowel: anatomic-radiographic correlation. Radiology 1979; 133:681–685.
83. Pasto ME, Deiling JM, O'Hara AE, Rifkin MD, Goldberg BB. Neonatal colonic atresia: ultrasound findings. Pediatr Radiol 1984; 14:346–348.
84. Gaines PA, Saunders AJS, Drake D. Midgut malrotation diagnosed by ultrasound. Clin Radiol 38:51–53.
85. Naik BR, Morday BG. Ultrasound diagnosis of gastroesophageal reflux. Arch Dis Child 1984; 459:366–379.
86. Dinkel E, Lehnart R, Troger J, Peters H, Dittrich M. Sonographic evidence of intraperitoneal fluid. An experimental study and its clinical significance. Pediatr Radiol 1984; 14:299–303.

PART 5

Computed Tomography

Paul Babyn, M.D.
David A. Stringer, B.Sc., M.B.B.S., F.R.C.R., FRCPC

The use of computed tomography (CT) in the evaluation of disorders of the pediatric abdomen has rapidly increased over the last decade.[1-5] Technologic advances, such as faster scan times and newer reconstructive algorithms, continue to help radiologists refine and expand the role of CT in the diagnostician's armamentarium.

The inherent advantages of CT, compared with plain radiography, are primarily its high spatial and high tissue-density discrimination. These advantages, coupled with axial tomographic techniques, have established it as the present-day primary imaging modality in oncology, multiple-organ trauma, and complicated inflammatory disease. CT is also helpful in the diagnosis of a wide spectrum of other conditions ranging from the evaluation of congenital anomalies to vascular disorders. The overall use of CT, however, will likely decrease given the present promise of magnetic resonance imaging (MRI), even though its eventual role has not yet been defined.

When deciding upon the appropriate course of investigations for a child, the radiologist must always strive to minimize both the child's exposure to radiation and the use of invasive procedures, while maximizing diagnostic potential. Because it requires the use of ionizing radiation, CT should not be considered a noninvasive test. The risks and discomfort associated with both oral and intravenous contrast enhancement for any child must be taken into account. Certainly, not all problems require a CT scan for their solution, so it is incumbent on all physicians not to become too complacent about its use. Close co-operation and communication between the attending clinician and the radiologist are vital if the investigation is to be tailored to the clinical problem and the patient. Blind adherence to a series of protocols can be costly, both physically for the patient because of the increased levels of radiation exposure and financially for the institution because of the additional expense.

Obtaining diagnostic images in children requires meticulous attention to technique. Degradation of the images caused by motion should be avoided. In those centers without ultrafast CT, sedation is often required. Before sedation is given (whether oral, intramuscular, or intravenous, depending on the institution), the patient must be adequately assessed for the impact of associated cardiac, airway, pulmonary, or central nervous system disease. Appropriate resuscitation equipment and monitoring devices (such as pulse oximeters and heating blankets) should be available.

The actual volume of oral contrast material administered is dependent on the age and weight of the patient, with increased contrast material needed for the primary evaluation of the gastrointestinal (GI) tract. We generally use a nonionic contrast agent diluted with water in a 20:1 ratio. The relative paucity of retroperitoneal fat found in children necessitates the use of intravenous contrast, as does the determination of the vascularity of a lesion. Fasting for a variable period (1 to 4 hours, depending on the age of the patient) is necessary to decrease the risk of vomiting after the administration of oral and intravenous contrast material.

The actual techniques of CT scanning vary depending on the type of equipment used, the clinical problem, and the individual patient. Table 1 shows the general guidelines for the evaluation of the abdomen. (See references 1 to 5 for more specific information.)

TABLE 1
Computed Tomography Technique for Pediatric Abdominal Imaging

Technique	Explanation
Extent of scan	From the level of the diaphragm superiorly down to iliac crests or through the pelvis, if necessary
Slice thickness and interval	Contiguous 1-cm cuts
Oral contrast	Given 20 minutes before scanning; amount dependent upon age and size of patient
Intravenous contrast	2 ml/kg administered as a bolus with dynamic scanning after one-half to two-thirds of the total volume given. Precontrast scans helpful for the initial evaluation of abdominal masses
Field of view	As small as possible to encompass patient

HEPATOBILIARY SYSTEM

CT may provide important information for the evaluation of either diffuse or focal disorders of the hepatic parenchyma, but it is perhaps of greatest benefit in the evaluation of patients with either focal hepatic masses or abdominal trauma. CT can rapidly define the character and anatomic extent of not only malignant hepatic lesions such as hepatoblastoma and hepatocellular carcinoma but also benign lesions such as cysts and abscesses. (For a consideration of the role of CT in hepatic trauma, see Abdominal Trauma.)

Diffuse disorders of the hepatic parenchyma examined here include cirrhosis, hemochromatosis, and metabolic disorders. In addition, the role of CT in liver transplantation and in abnormalities of the biliary system is discussed.

Normal Appearance and Anatomy

The normal appearance and anatomy of the liver do not change from infancy through adulthood. On nonenhanced scans, the hepatic parenchyma should be of uniform attenuation, slightly higher in density than the spleen. Throughout the liver, low-density linear or tubular structures representing the hepatic and portal veins should be evident. Immediately following the administration of the contrast material, the hepatic vasculature enhances to a much greater degree than does the normal parenchyma.

The classic anatomic division of the liver into right and left lobes, as demarcated by the falciform ligament and the fissure for the ligamentum teres, is no longer used. Instead, this can be divided into surgical subdivisions as shown in Figure 1. Further division of the hepatic lobar and segmen-

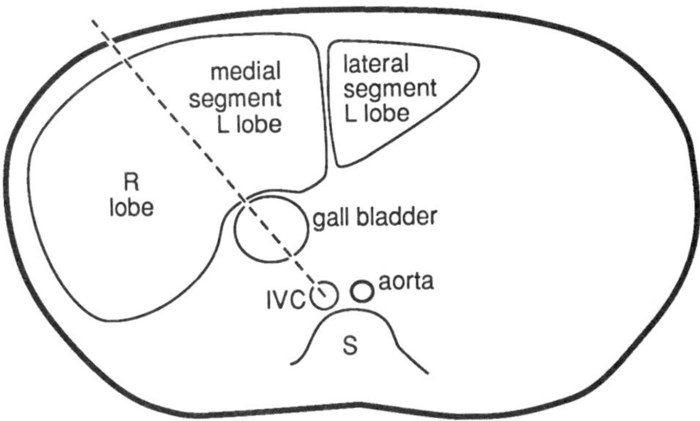

FIGURE 1 Surgical subdivision of the liver. The medial segment of the surgical left lobe lies to the right of the ligamentum teres and is demarcated by an oblique imaginary plane passing through the impression for the gallbladder and the inferior vena cava. (From Stringer.[69])

tal anatomy is possible with the use of the hepatic vasculature.[6] Accurate depiction of the anatomy is extremely important in the presurgical evaluation of hepatic neoplasms. A variable amount of fatty tissue that may be noted within the fissure of the ligamentum teres aids in the visualization of the underlying anatomy.

Normal intrahepatic bile ducts are not delineated in a CT scan in children. Occasionally, the extrahepatic bile duct, which should not measure more than 4 mm in diameter, is visible distally at the level of the pancreas.[3] The gallbladder appears as a pear-shaped structure of homogeneous fluid density along the inferior aspect of the liver. The normal gallbladder wall is thin and shows normal enhancement after intravenous administration of contrast material. This may be particularly evident if the hepatic parenchyma is decreased in density such as it is with fatty infiltration.

Beam-hardening artifacts, low-density areas seen adjacent to the inferior right ribs within the liver, should not be confused with focal hepatic lesions. Accessory hepatic veins and fissures may also be occasionally identified. Anomalies of lobar architecture, such as lobar agenesis, are quite rare.

Diffuse Hepatic Parenchymal Disease

CT scans can reveal diffuse abnormalities of the liver that may alter normal hepatic morphology or affect parenchymal attenuation.[7] Cirrhosis, with its diffuse parenchymal destruction and variable nodular parenchymal regeneration, can grossly distort the liver, making the hepatic outline appear lobulated in a CT study.[8] In addition, cirrhosis may cause a redistribution of normal hepatic volume or abnormally decreased liver volume, particularly in end-stage disease. Several investigators have described the relative enlargement of the caudate and lateral segment of the left lobe with atrophy of the right lobe apparent in both sonography and CT studies.[8,9] Changes in parenchymal attenuation may be delineated, particularly early on, if any fatty infiltration or fibrosis is present. The radiologist should also look for the secondary changes of portal hypertension, including splenomegaly, ascites, and collateral vein development (Fig. 2).

Portal vein thrombosis, a major cause of prehepatic hypertension, is frequently caused by neonatal omphalitis and complications of pancreatitis, neoplasm, or inflammation (Fig. 3). Most often the obstruction is chronic. A CT scan shows the multiple periportal and other collateral vessels that have formed. Occasionally, an acute thrombus may be identified as a linear low-density area, generally with an enhancing wall, in the expected position of the portal vein. Clot extension into the intrahepatic branches or superior mesenteric vein may also be seen and is often associated with inhomogeneous liver attenuation.[9]

Fatty infiltration, a nonspecific response to hepatocyte injury or metabolic derangement, is commonly seen in malnutrition, cystic fibrosis, storage disorders, chemotherapy, and cirrhosis (Fig. 4).[3,9,10] In a CT study, fatty infiltration may appear as either diffuse within the whole liver, geographic to a lobe or segment, or even more focal. With mild involvement, hepatic attenuation is diminished so that the normal liver-to-spleen attenuation ratio is reversed. More severe involvement may actually reduce the density below that of the hepatic vasculature. Focal fatty infiltration has occasionally been confused with solid tumors. The lack of mass effect and the normal-appearing hepatic vasculature through the region are helpful points of differentiation in the diagnosis of focal fatty infiltration.

Following radiation a low-density abnormality related to the radiation portal helps distinguish this condition.[11] Hepatic infarction is rare unless it is associated with hepatic artery thrombosis in liver transplantation. It may present with peripheral or central low-density areas that gradually become more sharply defined over time.[12]

Increased hepatic attenuation may be seen in children with increased iron deposition or glycogen-storage disease, or less

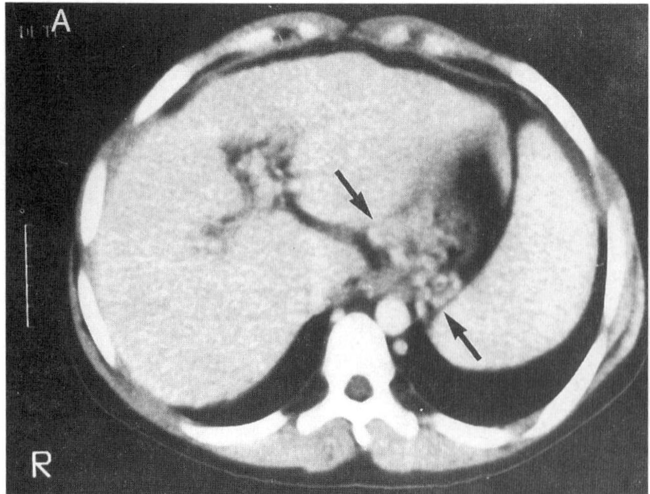

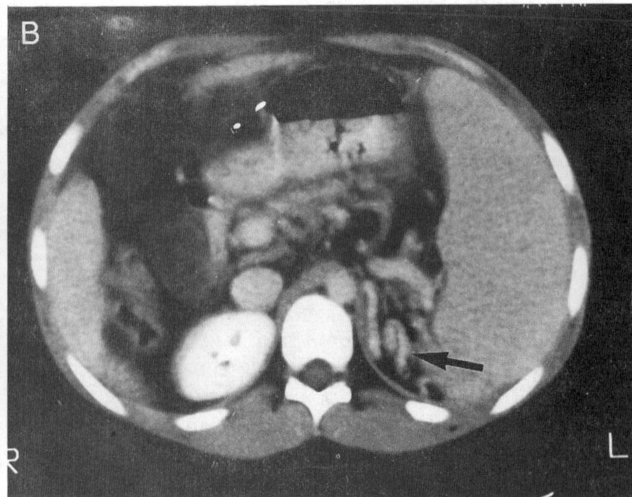

FIGURE 2 Portal hypertension with esophageal varices. Dynamic contrast-enhanced CT shows many collaterals *A*, adjacent to the gastroesophageal junction, (*between arrows*) and *B*, adjacent to the posteromedial part of the spleen (*arrow*). The spleen and liver are both enlarged in this child who has chronic active hepatitis.

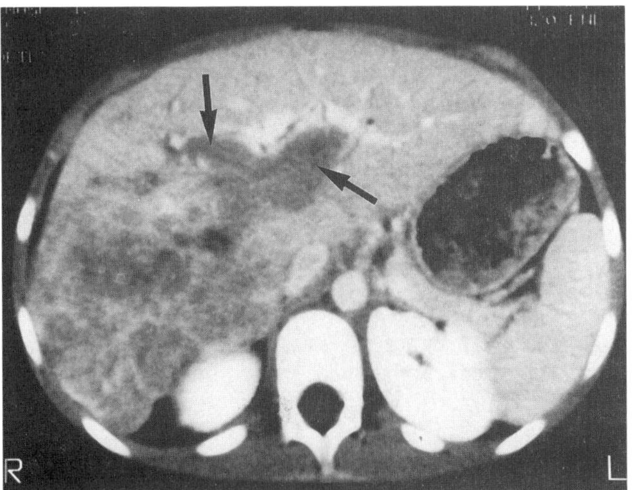

FIGURE 3 Hepatocellular carcinoma with portal vein tumoral thrombosis. Dynamic contrast-enhanced CT shows the hepatocellular carcinoma as multiple areas of decreased attenuation primarily in the right lobe of the liver and the involvement of left and right intrahepatic portal veins (*arrows*) by tumoral thrombosis. Adjacent enhanced vessels represent collaterals.

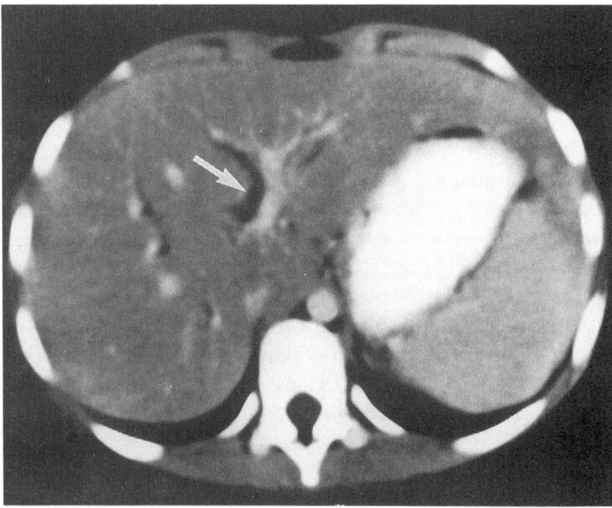

FIGURE 4 Fatty infiltration of the liver. CT shows a liver of markedly decreased attenuation, compared with the spleen, because of fat deposition. In addition, there is biliary duct dilatation (*arrow*), thought to be caused by sclerosing cholangitis in this child with ulcerative colitis.

commonly, after chemotherapy with cis-platinum[13] or hyperalimentation. Iron deposition leads to more markedly increased hepatic attenuation and is most often seen in children receiving long-term transfusion therapy for beta-thalassemia (Fig. 5).[14] Dual-energy CT scanning helps quantify the amount of iron present.[15] Both serial CT and MR scans can monitor the decrease in iron stores over time after chelation therapy. The appearance of the glycogen-storage diseases on a CT scan is variable.[16] Hepatic attenuation may be normal, decreased, or increased, depending on the relative amount of glycogen and fat. Increased glycogen deposition leads to increased attenuation, whereas fatty infiltration decreases hepatic attenuation. Associated hepatosplenomegaly or nephromegaly may be evident. Glycogen deposition may also be seen in the kidney, making the renal cortex appear dense. Hepatic adenomas, as found in type I glycogen storage disease, may appear hyperdense when there is surrounding fatty infiltration but more typically appear hypodense relative to the remaining liver. Serial sonographic evaluation is recommended for monitoring hepatic adenomas for subsequent malignant degeneration documented with any increase in size.[17]

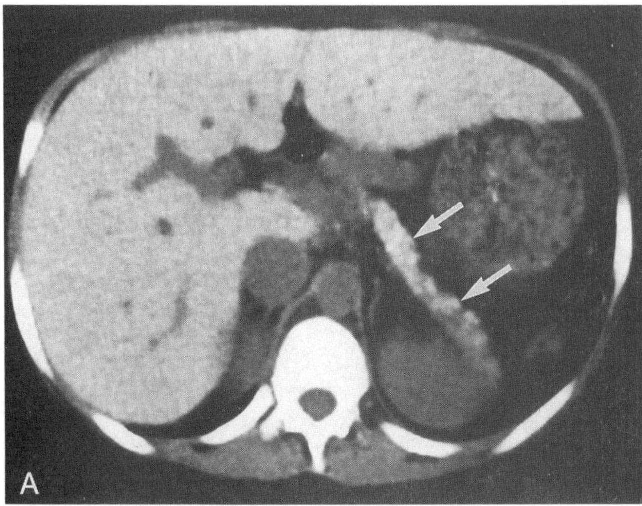

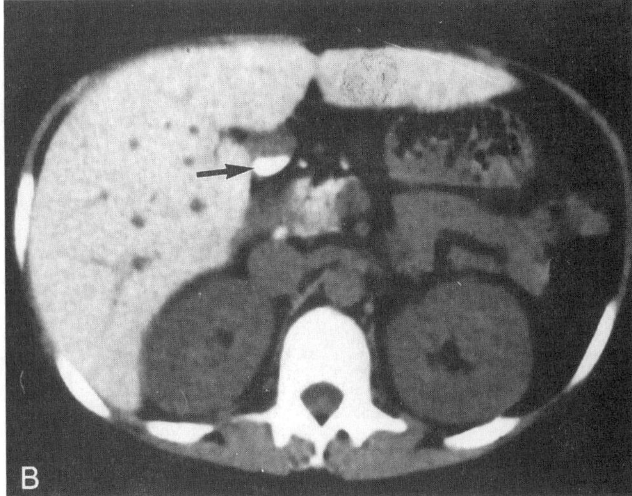

FIGURE 5 Iron deposition in a child with thalassemia. *A*, Nonenhanced CT shows very increased attenuation in the pancreas (*arrows*) and liver because of the iron deposition. *B*, On another slice, a small gallstone (*arrow*) is present.

Hepatic and Other Abdominal Masses

General Considerations for All Abdominal Masses

Abdominal masses can arise from anomalies in development, inflammation, neoplasm, or trauma.[18] A radiographic investigation of any mass lesion is designed to accomplish three primary objectives: to determine the site of the origin of the mass, to characterize the internal features of the mass, and to assess both the local effects on the surrounding organs and the distant spread of mass.

Sonography is our preferred initial modality for the assessment of abdominal masses because of its inherent advantages, particularly its ready availability and nonionizing nature. We reserve CT for situations in which additional anatomic or other tissue-specific information is needed.

Specific Features of Hepatic Masses

Although focal liver lesions account for a small minority of the abdominal masses seen in the pediatric population, the investigation of these lesions is a frequent indication for abdominal CT.[16,18–22] Overall, hepatic neoplasms are the third most common cause of solid abdominal tumors, after neuroblastoma and Wilms' tumor. Benign liver tumors account for one-third of hepatic neoplasms, with the vast majority of the malignant lesions being composed of hepatoblastomas and hepatocellular carcinomas.

In spite of the wide use of newer imaging modalities, there is still considerable overlap in the radiographic appearance of benign neoplastic or inflammatory lesions and that of malignant lesions. This overlap necessitates careful correlation of scanning results with clinical findings. With the significant exception of most benign vascular tumors in the younger age group, a specific diagnosis must almost always be confirmed by biopsy.

Benign Masses

Benign liver masses include abscesses, hematomas, cysts, and benign neoplasms.

Abscesses. Liver abscesses are infrequent. They are often seen in children who have a depressed immune system, and particularly in those who have chronic granulomatous disease or leukemia (Fig. 6). A CT scan reveals abscesses that are typically well-defined, low-density lesions with peripheral rim enhancement (Fig. 7).[23,24] Gas, although a diagnostic feature, is uncommonly seen. Pyogenic abscesses are more often solitary, whereas fungal disease is typically small and multiple. Both enhanced and nonenhanced scans may be necessary for the evaluation of suspected fungal abscesses because of their variable enhancement and attenuation (Fig. 8). Multiple-target lesions (so called because central areas are enhanced with a low-density periphery) are suggestive of fungal disease. Hydatid and amebic abscesses are rare and may be impossible to distinguish from other lesions, including bacterial abscesses, complicated cysts, hematomas, and cystic neoplasms.[25]

Benign Tumors. Benign tumors can be classified into two main groups according to their cell or origin, either mesen-

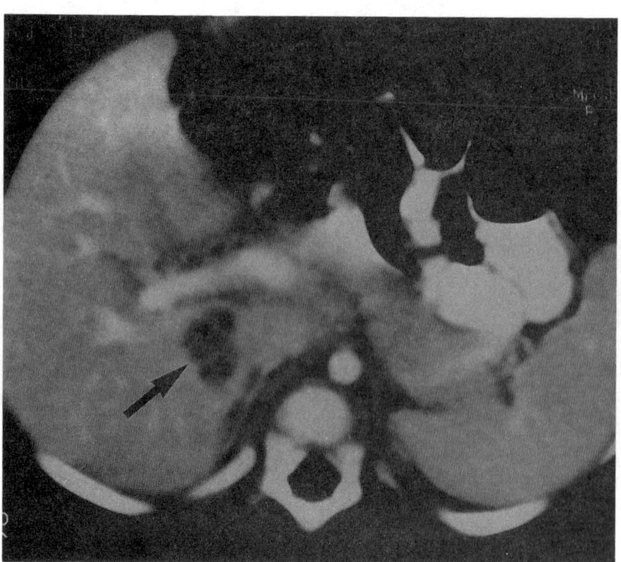

FIGURE 6 Pyogenic hepatic abscesses. Dynamic contrast-enhanced CT shows a septated lesion of decreased attenuation (*arrow*) in relation to the liver parenchyma in the posterior segment of the right lobe in a 10-month-old boy with chronic granulomatous disease.

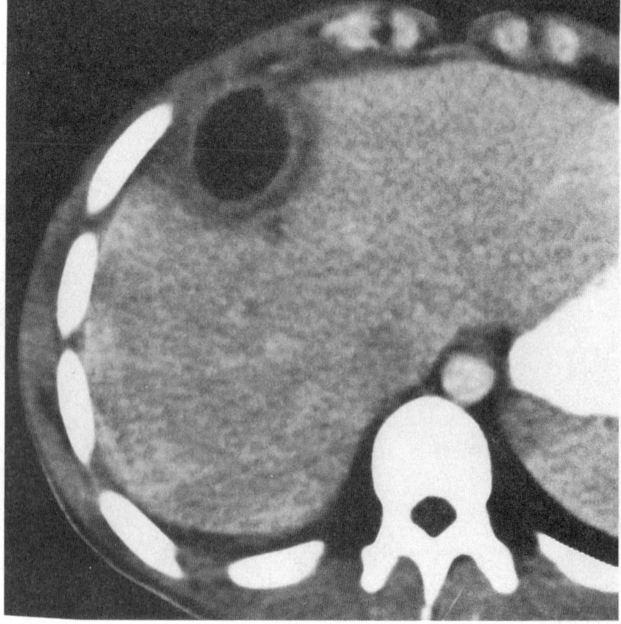

FIGURE 7 Pyogenic hepatic abscesses. Dynamic contrast-enhanced CT shows a well-defined region of decreased attenuation in the anterior part of the right lobe, with marked peripheral enhancement and surrounding edema.

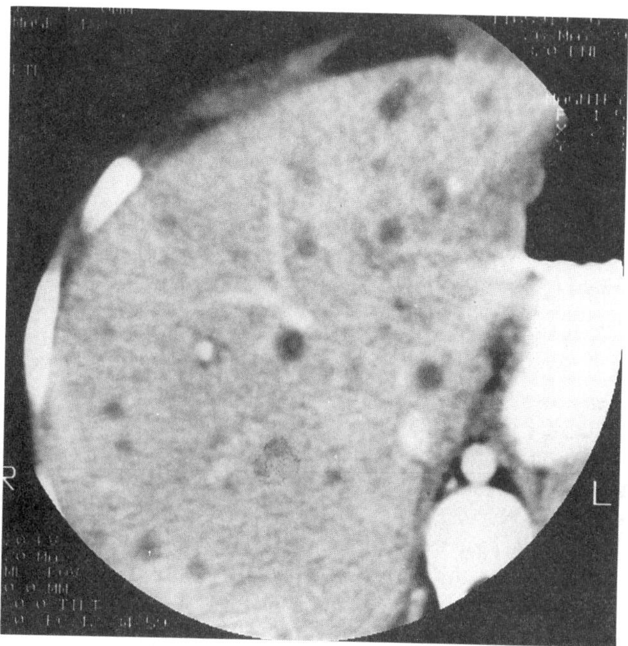

FIGURE 8 Fungal (*Candida*) hepatic abscesses. Dynamic contrast-enhanced CT shows multiple lesions of decreased attenuation in relation to the liver parenchyma. These were poorly seen on nonenhanced scans.

chymal or epithelial. Mesenchymal tumors include the vascular tumors, cavernous hemangiomas, and hemangioendotheliomas, as well as liver hamartomas. Epithelial tumors include congenital hepatic cysts, focal hyperplasia, and hepatic adenomas.

Hemangioendotheliomas and Hemangiomas. Hemangioendotheliomas are the most common symptomatic vascular liver tumors found in infancy.[16,18–20,26–28] Usually, they occur before 6 months of age in females who present with a palpable mass or liver enlargement. Not infrequently, the patient presents with congestive heart failure. Up to 45 percent of patients have associated cutaneous hemangiomas. On nonenhanced CT scans, these lesions are fairly well circumscribed and are less dense than the surrounding normal liver. They may be multifocal, diffusely involving the entire liver, or solitary lesions. Calcification, typically fine and speckled, was reported in 37 percent of patients in one series.[27] Following the administration of contrast material, intense peripheral or diffuse enhancement of the tumor, usually to a much greater degree than that of the surrounding liver, is evident (Fig. 9). Delayed scans may show a gradual filling-in of the hypodense central portion over time, similar to the opacification pattern described for adult hemangiomas. The caliber of the aorta distal to the hepatic artery origin may appear decreased.

Hemangiomas are usually asymptomatic and are often an incidental finding. They are generally much less common in infancy and childhood.[27]

Other Tumors. Mesenchymal hamartoma most likely represents a developmental anomaly of the bile ducts and mesenchymal tissue rather than a true neoplasm. It originates in the connective tissues adjacent to the portal tracts, causing progressive cystic degeneration and fluid accumulation. Typically, it presents within the first 2 years of life with abdominal swelling. The tumors are large and are more commonly seen in the right lobe with variably sized cystic spaces and intervening solid septa. On a CT scan, the lesion is well defined with low-attenuation areas corresponding to the cysts.[18,29,30] Calcification is not usually present. If a solid component is present, it may enhance with the administration of contrast material. The lesions may be exophytic, making them difficult to distinguish from other cystic abdominal masses, including loculated ascites.

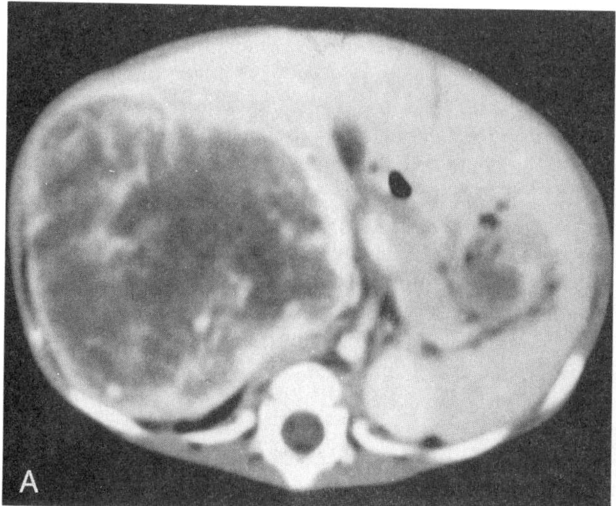

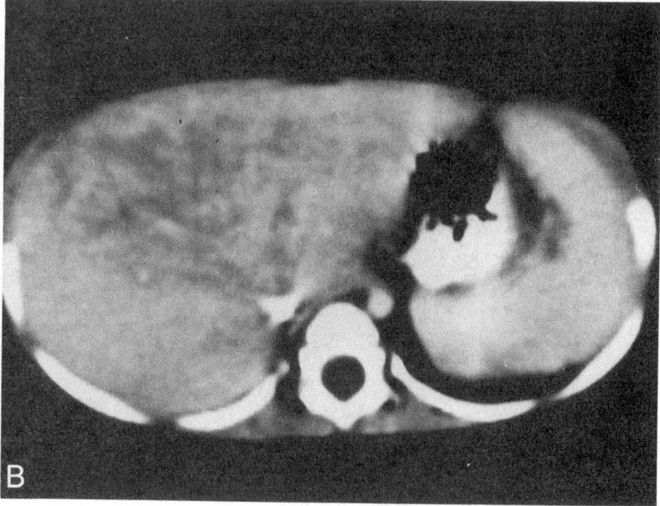

FIGURE 9 Hepatic hemangioendothelioma. *A*, Dynamic contrast-enhanced CT shows a large hepatic lesion of relatively low attenuation, which enhanced intensely peripherally. *B*, In another patient, a large relatively low-attenuation mass enhanced diffusely on dynamic contrast-enhanced CT.

Epithelial tumors are much less common than tumors of mesenchymal origin. Sonography is the preferred modality of investigation for congenital hepatic cysts. During a CT scan, they appear similar to other cysts, with uniform nonenhancing low attenuation (Fig. 10). Multiple cysts can be seen in polycystic kidney disease and tuberous sclerosis.

Hepatic adenomas are rarely seen in childhood. They are most often associated with glycogen storage disease, type I, or less commonly, type VI.[17] In glycogen storage disease, they are usually multiple and can occasionally be hyperdense if the surrounding liver shows fatty infiltration. Most often they are small discrete hypodense nodules with variable enhancement.[16,19,20] Intratumoral hemorrhage may be noted. Sonography and clinical correlation have been suggested for follow-up because malignant degeneration is thought to occur.[16,19,20]

Focal nodular hyperplasia presents as a palpable mass or an incidental finding. On the CT scan, it is typically of low attenuation, often with a central area of further hypodensity that represents the central scar observed pathologically. Calcification is not seen.[16,19,20]

Malignant Tumors

In the pediatric population, primary tumors of the liver are less frequent than metastases. Hepatoblastoma and hepatocellular carcinoma are the most frequent primary malignancies of the liver. They account for approximately 2 percent of all pediatric neoplasms.[31] Almost all patients with primary tumors present with hepatomegaly and abdominal distention. The age of the patient is normally the limiting factor in clinical radiologic analysis. Almost all cases of hepatoblastoma are found in patients under the age of 5 years, although rare presentations occur in adolescence or even in adulthood. Hepatocellular carcinoma is rarely seen in individuals under 3 years of age.

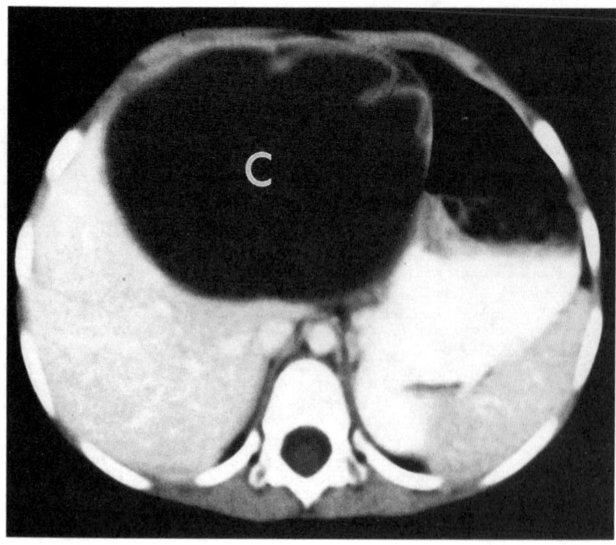

FIGURE 10 Isolated congenital hepatic cyst. A large cyst (C) on contrast-enhanced CT does not enhance and is of uniform low attenuation.

Hepatoblastoma was a term first used by Willis to describe a tumor of embryonal origin, histologically distinct from hepatocellular carcinoma, which may be epithelial or mixed mesenchymal-epithelial. Hepatoblastomas have been associated with hemihypertrophy, polycystic kidneys, and Beckwith-Wiedemann syndrome. Typically, hepatoblastoma is a solitary mass within the right lobe (Fig. 11) Less often it is composed of multiple nodular masses or may even have diffuse hepatic involvement. Coarse calcification, seen in association with osteoid masses, is often present in the tumor. On the CT scan the tumor is seen, both before and after enhancement, as a roughly spherical mass of less than normal hepatic density (Fig. 11). It may cause the liver surface to bulge. Septation within the tumor is best seen after the administration of contrast material. Occasionally, the scan may show peripheral enhancement that is suggestive of a vascular tumor. Small cystic spaces can be seen, but usually these can be readily differentiated from mesenchymal hamartoma.[32]

Hepatocarcinoma occurs infrequently before the age of 3 years, but it is the most common primary malignancy of the liver after the age of 5 years. Known risk factors for the development of hepatocellular carcinoma (HCC) include glycogen storage disease, hereditary tyrosinemia, biliary atresia, hepatitis, and the anabolic steroids used in the treatment of Fanconi's anemia. The CT scan appearance of HCC may be similar to that of hepatoblastoma, but it is more often multicentric, appearing to arise from within both lobes of the liver (Fig. 12). Nonenhanced scans demonstrate a low-density lesion with infrequent calcification. Enhancement is variable and may be peripheral. Typically, the enhancement is less than that of the surrounding normal parenchyma.[19-21] Tumor extension into the portal system is almost diagnostic of HCC. An important subtype of HCC is fibrolamellar carcinoma, which has a more favorable prognosis and normal alpha$_1$-fetoprotein. Fibrolamellar HCC more commonly arises within the left lobe.[33,34]

Other primary malignant liver tumors include undifferentiated sarcoma of the liver, as well as rhabdomyosarcoma of the biliary tree. Undifferentiated sarcoma is typically a large solitary mass seen in symptomatic children older than age 5 years. On the CT scan, it appears as a hypodense cystic mass with infrequent calcification, multiple septations, and variable amounts of enhancing tissue, often extending into the inferior vena cava and right atrium.[35] In children, rhabdomyosarcoma of the biliary tree is a rare tumor that may show dilatation of the biliary tree, displacement of the portal system, and most often a low-density mass.[36]

Metastases can occur with many childhood neoplasms.[18-22,37] The most frequent causes are neuroblastoma, leukemia, and lymphoma (Fig. 13). Often multiple lesions are seen, but large solitary metastases can occur (Fig. 14). Fortunately, the primary tumor is almost always known. Metastases are usually low-density lesions that show less enhancement than normal parenchyma on a CT scan. Neuroblastoma and Wilms' tumor can spread directly into the liver. Exclusion of hepatic involvement, or indeed of extrahepatic tumor origin, is often difficult with right upper quadrant extrahepatic masses because of their direct abutment against the hepatic parenchyma.

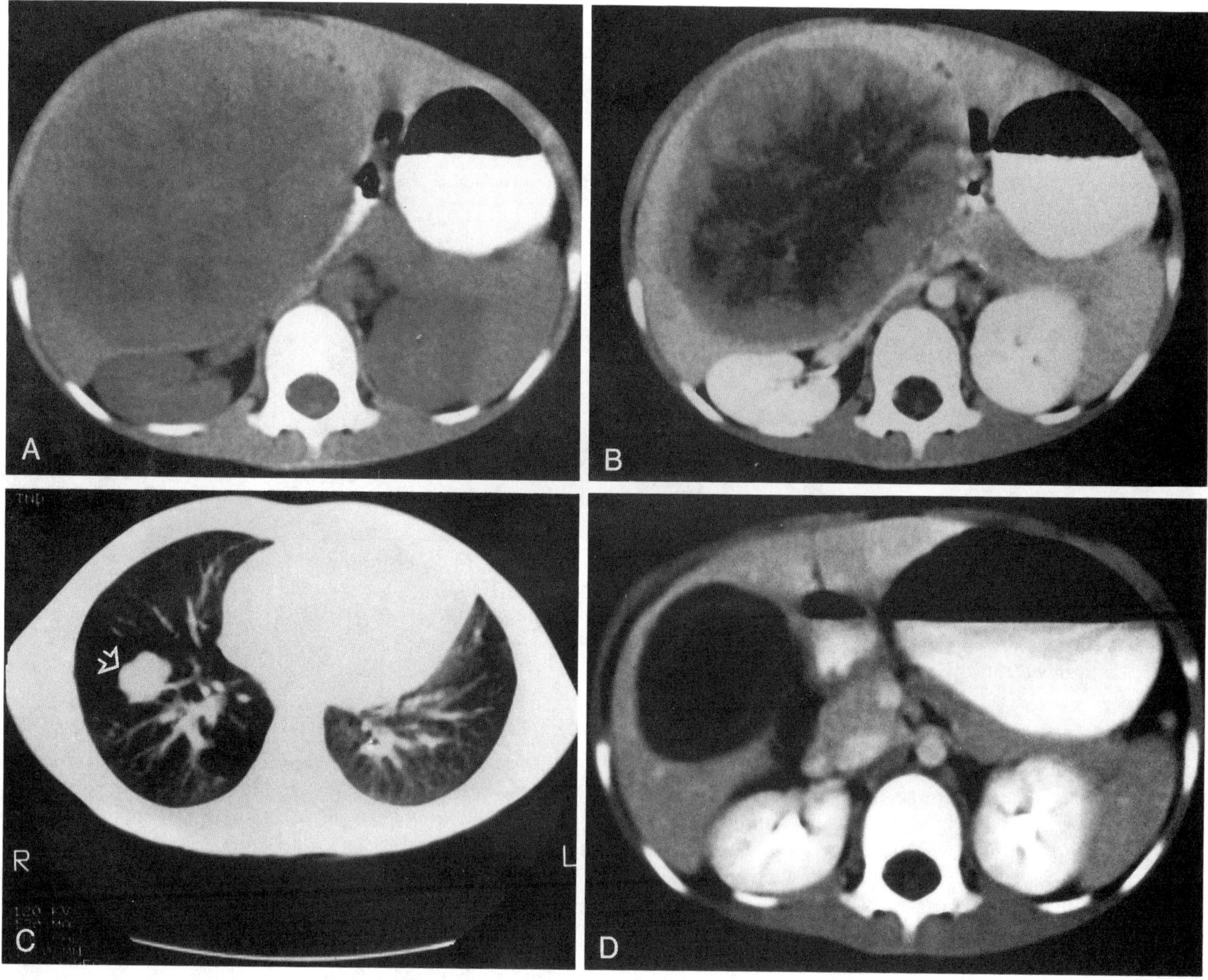

FIGURE 11 Hepatoblastoma. *A*, Nonenhanced CT shows a large mass of low attenuation replacing most of the right lobe of the liver, displacing normal midline structures and compressing the right kidney. *B*, Following intravenous contrast injection, there was some peripheral enhancement of the tumor; however, this enhancement was less than that of the adjacent normal liver. A central irregular area of markedly decreased attenuation probably represents necrosis. *C*, Chest CT showed a large right lung metastasis (*arrow*). *D*, There has been marked decrease in size and diminution in attenuation because of necrosis following chemotherapy prior to surgery.

Liver Transplantation

Liver transplantation has caused dramatic improvement in the initial survival of patients over the last few years. A successful liver transplantation program requires the co-ordinated commitment of professionals of several disciplines, including radiologists. Diagnostic imaging plays a vital role, both pre- and postoperative, in the management of these children.[38–41] Preoperatively, abdominal sonography and barium meal are used initially to identify potential vascular or gastrointestinal (GI) tract anomalies that may potentially contraindicate or complicate surgery. For example, biliary atresia, which we find to be the most common indication for liver transplantation, is occasionally associated with polysplenia. Vascular anomalies often associated with biliary atresia include interrupted inferior vena cava with azygous continuation, preduodenal portal vein, or anomalous hepatic artery supply. Intestinal malrotation may also be seen. Further evaluation of the portal vein or inferior vena cava by angiography, dynamic CT, or MRI may be warranted if initial sonography is not diagnostic. CT is useful in the evaluation of suspected malignancies in patients with metabolic disorders such as glycogen storage disease type I and tyrosinemia. CT also provides a rough guide to the recipients's hepatic volume. This aids in surgical planning

Postoperatively, CT is useful for the assessment of both acute and delayed complications.[39–41] It may reveal acute complications related to the technical difficulties of the surgery, including vascular occlusions of either the hepatic artery or the portal vein and any biliary obstructions or leaks at the anastomotic site. Often the coagulopathy arising from the pre-existing liver disease may compound postoperative

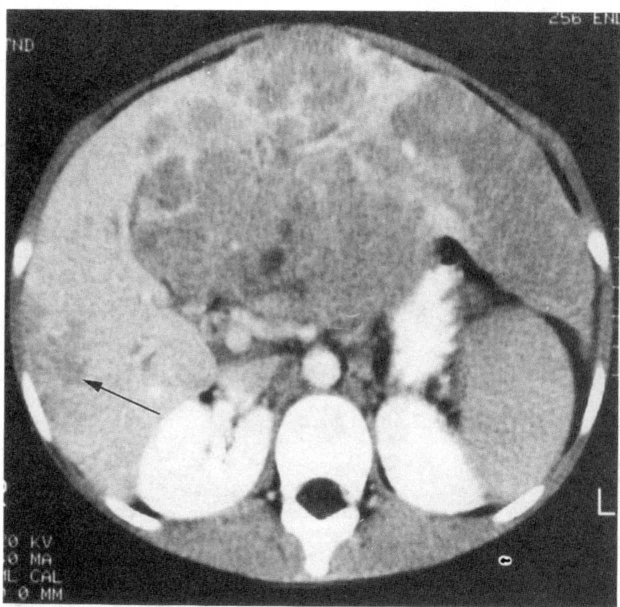

FIGURE 12 Hepatocellular carcinoma. Enhanced CT shows a relatively low-attenuation ill-defined diffuse mass filling the left lobe of the liver with involvement of the right lobe (*arrow*).

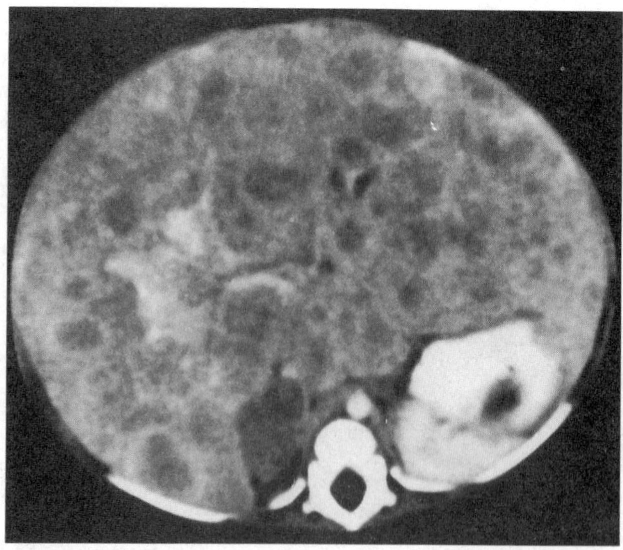

FIGURE 13 Metastasis from disseminated neuroblastoma. Enhanced CT shows multiple areas of low attenuation throughout the liver because of the involvement by a stage 4S neuroblastoma.

bleeding, with resultant fluid collections. Additionally, rejection of the allograft is a major concern. Postoperative infections may be localized in the liver or may be systemic. Hepatic artery thrombosis is, unfortunately, a more frequent complication in children, who have a 42 percent occlusion rate, than it is in adults. Hepatic artery thrombosis may manifest with massive necrosis of the liver or with more focal areas of necrosis and secondary abscess formation. Because the major arterial supply to the distal bile ducts is from the hepatic artery, biloma formation and stricture from bile duct ischemia may be found.

Sonography is the initial investigation of choice for the postoperative evaluation of the liver because it may be performed at the bedside with portable equipment. Sonography may reveal vascular compromise, reflected in areas of increased parenchymal echogenicity. Doppler evaluation of the hepatic artery or portal vein may document the presence of a thrombosis. CT is used to supplement the postoperative radiologic monitoring of liver transplant patients; it is able to detect both the biliary abnormalities and secondary changes of vascular occlusion.

On a CT scan, decreased attenuation of portions of the liver may reflect vascular compromise (Fig. 15). However, this problem may occasionally be confused with postbiopsy changes. Biliary dilatation, which can be easily seen by either sonography or CT, should be differentiated from the hypodense areas seen circumferentially around the main portal venous system and the intrahepatic inferior vena cava, which are thought to be secondary to the interruption of lymphatic drainage.[42] Dynamic CT may be helpful in documenting portal vein patency. Occasionally, high-attenuation areas within the donor aorta or inferior vena cava are seen in pediatric recipients. Autopsies suggest that these are intravascular thromboses with a variable degree of calcification.

The detection of liver rejection by CT remains controversial. In our experience, rejection is not reliably diagnosed by means of either CT or sonography; however, a periportal collar has proved to be a sensitive indicator of rejection.[43] This periportal collar is a low-attenuation circumferential region around multiple peripheral portal veins, not just the

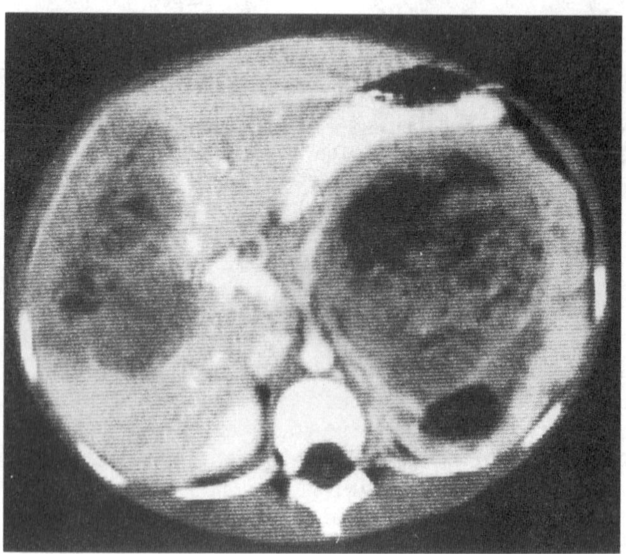

FIGURE 14 Metastasis from Wilms' tumor. CT shows a relatively well-defined low-attenuation mass in the right lobe of the liver. A central area of lower attenuation is present and is compatible with necrosis. In addition, there is a large mass of low attenuation arising from the left kidney, the primary Wilms' tumor.

main portal vein. This collar is presumed to occur secondary to lymphocytic infiltration and edema in the periportal region. However, this finding may also be seen in infectious cholangitis, graft necrosis, and nonspecific portal edema. CT is also helpful in the evaluation of fluid collections that may be perihepatic or located elsewhere in the abdomen. Extrahepatic abnormalities include associated adrenal hemorrhage and enlargement of the pancreas with pancreatitis, pneumatosis intestinalis, or focal bowel thickening, as well as splenic infarction.[44] Routine follow-up of transplant patients should be performed because of the high incidence of subsequent lymphoproliferative disorders.

Biliary System

The biliary system is rarely the primary indication for abdominal CT scanning. Almost always, sonography is satisfactory for the evaluation of jaundice, cholelithiasis, or other biliary tract anomalies. CT is reserved for the infrequent cases in which sonographic examination is inadequate because of technical problems caused by body habitus, bowel gas, or unusual pathology. Incidental note of gallstones may be made when the upper abdomen is scanned. These may appear as areas of increased or decreased attenuation within the surrounding bile, depending upon the relative calcium and cholesterol content. Choledocholithiasis is rare in the pediatric population. Increased attenuation of the gallbladder contents may be apparent after trauma because of hemobilia or vicarious excretion of contrast material from a prior angiography or other contrast study.

Sonography is the modality of choice for the evaluation of suspected choledochal cysts. If necessary, CT can be used to demonstrate the cystic dilatation of the extrahepatic biliary system and evaluate the intrahepatic bile ducts. In Caroli's disease, an uncommon problem, CT may show localized cystic areas representing biliary ectasia, communicating most often with a dilated intrahepatic biliary system. Children with periampullary masses or stricture formation may show dilatation of the proximal biliary system. Bile duct dilatation appears as hypodense, nonenhancing tubular structures, either anterior or posterior to the portal veins (Fig. 16).[45] There may or may not be associated jaundice, depending upon the degree of obstruction. CT may be particularly helpful for the delineation of the abnormality of neoplastic involvement caused by lymphadenopathy in the porta hepatis or actual tumor extension within the hepatoduodenal fissure compresses the common bile duct, causing proximal dilatation (Fig. 17).

PANCREAS

Sonography has revolutionized the radiologic evaluation of the pancreas in childhood. Because of its success, it remains the initial modality for the investigation of all pancreatic pathology with the exception of multiple organ trauma. CT is reserved for the few cases in which sonography is not satisfactory because of technical factors, that is, when overlying bowel gas is present or when a better definition of the anatomy is needed, as in the case of pancreatic neoplasms.

The pancreas is normally a comma-shaped organ that lies obliquely or, less often, transversely in the retroperitoneum (Fig. 18). In children, its borders are best defined by the opacification of the surrounding bowel and upper abdominal vasculature and , to a much lesser degree, by the amount of retroperitoneal fat present. The administration of oral and intravenous contrast material is therefore mandatory for an adequate examination. The uppermost portion of the pancreas

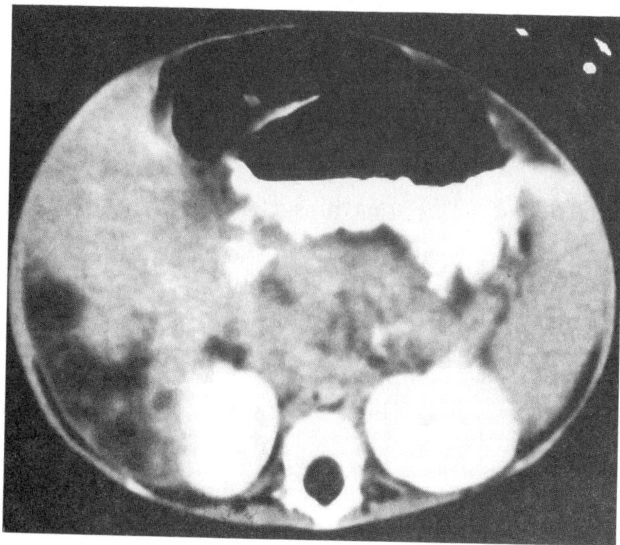

FIGURE 15 Focal necrosis in a liver transplant. Enhanced CT shows a peripheral ill-defined low-attenuation mass in the right lobe of the transplanted liver. The focal necrosis and low attenuation are due to the poor perfusion.

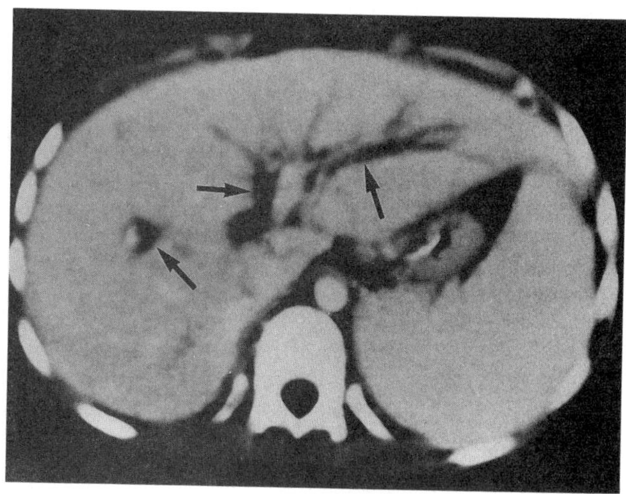

FIGURE 16 Common bile duct dilatation. Enhanced CT shows intrahepatic dilated bile ducts (*arrows*) as hypodense, nonenhancing tubular structures anterior and posterior to the intrahepatic portal veins. These ducts are of decreased attenuation relative to the contrast-enhanced liver and portal veins.

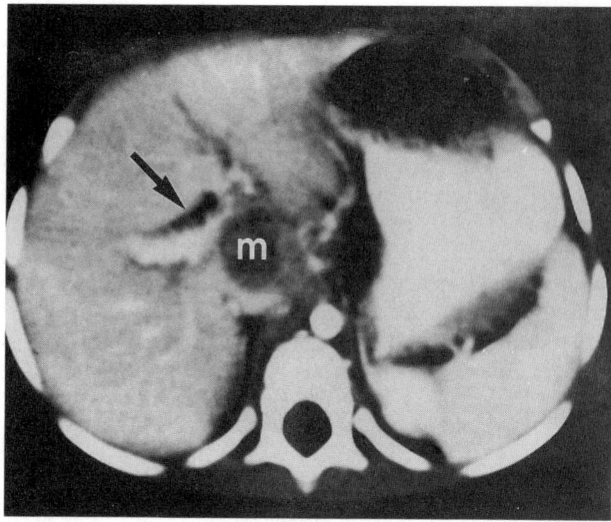

FIGURE 17 Neuroblastoma obstructing the common bile duct. Enhanced CT shows a dilated common hepatic duct (*arrow*) anterior to the right intrahepatic portal vein and a neuroblastoma mass (m) lying in the porta hepatis.

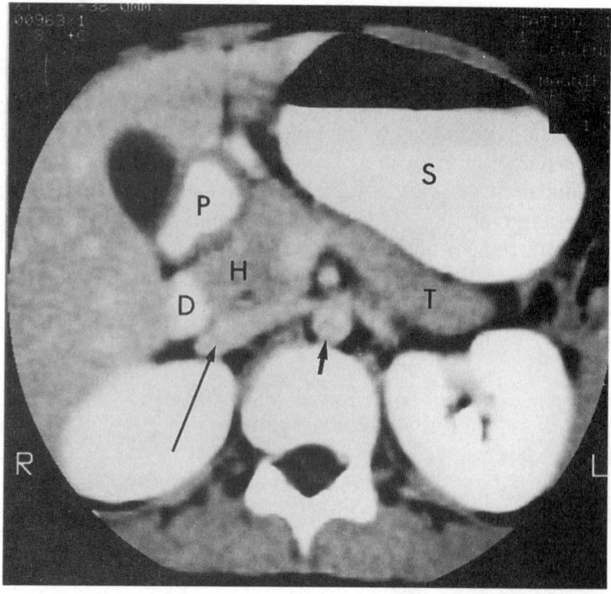

FIGURE 18 Normal pancreas. CT shows the body and tail (T) of the pancreas lying posterior to the stomach (S) and anterior to the splenic vein. The head of the pancreas (H) lies medial to the pylorus (P) and the duodenum (D). The inferior vena cava (*long arrow*), the aorta (*short arrow*), and the superior mesenteric artery are useful posterior landmarks. (From Daneman.[1])

is the pancreatic tail lying anterior and adjacent to the left kidney and splenic hilum. The pancreatic body and head lie more inferiorly. Posterior to the pancreatic body is the splenic vein and superior mesenteric vessels. The pancreatic neck is the portion of the pancreas that is anterior to the confluence of the splenic vein and superior mesenteric vein. The uncinate process of the pancreas may extend posteromedially to the superior mesenteric vein or artery. The right lateral aspect of the pancreatic head is nestled by the second and third portions of the duodenum, with the third and fourth portions of the duodenum extending below the pancreas.

The pancreas appears smooth in younger children.[46,47] The lobulation evident in later adolescence and adulthood develops gradually. The attenuation of the pancreas is homogeneous, just less than that of the liver. Increased pancreatic attenuation may be seen if iron deposition in thalassemia or other disorders is present. Focal increased attenuation from calcification may be secondary to chronic pancreatitis or cystic fibrosis. In cases of cystic fibrosis, the pancreas may also show parenchymal atrophy with prominent fatty replacement (Fig. 19) and, less commonly, macroscopic cyst formation.[47,48] Shwachman's syndrome may also reveal a fatty change in the pancreas.

Pancreatitis

Sonography also remains the modality most often utilized for the evaluation of pancreatitis. If CT is performed, it may show a spectrum of morphologic changes of the gland itself, including diffuse or focal enlargement, decreased attenuation secondary to edema, and blurring of the pancreatic outlines. CT can also easily visualize the complications of pancreatitis, such as pseudocyst formation (Fig. 20), abscess formation, or ascites. If it is extrapancreatic, a collection is usually located within the anterior pararenal space or lesser sac but may be found anywhere within the abdomen. If gas is identified within a collection, then an abscess must be suspected, and prompt drainage is required. Only 50 to 66 percent of pancreatic abscesses, however, show gas collections. Not all collections represent a pseudocyst. Pseudocysts can appear within days of pancreatic injury; however, they are usually more subacute and contain a thick fibrous wall. These can resolve spontaneously. If they persist, they may develop calcification in their periphery.

Pancreatic Neoplasms

Pancreatic tumors account for a very small percentage of all pediatric abdominal neoplasms. They can be broadly subdivided into functioning and nonfunctioning tumors.[46,49] Functioning tumors are of endocrine, islet cell origin and may be either benign or malignant. As is true for pancreatic neoplasms in general, benign functioning adenomas are much less commonly seen. Depending upon the active hormone secreted, these tumors may present with a variety of clinical features, including hypoglycemia (insulinoma), Zollinger-Ellison syndrome (gastrinoma), and water diarrhea (VIPoma), among others. Radiographically, these tumors can be difficult to detect and require almost the complete battery of imaging modalities available, including CT, angiography, and occasionally intraoperative sonography. In nesidioblastosis, not commonly found in neonates, pancreatic islet cells

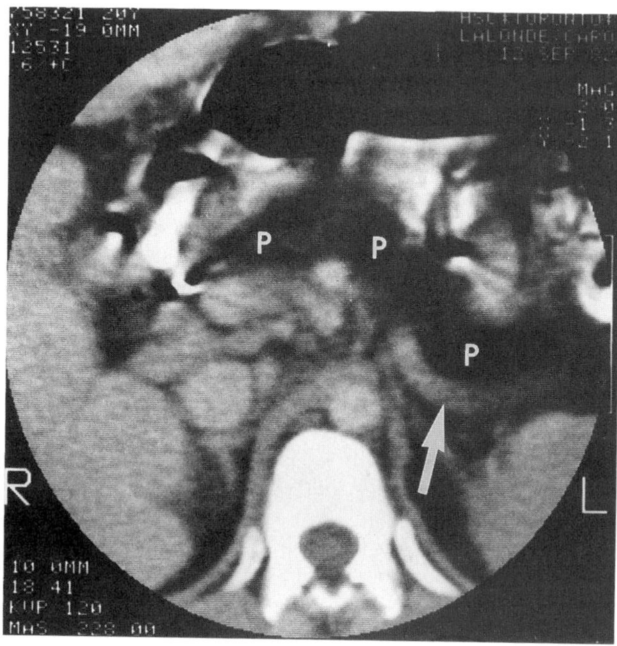

FIGURE 19 Pancreatitis in cystic fibrosis. Enhanced CT shows a small pancreas (P) of markedly decreased attenuation caused by fatty infiltration. It is just anterior to the splenic vein (*arrow*).

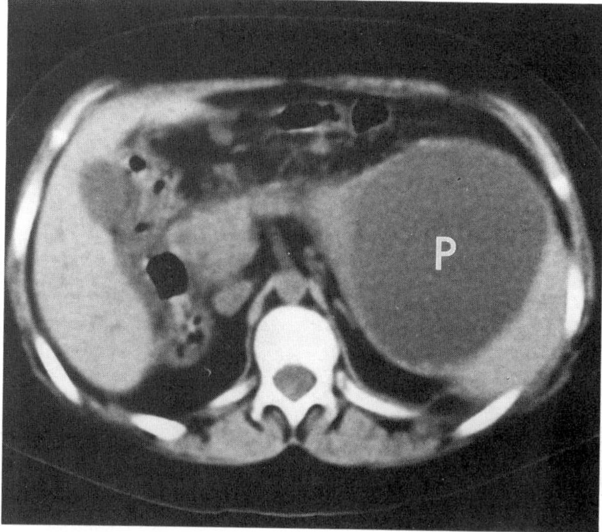

FIGURE 20 Pancreatic pseudocyst. CT demonstrates a mass of low attenuation (the pseudocyst—P) arising from the tail of the pancreas. There is a large quantity of fat present within the abdomen in this teenage girl who was receiving a high dose of steroids for an extended period of time for her renal transplants.

diffusely proliferate with secondary neonatal hypoglycemia; however, no distinctive radiologic features have been described to allow for preoperative diagnosis.

Nonfunctioning tumors may be of epithelial or nonepithelial origin and include adenocarcinomas, pancreatoblastomas, and solid and papillary epithelial neoplasms. Again, benign tumors are most uncommon in the pediatric population. These tumors most often present with a palpable mass and abdominal enlargement. Less frequent presentations include gastrointestinal obstruction, weight loss, and jaundice. Pancreatoblastoma or infantile carcinoma of the pancreas is usually found in the pancreatic head and shows inhomogeneous attenuation, reflecting the cystic and hemorrhagic areas within the tumor. Solid and papillary epithelial neoplasms (also known as papillary and cystic neoplasms or papillary cystic carcinomas) are uncommon tumors found chiefly in young females in adolescence and early adulthood. Often these tumors are first noted after minor abdominal trauma. Metastases are infrequent. CT typically shows a well-demarcated soft tissue mass containing low-attenuation areas of variable size, corresponding to hemorrhage and necrosis (Fig. 21).[50] Peripheral calcification may also be noted. Additional pancreatic tumors include metastatic lymphoma and neuroblastoma.

SPLEEN

Normal Appearance

Although CT can easily demonstrate the size, shape, and parenchyma of the spleen, primary evaluation of the spleen by abdominal CT is rarely indicated. Sonography is almost always satisfactory for the evaluation of splenic anatomy and pathology. Initial CT of the spleen is most often indicated for diffuse processes such as abdominal trauma or lymphoma. One should, however, be aware of the normal CT appearance because the spleen is included in almost every study of the upper abdomen.

With a CT scan, the normal spleen appears homogeneous in attenuation, located just slightly lower than the liver but higher than the adjacent kidney on nonenhanced scans.[1,3] Within the first few seconds of the scan, dynamic enhancement of the spleen may quickly show patch areas of decreased attenuation with a homogeneous blush apparent within 2 minutes.

It is important to be aware of normal variants such as prominent splenic lobulation, accessory spleens, splenic clefts, or recurrent spenules after a splenectomy (Fig. 22). For the unwary, these may simulate abdominal masses, lymphadenopathy, or even splenic laceration. Accessory spleens are most often located within the splenic hilum but are uncommon in younger children. They are more frequently visualized (10 to 30 percent) in adolescents and adults. Both accessory spleens and splenic lobules show normal splenic attenuation both before and after the administration of contrast material. Splenic ptosis, or a wandering spleen, may be seen even in the absence of previous abdominal surgery. Torsion of the splenic vascular pedicle may account for these cases. Streak artifacts from adjacent ribs or the gastric air-fluid level may also simulate splenic lesions.

Congenital anomalies of the spleen are not commonly evaluated with CT and are most often secondary to asplenia and polysplenia syndromes. An absence of the spleen is almost never isolated but instead is part of the asplenia syn-

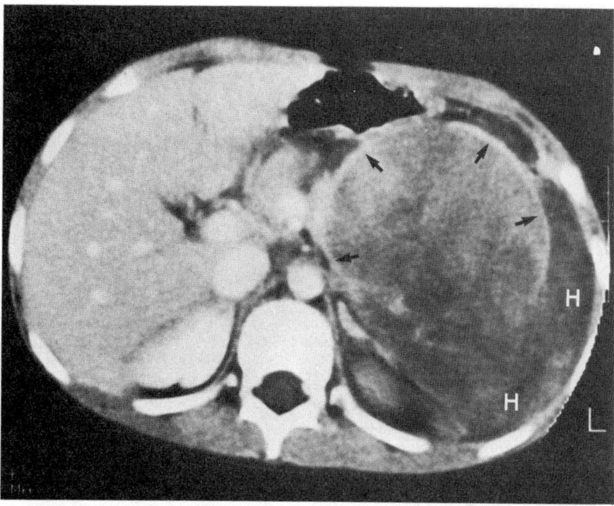

FIGURE 21 Solid and papillary epithelial tumor of the pancreas. Enhanced CT shows a mass of low attenuation arising from the tail of the pancreas with a slight enhancing rim (*arrows*). The mass had ruptured following a minor trauma. There was associated hemoperitoneum (H) laterally and posteriorly.

drome. In polysplenia, multiple small spleens may be noted. If children with these syndromes do undergo CT evaluation, then the radiologist must pay careful attention to the numerous anomalies often associated within the bowel, liver, kidneys, adrenals, and cardiovascular system.[1]

Splenic Pathology

Increased attenuation of the spleen may be diffuse, as seen in patients with thalassemia (usually to a lesser degree than that seen in the liver) or with the extensive calcification common in sickle cell disease. Focal areas of increased attenuation may represent calcification caused by granulomatous infection or abscess formation, trauma, or, more rarely, cyst formation. Focal areas of decreased attenuation are found in a wide gamut of lesions including neoplasms, abscesses, infarcts, hematomas, and cysts (Fig. 23).[51,52] Neoplasms are fortunately rare, except for lymphoma, which may show one or more focal areas of involvement or be more diffuse, revealing splenomegaly and overall normal attenuation. Abscesses may contain air and have an enhancing rim. Infarcts are typically peripheral wedge-shaped areas of low attenuation and are often associated with hematologic abnormalities. Splenic cysts may be congenital epidermoid cysts or pseudocysts, which are most likely post-traumatic in origin. Echinococcal cysts and cystic neoplasms, such as lymphangiomas, are less frequently encountered. Cysts are typically uniform in fluid density and well defined but may show trabeculae or wall calcification.

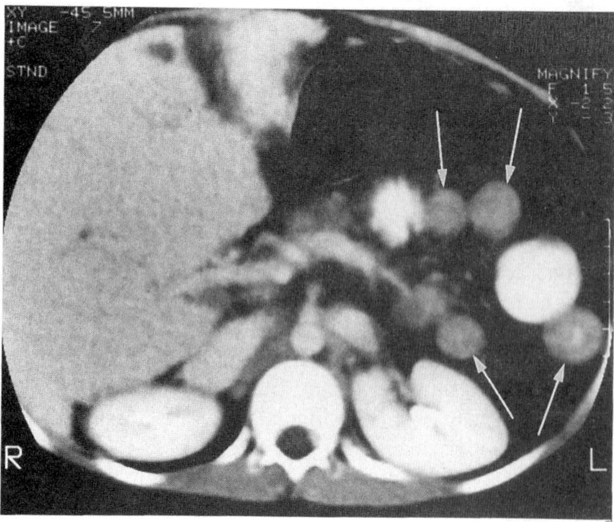

FIGURE 22 Accessory spleens after a splenectomy. Enhanced CT shows multiple small round opacities (*arrows*) lying anterior to the left kidney in a 13-year-old child after a splenectomy.

ALIMENTARY TRACT AND PERITONEAL CAVITY

Ascites

CT is not necessary for the initial investigation of suspected ascites. This is best left to sonography because small amounts of fluid can easily be outlined without radiation. CT, however, readily reveals ascites. Ascitic fluid is typically of low density (0 to 20 Hounsfield units). It tends to accumulate in the most dependent portions of the abdomen and pelvis. Initially, fluid is seen in the pelvis only. Increasing ac-

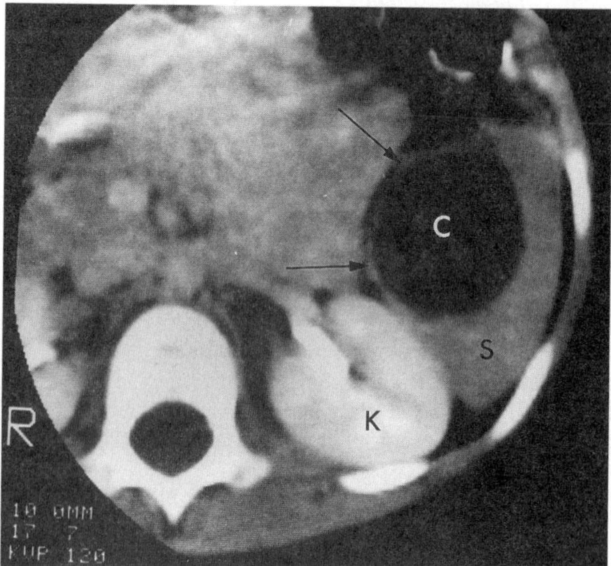

FIGURE 23 Splenic cyst. Contrast-enhanced CT shows a round mass of near-water-density material arising from the spleen (S) anterior to the kidney (K). There is a thin enhancing rim (*arrows*) around the medial aspect of the cyst (C).

cumulations of fluid anterior to the rectum are seen in the paracolic gutters, in the hepatorenal space, and in the area adjacent to the spleen. Massive fluid outlines the entire liver and spleen, as well as the falciform ligament (Fig. 24). CT cannot reliably differentiate among the various types of ascitic fluid, but may help to demonstrate the underlying etiology.

Mesentery

The CT appearance of the normal mesentery depends upon the amount of fat present to outline the mesenteric vessels. When visualized, the mesentery is usually sharply defined and homogeneous in attenuation. The mesentery can be involved in numerous pathologic conditions, including inflammatory bowel disease, neoplasms, trauma, and congenital cyst formation. Figure 25 demonstrates a mesenteric lymphangioma.

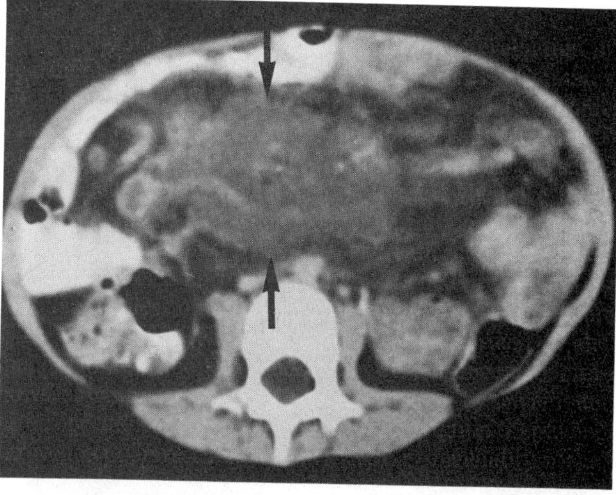

FIGURE 25 Mesenteric lymphangioma. There is a relatively low-attenuation mass (*between arrows*) arising in the mesentery and encasing an enhancing mesenteric vessel following intravenous contrast.

Adenopathy

Abdominal adenopathy may be seen in inflammatory or neoplastic conditions. Most commonly visualized in the periaortic region, it is homogeneous, like soft tissue in density, and often lobulated, or it appears as discrete nodules adjacent to the aorta and inferior vena cava (Figs. 26 and 27).

Alimentary Tract

CT is rarely necessary for imaging intraluminal abnormalities of the GI tract; these are best left to conventional contrast studies. The normal appearance of the alimentary tract often shows inhomogeneous, increased density within the stomach because of recent food ingestion.

CT can, however, be quite helpful in the assessment of abnormalities of the bowel wall, including extraintestinal spread. Fortunately, neoplasms of the alimentary tract are rare and include lymphoma, colonic polyps, and adenocarcinoma, as well as stomach adenocarcinoma (Fig. 27). CT plays a major role in the evaluation of the extraluminal spread of inflammatory bowel disease.

Although CT has been used for the evaluation of congenital anorectal malformations, MRI provides superior results.

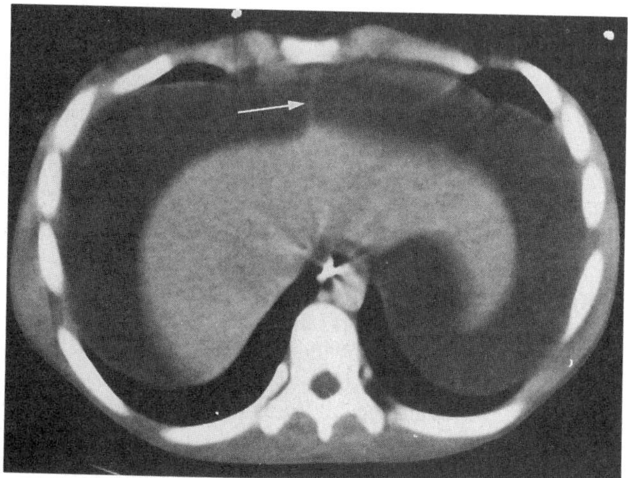

FIGURE 24 Ascites in a patient with disseminated malignant disease. There is a large amount of low-attenuation fluid lying around the liver and spleen, outlining the falciform ligament (*arrow*).

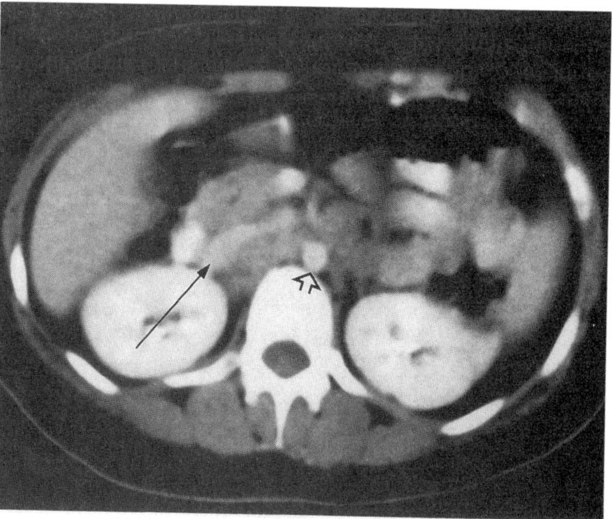

FIGURE 26 Hodgkin's disease. Multiple enlarged lymph nodes surround the aorta (*open arrow*) and inferior vena cava (*long arrow*) giving a lobulated appearance.

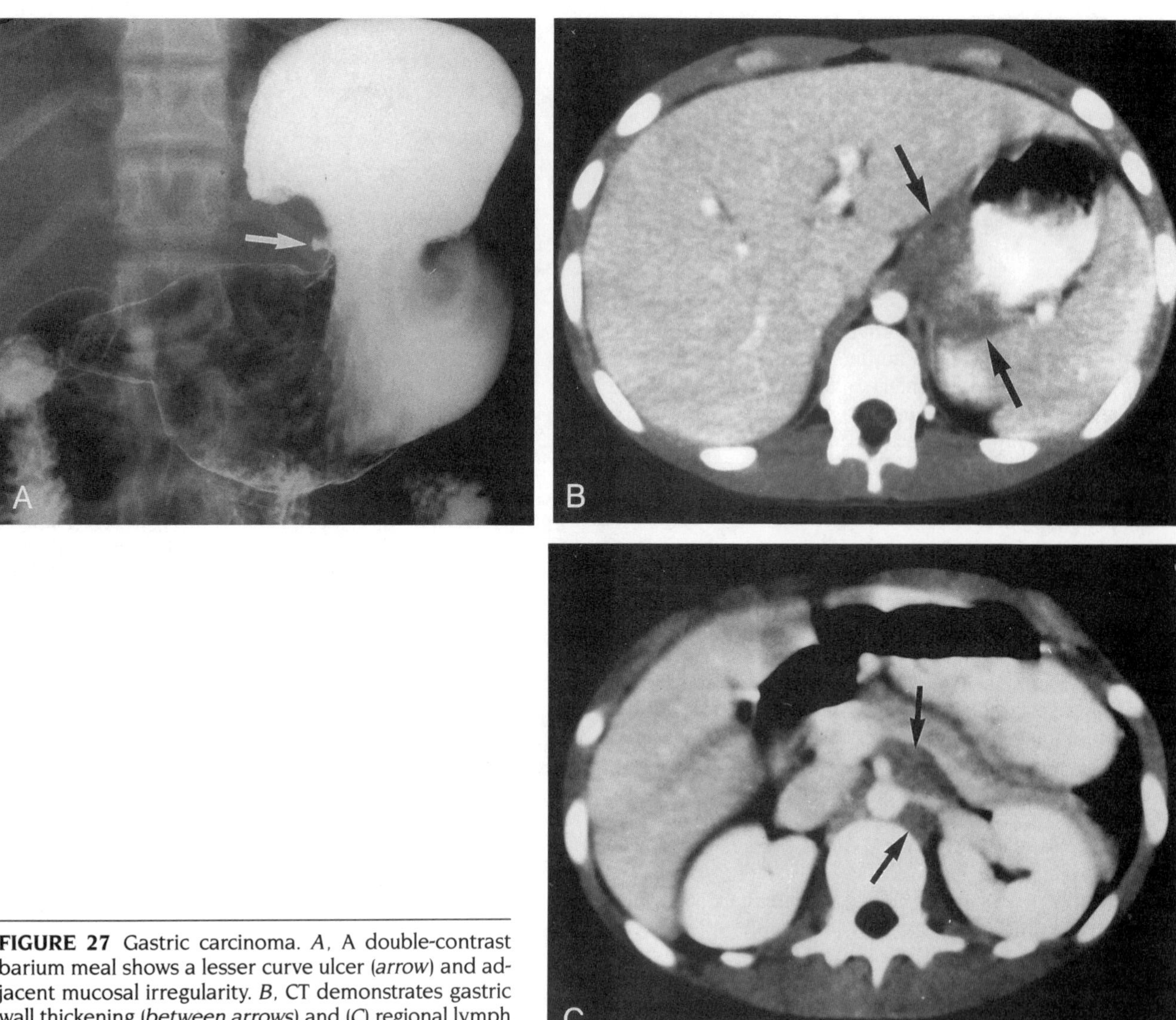

FIGURE 27 Gastric carcinoma. *A*, A double-contrast barium meal shows a lesser curve ulcer (*arrow*) and adjacent mucosal irregularity. *B*, CT demonstrates gastric wall thickening (*between arrows*) and (*C*) regional lymph node involvement (*arrows*).

Inflammation

The evaluation of children with suspected inflammatory disease of the abdomen is a daily occurrence. CT should not be used as the initial screening modality for suspected abdominal or pelvic inflammatory disease. Instead, CT is reserved for cases in which initial plain films, barium study, sonography, and/or nuclear medicine scanning are equivocal or inadequate or in which extraluminal pathology is suspected. CT, because of its greater anatomic definition, can localize inflammatory processes in areas in which sonography has limited application, such as in the retroperitoneum or in perirectal fat, and can better define widespread or multiple sites of involvement. CT is not limited by the presence of overlying extensive dressings used postoperatively. It may also be necessary for adequate aspiration of loculated collections.

As elsewhere in abdominal CT scanning, meticulous technique is necessary to achieve complete opacification of the bowel. Selectively rescanning a patient may be necessary if there is any concern about inadequate GI tract opacification after the administration of additional oral contrast material or after a delay to allow for better filling of the GI tract. This helps in the differentiation of fluid-filled bowel loops from abscesses. Abscesses may show a variable appearance on CT. Centrally, there is a typically low-attenuation area that fails to enhance with the administration of contrast material (Fig. 28). There may be air-fluid levels (Fig. 28), internal septations, or multiple cavities evident.[53-55] The abscess wall may not appear at all or may be well defined with marked enhancement, following the administration of contrast material. The appearance of the abscess wall seems to be characteristic of the response of the surrounding tissue rather than of the abscess itself. It is important to note that an air-fluid level may indicate the presence of a potential enteric fistula.

CT can be used to guide percutaneous drainage procedures, although we more commonly use sonography. CT is most use-

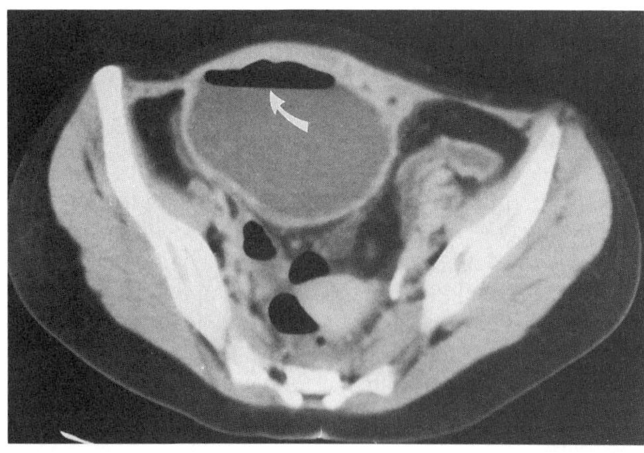

FIGURE 28 Crohn's disease with abscess formation. CT gives excellent delineation of an abscess resulting from a fistula from an involved bowel. The abscess contains an air-fluid level (*arrow*).

ful if bowel gas obscures the abscess from sonographic examination. Specific CT features, however, are not predictive of the eventual outcome of percutaneous drainage.

CT has recently been applied to the evaluation of periappendiceal abscesses and phlegmons.[56,57] Appendiceal abscesses are seen in 2 percent of patients with acute appendicitis. These patients may present with a palpable right lower quadrant mass, often referred to as an appendix mass. This may represent either a liquefied abscess or a phlegmon of inflamed omentum and adherent bowel loops. CT has proved valuable for the characterization of periappendiceal inflammatory masses and the determination of the relative size of their liquefied versus nonliquefied component, allowing accurate assessment of the size of the mass and aiding in the choice of therapy, regardless of whether it is antibiotic alone or in combination with percutaneous or surgical drainage.

Periappendiceal abscesses appear as low-density masses (less than 20 Hounsfield units) adjacent to the inferior aspect of the cecum. A CT scan can establish the specific diagnosis of periappendiceal abscess only if a calcified appendicolith is present. CT more adequately assesses the extent of the abscess, particularly the location of extraperitoneal spread or interloop abscesses. Also, CT is a more effective method of detecting an appendicolith than is a plain film examination. Postoperative abscesses can also be readily assessed with CT. They are generally found in the subphrenic or subhepatic region or along the flanks and in the pelvis.

Inflammatory bowel disease is another more recent indication for CT evaluation in adults and children.[58-60] CT is now considered the standard for the evaluation of the extraluminal components of the disease process. Abnormal wall thickness, greater than 3 mm, of either the small bowel or the colon can easily be assessed with adequate bowel opacification. The earliest radiographic changes of mucosal fold thickening may not, however, appear on a CT scan. With the development of more extensive changes, symmetric bowel wall thickening, usually between 5 and 15 mm, may be evident. Occasionally, a low-density zone or halo can be seen in the thickened bowel wall. It most likely represents submucosal edema or extensive submucosal fat accumulation. The normal sharp interface between the bowel wall and the fat density of the mesentery may become blurred as mesenteric density increases. This is secondary to fistulous tract formation and occurs with abscess or phlegmon formation as well. Mesenteric adenopathy may also be evident. In adults, the scan is most commonly obtained because of interloop separation, which is suggestive of a mesenteric mass. The most common CT finding is a fibrofatty proliferation in the mesentery. Complications of Crohn's disease, including abscess and fistula formation, can thus be evaluated. The fistulas can extend into the surrounding musculature, the bladder, or most commonly the small bowel. The radiologist looking for an enterovesical fistula must administer oral contrast material first and scan the patient without intravenous contrast. CT is helpful in the evaluation of the perirectal and perianal regions of chronic and acute abscesses. Extraintestinal disease, including fatty infiltration of the liver, evidence of pericholangitis, renal calculi, sacral osteomyelitis, or avascular necrosis of the femoral heads, may also be identified from the scan.

ABDOMINAL TRAUMA

The great preponderance of childhood abdominal trauma is blunt abdominal trauma, most often caused by motor vehicle and other accidents, falls, and child abuse. Dramatic advances in the management of blunt abdominal trauma have occurred over the last 15 years, facilitated in large part by the improved diagnosis afforded by CT. Many studies have now documented the superiority of CT over other imaging techniques in the evaluation of the severely injured child.[61-64] CT is well suited to the investigation of the child suspected of having multiple organ injuries because it provides an accurate overall assessment of the entire abdomen and pelvis. Unlike radionuclide studies, CT is not organ-specific, nor is it limited by overlying wounds or dressings as in sonography. The imaging sequence of patients with abdominal trauma is largely determined by the current clinical situation.

Following plain films (obtained primarily to exclude free intraperitoneal air), initial imaging with CT is recommended for children who are hemodynamically stable and suspected of having multiple intra-abdominal injuries or severe single-organ injury or who are undergoing CT scans of the head when concomitant abdominal injury is also likely. Clinically unrecognized hypovolemic shock may appear on CT with a flattened, empty inferior vena cava and dilated fluid-filled bowel.[61,63] Minimal or mild single-organ injury can be investigated with radionuclide scans or excretory urography, most often required for trace hematuria, as necessary. Urography also plays a role in the evaluation of severe trauma prior to operation to document the presence of two functioning kidneys. CT evaluation may also be needed if the findings of the initial study by another imaging modality are indeterminate.

Adequate CT examination for blunt abdominal trauma requires a commitment to detail. The study should be expedited as much as possible and preparations begun before the patient's arrival at the scanner. Careful patient monitoring is necessary throughout the study. We have found that an adequate examination requires the administration of both oral and intravenous contrast material. Oral contrast material allows a more accurate assessment of intramural bowel hematomas. Often a nasogastric tube is placed so that the instillation of the contrast material is straightforward. All tubes and overlying wires and electrocardiography pads should be withdrawn from the scan area to avoid streak artifacts through the images of the liver and spleen. Noncontrast scans are not needed. Scanning should be continued through the pelvis to evaluate the degree of hemoperitoneum present.

Visceral Injury

CT can depict the entire spectrum of abdominal injury from skeletal trauma to visceral disruption or bowel perforation. The liver is the most frequently injured organ in blunt abdominal trauma, followed closely by the spleen and then the kidney. Multiple organ trauma occurs in approximately 20 percent of cases and involves not only the intra-abdominal organs, but also the lower chest with lung contusions, lacerations, pleural effusions, and pneumothoraces.

Hepatic Injury

Hepatic parenchymal injury is variable in severity: it ranges from small hepatic lacerations to extensive fractures with life-threatening vascular injuries. During a CT scan, the injury appears as a predominantly hypodense, linear, round or stellate area and may occur in any portion of the liver (Fig. 29). A radiographic classification scheme has been proposed for children. It divides parenchymal injuries into superficial or deep, simple, and complex lesions.[65,66]

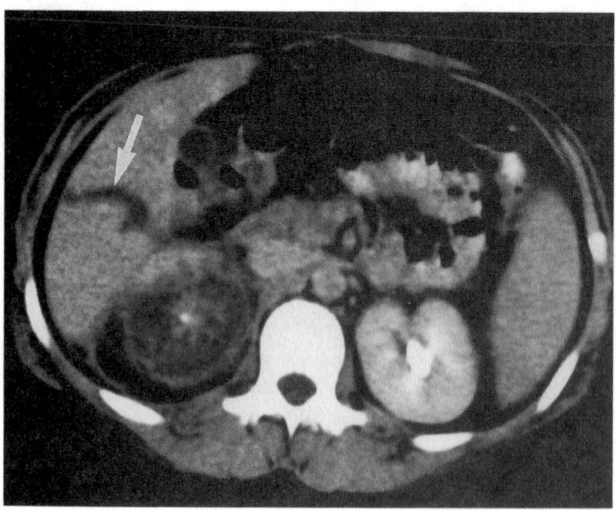

FIGURE 29 Hepatic and renal trauma. Enhanced CT shows an irregular linear area of decreased attenuation within the hepatic parenchyma (*arrow*) as well as marked decreased attenuation in the right kidney, which contains little contrast material because of vascular damage.

Simple lesions are usually well defined, focal, and superficial, involving the periphery of the liver. Complex lesions are more extensive and poorly defined, often stellate in outline, and deep or perihilar in location; they may be more frequently complicated in their course. Injury to the left lobe is more likely to be complex and associated with pancreatitis or duodenal injury. Fortunately, left lobe injury is significantly less common than right lobe trauma. Subcapsular hematomas often are associated with parenchymal injury and are hypodense or mixed-density peripheral lenticular collections that compress or flatten the underlying parenchyma. Tearing in the capsule leads to hemoperitoneum that can be quantitated by CT, depending upon the amount and distribution of fluid in the peritoneal spaces.

Associated injury to the biliary system can be seen with hematobilia, biloma formation, biliary duct laceration, or even free bile leakage. CT can show the increased density that represents hemorrhage in the gallbladder. Bile leakage can be confirmed with radionuclide studies.

The course of the complications of liver injury can be followed through to healing with either CT or preferably sonography. These studies monitor post-traumatic cyst formation, infection and, very occasionally, hepatic infarction. Calcification can also be seen occasionally.

Splenic Injury

The spleen is one of the most frequently injured organs in cases of abdominal trauma (Fig. 30). CT scanning may demonstrate a low-density intraparenchymal area representing a simple hematoma or splenic contusion.[67,68] Subcapsular hematomas can compress the underlying parenchyma, are lenticular in outline, and are similar to those previously described for the liver. Splenic lacerations may be linear or stellate and are frequently associated with intraperitoneal fluid. More severe injury to the spleen results in fragmentation and disruption of the spleen, often occurring with extensive hemoperitoneum. Associated injury to the left kidney and left lung base is commonly seen. Late complications of splenic injury include splenosis and pseudocyst formation.

Pancreatic Injury

Trauma is the most common cause of pancreatitis in childhood. CT can depict injuries ranging from focal or diffuse swelling to transection. Pancreatic lacerations or tears present with hypodense linear, often irregular areas within the gland. Peripancreatic fluid collections may be seen initially, as well a hemoperitoneum with later formation of pseudocysts, pancreatic abscesses, or pancreatic duct dilation.[63]

Gastrointestinal Injuries

The duodenum and proximal jejunum are the most commonly injured portions of the bowel with abdominal trauma. Bowel wall hematomas or even rupture can occur secondary

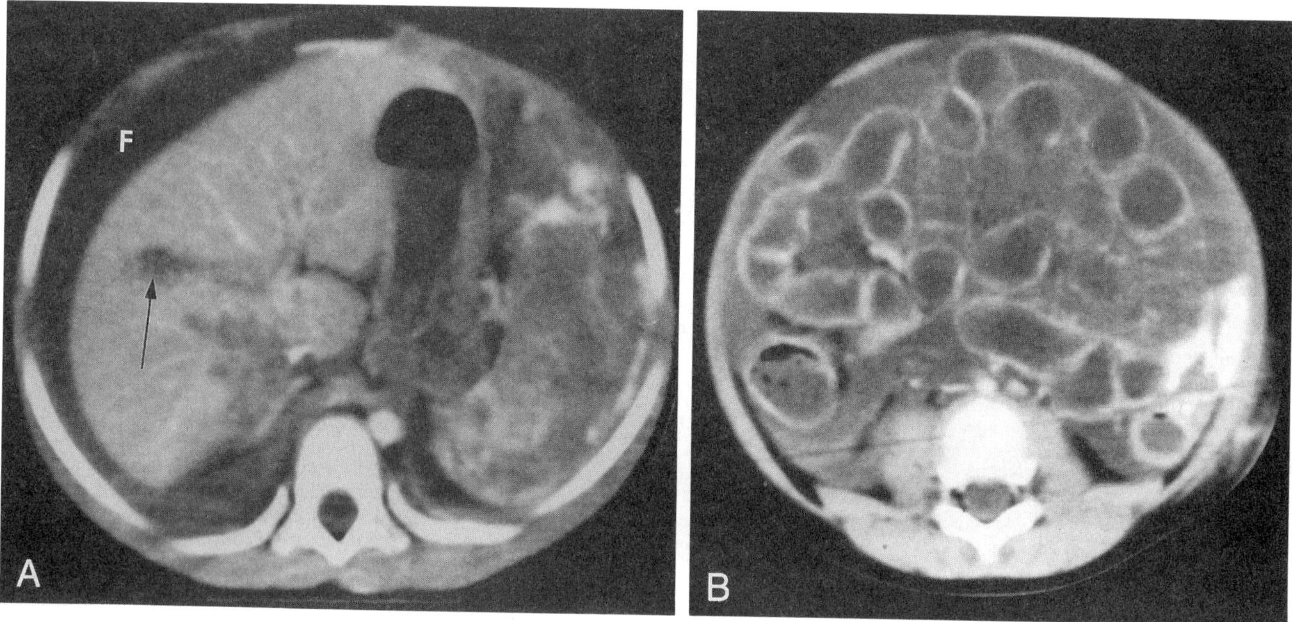

FIGURE 30 Hepatic and splenic trauma. *A*, CT shows an irregular area of decreased attenuation within the hepatic parenchyma (*arrow*) and fluid around the liver (F) as well as very disorganized attenuation in the ruptured spleen. *B*, A lower CT slice shows fluid around dilated fluid-filled loops of bowel and a narrow inferior vena cava compatible with hypovolemic shock.

to the compressive and shearing effect of the injury. Initially, the findings of the GI injury can be subtle. Wall hematomas may show eccentric luminal narrowing by a hypodense mass or fold thickening. Rupture of the bowel may show only minimal amounts of free intraperitoneal air or fluid (Fig. 31). Retroperitoneal air or contrast extravasation may be present. There may be associated mesenteric hemorrhage or pancreatic injury. Because CT scanning is unable to exclude bowel perforation, if clinically warranted, peritoneal lavage and/or upper GI contrast studies should be performed.

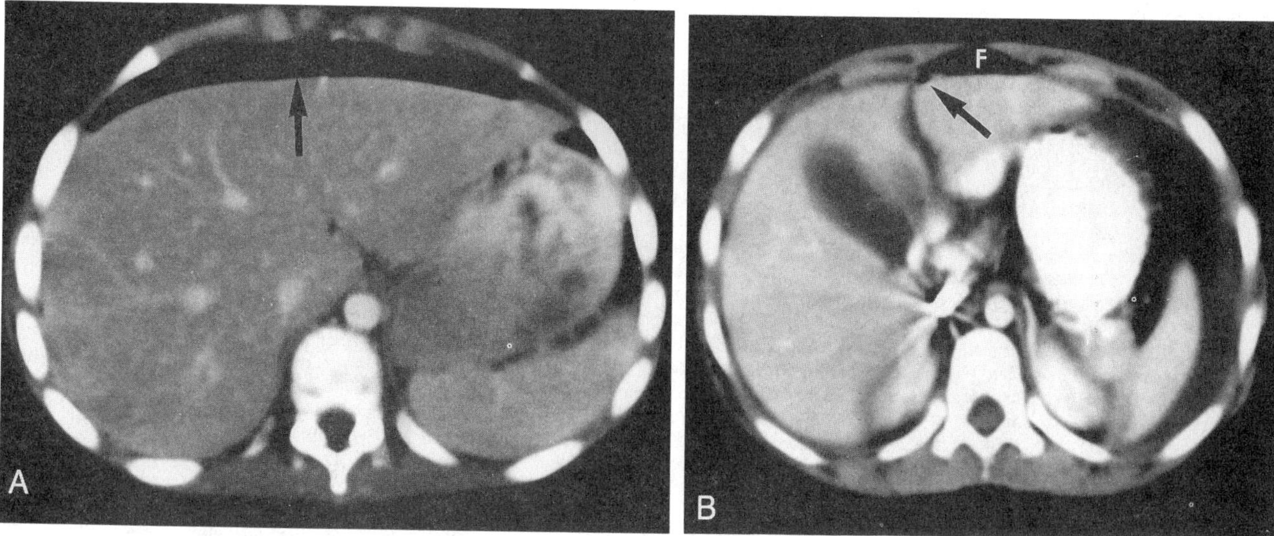

FIGURE 31 Bowel trauma with perforation. *A*, CT shows a large amount of free air anterior to the liver (*arrow*). *B*, In another patient, there is only a tiny amount of free air (*arrow*) adjacent to normal anterior abdominal wall fat (F). These findings are subtle; hence free air should be diligently sought because it heralds bowel perforation and requires urgent laparotomy.

REFERENCES

1. Daneman A. Paediatric body CT. New York: Springer-Verlag, 1987.
2. Friedman AC, ed. Radiology of the liver, biliary tract, pancreas and spleen. Baltimore: Williams & Wilkins, 1987.
3. Siegel MJ, ed. Paediatric body CT. New York: Churchill Livingstone, 1988.
4. Silverman FN, ed. Caffey's paediatric x-ray diagnosis: An integrated imaging approach, 8th ed. Chicago: Year Book Medical, 1985.
5. Riddlesberger MM. Evaluation of the gastrointestinal tract in the child. CT, MRI, and isotopic studies. Pediatr Clin North Am 1988; 35:281–310.
6. Pagani JJ. Intrahepatic vascular territories shown by computed tomography (CT). The value of CT in determining respectability of hepatic tumors. Radiology 1983; 147:173–178.
7. Weinreb JC, Cohen JM, Armstrong E, Smith T. Imaging the pediatric liver: MRI and CT. AJR 1986; 147:785–790.
8. Torres WE, Whitmire LF, Gedgaudas-McClees K, Bernardino ME. Computed tomography of hepatic morphologic changes in cirrhosis of the liver. J Comput Assist Tomogr 1986; 10:47–50.
9. Friedman AC, Johns T, Levy DW, Rindsberg S, Markle BM, Cirrhosis, other diffuse diseases, portal hypertension, and vascular diseases. In: Friedman AC, ed. Radiology of the liver, biliary tract, pancreas and spleen. Baltimore: Williams & Wilkins, 1987: 69.
10. Berger PE, Kuhn JP. Computed tomography of the hepatobiliary system in infancy and childhood. Radiol Clin North Am 1981; 19:431–434.
11. Unger EC, Lee, JK, Weyman PJ. CT and MR imaging of radiation hepatitis. J Comput Assist Tomogr 1987; 11:264–268.
12. Lev-Toaff AS, Friedman AC, Cohen LM, Radecki PD, Caroline DF, Hepatic infarcts: new observations by CT and sonography. AJR 1987; 149:87–90.
13. Aihara T, Fujioka M, Yamamoto K. Increased CT density of the liver due to the *cis* -diaminedichloro platinum (II). Pediatr Radiol 1987; 17:75
14. Long JA Jr, Doppman JL, Nienhus AW, Mills SR. Computed tomographic analysis of beta-thalassemic syndromes with hemochromatosis: pathologic findings with clinical and laboratory correlations. J Comput Assist Tomogr 1980; 4:159–165.
15. Leighton DM, de Campo JF, Matthews R. Sephton RG. Dual energy CT estimation of liver iron content in thalassemic children. Australas Radiol 1988; 32:214–219
16. Miller JH, Greenspoon BS. Integrated imaging of hepatic tumors in childhood. Part II. Benign lesions (congenital, reparative, and inflammatory). Radiology 1985; 154:91–100.
17. Brunelle F, Tamman S., Odievre M. Chaumont P. Liver adenomas in glycogen storage disease in children. Ultrasound and angiographic study. Pediatr Radiol 1984; 14:94–101.
18. Kirks DR, Merten DF, Grossman H, Bowie JD. Diagnostic imaging of pediatric abdominal masses: an overview. Radiol Clin North Am 1981; 19:527–534.
19. Boechat MI, Kangarloo H, Gilsanz V. Hepatic masses in children. Semin Roentgenol 1988; 23:185–193.
20. Smith WL, Franken EA, Mitros FA. Liver tumors in children. Semin Roentgenol 1983; 18:136–148.
21. Miller JH, Greenspan BS. Integrated imaging of hepatic tumors in childhood Part 1: Malignant lesions (primary and metastatic). Radiology 1985; 154:83–90.
22. Liu P, Daneman A. Stringer DA. Diagnostic imaging of liver masses in children. J Can Assoc Radiol 1985; 6:296–300.
23. Afshani E. Computed tomography of abdominal abscess in children. Radiol Clin North Am 1981; 19:515–526.
24. Francis IR, Glazer GM, Amendola MA, Trenkner SW. Hepatic abscesses in the immunocompromised patient: role of CT in detection, diagnosis, management, and follow-up. Gastrointest Radiol 1986; 11:257–262.
25. Merten DF, Kirks DR. Amebic liver abscess in children: the role of diagnostic imaging. AJR 1984; 143:1325–1329.
26. Lucaya J, Enriquez G, Amat L, Gonzalez-Rivero MA. Computed tomography of infantile hepatic hemangioendothelioma. AJR 1985; 144:821–826.
27. Dachman AH, Lichtenstein JE, Friedman AC, Hartman DS. Infantile hemangioendothelioma of the liver: a radiologic- pathologic-clinical correlation. AJR 1983; 140:1091–1096.
28. Ein SH, Stephens CA. Benign liver tumors and cysts in childhood. J Pediatr Surg 1974; 9:847–851.
29. Stanley P. Hall TR, Woolley MM, Diament MJ, Gilsanz V. Miller JH. Mesenchymal hamartomas of the liver in childhood; sonographic and CT findings. AJR 1986; 147:1035–1039.
30. Ros PR, Goodman ZD, Ishak KG, Dachman AH, Olmsted WW, Hartman DS, Lichtenstein JE. Mesenchymal hamartomas of the liver; radiologic-pathologic correlation. Radiology 1986; 158:619–624.
31. Weinberg AG, Finegold MJ. Primary hepatic tumors in childhood. Hum Pathol 1983; 14:512–537.
32. Dachman AH, Pakter RL, Ros PR, Fishman EK Goodman ZD, Lichtenstein JE. Hepatoblastoma: radiologic-pathologic correlation in 50 cases. Radiology 1987; 164:15–19.
33. Adam A. Gibson RN, Soreide O, et al. The radiology of fibrolamellar hepatoma. Clin Radiol 1986; 37:355–358.
34. Francis IR, Agha FP, Thompson NW, Deren DR. Fibrolamellar hepatocarcinoma: clinical radiologic, and pathologic features. Gastrointest Radiol 1986; 11:67–72.
35. Ros PR, Olmsted WW. Dachman AH, Goodman ZD, Ishak KG, Hartman DS. Undifferentiated (embryonal) sarcoma of the liver: radiologic-pathologic correlation. Radiology 1986; 160:141–145.
36. Geoffray A. Couanet D. Montagne JP, Leclere J, Flamant F. Ultrasonography and computed tomography for diagnosis and follow- up of biliary duct rhabdomyosarcomas in children, Pediatr Radiol 1987; 17:127–131.
37. Franken EA, Smith WL, Cohen MD, Kisker CT, Platz CE. Hepatic imaging in stage IV-S neuroblastoma. Pediatr Radiol 1986; 16:107–109.
38. Ledesma-Medina J, Dominguez R, Bowen A, Young LW, Bron KM. Pediatric liver transplantation. Part I: standardization of pre- operative diagnostic imaging. Radiology 1985; 157:335–339.
39. Dominguez R. Young LW, Ledesma-Medina J, et al. Pediatric liver transplantation. Part II: diagnostic imaging in post- operative management. Radiology 1985; 157:339–344.
40. Letourneau JG, Day DL, Frick MP, et al. Ultrasound and computed tomographic evaluation in hepatic transplantation. Radiol Clin North Am 1987; 25:323.
41. Letourneau JG, Day DL, Maile CW, Crass JR, Ascher NL, Frick MP. Liver allograft transplantation; post-operative CT findings. AJR 1987; 148:1099–1103.
42. Marincek B, Barbier PA, Becker CD, Mettler D, Ruchti C. CT appearance of impaired lymphatic drainage in liver transplants. AJR 1986; 147:519–523.
43. Wechsler RJ, Munoz SJ, Needleman L, et al. Periportal collar: a CT sign of liver transplant rejection. Radiology 1987; 165:57–60.
44. Solomon N, Sumkin J. Right adrenal gland haemorrhage as a complication of liver transplantation: CT appearance. J Comput Assist Tomogr 1988; 12:95–97.
45. Bret PM, de Stempel JV, Atri M, Lough JO, Illescas FF. Intrahepatic bile duct and portal vein anatomy revisited. Radiology 1988; 169:405–407.
46. Daneman A. Pediatric body CT. New York: Springer-Verlag, 1987: 107.
47. Boechat MI. Adrenal glands, pancreas, and retroperitoneal structures. In: Seigel MJ, ed. Pediatric body CT. New York: Churchill Livingstone, 1988: 177.
48. Daneman A, Gaskin K, Martin DJ, Cutz E. Pancreatic changes in cystic fibrosis: CT and sonographic appearances. AJR 1983; 141:653–655.
49. Kissane JM. Tumors of the exocrine pancreas in childhood. In: Humphrey GB, et al, eds. Pancreatic tumors in children. The Hague: Martinus Nijhoff, 1982: 99.
50. Oertel JE, Mendelsohn G, Compagno J. Solid and papillary epithelial neoplasms of the pancreas. In: Humphrey GB, et al, eds. Pancreatic tumors in children. The Hague: Martinus Nijhoff, 1982: 167.
51. Balcar I, Seltzer SE, Davis S, Geller S. CT patterns of splenic infarction: a clinical and experimental study. Radiology 1984; 151:723–729.
52. Dachman AH, Magiel D. Focal diseases. In: Friedman AC, ed. Radiology of the liver, biliary tract, pancreas and spleen. Baltimore: Williams & Wilkins, 1987: 947.
53. Afshani E. Computed tomography of abdominal abscesses in children. Radiol Clin North Am 1981; 19:515–526.
54. Jaques P, Mauro M, Safrit H, Yankaskas B, Piggott B. CT features of intraabdominal abscesses; prediction of successful percutaneous drainage. AJR 1986; 146:1041–1045.
55. Lundstedt C. Hederström E, Brisman J, Holmin T, Strand SE. Prospective investigation of radiologic methods in the diagnosis of intra-abdominal abscesses. Acta Radiol 1986; 27:49–54.
56. Jeffrey RB Jr, Tolentino CS, Federle MP, Laing FC. Percutaneous drainage of periappendiceal abscesses; review of 20 cases. AJR 1987; 149:59–62.

57. Jeffrey RB Jr, Federle MP, Tolentino CS. Periappendiceal inflammatory masses: CT-directed management and clinical outcome in 70 patients. Radiology 1988; 167:13–16.
58. Fishman EK, Jones B. Evaluation of Crohn's disease. In: Fishman EK, Jones B, eds. Computed tomography of the gastrointestinal tract. Baltimore: Churchill Livingstone, 1988: 147.
59. Jones B, Fishman EK. CT and other inflammatory bowel diseases. In: Fisherman EK, Jones B, eds. Computed tomography of the gastrointestinal tract. Baltimore: Churchill Livingstone, 1988: 109.
60. Riddlesberger MM. CT of inflammatory bowel disease in children. Pediatr Radiol 1985; 15:384.
61. Taylor GA, Fallat ME, Eichelberger MR. Hypovolemic shock in children: abdominal CT manifestations. Radiology 1987; 164:479–481.
62. Kuhn JP, Berger PE. Computed tomography in the evaluation of blunt abdominal trauma in children. Radiol Clin North Am 1981; 19:503–513.
63. Kaufman RA. CT of blunt abdominal trauma in children; a five-year experience. In: Siegel MJ, ed. Pediatric body CT. Baltimore: Churchill Livingstone 1988: 313.
64. Young JWR, Burgess AR. Use of CT in acute trauma victims. Radiology 1988; 166;903.
65. Stalker HP, Kaufman RA, Towbin R. Patterns of liver injury in childhood: CT analysis. AJR 1986; 147:1199–205.
66. Vock P, Kehrer B, Tschaeppeler H. Blunt liver trauma in children: the role of computed tomography in diagnosis and treatment. J Pediatr Surg 1986; 21:413–418.
67. Kaufman RA, Towbin R, Babcock DS, et al. Upper abdominal trauma in children: imaging evaluation. AJR 1984; 142:449–460.
68. Brick SH, Taylor GA, Potter BM, Eichelberger MR. Hepatic and splenic injury in children: role of CT in the decision for laparotomy. Radiology 1987; 165:643–646.
69. Stringer DA. Pediatric gastrointestinal radiology. Philadelphia: BC Decker, 1989.

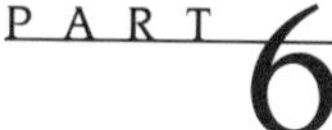

PART 6

Magnetic Resonance Imaging of the Gastrointestinal Tract

Mervyn D. Cohen, M.B., Ch.B., M.D., F.R.C.R., M.R.C.P.

With all its many organs and structures, the abdomen presents a fertile field to challenge and delight the magnetic resonance (MR) radiologist. The challenge presented by the abdomen has not yet been fully met. Recent advances in MR technology provide the tools for overcoming the problems of abdominal MR imaging (MRI) and provide us with the mechanism of obtaining good images of the abdominal structures. It is therefore most appropriate to review at this time the current status of MR abdominal imaging.

ADVANTAGES OF MAGNETIC RESONANCE AS AN IMAGING MODALITY

The advantages of MRI are as follows:

1. MRI uses no ionizing radiation. It is believed to be extremely safe, and no significant complications have yet been reported.
2. The patient is extremely comfortable, lying in a supine position on a padded table. It is not necessary to reposition the patient during the procedure.
3. MR machines have no moving parts. This removes a potential source of machine breakdown and down time.
4. MRI makes it possible to scan in any plane and produce true, not reconstructed, images. Being able to image in multiple planes is often extremely helpful. It permits better demonstration of the total extent of an abnormality. In addition, it often permits complete structures to be visualized on a single image. This is often not possible with other modalities.
5. Unlike CT, MRI does not produce streak artifacts from either bone or implanted metallic objects.
6. Like many other imaging modalities, MRI provides an anatomic map or photograph of internal body structures. Because of extremely high contrast resolution, adjacent soft tissue structures can be better identified with MRI than with any other imaging modality.
7. MRI imaging is good at visualizing the abdominal vessels. With CT or plain film radiographs, blood in the lumen of a vessel cannot be distinguished from the wall of the vessel. This can be achieved only by the injection of intravascular contrast agents. Because flowing blood produces little or no signal on the MR image, the lumina of blood vessels can clearly be identified, separate from their walls.
8. MRI has a potential for characterizing tissue, either by spectroscopic analysis or by evaluation of T1 and T2 relaxation times. The clinical usefulness of this new tissue information has not yet been fully evaluated.

DISADVANTAGES OF MAGNETIC RESONANCE IMAGING

A number of potential and real disadvantages are associated with MRI. As improvements in equipment design and manufacturing are made, many of the initial disadvantages are being overcome. The disadvantages are as follows:

1. MRI is expensive, and a fully installed unit costs between 1.5 and 3.5 million dollars.

2. It was originally thought that patients might find the confines of the machine to be claustrophobic and that they might refuse to be scanned. However, most patients, including children, tolerate the scanning procedure extremely well.
3. The signal that is detected from the body in MRI is weak, and scan time is long. Therefore, respiratory, cardiac, and peristaltic motion causes artifacts and is difficult to overcome.
4. Calcium cannot be directly visualized by MRI. Large areas of calcification in masses can be seen as a negative black area. MRI cannot detect small areas of calcium in body tissue.
5. It was initially thought that the presence of any metallic substance within the patient's body would be an absolute contraindication to MRI. This fortunately is now known to be untrue. Many metallic substances are not magnetic and therefore cause no problems. MRI can be successfully employed in patients with magnetic surgical clips, provided that they are in "safe" areas such as surgical scars.
6. Gradient coil switching is noisy. During scanning there is a loud and repetitious tapping noise, which some patients find uncomfortable.

TECHNIQUE

There are two fundamental reasons why MRI of the abdomen may be relatively poor. The first is the difficulty in distinguishing loops of bowel from adjacent tissues and from each other. Although some efforts have been made to develop contrast agents that can be utilized to opacify the bowel, this problem remains largely unresolved. The second problem in abdominal imaging is that of motion. Motion causes blurring and the development of artifacts that are superimposed on the image. The motion arises from respiration, cardiac pulsation transmitted through the diaphragm, aortic pulsation, and bowel peristalsis. Of these causes of motion, the most important by far is respiration. Because of their importance, it is appropriate to review, at this stage, some of the methods of reducing the effects of motion.[17]

Respiratory Gating. This is seldom used now, primarily because it is not completely effective in eliminating the effects of motion and also because it increases significantly the amount of time needed to image a patient.

Breath Holding.[16] It is now possible to utilize certain pulse sequences and obtain an image in 20 seconds or less. In co-operative patients, the utilization of these fast pulse sequences together with breath holding eliminates the effects of respiratory motion.

Signal Averaging. Instead of collecting a single set of data, two, four, or more sets of data can be collected from a single region of interest of the body. These signals can then be averaged, and this results in some improvement of the blurring artifacts caused by motion. This is a simple technique but results in a proportional increase in imaging time. Doubling the number of acquisitions doubles the imaging time. In general terms, the averaging of two or even four sets of data results in significant improvement in image quality. Collection of more data sets than this results in little further elimination of motion artifacts.

Specialized Inversion Recovery Pulse Sequences. If an inversion recovery sequence is chosen with a very short time to inversion, then tissues such as fat that have a relatively short T1 relaxation time and usually produce a strong signal on T1-weighted images can be made to produce a very low signal. The strong signal from moving fat in the abdominal wall is a major contributor to ghosting artifacts seen on abdominal images. By eliminating the signal from fat, the ghosting artifacts are significantly improved. The penalty that is paid for using this pulse sequence is that the images are somewhat noisier than with other pulse sequences.

Alteration of the Phasing Coding Axis in Abdominal Imaging. In MRI, structures are spatially located in the abdomen by coding along the x and y axes. Gradient fields are used to code along one axis and signal phase along the other. Most motion ghosting occurs in the plane of phase encoding. Therefore by phase encoding along the x axis (from side to side), one can reduce the artifact from the front to back movement of the abdominal wall, which is the major direction of excursion during breathing.

Short TE (Time to Echo), TR (Repetition Time) Pulse Sequences. The effect of motion is proportional to the time taken to acquire the image. By using spin-echo pulse sequences with short TE and short TR relaxation times, one can improve image quality. The TE should ideally be less than 20 msec and the TR less than 400 msec. The advantage of this pulse sequence is that it takes a short period of time. One therefore has the luxury of also doing multiple data acquisitions and averaging the results. The disadvantage of these pulse sequences is that if the TR is too short, then the overall signal strength falls, resulting in noisier images. In addition, these short TE/TR images are T1-weighted, whereas much pathology is best shown on T2-weighted images.

Phase Reordering. This method of motion suppression monitors respiration and instead of sequentially recording data, collects the data depending on the phase of the respiratory cycle. In simple terms, the computer, by knowing at what stage during the respiratory cycle data was collected, can locate its position and compensate for the motion. This technique does improve image quality, but it requires very complex computer manipulations and at the present time can be utilized effectively only for single slice imaging. It therefore may not be practical for routine use.

Nonlinear Magnetic Field Gradients. As mentioned before, gradient magnetic fields are utilized to locate the position of a structure in an image slice. When a structure moves, the computer loses track of its precise location. This technique, instead of using linear gradients, continually changes the gradient wave forms to compensate for movement. Advantages are that good images can be obtained with only a single signal average per view. Disadvantages are that the technique requires long TE and TR relaxation times and therefore is best used for T2 imaging. This is a highly promising technique that may become widely used.

Field-Echo Imaging. The major difference between this and conventional spin-echo imaging is that no 180-degree refocusing radiowave pulse is used to generate a signal. Instead the gradient fields are rapidly reversed to alter the rotation direction of the hydrogen atoms and produce a signal. With short tip angles and very short TE and TR relaxation times, images can be acquired very rapidly, in as little as 20 seconds. These field-echo images have slightly more noise than spin-echo images, but because of their very rapid acquisition and the significant improvement in motion artifact, the images are often extremely good.

INTERPRETING THE IMAGE

Image Slices. Like computed tomography (CT) scans, MR images are presented as a series of slices through a plane of the body. The slices can be varied in thickness, usually between 5 and 20 mm. They may be obtained in any plane.

Orientation of Images. The American College of Radiology asserts that MR images should all be viewed in a standard position. Transverse images should be positioned so that one is viewing the anatomic area from the patient's feet, coronal images should be positioned so that one is viewing them from the patient's front, and sagittal images should be viewed from the patient's left side.

Whiteness. The whiteness on the image is proportional to the strength of the signal received back from the body. The stronger the signal, the whiter the image. Strong-intensity signals (and therefore areas of high whiteness on the image) are received from regions with short T1 relaxation time, long T2 relaxation time, and high hydrogen ion concentration. Low-intensity signals are received from tissues with long T1 relaxation time, short T2 relaxation time, low hydrogen concentration, and fast-flowing blood.

The final intensity (whiteness) of an area of the body is the net result of all the previously mentioned factors in that region. Images can be created to emphasize either the T1 or the T2 characteristics of a tissue. This is done by altering the pulse sequence.

As examples of how these factors operate, air appears almost black on all images because it contains a very low concentration of hydrogen atoms. For a different reason, bone cortex appears almost completely black on all images. The highly dense nature of the bone inhibits the T1 recovery, so that the T1 relaxation times in bone are exceedingly long and energized hydrogen atoms cannot recover to be energized again. Fat has a high hydrogen concentration, a short T1 relaxation time, and a long T2 relaxation time. It therefore yields a strong signal and appears white on all images. Other tissues have intermediate T1 and T2 relxation times, and their intensity varies depending on whether the pulse sequence is chosen to emphasize the T1 or T2 characteristics of the tissue.

Grey Scales and Contrast. Grey scale ordering in CT and conventional radiography never changes. Bone always appears as the whitest tissue on images, followed by muscle, then fat, and then air, which always appears black. Unlike CT and conventional radiography, the grey scale ordering in MRI is highly variable and potentially confusing. Contrast and grey scales can be altered by changing the pulse sequences. The degree of whiteness or blackness of a tissue or organ depends on its T1 and T2 relaxation times and hydrogen concentration and also on whether the pulse sequence is chosen to emphasize T1 (T1-weighted) or T2 (T2-weighted) characteristics of the tissue. In conventional radiology, image contrast depends on only one factor, the differential absorption of x-rays by different tissues.

The choice of pulse sequences and imaging planes is wide. In general at least two different pulse sequences should be utilized, one with T1 weighting and the other with T2 weighting. In addition, it is probably advantageous to obtain images in at least two of the body planes in each patient.

CONTRAST AGENTS

Some oral contrast agents such as iron-containing or manganese-containing compounds have been utilized to opacify the bowel. A problem with these agents is that to obtain a desired effect, the local concentration of the agent is critical. However, following oral administration, the degree of dilution by bowel contents is unpredictable, so that clinical studies with these agents have been somewhat disappointing, and, as far as I am aware, they are not in routine clinical use. A recent report suggests that gadolinium in a 1-mmol of concentration is effective as an oral contrast agent.[31]

Intravenous contrast agents are being utilized in an experimental mode. The advantages of these agents are that they may potentially reduce scan time and, by altering contrast, they may enhance the visibility of a lesion. They have been utilized mainly to study liver lesions. The effect of gadolinium diethylenetriaminepenta-acetic acid (DTPA) on liver lesions has been somewhat unpredictable owing to varied diffusion of this agent through the liver. Recent work using a bolus injection of gadolinium followed fairly quickly by imaging suggests that this technique may result in improved contrast between pathology and normal liver. In a study of serial MR images after a bolus injection of gadolinium in patients with hepatocellular carcinoma, the degree of contrast enhancement following injection of gadolinium corresponded to the tumor vascularity.[22]

Another agent that has been experimentally used is ferrite iron oxide particles. These are selectively taken up by the reticuloendothelial system, causing a marked reduction in T2 relaxation time. This results in a very weak signal from normal liver. Diseased tissue, which lacks phagocytes, remains of high intensity with strong contrast between it and the normal tissue.

THE NORMAL ABDOMEN

All of the major abdominal structures, with the exception of bowel loops, can be well identified by MR. The size, location, and contours of the various organs are usually easily seen. Of the abdominal organs the liver normally has the shortest T1 and T2 relaxation times. The pancreas, spleen, renal cortex, and renal medulla, in this order, have increasing T1 and T2 relaxation times.

The aorta, inferior vena cava, and major branches of these vessels are readily seen on MR images. In the liver, the hepatic and portal veins are almost always seen. The signal intensity from bile varies depending on whether it is fresh bile or bile that has been stored in the gallbladder and concentrated. Fresh bile has high water content, whereas the signal from concentrated bile is dominated by its fat content. Normal bile ducts are usually not identified. Isolated bowel loops can sometimes be clearly identified, but mostly intestine is seen as a homogeneous nonspecific area. Fat in milk may produce a strong signal from the stomach on both T1 and T2 weighted images in babies.

PATHOLOGY

Liver and Gallbladder

The normal anatomy of the liver in children under 5 years of age has been found to be better depicted with MRI than with CT.[4] In this study the origin of the common hepatic artery from the celiac axis was identified in 74 percent of cases with MRI and 15 percent of cases with CT. MRI was better able to demonstrate the intrahepatic venous structures than CT. The segment of the inferior vena cava passing through the liver was identified in 100 percent of cases with MRI and 60 percent of cases with CT.

The liver is the most studied of all the abdominal tissues (Figs. 1 to 5). MRI has proved sensitive for the detection of a wide range of tumors, infections, obstructive lesions, and metabolic disorders, but the appearance has not been particularly specific. Most liver lesions are identified as focal or diffuse masses with prolonged T1 and T2 relaxation times causing them to be of lower intensity than normal liver on strongly T1-weighted images and higher intensity than liver on T2-weighted images. Liver tumors can be accurately visualized with MR, and there is promise that staging may be accurate as well. Stark found MRI to be more sensitive than CT for detection of liver metastases.[19] Itoh found MRI

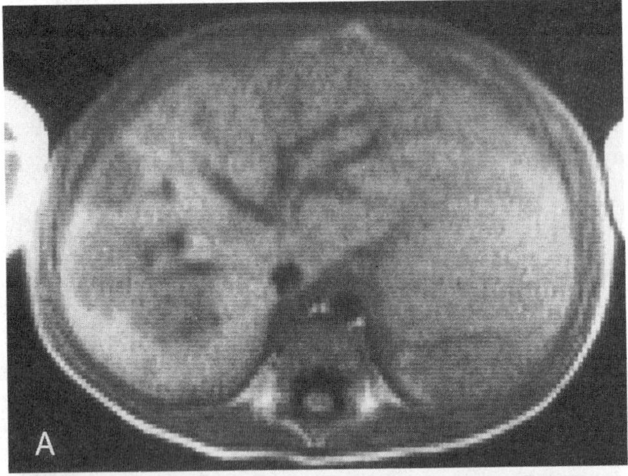

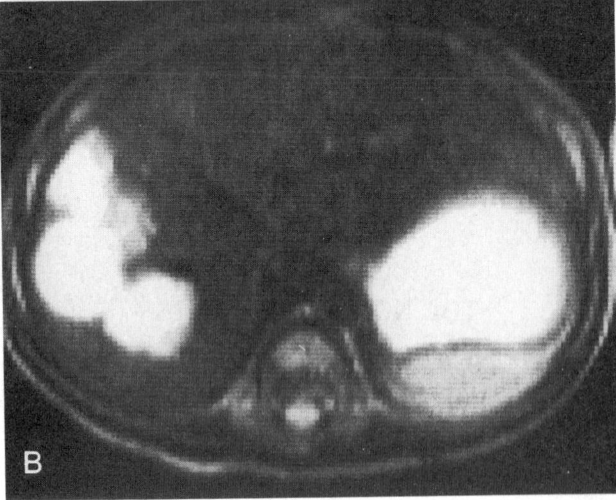

FIGURE 1 Cavernous hemangioma of the liver. *A*, T1-weighted image demonstrates well-marginated round homogeneous areas of low signal intensity in the right lobe of the liver. *B*, T2-weighted image shows characteristic appearance of cavernous hemangioma with well-defined margins and marked homogeneous increased signal intensity from the multiloculated lesions.

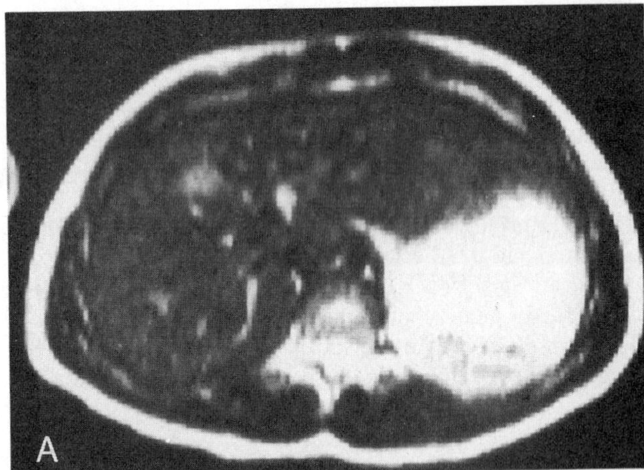

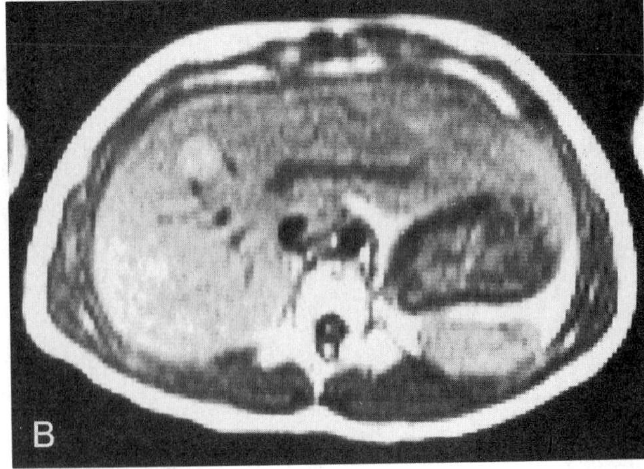

FIGURE 2 Hemochromatosis. *A*, The liver appears of normal intensity on this T1-weighted image. *B*, T2-weighted image shows marked reduction in the intensity of signal from the entire liver. In a normal individual, signal intensity should be stronger on the T2-weighted image than on the T1-weighted image. The reduction in signal intensity is due to the effect of the iron in the liver.

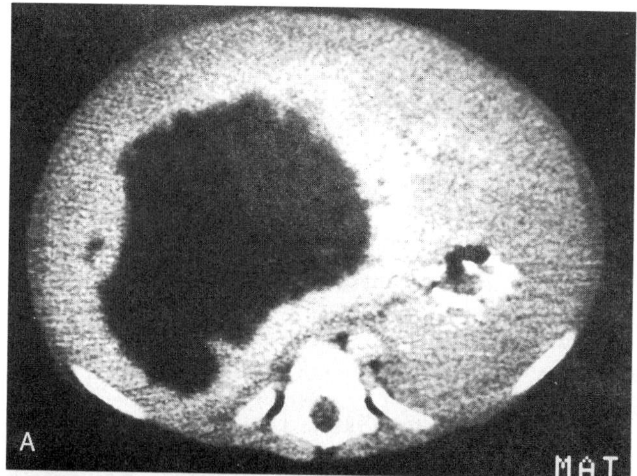

FIGURE 3 Hemangioendothelioma. *A*, CT scan following bolus injection of intravenous contrast demonstrates a large low-intensity liver lesion with a strongly enhancing periphery characteristic of this tumor. *B*, T1-weighted MR image shows a similar abnormality to the CT scan. The displaced portal vein is better demonstrated on the MR scan. *C*, A strongly weighted T2 image shows the central area of the lesion, which is necrotic fluid, to be of very strong intensity. The wall of the lesion is now of intermediate signal intensity.

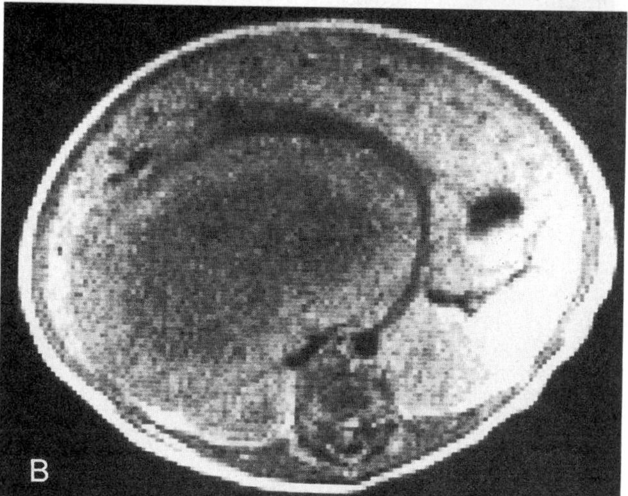

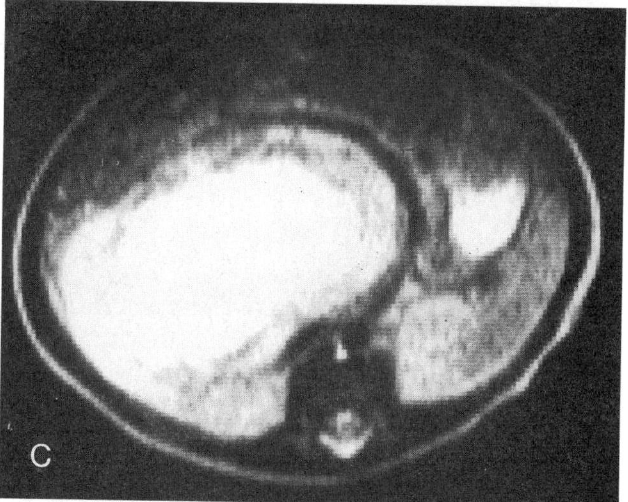

to be equivalent to CT in the detection of hepatocellular carcinoma; however, MRI was superior to CT in demonstrating the presence of a pseudocapsule and also tumor thrombi.[20] MRI can identify extension of tumor into the major hepatic vessels. Also, because of good visualization of portal and hepatic veins, segmental localization of the lesions should prove possible with MRI. In a study of 35 patients with pathologically proven liver tumors, MRI was found to be better than CT or sonography in the overall detection of tumors and evaluation of size, anatomic location, portal vein involvement, and secondary bile duct location.[21] While the appearance of many lesions in the liver is relatively nonspecific in MR images, cavernous hemangiomas can usually be definitively diagnosed (see Fig. 1). These lesions are seen as well-defined areas of low intensity on T1-weighted images, moderate intensity on intermediate images, and extremely strong signal—greater than that of fat and other tumors—on strongly T2-weighted images.[13] MRI is also highly sensitive for the detection of cavernous hemangiomas. In a study of 33 small lesions less than 3 cm in size, MRI was able to identify abnormality in 31 cases. Ultrasound was positive in 23 of the 33 cases, whereas CT was positive in 15 of 26 cases.[13]

Cavernous transformation of the portal vein can be identified with MRI. The MRI findings in this condition are multiple vascular structures seen in the region of the porta hepatis without identification of a normal portal vein.[9] The vascular structures are of low signal intensity on T1- and T2-weighted images because of flowing blood through the vessels. In addition, MRI is capable of demonstrating patency of collateral veins and the presence of associated varices and splenomegaly.[9]

MRI has been utilized experimentally to study metabolic disorders. Diffuse fatty infiltration of the liver may be extremely difficult to detect on conventional spin-echo images. Phase-contrast images, in which the signals from fat and water can be separately displayed, can readily detect fatty infiltration of the liver. In iron deposition diseases, changes in signal intensity in the liver are identified (see Fig. 2). The effects vary depending on the concentration of iron present. In a study of 15 children who required chronic blood transfusions for the management of sickle cell disease, MRI was able to identify iron overload in the liver. By evaluation of signal intensity on T1-weighted images, it was possible to separate out those patients with liver iron levels below or above 100 μg per milligram of liver tissue. In patients with liver iron greater than 100 μg per milligram, MRI was not able to quantitate the actual amount of iron present in the liver. All patients in this study had liver biopsies and direct measurement of the liver iron.[23]

Radiation produces changes in the liver that are detectable

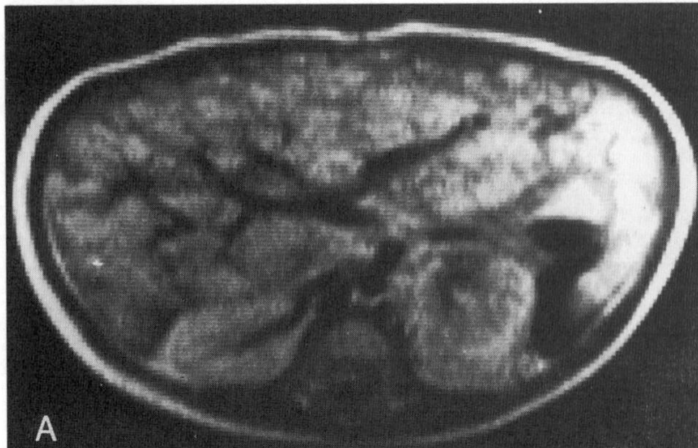

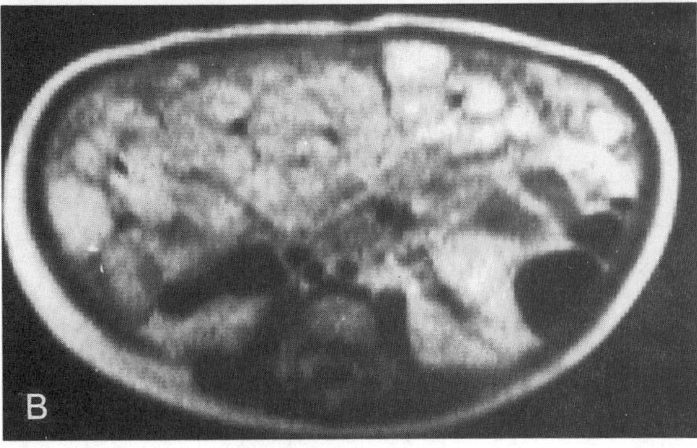

FIGURE 4 Diffuse neuroblastoma metastasis to the liver: 4S neuroblastoma. T1-weighted image (*A*) and T2-weighted image (*B*) show diffuse nodular abnormality distributed throughout both lobes of the liver.

by MRI. These are seen as areas of increased intensity in the liver on T2-weighted images. This increased intensity is due to increased water.[24]

In a recent report of MRI of the liver in 27 children, Weinreb[4] reported increased sensitivity for MRI compared with CT. Three lesions, missed by CT, were identified on MRI. MRI missed one case of fatty infiltration (but the authors did not utilize phase-contrast imaging). They also found that internal hepatic anatomy was better defined with MRI than with CT. This was particularly true in young children, those under the age of 5 years. Focal disease identified in the liver in this study[4] included hepatoblastoma, hemangioendothelioma, metastatic tumor, lymphoma, granulomas, and hamartoma. The findings in all the lesions were relatively nonspecific, with signal intensity compatible with increased T1 and increased T2 relaxations times in the area of pathology. Three liver lesions that were more clearly seen on MRI were small nodular metastasis from neuroblastoma, caseating granulomas, and nodular lymphomatous deposits.

Other recent reports in the literature also attest to the potential of MRI. Richards, in 27 patients with lymphoma, had seven patients with biopsy-proven diffuse hepatic involvement.[2] By actual measurement of T1 relaxation times of the liver, in comparison with normal individuals, MRI was able to detect abnormality in all seven cases. In this study there were a number of false-positive results.[2] Weinreb, however, found the opposite result. In a study of 13 patients with histologically proven lymphoma, MRI and CT identified focal abnormality in only one case. In the other 12 cases the MR image appeared normal. Calculated T1 and T2 relaxation times from areas of interest within the liver were also within normal limits.[18]

MRI has also been recently utilized by Day in the evaluation of vascular anatomy prior to liver transplantation.[5] She studied nine patients. Sonographic correlation was available in all nine patients, angiographic correlation in five, and pathologic correlation in seven. MRI was superior to sonography in two patients. In these patients, vessels were misidentified on the basis of sonography. These patients had azygous continuation of the inferior vena cava and a large collateral vein in the portal region. MRI was able to identify the portal vein in three patients in whom it was not clearly visualized with angiography. MRI missed one very small portal vein and another occluded by tumor.

Ferrucci in 142 patients found that MRI could identify 14 percent more liver metastases than CT.[6] He believes that the conventional T1-weighted image with TE = 30/TR = 500 does not have sufficient T1 weighting and that the lesions can be more readily seen utilizing a pulse sequence of TE = 20/TR = 300. This was also the experience of Reinig,[8] who reports that, utilizing a TE = 26/TR = 300 pulse sequence or an inversion recovery pulse sequence with a very short time to inversion (TI), MRI can identify more than 90 percent of liver metastases. A recent editorial, however, cautions against undue enthusiasm and concludes that MRI is not yet ready to be used for routine screening of liver metastases.[7]

There are several studies of MRI of the biliary system. The appearance of bile varies on both T1 and T2 pulse sequences.[11] This is because the T1 and T2 relaxation times of bile vary with its chemical composition and degree of concentration.[11] With concentration of bile the T1 decreases, resulting in an increased signal on T1-weighted images.[10] Concentrated bile therefore has a high signal intensity on both T1- and T2-weighted images, whereas fresh bile has a low signal on the T1-weighted images.[10] In one study of bile obtained from the gallbladder at surgery, 11 patients with acute cholecystitis, 41 patients with chronic cholecystitis, and 6 normal patients had no difference in the T1 and T2 relaxation times of the bile. In this study all the patients were fasting, and standard deviations between the different groups were large.[11] In another study patients with and without cholecystitis were studied after a 12-hour fast. In all the normal patients the signal on T1-weighted images was of intermediate or high intensity. In six of eight patients with acute cholecystitis there was decreased signal intensity in the bile on the T1-weighted image even after the 12-hour fast. This was due to the inability of the inflamed gallbladder to concentrate bile.[12]

In general MRI might prove highly valuable in evaluation of patients with portal hypertension.[14] MRI can show the presence or absence of portal vein occlusion and of collaterals, give some indication of flow, and identify the patency of operative shunts. In 23 cases of shunt for portal hypertension, MRI was able to demonstrate patency in 21 and thrombosis in two.[15]

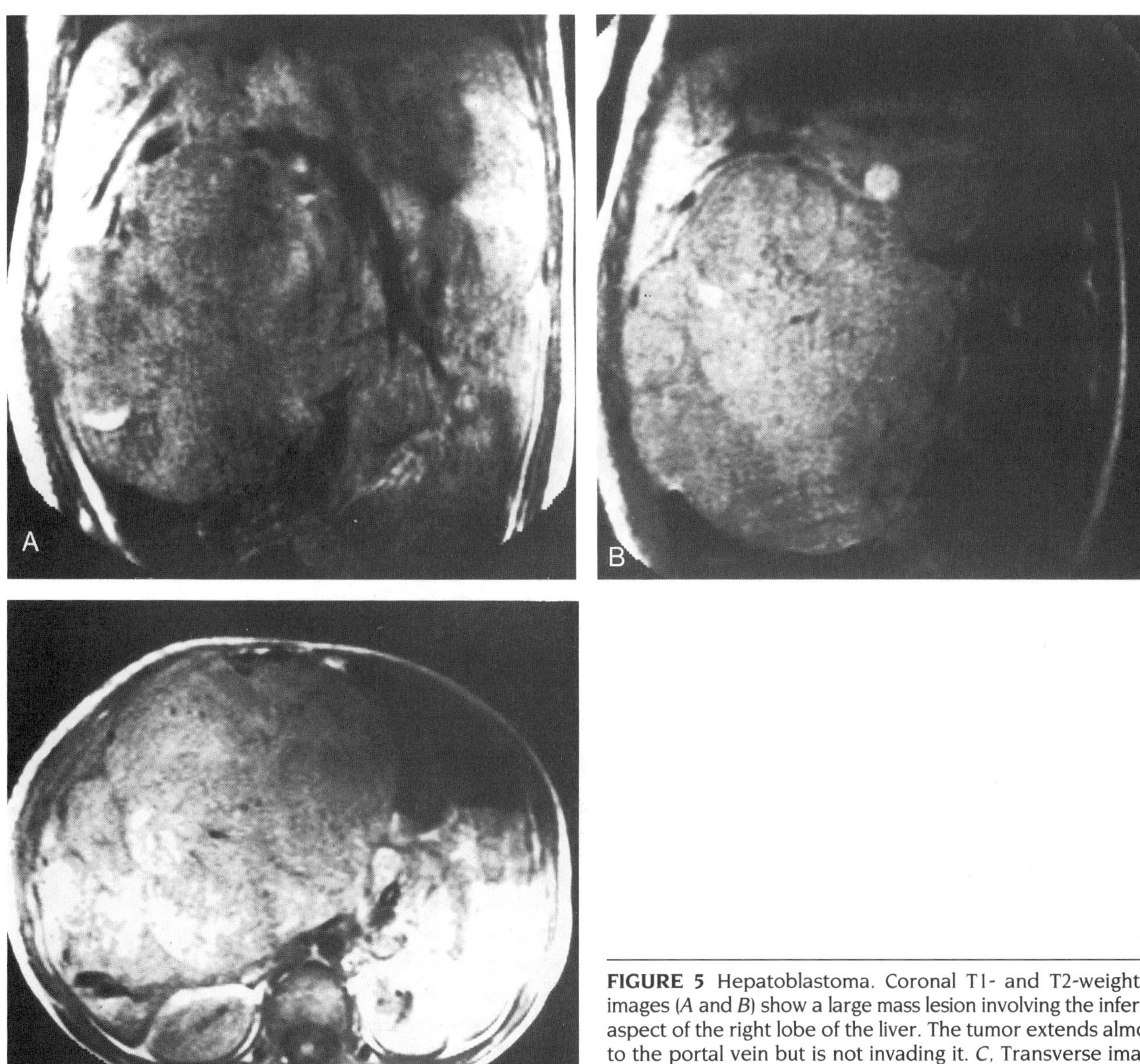

FIGURE 5 Hepatoblastoma. Coronal T1- and T2-weighted images (*A* and *B*) show a large mass lesion involving the inferior aspect of the right lobe of the liver. The tumor extends almost to the portal vein but is not invading it. *C*, Transverse image showing the very large lobulated tumor mass lying anterior to the right kidney.

Spleen

MRI is not being routinely utilized for splenic imaging. A wide variety of different disorders of the spleen have been visualized with MRI (Fig. 6). The overall sensitivity of MRI in detection of splenic lesions is not known, however. It may well be less than that in the liver. The reason for this is that many disorders have prolonged T1 and T2 relaxation times. The normal spleen also has relatively long T1 and T2 relaxation times, and this might make it more difficult to identify lesions in the spleen than in the liver. In one patient a lesion was isointense with the spleen on both T1- and T2-weighted pulse sequences.[25] In several other patients splenic lesions were identifiable only because of associated cystic change, necrosis, or hemorrhage within the lesion.[25] For many lesions the appearance in the spleen is relatively nonspecific. Splenic infarction in patients with sickle cell anemia does, however, produce a fairly specific abnormality.[3] Thirteen patients with known sickle cell disease were studied prospectively. Calculated T1 and T2 relaxation times for the splenic parenchyma in these patients were shorter than values obtained in the normal spleen. Iron deposition in the spleen causes reduction in signal intensity on T2-weighted images from the normal spleen. Infarcts show up as areas of strong signal against the low-intensity background of the rest of the spleen. One area in which splenic imaging may have potential is in the identification of involvement in Hodgkin's disease, but this issue is not yet settled.

In the spleen cavernous hemangiomas are well defined with low signal on T1-weighted images and very strong signal on T2-weighted images.[1]

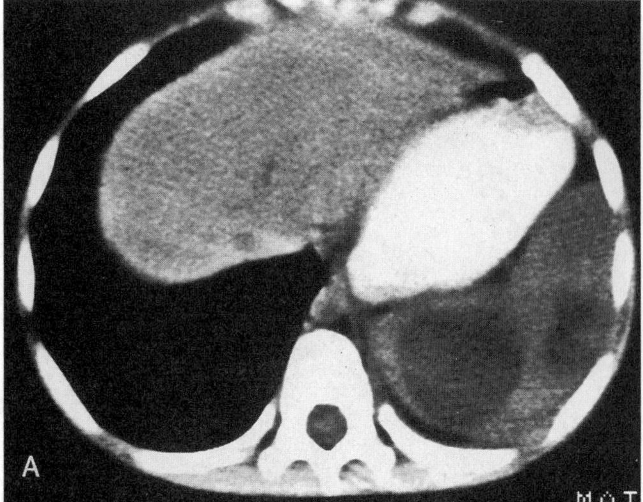

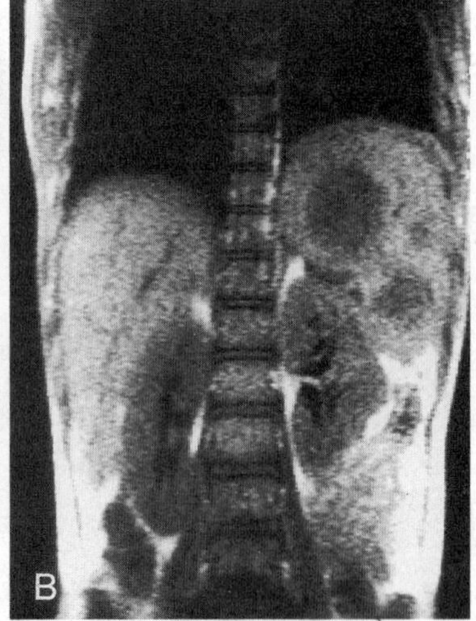

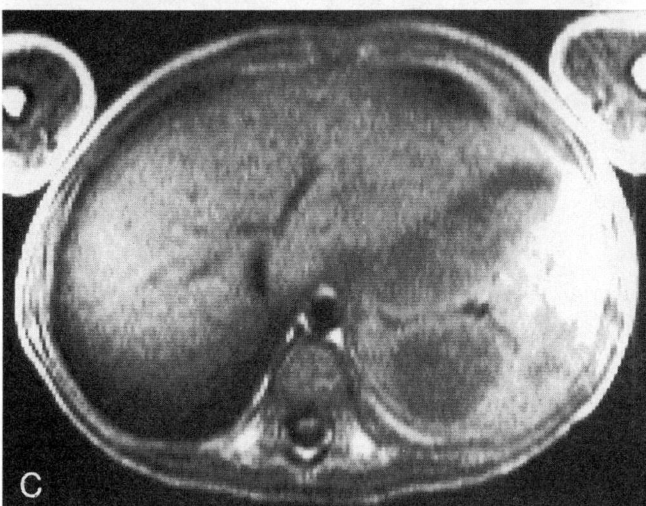

FIGURE 6 Splenic abscess. *A*, CT scan shows two low-intensity areas in the spleen. *B* and *C* are coronal and transverse T1-weighted MR images, both of which show multiple liver abscesses.

Pancreas

As with the spleen, MRI is not routinely utilized for pancreatic imaging. MRI can identify a wide range of pancreatic disorders, but sensitivity and specificity are not yet known. In patients with cystic fibrosis, the pancreas may appear normal or small. Infiltration of the pancreas with fat is seen as a strong signal from the pancreas on both T1- and T2-weighted images. In pancreatitis the gland is enlarged with increased T1 and T2 relaxation times. The margins are often poorly defined. Pancreatic pseudocysts can be identified. MRI can be utilized to monitor the change in size of the cyst with time. The cysts have very long T1 and T2 relaxation times, being of low intensity on T1-weighted images and strong intensity on T2-weighted images.

At the present time MRI is probably not the imaging modality of choice for screening for pancreatic disease.[26]

Bowel

MRI has been little utilized in the evaluation of intestine. There are isolated reports of the identification of abnormality in Crohn's disease, ulcerative colitis, lymphoma, and hemorrhage in the bowel wall.

In the evaluation of children with anorectal abnormalities MRI is proving extremely useful (Fig. 7). It can identify the levator muscles, which are seen as a low-signal band. The relationship of the muscles to the rectum and the extent of normal muscle present can be accurately evaluated in children with anal atresia.[27,28] In addition in these patients, MRI is useful for the detection of associated unsuspected abnormalities.[27,28]

A case report of a patient with an esophageal duplication cyst indicates that MRI can identify the presence of the cyst well. In the patient reported, the wall of the cyst was of low intensity on T1-weighted image, consistent with fibrosis. The signal intensity on the T1-weighted image from the fluid in the cyst was strong, suggesting the presence of blood within the fluid.[29]

In one patient with Morgagni hernia the lesion was identified with other modalities as well as MRI, but advantages of MRI were the ability to show continuity between fat in the hernia with omental fat and the ability of sagittal and coronal imaging planes to identify the defect within the diaphragm.[30]

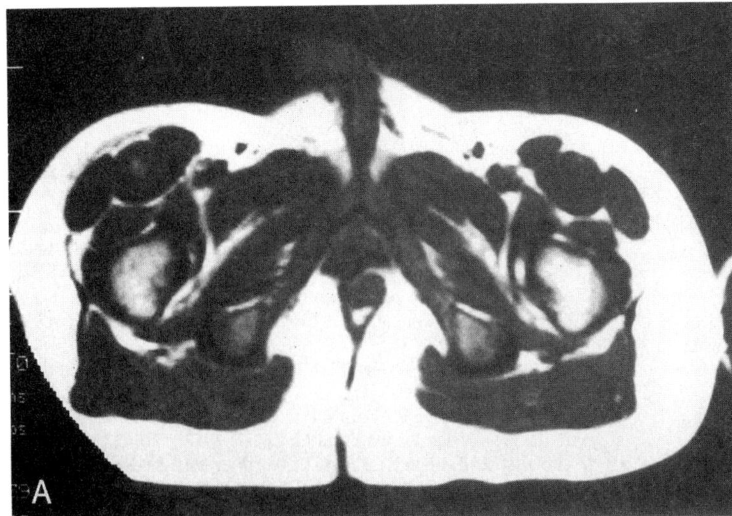

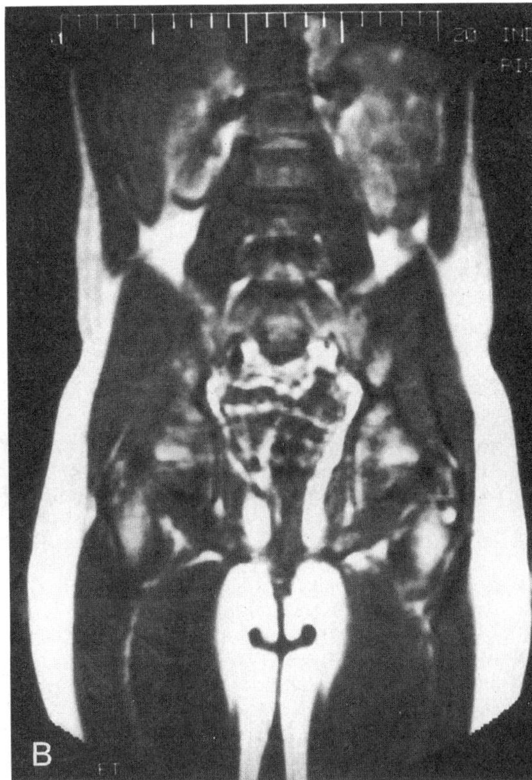

FIGURE 7 *A* and *B*, Anal atresia following pull-through procedure. The rectum is not lying in a normal position within the levator sling. Good muscle thickness is seen on the right side. The rectum lies to the left of the midline, probably out with the levator sling.

Abdominal Cavity

MRI is sensitive for detection of ascites. The fluid has very low intensity on T1 images and very high intensity on T2 images. Abscesses have been identified by means of MRI. With the recent developments in motion suppression and the power of MRI to manipulate contrast, MRI has the potential for becoming a sensitive method for screening the abdomen for the presence or absence of an abscess.

PERSPECTIVES

MRI has the widely reported virtues of being safe and noninvasive. It has the potential for achieving some degree of tissue characterization. The two additional major attributes of MRI are the ability to create images in any plane and its outstanding soft tissue contrast resolution. MRI also has the capability of excellent vessel visualization without the need for contrast injection.

Plain film radiographs provide an excellent overview of the abdomen and should still remain the initial screening test for any abdominal disease.

Sonography will probably remain the modality for use in many abdominal disorders. It does not image bone and will frequently have access to areas of the abdomen obscured by overlying gas. Field of view in sonography is also limited.

CT remains an excellent modality for abdominal imaging. It does require administration of oral and intravenous contrast media. Although spatial resolution is superior to that of MRI, there are more and more reports of greater sensitivity of MR for the detection of lesions in the abdominal soft tissues. This results from our ability to manipulate image contrast extensively with MRI. Another great advantage of MRI is its capability of imaging vessels well without the need for contrast agents. With CT it is difficult to consistently obtain superb images of the abdominal vessels.

MRI has great potential for making a major impact on abdominal imaging. Until recently, this was limited by motion. We now are able to largely overcome the effects of motion, and whether this will cause MRI to blossom into a modality that has unique applications remains to be determined. I predict that the initial impact of MRI will be on visualization, localization, and characterization of focal lesions in the liver and, to a lesser extent, the spleen. In the retroperitoneum, MRI may again provide unique information because of its excellent soft tissue contrast resolution. The unique role of MRI remains to be determined.

REFERENCES

1. Levine E, Wetzel LH, Neff JR. MR imaging and CT of extrahepatic cavernous hemangiomas. AJR 1986; 147:1299–1304.
2. Richards MA, Webb JA, Reznek RH, Davies G, Jewell SE, Shand WS, Wrigley PFM, Lister TA. Detection of spread of malignant lymphoma to the liver by low field strength magnetic resonance imaging. Br Med J 1986; 293:1126–1128.
3. Adler DD, Glazer GM, Aisen AM. MRI of the spleen: normal appearance and findings in sickle-cell anemia. AJR 1986; 147:843–845.
4. Weinreb JC, Cohen JM, Armstrong E, Smith T. Imaging the pediatric liver: MRI and CT. AJR 1986; 147:785–790.

5. Day DL, Letourneau JG, Allan BT, Ascher NL, Lund G. MR evaluation of the portal vein in pediatric liver transplant candidates. AJR 1986; 147:1027–1030.
6. Ferrucci JT. Leo J. Rigler lecture — MR imaging of the liver. AJR 1986; 147:1103–1116.
7. Bernardino ME (editorial). Focal hepatic mass screening: MR imaging or CT scanning? Radiology 1987; 162:282–283.
8. Reinig JW, Dwyer AJ, Miller DL, White M, Frank JA, Sugarbaker PH, Chang AE, Doppman JL. Liver metastasis detection: comparative sensitivities of MR imaging and CT scanning. Radiology 1987; 162:43–47.
9. Ros PR, Viamonte M Jr, Soila K, Sheldon JJ, Tobias J, Cohen B. Demonstration of cavernomatous transformation of the portal vein by magnetic resonance imaging. Gastrointest Radiol 1986; 11:90–92.
10. Dooms GC, Fisher MR, Higgins CB, Hricak H, Goldberg HI, Margulis AR. MR imaging of the dilated biliary tract. Radiology 1986; 158:337–341.
11. Loflin TG, Simeone JF, Mueller PR, Saini S, Stark DD, Butch RJ, Brady TJ, Ferrucci JT Jr. Gallbladder bile in cholecystitis: in vitro MR evaluation. Radiology 1985; 157:457–459.
12. McCarthy S, Hricak H, Cohen M, Fisher MR, Winkler ML, Filly RA, Margulis AR. Cholecystitis: detection with MR imaging. Radiology 1986; 158:333–336.
13. Itai Y, Ohtomo K, Furui S, Yamauchi T, Minami M, Yashiro N. Noninvasive diagnosis of small cavernous hemangioma of the liver: advantage of MRI. AJR 1985; 145:1195–1199.
14. Williams DM, Cho KJ, Aisen AM, Eckhauser FE. Portal hypertension evaluated by MR imaging. Radiology 1985; 157:703–706.
15. Bernardino ME, Steinberg HV, Pearson TC, Gedgaudas-McClees RK, Torres WE, Henderson JM. Shunts for portal hypertension: MR and angiography for determination of patency. Radiology 1986; 158:57–61.
16. Edelman RR, Hahn PF, Buxton R, Wittenberg J, Ferrucci JT, Saini S, Brady TJ. Rapid MR imaging with suspended respiration: clinical application in the liver. Radiology 1986; 161:125–131.
17. Wood ML, Runge VM, Henkelman RM. Overcoming motion in abdominal MR imaging. AJR 1988; 150:513–522.
18. Weinreb JC, Breteman L, Maravilla KR. Magnetic resonance imaging of hepatic lymphoma. AJR 1984; 143:1211–1214.
19. Stark DD, Wittenberg J, Butch RJ, Ferrucci JT Jr. Hepatic metastases: randomized, controlled comparison of detection with MR imaging and CT. Radiology 1987; 165:399–406.
20. Itoh K, Nishimura K, Togashi K, Fujisawa I, Noma S, Minami S, Sagoh T, Nakano Y, Itoh H, Mori K, Ozawa K, Torizuka K. Hepatocellular carcinoma: MR imaging. Radiology 1987; 164:21–25.
21. Curati WL, Halevy A, Gibson RN, Carr DH, Blumgart LH, Steiner RE. Ultrasound, CT, and MRI comparison in primary and secondary tumors of the liver. Gastrointest Radiol 1988; 13:123–128.
22. Ohtomo K, Itai Y, Yoshikawa K, Kokubo T, Yashiro N, Iio M, Furukawa K. Hepatic tumors: dynamic MR imaging. Radiology 1986; 163:27–31.
23. Hernandez RJ, Sarnaik SA, Lande I, Aisen AM, Glazer GM, Chenivert T, Martel W. MR evaluation of liver iron overload. J Comput Assist Tomogr 1988; 12:91–94.
24. Unger EC, Lee JKT, Weyman PJ. CT and MR imaging of radiation hepatitis. J Comput Assist Tomogr 1987; 11:264–268.
25. Hahn PF, Weissleder R, Stark DD, Saini S, Elizondo G, Ferrucci JT. MR imaging of focal splenic tumors. AJR 1988; 150:823–827.
26. Tscholakoff D, Hricak H, Thoeni R, Winkler ML, Margulis AR. MR imaging in the diagnosis of pancreatic disease. AJR 2987; 148:703–709.
27. Mezzacappa PM, Price AP, Haller JO, Kassner EG, Hansbrough F. MR and CT demonstration of levator sling in congenital anorectal anomalies. J Comput Assist Tomogr 1987; 11:273–275.
28. Pringle KC, Sato Y, Soper RT. Magnetic resonance imaging as an adjunct to planning an anorectal pull-through. J Pediatr Surg 1987; 22:571–574.
29. Lupetin AR, Dash N. MRI appearance of esophageal duplication cyst. Gastrointest Radiol 1987; 12:7–9.
30. Yeager BA, Guglielmi GE, Schiebler ML, Gefter WB, Kressel HY. Magnetic resonance imaging of Morgagni hernia. Gastrointest Radiol 1987; 12:296–298.
31. Laniado M, Kornmesser W, Hamm B, Clauss W, Weinmann H-J, Felix R. MR imaging of the gastrointestinal tract: value of Gd-DTPA. AJR 1988; 150:817–821.
32. Cohen MD. MRI of the gastrointestinal and musculoskeletal systems in children. Appl Radiol 1987; 16:50.

PART 7

Angiography

Patricia E. Burrows, M.D.

In the 1970s, abdominal angiography was a technique widely used in pediatric diagnosis to evaluate diseases ranging from abdominal masses to primary vascular disease. The present availability of less invasive cross-sectional imaging techniques and Doppler evaluation of the major vascular trunks has diminished and more clearly defined the need for angiographic techniques to investigate and treat gastrointestinal diseases. Currently, the most frequent indications for gastrointestinal angiography in children include the following:

1. The evaluation of hepatic blood supply and drainage prior to and following surgery in patients undergoing liver transplantation.
2. The determination of the nature and extent (resectability) of liver masses, as well as the vascular anatomy of the liver prior to surgery, combined with embolization in infants with congestive heart failure secondary to vascular masses (hemangiomas) of the liver.
3. The investigation of portal hypertension prior to a surgical shunting procedure.
4. The investigation and transcatheter treatment of gastrointestinal (GI) bleeding.
5. The presence of occlusive vascular disease as well as its treatment.

TECHNIQUES OF ANGIOGRAPHY

Gastrointestinal angiography involves selective catheterization of branches of the celiac trunk and mesenteric arteries combined with contrast injections recorded on serial x-ray images.

Patient Preparation

Gastrointestinal angiography is performed in the radiology angiography suite. Preshaped catheters are introduced percutaneously via the femoral artery. Although technically superior angiograms are obtained with complete motion control under general anesthesia, most examinations can be performed with sedation and local anesthesia. For sedation, we most frequently use a combination of 25 mg per milliliter meperidine, 6.25 mg per milliliter chlorpromazine, and 25 mg per milliliter promethazine, administered intramuscularly at a dose of 0.1 mL per kilogram up to a limit of 2 mL per kilogram. The blood pressure, heart rate, respiratory rate, and transcutaneous oxygen saturation of patients thus sedated are monitored throughout the examination. In addition, a rectal temperature probe is used to monitor body temperature in infants and in all patients under general anesthesia. Prevention of loss of body heat is especially important in infants and can be accomplished by the use of electrical water-heated warming blankets and radiant heaters. Patients must also be kept dry and, when necessary, their heads and extremities may be wrapped with a knit fabric or plastic cover. The quantity of flush solution and contrast material used must be regulated. Following the procedure, vital signs are monitored until the patient is alert, the puncture site is checked for bleeding or hematoma formation, and the pedal pulses are palpated to confirm femoral arterial patency.

Catheterization Technique

The Seldinger technique is used to introduce the catheters by percutaneous femoral arterial cannulation.[1] First the child's hips are elevated on a roll of towels or other material. After the skin is infiltrated with a local anesthetic, a tiny incision is made in the skin along the course of the palpable femoral artery, usually below the inguinal crease. A short beveled needle with a stylet is passed through the artery along a nearly horizontal course. The stylet is then removed and the needle withdrawn until pulsatile blood flow has been obtained. A flexible guide wire is advanced into the arterial system, and the needle is removed and exchanged for a catheter over the guide wire. Patients who weigh less than 15 kg are then anticoagulated with 100 units per kilogram of heparin to prevent femoral arterial thrombosis. With the recent development of thin-walled high-flow catheters most gastrointestinal angiography can be performed with 3- or 4-F catheters.

Aortography is usually performed before selective catheterization to outline the abdominal vascular distribution. In older children, aortography is accomplished with a high-flow multisidehole catheter exchanged over a guide wire for an endhole catheter that has been preshaped to catheterize selectively the desired vessel.[2] In small infants, catheter exchange should be avoided to minimize femoral arterial trauma. A 3-F multisidehole catheter is preshaped with a C or "cobra" curve. Following the aortic injection, the same catheter is used for selective angiography. In the first week of life, aortography and selective angiography can be performed via the umbilical artery.

Imaging Techniques

Angiography can be performed with a variety of imaging recording modalities. The three most commonly used techniques are conventional magnification film, 100- or 105-mm film, and digital subtraction angiography. Conventional magnification films give the highest spatial resolution, but they require a relatively high dosage of radiation and contrast material. Because of poor contrast resolution complicated by the superimposition of bowel gas, they produce relatively poor images of faintly opacified structures such as the portal vein. Magnification film technique is used when the visualization of small vessels or small areas of vascular irregularity is important, for example, in the investigation of vasculitis or tumors.

Exposing 100-mm film to the image intensifier produces a miniature image similar to that obtained with conventional film angiography, but only a small fraction of the radiation dosage is used. This technique is ideal for demonstrating vascular anatomy, especially if complete patient-motion control is not possible.

Digital subtraction angiography is performed by computer digitization and manipulation of image data obtained through the image intensifier. A number of mask images are made to include different phases of the respiratory and cardiac movement prior to the injection of contrast material. These masks are then computer-subtracted from postcontrast images, resulting in an image of only the opacified vascular structures. Digital subtraction angiography has lower spatial resolution than conventional magnification film technique, but has very high contrast resolution, making it possible to visualize structures with smaller amounts of contrast material. This characteristic permits the use of smaller catheters and half-strength contrast material (and therefore half the amount) and allows excellent visualization of vessels distal to an obstruction, abnormal parenchymal blushes, and venous structures. The radiation dose is lower than that used with conventional films but is higher than that used with 100-mm film. Digital subtraction angiography markedly shortens the examination time because the images are available on the television monitor immediately, whereas conventional and 100-mm film angiograms have to be processed before they can be viewed.

Digital subtraction angiography requires the absence of all motion except that caused by regular rhythmic respiratory and cardiac activity. Heavy sedation is necessary in infants and young children. Bowel motion must be arrested before each angiogram by the intravenous or intra-arterial administration of 0.1 to 0.5 mg of glucagon.

Contrast Material

Currently, only low-osmolarity nonionic contrast material is used for intravascular injection at The Hospital for Sick Children (HSC), Toronto. These agents have a lower incidence of allergic reaction than older ionic contrast agents and cause little or no pain during injection. The absence of pain is important because it helps to prevent the appearance of motion artifacts in the radiographs of sedated patients. Contrast agents with an iodine concentration of 300 to 320 mg per milliliter are used with conventional film or 100-mm film technique. With most digital subtraction angiography units, clearer images are obtained with a contrast medium of approximately 140 to 150 mg of iodine per milliliter. At this concentration, the nonionic contrast media are approximately iso-osmolar. If full-strength contrast medium is used with digital subtraction angiography, the quantity used per injection is usually one-half what would be used for film angiography.

Pharmacoangiography

Vasodilators given prior to contrast medium injection in the superior mesenteric artery improve the visualization of the portal vein.[3] Papaverine (0.6 to 1.0 mg per kilogram), Priscoline, or nitroglycerin can be injected approximately 30 seconds before the contrast medium injection.

Vasodilators have also been used to demonstrate the site of bleeding in patients with GI hemorrhage,[4] and vasoconstrictors, such as isoproterenol, can be used to control gastrointestinal bleeding when infused through a selective catheter.[5-7]

Complications of Angiographic Techniques

Significant complications of abdominal angiography in children are uncommon.[1] The most frequent complications involve the femoral artery puncture site and include femoral arterial spasm or thrombosis, bleeding, and, rarely arteriovenous fistula formation. Relief of femoral arterial spasm can sometimes be speeded by the injection of a small amount of nitroglycerin (10 to 20 μg in an infant) during the withdrawal of the catheter through the narrowed artery or by infiltration of lidocaine locally around the vessel. If pedal pulses cannot be palpated within 1 hour of catheter removal, systemic heparinization is instituted. Thrombolytic agents (e.g., streptokinase, urokinase) effectively dissolve ileofemoral thrombi resulting from cardiac catheterization,[8] but they are rarely required after diagnostic abdominal angiography. The use of heparin, small catheters, and minimal manipulation contributes to a low incidence of femoral arterial thrombosis.

Other complications include thromboembolism from the catheter tip and subintimal dissection vessels during selective catheterization.

DIAGNOSTIC ROLE OF ANGIOGRAPHY

Hepatic Masses

Angiography is used prior to operation in selected patients with hepatic masses to determine the resectability of the mass by partial hepatectomy. Angiography precisely defines the segmental distribution of tumor within the liver, based on the distribution of the hepatic arteries and veins, and the portal vein (Fig. 1).[2,9-11] At the same time, arteriography provides presurgical documentation of the anatomy of the arterial supply to the liver and tumor. In 55 to 65 percent of patients the celiac artery divides into three branches; the left gastric, splenic, and common hepatic arteries.[10] The remainder of the population have some anatomic variation, most commonly the origin of the hepatic or right hepatic artery from the superior mesenteric artery of the origin of the left hepatic artery from the left gastric artery (Fig. 2). The angiographic evaluation of the inferior vena cava and portal vein in patients with liver masses is indicated if noninvasive imaging cannot exclude their involvement.

Angiographic findings can be useful in distinguishing malignant from benign tumors in some but not all patients.[9,12,13] Angiographic techniques are also used occasionally to deliver arterial infusion of chemotherapeutic agents and to treat congestive heart failure in infants with hepatic hemangiomas by hepatic artery embolization.

Malignant Tumors

The angiographic findings in hepatoblastoma and hepatocellular carcinomas include the following: distortion and displacement of vessels (mass effect); hypervascularity; abnormal or bizarre appearance of feeding arteries with loss of tapering, caliber changes, and occlusions; tumor parenchymal blush; pooling or laking in sinusoidal spaces; hepatic artery–to–portal vein shunting; portal vein invasion or occlusion; and inferior vena caval or hepatic vein invasion (Figs. 2 and 3).[9,12-14] Following chemotherapy malignant tumors may appear relatively avascular.

The most important angiographic features necessary for predicting malignancy are the caliber changes and occlusions indicating the tumor has encased the vessel, hepatic vein and inferior vena caval invasion, and portal vein occlusion. Hepatic artery–to–portal vein shunting is much more common in malignant tumors than in benign masses, although it has been described in patients with hemangiomas.[15] We have seen apparent portal vein occlusion in one patient with a hemangioma.

Benign Liver Masses

Hemangiomas. The terminology of vascular liver masses includes the categories *cavernous hemangioma* and *hemangioendothelioma.*[16-22] In infants, the clinical behavior of the lesion does not necessarily have a good correlation with the histologic diagnosis.[16] In adults, the cavernous hemangioma presents as a mass lesion and has characteristic angiographic findings.[23] There is mild enlargement of the feeding hepatic arteries that appear to lead into dilated varix-like structures. The sinusoidal spaces fill early in the angiographic series and remain opacified for a long time without early filling of the veins. The portal system is reportedly not involved.[23]

In infants and children, areas of cavernous hemangioma and hemangioendothelioma are frequently seen in the same patient during histologic examination. Because lesions with both types of histology may have similar clinical behavior, including the tendency to regress, it is not possible to categorize the angiographic features according to the histologic terminology. Two major categories that have different angiographic features are those that present predominantly as mass lesions (Fig. 4) and those that are characterized by high-output cardiac failure (Figs. 5 and 6). Both categories may demonstrate other complications, including platelet con-

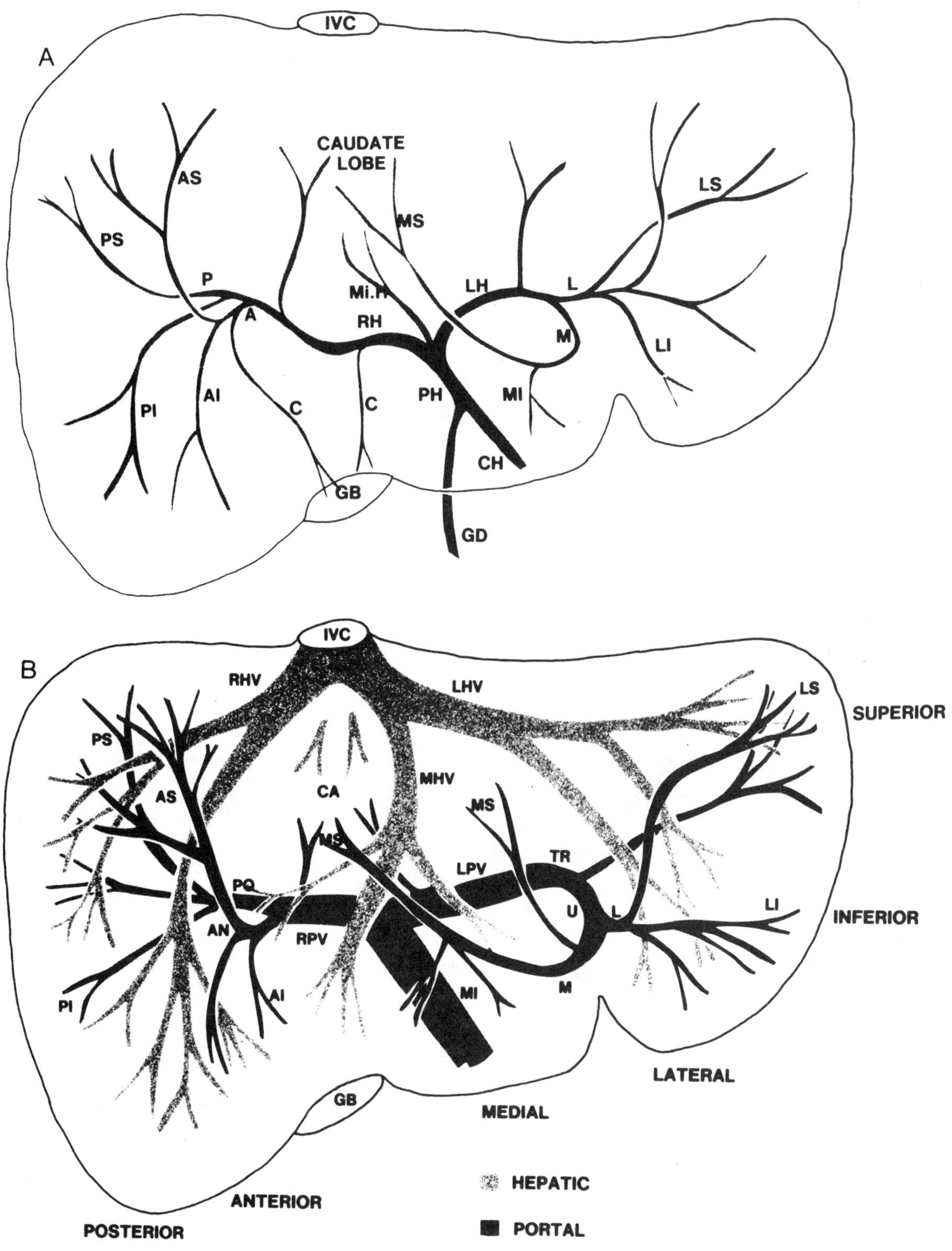

FIGURE 1 The normal vascular anatomy of the liver. These diagrams illustrate the most common pattern of the hepatic vascular supply and drainage. *A*, Hepatic arterial distribution. *B*, Portal and hepatic venous distribution. (A = anterior; AI = anteroinferior; AN = anterior; AS = anterosuperior; C = cystic, CA = caudate; CH = common hepatic; GB = gallbladder; GD = gastroduodenal; L = lateral; LH = left hepatic; LI = lateral inferior; LPV = left portal vein; LS = lateral superior; M = medial; MHV = middle hepatic vein; MI = medial inferior; MiH = middle hepatic; MS = medial superior; P = posterior; PH = proper hepatic; PI = posteroinferior; PO = posterior; PS = posterosuperior; RH = right hepatic; RPV = right portal vein; U = umbilical). (*A* and *B*, From Stanley[2]; © 1982, the Williams & Wilkins Co., Baltimore.)

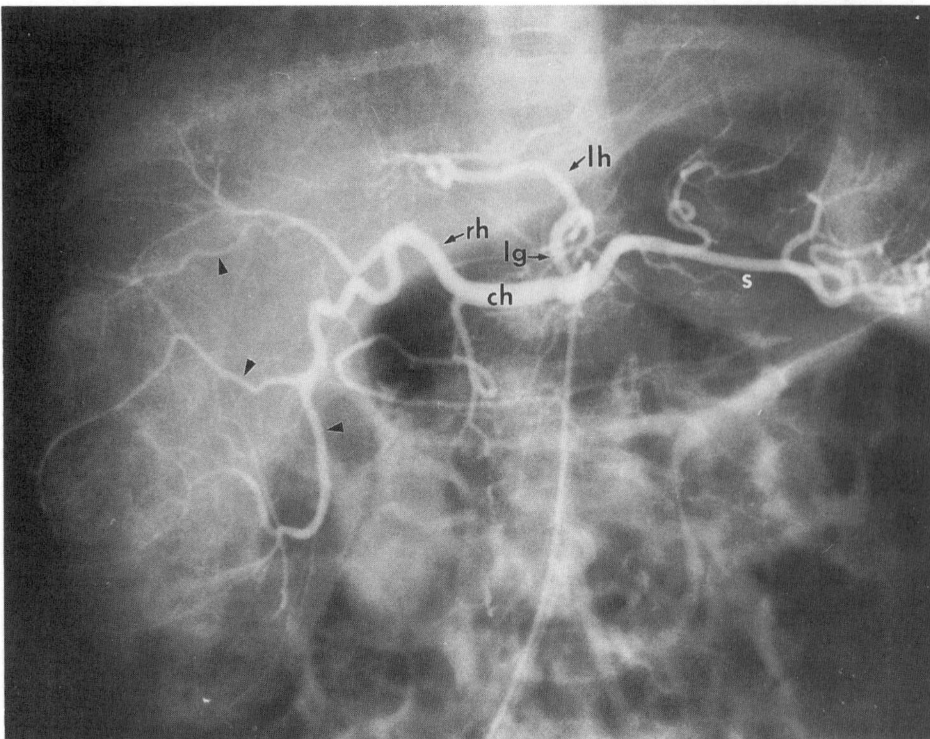

FIGURE 2 A celiac arteriogram, conventional technique, in a 4-month-old boy with a hepatoblastoma involving the right lobe. Note the caliber abnormalities of the feeding arteries (*arrowheads*) and the parenchymal blush. The left hepatic artery is a branch of the left gastric artery. (ch = common hepatic artery; lg = left gastric artery; lh = left hepatic artery; rh = right hepatic artery; s = splenic artery.)

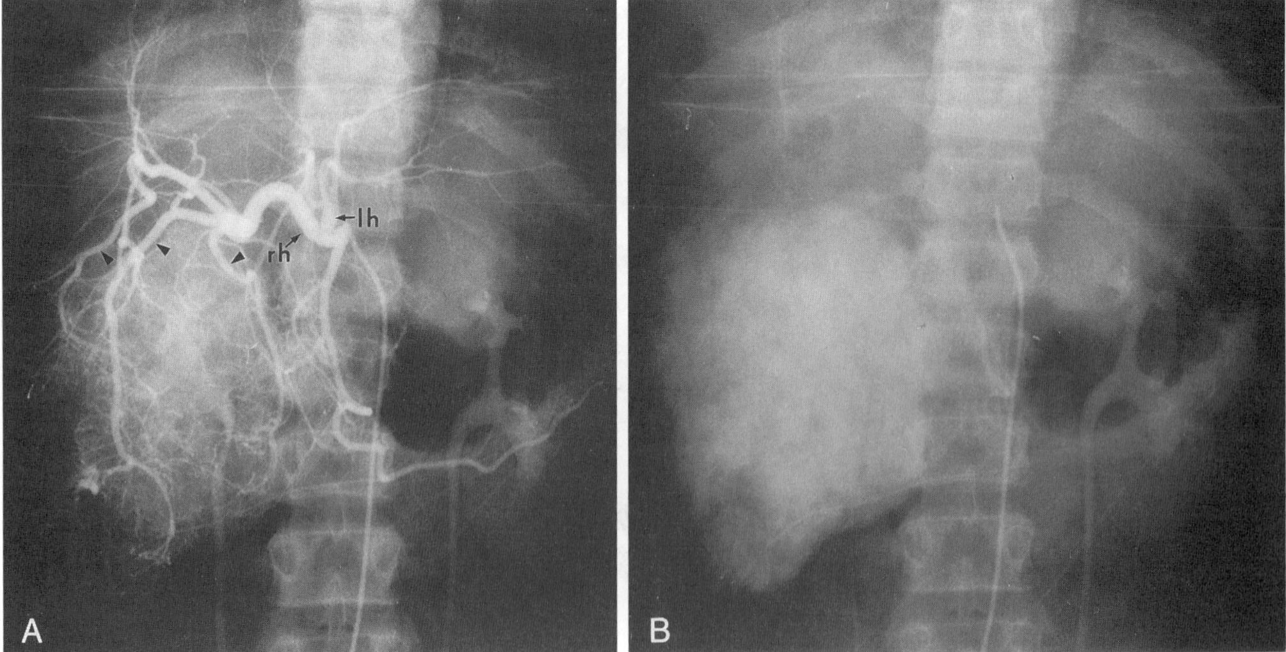

FIGURE 3 A selective common hepatic arteriogram in a 12-year-old boy with hepatocellular carcinoma involving the right lobe. *A*, The arterial phase shows enlargement of the feeding arteries (*arrowheads*) from the right hepatic artery and irregular tumor vessels within the mass. *B*, The capillary phase demonstrates an intense tumor blush, which is a characteristic of this type of tumor. (lh = left hepatic artery; rh = right hepatic artery.)

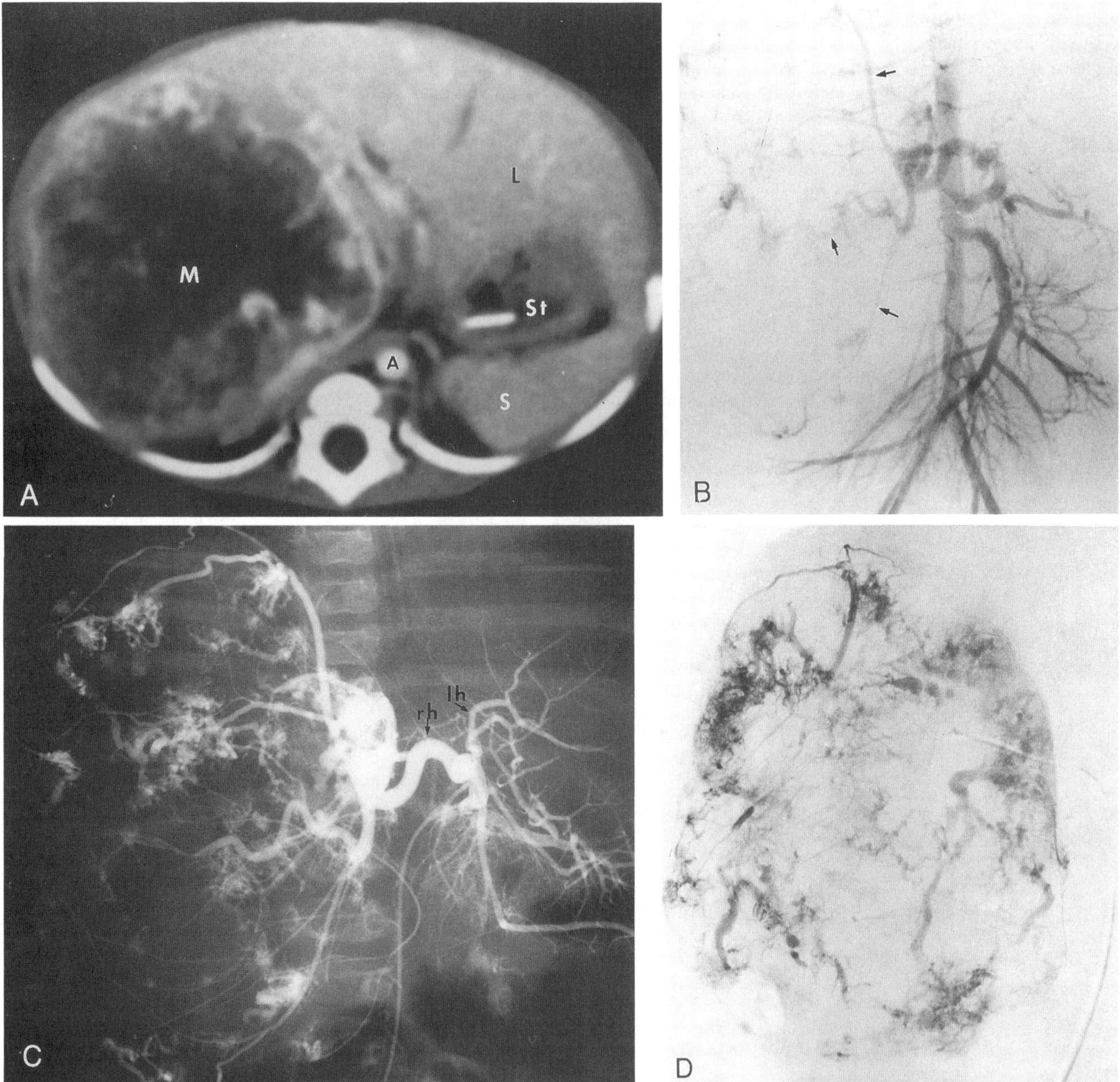

FIGURE 4 A large right hepatic hemangioma (hemangioendothelioma) in a 5-month-old boy with a cutaneous hemangioma and an enlarging abdominal mass but no symptoms of congestive heart failure. The angiographic findings are representative of the low-flow hemangiomas in children and are similar to those described in cavernous hemangiomas in adults. *A*, The axial CT image obtained through the liver following intravenous contrast administration shows a low-attenuation mass with peripheral enhancement, involving the right lobe and displacement of the stomach. *B*, The abdominal aortogram (conventional subtraction technique) shows no significant difference in the size of the abdominal aorta above and below the celiac axis. There is displacement of the celiac axis and superior mesenteric artery toward the left, and numerous abnormal branches from the right hepatic artery are seen (*arrows*). *C*, The selective celiac arteriogram (frontal projection) shows the early filling of sinusoidal vascular spaces from branches of the right hepatic artery. These branches appear stretched around the mass. *D*, The late phase of the right hepatic arteriogram (conventional subtraction technique) shows prolonged pooling of contrast material in the sinusoidal spaces at the periphery of the mass. Note the absence of opacification of hepatic veins, indicating no arteriovenous shunting. During surgery, hematoma was found to be the cause of the avascular center of this lesion. (A = aorta; L = liver; lh = left hepatic artery; M = mass; rh = right hepatic artery; S = spleen; St = stomach.)

sumption and hypofibrogenemia, hemolytic anemia, and rupture with hemorrhage.[16,17,21] Hepatic hemangiomas may be single or multiple, focal or diffuse. The lesions that present as increasing masses without congestive heart failure usually have angiographic features similar to those of the cavernous hemangiomas of adults: feeding hepatic arteries are normal in size or mildly enlarged, with loss of normal tapering. There is early, almost direct filling of adjacent sinusoidal spaces that may form a ring around an avascular center or may be separated by avascular areas (see Fig. 4). In some patients avascular areas have been shown to represent blood clot, although fibrosis is another possible explanation.[18] Contrast material typically persists without dilution in the sinusoidal spaces for 20 to 30 seconds or longer. There is no early filling of hepatic veins. In the presence of recent hemorrhage into the hemangioma, the hepatic arteries may appear stretched around a mass. In huge lesions, the stretching may produce narrowing, but irregular narrowing produced by vascular encasement in malignant tumors is generally not present.

Hemangiomas associated with congestive heart failure characteristically have enlargement of the aorta above the feeding arteries with rapid tapering of the distal abdominal aorta (Fig. 5).[17,20] The feeding hepatic arteries are dilated and tortuous, and there is early filling of the hepatic veins (Fig. 5*B*). The parenchymal phase may show a fine pattern of neovascularity with diffuse opacification of liver parenchyma, opacification of multiple discrete homogenous nodules, or collection of contrast material in sinusoidal spaces.[22] The lesions may be supplied by collateral vessels from adjacent tissues and organs, especially lumbar and intercostal, phrenic, renal, and mesenteric arteries.

The portal vein may also supply hemangiomas of the liver in infants.[17] Unfortunately, the incidence and significance of

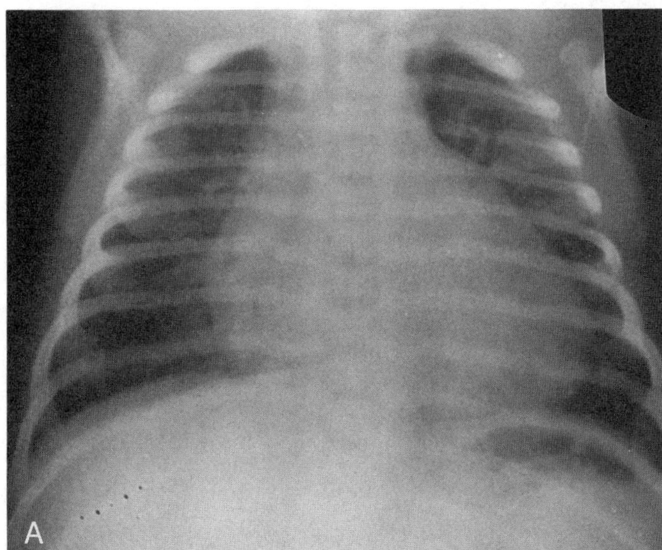

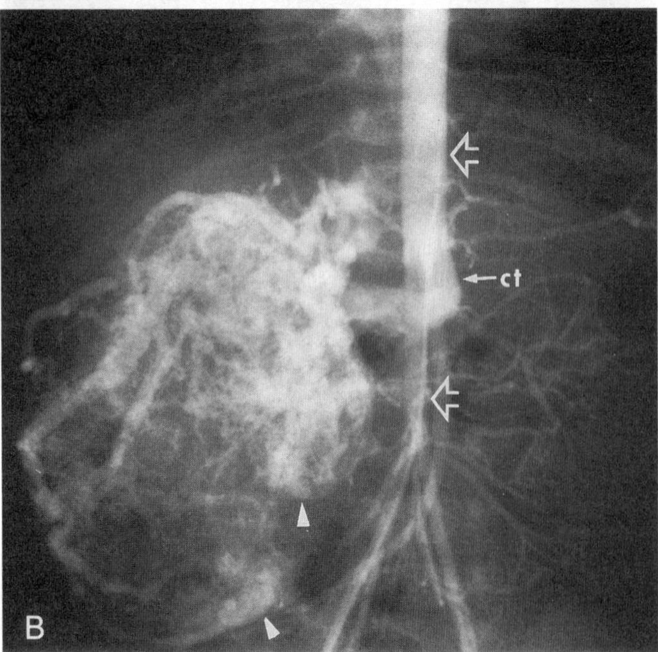

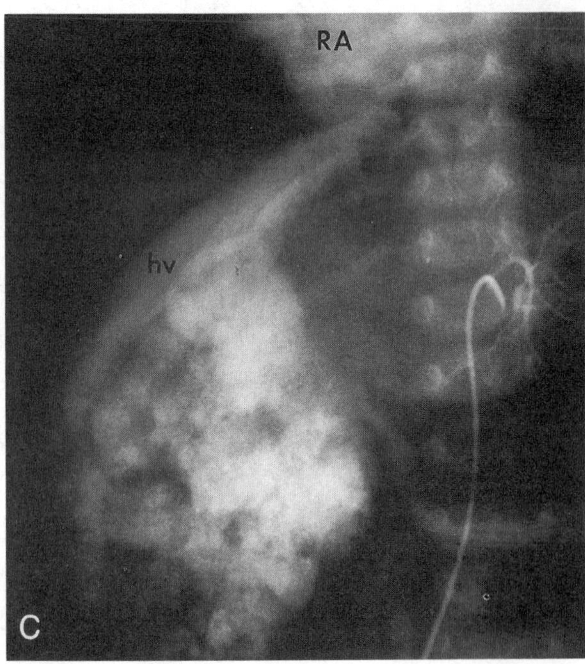

FIGURE 5 A high-flow hemangioma (hemangioendothelioma) in a 3-week-old boy with mild high-output congestive heart failure. *A*, The chest radiograph (frontal projection) shows cardiomegaly with increased pulmonary blood flow. Calcifications within the mass were seen on plain films of the abdomen (not shown). *B*, The abdominal aortogram demonstrates a marked difference in the size of the aorta (*open arrows*) above and below the celiac trunk, marked enlargement of the celiac trunk, hepatic artery and right hepatic artery branches, opacification of abnormal vascular spaces within the mass in the right lobe, and early filling of venous channels (*arrowheads*). *C*, The late phase of a selective celiac arteriogram shows contrast within large vascular spaces in the mass and opacification of huge hepatic veins. (ct = celiac trunk; hv = hepatic veins; RA = right atrium).

portal vein supply to these lesions are not known, since portal angiography has not been routinely performed in the past because of contrast medium limitations. Of the four infants at HSC whose portal veins were studied angiographically, all had portal vein involvement. Hepatic artery ligation or embolization may be less effective and is more likely to lead to hepatic ischemia and necrosis in the presence of portal vein supply of the tumor. Hepatic arteriovenous shunting may be present in patients with hemangiomas associated with congestive heart failure.[17,24] We have seen one patient with a portal vein–to–hepatic vein fistula that occurred with diffuse liver hemangiomatosis. Hepatic artery–portal vein fistulas described in one adult and four children with hepatic hemangiomas produced signs of portal hypertension rather than congestive heart failure.[15,25]

Angiosarcomas are rare malignant vascular tumors in children. They have been identified in a small number of children with recurrent liver masses that followed biopsy diagnosis of hemangioma and initial response to steroids.[26,27] Angiosarcomas appear as hypervascular masses with angiography, but demonstrate vascular encasement.

Focal Nodular Hyperplasia. Focal nodular hyperplasia is rare in children and is usually associated with other conditions such as sickle cell anemia, Fanconi's anemia, glycogen storage disease, and other lesions that produce scarring.[28] The lesion typically has a central fibrous area with radiating fibrovascular septae producing a well-circumscribed mass divided into multiple lobules. Two typical angiographic appearances have been described (Fig. 7).[29,30] The hepatic artery is usually enlarged. In one type, the arterial supply is from the periphery; circumferential arteries give off parallel penetrating arteries. Alternatively, an artery may penetrate the center of the mass and divide into multiple branches like the spokes of a wheel. The tumor usually has a dense parenchymal contrast stain with well-defined margins. The typical angiographic appearance is present in 82 percent to 90 percent of patients; 10 percent to 20 percent may be avascular or otherwise atypical. Arterial encasement, hepatic artery–to–portal vein shunting, and portal vein invasion are not present.

Hepatic Adenomas. Hepatic adenomas are usually hypervascular masses with a wide spectrum of angiographic appearances.[12] They may contain hypovascular areas caused by necrosis or hemorrhage. They usually do not have septations, but in many cases they are difficult to distinguish angiographically from focal nodular hyperplasia.

Hepatic Mesenchymal Hamartomas. Hepatic mesenchymal hamartomas are rare cystic lesions of the liver. The angiographic patterns vary, but they are usually hypervascular (Fig. 8).[2,9,31]

Portal Hypertension

In the investigation of children with portal hypertension, the goals of angiography are to confirm the diagnosis, to identify the point of obstruction, and to demonstrate the patterns of venous drainage of the spleen and bowel. Currently noninvasive imaging can usually demonstrate extrahepatic portal vein obstruction and the major portal vein collaterals; Doppler sonography can confirm hepatofugal flow in the portal vein. Angiography is reserved for patients in whom

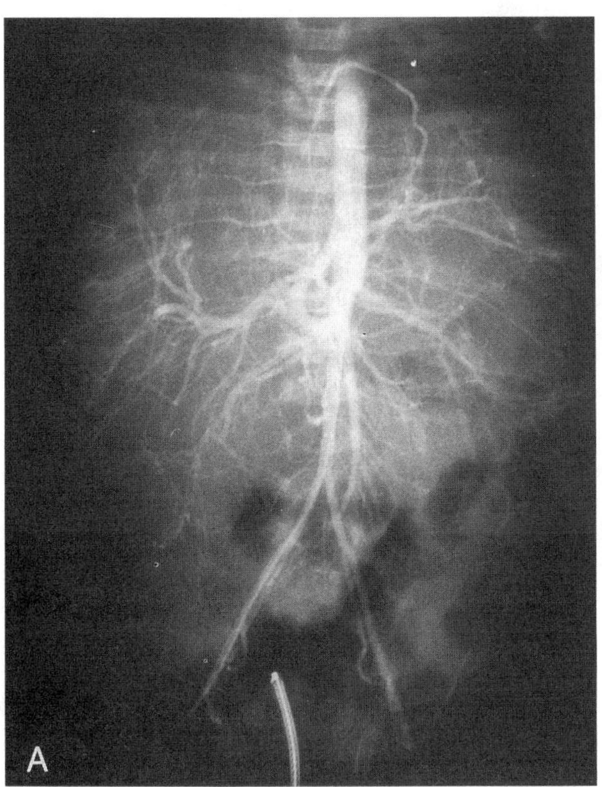

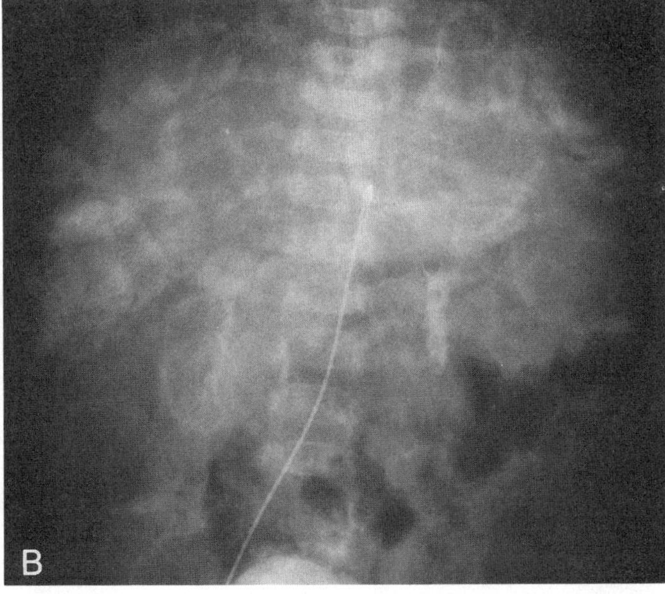

FIGURE 6 A diffuse hepatic hemangioma in a 2-month-old infant with multiple cutaneous hemangiomas and hepatomegaly. *A*, The abdominal aortogram shows a discrepancy in size between the aorta above and below the celiac axis, as well as enlargement of the hepatic arteries. *B*, Multiple areas of contrast staining with ring configuration are present on a selective hepatic arteriogram. This is one of several characteristic angiographic appearances of hepatic hemangiomas.

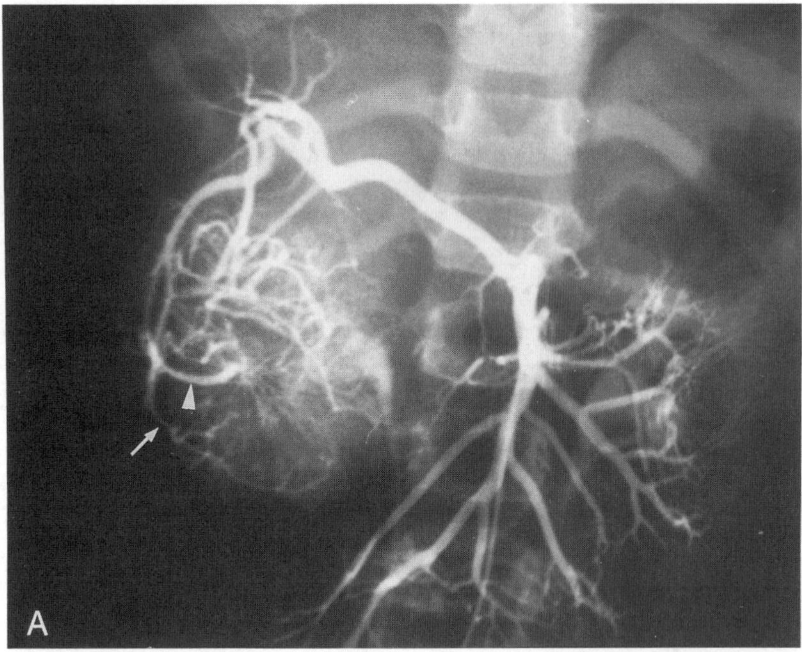

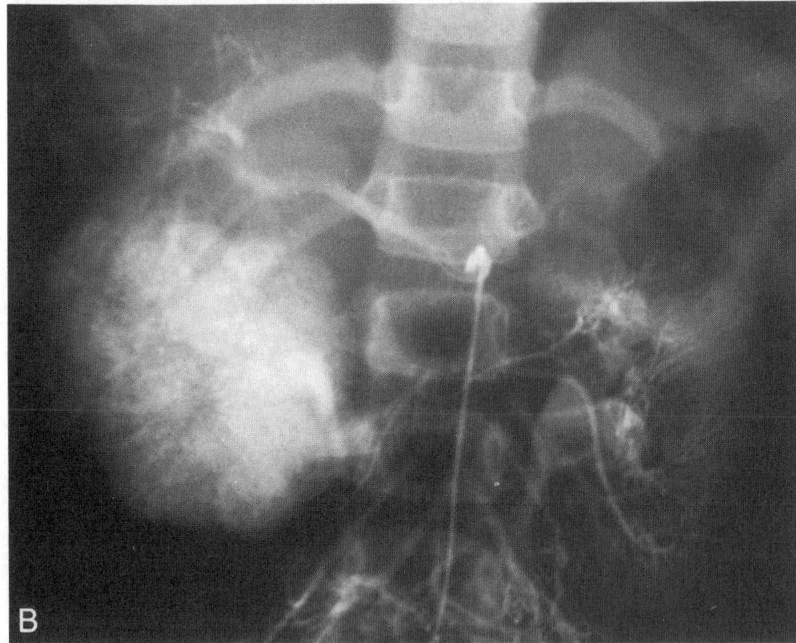

FIGURE 7 Focal nodular hyperplasia presenting as an asymptomatic abdominal mass with the origin of the right hepatic artery from the superior mesenteric artery in an otherwise healthy 3-year-old girl. *A*, The superior mesenteric arteriogram, early arterial phase, demonstrates enlarged branches supplying a mass in the inferior segments of the right lobe. Some feeding arteries (*white arrowhead*) enter the center of the mass and give rise to branches that radiate toward the periphery. Others (*white arrow*) give rise to feeding vessels that enter the mass from the periphery. *B*, The late phase of the arteriographic sequence shows the radial arrangement of the vessels and the radiolucent septae, which are characteristic of focal nodular hyperplasia. The mass appears to consist of several nodules.

noninvasive imaging is inconclusive, for preoperative assessment prior to portosystemic surgical shunt creation, and for postoperative assessment of portosystemic shunts.

Portal angiography can be performed indirectly after arterial injections or directly with direct splenoportography. Direct splenoportography gives superior visualization of the portal circulation, but it is currently used in children only after arterial portography has failed to outline a portal vein because of marked hepatofugal flow. The radiologist performs the technique on the patient under general anesthesia by inserting a 20- or 18-gauge needle and Teflon cannula into the splenic pulp during suspended respiration (Fig. 9).[32,33] Pressure measurements can then be made; pressures greater than 25 cm H_2O are diagnostic of portal hypertension. Twenty to 40 mL of contrast medium is injected by hand during serial filming of the abdomen. Relative contraindications to direct splenoportography include coagulopathy, low platelet count, and severe ascites.

Indirect portal arteriography usually requires a slow (over a 4 to 5 second period) injection of a large volume of contrast material (1.0 to 1.5 mL per kilogram) in the superior mesenteric artery, following an intra-arterial injection of a vasodilator.[3] Filming the abdomen must be continued over 24 to 30 seconds to demonstrate the obstructed portal venous

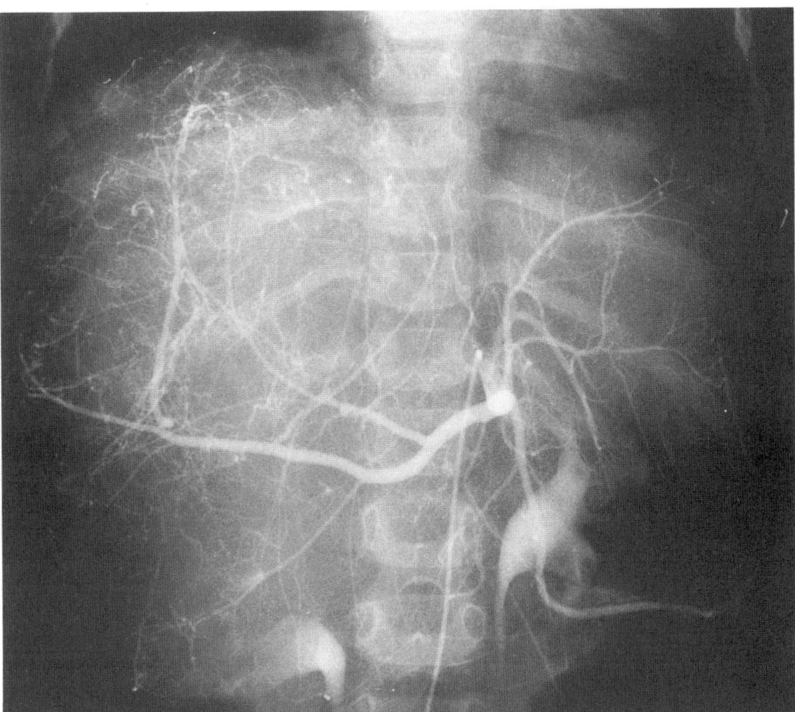

FIGURE 8 A hepatic hamartoma involving the right lobe in a 3-year-old child. A selective common hepatic arteriogram, frontal projection, shows a moderately hypervascular mass involving most of the right lobe of the liver. The tumor vessels are irregular; this lesion cannot be distinguished from a malignant tumor on the basis of the angiographic features.

drainage. Injection of contrast medium simultaneously into the superior mesenteric artery and splenic artery has also been used.

Percutaneous transhepatic and transjugular portal venography is frequently performed in adults, usually in conjunction with the embolization of gastroesophageal varices, but these techniques are infrequently used in children.

Angiographic findings in intrahepatic portal vein obstruction include hepatofugal flow with collaterals, usually through gastrocoronary-azygous, hemorrhoidal, retroperitoneal, and abdominal wall veins (Fig. 9).[3,32,33] The spleen is enlarged, and splenic vein opacification during splenic arteriography may be poor because of dilution from hepatofugal flow. Spontaneous portosystemic shunts often occur and produce opacification of the renal veins or the inferior vena cava. Hepatic arteriograms generally show hypervascularity, although a corkscrew pattern of vessels is present with hepatic cirrhosis.

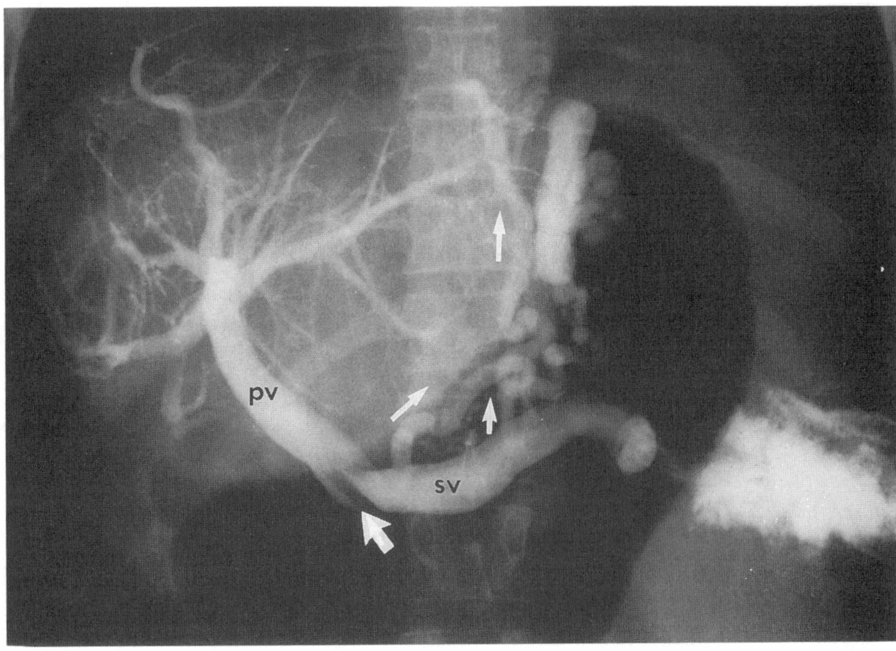

FIGURE 9 A direct splenoportogram in a 15-year-old with portal hypertension and gastroesophageal varices secondary to chronic hepatitis. In addition to a small portal vein, contrast opacifies varicose collateral veins along the lesser curvature of the stomach and the esophagogastric junction (*smaller white arrows*). The washout of contrast medium indicates the position of the superior mesenteric vein (*large white arrow*). (pv = portal vein; sv = splenic vein.)

Extrahepatic portal vein obstruction is most commonly caused by idiopathic portal vein thrombosis in childhood. The term *cavernous transformation of the portal vein* has been applied to this condition because of the appearance of multiple tortuous channels in the region of the porta hepatis (Fig. 10).[32,33] These tortuous channels are believed to represent biliary collaterals bypassing the portal vein thrombosis. These collaterals usually opacify an array of linear parallel, intrahepatic vessels, also thought to represent biliary collaterals. Occasionally, the intrahepatic portal veins appear relatively

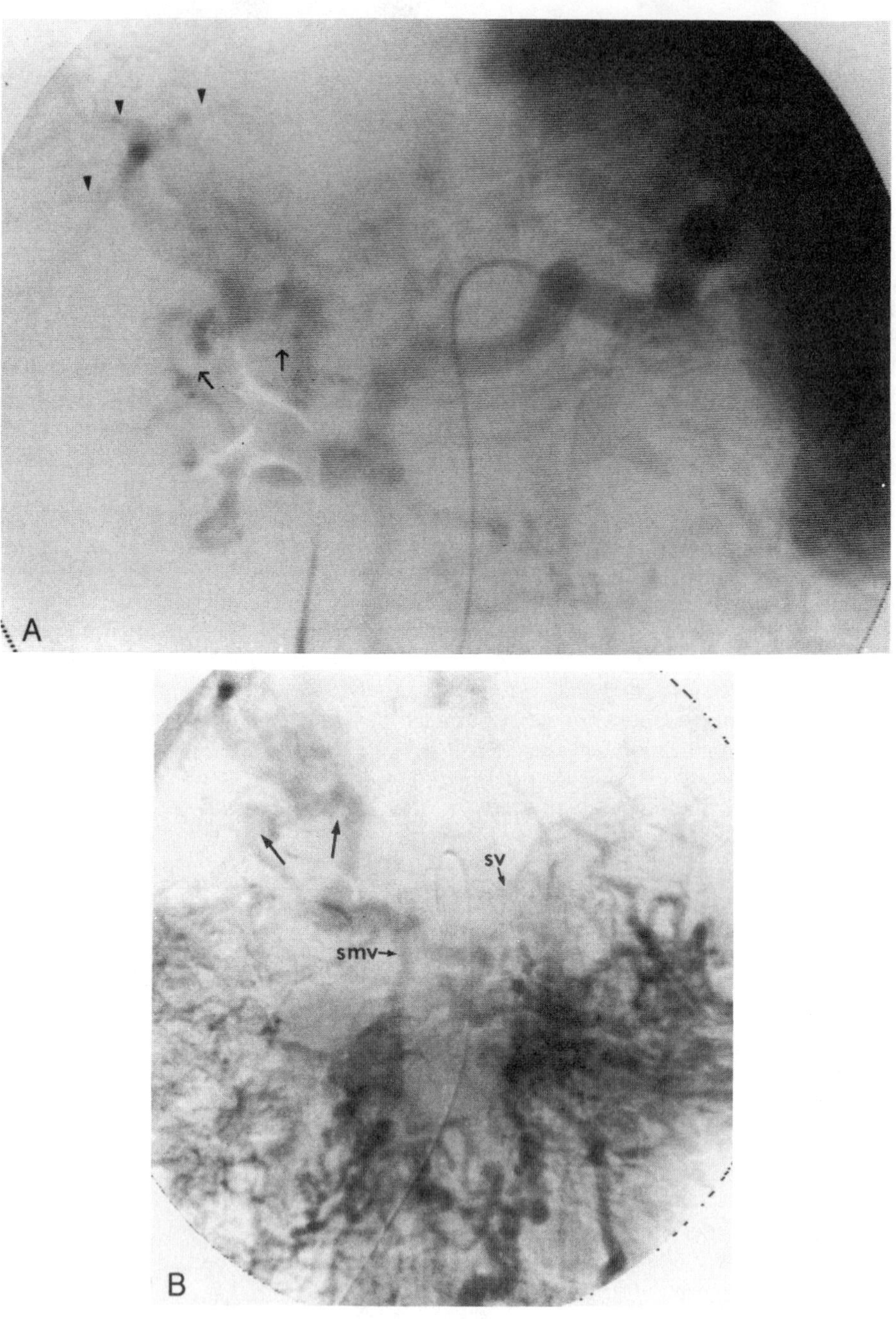

FIGURE 10 An arterial portography angiography (digital subtraction technique) in a 12-year-old girl who has idiopathic portal vein thrombosis and repeated gastrointestinal hemorrhages, in spite of numerous sessions of sclerotherapy. *A*, The venous phase of the splenic arterial injection shows opacification of a dilated splenic vein and reflux into the superior mesenteric vein. The portal vein is absent and is replaced by collateral channels (*arrows*), which most likely represent enlarged biliary veins connecting the superior mesenteric splenic vein confluence to the porta hepatis. Large coronary vein collaterals have been occluded by previous sclerotherapy, so collateral flow is now through many smaller vessels. The intrahepatic portal veins (*arrowheads*) are relatively normal. *B*, The venous phase of a high-volume contrast injection in the superior mesenteric artery shows tortuous dilated mesenteric veins and ultimate opacification of the peribiliary collaterals (cavernoma) (*arrows*). (smv = superior mesenteric vein; sv = splenic vein.)

normal, depending on the distal extent of the initial occlusive process. Portal blood flow is generally predominantly hepatopedal with idiopathic portal vein obstruction; there is some collateral flow to gastroesophageal veins.

Liver Transplantation

Angiography becomes necessary when noninvasive imaging modalities fail to unequivocally define the hepatic artery, portal vein, or caval anatomy before and after liver transplantation. Prior to transplantation, angiography is most frequently performed when the integrity or size of the portal vein is in question.[34,35] Angiographic demonstration of the portal vein is carried out in the same manner as in the investigation of portal hypertension (Figs. 11 and 12). Usually, superior mesenteric arteriography with an intra-arterial vasodilator will adequately demonstrate the portal vein, although some radiologists have resorted to direct splenoportography in patients with marked hepatofugal flow.[34]

Anomalies of the vascular anatomy may occur in as many as 25 percent of patients with biliary atresia, related to the association of this condition with abdominal heterotaxia and left isomerism.[35-39] Vascular anomalies include the absence of the hepatic segment of the inferior vena cava with azygous continuation, preduodenal portal vein, abdominal situs inversus or situs ambiguus with abnormal arborization of intrahepatic arteries and portal veins, separate drainage of the hepatic veins to the right atrium, common celiac-superior mesenteric arterial trunk, anomalous superior vena cava anatomy, polyspenia, and bowel malrotation.[35,39]

Following a portoenterostomy procedure, angiography frequently shows abnormal vascularity in the region of the porta hepatis. Prominent vascular collaterals may obscure the opacification of the portal vein during the venous phase of a superior mesenteric arteriogram. Hypoplasia of the portal vein has been found in children with biliary atresia (Fig. 12).[35,39] Absence of the hepatic artery and hypoplastic portal vein has been described in patients with arteriohepatic dysplasia.[35,39]

The use of angiography after liver transplantation is required if a sonographic or Doppler, study of liver ischemia, performed in the clinical setting, is abnormal or inconclusive,[35] if CT scanning or sonography demonstrates focal areas of inhomogeneity of the liver parenchyma,[40] and if there is severe gastrointestinal bleeding. Abnormal angiographic findings reported following liver transplantation include stenosis or occlusion of the hepatic artery, hepatic arteriovenous fistula or false aneurysm secondary to liver biopsy (Fig. 12*B*), bleeding from other adjacent abdominal vessels, stenosis or occlusion of the inferior vena cava, generally at the infrahepatic or suprahepatic anastomotic site, portal vein thrombosis, and splenic vein occlusion.[34,41]

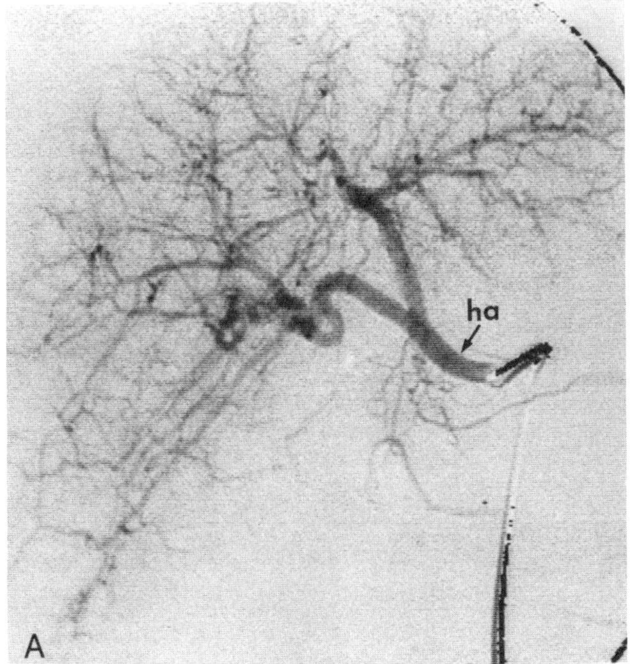

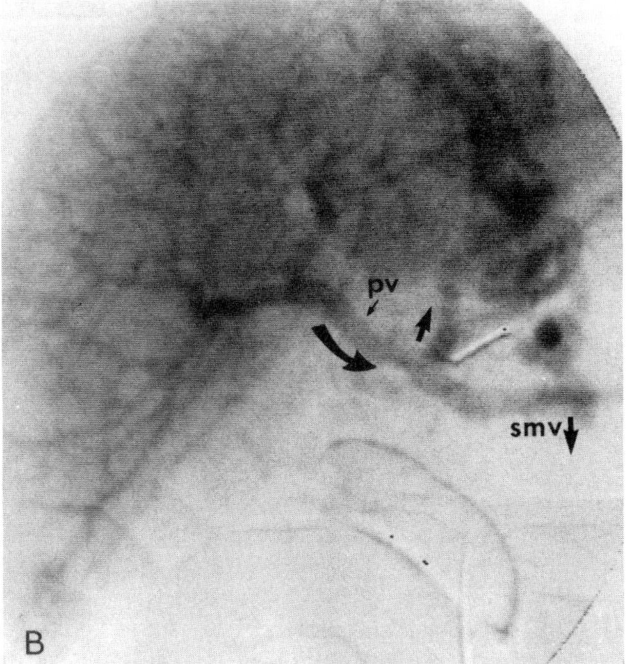

FIGURE 11 Angiography prior to liver transplantation (digital subtraction technique) in a 2-year-old with biliary atresia, cirrhosis, and previous attempted portoenterostomy. CT scans showed a spontaneous low-density area in the right lobe consistent with infarction. *A*, Hepatic arteriography. There is dilatation of the peripheral hepatic artery branches, except for a relatively avascular area in the right posteroinferior segment. *B*, On the late phase of the hepatic arteriogram, arterioportal shunting with marked hepatofugal flow (*curved arrow*) produces opacification of a small portal vein and collateral flow through the coronary vein (*upward-pointing arrow*) and superior mesenteric vein (*downward-pointing arrow*). Note the avascular area in the posteroinferior segment. (ha = hepatic artery; pv = portal vein; smv = superior mesenteric vein.)

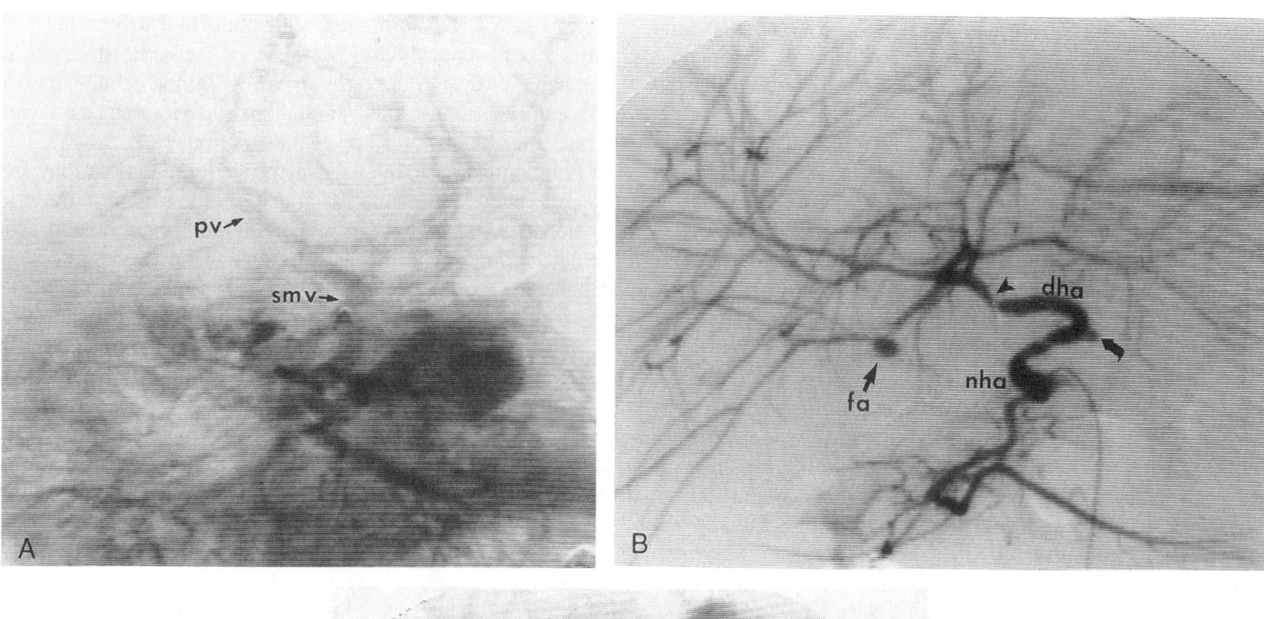

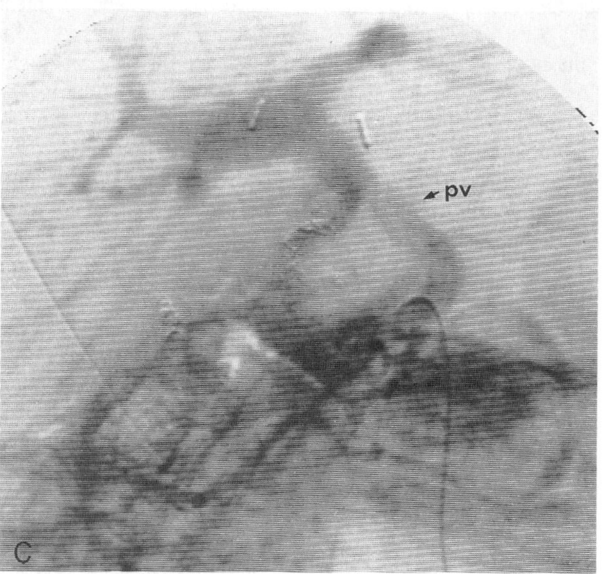

FIGURE 12 Angiography before and after liver transplantation in a 2-year-old girl with biliary atresia. The child developed significant gastrointestinal bleeding several days following surgery. *A*, The pretransplantation arterial portography was done because the portal vein could not be identified with certainty on sonographic examination. The venous phase of the postvasodilator superior mesenteric arterial contrast injection shows a patent but small portal vein with poor intrahepatic portal flow and extensive abdominal-wall collaterals. *B*, Hepatic angiography following liver transplantation shows a false aneurysm (fa) from the anteroinferior segmental branch, presumably secondary to percutaneous needle biopsy. Note the pseudostenosis caused by the surgical clip (*arrowhead*), which is superimposed on the hepatic artery and the ligated stump (*curved arrow*) of the donor gastroduodenal artery. *C*, The venous phase of the superior mesenteric arteriogram demonstrates patency of the portal vein. The surgical anastomosis had been augmented with an allograft venous patch. (dha = donor hepatic artery; fa = false aneurysm, nha = native hepatic artery; pv = portal vein; smv = superior mesenteric vein.)

Hepatic artery stenosis or occlusion may be related to the surgical technique when the problem occurs at the clamp (Fig. 13) or anastomotic (Fig. 14) sites. Obstruction occurs most frequently at sites of anastomosis between vessels of different size. Collaterals into the intrahepatic arteries have appeared within 6 weeks after hepatic artery thrombosis.[41]

The angiographic findings for some patients with allograft rejection include diffuse irregular narrowing of the hepatic artery, multiple areas of stenosis, decreased size of intrahepatic branches, and slow hepatic artery flow (Fig. 15).

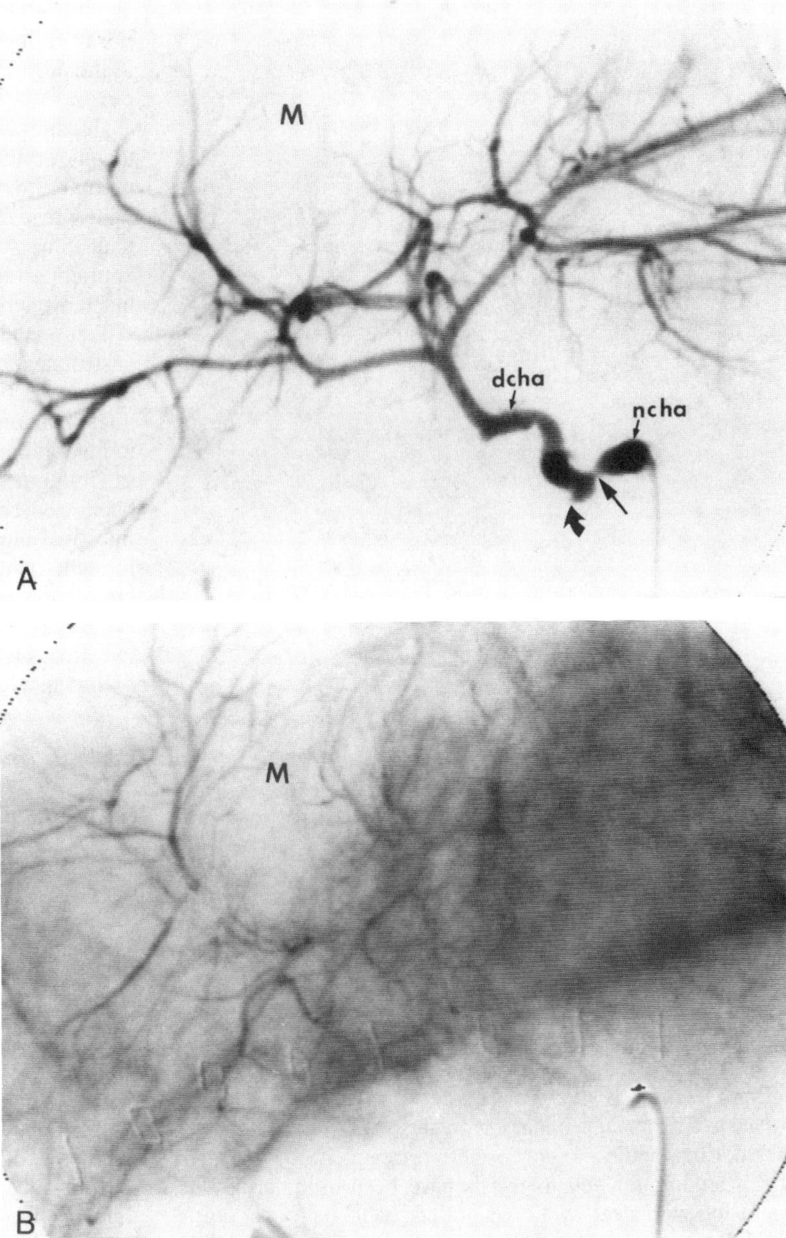

FIGURE 13 Hepatic-artery stenosis 3 weeks after liver transplantation. Hepatic enzymes were elevated and sonography showed a focal intrahepatic collection. *A* and *B*, The hepatic arteriogram (digital subtraction technique) shows the stenosis (*straight arrow*) proximal to the ligated native gastroduodenal artery (*curved arrow*), probably at a vascular clamp site. Note the avascular mass involving the right superior lobe. (dcha = donor common hepatic artery; M = mass; ncha = native common hepatic artery.)

Cardella[34] noted in some patients with chronic rejection a railroad-tracking pattern of vessels in the portal triad caused by hepatic artery–to–portal vein shunting.

Transcatheter interventional techniques used in the treatment of complications following liver transplantation have been described infrequently. Zajko et al[41] have used balloon angioplasty to relieve hepatic artery stenosis with partial success. Bleeding vessels have been embolized with gelatin sponge (Gelfoam).[34] The usefulness of thrombolytic agents in hepatic artery thrombosis has not been determined.

ROLE OF ANGIOGRAPHY IN TREATMENT

Vascular Interventional Techniques

Embolization

Transcatheter embolization techniques have been used to treat children with liver hemangiomas associated with congestive heart failure,[42–45] traumatic hemobilia (Fig. 16),[46] extrahepatic gastrointestinal bleeding,[47] and rarely malignant hepatic tumors.[48]

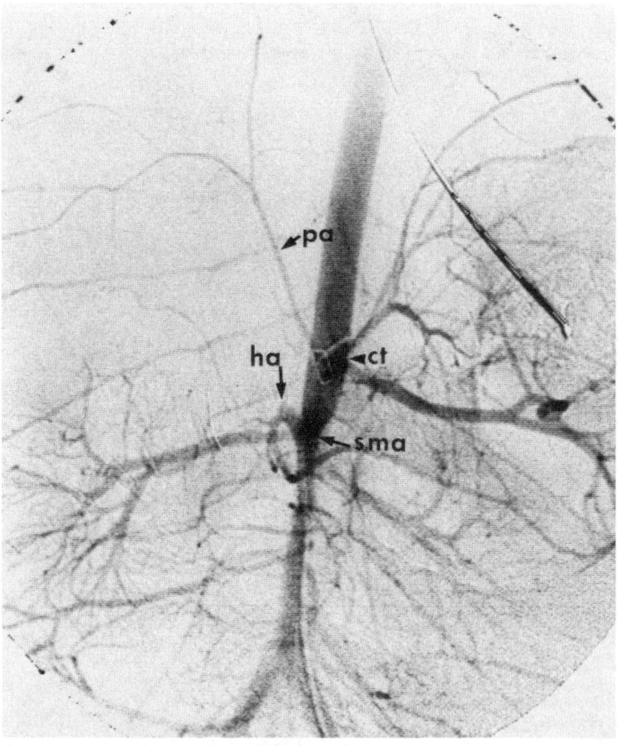

FIGURE 14 Hepatic arterial thrombosis 1 week after liver transplantation. The native hepatic artery arose from the superior mesenteric artery. An aortogram (digital subtraction technique) shows a stump arising from the proximal superior mesenteric artery but no flow into the liver. Hepatic arterial occlusion was confirmed with a selective superior mesenteric artery injection and at reoperation. (ct = celiac trunk; ha = hepatic artery; pa = phrenic artery; sma = superior mesenteric artery.)

Embolization of the hepatic arteries effectively controls congestive heart failure in some infants with liver hemangiomas not responding to corticosteroid treatment.[43–45] A variety of techniques and materials have been used: proximal occlusion with steel-wire coils or detachable balloons, polyvinyl alcohol particles, Gelfoam particles, and tissue adhesives. Proximal occlusion of the hepatic arteries theoretically has the disadvantage of permitting rapid revascularization through collaterals, but appears, from a small number of published cases,[43,45] to be as effective as hepatic artery ligation or particle embolization. Particle embolization theoretically permits more selective embolization of peripheral vessels supplying the lesions but carries a higher risk of complications, such as embolization of the pulmonary circulation, hepatic necrosis, gallbladder infarction, pancreatitis, and gastric or duodenal ulceration. Hepatic artery embolization may be ineffective in patients with diffuse hemangiomas who have extensive collateral supply to the liver from the adjacent abdominal wall, retroperitoneal, and bowel vessels. Little is currently known about the incidence of portal vein supply to these lesions. In a small number of patients at HSC, hepatic artery embolization of liver hemangiomas with extensive portal vein supply has been ineffective or has resulted in hepatic necrosis. If hepatic artery embolization is undertaken, it should be performed before the patient is moribund because portal vein perfusion may be inadequate to support the liver in the presence of systemic hypotension and reduced cardiac output.[45]

Hepatic artery embolization has become a widely used technique in the therapy of adult patients with inoperable primary or metastatic liver tumors.[49–51] No similar widespread experience is available for the treatment of malignant tumors in children although Ogita et al[48] reported encouraging results in two infants with mesenchymal hepatoblastoma who underwent chemoembolization.

Transcatheter techniques may be useful in the control of gastrointestinal hemorrhage.[5–7] We and others[46,47] have used embolization infrequently in the treatment of upper gastrointestinal hemorrhage, including gastric ulcers and traumatic hemobilia. In general, resorbable embolic material such as Gelfoam fragments are preferred. Embolization has also been used occasionally to treat children with lower gastrointestinal bleeding,[52,53] although embolization carries a significant risk of perforation because of the poor collateral circulation in the bowel. We have successfully used intra-arterial infusion of vasopressors to control lower gastrointestinal bleeding, usually in older children with advanced malignancy.

Balloon Angioplasty

Balloon angioplasty is infrequently used in the gastrointestinal vasculature of children. It may be required for superior mesenteric or celiac arterial stenosis caused by vasculitis, such as Takayasu's arteritis and hepatic arterial stenosis following liver transplantation.[41,54]

TRANSJUGULAR LIVER BIOPSY

A technique for biopsy of the liver through the internal jugular vein has been developed in adult patients for use when percutaneous needle biopsy is contraindicated, especially in the presence of noncorrectable coagulopathy.[55] The procedure involves cannulation of the internal jugular vein with a preshaped catheter. The catheter is advanced through the heart into the inferior vena cava; then pressure measurements in the inferior vena cava and hepatic vein, free and wedge positions, are taken. The catheter is then positioned in one of the hepatic veins, and a curved metal biopsy needle is passed beyond the tip of the venous catheter into the liver parenchyma. Any resulting parenchymal bleeding thus flows into the hepatic veins rather than into the peritoneal cavity. This technique makes available histologic information about patients in whom biopsy would otherwise be avoided. Other advantages of the technique include the availability of pressure measurements for the assessment of portal hypertension and the possibility of examination of the hepatic veins with contrast injections. Complications include bleeding at the puncture site, perforation of the inferior vena cava or heart, and hemoperitoneum. Clinically significant bleeding following biopsy occurs in approximately 0.35 percent of patients. The relatively large size of the system presently in use at this hospital (9 F) does not constitute a contraindication for use

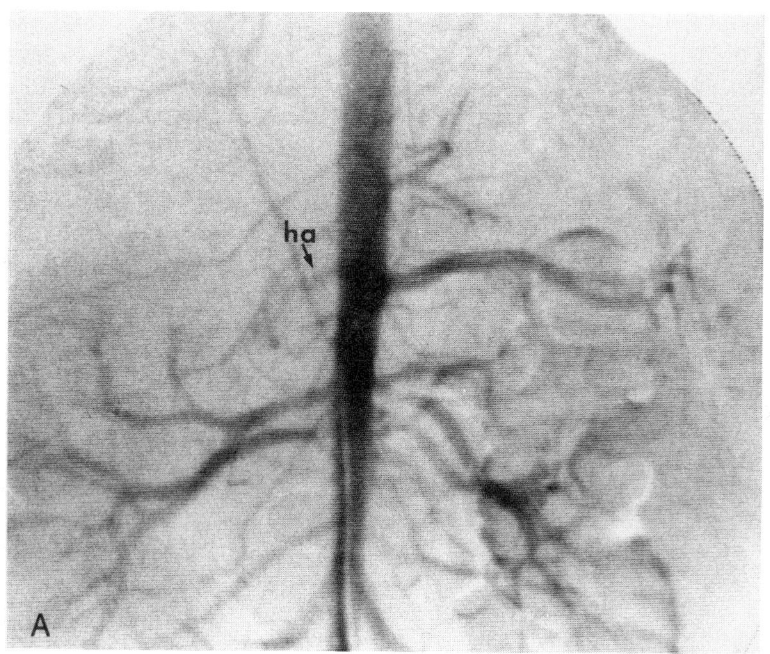

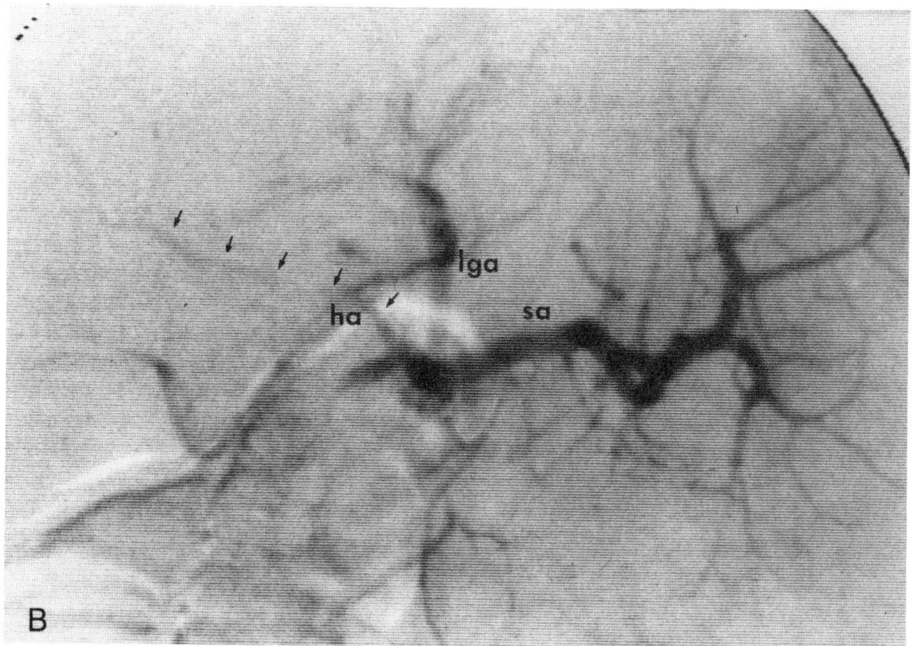

FIGURE 15 Severe allograft rejection. This 18-month-old received the liver of a newborn infant 2 weeks previously. Liver enzymes were elevated and biopsy findings suggested ischemia. On subsequent removal of the liver, the histology was consistent with severe rejection. *A*, The aortogram (digital subtraction technique) shows filling of the proximal hepatic artery but no flow toward the liver. *B*, Selective celiac angiography (oblique digital subtraction technique) demonstrates extremely slow flow in a small irregular allograft hepatic artery (*arrows*); these findings were consistent with rejection. (ha = hepatic artery; lga = left gastric artery; sa = splenic artery.)

in children. We have used this technique in patients who weigh as little as 14 kg and find the information provided for selected patients to be extremely useful. Although this procedure can be performed with sedation and local anesthesia, general anesthesia is commonly used for children.

SUMMARY

The role of angiography in the investigation and treatment of pediatric gastrointestinal disease has changed significantly in the past 10 to 15 years. In the presurgical investigation

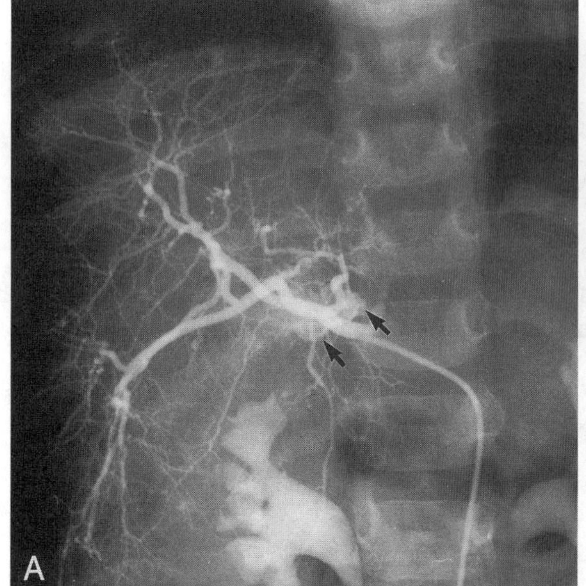

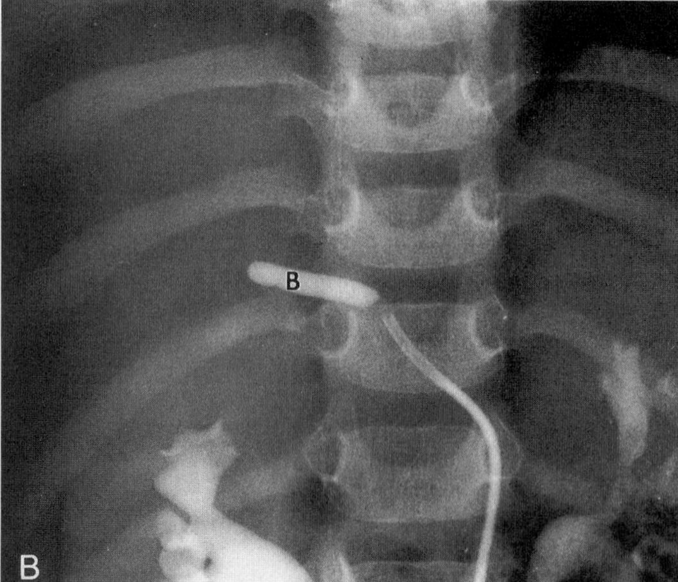

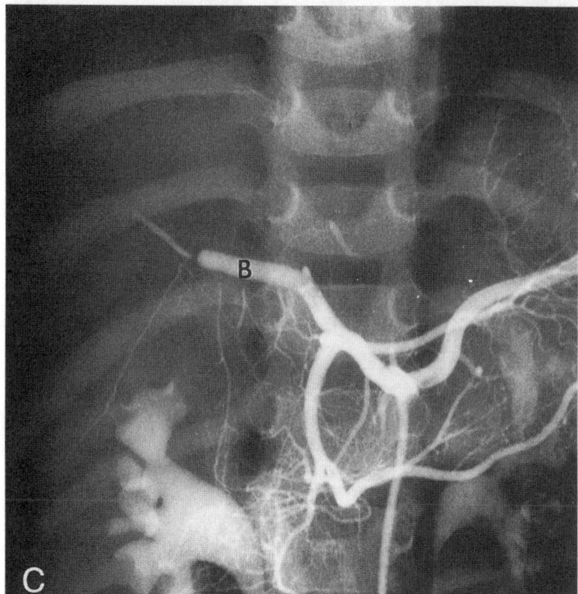

FIGURE 16 Transcatheter hepatic artery embolization for the treatment of traumatic hemobilia. *A*, Pre-embolization proper hepatic arteriography in a 4-year-old with severe hemobilia following closed abdominal trauma. There is extravasation of contrast material from the bifurcation of the proper hepatic artery (*arrows*). *B*, A contrast-filled silicone balloon (4-mm inflated diameter) has been detached in the hepatic artery. *C*, The hepatic arteriogram following embolization shows occlusion of the distal proper hepatic artery. There is some opacification of the hepatic artery distal to the balloon through small collaterals from the gastroduodenal artery. The hemobilia was controlled, and there were no hepatic ischemic complications. (B = detached balloon.)

of tumors, improved cross-sectional and Doppler imaging has made angiographic investigation only infrequently necessary. Angiography remains the gold standard for the delineation of vascular anatomy before and after liver transplantation and portacaval shunt surgery, but it is reserved for patients for whom noninvasive imaging has demonstrated an abnormality or is inconclusive. Constant improvements in the materials and techniques of interventional vascular procedures make this a developing area in pediatric gastrointestinal disease.

REFERENCES

1. Angiographic procedure. In: Stanley P, ed. Pediatric angiography. Baltimore: Williams & Wilkins, 1982: 1.
2. Stanley P, ed. Celiac axis arteriography. In: Pediatric angiography. Baltimore: Williams & Wilkins, 1982: 179.
3. Bron KM. Arterial portography. In: Abrams HL, ed. Abrams angiography: vascular and interventional radiology. 3rd ed, vol. 2. Boston: Little, Brown, 1983: 1605.
4. Rösch J, Keller FS, Wawrukiewicz AS, Krippaehne WW, Dotter CT. Pharmacoangiography in the diagnosis of recurrent massive lower gastrointestinal bleeding. Radiology 1982; 145:615–619.
5. Gastrointestinal bleeding. In: Reuter SR, Redman HC, Cho KJ, eds. Gastrointestinal angiography. 3rd ed. Philadelphia: WB Saunders, 1986: 282.
6. Ring EJ, Oleaga JA, Baum S. Current status of angiographic techniques in the management of gastrointestinal bleeding. J Clin Gastroenterol 1980; 2:99–103.
7. Gomes AS, Lois JF, McCoy RD. Angiographic treatment of gastrointestinal hemorrhage: comparison of vasopressin infusion and embolization. AJR 1986; 146:1031–1037.
8. Wessel DL, Keane JF, Fellows KE, Robichaud H, Lock JE. Fibrinolytic therapy for femoral arterial thrombosis after cardiac catheterization in infants and children. Am J Cardiol 1986; 58:347–351.
9. Tonkin IL, Wrenn EL Jr, Hollabaugh RS. The continued value of

angiography in planning surgical resection of benign and malignant hepatic tumors in children. Pediatr Radiol 1988; 18:35–44.
10. Vascular anatomy. In: Reuter SR, Redman HC, Cho KJ, eds. Gastrointestinal angiography. 3rd ed. Philadelphia: WB Saunders, 1986: 32.
11. Goldsmith NA, Woodburne RT. The surgical anatomy pertaining to liver resection. Surg Gynecol Obstet 1957; 105:310–318.
12. Freeny PC. Angiography of hepatic neoplasms. Semin Roentgenol 1983; 18:114–122.
13. Moss AA, Clark RE, Palubinskas AJ, De Lorimier AA. Angiographic appearance of benign and malignant hepatic tumors in infants and children. AJR 1971; 113:61–69.
14. Novy S, Wallace S, Medellin H, McBride C. Angiographic evaluation of primary malignant hepatocellular tumors in children. AJR 1974; 120:353–360.
15. Winograd J, Palubinskas AJ. Arterial-portal venous shunting in cavernous hemangiomas of the liver. Radiology 1977; 122:331–332.
16. Braun P, Ducharme JC, Riopelle JL, Davignon A. Hemangiomatosis of the liver in infants. J Pediatr Surg 1975; 10:121–126.
17. Slovis TL, Berdon WE, Haller JO, Casarella WJ, Baker DH. Hemangiomas of the liver in infants. Review of diagnosis, treatment and course. AJR 1975; 123:791–801.
18. Stanley P, Gates GF, Eto RT, Miller SW. Hepatic cavernous hemangiomas and hemangioendotheliomas in infancy. AJR 1977; 129:317–321.
19. McLean RH, Moller JH, Warwick WJ, Satran L, Lucas RV Jr. Multinodular hemangiomatosis of the liver in infancy. Pediatrics 1972; 49:563–573.
20. Dachman AH, Lichtenstein JE, Friedman AC, Hartman DS. Infantile hemangioendothelioma of the liver: a radiologic-pathologic-clinical correlation. AJR 1983; 140:1091–1096.
21. Leonidas JC, Strauss L, Beck AR. Vascular tumors of the liver in newborns. Am J Dis Child 1973; 125:507–510.
22. Pantoja E. Angiography in liver hemangioma. AJR 1968; 104:874–879.
23. Abrams RM, Beranbaum ER, Santos JS, Lipson J. Angiographic features of cavernous hemangioma of liver. Radiology 1969; 92:308–312.
24. Adler J, Goodgold M, Mitty H, Gordon D, Kinkhabwala M. Arteriovenous shunts involving the liver. Radiology 1978; 129:315–322.
25. Helikson MA, Shapiro DL, Seashore JH. Hepatoportal arteriovenous fistula and portal hypertension in an infant. Pediatrics 1977; 60:921–923.
26. Falk H, Herbert JT, Edmonds L, Heath CW Jr. Review of four cases of childhood hepatic angiosarcoma: elevated environmental arsenic exposure in one case. Cancer 1981; 47:382–391.
27. Kirchner SG, Heller RM, Kasselberg AG, Greene HL. Infantile hepatic hemangioendothelioma with subsequent malignant degeneration. Pediatr Radiol 1981; 11:42–45.
28. Markowitz RI, Harcke HT, Ritchie WG, Huff DS. Focal nodular hyperplasia of the liver in a child with sickle cell anemia. AJR 1980; 134:594–597.
29. Goldstein HM, Neiman HL, Mena E, Bookstein JJ, Appelman HD. Angiographic findings in benign liver cell tumors. Radiology 1974; 110:339–343.
30. Casarella WJ, Knowles DM, Wolff M, Johnson PM. Focal nodular hyperplasia and liver cell adenoma: radiologic and pathologic with differentiation. AJR 1978; 131:393–402.
31. Wendth AJ, Shamoun J, Pantoja E, Luther P, Frede T. Cystic hamartoma of the liver in a pediatric patient. Angiographic findings. Radiology 1974; 12:440.
32. Portal hypertension. In: Stanley P, ed. Pediatric angiography. Baltimore: Williams & Wilkins, 1982: 221.
33. Cirrhosis and portal hypertension. In: Reuter SR, Redman HC, Cho KJ, eds. Gastrointestinal angiography. 3rd ed. Philadelphia: WB Saunders, 1986: 382.
34. Cardella JF, Castaneda-Zuniga WR, Hunter D, Young A, Amplatz K. Angiographic and interventional radiologic considerations in liver transplantation. AJR 1986; 146:143–153.
35. Taylor KJ, Morse SS, Weltin GG, Riely CA, Flye MW. Liver transplant recipients: portable duplex US with correlative angiography. Radiology 1986; 159:357–363.
36. Teichberg S, Markowitz J, Silverberg M, et al. Abnormal cilia in a child with the polysplenia syndrome and extrahepatic biliary atresia. J Pediatr 1982; 100:399–401.
37. Lilly JR, Starzl TE. Liver transplantation in children with biliary atresia and vascular anomalies. J Pediatr Surg 1974; 9:707–714.
38. Starzl TE, Koep LJ, Halgrimson CG, et al. Fifteen years of clinical liver transplantation. Gastroenterology 1979; 77:375–388.
39. Starzl TE, Putnam CW. Experience in Hepatic Transplantation. Philadelphia: WB Saunders, 1969.
40. Segel MC, Zajko AB, Bowen A, et al. Hepatic artery thrombosis after liver transplantation: radiologic evaluation. AJR 1986; 146:137–141.
41. Zajko AB, Bron KM, Starzl TE, et al. Angiography of liver transplantation patients. Radiology 1985; 157:305–311.
42. Tegtmeyer CJ, Smith TH, Shaw A, Barwick KW, Kattwinkel J. Renal infarction: a complication of Gelfoam embolization of a hemangioendothelioma of the liver. AJR 1977; 128:305–307.
43. Kaufman SL, Kumar AAJ, Roland JMA, et al. Transcatheter embolization in the management of congenital arteriovenous malformations. Radiology 1980; 137:21–29.
44. Stanley P, Grinnell VS, Stanton RE, Williams KO, Shore NA. Therapeutic embolization of infantile hepatic hemangiomas with polyvinyl alcohol. AJR 1983; 141:1047–1051.
45. Burrows PE, Rosenberg HC, Chuang HS. Diffuse hepatic hemangiomas: percutaneous transcatheter embolization with detachable silicone balloons. Radiology 1985; 156:85–88.
46. Walter JF, Passo BT, Cannon WB. Successful transcatheter embolic control of massive hemobilia secondary to liver biopsy. AJR 1976; 127:847–849.
47. Filston HC, Jackson DC, Johnsrude IS. Arteriographic embolization for control of recurrent severe gastric hemorrhage in a 10-year-old boy. J Pediatr Surg 1979; 14:276–281.
48. Ogita S, Tokiwa K, Taniguchi H, Takahashi T. Intraarterial chemotherapy with lipid contrast medium for hepatic malignancies in infants. Cancer 1977; 60:2886–2890.
49. Takayasu K, Shima Y, Muramatsu Y, et al. Hepatocellular carcinoma: treatment with intraarterial iodized oil with and without chemotherapeutic agents. Radiology 1987; 162:345–351.
50. Clouse ME, Lee RGL, Duszlak EJ, et al. Peripheral hepatic artery embolization for primary and secondary hepatic neoplasms. Radiology 1983; 147:407–411.
51. Carrasco CH, Chuang VP, Wallace S. Apudomas metastatic to the liver: treatment by hepatic artery embolization. Radiology 1983; 149:79–83.
52. Meyerovitz MF, Fellows KE. Angiography in gastrointestinal bleeding in children. AJR 1984; 143:837–840.
53. Meyerovitz MF, Fellows KE. Typhlitis: a cause of gastrointestinal hemorrhage in children. AJR 1984; 143:833–835.
54. Odurny A, Sniderman KW, Colapinto RF. Intestinal angina: percutaneous transluminal angioplasty of the celiac and superior mesenteric arteries. Radiology 1988; 167:59–62.
55. Colapinto RF. Transjugular biopsy of the liver. Clin Gastroenterol 1985; 14:451–467.

PART 8

Interventional Radiology

Peter Liu, M.D.
David A. Stringer, B.Sc., M.B.B.S., F.R.C.R., FRCPC

Interventional radiology has become firmly established in the armamentarium of pediatric radiology in the last decade. In this discussion, we review the general considerations, indications, contraindications, and techniques of percutaneous biopsy, aspiration, and drainage. We also consider the removal of esophageal foreign bodies, nonvascular dilatation of the gastrointestinal (GI) and biliary tracts, percutaneous gastrostomy and jejunostomy, and percutaneous transhepatic cholangiography.

GENERAL CONSIDERATIONS

Percutaneous interventional techniques can be performed safely and effectively in children.[1-7] To achieve both adequate patient care and a high level of success, close consultation between the radiologist and the referring physicians and surgeons is essential. The following overview is based on our experience at The Hospital for Sick Children (HSC), Toronto.[7]

Preprocedural Planning

Preprocedural planning is crucial. The radiologist visits the patient and parents the day before the examination to explain the procedure and to secure an informed consent. The patient's history, including drug, allergy, and bleeding histories is obtained, and his or her bleeding parameters, including prothrombin time (PT), partial thromboplastin time (PTT), platelets, and hemoglobin, are verified. The patient is given nothing by mouth for at least 4 hours before the procedure; for patients older than 5 years of age, for at least 8 hours. If a patient is likely to undergo both aspiration and drainage, we prefer to have an intravenous line established. Those with abscesses or fluid collections, of course, may already have an established intravenous line for supportive and antibiotic therapy.

Sedation

The amount of sedation must be adequate to ensure the immobility and co-operativeness of the child during the procedure without undue side effects such as respiratory depression. The sedation protocol we have used for interventional radiology procedures for the last 6 years is the same as that used for cardiac catheterization and angiography for over 20 years. Younger patients under 30 kg are given catheter mixture No. 3 (CM3), 0.1 ml per kilogram to a maximum dose of 2 ml, intramuscularly half an hour before the procedure. CM3 consists of 25 mg per milliliter of meperidine, 6.25 mg per milliliter of chlorpromazine, and 6.25 mg per milliliter of promethazine. Because of bradycardiac effect and respiratory depression, CM3 is not given to infants less than 3 months of age. For older patients, approximately 1 mg per kilogram of meperidine combined with 0.5 mg per kilogram of promethazine is administered intramuscularly one-half hour before the procedure. Local anesthetic is also used at most puncture sites. Intravenous diazepam is occasionally given when supplemental sedation is needed during a lengthier procedure. In some instances, a child may require general anesthesia to successfully complete the procedure. In a recent series, we used general anesthesia in 2 of 43 patients.[7]

Temperature Control

Maintaining body temperature is critical for small infants. Most hospital rooms, especially those in the radiology department, are relatively cool to ensure the proper functioning of sensitive equipment. Raising the ambient room temperature for the procedure and using radiant warmers and heating pads help maintain the patient's body temperature. In addition to these precautions, one center[1] also wrapped the patient's trunk with commercial plastic films (Saran Wrap, Steri-drape). Exact temperature control is less critical for the older patient whose body size is larger.

Nursing

The pediatric nurse from the radiology department provides support for the patients and their families and assists the radiologist with the procedures. He or she may be able to reinforce and further clarify the procedure and explanation given by the radiologist and thus allay the fears of the patient and the family in a stressful situation. The nurse is also in constant attendance to help monitor the vital signs and to assist with the various procedure trays.

Antibiotic Coverage

Patients with a possible abscess should be started on intravenous antibiotics to control probable bacterial growth before the interventional procedures are performed. The antibiotics can be started 1 hour before the intervention[8] and may then be altered following the Gram stain and bacterial culture reports.

Imaging Guidance Systems

Interventional procedures may be performed under fluoroscopic, sonographic, or computed tomographic (CT) guidance. The advantages and disadvantages of the various guidance systems are listed in Table 1.[9]

It is generally easier and faster to perform interventional procedures with real-time sonography rather than with CT. Although sonography is the major imaging modality used for most of our cases (Fig. 1), it is occasionally supplemented by fluoroscopy. For some lesions containing gas bubbles, such as abscesses, or lesions containing calcium, fluoroscopy alone may be used for guidance (Fig. 2). Biplane fluoroscopy is recommended unless the exact depth of the lesion from the skin surface is known beforehand, possibly from a cross-sectional study such as sonography or CT.

However, for most cases, fluoroscopy alone is insufficient. We perform the majority of cases in a fluoroscopic suite equipped with portable sonographic equipment so that the operator may gain immediate access to fluoroscopy, if it is needed, without moving the patient. Such access is especially important for patients with lesions in upper abdomen because it may be desirable to know the level of the diaphragm.

In order to perform a biopsy on lesions less than 2 cm in size, especially those located well below the skin's surface, a biopsy-guide attachment may be used with the sonographic transducer probe so that more exact control of the needle can be achieved. The biopsy guide is not usually needed for larger lesions, since the free-hand method has proved successful.[7] CT control is reserved for tiny lesions that cannot be delineated by sonography or that are difficult to reach (Fig. 3).

In the future, magnetic resonance imaging (MRI) control may be used in selected cases, but so far we have had no need for this technique because ferromagnetic materials cannot be used.

Access-Route Planning

The principles of access-route planning are similar to those for adults: intervening bowel loops and vessels and contamination of sterile spaces (such as the pleural or peritoneal cavity) must be avoided, and, if possible, an extraperitoneal approach, the shortest path, and the dependent drainage should be used.

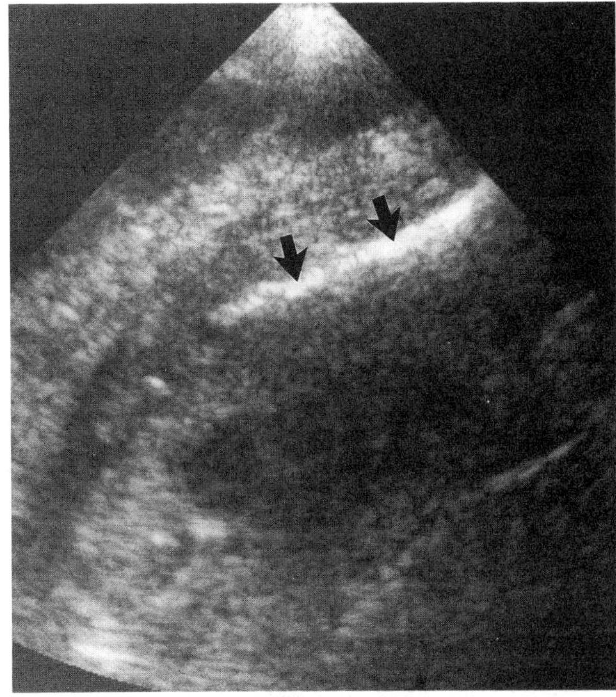

FIGURE 1 Five-year-old girl with right subphrenic collection. Sonography shows the catheter (*arrows*) in the echogenic collection.

A longer path to the target may be necessary to avoid certain structures. For example, to avoid the posterior pleural space, which extends down to the twelfth rib on the posterior midclavicular line, an angled cranial approach is often used to reach the lesions located high in the abdomen, such as some liver lesions. A direct, shortest-path approach in such a case may result in contamination of pleural space and pneumothorax (Fig. 4).[10]

Potential Complications

Any time a needle is introduced into a patient, there is a potential for injury to intra-abdominal organs, bowels, and vessels,[9,10] such as general sepsis, hemorrhage, bowel perforation, pneumothorax, and empyema (especially with any

TABLE 1
Advantages and Disadvantages of Guidance Systems

	Fluoroscopy	Sonography	Computed Tomography
Advantages	Availability Rapid localization Needle tip easy to identify Diaphragm easily seen	Rapid localization Flexible imaging Flexible patient positioning No radiation	Small lesions shown Needle tip easily seen Precise anatomic relationship revealed Precise target sampling No interference because of overlying bowel gas or bone
Disadvantages	Poor target visibility Radiation exposure	Needle difficult to see Limited anatomic information	Time-consuming Expensive Radiation exposure

Modified from Ferrucci et al.[9]

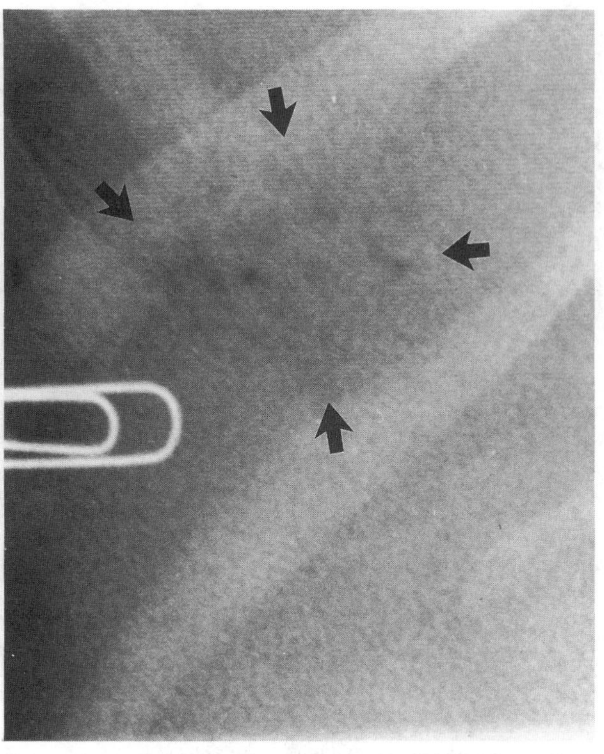

FIGURE 2 Seven-year-old boy with liver abscess following trauma. The abscess with gas bubble formation (*arrows*) was clearly shown on fluoroscopy and was used to guide the percutaneous puncture. (Paper clip was placed on patient's abdomen to locate lesion.)

transgression of the pleural cavity during drainage of subphrenic collections). Pancreatitis may occur with the biopsy of smaller pancreatic lesions.[11]

For percutaneous drainage, additional complications include the formation of sinus tracts and fistulas. During percutaneous biopsy, needle-tract dissemination of the tumor is also a possibility but is exceedingly rare with the smaller-gauge needle.[9,12]

SPECIFIC PROCEDURES

Percutaneous Biopsy

Indications and Contraindications

Percutaneous biopsy is performed for histologic identification of a solid mass.[1,2,7,13,14] The most common indications include the need to establish the diagnosis of an incurable tumor, documentation of metastatic or recurrent tumor, and staging for lymphoma. This procedure is especially valuable in children who are poor surgical risks. For a successful guided biopsy, the lesion must be accessible and should be detectable by an imaging modality.

The major contraindication to biopsy is a bleeding disorder. It should be corrected by the transfusion of appropriate clotting factors or platelets. Suspected echinococcal cysts are also a contraindication.[9,15]

Needle Selection

Depending on clinical circumstances, either small-bore (20- to 22-gauge) or large-bore (14- to 19-gauge) needles may be used for percutaneous biopsy. Some considerations in the needle selection include lesion size, access route, bleeding parameters, known primary malignancy, and the preference of the pathologist. The smaller-gauge needles tend to be safer because they may puncture the lumen of the bowel and vascular lesions with minimal risk, whereas the larger-gauge needles may cause complications. The larger-gauge needle usually yields more tissue specimen, enabling a more specific histologic diagnosis. The smaller-gauge needle may yield only enough tissue fragments for a cytologic study, the resulting tissue diagnosis may not be specific enough to formulate any meaningful conclusion about future therapy and treatment. Considerable expertise is needed for cytologic interpretation. It is wise to consult with the pathologist before the procedure is carried out to determine the amount of tissue sample needed.

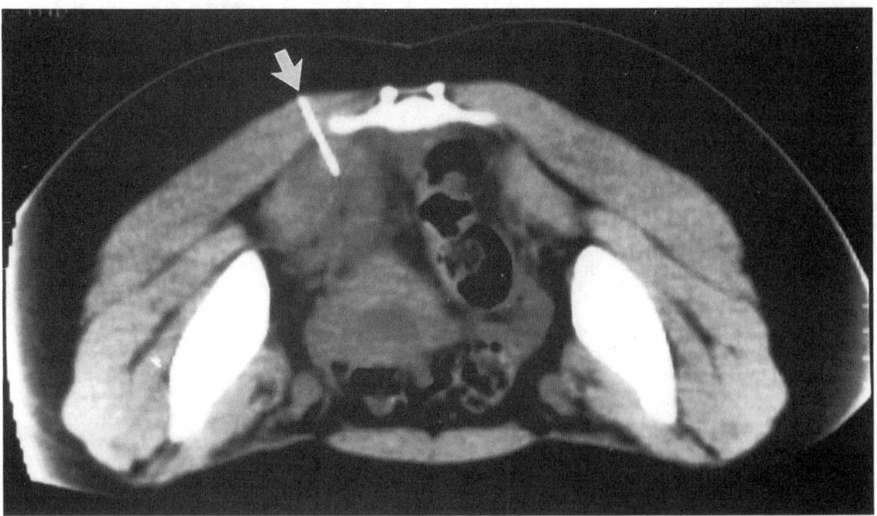

FIGURE 3 Thirteen-year-old girl with presacral inflammatory mass. Overlying bowel loops were avoided with CT guidance and a transgluteal approach. The patient was in a prone position for the biopsy. The white arrow indicates the biopsy needle.

Pediatric tumors are often small round cell tumors, such as lymphoma, rhabdomyosarcoma, Ewing's sarcoma, and neuroblastoma. To make a specific diagnosis such as Ewing's sarcoma rather than simply one such as a "round cell tumor," larger tissue samples are often needed for additional histologic analysis and staining. In contrast, adult tumors are often various types of carcinomas, which tend not to require as many cells to establish a pathologic diagnosis. Hence, in our hospital the pediatric pathologists prefer larger samples.

Because of its greater safety margin, multiple passes may be made with a thinner-gauge needle. In general, a minimum of three aspiration biopsies is recommended to ensure that adequate aspirates have been obtained for diagnosis. If a larger-gauge needle is used, one sample containing a significant piece of tissue from the lesion is usually sufficient, especially if thinner-gauge needles are used in the initial passes for localization and initial aspiration. No more than two passes should be made with larger-gauge needles because of the greater risk of bleeding.

Results

Our experience is similar to that of other centers[1,2,7,13,14]: The success rate of percutaneous biopsies is more than 90 percent in all series.

Percutaneous Aspiration and Drainage

Indications and Contraindications

The fluid collections that can be drained include abscess, hematoma, seroma, lymphocele, biloma, pancreatic pseudocyst, and loculated ascites.[9] The ideal conditions for draining fluid collections exist when they are unilocular and discrete, when they are in contact with the abdominal wall, and when they can be accessed extraperitoneally. Unfortunately, such ideal conditions are not always attainable; other common access routes include transperitoneal and transgluteal approaches. If necessary, transgastric and transhepatic approaches can also be used.

The major contraindications include the lack of an access route, frank peritonitis, uncontrolled coagulopathy, and echinococcal disease. Other contraindications include multiple or multilocular abscess, fungal abscess, necrotic infected tumor, and tiny collections.

Procedure

For most drainages, as in the case of percutaneous aspiration, an initial puncture with a 22-gauge spinal needle is made for localization. The initial puncture involves a minimal amount of aspiration to facilitate the subsequent placement of the catheter. An 18-gauge needle, placed in tandem beside the localizing needle, is used to make a second puncture, and the Seldinger technique (catheter over guide wire) is then employed to introduce an appropriately sized pigtail catheter.

The most commonly used pigtail catheters are 8.3 F and 10 F; we have found the prepackaged nephrostomy kit to be satisfactory. For pediatric patients, the dual-puncture Seldinger technique is safer because the collection is definitely identified before a large needle and catheter are introduced.

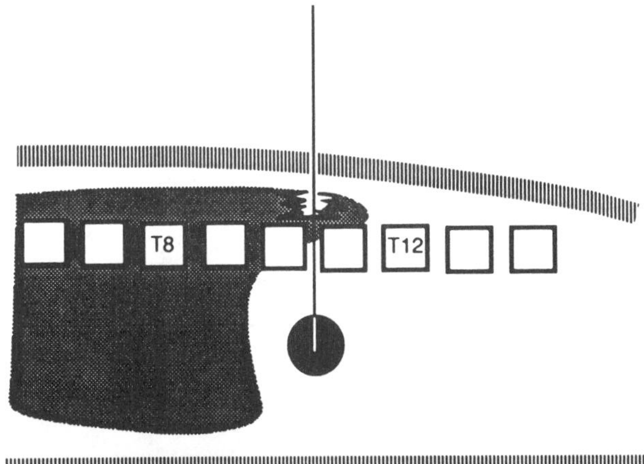

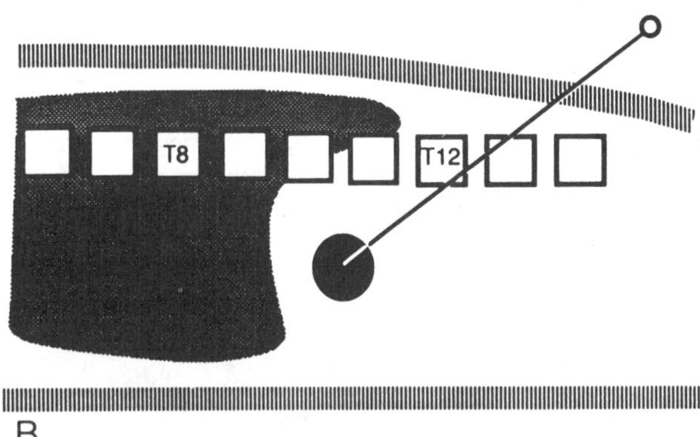

FIGURE 4 *A*, The most direct and shortest path to the lesion may result in contamination of pleural space and pneumothorax. *B*, An angled cranial approach avoids transgression of pleural space.

For large abdominal collections, especially those close to the abdominal wall, a single-puncture trocar technique may used be used because it is faster. However, the operator should be confident about reaching the lesion with the first and only pass before considering this method.

Postprocedural Care

After insertion, the catheter is connected to a Hemovac drain and irrigated at least twice daily with normal saline. As much of the fluid collection as possible is evacuated immediately after the placement of the catheter.

The radiologist's role should not end with the insertion of the catheter. Daily bedside rounds should be made and any catheter dysfunction evaluated and corrected, when necessary. Contrast studies may have to be performed to assess the catheter dysfunction. The radiologist should be continuously available for consultation after the procedure.

Typical responses to drainage include decreased fever, pain, and leukocytosis, decreasing amounts of drainage fluid, clear returns from irrigation, and decreased cavity size, as documented by the various imaging modalities.

Decisions about adjusting or removing the catheter should be made in conjunction with the clinicians. In most of the patients at HSC, the pigtail catheter was removed within 4 days (ranging from 1 to 7 days) of the percutaneous insertion. The major clinical improvement seems to be related to the initial decompression of the collection at the time of the procedure.

Hematomas and Pancreatic Pseudocysts

Pancreatic pseudocysts and hematomas are more difficult to treat than other fluid collections.[9,16-18] Pseudocysts often tend to recur if only simple aspiration and short-term drainage have been performed. An infected pseudocyst usually requires long-term drainage (over a 2-week period), and surgery is still required in up to one-third of the patients.[16] However, percutaneous drainage is useful as the initial therapy for symptomatic patients, because we have found that it results in a complete cure in most children; failing that, it is a useful temporizing measure to stabilize an ill patient before eventual surgery. On the other hand, percutaneous drainage is not useful if there are large blood clots because these are unlikely to drain even through large-caliber catheters. Furthermore, this lack of drainage may cause superimposed infection of the hematoma.[6] Therefore, catheter drainage of hematomas is not advisable.

Results and Current Status

Percutaneous drainage abscesses and fluid collection is now the treatment of choice for most patients; surgery is reserved for complex and difficult cases. Percutaneous drainage has been able to obviate surgery in more than 82 percent of the combined cases of seven published series.[1-7] The success rates of these various pediatric centers range from 78 to 92 percent. Percutaneous drainage has been described as "one of the major advances in modern abdominal surgery"[19] because it avoids the risks of general anesthesia and surgical operation, is better tolerated by patients, and results in financial savings to the consumer and the health care system.

Removal of Blunt Foreign Bodies from the Esophagus

Most swallowed foreign bodies are passed through the rectum without complications. Water may be given to hasten the passage of ingested foreign bodies impacted in the esophagus if no interventional treatment is desired.[20] Intravenous administration of glucagon to relax the gastroesophageal sphincter when the impaction occurs at the level of the distal esophagus has also been advocated.[21,22]

Endoscopy Versus Foley Balloon Catheter

If noninterventional methods fail or are not practical, there are currently two major methods of removing a blunt foreign body in the esophagus: (1) the traditional method, endoscopy[23] and (2) the more recent method, a Foley balloon catheter used under fluoroscopic control.[24-26] Good results have been obtained with both.

There is some controversy about which is the preferred approach. Proponents of endoscopy believe that it provides greater control of the patient's airway and thus reduces the risk of aspiration and airway obstruction during the procedure.[27,28] Endoscopy also reveals the presence of associated radiolucent foreign bodies.[29] Other large series[24-26] have shown the Foley catheter method to be equally successful without incurring any significant complication. Moreover, the Foley catheter method obviates the 1 percent complication rate of endoscopy and the risks of general anesthesia.

Contraindications and Precautions. The Foley catheter technique is reserved for blunt objects only; endoscopy should be used to remove a foreign body with sharp edges. Other contraindications to Foley catheter removal include the presence of the foreign body for longer than 72 hours, a full stomach, symptoms and signs suggestive of esophageal perforation, or the existence of an underlying esophageal disease or stricture. The last contraindication is relative, so a trial may be performed with extra care.

The Foley catheter method should be attempted only if a radiologist and a physician fully experienced in resuscitation and control of the airway are present in the fluoroscopic suite. All the appropriate equipment needed for the resuscitation and management of the airway obstruction should be immediately available in the room.

Procedure. A Foley catheter of appropriate length and size is usually inserted through the patient's mouth, although the nasal route has been used in some centers.[26] The patient is then placed in a semiprone oblique position, with the fluoroscopic table tilted head down by at least 15 degrees. Under fluoroscopic control, the tip of the Foley catheter is then passed beyond the impacted foreign body in the esophagus and the balloon inflated just distal to the foreign body (Fig. 5). Contrast agents are used to inflate the balloon so that it is visible fluoroscopically. The balloon should not be inflated any larger than the expected diameter of the esophagus.

With the balloon inflated, the catheter is pulled back until traction is felt when the balloon touches the foreign body. The catheter should be pulled back gently and quickly with one motion and the child immediately encouraged to cough out the foreign body from the hypopharynx. Blows with the heel of the hand to the back of the patient between the shoulder blades may also help in expelling the foreign body at this point. This is often the critical stage because, unless the foreign body is immediately removed from the pharynx, it may be swallowed back down the esophagus; worse, the foreign body may be aspirated into the airway, causing complete airway obstruction.

Other Methods of Removal

The Foley catheter method is especially useful for removing coins and other discoid objects. For removal of three-dimensional blunt foreign bodies, such as food boluses or hard spherical objects, especially in a patient with an underlying esophageal stricture, the basket extraction technique (similar to the popular bile stone basket extraction) has been advocated.[30] Magnetic techniques have also been used with metallic foreign bodies, but these require specialized equipment and are not widely used.[31]

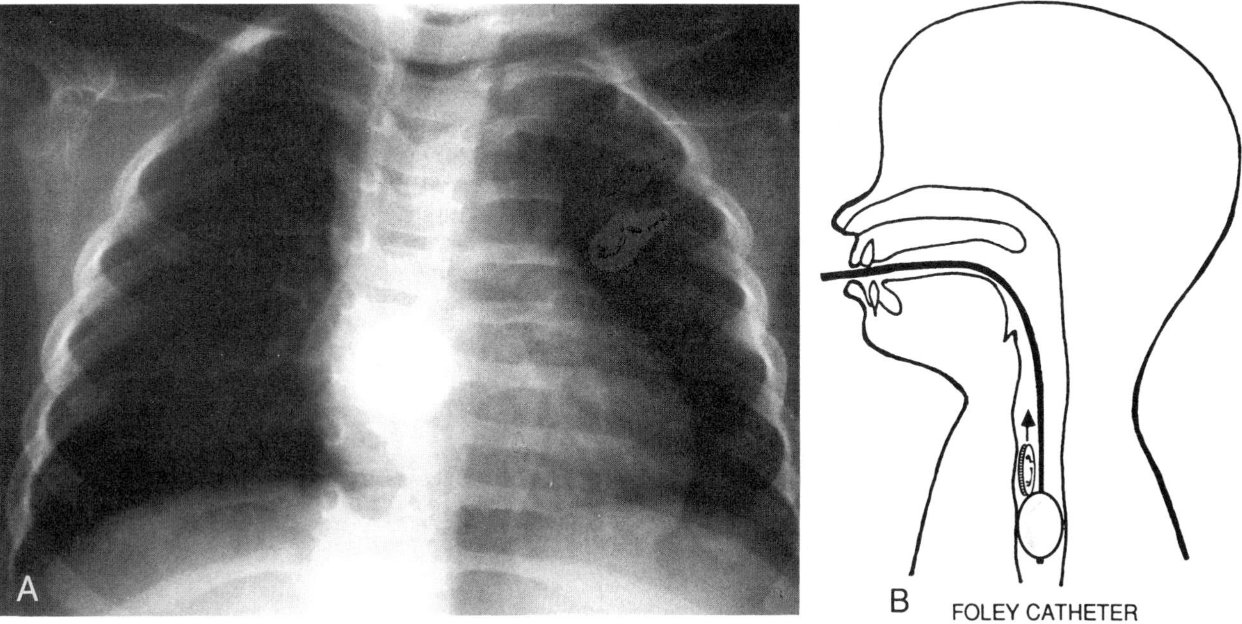

FIGURE 5 *A*, A plain chest radiograph reveals a swallowed penny in the distal esophagus. *B*, Schematic diagram showing the inflated balloon of the Foley catheter just distal to the penny. Successful removal of the penny was accomplished with the withdrawal of the Foley catheter.

Provided that proper precautions are taken, especially in the control of the airways, removing blunt foreign bodies in the esophagus with the Foley balloon catheter method would appear to be a viable alternative to endoscopy. There are currently excellent pediatric centers using either approach with success.

Nonvascular Stricture Dilatation

Recently, Gruntzig angioplasty balloon catheters have been used successfully to dilate esophageal, colonic, and biliary strictures.[32-39] At the present time, most of the reported experiences deal with the dilatation of esophageal strictures. Bougienage has traditionally been used to alleviate most of these strictures, but it carries a risk of perforation, as demonstrated in two adult series in which up to 8 percent of the patients suffered a perforation of the esophagus.[34,40] Although experience with the balloon catheter is less extensive to date, only a single case of esophageal perforation caused by balloon dilatation has been reported (it occurred in an adult who had a malignant stricture).[41]

The major indication for balloon catheter dilatation is a tight focal stricture of the esophagus. Its use is somewhat restricted by the size of the balloon. Gruntzig balloon catheters are available in balloon diameter sizes of 4 to 20 mm; the length varies from 4 to 15 cm. Strictures of a longer length (greater than 4 cm) are not as amenable to this balloon catheter technique because a sufficiently long balloon may not be available. In such cases, multiple sequential dilatation of a long stricture may be considered. If the stricture recurs, balloon dilatation may be repeated.

The principles of this balloon technique are simple but may be difficult to execute. A guide wire is initially passed across the stricture under fluoroscopic control. The balloon catheter is then advanced over the guide wire, and the balloon is positioned at the site of stricture. Inflation of this balloon results in a purely radial force against the narrowed segment, decreasing the risk to the patient (Fig. 6), unlike traditional bougienage, which transmits longitudinal and shearing forces and causes increased trauma to the esophagus and therefore increased risk of perforation.

Balloon catheter dilatation of GI strictures will most likely play an increasingly important role in the future.[42,43]

Percutaneous Gastrostomy and Gastrojejunostomy

When a patient requires enteric feeding, the traditional approach has been surgical gastrostomy, but this has a significant complication rate. A recent alternative, endoscopic-assisted gastrotomy,[44] also presents problems because it requires the service of a skilled endoscopist, it can be difficult to perform in patients with esophageal obstruction, and when performed in children it may require general anesthesia.

As a result, percutaneous gastrostomy and gastrojejunostomy have been rapidly gaining acceptance as methods of providing enteric alimentation in both children and adults.[45-53] These methods appear to be as effective as operative gastrostomy, are relatively simple to perform, avoid the risks of operative gastrostomy and general anesthesia, and appear to have fewer major complications than the operative method.

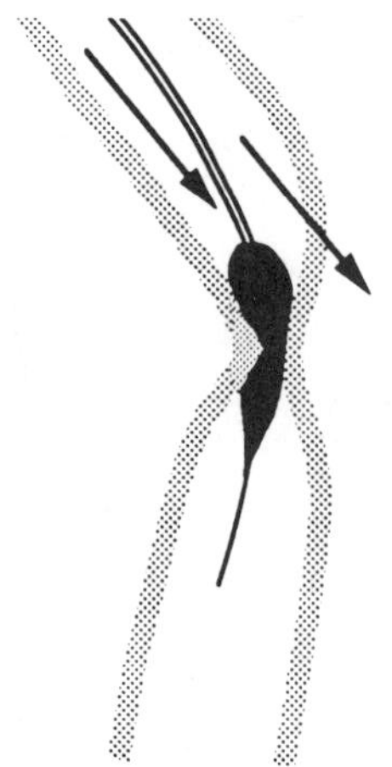

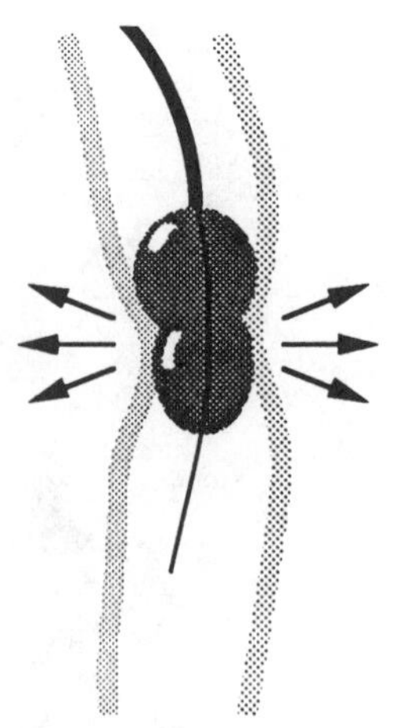

FIGURE 6 Traditional bougienage transmits longitudinal and shearing forces (*left*). Balloon dilatation results in a purely radial force against the narrowed segment, thus decreasing the risk of perforation (*right*).

Indications and Contraindications

The indications for gastrostomy are similar for both the surgical and percutaneous approaches. Gastrostomy is used to provide alimentation in patients with severe neurologic deficits from various causes, tumors of the head and neck, inability to swallow, and failure to thrive.

Contraindications to the percutaneous procedure include partial gastrectomy where there is a high gastric remnant above the costal junction, complete coverage of the gastric surface by the liver with no suitable access route, and ascites.

Procedure

Before the percutaneous procedure, the liver and colon are identified by sonography or CT to prevent inadvertent transgression. The lower edge of the left lobe of the liver is usually marked on the skin; any air in the bowel helps to localize the gut during fluoroscopy. A nasogastric tube is placed in the stomach so that air may be introduced for maximal gastric distention. Under aseptic conditions and local anesthesia, a needle is introduced into the body of the stomach, and its position is confirmed by the injection of a small amount of water-soluble contrast material. The Seldinger technique (catheter over guide wire) is used to place a catheter into the stomach or jejunum. The catheter is then well-secured to the skin to prevent its dislodgement. This retrograde approach to the introduction of the catheter is used with most percutaneous techniques, but the antegrade approach or placement has also been advocated.[49]

Enteric Alimentation

Enteric feeding may be started within 24 hours of the placement of the catheter, but the volume must be increased gradually. The amount is determined by consultation among the clinicians, the radiologist, and the clinical nutritional service.

Complications

Common findings after a percutaneous procedure include abdominal wall (33 percent) or gastric (17 percent) hematomas and pneumoperitoneum (56 percent). These tend to be self-limiting.[54] Pneumoperitoneum should be of concern only if it is increasing in size or is symptomatic. The presence of subcutaneous emphysema or free or loculated abdominal fluid collection should suggest possible complications.[54,55]

Peritoneal leakage with resulting peritonitis is an extremely serious complication of this percutaneous procedure. For this reason, the percutaneously introduced catheter is advanced to or beyond the duodenal jejunal flexure, making it difficult for the catheter to slip out. Within a short time (about 2 weeks), a fibrous tract is formed along the intraperitoneal portion of the catheter, preventing peritoneal leakage even if the catheter is dislodged. The reported complication rates for percutaneous procedures range from 0 to 4 percent, with peritonitis being the most common problem.[49] Since this finding compares favorably with the complication rates of 2 to 10 percent of surgical gastrostomies,[49] percutaneous gastrostomy and gastrojejunostomy will probably be the preferred approach in the near future.

Percutaneous Transhepatic Cholangiography

Indications and Contraindications

When an obstruction of the biliary tract is suspected in a child, the preferred screening modality is sonography. It either confirms or disproves the presence of biliary tract dilatation. It also shows the level of the obstruction and possibly its cause. In addition, sonography is noninvasive, does not involve ionizing radiation, and can be performed quickly and relatively inexpensively. In combination with CT, it can usually answer most clinical questions.

Percutaneous transhepatic cholangiography (PTC), which consists of the insertion of a needle through the liver into the biliary tract under radiologic guidance, is used when other techniques such as sonography have failed to solve a clinical problem.

PTC has a more limited role in pediatric than in adult cases. Its overall success rate in children is less than that in adults. In one study, only 50 percent of the cases were technically successful when normal-size intrahepatic ducts were present.[56] Furthermore, many pediatric patients require general anesthesia for this procedure. Endoscopic retrograde cholangiography (ERCP) is an alternative to PTC (see chapter on acute and chronic pancreatitis). However, PTC still has a role in selected cases because it can delineate the anatomy of the biliary tract clearly. It also helps to determine the patency of the biliary ducts if other results are equivocal.[57,58]

Although the use of a skinny needle (22-gauge or smaller) has significantly decreased the risk of bleeding, caution should still be taken in patients with bleeding disorders, and bleeding parameters should be corrected prior to the procedure if possible. Ascites, another relative contraindication, makes the procedure technically more difficult and also increases the risk of bleeding.

Procedure

Sonography is used first to find the porta, and its location is marked on the skin. Fluoroscopy is then used to locate the lowermost costovertebral angle, and its level is also marked on the skin. A 22-gauge 15-cm thin-walled needle is usually used. The puncture site is located on the lateral body wall in the midaxillary line or just anterior to it below the level of the costovertebral angle. A horizontal entry is made with the needle aimed at a point just superior to the porta. One quick thrust to the liver parenchyma is made to minimize any tearing of the liver tissue. Respiration is best suspended voluntarily or by the anesthetist at the time of the puncture. Once the point above the porta is reached, the stylet is taken out and water-soluble contrast material is injected as the needle is slowly withdrawn. When the bile ducts are opacified, appropriate spot films are obtained.

If the initial needle pass is unsuccessful, repeat passes may be made in a progressively caudal direction if care is taken to avoid the porta hepatis.[59] Up to six passes can probably be made safely in pediatric patients, although one survey from several adult centers suggests that as many as 12 to 14 passes may be made without significant complications.[60]

If the biliary ducts are obstructed and biliary drainage is needed, percutaneous biliary drainage may be done in the same session. Initially, a guide wire is introduced into the dilated biliary system, and the Seldinger technique is used to place the drainage catheter.

Complications

The incidence of serious complications seems to be low.[56-62] No complications were encountered in three of the larger pediatric series with a combined total of 30 patients.[56,58,61] In a large multi-institutional survey of predominantly adult patients (2,006 cases) treated with a fine, skinny needle (22-gauge or less), the incidence of serious complications was about 3.4 percent.[60] These complications include sepsis (1.4 percent), bile leakage (1.45 percent), intraperitoneal hemorrhage (0.35 percent), and death (0.2 percent). The incidence of pneumothorax was 0.1 percent (two patients), but neither patient required a chest tube.

PTC currently has a limited role in pediatrics. However, it still plays a role in selected cases because it can clearly delineate the anatomy of the biliary tract.

CONCLUSION

Many of the problems discussed here that have previously required surgery can now be satisfactorily dealt with by interventional radiology. However, a close rapport between the radiologist and the referring clinician is essential to ensure that these procedures are performed for the correct indications and are modified to suit the individual patient's problems.

REFERENCES

1. Towbin RB, Ball WS Jr. Pediatric interventional radiology. Radiol Clin North Am 1988; 26:419–440.
2. vanSonnenberg E, Wittich GR, Edwards DK, Casola G, Hilton SvW, Self TW, Keightley A, Withers C. Percutaneous diagnostic and therapeutic interventional radiologic procedures in children: experience in 100 patients. Radiology 1987; 162:601–605.
3. Towbin RB, Strife JL. Percutaneous aspiration, drainage, and biopsies in children. Radiology 1985; 157:81–85.
4. Diament MJ, Boechat MI, Kangarloo H. Interventional radiology in infants and children: clinical and technical aspects. Radiology 1985; 154:359–361.
5. Diament MJ, Stanley P, Kangarloo H, Donaldson JS. Percutaneous aspiration and catheter drainage of abscesses. J Pediatr 1986; 108:204–208.
6. Stanley P, Atkinson JB, Reid BS, Gilanz V. Percutaneous drainage of abdominal fluid collections in children. AJR 1984; 142:813–816.
7. Liu P, Daneman A, Stringer DA, Ein S. Percutaneous aspiration, drainage and biopsy in children. J Pediatr Surg 1989; 24:865–866..
8. Spies JB, Rosen RJ, Lebowitz AS. Antibiotic prophylaxis in vascular and interventional radiology: a rational approach. Radiology 1988; 166:381–387.
9. Ferrucci JT, Wittenberg J, Mueller PR, Simeone JF. Interventional radiology of the abdomen. 2nd ed. Baltimore: Williams and Wilkins, 1985.
10. Neff CC, Mueller PR, Ferrucci JT, Dawson SL, Wittenberg J, Simeone JF, Butch RJ, Papanicolaou N. Serious complications following transgression of the pleural space in drainage procedures. Radiology 1984; 152:335–341.
11. Mueller PR, Miketic LM, Simeone JF, Silverman SG, Saini S, Wittenberg J, Hahn PF, Steiner E, Forman BH. Severe acute pancreatitis after percutaneous biopsy of the pancreas. AJR 1988; 151:493–494.
12. Müller NL, Bergin CJ, Miller RR, Ostrow DN. Seeding of malignant cells into the needle track after lung and pleural biopsy. J Can Assoc Radiol 1986; 37:192–194.
13. Schaller RT Jr, Schaller JF, Buschmann C, Kiviat N. The usefulness of percutaneous fine-needle aspiration biopsy in infants and children. J Pediatr Surg 1983; 18:398–405.
14. Sabbah R, Ghandour M, Ali A, Lewall D. Tru-cut needle biopsy of abdominal tumors in children: a safe and diagnostic procedure. Cancer 1981; 47:2533–2535.
15. Bret PM, Fond A, Bretagnolle M, Valette PJ, Thiesse P, Lambert R, Labadie M. Percutaneous aspiration and drainage of hydatid cysts in the liver. Radiology 1988; 168:617–620.
16. Torres WE, Evert MB, Baumgartner BR, Bernadino ME. Percutaneous aspiration and drainage of pancreatic pseudocysts. AJR 1986; 147:1007–1009.
17. vanSonnenberg E, Wittich GR, Casola G, Stauffer AE, Polansky AD, Coons HG, Cabrera OA, Gerver PS. Complicated pancreatic inflammatory disease: diagnostic and therapeutic role of interventional radiology. Radiology 1985; 155:335–340.
18. Sacks D, Robinson ML. Transgastric percutaneous drainage of pancreatic pseudocysts. AJR 1988; 151:303–306.
19. Welch CE, Malt RA. Abdominal surgery (third of three parts). N Engl J Med 1983; 308:753–760.
20. Kushner DC, Cleveland RH. Removal of esophageal foreign bodies in childhood. In: Ferrucci JT, et al, eds. Interventional radiology of the abdomen. 2nd ed. Baltimore: Williams and Wilkins, 1985: 435.
21. Ferrucci JT, Long JA Jr. Radiologic treatment of esophageal food impaction using intravenous glucagon. Radiology 1977; 125:25–28.
22. Trenkner SW, Maglinte DDT, Lehman GA, Chernish SM, Miller RE,

Johnson CW. Esophageal food impaction: treatment with glucagon. Radiology 1983; 149:401–403.
23. Giordano A, Adams G, Boies L Jr, Meyerhoff W. Current management of esophageal foreign bodies. Arch Otolaryngol 1981; 107:249–251.
24. Campbell JB, Davis WS. Catheter technique for extraction of blunt esophageal foreign bodies. Radiology 1973; 108:438–440.
25. Campbell JB, Quattromani FL, Foley LC. Foley catheter removal of blunt esophageal foreign bodies. Experience with 100 consecutive children. Pediatr Radiol 1983; 13:116–119.
26. Rubin SA, Mueller DL. Removal of esophageal foreign bodies with a Foley balloon catheter under fluoroscopic control. Can Med Assoc J 1987; 137:125–127.
27. Healy GB. Removal of esophageal foreign bodies with a Foley catheter under fluoroscopic control. Can Med Assoc J 1988; 138:490.
28. Berdon WE. Editorial comment. Pediatr Radiol 1983; 13:119.
29. Stool SE, Deitch M. Potential danger of catheter removal of foreign body. Pediatrics 1973; 51:313–314.
30. Shaffer HA Jr, Alford BA, deLange EE, Meyer GA, McIlhenny J. Basket extraction of esophageal foreign bodies. AJR 1986; 147:1010–1013.
31. Volle E, Hanel D, Beyer P, Kaufmann HJ. Ingested foreign bodies: removal by magnet. Radiology 1986; 160:407–409.
32. Dawson SL, Mueller PR. Esophageal stricture dilatation. In: Ferrucci JT, et al, ed. Interventional radiology of the abdomen. 2nd ed. Baltimore: Williams and Wilkins, 1985: 429.
33. Maynar M, Guerra C, Reyes R, Major J, Garcia J, Facal P, Casteneda-Zuniga WR, Letourneau JG. Esophageal strictures: balloon dilatation. Radiology 1988; 167:703–706.
34. Sato Y, Frey EE, Smith WL, Pringle KC, Soper RT, Franken EA Jr. Balloon dilatation of esophageal stenosis in children. AJR 1988; 150:639–642.
35. Stringer DA, Pablot SM, Mancer K. Gruntzig angioplasty dilatation of an esophageal stricture in an infant. Pediatr Radiol 1985; 15:424–426.
36. Ball WS, Strife JL, Rosenkrantz J, Towbin RB, Noseworthy J. Esophageal strictures in children: treatment by balloon dilatation. Radiology 1984; 150:263–264.
37. Ball WS Jr, Seigel RS, Godlthorn JF, Kosloske AM. Colonic strictures in infants following intestinal ischemia: treatment by balloon catheter dilatation. Radiology 1983; 149:469–472.
38. Stringer DA. Gruntzig angioplasty balloon catheters in the treatment of bile duct stenosis. Ann Radiol 1984; 27:125–129.
39. Moore AV Jr, Illescas FF, Mills SR, Wertman DE, Heaston DK, Newman GE, Zuger JH, Salmon RB, Dunnick NR. Percutaneous dilatation of benign biliary strictures. Radiology 1987; 163:625–628.
40. Westdorp IC, Bartelsman JF, den Hartog Jager FC, Huibregtse K, Tytgat GN. Results of conservative treatment of benign esophageal strictures: a follow-up study in 100 patients. Gastroenterology 1982; 82:487–493.
41. LaBerge JM, Kerlan RK Jr, Pogany AC, Ring EJ. Esophageal rupture: complication of balloon dilatation. Radiology 1985; 157:156.
42. McLean GK, Cooper GS, Hartz WH, Burke DR, Meranze SG. Radiologically guided balloon dilatation of gastrointestinal strictures. Part I. Technique and factors influencing procedural success. Radiology 1987; 165:35–40.
43. McLean GK, Cooper GS, Hartz WH, Burke DR, Meranze SG. Radiologically guided balloon dilatation of gastrointestinal strictures. Part II. Results of long-term follow-up. Radiology 1987; 165:41–43.
44. Miller RE, Kummer BA, Tiszenkel HI, Kotler DP. Percutaneous endoscopic gastrostomy. Procedure of choice. Ann Surg 1986; 204:543–545.
45. vanSonnenberg E, Wittich GR, Brown LK, Tanenbaum LB, Campbell JB, Cubberley DA, Gibbs JF. Percutaneous gastrostomy and gastroenterostomy: 1. Techniques derived from laboratory evaluation. AJR 1986; 146:577–580.
46. vanSonnenberg E, Wittich GR, Cabrera OA, Quinn SF, Casola G, Lee AA, Princenthal RA, Lyons JW. Percutaneous gastrostomy and gastroenterostomy: 2. Clinical experience. AJR 1986; 146:581–586.
47. Wills JS, Oglesby JT. Percutaneous gastrostomy. Radiology 1983; 149:449–453.
48. Wills JS, Oglesby JT. Percutaneous gastrostomy: further experience. Radiology 1985; 154:71–74.
49. Towbin RB, Ball WS Jr, Bissett GS 3rd. Percutaneous gastrostomy and percutaneous gastrojejunostomy in children: antegrade approach. Radiology 1988; 168:473–476.
50. Ho CS. Percutaneous gastrostomy for jejunal feeding. Radiology 1983; 149:595–596.
51. Ho CS, Gray RR, Goldfinger M, Rosen IE, McPherson R. Percutaneous gastrostomy for enteral feeding. Radiology 1985; 156:349–351.
52. Keller MS, Lai S, Wagner DK. Percutaneous gastrostomy in a child. Radiology 1986; 160:261–262.
53. Gray RR, Ho CS, Yee A, Montanera W, Jones DP. Direct percutaneous jejunostomy. AJR 1987; 149:931–932.
54. Wojtowycz MM, Arata JA Jr, Micklos TJ, Miller FJ Jr. CT findings after uncomplicated percutaneous gastrostomy. AJR 1988; 151:307–309.
55. Wojtowycz MM, Arata JA Jr. Subcutaneous emphysema after percutaneous gastrostomy. AJR 1988; 151:311–312.
56. Franken EA Jr, Smith WL, Smith JA, Fitzgerald JF. Percutaneous cholangiography in infants. AJR 1978; 130:1057–1058.
57. Goldberg HI. Percutaneous transhepatic cholangiography and biliary drainage. In: Sleisenger MH, Fordtran JS, eds. Gastrointestinal Disease. 3rd ed. Philadelphia: WB Saunders, 1983: 1745.
58. Carty H. Percutaneous transhepatic fine needle cholangiography in jaundiced infants. Ann Radiol 1978; 21:149–154.
59. Mueller PR, Harbin WP, Ferrucci JT Jr, Wittenberg J, vanSonnenberg E. Fine-needle transhepatic cholangiography: reflections after 450 cases. AJR 1981; 136:85–90.
60. Harbin WP, Mueller PR, Ferrucci JT Jr. Transhepatic cholangiography: complications and use patterns of the fine-needle technique: a multi-institutional study. Radiology 1980; 135:15–22.
61. Chaumont P, Hamza R, Harry G. La cholangiographie transhepatique chez l'enfant. J Radiol Electrol Med Nucl 1975; 56:626–627.
62. Kreek MJ, Balint JA. "Skinny-needle" cholangiography—results of a pilot study of a voluntary prospective method for gathering risk data on new procedures. Gastroenterology 1980; 78:598–604.

PART 9

Radionuclide Diagnosis

Margaret A. Gainey, M.D.

The earliest available compounds in nuclear medicine resulted in high radiation doses, which effectively precluded their use in pediatric patients without malignant disease. A more widespread use of nuclear medicine imaging procedures has resulted from the availability of ^{99m}Tc-labeled radiopharmaceuticals, modern gamma camera detectors, and computers. The absorbed radiation doses from most nuclear medicine procedures, especially those employing ^{99m}Tc to examine the gastrointestinal (GI) tract in children, result in lower radiation exposures than from radiographic procedures such as fluoroscopy or computed tomography (CT) of the abdomen. Exceptions to this may occur with the use of a few relatively high dose nuclear medicine procedures such as ^{67}Ga-citrate or ^{111}In-labeled leukocyte scintigraphy. In all cases, imaging methods must be integrated to provide the needed information with a minimum of radiation exposure or potential harm to the individual patient.

Radionuclide imaging studies tend to have lower spatial resolution than that obtainable from conventional radiography, sonography, or CT. The poorer spatial resolution is usually offset by the greater sensitivity and the greater physiologic and/or quantitative information available with radionuclide techniques. For example, hepatobiliary scintigraphy allows evaluation of hepatocyte function, bile flow, and biliary drainage not provided by sonography or CT. To illustrate another example, the radionuclide technique for detection of ectopic gastric mucosa is far more sensitive than barium studies of the small bowel for the diagnosis of a Meckel's diverticulum.

Future developments in nuclear medicine will include additional ^{99m}Tc radiopharmaceuticals for imaging the GI tract, better cell labeling with ^{99m}Tc, improvements in monoclonal antibody techniques, and the eventual availability of truly physiologic imaging agents by the use of positron-emitting isotopes such as carbon, oxygen, and nitrogen in biologic compounds. These advances are predicted to increase the scope and specificity of nuclear medicine procedures in children as well as in adults.

GASTROESOPHAGEAL SCINTIGRAPHY

Gastroesophageal scintigraphy is a sensitive and noninvasive screening test for the detection of gastroesophageal reflux (GER).[1-4] After the administration of a small amount of radioactive material a gamma camera is used to monitor the distribution of the tracer within the esophagus and stomach. The presence of radioactivity within the esophagus during the period of observation is indicative of GER. Compared with simultaneous pH probe monitoring, the reported sensitivity of gastroesophageal scintigraphy is 65 to 79 percent.[5,6] Gastroesophageal scintigraphy does not require sedation or hospitalization. Although ambulatory probes for 24-hour pH monitoring are available, in some centers pH probe monitoring is still performed with sedation and hospitalization. Because of the presence of a probe in the esophagus and the possible effects of any sedation used during pH probe monitoring, gastroesophageal scintigraphy is considered a more physiologic technique. In addition, the gastric emptying data that can be obtained with gastroesophageal scintigraphy are not available with the pH probe techniques.

In comparison with barium studies of the upper GI tract, gastroesophageal scintigraphy permits longer observation times for the detection of reflux, at a considerably lower radiation dose than with barium fluoroscopic techniques.[7] Dosimetry estimates for gastroesophageal scintigraphy range from 0.07 cGy per 100 μCi in a 15-year-old to 0.93 cGy per 100 μCi in the newborn for the lower large intestine (critical organ), with gonadal doses of 0.01 cGy per 100 μCi or less in a 15-year-old to 0.10 cGy per 100 μCi or less in the newborn.[8] Dosimetry estimates for fluroscopy are more difficult to obtain; however, skin entrance doses of 1 to 2 cGy per minute and fluoroscopy times of 3 to 10 minutes are typical with equipment and practices commonly encountered (in our institution).

Unfortunately, neither gastroesophageal scintigraphy nor pH probe monitoring provides the anatomic information necessary to fully evaluate the pediatric patient. In the absence of other symptoms, the use of gastroesophageal scintigraphy without accompanying barium upper GI studies has at times been recommended in patients presenting with pulmonary disease or apneic spells.[9] This approach is not widely followed, particularly owing to fear of missing midgut malrotation or obstruction of the gastric outlet or duodenum. Furthermore, evaluation of swallowing and the function of the esophagus is usually desirable in these patients. Barium upper GI series and gastroesophageal scintigraphy are thus considered complementary procedures. Although techniques for the performance of barium studies in children are not well standardized, radionuclide studies have higher reported sensitivities (46 to 82 percent) than barium studies (15 to 75 percent) for the detection of reflux in referred patients in the same series.[1,3,10-12] When the results of barium upper GI series and gastroesophageal scintigraphy are combined, the sensitivity for the detection of reflux is improved but still is generally less than that of pH probe monitoring.

Infants and small children are typically fasted for 3 to 4 hours before the procedure. Older children may be kept fasting overnight. ^{99m}Tc–sulfur colloid is administered orally, or via nasogastric tube or gastrostomy where required. The typically administered activity is approximately 200 μCi to 1 mCi, or 7.4 to 37 MBq. The radionuclide may be diluted in a few milliliters of fluid for administration, followed by the feeding of an additional volume of nonradioactive fluid. Alternatively, the radioactivity may be diluted in a larger volume prior to administration. The latter method offers the potential advantage of imaging a constant concentration of activity but may result in inadequately administered activities or residual coating of the esophagus when delivered by the oral route.

A number of technical factors may affect the sensitivity of scintigraphy for the detection of reflux. The volume and type of fluid administered should mimic a normal feeding for the child. In our experience, especially with older children, the use of water or fruit juice results in rapid gastric emptying, which could theoretically reduce the severity and number of reflux episodes detected when compared with the use of milk or a similar (fat-containing) liquid feeding. Solid foods are not commonly administered when pediatric patients are being studied, although both labeled and unlabeled solids are routinely used in adults. Abdominal binders or maneuvers to increase the intra-abdominal pressure are unnecessary.

The supine position has been described as the most sensitive one for the detection of reflux, although prone or supine oblique positions may also be used. Most patients with reflux demonstrate episodes during the first 30 minutes of the examination. However, continuous data acquisition for a duration of 60 minutes is recommended as the method of choice in children. Reflux in some patients has been detected only during such longer acquisitions. In one series, reflux would have been missed in at least 25 percent of the cases if a 30-minute recording period had been used instead of a 1-hour period.[7] Imaging of the infant or child in the posterior projection (i.e., with the camera underneath the patient) is better tolerated than anterior imaging and facilitates patient care and monitoring during the procedure.

Computerized data acquisition should be performed to enhance the sensitivity of the technique and allow quantitation of the severity of the reflux. For a given camera/computer system and patient thickness, the detection of reflux is dependent on the isotope concentration in the stomach as well as on the volume and duration of reflux.[13] The image times (most often 0.1 to 0.5 sec per frame) should be sufficiently long to allow the detection of reflux and sufficiently short to separate individual reflux events. Regions of interest placed over the stomach, the esophagus, and a background area are used to generate time-activity curves. Spikes of increased activity in the esophageal curve indicate reflux (Fig. 1). Visual review of the acquired images allows detection of reflux confined to the most distal region of the esophagus, where higher background levels result from activity in the stomach, or when patient motion is excessive. Threshold levels in the computer display matrix should be adjusted to optimize the identification of small amounts of reflux.

DETECTION OF PULMONARY ASPIRATION

Many authors have advocated the use of gastroesophageal scintigraphy for the detection of pulmonary aspiration.[3,10-12,14,15] The summation of data frames and computer contrast enhancement techniques may improve the results. Delayed imaging obtained several hours and up to 24 hours after feeding has been recommended. The possibility of contamination must be excluded by the removal of clothing and linen, careful washing of the skin, and the use of imaging in multiple projections. The reported sensitivity of gastroesophageal scintigraphy for the detection of aspiration in children in these studies ranges from 5 to 40 percent of patients examined. These sensitivities are lower than the 29 to 75 percent sensitivities reported in some adult populations, although patient criteria and techniques differ.[16,17] Others have found

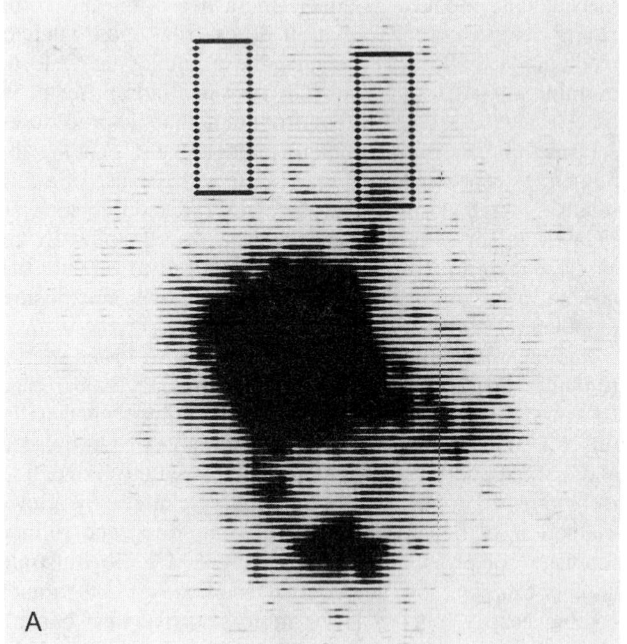

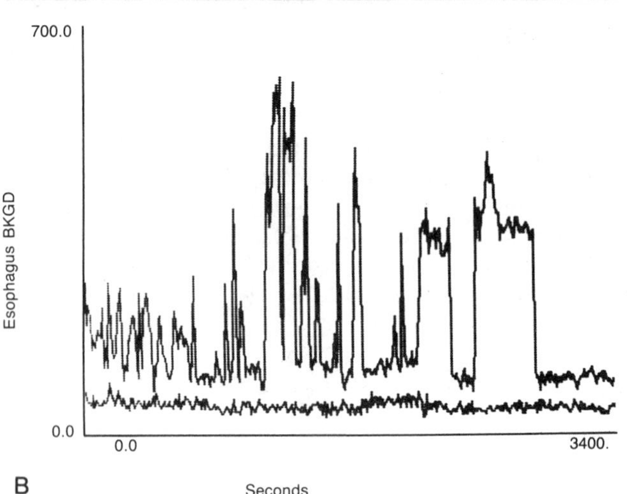

FIGURE 1 Gastroesophageal reflux. *A*, Regions of interest over the esophagus (*right rectangle*) and a background area (*left rectangle*) are used to generate *B*, time-activity curves, during gastroesophageal scintigraphy. Increased radioactivity in the esophagus from reflux appears as spikes of increased counts in the esophageal curve.

gastroesophageal scintigraphy unreliable for the detection of aspiration in children. In several series, aspiration has not been detected even when it has been strongly suspected.[1,18,19] Phantom studies have shown that small volumes of radioactivity (0.025 ml) may be detected using a concentration of ^{99m}Tc of 5 μCi per milliliter.[3] However, the actual activity concentration achieved in clinical situations may be several times lower than this owing to smaller amounts of administered activity, greater dilution of activity by gastric contents, and radioactive decay.

Recently, a more sensitive radionuclide method has been described for the detection of pulmonary aspiration.[20] The technique consists of placing 200 to 300 μCi of ^{99m}Tc–sulfur colloid in a small (less than 0.1 ml) volume directly onto the tongue. Computerized data acquisition is performed in the posterior projection with the patient in supine position for 1 hour. The mouth, chest, and stomach are included in the field of view. In a series of 27 patients with either recurrent pulmonary infections or abnormalities predisposing to aspiration of saliva, the sensitivity of the technique was 26 percent.[21]

Presumably, the greater concentration of radioactivity present with the "salivagram" described by Heyman et al[20,21] allows detection of small quantities of aspirated material, which are missed during imaging of the more dilute concentrations obtained with gastroesophageal scintigraphy. The procedure does not detect aspiration of refluxed material into the lungs but in fact detects the aspiration of saliva. Thus, GER is not evaluated by the technique, although gastroesophageal scintigraphy for reflux could be combined with the procedure. No attempt has yet been made to compare the sensitivity of the "salivagram" with other methods for the detection of aspiration.

ESOPHAGEAL SCINTIGRAPHY

Both qualitative and quantitative assessments of esophageal motility are readily performed using radionuclide techniques. The study may be useful in evaluating patients with swallowing dysfunction, anatomic abnormalities including strictures, and neuromuscular disorders of the esophagus. Commonly, it is performed as a part of the evaluation of patients with GER. Esophageal motility disorders have been described in more than 35 percent of patients with symptomatic reflux, a finding that may influence surgical antireflux procedures.[22] When obtained in conjunction with gastroesophageal scintigraphy for reflux, no additional radioactivity is required. The technique is a highly physiologic screening procedure that may in some cases preclude or help to determine the need for more invasive studies such as endoscopy.

For esophageal scintigraphy, the ^{99m}Tc–sulfur colloid dose is administered orally. Typically, the radioactivity is divided into one or more boluses in a small volume of milk or other liquid. Infants may be bottle fed, whereas older children may use a cup or a straw. With co-operative patients, dry swallowing on command or a nonradioactive liquid may be used after the initial radioactive bolus. Patients may be studied in the supine, semierect, or upright position. Although the upright position is more physiologic in the older child, the effect of gravity is increased and may mask subtle alterations in esophageal emptying.

Rapid-sequence computerized data acquisition permits quantitative analysis of esophageal transit. Time-activity curves are generated from regions of interest over two or more levels of the esophagus as well as the stomach. In normals, the bolus progresses rapidly toward the stomach. Higher count levels are normally recorded in the lower esophagus than in the upper esophagus, without build-up of radioactivity in any region of the esophagus. Following consecutive peristaltic waves, levels of activity return almost to baseline. Abnormal patterns may show delayed transit throughout the esophagus, suggesting a generalized motility disorder or a more focal delay in transit with increased count levels such as at the site of a stenosis.[23]

Transit of a bolus in the pharynx is rapid, requiring less than 1 second. Evaluation of pharyngeal motion is not usually attempted because of poor spatial resolution. The normal esophageal transit time is less than 10 seconds. The transit times for the upper, middle and lower portions of the esophagus are readily quantitated by this technique. There is a small, normal increase in esophageal transit time with increasing age, from 3.4 ± 1.0 seconds in infants to 4.6 ± 1.9 seconds at 8 to 16 years of age.[24] With GER or esophagitis, esophageal transit time is prolonged. Transit times as long as twice normal have been reported with severe reflux.[25] Improvement in esophageal transit times may be seen following successful therapy for esophagitis. With anatomic obstructions, focal hold-up of the tracer is seen above the obstruction, which results in slow esophageal transit.

GASTRIC EMPTYING

Measurement of gastric emptying is readily performed in children by using radionuclide techniques. For pediatric patients, as for adults, there is controversy over the use of liquids versus solid meals for studies of gastric emptying. The inaccuracies of the technique, problems of differential emptying of meal constituents, and difficulties with the radioactive labeling of both liquid and solid phases are well recognized. However, these limitations do not negate the usefulness of the procedure. Gastric emptying is readily measured in conjunction with the performance of gastroesophageal scintigraphy for reflux. Less commonly, it may be performed as an isolated procedure. Gastric emptying is calculated from regions of interest over the stomach, selected from the first and last data frames in a computerized acquisition. Activity in the bowel should be excluded from the regions. Background subtraction and correction for radioactive decay should also be performed. Gastric emptying (GE) is then expressed as a percentage of the initial counts in the stomach as follows:

$$GE = \frac{C_0 - C_{60} \times 100}{0.89} \div C_0$$

where C_0 is the initial activity in counts in the stomach region, C_{60} is the activity in counts in the stomach region at 60 minutes, and 0.89 is the correction factor for decay of the radionuclide (technetium) in 60 minutes. Similarly, the percentage of gastric residual (GR) is expressed as follows:

$$GR = \frac{C_{60} \times 100}{0.89} \div C_0$$

The potential error in estimating gastric counts from the single (usually posterior) projection alone is partially offset by the expression of GE and GR, since both C_0 and C_{60} are obtained from the same projection. Errors due to use of a single projection alone to estimate GE or GR may be as great as 20 percent.[26] The use of the geometric mean technique [(anterior counts × posterior counts)$^{1/2}$] requires count data in both the anterior and posterior projections but results in more accurate measurement of GE and GR.

Exact normal values for gastric emptying are difficult to determine in pediatric patients. Most gastric emptying studies are performed with the patient in the supine position, although older children may remain upright if gastroesophageal scintigraphy is not performed. The effect of the supine position (versus upright, prone, or prone oblique positions) on gastric emptying should be considered in comparing gastric emptying data. Similarly, the variations in meal composition and volumes require that normal values be established for each technique. Differences in the administered fluid or meal affect the rate and pattern of gastric emptying. In addition, there is variable precipitation of casein and thus the formation of solid material in which the radioactivity may be sequestered when milk is used for the "liquid" meal.[27]

It has been suggested that severe GER in infants is associated with significantly delayed gastric emptying.[28,29] In the data of Hillmeier et al, the mean gastric emptying at 1 hour was 20.5 ± 5.9 percent in infants with GER who had failure to thrive or pulmonary disease, compared with 44.3 ± 6.0 percent in infants with GER only. Other large series have not confirmed this finding but have demonstrated an age-related difference in gastric emptying, with faster emptying rates occurring in older children.[30-32] The age-related differences in gastric emptying are not accounted for by differences in the type of meal administered. Rosen and Treves found mean residuals at 1 hour of 54 percent in children less than 2 years of age and mean residuals of 30 percent in children older than 2 years. In the patients reported by DiLorenzo et al, older children presenting with GER had a significant delay in gastric emptying (mean residual activity at 60 minutes 41.6 ± 3.8 percent) when compared with those without reflux (28.7 ± 2.8 percent). An association between delayed gastric emptying and positive 24-hour pH probe testing has also been shown in a small number of patients reported by Seibert et al who had both negative gastroesophageal scintigraphy and negative 1-hour pH probe monitoring.[30]

HEPATOBILIARY SCINTIGRAPHY

Since the introduction of ^{99m}Tc–iminodiacetic acid (IDA) compounds in 1975, the imaging role of these agents in pediatric biliary tract disorders has become well established. Estimates of absorbed radiation doses for ^{99m}Tc-IDA agents are much lower than dose estimates for the ^{131}I rose bengal used previously. Refinements in the IDA group of radiopharmaceuticals have resulted in agents with lower renal clearance and higher concentrations within bile. In particular, compounds such as ^{99m}Tc-disofenin (DISIDA) allow better functional assessment of the liver and biliary structures even in the presence of siginificant hyperbilirubinemia.[33]

Patients are fasted for 3 to 4 hours before the study. The radiopharmaceutical is administered intravenously in a dose of 50 to 70 μCi per kilogram of body weight, with minimum doses of 500 to 1,000 μCi in infants. Gamma camera imaging is typically begun in the anterior projection, with the child in supine position beneath the camera. Sequential images of the liver, biliary system, and bowel are obtained with additional views in oblique and lateral projections as necessary to delineate the structures visualized. Images are obtained for up to 24 hours if excretion is delayed.

In normal children there is visualization of the liver, intrahepatic and extrahepatic ducts, gallbladder, and bowel within 1 hour after the injection. In normal neonates, intrahepatic and extrahepatic ducts are not seen because of their small size. With good extraction of the radiopharmaceutical by the hepatocytes, cardiac blood pool is cleared promptly. Renal excretion of the tracer is minimal when hepatocyte function is normal. Concentration of the material within the liver is usually maximal at 5 to 20 minutes after injection, with visualization of the gallbladder at 10 to 40 minutes after the injection.[34,35] Activity reaches the small bowel by 20 to 40 minutes after injection.

With elevated levels of serum bilirubin, the appearance time and quantity of excreted material are adversely affected. In patients with direct serum bilirubin levels greater than 10 mg per deciliter, ductal structures may not be visualized even in the absence of obstruction. Bowel activity is demonstrated with increased difficulty in the presence of severe hyperbilirubinemia, although diagnostic results may be achieved with direct bilirubin levels as high as 20 to 30 mg per deciliter.

In infants with biliary atresia there should be no demonstrable excretion of tracer into bowel, even after 24 hours (Fig. 2). Isolated case reports of biliary atresia with documented excretion into bowel have been published but are rare.[36-38] The finding of activity in bowel with biliary atresia is puzzling but may reflect the progressive nature of the disease, poor radiopharmaceutical labeling with free technetium in bowel, vicarious excretion of the labeled compound by the bowel, or misinterpretation of normal activity within the urinary tract. Hepatocyte uptake of the radiopharmaceutical is normal or nearly normal in the neonate with biliary atresia but deteriorates with increasing age. By 3 months of age hepatic damage may be sufficient to cause poor hepatocyte uptake, with prolonged visualization of cardiac blood pool and increased renal excretion of the tracer.

A variety of etiologies may cause a severe cholestatic jaundice in infants without extrahepatic obstruction, which must be differentiated from biliary atresia. These entities include viral and bacterial infections, inherited metabolic disorders such as alpha$_1$-antitrypsin deficiency or cystic fibrosis, cholestasis due to parenteral hyperalimentation, and idiopathic neonatal hepatitis. In infants with these disorders, hepatocyte uptake of the tracer varies from normal to severely impaired, since it is dependent on the degree of cholestasis and hepatocellular disease (Fig. 3). Scans demonstrate delayed

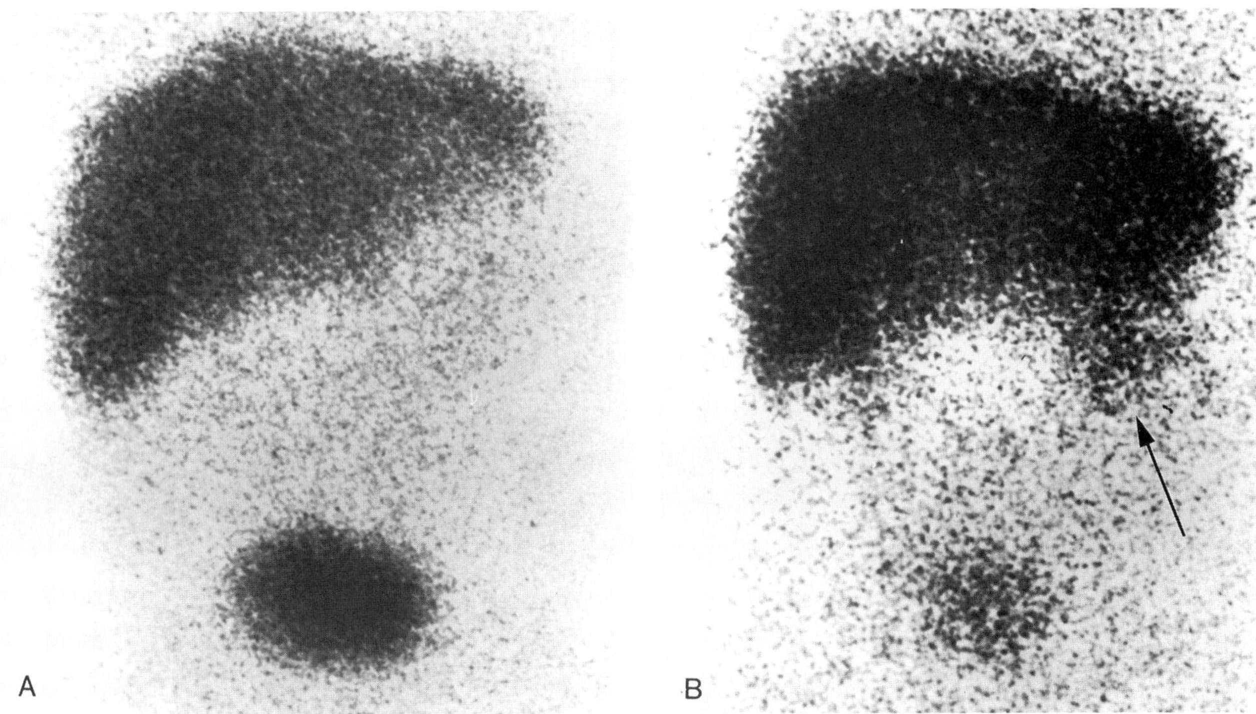

FIGURE 2 Biliary atresia. *A*, Early, and *B*, 24-hour delayed, hepatobiliary images, anterior projections. Activity persists in the liver without bowel visualization. Renal (*arrow*) and bladder activity should not be mistaken for excretion into gallbladder or bowel.

excretion of the tracer with diminished activity in the bowel, with or without visualization of the gallbladder.

The specificity of hepatobiliary scintigraphy in distinguishing biliary atresia from other causes of neonatal jaundice is improved greatly by the prior administration of phenobarbital in a total dose of 5 mg per kilogram per day for at least 5 days prior to the examination.[39] Visualization of tracer in the intestinal tract, with or without visualization of the gallbladder, indicates patency of the biliary ducts and thus virtually excludes biliary atresia. Absence of visualization of activity in the intestinal tract, when associated with poor hepatocyte uptake, is indicative of severe hepatocellular disease and thus is not specific for biliary atresia. Using these criteria, sensitivities on the order of 100 percent and specificities of up to 94 percent for the detection of biliary atresia can be achieved.[40,41]

Biliary tract abnormalities such as intrahepatic ductular hypoplasia or atresia (arteriohepatic dysplasia or Alagille's syndrome) may result in varying degrees of neonatal jaundice.[42,43] In patients with mild jaundice, the hepatobiliary scan may have a relatively normal appearance. In some cases, mild decrease in hepatic uptake without visualization of excretion into bowel may mimic biliary atresia.[44] If visualized, excretion into bowel allows exclusion of the diagnosis of extrahepatic biliary atresia in infants with ductal hypoplasia.[45] In older children with significant parenchymal liver disease, hepatocyte uptake of the tracer may be quite impaired whereas excretion into bowel is delayed but present.

Spontaneous perforation of the extrahepatic biliary ducts in infancy results in bile ascites or peritonitis. This serious condition is rarely encountered but is readily diagnosed by hepatobiliary scintigraphy.[46–48] The presence of excreted tracer in the peritoneal cavity provides noninvasive confirmation of the suspected diagnosis (Fig. 4). Leakage of bile may not be seen on early views, requiring delayed views beyond 1 hour to clearly demonstrate activity within ascitic fluid.

Hepatobiliary scintigraphy in bile plug syndrome (inspissated bile syndrome) in infants demonstrates absence of excretion of activity into the bowel, indicating obstruction.[49] Neither intrahepatic nor extrahepatic bile ducts are typically visualized, even when dilated. Ductal dilatation with occlusion at the site of the bile plug may be demonstrated on sonography or by cholangiography, allowing confirmation of the diagnosis.

Hepatobiliary scintigraphy is a useful adjunct in the diagnosis of suspected choledochal cysts. The excretion of activity into a choledochal cyst facilitates its differentiation from other cystic lesions occurring in the right upper quadrant (such as enteric duplications, pancreatic pseudocysts, and intrahepatic cysts). Dilated intrahepatic bile ducts (if present) will be demonstrated, with later filling of the extrahepatic bile ducts and the choledochal cyst due to stasis.[50,51] A choledochal cyst may initially be visualized as a photopenic area persisting for several hours after injection, with slow filling in with tracer depending on the size of the cyst and the degree of obstruction. Excretion into bowel may be delayed or absent.

Hepatobiliary scintigraphy is useful in patients with congenital dilatation of intrahepatic bile ducts (Caroli's disease). If sufficiently dilated, the intrahepatic ducts appear on early views as photopenic branching structures within the liver. Later views demonstrate excretion into the ducts with delayed

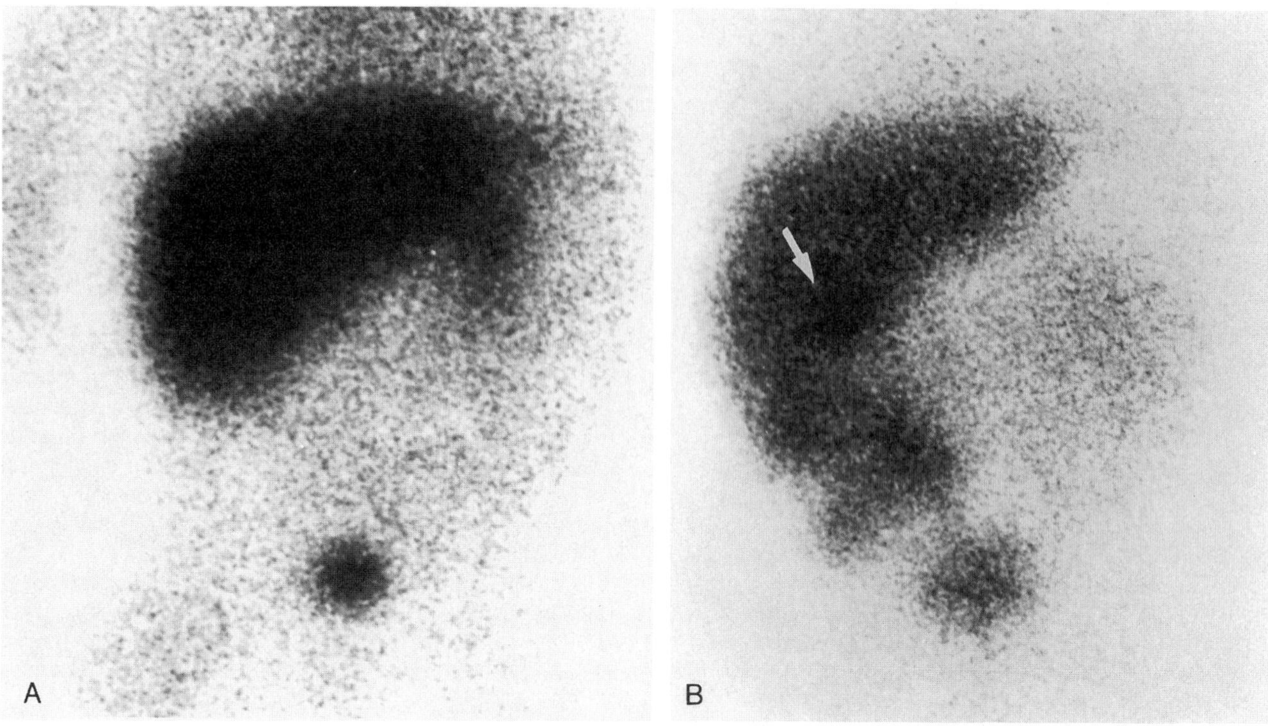

FIGURE 3 Neonatal hepatitis. *A*, Early hepatobiliary image shows prolonged cardiac and body blood pool activity due to impaired hepatocyte function. *B*, Delayed image demonstrates excretion into bowel and, in this case, gallbladder visualization (*arrow*).

drainage due to stasis and hepatic fibrosis if it is present.[52] Since there is no obstruction per se of the biliary tract in this disease, excretion of the tracer into bowel is demonstrated. If present, cholangitis and cirrhosis impair hepatocyte uptake of the tracer. Calculus formation within the ducts, a complication of Caroli's disease due to bile stasis, may result in ductal obstruction and thus absence of tracer excretion into bowel.

When sclerosing cholangitis is suspected, hepatobiliary scintigraphy also provides a noninvasive means of evaluating patients.[53–55] The primary or idiopathic form of the disease as well as the secondary form associated with inflammatory bowel disease has a scintigraphic pattern that may be distinguished from that in patients with isolated common bile duct obstruction or primary biliary cirrhosis. Patchy hepatic uptake may be seen on early views owing to varying degrees of segmental ductal obstruction and thus segmental variation in hepatocyte dysfunction (Fig. 5). Multiple focal areas of increased tracer accumulation corresponding to focally dilated ducts are visualized on routine views. Delayed isotope clearance from segments of the liver correspond to areas of more severe ductal stenosis and thus cholestasis. Single photon emission CT has been helpful in delineating the focal areas of bile stasis within the ducts.[56]

In addition, hepatobiliary scintigraphy also has a role in the evaluation of trauma to the liver or biliary tract. Both accidental and iatrogenic injury may result in intrahepatic bile collections or the free leakage of bile into the abdomen. The location and extent of bile leaks are readily evaluated with this technique.[57] Hepatobiliary scintigraphy is complementary to abdominal sonography or CT, allowing the confirmation of the nature of fluid collections suspected to contain bile. In addition, the integrity of anastomoses such as the portoenterostomy (Kasai procedure) for biliary atresia or biliary-enteric anastomoses may be readily determined.[58,59] The excretion of tracer into the bowel within 1 hour after injection excludes significant obstruction, even in the presence of postoperative biliary ductal dilatation. Prolonged tracer retention at a specific site in the biliary ducts or bowel will help to localize obstruction if it is present (Fig. 6). Unfortunately, incomplete obstruction may not be differentiated from severe hepatocyte damage in all cases. Postsurgical complications such as cholangitis result in impaired hepatocyte uptake of the tracer, impaired visualization of ductal structures, and impaired excretion of tracer into bowel without hold-up of the tracer at a specific site.

The role of hepatobiliary scintigraphy in the diagnosis and management of gallbladder disease in children, especially in infants, is less well established than in the adult. Scintigraphic visualization of the gallbladder implies patency of the cystic duct, which is useful in the attempt to exclude surgical gallbladder disease. However, nonvisualization of the gallbladder with hepatobiliary scintigraphy in no way proves the presence of surgical gallbladder disease. For example, hepatobiliary scintigraphy has shown nonvisualization of the gallbladder in infants with transient gallbladder distention who have not required cholecystectomy.[60] Follow-up scintigraphy, when performed, has been normal in these cases. This may

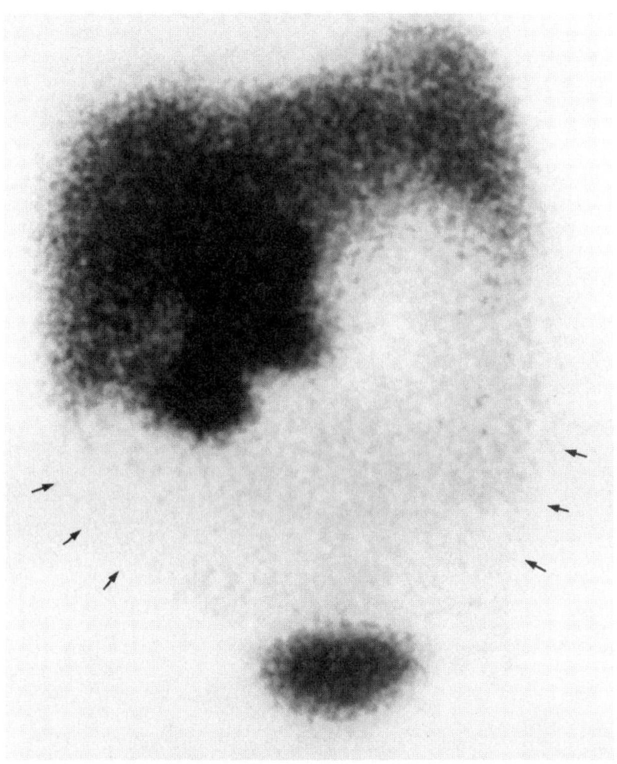

FIGURE 4 Idiopathic perforation of the common bile duct. Anterior hepatobiliary image of the abdomen at 3.5 hours demonstrates activity within ascitic fluid (*arrows*) as well as a focal collection of activity inferior to the liver. (Courtesy of S. Dadparvar, M.D., Hahnemann University.)

be explained by transient cystic duct obstruction due to edema. A number of other reports of acalculous cholecystitis, as well as incidental or transient cholelithiasis, in infants not requiring surgical treatment have appeared in the literature.[61,62] The association of stones or sludge in the biliary tract of neonates treated with furosemide or with total parenteral nutrition has also been recognized.[63,64] The increased frequency of these observations is attributable to the more widespread use of abdominal sonography as a screening procedure in the neonate. The role of radionuclide imaging in patients with these disorders, if any, has not yet been systematically evaluated. Beyond infancy, the greater frequency of acalculous cholecystitis in children than in adults may also limit the usefulness of hepatobiliary scintigraphy. As in infants, anatomic obstruction of the cystic duct may be transient and due to edema when it is present at all.

Visualization of the gallbladder by hepatobiliary scintigraphy excludes the presence of acute cholecystitis with cystic duct obstruction, but not the possibility of chronic cholecystitis without cystic duct obstruction. Gallbladder visualization has been reported to occur in 90 percent of minimally symptomatic patients with chronic cholecystitis. The remaining 10 percent of patients may show delayed visualization of the gallbladder or persistent nonvisualization, depending on the severity of the disease.[65,66] Delayed visualization of the gallbladder with an otherwise normal appearance of the hepatobiliary scan suggests the diagnosis of chronic cholecystitis. The visualization of intestinal activity before gallbladder activity in symptomatic patients may also suggest chronic cholecystitis, even when both the gallbladder and bowel are seen within 1 hour.[67]

Although failure to visualize the gallbladder may be the result of cystic duct obstruction, it is not diagnostic of either cholelithiasis or cystic duct obstruction per se. A number of other entities including prolonged fasting, total parenteral nutrition, severe hepatic parenchymal disease from any cause, and even severe systemic illness may result in failure to visualize the gallbladder on routine hepatobiliary scintigraphy.[68-70] In one series of adults, delayed imaging for up to 4 hours increased the frequency of gallbladder visualization and reduced the false-positive rate for the diagnosis of acute cholecystitis from 9.9 to 0.6 percent.[71] Delayed imaging for up to 24 hours after injection has been advocated by some authors, particularly in patients who have been fasting for more than 1 day.[72]

Low-dose morphine administration has been advocated to decrease the time required to visualize the gallbladder, improving the specificity of cholescintigraphy for the diagnosis of acute cholecystitis in adults from 83 to 100 percent without loss of sensitivity.[73,74] Treatment with cholecystokinetic agents in conjunction with hepatobiliary scintigraphy has also been advocated to improve gallbladder visualization in patients with chronic cholecystitis. Pretreatment with cholecystokinin facilitates earlier gallbladder visualization but decreases the sensitivity of the study to distinguish between chronic cholecystitis and the normal gallbladder. The infusion of cholecystokinin following hepatobiliary scintigraphy has also been advocated as an aid in the diagnosis of suspected cholecystitis in cases in which the gallbladder is visualized. Failure of the gallbladder to contract by more than 50 percent of its volume is suggestive either of a partial obstruction of the cystic duct or of acalculous or chronic cholecystitis.[75-77] Use of this agent in pediatric patients is not well described but may be appropriate in selected cases.

MECKEL'S DIVERTICULUM

The radionuclide detection of ectopic gastric mucosa with ^{99m}Tc-pertechnetate remains the primary noninvasive diagnostic tool for the diagnosis of Meckel's diverticulum in patients who present with lower GI bleeding. Standard barium radiographic examinations and arteriography both have poor sensitivities for the detection of this lesion.[78,79] Following the initial case reports in 1970, the success of the radionuclide technique has been confirmed by multiple authors.[80-83] In large pediatric series, surgically proven sensitivities as high as 85 percent and specificities as high as 95 percent for the detection of ectopic gastric mucosa have been reported.[84] When negative studies in patients with a different clinical diagnosis or no recurrence of bleeding but without surgery are included, sensitivities greater than 90 percent and specificities of 100 percent with overall accuracies of 99 percent can be achieved.[85]

The pertechnetate ion is metabolized in a manner similar to chloride or iodide ions in the body. ^{99m}Tc-pertechnetate is

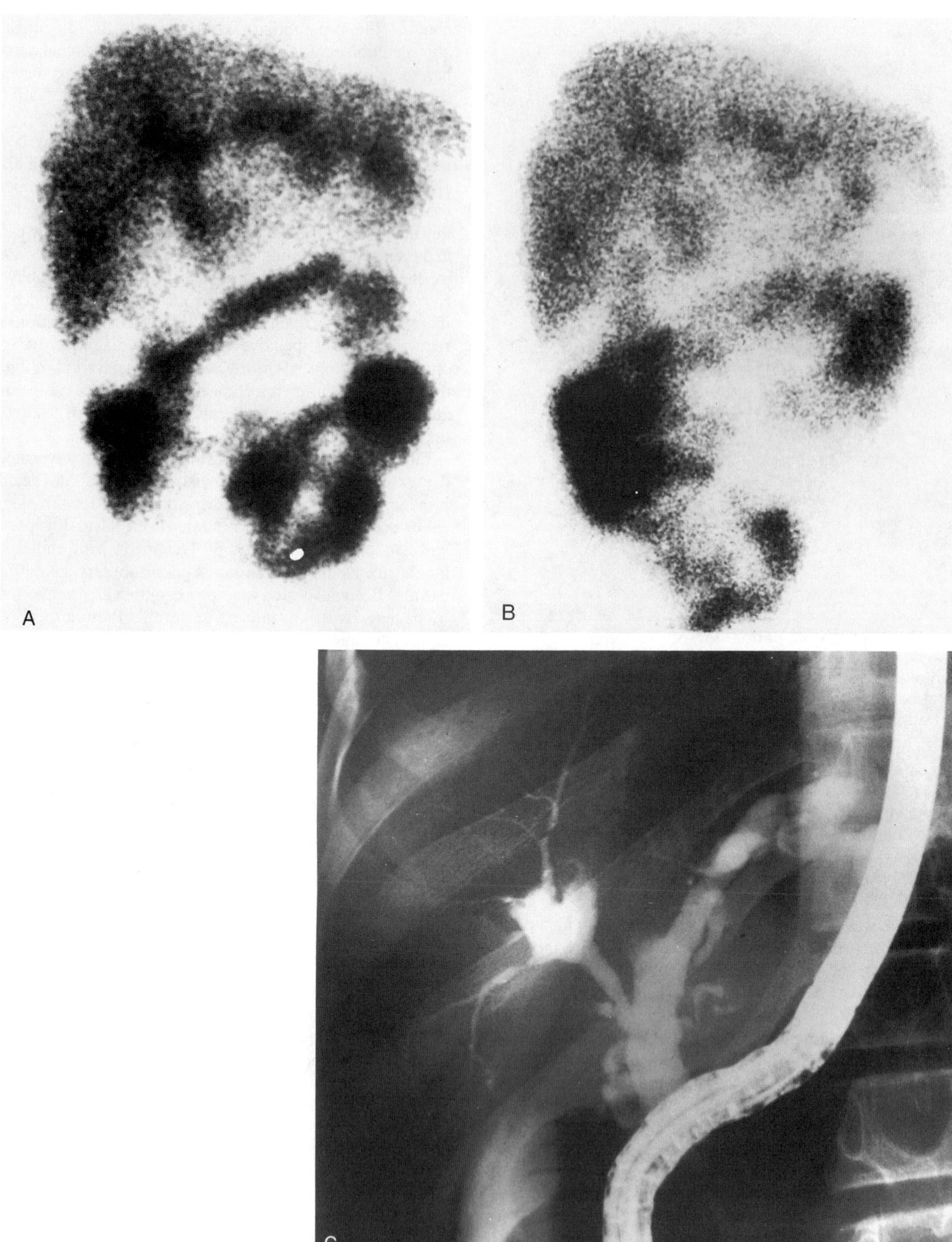

FIGURE 5 Sclerosing cholangitis. Hepatobiliary images at *A*, 1 hour, and *B*, 2 hours, show patchy hepatic uptake and slow clearance of activity from the liver with persistence of activity within nonuniformly dilated hepatic ducts. *C*, Note corresponding ductal irregularity and dilatation demonstrated on the retrograde cholangiogram.

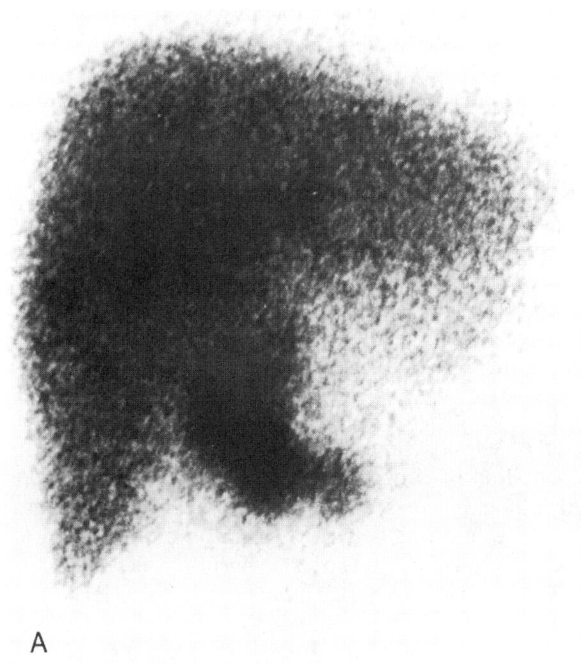

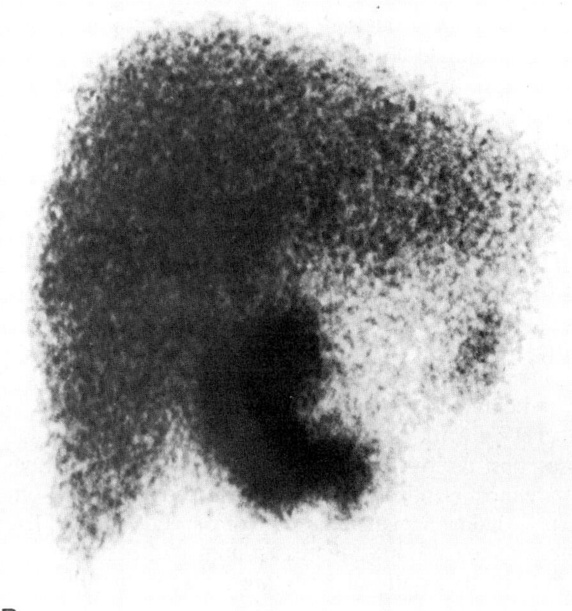

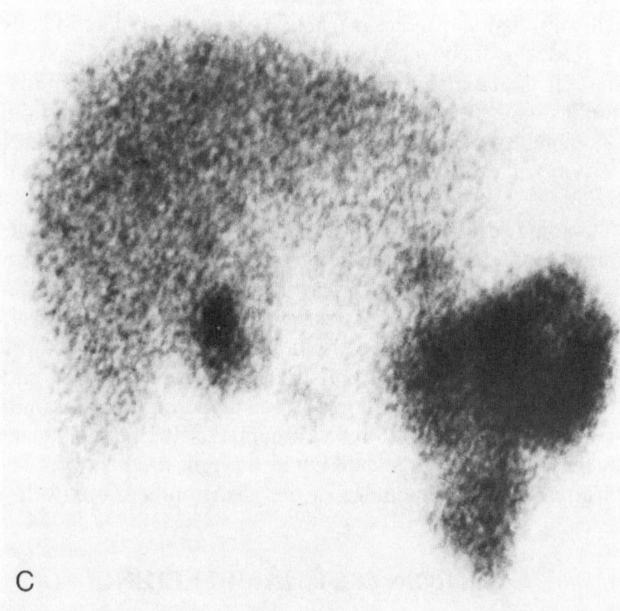

FIGURE 6 Partial common bile duct obstruction following cholecystectomy. Hepatobiliary images *A*, at 20 minutes, and *B*, at 45 minutes, show focal hold-up of activity in the dilated common bile duct, with *C*, eventual drainage into bowel by 90 minutes. Complete obstruction and extravasation are excluded on this examination.

thus concentrated in the thyroid, in the salivary glands, and in gastric mucosa.[86] Secretion of the pertechnetate ion is believed to occur within the mucin-secreting epithelial cells of gastric mucosa, although the precise mechanism and site remain unknown.[87] Since symptomatic Meckel's diverticula contain sufficient ectopic gastric mucosa to produce ulceration and bleeding, the amount of ectopic gastric mucosa is theoretically enough to permit visualization of the lesion with abdominal scintigraphy. Experimentally, at least 1.8 cm^2 of gastric mucosa is necessary for the lesion to be detected with usual gamma camera techniques.[88]

To perform the examination, ^{99m}Tc-pertechnetate in a dose of 200 μCi per kilogram of body weight (dose range 500 μCi minimum, 10 mCi maximum) is administered intravenously. Rapid-sequence imaging over the abdomen during the injection (angiographic phase) facilitates exclusion of an arteriovenous malformation, which may be seen as a focal hypervascular area that fades on later static images. In normal patients, serial static views of the abdomen demonstrate excretion of tracer via the kidneys into the ureters and urinary bladder. Normal gastric activity increases progressively during the first 30 minutes of the examination. Gastric emptying may be diminished by placing the patient in the supine left posterior oblique position during imaging or by nasogastric suction. An ectopic focus of gastric mucosa shows increasing activity in proportion to and in temporal sequence with increasing activity in the stomach (Fig. 7). Although typically seen as a stationary collection of abnormal activity in the right lower quadrant, the diverticulum may be visualized elsewhere in the abdomen and may show prominent motion.[89] Care should be taken to avoid misinterpreting normal body background in the testes, a hyperemic or menstruating uterus, or normal excreted material in the kidneys, ureters, or bladder as ectopic gastric mucosa. Images should be obtained in multiple projections and after bladder emptying to prevent missing a focus obscured by other normal structures.

A number of "false-positive" scans for Meckel's diverticulum have been reported. As would be expected, the technique does not allow discrimination between ectopic gastric mucosa in a Meckel's diverticulum and ectopic gastric mucosa in other locations such as Barrett's esophagus or a duplication of the bowel. Hydronephrosis, hydroureter, a pelvic kidney, and communicating urachal cysts may be mistaken for a Meckel's diverticulum.[90] Inflammatory bowel disease, abscesses, obstructed bowel loops, arteriovenous malformations, Peutz-Jeghers syndrome with intussusception, and some tumors including hemangiomas, sarcomas, and carcinoid have also been shown to have increased uptake of pertechnetate, which may be confused with Meckel's diverticulum.[91-94]

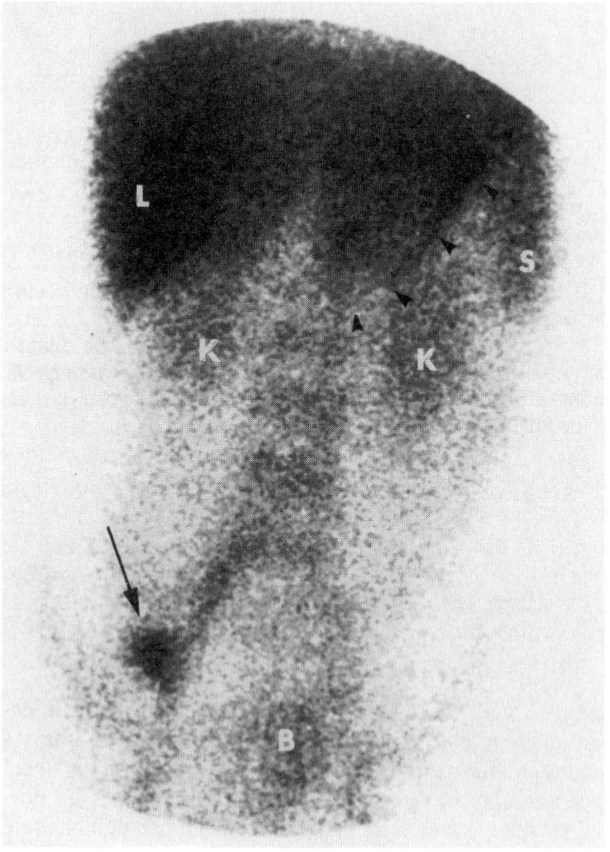

FIGURE 7 Meckel's diverticulum. ^{99m}Tc-pertechnetate image of the abdomen, anterior projection at 2 minutes. Note intense focal activity in the diverticulum (*arrow*). Fainter activity may be seen with smaller amounts of ectopic gastric tissue. Activity in the stomach (*arrowheads*), kidneys (K), bladder (B), and body background including the liver (L) and spleen (S) are normal findings.

Necrosis and hemorrhage within tumors with less vascularity and without gastric mucosa have also resulted in confusion of pertechnetate uptake with Meckel's diverticulum.[95]

False-negative examinations for ectopic gastric mucosa may result from failure to separate overlapping structures or obscuration of a small focus because of bowel hyperemia, dilution from hemorrhage, or excessive gastric emptying of normally excreted activity. Additional false-negative scans have been reported with hypofunctioning gastric mucosa in infants and due to atrophy, ischemia, or necrosis of the gastric mucosa within the lesions.[87,96,97]

The intravenous administration of glucagon delays gastric emptying but has an effective duration of action of only approximately 20 minutes. Glucagon also diminishes bowel peristalsis, which should theoretically diminish dilution and washout of activity from a Meckel's diverticulum. The prior administration of cimetidine inhibits gastric acid secretion and thus should increase the pertechnetate ion within the gastric mucosa, allowing better visualization of an ectopic focus and preventing interference from normally secreted gastric activity within the bowel.[98] Although most experience supports the beneficial effect of cimetidine, its use is not universally accepted, since it has also been argued that the drug would inhibit uptake of pertechnetate ions. Although pentagastrin stimulation of secretory activity by gastric mucosa cells increases pertechnetate uptake, the perceived risk of increasing GI hemorrhage diminishes its usefulness.[99] Animal studies have also shown early emptying of activity into the duodenum with this drug, which could result in small bowel activity interfering with visualization of the abnormal focus.[100]

Colonic irritants including laxatives for bowel preparation, and barium enema examinations should be avoided prior to abdominal scintigraphy, since they cause bowel hyperemia resulting in nonspecific increase of the tracer within bowel, which may obscure uptake within a small focus of ectopic gastric mucosa.[101] Food and irritating medications should also be avoided to minimize bowel hyperemia. Potassium perchlorate, often used to block uptake of the pertechnetate by the thyroid gland, should not be administered, since it interferes with tracer uptake in the gastric mucosa as well.

GASTROINTESTINAL BLEEDING

The scintigraphic diagnosis of GI bleeding in children may be accomplished by two techniques, using the intravenous administration of either ^{99m}Tc-labeled sulfur colloid or ^{99m}Tc-labeled red blood cells. The decision to use one technique versus the other is often dictated by the expectation of active bleeding at the time the examination is started, by the suspected rate of bleeding, and by the perceived requirement for delayed views. Both techniques have been shown to be more sensitive than arteriography in series of adult patients with GI bleeding and are less invasive.[102,103]

As little as 0.05 to 0.10 ml per minute of bleeding has been demonstrated experimentally using the sulfur colloid technique.[104] Rapid clearance of the material by the liver and spleen within a few minutes after injection reduces body background, allowing detection of small amounts of remaining extravasated material at the bleeding site. However, bleeding sites in patients with intermittent bleeding may be missed entirely with this procedure. Sites of bleeding adjacent to the liver and spleen may be obscured by the high levels of activity in these organs. The location of the bleeding site may be inferred from the appearance of the scan, although with small foci it may be difficult to distinguish small bowel from large bowel activity.

A dose of 200 μCi per kilogram of body weight of ^{99m}Tc–sulfur colloid (minimum 1 mCi, maximum 10 mCi) is administered intravenously with the child in the supine position. Views of the abdomen below the liver and spleen are obtained with the gamma camera every few minutes for the first 15 minutes. Oblique views of the abdomen may help to visualize sites obscured by the liver and spleen. If bleeding is detected, additional views may show progression of the activity and further help to define the bleeding site. Normal marrow activity will be visualized on the high count images obtained for the procedure. Ectopic or multiple spleens fail to move and should not be confused with a bleeding site. Repeat examinations may be performed as necessary but require the repeat administration of labeled sulfur colloid for each study.

^{99m}Tc-labeled red blood cells may be less sensitive than sulfur colloid techniques for the detection of bleeding, in some cases requiring as much as 30 to 60 ml of extravasated blood for the detection of bleeding.[105] Higher background levels of labeled red blood cells account for this lower sensitivity. Other authors have concluded that in vitro labeled red blood cells are far more sensitive than sulfur colloid for the detection of bleeding in the clinical setting, because of the intermittent nature of GI bleeding.[106] The red blood cell technique does allow the use of delayed views to detect intermittent bleeding, although peristaltic movement of extravasated material may lead to an erroneous impression of the exact location of the bleeding site. Breakdown of the labeled material over several hours may result in excretion of some ^{99m}Tc-pertechnetate into bowel as well as in bladder activity.

Autologous red blood cells may be labeled using in vivo or in vitro techniques.[102,107] In vitro labeling techniques are slightly more difficult to perform but have the advantage of better red blood cell tagging. The ^{99m}Tc dose for labeling is 200 to 250 μCi per kilogram (minimum 2 mCi, maximum 15 mCi), administered intravenously after nonradioactive stannous pyrophosphate for the in vivo technique or as labeled red blood cells with in vitro methods. With the child in the supine position, gamma camera views over the abdomen are obtained in posterior (anterior if possible) projections for approximately 1 hour after injection, with additional oblique and postvoid views as necessary to separate overlapping structures. If the site of bleeding is not identified, additional follow-up views of the abdomen should be obtained at intervals for at least 24 hours (Fig. 8). Computer enhancement techniques may improve detection of faint bleeding sites, prompting additional views or shorter intervals between follow-up views.

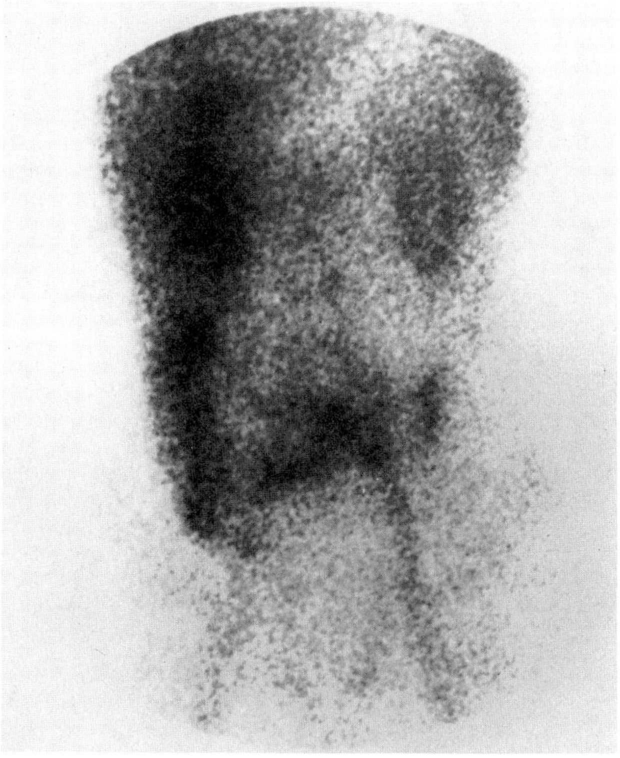

FIGURE 8 Gastrointestinal bleeding. Delayed ^{99m}Tc-labeled red blood cell image of the abdomen, anterior projection. There is abnormal activity in bowel above the pelvis and in the ascending colon. The presence of bleeding is well demonstrated, although the site of origin (in this case, the ileum) may be misinterpreted, owing to peristalsis.

LIVER AND SPLEEN

The role of scintigraphic imaging of the liver and spleen with ^{99m}Tc–sulfur colloid has changed dramatically since the introduction of real-time sonography, CT, and, more recently, magnetic resonance imaging (MRI) of the abdomen. Sulfur colloid imaging of the liver and spleen is now less often required as a primary modality to obtain structural information regarding these organs. However, the technique uniquely reflects the status of the reticuloendothelial system of the liver and spleen, thus retaining a physiologic imaging role.

The usual dose of ^{99m}Tc–sulfur colloid is 50 μCi per kilogram (minimum dose 500 μCi, maximum 3 to 5 mCi), administered intravenously. Rapid sequence (angiographic or flow phase) imaging over the abdomen during the injection may be performed, allowing qualitative estimation of blood flow to the liver and spleen as a whole. Because hepatic blood flow is primarily portal venous in origin rather than arterial, images demonstrate earlier and more intense activity within the spleen and kidneys than in the liver during the flow phase. Particularly in small children, both the temporal and spatial resolution of the flow study may not allow precise evaluation of flow to the liver from the hepatic artery. The relative hypo- or hypervascularity of focal lesions in the liver or spleen is more successfully assessed, provided that they are at least 1 to 2 cm in diameter. Particles of sulfur colloid, on the order of 0.5 to 1.0 μ in size, are phagocytized by the reticuloendothelial cells of the liver, spleen, and bone marrow. Following their intravenous administration, the particles are cleared rapidly from the bloodstream, with a typical half-time of less than 3 minutes. Owing to the greater concentration of reticuloendothelial tissue in the liver and spleen, bone marrow activity is not visualized in normal patients with routine techniques. Static views of the liver and spleen are obtained in multiple projections to allow better visualization of various areas within each organ and to separate overlapping areas. Adjacent normal or enlarged structures such as the gallbladder or kidney may produce extrinsic impressions on the organ contours. Three hundred and sixty degree rotational imaging with tomographic reconstruction (single photon emission CT, or SPECT) permits visualization of individual "slices" in multiple planes. SPECT improves the detection of focal lesions by removing overlying structures and by enhancing the contrast between normal and abnormal foci of activity in the liver and spleen. Because of the low doses of radioactivity typically administered and thus the time (up to 1 hour) required for the child to remain motionless, sedation may be necessary for younger patients undergoing SPECT imaging.

In conjunction with the evaluation of focal or diffuse disorders involving the liver and spleen, the confirmation of suspected hepatomegaly or splenomegaly with sulfur colloid imaging remains a useful determination in pediatric patients. Normal values must be correlated with the age, weight, and/or height of the child. Scintigraphic measurements of vertical liver span, correlated with sonographic data, have been published.[108] From the data of Holder et al, the scintigraphic dimension of the liver in centimeters measured halfway between the xiphoid and the right lateral margin of the liver is given by the formula:

$$\text{Scintigraphic dimension (cm)} = 5.47 + 0.114 \text{ height (inches)}$$

The scintigraphic normal values for maximum vertical liver dimension as well as maximum splenic dimension have also been reported.[109] The maximum vertical dimension (MVD) of the liver in centimeters related to age (A) in years is given by the following formula:

$$\text{MVD} = 8.8 + 0.46\text{A}$$

The correlation coefficient r was 0.89 in 66 children aged 0 to 19 years. Similarly, the maximum splenic dimension (MSD) is related to age (A) according to the formula:

$$\text{MSD} = 5.7 + 0.31\text{A}$$

Markisz et al correlated multiple hepatic and splenic parameters with age and weight in normal children.[110] Based on the mathematical model of a right cone with an elliptical base, much better correlation ($r = 0.94$) with weight has been found by using the triple product of liver height, width, and length rather than calculating actual liver volume. The scintigraphic correlation of linear splenic measurements with age or weight is poorer ($r = 0.70$). Correlation is improved using splenic volume as a function of either age or weight, assuming splenic volume to be a spheroid.

Congenital abnormalities including eventration of the diaphragm and upward displacement of the liver in diaphragmatic hernias are readily discernible on sulfur colloid imaging but may in most cases be evaluated sufficiently by sonography. Unusual liver configurations such as the symmetric or left-sided liver found in heterotaxia syndromes may be more readily diagnosed by scintigraphy. By injecting the ^{99m}Tc–sulfur colloid into both upper and lower extremity veins, anomalies and patency of the venae cavae can be confirmed. The presence of a normal spleen, malposition of the spleen, asplenia, or polysplenia (Fig. 9) can also be evaluated.[111] If splenic tissue is not clearly separable from the liver owing to overlap and similar intensities of uptake, spleen imaging with ^{99m}Tc-labeled heat-damaged red blood cells may be performed.[112]

Accessory splenic tissue is visualized as one or more areas of uptake in the left upper quadrant. Since these structures may be indistinguishable from tumor by sonography and CT, their uptake of sulfur colloid allows a specific diagnosis to be made. In the presence of a normal spleen, the detection of a smaller accessory spleen or spleens requires that very high count images be obtained. In suspected anatomic asplenia, sulfur colloid images may detect splenic tissue missed by screening with sonography. With functional asplenia such as that found in patients with sickle cell disease or cyanotic heart disease, the diminished or absent visualization of the

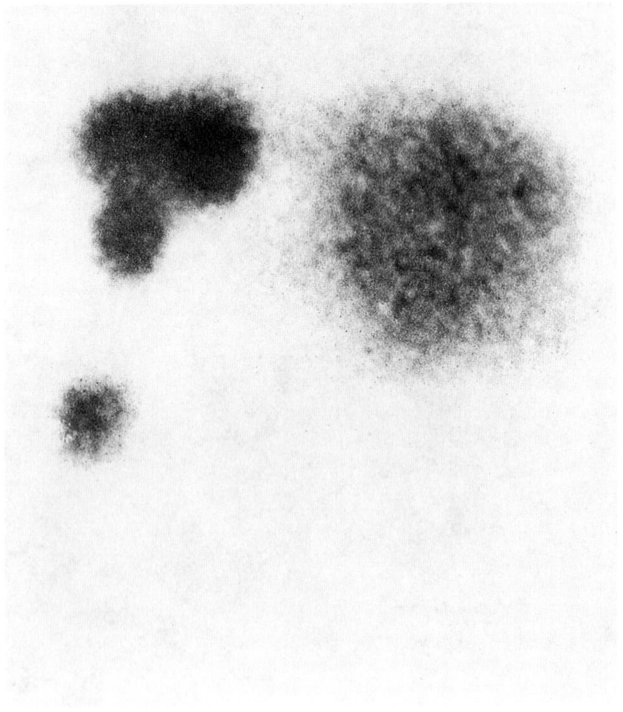

FIGURE 9 Polysplenia. Liver-spleen scan performed with ^{99m}Tc–sulfur colloid, posterior projection. Three small, rounded spleens show greater intensity of uptake than a fourth, more inferiorly positioned spleen. Demonstration of ectopic splenic tissue is more difficult in the presence of a normal, functioning spleen or spleens.

spleen reflects the status of that organ's phagocytic function.[113] Reversal of functional asplenia with treatment of the underlying disorder may also be demonstrated easily with sulfur colloid imaging. With splenosis following trauma or splenectomy, multiple nodules of activity may be demonstrated anywhere in the peritoneal cavity.[114]

In hepatic venous occlusion (Budd-Chiari syndrome), several scintigraphic patterns may be observed.[115] Typically, caudate lobe hypertrophy occurs with increased size and uptake in the caudate lobe accompanied by diffusely diminished uptake in the remainder of the liver. Patterns of segmental decrease in hepatic uptake, diffusely decreased hepatic uptake, and hypertrophy or preservation of a lobe other than the caudate are found less commonly. Both sonography and dynamic CT have also been advocated as screening techniques for this disorder.[116,117]

The greater anatomic detail and additional information about other structures possible with sonography, CT, and MRI limit the relative usefulness of radionuclide imaging of the liver and spleen in several other circumstances. For example, most focal or mass lesions are no longer routinely evaluated by sulfur colloid imaging of the liver and spleen. In large series of pediatric patients with blunt abdominal trauma, the use of CT resulted in fewer false positives and false negatives than with either scintigraphy or sonography.[118,119] This experience has been widely confirmed in the clinical setting. Radionuclide examination of the liver may still be useful in evaluating suspected areas of hepatic injury without infarction or hemorrhage, missed by other imaging techniques (Fig. 10). Rib, bowel gas, and other artifacts with sonography or CT may preclude evaluation of some areas of the liver and spleen or may produce an appearance difficult to distinguish from a small area of hemorrhage. CT of the abdomen in infants may result in poor-quality images of the liver and spleen and poor delineation of tissue planes due to their rapid respiratory motion and paucity of body fat. In such selected cases, sulfur colloid imaging will be more accurate. Exceptions to the general superiority of sonography and CT may also include the detection of early abscess formation, in which liquefaction and structural alteration in the liver have not occurred or may be delayed owing to an abnormal immune response. In patients for whom the use of intravenous iodinated contrast material is contraindicated, sulfur colloid flow and static images of the liver and spleen provide an alternative imaging method.

Vascular masses in the liver occurring in infancy are well suited to evaluation with radionuclide techniques. In the proper clinical setting, both liver biopsy and arteriography may be avoided in the management of hepatic hemangiomas or hemangioendotheliomas.[120,121] These lesions usually demonstrate increased perfusion during the angiographic phase and longer retention of activity in vascular spaces owing to either pooling or arteriovenous shunting. Owing to the absence of reticuloendothelial cells, these vascular masses show no uptake of activity on later sulfur colloid views. Hypervascular tumors in childhood such as hepatoblastomas and hepatomas show early increased flow without prolonged retention of activity during the flow phase. Because of the potential for overlap between the scintigraphic findings in hemangiomas of the liver and other lesions that have pronounced tumor vascularity and focal defects on delayed sulfur colloid views, the use of ^{99m}Tc-labeled red blood cells instead of sulfur colloid has been advocated in the infant or child with a suspected hemangiomatous liver lesion.[122] MRI of the liver has been described as an accurate technique for the diagnosis of hepatic hemangioma, although other lesions may also mimic the appearance of hemangiomas on MRI.[123,124]

Sulfur colloid imaging is frequently used as a screening tool for diseases with diffuse liver involvement. The primary scintigraphic findings in diffuse liver disease are diminished or inhomogeneous sulfur colloid uptake by the liver, with relatively increased sulfur colloid uptake in the spleen and increased bone marrow uptake with progressive disease (Fig. 11). Hepatic enlargement is frequently seen with early liver involvement, with variable progression depending on the specific disease and its severity. In screening for diffuse liver disease in the adult population, sulfur colloid imaging of the liver and spleen has been reported to have a higher sensitivity than either sonography or CT.[125,126] Other authors, however, have found a low overall sensitivity for sulfur colloid imaging in diffuse liver disease.[127,128]

Processes such as alpha$_1$-antitrypsin deficiency, cystic fibrosis, and congenital hepatic fibrosis resulting in cirrhosis eventually demonstrate diminished liver size with splenomegaly and markedly increased colloid within the spleen. Both hepatomegaly and splenomegaly are typically demonstrated with infiltrative disorders such as lymphoma and leukemia. Nonspecific patchy liver uptake, various degrees of hepatosplenomegaly, and marked uptake in lung as well as bone marrow have been described in histiocytosis X.[129] Inhomogeneous colloid uptake, focal liver defects, hepatomegaly, splenomegaly with increased colloid uptake, and wedge-shaped splenic infarcts have been described in Gaucher's disease.[130] Significant liver enlargement with uniform colloid distribution, a normal to minimally increased spleen size with normal to minimally increased colloid uptake, and prominent renal impressions due to nephromegaly are typical in young children with type I glycogen storage disease.[131] Older children demonstrate more heterogeneity in liver uptake with increased colloid shift to the enlarged spleen. The other types of glycogenoses may demonstrate the following: milder changes (type III), more severe liver involvement with early cirrhotic changes in the absence of renal enlargement (type IV), or hepatomegaly without splenomegaly (types VI or IX).[132] Focal liver defects in children with glycogen storage diseases may reflect the presence of adenomas.

^{67}Ga CITRATE AND ^{111}In-LABELED LEUKOCYTES

Unfortunately, the relative high radiation doses received by patients limit the applications of either ^{111}In white blood cell (wbc) or ^{67}Ga-citrate scanning in the pediatric age group. These techniques have been most widely applied in adult patients, although they are appropriate for pediatric patients in whom serious disease is suspected. There is greater experience with ^{67}Ga imaging than with ^{111}In wbc imaging in children.

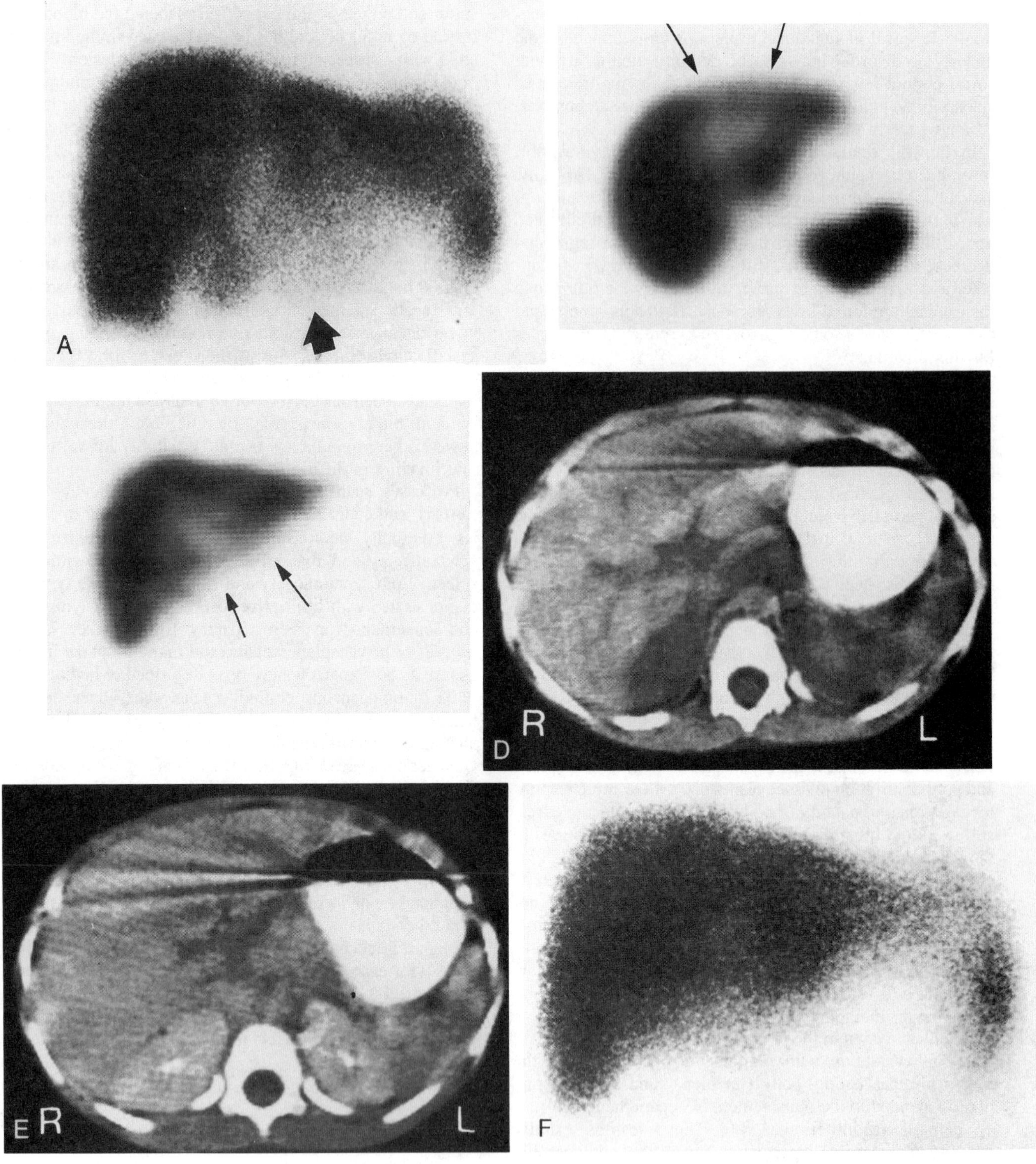

FIGURE 10 Hepatic contusion secondary to child abuse. ^{99m}Tc–sulfur colloid liver-spleen images in *A*, anterior projection, and after 360-degree tomography (SPECT) with reconstruction in *B*, the transaxial plane, and *C*, the coronal plane. Note diminished activity at the inferior aspect of the liver (*arrows*). SPECT images confirm the location of the contusion and exclude anatomic thinning. The lesion is not demonstrated on *D*, a precontrast CT view, or *E*, a postcontrast CT view. A spleen tip laceration (not shown) was present on both radionuclide and CT examinations. *F*, Follow-up sulfur colloid image of the liver, anterior projection, 3 months later is normal.

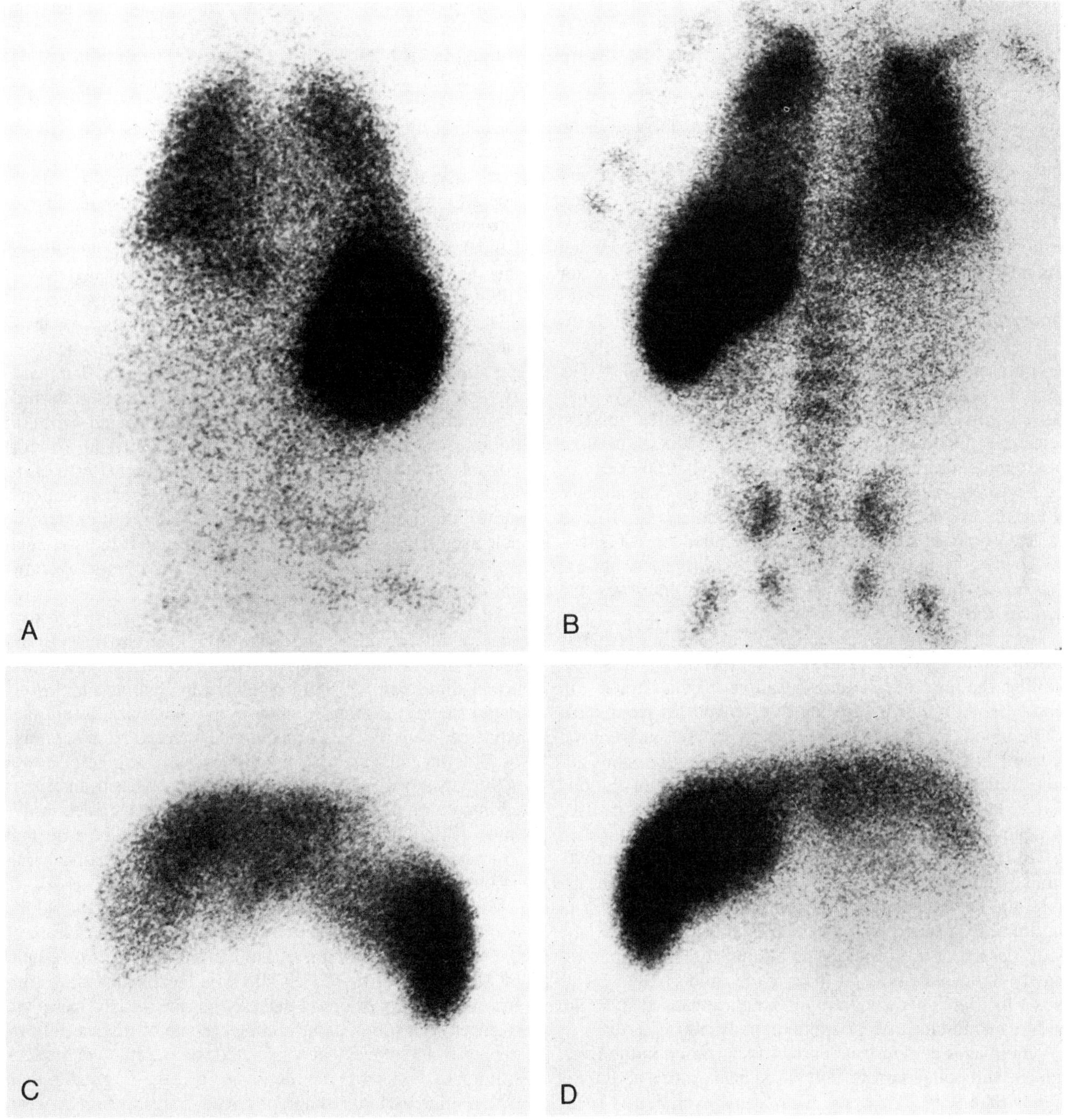

FIGURE 11 Hepatic failure secondary to fulminant enteroviral infection. *A*, Anterior image, and *B*, posterior image, ^{99m}Tc–sulfur colloid liver-spleen scan. There is minimal uptake in the liver with marked "colloid shift," i.e., increased activity in the spleen, lungs, and bone marrow, reflecting the diminished clearance of radioactive colloid particles by the reticuloendothelial cells in the liver. Follow-up images, *C*, anterior, and *D*, posterior, 3 weeks later show improvement in visualization of the liver, with residual relatively increased uptake in the spleen.

Based on extrapolations from adult data and actual measurements, dosimetry estimates for ^{67}Ga and ^{111}In wbcs in pediatric patients have been predicted to be similar.[133-137] Depending on the child's body weight and the dose administered, estimated pediatric radiation doses per procedure from ^{111}In wbcs are as follows: spleen, 4.1 to 42.0 cGy; liver, 0.7 to 4.2 cGy; marrow, 0.15 to 5.8 cGy; and whole body, 0.12 to 0.73 cGy. Attempts to measure biodistribution data for ^{111}In wbcs in pediatric patients have shown great variability in splenic uptake, which may be particularly high in cases of splenic hyperfunction or enlargement. The relatively high radiation dose from both procedures prevents their frequent use, as in the follow-up of inflammatory bowel disorders. In fact, some authors have argued that ^{111}In wbc techniques should be avoided in children because of their long life expectancy and the risk of chromosomal aberrations induced in the labeled lymphocytes.[138] Although chromosomal damage has been shown, survival and subsequent division of damaged cells have not been demonstrated.

There are several theoretical advantages of ^{111}In wbc imaging over ^{67}Ga-citrate imaging. The physical characteristics of the two radionuclides allow better images to be obtained with ^{111}In wbcs. Since ^{67}Ga is taken up by several tumors and noninfectious processes, ^{111}In wbcs are more specific for acute infection or inflammation than ^{67}Ga.[139,140] The significant uptake of ^{67}Ga in noninfected surgical wounds limits its use in the postoperative period, whereas ^{111}In wbc activity in noninfected surgical sites and wounds is minimal.[141] The normal excretion of ^{67}Ga by the colon and kidneys may cause confusion in the interpretation of abdominal images. Sequential abdominal views over 24 to 72 hours or, in older children, cathartic administration may be required before final interpretations of ^{67}Ga images can be made. The absence of normal excretion of ^{111}In wbcs by the kidneys or GI tract greatly simplifies the evaluation of abdominal sites of activity. Abscess-to-blood background ratios with ^{111}In wbcs are also much higher than with ^{67}Ga, which improves the chances for detecting lesions with ^{111}In wbcs.[142]

^{111}In wbc labeling can be accomplished for any pediatric patient, although cell labeling for the procedure is less simple than the intravenous administration of ^{67}Ga-citrate. ^{111}In wbc labeling requires separation of leukocytes from fresh whole blood, incubation of the wbcs with ^{111}In, and removal of free ^{111}In from the preparation prior to its intravenous administration. In the pediatric patient as little as 5 ml of blood may be labeled successfully. Fresh donor blood may be used in neutropenic patients.

^{111}In wbc images may demonstrate transient lung activity immediately after injection. At 24 hours after injection, the liver and spleen each contain approximately 25 percent of the administered activity, with the remainder in marrow and body tissues. The doses of ^{111}In administered are approximately 100 μCi for the first 10 kg of the child's body weight, plus 5 to 10 μCi per kilogram for weight greater than 10 kg, with a maximum dose of approximately 500 μCi.

^{67}Ga images demonstrate normal localization in the liver, spleen, and bone marrow. Soft tissue background activity is higher than with ^{111}In wbcs. Early renal excretion is seen, with normal visualization of the kidneys and urinary bladder. Bowel activity due to normal gallium excretion may remain visible for several days. Typical administered doses of ^{67}Ga-citrate are on the order of 50 μCi per kilogram, with a minimum dose of 500 μCi and maximum doses of 3 to 5 mCi.

The results of ^{111}In wbc scans in several large series of patients have shown an overall sensitivity of 80 to 96 percent and overall specificity of 90 to 99 percent.[141,143–148] Some pediatric patients are included in these reports. Small pediatric series have reported sensitivities of 77 to 81 percent and specificities of 94 to 100 percent.[134,135,149] By comparison, with ^{67}Ga scanning in occult inflammatory disease in children, reported sensitivities are 92 to 94 percent and specificities are 71 to 100 percent.[150,151]

The pitfalls and limitations of ^{111}In wbc and ^{67}Ga imaging are of potential significance in the pediatric patient.[152–155] Results of early views (a few hours after injection) are not sufficient to exclude the presence of an abscess. When no inflammatory focus is found, imaging must be repeated at 24 and 48 hours after injection. In instances in which the blood supply to the infected tissue is poor (such as infected cysts, hematomas, and abscesses), the scan may require 72 hours to become positive.[156] Malnutrition and a number of iatrogenic causes of impaired neutrophil function, including hemodialysis, hyperalimentation, hyperglycemia, hypocalcemia, and steroid administration, have been postulated to contribute to the occurrence of false-negative ^{111}In wbc scans.[144] ^{67}Ga appears to have better accumulation in relatively avascular sites than do ^{111}In wbcs. False-negative ^{111}In wbc scans are also more likely with subacute and chronic inflammatory sites of disease, in which case ^{67}Ga imaging is preferred.

Accumulation of ^{67}Ga-labeled or ^{111}In-labeled wbcs at noninfected sites of inflammation may be difficult (or impossible) to distinguish from clinically significant sites of infection or abscesses. The sites of intramuscular injections, indwelling drains, and catheters frequently result in identifiable accumulation of activity on the images. If intense, such activity may be particularly difficult to interpret in abdominal sites.

Diffuse peritonitis may result in intense ^{67}Ga or ^{111}In wbc activity throughout the abdomen. Bowel activity may also be seen with antibiotic administration, bowel ischemia, and bowel infarction.[153,157] ^{111}In wbcs accumulate at sites of GI hemorrhage, resulting in intense bowel activity. Swallowed white cell activity from expectorated material from the lungs or pharynx must also be remembered as a source of bowel activity. Surgical exploration of the abdomen has been reported in a child with cystic fibrosis and pulmonary infection.[152] Submandibular gland uptake of ^{111}In wbcs may be a normal finding in children but may result in radioactive saliva being swallowed.[158]

^{111}In-labeled wbcs have been used in children and adults to distinguish between active and inactive Crohn's disease of the small bowel or colon and to identify bowel involvement by ulcerative colitis.[149,159–161] ^{111}In wbc localization may confirm the activity of bowel disease; however, early views are required to avoid misinterpreting the site of disease following peristaltic movement of excreted wbcs. Although the sensitivity of ^{111}In wbcs for detecting disease is greater than with routine barium radiographic studies, distinction between types of inflammatory bowel disease is not reliable from the appearance of the scans. The use of ^{99m}Tc-labeled sucralfate to detect mucosal ulcerations has not been widely applied in assessing inflammatory bowel disease in children but has the advantage of lower absorbed radiation doses than ^{111}In-labeled wbcs.[162]

The normal accumulation of ^{67}Ga and ^{111}In wbcs in the liver and spleen makes detection of infected sites in or adjacent to these organs more difficult. Small abscesses within these organs and superficial foci overlying the liver and spleen are most likely to be missed. Careful correlation of ^{67}Ga or ^{111}In wbc images with sonography or CT improves the accuracy of interpretations in the upper abdomen. The use of ^{99m}Tc-sulfur colloid imaging of the liver and spleen, in combination with ^{67}Ga or ^{111}In wbc imaging, has been suggested to allow comparison of organ contours.[163,164] A more common problem occurs in evaluating a "cold" lesion within the liver or spleen on routine sulfur colloid views. Even mild ^{111}In wbc activity in such an area is strongly suggestive of an abscess. This finding is less reliable with gallium imaging because of its nonspecific uptake in other lesions. When interpreting wbc images, the possibility of activity in accessory spleens or regenerated splenic tissue should also be considered and not be mistaken for abscess activity.[153]

^{99m}Tc-LABELED LEUKOCYTES

There are several theoretical advantages of using ^{99m}Tc rather than ^{111}In as a white blood cell labeling agent, including technetium's shorter half-life and a photon energy more suitable for imaging. The potential for imaging inflammatory processes and abscesses at lower radiation absorbed doses associated with ^{99m}Tc is also of particular interest in pediatric patients. In addition, the earlier imaging possible with ^{99m}Tc wbcs may avoid the 24-hour or longer delay in diagnosis associated with the use of ^{111}In wbcs.

Imaging with ^{99m}Tc-labeled wbcs has not attained widespread clinical use. Preliminary reports of animal studies and reports of human use in patients with abscesses are promising.[165-169] An evaluation of ^{99m}Tc albumin colloid-labeled wbcs in 38 patients (including some children) with suspected appendicitis showed a sensitivity of 83 percent and a specificity of 100 percent, which is comparable to results with ^{111}In.[170] Further experience with this technique in pediatric patients will be necessary to determine its role in assessing inflammatory processes involving the GI tract.

REFERENCES

1. Arasu TS, Wyllie R, Fitzgerald JF, Franken EA, Siddiqui AR, Lehman GA, Eigen H, Grosfeld JL. Gastroesophageal reflux in infants and children: comparative accuracy of diagnostic methods. J Pediatr 1980; 96:798–803.
2. Fisher RS, Malmud LS, Roberts GS, et al. Gastroesophageal (GE) scintiscanning to detect and quantitate GE reflux. Gastroenterology 1976; 70:301–308.
3. Heyman S, Kirkpatrick JA, Winter HS, Treves S. An improved radionuclide method for the diagnosis of gastroesophageal reflux and aspiration in children (milk scan). Radiology 1979; 131:479–482.
4. Rudd TG, Christie DL. Demonstration of gastroesophageal reflux in children by radionuclide gastroesophagography. Radiology 1979; 131:483–486.
5. Seibert JJ, Byrne WJ, Euler AR, Latture T, Leach M, Campbell M. Gastroesophageal reflux—the acid test: scintigraphy or the pH probe? AJR 1983; 140:1087–1090.
6. Papanicolaou N, Abramson S, Winter H, Treves S. Simultaneous esophageal pH monitoring and radionuclide scintigraphy in the evaluation of pediatric patients for gastroesophageal reflux. (Abstract) Amsterdam: Society of European Pediatric Radiology, 1981.
7. Piepsz A, Georges B, Rodesch P, Cadranel S. Gastroesophageal scintiscanning in children. J Nucl Med 1982; 23:631–632.
8. Castronovo FP Jr. Gastroesophageal scintiscanning in a pediatric population: dosimetry. J Nucl Med 1986; 27:1212–1214.
9. Swischuk LE, Fawcett HD, Hayden CK, Isenberg JN. Gastroesophageal reflux: how much imaging is required? Radiographics 1988; 8:1137–1146.
10. Jona JZ, Sty JR, Glicklich M. Simplified radioisotope technique for assessing gastroesophageal reflux in children. J Pediatr Surg 1981; 16:114–117.
11. Macfadyen UM, Hendry GMA, Simpson H. Gastro-esophageal reflux in near-miss sudden infant death syndrome or suspected recurrent aspiration. Arch Dis Child 1983; 58:87–91.
12. McVeagh P, Howman-Giles R, Kemp A. Pulmonary aspiration studied by radionuclide milk scanning and barium swallow roentgenography. Am J Dis Child 1987; 141:917–921.
13. Paton JY, Cosgriff PS, Nanayakkara CS. The analytical sensitivity of Tc99m radionuclide 'milk' scanning in the detection of gastroesophageal reflux. Pediatr Radiol 1985; 15:381–383.
14. Boonyaprapa S, Alderson PO, Garfinkel DJ, Chipps BE, Wagner HJ Jr. Detection of pulmonary aspiration in infants and children with respiratory disease: concise communication. J Nucl Med 1980; 21:314–318.
15. Orellana P, Olea E, Pino C, Rossel M, Ceresa S, Gonzalez P, Otarola S, Astudillo S. Detection of pulmonary aspiration in children with gastroesophageal reflux. J Nucl Med 1985; 26:P10–P11.
16. Reich SB, Early WC, Ravin TH, Goodman M, Spector S, Stein MR. Evaluation of gastropulmonary aspiration by a radioactive technique: concise communication. J Nucl Med 1977; 18:1079–1081.
17. Crausaz FM, Favez G. Aspiration of solid food particles into lungs of patients with gastroesophageal reflux and chronic bronchial disease. Chest 1988; 93:376–378.
18. Thirunavukkarasu S, Siddiqui AR, Wyllie R, Eigen H, Franken EA, Wellman HN, Grosfeld JL, Fitzgerald JF. Usefulness of radionuclide studies in detection of gastroesophageal (GE) reflux and pulmonary aspiration in childhood. J Nucl Med 1979; 20:637.
19. Fawcett HD, Hayden CK Jr, Adams JC, Swischuk LE. Clinical efficacy of gastroesophageal reflux scintigraphy in childhood aspiration. Pediatr Radiol 1988; 18:311–313.
20. Heyman S. The radionuclide salivagram for detecting the pulmonary aspiration of saliva in an infant. Pediatr Radiol 1989; 19:208–209.
21. Heyman S, Respondek M. Detection of pulmonary aspiration in children by radionuclide "salivagram." J Nucl Med 1989; 30:697–699.
22. Fonkalsrud EW, Ament M, Berquist W. Surgical management of the gastroesophageal reflux syndrome in childhood. Surgery 1985; 97:42–48.
23. Heyman S. Esophageal scintigraphy (milk scans) in infants and children with gastroesophageal reflux. Radiology 1982; 144:891–893.
24. Guillet J, Wynchank S, Basse-Cathalinat B, Christophe E, Ducassou D, Blanquet P. Pediatric esophageal scintigraphy: results of 200 studies. Clin Nucl Med 1983; 8:427–433.
25. Guillet J, Basse-Cathalinat, Christophe E, Ducassou D, Blanquet P, Wynchank S. Routine studies of swallowed radionuclide transit in pediatrics: experience with 400 patients. Eur J Nucl Med 1984; 9:86–90.
26. Tothill P, McLoughlin GP, Heading RC. Techniques and errors in scintigraphic measurements of gastric emptying. J Nucl Med 1978; 19:256–261.
27. Parr N, Grime S, Jenkins S, Baxter J, Critchley M, Mackie C. The effects of pH on the distribution of radiolabels in milk—a source of error in gastric emptying tests? Nucl Med Commun 1986; 7:298–299.
28. Hillemeier AC, Lange R, McCallum R, Seashore J, Gryboski J. Delayed gastric emptying in infants with gastroesophageal reflux. J Pediatr 1981; 98:190–193.
29. Sty JR, Starshak RJ. The role of radionuclide studies in pediatric gastrointestinal disorders. Semin Nucl Med 1982; 12:156–172.
30. Seibert JJ, Byrne WJ, Euler AR. Gastric emptying in children: unusual patterns detected by scintigraphy. AJR 1983; 141:49–51.
31. Rosen PR, Treves S. The relationship of gastroesophageal reflux and gastric emptying in infants and children: concise communication. J Nucl Med 1984; 25:571–574.
32. DiLorenzo C, Piepsz A, Ham H, Cadranel S. Gastric emptying with gastroesophageal reflux. Arch Dis Child 1987; 62:449–453.
33. Chervu LR, Nunn AD, Loberg MD. Radiopharmaceuticals for hepatobiliary imaging. Semin Nucl Med 1982; 12:5–17.
34. Majd M, Reba RC, Altman RP, Hepatobiliary scintigraphy with 99mTc-Pipida in the evaluation of neonatal jaundice. Pediatrics 1981; 67:140–145.
35. Sty JR, Starshak RJ, Miller JH. Pediatric nuclear medicine. Norwalk: Appleton-Century-Crofts, 1983.
36. Williamson SL, Seibert JJ, Butler HL, Golladay ES. Apparent gut excretion of Tc-99m-DISIDA in a case of biliary atresia. Pediatr Radiol 1986; 16:245–247.
37. Manolaki AG, Larcher VF, Mowat AP, Barrett JJ, Portman NB, Howard LR. The prelaparotomy diagnosis of extrahepatic biliary atresia. Arch Dis Child 1983; 58:591–594.

38. Sty JR, Glicklich M, Babbitt DP, Starshak RJ. Technetium-99m biliary imaging in pediatric surgical problems. J Pediatr Surg 1981; 16:686–690.
39. Majd M, Reba RC, Altman RP. Effect of phenobarbital on 99mTc-IDA scintigraphy in the evaluation of neonatal jaundice. Semin Nucl Med 1981; 11:194–204.
40. Majd M. 99mTc-IDA scintigraphy in the evaluation of neonatal jaundice. RadioGraphics 1983; 3:88–99.
41. Gerhold JP, Klingensmith WC III, Kuni CC, Lilly JR, Silverman A, Fritzberg AR, Nixt TL. Diagnosis of biliary atresia with radionuclide hepatobiliary imaging. Radiology 1983; 146:499–504.
42. Alagille D, Odievre M, Gautier M, Dommergues JP. Hepatic ductular hypoplasia associated with characteristic facies, vertebral malformations, retarded physical, mental, and sexual development, and cardiac murmur. J Pediatr 1975; 86:63–71.
43. Rosenfield NS, Kelley MJ, Jensen PS, Cotlier E, Rosenfield AT, Riely CA. Arteriohepatic dysplasia: radiologic features of a new syndrome. AJR 1980; 135:1217–1223.
44. Summerville DA, Marks M, Treves ST. Hepatobiliary scintigraphy in arteriohepatic dysplasia (Alagille's syndrome); a report of two cases. Pediatr Radiol 1988; 18:32–34.
45. Markle BM, Potter BM, Majd M. The jaundiced infant and child. Semin Ultrasound 1980; 1:123–133.
46. So SK, Lindahl JA, Sharp HL, Cook AM, Leonard AS. Bile ascites during infancy: diagnosis using Disofenin Tc-99m sequential scintiphotography. Pediatrics 1983; 71:402–405.
47. Lilly JR, Weintraub WH, Altman RP. Spontaneous perforation of the extrahepatic bile ducts and bile peritonitis in infancy. Surgery 1974; 75:664–672.
48. Stringel G, Mercer S. Idiopathic perforation of the biliary tract in infancy. J Pediatr Surg 1983; 18:546–550.
49. Sty JR, Wells RG, Schroeder BA. Comparative imaging: bile plug syndrome. Clin Nucl Med 1987; 12:4489–4490.
50. Rosenthall L, Shaffer EA, Lisbona R, Pare P. Diagnosis of hepatobiliary disease by ^{99m}Tc-HIDA cholescintigraphy. Radiology 1978; 126:467–474.
51. Han BK, Babcock DS, Gelfand MH. Choledochal cyst with bile duct dilatation: sonography and ^{99m}Tc IDA cholescintigraphy. AJR 1981; 136:1075–1079.
52. Sty JR, Hubbard AM, Starshak RJ. Radionuclide hepatobiliary imaging in congenital biliary tract ectasia (Caroli disease). Pediatr Radiol 1982; 12:111–114.
53. Ament AE, Bick RJ, Miraldi FD, Haaga JR, Wiedenmann SD. Sclerosing cholangitis: cholescintigraphy with TC-99m-labeled DISIDA. Radiology 1984; 151:197–201.
54. Spivak W, Grand RJ, Eraklis A. A case of primary sclerosing cholangitis in childhood. Gastroenterology 1982; 82:129–132.
55. Werlin SL, Glichlich M, Jona J, Starshak RJ. Sclerosing cholangitis in childhood. J Pediatr 1980; 96:433–435.
56. Rodman CA, Keeffe EB, Lieberman DA, Krishnamurthy S, Krishnamurthy GT, Gilbert S, Eklem MJ. Diagnosis of sclerosing cholangitis with technetium 99m-labeled iminodiacetic acid planar and single photon emission computed tomographic scintigraphy. Gastroenterology 1987; 92:777–785.
57. Sty JR, Starshak RJ, Hubbard AM. Radionuclide hepatobiliary imaging in the detection of traumatic biliary tract disease in children. Pediatr Radiol 1982; 12:115–118.
58. Rosenthal L, Forseca C, Arzoumanian A, Hernandez M, Greenberg D. ^{99m}Tc-IDA hepatobiliary imaging following upper abdominal surgery. Radiology 1979; 130:735–739.
59. Miller JH, Sinatra FR, Thomas DW. Biliary excretion disorders in infants: evaluation using ^{99m}Tc-PIPIDA. AJR 1980; 134:47–52.
60. El-Shafie M, Mah CL. Transient gallbladder distension in sick premature infants: the value of ultrasonography and radionuclide scintigraphy. Pediatr Radiol 1986; 16:468–471.
61. Keller MS, Markle BM, Laffey PA, Chawla HS, Jacir N, Frank J. Spontaneous resolution of cholelithiasis in infants. Radiology 1985; 157:345–348.
62. Jacir NN, Anderson KD, Eichelberger M, Guzzetta PC. Cholelithiasis in infancy: resolution of gallstones in three of four infants. J Pediatr Surg 1986; 21:567–569.
63. Whitington PF, Black DD. Cholelithiasis in premature infants treated with parenteral nutrition and furosemide. J Pediatr 1980; 97:647–649.
64. Callahan J, Haller JO, Cacciarelli AA, Slovis TL, Friedman AP. Cholelithiasis in infants: association with total parenteral nutrition and furosemide. Radiology 1982; 143:437–439.
65. Freitas JE, Fink-Bennett DM. Asymptomatic cystic duct obstruction in chronic cholecystitis. (Abstract) J Nucl Med 1980; 21:P17.
66. Pare P, Shaffer EA, Rosenthall L. Nonvisualization of the gallbladder by Tc-99m–HIDA cholescintigraphy as evidence of cholecystitis. Can Med Assoc J 1978; 118:384–386.
67. Al-Sheikh W, Hourani M, Barkin JS, Clarke LP, Ashkar FS, Serafini AN. A sign of symptomatic chronic cholecystitis on biliary scintigraphy. AJR 1983; 140:283–285.
68. Shuman WP, Gibbs P, Rudd TG, Mack LA. PIPIDA scintigraphy for cholecystitis: false positives in alcoholism and total parenteral nutrition. AJR 1982; 138:1–5.
69. Kalff V, Froelich JW, Lloyd R, Thrall JH. Predictive value of an abnormal hepatobiliary scan in patients with severe intercurrent illness. Radiology 1983; 146:191–194.
70. Larsen MJ, Klingensmith WC, Kuni CC. Radionuclide hepatobiliary imaging: nonvisualization secondary to prolonged fasting. J Nucl Med 1982; 23:1003–1005.
71. Weissman HS, Sugarman LA, Badia JD, Freeman LM. Improving the specificity and accuracy of Tc-99m–IDA cholescintigraphy with delayed views. (Abstract) J Nucl Med 1980; 21:P17.
72. Zeman RK, Segal HB, Caride VJ. Tc-99m HIDA cholescintigraphy: the distended photon-deficient gallbladder. J Nucl Med 1981; 22:39–41.
73. Choy D, Shi EC, McLean RG, Hoschl R, Murrary IPC, Ham JM. Cholescintigraphy in acute cholecystitis: use of intravenous morphine. Radiology 1984; 151:203–207.
74. Kim EE, Pjura G, Lowry P, Nguyen M, Pollack M. Morphine-augmented cholescintigraphy in the diagnosis of acute cholecystitis. AJR 1986; 147:1177–1179.
75. Freeman LM, Sugarman LA, Weissman HS. Role of cholecystokinetic agents in ^{99m}Tc-IDA cholescintigraphy. Semin Nucl Med 1981; 11:186–193.
76. Spellman SJ, Shaffer EA, Rosenthall L. Gallbladder emptying in response to cholecystokinin. Gastroenterology 1979; 77:115–120.
77. Topper TE, Ryerson TW, Nora PF. Quantitative gallbladder imaging following cholecystokinin. J Nucl Med 1980; 21:694–696.
78. Dalinka MK, Wander JK. Meckel's diverticulum with emphasis on roentgenogaphic demonstration. Radiology 1973; 106:295–298.
79. Meguid MM, Wilkinson RH, Canty T, Eraklis AJ, Treves S. Futility of barium sulfate in diagnosis of Meckel's diverticulum. Arch Surg 1974; 108: 361–362.
80. Jewett TC, Duszynski DO, Allen JE. The visualization of Meckel's diverticulum with ^{99m}Tc-pertechnetate. Surgery 1970; 68:567–570.
81. Berquist TH, Nolan NC, Stephens DH, Carlson HC. Specificity of Tc-99m pertechnetate in scintigraphic diagnosis of Meckel's diverticulum: a review of 100 cases. (Abstract) J Nucl Med 1975; 16:515.
82. Gelfand MJ, Silberstein EB, Cox J. Radionuclide imaging of Meckel's diverticulum in children. Clin Nucl Med 1978; 3:4–7.
83. Ho JE, Konieczny KM. The sodium pertechnetate Tc99m scan: an aid in the evaluation of gastrointestinal bleeding. Pediatrics 1975; 56:34–40.
84. Sfakianakis GN, Conway JJ. Detection of ectopic gastric mucosa in Meckel's diverticulum and in other aberrations by scintigraphy: I. Pathophysiology and 10-year clinical experience. J Nucl Med 1981; 22:647–654.
85. Sfakianakis GN, Haase GM. Abdominal scintigraphy for ectopic gastric mucosa: a retrospective analysis of 143 studies. AJR 1982; 138:7–12.
86. Harper PV, Lathrop KA, Jiminez F, Fink R, Gottschalk A. Technetium-99m as a scanning agent. Radiology 1965; 85:101–108.
87. Berquist TH, Nolan NG, Stephens DH, Carlson HC. Radioisotope scintigraphy in diagnosis of Barrett's esophagus. AJR 1975; 123:401–411.
88. Priebe CJ Jr, Marsden DS, Lazarevic B. The use of 99m technetium pertechnetate to detect transplanted gastric mucosa in the dog. J Pediatr Surg 1974; 9:605–612.
89. Hegge FN. Prominent motion of a Meckel's diverticulum. (Letter) J Nucl Med 1978; 19:1087.
90. Schussheim A, Moskowitz GW, Levy LM. Radionuclide diagnosis of bleeding Meckel's diverticulum in children. Am J Gastroenterol 1977; 68:25–29.
91. Duszynski DO, Jewett TC, Allen JE: Tc 99m Na-pertechnetate scanning of the abdomen with particular reference to small bowel pathology. AJR 1971; 113:258–262.
92. Polga JP, Sargent J, Dickinson P. Positive intestinal scan caused by carcinoid tumor. J Nucl Med 1974; 15:365–366.
93. Duszynski DO, Anthone R. Jejunal intussusception demonstrated by ^{99m}Tc pertechnetate and abdominal scanning. AJR 1970; 104:724–732.

94. Case Records of the Massachusetts General Hospital (Case 37-1985). N Engl J Med 1985; 313:680–688.
95. Tauscher JW, Bryant DR, Gruenther RC. False positive scan for Meckel diverticulum. J Pediatr 1978; 92:1022–1023.
96. Moss AA, Kressel HY. Intestinal infarction: current problems and new methods of diagnosis using radionuclide scans. Appl Radiol Nucl Med 1976; 5:156–160.
97. Khettry J, Effmann E, Grand RJ, Treves S. Effect of pentagastrin, histalog, glucagon, secretin and perchlorate on the gastric handling of Tc-99m-pertechnetate in mice. Radiology 1976; 120:629–631.
98. Petrokubi RJ, Baum S, Rohrer GV. Cimetidine administration resulting in improved pertechnetate imaging of Meckel's diverticulum. Clin Nucl Med 1978; 3:385–388.
99. Treves S, Grand RJ, Eraklis AJ. Pentagastrin stimulation of technetium 99m uptake by ectopic gastric mucosa in a Meckel's diverticulum. Radiology 1978; 128:711–712.
100. Anderson GF, Sfakianakis GN, King DR, Boles ET Jr. Hormonal enhancement of technetium-99m pertechnetate uptake in experimental Meckel's diverticulum. J Pediatr Surg 1980; 15:900–905.
101. Martin GI, Kutner FR, Moser L. Diagnosis of Meckel's diverticulum by radioisotope scanning. Pediatrics 1976; 57:11–12.
102. McKusick KA, Froelich J, Callahan RJ, Winzelberg GG, Strauss HW. ^{99m}Tc red blood cells for detection of gastrointestinal bleeding: experience with 80 patients. AJR 1981; 137:1113–1118.
103. Alavi A, Ring EJ. Localization of gastrointestinal bleeding: superiority of ^{99m}Tc sulfur colloid compared with angiography. AJR 1981; 137:741–748.
104. Alavi A, Dann RW, Baum S, Biery DN. Scintigraphic detection of acute gastrointestinal bleeding. Radiology 1977; 124:753–756.
105. Dann R, Alavi A, Baum R, Baum S. A comparison of in vivo labeled red blood cells with Tc-sulfur colloid in the detection of acute gastrointestinal bleeding. (Abstract) J Nucl Med 1980; 21:P75.
106. Bunker SR, Lull RJ, Tanasescu DE, Redwine MD, Rigby J, Brown JM, Brachman MB, McAuley RJ, Ramanna L, Landry A, Waxman AD. Scintigraphy of gastrointestinal hemorrhage: superiority of ^{99m}Tc red blood cells over ^{99m}Tc sulfur colloid. AJR 1984; 143:543–548.
107. Pavel DG, Zimmer AM, Patterson VN. In vivo labeling of red blood cells with ^{99m}Tc: a new approach to blood pool visualization. J Nucl Med 1977; 18:305–308.
108. Holder LE, Strife J, Padikal TN, Perkins PJ, Kereiakes JG. Liver size determination in pediatrics using sonographic and scintigraphic techniques. Radiology 1975; 117:349–353.
109. Treves ST. Pediatric nuclear medicine. New York: Springer-Verlag, 1985.
110. Markisz JA, Treves ST, Davis RT. Normal hepatic and splenic size in children: scintigraphic determination. Pediatr Radiol 1987; 17:273–276.
111. Freedom RM, Treves S. Splenic scintigraphy and radionuclide venography in the heterotaxy syndrome. Radiology 1973; 107:381–386.
112. Ehrlich CP, Papanicolaou N, Treves S, Hurwitz RA, Richards P. Splenic scintigraphy using Tc-99m labelled heat denatured red blood cells in pediatric patients. J Nucl Med 1982; 23:209–213.
113. Spencer RP. Spleen imaging. In: Alavi A, Arger PH, eds. Multiple imaging procedures: abdomen. Orlando, FL: Grune & Stratton, 1980: 73.
114. Cukkingford GL, Surveyor I, Edis AJ. Demonstration of functioning heterotopic splenic autografts by scintigraphy. Aust NZ J Surg 1983; 53:343–351.
115. Picard M, Carrier L, Chartrand R, Franchebois P, Picard D, Guimond J. Budd-Chiari syndrome: typical and atypical scintigraphic aspects. J Nucl Med 1987; 28:803–809.
116. Powell-Jackson RP, Karani J, Ede RJ. Ultrasound scanning and ^{99m}Tc sulphur colloid scintigraphy in diagnosis of Budd-Chiari syndrome. Gut 1986; 27:1502–1506.
117. Mathieu D, Vasile N, Menu Y, Van Beers B, Lorphelin JM, Pringot J. Budd-Chiari syndrome: dynamic CT. Radiology 1987; 165:409–413.
118. Kaufman RA, Towbin R, Babcock DS, Gelfand MJ, Guice KS, Oldham KT, Noseworthy J. Upper abdominal trauma in children: imaging evaluation. AJR 1984; 142:449–460.
119. Brick SH, Taylor GA, Potter BM, Eichelberger MR. Hepatic and splenic injury in children: role of CT in the decision for laparotomy. Radiology 1987; 165:643–646.
120. Stanley P, Gates GF, Eto RT, Miller SW, Hepatic cavernous hemangiomas and hemangioendotheliomas in infancy. AJR 1977; 129:317–321.
121. Pereyra R, Andrassy RJ, Mahour GH. Management of massive hepatic hemangiomas in infants and children: a review of 13 cases. Pediatrics 1982; 70:254–258.
122. Miller JH. Technetium-99m labelled red blood cells in the evaluation of hemangiomas of the liver in infants and children. J Nucl Med 1987; 28:1412–1418.
123. Ferruci JT, Freeny PC, Stark DD, Foley WD, Mueller PR, May G, Burhenne HJ. Advances in hepatobiliary radiology. Radiology 1988; 168:319–338.
124. Brown RKJ, Gomes A, King W, Pusey E, Lois J, Goldstein L, Busuttil RW, Hawkins RA. Hepatic hemangiomas: evaluation by magnetic resonance imaging and technetium-99m red blood cell scintigraphy. J Nucl Med 1987; 28:1683–1687.
125. McClees EC, Gedgaudas-McClees RK. Screening for diffuse and focal liver disease: the case for hepatic scintigraphy. J Clin Ultrasound 1984; 12:75–81.
126. Drane WE, VanNess MM. Hepatic imaging in diffuse liver disease. Clin Nucl Med 1988; 13:182–185.
127. Henrikkson L, Kelter U. Ultrasonography and scintigraphy of the liver in focal and diffuse disease. Acta Radiol 1987; 28:165–168.
128. Jago JR, Gibson CJ, Diffey BL. Evaluation of subjective assessment of liver function from radionuclide images. Br J Radiol 1987; 60:127–132.
129. Schaub T, Ash JM, Gilday DL. Radionuclide imaging in histiocytosis X. Pediatr Radiol 1987; 17:397–404.
130. Israel O, Jerushalmi J, Front D. Scintigraphic findings in Gaucher's disease. J Nucl Med 1986; 27:1557–1563.
131. Miller JH, Gates GF, Landing BH. Scintigraphic abnormalities in glycogen storage disease. J Nucl Med 1978; 19:354–358.
132. Heyman S. Liver-spleen scintigraphy in glycogen storage disease (glycogenoses). Clin Nucl Med 1985; 12:839–843.
133. Thomas SR, Gelfand MJ, Burns GS, Purdom RC, Kereiakes JG, Maxon HR. Radiation absorbed-dose estimates for the liver, spleen, and metaphyseal growth complexes in children undergoing gallium-67 citrate scanning. Radiology 1983; 146:817–820.
134. Gainey MA, McDougall IR. Diagnosis of acute inflammatory conditions in children and adolescents using In-111 oxine white blood cells. Clin Nucl Med 1984; 9:71–74.
135. Gordon I, Vivian G. Radiolabelled leukocytes: a new diagnostic tool in occult infection/inflammation. Arch Dis Child 1984; 59:62–66.
136. Marcus C, Stabin MG, Watson EE. Pediatric radiation dose from 111-In leukocytes. (Letter) J Nucl Med 1986; 27:1220–1221.
137. Gainey MA, Siegel JA, Smergel EM, Jara BJ. Indium-111 labeled white blood cells: dosimetry in children. J Nucl Med 1988; 29:689–694.
138. Stringer DA. Imaging inflammatory bowel disease in the pediatric patient. Rad Clin North Am 1987; 25:93–113.
139. Edwards CL, Hayes RL. Tumor scanning with Ga-67 citrate. J Nucl Med 1969; 10:103–105.
140. Edeling CJ. Tumor imaging in children. Cancer 1976; 38:921–930.
141. McDougall IR, Baumert JE, Lantieri RL. Evaluation of 111-In leukocyte whole body scanning. AJR 1979; 133:849–854.
142. Thakur ML, Coleman RE, Welch MJ. Indium-111-labeled leukocytes for the localization of abscesses: preparation, analysis, tissue distribution, and comparison with gallium-67 citrate in dogs. J Lab Clin Med 1977; 89:217–228.
143. Thakur ML, Lavender JP, Arnot RN, Silvester DJ, Segal AW. Indium-111 labeled autologous leukocytes in man. J Nucl Med 1977; 18:1014–1021.
144. Ascher NL, Ahrenholz RL, Simmons RL, Weiblen B, Gomez L, Forstrom LA, Frick MP, Henke L, McCullough J. Indium 111 autologous tagged leukocytes in the diagnosis of intraperitoneal sepsis. Arch Surg 1979; 114:386–392.
145. Forstrom LA, Weiblen BJ, Gomez L, Ascher NL, Hoogland DR, Loken MK, McCullough J. Indium-111-oxine labeled leukocytes in the diagnosis of occult inflammatory diseases. In: Thakur ML, Gottschalk A, eds. Indium-111 labeled neutrophils, platelets, and lymphocytes. Proceedings of the Yale Symposium: Radiolabeled cellular blood elements. New York: Trivarium Publishing, 1981: 123.
146. Goodwin DA, Doherty PW, McDougall IR. Clinical use of indium-111 labeled white cells—an analysis of 312 cases. In: Thakur ML, Gottschalk A, eds. Indium-labeled neutrophils, platelets, and lymphocytes. Proceedings of the Yale Symposium: Radiolabeled cellular blood elements. New York: Trivarium Publishing, 1981: 131.
147. Carroll B, Silverman PM, Goodwin DA, McDougall IR. Ultrasonography and indium 111 white blood cell scanning for the detection of intraabdominal abscesses. Radiology 1981; 140:155–160.
148. Coleman RE, Welch DM, Baker WJ, Beightol RW. Clinical experience

using indium-111-labeled leukocytes. In: Thakur ML, Gottschalk A, eds. Indium-111 labeled neutrophils, platelets, and lymphocytes. Proceedings of the Yale Symposium: Radiolabeled cellular blood elements. New York: Trivarium Publishing, 1981: 103.
149. Vivian GC, Milla PJ, Gordon I. The value of indium-111 scanning in inflammatory bowel disease in childhood. (Abstract) J Nucl Med 1983; 24:P32.
150. Handmaker H, O'Mara RE. Gallium imaging in pediatricts. J Nucl Med 1977; 18:1057-1063.
151. Cox F, Hughes WT. Gallium 67 scanning for the diagnosis of infection in children. Am J Dis Child 1979; 133:1171-1173.
152. Crass JR, L'Heureux P, Loken M. False-positive 111-In-labeled leukocyte scan in cystic fibrosis. Clin Nucl Med 1979; 4:291-293.
153. Coleman RE, Welch DM. Possible pitfalls with clinical imaging of indium-111 leukocytes: concise communciation. J Nucl Med 1980; 21:122-125.
154. Wing VW, vanSonnenberg E, Kipper S, Bieberstein MP. Indium-111-labeled leukocyte localization in hematomas: pitfall in abscess detection. Radiology 1984; 152:173-176.
155. McAfee JG, Samin A. In-111 labeled leukocytes: a review of problems in image interpretation. Radiology 1985; 155:221-229.
156. Krieves DA, McDougall IR. Disparity between early and late In-111 white blood cell scans in a patient with proven abscess. Clin Nucl Med 1983; 8:243-245.
157. Gray HW, Cuthbert I, Richards JR. Clinical imaging with indium-111 leukocytes: uptake in bowel infarction. J Nucl Med 1981; 22:701-702.
158. Williamson SL, Williamson MR, Seibert JJ, Boyd CM, Latture T. Indium-111 leukocyte accumulation in submandibular gland saliva as a cause for false-positive gut uptake in children. Clin Nucl Med 1987; 12:867-868.
159. Saverymuttu SH, Peters AM, Hodgson HJ, Chadwick VS, Lavender JP, Indium-111 autologous leukocyte scanning: comparison with radiology for imaging the colon in inflammatory bowel disease. Br Med J 1982; 285:255-257.
160. Saverymuttu SH, Peters AM, Hodgson HJ, Chadwick VS, Lavender JP. Indium-111 leukocyte scanning in small-bowel Crohn's disease. Gastrointest Radiol 1983; 8:157-161.
161. Stein DT, Gray GN, Gregory PB, Anderson M, Goodwin DA, McDougall IR. Location and activity of ulcerative and Crohn's colitis by In-111-leukocyte scan: a prospective comparison study. Gastroenterology 1983; 84:388-393.
162. Dawson DJ, Khan AN, Miller V, Ratcliffe JF, Shreeve DR. Detection of inflammatory bowel disease in adults and children: evaluation of a new isotopic technique. Br Med J 1985; 291:1227-1230.
163. Fawcett HD, Lantieri RL, Frankel A, McDougall IR. Differentiating hepatic abscess from tumor: Combined ^{111}In white blood cell and ^{99m}Tc liver scans. AJR 1980; 135:53-56.
164. Datz FL, Luers P, Baker W. Improved detection of upper abdominal abscesses by combination of ^{99m}Tc-sulfur colloid and ^{111}In-leukocyte scanning. AJR 1985; 144:319-323.
165. Farid NA, White SM, Heck LL, Van Hove ED. Tc-99m labeled leukocytes: preparation and use in identification of abscess and tissue rejection. Radiology 1983; 148:827-831.
166. Rosenthall L, Arzoumanian A. A comparison of Tc-99m colloid labeled leukocytes and Ga-67 citrate for the disclosure of sepsis. Clin Nucl Med 1983; 8:340-343.
167. Kelbaek H, Fogh J, Gjrup T, Bulow K, Vestergaard B. Scintigraphic demonstration of subcutaneous abscesses with ^{99m}Tc-labeled leukocytes. Eur J Nucl Med 1985; 10:302-303.
168. Kelbaek H, Gjrup T, Fogh J. Anal abscess imaged with 99mTc-labeled leukocytes. Case report. Acta Chir Scand 1985; 151:485-486.
169. Sundrehagen E, Bengtsson AM, Bremer PO, Jacobsson H, von Krusenstierna S, Larrson S, Schnell PO, Svenberg T, Svenberg Appelgren P. A new method for granulocyte labeling with technetium-99m: preliminary results in abscess detection. J Nucl Med 1986; 27:555-559.
170. Butler JA, Marcus CS, Henneman PL, Inkelis SH, Wilson SE. Evaluation of Tc-99m leukocyte scan in the diagnosis of acute appendicitis. J Surg Res 1987; 42:575-579.

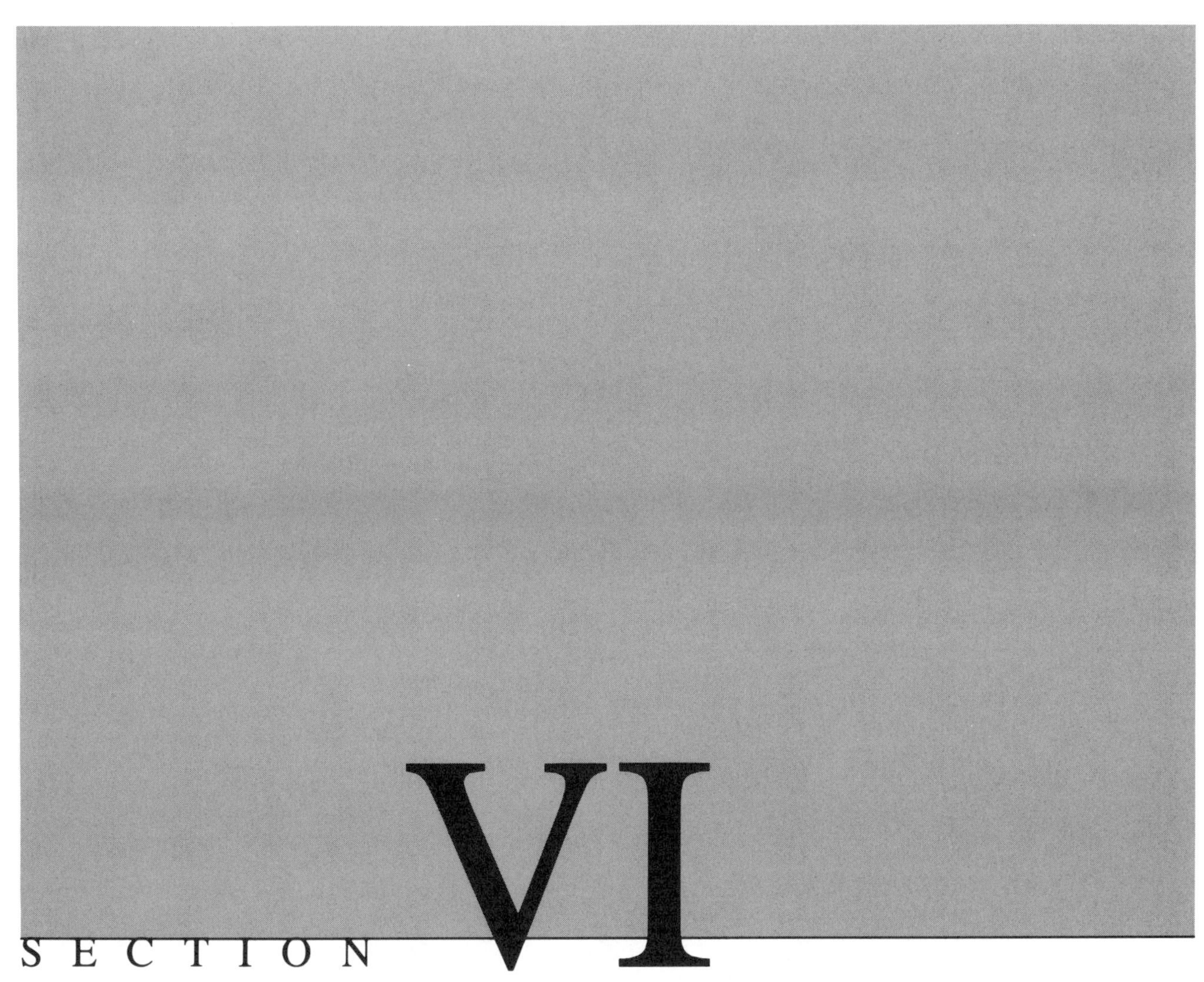

SECTION VI

Principles of Therapy

CHAPTER 40

Fluid Therapy of Diarrhea

PART 1

Developing Countries

Dilip Mahalanabis, M.B.B.S., F.R.C.P.

The approach to fluid management of gastrointestinal (GI) disorders, principally diarrhea, is sufficiently different in the industrialized world from that in developing countries that separate discussions of the two conditions are presented in this chapter. Clinicians involved in the management of these conditions have profited from each other's experience. Medical research in ion and water transport in the intestine provided the theoretical basis for oral rehydration solutions, and the practical experience of using oral rehydration therapy (ORT) has suggested its value in replacing intravenous rehydration in many acute and chronic diarrheal conditions. This part of the chapter provides information similar to that in Part 2; however, the discussions are complementary because of the difference in approach provided by the authors.

In many parts of the developing world, diarrheal attack rates are extremely high. Morbidity and mortality rates are devastating because of the severity and prevalance of enteric infection among young children. The enormity of the problem and the lack of sophisticated modern resources, combined with an improved understanding of how the intestine malfunctions during an episode of diarrhea, have prompted major advances in the treatment of the problem in the Third World. In fact, because of the initiative promoted by the World Health Organization (WHO) and other agencies, in which simple but rational approaches to treatment are used, treatment of acute diarrhea in many centers in the developing world has become superior to that practiced in our most modern developed world hospitals. Since the incidence of severe disease is much lower in the industrialized countries and mortality rates are low, less pressure has been felt to adopt these modern techniques.

The development of oral rehydration salts (ORS) solution for treatment of acute diarrhea is the major single therapeutic advance in the field of diarrheal diseases in recent years.[1] Ever since the demonstration in cholera patients[2–7] that an optimally constituted oral rehydration fluid could replace massive losses due to acute secretory diarrhea, a series of careful clinical trials and balance studies have established its usefulness in infants and children with acute diarrhea of diverse etiology.[8–17] An impressive demonstration of its practical usefulness under the most adverse field conditions occurred during a cholera epidemic among West Bengal refugee camps during the Bangladesh war.[18] In developing countries ORT is an essential component of primary care and a useful entry point for other child survival interventions. Appropriate feeding during and after diarrhea is part of optimum ORT. The ORS solution most widely used and recommended by WHO contains glucose (20 g) and three salts—sodium chloride (3.5 g), trisodium citrate dihydrate (2.9 g), and potassium chloride (1.5 g)—to be mixed in 1 liter of water. This formulation, optimal for rehydration of patients with dehydration due to acute diarrhea of any etiology,[19,20] has been found suitable for the replacement of ongoing diarrheal losses when appropriate amounts of the solution are administered along with other fluids, e.g., breast milk, diluted cow's milk, or formula and water, particularly in infants.[21,22] ORT alone can successfully rehydrate 90 percent of patients with dehydration due to acute diarrhea who previously would have received intravenous therapy. In recent years successful clinical trials of ORT in well-nourished children in developed countries have led to its wide acceptance.[23,24]

PHYSIOLOGIC BASIS OF ORAL HYDRATION

Intestinal Absorption of Sodium and Water—In Vitro Models

An understanding of the absorption of sodium from the mammalian intestine has been elucidated largely by in vitro experiments.[25] Water moves into and out of the gut lumen as an osmotic response to the net transport of electrolytes and organic solutes. Of these, sodium chloride and glucose are the most important. The postulated mechanisms by which sodium enters the enterocyte, stated in simple terms, are as follows:

1. Diffusion of the positively charged sodium ion down its "electrical" gradient accompanied by "electrically coupled" chloride absorption, mostly through a paracellular pathway.
2. Neutral sodium chloride (NaCl) co-transport. Electroneutral entry of sodium and chloride is believed to be the mechanism responsible for the absorption of most of the total sodium and chloride introduced daily into the small intestine. This process is inhibited by cholera toxin and by other enterotoxins responsible for secretory diarrhea, and probably during acute rotavirus diarrhea.
3. Sodium absorption coupled to absorption of organic solutes. Absorption of a variety of water-soluble organic solutes, notably glucose and amino acids, by the small intestine is coupled to the absorption of sodium, e.g., D-hexoses, amino acids, water-soluble vitamins.

These mechanisms, located in the luminal membrane, are thought to be capable of coupling the entries of sodium and other solutes. The flow of organic solute from the cell is directed along a concentration gradient and probably extruded through a carrier-mediated process. As discussed below, ORT exploits this organic solute–linked enhanced sodium absorption, which is robust and largely unaffected in some acute diarrheas (e.g., those due to *Vibrio cholerae*, enterotoxigenic *Escherichia coli*, enteropathogenic *E. coli*), but is impaired in rotavirus diarrhea.

Sodium entering cells by all the above mechanisms is actively extruded from the enterocyte into the intercellular and subcellular space by the ubiquitous Na^+, K^+-ATPase found in virtually every animal cell, the so-called sodium pump.

Intestinal Secretion

In the small intestine, crypt cells are believed to be largely secretory, whereas the more mature cells at or near the tip of the villi are largely absorptive. Chloride ion mediates intestinal secretion. Coupled NaCl entry in the basolateral membrane, combined with active extrusion of sodium by Na^+, K^+-ATPase, increases the Cl^- concentration within the crypt cells. Various secretory stimuli, via intracellular messengers such as cyclic nucleotides and calcium, reduce sodium and water absorption by inhibiting NaCl entry across the apical membrane and increase Cl^- exit from crypt cells to the lumen by increasing permeability to Cl^-. These two events lead to the blood-to-lumen flow of water.

Glucose-Linked Sodium Absorption—In Vivo Experiments

Of relevance to the clinical use of ORT are data from in vivo experiments, such as intestinal perfusion studies in animals and human volunteers,[26-31] which provide semiquantitative information on the magnitude of the effect of various organic solutes on the absorption of sodium and water. In addition to the mechanisms elucidated by in vitro studies discussed earlier, at the luminal concentrations attained by the organic solutes like glucose that are usually used in ORS formulations, sodium and chloride are absorbed (in vivo only) by an additional mechanism called "solvent drag."[27] Bulk flow of water between and through the enterocytes responding osmotically to solute transport events traps additional sodium and chloride molecules in the flowing stream and increases salt absorption.

Historically, in 1902, Waymouth Reid[32] from Scotland used dog intestinal loops (in vivo) to demonstrate enhanced sodium absorption in the presence of glucose by mammalian small intestine. In 1939, Barany and Sperber[33] confirmed these findings. In 1963 Schedl and Clifton,[34] using transintestinal intubation techniques in human volunteers, demonstrated a dramatic improvement in NaCl and water absorption from Ringer's solution in both the jejunum and ileum by adding 56 mmol of glucose per liter. Subsequent in vivo studies with normal human small intestine defined the quantitative relationships of glucose-linked enhanced sodium and water absorption.[26-31,35]

Glucose-Linked Sodium Absorption During Diarrheal Illness

In 1964, Robert Phillips[2] studied the effect of an orally administered glucose-containing electrolyte solution on the net intestinal balance of water and electrolytes in a few actively purging adult cholera patients. He demonstrated a positive balance for sodium and water absorption over a short period, having failed to do so earlier using a glucose-free electrolyte solution. Probably this is the first documented evidence that glucose-linked sodium absorption is retained during an acute diarrheal illness. Subsequent studies provided more definite evidence that during the phase of active purging in adult cholera patients, fluid and electrolyte losses were adequately replaced by an optimally constituted oral electrolyte solution containing glucose.[3-7] Radioactive tracer studies in cholera patients confirmed that 20 g per liter of glucose induced net absorption of sodium and water from the small intestine.[36] Carpenter et al[37] demonstrated that net sodium and water loss was reduced when glucose was added into the perfusion electrolyte solution in canine jejunal and ileal Thiry-vella loops challenged with crude cholera toxin.

Initial success of ORT for adult cholera patients was soon tested under controlled conditions in the treatment of children with cholera, in infants and small children with diarrhea induced by rotavirus, enterotoxigenic *E. coli*, and other etiologic agents.[8-17] It emerged as a powerful therapeutic tool able to correct dehydration due to acute diarrhea in all but the most severe cases and in all ages, irrespective of etiologic agents.

Composition of Oral Rehydration Fluids

An oral rehydration solution for the treatment of acute diarrhea should satisfy the conditions that govern net absorption of electrolytes and water by the intestine and at the same time should fulfill the need for fluid therapy in acute diarrheal illness. The conditions that govern net absorption of sodium and water by the intestine include the following: (1) the jejunum absorbs sodium (and water) at an enhanced rate when glucose is present; (2) the ileum actively absorbs sodium and chloride against a steep electrochemical gradient, even in the absence of glucose; (3) a glucose concentration of approximately 20 g per liter in a solution stimulates optimal absorption except in a very small number of severely affected patients who may develop temporary glucose malabsorption; (4) concentrations of glucose exceeding 20 g per liter may lead to its incomplete absorption and osmotic diarrhea; (5) after any fluid is ingested, isotonic osmolality is quickly equilibrated in the duodenal and jejunal lumen by the flow of water and/or solutes across the bowel wall; therefore, intake of an isosmotic oral rehydration fluid should create minimal disequilibrium.

Losses Due to Acute Diarrhea

A child with moderate to severe dehydration due to acute diarrhea may lose 8 to 12 mmol of sodium associated with an average water loss of 100 ml for each kilogram of body weight (10 percent of body weight).[19,20] Loss of chloride in diarrheal dehydration is closely linked to sodium loss and is of the same order of magnitude, its absorption being closely linked to sodium absorption. Potassium loss in diarrheal dehydration in infants and small children can be as high as sodium loss. Potassium is lost in the stool and in the urine as dehydration develops. Varying degrees of base deficit acidosis occur in diarrheal dehydration.

Since 1971, WHO has recommended an oral rehydration formulation (described earlier) to treat dehydration from diarrhea of any cause, including cholera, in all age groups. This formulation is generally prepacked in a dry form called "ORS," which is reconstituted when required. These ingredients are distributed by UNICEF in aluminum foil packets labeled "Oral Rehydration Salts." The composition of reconstituted Oral Rehydration Salts is shown in Table 1.

USE OF ORS IN DIARRHEA

The usefulness of ORS for the treatment of patients with dehydration in hospitals, clinics, and homes for infants as well as for older children and adults with acute diarrhea of diverse etiologies has been extensively documented. ORS composition (particularly its sodium concentration) is optimal for *rehydration*, i.e., replacement of salt and water deficit that has already occurred in a dehydrated child. Also, ORS has been found to be eminently suitable for the replacement of ongoing diarrheal stool losses in infants during *maintenance* therapy, provided that their additional water need is met by unrestricted breast-feeding, or in non–breast-feeding infants, water or dilute feeds after initial rehydration.

Formulations with sodium concentrations (e.g., 50 or 60 mmol per liter) lower than those constituting the WHO formulation have been shown to be quite efficient in treating most cases of diarrhea in infants[12,13,23,24]; they are not suitable for use in adults and older children with cholera and similar secretory diarrheas.

TABLE 1
Molar Concentration of Components of Oral Rehydration Salts Solution

	Millimoles per Liter of Water	
Component	Citrate-Containing Solution	Bicarbonate-Containing Solution
Sodium	90	90
Potassium	20	20
Chloride	80	80
Citrate	10	—
Bicarbonate	—	30
Glucose	111	111

Treatment Principles and Optimum Use of ORT

Fluids administered to a dehydrated child with acute diarrhea should (1) for rehydration—correct existing water and electrolyte deficits; (2) for maintenance—replace ongoing abnormal losses of water and electrolytes due to continuing diarrhea until diarrhea stops; (3) provide daily fluid requirements during rehydration and maintenance, particularly in infants; and (4) offer early appropriate feeding during fluid therapy.

In view of the adverse nutritional consequences of repeated attacks of acute diarrhea, particularly in infants and small children, we have added the fourth principle above to ensure that ORT use is compatible with early appropriate feeding.

Rehydration Therapy

Rehydration therapy is usually achieved orally with ORS solution, except in cases of severe dehydration, uncontrollable vomiting, or a serious complication that prevents successful oral therapy. An infant with unequivocal signs of dehydration may initially need an average amount of 100 ml of ORS solution per kilogram of body weight; usually this amount can be administered in 4 to 6 hours. Larger amounts may be required in some patients, whereas in others smaller quantities may suffice, but the needed amount can be judged adequately by the clinical response. In infants under 3 months, ORS solution is used only when the patient has overt signs of dehydration.

Maintenance Therapy

After the initial fluid and electrolyte deficit has been corrected, ongoing abnormal losses due to continuing diarrhea are replaced by ORS solution. If the diarrhea is severe, ORS solution is given at an average rate of 10 to 20 ml per kilogram of body weight per hour. In most patients, stool loss is moderate to mild and they are given (1) ORS 100 ml per kilogram per day until diarrhea stops, or (2) 10 ml ORS per kilogram of body weight for each diarrhea stool. Infants under 3 months are not given ORS during maintenace therapy when they receive other fluids discussed below. If they develop clinical signs of dehydration again, they are promptly rehydrated with ORS solution.

Normal Daily Fluid Requirements

These requirements are particularly important in infants. Breast milk, which meets this requirement because it is very low in solute load, should be commenced during rehydration and continued unrestricted during maintenance. Non-breast-fed infants should be given plain water (a minimum volume of half the amount of ORS solution already taken by the infant), usually over 2 to 3 hours, as soon as they are fully rehydrated and half-strength milk formulas as 3- to 4-hour feeds. Other traditional fluids appropriate for age (e.g., rice water, carrot soup, or weak tea) also fulfill this need adequately.

Method of Administration of ORS Solution

ORS solution is administered to infants by using a cup and spoon, a cup alone, or a feeding bottle. For weak small babies, a dropper or a syringe can be used to put small volumes of solution at a time into the mouth. For babies who cannot drink owing to fatigue or drowsiness but who are not in shock, a nasogastric tube can be used to administer the solution; a rate of 15 to 20 ml per kilogram per hour is well tolerated. Vomiting is common during the first hour or two of administration of ORS solution, but it usually does not prevent successful oral rehydration. Ideally, ORS solution should be administered by the mother herself. However, nonavailability of the mother or a close relative for administration of ORS solution can create a serious manpower problem in a hospital setting. Under these circumstances ORT has been successfully practiced using nasogastric drips, although this is not ideal.

DIETARY MANAGEMENT

During an episode of acute diarrhea, substantial amounts of nutrients can be absorbed; food itself may enhance the efficacy of the standard ORS. In a trial of soya-based formula in infants with diarrhea and dehydration,[38] significantly reduced stool output was demonstrated in a group fed liberally compared with a group given clear fluids and starved for 48 hours. In a metabolic study[39] of ORT, dehydrated children aged 3 to 36 months who received a full diet (110 kcal per kilogram per day) from the start of treatment, had a stool output similar to that of children who were starved for 48 hours. The former group had a significantly better nutritional outcome after 7 and 14 days of beginning therapy. In a clinical trial, a group of infants with acute diarrhea and dehydration treated with ORT and continued on breast-feeding was compared with a group in whom breast-feeding was withheld for 24 hours. The former group had a significantly reduced stool output and duration of diarrhea compared with the latter.[40] Therefore, recommendations for diet during and after diarrhea include the following:

1. Breast-fed infants should commence breast-feeding during the rehydration phase and continue unrestricted breast-feeding during maintenance.
2. Non–breast-fed infants should commence during maintenance therapy, milk normally consumed by the infant but diluted with an equal volume of plain water for 24 to 48 hours, after which full-strength formula feeding should resume.
3. Children aged 4 months and older should eat semisolids and solid foods; food should be started during maintenance therapy; the aim should be to achieve recommended daily calorie intake right from the first day of treatment.

COMPLICATIONS ASSOCIATED WITH ORS SOLUTION

Infants with Hypernatremic Dehydration

Many thousands of infants, including a large number of neonates with hypernatremic dehydration, have been treated with excellent results using ORS solution. These results are better than the best results reported with intravenous therapy.

Severe Malnutrition and ORT

Dehydration due to acute diarrhea in children with severe protein energy malnutrition (e.g., marasmus, kwashiorkor) has been managed with ORS solution as above. In children with kwashiorkor, rehydration therapy must be closely supervised because of the risk of increased edema and congestive heart failure (as with intravenous therapy).

PERSISTENT DIARRHEA AND ORT

The term *persistent diarrhea* is meant to define episodes of diarrhea that begin acutely but persist beyond the expected self-limited course of the disease. Many of these children fail to grow normally and may experience a significant decrease in nutritional status during and following the episode. Some may die. A large proportion of diarrhea-associated deaths in young children are in those with persistent diarrhea.[41]

Two broad clinical categories of persistent diarrhea are seen by pediatricians in the developing world. In the first are those who pass several liquid stools in a day but without much dehydration. This category is nevertheless important in that growth failure may occur, and adverse nutritional consequences may contribute to increased susceptibility to infections and increase the risk of death. The second group have severe and persistent watery diarrhea with dehydration. These two categories probably represent a spectrum of severity. For cases of mild to moderate severity, the use of ORT is still highly effective. In severe cases ORT may be ineffective, so parenteral fluid and electrolyte therapy is needed.

FUTURE OF ORT

Two general approaches to improving ORS are being studied.[42–47] The objective is to enhance the intestinal absorption of sodium and water by providing larger amounts of different types of organic solutes in the solution. In one approach glucose (20 g per liter) is replaced by a starch-based cereal powder (50 g per liter) such as cooked rice powder. In the second, chemically defined ingredients such as glucose polymers (maltodextrin) or amino acids are either combined with or used in place of glucose in the ORS preparation.

The theoretical advantage of using a starch-like material is that during digestion glucose is released slowly and promotes sodium absorption as it does in glucose ORS. Because of its polymeric structure, relatively large amounts of starch can be given without causing ORS to become hyperosmolar. If these amounts are given as glucose, the osmolality of the solution would be excessive and cause an outpouring of fluid into the intestine, which could make diarrhea more severe. The suggested use of amino acids and dipeptides is based on evidence that these can promote water and salt absorption by mechanisms that are distinct from the mode of action of glucose,[44,48,49] suggesting that they may provide an additional benefit when combined with glucose (or a polymer).

Cereal-Based ORS

Two recent studies,[50,51] in Egypt and India, have evaluated ORS containing cooked rice powder (50 g per liter) in place of glucose (20 g per liter) and have confirmed the greater efficacy of rice-based ORS reported earlier.[42,45] In these four studies, undertaken in children 4 months to 10 years of age, the rate of stool output in the first 24 hours was reduced by 13 to 42 percent, total stool output by 15 to 49 percent, ORS intake by up to 31 percent, and duration of diarrhea by 17 to 30 percent in groups receiving the rice-based ORS.

Further studies[50] are under way to evaluate the safety and efficacy of rice-based ORS in severely malnourished children and in infants under 4 months of age. The preparation of rice powder ORS is time-consuming and requires fuel. Therefore, studies have been initiated by WHO[50] to determine whether an ORS that contains precooked rice could be made sufficiently stable to be used in a prepackaged form like the glucose ORS.

Improved ORS Based on Defined Solutes

Glucose Plus Glycine (and Glycyl-Glycine)

Earlier studies[43,46] suggested that the addition of glycine to glucose ORS causes improved fluid absorption and reduces stool volume during acute diarrhea caused mostly by toxigenic bacteria (e.g., *V. cholerae 01*, enterotoxigenic *E. coli*). Glycyl-glycine was considered to be a substrate because of some experimental evidence that it enhances sodium absorption by a mechanism that is independent of that of glycine.[49] One recent study conducted in adults with severe cholera showed a 19 percent reduction in stool output in patients receiving the ORS containing glucose and glycine compared with those given standard ORS.[50] However, results from six other studies showed that the addition of glycine and in some studies glycyl-glycine to glucose ORS had no consistent beneficial effect on the rate of stool output, ORS intake, or duration of diarrhea in children under 3 years with acute diarrhea or in adults with noncholera diarrhea. Based on these results, it was concluded that although this approach may have some advantage in treating cholera and possible diarrhea caused by other toxigenic bacteria, it was no more effective than standard ORS for patients with diarrhea of more diverse etiology.

ORS Containing Glucose Polymers (Maltodextrin) and Amino Acid

By substituting maltodextrin for glucose in ORS solutions, it is possible to provide a source of glucose (in the form of medium-length polymers) equivalent in amount to that in standard ORS and to add an amino acid or dipeptide without the solutions becoming hyperosmolar. Several studies[50] suggest that an intermediate grade of maltodextrin plus glycine (and sometimes glycyl-glycine) has no beneficial effect compared with standard ORS.

WHO has also promoted several studies to evaluate an ORS containing 50 g per liter of a minimally hydrolyzed, more starchlike maltodextrin in place of glucose. This maltodextrin is of particular interest for inclusion in ORS because in addition to being readily soluble and relatively inexpensive, it is stable when stored under tropical conditions. Unfortunately, these studies have shown no significant benefit from ORS containing this type of maltodextrin in larger amounts.

L-Alanine Glucose ORS

Based on experimental evidence that L-alanine is highly effective in transporting sodium across the intestinal brush border membrane,[52] a recently conducted study[53] in adults and older children with cholera using a glucose and L-alanine ORS (16 g and 8 g per liter, respectively) compared with standard ORS demonstrated that such a solution promotes absorption; results indicated that experimental ORS was associated with 44 percent reduction in total stool output and 26 percent reduction in ORS requirement. In addition, 37 percent in the group treated with standard ORS required additional unscheduled intravenous therapy after starting oral rehydration, whereas only 4 percent needed it in the group receiving experimental ORS. These promising results led to further studies in young children with diarrhea, and the results are being awaited with interest.

Speculations on Improved ORS

The above study with L-alanine glucose ORS demonstrates convincingly that use of a suitable amino acid in ORS may substantially improve its absorption efficiency. The solution used was hyperosmolar. Ways to reduce osmolality, e.g., using a glucose polymer to replace glucose, may be considered to further improve its efficiency. In an experimental study[54] using transmissible gastroenteritis (TGE) virus–infected piglet jejunum, combined effect of L-alanine and D-glucose in stimulating sodium absorption exceeded the response to maximal stimulatory concentrations of either substrate alone. Data also confirmed that separate carrier systems for D-glucose and L-alanine are present in the jejunum in both healthy and TGE virus–infected piglet jejunum. Another amino acid of possible usefulness is glutamine, an important source of fuel energy for enterocytes. Recent in vitro experimental studies (M. Rhoads: unpublished data) indicate that glutamine is highly absorption-efficient and stimulates sodium and chloride absorption by small intestinal mucosa in rotavirus-infected piglets. In spite of many setbacks in research, we are hopeful that an improved ORS solution will eventually be developed.

INTRAVENOUS THERAPY

Under the following circumstances, ORT may not be adequate or intravenous therapy may be preferred:

1. In patients with dehydration with signs of shock, oral therapy may be too slow; these patients need rapid replacement of water and salts. After the initial 3 to 6 hours of rehydration intravenously, hydration can be adequately maintained with ORT.
2. In patients who cannot drink because of extreme fatigue, stupor, or coma, intravenous therapy is required. If the intravenous approach is not feasible, the oral solution can be given to such patients via nasogastric tube.
3. Patients with severe and persistent vomiting often require intravenous therapy, but if other clinical signs indicate improvement despite the vomiting, ORT can be successfully used.
4. Patients with severe watery diarrhea who are losing more than 10 ml per kilogram per hour may be unable to drink enough fluid to replace the continuing losses and may need intravenous therapy.
5. In the rare patient with acute diarrhea and temporary glucose malabsorption, oral therapy can cause a marked increase in watery diarrhea, in which the stool contains large amounts of glucose; stopping ORS solution leads to a prompt reduction of watery diarrhea.

When the use of ORT is optimal, intravenous therapy is limited to (1) rehydration of severely dehydrated patients and patients with complications and (2) rehydration and maintenance therapy of some severe cases of persistent diarrhea. For rehydration, a polyelectrolyte solution with a relatively high concentration of sodium is suitable, e.g., lactated Ringer's solution. In a small proportion of patients, particularly with persistent diarrhea, a maintenance polyelectrolyte solution with a low sodium concentration may also be required.

REFERENCES

1. Oral glucose/electrolyte therapy for acute diarrhoea. (Editorial) Lancet 1975; i:75–76.
2. Phillips RA. Water and electrolyte losses in cholera. Fed Proc 1964; 23:705–712.
3. Pierce NF, Banwell JG, Mitra RC, Caranos GJ, Keimowitz RI, Mondal A, et al. Oral maintenance of water-electrolyte and acid-base balance in cholera, a preliminary report. Indian J Med Res 1968; 56:640–645.
4. Pierce NF, Banwell JG, Mitra RC, Caransos GJ, Keimowitz RI, Mondal A, et al. Effect of intragastric glucose electrolyte infusion upon water and electrolyte balance in Asiatic cholera. Gastroenterology 1968; 55:333–343.
5. Hirschhorn H, Kinzie JL, Sechar DB, Northrup RS, Taylor JO, Ahmad SZ, et al. Decrease in net stool output in cholera during intestinal perfusion with glucose-containing solutions. N Engl J Med 1968; 279:176–181.
6. Nalin DR, Cash RA, Islam R, Molla M, Phillips RA. Oral maintenance therapy for cholera in adults. Lancet 1968; ii:370–373.
7. Pierce NF, Sack RB, Mitra RC, Banwell JG, Brigham KL, Fedson DS, et al. Replacement of water electrolyte losses in cholera by an oral glucose-electrolyte solution. Ann Intern Med 1969; 70:1173.
8. Mahalanabis D, Sack RB, Jacobs B, Mondal A, Thomas J. Use of an oral glucose electrolyte solution in the treatment of paediatric cholera—a controlled study. J Trop Pediatr Environ Child Health 1974; 20:82–87.
9. Hirschhorn N, Cash RA, Woodward WB, Spivey GH. Oral fluid therapy of Apache children with acute infectious diarrhea. Lancet 1971; ii:15.
10. Hirschhorn N, McCarthy BJ, Ranney B, Hirschhorn MA, Woodward ST, Lacapa A, Cash RA, Woodward WB. Ad libitum glucose electrolyte therapy for acute diarrhoea in Apache children. J Pediatr 1973; 83:562–571.
11. Nalin DR, Levine MM, Mata L, de Cespedes C, Vargas W, Lizano C, Loria AR, Simhon A, Mohs E. Comparison of sucrose with glucose in oral therapy of infant diarrhoea. Lancet 1978; ii:277–279.
12. Chatterjee A, Mahalanabis D, Jalan KN, et al. Evaluation of a sucrose/electrolyte solution for oral rehydration in acute infantile diarrhoea. Lancet 1977; i:133–135.
13. Chatterjee A, Mahalanabis D, Jalan KN, et al. Oral rehydration in infantile diarrhoea. Arch Dis Child 1978; 54:284–289.
14. Nalin DR, Levine MM, Mata L, de Cespedes C, Vargas W, Lizano C, Loria AR, Simhon A, Mohs E. Oral rehydration and maintenance of children with rotavirus and bacterial diarrhoea. Bull WHO 1979; 57:453–459.
15. Nalin DR, Harland E, Ramlal A, Swaby D, McDonald J, Gangarosa R, Levine M, Akierman A, Antoinee M, Mackenzie K, Johnson B. Comparison of low and high sodium and potassium content in oral rehydration solution. J Pediatr 1980; 97:848–853.
16. Patra FC, Mahalanabis D, Jalan KN, Sen A, Banerjee P. Is rice electrolyte solution superior to glucose electrolyte solution in infantile diarrhoea? Arch Dis Child 1982; 57:910–912.
17. Patra FC, Mahalanabis D, Jalan KN, Sen A, Banerjee P. Can acetate replace bicarbonate in oral rehydration solution for infantile diarrhoea? Arch Dis Child 1982; 57:625–627.
18. Mahalanabis D, Chowdhury AB, Bagchi NG, Bhattacharya AK, Simpson TW. Oral fluid therapy of cholera among Bangladesh refugees. Johns Hopkins Med J 1973; 132:197–205.
19. Darrow DC. The retention of electrolyte during recovery from severe dehydration due to diarrhoea. J Pediatr 1946; 28:515.
20. Mahalanabis D, Wallace CK, Kallen RJ, Mondal A, Pierce NF. Water and electrolyte losses due to cholera in infants and small children: a recovery balance study. Pediatrics 1970; 45:374.
21. Pizarro D, Posada G, Mata L, et al. Oral rehydration of neonates with dehydrating diarrhoea. Lancet 1979; ii:1209.
22. Pizarro D, Posada G, Mata L. Treatment of 242 neonates with dehydrating diarrhoea with an oral glucose-electrolyte solution. J Pediatr 1983; 102:153–156.
23. Santosham M, et al. Oral rehydration therapy of infantile diarrhoea: a controlled study of well-nourished children hospitalized in the US and Panama. N Engl J Med 1982; 306:1070–1076.
24. Vesikari T, Isolauri E. Glycine supplemented oral rehydration solutions for diarrhoea. Arch Dis Child 1986; 61:372–376.
25. Schultz SC. Sodium-coupled solute transport by small intestine: a status report. Am J Physiol 1977; 223:E249–E254.
26. Sladen GF, Dawson AM. Interrelationships between the absorption of glucose, sodium and water by the normal human jejunum. Clin Sci 1969; 36:119–132.
27. Fordtran JS. Stimulation of active and passive sodium absorption by sugars in the human jejunum. J Clin Invest 1975; 55:728–737.
28. Fordtran JS, Locklear W. Ionic constituents and osmolality of gastric and small intestinal fluids after eating. Am J Dig Dis 1966; 2:503–521.
29. Turnberg LA, Bieberdorf FA, Morawski SG, et al. Interrelationships of chloride, bicarbonate, sodium and hydrogen transport in the human ileum. J Clin Invest 1970; 49:557–567.
30. Turnberg LA, Fordtran JS, Carter NW, et al. Mechanism of bicarbonate absorption and its relationship to sodium transport in the human jejunum. J Clin Invest 1970; 49:548–556.
31. Modigliani R, Bernier JJ. Effects of glucose on net and unidirectional movements of water and electrolytes in the human small intestine. Biol Gastroenterol 1972; 5:165.
32. Reid EW. Intestinal absorption of solutions. J Physiol 1902; 28:241–256.

33. Barany EH, Sperber E. Absorption of glucose against a concentration gradient by the small intestine of the rabbit. Scand Arch Physiol 1939; 81:290.
34. Schedl HP, Clifton JA. Solute and water absorption by the human small intestine. Nature 1963; 199:1264–1267.
35. Malawar SJ, Enton M, Fordtran JS, Ingelfinger FJ. Interrelation between jejunal absorption of sodium glucose and water in man. (Abstract) J Clin Invest 1965; 44:1072.
36. Taylor JO, Kinzie J, Hare R, Hare K. Measurement of sodium flux in human small intestine. (Abstract) J Clin Invest 1968; 27:386.
37. Carpenter CCJ, Sack RB, Feeley JC, Steenberg RW. Site and characteristics of electrolyte loss and effects of intraluminal glucose in experimental canine cholera. J Clin Invest 1968; 47:1210–1220.
38. Santosham M, et al. Role of soy based lactose free formula during treatment of acute diarrhoea. Paediatrics 1985; 76:292–298.
39. Brown KH, Gastanaduy AS, Saavedra JM, et al. Effect of continual feeding on clinical and nutritional outcomes of acute diarrhoea in children. J Pediatr 1988; 112:191–200.
40. Khin Maung U, Nyunt-Nyunt-Wai, Myo-Khin, et al. Effect on clinical outcome of breast feeding during acute diarrhoea. Br Med J 1985; 290:587–589.
41. WHO. Persistent diarrhoea in children in developing countries. Report of a WHO meeting. WHO/CDD/88.27.
42. Patra FC, Mahalanabis D, Jalan KN, et al. Is oral rice electrolyte solution superior to glucose electrolyte solution in infantile diarrhoea. Arch Dis Child 1982; 57:910–912.
43. Nalin DR, Cash RA, Rahman M, et al. Effect of glycine and glucose on sodium and water absorption in patients with cholera. Gut 1970; 11:768–772.
44. Mahalanabis D, Patra FC. In search of a super oral rehydration solution: can optimum use of organic solute-mediated sodium absorption lead to the development of an absorption promoting drug? J Diar Dis Res 1983; 1:76–81.
45. Molla AM, Ahmed SM, Greenough WB. Rice-based oral rehydration solution decreases the stool volume in acute diarrhoea. Bull WHO 1985; 63:751–756.
46. Patra FC, Mahalanabis D, Jalan KN, et al. In search of a super solution: a controlled trial of glycine-glucose oral rehydration solution in infantile diarrhoea. Acta Paediatr Scand 1984; 73:18–21.
47. WHO. Control of Diarrhoeal Diseases. Fifth Programme Report 1984–1985. WHO/CCD/86.16.
48. Adibi SA, Fogel MR, Agarwal RM. Comparison of free amino acid and dipeptide absorption in the jejunum of sprue patients. Gastroenterology 1974; 67:586–591
49. Matthews DM. Absorption of peptides by mammalian intestine. In: Matthews DM, Payne JW, eds. Peptide transport in protein nutrition. Amsterdam and New York: North Holland/American Elsevier, 1975: 61.
50. WHO: CDD Sixth Programme Report 1986–1987, WHO/CDD/88.28 pp 42–46.
51. Bhan MK, Ghai OP, Khoshoo V, et al. Efficacy of mung bean (lentil) and pop rice based rehydration solution in comparison with the standard glucose electrolyte solution. J Pediatr Gastroenterol Nutr 1987; 6:392–399.
52. Mahalanabis D, Merson M. Development of an improved formulation of oral rehydration salts (ORS) with antidiarrhoeal properties: a "super ORS." In: Holmgren J, Lindberg A, Molby R, eds. Development of vaccines and drugs against diarrhoea. 11th Nobel Conference, Stockholm, 1985. Lund, Sweden: Student Litterateur, 1986.
53. Patra FC. Oral rehydration formula containing alanine and glucose for treatment of diarrhea: a controlled trial. Br Med J 1989; 298:1353–1356.
54. Rhoads MJ, McLeod JR, Hamilton JR. Alanine enhances jejunal sodium absorption in the presence of glucose: studies in piglet viral diarrhoea. Pediatr Res 1986; 20:879–883.

PART 2

Industrialized Countries

Julius G. Goepp, M.D.
Bert Hirschhorn, M.D.

An increased understanding of the pathophysiology of acute dehydrating diarrheal illness over the past two decades has resulted in a tremendous shift in the management of children with diarrhea. Widespread use of oral rehydration therapy (ORT) has contributed to a dramatic decline in morbidity and mortality from dehydration, the single largest cause of death in children worldwide. Increasing acceptance of the use of enteral or nutritional therapy has resulted in continued refinement of oral solutions and in the accumulation of considerable evidence that, in many situations, the combination of ORT and associated feeding is actually superior to intravenous treatment. Today, ORT is recommended by the World Health Organization (WHO) and by the American Academy of Pediatrics (AAP) as the treatment of choice for acute diarrhea in the great majority of children. Nevertheless, acceptance of this simple, inexpensive, and safe approach to the treatment of a potentially life-threatening condition has been quite slow in the industrialized world, in part because of inexperience with and lack of understanding of the principles and practices involved.

This discussion reviews currently accepted definitions and approaches to dehydration and rehydration, in the context of the pathophysiology of the gastrointestinal (GI) tract. Particular attention is paid to the use and composition of rehydration fluids in relation to the processes of intestinal secretion and absorption. The principles of fluid replacement for intravenous and oral therapy are recognized to be similar. Consideration is given to the nutritional implications of the early use of the gut in acute diarrhea and to a number of recently developed ORT solutions. Potential complications and problems encountered in the use of ORT as well as future developments in its composition and application are discussed.

DEFINITIONS

Dehydration

From a strictly physiologic standpoint, the terms *dehydration* and *rehydration* define pure water loss and replacement, respectively. Such pure losses, in fact, rarely occur in clinically meaningful quantities. In practice, the terms have come to be used to describe states of depletion and replacement of both body water and important electrolytes whose concentrations determine the volume of water in various physiologic compartments. In this discussion, *dehydration* is used to imply volume loss without regard to the specific composition of fluid involved, and *rehydration* to describe the process of volume repletion.

Volume loss may occur as the result of a number of disease entities including increased insensible losses through the skin and respiratory tree, and increased renal excretion, and by several routes including through the GI tract. This discussion is limited to GI losses.

The risk of rapid and profound dehydration is greater for pediatric patients than for adults. This difference arises chiefly because of the increased surface area relative to volume of the small patient, as well as from the greater tendency of children to become highly febrile; both factors contribute to considerably elevated insensible losses in young patients. Young children also consume a largely milk-based diet, which can create osmotic diarrhea in the infected intestine and exacerbate fluid loss in stool. The relatively higher protein content of milk results in a greater renal solute load. Finally, children with gastroenteritis have disproportionately more vomiting and diarrhea than have adults with similar illnesses.

The pathophysiology of dehydration is best understood by recognizing that sodium is the chief solute in extracellular fluid (ECF) and thus is the primary determinant of ECF volume. When ECF volume is reduced in acute dehydration, the total body sodium content is almost always reduced as well, regardless of measured serum sodium concentration. Restoration of circulating volume, therefore, requires concomitant sodium repletion. It has traditionally been taught that in acute dehydration, volume is lost chiefly from ECF. It is now clear that a substantial amount of intracellular fluid (ICF) is also lost in diarrhea following depletion of ICF potassium.[1] Since sodium moves from ECF to ICF to maintain electrical equilibrium, it can be seen that ECF sodium depletion in diarrhea occurs in two directions: out of the body in stool and into the intracellular compartment to replace potassium. This concept will be seen to have important implications when the role of potassium in replacement fluids is discussed below.

Serum sodium concentration in dehydration may be elevated, normal, or decreased, depending upon the rate of fluid loss, environmental conditions, the nature of fluids given for volume replacement, and the disease under consideration. Hypernatremia occurs in gastroenteritis, either as a result of water loss in excess of sodium loss or because of relative gain of sodium in excess of free water. The immediate renal response to a perceived volume deficit is stimulation of the renin-aldosterone system, which results in increased sodium retention and potassium excretion. In patients who are fed formulas that tend to produce or exacerbate osmotic diarrhea (e.g., milk) or under conditions that result in increased insensible fluid loss, hypernatremia may result. Potassium depletion and acidosis also tend to perpetuate hypernatremia. Excessive replacement of stool water losses with hypernatremic solutions has a similar effect. Hypernatremia resulting from oral rehydration solutions properly prepared and administered is a relatively infrequent occurrence.[1]

Isotonic dehydration is the most common situation in patients with gastroenteritis, resulting from roughly proportional losses of water and sodium in stool and an influx of sodium into cells proportional to ECF concentrations. A critical point in both hypernatremic and isotonic dehydration (as well as in hypotonic dehydration) is that in each case total body sodium is diminished.

When sodium loss is relatively greater than water loss or when water intake exceeds that of sodium, hyponatremic dehydration results. Such conditions are seen in patients with chronic or repeated diarrhea who have sustained chronic loss of potassium and are unable to maximize renal sodium retention mechanisms. The thirst mechanism in such patients will contribute to hyponatremia if salt-poor fluids are taken, as often occurs among children under conditions of poverty and malnutrition.

When dehydration is the result of excessive stool water and electrolyte loss, as in diarrhea, there is invariably a simultaneous loss of potassium from both intestine and kidneys. Under normal circumstances, stool potassium content is 50 to 90 mEq per liter. In diarrhea, although stool potassium concentration is usually less, the larger volume and more rapid transit of bowel contents may result in continued potassium losses. The primary source of potassium depletion, however, is renal, with aldosterone-stimulated retention of sodium and resultant potassium exchange. Such losses must be considered clinically when fluid repletion is undertaken.

Clinical dehydration is associated with a number of readily recognizable signs and symptoms. Taken in combination with appropriate history, such information may be used to provide an estimate of the degree of dehydration, usually expressed as a percentage of the total body weight depleted (Table 1). This figure may be arrived at directly if a recent fully hydrated weight is available. Plasma specific gravity is a further useful indicator of degree of dehydration but must be interpreted with caution in the infant because, for unclear reasons, plasma specific gravity is lower than in adults at the same proportional loss of weight. In general, clinical evidence of shock is interpreted as dehydration of approximately 10 percent of body weight in isotonic dehydration. Circulatory collapse may occur with relatively less volume loss in the hyponatremic patient, whereas in hypernatremia the opposite occurs: The circulation remains stable at greater levels of loss. The explanation of this phenomenon lies in the shifts of salt and water into or out of cells.

Rarely, under conditions of rapid fluid loss, as in infectious secretory diarrhea, changes in mucous membranes and skin turgor may not appear early in the course, when fluid shifts out of the interstitium have not occurred. Similarly, in hypernatremic dehydration, skin turgor changes may be seen only relatively late in the course.

TABLE 1
Clinical Indicators of Degree of Dehydration

Indicator	Estimated Degree of Dehydration As Percentage Loss of Healthy Weight		
	Less Than 5%	5–9%	10% and Greater
Fontanelle	Normal	Depressed	Deeply depressed
Skin elasticity	Normal	Possibly reduced	Markedly reduced
Mucous membranes	Moist	Sticky or dry	Very dry
Eyes	Normal	Slightly sunken	Deeply sunken
Urine output	Normal	Reduced	Absent
Extremities	Warm	Delayed capillary refilling	Cool, mottled
Mental status	Normal	Fussy to lethargic	Obtunded
Heart rate	Normal	Normal or increased	Rapid
Blood pressure	Normal	Orthostatic hypotension	Decreased or undetectable

Rehydration

Rehydration consists of the safe and rapid restoration of circulating volume. Fluid repletion may be accomplished by the direct intraveous administration of isotonic solutions or by the enteral route (orally or by nasogastric infusion). Regardless of the method employed, a similar approach should be taken: calculation of the fluid deficit (see below), initial replacement of losses (rehydration phase), and administration of adequate fluid for maintenance and replacement of ongoing losses (maintenance phase). Frequent clinical monitoring of the response to fluid therapy is vital.

The approach to fluid replacement advocated in this discussion differs significantly from that found in traditional pediatric texts (Table 2). Current teaching emphasizes slow repletion of fluid and sodium, with a prolonged period of "bowel rest" before initiation of feedings. By contrast, it has been found that aggressive, rapid replacement of losses (intravenous or oral) with a single polyelectrolyte solution containing substantial amounts of potassium and base provides successful therapy in the great majority of patients. This approach also stresses the resumption of enteral feeding as soon as appetite is restored. Such therapy has proved itself to be effective under extreme conditions in refugee camps as well as in well-equipped hospitals in developed countries.[1] Although this discussion is designed to provide the clinician with a physiologic basis for the use of ORT, it should be recognized that the principles and recommendations given may be applied equally well to fluid therapy by the intravenous route.

Both the intravenous and oral routes for rehydration have inherent advantages and disadvantages. Intravenous therapy provides a rapid initial response, with certainty and preci-

TABLE 2
Comparison of Two Approaches to Treatment of Dehydrating Diarrhea

	Traditional Teaching	Recently Developed
Physiologic model	Varying degrees of dehydration and tonicity require careful tailoring of fluid therapy	Within broad limits a simple and unified therapeutic approach may be taken
Speed of rehydration	24–48 hours	4–6 hours
Choice of initial rehydrating solution	Hypotonic with sodium content 30–60 mEq/L, especially for infants	Polyelectrolyte solution with sodium content 80–130 mEq/L for all ages
Use of potassium	Only after urination commences	In polyelectrolyte solution
Use of base	Only for severe acidosis	In polyelectrolyte solution
Use of oral fluids	Small infrequent sips of water in first 24 hours	Ad libitum intake of glucose-electrolyte solutions (at WHO recommendation)
Feeding	Fasting for 24–48 hours; careful reintroduction of food	Tolerated foods as soon as appetite restored (usually 6–24 hours) in small frequent amounts
Principal concerns	Overhydration, hypernatremia, persisting loose stools	Underhydration, hyponatremia, undernutrition

From Hirschhorn.[1]

sion of fluid administration. The patient as well as medical staff usually perceive intravenous replacement as an efficient and sophisticated treatment. Such technology, however, also demands trained personnel, expensive hardware, and premixed sterile fluids in bulky containers. Direct vascular access poses some danger of infection, excessively rapid rates of fluid administration, or administration of inappropriate fluids.

Oral or enteral rehydration, on the other hand, may be perceived as low-level technology and therefore as less effective. A potential for improper mixing and dispensing exists, although in large-scale studies such errors have been found to occur less frequently than expected. In busy tertiary-care settings, the use of oral fluids has been considered excessively time- and labor-consuming. The benefits of oral therapy, however, are considerable. The mixture may be transported compactly and manufactured cheaply and may be administered on the local level or even at home by people with minimal training. Therapy may be begun by the patient's family early in the course of illness, often eliminating the need for admission to a center for rehydration. The vast majority of patients in whom oral therapy is used do not require further treatment with intravenous solutions, even when the degree of dehydration was initially evident.[2] Those who do require intravenous resuscitation may be switched over to ORT in several hours if conscious and able to drink. It has been shown that the full spectrum of diarrheal dehydration responds well to a single oral solution,[1] which has greatly simplified treatment schemes.

ORAL REHYDRATION FLUIDS

Although the need for replacement of water and salt in severe dehydration was recognized by the early nineteenth century, it was the vast increase in our understanding of the intestinal pathophysiology of absorption and secretion in the past three decades that provided the first scientific basis of oral fluid therapy.[3,6] When appropriate quantities of glucose and sodium are presented to the intestinal co-transport systems, stimulated uptake of sodium and water by mucosal cells occurs. The discovery that the molecular mechanism for this effect remains intact in the intestines of patients with cholera allowed the first clinical use of a glucose-electrolyte oral solution in a large-scale trial.[4]

The specific composition of most oral solutions in common use today is the result of work done in a variety of experimental systems.[5] Glucose stimulation of water and sodium absorption occurs best at glucose concentrations of 56 to 140 mmol per liter. Higher glucose concentrations produce excessive osmolarity as well as less powerful stimulation of absorption. The compositions of oral rehydration solutions currently recommended by WHO are given in Table 3, along with other fluids commonly used for rehydration and maintenance in the industrialized nations. These fluids are often used as adjuncts to intravenous therapy. If used appropriately as indicated in the table, they may replace intravenous treatment during the appropriate therapeutic phase (with the exceptions of juice and Gatorade, which have excessively high sugar and low sodium concentrations).

The WHO ORS formula is considered appropriate for use in both rehydration and maintenance of patients with the full spectrum of types of dehydration, with a broad range of initial serum sodium values. In order to understand the rationale for using a single solution in a variety of clinical contexts, we now discuss each component of ORS separately and arrive at a basis for its inclusion in the existing quantity.

Sodium

The sodium concentration of ORS has been a source of great controversy since the inception of oral therapy.[1] Because dehydrated patients may be hyponatremic or hypernatremic or have normal serum sodium concentrations, it was initially believed by some that a number of solutions were needed to treat each category appropriately. An improved understanding of the pathophysiology of dehydrating diarrheas has led to the widespread acceptance of a single solution with a relatively high sodium concentration.

The normal physiologic responses to dehydration tend to produce hypotonicity: (1) elevation of levels of antidiuretic hormone (ADH) with resultant free water reabsorption in the renal collecting system; (2) thirst, which results in consumption of low-solute fluids. In the potassium-depleted state of many poorly nourished patients, hypokalemia may exacerbate hyponatremia by causing sodium to move into ICF to replace potassium, thus further depleting ECF sodium. Total body sodium is depleted from continued loss in stool, particularly in the secretory diarrheas such as cholera.

In such a situation, replacement of fluid with a solution resembling ECF (i.e., with fairly high sodium content) is clearly desirable, in order to rapidly replenish total body sodium, restore circulating volume, and abolish persistent stimuli for development of the hypotonic state.

The rationale for the use of an identical solution with regard to sodium content in the hypernatremic patient may be less evident. Again, it must be recognized that such a patient is deficient in total body sodium. Hypernatremia is perpetuated by hypokalemia, acidosis, and hypovolemia. Many hypernatremic patients have been fed a fairly concentrated formula that produces a high gut osmotic load, resulting in stool losses with high osmolality but relatively low sodium, which also tends to perpetuate hypernatremia. Thus, the appropriate response to hypernatremia is the abolition of the precipitating and perpetuating factors: (1) rapid restoration of circulating fluid volume with a solution similar in composition of ECF, (2) correction of acidosis by restoring perfusion as well as by titrating with base, (3) potassium repletion, and (4) reduction of the osmotic load presented to the gut. Rapid restoration of volume cannot be accomplished by significantly hypotonic solutions that provide excessive free water not contributing to intravascular volume. In practice, only solutions with sodium concentrations of 75 to 90 mEq per liter have been found adequate for the restoration of circulating volume with sufficient safety and rapidity to abolish hypoperfusion, acidosis, and continued deterioration.

Clearly, the administration of excessive amounts of sodium is dangerous. Several regimens attempted in the 1940s involved therapy with normal saline and added sodium bicarbonate, in the absence of potassium, which resulted in the

TABLE 3
Fluids Commonly Used for Rehydration

	Composition					
	CHO			K^+		
Fluid	(g/L)	(mmol/L)	Na^+	(mEq/L)	Cl^-	Base*
Rehydration						
Oral						
WHO ORS	20	111	90	20	80	30
Rehydralyte†	25	139	75	20	65	30
Intravenous						
0.9% NaCl‡	—	—	154	—	154	—
Ringer's lactate	0–10	0–56	130	4	109	28
Maintenance						
Pedialyte†	25	139	45	20	35	30
Lytren§	20	111	50	25	45	30
Apple juice	119	661	0.43	25	—	—
Gatorade	40	222	23.5	2.5	17	—

Various fluids in common use for rehydration and maintenance in infants and children with dehydrating diarrhea. Oral solutions listed under ''Rehydration'' may also be used for replacement of losses during maintenance, provided that adequate additional fluid as breast-milk formula is also taken. Juice and Gatorade are shown for comparison; neither is recommended for use because of high osmolarity.

*mEq potential bicarbonate; may be, e.g., citrate, acetate.

†Ross Laboratories.

‡20–30 mEq/L base; 20 mEq/L K^+ should be added.

§Mead-Johnson.

Adapted from Rowe PC, ed. The Harriet Lane handbook. 11th ed. Chicago: Year Book, 1987: 237.

complications of hypernatremia. Such fluid provided sodium concentrations as high as 177 mEq per liter, and mortality promptly diminished when sodium was lowered to 128 mEq per liter and potassium was added.

Even with today's standard 90 mEq of sodium per liter, transient overexpansion of ECF volume at a rate of 1 to 3 percent of total body weight is not an uncommon occurrence. It may be related to persistently increased renal tubular retention of sodium, and is of no clinical significance, provided that tissue acidosis and hypokalemia are corrected.

Chloride

A number of substances in addition to organic molecules such as glucose are necessary for the full effect of co-transport to be manifest. Chloride ion must be present in luminal fluid with sodium, presumably because of the importance of electroneutral sodium chloride absorption in small bowel water transport. Because of the presence of other anionic species in oral rehydration solutions (ORS), its chloride content is not isosmolar with sodium but is currently established at 80 mEq per liter.

Potassium

Attempts at rehydration with solutions deficient in potassium are often unsuccessful and may be unsafe. Total body potassium is depleted in diarrheal rehydration by several mechanisms: (1) continued potassium losses in stool, (2) shifts of intracellular potassium into ECF secondary to acidosis and water movement, (3) urinary potassium excretion under the influence of increased aldosterone as sodium is retained (probably the most important mechanism), (4) similar aldosterone effects on bowel potassium transport mechanisms.

Hypokalemia may also serve to perpetuate or exacerbate clinical deterioration by causing ileus with resultant decreased absorption and possibly by worsening both hyponatremia and hypernatremia (the former by movement of sodium into cells to replace potassium electrically, the latter by loss of water into nonmotile bowel segments).

The healthy child's requirement for potassium is 1 to 2 mEq per kilogram per day; under conditions of increased stool losses and dehydration, potassium needs to be replaced at a rate of about 4 to 6 mEq per kilogram per day, which results in a concentration in ORS of 20 to 30 mEq per liter.

Bicarbonate

Addition of alkali to intravenous fluids in cholera was attempted as early as 1832.[1] Subsequent rehydration schemes have, for the most part, included base in some quantity, in attempts to correct tissue acidosis. Sodium bicarbonate, lactate, and citrate have been the substances most commonly used, in varying proportions. The tremendous success of oral fluids containing bicarbonate, developed for use in cholera, led to the acceptance of sodium bicarbonate in 1980 as the standard base in WHO-recommended ORS. The concentration was 30 mEq of bicarbonate per liter. In 1984, the formulation was changed to provide 10 mEq of citrate per liter as trisodium citrate, which was found to have improved stability in storage. Citrate is hepatically metabolized to produce three bicarbonate ions per molecule.

It should be noted that the presence of base not only results in faster resolution of acidosis, but, in the case of bicarbonate, also stimulates sodium absorption independent of glucose or amino acid–linked systems.[6] The salts of other weak organic acids such as acetate, propionate, and butyrate also potentiate sodium and potassium absorption; this effect occurs not only in the small intestine but in the colon as well. With the exception of acetate, such agents have not been used in large-scale clinical trials to date.

Organic Constituents

The principle of successful ORT relies upon the presence in appropriate quantity of glucose or other organic molecules to be co-transported with sodium from the gut lumen to blood, with the accompanying obligate water flow. Glucose itself has been the most widely used and studied, although it is now clear that a number of other substrates are at least equally efficacious.[7]

Optimum stimulation of sodium co-transport has been found to occur at glucose concentrations approximately equimolar with sodium content of ORS. Higher concentrations are less stimulatory of absorption and produce undesirably high osmolality, actually exacerbating fluid loss.[5] At a concentration of 20 g per liter, glucose is present at 111 mmol per liter, close to the sodium concentration of 90 mEq per liter.

Disaccharides and oligosaccharides have the theoretical advantage of presenting a smaller osmotic load to the intestine by virtue of their larger molecular size. The most commonly used disaccharide, sucrose, is widely and cheaply available and is generally used in twice the gram quantity of glucose because it contains only one glucose residue per molecule.

The shorter oligosaccharides are broken down into their constituent simple sugars by enzymes in the intestinal brush border. Longer-chain oligosaccharides and polysaccharides require hydrolysis in the gut lumen by alpha amylase. A number of such substances have been studied with varying success as glucose substitutes in ORS (see below).

Shortly after the demonstration of the sodium-glucose co-transport phenomenon in the intestine, it was recognized that similar transport systems existed that made use of other organic substrates. Glycine was the first of the amino acids to be studied. Subsequently, it was shown that the other neutral amino acids alanine and leucine have similar effects on promotion of sodium and water absorption.[8] More recently, dipeptides and tripeptides have been used to further stimulate absorption, independent of the effects of their constituent amino acids.[7] In addition, the effects of the amino acids and peptides are independent of, and additive to, those of glucose on sodium absorption. Future ORS preparations will no doubt take advantage of these observations in maximally stimulating absorption.

Osmolality

The currently recommended ORT solution presents an osmolar load of 331 mOsm per liter to the intestine. Clearly, it is desirable to minimize the osmolarity of the administered fluid while maintaining maximal efficacy. Formerly, commercially prepared oral rehydration solutions were deficient in sodium, contained excessive glucose, and were hyperosmolar. These features tended to exacerbate diarrhea. The administration to the dehydrated patient of soft drinks, juices, or commercial glucose-electrolyte mixtures such as Gatorade is to be discouraged on similar grounds. Incorporation of complex carbohydrate or peptide molecules into ORS preparations may theoretically serve to increase effective substrate concentration, without imposing substantially greater osmotic load.[9] Although there is no evidence that purified, commercially prepared glucose polymers are beneficial in this respect, the use of rice powder and other unprocessed carbohydrate products has been shown to be effective.

ORAL REHYDRATION FORMULATION

WHO/UNICEF Recommendations

As of 1986, the World Health Organization recommended the use of a single ORS for use in essentially all types of dehydrating diarrheal illness (Table 3). Because wide variations in sodium and glucose concentrations have been found in home-prepared simple sugar-salt solutions, they are not currently recommended for therapy of patients with detectable degrees of dehydration or in areas where safe, prepackaged products are readily available.

Use in Diarrhea

WHO-recommended ORS should be used in the treatment of dehydration from diarrhea in two phases: initial replacement of the estimated deficit (rehydration phase) and maintenance of hydration with replacement of ongoing losses (maintenance phase). Appropriate feeding should begin as early in the second phase as possible.[12] Numerous studies have documented the safety and efficacy of the use of a single ORS in both phases.[1] A solution containing less sodium (50 to 70 mEq per liter) may be used in patients who are minimally dehydrated.

When intravenous fluids are readily available for use by those skilled in their administration, they may be considered superior in the early phases of treatment of the very sick child. In most of the industrialized world, for example, a premium is often placed on moving patients rapidly through an emergency department or clinic rather than engaging in more protracted efforts to use oral solutions and involving family members in their use. An initial bolus of isotonic intravenous fluid (normal saline or lactated Ringer's solution) may be repeated several times or may be followed by continuous intravenous fluid at a rate calculated to replenish losses in a certain amount of time. Alternatively, the initial intravenous bolus may be followed by oral fluid replacement. Such therapies are acceptable, provided that both the intravenous and oral fluids have appropriate glucose and electrolyte content (Table 3). The principles of the approach to rehydration and maintenance are identical, regardless of whether the oral or the intravenous route is chosen. A treatment algorithm showing the use of initial intravenous therapy followed by oral maintenance or of oral fluids alone is shown in Figure 1.

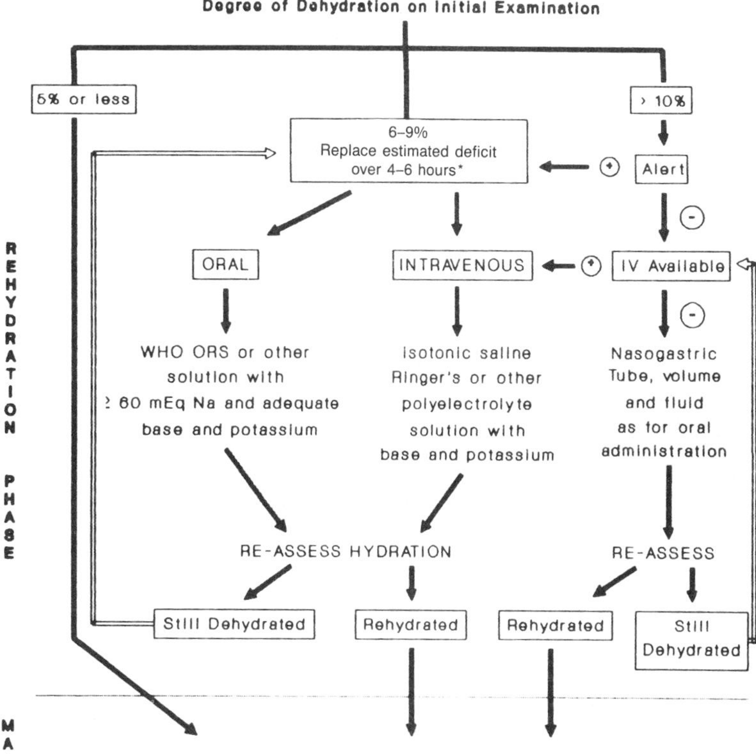

FIGURE 1 Treatment algorithm showing approach to rehydration of the dehydrated infant or child, beginning with either oral or intravenous therapy. The principles of volume repletion are identical in each case; the choice of therapy should depend upon availability of fluids and local practice. *Continue to replace ongoing losses with oral rehydration solution.

Rehydration Phase

The goal in this phase is the rapid restoration of circulating volume, with attendant abolition of the electrolyte imbalance and tissue acidosis. Contrary to the traditionally recommended time scale for intravenous fluid therapy (replacement of one-half the deficit over 8 hours and the balance over the next 16 hours), it has been found to be preferable to replace the entire volume deficit in the first 4 to 6 hours of treatment.[1] Provided that the fluid used contains glucose and electrolytes at or near the concentrations specified above, either the oral or intravenous route may be used. This phase is often accomplished in established rehydration centers or hospitals.

Calculation of the amount of fluid to be given in this phase is based on the patient's estimated healthy weight and the approximate percent of body volume lost. The latter figure is determined by clinical assessment and reference to established criteria (see Table 1). Healthy weight may be calculated by the formula: measured weight/(1 − percentage dehydration). Thus, a patient with estimated 10 percent dehydration who has a measured weight of 9.0 kg has a calculated healthy weight of 9.0/(1 − 0.1) = 10 kg. The volume to be given for replacement of his 1.0-kg deficit is then 1,000 ml of ORS, to be administered over a 4- to 6-hour period. Ongoing stool losses during the rehydration phase should be measured and added to the amount to be given.

The majority of dehydrated patients are able to consume the necessary quantity of fluid by taking small, frequent sips from a cup or spoon. Vomiting rarely precludes successful rehydration by this method if the fluid is administered steadily and in small doses. For example, if one 5-ml teaspoon of fluid is consumed each minute, an hourly rate of 300 ml is achieved, and significant vomiting related to volume of intake is unlikely. This "cup and spoon" method has enjoyed widespread success in the rehydration clinics of many developing countries and has proved successful in the emergency wards of busy United States and European centers as well.

In patients with intractable vomiting (more than four times per hour) or stool losses greater than 10 cc per kilogram per hour, or in those too lethargic to feed initially, fluid administration by nasogastric tube may be required. The calculated volume is given usually by continuous drip infusion, and the tube is removed and oral therapy begun as soon as the patient is able to drink.

In patients with frank hypovolemic shock, intravenous or intraosseous therapy should be given initially until pulse and blood pressure stabilize; the balance of the calculated deficit may then be given by the oral or nasogastric route. In areas where intravenous treatment is unavailable (or while a vein is being sought), the nasogastric method, if initiated early enough, may eliminiate or supplement intravenous treatment even for patients in shock.

At the end of the predetermined 4- to 6-hour rehydration period, the patient should be re-examined and weighed. If criteria for rehydration are not met (return to "healthy weight," disappearance of clinical signs noted on admission), a second rehydration phase is entered. The deficit is recalculated, and appropriate amounts of ORS are administered. Rarely, a third rehydration phase will be needed. Once criteria for rehydration have been fulfilled, maintenance therapy is begun.

Maintenance Phase

The goals of this phase are (1) maintenance of hydration by providing sufficient fluid for basal metabolic requirements, (2) replacement of ongoing fluid losses, and (3) institution of appropriate feeding to prevent additional caloric loss, and, potentially, to reduce stool volume and duration of diarrhea.

Maintenance fluid requirements may be calculated by any of a number of methods relying ultimately on basal metabolic rate and cellular glucose consumption. A general rule of thumb is that for the first 10 kg of body weight, a child requires 4 ml per kilogram per hour, 2 ml per kilogram per hour for the second 10 kg, and 1 ml per kilogram per hour for each kilogram over 20. Thus, a 24-kg child requires $40 + 20 + 4 = 64$ ml per hour for maintenance alone. Estimates should be revised upward in the case of patients with increased insensible losses, such as those with fever or elevated respiratory rates. This baseline fluid requirement should be met with breast milk, formula, or foods appropriate to age and culture. Usually, children may be fed ad libitum fluids in this phase and will be found to meet or exceed their calculated "maintenance requirement."

Replacement of ongoing losses should be performed by the administration of equivalent amounts of ORS. In a rehydration center or hospital, losses are measured by diaper weight. Because most patients are sent home after rehydration, ongoing losses must be estimated at home and replaced with a prescribed volume of ORS. Instead of estimating losses, a regimen of alternating feedings with ORS ad libitum has also been found to be effective.

Feeding

The institution of appropriate feedings early in the course of diarrheal illness has not been common practice. Traditional teaching by both professionals and the lay public has held that bowel rest provides most rapid resolution of symptoms. Recent data, however, support the notion that early feeding of patients with acute diarrhea does not worsen or prolong symptoms and may actually reduce stool output and duration of diarrhea,[13–15] possibly by maximizing the use of multiple channels for glucose:substrate co-transport. Transient, acquired lactase deficiency may occur, and lactose-free feedings are recommended where available but are not strictly necessary. Rice-based formulas or simply rice feedings begun as soon as rehydration is complete are another source of lactose-free carbohydrate. Current recommendations are that infants and children be allowed to begin regular feeding (with yogurt, milk, rice, formula, or other locally available food) immediately following the rehydration phase.

The regimen described above, involving an initial rehydration phase, followed by maintenance therapy at home, was devised initially for use in developing nations, where each center treats hundreds of patients daily. A similar system may be confidently recommended for use in clinics and hospital emergency departments in the industrialized world.

ASSOCIATED PROBLEMS AND COMPLICATIONS

Therapy of acute dehydration in diarrhea may be associated with complications either of the disease itself or of the treatment employed. Such problems may be encountered with both the intravenous and the enteral routes of rehydration, although the oral route has been relatively free of complications in a number of studies.[2] In the following discussion we focus attention on two of the most commonly discussed complicating factors seen in patients receiving oral therapy: hypernatremia and severe malnutrition. It must be stressed that both conditions, when seen, are usually present at the outset of treatment and rarely are the direct result of the use of oral therapy.

Hypernatremic Dehydration

Early reports of patients treated with oral rehydration fluids demonstrated an unacceptably high rate of hypernatremia and led to considerable concern in the medical community about the safety of such solutions.[1] These studies occurred during a period when many infants in the United States were being fed hyperosmolar formulas or feedings with a relatively high sodium content (e.g., boiled skimmed milk). Additionally, the early rehydration solutions were in many cases deficient in potassium and bicarbonate and may have thereby aggravated the hypernatremic state (see above). Large volume losses with a relatively low stool sodium content, such as might occur in lactose intolerance, can predispose the child to hypernatremia. These problems may be minimized by the administration of ORS of moderate tonicity, such as that currently in use, with adequate potassium and base content. Today, hypernatremic dehydration is most frequently seen in patients with particularly severe diarrhea.

Numerous studies have demonstrated that proper use of appropriately mixed ORS formulated as recommended by WHO results in rapid normalization of serum sodium in the overwhelming majority of patients, in spite of a wide range of initial sodium values. This response, even in hypernatremic patients, is probably related to the ability of the solution to rapidly replenish circulating volume and to "turn off" the stimuli that tend to perpetuate hypernatremia (e.g., hypokalemia, acidosis, physiologic elevation of aldosterone). Nonetheless, continued administration of ORS to patients with high initial serum sodium should be carefully monitored to assure gradual restoration of eunatremia.

The use of diluted ORS in hypernatremia or the alternate dosing with ORS and water is to be discouraged. The resulting solution actually perfusing the gut is one that contains inadequate sodium and glucose for optimal absorption and may in fact delay rehydration. Furthermore, excessively rapid drops in serum sodium from adminstration of hypotonic fluids may result in cerebral edema and convulsions.

Malnutrition

Although nutritional status has been shown to have little impact on the incidence of diarrhea, the duration of each episode is substantially increased in poorly nourished children, particularly with certain etiologic agents such as *E. coli* and *Shigella*.[12] Since each episode of diarrhea is usually accompanied by calorie-deficient feeding, a cycle is often begun in which prolonged illness results in poorer nutrition, which predisposes to still greater duration of disease and further caloric deprivation (Fig. 2).

A number of studies have demonstrated improved weight gain in children treated with ORT. Subsequently, it has been suggested that this effect may be related to the improved appetite accompanying the use of ORT, as well as to the more immediate improvement in hydration. Patients who are more rapidly rehydrated have earlier return of appetite and improve their food intake more readily than those who receive slower hydration.[12]

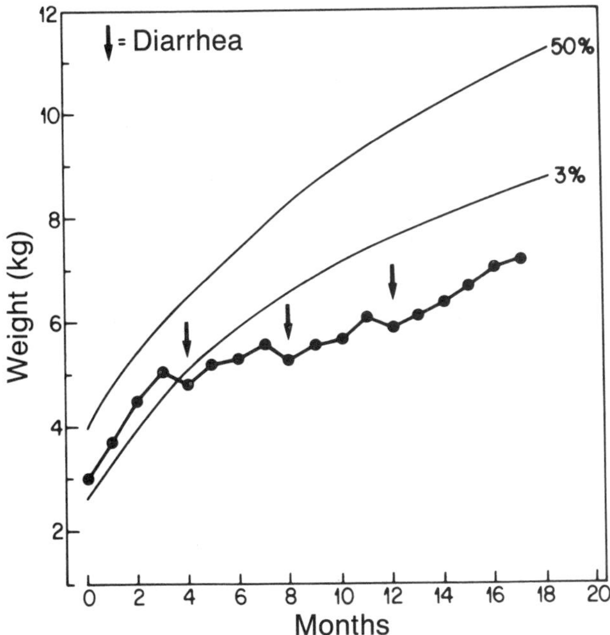

FIGURE 2 The cycle of diarrhea and malnutrition. Under current therapy, with each episode of disease, a malnourished child suffers substantial weight loss. Weight returns to premorbid value in about 1 month, leaving the child at a lower percentile. Subsequent illness perpetuates the cycle. With earlier introduction of appropriate feedings, the growth pattern would return to normal more rapidly.

Standard WHO ORS solution may be used successfully in acute diarrhea in patients with severe malnutrition. Many such patients, additionally, have become weak and anorexic secondary to chronic acidosis or anemia and supervening bowel infections or parasites. These patients may respond best to continuous nasogastric administration of ORS. About 1 to 2 percent of hospitalized patients do not tolerate glucose and have increased osmotic diarrhea. They may require glucose-free elemental feedings.

FUTURE OF ORAL REHYDRATION

Room for advancement remains in the production of oral rehydration solutions with improved efficacy, stability, and availability. Currently available ORS does not reduce the volume or duration of stool output. As discussed above, increasing concentrations of glucose in theory make possible increased salt and water co-transport but are not practical because of the limited capacity of the child's gut to absorb glucose, creating a higher osmotic load and consequently higher stool water content. Theoretically, this complication may be circumvented by using complex carbohydrates whose large molecular size contributes minimally to osmotic load while greatly increasing the availability of glucose molecules at the level of the intestinal brush border.[9] This approach depends upon the continued presence of pancreatic amylase and glucosidases in the gut lumen. To date, controlled clinical studies have not demonstrated any benefit from the use of purified complex carbohydrates such as glucose polymers. However, some cereal-based formulations (particularly those using rice) have been shown to reduce both the volume and duration of an episode of diarrhea and promote an earlier return of appetite.

Another theoretical approach has involved attempts to saturate co-transport systems in the intestinal epithelium. Amino acids have been shown to have an additive, noncompetitive effect, when present with glucose, on the stimulation of sodium absorption.[3] Future ORS formulations no doubt will attempt to take advantage of these effects in providing solutions whose net effect is to diminish stool output.

A number of substances have been explored for their usefulness as substrates in ORS. Because of their high content of carbohydrate polymers and ready availability, cereal grains have been widely used. Rice in various forms has been the most thoroughly tested cereal and so far appears superior in its effects on the reduction of stool output and duration. Other grains used have included maize, wheat, millet, and sorghum, as well as tubers, such as potatoes, and green bananas and plantains.[9]

A number of experimental ORS have been produced which use protein hydrolysates as a high molecular weight source of organic substrates.[7] Such formulations often lack stability, and the raw materials are not as readily available as the cereals.

Cereal- or protein-based solutions should increase fluid absorption over standard formulations and thus reduce net stool losses, but few carefully controlled studies have been performed to date. Although the formulations of such solutions vary greatly, they share relatively poor stability after preparation and rapid spoiling or settling.

In spite of these objections, such solutions hold considerable promise for the future. Any form of ORT which provides faster symptom resolution and decreased stool output will be speedily accepted by patients, parents, and healthcare workers, who may otherwise become disenchanted with solutions that simply maintain hydration.

More Stable Formulation

The importance of stability of ORT solutions was alluded to above. Early recognition of this problem led to the substitution of citrate for bicarbonate as the base in WHO ORS, and the result was improvement in the shelf life of the prepared packets and solution.

The more complex solutions are at increased risk of spoilage. Not only is the resulting fluid unpalatable, but the changes in chemical content and osmolarity reduce its utility as a therapy. Mixing these solutions in small batches and refrigerating unused fluids minimize the chance of spoilage.

Since most cereal-based solutions use a powdered or milled form of the grain, settling of the relatively large particles is a problem. Many solutions undergo nearly complete settling in about one-half hour and thus require frequent stirring to maintain standard compositions. A few solutions have recently been produced using finely milled rice, which results in an electrostatic suspension that remains mixed for about 24 hours. Such an approach relies upon relatively high technology for the milling and transportation of the powder. The addition of 1 percent pectin has also been shown to prolong the suspension of rice particles in some trials.

SUMMARY AND CONCLUSIONS

The approach to rehydration of the volume-depleted child has been discussed above. Certain vital points should be stressed in summary:

1. The physiologic consequences of volume depletion are profound and may begin to be manifest with as little as 2 percent volume loss.
2. In order to abolish pathologic responses to volume depletion, fluid must be replaced rapidly with isotonic solutions containing adequate potassium and base.
3. Recognition that mammalian bowel contains a powerful apparatus for absorption of sodium and water in conjunction with small organic molecules provided the basis for rapid fluid replacement using the gut.
4. Intravenous fluid therapy, while useful, is rarely necessary when oral solutions are available.
5. More rapid rehydration leads to earlier recovery of appetite and improved feeding. Furthermore, early feeding probably reduces duration and severity of diarrhea and enhances nutritional status.

Morbidity and mortality from dehydrating diarrhea have been dramatically reduced since the widespread introduction of oral rehydration therapy. A detailed understanding of the physiologic mechanisms involved occurred only after rapid distribution of the technology. Never an empiric therapy, the science of oral rehydration therapy is now well established. With current understanding of the molecular basis of intestinal secretion and absorption, it is evident that the system has yet to be fully exploited. The next generations of oral rehydration solutions may be designed as "drugs" to powerfully reverse the secretory consequences of disordered chloride channel regulation and result not only in rapid volume repletion, but actually in dramatic reduction of diarrheal symptoms.

REFERENCES

1. Hirschhorn N. The treatment of acute diarrhea in children. An historical and physiological perspective. Am J Clin Nutr 1980; 33:637–663.
2. Sharifi J, Ghavami F, Nowrouzi Z, Fouladvand B, Malek M, Rezaeian M, Emami M. Oral versus intravenous rehydration therapy in severe gastroenteritis. Arch Dis Child 1985; 60:856–860.
3. Powell D. Intestinal water and electrolyte transport. In: Johnson LR, ed. Physiology of the gastrointestinal tract. 2nd ed. New York: Raven Press, 1987: 1267.
4. Hirschhorn N, Kinzie J, Sachar D, Northrup R, Taylor J, Ahmad S. Decrease in net stool output in cholera during intestinal perfusion with glucose-containing solutions. N Engl J Med 1968; 279:176–182.
5. Sladen GE, Dawson AM. Interrelationships between the absorptions of glucose, sodium and water by the normal human jejunum. Clin Sci 1969; 36:119–132.
6. Donowitz M, Welsh J. Regulation of mammalian small intestinal secretion. In: Johnson LR, ed. Physiology of the gastrointestinal tract. 2nd ed. New York: Raven Press, 1987: 1351.
7. Mahalanabis D, Merson M. Development of an improved formulation of oral rehydration salts (ORS) with antidiarrhoeal and nutritional properties: a "super ORS." In: Holmgren J, Lindberg A, Mollby R, eds. Development of vaccines and drugs against diarrhea. 11th Nobel conference, Stockholm, 1985: 240.
8. Nalin DR. Oral therapy for diarrheal diseases. In: Dale CB, Northrup RS, eds. Symposium Proceedings: Cereal-based oral rehydration therapy: theory and practice. Washington: International Child Health Foundation, 1987: 24.
9. Greenough WB III. Status of cereal-based oral rehydration therapy. In: Dale CB, Northrup RS, eds. Symposium Proceedings; Cereal-based oral rehydration therapy: theory and practice. Washington: International Child Health Foundation, 1987: 29.
10. Molla AM, Sarber SA, Hossain M, Molla A. Rice-powder electrolyte solution as oral therapy in diarrhea due to *Vibrio cholerae* and *Escherichia coli*. Lancet 1982; i:1318–1319.
11. Nwoye LO, Uwagboe PE, Mdubuko GU. Evaluation of home-made salt-sugar oral rehydration solution in a rural Nigerian population. J Trop Med Hyg 1988; 91:23–27.
12. Santosham M. Nutritional aspect of ORT. In: Dale CB, Northrup RS, eds. Symposium Proceedings, Cereal-based oral rehydration therapy: theory and practice. Washington: International Child Health Foundation, 1987: 24.
13. Santosham M, Foster S, Reid R, et al. Role of soy-based, lactose-free formula during treatment of acute diarrhea. Pediatrics 1985; 76:292–298.
14. Brown KH, Gastanaduy AS, Saavedra J, Lembke J, Rivas D, Robertson A, Yolken R, Sack RB. Effect of continued oral feeding on clinical and nutritional outcome of acute diarrhea in children. J Pediatr 1988; 112:191–200.
15. Santosham M, Fayad IM, Hashem M, Goepp JG, Refat M, Sack RB. Is rice based oral rehydration solution more efficacious than "early feeding" with cooked rice for the treatment of acute diarrhea in infants? ; in press.

CHAPTER 41

Nutritional Therapy

PART 1

Introduction

John N. Udall Jr., M.D., Ph.D.

Optimal nourishment for children is important for several reasons. First, growth and development cannot proceed normally without adequate nutrition. Second, the development of some diseases has been linked to undernutrition and overnutrition. Finally, a sustained imbalance in the intake of certain nutrients may put some infants and children at risk of developing deficiency states.

To determine optimal nutrition for normal and hospitalized children, nutritional requirements must be estimated from established recommendations while undernutrition and overnutrition are avoided. To optimize health care for patients with compromised gastrointestinal function, it is important to consider not only the amounts of nutrients supplied and the composition of feedings but also the route of the feedings, i.e., enteral or parenteral.

The rate at which information concerning these aspects of nutritional therapy is being generated challenges even the most compulsive individuals attempting to keep abreast of current therapy. Still it is important to have a framework concerning nutritional requirements, undernutrition, overnutrition, and enteral and parenteral nutrition in order to effectively utilize nutritional therapy. These topics as they relate to gastrointestinal disease are covered in this discussion.

NUTRITIONAL REQUIREMENTS

Adequate nutrients for infants and children are necessary to maintain body mass, support activity, and allow for normal growth and development. Nutritional requirements are dependent on age, sex, body weight, and health or disease. It is difficult to assess requirements in the presence of disease when needs may be dramatically increased.

Recently, the tenth edition of the Recommended Dietary Allowances (RDA) was published and reviewed.[1] The RDA, which is established by the Food and Nutrition Board of the National Research Council and the National Academy of Sciences, is the standard by which an individual's diet is judged. It states that there is an increased need for protein, calories, and most nutrients early in life. The protein requirement for infants is 2.2 g per kilogram of body weight per day, and the requirement for adults is 0.8 g per kilogram of body weight per day.[2] Not only is the quantity of protein required for normal growth and development important, but also the quality of the protein ingested. Using nitrogen balance and growth as criteria, and most recently with the aid of studies of blood amino acid levels, the requirements of essential amino acids for children and adults have been estimated. Such estimates show wide variations among individuals and laboratories, but on careful analysis of published data, it is possible to arrive at values that are reasonably concordant and certainly relevant to utilization of dietary proteins of varying amino acid composition.[3] Estimates of the needs for essential amino acids suggest that additional quantities of essential amino acids are required during infancy compared with later in development.[4]

Energy requirements for infants are 108 kcal per kilogram of body weight per day, whereas for adults they are 36 kcal per kilogram of body weight per day.[2] Energy requirements should be provided by carbohydrates and lipids once protein needs are met. Young infants should receive 3 percent of their caloric intake in the form of essential fatty acids.[5] Infants and especially premature infants are at an increased at risk of essential fatty acid deficiency. Recent studies have shown that premature infants receiving intravenous nutrients and no essential fatty acids are prone to develop biochemical evidence of essential fatty acid deficiency within 2 weeks of birth.[6]

It is assumed that when an infant's or child's needs for proteins, calories, fats, and other nutrients are met he or she will grow at an acceptable rate.

UNDERNUTRITION AND OBESITY

Cicely Williams, an English pediatrician working in Africa in 1933, described a nutritional disease of childhood associated with the use of a maize diet.[7] Two years later she again described this condition using the term *kwashiorkor.*[8] One questions the progress that has occurred since her first description of protein calorie malnutrition (PCM), because it has been estimated that worldwide approximately 100 million children less than 5 years of age are severely or moderately undernourished.[9] In some rural areas as much as 75 percent of the population suffers from undernutrition. Worldwide undernutrition is responsible, directly or indirectly, for 53 percent of deaths of children under 5 years of age.[9]

We should not think that this problem of undernutrition exists only in Third World countries. Although in 1969 primary PCM was thought to be uncommon in the United States,[10] large numbers of children with PCM secondary to chronic disease can be identified in hospitals.[11] In 1980, a report of 14 cases of kwashiorkor and marasmic kwashiorkor in the United States was presented as a reminder that predisposing social and nutritional factors that can result in PCM do exist, even in affluent countries.[12]

It is of note that infants who are vigorously treated for PCM may develop hepatomegaly, abdominal distention, hypertrichosis, and eosinophilia, a condition known as "nutrition recovery syndrome."[13] More recently, hypophosphatemia has been described in this "nutrition recovery syndrome."[14] Health care workers should be aware of this syndrome when utilizing nutritional therapy for these undernourished patients.

Just as the scourge of PCM plagues underdeveloped countries, its counterpart, overnutrition or obesity, is the bane of developed countries. In the United States the prevalence of obesity has been estimated to be present in up to 40 percent of the population. The magnitude of the problem is staggering and challenges health care professionals because of the associated diseases, hypertension and diabetes, and an increased incidence of slipped capital femoral epiphyses and respiratory infections. We have not achieved the same success in the treatment of overnutrition as we have in the treatment of undernutrition, in part because of confusion that reigns in the lay literature. The confusion can be verified by a trip to any large bookstore where literally dozens of books on weight reduction, weight-reducing pills, newly contrived dietary foods, artificial sweetners, and information on surgical procedures for obesity are available for the weight-conscious individual.

One example of a newly contrived dietary food is aspartame. It is primarily composed of aspartic acid and phenylalanine and is 200 times sweeter than sugar.[15] The sweetener is used in small amounts which are calorically insignificant to sweeten beverages, desserts, breakfast cereals and chewing gum to mention a few products. Each year more than 100 million Americans consume products with aspartame.[15] Most of them believe that the artificial sweetener will help them lose weight, or at least avoid gaining weight. Little thought is given to the other variables which may be contributing to obesity. Still the search for miracle products goes on, and more recently, Simplesse (Nutra Sweet Company, Deerfield, IL), an all-natural fat substitute, has been produced from milk and egg protein. It is advertised as a "creamy, rich fluid with the texture of fat." Our willingness to develop products that may be shortcuts in maintaining ideal body weight is most likely short-sighted. We have a long way to go and much to learn before obesity can be treated effectively or, even better, prevented.

ENTERAL NUTRITION

It is well known that the gastrointestinal tract is well adapted to receive, digest, and absorb nutrients. As elementary as the concept of enteral nutrition would appear, the field has become a maze of confusion. The routes by which nutrients may be introduced into the intestine are varied. In addition, for those who cannot tolerate traditional diets there are multitudes of specialized formulas that contain varying mixtures of ingredients, some of which have been predigested or completely synthesized. Patients may tolerate one of these special formulas when traditional foods are not effectively digested or absorbed. Therefore, it behooves the health care provider involved in nutritional therapy to have a working knowledge of the indications for the various feeding routes and the variety of nutrients that are used.

PARENTERAL NUTRITION

Slightly more than 20 years ago Avery et al described 20 infants with intractable diarrhea.[16] Total parenteral nutrition by central venous lines was not available at that time, and of the 20 infants, 9 (40 percent) died. With the use of specialized formulas and total parenteral nutrition this 40 percent mortality figure has been decreased to 5 to 7 percent.[17] Indeed, children with a variety of diseases that compromise gastrointestinal function are being fed only by the intravenous route in the hospital or are sent home and maintained on total parenteral nutrition for months to years. The technology that has allowed this is indeed a most significant contribution to medicine.

As we have developed new routes by which to feed infants and children, new problems have arisen. Children who have been fed via central venous lines or gastrostomy tubes for long periods of time may refuse to eat when oral foods are eventually re-introduced. These children have been deprived of normal feeding experiences during sensitive periods of development and have poor feeding skills. They often cry, fight, gag, and vomit when attempts are made to put food in their mouths. This response frightens parents and discourages professionals who are trying to help the child make the transition back to oral feedings. Firm, consistent approaches to overcoming the child's resistance to eating food coupled with behavioral eating programs have been used to manage this problem.[18–21] Other problems are also associated with new feeding techniques and should be treated individually.

Our drive to improve nutritional therapy will undoubtedly continue, and investigators will more clearly define nutrient needs, deal more effectively with undernutrition and overnutrition, and develop improved enteral and parenteral formulations. This exciting and dynamic field of health care will continue to challenge us and stimulate health care workers to keep abreast of the latest developments. Parts of this chapter have been selected to cover nutritional therapies common to gastrointestinal disorders in pediatrics.

REFERENCES

1. Monsen ER. The 10th edition of the recommended dietary allowances: what's new in the 1989 RDSs? J Am Diet Assoc 1989; 89:1748–1752.
2. Recommended Dietary Allowances. 10th ed. Washington, D.C.: National Academy Press, 1989.
3. Human protein and amino acid requirements and their relevance to protein quality evaluation. In: Pallett PL, Young VR, eds. Nutritional evaluation of protein foods. Japan: The United Nations University, 1980.
4. Udall JN Jr, Kilbourne KA. Selected aspects of infant feeding. Nutrition 1988; 4:409–415.
5. Committee on Nutrition, American Academy of Pediatrics. Commentary on breast-feeding and infant formulas, including proposed standards for formulas. Pediatrics 1976; 57:278–285.
6. Friedman Z, Danon A, Stahlman MT, Oates JA. Rapid onset of essential fatty acid deficiency in the newborn. Pediatrics 1976; 58:640–649.
7. Williams CD. A nutritional disease of childhood associated with a maize diet. Arch Dis Child 1933; 8:423–433.
8. Williams CD. Kwashiorkor. A nutritional disease of childhood associated with a maize diet. Lancet 1935; ii:1151–1153.
9. Baker SS. Protein-energy malnutrition in the hospitalized pediatric patient. In: Walker WA, Watkins JB, eds. Nutrition in pediatrics. Boston: Little, Brown, 1985: 171.
10. Brown RE. Poverty and health in the United States. Clin Pediatr 1969; 8:495–498.
11. Merritt RJ, Blackburn GL. Nutritional assessment and metabolic response to illness of the hospitalized child. In: Suskind RM, ed. Textbook of pediatric nutrition. New York: Raven Press, 1981: 285.
12. Chase HP, Kumar V, Caldwell RT, O'Brien D. Kwashiorkor in the United States. Pediatrics 1980; 66:972–976.
13. Gómez F, Galván RR, Munõz JC. Nutritional recovery syndrome. Pediatrics 1952; 10:513–526.
14. Mezoff AG, Gremse DA, Farrell MK. Hypophosphatemia in the nutritional recovery syndrome. Am J Dis Child 1989; 143:1111–1112.
15. Farber SA. The price of sweetness. Tech Rev 1990; Jan:46–53.
16. Avery GB, Villavicencio O, Lilly JR, Randolph JG. Intractable diarrhea in early infancy. Pediatrics 1968; 41:712–722.
17. Rossi TM, Lebenthal E, Nord KS, Fazili RR. Extent and duration of small intestinal mucosal injury in intractable diarrhea of infancy. Pediatrics 1980; 66:730–735.
18. Blackman JA, Nelson CLA. Reinstituting oral feeding in children fed by gastrostomy tube. Clin Pediatr 1985; 24:434–438.
19. Geertsma MA, Hyams JS, Pelletier JM, Reiter S. Feeding resistance after parenteral hyperalimentation. Am J Dis Child 1985; 139:255–256.
20. Handen BL, Mandell F, Russo DC. Feeding induction in children who refuse to eat. Am J Dis Child 1986; 140:52–54.
21. Blackman JA, Nelson CLA. Rapid introduction of oral feedings to tube-fed patients. Develop Behav Pediatr 1987; 8:63–67.

PART 2

Nutritional Requirements

Russell J. Merritt, M.D., Ph.D.

An adequate diet is essential to maintain body mass, support activity and play, and allow growth and development of the infant and child. Dietary and nutrient adequacy can be evaluated by dietary history, examination of growth data, physical examination, and laboratory testing. Nutritional assessment and therapy are particularly important for the recognition, treatment, and prevention of nutritional complications of gastrointestinal (GI) diseases in infants and children.

Multiple factors may deprive the patient of the energy and nutrients required to maintain normal nutritional status. Anorexia is common in acute and chronic illness. Mechanisms of anorexia may include hormonal/metabolic alterations associated with the body's response to illness, early satiety, the presence of symptoms exacerbated by food ingestion, and depression. GI diseases may alter nutrient balance by decreasing absorption or increasing nutrient or macromolecule losses via the gut and, under certain circumstances, via urine or skin as well. Abnormal losses may provoke secondary pathophysiologic changes such as the hypoproteinemic edema associated with protein-losing enteropathy. Such pathophysiologic states are not induced by dietary deficiency; nonetheless, nutritional therapy may be beneficial.

Medications used to treat GI and liver disorders may also have effects on nutritional status. Mechanisms may include effects on appetite, gastric irritation, inhibition of nutrient absorption, diarrhea, constipation, or altered nutrient metabolism. Certain nutritional supplements may have adverse effects if administered at high dosage levels.

Specialized diets or formulas or feeding routes are required by some patients with GI and liver diseases. Poor palatability and undesirable hedonic properties of such diets and formulas may suppress appetite and lead to poor intake. Similarly, highly restrictive therapeutic diets may inadvertently lead to energy or nutrient deficiency. The use of enteral feeding tubes or intravenous catheters for feeding in early infancy may result in long-term feeding disorders and adverse developmental consequences for some children.

The above issues underscore the importance of sound, experienced, anticipatory nutritional management in patients with GI disorders. This discussion provides background regarding nutritional requirements, dietary and patient nutritional assessment, and the modification of nutritional needs in patients with GI disease.

NUTRITIONAL ASSESSMENT

The morbidity and potential mortality of primary malnutrition are well recognized. The morbidity and mortality of secondary malnutrition (that due to underlying disease or organ failure) have been increasingly recognized in hospitalized adults.[1-3] Growth failure and malnutrition are known to be characteristic of many pediatric GI diseases. More recently the reversibility of growth failure and malnutrition by optimal medical and nutritional therapy has been demonstrated for many of these conditions.[4-6] Therefore, monitoring nutritional status and growth and implementing nutritional therapy have become essential aspects of the care of patients with GI disease.

Because the growth process is sensitive to dietary deficiencies, growth monitoring is a basic aspect of pediatric nutritional assessment. This is most commonly performed by using the serial assessment of length or height, weight, and, in infancy, head circumference. The data are plotted on an appropriate reference standard, usually the growth charts produced by the National Center for Health Statistics (NCHS).[7] These charts are based on observations of healthy infants and children in the United States, made mostly in the 1960s and 1970s. Debate persists as to whether these should be considered optimal standards, in light of observation that infants who are breast-fed only grow somewhat more slowly than depicted on these charts, that there is a high prevalence of obesity in North American children, and that there remain some small racial differences in growth pattern.[8-12] Despite these concerns, the NCHS standards serve as a basic reference standard.[13]

Decreased weight for height (wt/ht) is considered an indicator of acute malnutrition, and decreased height for age (ht/age) is a marker for chronic malnutrition in association with low wt/ht.[14,15] One of the limitations of the current growth charts is that they provide no chart of wt/ht after the onset of puberty. This omission is related to the extreme variability of wt/ht during the pubescent years. Children with more advanced maturity are heavier as a result of the increase in muscle mass in males and fat mass in females that occurs during the adolescent years. The only tables available for wt/ht calculations in United States adolescents were published in 1925.[16]

Observed wt/ht and ht/age data can be expressed as a percentile value or as a percentage of the fiftieth percentile. This latter approach is helpful when an observation falls below the fifth percentile. Wt/ht values less than 90 percent of standard are considered low, and values below 70 percent are classified as indicating marasmus.[14] Morbidity and mortality are increased with substantial deficits in body mass.[17,18] Ht/age values below 95 percent of standard indicate stunting, and values below 85 percent are indicative of severe short stature.

Patients with low ht/age, but normal wt/ht may have hereditary short stature, constitutional growth delay, a congenital syndrome or other disease associated with short stature, hormone deficiency, inborn error of metabolism, chronic illness, maternal deprivation, a history of low birth weight, or a history of prior severe or prolonged malnutrition. Growth data should be optimally considered in the context of family members' height, growth history, and developmental patterns and the patient's medical history.

It is helpful to examine growth rate in selected patients. This may be useful in the absence of prior medical records or in comparing periods of growth, for example, on different therapies. Tables of growth rate and charts of growth rate are available and useful in these contexts.[19-21] Nevertheless, some caution must be exercised in interpreting growth rates for periods of time of much less than 1 year in school-age children.[22]

Knowledge of body composition may be of value in some circumstances. Some individuals may be obese but have wasting of lean tissue. Others may be overweight but not obese, as a result of increased lean body mass. Demonstration of adequate fat stores during growth failure suggests that current growth failure is probably not due to limited energy content of the diet. In order to assess body composition, various techniques have been developed to separately quantify the body's lean and fat compartments. The most useful bedside technique is the measurement of extremity circumferences and caliper-determined skin folds to define the fat and lean components. The measurements used most frequently are the mid–upper arm circumference and triceps skin fold. Percentile values are available for the American population.[23] The correlation of total body fatness with measurement of triceps skin fold is approximately 0.7.[24] Arm circumference is a particularly good indicator of future mortality in malnourished children.[27]

The other technique attaining clinical acceptance is the use of body impedance analysis (BIA) to estimate percentage of body fat.[25] This technique capitalizes on the observation that a weak electrical current passes readily through water and solute-containing body compartments but not as readily through body fat. The apparatus required is only modestly expensive and relatively simple to operate. When normal values become more clearly defined, this technique of body compartment analysis should prove to be clinically useful. Abnormalities in hydration status can invalidate results obtained by BIA.

Nutritional status is one of the factors that affect circulating concentrations of some serum proteins. Among the proteins that decrease in response to dietary protein deficiency are albumin, prealbumin, retinol-binding protein, fibronectin, collagen 1-c, and somatomedin-C.[26] As a result, these proteins are used as indicators of nutritional status, more specifically, "visceral" nutritional status.[27] Serum prealbumin has recently been used to assess adequacy of protein and energy intake in small preterm infants.[28] These proteins are modulated by other processes as well. Concentrations may fall owing to abnormal protein losses, such as in protein-losing enteropathy, or in response to infection or other metabolic stresses. This may be less true of fibronectin than the other visceral markers.[29] Some also decrease in response to limited energy intake or changes in the carbohydrate content of the diet.[30] As a consequence, concentrations of these nutritionally responsive serum proteins must be interpreted in light of the patient's overall medical and nutritional condition. Severe hypoalbuminemia is one of the hallmarks of kwashiorkor. Nutritional edema is always considered evidence of severe malnutrition. Hypoproteinemic edema occurs in some GI diseases such as cirrhosis or severe protein-losing enteropathy. As most of these children fail to normalize their serum proteins and clear their edema despite being provided with an adequate or increased protein intake, they cannot be considered to have nutritionally induced kwashiorkor. However, they still appear to be at increased risk of infectious complications due to local factors such as the presence of ascites or as a consequence of diminished serum protein concentrations.[31]

Parameters of immune function are also subject to nutritional influence.[32] In addition to protein-energy malnutrition, specific nutrients may alter lymphocyte or phagocyte function.[33] Total lymphocyte count depression has been used as a nonspecific indicator of protein-energy malnutrition. Depression of delayed hypersensitivity skin test responses has been found to reflect the severity of malnutrition and to have prognostic import for malnourished adult surgical patients.[34] Antigens used to test for nutritional anergy include tetanus and *Candida* extract. After starting a standard immunization series, almost all infants can mount at least a 2- to 3-mm reaction to the immunization antigens.[35] The size of the response increases with age. Demonstration of immune competence by means of an adequate lymphocyte count (generally greater than 1,500 per cubic millimeter) and skin test reactivity, may be particularly useful in deciding whether a borderline malnourished patient is ready to undergo a needed, but elective, surgical procedure.

ASSESSMENT OF DIET

The diet of the infant or child with GI symptoms needs to be assessed as to quantity and quality. Dietary recall is the simplest way of obtaining information in the context of an office visit. One can elicit a usual dietary pattern or 1-day recall. Such an approach usually provides some idea of the normalcy of the child's diet, but if quantitative information is needed a prospective food record is far preferable. Parents need to be carefully instructed on how to maintain the food record. All food and beverages are recorded with estimates of intake by weighing (usually impractical) or by using common household measures. A 3-day record is adequate for most clinical purposes. The diet record can then be analyzed using food composition tables or by computerized data bases for food composition.[36] Such data bases are marketed for use on personal computers. Analysis by a registered dietitian is preferable from the standpoint of expertise in interpretation and patient counseling. Analysis of the diet can indicate the adequacy of dietary energy or of specific nutrients in relation to estimated requirements appropriate for age and size. When a computerized system is used, it is essential to apply age-adjusted standards and to know how the reference standards for nutrient requirements were determined. Diet records are useful for calculation of the coefficient of fat absorption during a 72-hour fecal fat collection, evaluation of energy and nutrient adequacy of the diet in cases of failure to thrive, dietary evaluation of chronic diarrhea, or monitoring of dietary management of celiac disease, allergic gastroenteropathy, and hypercholesterolemia.

As the entire diet during early infancy may be infant formula, the energy and protein intakes are relatively simple to estimate. During later infancy many infants receive formula supplemented with commercially prepared infant foods. Four-ounce jars have an energy content of 40 to 140 kcal, depending on the food contained. If the infant is consuming a variety of goods, estimating the mean caloric contents per jar at 80 kcal—knowing that standard milks and formulas contain 20 kcal per fluid ounce—allows for a rapid office estimate of energy intake. Breast-milk intake estimation is more complex and requires premeal and postmeal weighings or use of deuterium dilution.[37]

The quality of the diet can be ascertained by estimating the number of servings per day from the modified four food groups.[38] These groups include milk and dairy products, meats and meat substitutes, breads and cereals, fruits and vegetables, fats and oils, and other foods (Table 1). This system of dietary analysis is structured to ensure that energy and most nutrient requirements will be met on a daily basis. These food groupings are also used for filling dietary prescriptions of a diet normal for a particular age. The recommended serving sizes increase with age.

Energy-Yielding Substrates—Carbohydrate, Lipid, and Protein

Biologic systems are dependent on an adequate supply of energy for survival and growth. In the animal kingdom this energy is derived quantitatively from ingested food rich in reduced carbon, i.e., carbohydrate, lipid, and protein—the last substrate also being the source of nitrogen and amino acids required for structural and enzymatic protein synthesis.

Lipid

Dietary lipid is the most energy-dense substrate. Dietary lipids are largely triglycerides from plant oils and animal fats, but also phospholipid-rich cell membranes, sterols, sphyngolipid, and other organic solvent–soluble organic molecules. The high-energy yield of dietary triglyceride is attributable to the highly reduced chemical structure of the fatty acids [$CH_3 - (CH_2)_n - COOH$] esterified to glycerol. The reduced carbon atoms are available for complete oxidative phosphorylation in the mitochondrial metabolic pathways terminating in CO_2 production.

Triglycerides (triacylglycerols) are also important for the specific fatty acids esterified to glycerol. Acyl groups of less than eight carbon atoms are considered short-chain fatty acids, those from eight to 12 medium-chain fatty acids, those from 16 to 20 long-chain fatty acids, and those above 20 very long chain fatty acids. Medium- and short-chain triglycerides are more readily absorbed from the intestine in the absence of bile acids, and the component fatty acids do not require acylation to carnitine to enter mitochondria for beta-oxidation.[39] Dietary triglyceride is catabolized for energy production via mitochondrial beta-oxidation. Much smaller amounts of complex lipids and fatty acids are metabolized by other oxidative mechanisms in microsomes, peroxisomes, and lysosomes.

In long-chain–containing triglycerides, the presence of unsaturated double bonds has important metabolic effects. Unsaturated fatty acids are identified by chain length, the number of unsaturated double bonds present, and the location of the first double bond from the methyl carbon (designated carbon 1) of the molecule (e.g., the notation C20:4,12 n6 for arachidonic acid indicates a *20*-carbon aliphatic fatty acid with the first of its *4* double bonds in the *n6* (or ω6) position). Not only is absorption affected by the presence and location of unsaturated fatty acids on the glycerol backbone,[40] but specific unsaturated fatty acids have unique metabolic effects.

TABLE 1
Food Groups and Serving Sizes*

Group	Foods	Daily Servings	1–3 Years	4–6 Years	7–10 Years	11–14 Years	15–18 Years	Key Nutrients Supplied
Milk and dairy products	Milk, yogurt, and milk-base soups	4	¼–½ C	½–¾ C	¾ C	1 C	1 C	
	Cottage cheese							Calcium
	Custard, milk pudding, and ice cream (but only after a meal		2-4 T	4-6 T	6 T	½ C	¾ C	Riboflavin
	Cheese (1 oz = 1 slice or 1″ cube)		⅓–⅔ oz	⅔–1 oz	1 oz	1¼ oz	1½ oz	Protein
Meat and meat alternatives	Beef, pork, lamb, veal, fish, and poultry; liver (every few weeks)	2	1 oz	1½ oz	4 T or 2 oz	3 oz	3 oz	
	Eggs		½	¾	1	1-3/week	1-3/week	Protein Niacin
	Peanut butter	2	2 T	3 T	3 T	3 T	4 T	Iron
	Cooked legumes, dried beans/peas		¼ C	⅜ C	½ C	¾ C	1 C	Thiamin
	Nuts†							
	Use additional servings of red meat, poultry, or fish if two servings of peanut butter, nuts, or legumes are not eaten daily.							
Fruits and vegetables	**Vitamin C source fruits, vegetables, and juices**							
	Citrus fruits, berries, melons, tomatoes, peppers, cabbage, cauliflower, broccoli, chiles, and potatoes	1	¼ C	¼ C	¼ C	½ C	1 C	Vitamin C
	Vitamin A source fruits and vegetables (deep green/yellow)							
	Melons, peaches, apricots, carrots, spinach, broccoli, squash, pumpkin, sweet potatoes, peas, beans (green, yellow, and lima), and Brussel sprouts	1	1-2 T	3-4 T	4-5 T	½ C	¾ C	Vitamin A
	Fruits‡	2	⅛ C	¼ C	½ C	¾ C	1 C	
	Vegetables		1-2 T	3-4 T	4-5 T	½ C	1 C	
Breads/cereals	Whole-grain, enriched, or restored breads		½ slice	¾ slice	¾–1 slice	1 slice	1½ slice	Thiamin Iron
	Cooked cereals, rice, and pasta	4	¼ C	⅓ C	½ C	½ C	1 C	Niacin
	Whole-grain or fortified ready-to-eat cereals		½ oz	¾oz	1 oz	1½ oz	2 oz	
Fats/oils	Butter, margarine, oils, mayonnaise, and salad dressings (1 T = 100 calories)	3	1 tsp	1 tsp	1 tsp	1 tsp	1 tsp	This group is a significant source of fats, for which there is no US RDA.
Other foods	Jams, jellies, soft drinks, candy, sweet desserts, salty snacks, gravies, olives, pickles, and catsup	Use in moderation		This group is a significant source of carbohydrates and fats, for which there is no US RDA.				

*Chart adapted from Endres J, Rackwell R. Food Nutrition and the Young Child. St. Louis: CV Mosby, 1980; and National Live Stock and Meat Board, 444 N. Michigan Ave., Chicago, IL, 60611.

†Nuts are not recommended for children under 5 years because they may cause choking.

‡Other fruits and vegetables not listed above.

Prostaglandins, leukotrienes, and thromboxanes all are derived from unsaturated 20-carbon fatty acids. The most important 20-carbon fatty acid precursors are the $\omega 3$, $\omega 6$, and $\omega 9$ fatty acids—eicosapentaenoic (EPA), arachidonic, and dihomo-gamma-linoleic acids, respectively. The resultant specific prostaglandin, thromboxane, and leukotriene products have different metabolic effects on the immune system, cholesterol metabolism, and inflammatory processes, including arteriosclerosis.[41,42] At present it appears that increasing the relative concentrations of long-chain and very long chain $\omega 3$ fatty acids in the diet can be potentially anti-inflammatory and protective against some forms of atherosclerosis.

Humans have the ability to elongate and desaturate dietary saturated and monounsaturated fatty acids. However, the polyunsaturated fatty acids linoleic[43,44] and probably linolenic[45] acids are essential dietary fatty acids. In the absence of dietary linoleic acid, skin lesions develop and growth is slowed. One to 5 percent of energy as linoleic acid appears adequate in most situations,[46] but malabsorption and energy deficiency may alter requirements.[47] Premature infants may need 10 percent of energy from linoleic acid in order to prevent biochemical evidence of deficiency.[48] Neurologic damage has been ascribed to linolenic acid deficiency in a parenterally nourished child. There is increasing evidence that the $\omega 3$ fatty acids—docosahexaenoic (DHA) and EPA—may be essential for optimal development of the nervous and visual systems. Visual disturbances have been reported in primates raised on diets deficient in these fatty acids,[49] and behavioral changes have been reported in $\omega 3$-deficient rats.[50] Human milk, but not the vegetable oils used in infant formulas, contains these fatty acids.[52] Humans probably have very limited ability to elongate and desaturate linolenic acid to EPA and DHA.

It has recently been proposed, with some evidence, that short-chain fatty acids, especially butyrate, may be essential to the structure and function of the colonic mucosa.[52] Dietary fiber is the usual dietary precursor of these fatty acids.

Carbohydrate

The general formula for dietary carbohydrate, $C_n(H_20)_n$, reflects its decreased potential for oxidation compared with fat. Dietary carbohydrates include simple sugars, disaccharides, oligosaccharides, starches, and fibers. Simple sugars and starches (after cooking) are nearly completely absorbed. Dietary fibers are digested and absorbed to a variable extent depending on the structure of the fiber.[53] Fiber may alter carbohydrate absorption by slowing gastric emptying and intestinal transit and delaying the hydrolysis of associated starches.[54,55]

Metabolism of absorbed carbohydrate ultimately occurs by way of the glycolytic pathway or the pentose shunt followed by oxidative phosphorylation in the Kreb's cycle. The body has a limited ability to store carbohydrate in the form of liver and muscle glycogen. Total stores are generally sufficient to meet no more than 12 to 24 hours of the body's energy requirement. Maintenance of normal levels of circulating glucose with more prolonged fasting requires gluconeogenesis from amino acids and the glycerol of triglyceride. When fasting is prolonged, the availability of fatty acid and ketone body substrates reduces the need for gluconeogenesis. Small amounts of dietary carbohydrate are also used to synthesize glycolipids and glycoproteins.

Protein

Dietary protein supplies essential amino acids, those which the body lacks the capacity to synthesize, and nonessential amino acids, which in addition to being supplied by the diet, can be synthesized from other amino acids or synthesized de novo. The basic chemical formula for amino acids is

$$\begin{array}{ccc} & & C^{-}OO^{-} \\ & & | \\ \overset{+}{N}H_3 & - & C - H \\ & & | \\ & & R \end{array}$$

Amino acids considered essential include valine, isoleucine, threonine, leucine, methionine, phenylalanine, tryptophan, histidine, and lysine.[56] Ingested amino acids may be used for protein synthesis, for energy production via oxidation, as precursors for other metabolic products, or for catabolism to the major nitrogen-containing waste products, ammonia and urea. Certain amino acids may become essential after premature birth, in some inborn errors of metabolism, in certain diseases, and during parenteral feeding.

Studies defining essential amino acid (EAA) requirements for healthy infants performed by Synderman and colleagues demonstrated that when a formula proved deficient, growth rate slowed and nitrogen balance became negative in response to the limiting amino acid.[57-60] Infants are thought to require a much higher percentage of total nitrogen from EAA than do adults or older children.[61] Recent stable isotope turnover studies of EAA in adults indicate depression of protein turnover and amino acid oxidation rates at currently recommended levels of some EAA. It has been claimed that such functional changes signal subclinical amino acid deficiency and that the percentage of total amino acids from EAA currently recommended for adults is too low, even though nitrogen balance is achieved at the currently recommended level.[62]

Amino acids thought to be nonessential or dispensable include glycine, alanine, serine, aspartic acid, asparagine, glutamic acid, and proline. Cysteine, taurine, tyrosine, and arginine may be synthesized to only a limited extent in the newborn or premature infant.[56] Taurine is a unique amino acid. It is not incorporated into peptides but plays a number of metabolic roles, including its use in bile acid conjugation and in processes in the central nervous system, the heart, and the retina.[56] Certain amino acids become essential only in disease states. Patients with liver disease, especially if fed intravenously, may have insufficient capacity for cysteine and tyrosine synthesis.[63] Arginine becomes essential in patients with urea cycle defects. Patients with cystic fibrosis may experience improved fat absorption with taurine supplementation and resultant enrichment of the bile acid pool with taurine-conjugated bile salts.[64] Glutamine appears to be required by the GI tract for its optimal integrity and function.[65] Its limited luminal availability during parenteral nutrition with glutamine-free solutions may be partly responsible for the atrophy of the intestinal mucosa seen with this mode of feeding. Enteral or parenteral replacement of glutamine in large doses enhances the integrity of colonic mucosa of laboratory animals under experimental conditions. The route of feeding may also affect the dispensability of some amino acids. Cysteine levels fall more rapidly with intravenous feeding devoid of cysteine than with the same synthetic diet given via the GI tract.[66]

After digestion, absorbed amino acids enter the circulating amino acid pool of the plasma and exchange with tissue amino acid pools, which may have a different amino acid composition.[67] The free amino acid pools make up less than 1 percent of the total amino acid content of the body.[68] Dietary amino acids are thought to contribute about one-third of the total daily amino acid flux in and out of protein-containing tissues.[68] The rest come from endogenous protein breakdown. Some tissues, such as the gut, contribute heavily to amino acid flux on the basis of rapid protein turnover. Others such as muscle—with its slower rate of protein turnover—contribute a large percentage of flux by virtue of the large mass of tissue involved.

The daily requirements for amino acids and nitrogen are largely functions of the quantity of catabolized essential amino acids and urinary and fecal nitrogen losses plus what is needed for growth.[61] The process of amino acid and nitrogen "replacement" is an inefficient one. Therefore, the daily amino acid nitrogen requirement is much higher than the nitrogen excretion observed on a protein-free diet.[61]

DETERMINING ENERGY, PROTEIN, AND NUTRIENT REQUIREMENTS

Estimates of nutritional requirements are developed by national and international scientific bodies such as the Committee on Dietary Allowances of the Food and Nutrition Board of the National Research Council of the National Academy of Sciences (United States) and by expert committees convened by the Food and Agriculture Organization (FAO) and the World Health Organization (WHO) of the United Nations.[61,69,70] The recommendations published by such groups are meant to be used to provide estimates of average daily energy and minimal nutrient requirements for almost all healthy individuals and for populations (Table 2). Some margin of safety is built into the calculation process to allow for the expected degree of individual biologic and environmental variability. It is recognized that there may be a range at the low end of the safe level of intake to which some degree of adaptation is possible.[71] Failure to meet estimated requirements on a given day is not an indicator of dietary inadequacy, as the estimated requirements are averages of intakes over time; for most individuals, minimal requirements (except for energy) will be less than the published estimates.

Energy

Energy needs are expressed in kilocalories (kcal) in the English measurement system and megajoules (mJ) in the metric system. One kcal is equal to 4.2 mJ. The kcal is the unit of heat required to raise 1 kg of water from 15° to 16°C. Human energy expenditure can be measured directly by measuring heat production in a total body calorimeter. It can also be estimated indirectly (indirect calorimetry) by measuring the volume of oxygen consumed, carbon dioxide produced, and urea excreted per unit time. The weight (and potential chemical energy content) of carbohydrate, fat, and protein completely oxidized to carbon dioxide and water can be calculated based on the stochiometry of the oxidation of these substrates.[72] The respiratory quotients, or ratio of the volume of CO_2 produced to volume of O_2 consumed (RQ), for carbohydrate, fat, and protein are 1, 0.7, and 0.8, respectively. In situations in which there is no net fat synthesis at the time of measurement (energy intake less than or equal to energy expenditure), the RQ is between 0.7 and 1.0. Deletion of the urea correction factor changes estimated energy expenditure by less than 1 percent under most circumstances.[72] Total daily energy expenditure includes basal (after an overnight fast) or resting metabolic expenditure, the energy required to synthesize new tissues for growth, and the energy expended in activity. Calorimetry does not measure the energy content of the new tissue synthesized. In the first months of life, energy expended on growth may be over one-third of total energy intake.

A newer method of indirect calorimetry utilizes isotope ratio mass spectroscopy to measure stable isotopes of hydrogen (^2H) and oxygen (^{18}O) in the "doubly labeled water" technique popularized for human use by Schoeller.[74] This technique takes advantage of the fact that hydrogen leaves the body only as water, but oxygen leaves as both water and CO_2. The difference between the turnover of ^{18}O and ^2H reflects CO_2 production. Serial urine samples, representative of body water, are obtained following equilibration and are assayed for ^{18}O and ^2H. The difference in disappearance rates is used to estimate oxygen consumption. An RQ of 0.85 is assumed. This technique has been used successfully in many age groups, including preterm neonates.[74] Potential advantages of this form of indirect calorimetry are that the estimate is not based on a single brief determination, energy consumption can be measured in the free-living state, and total energy expenditure is estimated, not just resting or basal metabolic energy expenditure. The energy content of new tissue synthesized during the interval is not detected with this method.

The energy value of dietary foodstuffs is determined by bomb calorimetry. The food is placed in the calorimeter and completely oxidized. The heat generated from the reaction is monitored during the process. Since the gross energy of a food measured by bomb calorimetry is not fully absorbable (e.g., dietary fiber), human in vivo experiments have been carried out to estimate the metabolizable energy (gross energy minus fecal energy loss) available from specific foods for humans. Food composition tables derived from such food analyses are readily available and contain detailed information on food energy content as well as other nutrients.[75,76]

Energy intake recommendations for infants, children, and adolescents in the United States have been derived from longitudinal intake studies of energy intake of normally growing children.[70] The recommended dietary allowance (RDA) values for energy are median values, as population-wide intakes at the upper end of the requirement spectrum would be expected to lead to obesity in most individuals. The observed tenth and ninetieth percentile energy intake data by age are also presented (Table 2). For infants, some investigators have suggested that lower intakes of energy may suffice,

TABLE 2
Suggested Intake Levels of Energy and Nutrients*

Age (yr)	0–0.5	0.5–1	1–3	4–6	7–10	Males 11–14	Males 15–18	Females 11–14	Females 15–18
Weight (kg)	6	9	13	20	28	45	66	46	55
Energy (kcal)	115/kg (95–145)	105/kg (80–135)	1,300 (900–1,800)	1,700 (1,300–2,300)	2,400 (1,650–3,300)	2,700 (2,000–3,200)	2,800 (2,100–3,900)	2,200 (1,500–3,000)	2,100 (1,200–3,000)
Protein (g)	13	14	16	24	28	45	59	46	44
Vitamin A (μg [RE])	375	375	400	500	700	1,000	1,000	800	800
Vitamin D (μg)	7.5	10	10	10	10	10	10	10	10
Vitamin E (mg [TE])	3	4	6	7	7	10	10	8	8
Vitamin K (μg)	5	10	15	20	30	45	65	45	55
Vitamin C (mg)	30	35	40	45	45	50	60	50	60
Thiamin (mg)	0.3	0.4	0.7	0.9	1.0	1.3	1.5	1.1	1.1
Riboflavin (mg)	0.4	0.5	0.8	1.1	1.2	1.5	1.8	1.3	1.3
Niacin (mg)	5	6	9	12	13	17	20	15	15
Pyridoxine (mg)	0.3	0.6	1.0	1.1	1.4	1.7	2.0	1.4	1.5
Folate (μg)	25	35	50	75	100	150	200	150	180
Vitamin B_{12} (μg)	0.3	0.5	0.7	1.0	1.4	2	2	2	2
Biotin (μg)	35	50	65	85	120	100–200	100–200	100–200	100–200
Pantothenic acid (μg)	2	3	3	3–4	4–5	4–7	4–7	4–7	4–7
Calcium (mg)	400	600	800	800	800	1,200	1,200	1,200	1,200
Phosphorus (mg)	300	500	800	800	800	1,200	1,200	1,200	1,200
Magnesium (mg)	40	60	80	120	170	270	400	280	300

Table continues on following page

at least in breast-fed infants.[77,78] The World Health Organization/Food and Agriculture Organization/United Nations University (WHO/FAO/UNU) committee has used the same methodology for children up to 10 years of age.[61] However, 5 percent has been added to the observed energy expenditure values, as, in the opinion of the committee, the energy expenditure of children in developed countries on whom the intake observations were made is suboptimal. For children between 10 and 17 years of age, the WHO/FAO/UNU committee has used the "factorial" method to calculate energy requirements. The WHO/FAO/UNU equations to estimate the basal metabolic rate (BMR) are 17.5 × weight (in kg) + 651 for males and 12.2 × weight + 746 for females aged 10 to 18 years.[61] (The term *resting metabolic expenditure* [RME] is sometimes used interchangeably with BMR. It is determined under less idealized conditions and may run up to 10 percent higher than the BMR.) The BMR may be substantially increased in malnourished individuals owing to a higher percentage of metabolically active lean tissue per unit of body weight. However, rates may also be decreased (by 15 to 30 percent) after prolonged energy deprivation. The estimated energy cost of growth is 5 kcal per gram of weight gain.[61]

Energy estimates for activity (based on observed activity patterns and measurement of the cost of a variety of physical activities) are then added to the estimates for basal and growth needs. The total energy requirement for boys is 1.6 to 1.75 × BMR and for girls is 1.5 to 1.65 × BMR.[61] Estimates of energy expenditure for BMR and growth versus total daily energy expenditure can be found in Figure 1. Much of the variability for energy expenditure among children is due to their remarkably different individual energy expenditures on physical activity.

TABLE 2 (Continued)

Age (yr)	0–0.5	0.5–1	1–3	4–6	7–10	Males 11–14	Males 15–18	Females 11–14	Females 15–18
Weight (kg)	6	9	13	20	28	45	66	46	55
Iron (mg)	6	10	10	10	10	12	12	15	15
Zinc (mg)	5	5	10	10	10	15	15	12	12
Iodine (μg)	40	50	70	90	120	150	150	150	150
Copper (mg)	0.5–0.7	0.7–1.0	1.0–1.5	1.5–2.0	2.0–2.5	2.0–3.0	2.0–3.0	2.0–3.0	2.0–3.0
Manganese (mg)	0.1–0.5	0.2–1.0	0.5–1.5	1.0–2.5	1.5–2.5	1.5–2.5	1.5–4.0	1.5–2.5	1.5–4.0
Fluoride (mg)	0.1–0.5	0.2–1.0	0.5–1.5	1.0–2.5	1.5–2.5	1.5–2.5	1.5–4.0	1.5–2.5	1.5–4.0
Chromium (mg)	0.01–0.04	0.02–0.06	0.02–0.08	0.03–0.12	0.05–0.20	0.05–0.20	0.05–0.20	0.05–0.20	0.05–0.20
Selenium (μg)	10	15	20	20	30	40	50	45	50
Molybdenum (mg)	0.03–0.06	0.04–0.08	0.05–0.10	0.06–0.15	0.10–0.30	0.15–0.50	0.15–0.50	0.15–0.50	0.15–0.50

*Conversion features:
1 μg retinol = retinol equivalent (RE) = 3.3 IU vitamin A.
1 μg beta-carotene = 0.5 RE.
10 μg cholecalciferol = 400 IU vitamin D.
1 mg d-alpha-tocopherol = 1 tocopherol equivalent (TE).
Based on 1980 RDA[70] and references 102 to 107.

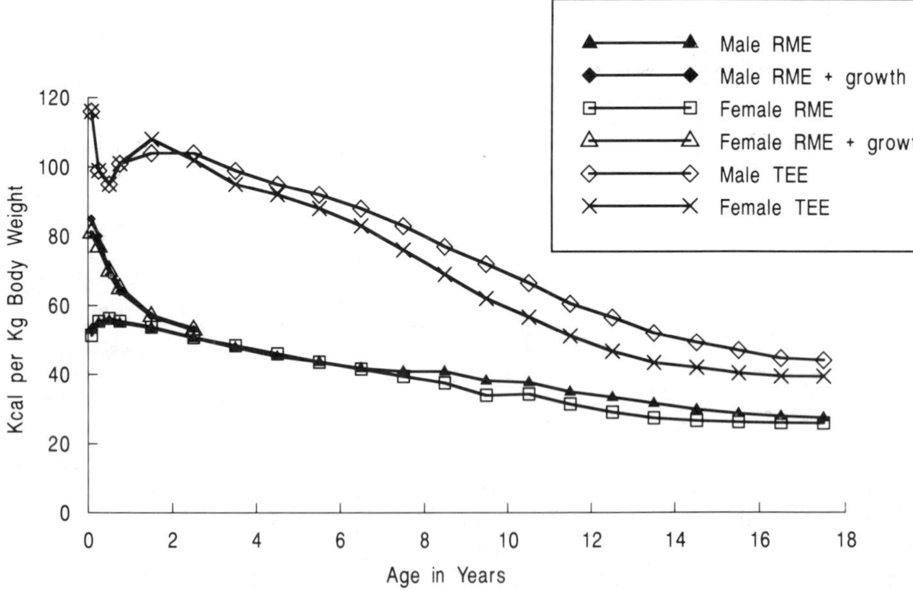

FIGURE 1 Energy requirements and expenditure by age (birth through 18 years). The figure depicts the basal metabolic rate (BMR) of males and females, the energy cost of growth to age 3 years (when energy expenditure on growth falls below 2 kcal per kilogram per day), and total energy requirement. Estimated fiftieth percentile body weights for age are from Hamill,[7] growth rates from Hamill[7] and Baumgartner et al,[20] BMR from the data of Talbot (1933), and calculations for the energy cost of growth and activity from Annex 7 of the WHO report.[61] It can be seen that during the first year of life energy requirements have a biphasic pattern, and there is a subsequent gradual decrease toward adult levels, despite the adolescent growth spurt. As noted in the text, recent studies suggest that total energy requirements for breast-fed infants may be less than depicted in the figure. RME = resting metabolic expenditure; TEE = total energy expenditure.

In children with GI illness, energy expenditure and requirements may be unchanged, decreased, or increased. Total energy requirements may be increased by malabsorption and situations that increase BMR. Most GI conditions do not increase BMR. In many conditions, the child's loss of well-being is sufficient to limit spontaneous activity and thus decrease daily energy expenditure. Chronic semistarvation decreases metabolic rate and also decreases activity. As a result, the metabolizable (absorbed and retained) energy requirement for maintenance in the sick child with GI disease is rarely greater than the mean recommended daily allowance. Febrile infectious complications, severe inflammation, as in necrotizing enterocolitis,[79] or anemia[80] may increase resting metabolic rate. In cystic fibrosis energy expenditure can also be increased by advanced pulmonary disease[81] and sympathomimetic medications used to treat bronchospasm.[82]

During nutritional repletion, high levels of energy intake may be needed in order to achieve transient "catch-up" growth. Rates exceeding 20 times the normal rate of growth for age can be observed during this rehabilitative process.[83] The optimal rate of growth during catch-up is not well defined, but over time the pattern tends to follow an exponentially decreasing rate.[84] When catch-up growth is stimulated, it is important to provide sufficient protein and noncaloric nutrients to assure adequate amino acids and micronutrients to optimize growth rates.[85] Nutrient deficiencies can limit growth or become symptomatic during nutritional rehabilitation.[86-88] Specific dynamic action or dietary-induced thermogenesis is also enhanced during high energy intakes. This postprandial increase in the metabolic rate is largely secondary to the metabolic cost of new tissue synthesis and is part of the 5 calories per gram required for new tissue synthesis. Calculation of 24-hour energy requirement for hospitalized pediatric patients needs to include resting energy expenditure, a factor for activity (usually 0.2 to 0.5 × BMR), plus energy for catch-up growth (5 calories per gram), when indicated. A further increase for fecal losses is needed when substantial malabsorption is present.

Protein

The observational approach has been used to develop estimates for protein requirements in the first 4 months of life by the most recent WHO/FAO/UNU committee, similar to the method used to estimate energy requirement for breast-fed infants. This may result in some overestimate of individual requirements.[89] For bottle-fed infants and for other age groups, nitrogen balance based on measured intakes, urinary and fecal nitrogen, and estimates for insensible nitrogen losses is used to estimate the protein allowance. This technique requires feeding various levels of protein to healthy infants or children on adequate energy intakes bracketing the suspected mean protein requirement level. The slope ratio technique permits identification of the mean level of protein intake for nitrogen maintenance and an estimate for the increment above maintenance intake which will result in sufficiently positive nitrogen balance to allow normal rates of nitrogen accretion (as determined from nitrogen accretion in carcass analysis studies). The mean intake values that achieve these goals are increased by two standard deviations to arrive at an estimate of safe protein intakes for almost all healthy children.

Correction for protein digestibility and quality is made for the diet of children less than 12 years of age when proteins other than milk, egg, meat, and fish are consumed. After 12 years of age only digestibility appears to materially affect protein utilization with standard mixed diets of many types. Digestibility and amino acid pattern are compared with a reference protein such as milk, egg, or protein of similar high quality. Digestibility is determined from in vivo human bioassay and chemical score by comparison of the milligrams of each essential amino acid per gram of protein relative to the comparable value for the reference protein. The essential amino acid present in lowest relative concentration is the limiting amino acid, and the chemical score (between 0 and 100) is the ratio of the limiting amino acid in the test protein to the reference[61]:

$$\text{Chemical score} = \frac{\text{mg amino acid in test protein}}{\text{mg amino acid in ref protein}} \times 100$$

For example, soya flour has a digestibility of 90 and a chemical score (methionine) of 74. The nutritional value (including digestibility and amino acid score) is 67 percent of that of milk, eggs, meat, or fish. The estimated protein requirement of a child receiving unsupplemented soya flour as his only source of dietary protein would be increased by 100/67 × the safe allowance level for his age.

In infants and children with GI disease, protein requirements may be increased by malabsorption (particularly pancreatic insufficiency), protein-losing enteropathy (common in mucosal diseases), and catabolic events such as infections.[90,91] The usual North American diet, providing 12 to 15 protein calories, is probably adequate for most of these situations. However, when using special formulas or total parenteral nutrition, provision of closer to 16 percent protein calories rather than the minimal level of 6 to 8 percent will provide protein sufficient to minimize negative nitrogen balance and enhance synthesis of visceral proteins to the extent possible. There is rarely indication to provide more than 4 gm of protein per kilogram per day. In the absence of renal disease or dehydration, a substantial rise in the serum urea nitrogen indicates that much of the dietary protein is entering catabolic pathways. When hypoproteinemia and edema are present in the face of adequate protein intake, salt restriction may be clinically more effective in controlling edema than a marked increase in protein intake.

Noncaloric Nutrients

The other nutrients essential in the human diet are required not as substrates for energy production or as precursors for protein synthesis, but for structural elements of cells and tissues, hormones, antioxidants, and enzyme components, cofactors, and regulators. These nutrients are organic lipid and water-soluble vitamins, electrolytes, minerals, and trace elements. Late nineteenth century and early twentieth century nutrition research identified and purified most of the known essential nutrients. This scientific progress led to the elimi-

TABLE 3
Vitamins: Absorption, Metabolism, Function, Assessment, Deficiency, and Toxicity

Vitamins[*]	Absorption[†]	Enhancement/ Inhibition[‡]	Metabolism[§]	Function	Assessment	Consequence of Deficiency	Toxicity
Vitamin A Retinol Beta-carotene—dietary precursor 1 IU vitamin A = 0.3 μg retinol RE = 1 μg retinol 1 mg beta-carotene = 0.5 mg retinol	(S)Proximal gut (M)Passive diffusion (E)Vitamin A 80% Beta-carotene 50%	Fat (+) Protein (+) Mineral oil—retinol (+) —carotene (−)	(S)90% stored in liver (1 to cells) (A)Circulates with PA and RBP (C)Excreted after hepatic glucuronidation in bile and in urine	Carbohydrate transfer to glycoprotein Retinal in rhodopsin and iodopsin Needed for cell proliferation Maintains epithelial integrity	Serum level-HPLC Absorption test Dark adaptation Liver biopsy concentration	Nyctalopia Xerophthalmia Bitot spots Phrynoderma ? Bronchopulmonary dysplasia after respiratory distress syndrome	Hepatomegaly/hepatic fibrosis Pseudotumor cerebri Teratogenesis Hypercalcemia Hyperlipidemia
Vitamin D Ergocalciferol (D_2) synthetic Cholecalciferol D_3 (endogenously synthesized) 40 IU = 1 μg	(S)Skin ultraviolet irradiation of 7-dehydrocholesterol (M)Dietary absorption Bile acid–dependent To lymphatics in chylomicrons	Fat (+) Bile acids (+)	(S)Stored in adipose tissue and concentrated in liver (A)25-hydroxylation in liver (A)1-hydroxylation in kidney (C)Biliary excretion	Regulates Ca/P absorption, bone resorption, and renal Ca, P excretion	Serum level of alk phos/Ca/P Radiographs Bone densitometry	Rickets/osteomalacia Dental caries Decreased serum Ca/P Increased alkaline phosphatase Increased urine phosphate/amino acid	Headache—increased ICP Bone pain/cortical hyperostosis Hypertension Hypercalciuria/ectopic calcification
Vitamin E Alpha-tocopherol 1 IU = 1 mg racemic alpha-tocopherol	(M)Bile acid–dependent (M)Transported by lymphatics (E)50% absorption	Fat (+) Bile acids (+)	(S)Liver is immediate reserve (S) Adipose tissue (C)Biliary excretion	Membrane antioxidant Inhibits peroxidation of unsaturated fatty acids Protects vitamin A during absorption	Plasma level-HPLC H_2O_2 hemolysis Tissue biopsy Breath pentane Blood malondialdehyde	Neurologic changes: decreased DTRs, wide-based gait, ocular palsy, spinocerebellar degeneration Anemia/hemolysis Altered prostaglandin synthesis	Prolonged PT/vitamin K antagonism In neonates, possible increased intraventricular hemorrhage, NEC, sepsis, hepatic toxicity with large IV doses
Vitamin K Phylloquinone Menadione (synthetic) μg	(S)Jejunum/ileum (M)Bile- and fat-dependent (E)Up to 80% absorption	Fat (+) Vitamin E (−)? Antibiotics (−)	(S)Liver/skin/muscle (A)Reduced to hydroquinone (A)Salvage via vitamin K cycle (C)Salvage via vitamin K cycle	Carboxylation of coagulation factors Affects bone formation	Prothrombin time Clotting factor levels	Coagulopathy/hemorrhagic disease of newborn Prolonged PT Abnormal synthesis of bone matrix	Shock, anaphylaxis with IV Hemolysis Water-soluble analogues associated with hyperbilirubinemia
Thiamine Vitamin B_1 mg	(S)Small intestine (M)Passive at high concentration (M)Active at low concentration	Carbohydrate (+) Alcohol (−) Thiaminase in fish (−)	(S)50% in skeletal muscle (A)Phosphorylated to co-enzyme (C)Urinary excretion	Oxidative phosphorylation Pentose phosphate shunt Aldehyde transferase Triosephosphate isomerase	Whole blood level Urine thiochrome RBC transketolase activity Microbiologic assay	Beriberi Cardiac failure/neuropathy Korsakoff's syndrome/Wernicke's encephalopathy Disrupted ATP synthesis Altered pentose phosphate shunt	Anaphylaxis from chronic parenteral administration Nausea/anorexia/lethargy—parenteral

TABLE 3 *(Continued)*

Vitamins*	Absorption†	Enhancement/ Inhibition‡	Metabolism§	Function	Assessment	Consequence of Deficiency	Toxicity
Riboflavin Vitamin B_2 mg	(S)Proximal gut (M)Active/saturable	Food (+) Bile (+) Metals as chelators (−) Galactoflavin (−)	(S)Little stored (A)Sequential phosphorylation by flavokinase and FAD synthetase	Oxidation/reduction reactions	Urinary excretion Erythrocyte concentration Erythrocyte glutathione reductase	Seborrheic dermatitis/cheilosis/glossitis Decreased fatty acid oxidation Altered vitamin B_6 activation to co-enzyme Decreased tryptophan to niacin conversion Personality changes Pure red cell cytoplasia of bone marrow	
Pyridoxine Vitamin B_6 Pyridoxal (PLP) Pyridoxamine mg	(M)Hydrolized by alkaline phosphatase (M)Nonsaturable uptake (M)Rephosphorylated by pyridoxal kinase		(S)Up to 90% in liver (C)Urine	Methyl donor system Sulfur amino acid conversion	Serum—RIA or microbiologic assay Schilling test dU suppression test	Dermatitis/glossitis/cheilosis Decreased serum transaminases Peripheral neuritis Irritability/convulsions Anemia	Convulsions Peripheral
Cyanocobalamin Vitamin B_{12} μg	(S)Terminal ileum (M)Diffusion/intrinsic factor mediated (M)Intake-dependent	Gastric acid (+) Trypsin (+)/bile (+) Reducing agents (−) Heavy metals (−)	(S)Concentrated in retina, adrenal, and pituitary glands (C)Excreted in urine as metabolites	Co-factor for hydroxylators Reducing agent Noradrenaline/carnitine synthesis Cholesterol catabolism	Serum HPLC Leukocyte conc Whole blood conc Urine conc	Macrocytic anemia/hypersegmented neutrophils Demyelination/posterior column signs CNS changes Acidosis/methylmalonic aciduria Lowers folate level	
Ascorbic acid Vitamin C mg	(M)Active/Na-dependent carrier-mediated (E)Up to 98%		(C)Salvage by biotinidase for neutralization (C)Urinary excretion	Coenzyme for carboxylases, decarboxylases, transcarboxylases	Serum—microbiologic assay Plasma lactate Urine organic acids Lymphocyte carboxylase	Scurvy Poor wound healing Hysteria, hypercheritosis, hemorrhagic signs, hematologic abnormalities Impaired hydroxylation and collagen synthesis	Altered glucose and creatinine assay
Biotin μg	(S)Proximal gut (M)Active transport (E)Biocytin readily absorbed	Avidin (−)	(S)Liver as polyglutamates (A)Active as tetrahydrofolate (C)Urine = bile excretion	Methyl donor RNA/DNA synthesis Amino acid conversion	RBC/serum level Microbiologic assay better than RIA	Multiple carboxylase deficiency Acidosis Dermatitis/alopecia Neurologic dysfunction, seizures, ataxia, depression	

TABLE 3 (*Continued*)

Vitamins*	Absorption†	Enhancement/ Inhibition‡	Metabolism§	Function	Assessment	Consequence of Deficiency	Toxicity
Folic acid Folate Folinic acid μg	(S)Proximal gut (M)Active greater than passive (E)Up to 90%	Glucose (+) Galactose (+) Zinc (−) Acidity (−) Alcohol (−)	(A)Phosphorylated to NAD and NADP (C)Oxidized to carboxamide and excreted in urine	Dehydrogenase activity as hydride acceptor Specific enzymes	Urine ratio of catabolites	Macroytic anemia/leukopenia Altered protein metabolism Impaired growth Diarrhea	Masks vitamin B_{12} deficiency Interferes with phenytoin anticonvulsant activity Reduces zinc absorption
Niacin Nicotinic acid Nicotinamide 1 mg = 1 niacin equivalent (NE)	(S)Proximal gut (M)Intestinal hydrolysis of pyridine nucleotides (M)Acid/amide by diffusion	Alkali with corn (+)	(A)Phosphorylated and conjugated with cysteine acetyl CoA to form coenzyme A (S)Hydroxylated and excreted in urine	Acetylation of alcohol or amines Carrier of acyl groups Pyruvate dehydrogenase complex	Urinary excretion Whole blood—RIA or microbiologic assay	Pellagra: dermatitis, diarrhea, dementia Glossitis/stomatitis/vaginitis Impaired absorption of vitamin B_{12}, fat, carbohydrate Histamine-fast achlorhydria	Flushing Burning, stinging hands Hepatotoxicity Peptic ulcer activation
Pantothenic acid mg	(M)As pantotheine after hydrolysis of CoA					Reduced ability to acetylate Anorexia and vomiting Postural hypotension Irascible personality Neuromuscular manifestations/increased DTRs	Calcium salt leads to diarrhea

*Entries under each vitamin are alternate names and units, respectively.
†(S) = site; (M) = method; (E) = efficiency.
‡(+) = enhancer; (−) = inhibitor.
§(S) = storage; (A) = activation; (C) = catabolism.
AA = amino acids; DTR = deep tendon reflexes; FAD = flavin adenine dinucleotide; HPLC = high-pressure liquid chromatography; ICP = increased intracranial pressure; NAD = nicotine adenine dinucleotide; NADP = nicotine adenine dinucleotide phosphate; PA = prealbumin; PLP = pyridoxal phosphate; PT = prothrombin time; PTH = parathyroid hormone; RBP = retinal-binding protein; RDW = red cell distribution width; RIA = radioimmunoassay; TSH = thyroid-stimulating hormone.

TABLE 4
Minerals and Trace Elements

Mineral/ Trace Element	Absorption*	Enhancement/ Inhibition†	Metabolism‡	Function	Assessment	Consequences of Deficiency	Toxicity
Calcium	(S)Total bowel/colon (M)Passive/active vitamin D–dependent (E)40–60%	Glucose/lactose (+) Alkaline pH (−) Phytates/fiber (−) Phosphate/oxalate (−)	Bone storage Urine excretion	Bone structure Cell metabolic regulator Nerve excitation threshold	Serum concentration Radiographs CT and photon densitometry	Increased serum 1,25-OH vitamin D Bone demineralization Tetany/seizures Cardiac arrhythmia	Nausea, vomiting Hypertension Polyuria Nephrocalcinosis (milk-alkali syndrome)
Chromium mg	(S)Jejunum (M)Facilitated diffusion (E)1%	Oxalates (+) Acidity (−) Mn/Fe (−) Phytates (−)	Urine excretion	Glucose tolerance factor Metabolism of nucleic acids May relate to iodine and thyroid function	Response to supplement	Glucose intolerance Neuropathy/encephalopathy Altered nitrogen metabolism Increased fatty acid level	No oral toxicity reported Inhalation related to bronchogenic cancer
Copper mg	(S)Proximal gut (M)Carrier-mediated (E)40%	High-dose zinc (−) Vitamin C (−) Heavy metals (−)	50% in bone/muscle Biliary excretion	Co-factor for superoxide dismutase, tyrosinase, cytochrome C oxidase Affects iron metabolism	Serum concentration Ceruloplasmin concentration Liver biopsy concentration Superoxide dismutase activity	Hypochromic anemia, neutropenia Hyperlipidemia/ hypercholesterolemia Skin depigmentation CNS dysfunction	Vomiting/diarrhea Hepatic necrosis Hemolysis Renal failure Coma/death
Fluoride	(E)50–80%	Milk products (−) Aluminum antacids (−)	Teeth/bone Urine	Cariostatic property Strengthens bone Decreases arterial calcification		Altered crystalline structure Increased dental caries Osteoporosis	Mottled enamel
Iron	(S)Proximal (M)Gut-regulated by stores transferrin-mediated (E)Up to 20%	Acidity (+) Protein (+) Ascorbic acid (+) Wheat bran (−) Tea/coffee (−)	Liver/bone marrow stores Bound to ferritin Some GI loss	Heme—synthesis Component of cytochromes	Hemoglobin/hematocrit RBC, indices, RDW Bone marrow aspirate for stainable iron	Hypochromic microcytic anemia Decreased heme synthesis Altered oxidative phosphorylation Decreased exercise tolerance Pica Inability to concentrate	Coagulopathy GI bleeding Shock Chronic use—arrhythmias
Iodine	(S)Gastric reduction to iodide (S)Proximal gut absorption (M)Absorbed as iodide or as iodo-amino acid complex (E)Highly efficient		Thyroid Oxidized by peroxidase Joined to tyrosine to form thyroid hormones Urine excretion	Incorporated into thyroxine	T_4/T_3/TSH Urinary iodide:creatinine ratio	Goiter Cretinism Increased TSH	Wolff-Chaikoff effect Thyrotoxicosis in chronically deficient

TABLE 4 *(Continued)*

Mineral/ Trace Element	Absorption*	Enhancement/ Inhibition†	Metabolism‡	Function	Assessment	Consequences of Deficiency	Toxicity
Magnesium	(S)Small bowel/small amount colon (M)Passive and facilitated diffusion (E)Up to 75%	Lactose (+) Fiber (−)	60% in bone 33% bound to plasma protein	Co-factor for hexokinase and phosphokinase Alters ribosomal aggregation in protein synthesis Increases nerve excitation threshhold	Plasma/serum concentration Loading test	Cardiac arrhythmia Neuromuscular hyperirritability Decreased PTH Hypocalcemia/hypokalemia Convulsions	Laxative effect Heart block Flaccid quadriplegia Respiratory paralysis Hypotension
Manganese	(S)Small bowel (E)Up to 10%	Enterohepatic circulation(+)	Biliary excretion	Mucopolysaccharide synthesis Pyruvate carboxylase co-factor Mitochondrial superoxide dismutase Cholesterol synthesis Cartilage/bone formation	Whole blood level	Decreased hair and nail growth Hair color ? Depressed clotting factors Dermatitis Weight loss	Inhalation secondary occupational exposure schizophrenic-like psychosis Parkinson's-like disease
Molybdenum	(S)Small intestine (E)Up to 80%	Excess Cu (−)	Incorporated into pterin structure Urinary excretion	Uric acid production Aldehyde oxidase Sulfite oxidase	No measure	Decreased xanthine oxidase activity Intolerance to sulfur-containing AA Growth retardation Tachypnea/tachycardia	Goutlike syndrome Antagonist of copper Hyperuricemia
Phosphorus	(S)Mid-small bowel (M)Na-dependent pump and diffusion (E)80% absorption	Vitamin D (+) Ca (−) Al (−)	85% in bone Urinary excretion—PTH regulation	Bone structure Glycogen deposition High-energy Acid-base balance Oxygen release—DPG	Serum concentration, P concentration, alkaline phosphatase Radiographs Densitometry (CT or photon)	Rickets Tissue hypoxia Hemolytic anemia Respiratory failure CNS abnormalities	Hypocalcemia Metastatic calcification Seizures
Selenium	(E)80%	Protein (+) Vitamins A, E, C (+)	Highest concentration in liver/kidney Urinary excretion	Glutathione peroxidase	Plasma concentration Glutathione peroxidase activity	Myositis with elevated CPK Cardiomyopathy Nail bed changes Increased susceptibility to vitamin E deficit Macrocytic anemia	Alopecia Garlic odor to breath Brittle nails Discolored teeth
Zinc	(M)Carrier-mediated, not energy-dependent (E)Up to 70%	Picolinic acid (+) Citrate (+) Phytate (−) Cu, Fe (−)	Stored as metallothionine Concentrated in retina/hair/bone/liver Excreted in stool via pancreatic secretion and in urine	Co-factor for more than 70 enzymes Cell replication Immune function Vision	Plasma concentration Serum alkaline phosphatase Urinary excretion Leukocyte concentration	Rash/skin lesions/poor wound healing Immune dysfunction, especially T cell Anorexia/dysgeusia Growth failure/negative nitrogen balance Hypogonadism/delayed puberty	Nausea/dyspepsia/vomiting Hypercholesterolemia Pancreatitis (with IV Zn) Anemia of copper deficiency

*(S) = site; (M) = mechanism; (E) = efficiency.
†(+) = enhancer; (−) = inhibitor.
‡Entries for each mineral describe activation and catabolism, respectively.

TABLE 5
Food Sources Rich in Vitamins and Minerals

I. Vitamins—Fat-Soluble
Vitamin A: fortified milk, egg, liver
Beta-carotene: dark green and yellow vegetables and fruits
Vitamin D: fortified milk, fish, egg yolk, sunlight
Vitamin E: cereal seed oil, nuts, soybeans, green leafy vegetables
Vitamin K: cow's milk, green leafy vegetables, pork, liver

II. Vitamins—Water-Soluble
Thiamin: meat, milk, whole grains, legumes
Riboflavin: meat, milk, egg, green vegetables, whole grains
Niacin: meat, fish, green vegetables, whole grains
Pyridoxine: meat, whole grains, soy beans
Vitamin B_{12}: meat, milk, egg
Ascorbic acid: citrus, tomato, cabbage, potato
Folate: green, leafy vegetables, cereals, oranges, liver
Biotin: liver, egg yolk, peanuts
Pantothenic acid: most foods

III. Minerals
Calcium: milk, cheese, greens, sardines
Phosphorus: meat, poultry, milk, egg, cheese
Magnesium: nuts, seafood, bran, green vegetables
Iron: liver, meat, seafood, grains

IV. Trace Metals
Zinc: seafood, liver, meat
Iodine: seafood, iodized salt
Copper: seafood, meat, legumes, chocolate
Manganese: nuts, whole grains
Fluoride: drinking water, tea
Chromium: meat, cheese, whole grains, yeast
Selenium: seafood, meat, whole grains
Molybdenum: meat, grains, legumes

nation of endemic nutritional deficiency diseases in industrialized nations but has not yet been adequately applied to other parts of the world. Previously common nutritional deficiency diseases now rarely seen in industrialized nations include beriberi, pellagra, scurvy, rickets, and cretinism. The prevalence of iron deficiency anemia[92] and dental caries[93] has also been reduced. The importance of trace elements in human nutrition has been appreciated only in the latter half of the twentieth century with the recognition of zinc, copper, selenium, and chromium deficiencies under special dietary and clinical conditions. The possible importance of specific nutrients in degenerative diseases including cancer, heart disease, and neurologic disorders is currently under scientific exploration.

The absorption, metabolism, and effects of dietary deficiency and excess of vitamins, minerals, and trace elements are presented in Tables 3 and 4. Most of these nutrients are found in a wide variety of food sources. Information on foods rich in specific nutrients can be found in Table 5. A listing of GI conditions that may be associated with specific nutrient deficiencies is compiled in Table 6. For detailed dietary counseling, most physicians find it advisable to have patients consult with a well-trained registered dietitian for implementation of dietary advice or a dietary prescription.

Recent work on nutritional requirements has focused on whether additional metabolic substrates may be essential for humans, especially under specific conditions such as disease states or intravenous feeding. Among the nutrients evaluated are carnitine, choline, and inositol. Each of these substances has important biologic functions and is required for normal metabolism. Diets based on a variety of foods provide generous quantities of these nutrients or their precursors. However, carnitine is present in limited quantity in vegan (and some hospital[94]) diets. Total parenteral nutrition does not provide carnitine or inositol. Lecithin, a precursor for choline, is present in intravenous lipid emulsions.

Signs of possible deficiency of these nutrients in humans have been described in specific clinical conditions. Findings in carnitine deficiency can include myopathy, cardiomyopathy, hepatomegaly, and hypoglycemia. Such findings have been reported in patients with inborn errors of metabolism, largely related to excessive renal losses of carnitine or defects in carnitine transport.[95] Cirrhotics[96] and premature newborn infants[97] have been found to have low plasma concentrations of carnitine. The peripheral neuropathy observed in diabetic patients has been claimed to improve with the administration of inositol.[98] The structural similarity of inositol to glucose and its impaired cellular uptake with hyperglycemia

TABLE 6
Potential Nutrient Deficiencies to Suspect in Gastrointestinal-Liver Diseases

			Vitamins					
	Energy	**Protein**	Fat-Soluble	Water-Soluble	**Electrolytes**	**Minerals**	**Trace Elements**	**Other**
Esophagitis							Fe	
Pyloric stenosis					+			
Peptic ulcer	+				+		Fe	
Cystic fibrosis	+	+	+	B_{12}	+	Mg	Fe, Zn, Se	EFA*, taurine
Cholestasis	+		+	B_{12}		Ca		
Cirrhosis		+					Fe, Zn	Carnitine*
								Cysteine*
Intractable diarrhea	+		+					Tyrosine
Celiac disease	+	+	+	B_{12}, folate				Branched-chain amino acid
Crohn's disease	+		+	B_{12}, folate	+	Mg	Fe, Zn, Cu, Se	Carnitine
								? Glutamine
Lactase deficiency		D			+	Mg	Fe, Zn	
Ulcerative colitis	+			Folate		Mg	Fe, Zn	
AIDS	+			B_{12}, B_6		Ca		
Prolonged total					+		Fe, Zn	
parenteral nutrition					+		Fe, Zn, Cu, Se	
						Ca, P	Fe, Zn, Cu, Se,	Taurine
							Cr, Mo	Carnitine
								? Glutamine
								EFA
								? Choline

*May become essential amino acids—see text.

is a postulated mechanism for this possible conditioned deficiency.

SUMMARY

Information on energy, protein, and micronutrient requirements of children and how they are determined has been presented. This information is important for understanding to what extent a given child is meeting nutritional requirements, recognizing deficiencies, and determining how requirements need to be modified in specific diseases. More detailed information on specific nutrients and pediatric nutritional requirements can be found in recent nutrition texts.[99–102]

REFERENCES

1. Bistrian BR, Blackburn GL, Halowell E, Heddle R. Protein status of general surgical patients. JAMA 1974; 230;858–860.
2. Bistrian BR, Blackburn GL, Vitale J, Cochran D, Naylor J. Prevalence of malnutrition in general medical patients. JAMA 1976; 235:1567–1570.
3. Weinsier RL, Hunker EM, Krumdieck C, Butterworth CE Jr. Hospital malnutrition—a prospective evaluation of general medical patients during the course of hospitalization. Am J Clin Nutr 1989; 32:418–426.
4. Kelts DB, Grand RJ, Shen GS, Watkins JB, Werlin SL, Boehme C. Nutritional basis of growth failure in children and adolescents with Crohn's disease. Gastroenterology 1979; 76:720–727.
5. Layden T, Rosenberg I, Nemchausky B, Elson C, Rosenberg I. Reversal of growth arrest in adolescents with Crohn's disease after parenteral alimentation. Gastroenterology 1976; 70:1017.
6. Levy L, Durie PR, Pencharz PB, Corey ML. Effects of long term nutritional rehabilitation on body composition in malnourished children and adolescents with cystic fibrosis. J Pediatr 1985; 107:225–230.
7. Hamill PV. National Center for Health Statistics: Growth charts for children birth–18 years, United States. Vital and Health Statistics, Series 11, No 165 DHEW Pub No (PHS) 78-1650; Nov, 1977.
8. Duncan B, Schaefer C, Sibley B, Fonseca NM. Reduced growth velocity in exclusively breast-fed infants. Am J Dis Child 1984; 138:309–313.
9. Breast-fed infants grow more slowly than infants fed formula and solids. Nutr Rev 1986; 44:168–169.
10. Gortmacher SL, Dietz WH, Sobel AM, Wehler CA. Increasing pediatric obesity in the United States. Am J Dis Child 1987; 141:535–540.
11. Ginsberg-Fellner F, Jagendorf LA, Carmel H, Harris T. Overweight and obesity in New York City. Am J Clin Nutr 1981; 34:2236–2241.
12. Garn SM, Clark DC. Nutrition growth, development and materation: findings from the ten-state nutrition survey of 1968–1970. Pediatrics 1975; 56:306–319.
13. Olness K, Yip R, Indritz A, Torjesen E. Height and weight status of Indo Chinese refugee children. Am J Dis Child 1984; 138:544–547.
14. Waterlow JC. Classification and definition of protein-calorie malnutrition. Br Med J 1972; 3:566–569.
15. Waterlow JC. Note on the assessment and classification of protein-energy malnutrition in children. Lancet 1973; ii:87–89.
16. Baldwin BT. Weight-height-age standards in metric units for American-born children. Am J Phys Anthropol 1925; 8:1–10.
17. Chen LC, Chowdhury AKM, Huffman SC. Anthropometric assessment of energy-protein malnutrition and subsequent risk of mortality among school-aged children. Am J Clin Nutr 1980; 33:1836–1845.
18. Graitcer PL, Gentry EM, Nichaman MZ, Lane JM. Routine anthropometric indicators of nutrition status and morbidity. J Trop Pediatr 1981; 27:292–298.
19. Roche AF, Himes JH. Incremental growth charts. Am J Clin Nutr 1980; 33:2041–2052.
20. Baumgartner RN, Roche AF, Himes JH. Incremental growth tables: supplementary to previously published charts. Am J Clin Nutr 1985; 107:317–329.
21. Tanner JM. Clinical longitudinal standard for height and height velocity for North American children. 1985; 1071:317–329.
22. Marshall WA. Evaluation of growth rate in height over periods of less than one year, Arch Dis Child 1971; 46:414–420.
23. Frisancho AR. New norms of upper limb fat and muscle areas for assessment of nutritional status. Am J Clin Nutr 1981; 34:2540–2545.
24. Durnin JVGA, Rahaman MM. The assessment of the amount of fat in the human body from measurements of skinfold thickness. Br J Nutr 1967; 21:681–689.
25. Khaled MA, McCutheon MJ, Reddy R, Pearman PL, Hunter GR, Weinsier RL. Electric impedance in assessing human body composition: the BIA method. Am J Clin Nutr 1988; 47:789–792.

26. Merritt RJ. Enteral feeding: who needs support? In: Ballistreri WF, Farrell HK, eds. Enterel feeding: scientific basis and clinical applications. Columbus: Ross Laboratories, 1988: 47.
27. Harvey KB, Moldawer LL, Bistrian BR, Blackburn GL. Biological measures for the formulation of a hospital prognostic index. Am J Clin Nutr 1981; 34:2013.
28. Maskowitz SR, Pereira G, Spitzer A, Heaf L, Amsel J, Watkins JB. Prealbumin as a biochemical marker of nutritional adequacy in premature infants. J Pediatr 1985; 102:749–753.
29. Sandstedt S, Cedarblad G, Larsson J, et al. Influence of total parenteral nutrition on plasma fibronectin in malnourished subjects with or without inflammatory response. JPEN 1984; 8:493.
30. Merritt RJ, Blackburn GL, Bistrian BR, Palombo J, Suskinor M. Consequences of modified fasting in obese pediatric and adolescent patients: effect of a carbohydrate-free diet on serum proteins. Am J Clin Nutr 1981; 34:2752–2755.
31. Cohn H, Fessel M. Spontaneous bacterial peritonitis in cirrhosis: variations on a theme. Medicine 1971; 60:161–197.
32. Neumann CG, Lawlor GJ, Steihm R, et al. Immunologic response in malnourished children. Am J Clin Nutr 1975; 28:89–104.
33. Beisel WR. Single nutrients and immunity. Am J Clin Nutr 1982; 35:S417–468.
34. Meakins JL, Pietsch JB, Bubernick O, et al. Delayed hypersensitivity: indicator of acquired failure of host defenses in sepsis and trauma. Ann Surg 1977; 186:241.
35. Franz ML, Carella JA, Galant SP. Cutaneous delayed hypersensitivity in a healthy pediatric population; diagnostic value of diphtheria-tetanus toxoids. J Pediatr 1976; 6:975–977.
36. Smith AE, Lloyd-Still JD. Value of computerized dietary analysis in pediatric nutrition. An analysis of 147 patients. J Pediatr 1983; 103:820–824.
37. Fjeld CR, Brown KH, Schoeller DA. Validation of the deuterium oxide method for measuring average daily milk intake in infants. Am J Clin Nutr 1988; 48:671–679.
38. Food, Home & Garden Bulletin #228, USDA, Science and Education Administration. Hassle-free guide to a better diet. 1979; Sept: 3–19.
39. Bach AC, Babayan VK. Medium chain triglycerides: an update. Am J Clin Nutr 1982; 36:950–962.
40. Tomarelli RM, Meier BJ, Weaver JR. Effect of positional distribution on the absorption of the fatty acids of human milk and infant formulas. J Nutr 1968; 95:583–590.
41. Robinson D, Tateno S, Patel B, Hirai A. Lipid mediators of inflammatory and immune reactions. JPEN 1988; 12:325–425.
42. Dyerberg J. Linolenate-derived polyunsaturated fatty acids and prevention of atherosclerosis. Nutr Rev 1986; 44:125–134.
43. Hansen AE, Wiese HF, Boelsche AN, et al. Role of linoleic acid in infant nutrition: clinical and chemical study of 428 infants fed on milk mixtures varying in kind and amount of fat. Pediatrics 1963; 31:171–192.
44. Friedman Z. Essential fatty acids revisited. Am J Dis Child 1980; 134: 397–408.
45. Holman RT, Johnson SB, Hatch TF. A case of human linolenic acid deficiency involving neurological abnormalities. Am J Clin Nutr 1982; 35:617–623.
46. Crawford MA, Hassam AG, Rivers JPW. Essential fatty acid requirements in infancy. Am J Clin Nutr 1978; 31:2181–2185.
47. Landow C, Kerner JA, Castillo R, Adams L, Whalen R, Lewiston NJ. Oral correction of essential fatty acid deficiency in cystic fibrosis. JPEN 1981; 5:501–504.
48. Farrell PM, Gutcher GR, Palta M, DeMets D. Essential fatty acid deficiency in premature infants. Am J Clin Nutr 1988; 48:220–229.
49. Neuringer M, Connor WE. N3 fatty acids in the brain and retina: evidence for their essentiality. Nutr Rev 1986; 44:285–294.
50. Lamptey MS, Walker BL. A possible essential role for dietary linelenic acid in the development of the young rat. J Nutr 1978; 106:86–93.
51. Putnam JC, Carlson SE, DeVoe PW, Barness LA. The effect of variations in dietary fatty acids on the fatty acid composition of erythrocyte phosphatidylcholine and phosphatidylethanolamine in human infants. Am J Clin Nutr 1982; 36:106–114.
52. Harig JM, Soergel KH, Komorowski RA, Woods CM. Treatment of diversion colitis with short-chain fatty acid irrigation. N Engl J Med 1989; 320:23–28.
53. Halloway WD, Tasman-Jones C, Lee SP. Digestion of certain factions of dietary fibers in humans. Am J Clin Nutr 1978; 31:927–930.
54. Nguyen KN, Welsh JD, Manion CU, Ficken UJ. Effect of fiber on breath hydrogen response and symptoms after oral lactose in lactose malabsorption. Am J Clin Nutr 1982; 35:1347–1351.
55. Anderson IH, Levine AS, Levitt MD. Incomplete absorption of the carbohydrate in all-purpose flour. N Engl J Med 1981; 15:891–892.
56. Laidlaw SA, Kopple JD. Newer concepts of the indispensable amino acids. Am J Clin Nutr 1987; 46:593–605.
57. Synderman SE, Pratt EL, Cheung MW, Norton P, Holt LE Jr. The phenylalamine requirement of the normal infant. J Nutr 1955; 56: 253–263.
58. Pratt EL, Synderman SE, Cheung MW, Norton P, Holt LE Jr. The threonine requirement of the normal infant. J Nutr 1955; 56:231–251.
59. Synderman SE, Norton PM, Fowler DJ, Holt LE Jr. The essential amino acid requirements of infants: lysine. AMA J Dis Child 1959; 97:175–185.
60. Synderman SE, Holt LE Jr, Smellie F, Boyer A, Westall RG. The essential amino acid requirements of infants: valine. AMA J Dis Child 1959; 97:186–191.
61. Report of Joint FAO/WHO/UNU Expert Consultation. Energy and protein requirements. Technical report series 724. Geneva: World Health Organization, 1985.
62. Young V. Kinetics of human amino acid metabolism: nutritional influences and some lessons. Am J Clin Nutr 1987; 46:709–725.
63. Rudman D, Kutner M, Ansley J, Jansen R, Chippon J, Bain RP. Hypotyrosinemia, hypocystinemia, and failure to retain nitrogen during total parenteral nutrition of cirrhotic patients. Gastroenterology 1981; 81:1025–1035.
64. Taurine supplementation in cystic fibrosis. Nutr Rev 1988; 46:257–258.
65. Souba WW, Smith RG, Wilmore DW. Glutamine metabolism by the intestinal tract. J Parenter Nutr 1985; 9:608–617.
66. Stegink LD, den Besten L. Synthesis of cysteine from methionine in normal adult subjects: effect of route of alimentation. Science 1972; 178:514–516.
67. Askanazi J, Carpentier YA, Michelsen CB, et al. Muscle and plasma amino acids following injury. Ann Surg 1970; 192:78–85.
68. Munro HN. Parenteral nutrition: metabolic consequences of bypassing the gut and liver. In: Greene HL, Hollidan MA, Munro HN, eds. Clinical nutrition update—amino acids, Chicago: American Medical Association, 1977; 140.
69. Scrimshaw NS. Shattuck lecture—Strengths and weaknesses of the committee approach—an analysis of past and present recommended dietary allowances for protein in health and disease. N Engl J Med 1976; 294:136–142, 198–203.
70. *The National Research Council* Recommended Daily Allowances, 9th ed. Washington, DC: National Research Council, 1980.
71. Beaton GH. Toward harmonization of dietary, biochemical, and clinical assessments: the meanings of nutritional status and requirements. Nutr Rev 1986; 44:349–358.
72. Weir JB de V. New methods for calculating metabolic rate with special reference to protein metabolism. J Physiol 1949; 109:1–9.
73. Roberts SB, Coward WA, Schlingenseipen KH, Nohria V, Lucas A. Comparison of the doubly-labeled water ($^2H2^{18}O$) method with indirect calorimetry and a nutrient-balance study for simultaneous determination of energy expenditure, water intake and metabolizable energy intake in preterm infants. Am J Clin Nutr 1986; 44:315–322.
74. Schoeller DA, van Santen E. Measurement of energy expenditure in humans by doubly-labeled water method. J Appl Physiol 1982; 53:955–959.
75. Adams CF. Nutritive value of American foods in common units. Agriculture Handbook 456. Washington, DC: Agricultural Research Service, United States Department of Agriculture, 1975.
76. Dennington JAT, Church HN. Food values of portions commonly used. 14th ed. New York: Harper & Son, 1985.
77. Poskitt EME. Energy needs in weaning period. In: Ballabriga A, Rey J, eds. Weaning: why, what and when? New York: Nestle Nutrition Vevey/Raven Press, 1987: 45.
78. Butte NF, Garza C, O'Brien Smith E, Nichols BL. Human milk intake and growth in exclusively breast-fed infants. J Pediatr 1984; 104:187–195.
79. Schafer L, Wesley JR, Tse Y, Dechert R, Coran AG, Bartlett RH. Effects of necrotizing enterocolitis on calculation of resting energy expenditure in infants with gastroschisis. (Abstract) JPEN 1986; 10:65.
80. Stockman JA III, Clark DA. Weight gain: a response to transfusion in selected preterm infants. Am J Dis Child 1984; 138:828–830.
81. Vaisman N, Pencharz PB, Corey M, Corey GJ, Hahn E. Energy expenditure of patients with cystic fibrosis. J Pediatr 1987; 111:496–500.
82. Vaisman N, Levy LD, Pencharz P, Tan YK, Soldin J, Corey GJ, Hahn E. Effect of salbutamol on resting energy expenditure in patients with cystic fibrosis. J Pediatr 1987; 111:137–139.

83. Ashworth A, Millward DJ. Catch-up growth in children. Nutr Rev 1986; 44:157–163.
84. Forbes G. A note on the mathematics of "catch-up" growth. Pediatr Res 1974; 8:929–931.
85. Whitehead RG. The protein needs of malnourished children. In: Poster J, Rolls BA, eds. Proteins in human nutrition. New York: Academic Press, 1973; 103.
86. Arroyave G. Interrelations between protein and vitamin A and metabolism. Am J Clin Nutr 1969; 22:1119–1128.
87. Golden MHN, Golden BE. Effect of zinc supplementation on the dietary intake, rate of weight gain, and energy cost of tissue deposition in children recovering from severe malnutrition. Am J Clin Nutr 1981; 34:900–908.
88. Castillo-Duran C, Uauy R. Copper deficiency impairs growth of infants recovering from malnutrition. Am J Clin Nutr 1988; 47:710–714.
89. Beaton GH, Chery A. Protein requirements of infants: a re-examination of concepts and approaches. Am J Clin Nutr 1989; 49:1403–1412.
90. Beisel WR. Magnitude of the most nutritional responses to infection. Am J Clin Nutr 1977; 30:1236–1247.
91. Raiha N, Boehm G. Protein and nitrogen metabolism in low-birth-weight infants. In: Stern S, ed. Feeding the sick infant. Nestle Nutrition Workshop Series, vol 11. New York: Nestle Nutrition Vevey/Raven Press, 1987: 63.
92. Progress towards the 1990 objectives for improved nutrition. MMWR 1988; 37:475–479.
93. Progress towards achieving the national 1990 objectives for fluoridation and dental health. MMWR 1988; 37:578–583.
94. Broquist HP. Vitamin-like molecules. Carnitine. In: Shils ME, Young VR, eds. Modern Nutrition in Health and Disease. 7th ed. Philadelphia: Lea & Febiger, 1988: 453.
95. Rebouche CJ, Engel AG. Carnitine metabolism and deficiency syndromes. Mayo Clin Proc 1983; 58:533–540.
96. Rudman D, Sewell CW, Ansley JD. Deficiency of carnitine in cachectic cirrhotic patients. J Clin Invest 1977; 60:716–723.
97. Borum PR: Possible carnitine requirement of the newborn and the effect of genetic disease on the carnitine requirement. Nutr Rev 1981; 39:385–390.
98. Salway JG, Finnegan JA, Barnett D, Whitehead L, Karunanayaka A, Payne RB. Effect of *myo*-inositol on peripheral-nerve function in diabetes. Lancet 1978; ii:1282–1284.
99. Grand RJ, Sutphen JL, Dietz WH, eds. Pediatric nutrition, theory and practice. Boston: Butterworth, 1987.
100. Walker WA, Watkins JB. Nutrition in pediatrics—basic science and clinical application. Boston: Little, Brown, 1985.
101. Forbes BB, Woodruff CW, eds. Pediatric nutrition handbook. 2nd ed. Oak Grove Village, IL: American Academy of Pediatrics, 1985.
102. Shills ME, Young VR. Modern nutrition in health and disease. Philadelphia: Lea & Febiger, 1988.
103. Olson JA. Recommended dietary intakes (RDI) of vitamin A in humans. Am J Clin Nutr 1987; 45:704–716.
104. Olson JA, Hodges RE. Recommended dietary intakes (RDI) of vitamin C in humans. Am J Clin Nutr 1987; 45:693–703.
105. Olson JA. Recommended dietary intakes (RDI) of vitamin K in humans. Am J Clin Nutr 1987; 45:687–692.
106. Herbert V. Recommended dietary intakes (RDI) of iron in humans. Am J Clin Nutr 1987; 45:679–686.
107. Herbert V. Recommended dietary intakes (RDI) of vitamin B_{12} in humans. Am J Clin Nutr 1987; 45:671–678.
108. Herbert V. Recommended dietary intakes (RDI) of folate in humans. Am J Clin Nutr 1987; 45:661–670.

PART 3

Protein Energy Malnutrition

Fernando E. Viteri, M.D., Sc.D.

Protein energy malnutrition (PEM) can be broadly separated in two categories: primary and secondary. Primary PEM is due to the inability of individuals and population groups to procure and consume the necessary foods for maintenance of health in their environment. Its origin is poverty and the exploitation of man by the more powerful. Secondary PEM is the consequence of a primary pathologic condition that either impairs the intake of food and its utilization or increases the losses or requirements of energy and protein so that metabolic needs are unattainable through the diet at the individual's disposal. Table 1 lists the more commonly found causes of secondary PEM. Often both types of PEM occur together, typically in the presence of infection (and diarrhea in particular) among the poor who live in environments with high rates of infection. Also, any nutrient deficiency except for energy decreases the efficiency of energy utilization, therefore increasing relatively the energy requirements, accounting for the characteristic weight loss and reduced growth velocities observed in all specific nutrient deficiencies.

PEM can also be acute or chronic. The former is rarely seen among primary PEM; populations and individuals suffering chronic PEM can suffer an acute aggravation of their chronic condition, e.g., during famines. War could be an exception, well-nourished populations being subjected to severe food scarcity. However, it must be recognized that throughout history, famine as seen in the Sahel, for example, affects the previously deprived populations and not those socioeconomically privileged.

Chronic primary PEM (henceforth called simply PEM) is prevalent throughout the developing world and among the underprivileged groups of industrial societies in which poverty and marked socioeconomic inequalities abound. The Subcommittee on Nutrition of the Administrative Coordinating Council of the United Nations, in a recent publication on the World's Nutritional Status, estimates that over 1 billion persons are suffering from mild to severe degrees of PEM.[1]

In this discussion, PEM is the chronic deficit of energy and/or protein intake that has led to a state of relative deple-

TABLE 1
Most Common Causes of Secondary Protein Energy Malnutrition

Decreased intake
- Appetite disorders (e.g., anorexia nervosa, bulimia)
- Anorexia due to chronic diseases: infections, endocrine, cardiorespiratory, renal, hepatic, neurologic, cancer
- Affective deprivation and depression
- Poor dentition and altered taste-smell functions
- Nausea and vomiting from chronic diseases, dehydration and electrolyte disturbances, hyperemesis gravidarum
- Dysphagia and/or obstruction from pharyngoesophageal and gastric diseases, pyloric stenosis, intestinal disorders (e.g., Crohn's disease, peptide ulcerations and scarring, diverticulosis) and biliary disease
- Intestinal parasites
- Restricted and imbalanced therapeutic diets
- Iatrogenic
- Substance abuse

Poor food digestion and absorption (reduced food utilization)
- Gastric diseases (atrophic gastritis, postresection pathology)
- Small bowel disease (short bowel syndrome, blind-loop syndromes, tropical and nontropical sprue, chronic diarrhea, gluten enteropathy, lymphoma)
- Pancreatic disease
- Liver and biliary disease
- Parasitic diseases

Increased nutrient losses
- Extensive burns
- Gastrointestinal fistulae
- Protein-losing enteropathy
- Chronic diarrhea
- Chronic gastrointestinal bleeding

Increased requirements and altered nutrient metabolism
- Inflammatory diseases
- Fever
- Cell proliferative diseases
- Endocrine diseases
- Congenital metabolic disorders
- Toxic states and substance abuse

tion of lean body mass and/or adipose mass or to functional limitations in order to preserve body mass. This definition requires (1) that there be evidence of chronic insufficient intake in relation to the individual's needs; (2) that body mass is inadequate for the individual's age, sex, and physiologic status; and (3) that in the presence of the first and absence of the second characteristic, there is evidence of functional limitations to preserve body mass (e.g., reduced spontaneous activity).

Other functional limitations are present among populations with chronic PEM, as observed in the areas of growth and development, defense mechanisms against infection, mental development and social behavior, reproductive performance, work capacity, and metabolic/physiologic reserves. Such limitations, if due to PEM, are associated with either loss of body mass or decreased energy expenditure and/or protein synthesis and turnover.[2]

DIRECT ETIOLOGIC MECHANISMS

Individuals who have higher requirements for energy and for both total nitrogen and essential amino acids relative to their body size are at greater risk of PEM. These are small children, adolescent boys, pregnant and lactating women in general and the adolescent in particular, and the elderly. Poor dietary practices and infectious processes are the most common direct etiologic mechanisms.

Poverty, some degree of ignorance about the adequacy of diets for specific conditions, such as during the process of weaning, and poor hygienic practices are indirect etiologic mechanisms. Often forgotten and very important indirect etiologic factors are poor mothering and the low social value of women among many cultures. This leads to low esteem for girls who, in the presence of scarce resources, are consciously or unconsciously discriminated against. They suffer reductions of their share of limited food in a household, negation of educational opportunities, and their "disposal" through early marriage, itself conducive to teen-age pregnancies in chronically undernourished girls and to low birth weight babies who begin their extrauterine life already undernourished.[3]

Poor Dietary Practices

In the developing world, over 95 percent of rural children are breast fed successfully up to about 3 to 4 months. After this age most children begin to exhibit growth faltering, and food complementation to breast milk is very often of poor nutritional quality (e.g., coffee and/or bush teas, small pieces of corn "tortilla," starchy gruels) and contaminated with coliform and other enteropathogenic bacteria.[4] Delayed introduction of food complements is not rare; by this time exexclusively breast-fed infants are already mildly to moderately undernourished. Breast-feeding, however, often continues for over 1 year. Ablactation is followed by the administration of locally prepared drinks that rarely include milk and that are either deficient in energy and protein (watery broths or herb teas) or prepared exclusively from starchy flours that provide only carbohydrates (typically Duryea corn starch). Solid foods are introduced very cautiously in terms of amounts and varieties. The result is children between 6 and 18 to 24 months of age who are growing very poorly and are thin and listless (chronic, moderate PEM) or who develop severe forms of PEM with the clinical pictures of marasmus, kwashiorkor, or a combination of both. The path to marasmus is one of simple, uncomplicated semistarvation; kwashiorkor is the result of protein deficits in the diet (e.g., feeding almost exclusively bananas, starch gruels, manioc, or cassava) after the child is weaned and is often precipitated further by toxic or infectious processes or by acute socioeconomic stress. In marasmus-kwashiorkor, the kwashiorkor component is superimposed on children already suffering from different degrees of marasmus. After this "critical age" when infant and child mortality takes its greatest toll, children tend to stabilize in terms of growth, and infections begin to diminish in both incidence and severity. A slow and most often incomplete nutritional recovery begins thanks to the child's reduced relative energy and protein requirements and his or her capacity to compete for the scarce family food supply.

The picture among the urban poor is frequently quite different; here, socioeconomic pressures and misguided directions for becoming more "modern" often result in a marked reduction in duration and frequency of breast-feeding, substituted by cow's milk preparations and formulae introduced by health personnel and by infant food companies whose advertising suggests that formula feeding is the "in thing to do." Unfortunately, the urban poor cannot afford adequate formula feeding, nor do they have the preparation and storage facilities to prevent bacterial contamination of bottles and their contents. Consequently, infants are frequently fed diluted and contaminated formula, leading to chronic energy deficiency and increased prevalence of infectious diseases, including diarrhea. Early PEM, mostly marasmus, is common under these circumstances.[5]

The diets of preschool-age children in poor underdeveloped societies are commonly devoid of animal proteins and are based on the available adult foods (mostly cereals and pulses) that are bulky and of low energy density. Some degree of energy deficit is common, particularly when children are fed only two to three times per day. Energy density can be easily increased by adding vegetable oils to porridges. A certain degree of protein deficiency also occurs among children being fed the adult-type diets because vegetable proteins are absorbed at only about 85 to 90 percent the rate of milk protein absorption, and their essential amino acid composition is unbalanced. Consequently, the nutritional value of such proteins is between 60 and 70 percent of that of milk. The complementary effect of mixtures of cereals and pulses in the right proportion of various amino acid–imbalanced vegetable proteins can yield a more balanced protein mixture. This, for example, is the case for corn- and bean-based diets in which between 40 and 60 percent of the protein is provided from each source. The biologic value of such protein mixtures increases to about 90 percent that of milk, although absorption still is 85 to 90 percent that of milk. A significant supplementary effect in protein quality is also obtained by the consumption of small amounts of animal proteins.

Unfortunately, neither the optimal proportions of staples nor the small amount of animal proteins and oil is usually consumed because of the cost of pulses, animal proteins, and oil, and because the common culinary preparation of pulses is not adequate for infant feeding. A simple sieve to prepare fine porridges and prolonged soaking of pulses in water before cooking are helpful for preparing nutritious and culturally accepted baby foods. Protein-deficient diets are the rule where the staples are starchy roots and fruits (e.g., yucca, cassava, tapioca, banana, plantain) because of the extremely low amount of protein in such foods. Poor-quality diets during adolescence, pregnancy, and lactation also pose limitations in energy and protein intakes in relation to their increased requirements.

The diet of the elderly is often inadequate because of the frequently observed isolation, poor capacity to acquire and cook adequate meals, reduced masticatory competency, reduced energy needs and appetite, and impaired sensory capacity. A higher ratio of protein to energy needs, characteristic of aging, can lead to predominant protein deficiency.[6]

Infectious Process

The relationship between repeated infections and PEM is well established among populations who live in areas where malaria and respiratory and diarrheal diseases are endemic. The importance of skin infections and communicable diseases of childhood, measles in particular, as precipitating causes of acute and severe PEM has also been amply documented.[7]

Besides the metabolic effects of infectious and inflammatory processes, to be described later, infections are accompanied by a significant reduction in food intake because of the anorexia typical of these processes and because most cultures restrict food from sick individuals and children in particular. Nutrient losses due to diarrhea and increased energy losses because of fever aggravate the already unfavorable nutritional situation. Malaria is particularly devastating to fetal nutrition because of its predilection for placental infection, and measles poses a special danger to vitamin A–deficient populations because it produces a keratitis that favors keratomalacia.

The commonly observed presence of various vitamin and mineral deficiencies in PEM enhances the effects of infection because they are often associated with reduced cell and humoral immunity. Recent reviews on this subject are abundant.[8]

CLINICAL PICTURE

The clinical picture of individuals suffering from PEM varies depending on their age at onset, the severity of the deficiency and its duration, the etiologic factors involved, and the predominant deficient nutrient.[9–12]

Mild to Moderate Protein Energy Malnutrition

PEM can occur in utero, giving rise to low birth weight (LBW) babies, both because of intrauterine growth retardation (small for gestational age [SGA]) and shortened gestational duration (preterm). The exact mechanisms by which these undesirable outcomes occur are not yet established, but in general it appears that smallness of mothers (short and/or underweight) because of their own impaired development as children and adolescents and insufficient pre-pregnancy weight are the main factors for SGA babies, most of whom are proportional or symmetric (small in all dimensions). Significant weight gain during pregnancy can partially or totally overcome the original disadvantage of these women.[13] On the other hand, famine during the last half of pregnancy will result in disproportional or asymmetric SGAs (basically babies with little subcutaneous fat).[14] The role of the placenta in intrauterine PEM is poorly defined as yet, but evidence of placental "insufficiency" exists.[15]

LBW babies begin their extrauterine life at a disadvantage, and proportional SGAs essentially never catch up fully. Therefore, these children are more prone to develop severe forms of PEM early in life.

Lactation performance of moderately malnourished mothers is adequate during early lactation, but often their infants begin to show diminished growth velocity before 4 to 6 months of age. These children's weight for age becomes progressively lower, and they appear lean and later clearly wasted unless adequate complementary food intake is implemented. Unfortunately, contamination of complementary feedings is a major problem among poor households, and weanling diarrhea and nutritional deterioration can follow.

Most children under these circumstances show a growth curve with alternating periods of poor growth and incomplete catch-up that leads to progressive retardation in both length and weight. This phase of progressive growth in a given channel or slow and incomplete catch-up occurs for the rest of their growth period. These children are somewhat stunted, may have adequate weight for their height, and are recognized as victims of simple, mild to moderate, chronic PEM.

Anthropometric parameters are used for the diagnosis of chronic mild to moderate PEM in population groups. The interpretation of these parameters for the diagnosis of PEM in a given child must be done with caution, because short, lean, healthy, and perfectly happy children are not undernourished. Their genetic make-up and other factors, pathologic or not, may define their growth characteristics. Short stature and/or low weight for height must alert the health personnel to the need for further investigations before a specific child is labeled as malnourished.

At the population level, height-for-age deficits reflect an early and prolonged period of PEM with or without chronic or repeated infections. If associated with small head circumference, it points to fetal or early (before 1 year of age) growth retardation, most probably associated with PEM. The use of height for age as a nutritional surveillance tool in school-age children therefore reflects mainly events that took place some years back in the life of the population. On the other hand, weight-for-height deficits and/or reduced arm circumference reflect the present "nutritional" condition of the population in question. Weight-for-age deficits alone reflect either present PEM (if associated with weight-for-height deficits) or some previous event no longer present (if weight for height is adequate). Chronic PEM may still be present, however, if only height for age is subnormal; under these circumstances the diagnosis of chronic and present PEM must be made on other grounds: inadequate intake, chronic repeated infections, apathetic and passive behavior, and the chronic undernutrition of the general population and even of domestic animals.

In the adult, chronic mild to moderate PEM is manifested mostly by low weight for height due to depleted adipose tissue reserves, although adiposities of 10 to 15 percent body weight in males and up to 20 percent in females do not exclude the possibility of chronic PEM if in order to preserve such body composition they diminish physical activity below their ideal activity level at work or leisure. Chronic PEM can be diagnosed without hesitation in adults and in the elderly if besides a decreased adipose mass, they exhibit a deficit in lean body mass and in muscle mass, weakness, apathy, decreased physical activity, and other functional impairments, including altered defense mechanisms.[16,17] Simply, adult lean male populations are not necessarily chronically undernourished if they are otherwise productive, physically fit, happy, and active. Adult female populations can be considered chronically undernourished if besides unsatisfactory weight for height before or during pregnancy and lactation their reproductive performance is suboptimal in terms of a high incidence of LBW and insufficient lactation (reduced growth velocity of their infants at or before 3 months of age). LBW prevalences as high as 60 percent have been reported in chronically undernourished populations.[18]

In undernourished populations the presence of other nutrient deficiencies is common.[11,19] The most prevalent associated deficiencies are those of fat-soluble vitamins (particularly A and D), B complex vitamins (particularly folate, niacinamide, pyridoxine, riboflavin), ascorbic acid, and minerals (especially iron, calcium, zinc). Some documentation of essential fatty acid deficiency is also available.

Severe Protein Energy Malnutrition

More severe forms of PEM are defined by specific signs and are recognized as marasmus when the predominant feature is marked emaciation in infants and children; kwashiorkor when edema, hepatomegaly, and skin lesions are evident;

TABLE 2
Main Clinical Characteristics of Severe Protein Energy Malnutrition Syndromes

	Marasmus	Kwashiorkor	Marasmus-Kwashiorkor
Age (months)	<18	12–60	9–36
Sex (M = male; F = female)	F > M	—	F > M
Growth faltering			
Stunting	+	+	++
Wasting	+++	+	++
Behavioral aspects			
Apathy	++	+++	+++
Irritability	+	+++	+++
Anorexia	−	+++	++
General appearance			
"Gravely ill"	++	+++	+++
Wasting	+++	−	+
Edema	−	+++	++
Skin and appendages			
Poor hair implantation	++	+	+++
Dry, lifeless hair	+	+++	+++
Depigmented hair	+	++	+++
Fragile, thin nails	++	++	+++
Dry, scaly skin	+	++	+++
Pellagroid lesions	−	+	+++
Ulcerations and fissures	−	++	+++
Petechia	−	+	++
Vital signs			
Hypothermia (<36 °C)	+++	++	+++
Hypotension	+	+	++
Slow pulse	++	+	++
Other physical signs			
Hepatomegaly	−	+++	++
Dehydration and diarrhea	+	+	++
Vitamin A deficiency	++	++	+++
Vitamin B complex deficiency	+	+++	++
Mucosal thinness	+	+++	+++
Paleness	+	+++	+++

and marasmus-kwashiorkor when the children are emaciated and also present the signs of kwashiorkor. This combined clinical picture is predominant in most parts of the world where severe PEM occurs. The presence of emaciation may be masked initially by edema but reappears early in the process of nutritional recovery as edema is lost. The main characteristics of these syndromes are listed in Table 2. These severe forms of PEM, although predominant in children, can occur in adults when social inequalities are profound and nutritional stresses and infections are exacerbated. Typical situations are famine and war.[20,21]

Classically, the natural history of marasmus is that of an LBW infant, born in poverty from an undernourished mother, who was either inadequately or not breast fed and/or was weaned at an early age. The course is usually protracted and uninterrupted by severe stresses in terms of infections and worsened feeding practices. The child "adapts" as well as possible to prolonged semistarvation and progresses to use all his or her body fat for energy purposes, losing little of his or her muscle mass as long as other energy sources supply progressively reduced energy needs. However, as internal fat sources for energy become depleted, the only alternative is to break down muscle at a rather fast rate. The child then becomes severely ill (French pediatricians called this a state of "decomposition") and is at severe risk of death.[11,22]

At the other extreme of severe PEM is the sugar-baby or "pure kwashiorkor" child who presents after weaning and has almost exclusively protein deficiency, induced by a force-fed carbohydrate diet, as described in Jamaica and certain regions in Africa.[9,23] These children are fat and have huge fatty livers, severe edema, skin lesions, dry discolored hair, and hypoalbuminemia. The course of kwashiorkor is acute and severe, leading to death if not properly treated.

Most forms of severe PEM follow a combined path in which some degree of wasting takes place as protein deficiency develops. Diets may not differ substantially from those of marasmic children, but generally the progressive adaptation to energy deficiency is upset by infection and stress or by the introduction of an exclusively carbohydrate diet.[9,11,22]

Figures 1 and 2 show Guatemalan children with severe PEM of marasmic and kwashiorkor types. Most often the process leading to severe PEM is progressive, dynamic, and of a mixed nature, involving both energy and protein deficiencies of different relative intensities and durations. All classifications of PEM are, therefore, somewhat arbitrary. The first attempt to classify "undernutrition" without differentiating between the relative contribution of energy or protein deficiencies was proposed by the Mexican school,[24] who clearly stated that for purposes of evaluating *risk of death among clinically undernourished children*, three degrees of severity of PEM should be recognized: first degree—when

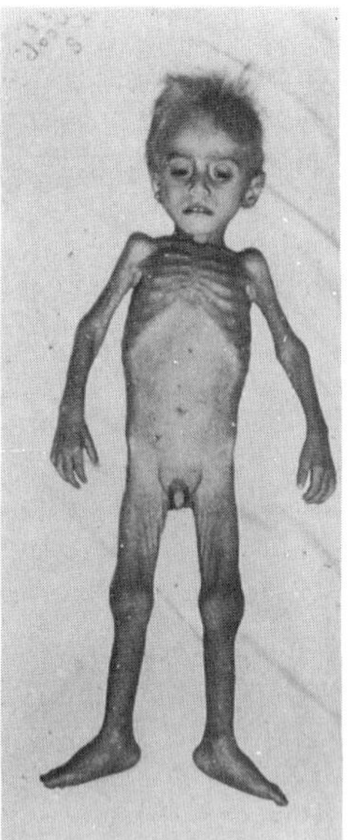
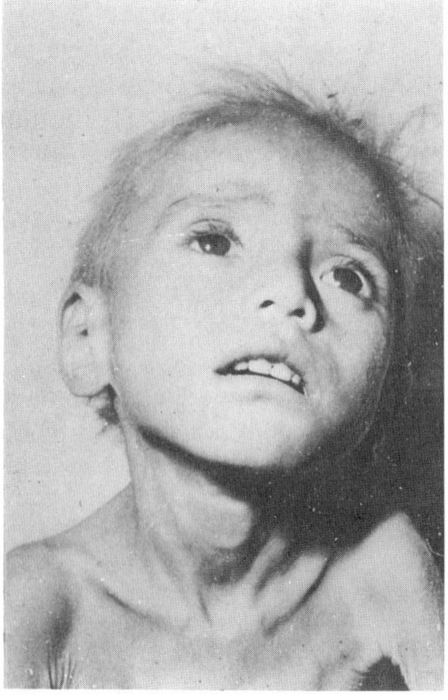

FIGURE 1 Marasmic child. Note extreme wasting, absence of edema or skin lesions, hair sparsity, misery, and corneal opacity. (From Viteri FE. Primary protein energy malnutrition: clinical, biochemical, and metabolic changes. In: Suskind RM, ed. Textbook of pediatric nutrition. New York: Raven Press, 1981: 189.)

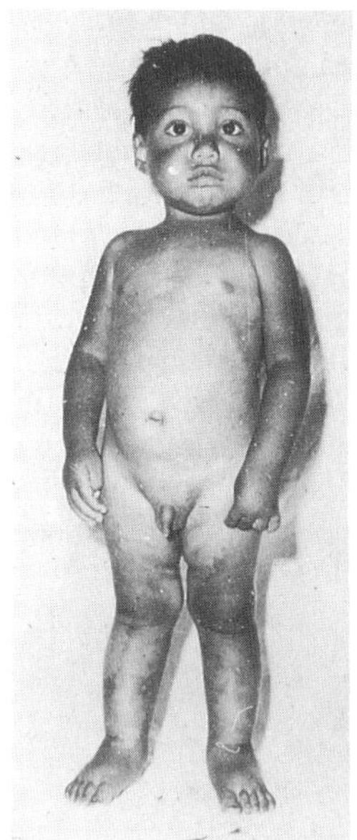
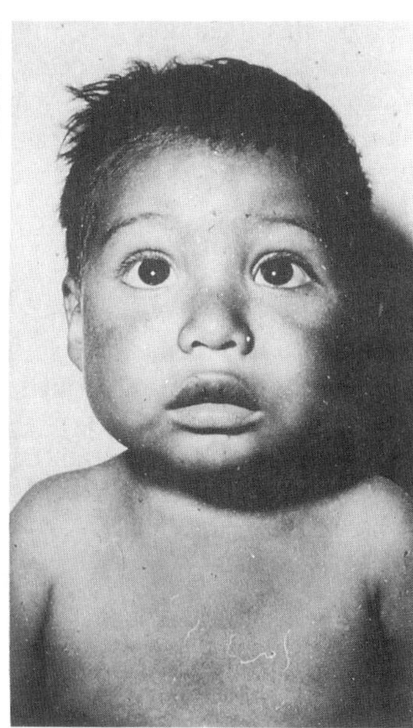

FIGURE 2 Kwashiorkor child. Note overall fatness, edema, moon facies, and skin lesions. (From Viteri FE. Primary protein energy malnutrition: clinical, biochemical, and metabolic changes. In: Suskind RM, ed. Textbook of pediatric nutrition. New York: Raven Press, 1981: 189.)

the weight for age of the clinically undernourished child was between 75 and 90 percent of the 50th percentile of the Boston standards; second degree—when weight for age was between 75 and 60 percent of the standard; and third degree—when weight for age was below 60 percent of standard or the child presented with edema. This classification was later used rather loosely for defining the presence and severity of PEM in populations, since older children were classified as chronically PEM when they were no longer currently undernourished, simply because of weight-for-age deficits. For example, an analysis of children discharged from the Instituto de Nutricion de Centro America y Panama (INCAP) metabolic ward indicated that 83 percent would be classified as second degree malnourished by the misapplied criteria of weight for age, even when all had creatinine height index (CHI) above 90,[25] indicative of full recovery of muscle (and protein mass) for the child's height, and had weight for height of 100 percent or greater, indicative of at least the "norm" of adipose mass when combined with a normal "protein mass." Later, the "Wellcome group" met and published the Wellcome classification of severe PEM,[26] which classified children with edema who weighed between 60 and 80 percent of the 50th percentile of the Boston standards for age as having kwashiorkor; if their weight with edema fell below 60 percent, they would fit the diagnosis of kwashiorkor-marasmus. In the absence of edema, the two weight-for-age groups would be diagnosed as underweight and marasmic, respectively. More recently, Waterlow proposed the widely

TABLE 3
Classification of Children with Protein Energy Malnutrition (PEM) by Height and Weight

Grade of Wasting (Percentage Expected Weight for Height)	Grade of Stunting (Percentage Expected Height for Age) 0 (>95)	1(95–90) 2(90–85) 3(<85)
0 (>90)	Normal	Progressive stunting residual of past PEM
1 (90–80)	Progressive wasting currently occurring	Progressively severe past and present malnutrition (stunting and wasting)
2 (80–70)		
3 (<70)		

Data from Waterlow[27] and Lancet 1973; ii:87–89.

accepted classification of PEM (Table 3), which considers the presence or absence of edema and both stunting (height-for-age deficit) and wasting (weight-for-height deficit).[27]

Discussion about the adequacy of a particular anthropometric standard for the classification of PEM among different genetic/ethnic groups has taken place. The World Health Organization (WHO), after considering different options and the scientific evidence about optimal growth patterns of different populations, has adopted the National Center for Health Statistics (NCHS) standards as a universal yardstick for evaluating growth of children throughout the world.[28]

When body weight, height, or age cannot be obtained with precision, the arm circumference by itself or related to head circumference, height, or arm skin fold has been proposed for the identification and classification of PEM of various degrees of severity. This simple measurement can be justified for its practicability under emergency situations; however, it is less sensitive and specific than other anthropometric measurements.[29]

Table 4 presents a summary of various biochemical findings in the major forms of severe PEM, compiled from a series of reviews on this subject.[10,11,30] The biochemical findings are the basis for or are compatible with a series of pathophysiologic mechanisms that have emerged in attempts to understand the basic adaptive mechanisms to undernutrition and marasmus and their failure under circumstances that lead to kwashiorkor or marasmus-kwashiorkor. These are presented in a simplified form below.

TABLE 4
Main Laboratory Findings in Severe Protein Energy Malnutrition Syndromes

Category of Finding	Marasmus	Kwashiorkor	Marasmus-Kwashiorkor
Serum			
Proteins	N-SR*	MR	R-MR
Albumin	N-SR	MR	R-MR
"Transport proteins"	SR	MR	MR
Urea	N-SR	MR	R-MR
"Amino acid ratio"	<3	>3.5	>3.5
Glucose	MR	N-R	R-MR
Ferritin	R-E†	E	E
"Acute phase" proteins	N-E	N-E	E
Lipids and fat-soluble vitamins	E-R	MR	MR
Blood			
Hemoglobin	N-R	R	R
White blood cells	N-R	R	R
T lymphocytes	N-R	R	R
Platelets	N	N-R	N-R
Red and white blood cells			
Selenium	—	R	R
Glutathione peroxidase	—	R	R
Glutathione	N	R	R
Pyruvic kinase	N	R	R
Liver cells			
Protein/DNA	N-R	R	R
Fat percentage	N-SE	ME	E-ME
Glycogen	N-R	R-E	R-E
AA recycling	—	E	E
Urea synthesis	R	R	R
Neoglucogenesis	E	R	R
Carbohydrate recycling	—	E	E
Muscle cells			
Noncollagen protein/DNA	N-R	R	MR
Creatine/g protein	N-R	R	R
Branched-chain AA transaminase	E	R	R
Branched-chain AA dehydrogenases	—	R	R
Urine			
Urea/24 hr	R	MR	MR
Creatinine/24 hr	SR-R	R-MR	MR
Ammonium ion	N	E	E
Titratable H^+	N	R	R
Osmolality	N	R	R
OH-proline	R	MR	MR
3-me-hystidine	R	MR	MR

*N = normal; SR = slightly reduced; R = reduced; MR = markedly reduced.
†E = elevated.
From references 9 to 12, 19, 30, and 54.

PATHOPHYSIOLOGIC MECHANISMS

The "natural," uncomplicated form of undernutrition is assumed to be the one developing chronically from semistarvation, with periods of more severe food restriction due to food scarcity, without major nutrient imbalances or severe concurrent infection. Widdowson and McCance[31,32] demonstrated that semistarvation in the adult rat produced body weight loss that was essentially parallel to liver and muscle weight losses, in contrast to a significantly higher loss of liver weight in acute starvation. In terms of total fat, protein, and water losses in starvation, the adult male rat exhibits equivalent losses of the three compartments, whereas adult female rats and pups protect protein and water losses at the expense of fat loss. Children with marasmus seem to protect both liver (visceral) and muscle protein losses while utilizing fat for energy purposes until the latter is exhausted. In this process, however, an adequate supply of glucose must be maintained for brain and erythrocyte metabolism. Studies on glucose turnover suggest that, in the fasting state, at least 8 percent is derived from amino acid catabolism in PEM children (compared to 16 percent in the well-fed state) while a seemingly constant 20 percent is provided by glycerol metabolism in PEM as in recovered children. Sixty to 70 percent of glucose is therefore derived from recycling products of glycolysis and alanine, depending on the underlying nutritional status.[33] Protein synthesis and catabolism are also reduced, and amino acid recycling is more efficient.[10] Muscle branched-chain amino acid transaminase appears to be especially sensitive to amino acid intake and circulating levels, thus diminishing muscle protein catabolism to a minimum during starvation. The active form of branched-chain keto-acid dehydrogenase is also responsive to the level of amino acid intake, increasing as these amino acids are available above a minimum level that seems to be fixed as the minimum obligatory nitrogen loss.[34] Amino acid oxidation is thus reduced to a minimum during semistarvation, but muscle supplies amino acids to the viscera with priority over other tissues. This visceral predominance and other body composition changes partly explain the relatively elevated state of hydration and increased oxygen consumption per unit of body weight characteristic of wasted children, in spite of the reduced basal energy expenditure per unit of height, or age, characteristic of starvation and semistarvation.[22,35,36]

These mechanisms of endogenous fat utilization, amino acid conservation, and interorgan redistribution are mediated by endocrine responses[37,38]: reduced food intake leads to reduced insulin levels that in turn facilitate lipolysis and reduce liver glycogen, lipogenesis, and amino acid incorporation into muscle (diminished "peripheral" protein synthesis). The gut beta-cytotrophic mechanism is also reduced in PEM, and insulin response is slow to various stimuli. The chronic stress of hunger plus hypoglycemia stimulates the production of cortisol, which appears elevated in its free form in plasma. Its clearance is also reduced. Glucagon plasma levels are normal or reduced. These endocrine changes enhance muscle amino acid release, neoglucogenesis, and glycogenolysis. Epinephrine levels are increased in relation to norepinephrine, also favoring glycogenolysis and lipolysis. At the same time, low amino acid levels impair liver somatomedin synthesis (parallel to decreased albumin synthesis), and consequently growth hormone secretion is augmented; thus, growth is markedly impaired, and urea synthesis is reduced while liver amino acid activation and recycling are increased. Lipolysis is favored and peripheral insulin sensitivity is reduced, partly due to hypokalosis, increased free-fatty acids, and cortisol. Starvation and semistarvation also reduce the peripheral production of tri-iodothyronine (T_3) and enhance the production of reverse T_3 from thyroxine (T_4), and these changes in turn diminish the production of thyroid-stimulating hormone (TSH). However, TSH response to thyrotropin-releasing hormone (TRH) is normal or elevated. The hypothalamo-hypophyseal axis thus appears preserved even though prolactin response to TRH is reduced, possibly in relation to excess body water. An incomplete blockage of adrenocorticotropic hormone (ACTH) secretion by dexamethasone and normal response to metyrapone, as well as the increased secretion of growth hormone and luteinizing hormone in response to decreased circulating testosterone in males and progesterone in females, also suggest primarily a target-organ dysfunction (adaptation?) with normal or even increased hypophyseal responsiveness.

These carefully concerted "adaptive" mechanisms in response to underfeeding are markedly disturbed by infectious processes and by the chronic administration of pure carbohydrate diets, often force fed as anorexia develops in children developing kwashiorkor. The so-called breakdown of adaptation leads to an acute aggravation of the nutritional status characterized by acute amino acid deficiency at the visceral level (including amino acid diversion from normal visceral utilization paths) and by marked alterations in lipid metabolism.

Infection, most probably through the effects of enhanced production of cytokines (i.e., interleukin 1, tumor necrosis factor) and altered prostaglandin metabolism (increased PgE), results in increased protein catabolism, substantial nitrogen loss, and enhanced specialized protein synthesis that diverts amino acids from the normal synthesis of albumin, transferrin, and other transport proteins toward that of acute-phase proteins, enzymes, complement, specific cell proliferation, and immunoglobulins. Antidiuretic hormone, TSH, ACTH, cortisol, aldosterone, and adrenomedullary functions are enhanced by infection. Glucagon and insulin production are also elevated, but peripheral insulin resistance, induced by hypokalosis, and slowed insulin clearance are the rule. T_4 and T_3 production and turnover are also elevated. Fat mobilization occurs but ketone body utilization is impaired (possibly because of relative hyperinsulinism), and the increased metabolic demands of infection must be met by increased glucose utilization. Neoglucogenesis at the expense of amino acids is markedly accelerated. Liver fat synthesis is increased, apolipoprotein synthesis is decreased, and lipoprotein lipases are inhibited by tumor necrosis factor, leading to fatty liver and hypertriglyceridemia, especially with gram-negative infections. These apparent undesirable effects of infection appear, however, essential for survival. The impaired production of interleukin 1 in severely undernourished patients with hypoalbuminemia indicates poor prognosis.

High intakes of almost exclusive carbohydrate diets also result in "dysadaptation," primarily because of the repeated stimulus to insulin production, and inhibition of glucagon, ACTH, growth hormone, and epinephrine release. Conse-

TABLE 5
Conditions That Carry Poor Prognosis in Severe Protein Energy Malnutrition

Age less than 6 months
Deficit in weight for height greater than 30 percent or in weight for age greater than 40 percent
Extensive exfoliative or exudative cutaneous lesions, ulcerations, or decubitus ulcers
Severe and persistent diarrhea, gastroenteric dilatation, gastrointestinal bleeding
Dehydration and electrolyte imbalances, especially hypokalosis, hypokalemia, and severe acidosis
Any manifestation of liver failure or necrosis
Hypothermia
Hypoglycemia
Severe, decompensated anemia with hypoxia
Signs of cardiorespiratory decompensation/failure
Intercurrent infections, particularly bronchopneumonia and measles
Petechial/hemorrhagic tendencies: generally indicative of septicemia or severe viral infections
Hypoproteinemia (less than 30 g per liter), hyperferritinemia (greater than 100 μg per liter), and signs of free radical damage
Stupor, comatous state, and other alterations of consciousness; muscle flaccidity

Modified after Torún and Viteri.[12]

quently, muscle amino acid outflow and lipolysis are markedly inhibited. Hypoalbuminemia and fatty liver ensue, the latter related to increased fat synthesis and decreased production of apolipoprotein B in the liver.

PROGNOSIS OF THE CHILD WITH SEVERE PROTEIN ENERGY MALNUTRITION

Short Term

Besides the already elevated risk of death among children being reared in environments where poverty is the rule, those with severe PEM and with greater body weight loss and edema (Gomez classification of third-degree undernutrition) are at even much higher risk. Particularly elevated risk is brought about by the acute effects induced by processes that lead to severe dysadaptation and that appear to favor formation and impaired disposal of free radicals, as well as several other commonly observed concomitant events and conditions brought about by the very nature of the environment where PEM is prevalent. Exposure to and ingestion of toxic factors and the mismanagement of PEM and associated illnesses (in particular diarrhea and respiratory infections) are common where PEM is endemic. Table 5 lists signs of poor prognosis among severely undernourished children.

Long Term

It has been suggested that once a child has been the victim of chronic severe PEM, the attainment of full development is not possible because of residual long-term histologic and functional impairments (e.g., pancreatic insufficiency), decreased cell numbers in different tissues, or simply missed developmental stages that are achievable only within a certain time margin in the process of growth.[39] The evidence for this irreversible type of damage from PEM is quite strong, but the precise partial contribution of nutritional deficits versus the negative effects of an unhealthy and smothering environment is far from clear. There is more evidence that the latter factor (of which PEM is only a part) is more responsible for hampered development; however, how critical are the negative effects of PEM (even if small in relative magnitude) within such an undesirable environment is not answerable at present.

FUNCTIONAL ABNORMALITIES IN SEVERE PROTEIN ENERGY MALNUTRITION

Severe PEM is characterized also by the presence of structural and functional alterations in different systems. What follows is a summary of many studies providing evidence that all functions explored in severe PEM have been found altered, particularly in children with kwashiorkor and marasmus-kwashiorkor.

Central and Peripheral Nervous System[10,40–43]

Early PEM, particularly that occurring in utero (especially prior to midpregnancy, before neuronal multiplication ceases) and during the first 6 months of life, has been found to produce an encephalic mass that is reduced in size and in glial and neuronal cellularity and that has defective myelinization and dilated ventricular volumes. The cerebellum with its greater cellularity appears to be more sensitive to severe PEM. Head circumference, as a proxy to encephalic mass, has been found permanently reduced in children with sustained PEM from early uterine life through early infancy. These findings are similar to those produced in experimental animals. Using transillumination and ultrasonic scanning, Engsner et al[40] found that brain size was reduced in severe PEM and that lateral ventricles were normal in marasmus and enlarged in kwashiorkor and kwashiorkor-marasmus; however, with nutritional recovery brain size rapidly increased and ventricular volumes returned to normal within a few months. In general, however, children who have had early PEM have reduced head circumference in relation to norms for age, but it is affected either less than or to about the same degree as stature. Enzymes involved in brain energy utilization have been found altered.

Functionally, the severely undernourished individual has depressed mental function and altered EEG, which recover substantially and promptly with nutritional recovery, particularly if accompanied by proper stimulation. Peripheral nerve conduction is also reduced in kwashiorkor and recovers fully with nutritional rehabilitation.

Long-term mental performance appears not to be hampered substantially by undernutrition itself even when it is early and severe. This statement is based on long-term follow-up of children who became malnourished because of war or secondary to cystic fibrosis. Rather, it is impaired by the general deprivation that accompanies poverty, including poor health and nutrition, lack of stimulation, and poor mothering. There is a consensus that the combination of early PEM and postnatal lack of stimulation is the worst combination for proper mental development.

Cardiorespiratory Functions[11,44,45]

Heart atrophy and reduced cardiac work and functional reserve are characteristic of severe PEM. The ease with which heart failure can be induced by increased cardiorespiratory loads (severe anemia, overhydration, rapid expansion of circulatory volume, hypermetabolic states, pulmonary infections) has been recognized by personnel caring for children with severe PEM. The presence of "wet lungs" with superimposed infection has been a frequent postmortem finding. Venous return and cardiocirculatory reflexes are impaired, causing postural hypotension.

Pulmonary ventilation is decreased because of weakness of respiratory muscles, diminishing further venous return and the child's capacity to compensate metabolic pH changes and CO_2 accumulation. Shallow tachypnea and peripheral collapse are ominous signs of uncompensated acidosis.

Renal Functions and Water and Electrolyte Metabolism[46,47]

Renal mass, plasma flow, and glomerular filtration rate are diminished in severe PEM, and the latter are aggravated by dehydration and forward failure. Tubular function is also impaired, as manifested by the child's inability to handle water, sodium, and acid loads. Tubular concentrating mechanisms are less responsive to vasopressin, and phosphaturia and aminoaciduria are frequent. Fatty infiltration and cloudy swelling of tubular cells plus evidence of pyelonephritis are commonly described at autopsy of children with kwashiorkor.

Total and extracellular water as percent of body weight or body solids are increased in PEM children even in the absence of clinical edema. However, greater increments in all compartments are observed in relation to the severity of edema and to markedly decreased serum albumin levels (usually below 25 g per liter) and plasma colloido-osmotic pressure. This state of overhydration increases temporarily during early treatment with high-energy intakes. Intracellular water is decreased in absolute amounts, defined as percent of the norm for well-nourished children of the same age and/or the same stature, reflecting a deficit in cell mass in severe PEM. In relation to cell solids, however, intracellular water is increased. Multiple mechanisms are probably involved in producing the overhydrated state, but the phenomenon is still poorly understood. Intracellular water is increased concomitantly to excessive intracellular sodium and hydrogen ions and to deficiencies of potassium, magnesium, noncollagen protein, and other compounds such as glycogen. This imbalance possibly reflects the demonstrated altered cell-membrane permeability (membranes leaky to cations), defective production of adenosine triphosphate (ATP) by the cells and inefficient sodium pump, diminished capacity for potassium retention (associated with decreased intracellular proteins and glycogen), altered physical state of intracellular water, peroxidation of membrane lipids (due to excess of free radical damage), and hypersecretion and/or enhanced sensitivity to antidiuretic hormones (associated with elevated levels of circulating ferritin).

The magnitudes of intracellular changes in electrolyte concentrations are remarkable: Muscle biopsies and circulating leukocytes show a threefold increase in sodium (values around 140 mEq per liter of cell water) and a 20 to 30 percent reduction in potassium (values around 250 mEq per kilogram of fat-free cell solids), and magnesium (values around 12 mEq per kilogram wet weight). With nutritional recovery these values return to normal, but the rate is slow, requiring several weeks to reach normality even when these minerals are administered in higher than normal amounts. Muscle potassium recovers in a fashion parallel to that of myofibrillar protein.[48,49]

All organs, including the brain, participate in the intracellular potassium deficiency. Muscle and circulating cells show deficient magnesium levels, while brain, heart, liver, and kidney have a normal Mg/N ratio. Bone magnesium is most probably decreased, since marked magnesium retention has been observed during recovery from PEM. Cadaver analyses, ^{40}K counting, and mineral retention levels in relation to nitrogen retention confirm the potassium and magnesium deficit.

Plasma is hypo-osmolar (values around 270 mOs per liter) and often hyponatremic (values around 120 to 130 mEq per liter). The lower sodium concentrations carry a poor prognosis. Potassium values in plasma are generally normal in spite of the marked deficit in total body, intracellular, and exchangeable potassium. Magnesium values in plasma are highly variable. Hypokalemia and hypomagnesemia can be responsible for severe functional cardiovascular, digestive, and muscular alterations and must be treated as emergencies but with extreme caution and close monitoring.

Hematologic and Immunologic Functions[22,50]

Anemia, defined as low hemoglobin (Hb) concentration below acceptable levels, is the rule in severe PEM of the kwashiorkor and marasmus-kwashiorkor types. Marasmic children often have normal or only slightly reduced Hb concentrations. The erythrocyte is most often normal in average size (MCV), although marked anisocytosis occurs, combining hypochromic microcytes and macro-ovalocytes with spherocytes and even some target cells. This variety of cells reflects the combination of the hematologic condition prior to PEM and that which is the consequence of the PEM process itself.

Functionally, PEM is characterized by a reduction of active tissue mass and therefore of the demand for tissue oxygen delivery. As the more acute types of PEM kwashiorkor and marasmus-kwashiorkor develop, the reduction in tissue oxygen needs takes place at faster rates than the average rate of red cell turnover, leading to a state of relative polycythemia and triggering an adaptation characterized by inhibition of erythropoietin production and a decrease in erythropoiesis until a new equilibrium between tissue oxygen needs and total oxygen transport is reached. The result is a lower Hb concentration, since vascular space and total blood volume are not reduced to the same degree. However, physiologically this is not a "true anemia," since the ratio of total circulating hemoglobin to basal or resting oxygen consumption is the same or higher than that found in normal, nonanemic, or fully recovered children, and there is no correlation between this ratio and Hb concentration in severe PEM. Reticulocyte counts are near zero among those with higher total circulating hemoglobin–to–oxygen consumption ratio, and if hypoxia occurs even in the face of untreated severe PEM, reticulocytosis occurs, reflecting the capacity of erythropoiesis to respond if needed. Moreover, in uncomplicated severe PEM the response to hematinics (iron, folate, vitamin B_{12}, tocopherol) is conditioned by the rate of increase in active tissue mass achieved by protein and energy administration. When severe anemia is present, it can usually be traced to a severe anemia prior to the development of PEM; however, mild iron deficiency may be obscured by the iron deposition that takes place during the relative polycythemic phase, when dying red cells are not being replaced. Severely PEM children have liver and bone marrow iron reserves in excess of non-PEM children of the same socioeconomic characteristics. Serum ferritin levels are also higher. These, however, may reflect not only increased iron stores but also the presence of infection.

Markedly elevated ferritin levels are prognostic of a poor outcome, and in conjunction with low levels of plasma tocopherol, ascorbate, and zinc, blood selenium and red cell glutathione and its peroxidase have been implicated as a source of free-radical damage and as one of the etiologic factors in edema formation in kwashiorkor and marasmus-kwashiorkor.[49] During recovery there is a marked red cell expansion, and low hematinic reserves may show up as deficiencies. This is particularly true of folate and vitamin E; iron becomes limiting usually later during recovery because of the previously expanded iron reserves.

Immunity in severe PEM is markedly compromised, since all of the natural barriers and defense mechanisms against bacterial, fungal, and viral infections are impaired.[8,51,52] To begin with, the epithelial barriers are damaged by discontinuity, ulcerations, cornification and hyperkeratosis, and decreased cell renovation. Vitamin A deficiency and its impaired transport further aggravate the consequences of PEM per se. The gastric acidity barrier is diminished to degrees that allow fungal and bacterial overgrowth in the stomach. Epithelial protective mechanisms are also impaired because of reduced secretion of mucus, lysozyme, and secretory IgA.

Marked deficiencies in the cell-mediated immunity system are well documented, including atrophy of thymic and lymphocyte germinating centers (including Peyer's patches); reduced circulating T lymphocytes affecting primarily the natural killer and helper subsets, leading to a predominance of null cells; and decreased functional responses to stimuli that normally induce T-cell activity, including proliferation, differentiation, and interleukin-1 and -2 production.[53] Secretion of thymic hormones is also impaired. A clinical manifestation of these alterations is obliteration of delayed skin hypersensitivity. Zinc deficiency, common in severe PEM with infection, is also responsible for impairment of these integrated cell systems.

In contrast to the very poor function of the above system, humoral immunity is generally preserved except for extremely severe PEM. B-cell counts are either normal or increased, and circulating levels of all immunoglobulins are often elevated. This may be related to decreased T-suppressor cell activity. The secretory component of IgA is, however, inadequate.

The phagocytic and complement systems are also defective in PEM. Polymorphonuclear leukocytes and macrophages are often reduced both in the circulation and in tissues. Chemotaxis, phagocytic capacity, hexose monophosphate shunt burst activity, and killing capacity have been found defective to different degrees. Some of these defects are probably associated with impaired T-cell functions as described above. The complement system is also reduced in PEM, and anticomplement activity is often detected in children who also have circulating endotoxins.

The degree of immune impairment present in moderate PEM is debatable, but some defects are demonstrated in multiple battery tests. The presence of other deficiencies such as zinc, iron, magnesium, selenium, and various vitamins among populations with mild to moderate PEM makes the interpretation of several of these findings difficult. What is well established is that the kwashiorkor and kwashiorkor-marasmic types of PEM are more severely affected than the marasmic type, and that with nutritional recovery immune functions recover fully and rather promptly.

Musculoskeletal System[48,53,54]

Muscle noncollagen nitrogen is markedly reduced in severe PEM, whereas collagen protein is preserved, most probably because of its very slow turnover rate. Creatinine, OH-proline, and 3-methyl-histidine excretion are reduced, except when acute infection accelerates muscle wasting. Muscle protein loss is essentially parallel to the degree of total body protein deficit and has important implications in terms of potassium metabolism and energy utilization, because the muscle's capacity to retain potassium is parallel to the myofibrillar protein mass. Muscle power and tone are decreased as muscle atrophy ensues.

The skeletal system is retarded in maturation in relation to chronologic age, and both long and membranous bones are markedly demineralized owing to the subperiosteal deposition of poorly mineralized bone and increased endosteal bone resorption, whereas ossification processes at cartilaginous ossification centers are markedly impaired.[55] Episodes of severe PEM leave their marks in the diaphyseal-epiphyseal junctions as lines of bone-growth detention. Rickets can develop during nutritional recovery and catch-up growth if the increased needs of vitamin D and calcium are not met. Horizontal dental enamel hypoplasia and subsequent caries at the base of the crown of incisors, canines, and early molars are frequently seen among populations that have a high prevalence of PEM and are more frequent among children who have had a severe bout of PEM.[56]

Digestive Function

In experimental animals, deficits of fetal and perinatal nutrition induced by reducing uterine blood supply, by specific maternal dietary deficits in protein and/or total diet during different periods of pregnancy and lactation, or by limiting lactation volumes are associated in the pups with impaired growth and development of the digestive apparatus and more specifically of the liver, exocrine pancreas, and gut (the distal small intestine more than the proximal one). Cellularity is decreased, cell size is smaller, intestinal villi are defective, and the timing of functional differentiation is delayed. Some functions are more affected than others; for example, the activity of brush border hydrolytic enzymes (specifically lactase and alkaline phosphatase) and pancreatic amylase and lipase are markedly reduced, whereas other digestive enzymes are very much preserved (enterokinase, maltase, trypsin, chymotrypsin, and carboxypeptidases). In spite of the widespread effects observed, present evidence indicates that with adequate subsequent nutrition functional recovery takes place, even though at different rates: Most functions compromised during fetal life recover if the pups can suckle amply from normally nourished mothers. The general interpretation of these experimental studies is that early PEM produces essentially fully reversible delayed maturation of function. However, the total size of digestive organs may be permanently reduced, together with the whole body size of the animal.[57]

After birth the growth and maturation of the small intestine are partially dependent on stimulation and nutrition provided by intraluminal food, independent of nutritional status. Consequently, the restriction of energy and/or protein intakes, even in well-nourished animals, is associated with impaired intestinal growth or even mucosal atrophy, manifested by blunted villi, reduced cell turnover and migration, and poor brush-border enzyme activity. These characteristics have also been described in children with PEM of different severity.[58]

Chronically undernourished children live in environments with high forces of infection because of poor sanitation. These children also have decreased gastrointestinal (GI) infection defense mechanisms, diminished GI motility, and impaired gastric acid secretory capacity that reduces the gastric barrier to bacterial contamination. All of these mechanisms favor the development of a chronically altered GI ecology in which bacterial overgrowth is the rule and overt infectious processes and diarrhea are common. This chronic situation is similar to what has been described as "tropical enteropathy" in adult populations of the developing world and results in morphologic and functional abnormalities evident even among "normal" children and adults living in contaminated environments. These include blunting of mucosal villi throughout the small intestine, cellular infiltration in the lamina propria, presence of "free" deconjugated primary and secondary bile acids, and slightly reduced absorption of D-xylose and fat.[59-61]

Superimposed on the chronic situation described above is the effect of severe PEM, characterized by further reductions in energy and/or protein intakes and often by recurrent diarrheal episodes. A summary of the salient features observed in the digestive system of severely PEM children follows:

Salivary glands are atrophied and buccal mucosa cell turnover is reduced. Lingual papillary atrophy is the rule.[9,11]

Gastric mucosal atrophy and reduced secretory capacity have been documented. However, this does not include the secretion of intrinsic factor, which appears to be preserved except in the most severe cases of PEM. Bacteria and fungi are commonly seen in gastric aspirates. Although gastric motility has not been accurately measured, gastric dilatation associated with potassium deficiency and diarrhea is common.

The small intestine presents general atrophy that includes all layers and the ganglionic plexus. Intestinal motility is reduced and irregular even when the child has diarrhea. Columnar epithelial cells flatten. Diarrhea is associated with increases in cellular infiltration in the lamina propria and with further mucosal atrophy, particularly in the distal small intestine. Bacterial counts throughout the gut and the proportion of free bile acids are increased. The mucosal mitotic index is reduced primarily when energy deficit is predominant (marasmic children) and in the presence of diarrhea.[62,63]

Electron microscopy[64] shows multiple nonspecific abnormalities in the microvilli and in the basal region; the brush border is generally flattened and may essentially disappear in very severe cases with diarrhea; lactase activity is reduced and lactose intolerance is common. However, PEM per se does not appear to enhance lactose intolerance when diarrhea is absent. A certain degree of milk intolerance can be seen in a few PEM children even after full recovery; its cause is unknown.[60]

Liver production of conjugated bile acids appears reduced, as is the bile-acid pool. Conjugated bile acids are more glycine than taurine conjugates, and the concentrations of free primary and secondary bile acids are abnormally increased, as is bacterial overgrowth throughout the gut. These alterations result in inadequate lipid micellarization and in mucosal cell damage.[60-62]

Other functional deficits observed in severe PEM include malabsorption of both purified triolein and purified oleic acid; malabsorption of vitamin A-palmitate (stimulated by a subsequent dose of fat), conjugated bile acids, D-xylose, and mannitol; decreased rate of glucose absorption; and essentially preserved vitamin B_{12} absorption (with or without intrinsic factor administration) and amino acid–nitrogen, although both may be malabsorbed in very severe PEM.[65-68] Superimposed diarrhea is translated in reduced absorption of all the nutrients and bile acids, and even fecal nitrogen excretion correlates with fecal volume. Protein-losing enteropathy has also been demonstrated in some children with PEM and diarrhea.

Enterocyte damage is also demonstrated by the altered permeability to simple sugars and disaccharides (reduced for the former and increased for the latter).[66] In spite of cell damage, the enterocyte's capacity to re-esterify absorbed fatty acids is normal, as are the pattern and time sequence of plasma chylomicronemia after a dose of fat. Since the absorption of triglycerides and fatty acids is similarly affected, fat malabsorption appears to be due mostly to faulty intraluminal events that affect both free and esterified fatty acids. Consequently, lipase deficit in the gut is not the preponderant factor in fat malabsorption, whereas events leading to cellular uptake of fat seem to be the main culprits (e.g., micellar formation and cell damage, possibly because of bacterial overgrowth and free bile acid toxicity to the enterocyte).

Functional recovery occurs at different rates as the child recovers from severe PEM: D-xylose, stimulated vitamin A palmitate, vitamin B_{12}, and amino acid–nitrogen absorption recover very rapidly, independent of the level of repletion of total body protein estimated by the creatinine height index;

fatty acid and triglyceride absorption and the rate of glucose absorption recover pari passu with total body protein. Even after full nutritional recovery, blunting of intestinal villi, some degree of bacterial overgrowth, and slight elevations of free bile acids often persist, but these abnormalities are not accompanied by detectable functional impairments above those associated with the chronically altered GI ecology (tropical enteropathy).[60,65]

Pancreatic acinar atrophy and scarcity of zymogen granules are the rule in severe PEM. The volume and enzymatic contents of pancreatic juice in response to food or secretin and pancreozymin stimulation are often reduced. As PEM becomes more severe, the activities of lipase, trypsin, chymotrypsin, and amylase are diminished, in that order.[9-11] Some degree of persistent pancreatic exocrine deficiency has been described even months after nutritional recovery; however, the functional significance of this persistent abnormality is unknown. On the other hand, lipase production can be rapidly stimulated in severe PEM children by feeding fat-rich diets while the children are still severely undernourished and receiving an initial diet providing only 0.7 g of protein and 80 kcal per kilogram of body weight.[69]

Pancreatic endocrine function apparently can also be affected by acute and chronic PEM as well as by the consumption of cyanoglucoside-rich foods (cassava, sorghum, ham, millet, lima beans, linseed, and maize) together with chronic protein-deficient diets. These practices result in malnutrition-related diabetes mellitus (MRDM), which affects young populations who develop diabetic complications by age 30. MRDM includes fibrocalculous pancreatic diabetes (FCPD) and protein-deficient diabetes mellitus (PDDM) or J type of diabetes.[70]

TREATMENT OF SEVERE PROTEIN ENERGY MALNUTRITION

Three stages of treatment are generally recognized: (1) resolving life-threatening conditions, (2) restoring nutritional status without abrupt changes in homeostasis, and (3) ensuring nutritional rehabilitation.[12,19,71]

Ideally, children should be treated and rehabilitated at home; however, the presence of complications, generally of infectious nature, the degree of severity, and the lack of confidence that the family will be able to follow recommendations force hospital admissions of PEM children. The main reasons for avoiding hospitalization are the risk of cross-infection, the emotional separation of the child, and the often negative results of aggressive therapeutic behavior, predominant in hospital wards, by upsetting the long-term nutritional metabolic homeostasis the undernourished child has slowly achieved. In this regard, an essential principle in the treatment of severe PEM is aggressive therapy for infectious complications in the face of relative patience (conservative attitude) in dietary and water-electrolyte therapy. The reason for patience is that the child has in play very delicate hormonal and metabolic mechanisms that have allowed him or her to survive during the progression of undernutrition. The severely PEM child is in a slowed catabolic state (except if in hypermetabolism because of infection) to which he or she has arrived through several days or weeks of adaptation. Functional reserves are minimal and easily overwhelmed. Thus, dietary and water-electrolyte therapy must first gently turn the slow catabolic state into a slow anabolic state that allows readaptation toward tissue synthesis that will become extremely high later, during nutritional rehabilitation.

Resolving Life-Threatening Conditions

Infection and dehydration are often obscured in severe PEM. Infection is often masked by the lack of fever and leukocytosis. Antibody titers can be low, and skin tests may be falsely negative. Flaccidity, hypothermia, obnubilation, impending circulatory collapse, and petechiae suggest a septicemic state. Careful clinical examination and complementary examinations can reveal a pneumonic process, favored by wet lungs if blood volume and osmotic pressure are rapidly increased by overenthusiastic rehydration and/or intravenous plasma or blood administration. Also common are otitis, urinary infections (often silent), and GI infections that may be initially diagnosed by a progressively increasing abdominal girth and decreased intestinal sounds prior to massive diarrhea. Early keratomalacia and meningeal signs should be carefully looked for. Any suspicion of bacterial infection should be investigated immediately and treated promptly and vigorously with antibiotics and other supportive measures suited to the suspected infection. Even though most PEM children have intestinal parasitism, very rarely does a complication develop that merits treatment before the child is in the phase of nutritional rehabilitation. In the presence of edema, the more reliable signs of dehydration are dry mucous membranes, low urinary output (less than 200 to 300 ml per day or spaced urinations), rapid and weak pulse, low blood pressure, and mental deterioration (which forewarns of impending circulatory collapse). Poor skin turgor can be falsely positive when the child is emaciated. It must be remembered that the severely PEM child is overhydrated, hypo-osmolar, and frequently slightly acidotic and that renal urine-concentrating and acid-secreting mechanisms are functioning poorly. Cell sodium is increased and potassium is decreased. Plasma electrolytes may reveal slight hyponatremia; potassium levels are usually normal. Because of hypoproteinemia and acidosis, these children have a relative tolerance to hypocalcemia, whereas a tetany-like syndrome is often due to magnesium deficiency and hypomagnesemia.

Rehydration and alimentation should be by the oral, nasogastric, or enteral route; parenteral rehydration and alimentation should be a last resort, when attempts to rehydrate by the former routes fail. The dangers of hyperosmolarity, blood volume expansion, poor insulin responses, and infection must guide a very cautious start of parenteral alimentation. A minimal urinary output of 200 ml per day should be achieved (micturition every 2 to 3 hours).

The rehydrating solutions should have an osmolality close to 280 mOsm per liter and provide 2 to 3 mEq of sodium and calcium, 1 mEq of magnesium, and 20 to 30 kcal per kilogram per day in a solution containing 50 g of glucose or sucrose per liter, until urine output is verified. If the kidneys are working, 6 mEq of potassium per kilogram per day should also be provided. This solution should be administered at an initial rate of 10 to 20 ml per kilogram of body weight per hour, and its rate and composition should be changed according to frequent evaluations. If diarrhea and/or vomiting persist, the lost volume should be replaced by a solution containing 35 mEq of sodium and 30 mEq of potassium per liter of 5 percent glucose. If diuresis is poor, potassium administration should proceed with caution or should be withheld until satisfactory renal function is restored.

Plasma should be administered only in cases with serum protein levels below 3 g per deciliter, anuria, and signs of impending collapse. Ten ml per kilogram in 2 hours should be administered intravenously, followed by the solutions and rates described above. Transfusions of whole blood or packed cells are indicated only when anemia is severe and there are signs of cardiorespiratory decompensation. In these cases, the volume should be just enough to control the problem and should be administered slowly. Raising hemoglobin levels more than 20 g per liter is risky, since heart failure can be induced because of limited cardiac reserve in the face of rapid blood volume expansion.

Occasionally marasmic children more than kwashiorkor children suffer from primary hypoglycemia. Repeated administration of sugar-containing solutions or repeated small feedings take care of the problem if it is not secondary to infection.

Ocular signs of vitamin A deficiency are a true emergency in PEM children. The routine oral administration of 100,000 units of water-miscible retinyl-acetate prevents acute corneal ulceration. If necessary, this dose can be repeated in 2 days or administered parenterally.

In our experience, rarely does hepatic failure occur in severely undernourished children. However, this syndrome is not uncommon in certain areas of Africa and the Caribbean where bush teas are frequently administered to these children. The usual therapy for this condition should be established, withholding the administration of high dietary protein to accelerate nutritional recovery until liver function is reestablished.

Restoring Nutritional Status

The transition from a very inadequate intake in quantity and quality to a diet tailored to achieve maximal recovery from PEM should be without abrupt changes and based on good-quality foods. Upon admission, intakes should provide between 80 and 100 percent of energy and protein requirements in a liquid diet based on the appropriate kind of milk considering the child's age, with sugar and vegetable oil added. This liquid diet should be administered at short intervals totaling about 100 ml per kilogram per day. Vitamin and mineral supplements are added to supply a safe excess above RDAs. Supplementary iron intake, however, is delayed until the child is already responding to progressive increments in protein and energy because of increased risk of septicemia when iron is administered earlier in the course of treatment.

This level of intake is maintained for 1 or 2 days, during which the tolerance to the diet is assessed. Generally this diet is provided to all children even when oral rehydration is proceeding. In this case, it can be alternated with the rehydration solution. Many kwashiorkor or marasmus-kwashiorkor children at first are anorexic or have difficulty in ingesting and retaining the diet. Gentle insistence in feeding the child by the nursing staff or the parents and relatives and a good dose of patience are essential at this stage. If diarrhea persists for the 2 days of this introductory diet and stools are of the fermentative type (acid, frothy, positive to the presence of reducing agents) and/or excess hydrogen is exhaled, lactose intolerance can be suspected and a synthetic low-lactose formula based on calcium caseinate, lactose-free milk, or formulated vegetable protein mixtures can be substituted for milk. Tolerance to milk-based formula will be tested again later in treatment with the hope of discharging the child consuming all the milk he or she can tolerate.

From the second day on, depending on tolerance and on weight changes, intakes should be increased every other day by making the formula more concentrated, to reach intakes four to five times the RDA for protein and up to three to four times the RDA for energy, plus abundant vitamins and minerals by the seventh to tenth day. Generally by the third or fourth day, anorexia has changed to a ravenous appetite and the child is tolerating a diet that provides about 2 g of protein and 120 kcal per kilogram per day. Faster increments can be tried to reach protein intakes of around 4 g per kilogram per day, which are sufficient to allow maximal recovery of lean body mass and intracellular potassium retention. Energy intakes can be a high as 250 to 300 kcal per kilogram per day, and weight gain can reach up to 25 times the normal rate for a child of similar age.

The edematous child's initial response may be loss of weight or stationary weight while edema is clinically disappearing. Abrupt weight losses should be viewed with care because of danger of hemodynamic decompensation, dehydration, and electrolyte imbalances.

The best signs of progress are mood changes: The child becomes interested in the environment and begins to smile, and he or she eats with tremendous appetite. Diarrhea stops, the child begins to recover strength and to catch up in weight and length. At this stage, and depending on the child's age, other foods can be progressively introduced to reach a normal diet as soon as possible. Nutritional rehabilitation is now on its way. By this time the child is receiving iron supplements, is treated for intestinal parasitism, is being immunized, if needed, and the tuberculin test is repeated.

Ensuring Nutritional Rehabilitation

This phase of treatment should take place outside the hospital under the direct care of those in charge of providing adequate nutrition and health to the child and under the supervision of adequately trained community personnel (e.g., health promoters, community health workers, primary health workers, auxiliary nurses). This phase should have a significant educational component and community involvement in order to prevent the development of new cases of severe PEM, while the child being rehabilitated serves as a training case. Traditional foods in adequate combinations should be the basis of the diet; physical, emotional, and mental stimulation is essential as soon as the child responds to the environment and should be incremented in this treatment phase. The follow-up of growth and health of the child should be ensured.

Food intake and growth rates are above normal until the child reaches his or her normal weight for height, when most often a diminution of appetite is apparent and the child tends to follow the growth channel defined by his or her height. The child by this time is probably stunted and catch-up in height, if it occurs, is a long-term process. As long as the child is healthy, active, and happy and follows height growth in a defined channel and weight for height are maintained, nutritional rehabilitation has been accomplished.

Treatment Outside the Hospital

Children with moderate and severe PEM without life-threatening complications can be treated and their nutritional status restored outside the hospital setting, ideally while the child remains at home. This requires, however, organized community involvement around the health and nutrition of the population. Several modalities of nutrition rehabilitation programs exist and have proved functional and efficient. These include nutrition education and rehabilitation services and food supplementation programs with or without direct supervision of food intake.

The most effective programs for nutritional recovery of PEM children include careful monitoring of dietary intake; prevention of infections; mental, emotional, and physical stimulation; and family and community involvement in the process of education that takes advantage of the dramatic changes that occur as their own children recover their health with food alone.

This process must also take into account the fact that the presence of one child with PEM of any degree of severity within a family qualifies that family as nutritionally at risk. Similarly, the presence of several families at risk qualifies the community as nutritionally at risk. Under this light, nutritional recovery of a child with PEM must be accompanied by actions leading to community and family prevention of undernutrition. This entails a multidisciplinary approach that includes food and nutrition surveillance within structured health and community development efforts.

REFERENCES

1. United Nations Administrative Committee on Coordination, Subcommittee on Nutrition (UNACC/SCN). First report on the world nutrition situation. Geneva: ACC/SCN, WHO, 1987.
2. Schürch B, Scrimshaw NS, eds. Chronic energy deficiency: consequences and related issues. Lausanne, Switzerland: IDECG-Nestlé Foundation, 1988.
3. Piwoz EG, Viteri FE. Studying health and nutrition behavior by examining household decision-making, intra-household resource distribution, and the role of women in these processes. Food Nutr Bull 1985; 7:1-31.
4. Chen LC, Scrimshaw NS, eds. Diarrhea and malnutrition. Interactions, mechanisms and interventions. New York: Plenum Press, 1983.
5. Mönckeberg F, ed. Desnutrición infantil. INTA, Universidad de Chile. Impresora Creces, 1988.
6. Munro HN, Suter PM, Russel RM. Nutritional requirements of the elderly. Annu Rev Nutr 1987; 7:23-49.
7. Mata LJ. The children of Santa María Cauqué: a prospective field study of health and growth. Cambridge, MA: MIT Press, 1978.
8. Myrvik QN. Nutrition and immunology. In: Shils ME, Young VR, eds. Modern nutrition in health and disease. Philadelphia: Lea and Febiger, 1988: 585.
9. Trowell HC, Davies JNP, Dean RFA. Kwashiorkor. London: Edward Arnold, 1954.
10. Alleyne GAO, Hay RW, Picou DI, Stanfield JP, Whitehead RG. Protein-energy malnutrition. London: Edward Arnold, 1977.
11. Viteri FE, Behar M, Arroyave G, Scrimshaw NS. Clinical aspects of protein malnutrition. In: Munro HN, Allison JB, eds. Mammalian protein metabolism. Vol 2. New York: Academic Press, 1964: 523
12. Torún B, Viteri FE. Protein-energy malnutrition. In: Warren KS, Mahmud AAF, eds. Tropical and geographical medicine. 2nd ed. New York: McGraw-Hill, 1988: 984.
13. Viteri FE, Schumacher L, Silliman K. Maternal malnutrition and the fetus. Semin Perinatol 1989; 13:236-249.
14. Stein Z, Susser M, Saenger G. Famine and human development: the Dutch hunger winter of 1944/45. New York: Oxford University Press, 1975.
15. Kretchmer N, Shumacher L, Silliman K. Biological factors affecting intrauterine growth. Semin Perinatol 1989; 13:169-179.
16. Viteri FE. Considerations of the effect of nutrition on the body composition and physical working capacity of young Guatemalan adults. In: Scrimshaw NS, Altschul AM, eds. Amino acid fortification of protein foods. Cambridge, MA: MIT Press, 1971: 350.
17. Solomons NW, Allen LH. The functional assessment of nutritional status: principles, practice and potential. Nutr Rev 1983; 41:33-50.
18. Puffer RR, Serrano CV. Patterns of birthweights. Washington, DC: Pan American Health Organization/World Health Organization, 1987.
19. Torún B, Viteri FE. Protein-energy malnutrition. In: Shils ME, Young VR, eds. Modern nutrition in health and disease. 7th ed. Philadelphia: Lea and Febiger, 1988: 746.
20. Stanier MW, Holmes EG. Malnutrition in African adults. Br J Nutr 1954; 8:155-164.
21. Scrimshaw NS. The phenomenon of famine. Annu Rev Nutr 1987; 7:1-21.
22. Viteri FE. Primary protein-energy malnutrition: clinical, biochemical and metabolic changes. In: Suskind RM, ed. Textbook of pediatric nutrition. New York: Raven Press, 1981: 189.
23. Waterlow JC. Fatty liver disease in infants in the British West Indies. MRC Spec Rep Ser No 263. London: HMSO, 1948.
24. Gomez F, Ramos-Galván R, Frenk S, Cravioto J, Chavez R, Vasquez J. Mortality in second and third degree malnutrition. J Trop Pediatr 1956; 2:77-83.
25. Viteri FE, Alvarado J. The creatinine height index: its use in the estimation of the degree of protein depletion and repletion in protein-calorie malnourished children. Pediatrics 1970; 56:696-706.
26. Wellcome Trust Working Party: Classification of infantile malnutrition. Lancet 1970; ii:302-303.
27. Waterlow JC. Classification and definition of protein-calorie malnutrition. Br Med J 1972: 3:566-569.
28. Waterlow JC, Buzina R, Keller W, Lane JM, Nichman MZ, Tanner JM. The presentation and use of height and weight data for comparing the nutritional status of groups of children under the age of ten years. Bull WHO 1977; 55:489-498.
29. Jelliffe EF, Jelliffe DB, eds. The arm circumference as a public health index of protein calorie malnutrition of early childhood. J Trop Pediatr 1969; 15:177-260.
30. Waterlow JC, Alleyne GAD. Protein malnutrition in children: advances in knowledge in the last ten years. Adv Prot Chem 1971; 25:117-241.
31. Widdowson EM, McCance RA. The effects of chronic undernutrition and of total starvation in growing and adult rats. Br J Nutr 1956; 10:363-373.
32. McCance RA, Strangeways WMB. Protein catabolism and oxygen consumption during starvation in infants, young adults and old men. Br J Nutr 1954; 8:21-32.
33. Kerr DS, Stevens CG, Robinson HM, Picou D. Hypoglycemia and the regulation of fasting glucose metabolism in malnutrition. In: Gardner LI, Amacher R, eds. Endocrine aspects of malnutrition. Santa Ynez, CA: The Kroc Foundation, 1973: 313.
34. Wohlheuter WM, Harper AE. Co-induction of rat liver branched chain α-keto acid dehydrogenase activities. J Biol Chem 1970; 245:2391-2401.
35. Keys A, Brozek J, Henschel A, Mickelsen O, Taylor HL. The biology of human starvation. Minneapolis: University of Minnesota Press, 1950.
36. Viteri RE, Pineda O. Effects on body composition and body function. In: Blix G, Hofvander Y, Vahlquist B, eds. Famine: a symposium dealing with nutrition and relief operations in times of disaster. Uppsala, Sweden: Almquist and Wisells; 1971: 25.
37. Gardner LI, Amacher P, eds. Endocrine aspects of malnutrition. Santa Ynez, CA: The Kroc Foundation, 1973.
38. Becker DJ. The endocrine responses to protein energy malnutrition. Annu Rev Nutr 1983: 3:187-212.

39. Bengoa JM. Significance of malnutrition and priorities for its prevention. In: Berg A, Scrimshaw NS, Call DA, eds. Nutrition, national development and planning. Cambridge, MA: 1971:104.
40. Engsner G, Habte D, Sjogren I, Vahlquist B. Brain growth in children with kwashiorkor. Acta Paediatr Scand 1974; 63:687–694.
41. Cravioto J, DeLicardie ER. Nutrition, the nervous system and behavior. Washington, DC: Pan American Health Organization/World Health Organization, 1972.
42. Winick M, Rosso P. Head circumference and cellular growth of the brain in normal and marasmic children. J Pediatr 1969; 74:774–778.
43. Pollitt E. A critical view of three decades of research on the effects of chronic energy malnutrition on behavioral development. In: Schürch B, Scrimshaw NS, eds. Chronic energy deficiency: consequences and related issues. Lausanne, Switzerland: IDECG–Nestlé Foundation, 1988: 77.
44. Viart P. Hemodynamic findings in severe protein calorie malnutrition. Am J Clin Nutr 1977; 30:334–338.
45. Viart P. Hemodynamic findings during treatment of protein calorie malnutrition. Am J Clin Nutr 1978; 31:911–926.
46. Klahr S, Alleyne GAO. Effects of chronic protein-calorie malnutrition on the kidney. Kidney Int 1973; 3:129–145.
47. Garrow JS, Smith R, Ward EE, eds. Electrolyte metabolism in severe infantile malnutrition. Oxford: Pergamon Press, 1968.
48. Nichols BL, Alvarado J, Hazelwood DF, Viteri RE. Clinical significance of muscle potassium depletion in protein-calorie malnutrition. J Pediatr 1972; 80:319–330.
49. Golden MHN. The consequences of protein deficiency in man and its relationship to the features of kwashiorkor. In: Blaxter K, Waterlow JC, eds. Nutritional adaptation in man. London: John Libbey, 1985: 169.
50. Viteri FE, Alvarado J, Luthringer DG, Wood RP, II. Hematological changes in protein calorie malnutrition. Vitam Horm 1968; 27:573–614.
51. Keusch GT. Nutrition and immune function. In: Warren KS, Mahmoud AAF, eds. Tropical and geographical medicine. New York: McGraw-Hill, 1984: 212.
52. Wade S, Parent G, Bleiberg-Daniel F, Maire B, Fall M, Schneider D, LeMoullac B, Dardenne M. Thymulin (Zn-FTS) activity in protein energy malnutrition: new evidence for interaction between malnutrition and infection on thymic function. Am J Clin Nutr 1988; 47:305–311.
53. Picou D, Halliday D, Garrow JS. Total body protein, collagen and non-collagen protein in infantile protein malnutrition. Clin Sci 1966; 30:345–351.
54. Waterlow JC, Cravioto J, Stephen JML. Protein malnutrition in man. Adv Protein Chem 1960; 15:131–238.
55. Garn SM, Guzman MA, Wagner B. Subperiosteal gain and endosteal loss in protein-calorie malnutrition. Am J Phys Anthrop 1969; 30:153–155.
56. Sweeney AE, Saffir AJ, de Leon R. Linear hypoplasia of deciduous incisor teeth in malnourished children. Am J Clin Nutr 1971; 24:29–31.
57. Lebenthal E, Young CM. Effects of intrauterine and postnatal malnutrition on the ontogeny of gut function. Prog Food Nutr Sci 1986; 10:315–335.
58. Levine GM, Deren JJ, Steiger E, Zinno R. Role of oral intake in maintenance of gut mass and disaccharidase activity. Gastroenterology 1974; 67:975–982.
59. Viteri FE, Schneider RE. Gastrointestinal functions in children with mild to severe protein-energy malnutrition and during recovery. Topics Paediatr 1980; 2:63–71.
60. Viteri FE, Schneider RE. Gastrointestinal alterations in protein-calorie malnutrition. Med Clin North Am 1974; 58:1487–1505.
61. Schneider RE, Contreras C, Viteri FE. Studies on the luminal events of lipid absorption in protein-calorie malnutrition (PCM) children; its relation with nutritional recovery and diarrhea. I. Capacity of the duodenal content to achieve micellar solubilization of lipids. Am J Clin Nutr 1974; 27:777–787.
62. Schneider RE, Viteri FE. Studies on the luminal events of lipid absorption in protein-calorie malnutrition (PCM) children; its relation with nutritional recovery and diarrhea. II. Alteration in the bile salts of the duodenal content. Am J Clin Nutr 1974; 27:788–796.
63. Schneider RE, Viteri FE. Some morphologic and functional alterations in the gastrointestinal tract in protein calorie malnourished children. Am J Clin Nutr 1972; 25:1092–1102.
64. Duque E, Lotero H, Bolanõs O, Mayoral LG. Enteropathy in adult protein malnutrition: ultrastructural findings. Am J Clin Nutr 1975; 28:914–924.
65. Viteri FE, Flores JM, Alvarado J, Behar M. Intestinal malabsorption in malnourished children and during recovery. Relationship between severity of protein deficiency and the malabsorption process. Am J Digest Dis 1973; 18:201–211.
66. Behrens RH, Lunn PQ, Northrop CA, Hanlon PW, Neale G. Factors affecting the integrity of the intestinal mucosa of Gambian children. Am J Clin Nutr 1987; 45:1433–1441.
67. Alvarado J, Vargas W, Diaz N, Viteri FE. Vitamin B_{12} absorption in protein-calorie malnourished children and during recovery: influence of protein depletion and diarrhea. Am J Clin Nutr 1973; 26:595–599.
68. James WPT. Intestinal absorption in protein calorie malnutrition. Lancet 1968; i:33–335.
69. Viteri FE, Contreras C, Schneider RE. Intestinal malabsorption in malnourished children and during recovery. Duodenal contents of lipase, nitrogen and micellar fat after fat stimulation. Arch Latinoam Nutr 1972; 2:613–627.
70. World Health Organization Study Group: Diabetes mellitus. Geneva: WHO, 1985.
71. Picou DM. Evaluation and treatment of the malnourished child. In: Suskind RM, ed. Textbook of pediatric nutrition. New York: Raven Press, 1981: 217.

PART 4

Obesity

William B. Weil Jr., M.D.

The traditional, historic concepts that a fat child is easily recognized, has become fat from overeating, will remain fat unless actively treated, and should respond to a calorie-restricted diet if it is adhered to are far too simplistic for what is now known about obesity. Yet there is no comprehensive contemporary concept in hand to replace these erroneous views of the problem of obesity in childhood.

Obesity, in fact, is a condition that is difficult to define and variable in its course, has important but uncertain effects, is multifactorial in etiology, and presents great difficulty in treatment. The problem is further complicated by our inability to distinguish specific etiologic factors in a specific child and a tendency for familial aggregation with the concomitant therapeutic difficulty of treating entire families.

DEFINITION

The definition of obesity, an excess of body fat, is complicated by two problems: how to measure body fatness and how to decide what is excessive.

Research Methods

Measurement of body fatness has been approached in three ways, each with its own advantages and disadvantages. The most precise method, direct carcass analysis, has been used for many experimental animals and on a few occasions on human bodies.[1] Basically the approach has been to weigh the entire carcass, then to dry and homogenize the entire animal. Once the carcass has been reduced to a dry homogeneous mass, an aliquot of dried, ground material is used for lipid extraction. The loss of weight resulting from the defatting process is used to calculate the total body lipid. While this method is laborious, it is relatively precise. However, the value obtained represents not only what is normally considered the body fat but also includes almost all other lipids in the body, many of them not ordinarily associated with adipose tissue. In addition, the lipid extraction method does not include the nonlipid constituents of adipose tissue, i.e., the cellular protein and fluid of the adipocytes and the supporting tissue of the fat lobules. Nevertheless the method has a precision that is useful when comparing groups of animals that have all been examined by the same procedure. Studies of dead human fetuses, newborns, and a few adults have provided information on the development of adipose tissue in the developing fetus[2] and over 25 years ago led to the conclusion that the newborn infant of the woman with diabetes is large primarily because of an increase in total body fat.[3] Because of changes in the social acceptability of such procedures, carcass analysis of human subjects is no longer feasible. In addition, it is unlikely to lead to any useful information that could not be obtained by other methodology.

The second set of methods is less direct but is applicable to living subjects and includes underwater weighing and the counting of naturally occurring total body ^{40}K. Both of these methods rely upon the assumption that lean (fat-free) tissue in the body has a constant density and that the density of the total body is lowered by an amount proportional to the amount of the lower-density fat that is present. The fat is also assumed to have a constant density. Because bone has a higher density than does muscle or the viscera, any variation in the proportion of bone to other "lean" tissue yields divergent results.[4] In addition, variation in the amount of air in the gastrointestinal (GI) tract or incomplete exhalation prior to submersion also causes variation in the results. Finally, it is obvious that in addition to requiring specialized equipment, this method is applicable only to individuals able to hold their breath long enough for the underwater weighing to take place.

The whole-body scintillation counting of ^{40}K obviates some of these problems but has its own limitations. The major assumption on which this method relies is that the amount of potassium in the lean body mass is a constant, in the range of 55 mEq K^+ per kilogram of lean body. Obviously the method would not be applicable to anyone who is potassium deficient. The ratio of ^{39}K to ^{40}K is also assumed to be constant, and this is probably quite reasonable. The method also assumes the absence of K^+ from fat. The amount of fat is calculated as the difference between actual weight and the weight of the lean body mass derived from the measurement of total body K^+. As with underwater weighing, any variation in the composition of the lean body mass alters the results. The major disadvantage of the method is the requirement for a large, expensive piece of equipment.[4]

Isotope dilution, neutron activation, and electrical impedance are other methods that lead to indirect determinations of total body fat.[4]

Clinical Methods

The third set of methods is more indirect, measures relative fatness rather than total fat, and has depended on the correlation with either underwater weighing or ^{40}K counting for validation. The basic method involves the estimation of subcutaneous fat thickness either by measurement of skin folds at specific locations—actually the measurement of a double layer of skin and subcutaneous tissues (the skin "fold")—or by measurement from imaging processes such as ultrasonography, radiography, computed tomography, or magnetic resonance imaging.[5] Currently, the most popular of these methods for measuring subcutaneous fat is that using skin fold calipers, which can now be obtained quite easily.[6]

Inherent in this methodology is the assumption that the amount of subcutaneous fat bears some regular relationship to the amount of fat in other body sites. In addition, there is considerable variation in the amount of subcutaneous fat over the surface of the body, and the pattern of distribution varies with age and sex and probably between individuals of the same sex and age as well. To overcome this shortcoming, many investigators measure skin folds at several locations (midtriceps, subscapular, iliac crest, and midabdomen) and sum the measurements in an unweighted manner.[7] However, there is no consensus as to whether the measurement of summed skin folds is any better as a measure of relative fatness than the values at one or two sites or weighted values prior to summing.[7] In any case, skin fold values are assumed to reflect a relative degree of adiposity and are generally not used to estimate total body fat. Tables with percentile distributions of triceps and subscapular skin folds for the United States population by age and sex have been published by the National Center for Health Statistics.[8]

Weight As a Measure of Adiposity

The least valuable but most commonly used measure of adiposity is weight or weight with some correction for height. Clearly measurement of weight will accurately reflect those individuals who are overweight if compared with appropriate standards. However, it has been demonstrated that excessive weight and excessive adiposity are not well correlated.[9] Roche reported correlations of about 0.3 for adiposity and weight in children.[10] Nevertheless, reports continue to be published equating overweight and adiposity. One common measure in adults is to use weight that is 20 percent above that expected for height and sex as a measure of excessive adiposity.[11] There have been comparable reports in the pediatric literature as well.[12] To improve on weight as a measure of adiposity, correction for height has been used in two ways. In the first method, the NCHS graphs of weight for height in preadolescent children have been utilized, and adiposity has been defined as weight for height that exceeds either the 85th or 95th percentile.[13] The second method of "correcting" weight for height has been the body mass index (BMI), which is calculated as weight in kilograms divided by the height in meters squared (wt/ht^2).[14] Although the use of height to modify the value for weight alone improves the correlation with adiposity to values in the range of 0.6 to 0.7, the correlation with triceps skin folds is in the range of 0.8.[10] All the measures using weight corrected for height are confounded by frame size. Dietz points out that BMI (wt/ht^2) correlates well with bony chest breadth (a measure of frame size; $r = 0.56 - 0.60$). "In addition the correlation coefficient of lean body mass with BMI approximates $r = 0.65$." He further states "in samples of children controlled for age, sex, height and triceps skinfold thickness, weight varied by 20 percent on either side of the mean for boys and girls aged six to eleven years old."[15]

The reason for detailing the issues of measurement of adiposity is that the preponderance of studies that form the basis of our current understanding of obesity are based on measures of weight or BMI, both of which may be quite misleading in identifying obesity, especially obesity of moderate degree and in young children and adolescents. Current research has focused more and more on skin fold thickness.

REFERENCE STANDARDS

The second problem in defining obesity, after some measure of adiposity has been selected, is to set some level of fatness above which persons can be said to be obese. The problem arises because degrees of adiposity have a unimodal distribution similar to that for many other biologic variables, being kurtotic and skewed to the higher values.[16] There are no biologic discontinuities among lean, normal, and fat persons. Thus, some level must be identified arbitrarily to separate persons who are obese from those who are not.

In general, two approaches have been used to establish levels of fatness that would define obesity. One approach has been to set some level independent of the distribution of the variable in the population. The use of 20 percent above expected weight for height and sex yields different proportions for the number of obese persons in a population, depending on the population examined and, more importantly, on the weight-for-height standard that is selected. A commonly used standard is that derived from the Metropolitan Life Insurance Company's data on longevity and weight.[17,18] These standards use an ideal weight for height related to the policyholders who live the longest. Since longevity is only one measure of healthiness and since life insurance policy owners do not form a representative sample of the United States population, there is appropriate concern about such a standard. The statement that "the average American is overweight" is based on this approach; the mean, median, and modal values for weight for the United States population are larger than the "ideal." Furthermore, in the life insurance data, the ideal weight for women is generally about 10 pounds less than for men. In the United States population the median weights for men and women of the same height and age are equivalent.[19]

The alternative approach in defining levels of adiposity that signify obesity is population based and uses some percentile level as the indicator for obesity. For example, many investigators using skin fold thicknesses have adopted the 85th percentile as indicating obesity and values above the 95th percentile indicating the "superobese."[16] In studies of children, population-based percentile boundaries are most commonly used.

PREVALENCE

The level at which one sets the cutoff for obesity determines the prevalence of the condition in the population being sampled. If one were to adopt the median value in a population, indicating that anyone with adiposity greater than the average was obese, there would be a prevalence of obesity of 50 percent. Similarly, by using the 85th percentile, 15 percent of the population on which the standards are based must be obese. Thus, any figures that indicate the prevalence of obesity in children and adults in the United States are arbitrary and depend on the criteria that one wishes to establish.

It is possible, however, to examine subgroups in the population to determine if they are more or less obese than one another or relative to the general population, as long as the criteria selected are valid for measuring adiposity. One can also examine whether one group or another is more or less overweight, provided that one does not confuse "overweightness" with obesity. Body mass index (BMI) or other corrections of weight for height, since they also correlate equally well with body frame and lean body mass as they do with body fatness, are equally suspect when they are used to define obesity per se. There is, however, enough of a correlation between BMI and weight-for-height values with adiposity that some useful information about the prevalence of obesity in groups can be obtained from these measures of weight, but applying these values to define obesity in specific individuals is not warranted. For single cases triceps or other skin fold thicknesses are more reliable.

Another problem arises when one examines populations cross-sectionally over a period of time. For example, Gortmaker et al examined data from the first and second Health and Nutrition Examination Surveys (HANES) in the 1970s and compared that population using the 85th percentile triceps skin fold figures for the same age group of children examined in the 1960s in the National Health Examination Survey (NHES). On this basis they concluded that obesity in children has increased in prevalence by 40 percent (15 to 21 percent) in children and adolescents.[20]

Secular trends of this type have been reported for heights and weights of children as well as adiposity.[21] Thus, over the past 50 years, children seem to be getting larger earlier and maturing earlier than they did in the recent past. The significance of such information is difficult to evaluate because it is not associated with any adverse change in health status for the group as a whole. In fact, by most measures one would consider the population of children to be healthier today than it was 50 years ago. For the period 1960 to 1987, the death rate for children 5 to 14 years of age declined from 64 per 100,000 population to 31.[22] This raises the question of whether it is appropriate to apply population-based standards obtained at one period of time to a subsequent population whose growth patterns and general health status have changed in the interim.

NATURAL HISTORY

The natural history of obesity in children involves attempts to answer one question: To what extent does obesity persist from any period of childhood into adult life? Two problems underlie the difficulty in obtaining a definitive answer to the question. A major problem is that many studies have used wt/ht values such as BMI rather than more direct measures of fatness, so that the results are better interpreted in terms of the extent to which overweight children become overweight adults. The other problem is that most studies have covered short periods of time and inferences have been drawn on the basis of overlapping periods of life. As an example of the difficulty created by such an approach, consider the possibility that over a period of 5 years, 50 percent of obese children would remain obese. If one started with a cohort of 1,000 obese 2-year-olds, 500 would be obese at 7 years of age, 250 at 12, and only 125 at 17. This would be less than the expected number (15 percent) in the general population. Yet at each 5-year interval it could be reported that the persistence of obesity was 50 percent. The unwary might then assume that of 1,000 obese children, 500 would be obese as adults. In fact, data from the Bogalusa Heart Study compared children at 1 and 7 years of age using the 80th percentile for subscapular skin folds. They found values as high as 40 percent in one group of children; i.e., of those above the 80th percentile at age 1 year, 40 percent were still above the 80th percentile at age 7 years.[23] By extrapolation, that would be 16 percent by age 13 and only 6 percent by age 19. Such extrapolations are not scientifically sound, but they do indicate that significant "tracking" for 6 years might become insignificant if the trend continued for 12 or 18 years.

Probably the most representative data are from the studies done in Tecumseh, Michigan, by Stanley Garn and others. Their data, which cover a 20-year period, do show evidence of tracking. About 25 percent of the initially obese children were also obese 20 years later.[24,25] Remembering that in any random population 15 percent would be obese because they used the 85th percentile as their cutoff level for obesity, this would indicate an obese child has a relative risk of about 1.7 of being obese 20 years later. However, several important points in these data need to be considered. (1) In general, individuals at the highest and lowest levels of adiposity both had a tendency to regress toward the mean. (2) Obese girls had a somewhat greater likelihood of being obese after 20 years than did obese boys. (3) Only 10 percent of obese boys were obese at each of four evaluations during the 20 years, and only 20 percent of the obese girls remained obese throughout the study. The remainder of the obese children had left their obese category sometime during the 20 years but had returned to that category by 20 years.[25]

Another issue of significance in the overall consideration of obesity is that the vast majority of obese adults were not obese as children. For example, in a study of Danish draftees using BMI, 68 percent of those found to have a BMI in excess of 31 on induction had not had elevated BMIs at 7 or at 13 years of age, and only 9 percent of those with elevated BMIs on induction had had elevated BMIs at 7 and at 13 years of age.[26] In a study of over 3,000 English children followed for 36 years, only 21 percent of obese 36-year-olds had been obese at age 11.[27]

Thus children who are obese, especially girls, are at higher risk of being obese as adults, but the majority of these obese children, 60 to 70 percent, will not be obese as adults, and the greatest proportion of obese adults were not obese as children.

Because these studies have grouped all obese children together, the data obscure the finding that there are criteria, in addition to sex, which alter the probability of adult obesity among obese children. The factors that increase the probability of adult obesity include the presence of other obese family members, especially if both parents are obese, and the degree and duration of obesity in the child.[28] Thus, the chance of the very obese child remaining obese as an adult is greater than that of the moderately obese child. If that obesity is maintained into adolescence from early childhood, the risk of adult obesity is also increased.

EFFECTS OF CHILDHOOD OBESITY

Examination of the relationship between obesity in childhood and other events occurring in the same time period are presented as either correlations or associations. There has been an understandable tendency to see these events as resulting from the obesity, and in some cases this is likely to be true. However, as with any correlation, it is not possible to determine which is cause and which is effect, or whether both may be the effects of some other cause, on the basis of correlation alone. An excellent example of this is in the relationships between growth and obesity.

Growth

In childhood, caloric intake must exceed other caloric expenditures if a child is to grow. Adding new tissue to the body requires about 4 kcal per gram, of which about 2.5 kcal is the energy equivalent of the tissue (20 percent fat, 80 percent lean) and another 1.5 kcal is required to create the tissue. Thus a child gaining 1 kg requires an intake of about 4,000 kcal in excess of other expenditures for that weight gain. The 1-month-old child gains about 15 g per day and thus needs an extra 60 kcal per day for this purpose. At age 5 years, it takes on the average about 6 months to gain a kilogram, or 22 kcal per day in excess of other expenditure. At age 15, a kilogram is gained about every 65 days, or 60 kcal per day. The percentage of energy intake needed for average growth represents about 20 percent of the 1-month-old's intake, 1 to 2 percent of the 5-year-old's intake, and 2 percent of the 15-year-old's. Thus except in infancy, a failure to grow because of a low caloric intake is rarely a problem unless the individual is on an energy-restricted diet for a period of many months. However, this becomes particularly significant in obese children who may be placed on such diets for a prolonged period or for nonobese children who restrict their own calories because of fear of obesity.[29]

It might be expected that children who consume energy greater than that required for their resting metabolic state, their dietary thermogenesis, physical activity, and average growth would be likely to grow at a rate greater than average. In addition, if the caloric excess is greater than can be utilized for the increased growth rate, energy will be stored as fat. That this does in fact occur appears to be borne out by the repeated observations that obese children, other than those whose obesity is endocrine or associated with other genetic or acquired conditions, are tall and have increased lean body masses for their respective age and sex. This observation has been used diagnostically to indicate that obese children who are tall for their age have obesity of exogenous origin, whereas those with primary endocrine disorders or other genetic syndromes are usually short for their age.[15]

Closely allied with the issue of growth is that of sexual maturation. It has been recognized that with increasing adiposity, there is earlier sexual maturation. With an earlier cessation of growth secondary to the earlier maturation, those obese children who had been taller than their age peers prior to maturation have an adult stature that fits a normal distribution. Thus, the increase in linear growth associated with adiposity is lost because growth ceases at an earlier age.

For some years it has been postulated that in girls it is the accumulation of a certain amount of body fat that triggers their menarche.[30] The girl who achieves that amount of fat earlier because of her adiposity will have menarche at an earlier age. Garn et al dispute this argument.[31] While recognizing the association between increasing body fatness and earlier menarche, their data suggest that it is the other way around: Girls who have an early menarche become fatter than girls with a later onset of menarche. Their studies, based on 16,000 subjects, do not indicate a mechanism for this phenomenon but they point out that the early maturers are fatter than the later maturers into the eighth decade of life.

Social-Behavioral Factors

The second major effect of obesity in childhood is in the social-behavioral area. Not only is there profound social stigmatization of the obese child and equally profound psychological differences between obese and nonobese children, but these effects are interactive. The social stigma increases the emotional problems of these children, which in turn tends to increase their isolation and the social discrimination.

According to Natalie Allon, "Stigmatization involves the rejection and disgrace which are connected with a condition viewed both as physical deformity and as a behavioral aberration."[32] Although some social approval remains for the "chubby" infant, negative social attitudes toward fatness become evident at some point during the preschool years. By the time that obese children reach kindergarten, there is already evidence of discrimination by their teachers.[33] Throughout their school years these children are treated negatively by their peers. They are usually the last to be chosen for games, and they are generally not found in the spontaneously arising leadership groups that characterize children in the pre-teen and teenage years. Allon characterizes the stigmatization of the obese in four areas: (1) in religion, as a sin; (2) in medicine, as a disease; (3) in crime, as a misdemeanor or "felony"; and (4) in esthetics, as ugliness. "The fat person often internalizes the social scorn and condemnation of overweight, so that he or she self-fulfills the prophecy of these four negative stigmas of fatness." Even children accept the dominant social view that obesity is the person's own responsibility based on a self-indulgent immorality. When asked about the likability of six children illustrated by line drawings (normal child, one with a leg brace, one in a wheelchair, one with a missing hand, one with a facial deformity, and an obese child) the obese child was least likable to the vast majority of children.[32] Educators equally discriminate against the obese child at all ages. High school recommendations and acceptances to college have been shown to be negatively fat-biased.[34]

Garn has shown that fat girls tend to marry downward in social class, whereas thin girls tend to marry upward. The adiposity of women in fact is negatively correlated with the educational level of their husbands; the higher the educational level of the man, the leaner his wife is likely to be. It is difficult to know how much of that relationship is based on social bias in the man or how much the self-image of the woman may contribute to selective mating.[35,36] Alternatively, some degree of this relationship may occur after marriage and result from social pressures on the women to conform to the image of their social class.

In any case, the self-image of obese individuals has often been noted to be negative. Allon, quoting Cahnman, indicates that many obese persons, full of "self-disparagement and self-hatred are trebly disadvantaged: (1) because they are discriminated against; (2) because they are made to feel that they deserve such discrimination; and (3) because they come to accept their treatment as just.... This self-fulfilling prophecy has been demonstrated among obese adolescent girls, who show their status as minority group members, with withdrawal, passivity, the expectation of rejection, and overconcern with self-image."[32]

As complex as the emotional response to obesity may be, it is of particular interest to those working with children that there is, at least in adults with childhood onset of obesity, a set of behavioral changes that accompany weight loss. In studies done by Jules Hirsch, hostile behavior and depression were more often noted after obese persons had lost weight than when they remained obese.[37] Others have also noted that childhood-onset obesity that continues into adulthood determines that individual's adult self-image. Weight reduction in this individual is associated with a loss of personal identity, leading Hirsch to conclude that "the psychological consequences of obesity are most clearly seen when weight is reduced."[37] The implications for treatment of obesity are obvious.

Hypertension

Hypertension has been associated with obesity in adults for many years. More recently it has become a concern with obese children. Much of the hypertension associated with obese children has been erroneous, secondary to the use of blood pressure cuffs that are too small. To obtain an appropriate blood pressure, it is necessary to have a cuff that is sufficiently large that the rubber bladder completely encircles the arm. This requires a cuff that is much larger than those customarily in use in pediatric clinics and offices. In fact, some children are sufficiently obese that an adult thigh cuff is necessary to obtain a bladder that is long enough to go completely around the arm. Only if this precaution is adhered to will the blood pressure readings in obese children be accurate.

Given the caveat on proper blood pressure cuff bladder size, there appears to be more hypertension in obese children than in those of normal fatness. Gortmaker et al, in reviewing the data from the National Health Examination Surveys (NHES) and the National Health and Nutrition Examination Surveys (NHANES) and using the 85th percentile of triceps skin fold for defining obesity and the 95th percentile to define the "superobese," noted an odds ratio for hypertension in children of 2.6 for elevated blood pressure in the obese and 3.4 for the superobese. For diastolic pressure the odds ratios were 1.6 and 1.9, respectively. For adolescents the systolic pressure odds ratios were 4.3 and 6.1 and for diastolic pressure were 3.8 and 5.3. If one examines the data in the reverse direction, children with elevated systolic pressure who were obese accounted for 32 to 48 percent of all children with hypertension. For adolescents 12 to 17 years of age, 36 to 49 percent of the systolic hypertension occurred among those who were obese.[20] In a smaller study from the University of Michigan on 72 obese adolescents, it was noted that blood pressure distribution was skewed one standard deviation to the right of normal. They also noted that weight loss resulted in decrease in blood pressure that was more marked if the weight loss resulted from combined diet and exercise than if it was accomplished by diet alone.[38]

It has also been noted that for children of the same age, there is a positive correlation between blood pressure and height.[39] Nevertheless, the correlations for hypertension with obesity, especially subscapular skin folds (evidence of truncal obesity) is greater than that for height.[40]

The Bogalusa study of 3,503 children and young adults (ages 5 to 24 years) also noted a clustering of other cardiovascular risk factors (fasting insulin levels and the ratio of low-density lipoprotein and very low density lipoprotein/high-density lipoprotein cholesterol) with hypertension in the upper tertile of fatness in these individuals.[41]

Hyperlipidemia

Although obesity and hyperlipidemia are reasonably correlated and hyperlipidemia and fatty streaks show a positive relationship, "obesity is related neither to fatty streaks nor raised lesions in agreement with the results of the International Atherosclerosis project."[42]

Endocrine Factors

The endocrine factors related to obesity in children include changes in insulin, growth hormone, and prolactin levels. Basal insulin levels were higher, and both growth hormone and prolactin responses to insulin were lower in 12 obese patients than in controls.[43] The abnormalities in carbohydrate metabolism have been recognized for over a decade. Martin and Martin[44,45] reported that 25 percent of the obese children they studied had impaired glucose tolerance.

In recent years the various consequences of obesity, including the endocrine abnormalities, have been related to the distribution of body fat in the adult. Obesity of the upper trunk relative to the obesity of the extremities (the android pattern) has been assessed by such measurements as the ratio of waist to hip circumferences and the relation between subscapular and triceps skin fold thicknesses. These differences in fat distribution have been shown to have considerable predictive value in adults.[46] Studies in children have confirmed that such a relationship also exists in the young. However, when controlled for overall body fatness, the correlation is no longer significant.[15] Although many of the endocrine abnormalities appear to be reversed with weight reduction, the continuance of normal values over time has yet to be determined.

Orthopedic Conditions

Although both slipped femoral epiphysis and Blount's disease (tibia vara) have been reported to be associated with obesity in the past, those relationships are not currently considered so clear-cut. For example, the obese boy with slipped femoral epiphysis is typically delayed in both osseous and gonadal development. These findings are in contrast to the common pattern of obesity, i.e., advanced bone age, increased stature, and early sexual maturation. Thus, it seems likely that these orthopedic complications are not directly related to typical patterns of obesity.

Respiratory Disease

Respiratory complications of obesity are of two types. Increased frequency of respiratory infections in young children with obesity was reported in the English literature in 1971,[47,48] but no subsequent studies have been identified. In the 1971 study, the prevalence of respiratory infections during a 6-month period was 40 percent in the infants who remained obese during the interval and 19 percent in the infants who remained nonobese during this time interval. Chandra has reviewed the relationship between nutritional status and immunodeficiency, but no clear-cut basis for increased rates of infection has emerged.[49]

The other respiratory problem is that of hypoventilation, also termed the Pickwickian syndrome. During mild exercise or sleep in some extremely obese children, there appears to be insufficient respiratory effort to maintain normal pulmonary function. The subsequent rise in Pco_2 is associated with drowsiness and somnolence. Untreated, this complication has led to cardiac failure and death. The exact mechanism for the syndrome, which is rare, is not fully understood, but small tidal volumes, decreased compliance, and low chemical ventilatory drive may all contribute to the process.[50]

Burns

It was reported in 1972 that fat boys were more likely to be burned than were normal boys, but no such relationship was present for girls.[51]

ETIOLOGY

The fundamental laws of physics make it clear that energy acquired = energy expended ± stored energy. If the difference between acquired and utilized nutrient energy in the human body is only 50 kcal per day on the positive side (less than a slice of dry toast), there will be a weight gain of 10 pounds in 1 year. Similarly, a net expenditure of 50 kcal per day in excess of absorption (about 5 minutes of walking) would result in a loss of 10 pounds of weight. Clearly it seems that obesity could result from a small consistent excess of food intake or a small, but consistent decrease in energy expenditure, or some combination of both mechanisms. In fact, it appears that there are data to support each of these possibilities. The major problem in validating the possibility is that the difference of 50 kcal represents about 2 percent of the energy consumed or expended by the older child and only 2 to 5 percent of such energy flows in the young child. These changes are well within the error of measurement in most studies. On the other hand, it seems likely that persons who become obese (infants, children, or adolescents) usually do so more rapidly than postulated above. Thus, the differences between intake and expenditure are often greater than 5 percent. It is also important to recognize that intake in excess of expenditure can arise when intake is above the mean for a group of persons of similar age and sex, at the mean, or even below the mean for normal weight persons as long as expenditure is less than intake at whatever level the intake is set.

Energy Intake

Animal studies have consistently demonstrated that increased food intake is associated with increasing adiposity in a variety of models of obesity. However, the data on human subjects are much more variable. While there is a common perception that obese individuals consume more energy than their peers, a number of studies have failed to demonstrate this difference. Stark and Lloyd, quoting work by Jung and James,[52] state that "obese children and adults do not appear to have higher food intakes or expend less energy in physical activity than their lean peers."[53] Johnson et al found that 28 obese girls consumed an average of 1965 kcal and their 28 controls consumed 2,706 kcal.[54] In a study of 248 French children, the correlation between energy consumption and subscapular skinfold thickness was −0.08 (n.s.).[55] Studies such as these have led Dietz to conclude that "multiple dietary histories from clinical patients fail to reveal substantial and consistent differences between either the frequency, pattern or types of foods consumed by obese children and adolescents."[15] In contrast, a study of 128 obese children in Egypt with 105 controls showed a mean caloric intake of 3,200 kcal in the obese children and 2,500 kcal in the controls.[56] However, in a study of 3- and 4-year-old children in England, the subjects, of comparable weight, were divided into two groups. One group had one or two obese parents and were thus considered to be at high risk for obesity. The other group, low risk, had no obese parents. Food intakes were measured by duplicate diet analysis for a 7-day period. The mean intake of the high-risk group was 1,103 kcal and of the low risk group 1,314 kcal ($P = 0.02$). When intakes were calculated on a body weight basis, the high-risk group's mean was 69 kcal per kilogram and the low-risk group 86 kcal per kilogram ($P = 0.002$).[57] Although overeating in relation to energy expenditure must be present, overeating in relation to normative data related to age, weight, and sex does not appear to be substantiated by the available data. In a 1988 review of the available data, Stunkard concluded, in reference to animal studies: "comparable evidence of the importance of diet in human obesity is lacking, but there is no reason to believe that diet is not also important in humans."[58] In what way is open to conjecture.

A possible explanation for the difficulty in finding consistent differences in the energy intakes of obese children is that, in general, they are studied only after they have become obese. It is conceivable that the differences in intake occur during the development of the obese state and, once obese, an equilibrium is reached and their food intake is no longer excessive. The small differences in energy consumption required to achieve weight gain (noted above) may also contribute to the lack of observed differences. An indirect support of this possibility is found in the French study, in which the authors note that a higher proportion of obese children were found in the lower social class, which, in their studies, had on average a greater caloric intake than did the groups of higher social class.[55]

One interesting and possibly relevant study on food intake is the work of Mattes et al on the caloric intake of normal-weight adults when one meal was altered in its caloric content. The change in caloric content of the mid-day meal was unknown to the participants. When the meal was reduced in calories by 66 percent, compensatory increases in other intake kept caloric balance unchanged. However, when the caloric value of the meal was increased by 66 percent, the reduction in other energy intake was insufficient to restore intake to baseline levels. The authors conclude "that humans compensate more readily for decreases than for increases in caloric intake."[59]

It also must be re-emphasized that if energy expenditure is stable, changes in food intake produce appropriate changes in weight. This topic has been carefully reviewed by Forbes in a re-examination of the studies of Neuman from 1902 and Gulick from 1922. Forbes states that "bodyweight does respond to modest as well as to profound alterations in energy intake.... The rather precise nature of the response... is a reminder of the central role of energy intake in weight homeostasis."[60]

The issue of food intake becomes further complicated today because of the changing patterns of food consumption that have been occurring in the past few years. An excellent review of these changes in dietary practices has been published by the National Dairy Council.[61]

In essence, the data on food intake are quite variable, and whether food intake is above or below the expected value for an individual at the time obesity is developing is unclear and is perhaps less important than that intake must exceed expenditure for fat storage to occur.

Energy Expenditure

Energy expenditures consist of four major categories: resting or basal metabolic rate, physical activity, thermogenesis associated with food consumption, and growth.

Resting metabolic rate (RMR), which amounts to about two-thirds of the total energy expenditure, is dependent to the greatest extent on lean body mass.[62] Obese children are known to have an increased lean body mass. In general, the weight gain associated with obesity has been shown to consist of about 80 percent adipose tissue and 20 percent lean body mass.[63] Other than an increase in RMR in proportion to the increased lean body mass associated with obesity, it has not been possible to demonstrate any differences between RMR expressed in terms of lean body mass in obese and nonobese adults.[62]

Physical activity accounts for about 25 percent of total energy expenditure but can vary widely between individuals and from time to time in the same individual. Because of this variability and the presumed ability that one has to alter this expenditure, attention has focused on changes in physical activity as a causative factor in obesity. In a series of studies by the group working with Jean Mayer, there appeared to be strong evidence that obese children were physically less active than their lean peers.[64] In a more recent study by Dietz and Gortmaker, it was noted that television viewing time was greater among children who subsequently became obese than among children who remained nonobese. Whether this increase in television viewing, which was associated with a 2 percent increase in prevalence of obesity for each additional hour per week of viewing time, was secondary to decreased activity and/or to the increased calories consumed while watching television is uncertain.[65] Nevertheless, there appears to be reduced energy expended in physical activity among those becoming obese. Further evidence supporting this view comes from a study of English children of obese and nonobese parents. The children, who were not obese when studied at age 4 to 5 years, were divided into high and low risk for obesity based on parental fatness. The high-risk group had lower overall energy expenditure, but the difference in energy expended for activity differed by about 35 percent.[66] In a study of infants less than 1 year of age, total energy expenditure of those found to become obese was 20 percent lower than for those who did not become obese. The authors state, "In the infants we studied, reduced expenditure of energy on physical activity appeared to be an important component of the low total energy expenditure."[67]

One of the possible differences in energy expended in physical activity between the obese and the lean is that resulting from small spontaneous movements. Differences in such energy losses between individuals can range from 100 to 900 kcal. Whether obese individuals have less spontaneous activity (fidgeting) than the lean remains conjectural.

The third component of energy expenditure is postprandial or dietary-induced thermogenesis. Although this represents a small component of total expenditure (5 to 10 percent), much attention has been focused on this element of energy loss, perhaps because of its relation to food intake. It has been postulated that individuals becoming obese have lower levels of dietary-induced thermogenesis (DIT) than nonobese persons. Schutz et al not only noted reduced glucose-induced thermogenesis in obese subjects (adults) but noted that the values fell still further after weight loss.[68] Dietz, quoting unpublished studies done by him and Bandini, was unable to document any differences between obese and lean adolescents in response to weight maintenance diet or to surfeit carbohydrate calories.[15]

In studies of vegetarians, traditionally not obese, their thermic response to food was lower than that of nonvegetarians—a difference in the wrong direction if changes in DIT were to be part of the explanation for obesity.[69]

In summarizing the studies on DIT, Sims and Danforth stated, "Of 24 studies in the last 15 years, only half give evidence of a thermic response (to food in the obese) differing from that of the lean."[70]

Closely allied with the energy expended in response to ingested food has been the energy that might be lost in "futile" cycles—reactions in which the only output was heat, such as with nonshivering thermogenesis in rats. Such reactions have been associated with brown fat, but the evidence for the presence of brown fat in the human organism and, if present, its role in obesity remain uncertain. In a similar direction, Na^+, K^+-ATPase activity in RBC has been examined. While differences were noted between obese and lean groups, there are also ethnic differences that may have accounted for the previous findings.[71,72] Studies have also been done on liver Na^+, K^+-ATPase, and in those studies the obese had greater hepatic activity than did the lean, an effect opposite to that predicted.[73]

The fourth type of energy expenditure is that associated with growth. This is the smallest component of total energy use and has not been identified as being different in lean and obese individuals, even though the caloric cost of creating a gram of tissue varies with the kind of tissue being produced. The usual growth tissue is about 20 percent fat, whereas the usual obese tissue is 80 percent fat. The caloric cost increases two- to threefold (4 to 10 kcal per gram) with differences in composition of this magnitude.

Studies of total energy expenditure, in which the four components have not been assessed separately, have generally shown lower overall energy utilization in obese persons compared to nonobese. The studies of Ravussin et al on American Indians demonstrated a correlation of −0.4 between energy expenditure and weight change over a 2-year period.[74] In another study of postobese women, their metabolic rates were about 15 percent lower than those of controls at various levels of activity.[75]

In summary, the energy expenditure of obese persons, including children, appears to be lower than that of nonobese. Much of this decrease may be in the physical activity component of energy use, and changes in other components remain controversial. Differences in energy intake are less easy to demonstrate but may be decreased as well, but not to the same extent as energy expenditure.

George Bray has developed a hypothetical model that integrates intake and expenditure into a "controlled nutrient system," with the brain as controller utilizing separate feedback systems for each of the major nutrients.[76] In Bray's model, obesity could result from perturbations in the system at various sites.

Genetics and Environment

Another method of examining the etiology of obesity is to consider factors that may be environmental in origin and those that may be genetic. There is good evidence that both environmental and genetic factors are operative, but the identification of specific mechanisms as being one or the other is not yet possible.

The strongest evidence of a role for environmental factors is the negative relationship between social class or educational level and obesity in women and a different relationship for children and men.[77] The relation between the education of a husband and the fatness of his wife, the correlations in adiposity between pets and owners, between adopted children and their adoptive parents in Tecumseh, between adopted children and their "natural" siblings, and between parents and children living together and those living separately all support environmental factors.[79,80] Other adoption studies noted opposite results.[81] Stunkard et al examined 540 Danish adoptees at an average 42 years of age. They divided the adoptees into four weight groups, and the correlation with biologic mothers was significant at a level of $P < 0.0001$ and for fathers $P < 0.02$. There was no significant correlation with the weight class of the adoptive parents.[82] Twin studies show evidence of high degrees of heritability for weight and BMI.[83-85]

Other etiologic factors that have not been identified as genetic or environmental but are related to the occurrence of obesity in children include (1) obesity in a first-degree relative, (2) being an only child, and (3) absence of one parent.[86]

For children at 24 months of age, determinants of skin fold thickness included (1) birth weight, (2) maternal weight, and (3) decreased duration of breast-feeding.

In spite of significant correlations, these factors combined explained only 10 percent of the variance in skin folds. Factors such as introduction of solid foods, maternal attitudes toward feeding, and infant temperament were not significant.[87,88]

In another study of infant feeding by Agras et al, it was found that a vigorous feeding style (sucking more rapidly, at higher pressure, longer sucking bursts, and shorter nonsucking intervals) was associated with greater adiposity.[89] It is of interest in their group that breast-feeding was protective against obesity only until age 6 months.

Thus it appears that many factors may be involved in the etiology of obesity in childhood. Some of these are genetic in origin and some environmental. If one were to speculate on the basis of existing data, it would seem reasonable to consider that energy expenditures are the more likely genetic factors and that these are altered into differing phenotypes by the interaction of environmental forces that have their primary effect on modifying energy intake.

TREATMENT

Education

Before undertaking any program to control obesity, individuals need a rather extensive educational program to understand what is being attempted and to become knowledgeable about the basic facts of nutrition. They need to know about essential nutrients and the caloric value of a wide variety of foods. In general, 1 kcal equals 1 kcal whether derived from fat, carbohydrate, or protein. Because of the higher caloric density of fat and at least a theoretical advantage in a greater reduction in fat calories than in carbohydrate or protein calories,[90] most diet counselors recommend diets that are based on about 10 percent of calories from protein, 65 percent of calories from carbohydrates, and 25 percent of calories from fat.

The advantage of exercise as an adjunct to calorie restriction needs to be clarified. Although some increase in energy expenditure occurs as a result of additional physical activity, the major advantages of exercise are psychological and possibly some preservation of lean body mass during weight loss.[91]

It also needs to be understood that weight loss followed by regaining of lost weight may be more harmful than maintaining existing weight. Prolonged loss of even modest changes is better than the yo-yo effect of repeated cycles of loss and gain.[93,94]

Education of parents of children at risk for obesity or with minimal existing obesity is most important. Prevention of obesity in children, although difficult, should be much more advantageous and safer than treatment programs.

One fairly extensive preventive-type education program instituted in New York schools was targeted at fourth through eighth graders. After 5 years the changes in the intervention group were small when compared to controls. There was no change in adiposity, but a small change of 1 to 2 mg per deciliter in total plasma cholesterol was noted.[95] A similar study with shorter follow-up, done in California, showed evidence of some decrease in triceps skin folds in girls but no change in boys.[96] One problem that has become apparent is that of parental overconcern with issues of weight control, which may lead to failure to thrive.[97] This problem is often seen in families in which one or both parents are obese and they are anxious to prevent their child from sharing their fate.

Diet

The traditional approach to obesity has been to reduce energy intake—calorie restricted diets. Diets have ranged from mild caloric restrictions of about 20 percent to total fasting. There is little doubt that restricting calorie intake to less than expenditures will produce weight loss. Millions of dollars are spent each year on the latest weight-reduction diets. Any of these diets that produce weight loss have one thing in common—ultimately they result in lowered caloric intakes. A popular alternative to traditional diets has been the very low calorie, "protein-sparing" diets. These are usually in liquid form and supply 50 to 75 g of protein and about 300 kcal. Whether there is any actual reduction in protein loss on such diets is uncertain. The majority of diets are aimed at producing relatively acute changes in weight. To accomplish losses of 5 pounds or more in a week almost always necessitates some degree of dehydration and excessive loss of lean body mass. One kilogram of idealized weight loss (800 g of fat, 50 g of protein, and 150 ml of body water) is equivalent to 7,400 kcal. If one were able to achieve a negative balance of 1,000 kcal per day, it is clear that weight loss would occur at a rate of about 2 pounds per week. This is considered the maximum rate of loss for any sustained effort at weighty reduction. With total fasting, a maximum of 5 pounds per week could occur unless the loss of lean body mass were in excess of 20 percent of the loss or dehydration also occurred.

In contrast, a loss of 1 pound a week can be accomplished with caloric restriction of about 500 kcal per day. This level of restriction can be accomplished for reasonably prolonged periods in individuals who are strongly motivated and will produce a weight loss of about 50 pounds in a year.

With any diet providing under 2,000 kcal per day, the possibility exists of creating vitamin or mineral deficiencies, especially vitamin A, iron, and calcium. Therefore, diets of 1,750 kcal or less should be supplemented appropriately.

Two problems inherent in calorie-restrictive diets are compliance (see below) and physiologic adaptation to the lower level of intake. These adaptations include reduced resting metabolic rate and thermogenic response to food and decreased activity. Thus, a caloric level producing weight loss initially has to be reduced further over time to continue a 500-kcal deficit between energy intake and expenditure. A diet of 1,750 kcal may ultimately need to be reduced to 1,250 to 1,500 kcal to continue a weight loss of 1 pound per week.

As much as one may be tempted to institute dietary restrictions leading to weight loss in children, this procedure has a serious risk. Weight reduction is inevitably accompanied by loss of lean body mass. In children who are growing and thereby needing to accrete lean body mass to accomplish that growth, the loss of lean body mass as part of a weight-reduction program necessarily reduces their rate of growth. In a society that places a high value on adult stature, the possibility of reducing ultimate adult height by prolonged weight-loss programs is a serious risk that must be considered.[98]

In general, although prevention of obesity should be the primary goal in working with children, treatment programs for children already obese should use weight maintenance rather than reduction as the major aim. If children who are obese can maintain their weight, ultimate growth in stature results in decreasing degrees of obesity over time. However, dietary modification is almost always necessary to achieve weight maintenance. Reduction in caloric intakes of 10 to 20 percent usually suffice to maintain existing weight. One exception to weight maintenance as a goal is the child with extreme obesity, especially if there is any evidence for respiratory compromise. In such cases even total fasting in a hospital environment may be indicated.

Exercise

Exercise has been the third component of most weight loss programs. As already mentioned, exercise programs have only a modest effect on increasing energy expenditure. Thirty minutes of aerobic exercises (calisthenics, swimming, brisk walking) expend about 3 to 4 kcal per kg.

Perhaps more important roles for exercise as part of a weight control program are the psychological sense of improved well being, the tendency of exercise to minimize the loss of lean body mass,[99] and the possibility that exercise may minimize the fall in resting metabolic rate that usually accompanies weight control when accomplished solely by caloric restriction.[100] Recent work suggests no difference in plasma lipids when weight loss occurs secondary to exercise or caloric restriction.

One of the important considerations in advocating an exercise program for children is the need to try to obtain full family participation in the effort. Obese children tend to respond more positively if other family members join together in any exercise program such as aerobics, swimming, skiing, running, and bicycling.

Behavior Modification

Behavior modification is increasingly recognized as a valuable adjunct to weight control measures in children. Most programs that have gained acceptance by demonstrating some degree of effectiveness are those that have combined education, energy intake limitation, exercise, and behavior modification. Programs such as Shapedown[101] are examples of this combined approach. Interestingly, one study suggests that adolescents do better when treated separate from their mothers than when treated together.[102]

Surgical Approach

Surgical interventions such as gastric stapling or intestinal bypass have rarely been utilized in the treatment of childhood obesity. However, in extreme cases, e.g., those with Pickwickian syndrome, there is some evidence that this can be effective. However, long-term follow-up of such cases has yet to be documented adequately.[103]

COMPLIANCE

The most discouraging aspect of the management of obesity in childhood has been the difficulty in generating long-term control of excessive adiposity. It is a common experience that programs utilizing only one or two of the treatment modalities discussed above are rarely successful in achieving weight control over the child's entire period of development. Even programs that contain all the nonsurgical treatment approaches have a low success rate for prolonged effectiveness. Recognizing that in the natural history of obesity only a small number of children will remain obese over a 20-year period, it seems reasonable to concentrate one's efforts on children who are at highest risk of continuing obesity. Such children can be recognized using the following two criteria: (1) skin fold thicknesses greater than the 95th percentile for age and sex, and (2) presence of obesity in one or both parents. If both parents are obese, the obese child's risk of obesity as an adult approaches 50 percent. If both criteria are present, the risk of adult obesity in the obese child exceeds 50 percent.[28]

SUMMARY

Obesity in children represents a degree of adiposity which is greater than the 85th percentile of skin fold thickness measured at the triceps and/or subscapular areas. The natural history of the condition indicates that the obese child has a relative risk of obesity as an adult of 1.7 (a normal-weight child has a risk of 1.0). Thus, the majority of obese children do not become obese adults, and most obese adults were not obese as children. However, if the child's skin fold thickness is greater than the 95th percentile or if one or both parents are obese, the relative risk is about 3.0; i.e., about 50 percent of such obese children will be obese as adults.

The most deleterious effect of obesity in childhood is on the psychological state of the child and the associated discrimination against him or her by peers, teachers, and other adults. Hypertension is the major medical problem associated with obesity in the young, but abnormal carbohydrate metabolism and other endocrine problems have also been observed. The obese child typically is tall for age but matures earlier and is therefore of expected stature as an adult.

Both genetic and environmental factors play an etiologic role. Total energy expenditure is reduced, even before the onset of obesity. Energy consumption may be quite variable but must exceed expenditures for adiposity to develop. It is postulated that the genetic influence may be exhibited in some aspect of energy expenditure and that energy intake may be more influenced by environmental factors.

Treatment programs in general have had limited success with high degrees of recidivism, but those programs with any consistent pattern of success have aimed at weight control, but not necessarily weight loss, and have combined nutrition education, dietary modification, increased physical activity, and behavior modification. Prevention efforts are more likely to be effective than treatment regimens, but regularly successful programs in either direction remain elusive.

REFERENCES

1. Pace N, Rathbun EN. Studies on body composition. J Biol Chem 1945; 158:685–692.
2. Poissonnet CM, LaVelle M, Burdi AR. Growth and development of adipose tissue. J Pediatr 1988; 113:1–9.
3. Fee BA, Weil WB. Body composition of infants of diabetic mothers by direct analysis. Ann NY Acad Sci 1963; 110:869–897.
4. Bandini LG, Dietz WH. Assessment of body fatness in childhood obesity: evaluation of laboratory and anthropometric techniques. J Am Diet Assoc 1987; 87:1344–1348.
5. Himes JH, Roche AF, Webb P. Fat areas as estimates of total body fat. Am J Clin Nutr 1980; 33:2093–2100.
6. Owen GM. Measurement, recording and assessment of skinfold thickness in childhood and adolescence: report of a small meeting. Am J Clin Nutr 1982; 35:629–638.
7. Garn SM, Sullivan TVE, Tenhave TR. The need for differential weightings with summed skinfold values. (Letter) Ecol Food Nutr 1987; 20:157–159.
8. U.S. Department of Health and Human Services. Basic data on anthropometric measurements and angular measurements of the hip and knee joints for selected age groups 1–74 years of age. Vital Health Stat 1981; 11:1–68.
9. Griffiths M, Rivers JPW, Hoinville EA. Obesity in boys: the distinction between fatness and heaviness. Hum Nutr Clin Nutr 1985; 39C:259–269.
10. Roche AF, Siervogel RM, Chumlea WC, Webb P. Grading fatness from limited anthropometric data. Am J Clin Nutr 1981; 34:2931–2838.
11. Weil WB. Obesity: a problem in perceptions. In: Infant child feeding. Orlando: Academic Press, Inc. 1981: 333.
12. Wolff OH. Obesity in childhood. A study of the birth weight, the height and the onset of puberty. Lancet 1955; ii:1908.
13. Kohrman AF, Weil WB. Obesity. Pract Pediatr 1984; 6:1–17.
14. Frankel HM. Determination of body mass index. JAMA 1986; 255:1292.
15. Dietz WH. Childhood obesity. Ann NY Acad Sci 1987; 499:47–54.
16. Garn SM, Bailey SM, Cole PE. Continuities and changes in fatness and obesity. In: Schemmel R, ed. Nutrition, physiology and obesity. Boca Raton, FL: CRC Press, 1980: 51.
17. Hutchinson JJ. Clinical implications of an extensive actuarial study of build and blood pressure. Ann Intern Med 1961; 54:90–96.
18. Simopoulos AP. The health implications of overweight and obesity. Nutr Rev 1985; 43:33–40.
19. U.S. Department of Health, Education, and Welfare: Weight by height and age for adults 18–74 years. Vital Health Stat 1979; 11:1–56.
20. Gortmaker SL, Dietz WH, Sobol AM, Wehler CA. Increasing pediatric obesity in the United States. Am J Dis Child 141:535–540.
21. Shear CL, Freedman DS, Burke GL, Harsha DW, Webber LS, Berenson GS. Secular trends of obesity in early life: the Bogalusa heart study. Am J Public Health 1988; 78:75–77.
22. U.S. Department of Health and Human Services. Annual summary of births, marriages, divorces, and deaths: United States, 1987; NCHS Monthly Vital Stat Rep 1988; 36:1–28.
23. Harsha DW, Smoak CG, Nicklas TA, Webber LS, Berenson GS. Cardiovascular risk factors from birth to seven years of age: the Bogalusa heart study. Pediatrics 1987; 80:779–783.
24. Garn SM. Family-line and socioeconomic factors in fatness and obesity. Nutr Rev 1986; 44:381–386.
25. Garn SM, LaVelle M. Two-decade follow-up of fatness in early childhood. Am J Dis Child 1985; 139:181–185.
26. Sorensen TIA, Sonne-Holm S. Risk in childhood of development of severe adult obesity: retrospective, population-based case-cohort study. Am J Epidemiol 1988; 127:104–113.
27. Braddon FEM, Rodgers B, Wadsworth MEJ, Davies JMC. Onset of obesity in a 36 year birth cohort study. Br Med J 1986; 293:299–303.
28. Garn SM. Continuity and changes in fatness in infancy through adulthood. Curr Probl Pediatr 1985; 15:1–47.
29. Lifshitz F. Nutritional dwarfing in adolescents. Growth Genet Hor 1987; 3:1–15.
30. Frisch RE. Fatness and fertility. Perspect Biol Med 1985; 28:611–633.
31. Garn SM, LaVelle M, Rosenberg KR, Hawthorne VM. Maturational timing as a factor in female fatness and obesity. Am J Clin Nutr 1986; 43:879–883.
32. Allon N. The stigma of overweight in everyday life. In: Bray GA, ed. Obesity in perspective. Washington, DC: US Government Printing Office, 1973.
33. Weil WB. Obesity in childhood. In: Children's blood pressure, report of the eighty-eighth Ross conference on pediatric research 1985; pp 103–109.
34. Dwyer J, Mayer J. The dismal condition: problems faced by obese adolescent girls in American society. In: Bray GA, ed. Obesity in Perspective, 1973: 103.
35. Garn SM, Socioeconomic level and fatness differences in husband-wife pairs. Hum Biol; in press.
36. Garn SM. Education of one spouse and the fatness of the other spouse. Am J Hum Biol 1989; 1:233–238.
37. Hirsch J. The psychological consequences of obesity. In: Bray GA, ed. Obesity in Perspective, 1973: 81.
38. Rocchini AP, Katch V, Anderson J, Hinderliter J, Becque D, Martin M, Marks C. Blood pressure in obese adolescents: effect of weight loss. Pediatrics 1988; 82:16–23.
39. Berchtold P, Jorgens V, Finke C, Berger M. Epidemiology of obesity and hypertension. Int J Obes 1981; 5:1–7.
40. Higgins MW, Hinton PC, Keller JB. Weight and obesity as predictors of blood pressure and hypertension. Presented at the Workshop on Juvenile Hypertension, 1983.

41. Smoak CG, Burke GL, Webber LS, Harsha DW. Srinivasan SR, Berenson GS. Relation of obesity to clustering of cardiovascular disease risk factors in children and young adults. Am J Epidemiol 1987; 125:364–372.
42. Newman WP, Freedman DS, Voors AW, Gard PD, Srinivasan SR, Cresanta JL, Williamson GD, Webber LS, Berenson GS. Relation of serum lipoprotein levels and systolic blood pressure to early atherosclerosis. N Engl J Med 1986; 314:138–144.
43. AvRuskin TW, Pillai S, Juan C. Decreased prolactin secretion in childhood obesity. J Pediatr 1985; 106:373–378.
44. Martin MM, Martin ALA. Obesity, hyperinsulinism and diabetes mellitus in children. J Pediatr 1973; 82:192–201.
45. Martin MM, Martin ALA. Obesity—a form of malnutrition. Med Ann DC 1973; 42:423–428.
46. Bjorntorp P. Classification of obese patients and complications related to the distribution of surplus fat. Am J Clin Nutr 1987; 45:1120–1125.
47. Tracey VV, De NC, Harper JR. Infantile obesity and respiratory infections. Nutr Rev 1971; 29:112–113.
48. Hutchinson-Smith B. Obesity and respiratory infection in children. (Letter) Br Med J 1971; 1:460–461.
49. Chandra RK. Immunodeficiency in undernutrition and overnutrition. Nutr Rev 1981; 39:225–231.
50. Riley DJ, Santiago TV, Edelman NH. Complications of obesity-hypoventilation syndrome in childhood. Am J Dis Child 1976; 130:671–674.
51. Wilmore DW, Pruitt BA. Fat boys get burned. Lancet 1972; ii:631–632.
52. Jung RT, James WPT. Obesity: is obesity metabolic. Br J Hosp Med 1980; 24:503–508.
53. Stark O, Lloyd JK. Some aspects of obesity in childhood. Postgrad Med J 1986; 62:87–92.
54. Johnson ML, Burke BS, Mayer J. Relative importance of inactivity and overeating in the energy balance of obese high school girls. Am J Clin Nutr 1956; 4:37–44
55. Rolland-Cachera MF, Bellisle F. No correlation between adiposity and food intake: why are working class children fatter? Am J Clin Nutr 1986; 44:779–787.
56. Darwish OA, Khalil MH, Sarhan AA, Ali HE. Aetiological factors of obesity in children. Hum Nutr Clin Nutr 1985; 39C:131–136.
57. Griffiths M, Rivers JPW, Payne PR. Energy intake in children at high and low risk of obesity. Hum Nutr Clin Nutr 1987; 41C:425–430.
58. Stunkard AJ. Obesity: risk factors, consequences and control. Med J Austral 1988; 148:S21–S28.
59. Mattes RD, Pierce CB, Friedman MI. Daily caloric intake of normal-weight adults: response to changes in dietary energy density of a luncheon meal. Am J Clin Nutr 1988; 48:214–219.
60. Forbes GB. Energy intake and body weight: a reexamination of two "classic" studies. Am J Clin Nutr 1984; 39:349–350.
61. National Dairy Council. Nutrition and modern lifestyles. Dairy Council Dig 1988; 59:1–6.
62. Owen OE. Resting metabolic requirements of men and women. Mayo Clin Proc 1988; 63:503–510.
63. Forbes GB. Lean body mass–body fat interrelationships in humans. Nutr Rev 1987; 45:225–231.
64. Bullen BA, Reed RB, Mayer J. Physical activity of obese and non-obese adolescent girls appraised by motion picture sampling. Am J Clin Nutr 1964; 14:211–223.
65. Dietz WH, Gortmaker SL. Do we fatten our children at the television set? Obesity and television viewing in children and adolescents. Pediatrics 1985; 75:807–812.
66. Griffiths M, Payne PR. Energy expenditure in small children of obese and non-obese parents. Nature 1976; 260:698–700.
67. Roberts SB, Savage J, Coward WA, Chew B, Lucas A. Energy expenditure and intake in infants born to lean and overweight mothers. N Engl J Med 1988; 318:461–466.
68. Schutz Y, Bessard T, Jequier E. Exercise and postprandial thermogenesis in obese women before and after weight loss. Am J Clin Nutr 1987; 45:1424–1432.
69. Poehlman ET, Arciero PJ, Melby CL, Babylak SF. Resting metabolic rate and postprandial thermogenesis in vegetarians and nonvegetarians. Am J Clin Nutr 1988; 48:209–213.
70. Sims EAH, Danforth E. Expenditure and storage of energy in man. J Clin Invest 1987; 79:1019–1025.
71. Mir MA, Charalambous BM, Morgan K, Evens PJ. Erythrocyte sodium-potassium-ATPase and sodium transport in obesity. N Engl J Med 1981; 305:1264–1268.
72. Beutler E, Kuhl W, Sacks P. Sodium-potassium-ATPase activity is influenced by ethnic origin and not by obesity. N Engl J Med 1983; 309:756–760.
73. Bray GA, Kral JG, Bjorntorp P. Hepatic sodium-potassium-dependent ATPase in obesity. N Engl J Med 1981; 304:1580–1582.
74. Ravussin E, Lillioja S, Knowler WC, Christin L, Freymond D, Abbott WGH, Boyce V, Howard BV, Bogardus C. Reduced rate of energy expenditure as a risk factor for body-weight gain. N Engl J Med 1988; 318:467–472.
75. Geissler CA, Miller DS, Shah M. The daily metabolic rate of the post-obese and the lean. Am J Clin Nutr 1987; 45:914–920.
76. Bray GA. Obesity—a disease of nutrient or energy balance? Nutr Rev 1987; 45:33–43.
77. Weil WB. Demographic determinants of obesity. Obesity and the family. Marriage Family Rev 1984; 7:21.
78. Garn SM, Bailey SM, Cole PE. Similarities between parents and their adopted children. Ecol Food Nutr 1977; 7:91–93.
79. Garn SM, Sullivan TV, Hawthorne VM. Effect of educational level on the fatness and fatness differences of husbands and wives. Clin Nutr 1989; 50:740–745.
80. Garn SM, LaVelle M, Pilkington JJ. Obesity and living together. Marriage Fam Rev 1984; 7:33–47.
81. Biron P, Mongeau JG, Bertrand D. Familial resemblance of body weight and weight/height in 374 homes with adopted children. J Pediatr 1977; 91:555–558.
82. Stunkard AJ, Sorensen TIA, Hanis C, Teasdale TW. Chakraborty R, Schull WJ, Schulsinger F. An adoption study of human obesity. N Engl J Med 1986; 314:193–198.
83. Borjeson M. The aetiology of obesity in children. Acta Paediatr Scand 1976; 65:279–287.
84. Stunkard AJ, Foch TT, Hrubec Z. A twin study of human obesity. JAMA 1986; 256:51–54.
85. Brook CGD, Huntley RMC, Slack J. Influence of heredity and environment in determination of skinfold thickness in children. Br Med J 1975; 2:719–721.
86. Wilkinson PW, Parkin JM, Pearlson J, Philips PR, Sykes P. Obesity in childhood: a community study in Newcastle Upon Tyne. Lancet 1977; i:350–352.
87. Kramer MS, Barr RG, Leduc DG, Biosjoly C, Pless IB. Infant determinants of childhood weight and adiposity. J Pediatr 1985; 107:104–107.
88. Dubois S, Hill DE, Beaton GH. An examination of factors believed to be associated with infantile obesity. Am J Clin Nutr 1979; 32:1997–2004.
89. Agras WS, Kraemer HC, Berkowitz RI, Korner AF, Hammer LD. Does a vigorous feeding style influence early development of adiposity? J Pediatr 1987; 110:799–804.
90. Dietz WH, Schoeller DA. Optimal dietary therapy for obese adolescents: comparison of protein plus glucose and protein plus fat. J Pediatr 1982; 100:638–644.
91. Ballor DL, Katch VL, Becque MD, Marks CR. Resistance weight training during caloric restriction enhances lean body weight maintenance. Am J Clin Nutr 1988; 47:19–25.
92. National Dairy Council. Diet, exercise, and health. Dairy Council Dig 1985; 56:1–6.
93. Weil WB. Current controversies in childhood obesity. J Pediatr 1977; 91:175–187.
94. National Dairy Council. Weight control: new findings. Dairy Council Dig 1988; 59:1–6.
95. Walter HJ, Hofman A, Vaughan RD, Wynder EL. Modification of risk factors for coronary heart disease. New Engl J Med 1988; 318:1093–1100.
96. Killen JD, Telch MJ, Robinson TN, Maccoby N, Taylor CB, Farquhar JW. Cardiovascular disease risk reduction for tenth graders—a multiple-factor school-based approach. JAMA 1988; 260:1728–1733.
97. Pugliese MT, Weyman-Daum M, Moses N, Lifshitz F. Parental health beliefs as a cause of nonorganic failure to thrive. Pediatrics 1987; 80:175–182.
98. Dietz WH, Hartung R. Changes in height velocity of obese preadolescents during weight reduction. Am J Dis Child 1985; 139:705–707.
99. Hill JO, Sparling PB, Shields TW, Heller PA. Effects of exercise and food restriction on body composition and metabolic rate in obese women. Am J Clin Nutr 1987; 46:622–630.
100. Ackerman S. The management of obesity. Hosp Pract 1983; 18:117–140.
101. Wood PD, Stefanick ML, Dreon DM, Frey-Hewitt B, Garay SC, Williams PT, Superko HR, Fortmann SP, Albers JJ, Vranizan KM, Ell-

sworth NM, Terry RB, Haskell WL. Changes in plasma lipids and lipoproteins in overweight men during weight loss through dieting as compared with exercise. N Engl J Med 1988; 319:1173–1179.
102. Brownell KD, Kelman JH, Stunkard AJ. Treatment of obese children with and without their mothers: changes in weight and blood pressure. Pediatrics 1983; 71:515–523.
103. VanItallie TB, Bray GA, Faloon WW, Mason EE, Sclafani A, Stunkard AJ. Symposium on surgical treatment of morbid obesity. National Institute of Arthritis, Metabolism, and Digestive Disease of the National Institutes of Health, 1978.

PART 5

Enteral Nutrition

Ana Abad Sinden, M.S., R.D.
Vivian L. Dillard, R.N., M.S.N., C.P.N.P.
James L. Sutphen, M.D., Ph.D.

Pediatric patients unable to tolerate adequate oral feeding may be nutritionally managed with enteral tube feeding. Commonly used enteral tube feeding routes include the nasogastric route, gastrostomy, nasojejunal, and jejunostomy. The nutritional goal for pediatric patients with chronic illness should be the provision of nutrients appropriate to their metabolic and physiologic limitations and capable of promoting continued growth and development. Although both enteral and parenteral nutrition can provide support to pediatric patients unable or unwilling to take in adequate oral feedings, recent data suggest that enteral tube feeding is the method of choice for a number of reasons: Enteral feedings are more economical, easier, and safer to administer than parenteral nutrition; they present fewer metabolic and infectious complications; and they promote the usual physiologic function of the gastrointestinal (GI) tract.[1-3] Initial attempts to achieve nutritional goals in malnourished pediatric patients should be via the oral route. Some common indications for enteral tube feedings include suck/swallow difficulties, cardiorespiratory distress, hypermetabolism, nutritional complications of prematurity, neurologic dysfunction, abnormalities of the head and neck, and esophageal dysmotility.[1,4] Although nasoenteric feedings are effective in the short-term support of these patients, long-term nutritional management of the child with a chronic nutrition-related disorder may require the placement of a feeding gastrostomy.

This discussion reviews the pathophysiologic mechanisms and nutritional aspects of various pediatric disorders that have been successfully managed with enteral feeding. Formula selection and modification as well as tube feeding techniques and equipment are presented. The administration and monitoring of pediatric enteral feedings and the management of common complications are also discussed.

TABLE 1
Conditions Under Which Enteral Feeding May Be Warranted

Preterm infants
Cardiorespiratory illness
Chronic lung disease
Cystic fibrosis
Congenital heart disease
Gastrointestinal disease and dysfunction
Inflammatory bowel disease
Short gut syndrome
Biliary atresia
Gastroesophageal reflux
Protracted diarrhea of infancy
Chronic nonspecific diarrhea
Renal disease
Hypermetabolic states
Burn injury
Severe trauma/closed head injury
Cancer
Neurologic disease/cerebral palsy

INDICATIONS FOR ENTERAL FEEDING: MANAGEMENT OF NUTRITION-RELATED DISORDERS

Table 1 lists conditions under which enteral feeding may be warranted.

Preterm Infants

A feeding method for preterm infants should be individualized to gestational age, birth weight, and medical status.[5] Preterm infants present a unique nutritional challenge owing to their GI immaturity; limited fluid tolerance; high requirements for specific nutrients such as protein, fat, calcium, and phosphorus; limited renal function; and predisposition to specific metabolic and clinical complications such as hypoglycemia and necrotizing enterocolitis.[4-6] As the coordination of sucking and swallowing appears at approximately 34 weeks' gestation, intragastric or jejunal feedings are often used before this time. These feedings may be useful beyond 34 weeks in selected infants unable to tolerate adequate oral feedings. As gastric bolus feedings may lead to abdominal distention and blood gas disturbances in neonates with limited gastric volume and cardiorespiratory distress,[5,7] continuous transpyloric feeding has been recommended as a better-tolerated alternative. A recent study, however, found that nasojejunal feedings resulted in lower rates of catch-up growth relative to nasogastric feedings, which may be partially attributable to a greater degree of fat malabsorption in infants fed nasojejunally.[8]

Cardiorespiratory Illness

Infants and children with cardiac and pulmonary disease often require enteral nutritional support during acute exacerbations of their primary disease as well as for nutritional rehabilitation of chronic secondary malnutrition. The etiology of growth failure in patients with bronchopulmonary dysplasia (BPD) is unclear but may be related to prolonged hypoxia, hypercapnia, increased oxygen dependency, elevated metabolic rates, inefficient suck and swallow mechanisms, poor appetite, decreased intake, and recurrent emesis with decreased gastric motility.[9-11] Nasogastric (NG) feedings of high-caloric-density, low-electrolyte formulas are often indicated in these infants.[9] Formula supplementation with equicaloric amounts of carbohydrate and fat increases caloric density without significantly increasing protein and mineral content. Children with cystic fibrosis (CF) also have elevated energy needs and poor intake, which result from their lung disease, malabsorption, chronic infections, debilitation, and fatigue.[12] Although behavior modification techniques and high-calorie oral supplementation should be instituted as routine components of a nutritional rehabilitation program, nocturnal NG feedings using elemental formulas have been promoted for children and adolescents who have failed these conservative measures.[12-14] Short-term NG feedings have resulted in increased caloric intake and significant weight gain for patients with CF, but long-term effectiveness is hampered by noncompliance.[13] Night-time gastrostomy feeding for long-term management is being advocated by some clinicians.[14]

Infants with congenital heart disease (CHD) are also at significant nutritional risk. The extent of their growth impairment depends upon their hemodynamic lesion and often results from inadequate caloric intake.[15] Growth failure resulting from poor intake and elevated energy expenditure may be caused by labored and rapid respiration, increased metabolic needs, reduced peripheral blood flow, tissue hypoxia, impaired absorption, and/or protein-losing enteropathy.[15-18] Owing to their elevated nutritional needs and limited fluid tolerance, these infants often require high-caloric-density formulas achieved through formula concentration to a maximum of 24 kcal per ounce. Concentration beyond 24 kcal per ounce may not allow enough free water for excretion of the renal osmotic load. Additional calories can be provided through carbohydrate or fat supplementation. The inability of some of these infants to achieve their nutritional needs despite these measures has prompted the limited use of NG feedings. Continuous NG feeding of infants with CHD has resulted in significant catch-up growth with effective nutrient absorption and only transient elevations in respiratory rate.[19]

Gastrointestinal Disease and Dysfunction

Pediatric patients with acute and chronic GI disease and dysfunction often benefit from enteral feeding regimens. The etiology of growth failure in children with Crohn's disease is multifactorial but is often related to inadequate nutrient intake. Elemental diets administered orally and nasogastrically have been clinically demonstrated to induce remission and produce a significant improvement in nutritional status.[20-23] Both continuous and intermittent elemental enteral nutrition have reversed growth failure. Clinical remission is more likely in Crohn's disease of the small bowel than of the colon.[23-25] The nutritional management of the infant with short bowel syndrome involves the initial use of total parenteral nutrition with gradually increasing amount of enteral feedings, which serve as a major stimulus to gut adaptation and regrowth. The period of transition to complete enteral feedings may take weeks to years depending upon the location and length of intestinal resection; however, parenteral nutrition must be continued until it is clinically evident that positive nitrogen balance and weight gain can be maintained or enteral nutrition alone.[26] Important considerations for provision of adequate enteral feedings include method of administration, volume osmolality, and nutrient quality (polymeric versus elemental). Polymeric nutrients are usually not well tolerated in the initial stages of the enteral feeding progression, whereas glucose and glucose polymers, medium-chain triglycerides (MCT), and hydrolyzed protein and dipeptides, which require less digestion, are more easily tolerated.[26]

Several other illnesses affecting GI function and nutritional status can be managed successfully with NG enteral feedings. Infants with biliary atresia frequently experience reduced intake associated with liver disease and infection.[27] Nutritional support with continuous NG feedings using an elemental formula rich in MCT can promote energy and nitrogen balance.[28,29] Infants with gastroesophageal reflux (GER) who have failed conventional therapy with thickened feeds and upright positioning and have subsequently experienced growth failure have been shown to benefit from continuous NG feeding with improved intake, reduction or cessation of vomiting, and catch-up growth.[30] Patients with favorable outcome demonstrated catch-up growth in the first week of enteral nutritional therapy, whereas those with poor response usually had other associated disorders, including chronic pulmonary disease, malabsorption, and cerebral palsy.[30] Children with chronic nonspecific or protracted diarrhea and malnutrition can also benefit from enteral tube feedings, if formula volume and concentration are advanced gradually.[31-33]

Postoperative Malnutrition

Enteral feeding for the postoperative pediatric patient has increased in recent years owing to improvements in enteral feeding products, equipment, and techniques.[1,34] Clinical studies have demonstrated that GI function can be adequately maintained with improved nitrogen balance and nutritional status in the postsurgical trauma patient.[34,35] Postsurgery pediatric patients may be managed via oral, enteral, or parenteral nutrition or a combination of these, depending upon the affected portion of the GI tract and the extent of surgery.[36] Certain patients with severe neurologic impairment or esophageal pathology may benefit from the placement of a feeding gastrostomy.[34] Gastrostomies and other enteral feeding routes are presented later in this discussion.

Renal Disease

Chronic renal failure in infants and children commonly results in growth failure and developmental delay, particularly in patients with congenital renal disease early in life.[37-39] The etiology of growth failure in these children is thought to be related to protein-calorie deficiency, renal osteodystrophy, chronic metabolic acidosis, and endocrine dysfunction.[37] Despite aggressive medical management and specialized formulas of high caloric density, poor growth and development often persist. Early nutritional intervention and dialysis can result in improved growth and development.[37,40] Nocturnal NG feedings over a period of 8 to 12 hours in patients with renal insufficiency have resulted in catch-up growth.[37,40]

Hypermetabolic States

Hypermetabolic states, e.g., severe head trauma or burn injury, often require specialized nutritional support. Metabolic effects associated with burn wounds that can lead to malnutrition include accelerated rate of energy expenditure, increased urine nitrogen excretion, and abnormal protein and glucose metabolism.[41] Complications of thermal injury may include sepsis, ileus, respiratory problems, or nutrient intolerance and often may preclude enteral nutritional support. We have found that when a burn patient has stabilized to the point of adequate GI function without other associated medical contraindications, continuous NG feeding with a high-calorie, high-nitrogen formula of low osmolality may be initiated. Enteral nutritional support is the preferred method for the nutritional management of children with uncomplicated severe head injuries.[42] Traumatized children can have protein and caloric requirements equivalent to those of severely burned patients. Certain pediatric cancer patients at high nutritional risk who have been screened for GI complaints, clotting function, and a strong family support structure may benefit from continuous NG feeding.[43]

Neurologic Disease and/or Impairment

The specific nutritional requirements and feeding approach for neurologically impaired children are highly variable and depend upon the degree of impairment, oral motor function, mobility, and muscular tone. These patients often require a high-caloric-density diet when oral intake is inadequate. Important considerations for the enteral feeding of these patients include method of feeding, risk of aspiration, formula caloric density, osmolality and fiber content, and effect of enteral feeding therapy on current and future oral-motor function and intake.[44]

NUTRITIONAL NEEDS OF THE ENTERALLY FED CHILD

Preterm Infant

Caloric requirements for normal intrauterine growth rates are estimated at 80 to 130 kcal per kilogram or higher, depending upon the infant's thermal environment, respiratory status, and metabolic stress.[4,5] Equally important for the promotion of appropriate weight gain is the ratio of protein content per 100 kcal consumed. Preterm infants require a minimum of 2.5 to 3.1 g of protein per 100 kcal to achieve an appropriate growth rate and body composition.[45] Intake of formulas with whey-to-casein ratios similar to that ratio in breast milk results in metabolic indices and plasma amino acid profiles closer to those of breast-fed infants.[46] Because of their GI immaturity, preterm infants demonstrate improved nutrient absorption when fed a mixture of MCT and long-chain unsaturated fatty acids and a mixture of lactose and glucose polymers as their fat and carbohydrate sources, respectively. Owing to the high accretion rates for calcium, phosphorus, and trace elements during the final trimester of gestation, preterm infants have elevated requirements for these nutrients.[4-6,47]

Infants and Children

The nutritional requirements of infants and children are outlined elsewhere. It must be emphasized that these recommended allowances are intended for healthy, active children and represent the average intake of nutrients that would maintain good health for an extended period.[48] As previously discussed, tube-fed children often have illnesses that result in malnutrition and inactivity and thus require adjusted allowances for energy and other nutrients. The specialized nutritional requirements of nutrition-related illnesses have been reviewed extensively in the literature.[9,12,15,20,26,28,34,41-44,49-53]

Particular attention should be given to the estimation of the energy and protein needs of the infant or child with failure to thrive. Catch-up growth, which should occur when the cause of growth impairment is removed, requires the provision of calories and protein in excess of normal needs.[54] Total energy needs may be 50 to 100 percent greater, with a proportional increase in protein requirement.[55] Estimated catch-up growth requirements can be calculated from the following equation[54]:

$$\frac{\text{kcal}}{\text{kg}} = \frac{\begin{pmatrix}\text{RDA kcal/kg} \\ \text{for weight age}\end{pmatrix} \times \begin{pmatrix}\text{ideal weight} \\ \text{in kilograms}\end{pmatrix}}{\text{actual weight in kilograms}}$$

where weight age is the age at which present weight is at fiftieth percentile and where ideal weight is the fiftieth percentile for age or ideal weight for height. (RDA = recommended daily allowance.) It is best to allow the child's appetite to be the determinant of intake whenever possible, as overfeeding during the initial stages of rehabilitation may be associated with edema.

Fluid balance is important in the pediatric tube-fed patient because several metabolic complications can be related to inadequate intake.[56] Fluid requirements can be calculated by estimating normal water requirements adjusted for specific disease-related factors; special consideration must be given to monitoring the fluid balance of children receiving high-calorie, high-protein formulas, those who have severe neurologic impairment, or those with emesis, diarrhea, fever, or polyuria.[56]

ENTERAL FORMULA SELECTION

Selecting an optimal infant enteral formula depends upon a number of factors, including diagnosis, associated nutritional problems and requirements, and GI function. Important formula factors include osmolality, renal solute load, caloric density, viscosity, and composition. Figure 1 presents an algorithm that identifies appropriate infant formulas based on indication for use. Table 2 lists and describes the nutrient sources in a variety of infant formulas.

Preterm Infant Formulas

Specialized formulas have been developed that are uniquely suited to the physiologic needs of the preterm infant. Physiologic factors in the preterm infant that call for alterations in their nutritional management include limited oral motor function, lactase deficiency, limited bile salt pool, decreased energy and nutrient stores, limited gastric volume, decreased intestinal motility, and limited renal function.[1,4] Several studies have demonstrated that preterm infant formulas, when used appropriately, can support the needs of the infant.[57-59]

There are various major differences between the nutrient content and composition of preterm and term infant formu-

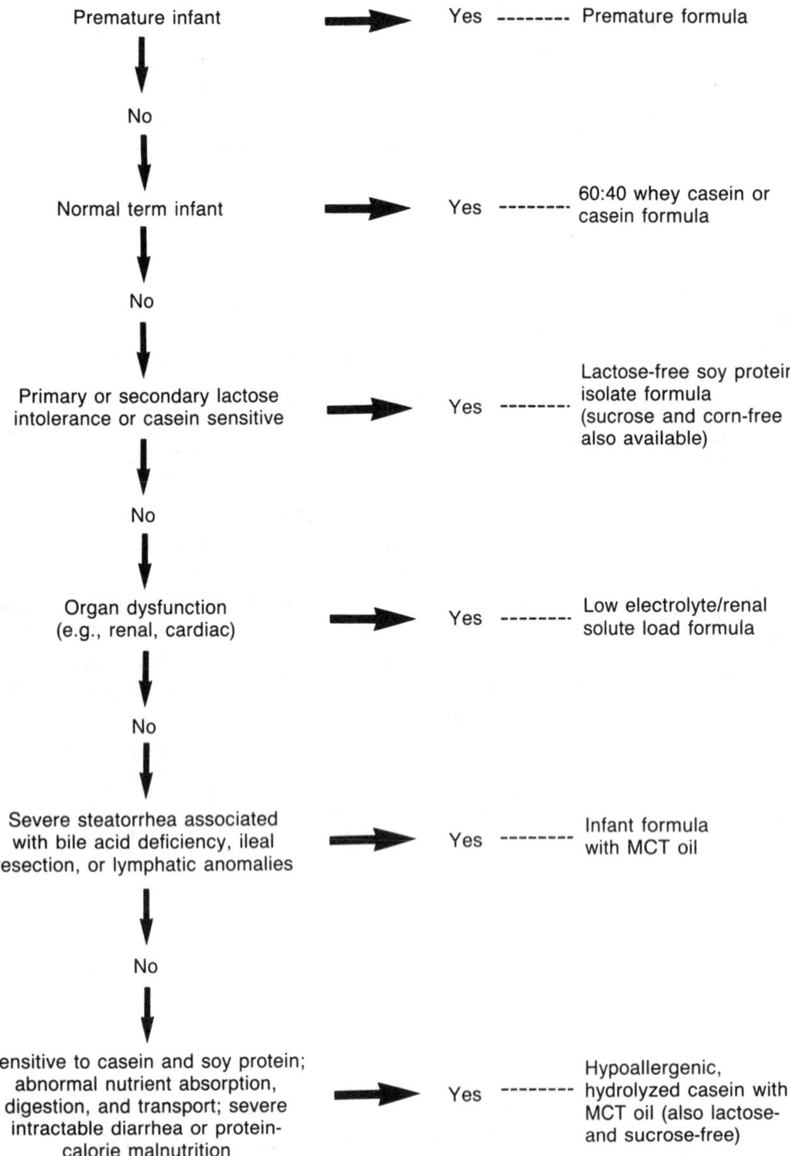

FIGURE 1 Algorithm for the selection of infant formulas based on digestive function. (Adapted from Wilson et al,[119] with permission.)

TABLE 2
Infant Formulas

Product Name	kcal/oz	Carbohydrate (gm/100 ml)	Fat (gm/100 ml)	Protein (gm/100 ml)	mOsm/kg	Nutrient Sources (Carbohydrate; Fat; Protein)
Preterm infant formulas						
Similac Special Care	24	8.6	4.4	2.2	300	Corn syrup solids, lactose; MCT oil, corn and coconut oil; nonfat milk, demineralized whey
Enfamil Premature	24	8.9	4.1	2.4	300	Same as above
"Preemie" SMA	24	8.6	4.4	2.0	268	Lactose, maltodextrins; MCT oil, coconut, oleic, oleo, soy oil; nonfat milk, demineralized whey
Term Infant Formulas*						
Similac	20	7.2	3.6	1.5	290	Lactose; soy, coconut oil; nonfat milk
Enfamil	20	6.9	3.8	1.5	278	Lactose; soy, coconut oil; nonfat milk, demineralized whey
SMA	20	7.2	3.6	1.5	300	Lactose; coconut, safflower, soy oils and oleo; nonfat milk, demineralized whey
Soy-Based Formulas†‡						
Isomil	20	6.8	3.6	2.0	250	Corn syrup solids, sucrose; soy and coconut oil; soy protein isolate, L-methionine
Prosobee	20	6.9	3.6	2.0	200	Corn syrup solids; soy and coconut oil; soy protein isolate, L-methionine
Nursoy	20	6.9	3.6	2.1	296	Sucrose; oleo, coconut, safflower, soy oils; soy protein isolate, L-methionine
Specialized formulas†‡						
Nutramigen	20	8.8	2.6	2.2	480	Sucrose, modified tapioca starch; corn oil; casein hydrolysate
Portagen	20	7.8	3.2	2.4	220	Corn syrup solids, lactose; MCT oil and corn oil; sodium caseinate
Pregestimil	20	9.1	2.7	1.9	350	Corn syrup solids, modified tapioca starch; corn oil and MCT oil; casein hydrolysate with amino acids
Good Start H.A.	20	7.4	3.4	1.6	265	Lactose, maltodextrins; palm oil, safflower oil, coconut oil; hydrolyzed whey
Alimentum	20	6.8	3.7	1.8	370	Tapioca starch, sucrose; MCT oil, safflower oil, soy oil; casein hydrolysate with amino acids

*Term infant formulas with the exception of SMA are also available in low-iron formulations. Term infant formulas are also available in 24 kcal per ounce ready to feed.
†Available as iron-fortified only.
‡Can be prepared to 24 kcal per ounce by adding less water to the concentrate or powder base.
MCT = medium-chain triglycerides.

las. Owing to the decreased intestinal lactase activity in the premature infant, the carbohydrate content of preterm infant formulas is a mixture of 40 to 50 percent lactose and 50 to 60 percent glucose polymers.[5,57] Preterm infants are often unable to digest and absorb the vegetable oils in term infant formula owing to their decreased bile salt pool; consequently, formulas utilize a fat blend containing between 10 and 50 percent of fat as MCT, which improves weight gain, nitrogen retention, and calcium absorption.[60,61] An elevated protein content and 60:40 whey-to-casein formulation promote a plasma amino acid profile closer to that of the breast-fed infant.[1,5] Increased amounts of sodium, calcium, and phosphorus accommodate for the increased urinary sodium losses seen in the preterm infant and promote bone mineralization closer to intrauterine rates.[4,5,62] The concentration of vitamin E in preterm infant formulas is three times the level recommended by the American Academy of Pediatrics (AAP) for full-term infants because of limited stores, wide variability in absorption, and susceptibility to hemolytic anemia.[58] Vitamin D content is also high in order to promote bone mineralization. However, if there is inadequate intake, supplementation with 400 IU of vitamin D may be recommended for some preterm infants.[5,57] Owing to the lower birthweight and initial hemoglobin concentration of preterm infants, iron has been added to preterm infant formulas, providing approximately 2 mg per kilogram of iron per day when fed at a level of 120 kcal per kilogram.[63] Because preterm infants are unable to consume adequate volumes and absorb all of their nutritional needs, multivitamin supplementation is generally recommended.[57]

Mature human milk is generally not recommended for use with the preterm infant, as it may be low in protein, sodium, calcium, and possibly other nutrients. Preterm human milk, however, which is higher in protein, sodium, chloride, magnesium, and iron than mature human milk, may be more suitable for the enteral feeding of the preterm infant.[57] Despite these advantages, preterm milk is still relatively deficient in calcium and phosphorus for the needs of the growing preterm infant.[4,57] Owing to the risk of developing osteopenia, rickets, and fractures from inadequate calcium deposition, premature infants should receive fortified human milk. Enfamil Human Milk Fortifier (Mead Johnson, Evansville, IN) has been developed to meet the nutritional needs of the premature infant. The addition of one packet of this product to 25 ml of human milk increases the caloric density by 4 kcal per ounce and also increases the levels of protein, calcium, phosphorus, and other minerals.

Term Infant Formulas

Standard infant formulas have been developed to meet the nutritional requirements of term infants during the first year of life. These formulas are prepared by diluting nonfat cow's milk to reduce the high protein content, adjusting the mineral content, and adding vegetable oils and carbohydrate to simulate the caloric distribution and digestibility of breast milk.[64,65] Similac (Ross Laboratories, Columbus, OH) contains nonfat cow's milk protein with a whey-to-casein ratio of 18:82; however, Enfamil and SMA (Wyeth, Philadelphia, PA) have a whey-to-casein ratio of 60:40. Despite these modifications, term infants grow equally well on whey-predominant or casein-predominant standard infant formulas.[64] Because term infants have lactase activity comparable or superior to that of adults, standard infant formulas contain lactose, which enhances calcium and iron absorption.[65] Standard infant formulas have replaced the butterfat of cow's milk with vegetable oils to simulate the ratio of polyunsaturated to saturated fats of breast milk. Vitamins and minerals are added to all infant formulas in accordance with the recommendations set by the AAP[66] and the Infant Formula Act of 1980.[67] Iron-fortified infant formula contains iron at a level that provides approximately 2 mg per kilogram for the infant consuming 120 kcal per kilogram.[64]

Standard infant formulas have a caloric density of 20 kcal per ounce, but pediatric patients with nutrition-related illnesses and malnutrition often require infant formulas with a caloric density of 24 kcal per ounce to meet their elevated energy needs. Concentrating a formula to a caloric density greater than 24 kcal per ounce should generally be avoided during the first year of life, as elevated renal solute load and osmolality may become a concern. The optimal formula osmolality for infants during their first year is close to that of breast milk, which ranges from 227 to 303 mOsm per kilogram of water.[1,66] Increased caloric densities can be achieved through formula supplementation with carbohydrate and fat modules in equicaloric distributions. Infants on high-caloric-density formulas need to be closely monitored for dehydration.[1]

Soy Infant Formulas

Except for carbohydrate and protein, soy protein formulas are similar in composition to standard infant formulas and follow the recommendations of the AAP.[66] The protein source in soy formulas, a refined soy protein isolate, is heat-treated for enhancement of protein digestibility and mineral bioavailability.[68] Zinc, however, appears to be less biologically available in soy formulas, which is possibly related to the presence of phytate.[64] Because soy protein has a lower biologic value than casein and whey, its concentration in soy formulas has been increased to 2.0 g per deciliter, and methionine has been added to improve protein quality. Carnitine, which plays an important role in the oxidation of long-chain fatty acids, is now added to soy formulas owing to its negligible amount in the unsupplemented product.[64,68] Soy formulas are lactose-free and contain corn syrup solids, sucrose, or a combination of these as their carbohydrate source.

Indications are numerous for the use of soy formulas in pediatric patients. The rare infant with primary lactase deficiency or galactosemia should be started on soy formulas. More important, these formulas can also be beneficial for the nutritional management of infants with secondary lactose intolerance following resolving gastroenteritis, protein-calorie malnutrition, or other causes of mucosal injury.[64] If sucrose intolerance also occurs following a bout of severe gastroenteritis, Isomil SF (Ross Laboratories) or Prosobee (Mead Johnson), which are both sucrose-free, is the formula of choice. Cow's milk protein sensitivity, which is considered the most common food sensitivity affecting children, is routinely managed with soy protein formulas. However, soy protein sensitivity may develop as well. Children with cow's milk allergy may demonstrate anemia and/or GI, dermatologic, respiratory, neurologic, or vascular symptoms. They should be taken off milk and then re-challenged with a milk feeding for establishment of a diagnosis.[70,71] Milk can generally be re-introduced into the diet within 6 months to 2 years, depending upon the severity of the milk sensitivity.[70]

Specialized Formulas

Nutramigen (Mead Johnson) is indicated for infants who have allergies to intact protein from either cow's milk or soy. The protein in Nutramigen consists of casein hydrolyzed to amino acids and polypeptides and charcoal-treated to decrease its allergenicity.[64] Nutramigen is essentially lactose-free and contains added sucrose (72 percent) and tapioca starch (28 percent) as the sources of carbohydrate and corn oil as the source of fat. Despite an osmolality of 480 mOsm per kilogram of water, Nutramigen is usually well tolerated by the term infant at a concentration of 20 kcal per ounce.[64] However, the cost is approximately twice that of standard infant formula.

Good Start H.A. (Carnation, Kansas City, MO), a recent addition to the line of specialized formulas, is marketed directly to consumers as a hypoallergenic formula. The protein in Good Start H.A. comes from whey hydrolyzed by heat treatment and enzyme modification to an average peptide length of 5.6 amino acids with an average molecular weight of 638 daltons. The product's hypoallergenicity has been tested in animal sensitization and challenge tests. Recent reactions reported to Good Start H.A. may question its hypoallergenicity. Now that multiple presumed hypoallergenic hydrolysate formulas exist, we can expect that their relative allergenicity will be the subject of case reports and prospective objective comparison trials. Good Start H.A. is composed of a carbohydrate blend of lactose (70 percent) and maltodextrins (30 percent). The fat component is a blend of palm oil (60 percent), high-oleic safflower oil (22 percent), and coconut oil (18 percent), with a resulting polyunsaturated-to-saturated fat ratio of 0.31, similar to that found in human milk (0.28 to 0.35). At a concentration of 20 kcal per ounce, Good Start H.A. has an osmolality of 265 mOsm per kilogram and a renal solute load of 100.6 mOsm per liter (Carnation product monograph). The cost of Good Start H.A. is approximately the same as that of standard infant formula.

Portagen (Mead Johnson), which contains 88 percent of its fat as MCT and 12 percent from corn oil, is indicated for use in the management of infants with steatorrhea due to a limited bile salt pool, e.g., biliary atresia and ileal resection. MCT is hydrolyzed rapidly in the intestinal lumen and is well absorbed even in the absence of bile salts.[64] Portagen contains sodium caseinate as its protein source and corn syrup solids (73 percent) and sucrose (25 percent) as carbohydrate sources. At the concentration of 20 kcal per ounce, Portagen has an osmolality of 220 mOsm per kilogram and is well tolerated in infants and young children with fat malabsorption.[64]

Pregestimil (Mead Johnson) is considered the most elemental of the specialized infant formulas and is routinely used for infants and young children with generalized malabsorption, e.g., short gut syndrome. Because of the elemental nature of both its protein and fat sources, Pregestimil is the formula of choice for use in infants with CF. Pregestimil contains casein hydrolysate with added L-cystine, L-tyrosine, and L-tryptophan as its protein source. Corn oil and MCT constitute 60 and 40 percent of the fat, respectively. Carbohydrate is provided by corn syrup solids (85 percent) and modified tapioca starch (15 percent). At a concentration of 20 kcal per ounce, Pregestimil has an osmolality of 350 mOsm per kilogram[64] and a cost of more than twice that of standard infant formula.

Another recent addition to the line of hypoallergenic formulas is Alimentum (Ross Laboratories). This product has a caloric distribution of 11 percent protein, 41 percent carbohydrate, and 48 percent fat. The protein is enzymatically hydrolyzed, charcoal-treated casein with 60 percent of the hydrolysate composed of free amino acids. A molecular weight profile of the hydrolysate in Alimentum has indicated that 99 percent of the hydrolysate has a molecular weight of less than 1,500 daltons. The hypoallergenicity of the formula has been tested through animal challenge tests and immunosorbent inhibition assays. The fat blend comprises MCT (50 percent), safflower oil (40 percent), and soy oil (10 percent). The carbohydrate fraction contains both tapioca starch and sucrose, which are digested and absorbed by separate mechanisms. Alimentum contains carnitine and taurine at the same level as that found in human milk. At present, Alimentum is available only in the ready-to-feed form at a concentration of 20 kcal per ounce and has an osmolality of 370 mOsm per kilogram with a renal solute load of 123 mOsm per liter (Ross product monograph).

Formula for Children One to Six Years of Age

Until now adult formulas have been used for the enteral nutritional support of children because a tube feeding formula for young children was not available. The primary disadvantages of using adult tube feeding formulas in young children are the elevated renal solute load and insufficient vitamin and mineral levels.[1,72] Dilution of the formulas to reduce renal solute load results in further reduction of the vitamin and mineral concentration.[72]

Pediasure (Ross Laboratories), a new formula, is designed to meet the specialized nutritional needs of the 1- to 6-year-old child. The product can be used for both enteral feedings and oral supplementation. The energy distribution of protein, carbohydrate, and fat is between that of infant and adult formulas. The vitamin and mineral concentrations in 1,100 ml of formula meet or exceed 100 percent of the RDAs for children 1 to 6 years of age. At a caloric density of 1 kcal per milliliter, the formula is useful for children with elevated metabolic needs or for those with fluid restrictions. The 1 kcal per milliliter caloric density permits some flexibility in dilution, still meeting 100 percent of the RDAs in 1,100 ml of 24 kcal per ounce formula.[72]

Pediasure contains 3.0 g of protein per 100 ml of formula with a calorie-to-nitrogen ratio of 208:1 and does not exceed protein intakes of greater than 18 percent of energy, the recommended limit for children under 4 years of age.[72,73] The fat component is a blend of 50 percent high oleic safflower oil, 30 percent soy oil, and 20 percent MCT oil. The carbohydrate content is a blend of corn syrup solids and sucrose.[72,74] The osmolality of 325 mOsm per kilogram of water reduces the osmotic intolerance often seen when using hypertonic formulas. With lower sodium, potassium, chloride, and protein levels than found in most adult enteral formulas, the estimated renal solute load is 200 mOsm per liter.[72] Children 7 years of age or older or those with highly specialized nutrient and metabolic needs may require enteral nutrition management with adult formulas.

Adult Enteral Tube Feeding Formulas

As with the selection of an infant formula, the selection of an optimal pediatric or adult enteral formula depends upon a number of factors such as GI function, nutrient metabolism capabilities, organ function, and diagnosis. Figure 2 is an algorithm for the selection of pediatric or adult formulas for children over 1 year of age based on GI function. Table 3 lists and describes the nutrient sources in a variety of adult formulas.

Blenderized Formulas

Commercially available blenderized diets consist of beef, eggs, milk, cereal, fruits and vegetables, and vegetable oils. These formulas, which contain a moderate to high level of

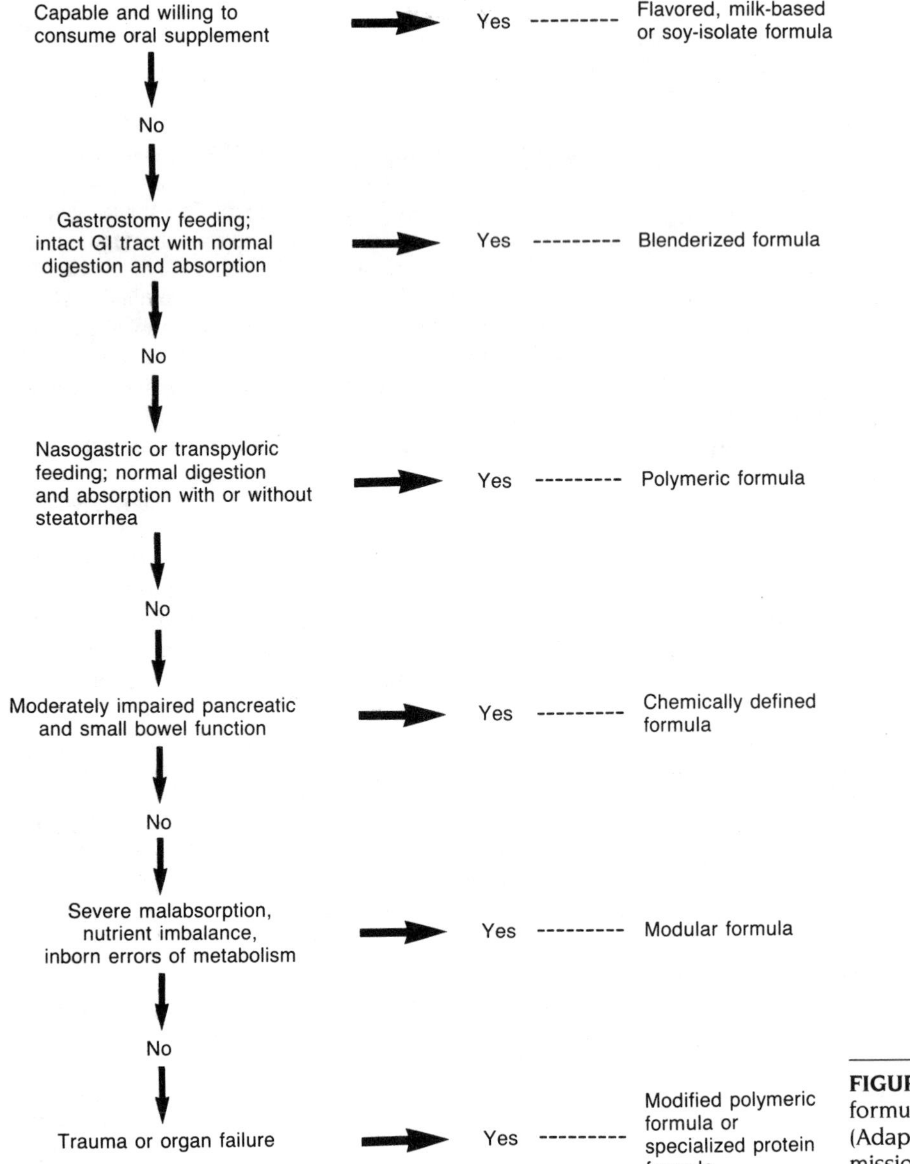

FIGURE 2 Algorithm for selection of adult formulas based on digestive function. (Adapted from Wilson et al,[119] with permission.)

residue, have osmolalities ranging from 300 to 435 mOsm per kilogram.[75] Blenderized feedings are beneficial for chronically ill patients who have normal digestive capabilities and require long-term enteral nutrition; however, they may not be well tolerated in the malnourished pediatric patient with compromised GI function.

Blenderized feedings can be prepared at home from milk, juices, cereals, and baby food.[1] Parents of neurologically impaired children who require long-term nutritional management through a feeding gastrostomy are often encouraged to prepare blenderized feedings at home because of their economical and psychosocial advantages. Care must be exercised for the provision of adequate free water with these often eclectic mixtures. A pediatric nutritionist can help the family design a blenderized feeding formula that will meet the child's specific nutritional needs.

Standard Hospital Tube Feeding Formulas

Standard tube feeding formulas have various properties that permit their use and tolerance by the nutritionally compromised patient. These standard formulas are polymeric, consisting of mixtures of protein isolates, oligosaccharides, vegetable oil, MCT, and added vitamins and minerals.[1] They can be further subdivided into categories based on their osmolality and nutrient composition and density. These formulas, most of which are lactose-free and low-residue, vary in osmolality from 300 to 650 mOsm per kilogram and in caloric density from 1.0 to 2.0 kcal per milliliter.[75] The isotonic formulas Osmolite (Ross Laboratories) and Isocal (Mead Johnson), which contain MCT oil, are often useful for individuals with a history of delayed gastric emptying, dumping syndrome, or osmotic diarrhea.[76] These isotonic

TABLE 3
Selected Adult Enteral Formulas*

Product Name	kcal/cc	Carbohydrate (gm/100 ml)	Fat (gm/100 ml)	Protein (gm/100 ml)	mOsm/kg	Volume to meet 100% U.S. RDA (cc)	Nutrient Sources (Carbohydrate; Fat; Protein)
Blenderized							
Compleat-B	1.07	13	4.3	4.3	405	1,500	Hydrolyzed cereal solids, fruits, vegetable, maltodextrin, lactose; beef, corn oil; beef, nonfat milk
Vitaneed	1.0	13	4.0	3.5	310	2,000	Maltodextrin, pureed fruits and vegetables; soy oil and beef; beef, sodium and calcium casein
Standard tube feeding formulas							
Ensure	1.06	14	3.7	3.7	450	1,887	Corn syrup, sucrose; corn oil; sodium and calcium caseinates, soy protein isolates
Enrich (with fiber)	1.1	16	3.7	4.0	480	1,391	Hydrolyzed corn starch, sucrose, soy polysaccharide; corn oil; same protein as Ensure
Isotonic tube feeding formulas							
Osmolite	1.06	14	3.8	3.7	300	1,887	Hydrolyzed corn starch; MCT, corn and soy oil; same protein as Ensure
Isocal	1.06	13	4.4	3.4	300	1,892	Maltodextrin; soy oil, MCT oil; same protein as Ensure
Renu	1.0	13	4.0	3.5	300	n/a	Maltodextrin, sucrose; soy oil; sodium and calcium caseinate
Precision Isotonic	1.0	15	3.0	3.0	300	1,560	Glucose, oligosaccharides, sucrose; soybean oil; egg white solids
High-caloric-density formulas†							
Ensure Plus	1.5	20	5.3	5.4	600	1,600	Corn syrup, sucrose; corn oil; same protein as Ensure
Sustacal HC	1.5	19	5.8	6.1	650	1,200	Corn syrup solids, sugar; soybean oil; calcium and sodium caseinates
Resource Plus	1.5	20	5.3	5.4	600	n/a	Maltodextrin, sucrose; corn oil; same protein as Ensure
Isotein HN	1.2	16	3.4	6.8	300	1,770	Maltodextrin, monosaccharides; soybean oil and MCT; delactosed lactalbumin
Magnacal	2.0	25	8.0	7.0	590	1,000	Maltodextrin, sucrose; soy oil; calcium and sodium caseinates
Elemental formulas							
Vital HN	1.0	19	1.1	4.2	460	1,500	Hydrolyzed corn starch, sucrose; safflower oil and MCT oil; di- and tripeptides, free amino acids
Tolerex	1.0	23	.15	2.0	550	1,800	Glucose oligosaccharides; safflower oil; free amino acids
Vivonex T.E.N.	1.0	21	.30	3.8	630	2,000	Maltodextrins, modified starch; safflower oil; free amino acids

Table continues on following page

tube feedings are the formulas of choice for general use with pediatric patients over 7 years of age owing to their low osmolality, caloric density, and moderate protein content. The low osmolality permits their use for both bolus intragastric and transpyloric continuous feedings. The isotonic formulas provide 100 percent of the United States RDA for adults and children over 4 years of age in approximately 1,900 ml. Children with significant fluid restriction may require vitamin and mineral supplementation. Tube feeding formulas with added fiber such as Enrich (Ross Laboratories), which range in osmolality from 300 to 480 mOsm per kilogram, are often useful for the management of patients with chronic constipation and diarrhea.[77] We have used fiber-containing formulas successfully for the long-term enteral support and bowel management of neurologically impaired children with chronic constipation.

Although high-calorie, high-nitrogen, hypertonic formulations are often well tolerated by the adult patient with elevat-

TABLE 3 *(Continued)*

Product Name	kcal/cc	Carbohydrate (gm/100 ml)	Fat (gm/100 ml)	Protein (gm/100 ml)	mOsm/kg	Volume to meet 100% U.S. RDA (cc)	Nutrient Sources (Carbohydrate; Fat; Protein)
Specialized formulas							
Trauma (high BCAA)							
Traum-Aid HBC	1.0	18	1.2	5.6	675	3,000	Maltodextrins; soybean oil and MCT; free amino acids (50% BCAA)
Stresstein	1.2	17	2.8	7.0	910	2,000	Maltodextrin; MCT, soybean oil; free amino acids (44% BCAA)
Hepatic (high BCAA, low AAA)							
Hepatic-Aid II‡	1.1	17	3.6	4.4	560	—	Maltodextrin, sucrose; soybean oil; free amino acids (46% BCAA)
Travasorb Hepatic	1.1	21	1.4	2.9	690	2,100	Glucose oligosaccharides; MCT, sunflower oil; free amino acids (50% BCAA)
Renal failure (high EAA)							
Amin-Aid‡	2.0	37	4.6	1.9	510	—	Maltodextrin, sucrose; soybean oil; free EAA plus histidine
Travasorb Renal	1.35	27	1.8	2.3	590	2,100	Same cholesterol and fat as Travasorb Hepatic; free amino acids

*Based on manufacturers' available literature.
†May also be used as oral supplements.
‡Does not contain vitamins or electrolytes.
BCAA = branched-chain amino acids; EAA = essential amino acids; MCT = medium-chain triglycerides.

ed metabolic needs, they are usually not tolerated by the pediatric patient, often leading to diarrhea, emesis, abdominal distention, and delayed gastric emptying.[1] We often observe that preteens and adolescents can tolerate high-calorie, hypertonic formulas when advanced slowly and administered via continuous NG feedings. These formulations, however, are generally not well tolerated when administered into the jejunum or in bolus feedings.[1] Children and adolescents with markedly elevated calorie and protein requirements secondary to severe trauma or burn injury are best managed with isotonic high-nitrogen formulations such as Isotein HN (Sandoz, Minneapolis, MN) and Travasorb MCT (Travenol Labs, Deerefield, IL).[41] These formulas, which contain MCT and glucose polymers, promote positive nitrogen balance while optimizing GI tolerance. However, because of the elevated protein levels in these formulas, hydration status must be closely monitored in pediatric patients.[1,78]

Elemental Formulas

Elemental formulas with predigested nutrients can be used for the nutritional support of pediatric patients with short gut syndrome, pancreatic insufficiency, inflammatory bowel disease, or other severe malabsorptive conditions. Predigested formulas have been used effectively for the continuous enteral feeding support of patients with Crohn's disease, CF, and short gut syndrome.[13,14,20,22,24,26] Nitrogen is more rapidly and effectively absorbed in both the healthy and compromised bowel in the form of dipeptides and tripeptides than from free amino acids[79-81]; therefore, emphasis in elemental product formulation is on the use of peptide formulas with supplemental free essential amino acids. Current research is focusing on the effect of variation of peptide length on nitrogen absorption and retention. Peptide-based formulations are also available in high-nitrogen varieties that provide a calorie-to-nitrogen ratio of 150:1 for the patient with severely compromised protein status.[79,82] Fats are provided from a blend of MCT oil and long-chain triglycerides, which provide the essential fatty acids. Both nutrient features promote improved GI tolerance in the compromised pediatric or adult patient. Several elemental products that contain free amino acids as their protein source also provide a high osmotic load, which may not be well tolerated by the pediatric patient. Owing to the high carbohydrate and extremely low fat content, fat supplementation for the prevention of essential fatty acid deficiency is often recommended when these products are used long term.[1] The only elemental formulas appropriate for young infants are Pregestimil and Alimentum (discussed above).

Specialized Enteral Formulas

Specialized nutritional formulas have been designed for the nutritional support of patients with specific diseases. Although emphasis has been placed on the use of these formulas, their advantage over standard tube feeding formulas for the management of diseases such as hepatic encephalopathy, renal failure, and trauma and sepsis remains controversial.[83] Formulas with elevated branched-chain amino acids (BCAA) and with lower calorie-to-nitrogen ratios are often advocated for use in adult patients with multiple trauma and sepsis.[83] Studies investigating the effectiveness of high BCAA formulations in humans are limited and inconclusive.[83,85] Although high BCAA formulas may be beneficial in the nutritional support of the adult patient in the first 7 days following traumatic injury, their effectiveness in pediatric patients is not accepted. Patients with hepatic diseases resulting in severe protein intolerance and hyperammonemia may develop hepatic encephalopathy, in part related to elevated levels of the aromatic amino acids (AAA) and the subsequent synthesis of false neurotransmitters.[86] Formulas of higher BCAA and lowered AAA content have been developed for the management of these patients; however, their effectiveness in the resolution of encephalopathic symptoms remains inconclusive.[83] Commercial formulations developed for the nutritional support of patients with acute renal failure have a low protein content provided as essential amino acids, are electrolyte-free, and contain no fat-soluble vitamins. These renal formulas may be used for short-term management in pediatric patients if vitamins, minerals, and electrolytes are supplemented as needed.

Oral Supplements

In the pediatric patient with normal intestinal function, we often advise a variety of high-calorie favorite foods that require minimal parental pressure for their successful administration. "Flavor fatigue" and control issues often severely limit the utility of commercial supplements. However, various flavored milk-based and polymeric formulas may be used as oral supplements for pediatric patients. Milk-based formulas are of moderate residue and high osmolality owing to their high lactose content. High-calorie and protein concentrations also may not be tolerated by the nutritionally compromised patient when taken in large volumes; thus, it is often recommended that they be taken in small frequent sips.[1] Oral supplements mixed with milk such as Carnation Instant Breakfast (Travenol Labs) are often better accepted by children than are the lactose-free commercial supplements. Flavored polymeric formulas that contain intact proteins, long-chain fatty acids, and simple carbohydrates are usually marketed as oral supplements because of their palatability. These products have osmolarities ranging from 450 to 600 mOsm per kilogram and are often not palatable for pediatric patients. Recent developments have focused on packaging these formulas in carton tetrapaks, improving the product's storage and utility characteristics as well as its palatability by reducing the "metallic" taste often detected in canned products. Some examples of milk-based and polymeric oral supplements include Sustacal (Mead Johnson), Meritene (Sandoz), Ensure Plus (Ross Laboratories), and Resource Plus (Sandoz).

Modular Components

Owing to the unique and often elevated nutritional requirements of the enterally fed pediatric patient, modification of enteral formulas with modular components is often necessary.[82] A variety of modular products are now available on the market including protein, fat, carbohydrate, and vitamin and mineral modules.[87] Modular protein products such as Casec (Mead Johnson) and Propac (Chesebrough-Pond, Greenwich, CT) may be used to increase formula protein density. Emulsified fat products such as Microlipid (Chesebrough-Pond) and Nutrisource MCT (Sandoz) may be added to tube feeding formulas, thus increasing formula caloric density without separating out of solution. Although these fat products are useful in tube feedings, they have a short shelf-life of between 24 and 72 hours. The addition of glucose polymers such as Polycose (Ross Laboratories) or Moducal (Mead Johnson) as a supplemental carbohydrate source can also increase formula caloric density while promoting GI tolerance. Both infant formulas and adult enteral formulas can be modified using modular components. When adding more than one modular component for maintenance of caloric distribution, we have found that a gradual and stepwise addition of each of these components individually promotes GI tolerance. Selection of appropriate nutrient modules depends upon the specific needs of the patient, the nutrient composition and digestibility of the module, and the availability of the product.[87]

TUBE FEEDING

When the requirement for enteral nutritional support has been established, the optimal route of delivering nutrients must be determined. Many practitioners recommend the placement of nasogastric or nasoduodenal feeding tubes when the estimated course of therapy will not exceed 1 to 3 months.[88] If the risk of aspiration is not significant, gastric feedings are preferable owing to the bactericidal effects of acid, the action of lingual lipase, and the ease of management. In addition, bypassing the pylorus negates its beneficial effects on control of the rate at which nutrients are presented to the duodenum.[89] If gastroesophageal reflux (GER) is present, aspiration is a significant risk, and the duration of tube feeding will be relatively short, transpyloric feeding is preferable to nasogastric feeding. An algorithm to aid the selection of enteral or parenteral feeding routes is presented in Figure 3.

Depending upon the family's capability and motivation, the use of a nasal tube may be feasible over a period longer than 2 to 3 months, obviating the need for surgical intervention to place a gastrostomy or jejunostomy device.[88,90] Tubes made of polyurethane and silicone rubber are soft and pliable and may be left in place for indefinite periods of time. Polyvinyl chloride tubes become stiff and nonpliable when left in place for more than a few days; however, they are useful for intestinal decompression or short-term feeding. They should be changed every 2 to 3 days to avoid skin necrosis or intestinal perforation.

Some feeding tubes made of polyurethane or silicone rubber have a tungsten or mercury weight at the tip that makes them useful for duodenal or jejunal feedings, e.g., Dobbhoff, Keofeed, Kangaroo. Tube sizes range from 5 to 12 F in outer diameter. Five to 8 F are appropriate sizes for most pediatric patients. The weight on tubes that are 7 or 8 F may be too great for easy passage in a young infant. The 5-F Keofeed (IVAC) tube has a weight that is nearly equivalent to the outer diameter of the tube and is useful for small in-

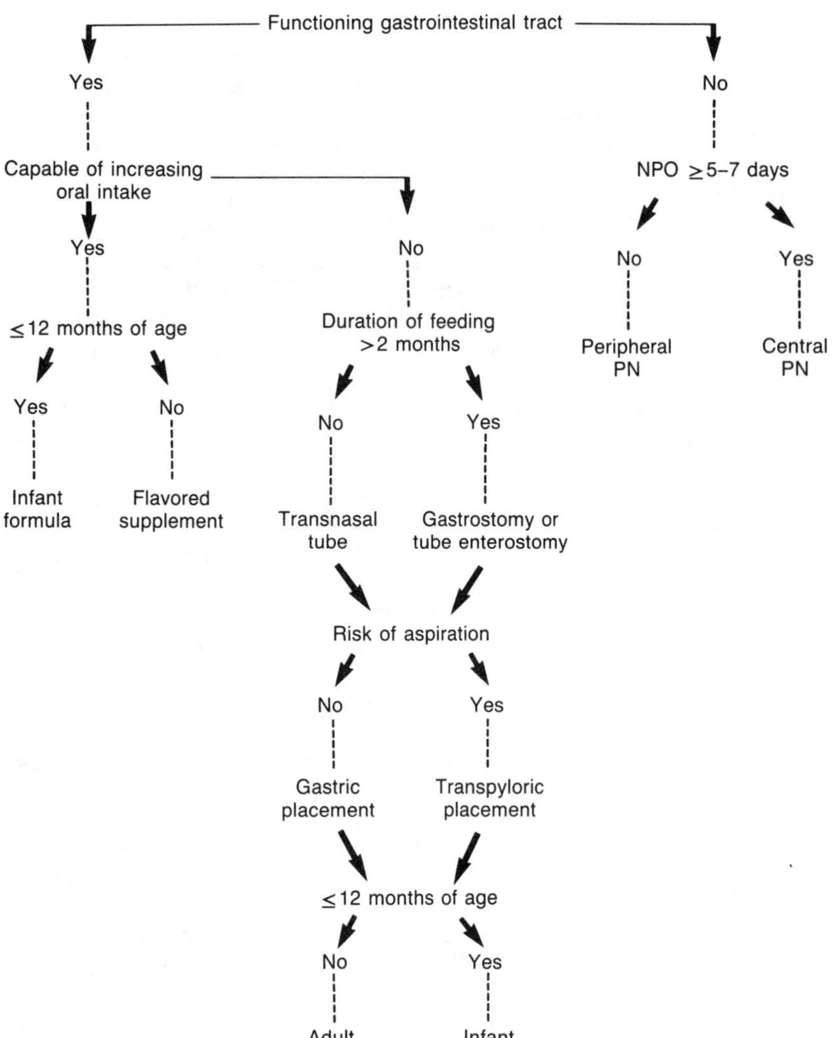

FIGURE 3 Algorithm for selection of enteral or parenteral feeding. (Adapted from Wilson et al,[119] with permission.)

fants. However, this tube is easily dislodged by coughing or vomiting. A less pliable 5-F polyurethane tube (Argyle) and a weighted tube placed in the distal duodenum or jejunum are options that circumvent displacement problems. The inner diameter of a polyurethane tube is larger than the equivalent size in the silicone tube, which makes them more practical in the smaller sizes, particularly when medications are given.

Children who require long-term tube feeding are candidates for placement of a gastrostomy tube. GER, which may occur in neurologically disabled children or even normal infants following gastrostomy tube placement, may necessitate an operative antireflux procedure (e.g., Nissen fundoplication). Although the procedure is effective in reducing GER, postoperative complications can be troublesome. Intractable retching episodes,[91] dumping syndrome,[92] continued problems with swallowing, impaired esophageal emptying,[93] slow feeding, and gas bloating have all been reported. Controversy currently exists over the necessity of an antireflux procedure in neurologically impaired children who require a feeding gastrostomy.[94]

Percutaneous endoscopic gastrostomy tubes can be placed without a laparotomy and often without general anesthesia.[95] In a series of 51 children, serious complications were less frequent than with traditional gastrostomy tube placement.[96] The most frequent complication of percutaneous endoscopic gastrostomies appears to be localized cellulitis, which can be managed by avoiding excessive tension on the outer bolster and by using antibiotics when necessary.[95] Percutaneous endoscopic gastrostomies are sometimes contraindicated after previous abdominal surgery, in the presence of an abdominal tumor, and when obesity complicates placement.

A common problem with all gastrostomies is migration of the tube through the ostomy site. Ultimately, the tip of the catheter contacts the pylorus where it occasionally induces retching as it passes in and out of the gastric outlet. Mechanical irritation of the stomach by the tube is often seen as well. These problems may be minimized by firmly attaching the tube and placing a mark on the tube or measuring the tube to detect inward migration. In addition, inserting the gastrostomy tube through the hole in a disposable feeding nipple, which is then secured to the skin, helps avoid inward migration. This technique also aids in preventing irritation of the ostomy site caused by movement of the tube. It is usually necessary to cut two or three small holes in the side of the nipple to allow for adequate aeration of the ostomy site.

The gastrostomy button is a feeding device that can be placed in an established gastrostomy tube site and has the advantage of being small and flush with the skin. The gastrostomy button cannot migrate through the pylorus, which, as discussed above, is a problem with conventional gastrostomy tubes. The button is also less prone to accidental removal.[97]

Feeding gastrostomies are generally contraindicated in the presence of delayed gastric emptying. If short-term enteral support is necessary and GER is significant, transpyloric feedings are an alternative. Placement of transpyloric nasoduodenal or nasojejunal tubes is more complicated than nasogastric tube placement and requires confirmation of position by radiograph or pH analysis of aspirates. In a group of 48 adult patients, 97 percent of the transpyloric tubes were, by radiograph, in proper position in 48 hours.[98] Placement of nasojejunal tubes can be facilitated by the use of fluoroscopy[99] and intravenous metoclopramide. In a pilot study, administering metoclopramide prior to tube insertion facilitated transpyloric intubation, compared with administering it after nasogastric insertion.[100] Feeding jejunostomies can also be placed endoscopically through existing gastrostomies.

Nasal transpyloric tubes may be easily displaced and are uncomfortable as a long-term approach to enteral nutritional support. Feeding jejunostomies overcome these difficulties and can be used for feedings in the immediate postoperative period.[101] They can be placed during an operative procedure and have been placed in adults using local anesthesia.[102] When tubes are placed beyond the pylorus, gastric decompression may be required to prevent distention that would impair small bowel motility or lead to aspiration.[99] Feeding jejunostomies generally do not tolerate large-bolus feeding over short intervals.

The transition from enteral feeding to full oral feeding can be prolonged. If infants and children are completely deprived of oral feeding during critical maturation phases, difficulties encountered when such feedings are resumed are not uncommon.[103] Reinstituting oral feedings in children who have been fed by means of a gastrostomy tube can evoke a resistant response, such as gagging, choking, and vomiting. An intensive inpatient program has been described that includes a preparation stage during which gastrostomy tube feedings are arranged to simulate oral feedings in timing and amount. The treatment stage, requiring 2 to 3 weeks on an inpatient basis and up to 2.5 years on an outpatient basis, involves managing feeding behaviors consistently and positively.[104] Continued oral stimulation may facilitate the transition to full oral feeding. Therapy sessions directed toward prevention of oral motor dysfunction and oral tactile defensiveness may ease the transition period.

CONTINUOUS VERSUS INTERMITTENT FEEDING

Two different methods are employed for delivery of enteral feedings. Intermittent bolus feedings deliver the formula over a period of time similar to that for an oral feeding, i.e., 10 to 20 minutes. This technique is simple, requires minimal supplies, and may facilitate the transition to home care. Intolerance of this method is indicated by gastric residuals, malabsorption, dumping syndrome, aspiration, or persistent regurgitation.[105] Bolus feeding is not well tolerated when feedings are delivered distal to the pylorus.

When there is intolerance of intermittent bolus feeding, continuous infusion is an alternative. Continuous enteral feeding is administered by infusion pump[106] and has been used successfully in clinical situations when bolus feeding has failed.[107,108] The basis of the success of continuous feeding is unclear. It may be related to a decrease in the nutrient load presented acutely to a compromised intestine, which may transiently overwhelm its absorptive capacity and lead to osmotic diarrhea. When compared with hourly bolus feeding in adult burn patients, continuous feeding resulted in fewer stools and reduced time to reach nutritional goals. Continuous feeding appears to be particularly beneficial when used for patients with impaired absorption, such as chronic diarrhea or short bowel syndrome.[107,109] For chronic diarrhea, the basis of the success of continuous feeding may be related to decreased gastric distention, which in turn affects the gastrocolic reflex.[107]

Continuous feeding requires an infusion pump to control the flow rate. If home enteral feeding is anticipated, pump selection depends upon the availability of the pump and administration sets plus accuracy, cost, and portability. The pump should be accurate within a range of no more than 20 percent[110] and preferably 10 percent.[111] The minimum size of the rate adjustment affects selection. Some pumps have rate adjustments of 5 to 25 ml per hour, which are too abrupt for young infants. Pumps should also have at least a 4-hour battery back-up and alarm systems for occlusion and empty bags and be simple to use and easy to clean. Ideally, a pump should be able to pump against a resistance of at least 12 psi to allow for use with small-bore tubes. However, the pump should trigger an alarm at a pressure of 25 to 30 to avoid rupturing the tube.[110,111]

Home Enteral Feeding

When initiating continuous feeding, consideration should be given to the long-range goals of nutritional therapy. Transition from continuous feeding to bolus or oral feeding can be prolonged. Home enteral nutrition may be an alternative when it is anticipated that continuous feeding will be required for more than 1 to 2 weeks. Successful home enteral feeding depends on detailed preparation for discharge, including a communication network in the community that links physicians, pharmacists, nurses, and social workers involved in the patient's care. Financial resources must be procured prior to discharge. Third-party payment conditions vary from state to state. In addition, arrangements for respite care should be made prior to discharge.

Successful home enteral feeding often requires the services of a home health care company. These companies provide the infusion pump, tubing, and formula. Home nursing care may be available through the same company. Those caring for a child and family in this situation must have experience in pediatrics in order to provide adequate information and support. Determining the agency's policies regarding indigent patients and long-term commitment to patients assists in selecting suitable companies. A meeting with parents and all interested parties prior to discharge is vital.

COMPLICATIONS OF ENTERAL FEEDING

Complications of enteral feeding are metabolic, mechanical, and gastrointestinal. Diarrhea is the most frequent complication (2 percent in adult patients).[112] In published studies of adults and children, diarrhea occurred in 10 to 30 percent.[1,113] Diarrhea in these groups is influenced by many variables, including antibiotics, malabsorption, malnutrition, osmolality of the formula, and fat intake. Hypoalbuminemia may contribute to poor tolerance owing to low oncotic pressure in the intestinal mucosa.[114,115] Examining stool for fat, reducing substances, and pH aids in determining the presence of malabsorption.[88]

In pediatrics, metabolic abnormalities are common in malnourished patients, especially those with renal disease or chronic diarrhea. Careful monitoring of serum potassium and phosphorus is required so that these elements can be appropriately replaced as lean body mass is created. Excessive losses due to diarrhea should be quantified whenever possible. Inadequate free water is often a problem if there are excess enteric or renal losses. In children with chronic illnesses, ongoing assessment of fluid, electrolyte, vitamin, mineral, and trace element status is necessary to prevent imbalances.

Mechanical complications are also common. The small-bore tubes can easily become clogged or kinked. Clogged feeding tubes can be a major problem, requiring repeated reinsertions. Newer enteral feeding tubes have wider openings to diminish clogging. Additional ports at the connection site allow for medication administration and flushing without interrupting the feeding. A comprehensive review of enteral tubes currently available is found elsewhere.[116]

To prevent clogging, liquid medications should be used whenever available. If medication in tablet form is necessary, it should be crushed to a fine powder. Adequate suspension in solution can sometimes be achieved by allowing the tablet to dissolve in water rather than attempting to dissolve the crushed tablet. Medications that congeal, such as Metamucil or cholestyramine, easily clog small-bore tubes and should be avoided when possible. If they are necessary, these medications should be administered and cleared quickly. Feeding tubes should be flushed with water before and after intermittent bolus feedings and periodically (every 4 to 6 hours) during continuous feeding. An investigation of nine nontoxic substances (including digestive enzymes, proteolytic enzymes, and cranberry juice) theoretically useful in clearing clogged feeding tubes demonstrated declogging with three substances after 4 hours. Successful declogging occurred with chymotrypsin, papain, and distilled water. Preventing feeding tubes from clogging appeared easier than attempting to clear them.[117] Other mechanical complications include irritation from transnasal tubes, which can produce sinusitis, otitis media, and nasopharyngeal and gastric irritation.[115]

Formula Advancement

Few controlled comparison studies of the many alternative feeding progression schedules are available. Feeding is usually initiated at a hypo-osmolar concentration that is gradually increased over 1 to 2 days to full concentration, followed by incremental increases in volume.[118] Alternatively, extremely small volumes of full-strength formula may be introduced and the volume slowly advanced. If the volume of residuals prior to the next bolus feeding is less than half of the previous feeding, the volume is increased by 25 to 30 percent. This method can also be used with continuous feeding by dividing the volume over the number of hours the feeding will be infused. During continuous infusions, residuals should be checked at least every 4 hours and preferably every 2 hours during the initial stages of advancement. If the volume of residual is greater than the volume infused over the previous 2 hours, the infusion is interrupted for 1 to 2 hours. If gastric residuals are not a problem, the rate of the feeding may be advanced by 1 to 5 ml per hour.[119] Significant gastric residuals may be more common during overnight infusion than with continuous feeding administered during waking hours.[88] In some situations, gastric emptying time may be prolonged during sleep.

SUMMARY AND CONCLUSIONS

We have discussed the indications for specialized enteral formulas and routes of administration. The enteral route is the preferred route of nutrient administration. Even in the face of relative compromise of the GI tract, specialized products and techniques promote positive nutrient balance. Partial use of the enteral route during parenteral nutrition prevents atrophy of the intestine and reduces the tendency toward cholestasis associated with intravenous feeding. If it is possible, the oral route is preferable, and appetizing, nutritious foods should be emphasized. Overwhelming factors related to nutrition, infection, and metabolism mandate initial consideration of the enteral route before parenteral feedings are instituted. Enteral feeding is cheaper, simpler, more effective, and safer than parenteral feeding.

REFERENCES

1. Wilson SE. Pediatric enteral feeding. In: Grand RJ, Sutphen JL, Dietz WH, eds. Pediatric nutrition. Boston: Butterworths, 1987: 771.
2. Heymesfield SB, Bethel RA, Ansley JD, Nixon DW, Rudman D. Enteral hyperalimentation: an alternative to central venous hyperalimentation. Ann Intern Med 1979; 90:63–71.
3. Bethel RA, Jansen RD, Heymsfield SB, Ansley JD, Hersh MD, Rudman D. Nasogastric hyperalimentation through a polyethylene catheter: an alternative to central venous hyperalimentation. Am J Clin Nutr 1979; 32:1112–1120.
4. Merritt RJ, Hack S. Infant feeding and enteral nutrition. Nutr Clin Pract 1988; 3:47–64.
5. Committee on Nutrition, American Academy of Pediatrics. Nutritional needs of the low-birth-weight infants. Pediatrics 1985; 75:976–986.
6. Ziegler EE, Biga RL, Fomon SJ. Nutritional requirements of the premature infant. In: Suskind RM, ed. Textbook of pediatric nutrition. New York: Raven Press, 1981: 29.
7. Patel BD, Dinwiddie R, Kumar SP, et al. The effects of feeding on

arterial blood gases and lung mechanics in newborn infants recovering from respiratory disease. J Pediatr 1977; 90:435–438.
8. Whitfield MF. Poor weight gain of the low birthweight infant fed nasojejunally. Arch Dis Child 1982; 57:597–601.
9. Sirois LW. Nutritional assessment and management of the infant with bronchopulmonary dysplasia. Nutr Support Serv 1984; 4:62–63.
10. Kurzner SI, Garg M, Bautista DB, Sargent CW, Bowman M, Keens TG. Growth failure in bronchopulmonary dysplasia; elevated metabolic rates and pulmonary mechanics. J Pediatr 1988; 112:73–80.
11. Markestad T, Fitzhardinge PM. Growth and development in children recovering from bronchopulmonary dysplasia. J Pediatr 1981; 98: 597–602.
12. Roy CC, Weber AM. A rational approach to meeting macro- and micronutrient needs in cystic fibrosis. J Pediatr Gastroenterol Nutr 1984; 3:S154–S162.
13. Bertrand JM, Morin CL, Lasalle R, Patrick J, Coates AL. Short-term clinical, nutritional, and functional effects of continuous elemental enteral alimentation in children with cystic fibrosis. J Pediatr 1984; 104:41–46.
14. Pencharz P, Hill R, Archibald L, Newth C. Energy needs and nutritional rehabilitation in undernourished adolescents and young adult patients with cystic fibrosis. J Pediatr Gastroenterol Nutr 3:S147–S153.
15. Rickard K, Brady MS, Greshman EL. Nutritional management of the chronically ill child. Pediatr Clin North Am 1977; 24:157–174.
16. Ehlers KH. Growth failure in association with congenital heart disease. Pediatr Ann 1978; 7:750–759.
17. Krauss AN, Auld PAM. Metabolic rate of neonates with congenital heart disease. Arch Dis Child 1975; 50:539.
18. Krieger I. Growth failure and congenital heart disease. Energy and nitrogen balance in infants. Am J Dis Child 1970; 120:497.
19. Yahav J, Avigad S, Frand M, Shem-Tov A, Barzilay Z, Linn S, Jonas A. Assessment of intestinal and cardiorespiratory function in children with congenital heart disease on high-caloric formulas. 1985; 4:778–785.
20. Seidman EG, Roy CC, Weber AM, Morin CL. Nutritional therapy of Crohn's disease in children. Dig Dis Sci 1987; 32:S82–S88.
21. O'Morain C, Segal AW, Levi AJ. Elemental diets in treatment of acute Crohn's disease. Br Med J 1980; 281:1173–1175.
22. Morin CL, Roulet M, Weber A. Continuous elemental enteral alimentation in children with Crohn's disease and growth failure. Gastroenterology 1980; 79:1205–1210.
23. Morin CL, Roulet M, Roy CC, Lapointe N. Continuous elemental enteral alimentation in the treatment of children and adolescents with Crohn's disease. JPEN 1982; 6:194–199.
24. Belli DC, Seidman E, Bouthillier L, Weber AM, Roy CC, Pletincx M, Beaulieu M, Morin CL. Chronic intermittent elemental diet improves growth failure in children with Crohn's disease. Gastroenterology 1988; 94:603–610.
25. Kirschner BS. Enteral nutrition in enteral bowel disease. In: Report of the 94th Ross Conference on Pediatric Research: Enteral feeding: scientific basis and clinical applications. 1988; 103–109.
26. Biller JA. Short small-bowel syndrome. In: Grand RJ, Sutphen JL, Dietz WH, eds. Pediatric nutrition theory and practice. Boston: Butterworths, 1987: 481.
27. Smith J, Horowitz J, Henderson JM, Heymsfield S. Enteral hyperalimentation in undernourished patients with cirrhosis and ascites. Am J Clin Nutr 1982; 35:56–72.
28. Kaufman SS, Murray ND, Wood P, Shaw BW, Vanderhoof JA. Nutritional support for the infant with extrahepatic biliary atresia. J Pediatr 1987; 110:679–685.
29. LeLeiko NS, Murray C, Munro HN. Enteral support of the hospitalized child. In: Suskind RM, ed. Textbook of pediatric nutrition. New York: Raven Press, 1981: 357.
30. Ferry GD, Selby M, Pietro TJ. Clinical response to short-term nasogastric feeding in infants with gastroesophageal reflux and growth failure. J Pediatr Gastroenterol Nutr 1983; 2:57–61.
31. Lo CW, Walker WA. Chronic protracted diarrhea in infancy: a nutritional disease. Pediatrics 1983; 72:786–800.
32. Larcher VF, Sheperd R, Francis DE, Harries JT. Protracted diarrhoea in infancy: analysis of 82 cases with particular reference to diagnosis and management. Arch Dis Child 1977; 52:597–605.
33. MacLean WC, Lopez de Romana G, Massa E, Graham GG. Nutritional management of chronic diarrhea and malnutrition: primary reliance on oral feeding. J Pediatr 1980; 97:316–323.
34. Cohen I, Wilson SE. Malnutrition in surgical patients. In: Grand RJ, Sutphen JL, Dietz WH, eds. Pediatric nutrition theory and practice. Boston: Butterworths, 1987: 651.
35. Moore EE, Jones TN. Nutritional assessment and preliminary report on early support of the trauma patient. J Am Col Nutr 1983; 2:45.
36. Greecher CP, Cohen IT, Ballantine TVN. Nutritional care of the surgical neonate. J Am Diet Assoc 1983; 82:654–656.
37. Strife CF, Quinlan M, Mears K, Davey ML, Clardy C. Improved growth of three uremic children by nocturnal nasogastric feedings. Am J Dis Child 1986; 140:438–443.
38. Betts PR, Magrath G. Growth pattern and dietary intake of children with chronic renal insufficiency. Br Med J 1974; 2:189–193.
39. Rizzoni G, Basso T, Setari M. Growth in children with chronic renal failure on conservative treatment. Kidney Int 1984; 26:52–58.
40. Warady BA, Kriley M, Lovell H, Farrell SE, Hellerstein S. Growth and development of infants with end-stage renal disease receiving long-term peritoneal dialysis. J Pediatr 1988; 112:714–719.
41. Kien CL. Nutrition in burn and trauma patients. In: Grand RJ, Sutphen JL, Dietz WH, eds. Pediatric nutrition theory and practice. Boston: Butterworths, 1987: 549.
42. Stool SE. Nutritional management after severe head injury in children. Nutr Support Serv 1983; 3:21–23.
43. Rickard KA, Grosfeld JL, Coates TD, Weetman R, Baehner RL. Advances in nutrition care of children with neoplastic diseases: a review of treatment, research, and application. J Am Diet Assoc 1986; 86:1666–1676.
44. Howard RB. Nutritional support of the developmentally disabled child. In: Suskind RM, ed. Textbook of pediatric nutrition. New York: Raven Press, 1983.
45. Kashyap S, Forsyth M, Zucker C, Ramakrishnan R, Dell RB, Heird WC. Effects of varying protein and energy intakes on growth and metabolic response in low birth weight infants. J Pediatr 1986; 108:955–963.
46. American Academy of Pediatrics, Committee on Nutrition. Nutritional needs of low-birth-weight infants. Pediatrics 1977; 60:519–530.
47. Pencharz PB. Nutrition of the low-birth-weight infant. In: Grand RJ, Sutphen JL, Dietz WH, eds. Pediatric nutrition theory and practice. Boston: Butterworths, 1987: 313.
48. Robbins S, Thorp JW, Wadsworth C. Tube feeding of infants and children. Aspen Monograph. Washington: Aspen, 1982: 1.
49. Motil KJ, Grand RJ. Nutrition in chronic inflammatory bowel disease. In: Grand RJ, Sutphen JL, Dietz WH, eds. Pediatric nutrition theory and practice. Boston: Butterworths, 1987: 465.
50. Eisenberg LD, Merritt RJ, Sinatra FR. Nutrition in hepatic disorders. In: Grand RJ, Sutphen JL, Dietz WH, eds. Pediatric nutrition theory and practice. Boston: Butterworths, 1987: 513.
51. Jaffe N. Nutrition in cancer patients. In: Grand RJ, Sutphen JL, Dietz WH, eds. Pedia.:ic nutrition theory and practice. Boston: Butterworths, 1987: 571.
52. Grupe WE. Nutrition in renal disease. In: Grand RJ, Sutphen JL, Dietz WH, eds. Pediatric nutrition theory and practice. Boston: Butterworths, 1987: 579.
53. Heymsfield SB, Andrews JS, Hood R, Williams PJ, Bagatell CJ. Nutrition and the heart. In: Grand RJ, Sutphen JL, Dietz WH, eds. Pediatric nutrition theory and practice. Boston: Butterworths, 1987: 597.
54. Peterson KE, Washington J, Rathburn JM. Team management of failure to thrive. J Am Diet Assoc 1984; 84:810–815.
55. Whitehead RG. Protein and energy requirements of young children living in developing countries to allow for catch-up growth after infections. Am J Clin Nutr 1977; 30:1545.
56. Vanlandingham S, Simpson S, Daniel P, et al. Metabolic abnormalities in patients supported with enteral tube feeding. JPEN 1981; 5:322–324.
57. Brady MS, Rickard KA, Ernst JA, Schreiner RL, Lemons JA. Formulas and human milk for premature infants: a review and update. J Am Diet Assoc 1982; 81:547–552.
58. Similac special care infant formula product handbook for the growing low-birth-weight infant. Columbus, OH: Ross Laboratories, 1980.
59. "Preemie" SMA low-birth-weight infant formula product handbook. Philadelphia: Wyeth Laboratories, 1981.
60. Tantibhedhyangkul P, Hashim SA. Medium chain triglyceride feeding in premature infants: effects on fat and nitrogen absorption. Pediatrics 1975; 55:359.
61. Andrews BF, Lorch V. Improved fat and calcium absorption in LBW infants fed a medium chain triglyceride containing formula. (Abstract) Pediatr Res 1974; 8:104.

62. Greer FR, Steichen JJ, Tsang RC. Effects of increased calcium, phosphorous, and vitamin D intake on bone mineralization in very low-birth-weight infants fed formulas with Polycose and medium chain triglycerides. J Pediatr 1982; 100:951–955.
63. Oski FA. Iron requirements of the premature infant. In: Tsang RC, ed. Vitamin and mineral requirements in preterm infants. New York: Marcel Dekker, 1985: 9.
64. Brady MS, Rickard KA, Fitzgerald JF, Lemons JA. Specialized formulas and feedings for infants with malabsorption or formula intolerance. J Am Diet Assoc 1986; 85:191–200.
65. Benkov KJ, LeLeiko NS. A rational approach to infant formulas. Pediatr Ann 1987; 16:225–230.
66. Committee on Nutrition. Commentary on breast-feeding and infant formulas, including proposed standards for formulas. Pediatrics 1976; 57:278.
67. United States Congress: Infant Formulas Act of 1980. Public Law 96-359, Sept 26, 1980.
68. Committee on Nutrition. Soy-protein formulas: recommendations for use in infant feeding. Pediatrics 1983; 72:359–363.
69. Leake RD, Schroeder KC, Benton DA, Oh W. Soy-based formula in the treatment of infantile diarrhea. Am J Dis Child 1974; 127:374.
70. Meeting the special feeding needs of infants with cow's milk and carbohydrate intolerance. Isomil product handbook. Columbus, OH: Ross Laboratories, 1985.
71. Goldman AS, Anderson DW, Sellars WA, et al. Milk allergy: I. Oral challenge with milk and isolated milk proteins in allergic children. Pediatrics 1963; 32:425–443.
72. Enteral nutrition support of children. Pediasure product handbook. Columbus, OH: Ross Laboratories, 1988.
73. Committee on Nutrition, American Academy of Pediatrics. Pediatric nutrition handbook. 2nd ed. Elk Grove Village, IL: American Academy of Pediatrics, 1985.
74. Kerzner B, Sloan HR, McClung HJS, Caniano D. Jejunal absorption of sucrose and glucose oligomers in the absence of pancreatic amylase. (Abstract) Pediatr Res 1983; 17:191A.
75. Bernard MA, Jacobs DO, Rombeau JL. Enteral feeding. In: Nutritional and metabolic support of hospitalized patients. Philadelphia: WB Saunders, 1986: 67.
76. Ensure, Ensure Plus and Osmolite. Product handbook. Columbus, OH: Ross Laboratories, 1980.
77. Enrich liquid nutrition with fiber. Product handbook. Columbus, OH: Ross Laboratories, 1983.
78. Taitz LS, Byers HB. High caloric osmolar feeding and hypertonic dehydration. Arch Dis Child 1972; 47:257.
79. Vital high nitrogen. Product handbook. Columbus, OH: Ross Laboratories, 1983.
80. Matthews DM, Adibi SA. Peptide absorption. Gastroenterology 1976; 71:151–161.
81. Adibi SA, Fogel MR, Agrawal RM. Comparison of free amino acid and depeptide absorption in the jejunum of sprue patients. Gastroenterology 1974; 67:586–591.
82. Reabilan product monograph. O'Brien Pharmaceuticals, Inc., 1988.
83. Skipper A. Specialized formulas for enteral nutrition support. J Am Diet Assoc 1986; 86:654–658.
84. Nuwer N, Cerra FB, Shronts EP, Lysne J, Teasley KM, Konstantinides FM. Does modified amino acid total parenteral nutrition alter immune response in high level surgical stress? JPEN 1983; 7:521.
85. Schmitz JE, Dolp R, Grunert A, Ahnfeld FW. The effect of solutions of varying branched-chain concentration on the plasma amino acid pattern and metabolism in intensive care patients. Clin Nutr 1982; 1:147.
86. Fischer JE. Amino acids in hepatic coma. Dig Dis Sci 1982; 27:97.
87. Smith JL, Heymsfield SB. Enteral nutrition support: formula preparation from modular ingredients. JPEN 1983; 7:280–288.
88. Moore MC, Greene HL. Tube feeding of infants and children. Pediatr Clin North Am 1985; 32:401–415.
89. Silk DB. Future of enteral nutrition. Gut 1986; 27(S1):116–121.
90. Guest JE, Murray ND, Antonson DL. Continuous nasogastric feeding in pediatric patients. Nutr Support Serv 1982; 2:34–41.
91. Sondheimer JM. Enteral feeding in infants and children with neurologic handicaps and developmental delay: questions needing answers. In: Report of the 94th Ross Conference on Pediatric Research: Enteral feeding: scientific basis and clinical applications. 1988: 123.
92. Caulfield ME, Wyllie R, Firor HV, Michener W. Dumping syndrome in children. J Pediatr 1987; 110:212–215.
93. Dedinsky GK, Vane DW, Black T, Turner MK, West KW, Grosfeld JL. Complications and reoperation after Nissen fundoplication in childhood. Am J Surg 1987; 153:177–182.
94. Gauderer MWL. Feeding gastrostomy or feeding gastrostomy plus antireflux procedure? J Pediatr Gastroenterol Nutr 1988; 7:795–796.
95. Ponsky JL, Gauderer MWL, Stellato TA. Percutaneous endoscopic gastrostomy. Arch Surg 1983; 118:913–914.
96. Mago H, Chen C, Wesson DE, Filler RM. Incisionless gastrostomy for nutrition support. J Pediatr Gastroenterol Nutr 1986; 5:66–69.
97. Gauderer MWL, Picha GJ, Izant RJ Jr. The gastrostomy "button"—a simple, skin-level, non-refluxing device for long-term enteral feedings. J Pediatr Surg 1984; 19:803–805.
98. Whatley K, Turner WW, Dey M, Meier DE. Transpyloric passage of feeding tubes. Nutr Support Serv 1983; 3:18–21.
99. Grant JP, Curtas MS, Kelvin FM. Fluoroscopic placement of nasojejunal feeding tubes with immediate feeding using a nonelemental diet. JPEN 1983; 7:299–303.
100. Whatley K, Turner WW, Dey M, Leonard J, Guthrie M. When does metaclopromide facilitate transpyloric intubation? JPEN 1984; 8:679–681.
101. Andrassy RJ, Mahour GH, Harrison MR, Muenchow SK, Mishalany HG, Woolley MM. The role and safety of early postoperative feeding in the pediatric surgical patient. J Pediatr Surg 1979; 14:381–385.
102. Freeman JB, Fairfull-Smith RJ. Feeding jejunostomy under local anesthesia. Can J Surg 1981; 24:511.
103. Illingworth RS, Lister J. The critical or sensitive period, with special reference to certain feeding problems in infants and children. J Pediatr 1964; 65:839–848.
104. Blackman JA, Nelson CLA. Reinstituting oral feedings in children fed by gastrostomy tube. Clin Pediatr 1985; 24:434–438.
105. Parathyras AJ, Kassak LA. Tolerance, nutritional adequacy, and cost-effectiveness in continuous drip versus bolus and/or intermittent feeding techniques. Nutr Support Serv 1983; 3:56–57.
106. Jones BJM, Payne S, Silk DBA. Indications for pump-assisted enteral feeding. Lancet 1980; i:1057–1058.
107. Parker P, Stroop S, Greene H. A controlled comparison of continuous versus intermittent feeding in the treatment of infants with intestinal disease. J Pediatr 1981; 99:360–364.
108. Hiebert JM, Brown A, Anderson RG, Halfacre S, Rodeheaver GT, Edlich RF. Comparison of continuous vs intermittent tube feedings in adult burn patients. JPEN 1981; 5:73–75.
109. Orenstein SR. Enteral versus parenteral therapy for intractable diarrhea of infancy: a prospective, randomized trial. J Pediatr 1986; 109:277–286.
110. Imbrosciano S, Kovach KM. Selecting the optimal enteral feeding pump. Nutr Support Serv 1986; 6:15–16.
111. Siguel EN. Use of pumps for enteral alimentation. Nutr Support Serv 1986; 6:40–43.
112. Cataldi-Betcher EL, Seltzer MH, Slocum BA, Jones KW. Complications occurring during enteral nutrition support: a prospective study. JPEN 1983; 7:546–552.
113. Gottschlich MM, Warden GD, Michel M, Havens P, Kopcha R, Jenkins M, Alexander JW. Diarrhea in tube-fed burn patients: incidence, etiology, nutritional impact and prevention. JPEN 1988; 12:338–345.
114. Ford EG, Jennings LM, Andrassy RJ. Serum albumin (oncotic pressure) correlates with enteral feeding tolerance in pediatric surgical patients. J Pediatr Surg 1987; 22:597–599.
115. Andrassy JR. Enteral feeding: complications and monitoring. In: Report of the 94th Ross Conference on Pediatric Research: Enteral feeding: scientific basis and clinical applications. 1988: 79.
116. Fagerman KE, Lysen LK. Enteral feeding tubes: a comparison and history. Nutr Support Serv 1987; 7:10–14.
117. Nicholson LJ. Declogging small-bore feeding tubes. JPEN 1987; 11:594–597.
118. Walker WA, Hendericks KM. Manual of pediatric nutrition. 1985.
119. Wilson SE, Dietz WH, Grand RJ. An algorithm for pediatric enteral alimentation. Pediatr Ann 1987; 16:233–240.

PART 6

Special Dietary Therapy for Specific Disease States

Lewis A. Barness, M.D.

Dietary therapy encompasses special diets for specific diseases discussed in this volume, rehabilitation diets for deficiency states, and recommended diets for large populations. The term *dietary therapy* in almost all instances is an overstatement. *Therapy* denotes treatment for a disease. Only rarely can one be truly treated for disease by diet. In many instances, however, nutritional alterations may beneficially affect the outcome of the disease, sometimes while other measures that more accurately are considered treatment are instituted. More commonly, as in some of the disease states discussed, healing occurs while the nutritional state is supported.

Failure to recognize nutritional needs during illness results in prolonging the illness and impeding recovery. Provision of optimal nutrition during illness is difficult owing to a combination of factors including limited knowledge of general as well as specific needs, changes in taste, metabolic changes including enzyme stimulation and enzyme deficiency, and changes in mental state. Frequently, it is necessary to determine the nutritional state of the child at diagnosis by obtaining a history with special reference to intake and excretion; by performing physical examinations including measurements of height, weight, blood pressure, skin folds, and arm circumference; and by determining serum chemical values, immunologic status, and frequently excretory products. Once the nutritional assessment has been completed, estimates are made of deficiencies or excesses and needs to bring all measures to normal. Parenteral or, preferably, enteral nutrition is then planned. After a short, finite period of time, the child is re-evaluated. If improvement is occurring, the same dietary measures are continued. If improvement is not noted, further corrections are necessary.

Certain caveats attend dietary therapy. Impatience to attain desired results may thwart recovery. Recommended dietary allowances (RDAs) as a basis of therapy may be inappropriate, since these have been developed for health maintenance of large healthy populations and not for individuals who are ill. Failure to follow results of diet alterations and lack of compliance with recommendations are further causes of frustration. Consuming food by mouth apparently has many advantages over other modes of providing nutrition. Nasogastric or gastrostomy tube feedings are preferable to parenteral alimentation if the intestinal tract is intact. For those fed parenterally, non-nutritive sucking may provide benefits for growth and development of the child.[1]

TABLE 1
Liver Disease: Dietary Therapy

Hepatocellular	Mild:	Diet as tolerated Sweetened fluids Electrolytes
	Severe:	Limit protein to <1 gm/kg Increase CHO Limit salt Neomycin, lactulose Sodium benzoate, arginine Vitamin K
Cholestatic	As above, plus:	MCT, fat-soluble vitamins Water-soluble vitamins

CHO = carbohydrate; MCT = medium-chain triglycerides.

NUTRITIONAL TREATMENT IN DISEASES OF THE LIVER

The many functions of the liver include glycogen storage and gluconeogensis from glycogen and amino acids, protein and lipid synthesis, and detoxification. Dietary treatment may be divided into that for hepatocellular disease and that for deficiency in excretory functions (Table 1).

Hepatitis represents an example of hepatocellular disease. In milder forms of cellular dysfunction, protein is usually well tolerated up to 2 g per kilogram per day, and normal amounts of fat and carbohydrates may be taken. Appetite, however, may be decreased and vomiting may occur. Acute viral hepatitis, an example of such hepatocellular disease, is usually self-limited.

If vomiting is frequent and profuse, sips of sweetened fluids may be attempted, followed by inclusion of some electrolytes. Ice cream, thin soups, or hard candies may be followed by vomiting. If simple methods do not suffice, parenteral fluids and foods are necessary.

In more severe forms, as in Reye's syndrome or severe viral hepatitis, protein intake is limited to 1 g per kilogram or less. Fatty foods are poorly tolerated. Increasing carbohydrates to 60 to 70 percent of the calories may be helpful. Studies and numerous trials indicate that high protein intake is associated with and may be the cause of encephalopathy.[2] In many, the serum ammonia level is increased and serum amino acids are unbalanced. On the other hand, low protein intake may result in even further depression of the already insufficient protein synthesis and may aggravate hypoalbuminemia, edema, ascites, and the child may stop eating.

The diet should contain the lowest amount of salt tolerated by the child in order to reduce water retention and edema. If serum electrolytes fall too precipitously, kidney function may decrease.

Ancillary measures useful in decreasing ammonia formation include administration of neomycin to decrease gastrointestinal (GI) bacterial fermentation, and lactulose, a nonabsorbable carbohydrate that increases intestinal mobility.

Increased amounts of dietary branched-chain amino acids may be beneficial. Some have found improvement in protein status using ketoacid derivatives of the branched-chain amino acids as substitutes for one-half of the quantity of these amino acids in the diet. Sodium benzoate and arginine, administered either orally or parenterally, effectively reduce serum ammonia if given early in the course of liver failure.[4]

Synthesis of one of the critical proteins, prothrombin, is decreased in hepatocellular disease, and supplemental vitamin K, usually delivered parenterally, may partially alleviate some bleeding tendencies. Otherwise, substitute measures may be required.

Although diets do not cure liver diseases, diets with least toxicity are associated with more rapid recovery in those with reversible diseases and may slow progression of deterioration in those with progressive disease.

Those with obstructive, cholestatic liver disease usually are burdened also with cellular disease. In addition to the recommendations above, these children also have absorptive errors, particularly of fats and fat-soluble vitamins.

Fat absorption may be increased by substituting up to half the fat as medium-chain triglycerides (MCTs) for the longer-chain triglycerides (LCTs). MCTs do not require bile salts for micelle formation and are more readily absorbed than LCTs.

Vitamin A deficiency is usually preventable with supplemental parenteral vitamin A, although production of retinol-binding protein may be limited. Vitamin D deficiency results in a definitive disease, hepatic rickets, which is poorly responsive to vitamin D but may respond to vitamin D metabolites such as 1,25-dihydroxycholecalciferol. Severe peripheral neurologic disease and occasional central neurologic disease are recognized as due to vitamin E deficiency.[5] This is preventable with adequate continuous supplemental vitamin E, but once neurologic damage is present, its chances of being reversed are poor. Variable absorption after oral administration of fat-soluble vitamins results in uncertain response. In any cholestatic liver disease likely to be long-lasting, these vitamins should be given parenterally.

Water-soluble vitamins and trace minerals may also be absorbed poorly. Usually twice the RDAs provide protection against deficiencies of these.

NUTRITIONAL TREATMENT IN DISEASE OF THE PANCREAS

Pancreatic diseases include those due to endocrine and those due to exocrine dysfunction.

Endocrine Dysfunction

The endocrine hormones of the pancreas are insulin, glucagon, somatostatin, vasoactive intestinal polypeptide, gastrin, pancreatic polypeptide, and others. Dietary treatment for deficiencies of any of these except for insulin is relatively uncommon. Definitive therapy usually involves removal of part of the pancreas.

Although the dietary treatment of insulin-dependent diabetes is an important part of its management, it is beyond the scope of this discussion. Growth and weight gain and avoidance of acidosis are important. Recent suggestions that dietary omega-3 fatty acids together with good diabetic control may avoid some of the complications of diabetes are encouraging and require further study.[6]

Tumor or hyperplasia of any of the endocrine pancreatic cells causes symptoms, the dietary treatment of which is largely supportive until the hypersecretive cells are definitely removed. This includes frequent administration of carbohydrate, together with pharmacologic agents to maintain normal glucose levels.

Exocrine Dysfunction

The exocrine functions of the pancreas include the digestive enzymes trypsin, lipase, and amylase. Defects of other enzymes of the pancreas occur more rarely.

Nutritional support requires great effort in children with cystic fibrosis of the pancreas. Dietary treatment is directed mainly against defects in the intestinal tract, although secondary benefits to the lungs and other organs may occur. Since any or all of the enzymes may be deficient, goals are combatting malabsorption and preventing dietary deficiencies (Table 2).

Caloric intake should approach 150 to 200 percent of the usual daily requirements of healthy children.[7] Protein should be easily absorbable. Vegetable proteins are not as well absorbed as those from animal sources. For those absorbing whole proteins poorly, hydrolyzed proteins or elemental diets are recommended. Pancreatic enzymes are given with each meal. Dietary fat may be increased and may be supplemented with MCT oils. Addition of taurine to the diet may improve fat absorption.[8] Essential fatty acids should provide 3 to 5 percent of the daily caloric intake. Carbohydrates are relatively well absorbed if diarrhea is controlled. Limiting dietary carbohydrates apparently is not beneficial.

Vitamin supplements must be given. Fat-soluble vitamins prepared in water-miscible forms, at least two times the RDA are recommended. Signs of vitamin A deficiency are not common, perhaps because of the common prescription of supplemental vitamin A. Rickets is not rare, perhaps because of a combination of vitamin D deficiency and increased cal-

TABLE 2
Pancreatic Disease (Exocrine Insufficiency): Dietary Therapy

Caloric intake 150–200% of normal
Hydrolyzed proteins, elemental MCT oils, taurine
Pancreatic enzymes
Fat-soluble vitamins
Minerals, salt

MCT = medium-chain triglycerides.

cium loss with fat excretion. Vitamin E supplements mitigate muscle weakness and promote a sense of well-being.[9] It may be necessary to supply vitamin K supplements periodically either by mouth or parenterally. Supplemental minerals including iron, calcium, zinc, and copper are recommended. Supplemental sodium chloride is necessary to compensate for the increased electrolyte losses through the skin.

Excessively rigorous changes in the diet may be self-defeating, since the diet may then become unpalatable. Even in the child with severe anorexia, providing favorite foods sometimes increases acceptance.

In those who develop pancreatic endocrine insufficiency as a complication of cystic fibrosis, diet may require modifications as in other diabetics. If liver disease and cirrhosis occurs, the dietary treatment above is not greatly modified, although hyperammonemia and bleeding due to hypoprothrombinemia become even greater problems.

NUTRITIONAL TREATMENT IN DISEASES OF THE INTESTINE

The diet may be considered to be treatment in some intestinal diseases, although even here diet is usually supportive while the disease runs its course. Diarrhea is defined as the passage of excessive amount of stool with an increased water content. It is the usual manifestation of intestinal diseases amenable to dietary therapy. Infants are especially sensitive to acute loss of intestinal fluid and electrolytes. In those with acute diarrhea, adequate calories undoubtedly hasten recovery, but this is not primary treatment. On the other hand, elimination of lactose from the diet of the lactose-deficient child or elimination of gluten from the diet of the child with celiac disease or dermatitis herpetiformis is definitive therapy.[10] Elimination of affective substances results in reversal of enteritis in cow's milk and soy protein enteropathy, and for children intolerant to other foods, elimination of those foods frequently relieves symptoms (Table 3).[11]

Children with toddler's diarrhea who are growing normally require no unusual dietary treatment. They usually suffer no nutrient deficiencies, and the diarrhea spontaneously subsides with no sequelae after 3 to 4 years. Malnutrition itself as in kwashiorkor may cause mucosal injury and is probably the most common cause of diarrhea worldwide. The decreased immunologic protection that occurs with malnutrition subjects the child's intestine to bacterial invasion. Trials in developing countries with oral rehydration solutions containing approximately equimolar concentrations of glucose and sodium, followed by early feedings of dilute lactose-containing milks[12] and rapidly progressing to full feedings followed by hypercaloric feeds, resulted in success in repairing mucosal injury, reversing diarrhea, and rehabilitating many malnourished children.[13] Treatment of infectious enteropathies may be completed by diet alone, but antibacterial or antiparasite medications may be required if specific agents are identified.

Children with chronic diarrhea of unknown cause or those with inflammatory bowel disease require accurate diagnosis.[14] Dietary treatment is secondary to specific treatment if a known disease is found and consists of alimentation with elemental diets together with all known micronutrients. If growth and weight gain cannot be achieved, these children benefit from parenteral nutrition.[15] Aggressive treatment as added protein, calories, iron, and folate may reverse some of the inflammation and foster adequate growth, particularly in children with Crohn's disease. Night feedings with liquid high-caloric-density, nutritionally balanced supplements, if tolerated without excessive diarrhea, improve linear growth rate and weight gain.[16] In any child with chronic diarrhea, in addition to supplying all micronutrients, zinc supplements for 5 to 10 days normalize zinc status and may hasten recovery.[17] Any child whose diarrhea persists more than 5 days should be given periodic vitamin K supplements. Vitamin K deficiency in children with diarrhea is due both to losses of precursors in the stool and to altered intestinal flora.

In children with short small bowel, parenteral nutrition may be required if the absorption surface is insufficient. Even in these children elemental diets[18] or, if elemental diets are not tolerated, non-nutritive sucking may stimulate gut growth.[1]

TABLE 3
Intestinal Malabsorption: Dietary Therapy

Specific intolerance	Gluten, lactose, cow's milk
General, acute	Fluids and electrolytes, followed early by usual feedings
General, chronic	Specific, if cause known Elemental diets, micronutrients Parenteral night feedings

NUTRITIONAL TREATMENT IN CONGENITAL HEART DISEASE

Nutritional maintenance in infants and children with congenital heart disease may be difficult. In children with congenital heart disease, dietary intervention may be necessary in three groups (Table 4). Children with congestive failure are improved if salt intake is limited. If such a diet is unpalatable to the child, it may be advantageous to provide salt to taste and treat edematous states with diuretics. Edema of the intestine may be responsible for decreased fat absorption found in some children with noncyanotic congenital heart disease. In children with cyanotic heart disease, other factors, particularly related to hypoxia, may be responsible for decreased fat absorption. For these, diets rich in unsaturated fats are helpful.

TABLE 4
Congenital Heart Disease: Dietary Therapy

Congestive heart failure	Restrict salt Unsaturated fats, total fat Diuretics Calories to 130% normal
Cardiomyopathy	Carnitine, iron
Small for gestational age	Increase caloric density Restrict salt Observe for dehydration

Some noncyanotic infants may have metabolic abnormalities due to hypoxia, acidosis, carnitine deficiency, and other metabolic abnormalities. After hypoxia is treated, electrolyte imbalances are corrected and arrhythmias treated. While first efforts are directed to the underlying abnormality, increasing fat in the diet up to 60 percent of the calories may lower CO_2 production and decrease respiratory distress. For those with cardiomyopathy due to carnitine deficiency, the cardiomyopathy may become asymptomatic with added dietary L-carnitine.[19] In many children with congenital heart disease, resting metabolic rate is increased. For these, caloric intakes of 130 to 160 percent of normal with normal protein intake for age may be necessary for growth. In children with cyanotic heart disease, iron status is carefully monitored, as iron deficiency even in the presence of plethora may cause heart failure and growth retardation.

The third group consists of children with congenital heart disease born small for gestational age. Such infants frequently benefit from formulas low in salt, with otherwise normal distribution of calories and caloric density of 80 to 90 kcal per deciliter instead of 60 to 70 kcal per deciliter. Infants fed such formulas must be observed for dehydration. Many such infants have other genetic or congenital anomalies.[20] Children with heart failure secondary to underlying illness are treated similarly. Children with GI disease such as kwashiorkor may develop beriberi due to deficiency of thiamine or other trace substance and require immediate supplements with these elements. Children with Williams' syndrome require monitoring of vitamin D metabolites; those with congenital thyroid abnormalities require that these be corrected.

For many of these children, no special dietary needs exist after successful correction of the heart lesion.[21] Whether surgery is successful or not, children should be observed periodically after surgical correction and dietary adjustments made if growth does not proceed normally.

NUTRITIONAL TREATMENT IN INBORN ERRORS OF METABOLISM

For many inborn errors, nutritional manipulations are the only treatments currently available. Even when genetic modification is available, until the infant or child is ready for such therapy, diet should be carefully monitored.

Disorders of Amino Acid Metabolism

Dietary treatment of almost all the disorders of amino acid metabolism involves the use of deficient or incomplete proteins.[22] Since all amino acids are required for the manufacture of new tissue and for growth, small amounts of complete protein must be fed together with the special diet. This requires careful monitoring for the rate of growth as well as blood levels of the amino acid in question.

Aminoacidopathies for which dietary treatment is available are listed in Table 5. Other aminoacidopathies may require no treatment or are asymptomatic. Organic acidemia may accompany several of the aminoacidopathies, and carnitine is added to the dietary requirement.[23]

TABLE 5
Amino Acid Disorders with Dietary Treatment

Amino Acid	Dietary Treatment
Phenylalanine	Phenylketonuria—decrease phenylalanine Biopterin deficiency—decrease phenylalanine. Add biopterin[25]
Tyrosinemia I and II	Decrease phenylalanine and tyrosine
Alkaptonuria	Decrease phenylalanine and tyrosine
Homocystinuria	See Table 7; decrease protein and methionine
Cystinosis[26]	See Table 7
Cystinuria[27]	Increase water, glutamine; decrease salt intake
Leucine-induced hypoglycemia	Decrease leucine, protein
Lysinuric protein intolerance	Decrease citrulline
Glutaric acid I	See Table 7; decrease protein, tryptophan, lysine
Urea cycle	Decrease protein intake to less than 1 gm/kg/day
Beta-alaninemia	See Table 7
Names not including the involved amino acid	
Maple syrup urine disease	See Table 7; decrease branched-chain amino acids
Isovaleric acidemia	Decrease leucine, protein; increase glycine
3-hydroxy 3-methyl glutaryl CoA lyase deficiency	Decrease leucine
3-Ketothiolase deficiency	Decrease protein
Propionic acidemia	See Table 7; decrease protein, isoleucine, valine, threonine, methionine
Methylmalonic acidemia	Same as for propionic acidemia
Hartnup's disease	Tryptophan malabsorption—see Table 7

From Goodman[22] and Brusilow et al.[24]

Since these diets in general require elimination of specific amino acids, other essential substances may also be eliminated. Care is necessary that vitamins and minerals are supplied in adequate amounts, usually according to RDA specifications.

Disorders of Carbohydrate Metabolism

Disorders of carbohydrate metabolism treatable by diet are listed in Table 6. Disorders of carbohydrate metabolism not treatable by dietary alterations include pyruvate dehydrogenase deficiency, lysosomal acid alpha-glucosidase deficiency (GSD-II), amylo 1, 4-1, 6 transglucosidase deficiency (GSD-IV), phosphofructokinase deficiency (GSD-VII), and higher-number glycogen storage diseases.

Several disorders involving carbohydrate metabolism and treatable by dietary alterations are included in Table 7.

If organic acidemia accompanies the disorders of carbohydrate metabolism, organic acids are excreted with carnitine metabolites, and L-carnitine is added to the dietary regimen.[23] Children with lactic acidosis may respond to supplements of thiamine.

TABLE 6
Carbohydrate Disorders with Dietary Treatments

Disease	Dietary Therapy
Sucrase-isomaltase deficiency	Elimination of sucrose
Lactose intolerance	Elimination of lactose
Glucose-galactose malabsorption	Fructose only permissible sugar
Galactosemia, galactokinase deficiency	Elimination of lactose, galactose
Hereditary fructose intolerance	Elimination of fructose, sucrose
Fructose-1,6-diphosphatase deficiency	Elimination of fructose, sucrose, sorbitol
Glycogen synthetase deficiency (GSD-0)	Frequent meals rich in protein, carbohydrates
Glucose 6-phosphatase deficiency (GSD-I)	Frequent feeds including uncooked starch; avoidance of galactose, fructose
Amylo-1,6-glucosidase deficiency (GSD-III)	High protein, frequent carbohydrate
Myophosphorylase deficiency (GSD-V)	Glucose during exercise
Liver phosphorylase deficiency (GSD-VI)	High protein
Ketotic hypoglycemia	Frequent feedings

From Stanley.[23]

Disorders of Lipid Metabolism

Two groups of disorders of lipid metabolism may be amenable to dietary intervention. The hypobetalipoproteinemias due to lack of carrier proteins for lipids are treated with large doses of vitamin E daily. If response is poor, vitamin E is given parenterally. Water-soluble forms of vitamin A and vitamin K, restriction of long-chain dietary fatty acids, and increased dietary MCTs may alleviate symptoms.

TABLE 7
Vitamin-Dependent Inborn Errors

Disease	Vitamin to Be Added in Pharmacologic Amounts
Darier	Vitamin A
Leigh	Thiamin, biotin
Thiamine-responsive anemia	Thiamine
Maple syrup urine disease	Thiamine (see Table 4)
Propionyl Co carboxylase deficiency	Biotin
Pyruvic carboxylase deficiency	Biotin
3-Methylcrotonyl carboxylase deficiency	Biotin
Acetyl CoA carboxylase deficiency	Biotin
Biotinidase deficiency	Biotin
Propionic acidemia	Biotin (?) (see Table 4)
Pyruvic kinase	Riboflavin
Glutaric acid I and II	Riboflavin (see Table 4)
Hartnup's disease	Niacin (see Table 4)
Cystathionuria	Pyridoxine
Homocystinemia I	Pyridoxine folate (see Table 4)
Homocystinemia II and III	Pyridoxine, B_{12}, folate, methionine
Vitamin B_6-dependent anemia	Pyridoxine
Xanthurenemia	Pyridoxine
Gyrate atrophy, choroid	Pyridoxine
Oxaluria	Pyridoxine
Beta-alaninemia	Pyridoxine
Formiminotransferase deficiency	Folate
Folate reductase deficiency	Folate
Methylmalonic acidemia	Vitamin B_{12} (see Table 4)
Chediak-Higashi syndrome	C
Vitamin D deficiency	D
Familial hypophosphatemia	D

From Stanley.[23]

The second group, the primary and secondary hyperlipoproteinemias, have received extensive publicity and manifold dietary recommendations in attempts to limit atherosclerotic events.[28] Whether any dietary intervention in childhood results in later amelioration of atherosclerotic events is controversial. Nonetheless, certain dietary recommendations seem harmless and relatively inexpensive.

The total dietary fat calories are limited to 30 percent of the diet after the age of 2 years.[29] The fatty acid composition is distributed as saturated 10 percent, monounsaturated 15 percent, and polyunsaturated 5 percent.[30-32] Diets high in unsaturated fats are easily oxidized. Such diets should contain antioxidants, and children consuming large quantities of unsaturated fatty acids may benefit from supplemental alpha-tocopherol. Oatmeal, beans, and popcorn provide a high-fiber intake. Fish oils[6] in the form of cold-water fish three or four times per week may prevent platelet adherence in atherosclerosis. Considerable debate focuses on the need to decrease dietary cholesterol.[33,34] Low cholesterol diets lower serum cholesterol by 10 to 25 percent in some individuals. Serum cholesterol levels are largely a result of endogenous metabolism. However, that human milk contains cholesterol, that cholesterol is necessary for myelin formation and hormone production, and that one of the usual sources of cholesterol for children is eggs suggest caution in recommending limitation of dietary cholesterol for children. Eggs are a source of lecithin, which is a precursor of acelylcholine, an important neurotransmitter. Except for secondary hyperlipoproteinemias as in analphalipoproteinemia (Tangier disease), further limitation of dietary cholesterol other than that obtained by limiting total fat intake is not apparently beneficial.

Children with familial hypertriglyceridemia improve with a diet causing weight reduction and carbohydrate limited to 45 percent of the diet. Omega-3 fatty acids obtained in cold-water fish effectively lower triglycerides but may also lower high-density lipoproteins.

Lipoprotein lipase deficiency and ApoC-II deficiency patients benefit symptomatically for limited periods from a diet with less than 20 percent of the calories as fat, mostly in the form of MCTs.

Carnitine is required for transport of long-chain fatty acids across the inner mitochondrial membrane. Deficiency of carnitine palmityl transferase is frequently treatable by dietary L-carnitine. D, L-carnitine should not be used and may be detrimental.[23]

For children at the present time, it seems appropriate to be cautious in dietary recommendations. Moderation in fat intake, sodium, distribution of fats, and elimination of nutritious foods seems pertinent.[35] If modifications are made in diet, growth and development should be monitored and children should proceed according to currently acceptable standards.

VITAMIN-DEPENDENT INBORN ERRORS OF METABOLISM

By definition, these are a group of disorders with an identifiable enzyme deficiency that respond completely or considerably, without additional treatment, to vitamin doses 100 to 10,000 times the usual recommended allowances. Those vitamin-dependent inborn errors for which dietary treatment is available are listed in Table 7.

As in other inborn errors, children with organic acidurias should be supplemented with L-carnitine; children with lactic acidosis may benefit from supplemental thiamine.

A mineral-dependent inborn error of metabolism amenable to dietary therapy is acrodermatitis enteropathica, which responds to zinc supplementation.

SUMMARY

Provision of adequate, nutritious diet is necessary for all children. Sick children are especially prone to dietary insufficiency because of increased requirements due to increased catabolism, alterations in enzyme activity, and modification in taste, smell, appetite, and emotional state. Care in selection of foods and supplementation may be necessary.

In some illnesses, such as diseases of the liver, pancreas, intestine, and congenital heart lesions, special dietary precautions are necessary to provide adequate support. Intestinal disease in the form of malabsorption is the model for increased losses that must be corrected. If possible, the oral route is preferable for dietary therapy.

True dietary therapy is necessary to correct losses and for those diseases in which a total diet may contain those elements that are the purported cause of the disease. This is especially obvious in those diseases caused by enzymatic deficiencies. Until genetic alterations become commonplace, diet manipulations remain the hallmark of treatment.

The effect of early dietary therapy as a prevention against later degenerative diseases is controversial. Until good evidence is developed, the prudent course is the recommendation of moderation. Regardless of the type of dietary therapy instituted, careful attention to accomplishing desired rates of growth and development is necessary.

REFERENCES

1. Marchini G, Lagercrantz H, Feuerberg Y, Winberg J, Uvnas-Moberg K. The effect of nonnutritive sucking on plasma insulin, gastrin and somatostation levels in infants. Acta Paediatr Scand 1987; 76:573–578.
2. Balistreri WF. Viral hepatitis: implications to pediatric practice. Adv Pediatr 1985; 32:287–320.
3. Freund H, Yoshimura N, Fischer JE. Chronic hepatic encephalopathy: long term therapy with a branched-chain amino acid-enriched elemental diet. JAMA, 1979; 242:347–349.
4. Batshaw ML, Brusilow S, Waber L, Blom W, Burton BK, Brubakk AM, Cann HM, Kerr D, Mamunes P, Matalon R, Myerberg D, Schafer IA. Treatment of inborn errors of urea synthesis: activation of alternative pathways of waste nitrogen synthesis and excretion. N Engl J Med 1982; 306:1387–1392.
5. Cynamon HA, Isenberg JN. Characterization of vitamin E status in cholestatic children by conventional laboratory standards and a new functional assay. J Pediatr Gastroenterol Nutr 1987; 6:46–50.
6. Kinsella JE. Dietary fish oils. Possible effects of n-3 polyunsaturated fatty acids in reduction of thrombosis and heart disease. Nutr Today 1986; Nov./Dec. 7–14.
7. Chase HP, Long MA, Labin MH. Cystic fibrosis and malnutrition. J Pediatr 1979; 95:337–347.
8. Belli DC, Levy E, Darling P, Leroy C, Lepage G, Giguere R, Roy CC. Taurine improves the absorption of the fat meal in patients with cystic fibrosis. Pediatrics 1987; 80:517–523.

9. Cynamon HA, Milov DE, Valenstein E, Wagner M. Effect of vitamin E deficiency on neurologic function in patients with cystic fibrosis. Pediatr 1988; 113:637-640.
10. Shmerling DH, Franck J. Childhood celiac diseases: A long-term analysis of relapses in 91 patients. J Pediatr Gastroenterol Nutr 1986; 5:565-569.
11. Proujansky R, Winter HS, Walker WA. Gastrointestinal syndromes associated with food sensitivity. Adv Pediatr 1988; 35:483-496.
12. Groothuis JR, Berman S, Chapman J. Effect of carbohydrate ingested on outcome in infants with mild gastroenteritis. J Pediatr 1986; 108:903-906.
13. Brown KH, Gastandauy AS, Saavedra JM, Lembcke J, Rivas D, Robertson AD, Yolken R, Sack RB. Effect of combined oral feeding on clinical and nutritional outcomes of acute diarrhea in children. J Pediatr 1988; 112:191-200.
14. Andres JM. Advances in understanding the pathogenesis of persistent diarrhea in young children. Adv Pediatr 1988; 35:483-496.
15. Ament ME, Barclay GN. Chronic diarrhea. Pediatr Ann 1982; 11: 124-131.
16. Mobil KJ, Grand RJ. Nutritional management of inflammatory bowel disease. Pediatr Clin North Am 1985; 32:447-470.
17. Sachdev HPS, Mittal NK, Mittal SK, Yadav HS. Controlled trial on utility of oral zinc supplementation in acute dehydrating diarrhea in infants. J Pediatr Gastroenterol Nutr 1988; 7:877-881.
18. Levine G, Dereu J, Yezdimer E. Small bowel resection: oral intake is the stimulus for hyperplasia. Dig Dis Sci 1976; 21:542-547.
19. Gilbert EF. Carnitine deficiency. Pathology 1985; 17:161-169.
20. Feldt RH, Stickler GB, Weidman WH. Growth of children with congenital heart disease. Am J Dis Child 1969; 117:573-579.
21. Rosenthal A. Care of the postoperative child and adolescent with congenital heart disease. Adv Pediatr 1983; 30:131-167.
22. Goodman SI. Inherited metabolic disease in the newborn: approach to diagnosis and treatment. Adv Pediatr 1986; 33:197-224.
23. Stanley CA. New genetic defects in mitochondrial fatty acid oxidation and carnitine deficiency. Adv Pediatr 1987; 34:59-88.
24. Brusilow SW, Batshaw ML, Waber L. Neonatal hyperammonemic coma. Adv Pediatr 1982; 29:69-103
25. Matalon R, Michals K. Hyperphenylalaninemia due to inherited deficiencies of tetrahydrobiopterin. Adv Pediatr 1986; 36:67-89.
26. Gahl WA. Cystinosis coming of age. Adv Pediatr 1986; 33:95-126.
27. Jaeger P, Portmann L, Saunders A, Rosenberg LE, Their SD. Anticystinuric effects of glutamine and of dietary sodium restriction. N Engl J Med 1986; 315:1120-1123.
28. Kwiterovitch PD. Biochemical, clinical, epidemiologic, genetic, and pathologic data in the pediatric age group relevant to the cholesterol hypothesis. Pediatrics 1986; 78:349-362.
29. American Academy of Pediatrics Committee on Nutrition. Prudent lifestyle for children: dietary fat and cholesterol. Pediatrics 1986; 78:521-525.
30. Grundy SM, Florentin L, Nix D, Whelan MF. Comparison of monounsaturated fatty acids and carbohydrates for reducing raised levels of plasma cholesterol in man. Am J Clin Nutr 1988; 47:965-969.
31. Carlson SE, DeVoe PW, Barness LA. Effect of infant diets with different polyunsaturated fat ratio on circulating high-density lipoprotein. J Pediatr Gastroenterol Nutr 1982; 1:303-309.
32. Barness LA. Cholesterol and children. JAMA 1986; 256:2871.
33. Bowman MB, Van Doren J, Taper LJ, Thye FW, Ritchie SJ. Effect of dietary fat and cholesterol on plasma lipids and lipoprotein fractions in normolipidemic men. J Nutr 1988; 118:555-560.
34. Katan MB, Berns MAM, Glatz JFC, Knuiman JT, Nobels A, DeVries JHM. Congruence of individual responsiveness to dietary cholesterol and to saturated fat in humans. J Lipid Res 1988; 29:883-892.
35. Committee on Nutrition, American Academy of Pediatrics. Toward a prudent diet for children. Pediatrics 1983; 71:78-80.

PART 7

Parenteral Nutrition

John A. Kerner Jr., M.D.

Intravenous nutrition is not a new concept. Various protein hydrolysates first became available more than 50 years ago. Glucose plus protein hydrolysates were successfully infused in the late 1930s by Elman and Weiner[1] in adult patients who either were postoperative or had unresectable carcinoma, and by Shohl and co-workers[2] in pediatric patients. Both groups demonstrated positive nitrogen balance but no significant weight gain.

In 1944 Helfrick and Abelson[3] infused 50 percent dextrose, 10 percent casein hydrolysate, and an homogenized emulsion of olive oil and lecithin in an alternating manner to a 5-month-old marasmic infant for 5 days via peripheral vein. This regimen provided 130 kcal per kilogram per day and a total volume of 150 ml per kilogram per day.[4] By the end of this period, "the fat pads of the cheek had returned, the ribs were less prominent, and the general nutritional status was much improved."[3] During the next 20 years parenteral nutrition (PN) in infants and children was unsuccessful, largely due to the inability of peripheral veins to tolerate the hyperosmolar infusates. Significant side effects, including allergic manifestations and marked elevations of body temperature, further complicated attempts at PN. Often there was inadequate provision of calories to allow the nitrogen to be utilized efficiently.

Intravenous fat preparations were also used. In fact, an entire symposium (Metabolism 1957; 591-831) was devoted to the experience gained in providing nutrition with an intravenous fat emulsion (Lipomul: Upjohn, Kalamazoo, MI). Despite the apparent benefits of the preparations, they were removed from general usage because of their instability, leading to the occurrence of a number of toxic side effects such as thrombosis, embolism, fever, vomiting, rash, eosinophilia, and thrombocytopenia.[5,6]

A group of surgeons at the University of Pennsylvania developed the techniques that provided the stimulus for the current widespread use of total parenteral nutrition (TPN). Dudrick, Wilmore, Vars, and Rhoades demonstrated in beagle puppies, and later in an infant, that the continuous intravenous infusion of hypertonic dextrose and amino acids through deep venous catheters could provide adequate caloric intake and allow normal growth and development.[7-9] They found that with slow infusions, the rapid blood flow through the superior vena cava diluted the hypertonic infusate, thereby preventing phlebitis and thrombosis.

The development of a safe intravenous fat preparation, Intralipid (Kabivitrum, Alameda, CA), was another major advance in PN. Earlier fat emulsions had not gained significant acceptance because of their serious toxic side effects. Fat emulsions now offer the dual advantage of high caloric density and isotonicity, thereby meeting caloric requirements without damaging peripheral veins. With the availability of fat emulsions and the technical advance of central venous nutrition, the physician now has alternatives for providing nutritional support to infants and children who cannot or should not be fed enterally.

In the mid-1970s protein hydrolysates were replaced by crystalline amino acid solutions. Their composition was more rigidly controlled than the hydrolysates, eliminating the risk of allergic reactions. The crystalline amino acid solutions high in arginine have resulted in a marked decrease in reported hyperammonemia in preterm infants. In the 1980s, crystalline amino acid solutions specifically designed for the unique needs of the neonate became available. Finally, appreciation of the vitamin and trace element requirements of neonates and older children led to the development of the infusible solutions designed to meet these needs. The spectrum of parenteral nutritional support in pediatrics now ranges from the provision of single nutrients—to meet either partial or total daily requirements—to the delivery of TPN.

Combination parenteral-enteral nutrition provides some nutrients enterally (those that can be digested and absorbed by the gastrointestinal [GI] tract) and the remainder parenterally.[10] Such a regimen is advantageous for the following patients: low birth weights (LBW) infants, who are able to tolerate limited enteral feedings; infants with intractable diarrhea, for whom the provision of small amounts of nutrients enterally stimulates the recovery of certain intestinal enzymes; and patients being "weaned" from TPN to a program of complete enteral nutrition (e.g., the infant with short bowel syndrome).

TABLE 1
Indications for Parenteral Nutrition in Pediatric Patients

Condition	Examples
Surgical gastrointestinal disorders	Gastroschisis, omphalocele, tracheoesophageal fistula, multiple intestinal atresias, meconium ileus and peritonitis, malrotation and volvulus, Hirschsprung's disease with enterocolitis, diaphragmatic hernia
Intractable diarrhea of infancy	
Inflammatory bowel disease	Crohn's disease, ulcerative colitis
Short bowel syndrome	
Serious acute alimentary diseases	Pancreatitis, pseudomembranous colitis, necrotizing enterocolitis
Severe malabsorption	Idiopathic villous atrophy
Chronic idiopathic intestinal pseudo-obstruction syndrome	
Gastrointestinal fistulas	Fistulas in Crohn's disease
Hypermetabolic states	Severe burns and trauma
Renal failure	
Low birth weight infants	Asphyxiated infants, very low birth weight infants, respiratory distress syndrome
Malignancies	Especially those receiving abdominal irradiation (causing radiation enteritis) or chemotherapy, which leads to severe nausea and intestinal dysfunction
Marrow and organ transplantation	
Special circumstances	Anorexia nervosa, cystic fibrosis, cardiac cachexia, hepatic failure, sepsis
Rare disorders	Congenital microvillous atrophy, chylothorax and chylous ascites, *Cryptosporidium*-induced secretory diarrhea

INDICATIONS FOR PARENTERAL NUTRITION

Although PN is potentially life-saving therapy and is now an accepted practice, increasing experience has demonstrated metabolic, mechanical, and infectious complications. Therefore, candidates for PN should be selected carefully and the indications considered diligently. The principal indications for PN are listed in Table 1.

PN is not indicated in patients with adequate intestinal function in whom nutrition may be maintained by oral, tube, or gastrostomy feedings, possibly using a defined formula (elemental diet) feeding.[11] Relative contraindications to PN are intended use for less than 5 days and the probability that a patient will die imminently because of his or her underlying disease.[12]

PN is supportive therapy for some illnesses and primary therapy for others. PN is supportive for burn patients, patients with protracted diarrhea and malnutrition, and patients with congenital GI anomalies. Studies have documented its worth as primary therapy for patients with GI fistulas, the short bowel syndrome, renal failure, and Crohn's disease. In addition, PN is now being suggested for use in malnourished oncology patients, patients with hepatic failure, malnourished patients before major surgery, patients with cardiac cachexia, and patients requiring prolonged respiratory support. Nutritional repletion in these patients has been associated with an apparent reduction of the incidence of sepsis, proper wound healing, and a return of normal skin test reactivity.[13]

PN is indicated for most patients who are unable to tolerate enteral feedings for a significant period of time.[14] Four or 5 days without adequate oral nutrition is usually sufficient indication for instituting some form of PN. Even 2 to 3 days without adequate nutritional intake for very low birth weight (VLBW) infants or infants with pre-existing nutritional depletion is likely to result in significant depletion of their limited endogenous stores.

Although PN is used to replenish the malnourished child, it may be started prophylactically in clinical situations in which prolonged starvation is expected, (e.g., following extensive intestinal surgery in the neonate[15] or following bone marrow transplantation in the older child). Other indications for PN include a recent loss of more than 10 percent of lean body weight with a concomitant inability to ingest sufficient nutrients to reverse this state and marginal nutritional reserves in a patient who is unable to ingest sufficient calories to prevent further negative nitrogen balance.

Infants receiving central vein TPN retain nitrogen and grow as well as normal infants fed either human milk or standard formulas. TPN has been directly credited with improving the survival of certain infants.[16] The mortality of patients with gastroschisis and intractable diarrhea has decreased to approximately 10 percent today from 75 to 90 percent before the development of TPN.[14] This drop in mortality has occurred without major changes in the medical aspects of therapy in these conditions and seems to be due solely to the prevention of starvation.[14] TPN is "supportive" therapy in these infants, providing normal nutrition until the GI tract is capable of functioning on its own.

Low Birth Weight Infants

LBW infants probably constitute the largest group of pediatric patients who receive parenteral nutrients.[4] In a review by Moyer-Mileur and Chan,[17] parenteral feeds in VLBW infants requiring assisted ventilation for more than 6 days led to a decrease in the percentage of weight loss from birth weight and a lesser amount of time required for recovery of birth weight than in those fed enterally or by a combination of enteral and parenteral feeds. Furthermore, a delay in enteral feeds increased the tolerance to subsequent enteral feeds in these infants. Tolerance was defined as absence of residuals, abdominal distention, or guaiac-positive, reducing substance–positive stools.[17] Another recent retrospective study presented conflicting data regarding the benefits and risks of parenteral nutrition.[18]

Limited data exist on the potential benefit of PN in the treatment of preterm infants. A controlled study[19] of peripheral TPN composed of casein hydrolysate, dextrose, and soybean emulsion in the 40 premature infants with respiratory distress syndrome (RDS) showed that TPN neither favorably altered the clinical course of the syndrome nor worsened an infant's pulmonary status. Among infants weighing less than 1,500 g, those who received TPN had a greater survival rate than did a control group (71 percent versus 37 percent).

Yu and co-workers[20] performed a controlled trial of TPN on 34 preterm infants with birth weights of less than 1,200 g. Infants in the TPN group had a greater mean daily weight gain in the second week of life and regained birth weight sooner than did control infants. Four in the milk-fed control group developed necrotizing enterocolitis (NEC), whereas none did in the TPN group.

The results of a study conducted by our group[21] of 40 infants who weighed less than 1,500 g at birth were in agreement with the two aforementioned controlled studies. We found no increased risk in using peripheral PN as compared with conventional feeding techniques, and we also found comparable growth in the two groups, with significantly increased skin fold thickness values in the peripheral PN group compared with the conventional feeding group.

In addition 59 infants weighing less than 1,500 g were randomly assigned either to a PN regimen via central catheter or to a transpyloric feeding regimen (mother's milk or SMA Gold Cap [Wyeth Laboratories, Philadelphia, PA]) via a Silastic nasoduodenal tube.[22] The authors postulated that some of the problems of enteral feeding in VLBW infants might be overcome if enteral nutrients were delivered beyond the pylorus.[23] The PN group had a higher incidence of bacterial sepsis. Conjugated hyperbilirubinemia occurred only in the PN group. In spite of the observations that 34 percent (10 of 29) of the infants in the transpyloric group failed to establish full enteral feeding patterns by the end of the first week of life and therefore had achieved lower protein energy intake than the PN group, no beneficial effect on growth or mortality was found in the PN group.

The authors concluded that "Parenteral nutrition does not confer any appreciable benefit and because of greater complexity and higher risk of complications should be reserved for those infants in whom enteral nutrition is impossible."[22] My colleagues and I agree with the comment of Zlotkin and co-workers: "Had peripheral-vein feeding been used rather than central venous alimentation, or had nasogastric gavage feeding been used in preference to transpyloric feeding, the morbidity and mortality would have declined and the results comparing TPN with enteral feeds would have been quite different."[24]

A classic study that remains a model for nutritional support in the VLBW infant was performed by Cashore and associates.[25] They described 23 infants who weighed less than 1,500 g in whom peripheral PN was begun on day 2 of life to *supplement* enteral feedings, thus allowing for adequate nutrition while avoiding overtaxing the immature GI tract. These infants regained their birth weight by the age of 8 to 12 days and achieved growth rates that approximated intrauterine rates of growth. Interestingly, infants weighing less than 1,000 g were still not taking all their nutrients enterally by 25 days of age.

A recent survey[26] of 269 neonatal intensive care units showed that TPN was used exclusively during the first week of life in 80 percent of infants weighing 1,000 g or less at birth. The others received a combination of parenteral and enteral feedings in the first week. As a general rule we, like Adamkin,[27] begin PN by 72 hours of age in neonates with a birth weight of less than 1,000 g in whom respiratory disease and intestinal hypomotility limit the safety of feedings in the first 1 to 2 weeks of life. In addition, premature infants, especially those who have respiratory distress syndrome and are incapable of full oral feeds, often receive PN because of their extremely limited substrate reserve, very rapid growth

TABLE 2
Complications of Incomplete Development of the Gastrointestinal Tract in the Low Birth Weight Infant

Incomplete development of motility
- Poor co-ordination of sucking and swallowing
- Aberrant esophageal motility
- Decreased or absent lower esophageal sphincter pressure
- Delayed gastric emptying time
- Poorly co-ordinated motility of the small and large intestine
  - Stasis
  - Dilatation

Delayed ability to regenerate new epithelial cells
- Decreased rates of proliferation
- Decreased cellular migration rates
- Shallow crypts
- Shortened villi
- Decreased mitotic indices

Inadequate host resistance factors
- Decreased gastric acidity
- Decreased concentrations of immunoglobulins in lamina propria and intestinal secretions
- Impaired humoral and cellular response to infection

Inadequate digestion of nutrients
- Decreased digestion of protein
  - Decreased activity of enterokinase
  - Trypsin activity low prior to 28 weeks' gestation
  - Decreased concentration of gastric hydrochloric acid and pepsinogen
- Decreased digestion of carbohydrates
  - Decreased hydrolysis of lactose
  - Decreased ability to actively transport glucose
  - Decreased activity of pancreatic amylase
- Decreased digestion of lipids
  - Decreased production and reabsorption of bile acids
  - Decreased activity of pancreatic lipase

Increased incidence of other problems that may indirectly lead to poor gastrointestinal function
- Hyaline membrane disease
- Intraventricular hemorrhage
- Patent ductus arteriosus
- Hypoxemic-ischemic states

Adapted from Sunshine P. Fetal gastrointestinal physiology. In: Eden RD, Boehm FH, eds. Assessment and care of the fetus: physiological, clinical, and medicolegal principles. East Norwalk, CT: Appleton and Lange, 1990: 93–112.

rate, and perceived susceptibility to irreversible brain damage secondary to malnutrition.[24]

To properly provide nutrition to the premature infant, one must have an understanding of the biochemical and physiologic processes that occur during the development of the GI tract. By 28 weeks of gestation the morphologic development of the GI tract in humans is nearly complete. Yet, as an organ of nutrition, the gut is functionally immature. Details of GI tract development have been described previously.[28-30] Further, complications due to the incomplete development of the GI tract in the LBW infant have been delineated superbly by Sunshine (Table 2).

Asphyxiated Infants

In an asphyxiated infant, in addition to the complications due to incomplete development of the GI tract, there is a superimposed insult to the gut from the asphyxia itself.

Most centers do not enterally feed an asphyxiated infant for the first 5 days to 2 weeks after the insult. This practice is extrapolated from animal data on cellular proliferation and migration. The intestinal mucosa of newborn and suckling rats has a very slow rate of cellular proliferation and migration compared with that of adult animals.[31] Although the turnover of intestinal epithelia in the adult jejunum is 48 to 72 hours, the rate in the 10-day-old animal is at least twice that long and in the 2- to 3-day-old animal it may be even longer.[32] In a study by Sunshine and colleagues[33] in the adult animal, labeled cells reached the tips of the villi within 48 hours. During the same period of time the labeled cells had migrated only one-eighth to one-fourth the length of the villi in the suckling animal. There are indications that this same slower rate of turnover of intestinal epithelia exists in the newborn human.[34]

Asphyxia per se may cause significant injury to the GI tract. Further, asphyxia may predispose an infant to develop NEC. Coupled with asphyxia, feeding the premature infant poses a significant risk for the development of neonatal NEC.

Necrotizing Enterocolitis

Because approximately 95 percent of patients with NEC have been fed, many nurseries have attempted to prevent the disease by delaying enteral feedings. In the excellent controlled study by Yu et al,[20] there was documented reduction of NEC in patients randomized to receive TPN and nothing enterally. Yet Walsh et al[35] pointed out that the lower incidence of NEC was confined to that study period. Once those assigned to receive TPN were fed, NEC subsequently was observed. It appeared that prolonging enteral feedings simply delayed the onset. Ostertag et al[36] showed that providing dilute enteral calories early (starting on day 1 of life) did not adversely affect the incidence of NEC comparison with a group given TPN until day 7 of life. The same investigators also showed that there was no protection against NEC in a group of premature infants weighing under 1,500 g who were given nothing by mouth for 2 weeks.[37] Book et al,[38] in a small prospective study, compared fast and slow feeding rates designed to attain complete enteral nutrition at 7 and 14 days, respectively. No difference in the incidence of NEC was found, yet large daily increases in feeds or large absolute daily volumes may contribute to the development of NEC.[39,40]

Further, Eyal et al[41] performed a 2-year study of the influence of feeding practices on the incidence of NEC. During the first year neonates were fed expressed breast milk on days 2 to 5 of life and were advanced at increments of 10 to 20 ml per kilogram per day. In the second year infants were first fed at 2 to 3 weeks of age. The incidence of NEC was 18 percent in the first year and 3 percent in the second year. In addition, in patients exposed to any risk factors that may lead to poor bowel perfusion, Brown and Sweet[42] have employed a regimen of prolonged periods of bowel rest to allow for recovery of the intestinal mucosa, while supplying all nutrients by the parenteral route. After a variable period of time (5 to 10 days), rigorous attention is paid to a slow progressive feeding regimen for these patients, with careful examination of gastric residua and reducing substances in the stool. By strict adherence to this regimen, they have shown a marked reduction and have nearly eliminated NEC in their institution.

The downside of prolonged periods of bowel rest is that bowel maturation may be delayed. There is evidence that enteral feeding may be the critical element that triggers postnatal gut maturation through release of gut peptide hormones.[43] Recent research in our laboratory confirms that intestinal development is arrested when animals receive TPN with no enteral nutrients but that resumption of intestinal maturation occurs on reintroduction of intraluminal nutrients.[44]

PARENTERAL NUTRIENT REQUIREMENTS

Calories (Energy)

Enteral caloric requirements for pediatrics are shown in Table 3. Infants generally require more enteral than parenteral calories.[45] General guidelines for caloric requirements on TPN are shown in Table 4. Circumstances that may increase caloric needs are shown in Table 5.

One may also calculate caloric requirements using published formulas. Many centers use the Harris-Benedict equations to determine basal energy expenditure (BEE) for children over 10 years of age.[46] A newer equation has been developed for infants.[47]

Boys: kcal/24 hr = 66.47 + (13.75 × W) plus (5.00 × H) + (6.76 × A)
Girls: kcal/24 hr = 655.10 + (9.56 × W) + (1.85 × H) − (4.68 × A)
Infants: kcal/24 hr = 22.10 + (31.05 × W) + (1.16 × H)

(W = weight in kg, H = height in cm, A = age in years)

TABLE 3
Caloric Requirements in Enteral Feedings

Preterm infant (kcal/kg/day)	
Basal requirements	40–50
Activity	5–15
Cold stress	0–10
Fecal losses	10–15
Specific dynamic action	10
Growth	20–30
TOTAL	85–130
Pediatrics (kcal/kg/day)	
Infants	
0.0–0.5 yr	117
0.5–1.0 yr	105
Children	
1–3 yr	100
4–6 yr	85–90
7–10 yr	80–85
11–14 yr	M 60–64/kg; F 48–55
15–18 yr	M 43–49/kg; F 38–40

Adapted from Hattner JAT, Kerner JA Jr. Nutritional assessment of the pediatric patient. In: Kerner JA Jr, ed. Manual of pediatric parenteral nutrition. New York: John Wiley & Sons, 1983: 28.

TABLE 4
Caloric Requirements on Total Parenteral Nutrition

Age (yr)	kcal/kg/day
0–1	90–120
1–7	75–90
7–12	60–75
12–18	30–60

Adapted from Wesley JR, et al, eds. Parenteral and enteral nutrition manual. Chicago: Abbott Laboratories, 1980: 17.

As shown in Table 5, metabolic factors such as fever, sepsis, burns, and growth failure significantly increase caloric requirements. One can allow for this increase by multiplying the BEE by a stress factor (1.25 for mild stress; 1.50 for nutritional depletion; 2.00 for high stress).[46]

In a controlled trial[48] of 14 premature appropriate-for-gestational-age infants, two isocaloric intravenous feeding regimens were compared. Each provided 60 kcal per kilogram per day, one via glucose alone and the other via glucose plus 2.5 g per kilogram per day of crystalline amino acids. Infants on the glucose-only regimen had a negative mean nitrogen balance, whereas those fed glucose plus amino acids had a positive balance. There was no significant weight gain in either group.

In a study of premature infants, Zlotkin and colleagues[49] found that intravenous intakes of 70 to 90 kcal per kilogram per day resulted in weight gain, and that energy intakes providing more than 70 kcal per kilogram per day (including intakes of 2.7 to 3.5 g per kilogram per day of protein) resulted in nitrogen accretion and growth rates similar to in utero values. In addition, earlier studies of adults suggested that additional stresses such as sepsis would increase caloric requirements by as much as 40 percent. More recent work,[50] however, has questioned such an increase, and it is probable that severe stress does not increase requirements by any more than 10 to 15 percent. The effect of stresses like sepsis on caloric requirements in preterm infants has not been critically studied. As in adults admitted to the intensive care unit and confined to their beds, premature infants' requirements for energy and physical activity may be reduced and hence may balance the increased needs due to the stress condition.[24]

It has been shown that portable indirect calorimetry (measurement of oxygen consumption and carbon dioxide production) gives a precise and easily obtained measurement of resting energy expenditure in the malnourished pregnant patient.[51] Recent studies of infants have been offered as arguments that indirect calorimetry provides a more accurate basis for calculating daily caloric needs than other clinical estimations.[52,53] The technology for providing indirect calorimetry in neonates has advanced dramatically, now allowing measurement even of infants on respirators. The cost of such equipment and the manpower required to run the machine and interpret the results, however, prevent its routine use. More studies are needed that seek to discover whether the use of indirect calorimetry significantly improves patient morbidity and mortality.

Fluid restrictions secondary to severe respiratory, cardiac, or renal disease may prevent the delivery of adequate

TABLE 5
Circumstances That Increase Caloric Requirements

Condition	Percentage Increase
1. Fever	12% for each degree above 37 °C
2. Cardiac failure	15–25%
3. Major surgery	20–30%
4. Burns	up to 100%
5. Severe sepsis	40–50%
6. Long-term growth failure	50–100%
7. Protein calorie malnutrition (PCM)	*

*A normal neonate needs approximately 80 kcal per kilogram per day for basal needs and 110 to 120 kcal per kilogram per day for growth. An infant with PCM needs 120 kcal per kilogram per day for basal needs and 150 to 175 kcal per kilogram per day for growth. An older child with PCM needs more than two times the basal energy requirement for growth to occur. (Suskind RM. Nutritional support of the secondarily malnourished child. A.S.P.E.N. Post Graduate Course. 6th Clinical Congress, San Francisco, February, 1982.)

In PCM patients, approximately 6 kcal are required for each gram of weight gain, at least during infancy. Thus, given the basal requirements for infants with PCM above, one can calculate the initial rate of weight gain during recovery from malnutrition. (Kerr D, et al. In: Gardner LI, Amacher P, eds. Endocrine aspects of malnutrition. Santa Ynez, CA: Kroc Foundation, 1973: 467.)

Modified from Wesley JR, et al, eds. Parenteral and enteral nutrition manual. Chicago: Abbott Laboratories, 1980: 17.

calories—even if the calories are given by central PN. Peripheral PN provides approximately 80 kcal per kilogram per day and therefore seems best suited for minimally stressed patients undergoing a limited course of PN for whom full growth and development is not the therapeutic goal. Central PN is indicated either for nutritional repletion of a seriously malnourished patient or when full growth and development are essential.

Balanced PN, including both fat and carbohydrate (as nonnitrogen calories), is the ideal regimen, especially for respiratory conditions (e.g., hyaline membrane disease). Such a regimen decreases the respiratory quotient, prevents excessive fluid administration, and may help to avoid fatty infiltration of the liver.

Fluids

Fluid requirements depend on hydration status, size, age, environmental factors (i.e., radiant warmers, phototherapy), and underlying disease.[55] Daily maintenance fluid requirements for pediatrics are outlined in Table 6. Premature babies have unique requirements.[46,54,56–58] Factors that increase or decrease their requirements are shown in Table 7. Further, excess fluid intake (greater than 150 ml per kilogram per day) in LBW infants may be associated with patent ductus arteriosus,[59] bronchopulmonary dysplasia,[60] necrotizing enterocolitis,[61] and intraventricular hemorrhage.[62,63] Recommended rates for the initiation of intravenous fluid intake in full-term and premature babies are shown in Table 8. Urine volume greater than 2 ml per hour and urine specify gravity less than 1.010 suggest an adequate state of hydration in a neonate free of renal disease.[56] Once the infant is in an incubator with approximately 50 percent humidity, an infant less than 1,000 g receives approximately 140 ml per kilogram per day by day 3 of life and 150 ml per kilogram per day by day 15.[58]

During parenteral nutrition, in order to provide adequate calories, fluids are given in excess of maintenance—especially

TABLE 6
Daily Maintenance Fluid Requirements

Body Weight (kg)	Amount of Fluid per Day
1–10	100 ml/kg
11–20	1,000 ml plus 50 ml/kg for each kilogram above 10 kg
>20	1,500 ml plus 20 ml/kg for each kilogram above 20 kg

TABLE 7
Water Requirements in Premature Infants

Factors increasing requirements
- Radiant warmers
- Conventional single-walled incubators
- Phototherapy
- An ambient temperature above the neutral thermal range
- Respiratory distress
- Any hypermetabolic problem
- Elevated body temperature
- Furosemide treatment
- Diarrhea
- Glycosuria (with associated osmotic diuresis)
- Intravenous alimentation

Factors decreasing requirements
- Heat shields
- Thermal blankets
- Double-walled incubators
- Placing the infant in relatively high humidity
- Use of warm humidified air via endotracheal tube
- Renal oliguria

Adapted from Kerner JA. Fluid requirements. In: Kerner JA, ed. Manual of pediatric parenteral nutrition. New York: John Wiley & Sons, 1983: 69.

TABLE 8
Initial Recommendations for Parenteral Fluid Therapy in Low Birth Weight Infants

Type of Bed	Weight (g)			
	600–800	801–1,000	1,001–1,500	1,501–2,000
Radiant warmer—volume (ml/kg/day)*	120	90	75	65
Incubator—volume (ml/kg/day)*	90	75	65	55
Either, with shield—volume (ml/kg/day)*	70	55	50	45

*Plus 30 percent with phototherapy.
Adapted from Pereira GR, Glassman M. Parenteral nutrition in the neonate. In: Rombeau JL, Caldwell MD, eds. Parenteral nutrition (Clinical nutrition, vol 2). Philadelphia: WB Saunders, 1986: 702.

if utilizing peripheral PN. One must be careful to avoid the complications stated above (relating to fluid excess) as fluids are advanced to achieve caloric goals. Underlying cardiac, renal, and respiratory diseases seriously challenge the clinician owing to the fluid restrictions involved. Utilizing 20 percent fat emulsion (instead of 10 percent) is one way to decrease total volume delivered to such infants. General guidelines for fluid management in PN in older infants and children are shown in Table 9.

Carbohydrate

The major source of nonprotein calories in PN is dextrose (D-glucose), which is provided in the monohydrate form for intravenous use—reducing its caloric yield to 3.4 kcal per gram rather than the 4 kcal per gram of enteral glucose or other carbohydrates. Dextrose contributes the majority of the osmolality of the PN solution. With peripheral PN, concentrations of dextrose above 10 percent are associated with an increased incidence of phlebitis (secondary to increased osmolarity) and thus a decreased "life span"of peripheral lines. Carbohydrates are initiated in a slow, stepwise fashion to allow an appropriate response of endogenous insulin and thus to prevent glucosuria (and subsequent osmotic diuresis). Specific guidelines for advancing glucose infusions have been described elsewhere.[64,65] Solutions containing greater than 20 percent glucose at 150 ml per kilogram per day may contribute to hepatic steatosis.[66] Glucose as the sole calorie source leads to greater water retention than when combined with intravenous lipids.[67] As mentioned previously, a balanced TPN solution, including both carbohydrate and fat (as non-nitrogen calories) may avoid (1) fatty infiltration of the liver, (2) water retention, and (3) worsening already severe respiratory compromise—in acutely ill ventilator-dependent patients, CO_2 production has been shown to be significantly higher with glucose as the entire source of nonprotein calories than when fat emulsion provides some of the total caloric load.[68]

TABLE 9
Fluid Recommendations for Parenteral Nutrition

Initial volume for patients free of cardiovascular or renal disease
- <10 kg = 100 ml/kg/day
- 10–30 kg = 2,000 ml/m^2/day
- 30–50 kg = 100 ml/hr (2.4 L/day)
- >50 kg = 124 ml/hr (3 L/day)

Volume may be increased by
- 10 ml/kg/day in infants until the desired caloric intake is achieved (to a maximum of 200 ml/kg/day, if tolerated).
- >10 kg: by 10 percent of initial volume/day until desired caloric intake is achieved (to a maximum of 4,000 ml/m^2/day, if tolerated).

Small premature infants have a poor glucose tolerance in the first days of life, and hyperglycemia (more than 125 mg per deciliter of sugar) occurs frequently. The infusion along with glucose of alternative carbohydrate sources such as galactose and fructose has enabled investigators to increase the total carbohydrate calories infused into the very premature infant while avoiding the development of hyperglycemia.[69,70] The potential side effects of these regimens, however, argue against their use at present.

Dextrose infusions are well tolerated by the neonate if the initial rate of administration does not exceed the hepatic rate of glucose production (6 to 8 mg per kilogram per minute). The premature infant may develop hyperglycemia even at lower rates of infusion.[56] An infusion rate of 7.5 mg per kilogram per minutes is equivalent to 11.3 percent dextrose at 96 ml per kilogram per day or 7.5 percent dextrose at 144 ml per kilogram per day.[71]

Insulin is usually not given to premature infants because of reports of highly variable responses: Some infants have developed profound hypoglycemia with minuscule insulin doses, and others have had no response. Vaucher and colleagues[72] suggested a possible benefit from continuous insulin infusion (through addition to the reservoir of the intravenous infusion set). Although the number of subjects was quite small, the researchers did document increased weight gain and increased tolerance of intravenous glucose in extremely premature hyperglycemic infants who received continuous insulin infusion. Theoretical considerations and practical limitations, such as the infiltration of peripheral intravenous lines, caused one reviewer to recommend the restriction of insulin use of this kind to investigative studies only.[73]

A recent innovative study[74] evaluated 10 critically ill VLBW infants who were treated with exogenous insulin through a continuous insulin infusion pump (Betatron II, Cardiac Pacemaker, Inc). Prior to insulin treatment, infants became hyperglycemic if glucose infusions exceeded 6 mg per kilogram per minute. The blood glucose levels normalized in all infants within 2 to 4 hours, with varying requirements for continuous insulin treatment. Tolerance to intravenous glucose increased from a mean of 7.4 mg per kilogram per minute to 11.2 mg per kilogram per minute with no glycosuria. Energy intake increased from 49.5 kcal per kilogram per day prior to insulin pump therapy to 70.4 kcal per kilogram per day afterward. The insulin pump was connected via a T connector into the three-way stopcock of a peripheral or umbilical catheter, allowing insulin to infuse concurrently with other intravenous solutions. Such technology suggests tremendous promise for improving energy intake and growth in critically ill VLBW infants. However, more careful studies are needed to evaluate the true benefits and potential risks, such as severe hypoglycemia, before this regimen becomes part of routine care. A very recent retrospective study concluded that insulin infusion improves glucose tolerance in VLBW infants and allows hyperglycemic infants to achieve adequate energy intake similar to that of infants who do not become hyperglycemic.[75] The authors mix their insulin in a separate solution with the same glucose concentration as other parenteral fluids. Albumin is added for a final concentration of 3.5 mg per milliliter to limit adsorption of insulin to plastic, and the tubing is flushed thoroughly. The insulin solution is infused via a reliable pump through a short length of tubing inserted "piggyback" into the infusion set for the PN fluids; it is placed as close to the patient as possible, between the patient and the in-line filter for the PN fluid.[75]

Protein

Problems with hyperammonemia and poor utilization of nitrogen commonly seen with protein hydrolysates have been alleviated by the introduction of purer, crystalline amino acid formulations. Hyperammonemia, seen with earlier solutions, now rarely occurs with the increased amounts of arginine and decreased quantities of glycine in the formulations. Hyperchloremic metabolic acidosis, another problem noted with earlier crystalline amino acid solutions, has been ameliorated by the substitution of acetate for chloride in the salts of lysine and the use of basic salts of histidine.[65] In addition to decreased toxicity, crystalline amino acids promote greater rates of nitrogen retention than protein hydrolysates. All amino acid formulations currently marketed consist of crystalline amino acids.[55]

Guidelines for amino acid requirements in PN are shown in Table 10. Preterm neonates given 2.5 to 3.5 g per kilogram per day of protein and approximately 80 kcal per kilogram per day achieve nitrogen retention at levels that approximate intrauterine nitrogen retention.[49] However, intakes greater than 2.5 to 3.0 g per kilogram per day may result in azotemia, especially in LBW infants.[4]

Until recently, no marketed amino acid solution appeared ideal for neonatal or pediatric use. The major solutions available were designed according to the requirements of normal, orally fed adult subjects and not infants and growing children. These solutions produce weight gain and positive nitrogen balance in the stable neonate or infant when adequate nonprotein calories are also provided. However, use of these solutions leads to high plasma concentrations of amino acids such as methionine, glycine, and phenylalanine (a cause for concern regarding safety) and to low plasma concentrations of amino acids such as the branched-chain amino acids, tyrosine, and cysteine (the basis of concern regarding efficacy).[76]

TABLE 10
Amino Acid Requirements of Parenterally Fed Infants and Children

Age Group	Amino Acids (g/kg/day)
Premature neonates	2.5–3.0
Infants, 0–1 yr	2.5
Children, 2–13 yr	1.5–2.0
Adolescents	1.0–1.5

Adapted from Zlotkin et al.[24]

Heird and colleagues found that free amino acid patterns of brain tissue from beagle puppies that received TPN were grossly abnormal compared with those of suckled puppies.[77] Brain weight and protein content of the TPN puppies were lower than those of controls. The abnormal free amino acid patterns of the TPN puppy brains reflected plasma amino acid levels. These findings led to the idea that completely normal plasma amino acid patterns should be an end-point for defining amino acid solutions used for TPN in neonates and infants.

Extensive research has led to the production of a new parenteral formula, TrophAmine (Kendall McGaw, Irvine, CA), which normalizes amino acid levels within the target range recommended by Wu (the values of 2-hour postprandial plasma amino acid concentrations in healthy, normal growing 30-day-old breast-fed term infants).[78] TrophAmine is unique in that it provides the essential amino acids (including taurine, tyrosine, and histidine) in adequate amounts as judged by the normalized plasma amino acid profile as well as providing aspartic acid, glutamic acid, and the dicarboxylic acids at appropriate levels. Studies of this product in preterm and term infants as well as in older children have recently been completed.

Helms and co-workers[79] compared TrophAmine with a standard amino acid formula (Freamine III: Kendall McGaw) in 25 neonates who required surgery for GI disease (mean birth weight was 1.37 + 0.23 kg in the TrophAmine group, 1.69 ± 0.72 kg in the Freamine III group). Infants were studied for periods of 5 to 21 days. PN was delivered via a central or peripheral catheter with a 100 mg per kilogram per day supplement of L-cysteine hydrochloride in both groups. The TrophAmine group had significantly greater weight gain and nitrogen retention than the Freamine III group. Neonates given TrophAmine had plasma amino acid concentrations within the postprandial neonatal target range.[78] Levels of methionine, glycine, and phenylalanine were above and tyrosine was below the range when Freamine III was used. There was no difference in serum albumin or direct bilirubin levels between the two groups.

An uncontrolled nonblind multicenter study[80] of the clinical, nutritional, and biochemical effects of intravenous administration of TrophAmine with a cysteine additive was conducted in 40 infants and children receiving only TPN for 5 to 21 days. Subjects ranged from 2.0 to 12.6 kg in weight. Each received 2.5 g per kilogram per day (121 mg per kilogram per day) of TrophAmine, 1.0 mmol per kilogram per day of L-cysteine hydrochloride, and approximately 110 kcal per kilogram per day of nonprotein calories. The subjects gained approximately 11 g per kilogram per day, and all were in positive nitrogen balance and had normalization of the plasma amino acid profile without adverse effects. Serial gamma-glutamyl transpeptidase (GGTP) values actually declined during the course of the study. Only one of the 31 subjects who received TPN for more than 10 days had an increase in direct bilirubin, despite a predicted incidence of cholestasis of 30 to 50 percent. TrophAmine has recently been shown to be equally efficacious in preterm infants.[81] The distinct decrease in cholestatic tendency with TrophAmine may be due to the presence of the solution of taurine, which results in "normal" plasma levels of taurine. Taurine deficiency has been proposed as a possible cause of cholestasis in patients receiving TPN for a prolonged period.[82] Overall imbalance of amino acids or toxicity of one or more amino acids elevated in plasma may also be responsible for hepatic dysfunction and cholestasis.[83] Thus, the normalization of plasma amino acids during PN, as demonstrated in this study, appears to be a desirable goal.

Of the *standard* amino acid solutions, Aminosyn (Abbott Laboratories, North Chicago, IL) has been our center's choice because of its low pH, which allows the addition of greater amounts of calcium and phosphate for growing preterm infants.[84] TrophAmine with the addition of cysteine hydrochloride has a lower pH than Aminosyn and allows even larger amounts of calcium and phosphorus to be added to the PN solution without precipitation.[85]

Aminosyn PF (Abbott Laboratories) has been released recently in an effort to meet the needs of preterm infants. A comparative study of Aminosyn PF and TrophAmine found TrophAmine superior.[86] Twenty-three preterm infants were studied. Nitrogen balance was better in the TrophAmine group; compared with the TrophAmine group, in whom all plasma amino acid levels were in the normal range, the Aminosyn PF group showed much lower levels of methionine and tyrosine. TrophAmine contains 60 percent essential amino acids. Aminosyn PF contains 50 percent essential amino acids. Helms' study is part of a larger multicenter study of the two formulations. In a preliminary report[87] of the multicenter study ($n = 87$), weight gain, nitrogen balance, and nitrogen retention were similar. Differences in aminograms reflected solution composition. Both Aminosyn PF and TrophAmine appeared to the authors to be better designed to meet the metabolic needs of the preterm infant than standard solutions.

Two other amino acid solutions for neonates have been studied. Neopham (modeled after the amino acid pattern found in human breast milk) was evaluated in 16 infants and children who received PN for at least 1 week. The daily nitrogen retention was comparable to that in eight infants receiving Aminosyn. Amino acid profiles were more normal with Neopham.[88] With a Japanese solution (PF-I-III), containing high concentrations of branched-chain amino acids, increased arginine and decreased glycine, phenylalanine, and methionine, no abnormal plasma amino acid patterns were seen at amino acid doses of 1.5 to 2.5 g per kilogram per day.[89]

In neonates, we start at 0.5 g per kilogram per day of amino acids and increase by 0.5 g per kilogram per day until we reach our desired goal. In older infants and children, we start at 1 g per kilogram per day and increase by 0.5 g per kilogram per day to the maximum dose.

The development of amino acid solutions *specific* to the needs of neonates may ultimately allow adequate growth to be maintained with protein and calorie intakes at lower amounts than have been previously described. In a preliminary study, Helms et al[90] reported positive nitrogen balance (greater than 200 mg per kilogram per day) and weight gain (greater than 10 g per kilogram per day) with low doses of TrophAmine (2 g per kilogram per day) and calories (50 kcal per kilogram per day) in preterm infants receiving PN. In the past, these results were achievable only with high-calorie and standard protein intakes.

Calorie-to-Nitrogen Ratio

To promote efficient net protein utilization (i.e., not to use the protein source exclusively as an energy source), approximately 150 to 200 nonprotein calories are required per gram of nitrogen:

1. Nitrogen content (grams) $= \dfrac{\text{protein (grams)}}{6.25}$
2. 1 g protein contains 0.16 g nitrogen
3. Therefore, 24 to 32 non-nitrogen calories must be supplied per gram of protein infused to yield a proper ratio of 150 to 200:1
   a. $\dfrac{\text{Non-nitrogen calories}}{\text{N(g)}} = \dfrac{24}{0.16} = \dfrac{150}{1}; \quad \dfrac{32}{0.16} = \dfrac{200}{1}$
   b. If 2 g per kilogram per day of protein as amino acids is supplied, then 48 to 64 kcal per kilogram per day of non-nitrogen calories must be supplied to ensure adequate protein utilization.
   c. If 2.5 g per kilogram per day of protein is supplied, then 60 to 70 kcal per kilogram per day of non-nitrogen calories must be supplied.

Fat

Intravenous fat (IVF) has become an integral part of the PN regimen. It not only provides a concentrated isotonic source of calories (the 10 percent solution supplies 1.1 kcal per milliliter; the 20 percent solution supplies 2.0 kcal per milliliter but also prevents or reverses essential fatty acid (EFA) deficiency. Patients who cannot tolerate large glucose loads can receive sufficient calories if IVF is added to the dextrose–amino acid regimen. The inclusion of fat with PN solutions infused through a peripheral vein can provide enough calories for growth in preterm neonates and infants who can tolerate fluid loads of 140 ml per kilogram per day.[25] In addition, continuous administration of IVF with the PN regimen prolongs the viability of peripheral intravenous lines in infants who may have limited venous access.[91]

EFA deficiency has been produced inadvertently in hospitalized infants and adults who were receiving nothing by mouth and fat-free TPN. Biochemical evidence of EFA deficiency has been noted in the serum of neonates as early as 2 days after initiating fat-free TPN.[92] Biochemical evidence of deficiency precedes clinical signs of deficiency—reduced growth rate, flaky dry skin, poor hair growth, thrombocytopenia, increased susceptibility to infections, and impaired wound healing.[92,93] EFA deficiency can be assessed by determination of the ratio of 5,8, 11-eicosatrienoic to arachidonic acid (triene-to-tetraene ratio). A ratio greater than 0.4 is generally assumed to be an early indicator of EFA deficiency.[93] An initial report[94] that topically applied sunflower seed oil reversed biochemical and clinical EFA deficiency in two neonates on fat-free PN could not be duplicated in a later study of 15 neonates[95] or 28 surgical patients from newborn to 66 years of age.[96]

Interestingly, 15 ml twice a day enterally of corn oil, sunflower oil, or safflower oil provides as much linoleic acid as 150 ml of 10 percent IVF at less than 5 percent of the cost. Many PN patients not on complete bowel rest tolerate such a regimen.[97]

EFA deficiency can be prevented by providing 2 to 4 percent of total calories as IVF (1 to 2 percent linoleic acid)—an IVF dose of 0.5 to 1.0 g per kilogram per day. Fat may frequently contribute 30 to 40 percent of total non-nitrogen calories, but should not exceed 60 percent. A suggested regimen for advancing IVF is shown in Table 11. IVF must be infused separately from any other PN solution, since these solutions may "crack" (disturb) the fat emulsion. IVF may be infused with dextrose amino acid solutions using a Y connector near the infusion site and beyond (proximal to) the Micropore filter. When administered in this way, the fat emulsion remains stable.

The rate of elimination and metabolic fate of IVF particles are the same as those of naturally occurring chylomicrons. Thus, clearance from the plasma is dependent upon the activity of lipoprotein lipase in the capillary endothelial cells, primarily in muscle and adipose tissue.

IVF should be infused over 24 hours whenever possible. Continuous IVF infusions (24 hours per day) are better tolerated than intermittent infusions (8 hours per day) by preterm infants.[98] Early studies argued against exceeding a rate of 0.15 g per kilogram per hour (3.6 g per kilogram per day).[93] Slower infusion rates are required for small-for-gestational-age (SGA) infants. Eighteen-hour infusions at a rate of 0.15 g per kilogram per hour with "6 hours off" to "assure cyclical regeneration of the enzyme systems involved in lipid metabolism" has also been suggested, especially if the patients have hyperglycemia associated with IVF use.[99] Brans et al showed that intermittent infusions (over 18 hours) greatly increased the fluctuations of plasma lipids and tended to elicit higher concentrations than continuous infusions (over 24 hours), especially at the higher daily rates of infusion.[100] Infusion rates of 0.12 g per kilogram per hour or less resulted in less elevation of plasma lipid levels than rates of 0.17 g per kilogram per hour or more.[100]

TABLE 11
Use of Intravenous Fat (10% Solutions)

	Premature or SGA Infants	Full-term AGA Infants	Older Children
Initial dose	0.5 g/kg/day (5 ml/kg/day)	1 g/kg/day (10 ml/kg/day)	1 g/kg/day (10 ml/kg/day)
Increase daily dose by	0.25 g/kg/day (2.5 ml/kg/day)	0.5 g/kg/day (5 ml/kg/day)	0.5 g/kg/day (5 ml/kg/day)
Maximum dose	3 g/kg/day (30 ml/kg/day)	4 g/kg/day (40 ml/kg/day)	2 g/kg/day (20 ml/kg/day)

SGA = small for gestational age; AGA = appropriate for gestational age.

Linoleic acid was previously thought to be the only essential fatty acid. Although the essentiality of linolenic acid in man has not been established, its presence in certain mammalian tissue such as the brain has led some investigators to speculate that it might be essential, especially in the developing neonate. On the other hand, there is the possibility that too much linolenic acid inhibits the conversion of linoleic to arachidonic acid. These concerns led to the development of Liposyn II (Abbott Laboratories), a blend of safflower oil (0.1 percent linolenic acid) and soybean oil (8.0 percent linolenic acid).

Currently used intravenous fat products are shown in Table 12. One study did clearly demonstrate that hypertriglyceridemia is more common in preterm infants who receive safflower oil–based as opposed to soybean oil–based intravenous fat.[101]

A recent study in neonates comparing Liposyn II and Intralipid found no difference in the incidence of hypertriglyceridemia between the two products.[101a] Two recent studies in neonates show that the plasma fatty acid profiles in the two products are comparable.[101b, 101c]

For optimum oxidation of fatty acids, carnitine is necessary.[93] Solutions currently used for intravenous alimentation contain no carnitine, although they contain all the precursor material required for its endogenous production. Infants maintained on PN solutions have decreased total plasma carnitine levels. Decreased tissue carnitine levels have also been found in neonates receiving TPN for more than 15 days. A recent study examined infants receiving long-term PN who were given a supplement of oral L-carnitine (50 mmol per kilogram per day); these infants achieved normal carnitine levels.[102] Another study of neonates[103] showed that intravenous administration of L-carnitine supplements resulted in normal plasma carnitine levels and lower peak triglyceride levels following delivery of a fat bolus (suggesting an enhanced ability to utilize exogenous fat for energy). Since other studies of supplemental carnitine[104] have not shown significant improvement in metabolism of fat emulsions, further research is needed in this area.

Recent reports suggest the benefit of adding medium-chain triglycerides (MCT) to intravenous preparations over using long-chain triglycerides (LCT) alone. Fifty-one neonates received Lipofundin MCT/LCT (50 percent MCT, 50 percent LCT) (B. Braun Medical) or conventional IVF. IVF was given over 20 hours. Triglyceride and fatty acid levels were not significantly different in the two groups. After 6 days of IVF, mean plasma cholesterol was 100 percent higher in the group receiving conventional IVF.[105] A second study of neonates showed elevation of triglycerides and free fatty acids in the MCT/LCT group.[106] Further studies are needed to evaluate the MCT/LCT regimen.

Finally, Canadian investigators are concerned that preterm infants lack transplacental accretion for eicosapentaenoic

TABLE 12
Intravenous Fat Emulsions (10 Percent)

	Intralipid	Liposyn*	Travamulsion	Soyacal	Liposyn II
Base	Soybean oil	Safflower oil	Soybean oil	Soybean oil	5% Safflower oil 5% Soybean oil
Glycerin content	2.25%	2.5%	2.25%	2.21%	2.5%
Osmolarity (mOsm/L)	280	300	270	280	320
Particle size (micron)	0.5	0.4	0.4	0.33	0.4
Fatty acid composition					
Linoleic	54%	77%	56%	49–60%	65.8%
Oleic acid	26%	13%	23%	21–26%	17.7%
Palmitic acid	9%	7%	11%	—	8.8%
Linolenic acid	8%	0.5%	6%	6–9%	4.2%
Stearic acid	—	2.5%	—	3–5%	3.4%

*No longer available.

(EPA) and docosahexaenoic acid (DHA). These fatty acids are essential for brain development but are not available in soybean-based IVF products. They designed a soy emulsion enriched with EPA and DHA and found no toxicity or biochemical abnormalities in piglets.[107]

Twenty percent IVF is indicated when there is a drastic need to restrict fluid volume (e.g., renal or cardiac compromise, chronic lung disease). The dose should not exceed 0.15 g per kilogram per hour. Four g per kilogram per day of 20 percent IVF caused *less* increase of plasma lipids than 2 g per kilogram per day of 10 percent IVF.[108] In another study, hyperlipidemia in TPN with 10 percent IVF but not 20 percent IVF was caused by an increase in lipoprotein X.[109] Twenty percent IVF has *twice* the amount of triglyceride (i.e., 20 g per deciliter) compared with the 10 percent IVF while having only the *same* amount of phospholipid. Phospholipid is believed to inhibit lipoprotein lipase—the main enzyme responsible for IVF clearance. Given this knowledge, one can appreciate why 20 percent IVF is cleared more rapidly than 10 percent IVF.

Electrolytes

The ranges of recommended daily intakes of electrolytes and minerals for PN solutions in pediatrics[110] are shown in Table 13. Calcium and phosphorus requirements change with age and are much greater in preterm infants than in term infants, older children, and adults.[111] Recommended amounts are shown in Table 14. During the last 6 to 8 weeks of gestation, calcium and phosphorus are incorporated into the bone matrix. Thus, premature infants are at risk for developing rickets and "handling" fractures. Radiographs should be periodically checked for evidence of early changes consistent with rickets. Calcium and phosphorus serum levels should be obtained weekly. The serum calcium level will be maintained at the expense of bone (demineralization), so a normal serum calcium does not necessarily mean that adequate amounts of calcium are being delivered. Serum phosphorus level does not fluctuate as rapidly and is a better indicator of total body stores (normal values[112] are shown in Table 15). Kovar et al[113] suggest screening for rickets in preterm infants with plasma alkaline phosphatase: Levels of up to five times the upper limit of the normal adult reference range are acceptable; a value of six times the upper limit of the adult reference range should prompt a radiograph to exclude rickets.

Calcium and phosphorus requirements for some patients may exceed the solubility of these two elements in PN solutions. This happens most frequently when patients are fluid restricted or have several other intravenous fluid lines. The maximum amounts of calcium and phosphorus that can be admixed in PN solutions are determined primarily by the pH of the solution,[114] which in turn is determined primarily by the amino acid product and concentration. Currently there are two amino acid products on the market designed for use in infants which have a low enough pH to allow adequate amounts of calcium and phosphorus for growth. They are

TABLE 13
Parenteral Provision of Electrolytes and Minerals

Electrolytes and Minerals	Daily Amount
Phosphate	0.5–2.0 mM/kg
Sodium	2.0–4.0 mEq/kg
Potassium	2.0–3.0 mEq/kg
Chloride	2.0–3.0 mEq/kg
Acetate	1.0–4.0 mEq/kg
Magnesium	0.25–0.5 mEq/kg
Calcium gluconate*	50–500 mg/kg

*Gluconate is the recommended calcium salt for use in parenteral nutrition solutions. Calcium chloride dissociates more readily than calcium gluconate solutions and can lead to precipitation problems with phosphate.

TABLE 14
Recommended Amounts of Calcium and Phosphorus

	Calcium Gluconate	Phosphate
Premature infants	300–500 mg/kg/day	1–1.5 mM/kg/day
Term infants	300–400 mg/kg/day	1–1.5 mM/kg/day
Older infants and children	100–200 mg/kg/day	1.0 mM/kg/day
Adolescent	50–100 mg/kg/day	0.5–1.0 mM/kg/day

TABLE 15
Normal Serum Phosphorus Levels

Premature	5.6–9.4 mg/dl
Term	5.0–8.9 mg/dl
Children	3.8–6.2 mg/dl
Adolescent	3.6–5.6 mg/dl
Adults	3.1–5.1 mg/dl

Adapted from Kempe CH, Silver HK, O'Brien D, Fulginiti VA, eds. Current pediatric diagnosis and treatment. Norwalk: Appleton and Lange, 1987: 1128–1136.

TrophAmine and Aminosyn PF. Of the other amino acid solutions designed for the use in adults, Aminosyn has the lowest pH and is probably a better choice than the others for use in children with active bone growth. Consult your pharmacy for information on institutional products and calcium phosphate precipitation curves.

Continuous infusion of calcium in the PN solution is preferable to bolus administration of calcium. With bolus administration, large amounts of calcium are lost in the urine.[115] Also, the potential tissue damage from line infiltration is much greater with concentrated calcium given as a bolus than with dilute calcium as a continuous infusion.

When daily calcium and phosphorus requirements were infused in two separate alternating 12-hour infusions, there were alternating periods of high and low serum concentrations of calcium and phosphorus depending on which solution was being infused.[116] Infusions of solutions containing both calcium and phosphorus resulted in stable calcium and phosphorus concentrations. Calcium concentrations of 50 mEq per liter and phosphate concentrations of 20 mmol per liter were compatible in solutions containing 2 percent TrophAmine, 10 percent dextrose, and 0.08 percent L-cysteine.[117] A subsequent study compared calcium-phosphorus solubility previously found with TrophAmine with results for similar Aminosyn PF solutions and showed that calcium-phosphorus solubility was less with Aminosyn PF.[118]

Vitamins

The Nutrition Advisory Group (NAG) of the Department of Food and Nutrition, American Medical Association (AMA), proposed guidelines for parenteral multivitamins that were sent to the FDA in December, 1975, and later published.[119] These guidelines indicated the need for separate adult and pediatric formulations. The FDA accepted the AMA adult formulation in 1979 (MVI-12: Armour Pharmaceutical, Blue Bell, PA). The pediatric formulation (MVI-Pediatric, Armour Pharmaceutical) was not approved until 1981. A distinguished subcommittee has recently re-evaluated parenteral vitamin requirements.[120] The committee's major recommendations were as follows:

1. The initial guidelines for stable term infants and children in the 1975 AMA report appear adequate to maintain blood levels of vitamins within acceptable ranges for short-term as well as long-term TPN.
2. MVI-Pediatric has been tested primarily in medically stable infants and children receiving TPN. Patients receiving oral supplements may need adjustments in the parenteral formulation.
3. There is an urgent need for a new formulation made specially for high-risk preterm infants.

Their specific recommendations for utilization of the existing vitamin preparation (1 vial of MVI-Pediatric per day for term infants and children and 40 percent of a vial per kilogram of body weight for preterm infants) and for a *new* formulation for preterm infants are both shown in Table 16.

Lipid-Soluble Vitamins

The lipid-soluble vitamins must be solubilized in an aqueous solution if they are to be provided in a single vitamin mixture. To solubilize them synthetic detergents such as poly-

TABLE 16
Suggested Intakes of Parenteral Vitamins in Infants and Children

		Preterm Infants (dose/kg body wt) (Maximum Not to Exceed Term Infant Dose)	
Vitamin	**Term Infants and Children (Dose per Day)***	Current Suggestions†	Best Estimate for New Formulation‡
Lipid-soluble			
A (μg)§	700.0	280.00	500.00
E (mg)§	7.0	2.80	2.80
K (μg)	200.0	80.00	80.00
D (μg)§	10.0	4.00	4.00
(IU)	400.0	160.00	160.00
Water-soluble			
Ascorbic acid (mg)	80.0	32.00	25.00
Thiamin (mg)	1.2	0.48	0.35
Riboflavin (mg)	1.4	0.56	0.15
Pyridoxine (mg)	1.0	0.40	0.18
Niacin (mg)	17.0	6.80	6.80
Pantothenate (mg)	5.0	2.00	2.00
Biotin (μg)	20.0	8.00	6.00
Folate (μg)	140.0	56.00	56.00
Vitamin B_{12} (μg)	1.0	0.40	0.30

*These guidelines for term infants and children are identical to those of the AMA (NAG) published in 1979.[119] MVI-Pediatric (Armour) meets these guidelines. Recent data indicate that 40 IU per kilogram per day of vitamin D (maximum of 400 IU per day) is adequate for term and preterm infants.[121] The higher dose of 160 IU per kilogram per day has not been associated with complications and maintains blood levels within the reference range for term infants fed orally. This dosage therefore appears acceptable until further studies using the lower dose formulation indicate its superiority.

†These represent a practical guide (40 percent of the currently available single-dose vial MVI-Pediatric (Armour) formulation per kilogram of body weight), which will provide adequate levels of vitamins E, D, and K but low levels of retinol and excess levels of most of the B vitamins. The maximum daily dose is one single-dose vial for any infant.

‡Because of elevated levels of the water-soluble vitamins, the current proposal is to reduce the intake of water-soluble vitamins and increase retinol as described in the committee's report.[120]

§700 μg RE (retinol equivalents) = 2,300 international units (IU); 7 mg alpha-tocopherol = 7 IU; 10 μg vitamin D = 400 IU.

Modified from Greene et al.[120]

sorbate have been used. Questions have recently been raised about the safety of these detergents given intravenously to preterm infants.[122,123] Either a safe agent should be documented or the European approach would be preferred. Vitalipid (Kabi vitrum, Stockholm) is a preparation containing vitamins A, D, E, and K dissolved in fractionated soybean oil and emulsified with fractionated egg phospholipids in the same manner that Intralipid is prepared. Infants requiring TPN receive water-soluble vitamins in the glucose amino acid solution and the lipid-soluble vitamins with IVF (devoid of synthetic emulsifiers). Such use has proved successful for years.

Intravenous vitamins may be lost through adsorption to plastic TPN bags and tubing or through light exposure. Vitamin A, for instance, is lost primarily because of its adherence to intravenous tubing and secondarily because of its biodegradation in the presence of light.[124] As much as 33 percent of riboflavin in the PN formulations is decomposed by exposure to ordinary light conditions.[125] Pyridoxine is also destroyed by direct sunlight.[126] Using radiolabeled vitamins, researchers found recently that only 31 percent of vitamin A, 68 percent of vitamin D, and 64 percent of vitamin E were actually delivered to the patient over a period of 24 hours.[127] The problem of vitamin loss (e.g., retinol loss) during TPN appears much more severe in the management of VLBW infants because of light intensity is higher in nurseries and smaller amounts of TPN solution remain exposed to the administration tubing for longer periods of time.[120]

Armour originally recommended that MVI-Pediatric doses be 5 ml per day for all patients weighing more than 3 kg and 3.25 ml per day for infants weighing less than 3 kg. Unfortunately, at the 3.25 ml dose, infants less than 1 kg displayed elevated vitamin E levels (greater than 3.5 mg per deciliter).[128] Such elevations have been associated with an increased incidence of necrotizing enterocolitis and sepsis.[129] The manufacturers subsequently modified their recommendations, suggesting that infants weighing less than 1 kg receive 1.5 ml per day of MVI-Pediatric. A this lower dosage vitamin E levels were less than 1 mg per deciliter in 44 percent of the infants less than 1 kg.[130] The American Academy of Pediatrics (AAP) has suggested that safe and effective blood levels of vitamin E are between 1 and 2 mg per deciliter.[131] Recent studies[130] show that 40 percent of a vial (2 ml = 2.8 mg alpha-tocopherol) per kg per day results in normal serum vitamin E levels within the range of 1.0 to 2.5 mg per deciliter. Using this dosage of 2 ml MVI-Pediatric per kilogram (to a maximum of 5 ml) per day, infants with birth weights between 450 and 1,360 g maintained adequate vitamin E levels[132]—this dose is recommended (Table 16). This recommended dose *may* be inadequate for *some* infants of 1,000 g or less. In a study presented at the 1990 ASPEN meeting, in neonates receiving 50 percent of a vial of MVI-Pediatric (a larger dose than recommended), 9 of 65 infants of 1,000 g or less at birth had vitamin E levels less than 1 mg per deciliter.[132a]

In addition, Green et al[133] have recently shown that VLBW infants (less than 1,000 g) who receive TPN for 1 month show a progressive decline in serum retinol, with half of such infants showing levels below 10 μg per deciliter (the level believed to result in clinical manifestations of vitamin A deficiency). His research team's observation was of significant importance in the light of two reports correlating a higher incidence of bronchopulmonary dysplasia (BPD) with low plasma retinol levels.[134,135] Shenai et al[136] subsequently performed a blind randomized trial to see if increased plasma retinol levels would alter the incidence of severity of BPD. The treatment group received approximately 400 to 450 μg per kilogram per day intramuscularly and an additional intravenous intake of 50 to 150 μg per kilogram per day for 4 weeks. The treatment group showed a significant increase in plasma retinol levels from 20.7 + 0.9 to 34 + 3.2 per deciliter. Additionally, the vitamin A–treated infants showed a significant reduction in the incidence of BPD compared with the control group.[136]

Seven infants (birth weight 450 to 1,360 g) recently had 40 percent of an MVI-Pediatric vial (280 μg retinol) per kilogram of body weight added to the IVF emulsion.[132] A significant rise in plasma retinol levels from 11.0 ± .76 μg per deciliter pretreatment to 19.2 ± .97 μg per deciliter was demonstrated after 19 to 28 days. The rise confirmed the benefit of adding fat-soluble vitamins to the IVF solution to avoid loss of vitamin onto the plastic tubing; the findings supported the previous European data using such an approach. The authors concluded, however, that 280 μg per kilogram per day was insufficient to raise blood levels of all infants into the normal range.[132] See Table 16 for current and theoretical recommendations for vitamin A intake.

MVI-Pediatric contains 200 μg per vial of phylloquinone (lipid-soluble vitamin K preparation). Since no deficiency states or toxicity has been reported with its use, the expert committee agreed to continue the recommendation as previously agreed to (Table 16). If one uses one vial of MVI-12, designed for patients greater than 11 years old to adulthood, the patient will need supplemental vitamin K, which can be given intravenously daily instead of a weekly intramuscular injection.[137] The study confirmed that regular addition of vitamin K to TPN regimens decreased the incidence of elevated prothrombin times—the vitamin K could be given *either* daily at 1 mg per day intravenously in the TPN solution or 10 mg intramuscularly weekly.[137]

Water-Soluble Vitamins

Deficiency of thiamin results in acute or chronic beriberi. A possible case of Shoshin (cardiac) beriberi determined by erythrocyte transketolase assay during TPN was reported in a 12-year-old girl who received TPN with inadequate amounts of thiamin.[138] As mentioned previously, riboflavin is inactivated by light, *especially phototherapy lights*.[139] Riboflavin deficiency involves primarily the epithelium (hyperemia and edema of the pharyngeal and oral mucous membranes, cheilosis, stomatitis, glossitis, seborrheic dermatitis) and normocytic anemia.[120] Such deficiency has not been described in children maintained on TPN. Recent findings of riboflavin-induced photohemolysis with excess riboflavin[140] indicate the importance of approximating normal blood levels of this vitamin.

The recommended parenteral dose of pyridoxine in full-term infants (1.0 mg per day) may be more than necessary but has not resulted in any toxicity or deficiency. For preterm infants receiving 40 percent of MVI-Pediatric (0.4 mg per kilogram per day), pyridoxine levels increased by more than 10-fold over cord blood and maternal levels; a lower dose of 0.18 mg per kilogram per day resulted only in twofold increases.[141] Another study by the same group also argued that the current dosage of pyridoxine for VLBW infants is excessive and recommended a newer formulation with a lower dosage.

The clinical syndrome resulting from biotin omission from TPN is characterized by scaly dermatitis, alopecia, pallor, irritability, and lethargy.[143] Biotin is currently included in MVI-Pediatric in doses adequate to prevent deficiency.

A multicenter study from the United States[144] and a second study from France[145] looked extensively at water-soluble vitamin determinations in term infants and children. Although the daily doses of vitamins were slightly different in the two studies, neither deficiency nor toxicity states were described; therefore, the 1975 AMA-NAG guidelines can remain unchanged for term infants and children.

Trace Elements

The first guidelines for intravenous administration of trace elements to pediatric patients were published in 1979.[146] An expert committee has recently updated the original recommendations (Table 16).[120]

Wolman and Ruz et al pointed out that persistent diarrhea or excessive GI fluid losses from ostomy sites may grossly increase zinc losses.[147,148] In adult balance studies the following *additional* zinc replacement is required: (1) 17.1 mg of zinc per kilogram of stool or ileostomy output, and (2) 12.2 mg of zinc per kilogram of small bowel fluid lost via fistula or stoma.

Selenium deficiency is now recognized as the major etiologic factor in Keshan disease, an often fatal cardiomyopathy affecting children and young women in a large geographical area of China.[149] Three similar cases of fatal cardiomyopathy were reported in adults on long-term PN who were found to be selenium-deficient[150-152]; three cases, including a child,[153] were reported in which selenium deficiency was associated with pain and tenderness of the skeletal muscles. In addition, selenium levels were low in four children receiving long-term TPN.[154] In the latter series, there was erythrocyte macrocytosis in three, loss of pigmentation of hair and skin in two, elevated transaminase and creatinine kinase in two, and profound muscle weakness in one. Intravenous supplementation with 2 μg per kilogram per day of selenium was begun in these children. Clinical and laboratory findings improved after long-term intravenous supplemental treatment.[154] A 27-month-old on long-term PN presented with regression of walking skills and tender skeletal myopathy affecting both legs only.[155] Plasma selenium level was low, 0.4 μg per deciliter (normal 6.3 to 12.6 μg per deciliter). Following intravenous repletion with sodium selenite there was complete disappearance of muscle pain and tenderness within 1 week; crawling and walking skills were regained within 6 weeks. A specific workshop on selenium requirements suggested 1.5 μg per kilogram per day.[156] Kelly et al[155] recommended 3.0 μg per kilogram per day for replacement and 1.5 μg per kilogram per day for maintenance. The recommendations in Table 17 are based on extrapolation from selenium intake in breast-fed infants, assuming 80 percent absorption.[120] There is no good evidence that selenium is required for short-term PN.

One case of molybdenum deficiency was reported in an adult on long-term PN.[157,158] Symptoms included tachycardia, tachypnea, vomiting, and central scotomas, with rapid progression to coma. The patient had an excellent clinical and biochemical response to 2.5 μg per kilogram per day of molybdenum.

TABLE 17
Recommended Intravenous Intakes of Trace Elements*

Element	Infants: Preterm† (μg/kg/day)	Infants: Term (μg/kg/day)	Children μg/kg/day (maximum μg/day)
Zinc	400.00	250 <3 mo 100 >3 mo	50.00 (5,000)
Copper‡	20.00	20.00	20.00 (300)
Selenium§	2.00	2.00	2.00 (30)
Chromium§	0.20	0.20	0.20 (5.0)
Manganese‡	1.00	1.00	1.00 (50)
Molybdenum§	0.25	0.25	0.25 (5.0)
Iodide	1.00	1.00	1.00 (1.0)

*When TPN is only supplemental or limited to less than 4 weeks, only zinc (Zn) need be added. Thereafter, addition of the remaining elements is advisable.

†Available concentrations of molybdenum (Mo) and manganese (Mn) are such that dilution of the manufacturer's product may be necessary. Neotrace (Lyphomed Co, Rosemont, IL) contains a higher ratio of Mn to Zn than suggested in this table (i.e., Zn = 1.5 mg and Mn = 25 μg in each milliliter).

‡Omit in patients with obstructive jaundice. (Manganese and copper are excreted primarily in bile.)

§Omit in patients with renal dysfunction.

Adapted from Greene et al.[120]

Iron

Intravenous iron (Fe) in PN regimens has continued to be controversial owing to concerns about the risks of adverse effects. Excess Fe is thought to enhance the risk of gram-negative septicemia. Fe has powerful oxidant properties and can enhance the demand for antioxidants, especially vitamin E; particular caution is needed in giving Fe to the preterm infant.[120] Fe dextran (Imferon: Fisons Corporation, Bedford, MA) has been recently added to TPN infusates in dilute form.[159] The author's inpatients and home PN patients received a daily dose of 0.5 mg (1 ml) with no adverse physiochemical or clinical effects.[159] At New England Deaconess Hospital, 2 mg of Fe as Fe dextran is given daily in the TPN solution. In over 10 years of use, averaging 250 patients per year, no reactions have been noted.[160] Porter et al[160] do agree that malnourished patients with low transferrin may be at risk receiving a substantial infusion of Fe in the free form, which may lead to stimulation of bacterial or fungal growth. In an otherwise stable patient who *cannot* take *any* oral Fe, starting at low doses of 0.5 mg Fe (as dilute Imferon) appears to be safe. Serum Fe, total iron-binding capacity, percent saturation, and ferritin should be followed to document repletion of iron stores. There is danger of adverse reactions, including death, when iron dextran is given intramuscularly or as a large infusion. Use of iron dextran in maintenance doses in TPN, however, appears to be safe; there have been *no* reports of reactions or deaths.[160]

Aluminum

Currently used TPN solutions are contaminated with aluminum (Al). Marked Al accumulation in bone can occur after only 3 weeks of TPN in infants. Al contributes to metabolic bone disease. Al impairment of bone matrix formation and mineralization may be mediated by its direct effect on bone cells or indirectly by its effect on parathyroid hormone and calcium metabolism. Its toxic effects are proportional to tissue Al load.[161] Intravenous calcium, phosphorus, and albumin solutions have high Al (greater than 500 μg per liter). Crystalline amino acids, sterile water, and dextrose water have low Al (less than 50 μg per liter).[161] Calcium gluconate can contribute up to 80 percent of the total Al load from TPN. Until regulatory guidelines are established, Al intakes should be measured when possible, especially in children at high risk for toxicity—the preterm infant, the infant or child with impaired renal function, and the patient on prolonged TPN (with no barrier to Al loading).[120]

ROUTE OF ADMINISTRATION

Central Versus Peripheral Vein

Ziegler and co-workers[162] compared the complication rates of children receiving nutrition via the peripheral veins; their findings are summarized in Table 18. Although infectious complications occurred in approximately 10 percent of the central-vein group and in none of the peripheral-vein group, morbidity related to the administration of solution (primarily in the form of soft-tissue sloughs) was more prevalent in the peripheral-vein group. Complications such as pleural effusions and thrombosis occurred in the central-vein group. The overall complication rate was higher in the central-vein group (20 percent versus 9.08 percent in the peripheral-vein group). However, when total days of therapy are considered in the complication incidence, the per diem complication rate between the two groups is not different.

The authors of this study acknowledge that the problem of venous accessibility is a deterrent to central venous nutrition in small infants. Their experience with percutaneous subclavian vein cannulation suggest that this technique is safe, allows repeated cannulation of the central venous system, and can be used in infants weighing as little as 600 g. Their data imply that *caloric need* is the primary determining factor for selecting the route of nutritional support. Peripheral-vein nutrient solutions are less calorically dense than central-vein solutions; therefore, centrally alimented patients may receive more calories and gain more weight on a daily basis. Furthermore, with frequent peripheral-vein infiltrations the number of calories actually infused is often less than was ordered. (If the patient is ordered to receive 100 kcal per kilogram over 24 hours and the intravenous line is out 30 percent of the time, the patient only receives 70 kcal per kilogram per day.) Since peripheral PN regimens maintain existing body composition, this routine of delivery is a reasonable choice for a normally nourished infant or child who is likely to tolerate an adequate enteral regimen in less than 2 weeks. Central PN is more reasonable choice for infants and older children, regardless of initial nutritional status, who will be intolerant of enteral feedings for longer than 2 weeks. It is difficult to maintain peripheral PN for more than 2 weeks; normal growth, rather than simply maintaining existing body composition, can be achieved with central but not peripheral PN.[4]

Heird has pointed out that pediatric patients who receive peripheral PN are not as likely to develop the characteristic cushingoid appearance as those on central PN.[4] In addition, the rate of weight loss immediately following cessation of PN is not excessive; the composition of the weight gain may not be hyperhydrated like that observed with central PN regimens.[4]

TABLE 18
Complications of Total Parenteral Nutrition

	Central Vein	Peripheral Vein
Number of patients	200.0	385.0
Mean duration (days)	33.7	11.4
Total days of therapy	6,629.0	4,389.0
Gained or maintained weight	82.5%	63.0%
Number of complications		
Infectious	21.0	0.0
Administration	7.0	32.0
Metabolic	12.0	3.0
Complication rate		
Total complications	40.0 (20.0%)	35.0 (9.1%)
Per patient day	0.604%	0.797%

Data from Ziegler et al.[162]

Central Venous PN

To achieve a high caloric intake, a hyperosmolar infusate should be delivered through a central, large-bore vein with high volume blood flow to minimize the risk of venous thrombosis and phlebitis. Silastic catheters have been used effectively in pediatric central venous PN for many years. They are adapted to the intravenous infusion system with a blunt needle. Complications with this method are leakage or perforation of the catheter. Silastic catheters are preferred to polyvinyl or polyethylene catheters; they have a high degree of flexibility and do not become rigid when in place for only a short time like polyvinyl catheters (which are associated with an increased likelihood of perforation of a vessel).

Two specially designed catheters for long-term PN are the Hickman and Broviac catheters. The catheter may be placed by either a cutdown incision or a percutaneous method.[163] It is possible to provide better catheter stability and to decrease the risk of infection by subcutaneously tunneling the catheter of choice to a distant exit site. After the catheter is placed, a separate incision is made on the chest or abdomen so that the distal end of the catheter can be directed through a subcutaneous tunnel between the two incisions. The catheter is then trimmed to an appropriate estimated length so that it will terminate in the superior vena cava. The Hickman and Broviac catheters differ from the traditional Silastic catheter in the following ways: (1) The portion of the catheter extending from the patient as well as the catheter neck is reinforced with Teflon in order to reduce the risk of cracking and breakage. (2) The distal end of the catheter has a Luer-Lok connector to enable snug insertion of intravenous tubing and to allow secure screw-capping of the catheter when not in use. (3) A Dacron cuff attached to the midportion of the catheter is placed subcutaneously at the catheter exit site; this stimulates the formation of dense fibrous adhesions that anchor the catheter securely and create a barrier for ascending bacteria. This process takes approximately 2 weeks, at which time the cutaneous sutures at the exit site can be removed.[4] The catheter is constructed so that it may be spliced if the external portion becomes cracked or cut or if the adapter piece disconnects. The manufacturer provides a special repair kit[164] that is essential to have on hand.

Placement of the central venous PN catheters is by either a percutaneous approach (using the internal jugular vein, subclavian vein, or femoral vein) or a cut-down technique (for the scalp, common facial, external jugular, brachial, cephalic, or inferior epigastric veins). Detailed descriptions of catheter placement appear elsewhere.[165,166]

Once the central venous catheter is inserted, it is advanced into the superior vena cava to its junction with the right atrium. It is desirable for the catheter to float in the superior vena cava instead of in the right atrium. Placement of the catheter in the atrium can stimulate cardiac arrhythmias or cause the catheter to incorporate itself into the endocardium. Cardiac tamponade can result from atrial perforation by the central venous catheter.[167,168] Cardiac tamponade occurs even with Silastic catheters.[169] Several groups believe that cardiac tamponade can be prevented if the catheter tip can be placed in the distal superior vena cava and not inside the cardiac chamber.[167,169]

After the insertion of any type of central venous catheter, chest films are mandatory to confirm proper placement and to rule out mechanical complications secondary to catheter placement. Each catheter type is radiopaque; catheter visualization can be made more distinct by injection with Renografin-60. Infusion of hypertonic PN solutions or fat emulsions should not be initiated until the film has been interpreted. During the interim, an isotonic solution should be infused slowly.

Depending on institutional protocol, central venous catheterization is performed either in the operating room or on the patient care unit. The placement of a central venous catheter to deliver PN can be facilitated by a nurse familiar with the procedure. The nurse will be expected to explain the procedure to the patient, to assemble the equipment, to assist the physician, to lend support to the patient, and to recognize and assist with any associated immediate complications (see Table 20).

Owing to the risk of septic complications, the catheter placement should be treated as an aseptic surgical procedure, requiring masks, gowns, and gloves. Complications can be minimized or prevented with strict sterile technique, proper equipment and lighting, appropriate patient preparation and positioning, and a nurse's assistance.[170]

Regular and meticulous care of the central PN catheter, particularly the catheter exit site, is essential for prolonged, safe, complication-free use. The dressing at the catheter site is changed at least three times per week.[4] Extensive nursing guidelines for catheter care as well as the techniques of setting up PN equipment are readily available.[170,171] Use of the catheter for purposes other than delivery of PN, particularly for blood transfusions and blood sampling, should be avoided.[4] PN teams using strict asepsis have reduced sepsis rates to 0 to 2 percent.[172]

For long-term venous access, the Broviac catheter continues to demonstrate a lower complication rate than the traditional Silastic catheter.[173] Long-term venous access can be safely accomplished even in the infant less than 1,000 g.[174] Interestingly, in a recent study by Sadig and co-workers,[175] the Broviac catheter–associated complications were compared in VLBW infants and older infants ($n = 48$). Sixty-nine percent of catheter-associated infections occurred in VLBW infants and only 20 percent in infants weighting more than 1,500 g. Seventy-eight percent (14/18) of these infections were successfully treated with antibiotics without catheter removal. The rate of thrombosis was also higher in VLBW infants.

Triple-lumen catheters are becoming available for pediatric use,[176] but their associated incidence of infection is not yet known. In addition, other new catheters are being developed[177] and will have to be critically evaluated before becoming part of routine care.

Umbilical Artery Catheters

In some nurseries umbilical arterial (UA) catheters are used for infusing parenteral nutrition. Few studies exist regarding the safety of this practice. Yu et al studied 34 infants with birth weight less than 1,200 g and randomly assigned them to TPN via UA catheters or enteral feeds.[20] The TPN group had better nitrogen balance, weight gain, less NEC, and unchanged mortality compared to the enterally fed group. No data on catheter-related complications were presented, although bacterial or fungal septicemia did not occur in either group in the study period.[20]

Higgs and co-workers[178] described a controlled trial of TPN versus formula feeding by continuous nasogastric drip. The study included 86 infants weighing from 500 to 1,500 g. The TPN, including glucose, amino acids, and fat emulsion, was administered by umbilical artery catheter for the first 2 weeks of life. There was no difference in neonatal morbidity or mortality between the two groups. Specifically, there was no difference in septicemia, although four of the 43 TPN babies had "catheter problems," described in the text only as "blockage" of the catheter.

Hall and Rhodes[179] delivered TPN to 80 infants by UA lines and to nine infants by indwelling umbilical venous catheters; these 89 infants were all "high-risk" infants unable to tolerate enteral feedings. Results were compared to those for 23 infants with tunneled jugular catheters for chronic medical or surgical problems preventing use of the GI tract. All infants studied ranged in weight from under 1,000 to over 2,500 g. As in the study of Higgs et al, Hall and Rhodes found that morbidity, mortality, and the common complications, such as infection and thrombosis, were similar in both groups.[179]

Hall and Rhodes concluded that TPN by indwelling umbilical catheters presents no greater risk than infusion through tunneled jugular catheters. However, careful analysis of the author's data raises questions about their conclusions. According to the authors, "Six deaths may have been catheter related."[179] Five of those deaths occurred in the umbilical artery catheter group; death resulted from the thrombosis of the aorta in one patient; candidal septicemia in two, streptococcal septicemia in one, and enterococcal septicemia in one. One death occurred in the jugular venous catheter group, with right atrial thrombosis, superior vena cava syndrome, and *Staphylococcus epidermidis* on blood culture.

Merritt[180] cautions against the use of umbilical arterial catheters for TPN, as this practice is associated with a high incidence of arterial thrombosis. Dr. Arnold Coran, a pediatric surgeon, strongly recommends that PN *not* be given through either umbilical arteries or umbilical veins.[181] PN through umbilical veins causes phlebitis, which may lead to venous thrombosis and portal hypertension. He is especially concerned about infusing PN solutions into a UA line, since this practice can lead to thrombosis of the aorta or iliac vessels. Furthermore, *severe damage can occur to an artery without being recognized*. There may even be thrombosis of the aorta without recognition. Only over an extensive period of time will the side effects of UA catheter use—such as inappropriate growth of one limb[181]—be known. Although the first three studies described earlier all claimed there were no short-term complications, they did not address the problem of long-term complications.

Coran states that if PN is required and peripheral veins are not usable of if peripheral vein delivery is inadequate to provide necessary calories, he would consider percutaneous subclavian vein catheterization, which he can perform successfully even in a 900-g infant.[181]

Like Coran and Merritt, we are reluctant to use umbilical catheters for the infusion of parenteral nutrients. We attempt to provide needed calories by peripheral vein. If more calories are needed or if PN must be provided for longer than 2 weeks, a central venous line is placed.[182]

INITIATING PN THERAPY

Prior to initiating PN, complete nutritional assessment including anthropometric measurements should be carried out to determine the potential need for nutritional repletion and to estimate caloric requirements (which will help dictate the route of administration utilized). Nutritional assessment techniques have bene reviewed elsewhere.[21,183–186] Skin fold thickness reference data are now available for preterm infants from 24 weeks' gestation on.[187] Mid-arm circumference data are also now available for preterm infants.[188–189] Using the mid-arm circumference–to–head circumference (MAC/HC) provides a "discriminative method for evaluation of intrauterine growth and a non-invasive technique for following somatic protein status in growing preterm infants."[188] If PN will be the therapy of choice, Merritt and Blackburn give guidelines to identify which patients require repletion therapy versus maintenance support:

Group 1 If serum albumin is less than 2.5 g per deciliter, transferrin level is less than 100 μg per deciliter (after 6 months), and the lymphocyte count is less than 1,000 per cubic millimeter (except in patients on chemotherapy or radiation therapy); or if the patient is anergic (beyond infancy and in patients not on steroids) in the presence of weight:height ratio greater than 2 standard deviations below normal or less than 80 percent of standard, arm muscle area below the fifth percentile, or creatinine height index (CHI) less than 60 percent of standard; or if the patient has marginal skeletal or visceral protein status and is markedly stressed. Group 1 definitely requires *repletion* therapy.[186]

Group 2 If serum albumin is less than 3 g per deciliter or the transferrin is less than 150 μg per deciliter, if the lymphocyte count is less than 1,500 per cubic millimeter, if the weight:height ratio is greater than 2 standard deviations below normal or less than 80 percent of standard, if the arm muscle area is below the fifth percentile, or if the CHI is less than 80 percent of standard. This group requires close monitoring for evidence of further nutritional depletion and at least *maintenance* nutritional support if full repletion is not feasible. If these patients also have sepsis secondary to surgery or major injury, they should be placed in Group 1.[186]

Group 3 If no nutritional deficits are documented, if the patient has no chronic disease, and if the patient will not encounter markedly stressful situations in the hospital. Normal patients who develop an infection undergo starvation, or undergo major surgery require repeat assessment in 1 to 2 weeks.[186]

Order Writing

PN solutions can be ordered using either of two basic formats, tailored or standardized. Tailored solutions are formulated specifically to meet the daily nutritional requirements of the individual patient, whereas standardized solutions are designed to provide a formulation that meets the majority of the nutritional needs of those patients with stable biochemical and metabolic parameters. Both of these order methods have advantages and disadvantages associated with their use. At Stanford University Hospital and the Children's Hospital at Stanford, we have had significant success using tailored solutions.

We designed a preprinted PN order sheet to save time for both the house staff and pharmacy personnel. In addition, the order sheet serves to avoid errors of omission, ensuring that all necessary nutrients are ordered. The order sheet provides the necessary input for a computer program written by Nick MacKenzie, M.D.[190] Required input includes the patients's weight (kg), total fluid intake for the day (ml per kilogram per day), the amount of fat emulsion (g per kilogram per day), fat concentration (10 or 20 percent), fluid volumes contributed by other parenteral lines or enteral feeds, desired protein intake via amino acids (g per kilogram per day), and the concentration of dextrose (percent). The doses of trace elements, vitamins, and electrolytes are ordered in amounts per day or amounts per kilogram per day. The computer performs all necessary calculations. (See order sheet in Figure 1). Protocol recommendations are provided in the right hand column of the order sheet for reference.

A. Please send TPN orders to the Pharmacy before 11:00 A.M. DAILY.

B. Order all additives on a 24-hours basis; i.e., mEq/Kg/day, mM/Kg/day, ml/day, ml/Kg/day.

PERIPHERAL ____ or CENTRAL ____ TPN LINE (check one) Today's DATE ____________

DUE DATE ___/___/___ (month day year) TIME DUE ________ (AM PM) Today's WEIGHT ____________ Kg

TOTAL FLUID INTAKE (ml/Kg/day) ____________ Next Bottle # ____________

AMOUNT OF FAT EMULSION (gm/Kg/day) ____________ Fat Concentration ____ 10% ____ 20% (check one)

How many IV or IA lines exist which will not be used for TPN? ____________

	Line		Line
Enter flow rates (ml/hr):	(1) ____	and % NaCl:	(1) ____
	(2) ____	(e.g., 0.45%)	(2) ____
	(3) ____		(3) ____

If taking enteral feeds, complete the following section (check one):

____ 1. Total fluids administered as parenteral and advancing enteral, i.e., "TPN + PO." (Additives are distributed assuming that the total fluids will be given parenterally)

____ 2. Total fluids administered as parenteral and fixed enteral. (Additives are distributed in parenteral fluids only; ignores electrolyte content of enteral fluids)

Enter Amount ________ (mls), Frequency: q ____ hrs, Calories/ml ____, Product Name ____________

Enter AMINO ACIDS (gm/Kg/day) † ____________ Enter DEXTROSE CONCENTRATION ____________ %

TODAY'S ADDITIVES			PROTOCOL RECOMMENDATION
TRACE ELEMENTS AND VITAMINS:			
1. PEDIATRIC TRACE ELEMENTS	____	ml/Kg/day	0.2 ml/Kg/day (weight < 20 Kg)
2. ADULT TRACE ELEMENTS	____	ml/day	5 ml/day (weight > 20 Kg)
3. ZINC (additional)	____	mcg/Kg/day	100 mcg/Kg/day — Premies Only
4. PEDIATRIC M.V.I.	____	ml/day	1.5 ml/day — infants < 1.5 Kg
			3.25 ml/day — infants > 1.5 Kg and < 3 Kg
			5 ml/day — infants > 3 Kg and children up to 11 yrs. of age
5. ADULT M.V.I. — 12 (or generic)	____	ml/day	10 ml/day — children > 11 yrs. of age
6. VITAMIN K	____	mg/day	0.5 mg/day — children > 11 yrs. of age
ELECTROLYTES AND MINERALS:			
1. PHOSPHATE*	____	mM/Kg/day	0.5-2 mM/Kg/day
2. SODIUM	____	mEq/Kg/day	2-4 mEq/Kg/day (Sodium from other IVs is included)
3. POTASSIUM	____	mEq/Kg/day	2-3 mEq/Kg/day
4. ACETATE* †	____	mEq/Kg/day	1-4 mEq/Kg/day
5. MAGNESIUM	____	mEq/Kg/day	0.25-0.5 mEq/Kg/day
6. CALCIUM GLUCONATE	____	mg/Kg/day	50-500 mg/Kg/day
7. HEPARIN	____	Units/ml	0.5-1 Unit/ml
8. INSULIN	____	Units/liter	
9. OTHER (specify)	____		
10. OTHER (specify)	____		

*NOTE: Balance of anions will be provided as chloride.

† Each 0.5 Gm/Kg/day of Amino Acids provides either 0.47 mEq/Kg/day of Acetate (TrophAmine) or 0.74 mEq/Kg/day of Acetate (Aminosyn)

____________________ RN ____________________ MD

FIGURE 1 Example of physician's orders for pediatric parenteral nutrition. (Adapted from Poole RL. Writing parenteral nutrition orders. In: Kerner JA Jr, ed. Manual of pediatric parenteral nutrition. New York: John Wiley & Sons, 1983: 236.)

The output of the computer program includes the following: (1) TPN and fat emulsion bottle labels; (2) mixing instructions for the pharmacy with calcium-phosphate precipitation curve data; and (3) a detailed nutritional summary including calorie:nitrogen ratio, kilocalories per kilogram per day, and percent of total calories vein as fat. The calcium-phosphate precipitation curve data and the calorie:nitrogen ratio are new modifications not available in the original program.[190]

The use of the order sheet and computer program has saved approximately 20 minutes of physician time per patient per day, time that was previously spent doing tedious, error-prone manual calculations. An additional 20 minutes per patient per day of pharmacy time is saved. Calculation and labeling errors have been eliminated by using the program.

For teenage patients, it may be best to use an adult standard solution. Preprinted order sheets and guidelines for the standard adult solution are readily available. We refer to Stanford University Hospital's "Adult TPN Handbook 1986/1987" written by Amy Andolina, R.N., Teresa Ponn, M.D., and Claudia Rupp, Pharm.D. (Chicago: Abbott Laboratories). More detailed explanations of order writing have appeared elsewhere.[11,46,185,191]

As mentioned previously, doses of carbohydrate, fat, and protein are gradually advanced to avoid overtaxing the metabolic capacities of the patient. The classic paper of Cashore et al[25] provides one such progression (Table 19).

Although cyclic TPN is well established for home TPN patients, its use in the hospital is limited. Faubion et al[192] described eight pediatric patients who received cyclic TPN in the hospital. Conditions necessary for instituting cyclic TPN included stable metabolic status, stable electrolytes, steady weight gain for at least 2 to 4 days on continuous TPN, and well-positioned central catheters. They described no major complications. We initially described cyclic TPN in five adolescent patients.[193] Like Faubion and co-workers, we believe that cyclic TPN provides a more normal and less stressful environment for the patient. The patients enjoy their freedom away from a constant TPN infusion as well as being given the autonomy to decide when their "time off" will be.[193] Cyclic TPN in hospital has become standard care at our center. Details of cycling have been published previously.[192,193]

TRANSITION FROM PARENTERAL TO ENTERAL NUTRITION

There is an approximately 50 percent decline in enteric mucosal mass in normal animals maintained on intravenous nutrition in positive nitrogen balance without enteric stimulation.[194] Pancreatic atrophy and impairment of function occurs as well.[195] All segments of the small intestine demonstrate a decrease in the rate of proliferation and migration of the epithelial cells in the parenterally fed animals versus animals enterally fed.[196] Numerous animal studies have demonstrated the positive impact that luminal nutrients have on maintaining the structural and functional integrity of the GI tract.[197-200] These trophic effects on the intestinal mucosa may be direct or may be mediated by the GI hormones. It is therefore desirable to maintain a small oral nutritional intake during PN whenever possible. In infants with intractable diarrhea, Greene and co-workers have demonstrated more rapid recovery of intestinal disaccharidases with the combination of PN plus elemental enteral feeds than with PN alone.[201] Recent research in our laboratory confirms that intestinal development is arrested when animals receive TPN with no enteral nutrients, but that resumption of intestinal maturation occurs on reintroduction of intraluminal nutrients.[202] Recent data suggest that, unlike the intestine and pancreas, the digestive function of the stomach is *not* impaired during TPN in the very preterm infant.[203] TPN has also been shown recently to cause decreases in both acid and pepsin in human infants.[204] When these infants are placed on constant-rate enteral infusion, these secretions return to normal.[204]

The transition from TPN to enteral feeding should be made very gradually, as the sudden cessation of PN may result in severe rebound hypoglycemia (secondary to high levels of insulin produced from high glucose intake). The transition period should be not less than 1 week and may extend over several weeks. Small volumes of dilute oral feedings are begun and then gradually increased to full strength. The volumes of feeds may then be cautiously increased while the volume of the PN is proportionally decreased. A recent publication from the University of Michigan Hospitals gives detailed guidelines for the transitional period.[205] Interestingly, one adult study of 48 patients showed that *none* of the patients had a symptomatic episode of hypoglycemia after *acute* discontinuation of TPN.[206] Some centers simply taper TPN down over 2 hours in adults, and one recent publication recommends "reducing the infusion rate by 50 to 70 percent for 30 to 60 minutes before discontinuation of PN. This is unnecessary if the patient is being fed enterally or orally when the infusion is discontinued."[12] No studies of acute discontinuation have been done in children; hence, the cautious tapering guidelines stated previously should be followed.

Many infants and children are reluctant to feed orally following prolonged PN for reasons that are not clear.[207] We have found that early involvement of oromotor therapists with these patients (in *advance* of their starting oral feedings) may prove extremely helpful.

TABLE 19
Total Daily Parenteral Nutrition Intake for Infants Weighing Less Than 1,500 Grams

Age (days)	Volume (ml/kg)	Fat (g/kg)	Protein (g/kg)	Carbohydrates (g/kg)	Calories (per kg)
1	65.0	0.0	0.0	6.5	26.0
2	100.0	2.0	2.0	8.0	60.0
3	115.0	2.5	2.0	9.0	71.0
4	125.0	3.0	2.5	9.5	81.0
5+	140.0	3.5	3.0	10.5	93.0

Adapted from Cashore et al.[25]

COMPLICATIONS

Patients receiving PN are at risk for developing technical, infectious, and metabolic complications. These complications can be avoided or minimized only by regular monitoring, strict asepsis, and a multidisciplinary nutrition support team including a physician, pharmacist, nutrition support nurse, and nutritionist.[208] Complications are fewer when PN protocols are administered by those familiar with the technique.[209]

Technical Complications

Possible complications at the time of the catheter insertion are depicted in Table 20. Complications related to ongoing

TABLE 20
Possible Complications at the Time of Catheter Insertion

Pneumothorax	Catheter embolism
Hemothorax	Catheter malposition
Hydromediastinum	Thoracic duct laceration
Subclavian artery injury	Cardiac perforation and tamponade
Subclavian hematoma	Brachial plexus injury
Innominate or subclavian vein laceration	Horner's syndrome
Arteriovenous fistula	Phrenic nerve paralysis
Air embolism	Carotid artery injury

use of the catheter are shown in Table 21. Detailed descriptions of such complications are readily available.[165,166,170,171,210]

Heparin

Because of the desire to prevent thrombosis, many centers use heparin prophylactically in their PN solutions in the concentration of *one unit per milliliter.* The heparin tends to reduce the formation of a fibrin sheath around the catheter and possibly reduces phlebitis with peripheral PN solutions. Grant firmly states, "the addition of 1000 units of heparin per liter of solution completely eliminates catheter clotting (500 units of heparin per liter is inadequate)."[211] *No controlled* studies have conclusively demonstrated the benefit of heparin in PN.

Besides prophylaxis against thrombosis, the use of heparin in PN solutions may have additional benefits. A controlled trial has shown that heparin reduces the incidence of catheter-related sepsis.[212] Heparin also stimulates the release of the enzyme lipoprotein lipase and has been suggested as an agent to help enhance clearance of IVF. Heparin was shown to decrease total lipid levels and turbidity when given as a single injection of 50 to 100 U per kilogram to SGA infants.[213] Neonates receiving bolus doses of heparin (10 U per kilogram) in addition to heparin (1 U per milliliter) mixed with the PN solution had significantly lower triglyceride concentrations than patients receiving only the bolus dose (10 U per kilogram).[214] In a study of 21 preterm infants receiving TPN with heparin (1 U per millileter), the patients were given Intralipid, 1, 2, and 3 g per kilogram per day over 15 hours on days 1, 2, and 3, respectively.[215] Considerable intravascular lipolysis occurred, but, even so, lipemia was not prevented. The authors were concerned that the intravascular lipolysis probably exceeds the free fatty acid (FFA) disposal capacity of premature infants. The rise in plasma FFA to 2.0 μmol per milliliter warrants caution in the combined use of Intralipid (at rates exceeding 2 g per kilogram per day) and low levels of heparin in premature infants managed on PN.[215] The study also showed that while FFA and triglyceride levels returned to preinfusion levels 9 hours after stopping the infusion of Intralipid (1, 2, or 3 g per kilogram per day), there was a cumulative increase in plasma cholesterol and glucose.[215] One unit of heparin per milliliter of PN solution seems safe for full-term infants on up to adults. In premature babies, no definitive guidelines are available. In our intensive care nursery we routinely give 0.5 ml heparin per milliliter of TPN solution. Further studies are needed to define the safe level of heparin for preterm infants receiving PN.

TABLE 21
Possible Complications Related to Use of the Catheter

Venous thrombosis
Superior vena cava syndrome
Pulmonary embolus
Catheter dislodgment
Perforation and/or infusion leaks (pericardial, pleural, mediastinal)

Catheter-Associated Infection

The major catheter-related complication is infection. Such infections usually result from improper care of the catheter, especially the failure to follow meticulously the requirement for frequent changes of dressing covering the catheter exit site. Merritt and Mason have recently reviewed the entire issue of catheter-associated infections[216] and have stated criteria for the diagnosis of catheter-related sepsis (Table 22). Their review points out that the majority of catheter-related infections can be treated with the catheter in situ, as a recent prospective study reported.[217] *Staphylococcus epidermidis* is the most frequent organism encountered. Schropp and coworkers have demonstrated the importance of initial therapy through the line with vancomycin in suspected catheter sepsis.[218] Gentamicin is usually added to the initial regimen,[219] pending final culture report and sensitivities. Lack of defervescence of fever and continued positive blood cultures for 2 to 4 days despite antibiotics are indications for catheter removal.[220] Otherwise antibiotics should be continued for 14 to 21 days.[220] The complete cure of catheter sepsis in patients treated with antibiotics through the infected lumen has occurred in 75 percent of patients[218] and 86 percent of patients[219,220] in recent studies. When continued use of a Broviac or Hickman catheter is desired, a trial of antibiotic therapy should be attempted before catheter removal.[219] The GI tract may be a source of microbial seeding of the catheter.

TABLE 22
Criteria for the Diagnosis of Catheter-Related Sepsis

1. Positive blood cultures (two or more) from the catheter and peripheral sites with the same organism isolated from the catheter tip upon removal.
2. Persistently positive blood cultures from the catheter and negative cultures from peripheral sites associated with clinical signs of sepsis.
3. Quantitative blood cultures simultaneously collected from the catheter and peripheral sites which show a concentration of organisms 5 to 10 times greater in the catheter sample than in the peripheral sample.
4. Infection at the exit site or tunnel wound due to the same organism as isolated from blood culture.

Modified from Merritt and Mason.[216]

There is considerable interest in therapies that maintain or improve the integrity of the gut.[216] Therefore, the role of glutamine in preventing gut atrophy in parenterally fed, enterally fasted patients needs to be further explored,[221] since gut atrophy may foster increased intestinal permeability of bacterial pathogens.

TABLE 23
Potential Metabolic Complications of Parenteral Nutrition

Complication	Possible Etiology
Disorders related to metabolic capacity of the patient	
Congestive heart failure and pulmonary edema	Excessively rapid infusion of the PN solution
Hyperglycemia (with resultant glucosuria, osmotic diuresis, and possible dehydration)	Excessive intake (either excessive dextrose concentration or increased infusion rate) Change in metabolic state (e.g., sepsis, surgical stress, use of steroids) Common in low birth weight infants if dextrose load exceeds their ability to adapt
Hypoglycemia	Sudden cessation of infusate
Azotemia	Excessive administration of amino acids or protein hydrolysate (excessive nitrogen intake)
Electrolyte disorders Mineral disorders Vitamin disorders Trace element disorders	Excessive or inadequate intake
Essential fatty acid deficiency	Inadequate intake
Hyperlipidemia (increased triglycerides, cholesterol, and free fatty acids)	Excessive intake of intravenous fat emulsion
Disorders related to infusate components	
Metabolic acidosis	Use of hydrochloride salts of cationic amino acids
Hyperammonemia	Inadequate arginine intake, ? deficiencies of other urea cycle substrates, ? plasma amino acid imbalance, ? hepatic dysfunction
Abnormal plasma aminograms	Amino acid pattern of infusate
Miscellaneous	
Anemia	Failure to replace blood loss; iron deficiency, folic acid and vitamin B_{12} deficiency; copper deficiency
Demineralization of bone; rickets	Inadequate intake of calcium, inorganic phosphate, and/or vitamin D
Hepatic disorders Cholestasis Biochemical and histopathologic abnormalities	Prematurity; malnutrition: sepsis, ? hepatotoxicity due to amino acid imbalance; exceeding non-nitrogen calorie:nitrogen ratio of 150:1 to 200:1, leading to excessive glycogen and/or fat deposition in the liver; decreased stimulation of bile flow; nonspecific response to refeeding
Eosinophilia	Unknown

Modified from Heird WC. Total parenteral nutrition. In: Lebenthal E, ed. Textbook of gastroenterology and nutrition in infancy. New York: Raven Press, 1981: 662.

Catheter Occlusion

An 11-month-old infant on TPN developed superior vena cava syndrome, with head and neck swelling, secondary to a thrombus at the catheter tip occluding the superior vena cava. A 48-hour infusion of urokinase (4,400 units per kilogram per hour) resulted in clinical and radiographic evidence of clearance of the thrombus.[222] Glynn et al[223] have described using urokinase in 20 adults, with and without antibiotics, for thrombosis and associated infection occurring in implanted Silastic catheters. As the infected thrombotic clot is dissolved by the urokinase, antibiotics are able to reach the "hiding organisms."[223] No comparable studies have been done in pediatric patients, but urokinase (e.g., Abbokinase: Abbott Laboratories) has been used successfully in pediatric patients to clear central venous lines occluded by thrombi.[224]

Six pediatric patients with occlusion of central venous catheters by calcium phosphate crystals were successfully treated by irrigating their catheters with a hydrochloric acid and heparin solution.[225] Temporary febrile reactions occurred in three cases, but no serious complications were encountered. Such treatment needs further documentation. In the meantime, clinicians can minimize such precipitation by closely watching that concentrations of calcium and phosphorus fall well within standard solubility curves.

Metabolic Complications

Potential metabolic complications in patients on PN are shown in Table 23. As Heird has pointed out, these complications are of two general types: (1) those resulting from the patient's limited metabolic capacity for the various components of the PN infusate; and (2) those secondary to the PN infusate per se.[4]

Use of Intravenous Fat

The incidence of complications associated with the use of IVF is low, although the list is long (Table 24). If the IVF infusion exceeds its maximal clearance rate, hyperlipidemia occurs, which may then cause the potential complications shown in Table 25. Thus, careful monitoring of the use of IVF emulsions is essential. "Turbidity checks" (visual inspection of centrifuged hematocrit tubes to assess plasma lactescence) have been ineffective in estimating lipid concentrations in plasma.[226] Thus, several investigators[227,228] have advocated the use of a micronephelometer to measure the plasma light-scattering index (LSI), a more accurate measure of plasma turbidity. The LSI has a strictly linear correlation with IVF concentration in serum or saline[226]; the test can be performed easily and rapidly on a very small sample of capillary blood (50 μl). The advocates of nephelometry use cite the work of Forget et al,[229] who observed that IVF concentrations determined by a Thorp micronephelometer (Scientific Furnishings Ltd., Poynton, Cheshire, England) which exceeded 100 mg per deciliter were associated with hypertriglyceridemia, hypercholesterolemia, hyperphospholipidemia, and hyper pre-beta-lipoproteinemia in five patients studied. In contrast, Schreiner et al,[226] using a common

TABLE 24
Actual or Theoretical Complications with Intravenous Fat (IVF) Use

1. Impaired utilization of glucose
2. Acute hypersensitivity reaction
3. Transient sinus bradycardia
4. Increased concentrations of IVF in plasma can interfere with biochemical tests, leading to spurious hyperbilirubinemia when determined by certain direct spectrophotometric methods and spurious hyponatremia caused by the space-occupying effect of fat (these inaccurate readings can be corrected by prior ultracentrifugation)
5. Decreased concentrations of ionized calcium in serum
6. Pulmonary vasculitis induced by *Malassezia furfur*
7. Hemolysis (described in three cases of adult patients)
8. Arachidonic acid deficiency occurring in spite of the high linoleic acid content of IVF
9. Altered rates of synthesis of prostaglandins that might lead to abnormalities of platelet function and pulmonary function
10. Agglutination of Intralipid by sera of acutely ill patients

laboratory fluorometer set up as a nephelometer, found that the plasma LSI was a poor predictor of hyperlipidemia and did not correlate with serum triglycerides, cholesterol, or FFAs.

We studied the usefulness of nephelometry and chose to use the Thorp micronephelometer, the machine used both by Forget et al[229] and by the pioneers of IVF monitoring. Twenty-three infants in our intensive care nursery receiving 0.25 to 2.5 g per kilogram per day IVF by continuous infusion were tested simultaneously for IVF levels ($n = 58$; range 18 to 150 mg per deciliter), serum FFA: albumin molar ratios ($n = 58$; range 0 to 5.18), serum triglycerides ($n = 54$; range 33 to 305 mg per deciliter), serum cholesterol ($n = 34$; range 85 to 304 mg per deciliter), and serum turbidity.[230] We found a positive correlation between IVF level and triglycerides ($r = 0.406$; $P < 0.01$), but the IVF level did not reliably predict elevated triglycerides. Of seven triglyceride determinations above 200 mg per deciliter, only one had an elevated IVF level (greater than 100 mg per deciliter). No correlation was found between IVF level and cholesterol or FFA:albumin molar ratio. Serum turbidity was also a poor predictor of hyperlipidemia.[230] We, like Schreiner and coworkers,[226] concluded that monitoring IVF use with either IVF levels or turbidity checks does not accurately provide information regarding hyperlipidemia; therefore, one must regularly monitor serum triglycerides, cholesterol, and fatty acids when using IVF.

TABLE 25
Potential Hazards of the Hyperlipidemia Resulting from Failure to "Clear" Intravenous Fat

Major
- Impairment of pulmonary function
- Deposition of pigmented material in macrophages (which may lead to diminished immune responsiveness)
- Displacement of albumin-bound bilirubin by plasma free fatty acids (which may lead to kernicterus)

Minor
- Possible risk of coronary artery disease
- Fat overload syndrome (hyperlipemia, fever, lethargy, liver damage, coagulation disorders), encountered infrequently in infants and children

Altered Pulmonary Function. Following boluses of IVF to neonates, several investigators have demonstrated significant drops of Pa_{O_2} without alternation in other pulmonary function tests.[231,232] McKeen et al[233] found that administering IVF doses of 0.25 g per kilogram per hour to sheep caused (1) an increase in pulmonary artery pressure, (2) a decrease in arterial oxygen tension (Pa_{O_2}), and (3) an increase in pulmonary lymphatic flow. Identical findings recently have been described with doses of only 0.125 g per kilogram per hour.[234]

The use of IVF in patients with pulmonary compromise has yielded conflicting results. Because fat emboli were found in pulmonary capillaries during postmortem examinations of neonates who received Intralipid, the infusion of IVF in neonates was postulated to further alter pulmonary function.[235,236] Yet, the fat deposition in the pulmonary microcirculation also occurred in babies who never received IVF.[236] Shroeder et al[237] found *no* pulmonary fat accumulation in 22 infants, 13 of whom received Intralipid, when lungs were fixed in situ immediately after death; they attributed the previous findings to artifact secondary to delayed fixation of the lungs. Yet, Shulman et al[238] reviewed the histopathology and clinical course of 39 hospitalized infants who died during a 2-year period. Thirteen had received no IVF; 26 had received IVF. All 39 had lipid in pulmonary macrophages, chondrocytes, and interstitial cells. However, the incidence of pulmonary vascular lipid deposition in the group given IVF was significantly greater than in the other group. The grade of pulmonary vascular lipid depositions in the IVF group correlated positively with the percentage of the infants' lives during which lipids were administered and with mean intake; there was no correlation with the peak serum triglyceride level or the frequency of elevated triglycerides.[238] Experimental animal studies have shown that lipid-induced hypoxemia can be prevented with indomethacin.[233] Interestingly, Hageman et al[239] noted that in rabbits there were no blood gas or prostaglandin changes in lipid-infused normal animals. However, when the rabbits' lungs were damaged with oleic acid and then infused with IVF, significant deterioration in gas exchange occurred. Furthermore, these changes were blocked by indomethacin (implying prostaglandin-mediated effects of IVF). Brans et al[240] recently found that oxygen diffusion in the lungs of premature infants was not affected by the infusion of up to 4 g per kilogram per day of Intralipid over 24 hours. A very recent study[241] is quite disturbing. Forty-two neonates (less than 1,750 g birth weight) were randomly assigned to PN with or without IVF for 5 days in the first week of life. Chronic lung disease was increased in duration and tended to be more severe after lipid administration. Five IVF patients developed stage 3 BPD versus none of the control group. Seven IVF infants were discharged home on O_2 versus none in the control group. Other centers have administered IVF in similar manner in the first week of life (beginning at 0.5 g per kilogram per day, increased to a maximum of 2.5 g per kilogram per day) without reporting such findings. Further, many centers avoid IVF during the first week of life in LBW infants owing to hyperbilirubinemia. Careful controlled studies are needed to corroborate the findings of Hammerman et al.[241] In the meantime, one should use IVF cautiously in all LBW infants with respiratory or cardiovascular disease and reconsider the use of IVF in the first week of life in such infants.

Risk of Kernicterus. Although the IVF emulsions themselves have been shown not to displace bilirubin from albumin circulating in plasma,[242,243] there has been concern that liberation of FFAs during hydrolysis of IVF might displace albumin-bound bilirubin. If infants are icteric, the use of IVF emulsions has been considered hazardous if, indeed, unbound or free bilirubin might potentially increase the risk of kernicterus. Andrew et al[244] recommended that a safe method for monitoring and preventing such complications would be to maintain an FFA-to–serum albumin molar ratio (FA:SA) at 6 or less. Using a simplified method to measure the FA:SA, we found that in preterm infants receiving 0.5 to 3.3 g per kilogram per day of continuous IVF infusions in the second week of life, the mean ratio was only 1.1 (range 0 to 5).[245] If, on the other hand, bolus infusions are utilized or if IVF is administered in the first week of life, the FA:SA might exceed 6[244] and such infants might be at risk. Recent data suggest that premature infants can have FA:SA ratios greater than 10.[246] Spear et al[247] studied 20 premature infants (26 to 37 weeks' gestational age) given 1, 2, and 3 g per kilogram IVF over 15 hours on successive days. Infants less than 30 weeks' gestation had significant increases in FA:SA with each increase in lipid dose, whereas infants greater than 30 weeks tolerated the IVF without increase in FA:SA. Infants whose FA:SA was greater than 4.0 were significantly more premature; such elevations occurred at both 2 and 3 g per kilogram per day. 1 g per kilogram per day IVF over 15 hours resulted in minimal risk of decreased bilirubin binding.[247] Therefore, in icteric infants, it is crucial to monitor the fatty acid-to-serum albumin molar ratio if they are receiving IVF. The American Academy of Pediatrics recommends that infants with bilirubin levels of 8 to 10 mg per deciliter (assuming an albumin concentration of 2.5 to 3.0 mg per deciliter) should receive *only* the amount of IVF required to meet essential fatty acid requirements (0.5 to 1.0 g per kilogram per day).[248]

Sepsis. A recent study[249] confirms previous observations that septic infants can develop significant elevations in triglyceride levels. A sudden rise in triglycerides not associated with an increase in IVF dose should make caregivers suspicious of sepsis. Dahlstrom and co-workers also argue that the dose of IVF be lowered during acute illness.[250] In a 1-year prospective study of 15 children on home TPN, they noted that acutely sick children had significantly increased serum triglyceride levels and prothrombin and partial thromboplastin values compared to times when they were well. Their monocyte activation and complement factors remained normal even with acute illness.[250]

Thrombocytopenia. There is a reluctance to use IVF in patients with low platelet counts, based on reports of varying degrees of thrombocytopenia with earlier IVF preparations and on one case report with Intralipid. Many anecdotal reports of thrombocytopenia may well be secondary to an underlying condition (e.g., sepsis) rather than to IVF. Cohen et al[251] could not implicate IVF as a cause of thrombocytopenia in any of the 128 patients studied. In addition, 10 of the patients had established thrombocytopenia secondary to sepsis or bone marrow suppression by cancer chemotherapy. In all 10, platelet counts actually rose with IVF use, concomitant with the improvement of the septicemia state or with marrow recovery after cessation of chemotherapy. Interestingly, TPN *without* IVF may lead to EFA deficiency, which in turn may cause thrombocytopenia and platelet dysfunction. A recent study in ill neonates also failed to document any association between IVF and thrombocytopenia.[252] Goulet et al[253] have the only documented association of IVF with thrombocytopenia. Seven patients on home TPN receiving 1 to 2 g per kilogram per 24 hours over 3 to 18 months developed recurrent thrombocytopenia. Platelet lifespan was reduced. Sea blue histiocytes containing granulations and hemophagocytosis were seen on bone marrow smears. Scans taken after injection of autologous erythrocytes labeled with ^{99m}Tc showed bone marrow sequestration of these cells. The authors concluded that long-term IVF administration induces hyperactivation of the monocyte-macrophage system.[253]

Elevated Triglycerides. Finally, it should be noted that elevated triglycerides can occur in preterm babies solely on enteral feedings.[254,255] Recently, two preterm babies with severe bronchopulmonary dysplasia had profound triglyceride elevations (352 to 2,142 mg per deciliter) receiving formula feedings.[256] The significance and etiology of this finding are as yet unknown and point to an important need for further research in this area.

Recommendations

1. Patients receiving IVF should have laboratory specimens for total bilirubin, sodium, and calcium ultracentrifuged to avoid spurious laboratory values.
2. All patients receiving IVF should have triglyceride and cholesterol determinations at least weekly. If either value is elevated, the IVF dose should be adjusted appropriately.
3. A serum triglyceride level should be obtained 24 hours after an incremental increase in IVF dose to be sure that the patient can tolerate this new dose.
4. A sudden elevation in triglyceride level at an IVF dose previously tolerated should raise the suspicion of sepsis.
5. A determination of the free fatty acid–to–serum albumin molar ratio (FA:SA) should be performed twice weekly on infants with any elevation of indirect bilirubin who are receiving IVF. Ideally, the FA:SA should be kept below 4 (the level at which no free bilirubin is generated in a number of in vitro studies).
6. Any infant with respiratory or cardiac disease should have frequent monitoring of Pa_{O_2} or transcutaneous O_2 and any fall in this value should result in an appropriate decrease in the IVF dose.
7. We attempt to keep the serum triglyceride below 150 mg per deciliter (our laboratory normal values: 30 to 200 mg per deciliter), the cholesterol below 250 mg per deciliter (normal: 120 to 280 mg per deciliter), and the FA:SA below 4.
8. Monitor platelet count and protime weekly during hospitalizations.

Use of Carbohydrate

If urine glucose by Keto-Diastix (Ames Company, Elkhart, IN) is 1/4 percent (250 mg per deciliter) or greater, monitor Dextrostix (if Dextrostix is elevated, confirm with a blood glucose). The dextrose content of the solution may need to be decreased to prevent osmotic diuresis. A systematic review of all possible etiologies for glucosuria includes (1) use of steroids, (2) use of other medications, (3) dietary indiscretions, (4) error in the PN delivery rate, and (5) possible sepsis.

Use of Protein

Amino acid infusions of greater than 2.5 g per kilogram per day can result in increased blood urea nitrogen (BUN), increased ammonia production, and metabolic acidosis, especially in LBW infants who have limited tolerance.[257,258] Patients with kidney or liver disease are also at increased risk for developing acidosis while receiving PN. Thus, frequent monitoring of serum electrolytes, blood pH, BUN, and NH_3 is indicated.

Recommendations. Ideally, with each increase in amino acid amount, a BUN should be obtained to be sure that the increase in protein is tolerated.

If possible, blood NH_3 determinations should be performed one or two times weekly to monitor for protein intolerance and possibly for early evidence of sepsis.[259]

A 24-hour urine collection for urine urea nitrogen (UUN) is necessary to determine nitrogen balance and should be determined weekly during a course of PN until positive nitrogen balance is seen consistently. The UUN is measured in milligrams per 100 ml.

$$N_2 \text{ balance} = \frac{\text{grams of protein (intake)}}{6.25} - (\text{UUN} + 3)$$

The protein intake should include grams of protein provided by oral or enteral feeds plus that provided by intravenous amino acids. Dividing by 6.25 converts the protein intake into grams of nitrogen. The UUN in this equation is expressed in grams (e.g., if UUN = 500 mg per 100 ml or 5,000 mg per liter and the patient's 24-hour urine is 2 liters, UUN = 10,000 mg or 10 g per 24 hours). The constant of 3 in the equation corrects for nonurea nitrogen losses (approximately 2 g per day), fecal losses (approximately 1 g per day), and skin, hair, and nail losses (approximately 0.2 g per day). This constant has been established in adult balance studies. It is not clear that the same constant can be used in premature infants or young children.

Osteopenia of Prematurity

Premature infants are subject to a unique condition, "osteopenia of prematurity" or "rickets of prematurity," a frequently occurring but poorly defined metabolic bone disease associated with decreased bone mineralization. In most cases, decreased bone mineralization is subclinical; this condition is diagnosed only after the development of bone fractures or overt rickets.[260] Geggel et al[261] have advocated monitoring premature infants for the development of rickets by detecting generalized aminoaciduria (by performing urinary amino acid screens), which is an early sensitive index of vitamin D deficiency and which precedes changes in serum calcium, phosphorus, or alkaline phosphatase values. Experts now believe that a deficiency of calcium and phosphorus is more likely than a defect in vitamin D metabolism to be the cause of osteopenia in preterm infants.[262] Kovar et al,[113] as described earlier, suggest screening for rickets in preterm infants with plasma alkaline phosphatase: Levels of up to five times the upper limit of the normal adult reference range are acceptable; a value of six times the upper limit of the adult reference range should prompt a radiograph to exclude rickets. Serial infant-adapted photon absorptiometry can help physicians follow the bone mineral content of preterm infants; unfortunately, this study is not routinely available.

Hepatic Dysfunction

The development of liver disease during TPN was first reported in 1971 in a preterm infant.[263] At autopsy, the infant's liver revealed cholestasis, bile duct proliferation, and early cirrhosis. Hepatic dysfunction remains one of the most common and most serious complications of TPN. The spectrum of TPN-associated liver complications is depicted in Table 26 and has recently been reviewed.[264,265] Cholestasis is especially prevalent in very premature infants and in infants on TPN for longer than 2 weeks.

Hepatomegaly with mild elevation of serum transaminases in the absence of cholestasis may result from hepatic accumulation of lipid or glycogen secondary to either excess carbohydrate calories or an inappropriate non-nitrogen calorie: nitrogen ratio. Fatty infiltration of the liver as a result of excessive caloric intake is readily reversible in nearly all instances by reduction of total calories administered and, if necessary, alteration of the non-nitrogen calorie-to-nitrogen ratio.[266]

Abnormal liver function tests are not uncommon in patients on PN for long periods of time. Those with chronic intestinal conditions complicated by infection or bacterial over-

TABLE 26
Total Parenteral Nutrition–Associated Liver Complications

Hepatomegaly
Hepatic dysfunction
Elevated blood ammonia
Elevated transaminases (SGOT and SGPT)
Cholestasis
Fatty infiltration of the liver
Damage to hepatocytes
Overt liver disease
Fibrosis
Bile duct proliferation
Cirrhosis

growth are particularly susceptible to hepatic complications. In most of these patients, elevated liver enzymes improve with the initiation of partial enteral alimentation.[266]

A small percentage of infants and children go on to develop chronic liver disease associated with poor growth[267] and even cirrhosis[268] and hepatic failure.[269] A recent follow-up study of patients on long-term PN documented a wide variety of complications, but all of them except liver dysfunction proved to be temporary.[269a] In this series, 57.6 percent of the children showed liver dysfunction during PN, and some of them showed long-term abnormalities after its cessation (see Chapter 28, Part 20).

Recommendations. If the serum glutamic-oxaloacetic transaminase (SGOT; AST) or serum glutamic-pyruvic transaminase (SGPT; ALT) rises in association with a normal or nearly normal direct bilirubin and alkaline phosphatase, check the total caloric intake and the calorie-to-nitrogen ratio. Reduce the caloric intake and/or decrease the non-nitrogen calorie-to-nitrogen ratio, which ideally should be 150 to 200:1.

Monitor for early evidence of cholestasis: Use either the GGTP, 5′-nucleotidase, or serum bile acids, or, if the above tests are not easily obtainable, measure the direct bilirubin on a weekly basis.

Increased Risk of Gallstones

Long-term administration of PN increases the risk of gallstones in patients of all ages[270-277]; children with ileal disease or resection are at particularly high risk.[276] In one adult series there was a twofold increase in gallbladder disease in patients who received no oral intake during PN as opposed to those who had oral supplementation in addition to PN[275]; the gallbladder disease appears to be secondary to bile stasis.

Clinically, gallbladder disease can be detected by the demonstration of "sludge" or a stone (or stones) in a patient with liver function tests consistent with cholestasis. Messing et al[274] demonstrated "sludge" in 6 percent of cases in the first 3 weeks of TPN; the incidence increases to 50 percent between the fourth and sixth weeks and reaches 100 percent after 6 weeks.

Roslyn et al[276] recommend periodic ultrasonography in children on prolonged PN, especially if they have an ileal resection or underlying ileal disease. They advise clinicians to suspect cholecystitis in any child on TPN who complains of abdominal pain.

A recent review[278] of 246 infants and children receiving PN for more than 4 weeks revealed significant biliary disease. In 68 who died there were postmortem or ultrasound studies available in 16; of the 178 survivors, 68 had adequate abdominal ulrasonographic findings. Eleven of the 84 patients studied had cholelithiasis. Six required cholecystectomy for relief of chronic abdominal pain, pancreatitis, or empyema of the gallbladder. One had cholecystotomy. Two of the remaining four are asymptomatic; one has abdominal colic, and one expired of hepatic insufficiency related to PN. The authors recommend routine abdominal ultrasonography for those on PN for longer than 30 days as well as for any patient on PN who presents with abdominal pain. They argue for early elective cholecystectomy for PN-associated cholelithiasis,[278] but many centers elect to watch asymptomatic patients, and several have actually described spontaneous resolution of stones.

MONITORING PN

The suggested schedule for chemical and anthropometric monitoring is shown in Table 27. Such monitoring should allow detection of metabolic complications in sufficient time to permit alteration of the PN infusate with resultant correction of any abnormality. More detailed descriptions of monitoring are readily available.[4,46,170,185,279]

PSYCHOSOCIAL ASPECTS OF PN

When infants are parenterally fed for longer than 2 months, they may become increasingly withdrawn and isolated and demonstrate impaired intellectual and emotional develop-

TABLE 27
Essentials of Monitoring in Patients on Parenteral Nutrition

I. **Prior** to initiating PN, you must obtain baseline laboratory values, ideally including
   A. General survey panel (GSP) (contains glucose, renal functions, liver function, albumin, calcium, phosphorus)
   B. Direct bilirubin
   C. Serum magnesium
   D. Serum trigycerides (should be obtained **fasting**)
   E. Electrolytes
   F. CBC with platelet count, prothrombin time
   G. Urinalysis

   In patients you expect to be on PN for 1 month or more
   H. Serum zinc, copper, vitamin B_{12}, folate

   Optional:
   I. 24-hr urine for urea nitrogen (UUN)—used to determine nitrogen balance
   J. Serum prealbumin; somatomedin-C
   K. Blood NH_3

   Also order nutritional consult to obtain anthropometric measurements (e.g., triceps skin fold thickness, mid-upper arm circumference)

II. **Ongoing monitoring**
   A. GSP, direct bilirubin, magnesium weekly
   B. Electrolytes—initially daily or qod; when stable weekly
   C. Calcium, phosphorus—initially two times per week (i.e., Mon.-Thurs. or Tues.-Fri.); when stable—weekly (run on GSP so they do not have to be ordered separately)
   D. Triglycerides—within 24 hr of each increase in dose of IV fat; then weekly
   E. BUN—within 24 hr of each increase in dose of IV amino acids
   F. Anthropometrics every 2 weeks
   G. 24-hr urine for urea nitrogen—weekly (optional)
   H. Serum zinc, copper, vitamin B_{12}, folate—monthly
   I. CBC with platelet count, prothrombin time—weekly
   J. Blood NH_3—weekly (optional)
   K. Prealbumin—weekly (optional)
   L. Somatomedin-C every 2 weeks (optional)

ment[11] unless aggressive measures are taken to prevent these disorders—utilizing a trained mental health worker. Our early experience identified that children receiving PN therapy have unique psychosocial needs, related to their not feeling "normal" owing to their inability to eat regularly like their peers.[280] The attempt to promote a healthy adaptation to PN is finally beginning to receive the attention it deserves.[281,282] Finally, a recent paper has shown that an educational booklet about TPN decreased parental anxiety and increased satisfaction with patient care more successfully than did verbal communication.[283] The authors speculated that such a booklet may reduce parentally induced anxiety in the child and facilitate parent-hospital staff interactions.[283] The hospital team is not immune from stresses related to TPN. Patients who have had massive small bowel resection or who have diseases such as congenital microvillous atrophy can survive only with the aid of TPN. Exposing the patient, the family, and themselves to the unpleasant consequences of treatment that may extend for years is often extremely difficult.[11] The decision to begin such therapy requires intense discussion, including mental health workers and a representative of the family's religion.

PRACTICAL ISSUES

The approach to interrupting TPN therapy for drug administration differs from hospital to hospital[284,285] and should be carefully discussed with the pharmacy by the hospital's TPN committee. Acyclovir, amphotericin B, metronidazole, and Septra *cannot* be given with the TPN solution. They may be given in D_{10} with the TPN turned off. Other antibiotics, compatible or incompatible with TPN, should be given by intravenous push, if possible. The pharmacist should be consulted for guidelines on specific antibiotics.

SUMMARY

Parenteral nutrition remains a therapy in evolution. Since the publication of *Manual of Pediatric Parenteral Nutrition*,[286] a new technology for the provision of continuous insulin to VLBW infants has appeared. New amino acid solutions (e.g., TrophAmine, Aminosyn PF) have been designed for the preterm infant. A new fat solution has been released (Liposyn II), and solutions containing MCT oil are being developed. A new pediatric multivitamin (MVI-Pediatric) has also been released. A recent revision of AMA expert guidelines has been published on the use of vitamins, trace elements, calcium, phosphorus, and magnesium. Oral and intravenous preparations of L-carnitine have become available. New technology to help better access caloric needs has been designed.[287] Standards for nutritional support in hospitalized pediatric patients have been established.[288] Finally, alternative routines of nutrient delivery are being considered.[289,290] The practitioner is strongly urged to keep up aggressively with the latest literature so that his or her patients may continue to receive state-of-the-art care.

REFERENCES

1. Elman R, Weiner DO. Intravenous alimentation with special reference to protein (amino acid) metabolism. JAMA 1939; 112:796–802.
2. Shohl AT, Butler AM, Blackfan KD, et al. Nitrogen metabolism during the oral and parenteral adminstration of the amino acids of hydrolyzed casein. J Pediatr 1939; 15:469–475.
3. Helfrick FW, Abelson NM. Intravenous feeding of a complete diet in a child. J Pediatr 1944; 25:400–403.
4. Heird WC. Parenteral nutrition. In: Grand RJ, Sutphen JL, Dietz WH, eds. Pediatric nutrition. Boston: Butterworths, 1987: 747.
5. Forbes AL. Incidence of reactions to an intravenous fat emulsion administered at two different rates. Metabolism 1957; 6:645–649.
6. Lehr HL, Rosenthal O, Rownsley HM, et al. Clinical experience with intravenous fat emulsions. Metabolism 1957; 6:666–672.
7. Dudrick SJ, Wilmore DW, Vars HM. Long-term total parenteral nutrition with growth in puppies and positive nitrogen balance in patients. Surg Forum 1967; 18:356–357.
8. Dudrick SJ, Wilmore DW, Vars HM, et al. Long-term total parenteral nutrition with growth, development and positive nitrogen balance. Surgery 1968; 64:134–142.
9. Wilmore DW, Dudrick SJ. Growth and development of an infant receiving all nutrients exclusively by vein. JAMA 1968; 203:140–144.
10. Coran AG. Profiles in nutritional management: the infant patient. Chicago, Medical Directions, 1980: 3.
11. Booth IW, Shaw V. Parenteral nutrition. In: Milla PJ, Muller DRR, eds. Harries' pediatric gastroenterology. 2nd ed. Edinburgh: Churchill Livingstone, 1988; 558.
12. Weinsier RL, Heimburger DC, Butterworth CE. Handbook of clinical nutrition. St. Louis: CV Mosby, 1989: 221.
13. Reimer SL, Michener WM, Steiger E. Nutritional support of the critically ill child. Pediatr Clin North Am 1980; 27:647.
14. Levy JS, Winters RW, Heird WC. Total parenteral nutrition in pediatric patients. Pediatr Rev 1980; 2:99.
15. Filler RM. Parenteral support of the surgically ill child. In: Suskind RM, ed. Textbook of pediatric nutrition. New York: Raven Press, 1981: 341.
16. Candy DCA. Parenteral nutrition in paediatric practice: a review. J Hum Nutr 1980; 34:287.
17. Moyer-Mileur L, Chan GM. Nutritional support of very-low-birth-weight infants requiring prolonged assisted ventilation. Am J Dis Child 1986; 140:929–932.
18. Unger A, Goetzman BW, Chan C, et al. Nutritional practices and outcome of extremely premature infants. Am J Dis Child 1986; 140:1027.
19. Gunn T, Reaman G, Outerbridge EW. Peripheral total parenteral nutrition for premature infants with the respiratory distress syndrome: a controlled study. J Pediatr 1978; 92:608.
20. Yu VYH, James B, Hendry P, et al. Total parenteral nutrition in very low birthweight infants: a controlled trial. Arch Dis Child 1979; 54:653.
21. Kerner JA, Hattner JAT, Trautman MS, et. al Postnatal somatic growth in very low birth weight infants on peripheral parenteral nutrition. J Pediatr Perinat Nutr. 1988; 2:27–34.
22. Glass EJ, Hune R, Lang MA, et al. Parenteral nutrition compared with transpyloric feeding. Arch Dis Child 1984; 59:131.
23. Dryburgh E. Transpyloric feeding in 49 infants undergoing intensive care. Arch Dis Child 1980; 55:879.
24. Zlotkin SH, Stallings VA, Pencharz PB. Total parenteral nutrition in children. Pediatr Clin North Am 1985; 32:381.
25. Cashore WJ, Sedaghatian MR, Usher RH. Nutritional supplements with intravenously administered lipid, protein hydrolysate, and glucose in small premature infants. Pediatrics 1975; 56:8.
26. Churella HR, Bachhuber BS, MacLean WC. Survey: methods of feeding low-birth-weight infants. Pediatrics 1985; 76:243–249
27. Adamkin DA. Nutrition in very very low birth weight infants. Clin Perinatol 1986; 13:419–443.
28. Grand RJ, Watkins JB, Torti FM. Development of the human gastrointestinal tract. Gastroenterology 1976; 70:790–810.
29. Lebenthal E, Lee PC. Interactions of determinants in the ontongeny of the gastrointestinal tract: a unified concept. Pediatr Res 1983; 17:19–24.
30. Milla PJ. Development of intestinal structure and function. In: Tanner MS, Stocks RJ, eds. Neonatal gastroenterology— contemporary issues. Newcastle upon Tyne: Intercept, 1984: 1.
31. Koldovsky O, Sunshine P, Kretchmer N. Cellular migration of intes-

tinal epithelia in suckling and weaned rats. Nature 1966; 212:1389–1390.
32. Herbst JJ, Sunshine P. Postnatal development of the small intestine of the rat. Pediatr Res 1969; 3:27.
33. Sunshine P, Herbst JJ, Koldovsky O, Kretchmer N. Adaptation of the gastrointestinal tract to extrauterine life. Ann NY Acad Sci 1971; 176:16–29.
34. Herbst JJ, Sunshine P, Kretchmer N. Intestinal malabsorption in infancy and childhood. Adv Pediatr 1969; 16:11.
35. Walsh MC, Kliegman R, Fanaroff A. Necrotizing enterocolitis: a practitioner's perspective. Pediatr Rev 1988; 9:219–226.
36. Ostertag SG, LaGamma EF, Reisen CE, Ferrentino RL. Early enteral feeding does not affect the incidence of necrotizing enterocolitis. Pediatrics 1986; 77:275–280.
37. LaGamma E, Ostertag S, Birnbaum H. Failure of delayed oral feedings to prevent necrotizing enterocolitis. Am J Dis Child 1985; 139: 385–389.
38. Book LS, Herbst JJ, Jung AL. Comparison of the fast-and-slow feeding rate schedules to the development of necrotizing enterocolitis. J Pediatr 1976; 89:463–466.
39. Goldman HI. Feeding and necrotizing enterocolitis. Am J Dis Child 1980; 134:553–555.
40. Anderson DM, Rome ES, Kleigman RM. Relationship of endemic necrotizing enterocolitis to alimentation. Pediatr Res 1985; 19:331A.
41. Eyal F, Sagi E, Avital A. Necrotizing enterocolitis in the very low birth weight infants: expressed breast milk feeding compared with parenteral feeding. Arch Dis Child 1982; 57:274–276.
42. Brown E, Sweet A. Neonatal necrotizing enterocolitis. Pediatr Clin North Am 1982; 29:114–170.
43. Aynsley-Green A. Metabolic and endocrine interrelation in the human fetus and neonate. Am J Clin Nutr 1985; 41:399–417.
44. Feng JJ, Kwong LK, Kerner JA, et al. Resumption of intestinal maturation upon reintroduction of intraluminal nutrients: functional and biochemical correlations. Clin Res 1987; 35:228A.
45. Reichman B, Chessex P, Putet G, et al. Diet, fat accretion, and growth in premature infants. N Engl J Med 1981; 305:1495–1500.
46. Wheeler N. Parenteral nutrition. In: Kelts DG, Jones RD, eds. Manual of pediatric nutrition. Boston: Little, Brown, 1984: 151.
47. Caldwell MD, Kennedy CC. Normal nutritional requirements. Surg Clin North Am 1981; 61:491–498.
48. Anderson TL, Muttart CR, Bieber MA, et al. A controlled trial of glucose versus glucose and amino acids in premature infants. J Pediatr 1979; 94:947.
49. Zlotkin SH, Bryan MH, Anderson CH. Intravenous nitrogen and energy intakes required to duplicate in utero nitrogen accretion in prematurely born human infants. J. Pediatr 1981; 99:115.
50. Baker JP, Detsky AS, Stewart S, et al. Randomized trial of total parenteral nutrition in critically ill patients: metabolic effects of varying glucose-lipid ratios as the energy source. Gastroenterology 1984; 87:53.
51. Landon MB, Gabbe SG, Mullen JL. Total parenteral nutrition during pregnancy. Clin Perinatol 1986; 13:57.
52. Mendeloff E, Wesley JR, Dechert R, et al. Comparison of measured resting energy expenditure versus estimated resting expenditure in infants. JPEN 10 (suppl) 1986; 1:6S.
53. Schafer L, Wesley JR, Tse Y, et al. Effects of necrotizing enterocolitis (NEC) on calculation of resting energy expenditure (REE) in infants with gastroschisis. JPEN 10 (suppl) 1986; 1:6.
54. Adamkin DH. Total parenteral nutrition in hyaline membrane disease. In: Lebenthal E, ed. Total parenteral nutrition: indications, utilization, complications, pathophysiologic considerations. New York: Raven Press, 1986: 305.
55. Cochran EB, Phelps SJ, Helms RA. Parenteral nutrition in pediatric patients. Clin Pharmacol 1988; 7:351–366.
56. Pereira GR. Glassman M. Parenteral nutrition in the neonate. In: Rombeau JL, Caldwell MD, eds. Parenteral nutrition (Clinical nutrition, vol 2). Philadelphia: WB Saunders, 1986: 702.
57. Hay WW Jr. Justification for total parenteral nutrition in premature and compromised newborn. In: Lebenthal E, ed. Total parenteral nutrition: indications, utilization, complications, and pathophysiologic considerations. New York: Raven Press, 1986: 277.
58. Pittard WB, Levkoff AH. Parenteral nutrition for the neonate. In: Tsang RC, Nichols BL, eds. Nutrition during infancy. Philadelphia: Hanley and Belfus, 1988: 327.
59. Bell EF, Warburton D, Stonestreet BS, et al. Effect of fluid administration on the development of symptomatic patent ductus arteriosus and congestive heart failure in premature infants. N Engl J Med 1980; 302:598–604.
60. Brown ER, Start A, Sosenko I, et al. Bronchopulmonary dysplasia: possible relationship to pulmonary edema. J Pediatr 1978; 92:982–984.
61. Goldman HI. Feeding and necrotizing enterocolitis. Am J Dis Child 1980; 134:553–555.
62. Goldberg RN, Chung D, Goldman SL, et al. The association of rapid volume expansion and intraventricular hemorrhage in the preterm infant. J Pediatr 1980; 96:1060–1063.
63. Kerner JA. Fluid requirements. In: Kerner JA, ed. Manual of pediatric parenteral nutrition. New York: John Wiley and Sons, 1983: 69.
64. Kerner JA Jr. Carbohydrate requirements. In: Kerner JA Jr, ed. Manual of pediatric parenteral nutrition. New York: John Wiley and Sons, 1983: 79.
65. Committee on Nutrition, American Academy of Pediatrics, Parenteral nutrition. In: Forbes GB, Woodruff CW, eds. Pediatric nutrition handbook. 2nd ed. Chicago: American Academy of Pediatrics, 1985: 154.
66. Committee on Nutrition, American Academy of Pediatrics. Commentary on parenteral nutrition. Pediatrics 1983; 71:547.
67. Macfie J, Smith RC, Hill GL. Glucose or fat as a non-protein energy source? A controlled clinical trial in gastroenterological patients requiring intravenous nutrition. Gastroenterology 1981; 80:103–107.
68. Askanazi J, Nordenstrom J, Rosenbaum SH, et al. Nutrition for the patient with respiratory failure: glucose vs fat. Anesthesiology 1981; 54:373.
69. Sparks JW, Avery GB, Fletcher AB, et al. Parenteral galactose therapy in the glucose-intolerant premature infant. J Pediatr 1982; 100:255.
70. Rigo J, Senterre J. Parenteral nutrition in the very-low-birth-weight infant. In: Kretchmer N, Minkowski A, eds. Nutritional adaptation of the gastrointestinal tract of the newborn. New York: Nestle, Vevey/Raven Press, 1983: 191.
71. Yu VYH, James BE, Hendry PG, et al. Glucose tolerance in very low birth weight infants. Aust Paediatr J 1979; 15:150.
72. Vaucher YE, Walson PD, Morrow G. Continuous insulin infusion in hyperglycemic, very low birth weight infants. J Pediatr Gastroenterol Nutr 1982; 1:211.
73. Schwartz R. Should exogenous insulin be given to very low birth weight infants? J Pediatr Gastroenterol Nutr 1982; 1:287–288.
74. Ostertag SG, Jovanovic L, Lewis B, et al. Insulin pump therapy in the very low birth weight infant. Pediatrics 1986; 78:625.
75. Binder ND, Raschko PK, Benda GI, Reynolds JW. Insulin infusion with parenteral nutrition in extremely low birth weight infants with hypoglycemia. J Pediatr 1989; 114:273–280.
76. Winters RW, Heird WC, Dell RB, et al. Plasma amino acids in infants receiving parenteral nutrition. In: Greene HL, Holliday MA, Munro H, eds. Clinical nutrition update: amino acids. Chicago: American Medical Association. 1977: 147.
77. Heird WC, Malloy MH. Brain composition of beagle puppies receiving total parenteral nutrition. In: Itka V. ed. Nutrition and metabolism of the fetus and infant. The Hague: Nijhoff Publishers, 1979: 365.
78. Wu PYK, Edwards NB, Storm MC. Characterization of the plasma amino acid pattern of normal term breast-fed infants. J Pediatr 1986; 109:347.
79. Helms RA, Christensen ML, Mauer EC, et al. Comparison of a pediatric versus standard amino acid formulation in preterm neonates requiring parenteral nutrition. J Pediatr 1987; 110:466.
80. Heird WC, Dell RB, Helms RA, et al. Amino acid mixture designed to maintain normal plasma amino acid patterns in infants and children requiring parenteral nutrition. Pediatrics 1987; 80:401.
81. Heird WC, Hay W, Helms RA, et al. Pediatric parenteral amino acid mixture in low birth weight infants. Pediatrics 1988; 81:41.
82. Cooper A, Betts JM, Pereira GR. Taurine deficiency in the severe hepatic dysfunction complicating total parenteral nutrition. J Pediatr Surg 1984; 19:462.
83. Kerner JA Jr. Metabolic complications. In: Kerner JA Jr, ed. Manual of pediatric parenteral nutrition. New York: John Wiley & Sons, 1983: 199.
84. Poole RL, Rupp CA, Kerner JA. Calcium and phosphate in neonatal parenteral solutions. JPEN 1983; 7:358.
85. Fitzgerald KA, MacKay MW. Calcium and phosphate solubility in neonatal parenteral nutrient solutions containing TrophAmine. Am J Hosp Phar 1986; 43:88.
86. Helms RA, Johnson MR, Christensen ML, et al. Evaluation of two

pediatric amino acid formulations. (Abstract) JPEN 1988; 12:4.
87. Adamkin DH, McClead R, Marchildon M, Desai N, O'Neal W, Benawra R, McCulloch K. Multicenter comparative evaluation of Aminosyn-PF (A) and TrophAmine (T) in preterm infants. (Abstract) JPEN 1989; 13:18.
88. Coran AG, Drongowski RA. Studies on the toxicity and efficacy of a new amino acid solution in pediatric parenteral nutrition. JPEN 1987; 11:368–377.
89. Imura K, Okada A, Fukui Y, Kawahara H, Yagi M, Kubota A, Kanava S, Kamata S, Nagata Y. Clinical studies on a newly devised amino acid solution for neonates. JPEN 1988; 12:496–504.
90. Helms RA, Johnson MR, Christensen ML, Fernandes E. Altered caloric and protein requirement in neonates receiving a pediatric amino acid formulation. (Abstract) Pediatr Res 1987; 21:429A.
91. Phelps SJ, Cochran EC, Kamper CA. Peripheral venous line infiltration in infants receiving 10% dextrose, 10% dextrose/amino acids, 10% dextrose/amino acids/fat emulsion. (Abstract) Pediatr Res 1987; 21:67A.
92. Friedman Z, Danon A, Stahlman MT, et al. Rapid onset of essential fatty acid deficiency in the newborn. Pediatrics 1976; 58:640.
93. Kerner JA Jr. Fat requirements. In: Kerner JA Jr, ed. Manual of pediatric parenteral nutrition. New York: John Wiley & Sons, 1983: 103.
94. Friedman Z, Shochat SJ, Maisels JM, et al. Correction of essential fatty acid deficiency in newborn infants by cutaneous application of sunflower seed oil. Pediatrics 1976; 58:650–654.
95. Hunt CE, Engel RR, Modler S, et al. Essential fatty acid deficiency in neonates: inability to reverse deficiency by topical applications of EFA-rich oils. J Pediatr 1978; 92:603–607.
96. O'Neill JA, Caldwell MD, Meng HC. Essential fatty acid deficiency in surgical patients. Ann Surg 1977; 185:536.
97. Pelham LD. Rational use of intravenous fat emulsions. Am J Hosp Pharm 1981; 38:198.
98. Kao LC, Cheng MH, Warburton D. Triglycerides, free fatty acids, free fatty acids/albumin molar ratio, and cholesterol levels in serum of neonates receiving long-term lipid infusions: controlled trial of continuous and intermittent regimens. J Pediatr 1984; 104:429.
99. Das JB, Joshi ID, Philippart AI. Depression of glucose utilization by Intralipid in the post-traumatic period: an experimental study. J Pediatr Surg 1980; 15:739–745.
100. Brans YW, Andrews DS, Carrillo DW, Dutton EP, Menchaca EM, Puleo-Scheppke BA. Tolerance of fat emulsions in very-low-birth-weight infants. Am J Dis Child 1988; 142:145–152.
101. Cooke RJ, Burckhart GJ. Hypertriglyceridemia during the intravenous infusion of a safflower-oil based fat emulsion. J Pediatr 1983; 103:959.
101a. Nizar L, Vyhmeister N, Fisher L, Grill B. The risk of hypertriglyceride increases with the duration of intravenous fat administration. (Abstract) Clin Res 1990; 38:191A.
101b. Grill B, Yoon S, Fisher L, et al. Prospective comparison of two intravenous lipid emulsions in premature infants: effects on plasma fatty acids. (Abstract) JPEN 1990; 14:115.
101c. Malkani A, Abraham S, Hartman G, et al. Evaluation of a new fat emulsion (Liposyn II) in neonates. (Abstract) Clin Res 1990; 38:190A.
102. Helms RA, Whitington PF, Mauer EC, et al. Enhanced lipid utilization in infants receiving oral L-carnitine during long-term parenteral nutrition. J Pediatr 1986; 109:984.
103. Helms RA, Borum PR, Hay WW, et al. Intravenous (IV) carnitine during parenteral nutrition (PN) in neonates. JPEN 1987; 11(suppl):9.
104. Stahl GE, Spear ML, Hamosh M. Intravenous administration of lipid emulsions to premature infants. Clin Perinatol 1986: 13:133.
105. Lima LAM, Murphy JF, Stansbie D, Rowlandson P, Gray OP. Neonatal parenteral nutrition with a fat emulsion containing medium chain triglycerides. Acta Paediatr Scand 1988; 77:332–339.
106. Bientz J, Frey A, Schirardin H, Bach AC. Medium chain triglycerides in parenteral nutrition in the newborn: a short-term clinical trial. Infusionstherapie 1988; 15:96–99.
107. Van Aerde J, Chan G. Eicosapentaenoic (EPA) and docasahexaenoic acid (DHA)-enriched intravenous (IV) fat emulsions for the neonate. (Abstract) Clin Res 1989; 37:209.
108. Haumont D, Richelle M, Dahlan W, Elwyn DH, Deckelbaum RJ, Carpentier YA. Four g/kg/day Intralipid (IL) increases plasma lipids less than 2 g of 10%. (Abstract) JPEN 1989; 13:5S.
109. Tashiro T, Sanada M, Mashima Y, Yamamori H. Lipoprotein metabolism during TPN with Intralipid 10% vs 20%. (Abstract) JPEN 1989; 13:7S.
110. Poole RL. Electrolyte and mineral requirements. In.: Kerner JA Jr, ed. Manual of pediatric parenteral nutrition. New York: John Wiley & Sons, 1983: 129.
111. Vileisis RA. Effect of phosphorus intake in total parenteral nutrition infusates in premature neonates. J Pediatr 1987; 110:586–590.
112. O'Brien D, Hammond KB. In: Kempe CH, Silver HK, O'Brien D, eds. Current pediatric diagnosis and treatment. Los Altos: Lange Medical, 1978: 1045.
113. Kovar I, Mayne P, Barltrop D. Plasma alkaline phosphatase activity: a screening test for rickets in preterm neonates. Lancet 1982; i:308–310.
114. Poole RL, Rupp CA, Kerner JA. Calcium and phosphorus in neonatal TPN solutions. JPEN 1983; 7:358–360.
115. Goldsmith MA, et al. Gluconate calcium therapy and neonatal hypercalciuria. Am J Dis Child 1981; 135:538.
116. Kimura S, Nose O, Seino Y. Effects of alternate and simultaneous administration of calcium and phosphorus on calcium metabolism in children receiving total nutrition. JPEN 1986; 10:513–516.
117. Fitzgerald KA, McKay MW. Calcium and phosphate solubility in neonatal parenteral nutrient solutions containing TrophAmine. Am J Hosp Pharm 1986; 43:88–93.
118. Fitzgerald KA, McKay MW. Calcium and phosphate solubility in neonatal parenteral nutrient solutions containing Aminosyn PF. Am J Hosp Pharm 1987; 44:1396–1400.
119. American Medical Association, Department of Foods and Nutrition. Multivitamin preparations for parenteral use: a statement by the Nutrition Advisory Group 1975. JPEN 1979; 3:258–265.
120. Greene HL, Hambidge KM, Schanler R, Tsang RT. Guidelines for the use of vitamins, trace elements, calcium, magnesium, and phosphorus in infants and children receiving total parenteral nutrition: report of the subcommittee on pediatric parenteral nutrient requirements from the committee on clinical practice issues of the American Society for Clinical Nutrition. Am J Clin Nutr 1988; 48:1324–1342.
121. Koo WK, Tsang RC, Succo PP, et al. Vitamin D requirements in infants receiving parenteral nutrition. JPEN 1987; 11:172–177.
122. Alade SL, Brown RE, Paquet A. Polysorbate 80 and E-ferol toxicity. Pediatrics 1986; 77:593–597.
123. MacDonald MG, Getson PR, Glasgow A, et al. Propylene glycol: increase of seizures in low birth weight infants. Pediatrics 1987; 79:622–625.
124. Shenai JP, Stahlman MT, Chytil F. Vitamin A delivery from parenteral alimentation solution. J Pediatr 1981; 99:661.
125. Ostrea EM, Greene CD, Balum JE. Decomposition of TPN solutions exposed to phototherapy. J Pediatr 1982; 100:669.
126. Chen MF, Boyce HW Jr, Triplett L. Stability of the B vitamins in mixed parenteral nutrition solutions. JPEN 1983; 7:462.
127. Gillis J, Jones G, Pencharz P. Delivery of vitamins A, D, and E in parenteral nutrition solutions. JPEN 1983; 7:11.
128. Kerner JA Jr, Poole Rl, Sunshine P, et al. High serum vitamin E levels in premature infants receiving MVI® -Pediatric. J Pediatr Perinat Nutr 1987; 1:75.
129. Johnson L, Bowen FW, Abbasi S, et al. Relationship of prolonged pharmacologic serum levels of vitamin E to incidence of sepsis and necrotizing enterocolitis in infants with birth weight 1,500 grams or less. Pediatrics 1985; 75:619–638.
130. Phillips B, Franck LS, Greene HL. Vitamin E levels in premature infants during and after intravenous multivitamin supplementation. Pediatrics 1987; 80:680–683.
131. Poland RL. Vitamin E: what should we do? Pediatrics 1986; 77:787–788.
132. Baeckert PA, Greene HL, Fritz I, Oelberg DG, Adcock EW. Vitamin concentrations in very low birth weight infants given vitamins intravenously in a lipid emulsion: measurement of vitamins A, D, and E and riboflavin. J Pediatr 1988; 113:1057–1065.
132a. Spalding KA, D'Harlingue A, Cheng S, et al. Fifty percent of a vial of MVI-Pediatric is sufficient to maintain accepted serum vitamin E levels in infants of $\leq$1000 g. (Abstract) JPEN 1990; 14:115.
133. Greene HL, Phillips BL, Franck L, Fillmore CM, Said HM, Murrell BS, Courtney-Moore ME, Briggs R. Persistently low blood retinol levels during and after parenteral feeding of very low birth weight

infants—examination of losses into IV administration sets and a method of prevention by addition to a lipid emulsion. Pediatrics 1987; 79:894–900.

134. Hustead VA, Gutcher GR, Anderson SA, et al. Relationship of vitamin A (retinol) status to lung disease in the preterm infant. J Pediatr 1984; 105:610–615.

135. Shenai JP, Chytil F, Stahlman MT. Vitamin A status of neonates with bronchopulmonary dysplasia. Pediatr Res 1985; 19:185–187.

136. Shenai JP, Kennedy KA, Chytil F, Stahlman MT. Clinical trial of vitamin A supplementation in infants susceptible to broncho-pulmonary dysplasia. J Pediatr 1987; 111:269–277.

137. Schepers GP, Dimitry AR, Eckhauser FE, Kirking DM. Efficacy and safety of low-dose intravenous versus intramuscular vitamin K in parenteral nutrition patients. JPEN 1988; 12: 174–177.

138. La Selve P, Demolin P, Holzapfel L, Blanc PL, Teyssier G, Robert D. Soshin beriberi: an unusual complication of prolonged parenteral nutrition. JPEN 1986; 10:102–103.

139. Fritz I, Said H, Harris C, Murrell J, Greene HL. A new sensitive assay for plasma riboflavin using high performance liquid chromatography. (Abstract) J Am Coll Nutr 1987; 6:449.

140. Brown MC, Roe DA. Role of riboflavin in drug-induced photohemolysis. (Abstract) Clin Res 1988; 36:755.

141. Greene HL, Baekert PA, Murrell J, Oelburg DG, Adock EW III. Blood pyridoxine levels in preterm infants receiving TPN. JPEN; in press.

142. Greene H, Smith R, Murrell BS, Powers J, Baeckert P. HPLC measurement of pyridoxine vitamers in infants receiving total parenteral nutrition. (TPN) (Abstract). JPEN 1989; 13:5S.

143. Mock DM, DeLorimer AA, Liebman WM, Sweetman L, Baker H. Biotin deficiency: an unusual complication of parenteral alimentation. N Engl J Med 1981; 304:820–823.

144. Moore MC, Greene HL, Phillips B, et al. Evaluation of a pediatric multiple vitamin preparation for total parenteral nutrition in infants and children, I. Blood levels of water-soluble vitamins. Pediatrics 1986; 77:530–538.

145. Marinier E, Gorski AM, Potier de Courcy G, et al. Blood levels of water soluble vitamins in pediatric patients on total parenteral nutrition using a multivitamin preparation. JPEN 1989; 13:176–184.

146. Shils ME, Burke AW, Greene HL, Jeejeebhoy KN, Prasad AS, Sandstead HH. Guidelines for essential trace element preparations for parenteral use. JAMA 1979; 241:2051–2054.

147. Wolman SL, Anderson GH, Marliss EB, Jeejeebhoy KN. Zinc in total parenteral nutrition: requirements and metabolic effects. Gastroenterology 1979; 76:458–467.

148. Ruz M, Solomons N. Fecal zinc excretion during oral rehydration therapy for acute infectious diarrhea. (Abstract) Fed Proc 1987; 46:748.

149. Keshan Disease Research Group, Chinese Academy of Medical Sciences, Beijing. Observations on effect of sodium selenite in prevention of Keshan disease. Chin Med J 1979; 92:471–476.

150. Johnson RA, Baker SS, Falton JT, et al. An occidental case of cardiomyopathy and selenium deficiency. N Engl J Med 1981; 304:1210–1212.

151. Fleming RC, Lie JT, McCall TJ, et al. Selenium deficiency and fatal cardiomyopathy in a patient on home parenteral nutrition. Gastroenterology 1982; 83:689–693.

152. Quercia RA, Korn S, O'Neill D, et al. Selenium deficiency and fatal cardiomyopathy in a patient receiving long-term home parenteral nutrition. Clin Pharmacol 1984; 3:531–535.

153. Kien CL, Ganther HE. Manifestations of chronic selenium deficiency in a child receiving total parenteral nutrition. Am J Clin Nutr 1983; 37:319–328.

154. Vinton NE, Dahlstrom KA, Strobel CT, Ament ME. Macrocytosis and pseudoalbinism: manifestations of selenium deficiency. J Pediatr 1987; 111:711–717.

155. Kelly DA, Coe AW, Shenkin A, Lake BD, Walker-Smith JA. Symptomatic selenium deficiency in a child on home parenteral nutrition. J Pediatr Gastroenterol Nutr 1988; 7:783–786.

156. Levander OA, Burk RF. Report on the 1986 ASPEN Research Workshop on Selenium in Clinical Nutrition. JPEN 1986; 10:545–549.

157. Abumrad NN, Schneider AJ, Steel D, Rogers LS. Amino acid intolerance during prolonged total parenteral nutrition reversed by molybdate therapy. Am J Clin Nutr 1981; 34:2551–2559.

158. Abumrad NN. Molybdenum—is it an essential trace metal? Bull NY Acad Med 1984; 60:163–171.

159. Wan KK, Tsallas G. Dilute iron dextran formulation for addition to parenteral nutrient solutions. Am J Hosp Pharm 1980; 37:206–210.

160. Porter KA, Blackburn GL, Bistrian BR. Safety of iron dextran in total parenteral nutrition: a case report. J Am Coll Nutr 1988; 7:107–110.

161. Koo WW, Kaplan LA. Aluminum and bone disorders: with specific reference to contamination of infant nutrients. J Am Coll Nutr 1988; 7:199–214.

162. Ziegler M, Jakobowski D, Hoelzer D, et al. Route of pediatric parenteral nutrition: proposed criteria revision. J Pediatr Surg 1980; 15:472.

163. Rubenstein R, Michalak J, Stegman R, et al. Hickman catheter insertion via the percutaneous subclavian route. Nutr Support Serv 1982; 2:9.

164. Pollack PF, Kaddan M, Byrne WG, et al. 100 patient years' experience with the Broviac silastic catheter for central venous nutrition. JPEN 1981; 5:34.

165. Jewett TC Jr. Techniques with catheters and complications of total parenteral nutrition. In: Lebenthal E, ed. Total parenteral nutrition: indications, utilization, complications, and pathophysiological considerations. New York: Raven Press, 1986: 185.

166. Grant JP. Catheter access. In: Rombeau JL, Caldwell MD, eds. Parenteral nutrition. (Clinical nutrition, vol 2) Philadelphia: WB Saunders, 1986: 306.

167. Agarwal KC, Khan MAA, Falla A, Amato JJ. Cardiac perforation from central venous catheters: survival after cardiac tamponade in an infant. Pediatrics 1984; 73:333–338.

168. Collier PE, Ryan JJ, Diamond DL. Cardiac tamponade from central venous catheters—report of a case and review of the English literature. Angiology 1984; September 595–600.

169. Leibovitz E, Ashkenazi A, Levin S, Nissim F. Fatal cardiac tamponade complicating total parenteral nutrition via a silastic central vein catheter. (Letter) J Pediatr Gastroenterol Nutr 1988; 7:306–307.

170. Morrow AI, Poirier-Kerner L, Andolina AS, Walsh ME. Nursing care of the pediatric patient on parenteral nutrition. In: Kerner JA Jr, ed. Manual of pediatric parenteral nutrition. New York: John Wiley & Sons, 1983: 239.

171. Forlaw L, Torosian MH. Central venous catheter care. In: Rombeau JL, Caldwell MD, eds. Parenteral nutrition. (Clinical nutrition, vol 2) Philadelphia: WB Saunders, 1986: 306.

172. Maki DG. Nosocomial bacteria. An epidemiologic overview. Am J Med 1981; 70:179.

173. Yokoyama S, Fujimoto T, Tajima T, Mitomi T, Yabe H, Kato S. Use of Broviac/Hickman catheter for long-term venous access in pediatric cancer patients. Jpn J Clin Oncol 1988; 18:143–148.

174. Warner BW, Gorgone P, Schilling S, Farrell M, Ghory MJ. Multiple purpose central venous access in infants less than 1,000 grams. J Pediatr Surg 1987; 22:9.

175. Sadig HF. Broviac catheterization in low birth weight infants. Incidence and treatment of associated complications. Crit Care Med 1987; 15:47–50.

176. Weese JL, Trigg ME. Triple lumen venous access for pediatric bone marrow transplantation candidates. J Surg Oncol 1987; 36:55–57.

177. Superina RA, Wesson DE, Bahoric A, Filler RM. Evaluation of a new catheter for total parenteral nutrition. J Pediatr Gastroenterol Nutr 1988; 7:657–661.

178. Higgs SC, Malan AF, Heese H DeV, et al. A comparison of oral feeding and total parenteral nutrition in infants of very low birthweight. S Afr Med J 1974; 48:2169.

179. Hall RT, Rhodes PG. Total parenteral alimentation via indwelling umbilical catheters in the newborn period. Arch Dis Child 1976; 51: 929–934.

180. Merritt RJ. Neonatal nutritional support. Clin Consul Nutr Support 1981; 1:10.

181. Coran AG. Parenteral nutritional support of the neonate. Tele Session (a group telephone workshop) New York: Tele Session Corporation, August 17, 1981.

182. Kerner JA. The use of umbilical catheters for parenteral nutrition. In: Kerner JA, ed. Manual of pediatric parenteral nutrition. New York: John Wiley and Sons, 1983: 303.

183. Hattner JAT, Kerner JA Jr. Nutritional assessment of the pediatric patient. In: Kerner JA Jr, ed. Manual of pediatric parenteral nutrition. New York: John Wiley and Sons, 1983; 19.

184. Ney D. Nutritional assessment. In: Kelts DG, Jones RD, eds. Manual of pediatric nutrition. Boston: Little, Brown, 1984: 99.

185. Walker WA, Hendricks K. Manual of pediatric nutrition. Philadelphia: WB Saunders, 1985.
186. Merritt RJ, Blackburn GL. Nutritional assessment and metabolic response to illness of the hospitalized child. In: Suskind RM, ed. Textbook of pediatric nutrition. New York: Raven Press, 1981: 285.
187. Vaucher YE, Harrison, GG, Udal JN, et al. Skinfold thickness in North American infants 24–41 weeks gestation. Hum Biol 1984; 56:713.
188. Sasanow SR, Georgieff MK, Pereira GR. Mid-arm circumference and mid-arm/head circumference ratios: standard curves for anthropometric assessment of neonatal status. J Pediatr 1986; 109:311.
189. Georgieff MK, Sasanow SR, Mammel MC, et al. Mid-arm circumference/head circumference ratios for identification of symptomatic LGA, AGA, and SGA newborn infants. J Pediatr 1986; 109:316.
190. MacKenzie N. TPN PGM: A computer program to help provide PN in pediatric patients. In: Kerner JA Jr, ed. Manual of pediatric parenteral nutrition. New York: John Wiley and Sons, 1983; 345.
191. Poole RL. Writing parenteral nutrition orders. In: Kerner JA Jr, ed. Manual of pediatric parenteral nutrition. New York: John Wiley & Sons, 1983: 233.
192. Faubion WC, Baker WL, Iotl BA, et al. Cyclic TPN for hospitalized pediatric patients. Nutr Supp Serv 1981; 1:24.
193. Kerner JA Jr. Cyclic TPN for hospitalized pediatric patients. In: Kerner JA Jr, ed. Manual of pediatric parenteral nutrition. New York: John Wiley & Sons, 1983: 307.
194. Williamson RCN. Intestinal adaptation. N Engl J Med 1978; 298:1444.
195. Hughes CA, Prince A, Dowling RH. Speed of change in pancreatic mass and in intestinal bacteriology of parenterally fed rats. Clinical Science 1980; 59:329–336.
196. Heird WC. Effects of total parenteral alimentation on intestinal function. In: Gastrointestinal function and neonatal nutrition. Columbus, OH: Ross Laboratories, 1977.
197. Levine GM, Deven JJ, Steiger E, Zinno R. Role of oral intake on maintenance of gut mass and disaccharidase activity. Gastroenterology 1974; 67:975.
198. Eastwood GL. Small bowel morphology and epithelial proliferation in intravenously alimented rabbits. Surgery 1977; 82:613.
199. Feldman EJ, Dowling RH, McNaughton J, Peters TJ. Effects of oral versus intravenous nutrition in intestinal adaptation after small bowel resection in the dog. Gastroenterology 1976; 70:712.
200. Johnson LR, Copeland, EM, Dudrick ST, Lichtenberger LM, Castro GA. Structural and hormonal alterations in the gastrointestinal tract of parenterally fed rats. Gastroenterology 1975; 68:1177.
201. Greene HL, McCabe DR, Merenstein GB. Protracted diarrhea and malnutrition in infancy: changes in intestinal morphology and disaccharidase activities during treatment with total intravenous nutrition or oral elemental diets. J Pediatr 1975; 87:695.
202. Feng JJ, Kwong LK, Kerner JA, et al. Resumption of intestinal maturation upon reintroduction of intraluminal nutrients: functional and biochemical correlations. (Abstract) Clin Res 1987; 35:228A.
203. Mehta NR, Liao TH, Hamosh M, Smith YF, Hamosh P. The effect of total parenteral nutrition on lipase activity in the stomach of very low birth weight infants. Biol Neonate 1988; 53:261–266.
204. deAngelis GL, Poitevin C, Cezard JP, Vatier J, Foucaud P, Navarro J. Gastric pepsin and acid secretion during total parenteral nutrition and constant-rate enteral nutrition in infancy. JPEN 1988; 12:505–508.
205. Braunschweig CL, Wesley JR, Mercer N. Rationale and guidelines for parenteral and enteral transition feeding of the 3 to 30 kg child. J Am Diet Assoc 1988; 88:479–482.
206. Wagman LD, Miller KB, Thomas RB, Newsome HH, Weir GC. The effect of acute discontinuation of total parenteral nutrition. Ann Surg 1986; 204:524–529.
207. Geertama MA, Hyams JS, Pelletier JM, Reiter S. Feeding resistance after parenteral hyperalimentation. Am J Dis Child 1985; 139:255–256.
208. Poole RL, Kerner JA Jr. The nutrition support team. In: Kerner JA Jr, ed. Manual of pediatric parenteral nutrition. New York: John Wiley & Sons, 1983: 281.
209. Nehme AL. Nutritional support of the hospitalized patient. The team concept. JAMA 1980; 243:1906–1908.
210. Kerner JA Jr. Technical complications. In: Kerner JA Jr, ed. Manual of pediatric parenteral nutrition. New York: John Wiley & Sons, 1983: 193.
211. Grant JP. Administration of parenteral nutrition solutions. In: Grant JP, ed. Handbook of total parenteral nutrition. Philadelphia: WB Saunders, 1980: 103.
212. Bailey MJ. Reduction of catheter-associated sepsis in parenteral nutrition using low-dose intravenous heparin. Br Med J 1979; 1:1671–1673.
213. Gustafson A, Kjellmer I, Olegard R, et al. Nutrition in low birth weight infants. II. Repeated intravenous injections of fat emulsion. Acta Paediatr Scand 1974; 63:177.
214. Zaiden H, Dhanireddy R, Hamosh M, et al. Effect of continuous heparin administration of Intralipid® clearing in very low-birth-weight infants. J Pediatr 1982; 101:599–602.
215. Berkow SE, Spear ML, Stahl GE, Gutman A, Polin RA, Pereria GR, Olivecrona T, Hamosh P, Hamosh M. Total parenteral nutrition with Intralipid in premature infants receiving TPN with heparin: effect on plasma lipolytic enzymes, lipids, and glucose. J Pediatr Gastroenterol Nutr 1987; 6:581–588.
216. Merritt RJ, Mason W. Catheter associated infections—1988. Nutrition 1988; 4:247–250.
217. Flynn P, Shenep J, Stokes D, et al. In situ management of confirmed central venous catheter-related bacteremia. Pediatr Infect Dis 1987; 6:729.
218. Schropp KP, Ginn-Pease ME, King DR. Catheter-related sepsis: a review of the experience with Broviac and Hickman catheters. Nutrition 1988; 4:195–200.
219. Nahata MC, King DR, Powell DA, Marx SM, Ginn-Pease ME. Management of catheter related infections in pediatric patients. JPEN 1988; 12:58–59.
220. Wang EEL, Prober CG, Ford-Jones L, Gold R. The management of central intravenous catheter infections. Pediatr Infect Dis 1984; 3:110–113.
221. Jacobs, D, Evans DA, O'Dwyer ST, et al. Trophic effects of glutamine enriched parenteral nutrition on colonic mucosa. (Abstract) JPEN 1988; 12:6S.
222. Wilson CM, Merritt RJ, Thomas DW. Successful treatment of superior vena cava syndrome with urokinase in an infant. JPEN 1988; 12:81–83.
223. Glynn MFX, Langer B, Jeejeebhoy KN. Therapy for thrombotic occlusion of the long-term intravenous alimentation catheters. JPEN 1980; 4:387.
224. Winthrop AL, Wesson DE. Urokinase in the treatment of occluded central venous catheters in children. J Pediatr Surg 1984; 19:536–538.
225. Breaux CW Jr, Duke D, Georgeson KE, Mestre JR. Calcium phosphate crystal occlusion of central venous catheters used for total parenteral nutrition in infants and children: prevention and treatment. J Pediatr Surg 1987; 22:829–832.
226. Schreiner RL, Glick MR, Nordschow CD, Gresham EL. An evaluation of methods to monitor infants receiving intravenous lipids. J Pediatr 1979; 94:197–200.
227. Bryan H, Shennan A, Griffin E, Angel A. Intralipid® —its rational use in parenteral nutrition of the newborn. Pediatrics 1976; 58:787–790.
228. Filler RM, Takada Y, Carreras T, Heim T. Serum Intralipid® levels in neonates during parenteral nutrition: the relation to gestational age. J Pediatr Surg 1980; 15:405–410.
229. Forget PP, Fernandes J, Begemann PH. Utilization of fat emulsion during total parenteral nutrition in children. Acta Paediatr Scand 1975; 64:377–384.
230. D'Harlingue AD, Hopper AO, Stevenson DK, Shahin SM, Kerner JA. Limited value of nephelometry in monitoring the administration of intravenous fat in neonates. JPEN 1983 7:55–58.
231. Pereira GR, Fox WW, Stanley CA, Baker L, Schwartz JG. Decreased oxygenation and hyperlipemia during intravenous fat infusions in premature infants. Pediatrics 1980; 66:26–30.
232. Sun SC, Ventura C, Verasestakul S. Effect of Intralipid® -induced lipemia on the arterial oxygen tension in preterm infants. Resuscitation 1978; 6:265–270.
233. McKeen CR, Brigham KL, Bowers RE. Pulmonary vascular effects of fat emulsion infusion in unanesthetized sheep. J Clin Invest 1978; 61:1291–1297
234. Teague WG, Braun D. Goldberg RB, Bland RD. Intravenous lipid infusion increases lung fluid filtration in lambs. (Abstract) Pediatr Res 1984; 18:313.
235. Barson AJ, Chiswick ML, Doig MC. Fat embolism in infancy after intravenous fat infusions. Arch Dis Child 1978; 53:218–223.
236. Hertel J. Tystrup I, Andersen GE. Intravascular fat accumulation after Intralipid® infusion in the very low-birth-weight infant. J. Pediatr 1982; 100:975–976.
237. Shroeder H, Paust H, Schmidt R. Pulmonary fat embolism after Intralipid® therapy—a post-mortem artifact? Acta Paediatr Scand

1984; 73:461–464.

238. Shulman RJ, Langston C, Schanler RJ. Pulmonary vascular lipid deposition after administration of intravenous fat to infants. Pediatrics 1987; 79:99–102.

239. Hageman J, McCulloch K, Gora P, Olsen E, Pachman L, Hunt C. Intralipid® alterations in pulmonary prostaglandin metabolism and gas exchange. Crit Care Med 1983; 11:794–798.

240. Brans YW, Dutton EB, Andrew DS, et al. Fat emulsion tolerance in very low birth weight neonates: effect on diffusion of oxygen in the lungs and on blood pH. Pediatrics 1986; 78:79–84.

241. Hammerman C. Aramburo MJ. Decreased lipid intake reduces morbidity in sick premature neonates. J Pediatr 1988; 113:1083–1088.

242. Thaler MM, Pelger A. Influence of intravenous nutrients on bilirubin transport. III. Emulsified fat infusion. Pediatr Res 1977; 11:171–174.

243. Thaler MM, Wennberg RP. Influence of intravenous nutrients on bilirubin transport. II. Emulsified lipid solutions. Pediatr Res 1977; 11:167–171.

244. Andrew G, Chan G, Schiff D. Lipid metabolism in the neonate. II. The effect of Intralipid® on bilirubin binding *in vitro* and *in vivo*. J Pediatr 1976; 88:279–284.

245. Kerner JA Jr, Cassani C, Hurwitz R, Berde CB. Monitoring intravenous fat emulsions in neonates with the fatty acid/serum albumin molar ratio. JPEN 1981; 5:517–518.

246. Kao LC, Chen MH, Warburton D. Triglycerides, free fatty acids, free fatty acids/albumin molar ratio, and cholesterol levels in serum of neonates receiving long-term lipid infusions: controlled trial of continuous and intermittent regimens. J Pediatr 1984; 104:429–435.

247. Spear ML, Stahl GE, Paul MH, et al. The effect of fifteen hour fat infusions of varying dosage on bilirubin binding to albumin. JPEN 1985; 9:144–147.

248. American Academy of Pediatrics, Committee on Nutrition. Use of intravenous fat emulsions in pediatric patients. Pediatrics 1981; 68:738.

249. Park W, Paust H, Schroder H. Lipid infusion in premature infants suffering from sepsis. JPEN 1984; 8:290–292.

250. Dahlstrom KA, Goulet OJ, Roberts RL, Ricour C, Ament ME. Lipid tolerance in children receiving long-term parenteral nutrition: a biochemical and immunologic study. J Pediatr 1988; 113:985–990.

251. Cohen IT, Dahms B, Hays DM. Peripheral total parenteral nutrition employing a lipid emulsion (Intralipid®): complications encountered in pediatric patients. J Pediatr Surg 1977; 12:837.

252. Stern ST, Christensen RD. Intralipid® and thrombocytopenia in ill neonates. (Abstract) Clin Res 1985; 33:134.

253. Goulet O, Girot R, Maier-Redelsperger M, Bougle D, Virelizier JL, Ricour C. Hematologic disorders following prolonged use of intravenous fat emulsions in children. JPEN 1986 10:284.

254. Ritthamel-Weinstein MR, Haugen K. Hypertriglyceridemia in an infant with bronchopulmonary dysplasia. Nutr Clin Pract 1987; 2:112–116.

255. Greer FR, McCormick A, Kashyap ML, Glueck EJ. Late hypertriglyceridemia in very low birth weight infants fed human milk exclusively. J Pediatr 1987; 111:466–469.

256. Wareham JA, Ferlauto JJ, Wells DH, Newell RW. Hypertriglyceridemia in infants with bronchopulmonary dysplasia. J Pediatr 1989; 114:458–460.

257. Johnson JD, Albritton WL, Sunshine P. Hyperammonemia accompanying parenteral nutrition in newborn infants. J Pediatr 1972; 81:154–161.

258. Kelts D, Jones E. Selected topics in therapeutic nutrition. Curr Prob Pediatr 1983; 12:24–45.

259. Thomas DW, Sinatra FR, Hack SL, Smith TM, Platzker ACG, Merritt RJ. Hyperammonemia in neonates receiving intravenous nutrition. JPEN 1982; 6:503–506.

260. Greer FR, Steichen JJ, Tsang RC. Effects of increased calcium, phosphorus, and vitamin D intake on bone mineralization in very-low-birth-weight infants fed formulas with Polycose and medium-chain triglycerides. J Pediatr 1982; 100:951–955.

261. Geggel RL, Pereira GR, Spackman TJ. Fractured ribs: unusual presentation of rickets in premature infants. J Pediatr 1978; 93:680–682.

262. Tsang RC. The quandry of vitamin D in the newborn infant. Lancet 1983; i:1370-1372.

263. Peden VH, Witzleben DL, Skelton MA. Total parenteral nutrition. J Pediatr 1971; 78:180–181.

264. Sinatra FR. Cholestasis in infancy and childhood. Curr Prob Pediatr 1982; 12:6–54.

265. Sax HC, Bower BH. Hepatic complications of total parenteral nutrition. JPEN 1988 12:615–618.

266. Thaler MM. Liver dysfunction and disease associated with total parenteral alimentation. In: ASPEN 6th Clinical Congress. San Francisco: American Society for Parenteral and Enteral Nutrition, 1982: 67.

267. Marino L. Hack M, Dahms B. Two year follow-up: growth and neonatal PN-associated liver disease. JPEN 1981; 5:569.

268. Kibort PM, Ulich TR, Berquist WE, Lewin KJ, Ament ME. Hepatic fibrosis and cirrhosis in children on long-term parenteral nutrition. (Abstract) Clin Res 1982; 30:115.

269. Hodes JE, Grosfeld JL, Weber TR, Schreiner RI, Fitzgerald JF, Mirkin LD. Hepatic failure in infants on total parenteral nutrition (TPN): clinical and histopathologic observations. J Pediatr Surg 1982; 17:463–468.

269a. Suita S, Ikeda K, Nagasaki A, Hayashida Y, Kaneko T, Hamano Y, Nakata M, Fung KC. Follow-up studies of the children treated with long-term intravenous nutrition (IVN) during the neonatal period. J Pediatr Surg 1982;17:37–42.

270. Benjamin DR. Cholelithiasis in infants: the role of total parenteral nutrition and gastrointestinal dysfunction J. Pediatr Surg 1982; 17:386–389.

271. Boyle RJ, Sumner TE, Volberg FM. Cholelithiasis in a 3-week-old small premature infant. Pediatrics 1983; 71:967–969.

272. Callahan J, Haller JO, Caccirelli AA, Slovis TL, Friedman AP. Cholelithiasis in infants: association with total parenteral nutrition and furosemide. Radiology 1982; 143:437–439.

273. Holzbach RT. Gallbladder stasis: consequence of long-term parenteral hyperalimentation and risk factor for cholelithiasis. Gastroenterology 1983; 84:1055–1058.

274. Messing B. Bories C, Kunstlinger F, Bernier JJ. Does total parenteral nutrition induce gallbladder sludge formation and lithiasis? Gastroenterology 1983; 84:1012–1019.

275. Roslyn JJ, Pitt HA, Mann LL, Ament ME, DenBesten L. Gallbladder disease in patients on long-term parenteral nutrition. Gastroenterology 1983; 84:148–154.

276. Roslyn JJ, Berquist WE, Pitt HA, Mann LL, Kangarloo H, DenBesten L, Ament ME. Increased risk of gallstones in children receiving total parenteral nutrition. Pediatrics 1983; 71:784–789.

277. Whitington PF, Black DD. Cholelithiasis in premature infants treated with parenteral nutrition and furosemide. J Pediatr 1980; 97:647–649.

278. King DR, Ginn-Pease ME, Lloyd TV, Hoffman J, Hohenbrink K. Parenteral nutrition with associated cholelithiasis: another iatrogenic disease of infants and children. J Pediatr Surg 1987 22:593–596.

279. Kerner JA Jr. Monitoring of pediatric parenteral nutrition in the hospital and at home. In: Lebenthal E, ed. Total parenteral nutrition: indications, utilization, complications, and pathophysiological considerations. New York: Raven Press, 1986: 231.

280. Walsh ME. Psychosocial aspects of pediatric parenteral nutrition. In: Kerner JA Jr, ed. Manual of pediatric parenteral nutrition. New York: John Wiley & Sons, 1983: 271.

281. Berry RK, Jorgensen S. Growing with home parenteral nutrition: adjusting to family life and child development. Pediatr Nurs 1988; 14:43–45.

282. O'Conner MJ, Ralston CW, Ament ME. Intellectual and perceptual-motor performance of children receiving prolonged home total parenteral nutrition. Pediatrics 1988; 81:231–236.

283. Laine L, Shulman RJ, Bartholomew K, Gardner P, Reed T, Cole S. An educational booklet diminishes anxiety in parents whose children receive total parenteral nutrition. Am J Dis Child 1989; 143:374–377.

284. Burke WA. A pragmatic approach to interrupting TPN therapy for drug administration. Nutr Supp Serv April 1985; 45–46.

285. Robinson LA, Burch KJ. Using a central line for both TPN and drug infusion. Nutr Supp Serv April 1985; 46–47.

286. Kerner JA Jr, ed. Manual of pediatric parenteral nutrition. New York: John Wiley & Sons, 1983.

287. Foster GD, Knox LS, Dempsey DT, Mullen JL. Caloric requirements for total parenteral nutrition. J Am Coll Nutr 1987; 6:231–253.

288. American Society for Parenteral and Enteral Nutrition. Standards for nutrition support—hospitalized pediatric patients. Nutr Clin Pract 1989; 4:33–37.

289. Wenner WJ Jr, Kerner JA Jr. The addition of amino acids to the peritoneal dialysate in acute renal failure. J Perinatol 1986; 6:342–343.

290. Merritt RJ, Atkinson JB, Whalen TV, Thomas DW, Sinatra FR, Roloson GI. Partial peritoneal alimentation in an infant. JPEN 1988; 12:621–625.

PART 8

Home Total Parenteral Nutrition

Marvin E. Ament, M.D.

Home total parenteral nutrition (HTPN) is a technique for providing all the body's nutritional needs through a central venous catheter at home. The technique was first described by Dr. Belding Scribner of the University of Washington in 1970.[1] Scribner referred to HTPN by the name "the artificial gut." The first patients he put on this system had Crohn's disease with short bowel syndrome or diffuse small bowel disease. Other early pioneers in the development and modification of this technique, in both children and adults, were Dr. Jeejeebhoy in Toronto, Dr. Steiger of the Cleveland Clinic, Dr. Salassol in France, Dr. Fleming in Rochester, Dr. Shils in New York City, and ourselves in Los Angeles.[1-6]

The first to place pediatric patients on HTPN were Drs. Scribner, Broviac, and Ament in 1971. One patient was a 9-year-old girl with diffuse mast cell disease in whom the intestinal lining was replaced with a flat intestinal mucosa with poor absorption and increased secretion; the other was a 3-year-old boy with end stage acrodermatitis enteropathica. Both patients received HTPN for up to 3 years before they died of complications of their basic illnesses.

The reason for developing techniques of intravenous nutritional support at home was that some patients were being kept hospitalized solely to receive intravenous fluid and nutrients—protein, carbohydrate, fat, vitamins, minerals, and trace elements—thus preventing them from normalizing their lives.

Over the past two decades, HTPN has been greatly expanded and has come to be accepted as a useful supportive and therapeutic technique for a variety of gastrointestinal (GI) diseases and conditions. In the United States, more than 3,000 patients are reported to be on HTPN, and of this group, between 10 and 20 percent are infants and children less than 18 years of age.

INDICATIONS FOR HOME TOTAL PARENTERAL NUTRITION

HTPN is indicated for any patient whose only reason for remaining in the hospital is to receive parenteral support and who does not require nursing support beyond the capability of the family members. We believe that a patient should require a minimum of 30 days of parenteral support at home to justify the time and expense involved in training the family members and establishing the program.

The most common indications for HTPN in children are listed in Table 1 and are documented by many investigators.[7-18] In some patients, the purpose of the TPN is to provide nutrition while the infant gains weight and grows and while the short small intestine adapts to enteral support. In others, the length of time of support is indefinite because the intestine is too short, damage to the mucosal lining is irreversible, or, in the rarest instances, the villi fail to develop because of a congenital defect. Some patients require complete support, others partial support, and still others intermittent support.

Other indications occur among oncology patients, who typically need support for mucositis in graft-versus-host disease (GVHD), for idiopathic nausea, for anorexia, and for vomiting after or during chemotherapy and radiotherapy. Ménétrier's disease, intestinal lymphangiectasia, and idiopathic chylous ascites are three less commonly seen conditions in which HTPN may be useful to control the diarrhea, malabsorption, protein-losing enteropathy, and abdominal distention seen with those conditions. Recently, partial or complete HTPN or both have been utilized to improve the nutritional status of infants and children waiting for orthotopic liver transplantation. Recently we have supported children with AIDS at home because of intractable diarrhea and/or pancreatitis.

TABLE 1
Common Indications for Home Total Parenteral Nutrition in Children

Short bowel syndrome
- Secondary to jejunoileal atresia
- Secondary to necrotizing enterocolitis
- Secondary to midgut volvulus with strangulation
- Associated with gastroschisis
- Congenital short bowel
- Secondary to Crohn's disease

Intestinal motility disorders
- Chronic intestinal pseudo-obstructive syndromes (neuropathic, myopathic, unknown)
- Secondary to chemotherapy and radiation therapy

Intractable diarrhea
- Failure of enteral nutrition
  - Refractory sprue
  - Autoimmune mucosal disease
  - Crohn's disease
  - Intestinal lymphangiectasia
  - Hypoplastic villous syndrome
  - Secretory tumors, etiology unknown

Ascites
- Intractable chylous ascites

Other
- Cystic fibrosis
- Preorthotopic liver transplantation

Cancer-related
- After bone marrow transplantation—graft-versus-host disease
- Radiation damage to intestine with obstruction and/or diarrhea
- Diarrhea, anorexia, vomiting secondary to chemotherapy

Acquired immunodeficiency syndrome

CONTRAINDICATIONS TO HOME TOTAL PARENTERAL NUTRITION

There are no absolute contraindications to HTPN; however, it should not be utilized when there is no parent or family member dedicated to learning and performing the daily techniques for a successful program or when the parent(s) or other family members do not have sufficient intelligence to learn.

SITE OF VENOUS ACCESS

The intravenous site most commonly used to gain access to the superior vena cava for TPN has been the infraclavicular subclavian vein.[19] This vein may be cannulated by either the supraclavicular or the infraclavicular approach. In either situation, the exit site is on the anterior chest wall. The main advantages of this location are (1) easy maintenance of a sterile dressing and (2) easy mobility of the patient. The internal jugular vein has also been used for access to the superior vena cava. Such catheters often exit from the neck on the anterior chest wall using a "tunneling" technique.[20] The brachiocephalic vein has also been used to place catheters into the superior vena cava. Catheterization of the femoral and saphenous veins has also been used. These catheters are threaded into the iliac veins and then to the vena cava.[21] Catheters placed through the femoral saphenous area are typically placed either below the renal veins or just below the diaphragm. In rare cases in which all venous access sites have been used, placement of a catheter through the azygos vein has been done and/or a thoracotomy with direct placement of the catheter in the superior vena cava has been utilized.[22] In our experience with children, azygos vein placement has been utilized only twice in 20 years and placement of the catheter by thoracotomy only once.

LONG-TERM VENOUS ACCESS DEVICES

Broviac and Hickman right atrial access* catheters have been utilized in all the sites mentioned, specifically for long-term venous access. These catheters, which are flexible and nonbrittle, carry a decreased risk of developing a thrombus.[23,24] They have a Dacron cuff placed at their midpoints, which allows the catheter to become adherent to the chest or the abdominal wall once implanted. The Dacron cuff serves as a foreign body, and the reaction around it makes it adherent. This process usually takes 7 to 14 days. The newer forms of these catheters have a temporary dissolvable cuff impregnated with silver salts (Vitacuff: Vitaphore Corporation, San Carlos, CA) that serves as a barrier to micro-organisms migrating up along the catheter from the site where it enters the subcutaneous tunnel. Such devices protect the catheter against infection until the Dacron cuff becomes adherent and the tissue around the catheter forms a seal along its course. An advantage of the Broviac and Hickman catheters is the Luer lock at their proximal end, which allows them to be capped off following use and filled with a heparin solution to prevent thrombosis. These catheters have been reported to last for weeks to as long as 15 years without requiring removal (personal observations).[21,23]

The Broviac catheter is made in sizes for both infants and children, whereas the Hickman catheter was meant for older children and adults. Early in this decade, Broviac and Hickman catheters with double lumens were developed for access to the right atrium.[25] These catheters provided two separate ports for entry into the right atrium for the purpose of allowing simultaneous administration of parenteral nutrition solutions and antibiotics or other fluids. Use of these catheters involved considerably more work for the nursing personnel in the hospital and for the patients and their families at home. Although triple lumen catheters have been developed for the adults on both an inpatient and outpatient basis, their use is highly limited.

A totally implantable venous and arterial access system was developed early in the 1980s for the treatment of cancer patients with chemotherapy. This device (Infuse-a-port: Intermedics Infusaid Corporation, Norwood, MA) consists of a silicone rubber catheter connected to a subcutaneously placed molded plastic injection port or reservoir. Venous access is gained through the subclavian vein and into the right atrium, using the silicone rubber catheter.[26] The catheter is attached to the reservoir, which is implanted subcutaneously and sutured to muscular fascia for stability. Entry into the venous system is achieved with the use of a specially deflected pointed Huber needle, used to prevent coring of the self-sealing subcutaneous reservoir. A similar device, called a Port-a-cath (Pharmacia Laboratories, Piscataway, NJ), has also been reported.

These systems have been used for the administration of drugs, blood products, and parenteral nutrition. Long-term daily use of these systems for parenteral nutrition is not as well established. Complications in using the implanted catheter systems can be categorized into five groups: (1) venous thrombosis (16 percent), (2) catheter migration (8 percent), (3) infection (9 percent), (4) extravasation (6 percent), and (5) withdrawal occlusion (14 percent).[27] These implanted catheters have been reported to be used for up to 5 months for a variety of purposes.[22] No study has compared the totally implanted catheter system with other types of implanted catheter systems in a prospective control, randomized fashion.

The tip of all catheters or access devices should be in the superior vena cava, just above its entrance to the right atrium or just below the diaphragm if inserted through the inferior vena cava to minimize risk of thrombosis and cardiac tamponade.

PREVENTION OF CATHETER-RELATED SEPSIS

Catheter Insertion and Care

Central venous catheters inserted and cared for using aseptic or clean technique have been shown to have acceptably low levels of infectious complications, although the level does vary among studies. A catheter insertion for parenteral nutri-

*A recent FDA task force suggested that "the catheter tip should not be placed in, or allowed to migrate into the heart."

tion is considered elective and should be performed under optimal conditions. Catheters should be inserted using an aseptic surgical procedure. Following placement of the catheter and on a daily or every-other-day basis, the site of the catheter insertion should be cleaned with 70 percent alcohol followed by a povidone-iodine surgical scrub and/or solution. The povidone-iodine, if used, should remain on the skin. The sustained release of free iodine from povidone-iodine seems to have an antibacterial effect.[27] Chlorhexidine, 0.5 percent in 75 percent isopropyl alcohol, has been promoted for use as a skin disinfectant.[29] For cleaning the skin, it should always be applied with a circular friction motion, progressing from the potential insertion site to peripheral and adjacent sites. Patients who are allergic to iodine can be prepped with either 70 percent alcohol solution for 5 minutes or chlorhexidine solution. Once the catheter has been placed, sutures may be used to prevent motion of the catheter in the cutaneous exit site and to prevent dislodgment. Sutures may be difficult to keep sterile on a long-term basis and may form an abscess very close to the catheter-skin junction. Sutures should be removed once a catheter has had an opportunity to become fixed in place. Before the catheter is dressed, a topical ointment is often applied to the catheter-skin junction. The use of ointment in parenteral nutrition catheter care is controversial. One study in which subjects were randomized to placebo ointment of a petroleum base versus antibiotic ointment containing polymixin B, zinc bacitracin, and erythromycin sulfate has been done[30] Interestingly, there seems to be no difference between the placebo group and the antibiotic ointment group. This suggests that antibiotic ointments need not be used once a catheter site is appropriately cleaned and that the most important factor is antiseptic skin preparation.

Solution Preparation and Delivery

Solutions used for TPN have been documented as supporting the growth of multiple organisms. Therefore, infected solutions may lead to contaminated catheters. To prevent contamination by a variety of pathogens, sterile preparation and administration of amino acid and dextrose solutions and intravenous fat emulsions must be observed. The solutions should be prepared in an aseptic fashion using laminar flow hoods with double filtration to prevent the passage of microorganisms and particulate matter into the solutions. It is unlikely that catheters will become contaminated from the solutions if they are prepared in this manner. To ensure patient safety, we believe that batches of solutions should be cultured and tested for pyrogens in a routine fashion before they are dispensed.

Fat emulsions are typically sterile but may become contaminated if they are allowed to hang for more than 24 hours.[32]

Use of In-Line Filters

The use of in-line filters in parenteral nutrition at home is controversial.[33] No studies show that in-line filters significantly reduce the incidence of catheter infection and sepsis in HTPN. Because of our personal experience with filters breaking and leaking, we have not used them for 1½ decades. If the solutions are double filtered at the time of manufacturing or compounding, it is unlikely that filters would be useful at the time the solutions are infused. Since at the present time there is no study supporting the usefulness of filters in patients receiving HTPN parenteral nutrition, we do not use them.

Dressing Changes—Frequency and Materials

Dressing materials and frequency of dressing changes in parenteral nutrition have been the subject of controversy since parenteral nutrition was first described. Studies indicate that when carefully thought out protocols are followed without variation, the rate of infection of central venous catheters for parenteral nutrition is acceptably low.[33] When violations in established protocols occur, infection rates increase dramatically. If the predominant infecting agents in central venous catheters used for parenteral nutrition are organisms commonly found on the skin, it could be argued that daily dressing changes would help to prevent catheter-related infection. Most protocols use dressing changes with traditional gauze and tape. Studies have been done that indicate there is a 3.5 percent incidence of positive skin cultures involved with daily dressing changes,[34] although they may be valuable in patients at high risk for septic complications. Other studies have been done comparing standard gauze and tape dressing with the use of the new semipermeable clear adhesive-backed membrane dressings. Such studies have shown a numerically higher sepsis rate in those using the semipermeable membrane dressing once weekly, but the difference is not statistically significant.[35] Studies have been done to compare effectiveness of the semipermeable dressing changes done on a weekly basis with that of every-other-day gauze and tape dressing changes. The results of these studies appear to show that the latter is as effective as the former.[36]

Catheter Intravenous Tubing Connection

There is no question that contamination of central venous catheters occurs inadvertently in patients on HTPN when the central line is either opened or disconnected from the intravenous tubing at the end of the infusion time. This is the time of greatest risk of catheter contamination.[37]

Subcutaneous Tunnels

There is no evidence of a difference in sepsis rate between those catheters inserted by the direct insertion technique and those which are tunneled. The prevention of TPN catheter sepsis is best achieved by strict adherence to an aseptic or clean nursing procedure. In the care of long-term catheters, as in the care of short-term catheters, an adherence to established protocol seems to be emerging as the determining factor in catheter-related sepsis.

MECHANICAL DAMAGE

Broviac and Hickman catheters may become damaged at their external segment from repeated clamping and unclamping of their male adaptor pieces. Sterile technique must be observed when repairing these catheters. Broken or disconnected catheters may be repaired utilizing catheter-specific repair kits available from each catheter manufacturer. New ends are spliced to the damaged catheter according to the manufacturer's directions.[38] Our experience indicates that catheters may be repaired three or four times without losing effectiveness. It is important that the total length of the catheter not be increased to avoid interference with handling the catheter and to allow for sufficient heparin and saline solution to flush the catheter.

TOTALLY IMPLANTABLE CATHETERS

Methods for caring for the totally implanted catheter have been described. The skin surface over the implanted hub is scrubbed with povidone-iodine solution. The self-sealing chamber is palpated with gloved fingers and injected with a special nonchlorine Huber needle using sterile technique. Infusions can be either continuous or intermittent. The self-sealing chamber is injected with a special nonchlorine right-angle needle using sterile technique and is secured with a clear plastic adhesive dressing after application of antibiotic ointment. The infusion set can then be attached to the needle. Because these devices are so new, few data exist concerning long-term use for patients receiving parenteral nutrition.

REMOVAL OF LONG-TERM CATHETERS

Removal of long-term catheters should be done by someone who is familiar with the procedure. Following the resection of the Dacron cuff holding the catheter in place by lysing adhesions around it, a firm and constant traction must be used for its removal. The most serious complications that can occur with removal of the catheter are related to retained catheter remnants. Catheters that become calcified and cannot be pulled out should be left in place, and not removed surgically under general anesthesia.

THROMBUS AND CATHETER OCCLUSION

Thrombosis is a complication of both short-term and long-term catheter use.[39] All catheters are foreign bodies within blood vessels, and they have the potential to form thrombus around the catheter, within the lumen of the vein. A number of factors have been identified as carrying risk of thrombosis in the great vein. These include volume depletion, any physical factor that hinders blood flow, any other thrombogenic stimuli (including infection), and any other hypercoagulable state. If the thrombus becomes seeded by bacteria or fungi, it may provide a constant source of infection to the bloodstream. It has been demonstrated that microemboli and pulmonary emboli may result from untreated great vein thrombosis.

CATHETER OCCLUSION

Heparin flushes have been used to prevent occlusion, and urokinase has been reported for clearing the occluded catheter.[40,41] Patency in long-term catheters is generally maintained with intermittent "flushes" of heparinized solution into the catheter. Protocols to maintain patency vary among institutions. Heparin concentrations ranging from 10 units per milliliter to 1,000 units per milliliter and volumes of flushed solution ranging from 1.5 to 10 ml used twice daily to once weekly have been reported.[24] Minimum requirements for heparin flush concentrations, volume, and frequency have not been established.

If a long-term central venous catheter does become occluded or gives indication of the infusion slowing, infusing 2.5 ml of urokinase, which is 2,500 IU per milliliter of saline, slowly into the occluded catheter should be done and the catheter capped off. The urokinase should be allowed to remain in place for 3 hours and then aspirated back. Twenty-five milliliters of flushing solution containing 100 U of heparin can then be used to clear the catheter. Seventy-seven percent of acutely occluded catheters may be restored to patency by injection of a fibrinolytic agent.[45] If the catheter cannot be filled because occlusion is complete, it must be removed. A continuous low-dose urokinase infusion is given over 24 to 30 hours for "clogged" catheter unresponsiveness. We have used this technique successfully.

CHARACTERISTICS OF DIFFERENT CATEGORIES OF PATIENTS ON HOME TOTAL PARENTERAL NUTRITION

Table 2 lists the initial diagnoses made at the time HTPN is started, based on the UCLA experience. Short bowel syndrome is still the most frequent condition associated with the

TABLE 2
Initial Diagnosis at Time of Starting Home Total Parenteral Nutrition Treatment (UCLA Experience)

Disorder	Number
Short bowel syndrome	
Intestinal atresia	8
Volvulus	8
Necrotizing enterocolitis	6
Congenital	3
Trauma (surgery)	4
Omphalocele	1
Gastroschisis	3
Exomphalos	1
Crohn's disease	20
Ulcerative colitis	2
Idiopathic intestinal pseudo-obstruction syndrome	10
Malignancy	
Lymphohistiocytosis	1
Acute lymphoblastic leukemia	1
Neuroblastoma	2
Leiomyosarcoma of stomach	1
Histiocytosis	1
Adenocarcinoma of esophagogastric junction	1
Rhabdomyosarcoma	1
Arrhenoblastoma	1
Lymphoma of stomach	1
Intractable diarrhea of infancy	15
Miscellaneous (including 3 with AIDS)	11

need for HTPN in infants and children.[8,11,18] It occurs because of either congenital intestinal atresias or malrotation volvulus with strangulation, or it can develop secondary to resection performed because of necrotizing enterocolitis (NEC). In recent years, because of increasing sophistication in the management of infants with prematurity and NEC, fewer of these infants are having massive intestinal resections resulting in serious short bowel syndromes. We have, therefore, seen a decline in the incidence of this condition. Only rare youngsters may have congenital short intestine.[42]

Crohn's disease in the pediatric age group rarely leads to multiple and massive intestinal resections; however, there is an occasional patient in whom this occurs. In addition, some patients have diffuse small bowel disease that is refractory to medical management although they are uncommon.[8,43,44] In recent years, because of increasing sophistication in the use of the medications for management of Crohn's disease, including corticosteroids, immunosuppressive agents such as 6-mercaptopurine, antibiotics such as metronidazole, and the newer anti-T-cell agent cyclosporine, fewer patients are proving to be refractory to medical management. It is hoped that this will reduce the number of pediatric patients who undergo major intestinal resections.

Chronic intestinal pseudo-obstruction syndrome is another condition in which HTPN has made the difference between life and death.[8,45,46] These chronic motility disorders can present in the neonatal period, during infancy, or later in childhood. Affected youngsters have either a defect in the intramural plexus of nerves or a degenerative or congenital defect in the development of their smooth muscles. Children with the congenital form of disease are often misdiagnosed as having total aganglionosis because they develope bilious vomiting and microcolon. Many are operated on two or three times before the condition is recognized. Typically, they are operated on for obstruction and are given an ileostomy to relieve the presumed obstruction, but the intestinal contents fail to be delivered through the ostomy. They often undergo a second operative procedure to explore for adhesions before the physician becomes aware of the lack of intestinal motility. Some children with this condition who require TPN do not become symptomatic until later in life. Rare infants with pseudo-obstruction at birth improve and on rare occasions ultimately do well without parenteral nutrition. We have seen two premature infants with all the classic features of pseudo-obstruction syndrome who by 6 months of age were eating normally. This is why it is imperative to support infants who have such syndromes until they can be fed enterally or by mouth. Rare infants develop intestinal obstruction secondary to prior intra-abdominal surgeries leading to intestinal resection.

Some youngsters develop intractable diarrhea in the first days of life. A major portion of these youngsters may have hypoplastic microvillous syndrome.[47] They have intestinal villi that fail to develop normally and have defective enterocyte and microvillous formation. These cases are rare, and most are familial. Most of these patients do not improve with the passage of time. Typically they have diarrhea from birth and have difficulty with even the simplest of nutrients. If a physician recognizes this type of condition shortly after birth, the youngster should have an upper GI and small bowel series as well as intestinal biopsies performed to confirm the diagnosis. This is one reason why such studies should be done for infants who develop diarrhea even with feeding of dextrose and electrolytes.

Occasional children who are exquisitely sensitive to milk and soy formula proteins develop massive diarrhea with intractable symptoms. Some require weeks to months for healing of the intestinal mucosa. Occasional patients may require long-term parenteral support at home. They typically are recognizable by the inflammatory changes seen in their small intestinal biopsies, by their usual family history for intestinal allergies and atopy, and by their septic condition at presentation.

In recent years, we have had an increasing number of youngsters with intra-abdominal malignancies who require HTPN because of damage to the intestine from radiotherapy and intra-abdominal operative procedures. In some, the need for parenteral nutrition is temporary; in others it is lifelong.[8] Others have obstruction to the intestinal tract and intra-abdominal and intra-intestinal malignancies. Some of these patients may benefit from chemotherapy. In such youngsters, parenteral support at home may allow them to survive while these therapies are attempted.

With the development of techniques for bone marrow transplantation, an increasing number of youngsters have developed GVHD.[48] The intestinal manifestations of this condition are fever, skin rash, mucositis, and diarrhea. Such patients often require weeks or months of parenteral support until the GVHD resolves. An increasing number are being sent home, since their only requirements are for fluid and nutritional support until the disease resolves.

Patients with immunodeficiency disorders of the combined type or those with selective IgA deficiency may require prolonged parenteral support because of intractable diarrhea. In some of these youngsters, a severe mucosal lesion develops for which no specific cause can be found. Such patients should be carefully evaluated for giardiasis, strongyloidiasis, cryptosporidiosis, cytomegalovirus, and chronic rotavirus excretion.[33] Many of these conditions are treatable and result in improved digestion and absorption, whereas there is no specific treatment for some. Occasionally HTPN is used in immunodeficient patients to support them until bone marrow transplantation becomes feasible. Children with AIDS have been supported with HTPN because of chronic pancreatitis and intractable abdominal pain as well as intractable diarrhea with no specific agent other than the AIDS virus or *Cryptosporidium* parasite. Management of such patients does not differ from management of those who do not have AIDS.

Cystic fibrosis is another condition in which placement of a Broviac catheter may be used to support nutrition as well as to provide home antibiotics.[48a] We have often wondered whether patients with cystic fibrosis should be started on parenteral support sooner rather than later in order to improve their condition before damage has occurred.

Intestinal lymphangiectasia is typically thought of as a condition that can be managed by dietary means. However, a substantial number of affected patients do not benefit from low-fat diets with medium-chain triglycerides. Their ascites persists, as do their diarrhea and malabsorption. Some of these patients may benefit from parenteral support on a long-term basis at home.[48b]

IMPLEMENTATION OF HOME TOTAL PARENTERAL NUTRITION

Preparing a Patient for Home Total Parenteral Nutrition

The physician who decides to place a pediatric patient on a HTPN program should discuss with the parents what can be accomplished by such a program. Both the benefits and the risks to the patients should be discussed. The duration of the HTPN should also be presented. Complications and the possibility of death from infection should be mentioned. If a patient has had an intestinal resection, the physician may indicate that the youngster may achieve intestinal adaptation if supported for a sufficient length of time. However, it is an established fact that a youngster who has infarction or atresia of the entire jejeunum and ileum may never adapt and will be on HTPN for the rest of his or her life. Ninety percent of children who have at least 25 cm of small intestine and an ileocecal valve eventually are able to discontinue parenteral support.[49] Those children who have an intact ileocecal valve and 15 to 20 cm of small bowel may ultimately adapt completely, but they may have only partial adaptation.[49,50] Children with pseudo-obstruction may not adapt at all or may have partial adaptation requiring parenteral support only a part of each week. For children with intractable diarrhea, the duration of time for the HTPN depends on the lesion responsible for the diarrhea. The physician must be as straightforward as possible in presenting this information to the parents. The potential for complications of TPN, including catheter infection and sepsis, thrombosis of the catheter, hypoglycemia from stopping the infusion too rapidly, bleeding from separation of the catheter from the intravenous tubing, and unknown and unforeseen metabolic complications, should be presented. Further, details describing how a child on HTPN may affect the whole family's life should be presented.

Establishing a Patient on a Home Total Parenteral Nutrition Program

After a decision has been made to place a patient on HTPN, the surgical consultant should place a Broviac or Hickman venous catheter in the external or internal jugular, femoral, saphenous, or subclavian vein. In female infants and children, the femoral saphenous vein placement may be used because of parents' concern about the cosmetic effect of placing a catheter on the anterior chest wall. Catheters placed in the lower extremities with an exit site on the abdominal wall do not necessarily have a greater risk of becoming infected.[21]

The size of the Broviac catheter used depends in part on the size of the child and the major vein as well as the purposes for which the central catheter will be used. A Hickman catheter is a larger version of the Broviac catheter and may be chosen if it is going to be used for administration of blood and blood products as well as to sample from it and give TPN.[23,24] A Hickman catheter can be used in a child of school age.[24] It has a greater internal as well as external diameter and is typically used for four purposes: (1) TPN, (2) administration of blood products, (3) taking blood samples, and (4) giving chemotherapy. The Broviac catheter is smaller than the Hickman and is designed specifically for infants and young children, as already discussed. The physician should be aware that there is an infant Broviac catheter as well as a standard Broviac catheter.[21] Both have screw caps and Luer locks. In addition, in school-age children, dual-lumen catheters may be used, especially for those who undergo chemotherapy as well as require parenteral support. However, the use of a dual-lumen catheter for home care increases the work of the parent or health care worker who must look after the catheter.

Planning Solutions for Home Use

The determination of the patient's nutritional requirements is based on the expected weight and height of the patient according to age and sex (Table 3).[51] Fluid requirements are determined by the patient's clinical condition as well as by anthropometric measurements. We try to provide 25 percent of the energy calories in the form of a 20 percent fat emulsion to decrease the risk of liver dysfunction.[51a,51b] The remainder of the energy calories are derived from glucose. The determination of electrolytes, trace metals, and vitamins to be added is based on the patient's weight and height. Additional electrolytes and minerals may be necessary depending on the patient's losses. If the patient has excessive losses from ostomy because of diarrhea, they may be supplied via a replacement solution. Pediatric multivitamin infusion may be used for children less than 3 years of age.[52] In those older than 3 years, a multiple vitamin solution for adults suffices.[53] Vitamin K is present only in the pediatric multiple vitamin infusion. In those older than age 3 in whom an adult multiple vitamin infusion is used, vitamin K may be provided at the discretion of the physician. Vitamin K becomes necessary only in those individuals who receive antibiotics frequently. Otherwise, the natural production of vitamin K in the distal small bowel and colon is sufficient for the production of vitamin K–dependent coagulation factors.

TABLE 3
Recommended Energy and Protein Intakes

Age (yr)	Energy (mean) (kcal/kg)	Kcal/day (mean)	Protein (g/kg)	Protein (g/day)
Infants and children				
0.–0.5	115	300	2.2	
0.5–1	105	600	2.0	
1–3	100	1,300	1.8	
4–6	85	1,700	1.5	
7–10	85	2,400	1.2	
Adolescents				
Boys				
11–14		2,800		45
15–18		3,000		56
Girls				
11–14		2,400		46
15–18		2,100		46

TABLE 4
Typical Infant/Child Home Total Parenteral Nutrition with Vitamin Ingredients

Final Concentrations	Infants	Children
Neonatal amino acids (TrophAmine, Kendall-McGaw)	2%	
Balanced amino acids		3.5–4.25%
Dextrose*	10–25%	10–25%
Sodium	30 mEq/L	35 mEq/L
Potassium	25 mEq/L	30 mEq/L
Calcium	10 mEq/L	5 mEq/L
Magnesium	10 mEq/L	10 mEq/L
Phosphate	7.5 mmol/L	10 mmol/L
Chloride	30 mEq/L	35 mEq/L
Acetate	27 mEq/L	64 mEq/L
Zinc	2 mg/L	2 mg/L
Copper	1 mg/L	1 mg/L
Selenium	20 μg/L	20 μg/L
Chromium	2 μg/L	2 μg/L

Pediatric multivitamin

Vitamin	Term Infants and Children (dose per day)	Preterm Infants (dose/kg body wt) (maximum not to exceed term infant dose): Current Suggestions	Best Estimate for New Formulation
Lipid-soluble			
A (μg)	700.0	280.00	500.00
E (mg)	7.0	2.80	2.80
K (μg)	200.0	80.00	80.00
D (μg)	10.0	4.00	4.00
Water-soluble			
Ascorbic acid (mg)	80.0	32.00	25.00
Thiamin (mg)	1.2	0.48	0.35
Riboflavin (mg)	1.4	0.56	0.15
Pyridoxine (mg)	1.0	0.40	0.18
Niacin (mg)	17.0	6.80	6.80
Pantothenate (mg)	5.0	2.00	2.00
Biotin (μg)	20.0	8.00	6.00
Folate (μg)	140.0	56.00	56.00
Vitamin B_{12} (μg)	1.0	0.40	0.30

*Higher concentrations may be used if there is reason to restrict fluid volume. D_{30} and D_{35} may be used.

Table 4 indicates the typical ingredients of an HTPN solution. The concentration of dextrose used depends in part on the calories to be delivered. It is more typical to use a 20 or 25 percent dextrose solution. However, rare patients, because of their cardiopulmonary status, may not tolerate such solutions. More concentrated solutions containing 30 or 35 percent dextrose may be necessary.

Infusion Time

Initially, a patient is established on a 24-hour infusion in the hospital. Once the maximal concentration of dextrose solution and the maximal amount of fat to be used are reached, the number of hours of support is decreased by 1 to 2 hours per day. The rate of administration is increased, but the volume administered remains constant. Gradually, over a period of 7 days, the number of hours of infusion is decreased to 10 to 17 hours per day. The younger the infant, the more hours the infusion is allowed to run. In school-age children, most infusions are given during a 10-hour infusion period. This allows the patient a maximal amount of time to be free of attachment to an infusion system.

Ending the Infusion

At the end of the infusion, the rate of administration is reduced twice by 50 percent over a period of 30 minutes. Occasional patients may require the infusion rate to be reduced by 25 percent every 15 minutes over 1 hour. This is to reduce the risk of hypoglycemia.

Some school-age children are able to participate in and perform a portion of their care. Most of junior high school age have been trained to do their own care, except for the hanging of the plastic bags containing their solution. Most teenagers, unless they are critically ill, can perform all the care required for their support.

In the care of the infant, it is the parent(s) who is required to learn the techniques of HTPN. The parent(s) should be given written booklets on the techniques of HTPN care. They should either be shown a videotape of how the techniques are performed or be given demonstrations by nurses. They should work on a mannequin under supervision until their techniques are perfected. Only after they have shown their ability to work on their own using a mannequin without problem would they be allowed to work on their own child.

The amount of time necessary to train parents for HTPN is variable. The typical period of time to teach parents catheter and line care as well as infusion care varies from as little as 5 days to as much as a month. The average parent requires 10 days of lessons and practice to perfect these techniques. Once parents have demonstrated mastery in the use of catheter and infusion pump, they should be allowed to do the techniques independently while in the hospital. This gives them the confidence necessary to allow independent function at home. Parents need to be taught the problems and complications that they may encounter at home such as fever, separation of catheter from intravenous tubing, bleeding from the catheter, hypoglycemia, and management of fever.

Planning Discharge

Most families, unless they live in remote areas, receive their solutions premixed. Premixed solutions require refrigeration and have a variable storage life, depending on the conditions under which they have been mixed and on the testing that is done to substantiate their purity. Some proprietary HTPN companies provide solutions every 2 days, some for a week at a time, and others for up to 2 to 4 weeks.

Families should be aware that solutions provided in small volumes or lots are more likely supplied by companies with less stringent techniques of sterility. Families able to obtain large volumes of solution for storage must have adequate refrigeration space. Prior to discharge, a social worker should try to make a home visit to assess the cleanliness and amount of space available for storage of supplies. Most families typically take home 1 to 4 weeks' worth of supplies. Solutions are almost always delivered directly to the home.

At the time of discharge, the patients' families are given telephone numbers of individuals to call in case of emergency. Ideally, they have phone numbers of physicians available 24 hours a day in case of complications.[53] They must have access 24 hours a day to the home health care agencies in order to obtain help with regard to the solutions and infusion pumps, should problems develop.

Ongoing Care—Nutritional Reassessment

In is important to follow infants and children closely. After discharge from the hospital, the patient should be seen within 1 week. At that and subsequent visits, anthropometric measurements are taken, and the nutritional support is recalculated to determine if there is a need to change any of the nutrients. Before discharge the patient's family should be given a copy of the prescription their child is receiving. They should be instructed to bring this and any subsequent changes in their formula to each clinic visit. In this way, they will become familiar with what their child is receiving and also provide for the physician a check on what is being received each time they are seen.

Pediatric patients differ from adults in that their weight and height are constantly changing until they complete puberty. This is the reason for the continuous attention given to anthropometric determinations and for following the patient along growth channels. At each visit the infant or child should have his or her height and weight measured and plotted on growth channels. In the infant it is especially important to measure head circumference at specific intervals. After the initial visit, subsequent visits may be done on an every-2-week basis for 1 month. If the patient appears stable during the next month, subsequent visits should be on a monthly basis through the first year of life and every 2 or 3 months thereafter for the remainder of the second year. We believe that throughout childhood quarterly visits are absolutely necessary to monitor growth and weight gain. Laboratory tests performed at each visit should consist of a complete blood count, electrolytes, calcium, magnesium, total proteins, albumin, and prealbumin. Trace metal determinations should be done at least yearly. Liver function tests should be done quarterly or twice a year after infancy. Such determinations are necessary for the optimal management of the patient. Fat-soluble vitamin determinations should also be done at least twice a year.

At each visit, besides a review of what the patient is receiving and a discussion of whether there are problems relating to the catheter or the infusion pump, the physician should do a general pediatric evaluation of the patient with an emphasis on the developmental aspects of the child's progress.

HTPN patients who have some function of the intestine should be encouraged to feed as much as they possibly can. From the beginning, even small amounts of feeding should be given by mouth, in order to ensure maximal stimulation of the GI tract for its growth.[11,18,50,54] Even infants who have no chance of ultimately living without parenteral nutrition should be given at least 5 percent of their caloric requirements orally. Failure to initiate feeding orally can result in serious problems at a later age when attempts are made to socialize the infant or child through feeding.

Duration of Therapy

In our experience, 120 pediatric patients have received parenteral nutrition at home for over 100,000 days of therapy. The mean per patient has been nearly 1,000 days.[80] The longest period for any patient has been well over 12 years.[55] Half of the 25 pediatric patients we are currently following have received parenteral support at home for 8 or more years. The typical catheter remains in place for well over 700 days. Some patients have utilized the same catheter for as long as 6 years. The average patient during the first decade of life typically has a catheter changed every 5 to 6 years. Twenty

TABLE 5
Catheter Removal Due to Complications

Type of Complication	Number Removed
Infection	76
Occlusion	42
Breakage	9
Pulled out	3

percent of all patients on long-term TPN support have had more than four catheters.[8] Table 5 lists the number of removals for each type of complication.

COMPLICATIONS OF HOME TOTAL PARENTERAL NUTRITION

Sepsis

Sepsis is the most serious and frequent complication for infants and children on HTPN,[8] just as it is for adults.[56,57] In all instances, complications are usually due to some known or unsuspected break in the technique in which the patient or parents were instructed. In infants and preschool children, fever can occur not only from breaks in the technique of administering the parenteral nutrition but also from usual childhood illnesses. Physicians who care for children on HTPN must carefully examine them each time a fever develops to try to identify its source. If there is no recognizable source, the most likely possibility is either a catheter infection or a viral infection. Each time a patient develops fever a careful history must be taken to determine if there are any simple explanations for the fever. Parents are always asked to bring the child for an examination, which must be done carefully. The parents must be questioned concerning the routine they have used for catheter care in administering the solution. They should be asked if they are aware of any lapse in technique that may have occurred. If there is no obvious source of infection, the patient should have blood cultures taken from the catheter and the peripheral vein. Cultures should be done for aerobes, anaerobes, and fungi. A CBC with differential count and a urinalysis should be done. Other tests depend on the clinical findings and suspicions of the examining physician. *If a specific source of infection is identified, the patient should be treated appropriately.* This may necessitate the initiation of antibiotics given intravenously at first in the hospital and then at home. Since most of the patients on HTPN cannot effectively absorb all antibiotics, the intravenous route is most commonly utilized.

If the antibiotics are given at home, we typically attempt to choose those that can be given either every 8 or 12 hours. As soon as the parents are taught the technique for administering the antibiotics and the patient is afebrile, the child may be sent home. Once the parents have learned the techniques for administering all the antibiotics, they can be applied in the future if a similar problem occurs.

If no obvious source of infection is found, a white blood cell count is obtained. If it is elevated or there is a shift to the left with increased numbers of band forms, antibiotic coverage may be started to treat the suspected infection in the catheter. Since the most common organisms are either *Staphylococcus aureus* or *Staphylococcus epidermidis* (Table 6), vancomycin should be started.[39] If no specific organism is found, we typically use a combination of vancomycin and gentamicin. We typically treat patients such as this for 14 days and then discontinue the antibiotics. If a specific organism is found that we believe is responsive to antibiotics, the treatment typically is given for 1 month. As a general rule, fungi and gram-negative infections cannot be as effectively treated while leaving the catheter in place. In situations such as this the catheter must be removed. A new central venous catheter may be replaced after a patient has been afebrile for 72 hours and blood cultures no longer contain the infectious organism. In our experience, more than a majority of the patients have never had a catheter infection. However, of those who have had them, some patients have repeated catheter infections. Ten percent of our patients have had four to six infections. One fifth of all infections occur at the catheter insertion site. In the most recent experience, there has been a dramatic reduction in infections at the insertion site. We believe that this is due to a change in the structure of the new Broviac and Hickman catheters with a silver-impregnated antibiotic cuff proximal to the Dacron cuff. This prevents access of bacteria growing up along the catheter. Three-fourths of the infections have been either *Staphylococcus aureas* or *Staphylococcus epidermidis*. *Candida* species account for 12 percent, *Pseudomonas aeruginosa* 10 percent, *Eschericha coli* 3 percent, and group D streptococci and *Klebsiella* species smaller percentages.[8] Positive blood cultures from the central line were obtained in over 80 percent of those in whom sepsis was suspected. Eighty-six percent of patients with positive central line cultures have positive concomitant peripheral blood cultures. Interestingly, we could not find a direct correlation between the total white blood count and the percentage of band forms in those with positive cultures.[8]

Cholelithiasis, Cholecystitis, and Chronic Liver Disease

Cholelithiasis or biliary sludge has been documented in over 10 percent of all patients on long-term TPN.[58,59] This is a dramatic incidence when compared with the rare find-

TABLE 6
Organisms Responsible for Infection in Catheter and at Catheter Insertion Site

Organism Cultured	Number of Times Cultured
Staphylococcus aureus	42
Staphylococcus epidermidis	33
Candida albicans	18
Candida tropicalis	4
Pseudomonas aeruginosa	10
Escherichia coli	6
Group D *Streptococcus*	1
Klebsiella species	1
Streptococcus viridans	1
Pityrosporum orbiculare	1

ing of gallstones in healthy children. It is said that gallstones are found in only 1 out of 15,000 infants and children coming to postmortem examination. It is our belief that those who become symptomatic with recurrent right upper quadrant and midepigastric pain should undergo cholecystectomy. The development of the gallstone is secondary to stasis and an imbalance in chemical composition of the bile because of the short bowel syndrome. It is possible that by more frequent feeding of those infants and children, there would be a lesser incidence of biliary sludge and stones. We do not know whether lithotripsy or the feeding or chenodeoxycholic or ursodeoxycholic acid to such infants and children would reduce the incidence of cholelithiasis.[60,61]

Serious life-threatening liver disease had been a rare occurrence in our patients on HTPN, although it has been reported in early infancy, especially in preterm infants on TPN.[62,45] Over the period of nearly two decades we have had only five children who developed serious and progressive chronic liver disease. The cause of the liver disease in these patients may be a variety of factors, including one or more blood transfusions, one or more episodes of sepsis, and/or as a complication of multiple drug therapy over a period of years. Interestingly, we have seen significantly less liver disease in recent years. This may be secondary to an improvement in parenteral nutrition solutions. The development of special amino acid solutions specifically formulated for infants may be the reason for this decrease in frequency of chronic liver disease as well as a change in our protocol on initiating enteral nutrition sooner.[46]

Metabolic Abnormalities

Fluids and Electrolytes

Significant abnormalities in fluid and electrolyte balance requiring rehospitalization virtually never occur.[8] This, we believe, is secondary to the careful training provided to parents and the meticulous attention paid to such balance before patients leave the hospital and at subsequent visits. Fat overload syndromes do occur if patients are given excessive quantities of lipid emulsion, usually greater than 3 g per kilogram. During hospitalization and before the patient leaves the hospital, fasting triglyceride determinations should be done before lipid emulsion is given to check that it is effectively cleared. Overload occurs when lipid is given too rapidly or dose is greater than can be cleared.

TABLE 7
Recommended Intravenous Intakes of Trace Elements

Element	Infants (μg/kg/days)		Children (μg/kg/day) [maximum μg/day]
	Preterm	Term	
Zinc	400.00	250 <3 mo 100 >3 mo	50.00 [5,000]
Copper*	20.00	20.00	20.00 [300]
Selenium†	2.00	2.00	2.00 [40]
Chromium†	0.20	0.20	0.20 [5]
Manganese*	1.00	1.00	1.00 [50]
Molybdenum†	0.25	0.25	0.25 [5]
Iodide	1.00	1.00	1.00 [1]
Iron (see text)			
Fluoride (see text)			

*Omit in patients with obstructive jaundice.
†Omit in patients with renal dysfunction.

Trace Elements

During the past 15 years, a variety of trace element deficiencies have been described in patients on long-term TPN. Such deficiencies no longer need occur, since it is now recognized that zinc, copper, selenium, and chromium should be supplied to patients (Table 7).[63-66]

Zinc deficiency is characterized by loss of hair including eyebrows and eyelashes, photophobia, a yellow crusting eruption at the acral portions of the extremities and around the mouth, nose, and ears, as well as bullous eruption at the bases of the fingers, toes, anus, and genitalia. Such a condition should no longer occur, since zinc is routinely added to parenteral nutrition solutions. However, it is important to recognize that more than normal zinc supplementation is required in patients who have massive diarrhea and malabsorption.

Copper deficiency also is highly uncommon and has rarely been reported.[64] It is characterized by iron deficiency anemia, leukopenia with neutropenia, and thrombocytopenia. Rarely it is associated with thin, kinky hair.

Selenium deficiency has only recently been recognized in pediatric patients.[65] It is characterized by decrease in hair and skin pigmentation.[50] Patients with selenium deficiency may also present with macrocytosis, cerebellar ataxia, and loss of muscle strength.[66,67] Cardiac arrhythmias and heart failure have been described in adults but not in children. A myopathy in which the patients have decreased muscle strength and transaminitis has also been described. Table 7 indicates the amount of supplementation necessary to avoid such deficiencies. There are a variety of other trace metals, but it is not clear whether they should be supplemented. These include fluoride, manganese, and cobalt. There is no question that other trace metals should be added to the parenteral nutrition solutions, but the documentation is not available.

Vitamin deficiency has not been apparent in most individuals reported on HTPN. It is exceedingly uncommon and should not occur if the infants and children are provided with the appropriate supplementation. The multiple vitamin preparations should be added to the TPN solutions just before administration to minimize losses while the solution is hanging.

Renal Disease

Recent studies have led us to believe that long-term TPN is correlated with a reduction in renal function. We have found that this correlation is strictly with parenteral nutrition and not with multiple courses of antibiotics for infection. We are concerned about the significance of this for the long term but at this point do not know the basis for it.

Bone Disease

Although pathologic factors have been an extremely rare occurrence in patients on HTPN, it is characteristic of most patients to have demineralization of the spine and the long bones.[69] Such abnormalities are present in most patients, but the etiology is unclear. Although studies have been done measuring calcium, phosphorus, magnesium, and vitamin D levels, there have been no consistent abnormalities found in these tests to explain the demineralization. A number of factors have been considered that may contribute to the decreased mineralization. Deficiencies in fluoride, boron, and silicone could be contributing factors.

Developmental Delay and Social Problems

Most patients in HTPN programs that start in infancy develop more slowly because of a prolonged hospitalization prior to discharge.[70] However, if patients are promptly discharged from the hospital and are successfully managed at home without rehospitalization, the best chance for developing in a completely normal fashion is provided. The more patients are hospitalized for complications, the greater the risk that their development will be slowed by being taken out of the home environment. In general, those of our patients who have been tested by standard developmental tests for infants and children have shown normal or nearly normal intelligence and motor function.[71]

Despite these observations these children are likely to have some difficulties because they are special. Parents often prevent them from fully participating in physical activities because of their fear of harm resulting from the presence of the central venous catheter. Some of these children seem to have poor muscle development without a clear explanation. The majority of children on long-term parenteral nutrition have deficits in perceptual-motor performance; this is particularly true for the older children. Social class was highly associated with verbal and nonverbal intelligence.[71]

LONG-TERM NUTRITIONAL STATUS

Children receiving long-term TPN can obtain and maintain normal height, weight, and other anthropomteric measurements of nutritional status. Patients who receive almost all nutrition parenterally may achieve more normal nutritional status because there is a propensity to underestimate the amount of parenteral nutrition needed by patients who ingest more than 30 percent of their nutrients.[72,73]

TABLE 8
TPN and Non-TPN–Associated Mortality in 31 Patients on Home Total Parenteral Nutrition

	Number
TPN-related	
Liver failure	2
Catheter-related sepsis	9
Improper administration of TPN	1
Pulmonary edema	1
SUBTOTAL	13
Non-TPN–related	
Sepsis	5
Malignancy	5
Cytomegalovirus hepatitis	1
Cystic fibrosis	2
Aspiration syndrome	1
Pneumonia	1
Accidental	1
Unknown	2
SUBTOTAL	18

MORTALITY

HTPN does have associated risks, and death is one of them (Table 8). Sepsis is the number one cause of death in patients on HTPN. In most instances, there is delay on the part of the parents in bringing the febrile infant or child to the physician. However, on occasion, failure of the physician to recognize the early signs of sepsis or a fulminant septic course may be responsible. Mechanical problems such as overly rapid administration of TPN fluids has occurred once in our experience. Liver failure as the primary cause of death is uncommon.

CONCLUSIONS

HTPN for infants and children is a well-established technique for supplying all or part of their nutritional needs for as long as necessary to sustain normal weight gain and growth through long-term venous access devices. Theoretically it should be possible to provide this support, if necessary, for an entire life span. The techniques for this support can be mastered by most parents and teenagers and it may be done without serious complications in many.

HTPN is expensive, but it is substantially less expensive than keeping a patient hospitalized for equivalent care. A typical child receiving HTPN may have direct and indirect costs of $50,000 to $75,000 per year. In most states government financial support is provided if insurance does not cover the cost.

Mortality in HTPN for those who do not have terminal diseases is most commonly secondary to infection of the central venous catheter, a preventable complication.

Since HTPN as a technique has been available for less than 2 decades, all of its long-term consequences have not been defined.

Acknowledgments

I would like to thank Laurie Reyen, R.N., M.N., Clinical Nurse Specialist, and William Guss, Pharm.D., Pharmacist Specialist in Nutrition Support, for their contributions in the preparation of the manuscript and for their support in care of these patients on HTPN.

REFERENCES

1. Scribner BH, Cole JJ, Christopher TG. Long-term total parenteral nutrition. JAMA 1970; 212:457.
2. Jeejeebhoy KN, Zohrab WJ, Langer B, et al. Total parenteral nutrition at home for 23 months without complications and with good rehabilitation. A study of technical and metabolic features. Gastroenterology 1973; 65:811.
3. Salassol C, Joyeux H, Etco L, et al. New techniques for long-term intravenous feeding and artificial gut in 75 patients. Ann Surg 1974; 179:519.

4. Fleming CR, McGill DB, Berkner S. Home parenteral nutrition as primary therapy in patients with extensive Crohn's disease of small bowel and malnutrition. Gastroenterology 1977; 73:1077.
5. Shils M. A program for total parenteral nutrition at home. Am J Clin Nutr 1975; 28:1429.
6. Strobel CT, Byrne WJ, Fonkalsrud EW, Ament ME. Home parenteral nutrition: results in 34 pediatric patients. Ann Surg 1978; 188:394.
7. Wesley JR. Home parenteral nutrition: indications, principles, and cost-effectiveness. Compr Ther 1983; 9:29–36.
8. Vargas JH, Ament ME, Berquist WE. Long-term home parenteral nutrition in pediatrics: ten years of experience in 102 patients. J Pediatr Gastr Nutr 1987; 6:L24–32.
9. Mughal M, Irving M. Home parenteral nutrition in the United Kingdom and Ireland. Lancet 1986; 2:383–387.
10. Wolfe BM, Beer WH, Hayashi JT, Halsted CH, Cannon RA, Cox KL. Experience with home parenteral nutrition. Am J Surg 1983; 146:7–14.
11. Grosfeld JL, Rescorla FJ, West KW. Short bowel syndrome in infancy and childhood. Analysis of survival in 60 patients. Am J Surg 1986; 151:41–46.
12. Cochran WJ, Klish WJ, Brown MR, Lyons JM, Curtis T. Chylous ascites in infants and children: a case report and literature review. J Pediatr Gastroenterol Nutr 1985; 4:668–673.
13. Postuma R, Moroz SP. Pediatric Crohn's disease. J Pediatr Surg 1985; 20:478–482.
14. Stokes MA, Irving MH. How do patients with Crohn's disease fare on home parenteral nutrition? Dis Col Rectum 1988; 31:454–458.
15. Pitt HA, Mann LL, Berquist WE, Ament ME, Fonkalsrud EW, DenBesten L. Chronic intestinal pseudo-obstruction. Management with total parenteral nutrition and a venting enterostomy. Arch Surg 1985; 120:614–618.
16. Ling LJ, Hersenson MB, Young S, Traisman HS. Home parenteral nutrition in a child with Menetrier disease. Eur J Pediatr 1986; 144:505–507.
17. Skehan AM, Fitzgeral RJ. Home parenteral nutrition in childhood. Ir Med J 1986; 79:253–254.
18. Taylor CJ, Manning D. Home parenteral nutrition in infantile short bowel syndrome. Acta Paediatr Scand 1986; 75:866–867.
19. Yotta D. Supraclavicular subclavian venipuncture and catheterization. Lancet 1965; ii:614.
20. Benotti PN, Bothe A, Miller JDB, et al. Safe cannulation of the internal jugular vein for long-term hyperalimentation. Surg Gynecol Obstet 1977; 144:574.
21. Maksimak M, Ament ME, Fonkalsrud EW. Comparison of the pediatric Silastic catheter with a standard No. 3 French Silastic catheter for central venous alimentation. J Pediatr Gastroenterol Nutr 1982; 1:227.
22. Lammermeier D, Steiger E, Cosgrove D, Zelch M. Use of intercostal vein for central venous access in home parenteral nutrition: a case report. JPEN 1986; 10:659.
23. Broviac JW, Cole JJ, Scribier BH. A silicone rubber catheter for prolonged parenteral nutrition. Surg Gynecol Obstet 136; 1973:606.
24. Hickman RO, Buckner CD, Cliff R, et al. A modified right atrial catheter for access to the venous system in marrow transplant recipients. Surg Gynecol Obstet 1979; 148:871.
25. Sanders JE, Hickman RO, Aker S, et al. Experience with double lumen right atrial catheters. JPEN 1982; 6:95.
26. Ecoff L, Barone RM, Simons RM. Implantable infusion port (Port-a-Cath). J Natl Intraven Ther Assoc 1983; 6:406.
27. Lokich JJ, Bothe A, Benotti P, et al. Complications and management of implanted venous access catheters. J Clin Oncol 1985; 3:710.
28. Peterson AF, Rosenberg A, Alatary SP. Comparative evaluation of surgical scrub preparations. Surg Gynecol Obstet 1978; 146:63.
29. Lowbury EJL, Lilly HA. The effect of blood on disinfection of surgeon's hands. Br J Surg 1974; 61:19.
30. Norden CW. Application of antibiotic ointment to the site of venous catheterization. A controlled trial. J Infect Dis 1969; 120:611.
31. Brier KL, Latiolais CJ, Schneider PJ, et al. Effects of laminar air flow and clean room dress on contamination rates of intravenous admixtures. Am J Hosp Pharm 1981; 38:1144.
32. Crocker KS, Noja R, Filibeck DK, et al. Microbial growth comparisons of five commercial parenteral lipid emulsions. JPEN 1984; 8:391.
33. Goldman DA, Maki DG. Infection control in total parenteral nutrition. JAMA 1983; 223:1360.
34. Jarrard MM, Olsen CM, Freeman JB. Daily dressing change effects on skin flora beneath subclavian catheter dressings during total parenteral nutrition. JPEN 1981; 4:391.
35. Powel C, Regan C, Fabri PJ, et al. Evaluation of Opsite catheter dressings for parenteral nutrition. A prospective randomized study. JPEN 1982; 6:43.
36. Nehme AE, Trigger JA. Catheter dressings in central venous parenteral nutrition. A prospective randomized comparative study. Nutr Support Serv 1984; 4:42.
37. Sitges-Serra A, Linares J, Perez JL. A randomized trial of the effect of tubing changes on hub contamination and catheter sepsis during parenteral nutrition. JPEN 1985; 9:322.
38. Bjeletich J, Hickman RO. The Hickman indwelling catheter. Am J Nurs 1980; 80:62.
39. Glynn MGY, Langer B, Jeejeebhoy KN. Therapy for thrombotic occlusion in long-term intravenous alimentation catheters. JPEN 1980; 4:87.
40. Bailey MJ. Reduction of catheter associated sepsis in parenteral nutrition using low-dose intravenous heparin. Br Med J 1979; 1:1671.
41. Hurtubise MR, Bottino JC, Lawson M, et al. Restoring patency of occluded central venous catheters. Arch Surg 1980; 115:212.
42. Dorney SF, Byrne WJ, Ament ME. Case of congenital short small intestine: survival with use of long-term parenteral feeding. Pediatrics 1986; 77:386–389.
43. Seidman EG, Roy CC, Weber AM, Morin CL. Nutritional therapy of Crohn's disease in childhood. Dig Dis Sci 1987; 32(12 suppl):825–888.
44. Amarnath RP, Fleming CR, Perrault J. Home parenteral nutrition in chronic intestinal diseases: its effect on growth and development. J Pediatr Gastroenterol Nutr 1987; 6:89–95.
45. Vargas JH, Sachs P, Ament ME. Chronic intestinal pseudo-obstruction syndrome in pediatrics. J Pediatr Gastroenterol Nutr 1988; 7:323.
46. Warner E, Jeejeebhoy KN. Successful management of chronic intestinal pseudo-obstruction with home parenteral nutrition. JPEN 1985; 9:173–178.
47. Cutz E, Rhoads JM, Drumm B, et al. Microvillus inclusion disease: an inherited defect of Brush-Border assembly and differentiation. N Engl J Med 1989; 320:646–651.
48. Weisdorf SA, Salati LM, Longsdorf JA, Ramsay NKC, Shrep HL. Graft versus host disease of the intestine: a protein losing enteropathy characterized by fecal alpha-l-antitrypsin. Gastroenterology 1983; 85:1076.
48a. Skeie B, Askanazi J, Rothkopf M, et al. Improved exercise tolerance with long-term parenteral nutrition in cystic fibrosis. Crit Care Med 1987; 15:960–962.
48b. Asch MJ, Sherman NJ. Total parenteral nutrition in management of refractory chylous ascites. J Pediatr 1979; 94:260–262.
49. Dorney SF, Ament ME, Berquist WE, Vargas JH, Hassal E. Improved survival in very short small bowel of infancy with use of long-term parenteral nutrition. J Pediatr 1985; 107:521–525.
50. Postuma R, Moroz S, Friesen F. Extreme short-bowel syndrome in an infant. J Pediatr Surg 1983; 18:264–268.
51. Queen PM, Wilson SE. Growth and nutrient requirements of infants and children. In: Grand RT, Sutphen JL, Dietz WH Jr, eds. Pediatric Nutrition. Boston: Butterworths, 1987.
51a. Meguid MM, Schimmel E, Johnson WC. 1982 Reduced metabolic complications in total parenteral nutrition using fat to replace 1/3 of glucose calories. JPEN 1982; 6:304–307.
51b. McDonald AT, Phillips MJ, Jeejeebhoy KN. Reversal of fatty liver by Intralipid in patients on total parenteral alimentation. Gastroenterology 1973; 64:885.
52. Moore MC, Greene HL, Phillips B, et al. Evaluation of a pediatric multiple vitamin preparation for total parenteral nutrition in infants and children. I. Blood levels of water soluble vitamins. Pediatrics 1986; 77:530.
53. Kun S, Warburton D. Telephone assessment of parents' knowledge of home-care treatments and readmission outcomes for high-risk infants and toddlers. Am J Dis Child 1987; 141:888–892.
54. Nuutinen LS, Luoma PV, Lahtela JT, Nuutinen O. Combined oral and home parenteral nutrition for the short bowel syndrome. Ann Chir Gynaecol 1985; 74:32–35.
55. Personal observation.
56. Riella MC, Scribner BH. Five years experience with a right atrial catheter for prolonged parenteral nutrition at home. Surg Gynecol Obstet 1976; 143:205.
57. Begala JE, Maher K, Cherry JD. Risk of infection associated with the use of Broviac and Hickman catheters. Am J Infect Control 1982; 10:17.

58. Pitt HA, King W, Mann LL, Roslyn JJ, Berquist WE, Ament ME. Prolonged parenteral nutrition increases the risk of cholelithiasis. Am J Surg 1983; 145:106.
59. Roslyn JJ, Berquist WE, Pitt HA, Mann LL, Kangharloo H, DenBesten L, Ament ME. Increasing risk of gallstones in children receiving total parenteral nutrition. Pediatrics 1983; 71:784.
60. Mulley AC Jr. Shock wave lithotripsy. Assessing a slam-bang technology. N Engl J Med 1986; 314:845.
61. Tint GS, Salen F, Chazen P. Symptomatic gallstones are likely to recur after dissolution with ursodeoxycholic acid (UDCA) but this may be prevented by low-dose UDCA. Gastroenterology 1987; 92:187.
62. Wesson DE, Rich RH, Zlotkin SH, Pencharz PB. Fat overload syndrome causing respiratory insufficiency. J Pediatr Surg 1984; 19:777–778.
63. Arakawa T, Tamara R, Igarashi Y, et al. Zinc deficiency in two infants during total parenteral nutrition for diarrhea. Am J Clin Nutr 1976; 29:197.
64. Kadowaki H, Ouchi M, Kaga M, Motegi T, Yanagawa Y, Hayakawa H, Hashimoto G, Furuya K. Problems of trace elements and vitamins during long-term total parenteral nutrition: a case report of idiopathic intestinal pseudo-obstruction. JPEN 1987; 11:322–325.
65. Vinton NE, Dahlstrom KA, Strobel CT, Ament ME. Macrocytosis and pseudoalbinism: manifestations of selenium deficiency. J Pediatr 1987; 111:711.
66. Dahlstrom KA, Ament ME, Medhin MG, Meurling S. Serum trace elements in children receiving long-term parenteral nutrition. J Pediatr 1986; 109:625.
67. Kelly DA, Coe AW, Shenkin A, Lake BD, Walker-Smith JA. Symptomatic selenium deficiency in a child on home parenteral nutrition. J Pediatr Gastroenterol Nutr 1988; 7:783–786.
68. Moukarzel A, Ament M, Vargas J, et al. True glomerular filtration rate of children on long term parenteral nutrition (PN). Clin Res 1990; 38:190A.
69. Moukarzel A, Ament ME, Vargas J, et al. Parenteral nutrition bone disease in children. Clin Res 1990; 38:190A.
70. Ralston CW, O'Connor MJ, Ament M, Berquist WE, Parmelee AH Jr. Somatic growth and developmental functioning in children receiving prolonged home total parenteral nutrition. J Pediatr 1984; 105:842–846.
71. O'Connor MJ, Ralston CW, Ament ME. Intellectual prolonged home total parenteral nutrition. Pediatrics 1988; 81:231–236.
72. Dahlstrom KA, Strandvik B, Kopple J, Ament ME. Nutritional status in children receiving home parenteral nutrition. J Pediatr 1985; 107:219–224.
73. Lin CH, Rossi TM, Heitlinger LA, Lerner A, Riddlesberger MM, Lebenthal E. Nutritional assessment of children with short-bowel syndrome receiving home parenteral nutrition. Am J Dis Child 1987; 141:1093–1098.
74. Geggel HS, Ament ME, Heckenlively JR, Martin DA, Kopple JD. Nutritional requirement for taurine in patients receiving long-term parenteral nutrition. N Engl J Med 1985; 312:142–146.
75. Bowyer BA, Fleming CR, Ilstrup D, Nelson J, Reek S, Burnes J. Plasma carnitine levels in patients receiving home parenteral nutrition. Am J Clin Nutr 1986; 43:85–91.
76. Geggel HS, Ament ME, Heckenlively JR, Martin DA, Kopple JD. Nutritional requirements for taurine in patients receiving long-term parenteral nutrition. N Engl J Med 1985; 312:142.
77. Vinton NE, Laidlaw SA, Ament ME, Kopple JD. Taurine concentrations in plasma, blood cells, and urine of children undergoing long-term total parenteral nutrition. Pediatr Res 1987; 21:399–403.

CHAPTER 42

Drug Therapy

PART 1

Principles of Pediatric Therapeutics

Eli Zalzstein, M.D.
Stephen P. Spielberg, M.D., Ph.D.

Although pediatric pharmacology has developed rapidly in recent years, there are still major gaps in our understanding of the handling of and response to therapeutic agents in children. Children were described as "therapeutic orphans" more than 20 years ago, owing to the lack of pediatric studies on the vast majority of marketed drugs.[1,2] Considerable progress has been made in recent years in providing a rational basis for use of medications in children, encouraged by the pediatric clinical pharmacology community and organizations such as the Committee on Drugs of the American Academy of Pediatrics. Nonetheless, most drugs currently marketed still do not have labeling with evidence of proof of safety and efficacy in children. Regulatory agencies allow marketing of compounds without such information as long as an appropriate disclaimer is present in the labeling.

This situation is particularly interesting, since tragedies in pediatric therapeutics have established the current regulatory milieu under which drugs are developed. Thus, the deaths of several hundred children from elixir of sulfanilamide in the 1930s led to the Pure Food and Drug Act of 1938, establishing the US Food and Drug Administration in its present form.[3] The thalidomide tragedy of the 1950s led to the Kefauver-Harris Amendments to the Act in 1960.[4,5] Adverse drug effects in the developing fetus and in children continue to be noted to the present. Our need for increased knowledge in the area of developmental pharmacology and for continued vigilance in the use of medications in children remains. Here we briefly examine some of the effects of growth and development on the handling of medications. We then discuss some special considerations about administration of drugs to infants and small children. Finally, we review pediatric adverse drug reactions and suggest areas that require careful attention in initiating therapy with new drugs in children.

EFFECTS OF GROWTH AND DEVELOPMENT ON THE HANDLING OF DRUGS

From a pharmacologic point of view, the child is a continuously changing and developing organism. Rational dosing of children, from 600-g premature infants through adolescents, must take into consideration a variety of changing variables. Since many of the processes involved in the handling of drugs change at variable times during development and can be influenced by a wide variety of environmental factors, individualized dosing in the pediatric population is often more difficult than among adults.

In the broadest context many physiologic variables tend to be proportional to body surface area as opposed to weight. The ratio of body surface area to weight decreases threefold from a 2-kg child through a 70-kg adult. Ideally, dosing by body surface area would in many circumstances be more accurate than using weight as a basis. However, in a practical sense, most compounds are dosed on a milligram per kilogram basis. Weight can be measured directly, whereas surface area requires calculation with potential introduction of errors. In addition, determining a loading dose to achieve a specific concentration in plasma rapidly requires calculation of drug dose as milligrams per kilogram.

Absorption

The maturation of the gastrointestinal (GI) system is discussed in detail throughout this text. Many of the maturational changes in secretion of gastric acid,[6-8] bicarbonate and enzyme secretion by the pancreas,[9,10] and small intestinal surface area and cell maturation[8,11,12] can influence the absorption of drugs. Age- or disease-dependent changes in transit time can have a marked effect on drug absorption, particularly for sustained-release preparations. Similarly, other environmental factors such as food[13-18] can affect the absorption of a variety of therapeutic agents. The practical issue with respect to all of these changes in the GI system is that adult bioavailability studies simply cannot be extrapolated to children. Data must be obtained in specific age groups in order to provide appropriate dosing guidelines. This includes consideration of the specific preparations used for pediatric drug delivery, including suspensions, solutions, and microencapsulated products. Many drugs suitable for administration to adults are not suitable for children and require development of specific formulations for children of different ages. Bioavailability of compounds can also be influenced by the state of maturation of hepatic drug metabolism enzymes and hepatic extraction of compounds. For compounds that undergo "high first-pass effects," the relative state of maturation of the liver becomes even more important.

The large surface area of small infants compared with their weight has consequences for percutaneous absorption of drugs. Skin permeability to drugs is often increased in the newborn and, since a larger relative surface area may be covered with a medication, the systemic dose administered to that child may produce toxic effects.

Distribution

Once absorbed, compounds distribute in the body depending on their physicochemical characteristics. A drug's volume of distribution (Vd) is defined as the volume in which a dose must distribute to achieve a specific plasma concentration:

$$\text{Vd (L/kg)} = \frac{\text{Dose (mg/kg)}}{\text{Plasma concentration (mg/L)}}$$

Many parameters, including changes in body composition, can alter the Vd of a drug. For example, there are marked changes in the body's water content and distribution with age.[19-23] Total body water content is 80 to 90 percent in the premature infant, 70 to 80 percent in the term infant, and 50 to 60 percent in adults. Similarly, extracellular water decreases from 40 to 60 percent in the premature to perhaps 20 percent in the adult. These marked changes in water composition can alter the Vd of many drugs. For example, the Vd of gentamicin is approximately 0.5 L per kilogram in the premature and 0.3 L per kilogram in adults. Changes in Vd alter the choice of a loading dose of a drug to achieve a therapeutic plasma concentration; the larger the Vd, the more drug on a milligram per kilogram basis must be administered to achieve the same plasma concentration.

There are significant changes in fat content of the body with age, even with gestational age, varying from 1 percent in the premature infant to 15 percent of body weight at term. There may also be marked changes in relative sizes of organs with age. The effects of these maturational changes on drug distribution have not been systematically studied. However, when drugs are administered into a specific compartment, the effects of growth and development may be quite different. For example, the volume of cerebrospinal fluid does not vary with weight or surface area; it changes proportionately much less from a child to an adult. This has important consequences for intrathecal dosing of medications.

Plasma Protein Binding

The extent of binding of a drug to plasma proteins can influence the availability of the drug to act at biologically important sites. In general, acidic drugs tend to be bound to plasma albumin, whereas basic drugs are bound primarily to alpha$_1$-acid glycoproteins and lipoproteins.[24-27] Total plasma protein, albumin, and alpha$_1$-acid glycoprotein are all decreased in the newborn, and affinity of the proteins for binding specific drugs may also be somewhat decreased. This may influence the free fraction of drug in neonatal serum compared to that in older children or adults. Of even more importance, however, are potential interactions between drugs and endogenous substances, particularly bilirubin. Such drug-bilirubin interactions have been known for a long time, first noted in the case of neonatal sulfonamide use.[28] The increased burden of bilirubin as a result of catabolism of hemoglobin in the newborn, coupled with decreased hepatic conjugation capacity, acidosis, and increased penetration of the central nervous system by bilirubin, all place the newborn at increased risk of bilirubin toxicity and kernicterus as a result of displacement of bilirubin from albumin-binding sites by drugs. It is important to consider protein binding and potential bilirubin displacement by any new medication being used in the newborn.

Metabolism

Hepatic metabolism of drugs is a major mechanism of drug elimination. Enzymatic conversion of drugs to more polar and more easily excreted metabolites is generally divided into phase I and phase II processes. Phase I includes oxidation and reduction reactions. The major pathways for the majority of drugs we use are dependent on the cytochrome P-450 superfamily of enzymes. Phase II reactions are conjugations of products of phase I metabolism or the parent compounds themselves to glucuronide, sulfate, glycine, and glutathione. Nearly all of the enzymatic pathways are immature in the newborn, particularly so in the premature. Activities, however, may be influenced by environmental factors such as inducing substances (e.g., phenobarbital for glucuronidation and some types of cytochromes P-450; cigarette smoke and compounds such as polychlorinated biphenyls (PCBs) for other types of cytochromes P-450[29]). Severe limitation in glucuronidation capacity was first noted in the "grey baby syndrome" caused by chloramphenicol.[30,31] Exceedingly high serum concentrations of chloramphenicol resulted from the extrapolation of adult doses down to the newborn. Inability to glucuronidate the compound leads to a marked increase in the half-life of the drug from adult values of perhaps 4 hours up to 24 hours. It was found that newborns treated with chloramphenicol for sepsis prophylaxis following premature rupture of membranes had significantly higher mortality than babies who were treated with the remaining antibiotics then available, penicillin and streptomycin, or babies who received no antibiotics at all.[30] This tragedy again emphasizes the need for controlled clinical studies in populations of children who will be exposed to new compounds and the need for careful monitoring of serum concentrations of compounds that exhibit significant blood level–related toxicities.

Another consequence of limited metabolism by some pathways in the newborn is shunting of metabolism toward metabolites not seen routinely in the adult population. For example, theophylline is normally metabolized by cytochrome P-450 to a variety of oxidative metabolites. In the premature infant, however, owing to extremely limited oxidative metabolism, some of the drug is methylated to caffeine.[32,33] Since caffeine has a half-life considerably greater than that of theophylline, and both compounds are pharmacologically active, one has to take into consideration the accumulation of caffeine in the premature treated with theophylline. In older children or adults, oxidative pathways are more important than the methylation pathway, and essentially no caffeine is formed.

Beyond the newborn period, there is rapid maturation of most of the drug-metabolizing pathways. This occurs with normal growth and development and can be influenced by a variety of factors, including exposure to enzyme-inducing or inhibiting medications. Rates of maturation vary considerably from child to child. Monitoring of drugs with narrow therapeutic ranges (serum concentration associated with toxicity/serum concentration associated with efficacy) is critical to safe use of such drugs in this age group. In general, rates of drug clearance by metabolism are *greater* in children beyond the first year of life, up until the time of puberty, than in adults. For example, children may require 20 to 40 mg per kilogram per day of theophylline to maintain therapeutic serum concentrations, whereas the same person as an adult might only require 12 to 16 mg per kilogram per day. This increased rate of clearance among children is frequently unrecognized and, without appropriate studies of new medications in this age group, underdosing can result, analogous to the situation of overdosing in the newborn.

Treatment of adolescents is always a difficult problem, with increased issues of compliance and other complex psychosocial issues. In addition, there are marked pharmacologic changes occuring at about the time of puberty. In the case of drugs that undergo oxidative metabolism such as theophylline, there is dramatic down-regulation of the cytochrome P-450 enzymes, occurring at somewhat earlier Tanner stages in girls than in boys.[34,35] Such changes can be rather abrupt and can lead to dramatic increases in serum concentrations of drugs in patients maintained on constant milligram per kilogram doses. While toddlers probably exhibit greater variability in the handling of most drugs than adults (and therefore therapeutic monitoring of drugs is important in toddlers), the significant changes in metabolism occurring at puberty make it an even more critical period during which to monitor carefully patients on chronic therapy for any disease. The decrease in hepatic metabolism occurring at puberty then remains reasonably stable through adult life, allowing for the effect of variables of diet, other drugs, and disease state.

RENAL ELIMINATION OF DRUGS

Renal elimination of drugs follows a pattern somewhat similar to that of hepatic metabolism. Both glomerular filtration and renal tubular secretion of drugs are extremely limited in the premature and less so in the term infant. Maturation occurs quickly and variably among children and can be influenced by exogenous variables such as exposure to drugs.[36-39] In a practical sense, it is important to recognize the variability in rates of maturation, as well as to consider the developing neonate and child as a continuously changing organism. Renal clearance exceeds that in adults and decreases at puberty.

In summary, the newborn—particularly the premature—can be viewed as having very limited clearance of drugs by either renal or hepatic mechanisms. The toddler through prepuberty exhibits drug clearance by most mechanisms which exceeds that of adults and thus requires higher dosing of most drugs on a milligram per kilogram per day basis. At puberty, down-regulation of clearance mechanisms occurs at variable times and to a variable extent and can lead to large decreases in dosage requirements. Because of all these considerations, it is mandatory to obtain good kinetic and pharmacodynamic data in children of various ages before medications can be rationally used in these age groups. Appropriate use of therapeutic drug monitoring can be helpful in individualizing doses, particularly for drugs with narrow therapeutic indices. Particular caution has to be observed in patients being treated for chronic illness as they mature from newborn to toddler and through puberty.

SPECIAL CONSIDERATIONS IN ADMINISTRATION OF MEDICATIONS TO CHILDREN

The predicament of the "therapeutic orphan," because so many medications are not tested for safety and efficacy in various age groups of children, is made worse by the frequent lack of availability of appropriate pediatric dosage forms. Often the concentrations of intravenous medications available for adult use are inappropriate for small infants, since dosing would require that volumes under 0.1 ml be given. Inaccuracy of measurement of small volumes has been a major problem in the treatment of children with a variety of adult intravenous preparations. This becomes even more important for unstable preparations in which dilution of the product might cause precipitation of the drug, leading to further complications in administration. Increasingly we are recognizing the need for specific pediatric preparations of parenteral medications in concentrations appropriate for use in children.

While we generally view the intravenous route of administration as assuring delivery of drugs to patients, several investigators have demonstrated that the situation, particularly in small infants, is not so simple.[40,41] When intravenous fluid administration rates are very low, such as frequently occurs in the nursery, or if medications are administered many milliliters away from the patient, delivery of drug will be delayed or the drug may never reach the patient. In such situations, when peak concentration would normally be expected in adults in 0.5 hour and the trough at 6 hours, it may take fully 6 hours for the drug to reach the patient. This has led to much confusion about the use of therapeutic drug monitoring and may be responsible for failure of efficacy or for toxicity. Similarly, at very slow administration rates, medications that do not readily mix with intravenous solutions and have densities different from that of the solution being administered to the patient can "settle out" at the bottom of loops of intravenous tubing and never reach the patient.[41] New techniques are being developed to assure proper drug delivery of small volumes of medications to small infants, including the use of pumps that administer medication at a controlled rate distally in the intravenous line, and thus directly to the patient. Technical problems such as these are sufficient to place some doubt regarding older kinetic data, and interpretation of kinetic studies in the newborn must take into account the precise method of administration of the drugs in question.

Mention has been made regarding percutaneous absorption of drugs and the greater surface-to-volume ratio in small children than in adults. This can be of importance, for example, in the use of topical steroids over a large surface area in a child, which can lead to significant serum concentrations of steroids and resultant toxicity. The same is true for almost any substance applied to a large area of skin in small children.

There are several difficulties associated with oral preparations of medications for children. Studies done on bioavailability of medications in which adult preparations are crushed and suspended in water may provide erroneous data compared to a marketed preparation specifically designed for pediatric use. We frequently have to make extemporaneous preparations of medications in pediatric hospital pharmacies because no preparations are available commercially, and issues of stability and bioavailability are very real under these circumstances. When commercial preparations are available, studies must be undertaken with these specific preparations. Medications usually contain a variety of excipients, suspending agents, coloring agents, and flavorings, and attention has to be paid to pharmacologic and toxicologic effects of the entire product, including the specific medication to be administered.

Considerable interest has recently been paid to microencapsulation techniques that place medication in coated particles. This removes the issue of bad taste, which creates a major compliance problem for many pediatric preparations and, depending on composition of the "beads," can produce a sustained-release preparation. Here again, however, it is necessary to study such preparations in children prior to making dosing recommendations. Infants with rapid intestinal transit, either developmentally or because of a disease state, can end up passing most of the "time-release pills" in stool without absorbing the drug. Sustained-release preparations make good sense in pediatrics for many medications whose clearance may be more rapid than in adults, and the sustained-release product may produce "smoother" serum concentration curves. However, this has to be demonstrated for specific products in children, and data cannot simply be extrapolated from studies in adults.

SPECIAL ADVERSE REACTION CONSIDERATIONS IN CHILDREN

Some of the major adverse reactions that have occurred in the pediatric population have been associated with pharmacokinetic differences between children and adults. Such was the case with chloramphenicol-induced "grey baby syndrome." Others have resulted from the unique pathophysiology of the newborn together with pharmacokinetic considerations, such as sulfonamide-induced kernicterus. Our expanding knowledge of kinetics and the handling of drugs in children of different ages has provided a rational starting point for studying new pharmaceutical entities in the pediatric population. However, other considerations have to be taken into account, including so-called "inactive" ingredients in drug preparations as well as unique effects that drugs can have on a growing and developing organism.

Recognition of a major problem with excipients in pediatrics was made in the 1930s with the tragedy of the elixir of sulfanilamide.[28] In these patients renal failure resulted from the ethylene glycol vehicle, not from the sulfanilamide. Despite the early recognition that "inactive" ingredients may be toxic in the pediatric population, problems have continued to arise to the present time. For example, 50 years following the sulfanilamide story, the "gasping syndrome" associated with excessive use of benzyl alcohol–containing intravenous preparations in newborns was described.[42–44] Although the amounts of benzyl alcohol in intravenous medications generally pose no problem for adults, use of such preparations in the newborn can lead to accumulation of benzoic acid with resultant toxicity. More recently, questions have been raised about toxicity of a new parenteral vitamin E preparation containing polysorbate 80.[45–48] Although it is uncertain if the toxicity resulted directly from the polysorbate, it is clear that we must still be cautious about introduction of any new pharmaceutical preparations in the newborn. Similarly, allergic reactions can occur to a number of components within medications, including dyes and flavoring agents. Since we frequently deal with liquid preparations in pediatrics, such issues become all the more important.

Several types of adverse drug effects become manifest because children are growing and developing. Thus, corticosteroid toxicity in children undergoing chronic treatment can include growth failure as well as all of the other side effects noted in adults. Another example is the deposition of tetracycline in developing teeth, with resultant staining. Increasingly, there is the recognition that many medications may interfere with cognitive development and learning in children. For example, in a recent study, phenobarbital was demonstrated to have significantly more effect on cognitive development and more adverse effects on behavior than valproic acid.[49] Since we are dealing with a continuously developing and growing child, great emphasis must be placed on the need for longitudinal studies of any medication used chronically in children, and particular attention must be paid to neurodevelopmental issues.

SUMMARY

We have learned a great deal about age-dependent differences in pharmacokinetics, absorption, distribution, metabolism, and renal excretion of drugs. Information is slowly beginning to accumulate about age-dependent differences in receptors and in pharmacodynamics. Consideration of development of a new drug in the pediatric population requires not only consideration of optimal dosing regimens based on kinetics but also appreciation of the precise nature of the preparations used, concentrations of intravenous drugs, excipients and other agents present in both intravenous and oral formulations, and vigilance with respect to unforeseen idiosyncratic adverse effects.

REFERENCES

1. Shirkey HC. Therapeutic orphans—everybody's business. Drug Intell 1968; 2:323-327.
2. Shirkey HC. Therapeutic orphans: who speaks for children. South Med J 1970; 63:1361-1363.
3. Geiling EMK, Cannon PR. Pathologic effects of elixir of sulfanilamide (diethylene glycol) poisoning. JAMA 1938; 111:919-926.
4. McBride WG. Thalidomide and congenital abnormalities. Lancet 1961; ii: 1358.
5. Lenz W. Thalidomide and congenital abnormalities. Lancet 1962; i: 45.
6. Avery GB, Randolph JG, Weaver T. Gastric acidity in the first day of life. Pediatrics 1966; 37:1005-1007.
7. Euler AR, Byrne WJ, Meis PJ, Leake RD, Ament ME. Basal and pentagastrin-stimulated acid secretion in newborn human infants. Pediatr Res 1979; 13:36-37.
8. Grand RJ, Watkins JB, Torti FM. Development of the human gastrointestinal tract. A review. Gastroenterology 1976; 70:790-810.
9. Zoppi G, Andreotti G, Payno-Ferrara F, Nyai DM, Gaburro D. Exocrine pancrease function in premature and full-term neonates. Pediatr Res 1972; 6:880-886.
10. Lieberman J. Proteolytic enzyme activity in fetal pancreas and meconium. Gastroenterology 1966; 50:183-190.
11. Scammon RE, Kittleson JA. The growth of the gastrointestinal tract of the human fetus. Proc Soc Exp Biol Med 1926; 24:303-307.
12. Lipkin M. Proliferation and differentiation of gastrointestinal cells. Physiol Rev 1973; 53:891-915.
13. Melander A, Danielson K, Hanson A, Jansson L, Renup C, Schersten B, Thulin T, Walin E. Reduction of isoniazid bioavailability in normal men by concomitant intake of food. Acta Med Scand 1976; 20:93-97.
14. Neu HC. Antimicrobiol activity and human pharmacology of amoxicillin. J Infect Dis 1974; 129(Suppl):123-131.
15. Melander A, Kahlmeter G, Kamme C, Ursing B. Bioavailability of metronidazole in fasting and non-fasting healthy subjects and in patients with Crohn's disease. Eur J Clin Pharmacol 1977; 12:69-72.
16. Jordan MC, Moine J, Kirby W. Clinical pharmacology of pirampicillin as compared with ampicillin. Antimicrob Agents Chemother 1970; 2:438-441.
17. Bates TR, Segueiras, Tembo AV. Effect of food on nitrofurantoin absorption. Clin Pharmacol Ther 1974; 16:63-68.
18. Kappas A, Anderson KE, Conney AH, Alveras AP. Influence of dietary protein and carbohydrate on antipyrine and theophylline metabolism in man. Clin Pharmacol Ther 1976; 20:643-653.
19. Wettrell G, Andersson KE, Nyberg L. Effect of exchange transfusion on the elimination of digoxin in neonates. Eur J Clin Pharmacol 1976; 10:25-29.
20. Cassady G. Plasma volume studies in low birth weight infants. Pediatrics 1966; 38:1020-1027.
21. Usher R, Shepherd M, Lind J. The blood volume of the newborn infant and placental transfusion. Acta Pediatr Scand 1963; 52:497-512.
22. Friis-Hansen B. Body water compartment in children: changes during growth and related changes in body composition. Pediatrics 1961; 28:169-181.
23. Brans YW, Milstead RR, Bailey PE, Cassady G. Blood-volume estimates in Coombs-test positive infants. N Engl J Med 1974; 290:1450-1452.
24. Craig WA, Welling PG. Protein binding of antimicrobials. In: Gibaldi M, Prescott L, eds. Handbook of clinical pharmacokinetics. New York: Adis Health Science Press, 1983: 55.
25. Ehrnebo M, Agurell S, Jalling B. Age differences in drug binding by plasma protein: studies on human fetuses, neonates and adults. Eur J Clin Pharmacol 1971; 3:189-193.
26. Rane A, Lude PK, Jalling B, Yaffe SJ, Sjoqvist F. Plasma protein binding of diphenylhydantoin in normal and hyperbilirubinemic infant. J Pediatr 1971; 78:877-882.
27. Piasky KM. Disease-induced changes in the plasma binding of basic drugs. Clin Pharmacokinet 1980; 5:246-262.
28. Silverman WA, Anderson DH, Blanc WA, et al. A difference in mortality rate and incidence of kernicterus among premature infants allotted to two prophylactic antibacterial regimens. Pediatrics 1956; 18:614-625.
29. Okey AB, Roberts EA, Harper PA, Denison MS. Induction of drug-metabolizing enzymes: mechanisms and consequences. Clin Biochem 1986; 19:132-141.
30. Weiss CF, Glazko AJ, Weston JK. Chloramphenicol in the newborn infant: a physiological explanation of its toxicity when given in excessive doses. N Engl J Med 1960; 262:787-794.
31. Kent SP, Wideman GL. Prophylactic antibiotic therapy in infants born after premature rupture of membranes. JAMA 1959; 171:1199-1203.
32. Boutroy MJ, Vert P, Royer RJ, Monin P, Royer-Morrot MJ. Caffeine, a metabolite of theophylline during the treatment of apnea in the premature infant. J Pediatr 1979; 94:996-998.
33. Tserng KJ, King KC, Takieodine FN. Theophylline metabolism in premature infants. Clin Pharmacol Ther 1981; 29:595-600.
34. Lambert GH, Schoeller DA, Kotake AN, Flores C, Hay D. The effect of age, gender and sexual maturation on the caffeine breath test. Devel Pharmacol Ther 1986; 9:375-388.
35. Lambert GH, Kotake AN, Schoeller D. The CO_2 breath test as monitors of the cytochrome P-450 dependent mixed function monoxygenase system. In: MacLeod, Okey, Spielberg, eds. Developmental pharmacology. New York: Alan R. Liss, 1983: 119.
36. Potter EL. Development of the human glomerulus. Arch Pathol 1965; 80:241-255.
37. MacDonald MS, Emery JL. The late intrauterine and postnatal development of human renal glomeruli. J Anat 1959; 93:331-340.
38. Leak RD, Trygstad CW, Oh W. Inulin clearance in the newborn infant: relationship to gestational and postnatal age. Pediatr Res 1976; 10:759-762.
39. Calcagno PL, Rubin MI. Renal extraction of PAH in infants and children. J Clin Invest 1963; 42:1632-1639.
40. Roberts RJ. Intravenous administration of medication in pediatric patients, problems and solutions. Pediatr Clin North Am 1981; 28:23-34.
41. Rajchgot P, Radde IC, MacLeod SM. Influence of specific gravity on intravenous drug delivery. J Pediatr 1981; 99:658-661.
42. Gershanik JJ, Boecler G, Ensley H, McCloskey S, George W. The gasping syndrome and benzyl alcohol poisoning. N Engl J Med 1982; 307:1384-1388.
43. Hiller JL, Benda GI, Rahatzad M, Allen JR, Culver DH, Carlson CV, Reynold JW. Benzyl alcohol toxicity: impact on mortality and intraventricular hemorrhage among very low birth weight infants. Pediatrics 1986; 77:500-506.
44. Benda GI, Hiller JL, Reynolds JW. Benzyl alcohol toxicity: impact on neurologic handicaps among surviving very low birth weight infants. Pediatrics 1986; 77:507-512.
45. Alade SL, Brown RE, Paquet A. Polysorbate 80 and E-Ferol toxicity. Pediatrics 1986; 77:593-597.
46. Unusual syndrome with fatalities among premature infants: association with new intravenous vitamin E product. MMWR 1984; 33:198-199.
47. Bodenstein CH. Intravenous vitamin E and deaths in the intensive care unit. (Letter) Pediatrics 1984; 73:733.

48. Lorch V, Murphy MD, Hoersten LR, Harris E, Fitzgerald J, Sinha SW. Unusual syndrome among premature infants: association with a new intravenous vitamin E product. Pediatrics 1985; 75:598–602.
49. Vining EP, Mellits ED, Dorsen MM, Cataldo MF, Quaskey SA, Spielberg SP, Freeman JM. Psychologic and behavioral effects of antiepileptic drugs in children: a double-blind comparison between phenobarbital and valproic acid. Pediatrics 1987; 80:165–174.

PART 2

Pharmacologic Treatment of Inflammatory Bowel Disease

Anne M. Griffiths, M.D., FRCPC

Drugs constitute the mainstay of treatment of ulcerative colitis and Crohn's disease, although nutritional therapy is becoming an increasingly used alternative in the latter. Controlled clinical trials are the best means of validating treatment in conditions with such variable natural history and potential to remit spontaneously. This chapter reviews the pharmacologic agents currently used in inflammatory bowel disease, systematically discussing the pharmacokinetics, mode of action, clinical use, limitations, and toxicity of each. Such data are usually established among adults; there are few specifically pediatric studies. Table 1 provides a guide to drug selection, based on the nature and localization of disease.

SULFASALAZINE

The therapeutic efficacy of sulfasalazine, or salicylazosulfapyridine, in ulcerative colitis was rather fortuitously discovered over 40 years ago. Dr. Nanna Svartz encouraged the development of such a combination of a salicylate with its

TABLE 1
Pharmacologic Treatment of Inflammatory Bowel Disease

	Treatment of Active Disease	Maintenance of Remission
Ulcerative colitis	Sulphasalazine[11,12] Oral 5-ASA (Asacol[36] Dipentum,[37] Pentasa)* Corticosteroids[12,58] 5-ASA enemas (left-sided disease)[51,52] Cortenemas (distal disease)[68]	Sulphasalazine[14–16] Oral 5-ASA (Pentasa,[39] Asacol,[38,41] Dipentum[37]) 5-ASA enemas[54]
Crohn's disease		
Small bowel only	Corticosteroids[19,21] ?Oral 5-ASA (especially Pentasa or Salofalk)* 6MP[81]/?azathioprine†	?6MP/azathioprine[83]
Colon only	Sulphasalazine[19,21] ?Oral 5-ASA (Pentasa, Asacol, Dipentum)* Metronidazole[20] Corticosteroids[21] ?5-ASA enemas* 6MP[81]/?azathioprine†	?6MP/azathioprine[83]
Ileocolonic	(same as for small bowel *and* colon)	?6MP/azathioprine[83]
Perianal	Metronidazole[73] 6MP[82]/?azathioprine	

*Not subjected to controlled clinical trial.
†For treatment of chronically active disease.
5-ASA = 5 aminosalicylic acid; 6MP = 6-mercaptopurine.

anti-inflammatory properties and a sulfa drug with its antibacterial action. Although early trials did not establish the intended beneficial effect in rheumatoid arthritis, patients with arthritis associated with colitis, when given sulfasalazine, experienced substantial improvement in their bowel symptoms as well as their joints.[1]

Sulfasalazine is an acid azo compound of 5-aminosalicylic acid and sulfapyridine.[2,3] Sulfasalazine is absorbed from the upper intestinal tract. The maximum blood concentration is reached 3 to 5 hours after ingestion. Most returns to the gastrointestinal (GI) tract in bile. There is net absorption of only 10 to 20 percent, the remainder reaching the colon intact. Colonic bacteria cleave the diazo bond, liberating sulfapyridine and 5-aminosalicylic acid. Variations in intestinal flora and colonic transit time may influence this critical step. Sulfapyridine is largely (95 percent) absorbed, whereas two-thirds of the released 5-aminosalicylic acid stays in the colon to be excreted in the feces.

The absorbed sulfapyridine, like other sulfonamides, undergoes acetylation, hydroxylation, and glucuronidation in the liver and is excreted in the urine in the form of these metabolites or in its free form. The efficiency of acetylation is genetically determined. Slow acetylators have higher serum (and urine) levels of free sulfapyridine than do rapid acetylators.

The pioneer experiments of Azad Khan in Truelove's laboratory[4] and subsequent corroborative studies[5,6] have established 5-aminosalicylic acid as the therapeutically active component of sulfasalazine. The important action occurs locally. Sulfapyridine functions only as the carrier responsible for the delivery of the active moiety to the colon. The exact means by which 5-aminosalicylic acid impedes the inflammatory process in the intestinal mucosa is uncertain. Most significance is currently attributed to its interference, via the cyclo-oxygenase and lipoxygenase pathways of arachidonic acid metabolism, with prostaglandin and more importantly leukotriene biosynthesis.[7,8] Further modification of neutrophil-mediated tissue damage via interference with oxygen free radical production and myeloperoxidase activity may also be important.[9,10]

Sulfasalazine has been demonstrated in controlled trials to be useful in the treatment of active ulcerative colitis[11-13] and in the maintenance of remission.[14-16] These studies in adults suggest that a 60 to 70 percent response rate can be anticipated in the treatment of mild and moderate attacks of ulcerative colitis and that maintenance treatment reduces the 60 to 70 percent natural relapse rate to approximately 30 percent. In the treatment of active disease, resolution of symptoms, where achieved, occurs after a mean time of 3 to 4 weeks. Optimum dose represents a balance between efficacy and toxicity, both of which are dose-dependent. Reviews of treatment in adults generally cite a total daily dose of 4 g divided into four doses only for the treatment of active disease and a reduced dose of 2 g daily as optimal for maintenance of remission.[17] For children and adolescents who have not reached adult size, a therapeutic dose range of 50 to 75 mg per kilogram per day is generally advised.[18] A gradual increase from an initial low dose to maximum over a week may be rewarded with better tolerance and identify drug allergy early. Oral sulfasalazine is often used in addition to systemic corticosteroids in treating acute attacks of ulcerative colitis, but there have been no controlled trials to document such an adjunctive effect.

The role of sulfasalazine for treating Crohn's disease is less clear-cut. The American National Cooperative Crohn's Disease Study (NCCDS) demonstrated clinical response to a daily dose of 1 g per 15 kg body weight (maximum 5 g) in active ileocolic and colonic disease but not when disease was confined to the small bowel.[19] The Cooperative Crohn's Disease Study in Sweden[20] and the European Cooperative Crohn's Disease Study (ECCDS)[21] likewise found small bowel disease to be refractory to treatment with sulfasalazine. This is generally attributed to the important role of colonic bacteria in liberating the therapeutically active 5-aminosalicylic acid moiety from the parent drug. A small double-blind placebo-controlled trial conducted in adults in Holland with a higher dose of 4 to 6 g daily stands alone in finding sulfasalazine effective in reducing inflammatory activity irrespective of the intestinal localization of disease.[22] It is argued in this report that patients with small bowel Crohn's disease may have bacterial overgrowth, which facilitates cleavage of the diazo bond before the colon is reached. Both the NCCDS (using 0.5 g per 15 kg body weight, maximum 2.5 g daily) and the ECCDS (using 3 g daily) failed to find a beneficial effect for sulfasalazine in reducing the relapse rate among patients with inactive Crohn's disease.

Unfortunately, many patients with acute ulcerative colitis or Crohn's disease, particularly involving the small bowel, fail to respond to sulfasalazine. Furthermore, 20 to 25 percent of treated patients experience adverse drug reactions that either limit its dosage or preclude its use entirely.[23,24] Most undesirable effects, both dose-related and idiosyncratic, seem attributable to the sulfapyridine component.[25]

A serum total sulfapyridine concentration of greater than 50 μg per milliliter has been associated with the onset of dose-dependent side effects.[25] These include nausea, vomiting, headaches, and mild hemolysis. The dose of sulfasalazine at which such reactions occur varies between individuals, partly reflecting acetylator status and its effect on sulfapyridine metabolism.[25] Dyspeptic symptoms may resolve with the use of an enteric-coated preparation. Temporary interruption in therapy followed by a more gradual increase in dosage may avoid a recurrence of dose-dependent adverse effects. Glucose-6-phosphate dehydrogenase deficiency aggravates hemolysis and is therefore a contraindication to sulfasalazine administration.

Idiosyncratic adverse reactions demand cessation of therapy rather than dose reduction. These, fortunately, are much less common than the dose-dependent effects and usually occur at the initiation of therapy.[23] Fever, various exanthems including a severe exfoliative dermatitis, Stevens-Johnson syndrome, pulmonary complications, hepatotoxicity, pancreatitis, an exacerbation of colitic symptoms,[26] and, very rarely, agranulocytosis have all been reported. A known hypersensitivity to sulfonamides is a contraindication to sulfasalazine therapy. Sulfasalazine is now recognized to reversibly impair male fertility.[27] Sperm morphology and motility revert to normal after discontinuation of the drug.[28] Sulfasalazine impedes folate absorption[29] but not significantly enough to justify routine supplementation.[17]

ORAL 5-AMINOSALICYLIC ACID

The recognition of oral 5-aminosalicylic acid (5-ASA) as the therapeutically active component of sulfasalazine led to attempts to eliminate the sulfa carrier, thereby improving tolerance. Alternate delivery systems have been developed to facilitate transport and release of 5-ASA distally. 5-ASA ingested in a nonprotected form is rapidly absorbed in the proximal small intestine.[30] The plethora of oral 5-ASA analogues now available differ importantly with respect to the mechanism[31-35] and site of 5-ASA release; this in turn determines their potential usefulness. Similarly, lack of response may indicate inadequate release, necessitating use of a different preparation.

Table 2 lists the oral 5-ASA preparations currently in clinical use. Availability varies in different parts of the world. These analogues are best understood in three groups. First, *olsalazine*, in which 5-ASA is attached to a second molecule of itself, depends, like sulfasalazine, on bacterial cleavage of the azo bond. Second, the delayed-release preparations, known collectively as *mesalazine*, employ different acrylic-based resins, designed to break at a set pH, thereby making 5-ASA available to the intestinal mucosa. Finally, the timed-release formulation *Pentasa* contains 5-ASA in microgranules coated with a semipermeable membrane of ethyl cellulose. Release occurs continually but at a rate affected by pH. In aqueous solution ethyl cellulose has amphoionic properties that allow dissolution in acid and alkaline media.

The site of intestinal release of 5-ASA can be predicted to be colon for olsalazine, distal ileum or right colon for some mesalazine preparations (Asacol, Rowasa), mid-small bowel for others (Salofalk, Claversal), and continually throughout the gut, beginning in the proximal intestine, for timed-release 5-ASA (Pentasa). A mean of 19 percent (range 8 to 28 percent) of the ingested dose of Pentasa is still in the nonreleased form in ileostomy effluents.

The fate of 5-ASA released from any of these delivery systems is similar. Acetylation may occur in the intestinal mucosa. Both 5-ASA and acetyl-5-ASA (Ac-5-ASA) are recovered from feces. Whether both are therapeutically active has not been verified. Absorbed 5-ASA may also be acetylated in the liver uninfluenced by acetylator phenotype. Ac-5-ASA predominates over free 5-ASA in the circulation. Acetylated 5-ASA is greater than 80 percent bound to plasma proteins and secreted into the urine by the renal tubules. Renal clearance rates exceed glomerular filtration rates.

The percentage of systemic absorption varies with the different delivery systems, being greatest (60 percent) for Pentasa (35 percent by the small intestine plus 25 percent by the colon). Plasma Ac-5-ASA is detectable 30 minutes after ingestion of Pentasa and peaks within 2 to 5 hours. With Asacol and Rowasa 5-ASA and Ac-5-ASA become detectable in plasma 2 hours after ingestion. Percentage absorption determined by urinary recovery averages 34 to 44 percent, seemingly lower at higher doses, perhaps suggesting a limit to the colon's absorptive capacity. With the other mesalazine preparations (Salofalk and Claversal), 5-ASA appears in plasma 1 hour after ingestion. Absorption averages 44 percent. Systemic absorption of 5-ASA and Ac-5-ASA from olsalazine has been estimated to vary between 20 and 40 percent.

5-ASA formulations provide an alternative to sulfasalazine in the acute treatment of mild to moderate ulcerative colitis[37,38] and in the maintenance of remission.[39-42] The main advantage they offer is reduced toxicity. No studies suggest increased efficacy. The results of a number of clinical trials conducted in adults have now been published. No studies among children have as yet been completed. The efficacy of mesalazine (Asacol),[38,41] timed-release 5-ASA (Pentasa),[39] and olsalazine (Dipentum)[37] in maintaining remission has been found to be comparable to that of sulfasalazine. In a recent double-blind trial, olsalazine was significantly more effective than placebo in treating active disease,[37] but the

TABLE 2
Oral 5-ASA Analogues

Generic Name	Trade Name	Dosage Form	Formulation	Release Mechanism	Site of Release	Absorption
Olsalazine or disodium azodisalicylate	Dipentum	250-mg capsules	Two 5-ASA molecules in diazo linkage	Bacterial cleavage of diazo bond	Colon	20–40%
Mesalazine or mesalamine	Asacol Rowasa	400-mg tablets	5-ASA in acrylic resin coating (Eudragit S)	pH-dependent breakdown of resin	pH>7.0, i.e., distal ileum or right colon	34–44%
Mesalazine or mesalamine	Salofalk Claversal	250-mg tablets	5-ASA in ethyl cellulose membrane and acrylic resin (Eudragit L)	pH-dependent breakdown of resin	pH>5.6, i.e, from mid-small bowel distally	44%
Timed-release 5-ASA	Pentasa	250-mg tablets	5-ASA in microgranules coated with ethyl cellulose membrane	Timed release	Throughout small intestine and colon	60%

5-ASA = 5-aminosalicylic acid.

overall 35 percent response rate with olsalazine is rather disappointing. This study suggested a dose-response relationship, as did another double-blind placebo-controlled trial employing Asacol.[36] Therapy with 4.8 g daily resulted in complete response in 24 percent and partial response in 50 percent.[36] These studies suggest that the optimal dose of 5-ASA analogues has yet to be determined. This must certainly be true for children. The originally recommended dose of 30 mg per kilogram per day based on extrapolation from experience with sulfasalazine need not be considered a maximum. Doses of 50 to 60 mg per kilogram per day may often be required.

Studies of 5-ASA analogues in Crohn's disease are few. Pentasa, by virtue of its release profile, has the most potential to extend the scope of usefulness to small intestinal disease. The only open study published to date showed an improvement in 72 percent of a small group of patients with ileitis or ileocolitis treated for 6 weeks.[42] A double-blind trial of Salofalk versus sulfasalazine in treatment of 30 patients with active Crohn's disease (ileitis, ileocolitis, and colitis) documented comparable clinical improvement with both (87 percent versus 80 percent), but corticosteroids were necessary in nearly half of each group.[43] Certainly the efficacy of oral 5-ASA in Crohn's disease, although attractive, has yet to be well established, and again studies are needed to ascertain optimal doses.

It would appear from the now sizeable world experience with new 5-ASA formulations that the promise of diminished toxicity has been fulfilled.[45] 5-ASA is in general well tolerated by patients intolerant to sulfasalazine, although occasionally the same adverse reaction is observed.[40] Side effects are difficult to verify in open trials, and double-blind placebo-controlled trials suggest a very low incidence.[38,41,42] An exacerbation of colitic symptoms[45] and hair loss have been reported with 5-ASA.[46] In an open trial 12.5 percent of patients stopped olsalazine because of diarrhea,[40] but this side effect was not encountered significantly in a placebo-controlled trial.[37] In vitro studies suggest that the 5-ASA dimer is a potent secretagogue in the distal ileum.[47]

5-ASA is nephrotoxic in rats, but at doses that are 10 to 30 times higher than those given to man, resulting in plasma concentrations far higher than obtained in inflammatory bowel disease patients.[33] This potential needs to be borne in mind, however, particularly with the current trend to increase the administered dose.

Enemas containing 4 g of 5-ASA in a 60-ml suspension are available for rectal administration. ^{99m}Tc labeling studies in adults have demonstrated retrograde spread to the descending colon, and to the splenic flexure when the volume is increased to 100 ml.[48] Suppositories of 250 mg, well tolerated by even the youngest patients, have been similarly documented to distribute 5-ASA to the sigmoid colon and rectum.[49]

Absorption from the distal colon is slow and incomplete, implying a predominantly topical action.[51] Dose strength does not affect the rate of absorption, which is constant during the time that the enema is retained. This suggests a rate-limiting factor related either to drug solubilization or directly to the absorptive capacity of the distal bowel. Plasma levels reach a peak within 3 to 6 hours and are negligible after 24 hours. Most of the drug is present in the acetylated form and eliminated as such via the kidney. Total urinary recovery rates vary between only 7 and 20 percent of the administered dose, dependent directly on enema retention time. Higher-volume (lower-concentration) enemas may be held longer and consequently more completely absorbed.

The development of 5-ASA enemas has been an important advance in the management of distal and left-sided ulcerative colitis. Campieri et al found a 15-day course of nightly 5-ASA 4-g (100-ml) enemas more effective than 100-mg (100-ml) hydrocortisone enemas in the treatment of acute disease in 86 patients studied in double-blind fashion.[51] Topical therapy may be used alone as the first-line treatment of distal disease. North American studies and reports, however, emphasize the role of 5-ASA enemas in the management of the refractory patient. Efficacy rates average 50 to 75 percent in this category of patients with distal disease who have failed to respond to sulfasalazine, oral corticosteroids, or steroid enemas.[52] Relapse rate is high after cessation of therapy. Clinical studies have not yet determined whether a maintenance schedule of less frequent than nightly enemas[53] might be an effective and acceptable means of sustaining remission. There is no published experience with the use of topical 5-ASA therapy in Crohn's disease with left colonic involvement.

No information is currently available concerning the distribution or safety of 4-g 5-ASA enemas in children. The low systemic absorption suggests that the adult dosage should be safe. Comparative pharmacokinetic studies with different strength enemas are currently being conducted in young patients to determine whether lower dose formulations are preferable.

CORTICOSTEROIDS

Corticosteroids continue to be a mainstay of treatment of inflammatory bowel diseases. Their mode of action in these disorders is not precisely known but presumably relates to their inhibition of cell-mediated immunity and their anti-inflammatory effects.[54] The latter include decreased capillary permeability, impaired neutrophil and monocyte chemotaxis, and stabilization of lysosomal membranes. Release of arachidonate from phospholipids is blocked, meaning that less substrate is available for prostaglandin and leukotriene synthesis.

The commercially available glucocorticoids differ with respect to duration of action, relative glucocorticoid potency, and relative mineralocorticoid activity.[54] Oral prednisone in North America, the comparable prednisolone in Britain, and the slightly more potent methylprednisolone in Europe are favored in the treatment of Crohn's disease and ulcerative colitis. They offer the advantage of minimal mineralocorticoid effects unlike parenteral hydrocortisone used in the management of acute severe colitis. A discussion of the pharmacokinetics and toxicity of prednisone is given in Part 4 of this chapter.

In treating inflammatory bowel disease one must bear in mind the possibility of reduced absorption in patients with active Crohn's disease of the small intestine.[55] The concept that the effects of corticosteroids at the tissue level outlast drug concentrations in serum[54] is important to the derivation of treatment regimens. Intermittent rather than sustained high blood levels, as long as therapeutically efficacious, are preferable, by virtue of causing fewer side effects and less suppression of the hypothalamic-pituitary-adrenal axis. Alternate-day therapy is associated with fewer side effects in general and, importantly in children, does not inhibit linear growth.[56] Daily corticosteroids interfere with somatomedin activity, whereas alternate-day steroids do not.[57]

The classic controlled trial reported by Truelove and Witt in 1955[58] established the efficacy of oral corticosteroids in active ulcerative colitis. Clinical improvement was achieved in 70 percent of a group of patients with all grades of disease severity. Steroid use in active Crohn's disease of the ileum alone or ileum plus colon has been validated by the NCCDS[20] and ECCDS.[21] Disease confined to the colon, which was relatively refractory to glucocorticoid treatment in the former trial, appeared to benefit from combination therapy with sulfasalazine in the European study. Few attempts have been made to establish a relationship between dose and response in active disease.[59] The NCCDS titrated the dose of prednisone to the level of disease activity within a daily dose range of 0.25 to 0.75 mg per kilogram (maximum 60 mg). One study in adults with ulcerative colitis found little therapeutic benefit but greater toxicity with 60 mg versus 40 mg daily, whereas both were more effective than 20 mg.[60] A once-daily dose of prednisone appeared as effective as the same total dose divided throughout the day in the treatment of active colitis.[61]

Our practice for both active ulcerative colitis and active Crohn's disease has been to give prednisone 1 mg per kilogram once daily (maximum 40 to 60 mg) for 4 to 6 weeks, with subsequent tapering of the daily dose by 5 mg at weekly intervals. Others employ shorter full-dose therapy and more rapid tapering.

There is little justification from longitudinal placebo-controlled trials for the use of low-dose (less than 20 mg prednisone daily in adults) corticosteroids to prevent relapse in patients with inactive Crohn's disease[19] or ulcerative colitis.[62,63] One study in ulcerative colitis using a higher dose suggested a beneficial effect, but that was at the expense of significant side effects.[64] There are, however, patients with both conditions who have chronically active disease requiring continued corticosteroid suppression. In prepubertal patients any such long-term therapy should be with alternate-day steroids, which do not impede linear growth.

The use of corticosteroids in the setting of acute severe colitis deserves special attention. Parenteral steroids are generally employed in conjunction with bowel rest, although their superiority over oral glucocorticoids has not been tested. Controversy exists as to whether ACTH is more effective than hydrocortisone. Based on the most recent double-blind trial[65] comparing the two drugs given by continuous intravenous infusion and earlier studies,[66,67] there is no reason to consider the use of ACTH in patients with severe ulcerative colitis already on oral steroid therapy. However, for patients presenting without prior steroid use, the possibility remains that ACTH may be more effective.[65] ACTH makes pharmacologic concentrations of corticosteroids available to body tissues; there may be benefit to the mixture of glucocorticoids, mineralocorticoids, and androgens released.

Corticosteroid retention enemas are of proven efficacy in the treatment of distal and even left-sided ulcerative colitis[68] and are often used as adjunctive therapy in more extensive disease. Suppositories and foam preparations are of value in proctitis. The most commonly used enemas (hydrocortisone hemisuccinate or acetate and prednisolone 21-phosphate) are systemically absorbed, with the potential therefore for systemic side effects (and therapeutic effects) as well as local action. Of interest are two other groups of rectally instilled steroids: the poorly absorbed group with low systemic activity (e.g., prednisone meta-sulfobenzoate or beclomethasone dipropionate) and the absorbable tixocortol[69] pivalate, which has only local and no systemic effects by virtue of its rapid elimination. Tixocortol appears of comparable efficacy to hydrocortisone in clinical trials to date.[70,71]

METRONIDAZOLE

Metronidazole has been in clinical use as an antibacterial and antiprotozoal agent since 1960. It is usually well absorbed after oral administration; peak levels are achieved within 1 hour. The serum half-life of the drug is about 8 hours, and it penetrates well into all tissues and mucosal surfaces.

Metronidazole consists of an imidazole ring bearing a nitro group. Intermediates formed during partial reduction of the nitro group appear to be vital to all the biologic actions of the drug.[72] Oxidation of side chains and glucuronidation take place in the liver. Both unchanged metronidazole and several metabolites are excreted in the urine. Bacteria in the gut are also able to split the imidazole ring, giving rise to different intermediate products, which may have their own activity.

Apart from prior isolated observations, Bernstein et al in 1980 published the first report of the efficacy of metronidazole in chronic perineal Crohn's disease.[73] Eighty-three percent of 21 consecutive patients with a variety of perianal fistulas, rectovaginal and rectolabial fistulas, and unhealed perineal wounds experienced advanced or complete healing with administration of 20 mg per kilogram per day in three to five divided doses over 2 to 4 months. Subsequent follow-up[74] for as long as 36 months indicated that, although perianal disease seldom relapsed on full-dose therapy, reduction in dose or cessation of therapy was often associated with exacerbation. Metronidazole could be successfully discontinued in only 28 percent of patients. Reinstitution of the drug in those whose disease recurred was again associated with rapid healing.

Metronidazole is also used in the treatment of active intestinal Crohn's disease. Early reports of its usefulness have been followed by the larger Swedish co-operative study reported by Ursing and colleagues.[20] Metronidazole (0.8 g per day) was found to be at least as effective as sulfasalazine (3 g per day) in this double-blind crossover trial. Both drugs showed a less pronounced effect when the disease was located solely in the small intestine. The time required for a clinical improvement in the majority of patients was 1 month. Metronidazole has not been assessed in the treatment of ulcerative colitis.

The mode of action of metronidazole in Crohn's disease is uncertain. Its well-known antimicrobial effects against anaerobic bacteria may be important, but neither healing of perianal lesions nor improvement in clinical disease activity always correlates with reduction of *Bacteroides* and other anaerobic species.[74] Speculation as to an alternate mechanism of action has focused on the possible immunosuppressive action of metronidazole and on its influence on leukocyte chemotaxis.

Side effects of metronidazole include metallic taste, glossitis and furry tongue, dark urine, and occasional anorexia, nausea, and vomiting. Adolescents should be warned that it has a disulfiram-like effect with alcohol ingestion.[72]

Of more concern is the issue of peripheral neuropathy, which appears to be related to dosage and duration of therapy. It is stated to occur in adults only after a cumulative dose of greater than 30 g.[75] Metronidazole given in relatively low dose over 4 months as part of the Swedish co-operative study was associated with minor paresthesias on specific questioning in only two of 78 patients.[20] In contrast, Brandt et al noted paresthesias in 50 percent of their patients treated with 20 mg per kilogram per day for 6 months.[74] In some these were alleviated simply by dose reduction. Objective electrophysiologic testing of sural nerve function in children and adolescents documented a high (54 percent) prevalence of peripheral sensory neuropathy.[76] Metronidazole had been administered for a mean of 7 months (range 4 to 11 months) at a dose of 10 to 33 mg per kilogram per day (mean 19 mg per kilogram per day) at the time of these nerve conduction studies. Experimental studies suggest that metronidazole or a metabolite binds to neuronal RNA, thereby inhibiting protein synthesis and resulting in axonal degeneration.[77] Electron microscopic studies of human sural nerve biopsies in two patients have shown loss of myelinated fibers and wallerian degeneration.[78] Clinical experience to date suggests that paresthesias always resolve, albeit at times very slowly over up to 2 years, following discontinuation of the drug.[74-76] The course of the peripheral neuropathy in the face of continued therapy is not known.

Another concern with long-term metronidazole therapy arises from its potential mutagenic and carcinogenic effects. Metronidazole has been shown to be mutagenic for a variety of bacteria and carcinogenic for mice and rats.[72] The available long-term follow-up studies on humans previously exposed to metronidazole are not completely reassuring as, in general, use was short-term in the setting of a specific infection. No increase in the frequency of chromosomal aberrations with metronidazole was detected during the course of the Swedish co-operative study,[20] although an earlier report by the same group had raised that concern.[79]

AZATHIOPRINE AND 6-MERCAPTOPURINE

Azathioprine is a chemical analogue and consequently an antagonist of the physiologic purines. It is metabolized in vivo to mercaptopurine. Both drugs have immunosuppressive activity. Their related structure and metabolism lead one to anticipate similar clinical effects, but few direct comparative studies exist.

The NCCDS[19] found azathioprine no more effective than placebo in treating active disease or in maintaining remission. This and other negative studies are criticized by failure either to continue therapy for long enough[80] or to employ the optimal dosage (2 mg per kilogram per day). The strongest validation of 6-mercaptopurine (6MP) comes from the long-term randomized double-blind placebo-controlled crossover trial of Present et al.[81] Sixty-seven percent of chronically ill patients experienced improvement in their disease with 6MP at a dose of 1.5 mg per kilogram per day. The mean time until clinical improvement was 3.1 months (range 1 to 9 months). The same group of investigators has also reported on the specific usefulness of this drug in perianal and enteric fistulous disease.[82] Furthermore, O'Donoghue et al found a significantly increased risk of disease recrudescence when azathioprine therapy was withdrawn from patients who had achieved remission through its use.[83]

Those who have questioned the role of azathioprine and 6MP in the treatment of inflammatory bowel disease[84] have done so in part because of conflicting results of clinical trials and in part because of apprehension about long-term toxicity. The latter concern particularly influences pediatric gastroenterologists. Kinlen et al have estimated the risk of malignant disease in patients given azathioprine for nontransplant noncancer indications to be increased 1.6-fold.[85] Although small, such a risk must figure in decisions to treat young patients with inflammatory bowel disease

Short-term toxicity is more easily documented. Overall, about 10 percent of patients need to stop the drug.[81] Although intermittent leukopenia is common, significant bone marrow depression should not supervene, provided that dosage and monitoring are appropriate. White blood cell counts are checked at weekly intervals initially until stability is assured. The incidence of superinfections in adult patients with inflammatory bowel disease taking 6MP has been reported by the Present group to be less than 2 percent. The most common early adverse reaction is pancreatitis, with an incidence of 3.25 percent.[86] It almost always occurs within the first few weeks of starting therapy and resolves with its discontinuation. Other less common reactions include fever, joint pains, and hepatitis.

In spite of these problems, most regard azathioprine and 6MP as effective adjunctive treatments, justified in the management of patients with extensive, chronically active Crohn's disease,[84] even in a pediatric population. Their use may allow reduction of an otherwise intolerably high dose of steroids. Their use in young patients with ulcerative colitis cannot be endorsed in the same way because of the alternative of cure offered by colectomy. Chronic localized Crohn's disease is also preferably treated by resection, even though it is not curative. Our practice in a select subgroup of children and adolescents with chronic, severe steroid-dependent ileocolonic or colonic Crohn's disease is to employ azathioprine or 6MP, if beneficial, for 12 to 18 months and then to attempt discontinuation.

FUTURE DIRECTIONS

The observed effectiveness of anti-inflammatory and immunosuppressive drugs in ulcerative colitis and Crohn's disease may serve as a clue to the etiology and pathogenesis of these disorders. Research into the mechanism of action of sulfasalazine and 5-aminosalicylic acid has led to an understanding of the pathophysiology of intestinal inflammation. As this work continues, specific inhibitors of individual leukotrienes may prove to be useful pharmacologic agents. Recently, cyclosporine has been introduced into the therapeutic armamentarium for Crohn's disease. The response rate of acute disease in open trials has been encouraging.[87,88] Cyclosporine allows the expansion of suppressor T-lymphocyte populations while selectively inhibiting helper T-lymphocyte production of interleukin-2 essential for B-lymphocyte and cytotoxic T-lymphocyte differentiation and proliferation.[89] Again, confirmation of its benefit in the chronic inflammatory bowel diseases may eventually lead to a better elucidation of the immune regulatory dysfunction, thought to be important at least in their perpetuation.

REFERENCES

1. Svartz N. Salazopyrin, a new sulfanilamide preparation. Acta Med Scand 1942; 110:557–590.
2. Schroeder H, Campbell DES. Absorption, metabolism and excretion of salicylazosulfapyridine in man. Clin Pharmacol Ther 1972; 13: 539–551.
3. Goldman P, Peppercorn MA. Drug therapy. Sulfasalazine. N Engl J Med 1975; 293:202–203.
4. Azad Khan AK, Piris J, Truelove SC. An experiment to determine the active therapeutic moiety of sulphasalazine. Lancet 1977; ii:892–895.
5. Van Hees PAM, Bakker JH, van Tongeren JHM. Effect of sulphapyridine, 5-aminosalicylic acid and placebo in patients with idiopathic proctitis: a study to determine the active therapeutic moiety of sulphasalazine. Gut 1980; 21:632–635.
6. Klotz U, Maier K, Fischer C, Heinkel K. Therapeutic efficacy of sulfasalazine and its metabolites in patients with ulcerative colitis and Crohn's disease. N Engl J Med 1980; 303:1499–1502.
7. Stenson WF, Lobos E. Sulfasalazine inhibits the synthesis of chemotactic lipids by neutrophils. J Clin Invest 1982; 69:494–497.
8. Donowitz M. Arachidonic acid metabolites and their role in inflammatory bowel disease. Gastroenterology 1985; 88:580–587.
9. Miyachi Y, Yoshioka A, Imamura S, Niwa Y. Effect of sulphasalazine and its metabolites on the generation of reactive oxygen species. Gut 1987; 28:190–195.
10. von Ritter C, Grisham MB, Granger DN. Sulfasalazine metabolites and dapsone attenuate formyl-methionyl-leucyl-phenylalamine induced mucosal injury in rat ileum. Gastroenterology 1989; 96:811–816.
11. Baron JH, Connell AM, Lennard-Jones JE. Sulphasalazine and salicylazosulphadimine in ulcerative colitis. Lancet 1962; i:1094–1096.
12. Truelove SC, Watkinson G, Draper G. Comparison of corticosteroid and sulfasalazine therapy in ulcerative colitis. Br Med J 1962; 2:1708–1711.
13. Dick AP, Grayson JJ, Carpenter RG. Controlled trial of sulfasalazine in the treatment of ulcerative colitis. Gut 1964; 5:437–442.
14. Dissanayake AS, Truelove SC. A controlled therapeutic trial of long-term maintenance treatment of ulcerative colitis with sulfasalazine. Gut 1973; 14:923–962.
15. Misiewicz JJ, Lennard Jones JE, Connell JE. Controlled trial of sulfasalazine in maintenance therapy for ulcerative colitis. Lancet 1965; i:185–188.
16. Riis P, Anthonisen P, Wilff HR, Falkenborg O, Bonnevie O, Burder V. The prophylactic effect of salazosulphapyridine in ulcerative colitis during longterm treatment. A double-blind trial on patients asymptomatic for one year. Scand J Gastroenterol 1973; 8:71–74.
17. Azad Khan Ak, Howes DT, Piris J, Truelove SC. Optimum dose of sulphasalazine for maintenance treatment in ulcerative colitis. Gut 1980; 21:232–240.
18. Goldstein PD, Alpers DH, Keating JP. Sulfapyridin metabolites in children with inflammatory bowel disease receiving Sulfasalazine. J Pediatr 1979; 95:638–640.
19. Sumers RW, Switz DM, Sessions JT, Becktel JM, Best WR, Kern F, Singleton JW. National cooperative Crohn's disease study: results of drug treatment. Gastroenterology 1979; 77:847–869.
20. Rosen A, Ursing B, Alm T, Barany F, Bergelin I, Ganrot-Norlin K, Hoevels J, Huitfeldt B, Jarnerot G, Krause U, Krook A, Lindstrom B, Nordle O. Comparative study of metronidazole and sulfasalazine for active Crohn's disease. The cooperative Crohn's disease study in Sweden. II. Result. Gastroenterology 1982; 83:550–562.
21. Malchow H, Ewe K, Brandes JW, Goebell H, Ehms H, Sommer H, Jesdnisky H. European cooperative Crohn's disease study: results of drug treatment. Gastroenterology 1984; 86:249–266.
22. Van Hees PAM, Van Lier HJJ, Van Elteren PH, Driessen WMM, van Hogezend RA, Ren Velde GPM, Bakker JH, van Tongeran JHM. Effect of sulfasalazine in patients with active Crohn's disease. A controlled double-blind study. Gut 1981; 22:404–409.
23. Taffet SL, Das KM. Sulfasalazine. Adverse effects and desensitization. Dig Dis Sci 1983; 28:833–842.
24. Collins JR. Adverse reactions to salicylazosulfapyridine (Azulfidine) in the treatment of ulcerative colitis. South Med J 1968; 61:354–358.
25. Das KM, Eastwood MA, McManus JPA, Sircus W. Adverse reactions during salicylazosulfapyridine therapy and the relation with drug metabolism and acetylator phenotype. N Engl J Med 1973; 289:491–495.
26. Werlin SL, Grand RJ. Bloody diarrhea—a new complication of sulfasalazine. J Pediatr 1978; 92:450–451.
27. Birnie GG, McLeod T, Watkinson G. Incidence of sulfasalazine induced male infertility. Gut 1981; 22:452–455.
28. Toth A. Reversible toxic effect of salicylazosulfapyridine on semen quality. Fertil Steril 1979; 31:538–540.
29. Franklin JL, Rosenberg IH. Impaired folic acid absorption in inflammatory bowel disease: effects of salicylazosulfapyridine. Gastroenterology 1973; 64:517–523.
30. Nielsen OH, Bondesen S. Kinetics of 5-aminosalicylic acid after jejunal instillation in man. Br J Clin Pharmacol 1983; 16:738–740.
31. Friedman G. Sulfasalazine and new analogues. Am J Gastroenterol 1986; 81:141–144.
32. Bondesen S, Rasmussen SN, Rask-Madsen J, Nielsen OH, Lauritsen K, Binder V, Hansen SH, Hvidberg EF. 5-Aminosalicylic acid in the treatment of inflammatory bowel disease. Acta Med Scand 1987; 221:227–242.
33. Rasmussen SN, Bondesen S, Hvidberg EF, Hansen SH, Binder V, Halskov S, Flachs H. 5-Aminosalicylic acid in a slow-release preparation: bioavailability, plasma level and excretion in humans. Gastroenterology 1982; 83:1062–1070.
34. Dew MJ, Hughes PJ, Lee MG, Evans BK, Rhodes J. An oral preparation to release drugs in the human colon. Br J Clin Pharmacol 1982; 14:405–408.
35. Van Hogezand RA, Van Hees PAM, Zwanenburg B, van Rossum JM, van Tongeren JHM. Disposition of disodium azodisalicylate in healthy subjects. Gastroenterology 1985; 88:717–722.
36. Schroeder KW, Tremaine WJ, Ilstrup DM. Coated oral 5-aminosalicylic acid for mildly to moderately active ulcerative colitis. A randomized study. N Engl J Med 1987; 371:1625–1629.
37. Meyers S, Sachar DB, Present DH, Janowitz HD. Olsalazine sodium in the treatment of ulcerative colitis among patients intolerant of sulfasalazine. Gastroenterology 1987; 93:1255–1262.
38. Dew MJ, Hughes P, Harries AD, Williams C, Evans BK, Rhodes J. Maintenance of remission in ulcerative colitis with 5-aminosalicylic acid in high dose by mouth. Br Med J 1983; 287:23–24.
39. Mulder CJ, Tytgat GNJ, Weterman IT, Dekker W, Blok P, Schrijner M, van der Heide H. Double blind comparison of slow-release 5-aminosalicylate and sulfasalazine in remission maintenance in ulcerative colitis. Gastroenterology 1988; 95:1449–1453.
40. Sandberg-Gertzen H, Jarnerot G, Kraaz W. Azodisal sodium in the treatment of ulcerative colitis. A study of tolerance and relapse-prevention properties. Gastroenterology 1986; 90:1024–1030.
41. Riley SA, Mani V, Goodman MJ, Herd ME, Dutt S, Turnberg LA. Comparison of delayed-release 5-aminosalicylic acid (mesalazine) and sulfasalazine as maintenance treatment for patients with ulcerative colitis. Gastroenterology 1988; 94:1383–1389.
42. Rasmussen SN, Binder V, Maier K, Bondesen S, Fischer C, Klotz U, Hansen SH, Hvidberg EF. Treatment of Crohn's disease with peroral 5-aminosalicylic acid. Gastroenterology 1983; 85:1350–1353.
43. Maier K, Fruhmorgen P, Bode CJ. Successful management of chronic

inflammatory gut disease with oral 5-aminosalicylic acid. Dtsch Med Wochenschr 1986; 95:1677–1683.
44. Peppercorn MA. Update on the aminosalicylic acid: a promise fulfilled. Gastroenterology 1988; 95:1672–1683.
45. Austin CA, Caun PA, Jones TH, Holdsworth CD. Exacerbation of diarrhea and pain in patients treated with 5-aminosalicylic acid for ulcerative colitis. Lancet 1984; 1:917–918.
46. Kutty PK, Raman KRK, Hawken K. Hair loss and 5-ASA enemas. Ann Intern Med 1982; 97:785–786.
47. Pamukcu R, Hanauer S, Chang EB. Effect of disodium azodisalicylate on electrolyte transport in rabbit ileum and colon in vitro. Gastroenterology 1988; 95:975–981.
48. Campieri M, Lanfranchi GA, Bazzocchi G. Retrograde spread of 5-aminosalicylic acid enemas in patients with active ulcerative colitis. Dis Colon Rectum 1986; 29:108–110.
49. Williams CN, Haber G, Aquino JA. Double-blind placebo-controlled evaluation of 5-ASA suppositories in active distal proctitis. Dig Dis Sci 1987; 32:71S–75S.
50. Campieri M, Lanfranchi GA, Boschi S. Topical administration of 5-aminosalicylic acid enemas in patients with ulcerative colitis. Studies on rectal absorption and excretion. Gut 1985; 26:400–405.
51. Campieri M, Lanfranchi GA, Bazzocchi G. Treatment of ulcerative colitis with high-dose 5-aminosalicylic acid enemas. Lancet 1981; ii:270–271.
52. Barber GB, Lee DE, Antarioli DA, Peppercorn MA. Refractory distal ulcerative colitis responsive to 5-aminosalicylate enemas. Am J Gastroenterol 1985; 80:612–614.
53. Biddle WL, Greenberger NJ, Swan JT. 5-Aminosalicylic acid enemas: effective agent in maintaining remission in left-sided ulcerative colitis. Gastroenterology 1988; 94:1075–1079.
54. Axelrod L. Glucocorticoid therapy. Medicine 1976; 55:39–65.
55. Shaffer JL, Williams SE, Turnberg LA, Houston JB, Rowland M. Absorption of prednisolone in patients with Crohn's disease. Gut 1983; 24:182–186.
56. Soyka LF. Alternate-day corticosteroid therapy. Adv Pediatr 1972; 19:47–70.
57. Elders JM, Wingfield BS, McNatt Ml, Clarke JS, Hughes ER. Glucocorticoid therapy in children. Effect on somatomedin secretion. Am J Dis Child 1975; 129:1393–1396.
58. Truelove SC, Witt LJ. Cortisone in ulcerative colitis: final report of a therapeutic trial. Br Med J 1955; 2:1041–1048.
59. Lennard-Jones JE. Toward optimal use of corticosteroids in ulcerative colitis and Crohn's disease. Gut 1983; 24:177–181.
60. Baron JH, Connell AM, Kanaghinis TG, Lennard-Jones JE, Jones FA. Out-patient treatment of ulcerative colitis: comparison between three doses of oral prednisone. Br Med J 1962; 2:441–443.
61. Powell-Tuck J, Boun RL, Lennard-Jones JE. Comparison of oral prednisolone given as single or multiple daily doses for active proctocolitis. Scand J Gastroenterol 1978; 13:833–837.
62. Truelove SC, Witts LH. Cortisone and corticotrophin in ulcerative colitis. Br Med J 1959; 1:387–394.
63. Lennard-Jones JE, Misiewicz JJ, Connell AM, Baron JH, Avery-Jones F. Prednisone as a maintenance treatment for ulcerative colitis in remission. Lancet 1965; i:188–189.
64. Spencer JA, Kirsner JB, Milynaryk P, Reed PI, Palmer WL. Immediate and prolonged therapeutic effects of corticotrophin and adrenal steroids in ulcerative colitis. Gastroenterology 1962; 42:113–128.
65. Meyers S, Sachar DB, Goldberg JD, Janowitz HD. Corticotrophin versus hydrocortisone in the intravenous treatment of ulcerative colitis. Gastroenterology 1983; 85:351–357.
66. Powell-Tuck J, Bucknell NA, Lennard-Jones JE. A controlled comparison of corticotropin and hydrocortisone in the treatment of severe proctocolitis. Scand J Gastroenterol 1977; 12:971–975.
67. Kaplan HP, Portnoy B, Binder HJ, Amatruda T, Spiro H. A controlled evaluation of intravenous adrenocorticotropic hormone and hydrocortisone in the treatment of acute colitis. Gastroenterology 1975; 69:91–95.
68. Truelove SC. Treatment of ulcerative colitis with local hydrocortisone hemisuccinate sodium: a report on a controlled therapeutic trial. Br Med J 1958; 2:1072–1077.
69. Larochelle P, Du Soich P, Bolte E, Leborier J, Goyer R. Tixocortol pivalate, a corticosteroid with no systemic glucocorticoid effect after oral, intrarectal and intranasal application. Clin Pharmacol Ther 1983; 33:343–350.
70. Levinson RA. Intrarectal treatment of ulcerative colitis with tixocortol pivalate, a topical, non-systemic anti-inflammatory steroid, comparison with hydrocortisone enema. Gastroenterology 1986; 90:1520.
71. Hanauer SB, Kirsner JB, Barrett WE. The treatment of left-sided ulcerative colitis with tixocortol pivalate. Gastroenterology 1986; 90:1449.
72. Goldman P. Metronidazole. N Engl J Med 1980; 303:1212–1218.
73. Bernstein LH, Frank MS, Brandt LJ, Boley SJ. Healing of perineal Crohn's disease with metronidazole. Gastroenterology 1980; 79:357–365.
74. Brandt LJ, Bernstein LH, Boley SJ, Frank MS. Metronidazole therapy for perineal Crohn's disease: a follow-up study. Gastroenterology 1982; 83:383–387.
75. Karlsson IJ, Hamlyn AN. Metronidazole neuropathy. Br Med J 1977; 3:832.
76. Duffy LN, Daum F, Fisher SE, Selman J, Vishnubhakat SM, Aiges HW, Markowitz JF, Silverberg M. Peripheral neuropathy in Crohn's disease patients treated with metronidazole. Gastroenterology 1985; 88:681–684.
77. Bradley WG, Karlsson IJ, Rassol CG. Metronidazole neuropathy. Br Med J 1977; 3:610–611.
78. Said G, Goasguen J, Laverdant C. Polyneurites au cours des traitements prolonges par le metronidazole. Rev Neurol (Paris) 1978; 134:515–521.
79. Mitelman F, Hartley-Asp B, Ursing B. Chromosome aberrations and metronidazole. Lancet 1976; ii:802.
80. Korelitz Bl, Present DH. Shortcomings of the NCCDS: the exclusion of azathioprine without adequate trial. Gastroenterology 1981; 80: 193–196.
81. Present DH, Korelitz Bl, Wisch N, Glass JL, Sachar DB, Pasternack BS. Treatment of Crohn's disease with 6-mercaptopurine. A long-term randomized double-blind study. N Engl J Med 1980; 302:981–988.
82. Korelitz BL, Present DH. Favorable effect of 6-mercaptopurine on fistulae of Crohn's disease. Dig Dis Sci 1985; 30:58–64.
83. O'Donoghue DP, Dawson AM, Powell-Tuck J, Boun RL, Lennard-Jones JE. Double-blind withdrawal trial of azathioprine as maintenance treatment for Crohn's disease. Lancet 1978; ii:955–957.
84. Ginsberg AL, ed. The azathioprine controversy. Lennard-Jones JE, Jones vs. Singleton JW. Dig Dis Sci 1981; 26:364–371.
85. Kinlen LJ, Sheil AGR, Peto J, Doll R. Collaborative United Kingdom-Australasian study of cancer in patients treated with immunosuppressive drugs. Br Med J 1979; 2:1461–1466.
86. Haber CJ, Meltzer SJ, Present DH, Korelitz BL. Nature and course of pancreatitis caused by 6-mercaptopurine in the treatment of inflammatory bowel disease. Gastroenterology 1986; 91:982–986.
87. Brynskov J, Binder V, Riis R. Clinical experience with cyclosporine in chronically-active, therapy resistant Crohn's disease. A pilot study. Gastroenterology 1987; 92:1330.
88. Peltekian KM, Williams CN, MacDonald AS, Roy PD, Czolpinska E. Open trial of cyclosporine in patients with severe active Crohn's disease refractory to conventional therapy. Can J Gastroenterol 1988; 2:5–11.
89. Cohen DJ, Loertscher R, Rubin MF, Tilney NL, Carpenter CB, Strom TB. Cyclosporine: a new immunosuppressive agent for organ transplantation. Ann Intern Med 1984; 101:667–682.

PART 3

Treatment of Acid-Peptic Disease

Thomas A. Shaw-Stiffel, M.D., C.M., FRCPC, F.A.C.G.
Eve A. Roberts, M.D., FRCPC

Acid-peptic disease encompasses a heterogeneous group of disorders affecting the upper gastrointestinal (GI) tract, all characterized by localized injury to the mucosa and underlying tissues. Initially applied only to gastric and duodenal ulcers, this generic term now includes reflux esophagitis, acute erosive gastroduodenal injury, and the Zollinger-Ellison syndrome. Recent evidence suggests that these disorders result from a critical imbalance in several *aggressive* and *defensive* mucosal factors.[1,2] The wide variety of drugs useful in the management of acid-peptic disease can thus be classified according to which of these factor(s) is modified to help restore mucosal integrity (Table 1).

Initial treatment strategies with antacids or the H_2-receptor antagonists were designed to reduce intragastric acid, the major aggressive mucosal factor. More potent H_2-antagonists, antimuscarinics such as pirenzepine, and the proton-pump inhibitor omeprazole, were also developed with this in mind. However, numerous problems including bacterial overgrowth, nosocomial infections, and the potential risk of carcinogenesis, have recently warranted a reexamination of the role of excessive acid suppression, especially in children. Agents that directly enhance mucosal defense factors instead, such as the prostaglandin analogues and the coating agents sucralfate and colloidal bismuth subcitrate (CBS), avoid many of these problems. CBS may also reduce duodenal ulcer relapse rates, a unique property possibly related to its ability to eradicate *Campylobacter pylori*, a spiral gram-negative bacterium often associated with several of these disorders.[3,4]

The intent of this chapter is to discuss in detail the pharmacologic aspects of these agents, particularly their chemical structure, mechanism of action, relevant pharmacokinetic

TABLE 1
Treatment of Acid-Peptic Disease in Children

Class	Mechanism	Name	Widely Used in Children?	Side Effects	Comments
Antacids	Neutralize gastric acid	(Numerous)	Yes	Milk-alkali syndrome Sodium retention Drug adsorption Diarrhea	Problems with compliance
H_2-blockers	Block gastric histamine H_2-receptors	Cimetidine Ranitidine Famotidine Nizatidine Roxatidine	Yes Yes No No No	Confusion (c) Drug interactions (c)	Effective Important side effects
Substituted benzimidazole	Block Ha^+,K^+-ATPase in parietal cell secretory apparatus	Omeprazole	No	Hypergastrinemia Drug interactions Carcinoid tumors in laboratory animals	Neoplastic potential with chronic use
Tricyclics	Block muscarinic cholinergic activity	Pirenzepine Trimipramine	No No	Anticholinergic effects	Frequent side effects
Prostaglandin analogues	Suppress gastric acid secretion via parietal cell membrane receptors Decrease gastrin production Mucosal protection	Misoprostol Enprostil	No No	Diarrhea	No increased efficacy over H_2-blockers in peptic ulcer disease Possibly beneficial as prophylaxis against NSAID-induced gastritis
Coating agent	Coat inflamed mucosa Increase prostaglandin production	Sucralfate	Yes	Drug adsorption	Tablets hard to administer
Bismuth	Coat mucosa Increase prostaglandins	CBS Pepto-Bismol	No Yes	Staining of teeth Al absorption in chronic renal failure (CBS) Drug adsorption	Effective for infection-induced peptic ulcer Contains salicylate (pb)

NSAID = nonsteroidal anti-inflammatory drug; CBS = colloidal bismuth subcitrate; c = cimetidine; pb = Pepto-Bismol.

TABLE 2
Antacid Neutralization

$NaHCO_3 + HCl \rightarrow NaCl + H_2O + CO_2$ (sodium bicarbonate)
$CaCO_3 + 2HCl \rightarrow CaCl_2 + H_2O + CO_2$ (calcium carbonate)
$Al(OH)_3 + 3HCl \rightarrow AlCl_3 + 3H_2O$ (aluminum hydroxide)
$Mg(OH)_3 + 2HCl \rightarrow MgCl_2 + 2H_2O$ (magnesium hydroxide)

and pharmacodynamic data, as well as important side effects. Their clinical efficacy is reviewed here only within this context. Studies in children are discussed whenever possible, as are recent investigations in adults pertinent to pediatric acid-peptic disease. All too often, they are the only data available, since very few studies have specifically addressed the use of these drugs in children. Furthermore, as with any medication in pediatrics, the risks and benefits of each drug must be balanced carefully before it is prescribed.

ANTACIDS

Antacids have been used empirically in the treatment of acid-peptic disease for centuries. Judging from the extent of media advertising, few other remedies used by the general public are still as popular. In pediatrics, where tablet formulations are difficult to administer, liquid antacids continue to be the mainstay therapy. The main purpose of these agents is to neutralize gastric acid by reacting with HCl to form water and an insoluble salt, as shown for the four main antacids in Table 2.[5,6] Absolute neutrality is not required since, above pH 3.5, little free acid is available.[6,7] Antacids also inactivate pepsin by alkalinization above pH 6,[5,8] while aluminum-containing antacids directly adsorb pepsin at a pH greater than 3,[9] bind bile salts,[10] and enhance mucus production.[5] However, "coating" properties similar to those of sucralfate have not yet been documented.

The relative safety, solubility, and degree of acid neutralization unique to each antacid are determined by their constituent metallic cations and basic anions.[5] The most commonly used base is hydroxide (OH^-), but others include bicarbonate, carbonate, trisilicate, and citrate. Aluminum and magnesium are the metallic cations most frequently combined with hydroxide. Although aluminum hydroxide and magnesium hydroxide are poorly soluble, they react sufficiently well with H^+-ion to produce effective neutralization.[11] Other antacids and their combinations have their own unique properties as shown in Table 3. The in vitro potency or acid-neutralizing capacity (ANC) of each antacid is determined by the amount of 0.1 N HCl (100 mEq H^+ per liter) that can be added to 1 ml of liquid antacid over a 2-hour period without lowering pH below 3.0. The ANC has been shown to correlate well with in vivo potency in ulcer patients.[11]

By raising gastric pH, antacids might be expected to enhance gastrin release by antral G cells and consequently to increase acid secretion. However, recent studies using standard doses of a combination antacid (Al/Mg) taken chronically have shown no such effect.[7,12,13] Although acid secretion may be minimally stimulated during antacid therapy, it may persist temporarily after treatment is stopped and lead to an apparent "acid-rebound" effect.[14] Once thought to be clinically significant with calcium carbonate,[15] this effect has recently been questioned.[12] GI motility may also be altered indirectly by antacids. Alkalinization of gastric contents enhances gastric emptying and increases lower esophageal sphincter pressure.[16,17] However, aluminum-containing antacids may relax both gastric and small intestinal smooth muscle by interfering with calcium influx, thus actually slowing gastric emptying and intestinal transit.[5,18] Magnesium tends to have the reverse effect. Its laxative action is mediated by osmosis and perhaps indirectly by cholecystokinin.[5] As a result, aluminum and magnesium antacids are usually combined together in an attempt to avoid these adverse effects on motility.[19,20]

Systemic absorption of the antacids and their components varies considerably. Sodium bicarbonate and sodium citrate are rapidly absorbed and frequently cause metabolic alkalosis, whereas aluminum, magnesium, and calcium ions are minimally absorbed. Nevertheless, the insoluble salts that result from neutralization of intragastric acid (e.g., $AlCl_3$, $MgCl_2$, $CaCO_3$) may still undergo significant absorption during transit through the small intestine. About 5 percent of the magnesium present in antacids is absorbed and rapidly excreted in the urine.[21] Thus, toxic plasma concentrations rarely occur except in patients with renal failure. When treated with the aluminum-containing antacids, these patients may also have elevated plasma aluminum levels, occasionally in excess of 300 μg per liter (about 15 times normal) and often associated with toxic encephalopathy. Even in normal subjects, aluminum concentrations may double despite standard doses of antacid, and levels up to 10 times normal have been reported. The calcium-containing antacids rarely cause hypercalcemia, again with the notable exception of uremic patients.[5,7,12]

TABLE 3
Properties of Commonly Used Antacids

Name	ANC (mEq H^+ per ml Antacid)	Buffering Capacity	Sodium Content (mEq Na/15 ml)
Liquid—high potency			
Gelusil II	6.0	20	0.18
Maalox TC	5.7	17	0.11
Mylanta II	5.3	20	0.15
Maalox Plus	—	37.5	0.18
Liquid—normal potency—Al/Mg			
Gelusil	2.8	44	0.10
Maalox	3.0	—	0.20
Mylanta	2.9	40	0.10
Riopan	2.5	37.5	0.04
Liquid—normal potency—Aluminum			
Amphojel	1.7	20	0.3
Alternagel	3.8	—	0.1
Tablets			
Amphojel	23		
Gelusil II	23		
Maalox No. 2	22		
Mylanta II	23		
Tums ($CaCO_3$)	10		
Rolaids (Al/Na carbonate)	8		

Modified from references 4 and 5.

TABLE 4
Important Side Effects of the Antacids

pH-Dependent	Composition-Dependent
Metabolic alkalosis	Altered bowel motility
Milk-alkali syndrome	Gastric bezoars
Hypercalcemia	Hypophosphatemia
Hypercalciuria	Hypermagnesemia
Nephrocalcinosis	Congestive heart failure (Na)
Nephrolithiasis	Encephalopathy (Al)
Upper GI tract bacterial overgrowth	

Other side effects, either pH- or composition-dependent, have been reported with the antacids (Table 4). Tums (mostly calcium carbonate) and Rolaids (dihydroxy-aluminum sodium carbonate) when used in excess may lead to increased acid production.[5] Calcium carbonate may also cause the milk-alkali syndrome and rarely gastric bezoars.[22] Altered bowel motility, cation toxicity, and sodium retention occur not infrequently with Al/Mg preparations. A number of drug interactions are also associated with the antacids and are documented in Table 5.[5,23] They may also impair the absorption of cimetidine,[24] ranitidine,[25] digoxin,[26] chlorpromazine,[27] and glucocorticoids,[28] either by direct interaction with the drug or by pH-dependent changes in absorption. Magnesium hydroxide may enhance the absorption of bishydroxycoumadin.[29]

The clinical efficacy of the antacids in treating duodenal ulcer has been shown in many trials.[4,12,30] Based on studies in adults by Peterson et al done in the 1970s,[31,32] antacids have usually been prescribed seven times a day: 1 and 3 hours after meals and at bedtime. Using this antacid regimen, duodenal ulcer healing rates in adults were 78 percent at 4 weeks compared to 45 percent with placebo.[31] The acid-neutralizing capacity of this regimen was 1,008 mmol per day, a high level thought necessary to maintain intragastric pH elevated throughout the day and to keep the H^+-ion duodenal load at a minimum. Antacids taken with meals remain in the stomach longest. By three hours after meals the pH begins to fall as antacid is fully consumed or absorbed and food buffers leave the stomach. Antacids taken only at bedtime are rapidly emptied from the stomach, and nocturnal acid neutralization is inadequate unless anticholinergic agents are also used.[32]

TABLE 5
Important Drug Interactions with Antacids

Effect	Antacid Component: $Al(OH)_3$	$Mg(OH)_2$	$NaHCO_3$
Depressed drug level or effect	Aspirin Chlordiazepoxide Chlorpromazine Isoniazid Propranolol Phosphorus Vitamin A Tetracycline	Aspirin Cimetidine Digoxin Chlordiazepoxide Tetracycline	Iron Tetracycline
Enhanced drug level or effect	Levodopa Quinidine	Levodopa Dicumarol Sulfonamides Quinidine	Amphetamine Sulfonamides Naproxen

Recent studies have suggested that patients who secrete normal amounts of acid require individual antacid doses with 40 to 80 mEq of buffer, whereas those who secrete more than 20 mEq H^+ per hour need 80 to 160 mEq.[4,30,32] The clinical relevance of this remains unclear, as differentiating patients who are "hypersecretors" from normals is often difficult. Furthermore, other studies in adults have documented excellent healing rates of duodenal ulcers with doses as low as 280 mEq per day.[33,34] Even a regimen using one tablet of an Al/Mg antacid 1 hour after meals and at bedtime (120 mmol per day) resulted in healing rates similar to those with cimetidine 800 mg at bedtime.[35] These results have not yet been confirmed in children.

Controversy persists as to whether tablet formulations are as effective as the liquid ones in terms of both ANCs and healing rates.[36] Liquid formulations are obviously more convenient for use in children. Recommended doses have been 1 ml per kilogram at 1 and 3 hours after meals, with 2 ml per kilogram at bedtime.[1,37,38] Antacids are also the preferred agents below 2 years of age. Combining antacids with various other agents such as the tricyclics and the H_2-receptor antagonists has shown no advantage in adults except with pirenzepine.[30] A reduced dose of antacid in this combination may thus result in similar healing rates but with fewer side effects.

Several studies have also shown the utility of antacids in the treatment of gastric ulcer.[39,40] Reflux esophagitis responds well to antacids, owing both to their acid-neutralizing activity and to their ameliorative effects on lower esophageal pressure and gastric emptying, as discussed earlier. Antacids appear to reduce the number, duration, and magnitude of reflux episodes to the same degree as cimetidine and ranitidine.[7,30] Their use in the treatment of reflux disease in pediatrics is thus well established.[1] In adults, antacids are also more effective than the H_2-antagonists in preventing hemorrhage from stress-related gastric ulceration.[41] An intragastric pH consistently above 3.5 appears crucial. The role of antacids for stress ulceration in children, however, has not been studied systematically.

H_2-RECEPTOR ANTAGONISTS

In response to various physiologic stimuli, histamine is released by mast cells in the fundic mucosa and acts upon nearby parietal cells to stimulate acid secretion. Its action is mediated by specific H_2-receptors on the parietal cells that activate adenyl cyclase and second messenger cyclic AMP.[1,3] H_2-antagonists block histamine binding to these receptors competitively, resulting in potent but reversible suppression of acid secretion.[42] Although these receptors are found elsewhere in the body, their role outside the GI tract appears to be of minor importance.[3] In the early 1970s, successive modifications of the histamine molecule led to the first drug

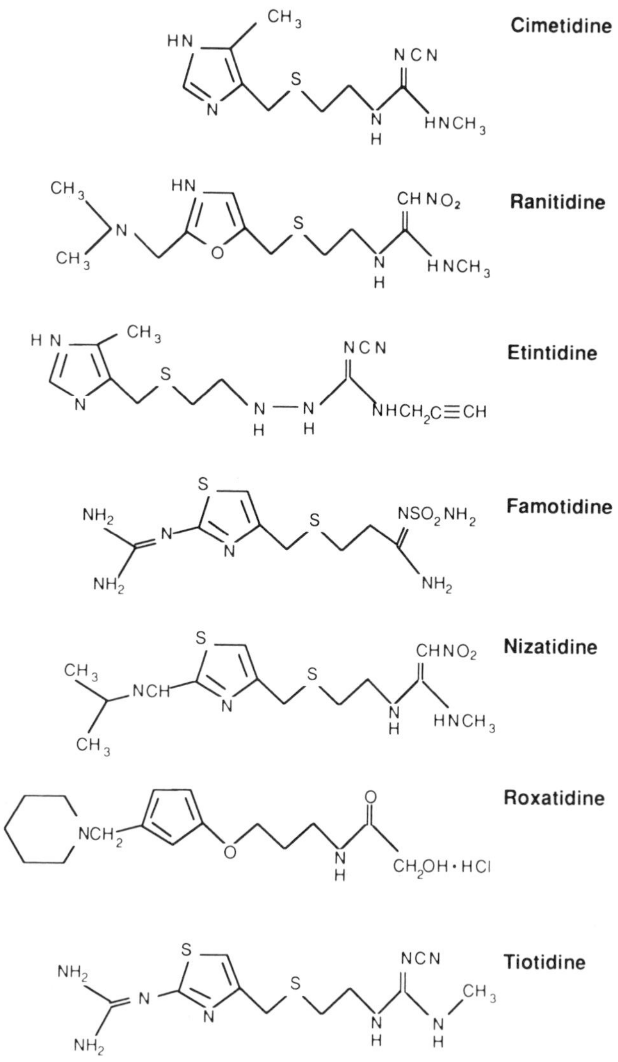

Cimetidine

Ranitidine

Etintidine

Famotidine

Nizatidine

Roxatidine

Tiotidine

FIGURE 1 Chemical structures of the H_2-receptor antagonists.

with potent H_2-blocking activity, burimamide. Further changes to the molecule while retaining the imidazole ring resulted in cimetidine.[43] Other H_2-antagonists now under development, oxmetidine and etintidine, also share this imidazole ring, whereas ranitidine has instead an alkyl furan ring.[3] The imidazole ring thus does not appear to be essential for antisecretory activity. Other agents have been developed lately with even more powerful and prolonged antisecretory properties. They include famotidine, nizatidine, roxatidine, tiotidine, loxtidine, and lamtidine (Fig. 1).

The H_2-antagonists inhibit basal, stimulated, and nocturnal acid secretion. Both the volume of gastric juice and its acid concentration are reduced significantly. Pepsin secretion by the chief cells is also suppressed through an unknown mechanism. Effects on intrinsic factor secretion and GI motility are insignificant.[5] Despite differences in potency between cimetidine and ranitidine, both are equivalent in terms of acid suppression clinically, raising gastric pH to above 3.5 within 30 minutes and persisting for 3 to 4 hours.[5] Some

TABLE 6
Cimetidine Pharmacokinetics in Children and Adults

Group	$\beta\ t_{1/2}$ (hr)	k_{el} (hr^{-1})	V_D (L/kg)	Cl_p (ml/kg/hr)	Recommended Dosing
Premature neonates	2.6	0.26	0.95	26	4 mg/kg q12h
Children (ages 1–12)	1.44	0.52	2.13	14.21	24 mg/kg/day
Adults					
Peptic ulcer disease	1.79	—	1.39	9.07	5–10 mg/kg
Multiple trauma	2.27	—	1.66	9.12	40 mg/kg/day
Healthy	1.5	—	1.12	9.17	1.4 mg/kg/day

Modified from references 45 to 48, and 63.

studies have documented a direct relationship between the plasma concentrations of H_2-antagonists and the inhibition of gastric activity,[44,45] whereas others including one in children have not.[46,47]

Limited data concerning the pharmacokinetics of the H_2-antagonists exist in children.[46,48-50] Basic parameters for cimetidine have been assessed in only a few studies and are shown in Table 6. Similar data for adults are included for comparison.[47,51,52] Oral absorption of cimetidine and ranitidine is complete within 90 minutes.[53,54] The bioavailability of cimetidine has not yet been studied in children but ranges from 63 to 78 percent in adults.[3] A significant first-pass effect reduces the bioavailability of ranitidine to as low as 39 percent.[3,54] In adults, both cimetidine and ranitidine exhibit biexponential elimination curves after intravenous administration and bimodal curves after oral ingestion.[55-57] This pharmacokinetic feature most likely relates to pH-dependent alterations in gastric emptying, and its clinical significance remains unclear.

Drug distribution of the H_2-antagonists in children has also received little attention. In one recent study, the apparent volume of distribution ranged from 1 to 2 L per kilogram, somewhat higher than that in adults.[46,47,51,53] Cimetidine distributes primarily in total body water, namely to skeletal muscle, and dosage calculations should therefore be based on ideal body weight. Placental transfer may occur and cimetidine has been found in breast milk.[58,59] Cimetidine is excreted in the urine, mostly unchanged, via active tubular secretion. However, it does undergo some hepatic metabolism. The main metabolites—sulfoxide, glucuronide, and guanyl-urea—are inactive and excreted by the kidney.[60] On the other hand, ranitidine undergoes mostly renal excretion and very limited metabolic conversion.[61] Another H_2-antagonist, roxatidine, is desacetylated following absorption and then undergoes further hepatic metabolism.[62]

The total body clearance of cimetidine appears to be higher in younger age groups and is associated with a shorter elimination half-life (Table 7).[46,48,49] Premature neonates, however, may clear this drug somewhat more slowly until renal development reaches adult capacity at about 2 weeks of age.[49,63] During this period cimetidine metabolites may accumulate, but the clinical significance of this is unknown.[49]

TABLE 7
Some Important Side Effects of Cimetidine

Altered absorption of drugs due to changes in gastric pH (e.g., ketoconazole, acetylsalicylic acid)
Inhibition of drug metabolism via hepatic cytochromes P-450 (e.g., theophylline, warfarin, phenytoin, diazepam)
Inhibition of renal tubular drug secretion (e.g., procainamide)
Antiandrogenic effects (e.g., gynecomastia, impotence)
Mental confusion, particularly in children and elderly individuals
Cholestatic hepatitis
Interstitial nephritis
Polymyositis
Leukopenia, thrombocytopenia, agranulocytosis (rare)
Bradycardia, hypotension (only following rapid IV infusion)

In patients with cystic fibrosis, the clearance of cimetidine may[64] or may not[65] be increased, although both studies lacked adequate controls. The exact mechanism here remains unclear, but is probably related to altered hepatic metabolism rather than to increased renal excretion.

A recent study has shown that the pharmacokinetic data for ranitidine in a group of children aged 3.5 to 16 years with either duodenal or gastric ulcers are similar to those for ranitidine in adults.[66] Oral and intravenous data were equivalent. Bioavailability ranged from 22 to 96 percent. No adverse clinical or laboratory effects were documented with either formulation. To achieve greater than 90 percent suppression of gastric acid, a relatively narrow therapeutic range of 40 to 60 ng per milliliter was required, in contrast to adults, in whom this range varies considerably.[61] The recommended oral dose to attain this degree of suppression was found to be 1.25 to 1.90 mg per kilogram every 12 hours.[66] In another study, a dose of 2.0 to 2.5 mg per kilogram was shown comparable to the adult dose of 150 mg twice a day, and pharmacokinetic parameters in patients aged 6 to 10 were essentially similar to those in children aged 11 to 16 and in normal adults.[67]

Over 100 studies in adults as well as children have shown that cimetidine and ranitidine are more effective than placebo in healing duodenal and gastric ulcers.[3,4,44,68] Single bedtime doses (800 mg cimetidine and 300 mg ranitidine) heal duodenal ulcers in adults as well as multiple daily doses with improved compliance,[3,44] but there have been no studies to confirm this in children. Numerous studies in adults have also documented the effectiveness of these agents in reflux esophagitis, Zollinger-Ellison syndrome, and stress-induced ulceration.[1,3] In critically ill children, cimetidine doses of 24 mg per kilogram per day administered in divided doses every 4 to 6 hours are recommended for prophylaxis. Gastric pH should be maintained above 4.[47] Cimetidine may be added directly to intravenous hyperalimentation or enteral feeds.[3] Newer agents have recently been introduced such as famotidine,[69] nizatidine,[70,71] etintidine,[72] and roxatidine acetate.[62] Their potencies are equal to or greater than that of ranitidine. As would be expected, they have shown considerable promise in the treatment of acid-peptic disease in adults, but their role in pediatrics remains unclear.

Of all the H_2-receptor antagonists, cimetidine has been the one most reported to have significant side effects[1,3,44] (Table 7). These include agranulocytosis,[73] mental confusion,[74] antiandrogenic effects (e.g., gynecomastia, impotence),[75,76] and minor changes in aminotransferases and creatinine.[3,5,43] The antiandrogenic effects result from cimetidine's displacement of dihydrotestosterone from androgenic binding sites.[76] The absorption of drugs such as ketoconazole[77] and acetylsalicylic acid[78] may also be altered by changes in gastric pH. Cimetidine-induced cholestasis is rare.[79] In general, chronic renal failure significantly prolongs cimetidine and ranitidine plasma clearance, whereas hepatic disease—unless severe—has little effect on the clearance of either drug.[3] Appropriate dose adjustments are thus required depending on the severity of renal or hepatic disease. The H_2-antagonists are not recommended for use during pregnancy or breast-feeding.[5]

An important pharmacologic effect of cimetidine is its direct inhibition of hepatic cytochrome P-450 monooxygenases, which are crucial in drug metabolism.[80,81] Depending on their chemical structure, drugs can bind to the cytochrome P-450 in at least two ways: via the lipoprotein moiety (high-affinity site) or directly to the iron atom attached to the protoporphyrin ring (low-affinity site). Cimetidine binds at both sites, whereas ranitidine binds only to the low-affinity site. Cimetidine also binds more avidly than ranitidine, resulting in greater inhibition.[81-83] The imidazole ring appears to be the active site at which cimetidine binds to these P-450 moieties.[83-85] Cimetidine has been shown to inhibit the metabolism of warfarin,[86] phenytoin,[87] diazepam,[88] theophylline,[89] and many other drugs.[85,90,91] The other H_2-antagonists to date have had minimal or no similar effects.[3,69,85] Controversy surrounds possible alterations in hepatic blood flow due to cimetidine and the impairment in metabolism of such high-extraction-ratio drugs such as propranolol.[92] This effect on hepatic blood flow now appears improbable. Intravenous boluses of cimetidine should be administered slowly to prevent hypotension or serious cardiac arrhythmias.[3]

OMEPRAZOLE

The substituted benzimidazoles form part of a new class of highly potent antisecretory agents.[93-95] Omeprazole has been the most thoroughly investigated to date. Other similar compounds include timoprazole and picoprazole. These agents act by binding to the proton-pump enzyme, H^+,K^+-ATPase, located adjacent to the parietal cell's apical secretory apparatus. Their antisecretory activity is highly potent for a number of reasons. First, the enzyme they inhibit, H^+,K^+-ATPase, mediates the final, critical step in gastric acid formation.[94,96] As well, within the highly acidic milieu of the tubulovesicles surrounding the secretory canaliculi, these drugs become protonated and are thus prevented from diffusing out through lipid membranes.[97] Once protonated, these drugs also bind irreversibly to H^+,K^+-ATPase, further prolonging their antisecretory effect.[98,99]

As a result, omeprazole markedly reduces both basal acid secretion and that stimulated by gastrin, acetylcholine, histamine, and cyclic AMP.[100] When given in an adult dose of 30 mg per day, it suppresses H^+ activity by 95 percent, especially at night. This suppression is considerably more than that with ranitidine (69 percent with 300 mg per day) or cimetidine (48 percent with 1 g per day).[101] Moreover, even though its serum half-life is only about 60 minutes, intragastric acidity is still suppressed (by 26 percent) 7 days after omeprazole is discontinued.[102] Omeprazole also decreases pepsin output[103] and may have some mucosal protective activity, although it remains unclear whether this effect is prostaglandin-mediated.[104]

Omeprazole degrades rapidly in solutions with a low pH, and it is thus delivered in granules within a gel capsule to protect it from gastric acid.[105] This formulation likely explains the progressive rise in bioavailability over the first 3 to 4 days of oral use, as gastric acidity is gradually neutralized. There is no correlation between plasma omeprazole levels and the suppression of gastric acid; despite its short half-life, omeprazole reduces gastric acid secretion for well over 24 hours.[106] Food, but not antacids, may delay the absorption of omeprazole and the drug should therefore be taken on an empty stomach. Omeprazole distributes rapidly, mostly in extracellular water, throughout many organs excluding the brain. It is highly protein-bound. The metabolism and excretion of omeprazole and its three metabolites (hydroxy, sulfone, and sulfide) remain poorly defined, but it appears that minimal parent compound is excreted in the urine. Its terminal half-life is 0.5 to 1.5 hours.[107] There appears to be no change with hemodialysis or chronic renal failure.[108]

Several controlled clinical trials[109,110] have confirmed the superior healing rates of duodenal ulcers with omeprazole (20 to 40 mg orally once daily before breakfast), including those refractory to therapy with the H_2-receptor antagonists.[111] Healing rates approach 100 percent at 4 weeks even with lower doses. Symptomatic relief is achieved equal to or better than that with ranitidine or cimetidine. Relapse rates are similar.[112] Gastric ulcers may respond better to omeprazole than to other agents, contrary to earlier reports.[113] Omeprazole has also shown considerable success in treating Zollinger-Ellison syndrome resistant to H_2-receptor antagonists; doses of 60 to 120 mg per day were used for up to 4 years without apparent complications.[114] There are no other data regarding maintenance therapy.

Omeprazole has also proved to be especially useful in the treatment of reflux esophagitis. Total reflux time is significantly reduced concomitantly with decreased gastric volume and acid concentration. A recent double-blind study has shown dramatic healing rates assessed at endoscopy after only 4 weeks of omeprazole (up to 81 percent) as compared to those with ranitidine (less than 27 percent). In addition, symptoms were relieved more rapidly and more fully with omeprazole. Predictably, Barrett's ulcers and grade 4 esophagitis remained rather resistant to therapy, with less than 50 percent responding after 4 weeks.[115] Larger doses (40 mg) appear to induce endoscopic and histologic healing as well as symptomatic relief more quickly than 20 mg, and, with these higher doses, intraesophageal pH can be normalized in all patients. Relapse occurs rapidly, however, after omeprazole is stopped.[115] No effect on gastric motility or lower esophageal sphincter pressure has yet been reported.

The major problem with this drug has been the consistent rise in basal and postprandial serum gastrin levels to about four times normal.[116] However, these levels are not as elevated as those reported in pernicious anemia or the Zollinger-Ellison syndrome. This phenomenon appears related to omeprazole's profound acid inhibition rather than to any direct stimulation of gastrin release.[95,100] As gastrin has important trophic effects, the occurrence of enterochromaffin-like cell tumors and carcinoids in rodents comes as no surprise.[117] These tumors have been reported in patients with marked hypergastrinemia due to pernicious anemia but not as yet with omeprazole.[118] Concerns about hypochlorhydria-related bacterial overgrowth and carcinogenesis with *N*-nitroso compounds have also been raised.[119] In addition, omeprazole may inhibit the cytochrome P-450 microsomal system, thereby altering the clearance of certain drugs.[120] Recently this drug has also been reported to inhibit adrenal cortical steroidogenesis and to reduce protein-bound cobalamin absorption.[121,122] These features have therefore tempered enthusiasm for using omeprazole in children.

PIRENZEPINE

Although effective in reducing gastric acid and pepsin secretion, "classic" anticholinergic agents have frequent atropine-like side effects such as blurred vision, tachycardia, and dry mouth. Gastric emptying and lower esophageal sphincter pressure may also be adversely affected. Pirenzepine instead acts directly on the M1 postganglionic receptors, thereby inhibiting muscarinic cholinergic activity and avoiding most of the side effects associated with general (M1 and M2) receptor antagonists.[123] Pirenzepine suppresses gastric acid secretion both in the basal state and after stimulation, in normal subjects as well as in those with duodenal ulcers,[124] and it acts synergistically with the H_2-antagonists.[125] Pirenzepine also reduces pepsin output significantly.[126] Its chemical structure is similar to that of the tricyclic antidepressants, as well as histamine and cyproheptadine, a serotonin antagonist.[127]

Pirenzepine may have mucosal protective properties similar to those of the prostaglandin analogues and it may thus protect against nonsteroidal anti-inflammatory drug (NSAID)–induced or stress-induced gastric lesions.[128] It has no apparent effects on lower esophageal sphincter function or small bowel motility, although gastric emptying of liquids may be somewhat delayed.[129] Preliminary data show that this agent may also enhance appetite to a greater extent than cyproheptadine.[127] After oral administration, about 25 percent of the drug is absorbed, with peak plasma levels achieved in about 4 hours. It distributes widely to various organs including the liver, kidney, intestine, and salivary glands.[130] Only 12 percent of pirenzepine is protein-bound. Its half-life is about 11 hours, and most of it is excreted in the urine unchanged. A small amount is transformed in the liver to an inactive metabolite.[131] Because of its hydrophilic properties, pirenzepine does not cross the blood-brain barrier or the placenta.[132]

Clinical studies with this drug have been confined to adults.[133] Pirenzepine promotes the healing of both duodenal and gastric ulcers better than placebo and is equivalent to cimetidine in this respect.[134] Symptom relief and relapse rates are also similar to those with cimetidine. Pirenzepine has also been used to treat reflux esophagitis and nonulcer dyspepsia[134,135] with limited success. Despite this agent's apparent selectivity for M1 receptors, up to 50 percent of patients on normal doses may develop anticholinergic side effects, dry mouth being the most common.[134,136] For the most part, however, these are minor compared to those associated with classic anticholinergics. No important drug interactions or other notable adverse effects have been reported,[136] but clinical experience remains limited, particularly in children.

PROSTAGLANDIN ANALOGUES

Since the naturally occurring prostaglandins (PGs) are rapidly degraded by the GI mucosa, chemical modifications were necessary to produce more stable, longer-acting analogues that still retain their unique biologic effects.[137] The two agents most studied to date are analogues of PGE_1 (misoprostol) and PGE_2 (enprostil). They initially showed considerable promise in the treatment of acid-peptic disease, with animal studies documenting their dramatic ability to protect the gastric mucosa against a wide variety of noxious agents, including concentrated ethanol and even boiling water.[95,138] However, studies in humans have not confirmed any clear advantage of the PG analogues over the H_2-receptor antagonists, and their clinical efficacy is now attributed primarily to their antisecretory activity. The PG analogues bind to specific receptors on the parietal cell membrane, distinct from those at which the H_2-antagonists act and prevent the activation of adenylate cyclase by histamine, thereby inhibiting cyclic AMP–mediated acid production.[139,140] This process appears dependent on guanidine triphosphate as well.[141]

Studies in humans have shown that both enprostil[142] and misoprostol[143] are intermediate inhibitors of acid secretion, equivalent to cimetidine but less potent than ranitidine. Enprostil also reduces nocturnal pepsin output by up to 85 percent in duodenal ulcer patients.[142] The release of intrinsic factor may also be suppressed by these agents.[143] Despite a significant reduction in acid secretion, misoprostol does not elevate either basal or postprandial serum gastrin levels,[144] whereas enprostil actually suppresses these levels in healthy volunteers and in patients with inactive duodenal ulcers, antral G-cell hyperfunction, pernicious anemia, or Zollinger-Ellison syndrome. This phenomenon suggests that some PG analogues may also directly inhibit the release of gastrin by G cells.[95] As a result, acid suppression is associated with normal or lowered gastrin levels, in contrast to the H_2-receptor antagonists and omeprazole.

TABLE 8
Effects of the Prostaglandin Analogues on Mucosal Protection

↑ Gastric mucus secretion
↑ Bicarbonate secretion
↑ Mucosal blood flow
↑ Epithelial regeneration
↓ Gastric acid secretion

In addition to blocking acid secretion and gastrin production, these agents may also directly enhance *mucosal protection* (the more precise term that has replaced *cytoprotection*).[145] In animals, PGs protect the mucosa against damage from such noxious agents as bile, ethanol, NSAIDs, and prednisolone, as well as against ulceration caused by sepsis and stress.[146] In man, misoprostol can also minimize the mucosal injury caused by ethanol and NSAIDs.[147-149] The various ways in which these agents are thought to enhance mucosal protection are listed in Table 8. Several of these effects have been documented with misoprostol,[150] whereas few have been shown for enprostil.[151]

At present, pharmacokinetic data for misoprostol and enprostil derive from studies in animals and healthy adult volunteers only.[152,153] Following oral doses, misoprostol is rapidly absorbed and de-esterified to its acid form, peak concentrations being reached in 30 to 60 minutes. This free acid metabolite remains as potent as the parent drug in inhibiting acid secretion. It is 85 percent protein bound. Binding is not affected by age or other drugs. Further metabolism occurs via oxidation of the side-chain followed by reduction to PGF analogues. This process likely takes place in the liver and kidney. Biphasic elimination occurs with a terminal half-life of about 1.5 hours. By 8 hours, 90 percent of a single oral dose is excreted, mostly in the urine. No parent drug is recovered.[143,152] Limited data exist for enprostil. Peak concentrations occur at 30 to 60 minutes as with misoprostol, but the elimination half-life is much longer at 34 hours. Renal excretion again predominates.[151,153]

In terms of clinical efficacy, both misoprostol (200 μg orally four times a day) and enprostil (35 μg orally twice a day) are equivalent to cimetidine in the healing of duodenal ulcers.[95,154,155] They may be less effective than ranitidine in this regard.[143,151] In addition, ulcer pain, especially at night, does not respond as well to the PG analogues as to the H_2-receptor antagonists, and it may in fact be worsened temporarily.[155] In the treatment of gastric ulcers, misoprostol and enprostil have been equivalent to cimetidine in terms of healing and the relief of symptoms.[143,152] The PG analogues appear to have no role in preventing duodenal ulcer recurrence.[151] In patients with reflux esophagitis, a recent study showed that enprostil (35 μg twice a day) led to a significant early improvement endoscopically, but healing rates over a 12-week period were no better than with placebo.[156] The natural PGs decrease lower esophageal sphincter pressure in animals and may thus theoretically worsen esophagitis.[7] However, in humans, the synthetic analogues appear to have no such effect.[157] A recent study showed that misoprostol may also improve nutrient absorption in cystic fibrosis patients with steatorrhea.[7]

The PG analogues have no apparent effects on cytochromes P-450, unlike cimetidine.[158,159] Apart from a possible interaction with propranolol, no major drug interactions have been reported so far.[160] However, at least 15 percent of subjects on these agents complain of diarrhea (usually mild) and other symptoms of GI upset due to enhanced small bowel motility.[143,151] Furthermore, the PG analogues are contraindicated during pregnancy or in women at risk of becoming pregnant, since misoprostol enhances spontaneous abortion rates through its effects on uterine contractility. Enprostil may be less prone to this side effect.[160] There are reports that misoprostol may impair glucose tolerance, whereas enprostil may have the reverse effect.[161] Thus these two PG analogues have important similarities as well as differences in their pharmacology and adverse effects.

SUCRALFATE

The coating agent sucralfate is a basic aluminum salt of sucrose sulfate. At an acid pH, it polymerizes to form a white, paste-like substance that adheres selectively to ulcers or erosions. This has been shown to occur both in vitro and in vivo, for both duodenal and gastric ulcers, even up to 1 month after healing is complete. The affinity of sucralfate for these sites depends on an electrostatic attraction between the negatively charged sucralfate polyanions and the positively charged protein moieties exposed by the inflamed mucosa.[162] At these specific sites, sucralfate acts as a protective barrier by slowing the back-diffusion of acid, pepsin, and bile salts.[163,164] It also directly inhibits the binding of pepsin to ulcer protein and adsorbs free bile salts much as cholestyramine does.

Other important effects include increased bicarbonate and mucus production,[165] enhanced epithelial cell renewal,[166] and the restoration of a normal transmucosal potential difference.[167] In addition, sucralfate protects the gastric mucosa against damage induced by ethanol, bile acids, and NSAIDs[168] and prevents stress ulceration in critically ill patients.[169] These effects appear mediated by enhanced PGE_2 production[170] or perhaps epidermal growth factors.[171] Despite its $Al(OH)_3$ components and some minor acid-buffering capability, sucralfate does not increase gastric pH, nor does it act as an antacid at usual therapeutic doses.[163,167] In addition, sucralfate has no apparent effects on gastric acid secretion, gastrin release, or upper GI motility.[18,163] Thus, hypochlorhydria and concomitant bacterial overgrowth do not occur.[172] Sucralfate may also have inherent antibacterial activity.[173]

Minimal if any sucralfate is absorbed after oral administration. Following a single 1-gram dose of ^{14}C-labeled sucralfate, only 0.5 to 2.2 percent of total radioactivity was excreted in urine over a 4-day period, with most excreted in the first 4 hours.[174] Aluminum absorption was not found to be significantly different from controls in patients with gastric or duodenal ulcers on sucralfate (4 g daily for up to 10 weeks).[175] In another study using normal subjects, only transient increases in blood aluminum concentrations were noted with full-dose sucralfate, whereas bone aluminum levels remained normal even after 2 months.[176] In the presence of severely impaired renal function, however, blood aluminum levels may rise slightly but not more than in patients on usual therapeutic doses of the $Al(OH)_3$-containing antacids.[168]

Sucralfate is relatively free of side effects, the only major one being constipation. This occurs in about 2 to 3 percent of patients, whereas nausea and headaches occur much less frequently.[163,168] Hypophosphatemia may also result from sucralfate's action as a phosphate binder.[177] Enhanced aluminum accumulation may be a problem in uremia, as mentioned earlier. In addition, the absorption of certain drugs such as warfarin,[178] digoxin,[179] and phenytoin[180] may be decreased when sucralfate is given concurrently. This effect is minimized by taking the drugs at least 2 hours apart.

Several studies in adults have shown that sucralfate (1 g orally before meals and at bedtime) is significantly better than placebo and equivalent to cimetidine or ranitidine in the healing of duodenal and gastric ulcers.[181] Recently, a dose of 2 g orally twice a day has been shown to be as effective as the usual dose of 1 g three times a day.[182] Healing rates of gastric ulcers are, however, slower than those of duodenal ulcers, as has been reported for other drugs. Preliminary evidence suggests that sucralfate may also heal duodenal ulcers resistant to H_2-receptor antagonists. Maintenance therapy with sucralfate decreases the recurrence rate not only of duodenal ulcers (1 g twice a day) and but also of gastric ulcers (1 g every morning and 2 g at bedtime).[183] A single nocturnal dose of 2 g is equally effective for either type of ulcer.[184] Concomitant therapy with sucralfate may also protect against NSAID-induced gastric lesions[185] and relieve nonulcer dyspepsia.[186]

Sucralfate is significantly superior to placebo in the treatment of reflux esophagitis[187] and is comparable to the alginate/antacid combinations or the H_2-receptor antagonists in terms of symptom relief and endoscopic healing.[188] Whether sucralfate coats the inflamed esophagus during its initial passage or after polymerization in the stomach remains unclear. Sucralfate can also prevent stress ulceration in critically ill patients.[172] The lack of acid suppression and concomitant bacterial overgrowth may prove to be a significant advantage of sucralfate in this respect, with a lower incidence of nosocomial infections as compared to the H_2-receptor antagonists.[173] Sucralfate is thus particularly well-suited for maintenance therapy in children owing to the infrequent association with bacterial overgrowth and possible nitrosamine-induced carcinogenesis. A new sucralfate suspension is expected to improve compliance compared to that with the previously large tablets,[189] especially in children.

COLLOIDAL BISMUTH SUBCITRATE

Bismuth-containing compounds have been available for many years. However, only recently has one of these compounds, colloidal bismuth subcitrate (CBS), or De-Nol, demonstrated efficacy in the treatment of acid-peptic disease equal to that of the H_2-receptor antagonists. CBS also dramatically reduces the recurrence rate of duodenal ulcers following initial therapy. It is a stable complex salt of bismuth and citric acid, highly soluble in water, that precipitates at a pH less than 5 and in gastric juice at optimum pH 3.5.[190] Following precipitation, CBS is deposited preferentially in ulcer craters or over eroded mucosa, where it combines with exposed protein moieties to form a glycoprotein-bismuth complex. This chelate provides a protective layer against acid and pepsin specifically at sites where damage has occurred, much as sucralfate does. This property appears unique to CBS as compared to the other bismuth salts.[191] Other effects of CBS include increased mucosal bicarbonate secretion, the prevention in rats of damage induced by ethanol, aspirin, or stress, and the restoration in humans of normal epithelial morphology,[192,193] all associated with enhanced PGE_2 production.[192] CBS also directly inactivates pepsin and conjugated bile acids.[194] Unlike the H_2-receptor antagonists and omeprazole, CBS has no effects on gastric acid secretion or gastrin release.[195,196]

Although the exact role of *C. pylori* in acid-peptic disease remains unclear, there appears to be a strong link between the presence of this organism in the stomach and both primary acute antral gastritis and duodenal ulcers, particularly in older children.[197-200] In this regard, CBS may work by inhibiting the growth of *C. pylori* both in vivo and in vitro,[201] in contrast to the H_2-receptor antagonists. Recent studies using electron microscopy reveal multiple cytopathic changes in these organisms directly related to this drug.[202] Moreover, CBS restores normal mucus composition[203] and counteracts the deleterious effects of *C. pylori* on mucus viscosity and H^+ ion back-diffusion.[204] This ability of CBS both to inhibit growth of *C. pylori* and to reverse its adverse consequences may well prove to be one of its most important therapeutic effects.

In earlier clinical studies using CBS, proper double-blinding was a major methodologic problem because of its strong characteristic taste and smell. This problem has been mostly avoided with the coated tablets. In several recent studies, the healing rates of uncomplicated duodenal[203,204] and gastric ulcers[203,205] with CBS have been significantly better than those with placebo. The usual dose is 480 mg Bi_2O_3 daily for 4 to 8 weeks in two to four daily doses. These healing rates have also been comparable to those with cimetidine[202,206] and ranitidine.[207-209] As well, CBS tablets whether given twice or four times daily[210] heal duodenal ulcers to the same extent, although eradication of *C. pylori* infection may not be as complete using the former. Cimetidine combined with CBS to treat duodenal ulcer may also enhance early healing at 4 weeks, compared to that when either agent is used alone.[211] Furthermore, duodenal ulcers resistant to the usual doses of H_2-receptor antagonists have been shown to respond well to CBS alone.[212]

A remarkable feature of CBS is its specific ability to reduce the relapse rates of duodenal ulcer following acute therapy, as confirmed in a recent meta-analysis of more than 25 trials.[213] Rates of only 39 to 76 percent occur with CBS after 1 year, compared to those of 60 to 100 percent with the H_2-receptor antagonists.[206,207] However, the clearance of *C. pylori* from the stomach appears to be essential. In a recent study by Goodwin et al,[214] duodenal ulcer patients in whom *C. pylori* was cleared completely with CBS alone or in combination with tinidazole had better initial healing rates (93 percent versus 61 percent), and, in particular, lower relapse rates after 12 months (20 percent versus 74 percent) than those in whom *C. pylori* persisted. Other studies have found similar results.[215] However, it now appears that CBS may simply delay recurrence since, at 2 years, ulcers relapse regardless of initial therapy.[216] Whether gastroduodenal accumulation of bismuth plays a role remains to be determined.[217] Chronic antral gastritis and nonulcer dyspepsia, when associated with the presence of *C. pylori*, also show significant improvement with CBS both endoscopically and symptomatically.[218] However, early relapse occurs unless *C. pylori* is completely eradicated, which usually requires the use of an antimicrobial agent as well.[4,219] A combination of Pepto-Bismol (bismuth subsalicylate) and ampicillin has been used at our institution with considerable success, but the results of controlled trials are eagerly awaited.

The main formulations of CBS are chewable tablets or coated tablets[220,221]; the solution is no longer readily available. Coated tablets in particular reduce the unpleasant taste and smell, as well as the black discoloration of the tongue and teeth. Compliance is thus improved. In contrast to the situation with other bismuth-containing compounds, only a small amount of the bismuth in CBS is soluble,[7] so that absorption is usually minimal. Although peak plasma bismuth concentrations vary widely, they rarely exceed 50 μg per liter, even after 4 weeks of use. In a recent report, both CBS and bismuth subsalicylate exhibited similar peak concentrations of bismuth and time for the peak in gastric mucosa, gastric juice, and plasma.[222] Most of the ingested bismuth is excreted in stool as bismuth sulfide.[221]

At present, the disposition of bismuth in humans remains poorly understood. Any absorbed bismuth appears to be excreted in the urine, and thus cautious use of CBS is warranted in all patients with renal dysfunction.[223] A persistently elevated urinary excretion of bismuth in normal subjects, even several weeks after CBS is discontinued, suggests that significant tissue accumulation can occur.[221] This might explain the unique ability of CBS to reduce ulcer relapse rates up to 1 year after initial therapy. However, a recent report showed that gastroduodenal accumulation of CBS was not significant after 8 weeks,[217] even though plasma bismuth levels were elevated sevenfold. In another trial, CBS was used continually for 6 months without any apparent adverse effects.[224]

So far, there are no reports of any major adverse systemic effects with short-term use, except for a toxic encephalopathy. Only a single report of this exists for CBS when it was prescribed in high doses for a prolonged period.[225,226] Whether children or fetuses are more susceptible is not known. Until further data are available, the use of CBS during pregnancy should be avoided. CBS may also chelate certain drugs such as tetracycline, iron, or calcium, and antacids and food given concurrently may impair the in vivo precipitation of CBS.[221] Reye's syndrome is another potential problem with bismuth subsalicylate, although there have been no reports to date. CBS is not yet approved for use in the United States or Canada.

REFERENCES

1. Nord KS. Peptic ulcer disease in the pediatric population. Pediatr Clin North Am 1988; 35:117–140.
2. Drumm B, Rhoads JM, Stringer DA, Sherman PM, Ellis LE, Durie PR. Peptic ulcer disease in children: etiology, clinical findings, and clinical course. Pediatrics 1988; 82 (2):410–414.
3. Debas HT, Mulholland MW. Drug therapy in peptic ulcer disease. Curr Prob Surg 1989; 26:1–54.
4. Peterson WL, Richardson CT. Pharmacology and side effects of drugs used to treat peptic ulcer. In: Sleisinger MH, Fordtran JS, eds. Gastrointestinal disease—pathophysiology, diagnosis, management. 3rd ed. Philadelphia: WB Saunders, 1983: 708.
5. Harvey SC. Gastric antacids, miscellaneous drugs for the treatment of peptic ulcers, digestants, and bile acids. In: Gilman AG, Goodman LS, Rall TW, Murad FM, eds. The pharmacological basis of therapeutics. 7th ed. Toronto: Collier Macmillan Canada, 1985: 980.
6. Morrissey JF, Barreras RF. Antacid therapy. N Engl J Med 1974; 290:550–554.
7. Scarpignato C. Pharmacological bases of the medical treatment of gastroesophageal reflux disease. Dig Dis 1988; 6:117–148.
8. Berstad A. Antacids and pepsin. Scand J Gastroenterol 1982; 17 (suppl 75): 13–15.
9. Goldberg HI, Dodds WJ, Gee S, Montgomery C, Zboralske FF. Role of acid and pepsin in acute experimental esophagitis. Gastroenterology 1969; 56:223–230.
10. Clain JE, Malagelada J-R, Chadrick VS, Hofmann AF. Binding properties in vitro of antacids for conjugated bile acids. Gastroenterology 1977; 73:556–559.

11. Fordtran J, Morawski S, Richardson C. In vivo and in vitro evaluation of liquid antacids. N Engl J Med 1973; 288:923–928.
12. Texter EC Jr. A critical look at the clinical use of antacids in acid-peptic disease and gastric acid rebound. Am J Gastroenterol 1989; 84:97–108.
13. Peters MN, Feldman M, Walsh JH, Richardson CT. Effect of gastric alkalinization on serum gastrin concentrations in humans. Gastroenterology 1983; 85:35–39.
14. Fordtran JS. Acid rebound. N Engl J Med 1968; 279:900–905.
15. Levant JA, Walsh JH, Isenberg JI. Stimulation of gastric secretion and gastrin release by single oral doses of calcium carbonate in man. N Engl J Med 1973; 289:555–559.
16. Higgs RH, Smyth RD, Castell DO. Gastric alkalinization: effect on lower esophageal sphincter pressure and serum gastrin. N Engl J Med 1974; 291:486–488.
17. Hurwitz A, Robinson RG, Vats TS, Whittier FC, Herrin WF. Effects of antacids on gastric emptying. Gastroenterology 1976; 71:268–273.
18. Marano AR, Caride VJ, Prokop EK, Troncale FJ, McCallum RW. Effect of sulcrafate and of aluminum hydroxide gel on gastric emptying of solids and liquids. Clin Pharm Ther 1985; 37:629–632.
19. Strom M. Antacid side-effects on bowel habits. Scand J Gastroenterol 1982; 17(suppl 75):54–56.
20. Herzog P, Grendahl T, Linden J, van den Schmitt KF, Holtermuller K-H. Adverse effects of high-dose antacid regimen: results of a randomized, double-blind trial. Gastroenterology 1981; 80:1173–1179.
21. Brannan PG, Vergne-Marini P, Pak CYC, Hull AR, Fordtran JS. Magnesium absorption in the human small intestine. Results in normal subjects, patients with chronic renal disease, and patients with absorptive hypercalciuria. J Clin Invest 1976; 57:1412–1420.
22. Portuguez-Malavsai A, Aranda JV. Antacid bezoar in a newborn. Pediatrics 1979; 63:679–680.
23. Hurwitz A. Antacid therapy and drug kinetics. Clin Pharmacokinet 1977; 2:269–280.
24. Steinberg WM, Lewis JH, Katz DM. Antacids inhibit absorption of cimetidine. N Engl J Med 1982; 307:400–404.
25. Mihaly GW, Marino AT, Webster LK, Jones DB. High dose antacid (Mylanta II) reduces bioavailability of ranitidine. Br Med J 1982; 285:998–999.
26. Brown DD, Juhl RP. Decreased bioavailability of digoxin due to antacids and kaolin-pectin. N Engl J Med 1976; 295:1034–1037.
27. Fann WE, Davis JM, Janowsky DS. Chlorpromazine: effects of antacids on its gastrointestinal absorption. J Clin Pharmacol 1973; 13:388–390.
28. Uribe M, Casian C, Rojas S. Decreased bioavailability of prednisone due to antacids in patients with chronic active liver disease and in healthy volunteers. Gastroenterology 1981; 80:661–665.
29. Ambre JJ, Fisher LJ. Effect of coadministration of aluminum and magnesium hydroxides on absorption of anti-coagulants in man. Clin Pharmacol Ther 1973; 14:231–237.
30. Lanza FL, Sibley CM. Role of antacids in the management of disorders of the upper GI tract: review of clinical experience 1975-85. Am J Gastroenterol 1987; 82:1223–1241.
31. Peterson WL, Sturdevant RAL, Frankl HD, Richardson CT, Isenberg JI, Elashoff JD, Sones JQ, Gross RA, McCallum RW, Fordtran JS. Healing of duodenal ulcer with an antacid regimen. N Engl J Med 1977; 297:341–345.
32. Peterson WL, Barnett C, Feldman M. Richardson CT. Reduction of twenty-four hour gastric acidity with combination drug therapy in patients with duodenal ulcer. Gastroenterology 1979; 77:1015–1022.
33. Berstad A, Weberg R. Antacids in the treatment of gastroduodenal ulcer. Scand J Gastroenterol 1986; 21:385–391.
34. Kumar N, Vij JC, Karol A, Anand BS. Controlled therapeutic trial to determine the optimum dose of antacids in duodenal ulcer. Gut 1984; 25:1199–1202.
35. Weberg R, Aubert E, Dahlberg O, Dybdahl J, Ellekjaer E, Farup PG, Hovdenak N, Lange O, Melsom M, Stallemo A, Vetnik KR, Berstad A. Low-dose antacids or cimetidine for duodenal ulcer? Gastroenterology 1988; 95:1465–1469.
36. Sturdevant RAL, Isenberg JI, Secrist D, Ansfield JJ. Antacid and placebo produced similar pain relief in duodenal ulcer patients. Gastroenterology 1977; 72:1–5.
37. Grybosski JD. Pain and peptic ulcer disease in children. J Clin Gastroenterol 1980; 2:277–279.
38. Christie DL, Ament ME. Diagnosis and treatment of duodenal ulcer in infancy and childhood. Pediatr Ann 1976; 5:672–677.
39. Isenberg J, Elashoff J, Sandersfeld M, Peterson W. Double-blind comparisons of cimetidine and low-dose antacid versus placebo in the healing of benign gastric ulcer. Gastroenterology 1982; 82:1090.
40. Englert E, Freston JW, Graham DY, Finkelstein W, Kruss DM, Priest RJ, Raskin JB, Rhodes AI, Wenger J, Wilcox LL, Crossley RJ. Cimetidine, antacid and hospitalisation in the treatment of benign gastric ulcer. A multicenter double blind study. Gastroenterology 1978; 74:416–425.
41. Pribe HJ, Skillman JJ, Bushnell LS, Long PC, Silen W. Antacid versus cimetidine in preventing acute gastrointestinal bleeding. A randomized trial in 75 critically-ill patients. N Engl J Med 1980; 302:426–430.
42. Brimblecombe RW. Characterization and development of cimetidine as a histamine H_2-receptor antagonist. Gastroenterology 1978; 74: 339–347.
43. Freston JW. Cimetidine. I. Developments, pharmacology, efficacy. Ann Intern Med 1982; 97:573–580.
44. Gugler R, Fuchs G, Dieckmann M, Somogyi AA. Cimetidine plasma concentration-response relationships. Clin Pharm Ther 1981; 29: 744–748.
45. Burland WL, Duncan WAM, Hesselbo T, Mills JG, Sharpe PC. Pharmacological evaluation of cimetidine, a new histamine H_2-receptor antagonist, in healthy man. Br J Clin Pharmacol 1975; 2:481–486.
46. Chin TWF, MacLeod SM, Fenje P, Baltodano A, Edmonds JF, Soldin SJ. Pharmacokinetics of cimetidine in critically-ill children. Pediatr Pharmacol 1982; 2:285–292.
47. Pancorbo S, Bubrick MP, Chin TWF, Miller KW, Onstad G. Cimetidine dynamics after single intravenous doses. Clin Pharmacol Ther 1981; 29:744–748.
48. Chattriwalla Y, Colon AR, Scanlon JW. The use of cimetidine in the newborn. Pediatrics 1980; 65:301–302.
49. Ziemniak JA, Wynn RJ, Aranda JV, Zarowitz BJ, Schentag JJ. The pharmacokinetics and metabolism of cimetidine in neonates. Dev Pharmacol Ther 1984; 7:30–38.
50. Somogyi A, Becker M, Gugler R. Cimetidine pharmacokinetics and dosage requirements in children. Eur J Pediatr 1985; 144:72–76.
51. Bodemar G, Norlander B, Walan A. Pharmacokinetics of cimetidine after single doses and during continuous treatment. Clin Pharmacokinet 1981; 6:306–315.
52. Ostro MJ. Pharmacodynamics and pharmocokinetics of parenteral histamine (2)-receptor antagonists. Am J Med 1987; 83(suppl 6A):15–22.
53. Lebert PA, Mahon WA, MacLeod SM, Soldin SJ, Vandenberghe HM. Ranitidine kinetics and dynamics: II. Intravenous dose studies and comparison with cimetidine. Clin Pharmacol Ther 1981; 30:545–550.
54. Brogden RN, Carmine AA, Heel RC, Spreight TM, Avery GS. Ranitidine: a review of its pharmacology and therapeutic use in peptic ulcer disease and other allied diseases. Drugs 1982; 24:267–303.
55. Bogues K, Dixon GT, Fowler P, Jenner WN, Maconochie JG, Martin LE, Willoughby BA. Pharmacokinetics and bioavailability of ranitidine in humans. Br J Pharmacol 1981; 763:275–276.
56. Grahnen A, von Bahr C, Lindstrom B, Rosen A. Bioavailability and pharmacokinetics of cimetidine. Eur J Clin Pharmacol 1979; 16: 335–340.
57. Miller R. Pharmacokinetics and bioavailability of ranitidine in humans. J Pharm Sci 1984; 73:1376–1379.
58. Howe JP, McGowan WA, Moore J. The placental transfer of cimetidine. Anesthesia 1981; 36:371–375.
59. Somogyi A, Gugler R. Cimetidine excretion into breast milk. Br J Clin Pharmacol 1979; 7:627–628.
60. Taylor DC, Cresswell PR, Barlett DC. The metabolism and elimination of cimetidine, a histamine H_2-receptor antagonist in the rat, dog, and man. Drug Metab Dispos 1978; 6:21–29.
61. Roberts CJ. Clinical pharmacokinetics of ranitidine. Clin Pharmacokinet 1984; 9:211–221.
62. Bonfils S, Classen M, Langman MJS, eds. Symposium on roxatidine acetate. Drugs 1988; 35(suppl 3):1–142.
63. Aranda JV, Outerbridge EW, Schentag JJ. Pharmacodynamics and kinetics of cimetidine in a premature newborn. (Letter) Am J Dis Child 1983; 137:1207.
64. Ziemniak JA, Assael BM, Padoan R, Schentag JJ. The bioavailability and pharmacokinetics of cimetidine and its metabolites in juvenile cystic fibrosis patients: age related differences as compared to adults. Eur J Clin Pharmacol 1984; 26:183–189.
65. Bradbear RA, Shepherd RW, McGuffie C, Grice J, Roberts RK. The kinetics of oral cimetidine in children with cystic fibrosis. Br J Clin Pharmacol 1981; 12:248–249.

66. Blumer JL, Rothstein FC, Kaplan BS, Yamashita TS, Eshelman FN, Myers CM, Reed MD. Pharmacokinetic determination of ranitidine pharmacodynamics in pediatric ulcer disease. J Pediatrics 1985; 107:301–306.
67. Leeder JS, Harding L, MacLeod SM. Ranitidine pharmacokinetics in children. Clin Pharmacol Ther 1985; 37:201.
68. Nord KS, Rossi TM, Rosenthal E. Peptic ulcer disease in children. Compr Ther 1983; 9:18–25.
69. Smith JL, Gamal MA, Chremos AN, Graham DY. Famotidine, a new H_2 receptor antagonist. Dig Dis Sci 1985; 30:308–312.
70. Simon B, Cremer AN, Dammann HG, Hentschel E, Keohane PP, Mulder H, Mullen P. 300 mg nizatidine or 300 mg ranitidine at night in patients with duodenal ulcer. Scand J Gastroenterol 1987; 22(suppl 136):61–70.
71. Merton DM. Pharmacology and toxicology of nizatidine. Scand J Gastroenterol 1987; 22(suppl 136):1–8.
72. Brater DC, Meyers WM Jr, Dandekar KA. Clinical pharmacology of etintidine in patients with duodenal ulcer. Eur J Clin Pharmacol 1982; 23:495–500.
73. Freston JW. Cimetidine and agranulocytosis. Ann Intern Med 1979; 90:264–265.
74. McMillan MA, Amelis D, Siegel JH. Cimetidine and mental confusion. N Engl J Med 1978; 298:284–285.
75. McGuigan JE. Side effects of histamine H_2-receptor antagonists. Clin Gastroenterol 1981; 12:819–838.
76. Delitala G, Stubbs WA, Wass JAH, Jones A, Williams S, Besser GM. Effects of the H_2-receptor antagonist cimetidine on pituitary hormones in man. Clin Endocrinol 1979; 11:161–167.
77. Van der Meer JWM, Kenning JJ, Scheijgrond HW, Keykants J, Van Cutsem J, Brugmans J. The influence of gastric acidity on the bioavailability of ketoconazole. J Antimicrob Chemother 1980; 6:552–554.
78. Khoury W, Gerasi K, Askari A, Johnson M. The effect of cimetidine on aspirin absorption. Gastroenterology 1979; 76:1169.
79. Lilly JR, Hitch DC, Javitt NB. Cimetidine cholestatic jaundice in children. J Surg Res 1978; 24:384–387.
80. Somogyi A, Gugler R. Drug interactions with cimetidine. Clin Pharmacokinet 1982; 7:23–41.
81. Puurunen J, Sotaniemi E, Pelkonen O. Effect of cimetidine on microsomal drug metabolism in man. Eur J Clin Pharmacol 1980; 18:185–187.
82. Bell JA, Gower AJ, Martin LE, Mills ENC, Smith WP. Interaction of H_2-receptor antagonists with drug metabolizing enzymes. Biochem Soc Trans 1981; 9:113–114.
83. Rendic S, Kajfez F, Ruf HH. Characterization of cimetidine, ranitidine and related structures. Interaction with cytochrome P-450. Drug Metab Dispos 1983; 11:137–142.
84. Rendic S, Sundic V, Toso R. Interaction of cimetidine with liver microsomes. Xenobiotica 1979; 9:555–564.
85. Mitchard M, Harris A, Mullinger BM. Ranitidine drug interactions—a literature review. Pharmacol Ther 1987; 32:293–325.
86. Serlin MJ, Sibeon RG, Mossman S, Breckenridge AM, Williams JRB, Atwood JL, Willoughby JMT. Cimetidine interaction with oral anticoagulants in man. Lancet 1979; ii:317–319.
87. Bartle WR, Walker SE, Shapero T. Dose-dependent effect of cimetidine on phenytoin kinetics. Clin Pharmacol Ther 1983; 33:649–655.
88. Klotz U, Reimann I. Delayed clearance of diazepam due to cimetidine. N Engl J Med 1980; 302:1012–1014.
89. Roberts RK, Grice J, Wood L, Petroff V, McGuffie C. Cimetidine impairs the elimination of theophylline and antipyrine. Gastroenterology 1981; 81:19–21.
90. Desmond PV, Patwhardhan RV, Schenker S, Speeg KV. Cimetidine impairs the elimination of chlordiazepoxide (Librium) in man. Ann Intern Med 1980; 93:266–268.
91. Breen KG, Bury R, Desmond PV, Mashford ML, Morphett B, Westwood B, Shaw RG. Effects of cimetidine and ranitidine on hepatic drug metabolism. Clin Pharmacol Ther 1982; 31:297–300.
92. Feely J, Wilkinson GR, Wood AJJ. Reduction of liver blood flow and propranolol metabolism by cimetidine. N Engl J Med 1981; 304:692–695.
93. Wallmark B, Lorentzon P, Larsson H. The mechanism of action of omeprazole—a survey of its inhibitory actions *in vitro*. Scand J Gastroenterol 1985; 20(suppl 108):37–52.
94. Sachs G. Pump blockers and ulcer disease. N Engl J Med 1984; 310:785–786.
95. McColl KEL. Assessment of two new therapies for peptic ulcer disease: Omeprazole and the prostaglandin analogues. Dig Dis 1988; 6:65–75.
96. Berglindh T, Sachs G. Emerging strategies in ulcer therapy: Pumps and receptors. Scand J Gastroenterol 1985; 20(suppl 108):7–14.
97. Brandstrom A, Lindberg P, Junggren U. Structure and activity relationships of substituted benzimidazoles. Scand J Gastroenterol 1985; 20(suppl 108):15–22.
98. Wallmark B, Branstrom A, Larsson H. Evidence for acid-induced transformation of omeprazole into an active inhibitor of (H^+ + K^+) ATPase within the parietal cell. Biochim Biophys Acta 1984; 778:549–558.
99. Keeling DJ, Fallowfield C, Milliner KJ, Tingley SK, Ife RJ. Studies on the mechanism of action of omeprazole. Biochem Pharmacol 1985; 34:2967–2973.
100. Londong W, Londong V, Cederberg C, Steffen H. Dose-response study of omeprazole on meal-stimulated gastric acid secretion and gastrin release. Gastroenterology 1983; 85:1373–1378.
101. Walt RP, Gommes M de FA, Wood EC, Logan LH, Pounder RE. Effect of daily oral omeprazole on 24-hr intragastric acidity. Br Med J 1983; 287:12–14.
102. Pounder RE, Sharma BK, Walt RP. Twenty-four hour intragastric acidity during treatment with oral omeprazole. Scand J Gastroenterol 1986; 21(suppl 118):108–116.
103. Kittang E, Aasland E, Schjonsby H. Effect of omeprazole on the secretion of intrinsic factor, gastric acid and pepsin in man. Gut 1985; 26:594–598.
104. Konturek SJ, Brzozowski T, Radecki T. Protective action of omeprazole, a benzimidazole derivative, on gastric mucosal damage by aspirin and ethanol in rats. Digestion 1983; 27:159–164.
105. Clissold SP, Campoli-Richards DM. Omeprazole—a preliminary review of its pharmacodynamic and pharmacokinetic properties, and therapeutic potential in peptic ulcer disease and Zollinger-Ellison syndrome. Drugs 1986; 32:15–47.
106. Naesdal J, Bodemar G, Walan A. Effect of omeprazole, a substituted benzimidazole, on 24-hr intragastric acidity in patients with peptic ulcer disease. Scand J Gastroenterol 1984; 19:916–922.
107. Howden CW, Meredith PA, Forrest JAH, Reid JL. Oral pharmacokinetics of omeprazole. Eur J Clin Pharmacol 1984; 26:641–643.
108. Howden CW, Payton CD, Meredith PA, Hughes DMA, Macdougall AL, Reid JL, Forrest JAH. Antisecretory effect and oral pharmacokinetics of omeprazole in patients with chronic renal failure. Eur J Clin Pharmacol 1985; 28:637–640.
109. Huttemann W, Rotner HG, duBosque G, Rehner M. Hebbeln H. 20 versus 30 mg omeprazole once daily: effect on healing rates in 115 duodenal ulcer patients. Digestion 1986; 33:117–120.
110. Archambeault AP, Pare P, Bailey RJ, Navert H, Williams CN, Freeman HJ, Baker SJ, Marcon NE, Hunt RH, Sutherland L, Kepkay DL, Saibil FG, Hawken K, Farley A, Levesque D, Ferguson J, Westin JA. Omeprazole (20 mg daily) versus cimetidine (1200 mg daily) in duodenal ulcer healing and pain relief. Gastroenterology 1988; 94:1130–1134.
111. Tytgat GNJ, Lamers CBHW, Wilson JA, Hameeteman W, Jansen JBMJ, Wormsley KG. 100 percent healing with omeprazole of peptic ulcers resistant to histamine H_2-receptor antagonists. Gastroenterology 1985; 88:1620.
112. Lauritsen K, Rune SJ, Bytzer P, Kelbaek H, Jensen KG. Effect of omeprazole and cimetidine on duodenal ulcer. N Engl J Med 1985; 312:958–961.
113. Walan A, Bader J-P, Classen M, Lamers DBHW, Piper DW, Rutgersson K, Eriksson S. Effect of omeprazole and ranitidine on ulcer healing and relapse rates in patients with benign gastric ulcer. N Engl J Med 1989; 320:69–75.
114. Lloyd-Davies KA, Rutgersson K, Solvell L. Omeprazole in Zollinger-Ellison syndrome: four-year international study. Gastroenterology 1986; 90:1523.
115. Hetzel DJ, Dent J, Reed WD, Laurence BH. Healing and relapse of severe peptic esophagitis after treatment with omeprazole. Gastroenterology 1988; 95:903–912.
116. Festen HPM, Thijs JC, Lamers CBHW, Jansen JMBJ, Pals G, Frants RR, Defize J, Meuwissen SGM. Effect of oral omeprazole on serum gastrin and serum pepsinogen I levels. Gastroenterology 1984; 87:1030–1034.
117. Larsson H, Carlsson E, Mattson H, Lundell L, Sundler F, Sundell G, Wallmark B, Watanabe T, Hakanson R. Plasma gastrin and gastric

enterochromaffin-life cell activation and proliferation. Studies with omeprazole and ranitidine in intact and antrectomized rats. Gastroenterology 1986; 90:391–399.
118. Borch K, Renvall H, Liedberg G, Andersen BN. Relations between circulating gastrin and endocrine cell proliferation in the atrophic gastric fundic mucosa. Scand J Gastroenterol 1986; 21:357–363.
119. Sharma BK. Santana IA, Wood EC, Walt RP, Pereira M, Noone P, Smith PLR, Walters CL, Pounder RE. Intragastric bacterial activity and nitrosation before, during, and after treatment with omeprazole. Br Med J 1984; 289:717–719.
120. Gugler R, Jensen JC. Omeprazole inhibits oxidative drug metabolism. Gastroenterology 1985; 89:1235–1241.
121. Dowie LJ, Smith JE, MacGilchrist AJ, Fraser R, Honour JW, Kenyon CJ. In vivo and in vitro studies of the site of inhibitory action of omeprazole on adrenocortical steroidogenesis. Br J Pharmacol 1988; 93:288P.
122. Festen H, Tertoolen J. Malabsorption of protein-bound but no unbound cobalamin during treatment with omeprazole. Gastroenterology 1988; 94:A125.
123. Hammer R, Berrie CP, Birdsall NJ, Burgen ASV, Hulme EC. Pirenzepine distinguishes between different subclasses of muscarinic receptors. Nature (Lond) 1980; 283:90–92.
124. Bianchi-Porro G, Prada A, Petrillo M, Grossi M. Inhibition of pentagastrin and insulin-stimulated gastric secretion by pirenzepine in healthy and duodenal ulcer subjects. Scand J Gastroenterol 1979; 14(suppl 57):63–69.
125. Londong W, Londong V, Ruthe C, Weizert P. Complete inhibition of food-stimulated gastric acid secretion by combined application of pirenzepine and ranitidine. Gut 1981; 22:542–548.
126. El Sabbagh HN, Prinz RA, Welburn RB, Baron JH. Influence of intravenous pirenzepine on gastric acid and pepsin in man. Scand J Gastroenterol 1980; 15(suppl 66):73–77.
127. Heathcote BV. Classification of antimuscarinic substances. Scand J Gastroenterol 1982; 17(suppl 72):271.
128. Konturek SJ, Brzozowski T, Radecki T, Piastucki I. Gastric cytoprotection by pirenzepine. Role of endogenous prostaglandins. Scand J Gastroenterol 1982; 17(suppl 72):255–260.
129. Soffer EE, Kumar D, Mridha K, Das-Gupta A, Britto J, Wingate DL. Effect of pirenzepine on oesophageal, gastric, and enteric motor function in man. Scand J Gastroenterol 1988; 23:146–150.
130. Hammer R, Koss FW. The pharmacokinetic profile of pirenzepine. Scand J Gastroenterol 1979; 14(suppl 57):1–6.
131. Bozler G, Hammer R. An international pharmacokinetic study on pirenzepine following a single oral dose. Scand J Gastroenterol 1980; 15(suppl 66):27–33.
132. Jaup BH, Blomstrand C. Cerebro-spinal fluid concentrations of pirenzepine after therapeutic dosage. Scand J Gastroenterol 1980; 15(suppl 72):35–37.
133. Texter EC, Reilly PA. The efficacy and selectivity of pirenzepine. Review and commentary. Scand J Gastroenterol 1982; 17(suppl 72):237–246.
134. Giorgi-Conciato M, Daniotti S, Ferrari PA, Gaetani M, Petrin G, Sala P, Valentini P. Efficacy and safety of pirenzepine in peptic ulcer and in non-ulcerous gastroduodenal diseases. A multicenter controlled clinical trial. Scand J Gastroenterol 1982; 17(suppl 81):1–42.
135. Dal Monte PR, D'Imperio N, Accardo P, Daniotti S. Pirenzepine in non-ulcer dyspepsia. A double-blind, placebo controlled trial. Scand J Gastroenterol 1982; 17(suppl 72):247–250.
136. Carmine AA, Brogden RN. Pirenzepine. A review of its pharmacodynamic and pharmacokinetic properties and therapeutic efficacy in peptic ulcer disease and other allied diseases. Drugs 1985; 30:85–126.
137. Dajani EZ, Driskill DR, Bianchi RG, Collins PW, Pappo R. Influence of the position of the side chain hydroxy group on the gastric antisecretory and antiulcer actions of E_1 prostaglandin analogs. Prostaglandins 1975; 10:733–745.
138. Hawkey CJ, Rampton DS. Prostaglandins and the gastrointestinal mucosa: are they important in its function, disease, or treatment? Gastroenterology 1985; 89:1162–1188.
139. Allison AC, Kowalski WJ, Strulovici B. Effects of enprostil on platelets, endothelial cells, and other cell types, and second messenger systems by which these effects are mediated. Am J Med 1986; 81(suppl 2A):34–39.
140. Bauer RF. Misoprostol: preclinical pharmacology. Dig Dis Sci 1985; 30(suppl):118S–125S.
141. Shimizu N, Nakamura T. Prostaglandins as hormones. Dig Dis Sci 1985; 30(suppl):109S–113S.
142. Deakin M, Ramage J, Paul A, Gray SP, Billings J, Williams JG. Effect of enprostil, a synthetic prostaglandin E2 on the 24 hour intragastric acidity, nocturnal acid and pepsin secretion. Gut 1986; 27:1054–1057.
143. Monk JP, Clissold SP. Misoprostol—a preliminary review of its pharmacodyanamic and pharmacokinetic properties, and therapeutic efficacy in the treatment of peptic ulcer disease. Drugs 1987; 33:1–30.
144. McGuigan JE, Chang Y, Dajani EZ. Effect of misoprostol, an antiulcer prostaglandin, on serum gastrin in patients with duodenal ulcer. Dig Dis Sci 1986; 31(suppl):120S–125S.
145. Miller TA. Protective effects of prostaglandins against gastric mucosal damage: current knowledge and proposed mechanisms. Am J Physiol 1983; 245:G601–G623.
146. Liss RH, Letourneau RJ, Schepsis JP. Evaluation of cytoprotection against ethanol-induced injury in gastric mucosa pretreated with misoprostol, cimetidine, or placebo. Dig Dis Sci 1986; 31(suppl):108S–114S.
147. Cohen MM, Clark L, Armstrong L, D'Souza J. Reduction of aspirin-induced fecal blood loss with low-dose misoprostol tablets in man. Dig Dis Sci 1985; 30:605–611.
148. Hunt JN, Smith JL, Jiang CL, Kessler L. Effect of synthetic prostaglandin E1 analog on aspirin-induced gastric bleeding and secretion. Dig Dis Sci 1983; 28:897–902.
149. Lanza FL. A double-blind study of prophylactic effect of misoprostol on lesions of gastric and duodenal mucosa induced by oral administration of tolmetin in healthy subjects. Dig Dis Sci 1986; 31(suppl): 131S–136S.
150. Russell RI. Protective effects of the prostaglandins on the gastric mucosa. Am J Med 1986; 81(suppl 2A):2–4.
151. Goa KL, Monk JP. Enprostil—a preliminary review of its pharmacodynamic and pharmacokinetic properties, and therapeutic efficacy in the treatment of peptic ulcer disease. Drugs 1987; 34:539–559.
152. Schoenhard G, Oppermann J, Kohn FE. Metabolism and pharmacokinetic studies of misoprostol. Dig Dis Sci 1985; 30(suppl):126S–128S.
153. Stanski DR, Burch PG, Tomlinson R, Sevelius H. Disposition of a synthetic dehydroprostaglandin E2 analog in man. Clin Pharmacol Ther 1982; 31:273.
154. Carling L, Unge P, Almstrom C, Cronstedt P, Ekstrom P, Hagg S, Hansson B. Enprostil and cimetidine: comparative efficacy and safety in patients with duodenal ulcer. Scand J Gastroenterol 1987; 22:325–331.
155. Winters L, Willcox R, Ligny G, Barbier P, Deltenre M. Comparison of enprostil and cimetidine in active duodenal ulcer: summary of pooled European studies. Am J Med 1986; 81(suppl 2A):69–74.
156. Kanuer CM. The efficacy of enprostil in reflux esophagitis. Dig Dis Sci 1986; 31(suppl):215S.
157. Moore JG, Alazraki N, Clay GD. Effect of synthetic prostaglandin E1 analog on gastric emptying of meals in man. Dig Dis Sci 1986; 31(suppl):16S–20S.
158. Bynum L, Gross G. Use of enprostil in asthmatics taking theophylline. Clin Pharm Ther 1986; 39:184.
159. Reilly CS, Biollaz J, Koshakji RP, Wood AJJ. Enprostil, in contrast to cimetidine, does not inhibit propranolol metabolism, Clin Pharm Ther 1986; 40:37–41.
160. Herting RI, Clay GA. Overview of clinical safety with misoprostol. Dig Dis Sci 1985; 30(suppl):185S–193S.
161. Schwartz K, Zaro B, Reynolds J, Saito T, Duffy J, Hunt J, Senelius H. Effects of enprostil, a potent prostaglandin analogue, on carbohydrate metabolism in normal subjects. Clin Res 1986; 34:554A.
162. Richardson CT. Sucralfate. Ann Intern Med 1982; 97:269–271.
163. Nagashima R. Mechanism of action of sucralfate. J Clin Gastroenterol 1981; 3(suppl 2):117–127.
164. Samloff IM. Inhibition of peptic aggression by sucralfate. The view from the ulcer crater. Scand J Gastroenterol 1983; 18(suppl 83):7–11.
165. Crampton JR, Gibbons LC, Rees W. Effects of sucralfate on gastroduodenal bicarbonate secretion and prostaglandin E_2 metabolism. Am J Med 1987; 83(suppl 3B):14–18.
166. Konturek SJ, Kwiecien N, Obtulowicz W, Oleksy J. Gastroprotection by sucralfate against acetylsalicylic acid in humans. Role of endogenous prostaglandins. Scand J Gastroenterol 1987; 22(suppl 140):19–22.
167. Harrington SJ, Schlegel JF, Code CF. The protective effect of sucralfate on the gastric mucosa of rats. J Clin Gastroenterol 1981; 3(suppl 2):129–134.
168. Brogden RN, Hill RC, Speight TM, Avery GS. Sucralfate. A review

of its pharmacodynamic properties and therapeutic use in peptic ulcer disease. Drugs 1984;27:194–207.

169. Bresalier RS, Grendell JH, Cello JP, Meyer AA. Sucralfate suspension *versus* titrated antacid for the prevention of acute stress-related gastrointestinal hemorrhage in critically ill patients. Am J Med 1987; 83(suppl 3B):110–116.

170. Tarnawski A, Hollander D, Gergely H. The mechanism of protective, therapeutic and prophylactic actions of sucralfate. Scand J Gastroenterol 1987; 22(suppl 140):7–13.

171. Nexo E, Poulsen SS. Does epidermal growth factor play a role in the action of sucralfate? Scand J Gastroenterol 1987; 22(suppl 127):45–49.

172. Tryba M. Risk of acute stress bleeding and nosocomial pneumonia in ventilated intensive care unit patients: sucralfate versus antacids. Am J Med 1987; 83(suppl 3B):117–124.

173. Tryba M, Mantey-Stiers F. Antibacterial activity of sucralfate in human gastric juice. Am J Med 1987; 83(suppl 3B):125–127.

174. Giesing D, Lonsaan R, Runsen D. Absorption of sucralfate in man. Gastroenterology 1982; 82:1066.

175. Kinoshita H, Kumaki K, Nakano H, Tsuyama K, Nagashima R, Okuda M, McGraw B. Plasma aluminum levels of patients on long term sucralfate therapy. Res Commun Chem Pathol Pharmacol 1982; 35: 515–518.

176. Bolin TD, Davis AE, Duncombe VM, Billington B. Role of maintenance sucralfate in prevention of duodenal ulcer recurrence. Am J Med 1987; 83(suppl 3B):91–94.

177. Leung AC, Henderson IS, Halls DJ, Dobbie JW. Aluminium hydroxide versus sucralfate as a phosphate binder in uremia. Br Med J 1983; 286:1379–1381.

178. Mungall D, Talbert RL, Phillips C, Jaffe D, Ludden TM. Sucralfate and warfarin. Ann Intern Med 1983; 98:557.

179. Giesing DH, Lanman RC, Dimmitt DC, Runsen DJ. Lack of effect of sucralfate on digoxin pharmacokinetics. Gastroenterology 1983; 84:1165.

180. Lacz JP, Groschang AG, Giesing DH, Browne RK. The effect of sucralfate on drug absorption in dogs. Gastroenterology 1982; 82:1108.

181. Martin F, Farley A, Gagnon M, Bensemana D. Comparison of the healing capacities of sucralfate and cimetidine in the short-term treatment of duodenal ulcer: a double-blind randomised trial. Gastroenterology 1982; 82:401–405.

182. Marks IN, Wright JP, Glinsky NH. A comparison of sucralfate dosage schedule in duodenal ulcer healing. J Clin Gastroenterol 1986; 8:419–423.

183. Glise H, Carling L, Hallerbaeck B, Hallgren T, Kagevi I, Solhaug JH, Svedberg L-E, Waehlberg L. Relapse rate of healed duodenal, prepyloric, and gastric ulcers treated either with sucralfate or cimetidine. Am J Med 1987; 83(suppl 3B):105–109.

184. Marks IN, Girdwood AH, Wright JP, Newton KA, Gilinsky NH, Kalvaria I, Burno DG, O'Keefe SJ, Tobias R, Lucke W. Nocturnal dosage regimen of sucralfate in maintenance treatment of gastric ulcer. Am J Med 1987; 83(suppl 3B):95–98.

185. Caldwell JR, Roth SH, Wu WC, Semble EL, Castell DO, Heller MD, Marsh WH. Sucralfate treatment of non-steroidal anti-inflammatory drug-induced gastrointestinal symptoms and mucosal damage. Am J Med 1987; 83(suppl 3B):74–82.

186. Kairoluoma MI, Hentilae R, Alavaikko M, Kellosalo J, Stahlberg M, Jalovaara P, Olsen M, Jaevernsivu P, Laitinen S. Sucralfate versus placebo in the treatment of non-ulcer dyspepsia. Am J Med 1987; 83(suppl 3B):51–55.

187. Eisborg L, Beck B, Studgaard M. Effect of sucralfate on gastroesophageal reflux in esophagitis. Hepatogastroenterology 1985; 32: 181–184.

188. Tytgat GN. Clinical efficacy of sucralfate in reflux esophagitis: comparison with cimetidine. Am J Med 1987; 83(suppl 3B):38–42.

189. Williams RM, Orlando RC, Bozymski EM, Readling RD, Castell DO, Ronfail WM, Rick GG, Rubin SE, Sinar DR. Multicenter trial of sucralfate suspension for the treatment of reflux esophagitis. Am J Med 1987; 83(suppl 3B):61–66.

190. Wieriks J, Hespe W, Jaitly KD, Koekkoek PH, Lavy U. Pharmacological properties of colloidal bismuth subcitrate (CBS, De-Nol). Scand J Gastroenterol 1982; 17(suppl 80):11–16.

191. Koo J, Ho J, Lam SK, Wong J, Ong GB. Selective coating of gastric ulcer by tripotassium dicitrato bismuthate in the rat. Gastroenterology 1982; 82:864–870.

192. Konturek SJ, Bilski J, Kwiecien N, Obtulowicz W, Kopp B. De-Nol stimulates gastric and duodenal alkaline secretion through prostaglandin dependent mechanism. Gut 1987; 28:1557–1563.

193. Konturek SJ, Radecki T, Piastucki I, Drozdowicz D. Advances in the understanding of the mechanism of cytoprotective action by colloidal bismuth subcitrate. Scand J Gastroenterol 1986; 21(suppl 122):6–10.

194. Konturek SJ, Radecki T, Piastucki I, Drozdowicz D. Studies on the gastroprotective and ulcer healing effects of colloidal bismuth subcitrate. Digestion 1987; 37(suppl 2):8–15.

195. Moshal MG, Gregory MA, Pillay C, Spitaels JM. Does the duodenal cell ever return to normal? A comparison between treatment with cimetidine and De-Nol. Scand J Gastroenterol 1979; 14(suppl 54):48–51.

196. Baron JH, Barr J, Batten J, Sidebotham R, Spencer J. Acid, pepsin and mucus secretion in patients with gastric and duodenal ulcer before and after colloidal bismuth subcitrate (De-Nol). Gut 1986; 27:486–490.

197. Rauws EA, Langenberg W, Houthoff HJ, Zanen HC, Tytgat GN. *Campylobacter pyloridis*-associated chronic active antral gastritis. Gastroenterology 1988; 94:33–40.

198. Dooley CP, Cohen H. The clinical significance of *Campylobacter pylori*. Ann Intern Med 1988; 108:70–79.

199. Drumm B, O'Brien A, Cutz E, Sherman P. *Campylobacter-pyloridis* associated primary gastritis in children. Pediatrics 1987; 80:192–195.

200. Drumm B, Sherman P, Cutz E, Karmali M. Association of *Campylobacter-pyloridis* on the gastric mucosa with antral gastritis in children. N Engl J Med 1987; 316:1557–1561.

201. Tytgat GN, Rauws E, Langenberg ML. The role of colloidal bismuth subcitrate in gastric ulcer and gastritis. Scand J Gastroenterol 1986; 21(suppl 122):22–29.

202. Armstrong JA, Wee SH, Goodwin CS, Wilson DH. Response of *Campylobacter pyloridis* to antibiotics, bismuth and an acid-reducing agent *in vitro*—an ultrastructural study. J Med Microbiol 1987; 24:343–350.

203. Lee SP, Nicholson GI. Increased healing of gastric and duodenal ulcers in a controlled trial using tripotassium dicitrato-bismuthate. Med J Austral 1977; 1:808–812.

204. Wilson P, Alp MH. Colloidal bismuth subcitrate tablets and placebo in chronic duodenal ulceration: a double-blind, randomised trial. Med J Austral 1982; 1:222–223.

205. Glover SC, Cantlay JS, Weir J, Mowat NA. Oral tripotassium-dicitratobismuthate in gastric and duodenal ulceration: a double-blind controlled trial. Dig Dis Sci 1983; 28:13–17.

206. Hamilton I, O'Connor HJ, Wood NC, Bradbury I, Axon AT. Healing and recurrence of duodenal ulcer after treatment with tripotassium dicitrato bismuthate (TDB) tablets or cimetidine. Gut 1986; 27:106–110.

207. Ward M, Halliday C, Cowen AE. A comparison of colloidal bismuth subcitrate tablets and ranitidine in the treatment of chronic duodenal ulcers. Digestion 1986; 34:173–177.

208. Lee FI, Samloff IM, Hardman M. Comparison of tri-potassium dicitrato bismuthate tablets with ranitidine in healing and relapse of duodenal ulcers. Lancet 1985; ii:1299–1302.

209. Parente F, Lazzaroni M, Petrillo M, Bianchi Porro G. Colloidal bismuth subcitrate and ranitidine in the short-term treatment of benign gastric ulcer: an endoscopically controlled trial. Scand J Gastroenterol 1986; 21(suppl 122):42–45.

210. Lazzaroni M, Parente F, Prada A, Bianchi Porro G. Colloidal bismuth subcitrate as coated tablets: four times *versus* twice daily dosage in duodenal ulcer. Scand J Gastroenterol 1986; 21(suppl 122):51–53.

211. Salmon PR. Combination treatment; colloidal bismuth subcitrate with H_2-antagonists. Digestion 1987; 37(suppl 2):42–46.

212. Bianchi Porro G, Parente F, Lazzaroni M. Tripotassium dicitrato bismuthate (TDB) *versus* two different dosages of cimetidine in the treatment of resistant duodenal ulcers. Gut 1987; 28:907–911.

213. Dobrilla G, Vallaperta P, Amplatz S. Influence of ulcer healing agents on ulcer relapse after discontinuation of acute treatment: a pooled estimate of controlled clinical trials. Gut 1988; 29:181–187.

214. Goodwin CS, Marshall BJ, Blincow ED, Wilson DH, Blackbourn S, Phillips M. Prevention of nitroimidazole resistance in *Campylobacter pylori* by coadministration of colloidal bismuth subcitrate: clinical and *in vitro* studies. J Clin Pathol 1988; 41:207–210.

215. Coghlan JG, Gilligan D, Humphries H, McKenna D, Sweeney E, Keane C, O'Morain C. *Campylobacter pylori* and recurrence of duodenal ulcers—12-months follow-up study. Lancet 1987; ii:1109–1111.

216. Lane MR, Lee SP. Recurrence of duodenal ulcer after medical treatment. Lancet 1988; i:1299–1300.

217. Lambert JR, King RG, Way DJ, Korman MG, Hansky J. Accumula-

tion of bismuth in gastric mucosa after D-Nol therapy—fact or fiction. Gastroenterology 1989; 96:A284.
218. Marshall BJ, Armstrong JA, Francis GJ, Nokes NT, Wee SH. Antibacterial action of bismuth in relation to *Campylobacter pyloridis* colonisation and gastritis. Digestion 1987; 37(suppl 2):16–30.
219. Rauws EAJ, Langenberg W, Houthoff HJ, Zaven HC, Tytgat GNJ. *Campylobacter pylori* associated gastritis—a prospective study of its prevalence and the effects of antibacterial treatment. Gut 1988; 94:33–40.
220. Hollanders D, Morrissey SM, Mehta J. Mucus secretion in gastric ulcer patients treated with tripotassium dicitrato bismuthate (De-Nol). Br J Clin Pract 1983; 37:112–114.
221. Wagstaff A, Benfield P, Monk JP. Colloidal bismuth subcitrate—a review of its pharmacodynamic and pharmacokinetic properties, and its therapeutic use in peptic ulcer disease. Drugs 1988; 36:132–157.
222. Lambert JR, Way DJ, King RG, Eaves ER, Lianeas K, Wan A. De-Nol versus peptobismol—bismuth pharmacokinetics in the human gastric mucosa. Gastroenterology 1989; 96:A284.
223. Dekker W, Reisma K. Double-blind controlled trial with colloidal bismuth subcitrate in the treatment of symptomatic duodenal ulcers, with special references to blood and urine bismuth levels. Ann Clin Res 1979; 11:94–97.
224. Bianchi Porro G, Lazzaroni M, Cortvriendt WRE. Maintenance therapy with colloidal bismuth subcitrate in duodenal ulcer disease. Digestion 1987; 37(suppl 2):47–52.
225. Weller MP. Neuropsychiatric symptoms following bismuth intoxication. Postgrad Med J 1988; 64:308–310.
226. Bader JP. The safety profile of De-Nol. Digestion 1987; 37(suppl 2):53–59.

PART 4

Drug Therapy for Liver Disease

Eve A. Roberts, M.D., FRCPC

Although hepatology has been regarded for years as the domain of the therapeutic nihilist, drug therapy is potentially curative in various childhood liver diseases. Drug treatment of the consequences of severe chronic liver disease, such as pruritus, vitamin deficiencies, and hepatic encephalopathy, is also a major consideration in the medical management of children with chronic liver diseases. It is now becoming clear that innovative antiviral treatments may be useful in treating some types of infective hepatitis. Pharmacologic and developmental aspects of such drug therapy are important. Nutritional management of liver disease and primary prophylaxis against infective hepatitis will not be considered here. For detailed discussion of the clinical features of specific liver diseases, the reader should refer to the appropriate chapter elsewhere in this textbook.

TREATMENT OF AUTOIMMUNE CHRONIC ACTIVE HEPATITIS

Autoimmune chronic active hepatitis (AICAH) is a chronic inflammatory disease of the liver, presumed to be of immune origin and associated with the presence of non–organ-specific autoantibodies. As its histopathology is not specific, other causes of "chronic active hepatitis" (namely virus infection, drug hepatotoxicity, Wilson's disease, $alpha_1$-antitrypsin deficiency) must be excluded. Although it may have an insidious onset, AICAH frequently presents in children as an acute hepatitis with jaundice, anorexia, and sometimes ascites. In children AICAH tends to progress rapidly to cirrhosis, often present at the time of diagnosis.[1] However, treatment can lead to clinical and biochemical improvement, and decompensated liver function may not develop for some time.

For nearly 20 years, the treatment of AICAH has involved immunosuppression, and the mainstay of this treatment is oral corticosteroids.[2–6] Early studies in adults established the efficacy of prednisolone or prednisone in low maintenance doses[3] or combined with azathioprine[4] and the ineffectiveness of azathioprine as sole initial treatment.[5] Despite their evident shortcomings (including failure to exclude hepatitis B–induced chronic active hepatitis, small study numbers, and erratic dose schedules), these studies form the basis for treating AICAH with steroids. A follow-up study from the Royal Free Hospital[7] attested to the efficacy of corticosteroids to diminish morbidity and prolong life in adults with AICAH. Late results from the Mayo Clinic study, however, suggest that true cures are few and tenuous.[8,9]

Prednisone is a synthetic glucocorticoid of intermediate potency. In itself prednisone has no glucocorticoid activity: It must first be converted, in the liver, to *prednisolone*, the active form, by 11-beta-hydroxylation (Fig. 1). The liver also produces the major transport proteins for prednisolone, both *transcortin* with high affinity but low capacity and *albumin* with lower affinity but high capacity. The liver is partly responsible for inactivation and excretion of prednisolone via reduction of the A ring. Quantitative studies of prednisone and prednisolone pharmacokinetics have become possible with the development of radioimmunoassays and high-pressure liquid chromatography assays of these chemicals in serum. However, serum concentrations do not measure biologic activity directly. Effects of corticosteroids at the tissue level tend to last longer than the serum concentrations. These biologic effects vary with each synthetic glucocorticoid. They appear to depend upon free drug concentration, characteristics of glucocorticoid receptor binding and function, and possibly special tissue characteristics. Meikle and Tyler[10] attempted to find a predictable relationship between the elimi-

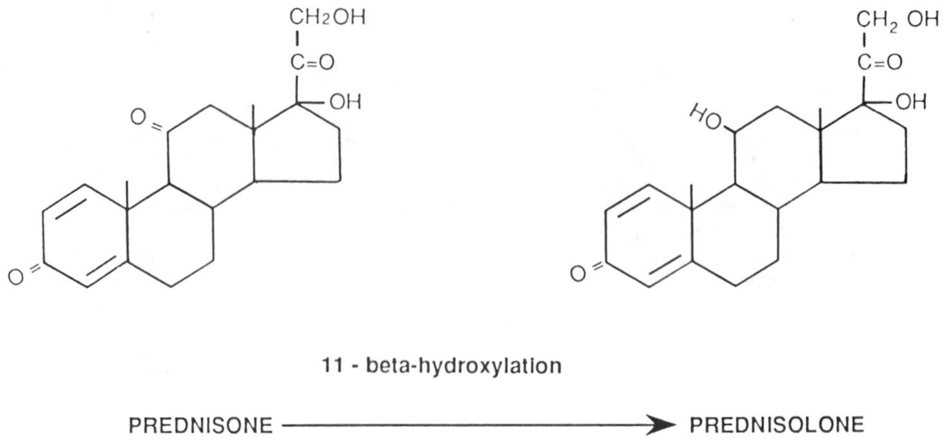

FIGURE 1 Activation of prednisone in the liver.

nation half-life and biologic half-life of various glucocorticoids. As an estimate, the biologic half-life is approximately twice the elimination half-life in adults. Although little is known about glucocorticoid receptor function in children, this formulation may also have general validity in pediatric therapeutics with corticosteroids.

The majority of pharmacokinetic studies regarding prednisone have been performed in adults. Both prednisone and prednisolone are promptly and completely absorbed from the gastrointestinal (GI) tract in most individuals,[11-13] and liver disease appears to make no difference to absorption. Some people have trouble absorbing prednisone or prednisolone, perhaps because of intestinal disease[13]; this has been found in children as well.[14] Simultaneous ingestion of food delays absorption but does not reduce total absorption of the prednisone dose.[15,16] Typical adult doses of antacids taken simultaneously with prednisone interfere with bioavailability. The serum curve of prednisolone concentrations is displaced downward and to the right, indicating delayed peak concentrations and smaller total prednisolone dose attained. The mechanism of this effect, possibly absorption of prednisone to antacid in the GI tract, is not known.[17] When smaller doses of antacid are used, there is no apparent change in absorption.[18]

Whether prednisone or prednisolone is administered, the pharmacokinetics of the active drug, prednisolone, are of greater interest. The elimination of prednisolone *in normals* appears to follow dose-dependent kinetics.[19] This may be due to nonlinearity of protein binding.[20] The elimination half-life has been estimated in several studies in adults after either oral or intravenous administration of prednisone or prednisolone. It appears to be 3 to 4 hours in normal adults.[10,11,21] In children the apparent elimination half-life is *much shorter* at 2.2 hours, with a range of 1.2 to 3.5 hours in 22 children studied. None of these had liver disease, but some were already taking corticosteroids at the time of study.[14] Thus prednisolone appears to be like many other drugs—metabolized more rapidly in children than in adults.

An important and frequently debated question is whether *prednisone* should be used at all for treating liver disease. Since prednisone has to be converted to prednisolone in the liver and since the liver is diseased, it might be better to use *prednisolone* right from the start. This has been studied in adults only. In the presence of active liver disease, the peak plasma concentration of prednisolone appears later after taking prednisone than after taking prednisolone,[11,13,21] but hepatic inactivation of prednisolone is also slower.[22] There has been only one study to the contrary[23] in which adults with severe liver disease had much lower serum prednisolone concentrations during the first 4 hours after oral prednisone was given. However, these patients were not studied long enough to determine rate of elimination. In patients with hypoalbuminemia the concentration of free prednisolone, which is the pharmacologically active agent, is higher.[11,21] Whether this free concentration is higher because of the hypoalbuminemia per se or because these patients have the lowest hepatic capacity for inactivating prednisolone is uncertain, but the latter possibility seems more likely. Patients with hypoalbuminemia associated with nephrotic syndrome and no liver disease have high free fractions of prednisolone, but the mean concentration of free prednisolone is the same as in controls; prednisolone clearance in these patients is higher than in controls.[24] In liver disease the impaired inactivation mechanisms appear to compensate for diminished drug activation.

Thus, there seems to be no justification for preferring prednisolone to prednisone routinely.[21] However, some individuals (both patients and *controls* in one study) have low serum prednisolone concentrations after administration of prednisone: These observations suggest that some people convert prednisone to prednisolone slowly, perhaps on the basis of an inherited enzymic polymorphism.[25] Formal pharmacokinetic studies may be helpful in children who fail to benefit from apparently adequate doses of prednisone because these children may be unable to 11-hydroxylate prednisone adequately owing to genetic factors or disease severity. Green et al[14] showed that a serum prednisolone concentration greater than 19 μg per deciliter (achieved at a dose of prednisolone of 0.5 mg per kilogram) was sufficient to block temporarily somatomedin secretion and cell-mediated immunity tested in vitro. This drug concentration was exceeded in most adult patients with liver disease taking prednisone or prednisolone.[21]

Prednisone and prednisolone are metabolized in part by hepatic cytochromes P-450. Prednisone may have some capacity to induce these hepatic drug-metabolizing enzymes:

thus, it was surprising to find that there was no change in D-glucaric acid administration after subchronic dosing with prednisolone.[26] The same investigators found no change in galactose elimination or bromsulphthalein disposition. Although the study is possibly flawed by too short a treatment period with prednisolone, it is generally accepted that prednisone and prednisolone do not change quantitative biochemical tests of liver function in themselves. By contrast, the elimination of prednisolone is accelerated when hepatic enzyme induction occurs after treatment with stronger inducing chemicals than prednisolone. This has been shown after administration of phenytoin,[27] phenobarbital,[28] and rifampicin.[29] This phenomenon has even been observed in a patient with severe liver disease.[22] The extend of this effect is probably partly dependent on the individual's susceptibility to induction of certain cytochromes P-450; however, such induction can occur in the presence of chronic liver disease.

In general, corticosteroids affect cellular metabolism and have important anti-inflammatory and immunosuppressive effects.[30] Steroids enhance hepatic gluconeogenesis. They also generate a degree of insulin resistance in peripheral tissues. Glucose intolerance may thus develop. They enhance catabolism and thus lead to muscle wasting and myopathy. Finally, they depress long-chain fatty acid synthesis, resulting in increased plasma concentrations of free fatty acids and glycerol. Because corticosteroids are needed for the activity of lipolytic hormones such as catecholamines, glucagon, and growth hormone, there tends to be mobilization of fat from peripheral fat stores sensitive to these hormones. This may account in part for the redistribution of fat to the trunk.[31]

With respect to anti-inflammatory effects, corticosteroids have major effects on neutrophils. Neutrophils are increased in number, but chemotaxis (although not bactericidal function) is severely impaired. Monocyte function is also affected: chemotaxis, ability to respond to lymphokines, and bactericidal activity are also decreased.[32] Corticosteroids interfere with capillary permeability so that less local edema forms at a site of inflammation. This further limits accumulation of inflammatory cells. Moreover, corticosteroids reduce the ability of white blood cells to stick to capillary membranes and pass through them. Not only capillary but also lysosomal membranes are stabilized by corticosteroids.[30]

The immunosuppressive effects of corticosteroids involve mainly cell-mediated immunity rather than antibody production. The number of circulating lymphocytes, particularly T lymphocytes, and monocytes is reduced transiently. There is also reduced T-cell cytotoxicity. These effects may be mediated more through direct membrane effects of corticosteroids than via the cellular glucocorticoid receptor.[32] Serum concentrations of complement components are variably reduced.[32] The important effect of corticosteroids in AICAH appears to be restoration of suppressor T-cell activity, possibly by restoring responsiveness to interleukin-2.[34,35]

Corticosteroids have major effects on the skeleton: They inhibit long bone growth *and* epiphyseal closure. The outcome is typically growth inhibition during treatment, with catch-up growth when treatment is discontinued.[36] In some patients supranormal growth velocity has been observed when alternate-day dosing is begun; daily, but not alternate-day, steroid administration interferes with somatomedin activity, although other factors may be involved.[37] Corticosteroids may interfere with calcium homeostasis and possibly with vitamin D metabolism.[38] Another structural effect of corticosteroids is to impair collagen synthesis.[39,40] This may be important in preventing scar formation in areas of inflammation.

Most of the adverse side effects of corticosteroids can be predicted from their metabolic actions. Diabetes mellitus, myopathy, hyperlipidemia, growth retardation, osteoporosis, and susceptibility to opportunistic infections are among the most notable. Cosmetic changes, including "moon face," truncal obesity, hirsutism, acne, and cutaneous striae, are particularly troublesome to any teenager. There is a slightly higher incidence of peptic ulcer disease in persons taking steroids chronically.[41] Systemic hypertension may occur. Pseudotumor cerebri has been encountered in children. Exacerbation of clinically inapparent infections, such as tuberculosis or strongyloidiasis, may occur.

Azathioprine, a thiopurine, differs greatly from prednisone. It was developed as a prodrug for 6-mercaptopurine (6MP), since azathioprine comprises 6MP linked to an imidazole moiety (Fig. 2). Its pharmacology is in many respects identical to that of 6MP.[42] 6MP is metabolized to several active compounds, including 6-thioinosinic acid and, eventually, 6-thioguanine nucleotides. The splitting of azathioprine to 6MP is mediated by sulfhydryl groups on glutathione or cellular proteins, via thiolysis. Azathioprine can also be hydroxylated first before the imidazole moiety is cleaved: This forms 8-hydroxy-6MP and ultimately, via xanthine oxidase, 6-thiouric acid.[42] Allopurinol, which inhibits xanthine oxidase, increases toxicity of azathioprine.[43] However, azathioprine actually has multiple metabolites, and some of these metabolites besides 6MP may be active. For example, one other major metabolite is the product of cleaving the molecule so that the sulfur stays with the imidazole moiety.[44] All metabolites are produced primarily in the liver. It is theorized that hepatic metabolism must be relatively intact for azathioprine to work. Urinary metabolite profiles in patients with liver disease are like those in normals.[44] However, early studies suggested that the immunosuppressive effect of azathioprine was less for a given dose in patients with severe liver disease; it is not clear from the data that this was due to inadequate hepatic metabolism.[45]

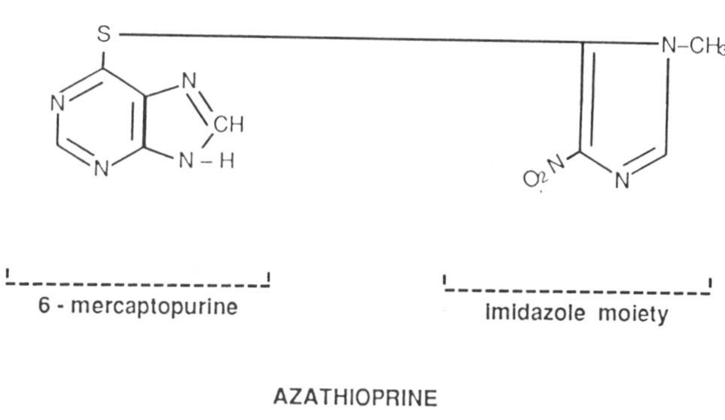

FIGURE 2 Chemical structure of azathioprine. 6-Mercaptopurine is linked to an imidazole moiety. (Modified from Davis et al.[51])

The absorption and inactivation of azathioprine have not been studied in children. In adults azathioprine has been shown to be rapidly absorbed from the GI tract,[45] somewhat better than 6MP. There is no predictable relationship between the dose of azathioprine and the resulting serum concentrations of 6MP.[43] The apparent pharmacokinetics of azathioprine, based on studies of ^{35}S-azathioprine, are essentially the same in normal adults and patients with severe liver disease.[45] Elimination is mostly renal, but little azathioprine or 6MP is excreted unchanged.

The mechanism of action of azathioprine remains uncertain. 6MP is capable of interfering with cellular metabolism by various means: by interfering with purine nucleotide synthesis or interconversion or by being incorporated into cellular RNA or DNA.[42] With respect to immunosuppressive action, azathioprine may differ substantially from 6MP. Azathioprine is more potent than 6MP in inhibiting the human mixed lymphocyte reaction, by apparently a different mechanism.[46,47] The cleaved imidazole moiety may contribute to the immunosuppressive effects of azathioprine.[42] It may also contribute to its toxicity.

Side effects of azathioprine include bone marrow suppression, susceptibility to opportunistic infections, pancreatitis, and hepatotoxicity.[48] Leukopenia can be correlated with high levels of 6-thioguanine nucleotides in red blood cells.[43,49] It is now apparent that susceptibility to azathioprine myelotoxicity is influenced by a genetic polymorphism for the enzyme thiopurine methyltransferase: Individuals with the low-activity allele for this detoxifying enzyme (which converts 6MP to 6-methyl-MP) are more likely to have high levels of 6-thioguanine nucleotides in erythrocytes.[50] Some patients develop nausea, vomiting, headache, and fever, possibly related to the imidazole moiety.[51] Structural changes in chromosomes of blood-forming cells have been observed during azathioprine treatment; however, it has been difficult to estimate the increased risk of developing malignancy during prolonged treatment with the drug. Several studies of long-term use of azathioprine in adults with chronic liver disease have failed to show any increased incidence of malignancy. In one study to the contrary, death from malignancies was more common in patients with chronic liver disease treated with azathioprine than in those treated with prednisone, but the differences did not reach statistical significance.[52] Depressed fertility is a side effect of related immunosuppressants; teratogenicity is at least a theoretical risk. These considerations are all very apposite when proposing to treat children and adolescents with this drug for years.

Treatment regimens in children with AICAH vary from study to study. The consensus is to begin with large daily doses of prednisone and taper the dose over the first 2 to 3 months as symptoms and laboratory findings improve. Corticosteroids may be used alone initially,[1,53,54] with azathioprine added only if response to steroids is considered unsatisfactory. Alternatively, a combination of prednisone and azathioprine may be used from the beginning.[55] Since the majority of patients tend to require both drugs,[1] the latter approach may have more merit. This type of regimen was also found to be effective in adults.[4] Younger children appear to need higher doses of prednisone than older ones; this may reflect accelerated drug metabolism in younger children. Opinion about the efficacy of alternate-day dosage of corticosteroids in childhood AICAH remains divided.

It has been difficult to identify features at clinical presentation which will reliably predict response to treatment. In children, however, retrospective review of treatment efficacy suggests that early initiation of treatment is an important determinant of favorable outcome. Early initiation of treatment may have accounted for the favorable results reported by Arasu et al[54] in which all patients responded to treatment and none died. In another study, treatment was stopped in 5 of 13 children with AICAH diagnosed before 6 months' duration of disease, and a further 5 of 13 were well-controlled on treatment; one died, however, 1 week into treatment with a total duration of illness of 4 weeks.[1] Childhood AICAH appears to be a more rapidly progressive process than the disease in adults. The chronologic criterion of 6 months' duration (derived from experience with the adult disease) should not be applied to children. Delay in diagnosis and treatment appears to be detrimental.

Another difference between AICAH in children and adults may be that children can attain a prolonged clinical and biochemical remission. During this time drug treatment can be stopped. Such remission was reported in 28 percent[1] and in 73 percent[54] of patients in two childhood studies; this is quite different from the emerging pattern in adults, in whom relapse is common in some prolonged longitudinal studies.[8,56] By contrast in a further series of childhood AICAH, relapse was common in the rare patient in whom treatment could be withdrawn.[55] Clearly, more observations are needed before childhood AICAH can be regarded as a "curable" liver disease. Moreover, the prevailing tendency to cirrhosis militates against true cure.

Although azathioprine has been shown in two studies to be ineffective as sole initial treatment for AICAH,[5,57] recent observations in adults suggest that it may be effective as prolonged treatment. Stellon et al[58] reported no difference in effectiveness between prednisolone plus azathioprine and azathioprine alone (at dose of 2 mg per kilogram per day) in maintaining remission previously established with corticosteroids and azathioprine. Continued treatment with azathioprine after stopping prednisone has been reported in children.[55] The actual safety of prolonged use of azathioprine in children still remains to be proven.

Penicillamine has been investigated as a possible alternative treatment for AICAH,[59,60] but it is not used routinely. It may be immunoregulatory and it may also interfere with fibrogenesis. However, as with other autoimmune diseases, the side effects of penicillamine were so severe that they outweighed any apparent therapeutic benefit. Penicillamine has been shown in a prospective trial to be of no benefit in treating primary sclerosing cholangitis,[61] which may present in children looking clinically like AICAH.[62]

TREATMENT OF WILSON'S DISEASE

Wilson's disease is an inherited metabolic disease characterized by accumulation of copper in various tissues, notably the liver and parts of the brain, with progressive hepatic dysfunction and/or neurologic degeneration. The pathogenesis of this disease is not known but seems to be a primary hepatic abnormality in the disposition of copper. Copper is not excreted in bile efficiently.[63,64] Because the handling of copper

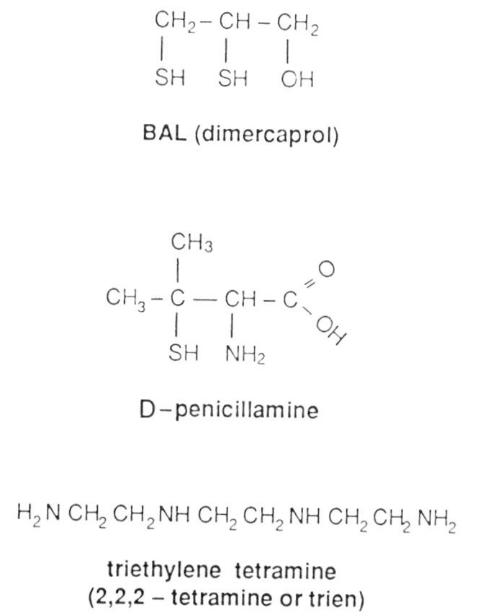

$CH_2-CH-CH_2$ (SH, SH, CH)

BAL (dimercaprol)

$CH_3-C(CH_3)(SH)-CH(NH_2)-C(=O)OH$

D-penicillamine

$H_2N\,CH_2\,CH_2NH\,CH_2\,CH_2NH\,CH_2\,CH_2\,NH_2$

triethylene tetramine
(2,2,2 - tetramine or trien)

FIGURE 3 Chemical structures of treatments for Wilson's disease. Dimercaprol and penicillamine are similar. The very different structure of trien is consistent with a different chemical mechanism of copper chelation.

in Wilson's disease is similar to that in the fetus, it has also been hypothesized that developmental switching of copper disposition does not occur in Wilson's disease.[65] Wilson's disease was uniformly fatal or incapacitating until D-penicillamine was introduced in 1956 as oral treatment.[66] It remains the first-line treatment. Life-long treatment halts the progression of disease in most patients who tolerate it.

Penicillamine was actually first detected as a breakdown product of penicillin—hence its name—but it is in fact the sulfhydryl-bearing amino acid cysteine doubly substituted with methyl groups (Fig. 3). Walshe[67] established that it was partly excreted in urine with the sulfhydryl group intact; he speculated that it could function as a chelator, because like dimercaprol (British anti-lewisite, or BAL) it had a free sulfhydryl group, and showed that its chelating potential disappeared when the sulfhydryl group was not present, as in tetramethylcystine. Detailed pharmacokinetic studies were not possible until recently, when improvements in chromatography have permitted direct analysis of penicillamine and its metabolites.

Penicillamine is rapidly absorbed from the GI tract. Uptake may occur by an unusual mechanism: disulfide binding to the enterocyte membrane followed by pinocytosis.[68] Like certain other drugs used frequently in children, notably phenytoin and cimetidine, penicillamine shows a double-peaked curve for intestinal absorption.[68-70] The reason for this absorption pattern is not known; simultaneous administration of food seems to interfere with this pattern of absorption.[70] However, a meal taken with penicillamine decreases absorption of the drug overall by about half.[70,71] In other studies, the overall bioavailability was estimated between 40 and 70 percent.[69,72] Once absorbed, penicillamine circulates mostly bound to plasma proteins; of the 20 percent that is unbound, 6 percent is free penicillamine and the rest is mostly penicillamine disulfide (tetramethylcystine) or cysteine-penicillamine disulfide. These would be predicted to be inactive, since they lack a free sulfhydryl group. Excretion of penicillamine is largely urinary, with fecal excretion accounting for approximately 16 percent of the total. In addition to these metabolites, a methylated metabolite, S-methyl-D-penicillamine, is also found. S-methylation occurs in the liver; this metabolite is more common in rheumatoid arthritis than in Wilson's disease. Estimates of the elimination half-life of penicillamine are unsatisfactory, partly on technical grounds and partly because of considerable interindividual variation. The half-life of penicillamine is on the order of 1.7 to 7 hours.[68,70,72] However, penicillamine metabolites are sometimes still detectable in urine months after stopping the drug.[73]

The major therapeutic effect of penicillamine in Wilson's disease is to promote urinary excretion of copper.[74] Chronic treatment is thought to lead to removal of excess stored copper and to keep it from reaccumulating. Recent studies showing that penicillamine induces hepatic metallothionein in mice and rats[75,76] have led to speculation that penicillamine acts by inducing metallothionein in individuals with Wilson's disease.[77] Copper complexed with metallothionein is nontoxic. This mechanism would account for detoxification without a totally negative body copper balance; however, it has not been proved in humans yet. Penicillamine can be used as a chelating agent for other heavy metals.[68] It has also been used to treat cystinuria. In general penicillamine has not been effective for cholestatic liver disease characterized by hepatic copper accumulation. Penicillamine was not beneficial in a small series of infants with idiopathic chronic cholestatic syndromes,[78] but it reduced mortality in preicteric cases of Indian childhood cirrhosis.[79] Penicillamine also has other pharmacologic effects that may be important in treating various liver diseases. It interferes with collagen cross-linking[80] and thus may interfere with fibrosis. It also has some immunosuppressant actions.[81,82]

Penicillamine is still the standard treatment for Wilson's disease. Many retrospective studies attest to its effectiveness.[83-85] However, a small number of patients do not respond to penicillamine or any other treatment and require liver transplant because of liver failure. Penicillamine is usually ineffective in patients presenting with fulminant liver failure and intravascular hemolysis[86]; for these patients liver transplantation may be life-saving.[87] If penicillamine treatment is stopped without substituting another form of decoppering treatment, then the previously stable patient may develop severe, often irreversible, hepatic decompensation[88]; thus, compliance is an important issue, especially with adolescents. Patients who present with neurologic disease may experience transient neurologic deterioration during the early months of treatment with penicillamine[89]; the mechanism of this clinical response is not known. Recently liver transplantation has also been proposed as effective treatment for neurologic disease totally unresponsive to chronic chelator treatment.[90]

Penicillamine has important side effects, most of which have become apparent when it is used to treat diseases other than Wilson's disease.[91] Adverse reactions involving the skin include various types of rashes, pemphigus, and elastosis perforans serpiginosa.[92] Other side effects include thrombocytopenia, proteinuria, GI upset, arthralgias, and dysgeusia. Rarely, severe global bone marrow depression has occurred. Nephrotic syndrome is the major severe nephrotoxicity.[85]

Systemic disease similar to lupus erythematosus[93] or Goodpasture's syndrome[85] have been reported, as well as a myasthenia syndrome. Infants have been born normal after continued use of penicillamine during pregnancy, but one newborn had a peculiar Ehlers-Danlos–like syndrome, apparently due to abnormal collagen formation.[94] It has been speculated that these side effects are less common in Wilson's disease because the reactive sulfhydryl group combines with copper rather than with body tissues. Clearly, these severe side effects require cessation of treatment. A problem seen early in treatment in approximately 20 percent of patients with Wilson's disease is the so-called hypersensitivity reaction to penicillamine, with rash, fever, arthralgia, and malaise.[95] This can usually be treated by restarting the penicillamine at small and gradually increasing doses with corticosteroid cover.[85,89]

The usual next alternative for people who manifest severe toxicity from penicillamine is triethylene tetramine dihydrochloride (2,2,2-tetramine), known by its official short name *trien* or as *trientine*. It was introduced in 1969 and has since been found to be effective in treating Wilson's disease in patients who become intolerant of penicillamine either early (in the first few weeks) or late (after several years).[96,97] This implies that trien is effective both in mobilizing excess copper and in maintaining remission after the patient is "decoppered." Trien has also been used safely as a substitute for penicillamine during pregnancy in patients with Wilson's disease, with no obvious adverse effect on the infant in a small series. The fetus does not appear to become copper-depleted on this regimen.[98]

Trien is one of a chemical family of chelators. It does not have sulfhydryl groups. Copper is chelated by forming a stable complex with the four constituent nitrogens in a planar ring (Fig. 3). A related compound, 2,3,2-tetramine, is actually a more effective chelator than trien for structural reasons, but its safety in humans is entirely unknown.[99,100] Trien itself has not been studied in detail pharmacologically, and little is known about its pharmacokinetics. It is poorly absorbed from the GI tract, and what is absorbed its metabolized and inactivated.[98] It has been found to have little clinically important toxicity in Wilson's disease apart from inducing iron deficiency, presumably on the basis of chelating iron in the GI tract. Adverse effects due to penicillamine resolve and do not recur during treatment with trien. However, trien is capable of causing adverse effects of its own, as seen in patients with primary biliary cirrhosis: These included hemorrhagic gastritis, loss of taste, and rashes.[101]

The relative potency of trien compared to penicillamine is an important practical question. In patients not previously treated, both penicillamine and trien can cause the same extent of cupruresis, although a higher dose of trien is required.[102] Subsequent studies in laboratory animals do not support the conclusion that penicillamine is stronger on a molar basis than trien.[100,103] It is likely that these two agents differ in their mechanisms of chelating copper. Trien forms a small molecular complex with copper, whereas the penicillamine-copper complex is polymeric. Trien competes for copper bound to albumin, whereas penicillamine does not.[103] Trien tends to cause serum copper to rise initially, whereas penicillamine leads to a fall in serum copper.[104] Trien and penicillamine may mobilize different pools of body copper. In particular, trien may mobilize copper from tissues better than penicillamine; whereas penicillamine promotes excretion of copper in the plasma compartment.[103] These findings, obtained mostly in laboratory animals, are somewhat disputed and difficult to extrapolate to humans. They raise the possibility of using the two drugs together for a synergistic effect.

With either chelator, it is important to *customize* chelator treatment to the needs of each patient by measuring urinary copper excretion during treatment and adjusting the dose of chelator accordingly, weighing the clinical severity and potential for dose-related side effects. This is clearly more important early in treatment than later when much excess copper has been removed. This same consideration applies to treatment modalities currently being developed.

The most recent innovation in the treatment of Wilson's disease is zinc supplementation. Zinc competes with copper for absorption from the GI tract. Although zinc was used to treat Wilson's disease by Schouwink in Holland in the early 1960s,[105] it has gained attention as an alternative treatment modality only recently. The observation that treating patients with sickle cell anemia with zinc caused them to develop clinically apparent copper deficiency[106] led Brewer and colleagues to treat patients with Wilson's disease with zinc.[107] Their initial regimen of zinc acetate (equivalent to 25 mg elemental zinc) orally every 4 hours during the day, with twice the dose at bedtime and no food taken for 1 hour before or after each dose was unwieldy, but it led to a negative total body copper balance. Further studies have shown that 50 mg elemental zinc three times daily (still with no food for 1 hour before or after the dose) is an equally effective regimen.[108] Effectiveness of zinc treatment involves complicated balance studies because copper is lost mainly in the stool, not the urine. Brewer's group has shown that effectiveness can be monitored by measuring urinary copper excretion in 24 hours, which reflects residual total body copper load, and free plasma copper, which falls with effective treatment.[109] They have developed a test to measure radiocopper absorption, which is extremely low when zinc treatment is effective.[110]

Brewer and colleagues have used zinc mainly in patients intolerant of penicillamine or after stabilization on penicillamine. Their clinical experience is mostly with adults. More extensive clinical use of zinc for treating Wilson's disease has been reported by Hoogenraad and colleagues: 25 patients treated since 1977 and two patients treated since 1958.[105] The regimen for adults was 200 mg of zinc sulfate (equivalent to 45 mg elemental zinc) orally 30 minutes before meals three times daily, with half that dose used for children. Of these 27 patients, nine (including six children) were treated solely with zinc, and all improved except one who presented with subfulminant liver failure. Other patients who received penicillamine first and then were changed to zinc treatment also were well clinically, irrespective of whether penicillamine treatment had been stopped prematurely because of intolerance or not. No adverse effects attributable to the zinc treatment were found. Transient neurologic deterioration was not seen with zinc treatment. Two patients resumed penicillamine because they found its dosage schedule more convenient.

The mechanism of action of zinc in Wilson's disease is entirely different from that of chelators. Zinc treatment interferes with uptake of copper from the GI tract. The mechanism is more complicated than simple competitive interference for uptake. It is postulated that excess zinc induces metallothionein in enterocytes. This metallothionein, however, has greater affinity for copper than for zinc and thus preferentially binds copper present in the GI tract. Once bound, the copper is not absorbed, and the metallothionein-bound copper is lost into the fecal contents as enterocytes are shed in normal turnover.[109] Copper enters the GI tract from the diet and from saliva and gastric secretions; thus, it is possible that zinc treatment might mobilize endogenous copper.[107] Studies in rats show that pharmacologic doses of zinc can indeed elevate concentrations of enterocyte metallothionein.[111] Patients who have received penicillamine chronically may be absolutely zinc deficient, and treatment with zinc may not be effective until total body zinc stores are repleted.[107] An important unanswered question is whether or not zinc treatment induces levels of hepatic metallothionein. Patients treated with zinc chronically have been found to have higher concentrations of hepatic copper late in treatment, despite being well clinically.[105,112] It is possible that this copper is complexed to hepatic metallothionein and is thus detoxified, but that has not been proven. Although the data can be interpreted as showing no major reaccumulation of copper in the liver, based on conjectures of how much copper might be stored in the liver without any treatment,[112] these findings are problematic.

Ostensibly zinc should be relatively safe because it is not a xenobiotic. Studies have shown that with chronic treatment both the urinary excretion and the hepatic accumulation of zinc plateau.[105,119,112] The major adverse effect has been abdominal pain, probably due to gastritis. This can be minimized by using the acetate or gluconate salt of zinc rather than the sulfate. It is probably less likely to occur if the zinc is taken with food, but food interferes greatly with zinc absorption[113] and effectiveness of treatment. Other long-term effects in humans are uncertain, but studies in laboratory animals suggest that high doses of zinc may be immunosuppressive and depress polymorphonuclear leukocyte chemotaxis.[114] Zinc may also interfere with bone formation, as has been demonstrated in rats.[115]

The clinical data on using zinc in children are limited. In addition to those children included in Hoogenraad's series, three other children are reported with favorable outcomes.[116,117] One of these presented with ascites and coagulopathy and was treated only with zinc.[116] It is probably premature to assess the effectiveness of this drug in children, especially with the variability in dosage regimens used. In any case, there are foreseeable practical problems in getting a child to take any medication regularly three times a day away from snacks and meals. Compliance is an important consideration in treating Wilson's disease in children and may be difficult to ensure with penicillamine on a twice-daily regimen. It is also possible that children may be more susceptible to the adverse effects of zinc, notably with respect to bone formation.

In summary, zinc may be an effective treatment for Wilson's disease, but its place among currently available treatments remains disputed. Experience with this drug in children is quite limited. An effective dose and dosage schedule likely to promote compliance to treatment have not been established for children. Little is known about long-term toxicities in patients treated from childhood onward. It is not yet clear how to monitor the effectiveness of zinc treatment conveniently and reliably. The significance of increasing hepatic copper in some patients during chronic zinc treatment remains uncertain. The present consensus is that zinc has not yet been proved to be the modern first-line drug of choice.[118] It may be appropriate for treating patients already stabilized by standard chelator treatment, particularly if drug intolerance develops. Further studies are needed to clarify questions about when to use zinc in Wilson's disease.

There are several other alternative treatments that have had only limited use or are frankly experimental. The most interesting of these is sodium tetrathiomolybdate, which is known both to interfere with intestinal copper absorption and to bind tightly to copper in plasma. Extensive clinical studies are not yet available. It may have untoward effects on bone development and thus be unsuitable for children.[119] Unithiol, a water-soluble analogue of dimercaprol, has been reported by Walshe as effective treatment in one patient who tolerated neither penicillamine nor trien.[120] This compound is not metabolized, is somewhat fat-soluble, crosses the blood-brain barrier, and is capable of inducing the same magnitude of cupruresis in Wilson's disease as penicillamine. Unfortunately it can have major side effects including leukopenia and GI intolerance and probably will not be a major therapeutic modality in this disease.

TREATMENT OF CHRONIC VIRAL HEPATITIS

Although hepatitis A is a self-limited hepatic infection that almost always resolves spontaneously without sequelae, hepatitis B and hepatitis non-A, non-B (NANB) virus infections can be chronic and cause severe liver disease. Most efforts to find effective drug treatments for hepatitis have been aimed at chronic hepatitis B infection because it is common (and thus a pressing world health problem) and because the virology of hepatitis B is well understood. Some of these therapeutic innovations may be applicable to NANB hepatitis, although pertinent studies are lagging owing to difficulties in specific diagnosis.

In hepatitis B infections hepatocytes are killed by the body's immune response to the virus, not by the virus itself. Approximately 10 percent of acutely infected adults fail to clear the virus; this may be because of faulty immune response. The observation that corticosteroid treatment of acute hepatitis B virus (HBV) hepatitis tends to interfere with viral clearance and promote development of the carrier state supports this hypothesis. Inability to produce interferons may also be a factor leading to chronic HBV infection in adults.[121] The majority of infants infected at birth fail to clear hepatitis B virus. The reason is not known, but it is believed that several factors may contribute. Maternal anti-HBc/IgG crossing the placenta may blunt the infant's immune response to HBV[122]; the infantile immune system is relatively underdeveloped, and moreover HBV viral proteins present early in life may be regarded as nonforeign.[123] Many studies have now shown that the best way to treat these infants is to protect them prospectively, that is, by providing passive and active immunity with hepatitis B immune globulin and hepatitis B surface antigen (HBsAg) immunization (with either the human plasma-derived or recombinant HBsAg vaccine).[124,125] The impressive response of infants to active immunization casts some doubt on the notion that the inadequacy of the infantile immune response is the simple reason for failure to clear HBV in perinatal infection.[126]

For the patient chronically infected with HBV, the natural history of the disease dictates therapeutic interventions.[127] In chronic infection HBV replicates in hepatocytes for an indefinite period; during this time hepatitis B e antigen (HBeAg) and HBV DNA may be found in the patient's blood. At some point the viral DNA integrates with the host DNA: HBV DNA is then no longer found in the blood and ordinarily the patient elaborates anti-HBe, the antibody to the HBV "e" determinant. After this integration, parenchymal liver disease usually improves; however, the risk for oncogenesis rises. Antiviral treatments are appropriate before HBV DNA integrates into the host DNA. Anti-inflammatory treatments, if they have any role at all, are probably best reserved for disease after viral replication has ended.

Antiviral Treatment

The immediate goal for antiviral treatment is to stop HBV replication in hepatocytes. Ongoing viral replication is associated with progressive severe parenchymal damage and ultimately with cirrhosis; infectivity remains high. While clearly the preferred outcome of antiviral treatment is to lose HBsAg expression and to develop anti-HBs antibodies, the usual and currently accepted successful outcome is to lose HBeAg positivity and develop anti-HBe antibodies, along with HBV DNA no longer detectable in the blood. Whether this outcome predisposes to development of hepatocellular carcinoma is a moot point. It is contended that hepatocellular carcinoma is less likely to occur in the absence of cirrhosis.[128] Further experience with antiviral treatments for chronic hepatitis B infection should clarify this important question, especially because preventing hepatocellular carcinoma is also a reasonable goal for antiviral treatment in chronic hepatitis B disease. However, being a "healthy carrier" of HBV, even with HBV DNA integrated in host DNA, is undoubtedly better than being chronically unwell with progressive liver disease. For a child or adolescent the implications for normal growth and psychosocial development are enormous.

ARA-A (vidarabine) is a purine nucleoside. It is relatively insoluble in water so that intravenous infusion in large fluid volumes is mandatory. Its 5-monophosphate ester *ARA-AMP* is much more water-soluble and thus can be administered intramuscularly as well as intravenously.[129] Both are active against many DNA viruses. ARA-A and ARA-AMP have similar pharmacokinetic characteristics.[130] The major metabolite of each is arabinofuranosylhypoxanthine (ARA-Hx). Thus, metabolism involves the adenine moiety, which is deaminated. This does not involve the cytochromes P-450.[131] Metabolism is so rapid that after giving ARA-A intravenously only ARA-Hx is detected in serum samples.[131,133] The elimination half-life for ARA-Hx after ARA-A intravenously was found to be approximately 2 to 5 hours.[132] In one study the half-life of radiolabeled ARA-AMP given intravenously was 3.5 to 6 hours. In another pharmacokinetic study, mainly in adults, only the major metabolite and small amounts of ARA-A were detected in serum after intravenous or intramuscular administration of ARA-AMP; the time from intramuscular injection to peak metabolite concentration was 3 hours.[133] Excretion is mostly renal, and ARA-Hx is the major urinary metabolite. ARA-AMP can cross the blood-brain barrier.[133] Toxicities are dose-related and correspond to high concentrations of metabolite. Renal disease and possibly older age predispose to toxicity.[130]

The major toxicity with ARA-A and ARA-AMP in patients with liver disease has been neurotoxicity: a peripheral neuropathy affecting predominantly the lower limbs with pain, causalgia, and sensory abnormalities. Nerve conduction tests are abnormal. Other patients have myalgias. These problems tend to develop late in treatment and may not resolve for weeks after treatment has been stopped.[129] Ataxia and intentional tremors have also been observed in patients with liver disease. Other toxicities have included nausea and vomiting, diarrhea, leukopenia, thrombocytopenia, and the syndrome of inappropriate antidiuretic hormone secretion.[131]

Both ARA-A and ARA-AMP have been shown to inhibit HBV replication in humans, and some individuals have lost HBeAg and elaborated anti-HBe after treatment.[134,135] In at least one study the spontaneous loss of HBeAg in controls was high enough to render the pharmacologic effect of ARA-AMP undistinguished.[136] These drugs have not been used in children.

Interferons were discovered about 30 years ago in the course of studies on viral interference.[137,138] They are small molecules of molecular weight approximately 20,000 daltons

TABLE 1
Summary of Interferons

	IFN-alpha	IFN-beta	IFN-gamma
Former name	Leukocyte	Fibroblast	Immune
Number of types	>15	1	1–2
Source	Lymphocytes, macrophages	Fibroblasts, epithelial cells	T lymphocytes
Inducer	Virus, dsRNA	Virus, dsRNA	Foreign antigens, mitogens
pH stable	Yes	Yes	No
Gene on chromosome*	9	9	12
Receptor gene on chromosome*	21	21	21
Glycosylation†	Yes	No	No
Functional unit	Monomer	Dimer	Trimer
Hydrophobicity	±	+	+
Catabolism of exogenous IFN	Renal	Hepatic	Hepatic

*All chromosome locations human.
†Glycosylation refers to natural, not recombinant, IFN.
Based on references 138 and 140.

elaborated by various cells. There are three main types (Table 1). Nomenclature is in a state of flux. Alpha-interferon (IFN-alpha) is produced by leukocytes; other sources include virally stimulated continuous lines of human lymphoblastoid cells and more recently *Escherichia coli* using recombinant DNA technology. Natural IFN-alpha is not glycosylated; it is less hydrophobic than other interferons. Beta-interferon (IFN-beta) is produced by human fibroblasts and epithelial cells. IFN-alpha and IFN-beta compete for the same cell membrane receptor. Gamma-interferon (IFN-gamma) is somewhat different from the other interferon classes physicochemically and is in fact a lymphokine; it has immunomodulatory activity not found in the other interferons.

Although much has been discovered about the effects and mechanism of action of interferons, much remains unknown. It is clear that interferons are part of a complex system governing cellular responses. Effects on cell proliferation, cell differentiation, antigen expression, and modulation of immune response have given interferons a role in treatment of neoplasia.[139] The main argument for using interferons to treat hepatitis arises from their action of interfering with viral infection. IFN activates 2′, 5′-oligoadenylate synthetase (2′, 5′-AS), which leads to the formation of oligonucleotides from ATP and which in turn, in the presence of double-stranded RNA, activates ribonucleases that inhibit viral replication.[140] IFN also activates a protein kinase, which leads to phosphorylation and inactivation of a co-factor needed for viral replication.[137] IFN also interferes with the enveloping mechanism of enveloped viruses, which may be important for hepatitis B. With respect to immunologic effects, IFN-alpha increases T-cell and NK-cell cytotoxicity and enhances cell surface expression of HLA antigens and beta$_2$-microglobulin on hepatocytes and lymphocytes.[140]

The pharmacokinetics of large parenteral doses of IFN-alpha are different from those of endogenously produced interferons. Small amounts of interferon have only brief local concentrations; the large amounts of interferon produced during viral infection spill into the circulation but are cleared quickly. IFN-alpha given by intravenous bolus undergoes rapid renal clearance, with tubular reabsorption and catabolism. If IFN-alpha is given intramuscularly, plasma concentrations persist longer, with peak concentration at 1 to 6 hours and stable concentrations for about 6 to 12 hours. In one study peak concentration after intramuscular injection was higher on day 18 than on day 1.[141] IFN-beta and IFN-gamma have different pharmacokinetic features from IFN-alpha, notably insignificant plasma concentrations even after intramuscular administration and predominantly hepatic metabolism. Differences in hydrophobicity are thought to account for these pharmacokinetic disparities.[138]

The major side-effects of interferons are fever, headache, anorexia,[141] and myalgia. In fact, interferons are thought to be responsible for the "flu-like syndrome" of viral influenza: These flu-like reactions have also been observed in children receiving IFN-alpha.[142] Transient leukopenia typically occurs after beginning treatment, without increased incidence of infections.[140] With prolonged use, interferon is somewhat myelosuppressive. Fatigue and irritability are also common side effects. Some side effects are clearly dose-dependent. At high doses, not appropriate for treating viral hepatitis, major depression of myocardial and central nervous system function has occurred, causing hypotension, coma, or confusion.[140] Interestingly, children with trisomy 21 are more sensitive to effects of interferons, apparently because they have more gene copies for the IFN cell surface receptors.[138]

Interferon has important effects on the activity of cytochromes P-450. It has been known for some time that viral infections can depress the activity of cytochromes P-450.[143,144] Agents that are known to induce interferons and certain immunoregulators such as endotoxin have been shown to depress cytochromes P-450.[145] Autologous, but not heterologous, IFN has been shown to impair hepatic drug metabolism in rats.[146] Recombinant IFN-alpha has been shown to inhibit antipyrine[147] and theophylline[148] clearance in humans. This may be particularly relevant to children because viral infections in children, but not in the elderly, may lead to theophylline toxicity.[144] Thus changes in hepatic drug metabolism due to interferon may be clinically important in children.

There is a comparatively broad experience with interferons for treatment of chronic hepatitis B infection. Studies with recombinant IFN-alpha in adults have extended and largely confirmed early results with leukocyte or lymphoblastoid interferon,[149,150] but not all have shown advantage over the spontaneous conversion from replicating virus to integrated viral DNA stage.[151] It appears that 12 weeks of treatment is necessary and that it is less likely to work in homosexuals than in heterosexuals.[122] IFN-alpha has been used in children.[142,152,153] In a well-designed, although small, study[142] in Oriental children, recombinant alpha$_2$-IFN (10 million units per square meter given three times per week for 12 weeks) led to a drop in blood HBV DNA in all 12 patients only while the medication was being given; two of these 12 permanently lost detectable HBV DNA in their blood and became anti-HBe–positive. Two control patients also seroconverted similarly during the same time. Thus interferon treatment was not advantageous. IFN treatment in adult Chinese patients has also shown a low response rate in one study.[154] In a Spanish study of Caucasian children, the same drug showed approximately the same long-term effect.[153] Others have noted that perinatally infected individuals do not respond well to interferon.[122] Thus, although IFN-alpha appears to be safe to administer to children, it does not appear in these small studies to promote a course much different from the natural history of the disease. In scattered anecdotal reports, when interferon treatment was successful in a child with membranous nephropathy associated with chronic hepatitis B infection, the nephropathy also improved.[152,155,156]

IFN-beta appears to be less effective than IFN-alpha, apparently because it disappears more rapidly. It is not clear whether this rapid disappearance is due to chemical instability or to more active degradation mechanisms. IFN-gamma is currently being studied as treatment for chronic hepatitis B disease. Regimens combining various antiviral drugs are also being investigated, although as yet not in children.

There is growing evidence that IFN-alpha may be effective in NANB hepatitis.[157,158] Extensive clinical studies in adults are underway. These are limited by the lack of specific virologic markers for NANB infection. No formal studies have been performed in children as yet.

Acyclovir interferes with the activity of herpes virus thymidine kinase and has proved to be effective treatment for herpes viruses and of limited use for related viruses. At high doses it interferes with HBV replication, but these doses can be nephrotoxic.[159] Acyclovir shows more promise used together with IFN-alpha.[160] Large studies have not been performed in children. One child recovered from HBV-associated glomerulonephritis with resolution of nephrotic syndrome and with conversion of HBeAg to anti-HBe after treatment with interferon plus acyclovir.[156]

Prednisone in Chronic Hepatitis B

The value of prednisone treatment in chronic hepatitis B remains highly disputed.[161,162] Many studies in adult patients have shown little or no benefit[163,164]; others suggest that steroids may be detrimental.[165] These must be reinterpreted now in light of several confounding factors: presence or absence of replicating HBV and immune status, particularly those perinatally infected and homosexuals. Recent studies in children are similar. A small prospective study of Italian children with moderately severe chronic active hepatitis who varied in mode of presentation and HBeAg showed no benefit or detriment from prednisone plus azathioprine over 2 years.[166] A large retrospective study of Italian children with HBV-associated chronic active hepatitis found that deterioration was more frequent in *un*treated patients.[167] This study has many of the inevitable design faults of multicenter retrospective studies; interestingly, few children in any group developed cirrhosis or lost HBsAg. Another similar Italian retrospective study (in which untreated patients tended to have milder liver disease than treated) found no deterioration on immunosuppression but a tendency not to convert from HBeAg to anti-HBe if treated.[168] It is possible that children with ongoing hepatic inflammation but no evidence of replicating HBV may improve with corticosteroid treatment,[164,169] but this hypothesis requires further investigation. Continued caution in using corticosteroids for treating chronic hepatitis B infection certainly seems appropriate.

TREATMENT OF COMPLICATIONS OF CHRONIC LIVER DISEASE

Pruritus

Pruritus, which is akin to pain, is one of the most distressing complications of chronic cholestatic liver disease. In children it may interfere with sleeping and eating and limit play and social interactions essential for normal growth and development. The mechanism of this pruritus remains unknown. There are few effective treatments. Covering the skin, using cotton socks as mitts on the hands during naps, humidifying the air, applying lubricating skin creams, and adding oil to bath water may help. Antihistamines usually provide limited benefit, although there is individual variation.

Cholestyramine is the major pharmacologic intervention. It is a nonabsorbable ion resin that binds bile salts irreversibly in exchange for chloride ions.[170] The bile salts are then excreted in the feces. The affinity of cholestyramine is greater for dihydroxy than for trihydroxy bile salts. This augmented fecal excretion of bile salts causes temporary contraction in the total bile salt pool and leads to further synthesis of bile acids.[171] Thus cholestyramine is capable of acting as a cholegogue. It is not certain whether its therapeutic effect depends on removing bile salts from the liver, affecting their hepatic metabolism, or reducing the concentration of bile salts in the systemic circulation. Cholestyramine relieves pruritus only when extrahepatic bile duct obstruction is incomplete.[172] In patients with intrahepatic bile duct paucity syndromes, chronic administration of cholestyramine has been shown to lead to resolution of pruritus, decrease in serum bile acid concentrations, and onset of more normal growth.[173]

Other chemicals besides bile salts may bind to cholestyramine. These include thiazide diuretics, phenobarbital, digoxin, and fat-soluble vitamins.[170,174,175] The potential for binding of vitamins D and E is particularly important in children with chronic cholestasis, who are very susceptible to these deficiencies. The absorption of folic acid may also be reduced during cholestyramine treatment so that the child may develop macrocytosis.[175] Dosage schedules should be arranged to avoid giving cholestyramine and oral vitamin supplements at the same time. Infants taking cholestyramine are at risk for developing metabolic acidosis with hypernatremia[176,177]; this occurs when the large chloride load derived from the resin is greater than the infantile kidneys can excrete. Occasionally an infant develops intestinal obstruction due to cholestyramine; cholestyramine ordinarily should not be mixed with formula, and extra fluids should be given to these infants.[178] Although cholestyramine is said to have an unappealing taste, many children take it without difficulty, and its flavor can be disguised with fruit juice or applesauce.

Rifampicin is a rifamycin type of antibiotic that has been proposed as an alternative treatment for intractable pruritus in cholestatic liver disease. Recent studies suggest that it may be effective.[179,180] The antipruritic effect may be due to changes in hepatic metabolism of bile acids.[181] Rifampicin can have major side effects, such as thrombocytopenia. As it may affect hepatic vitamin D metabolism adversely in children, its overall usefulness in childhood cholestatic liver disease may be limited.[182]

Fat-Soluble Vitamin Deficiencies

Vitamin E (alpha-tocopherol) is a very lipophilic compound that functions as an antioxidant to protect against cellular membrane damage.[183] Its absorption is critically dependent upon the concentration of intraluminal bile salts in the small intestine.[184,185] Vitamin E deficiency was first recognized as a clinically important complication of abetalipoproteinemia. More recently it has been recognized as a major complication of chronic cholestatic liver disease in adults and children.[186] Hemolytic anemia may also develop. Importantly, deficiency manifests itself as neurologic dysfunction characterized by areflexia, ataxia, loss of proprioception and vibratory sense, dysdiadochokinesis, eye movement disorders, and retinal abnormalities.[187,188] The lesion involves demyelination of peripheral nerves.[189] Prompt and adequate repletion of vitamin E may reverse the neurologic abnormalities,[190,191] but long-established neurologic disease is usually irreversible. Thus, effective prophylaxis by vitamin E supplementation is extremely important.

Current prophylaxis in North America most commonly involves the use of a water-soluble preparation of vitamin E because the ordinary vitamin E in oil or vitamin E–rich oils (such as wheat germ oil) are not adequately absorbed. Vitamin E acetate (dl-alpha-tocopherol acetate) is water-soluble; the acetate must be removed by the liver. Studies in a newborn (noncholestatic) rabbit model have shown that intravenous alpha-tocopherol acetate is not completely converted to alpha-tocopherol.[192] It is not known whether alpha-tocopherol acetate is an effective as vitamin E biologically. Moreover, the absorption of this water-soluble preparation in the presence of cholestasis may be less than expected. Thus, the overall effectiveness of this preparation remains somewhat in doubt. An alternative approach to oral treatment is to use the oil-soluble preparation of vitamin E in a sufficiently high dose to overcome the absorption inefficiency. However, this has not been subjected to rigorous testing of its effectiveness. Recently a different formulation of oral vitamin E has been investigated. This is D-alpha-tocopheryl polyethylene glycol succinate (TPGS). In TPGS the vitamin E is linked via a succinate linkage to polyethylene glycol, which readily passes through the intestinal epithelium. TPGS is thus a prodrug in which the vitamin E is absorbed passively in conjunction with the polyethylene glycol. The efficacy of TPGS was compared some years ago to that of alpha-tocopherol acetate for vitamin E supplementation in newborn infants: TPGS was free of toxicity in this patient group.[193] TPGS has been administered to children with chronic cholestatic liver disease and found to be efficacious for treating vitamin E deficiency.[194,195]

Vitamin E for intramuscular injection is used mostly in Europe.[196] Recent studies have shown that intramuscular vitamin E can reverse the neuropathy of the deficiency state.[197] Vitamin E prepared for intravenous use, as in TPN solutions, has not been used for routine vitamin E supplementation in chronic liver disease. There has been toxicity in low birth weight premature infants with one intravenous formulation of vitamin E, but this was due to the excipient (polysorbate-80), not the vitamin itself.[198,199]

Vitamin D deficiency may be severe in children and adults with chronic cholestatic liver disease.[200,201] Intraluminal bile salts are required for adequate absorption of vitamin D from the intestinal tract, and 25-hydroxylation of vitamin D occurs in the liver. The requirement for bile salts appears to be less stringent for intestinal absorption of vitamin D than vitamin E.[185,202] Whether severe hepatic disease interferes with 25-hydroxylation extensively enough to be clinically significant is uncertain.[203] However, rickets may develop in severe childhood cholestasis and subnormal serum concentrations of 25-hydroxyvitamin D are frequently found.[204,205] Florid rickets is more likely to occur in infants with unabating cholestasis, such as in Byler's disease or in unsuspected extrahepatic biliary atresia. In addition, osteoporosis is common, affecting 62 percent of children with various types of chronic liver disease in one series.[204]

Effective treatment requires circumventing the intestinal malabsorption. Large doses of oral vitamin D may suffice as prophylaxis against this vitamin deficiency, but their efficacy is not totally reliable. Oral administration of the more polar 25-hydroxyvitamin D may be more effective.[202] For severe disease parenteral treatment is required. Either vitamin D or 25-hydroxyvitamin D may be given; effectiveness is monitored by serum 25-hydroxyvitamin D concentrations and clinical and radiologic improvement. A more novel approach is to use sunlamp therapy; this has been shown to be effective as treatment for florid rickets.[206] Jaundice does not appear to interfere with the light-dependent production of vitamin D in the skin.

Vitamin A deficiency leads to visual deficits in children,[187] but the clinical diagnosis of night blindness can be difficult to establish in young children. Vitamin A deficiency can also lead to skin disorders and cheilosis. However, vitamin A is also potentially toxic to the liver and can cause severe fibrosis due to activation of Ito cells.[207] Thus, supplementation of this fat-soluble vitamin in chronic cholestasis, although important, has to follow a middle course with regard to dosage.

Vitamin K is necessary for the production of clotting Factors II, VII, IX, and X. Vitamin K is produced mostly by the intestinal flora; it is malabsorbed when there is cholestasis. However, vitamin K has other roles. It is necessary for the production of osteocalcin (Gla protein), which has a role in bone calcification.[208,209] Vitamin K–dependent proteins are produced in certain other extrahepatic tissues, including kidney, lung, and testis,[210] and vitamin K may also have a role in the synthesis of brain sphingolipids.[211] It is not known whether vitamin K deficiency may affect bone mineralization or nervous system development in children with chronic cholestatic liver disease. Adult patients with cholestatic liver disease have been found to have low osteocalcin concentrations.[212] The high prevalence of osteoporosis[204] and neurodevelopmental delay[213] in these children is well recognized. Whether these abnormalities relate to lack of vitamin K as well as of vitamins D and E, respectively, is not known. The importance of supplementation of vitamin K beyond that required for adequate coagulation capability has not been determined.

Hepatic Encephalopathy

Hepatic encephalopathy is a metabolic encephalopathy associated with severe liver disease. Chronic hepatic encephalopathy results in abnormal behavior with confusion, inattention, and distraction; it is difficult to diagnose in young children but results in forgetfulness and inappropriate behavior in older children. Wakefulness at night and day-time drowsiness ("day-night reversal") may occur. Acute encephalopathy accompanies acute liver failure; lethargy and confusion progress rapidly to stupor and coma. Although the full mechanism of hepatic encephalopathy is unknown, one component appears to be that the liver fails to remove endogenous toxins, such as ammonia, from the GI tract. Most drug treatment is designed to limit ammonia absorption. The principal drugs for hepatic encephalopathy are neomycin and lactulose.

Neomycin is an aminoglycoside antibiotic. It is poorly absorbed from the GI tract and is active against much of the GI flora. It reduces the number of bacteria and inhibits bacterial ureolysis so that less ammonia is produced. Enough neomycin is absorbed after oral administration, on the order of 1 to 3 percent of a single dose,[214] that nerve deafness and nephrotoxicity can develop with prolonged chronic use. Malabsorption of fats and other nutrients can also develop; penicillin and digoxin are also prone to malabsorption.[215] In general, neomycin should be used for only limited periods of 1 to 2 weeks maximum.

Lactulose is a ketoanalogue of lactose.[216] It is hardly absorbed when taken orally, and it is not hydrolyzed by brush-border enzymes.[217] In the colon it is metabolized by bacteria to lactic, formic, and acetic acids, which cause an osmotic diarrhea and drop the stool pH. There are several theories for its effectiveness in treating hepatic encephalopathy. Although lactulose leads to changes in the complement of colonic flora, these changes do not correspond to clinical improvement.[218] Likewise, its laxative effect in itself does not explain its effectiveness.[219] Ion-trapping in the colonic contents may partly explain its effect: In the acidic stool ammonia becomes the charged species ammonium and cannot traverse the mucosa. Thus there is less *ammonia absorption*. Recent studies suggest that lactulose also leads to less *ammonia production* by directly affecting bacterial ammonia metabolism.[218]

Lactulose should be given in a dose sufficient to produce a few soft or mushy stools daily with a pH of 5.5 or less. It is not necessary to cause severe diarrhea to ensure effectiveness. In small children there is a tangible risk of dehydration and hypokalemia with overly aggressive treatment. Some patients nevertheless complain of gassiness and abdominal cramps. Lactulose, unlike neomycin, can be used for prolonged courses. Lactulose should not be given to persons with galactosemia.[216]

Neomycin and lactulose can be used simultaneously. Neomycin in fact does *not* eradicate all colonic bacteria and thus render lactulose ineffective. The effects of lactulose and neomycin on bacterial ureolysis appear to be additive.[220] Neomycin does not change lactulose metabolism by colonic bacteria insofar as there is no change in stool pH. Interindividual differences in colonic flora may explain differences in response to these drugs, whether used separately or together.

Sodium benzoate has achieved some prominence as an effective treatment for encephalopathy associated with urea cycle disorders.[221] In recent studies,[222,223] lactulose and sodium benzoate (10 g daily by mouth) were compared in adults with cirrhosis and chronic portosystemic encephalopathy. In one study patients improved on treatment, comparable to effective conventional therapy. These authors found sodium benzoate alone better than sodium phenylacetate alone, although some patients responded better to a combination of the two drugs.[222] In a study comparing lactulose and sodium benzoate, improvement in serum ammonia and performance of number connection tests were approximately the same in both groups. The patients receiving sodium benzoate did not have any change in bowel habit. The effectiveness of sodium benzoate was paralleled by increased urinary excretion of hippurate. Sodium benzoate may thus have a wider application in chronic hepatic encephalopathy, and it may be particularly useful in children and adolescents noncompliant with lactulose because of diarrhea. Risks for toxicity from chronic use of sodium benzoate in these children remain unknown. Intravenous sodium benzoate may be toxic to infants, and thus this proposed treatment is not suitable for them.

Acute Liver Failure

For some years corticosteroids were thought to be beneficial in treating fulminant viral hepatitis. Several controlled clinical trials have now been conducted, and although their designs are different and patient numbers small, it is clear that corticosteroids have no role in treatment of fulminant viral hepatitis[224,225] or severe acute hepatitis.[226] The one study of fulminant liver failure in children also showed no benefit.[227] Whether interferon is beneficial in acute liver failure is not known.[228] Prostaglandin E may be effective treatment in fulminant hepatic failure. In an inbred strain of mouse which develops fulminant liver failure when infected with murine hepatitis virus, prostaglandin E_2 reversed the severe course of hepatitis. Preliminary data in humans suggest that a continuous infusion of prostaglandin E_1 may lead to recovery from acute liver failure. However, data from a controlled trial of PGE_1 are needed, and even then its usefulness in infants and children may remain uncertain.

SUMMARY

In liver disease, drug treatment may be aimed at primary treatment of the liver disease itself or at the consequences of liver disease. This encompasses a highly diverse group of drugs. The disposition of these drugs may be different in children and adults. The pharmacology is complicated in some instances by the effect of liver damage on the metabolism and disposition of the drug. Chronic treatment may be life-long in children and include important periods of growth and development; this puts special constraints on defining acceptable side effects. As new drug treatments are developed, these considerations will remain important with respect to treating childhood liver disease.

REFERENCES

1. Vegnente A, Larcher VF, Mowat AP, Portmann B, Williams R. Duration of chronic active hepatitis and the development of cirrhosis. Arch Dis Child 1984; 59:330–335.
2. Read AE, Sherlock S, Harrison CV. Active "juvenile" cirrhosis considered as part of a systemic disease and the effect of corticosteroid therapy. Gut 1963; 4:378–393.
3. Cook GC, Mulligan R, Sherlock S. Controlled prospective trial of corticosteroid therapy in active chronic hepatitis. Q J Med 1971; 40:159–185.
4. Soloway RD, Summershill WHJ, Baggenstoss AH, Gear MG, Gitnick GL, Elvebock LR, Schoenfield LJ. Clinical biochemical and histological remission of severe chronic active liver disease: a controlled study of treatments and early prognosis. Gastroenterology 1972; 63:820–833.
5. Murray-Lyon IM, Stern RB, Williams R. Controlled trial of prednisone and azathioprine in active chronic hepatitis. Lancet 1973; i:735–737.
6. Schaffner F. Autoimmune chronic active hepatitis: three decades of progress. In: Popper H, Schaffner F, eds. Progress in liver diseases. Vol VIII. New York: Grune & Stratton, 1986: 485.
7. Kirk AP, Jain S, Pocock S, Thomas HC, Sherlock S. Late results of the Royal Free Hospital prospective controlled trial of prednisolone therapy in hepatitis B surface antigen negative chronic active hepatitis. Gut 1980; 21:78–83.
8. Czaja AJ, Davis GL, Ludwig J, Taswell HF. Complete resolution of inflammatory activity following corticosteroid treatment of HBsAg-negative chronic active hepatitis. Hepatology 1984; 4:622–627.

9. Czaja AJ, Beaver SJ, Shiels MT. Sustained remission after corticosteroid therapy of severe hepatitis B surface antigen-negative chronic active hepatitis. Gastroenterology 1987; 92:215–219.
10. Meikle AW, Tyler FH. Potency and duration of action of glucocorticoids. Am J Med 1978; 63:200–207.
11. Powell LW, Axelsen E. Corticosteroids in liver disease: studies on the biological conversion of prednisone to prednisolone and plasma protein binding. Gut 1972; 13:690–696.
12. Uribe M, Schalm SW, Summershill WHJ, Go VLW. Oral prednisone for chronic active liver disease: dose responses and bioavailability studies. Gut 1978; 19:1131–1135.
13. Davis M, Williams R, Chakraborty J, English J, Marks V, Ideo G, Tempini S. Prednisone or prednisolone for the treatment of chronic active hepatitis? A comparison on plasma availability. Br J Clin Pharmacol 1978; 5:501–505.
14. Green OC, Winter RJ, Kawahara FS, Phillips LS, Lewy PR, Hart RL, Pachman LM. Pharmacokinetic studies of prednisone in children. Plasma levels, half-life values, and correlation with physiologic assays for growth and immunity. J Pediatr 1978; 93:299–303.
15. Uribe M, Schalm SW, Summershill WHJ, Go VLW. Effect of liquid diet on serum protein binding and prednisolone concentrations after oral prednisone. Gastroenterology 1976; 71:362–364.
16. Uribe M, Go VLW. Corticosteroid pharmacokinetics in liver disease. Clin Pharmacokinet 1979; 4:233–240.
17. Uribe M, Casian C, Rojas S, Sierra J, Go VLW. Decreased bioavailability of prednisone due to antacids in patients with chronic active liver disease and in healthy volunteers. Gastroenterology 1981; 80:661–665.
18. Tanner AR, Caffin JA, Halliday JW, Powell LW. Concurrent adminstration of antacids and prednisone: effect on serum levels of prednisolone. Br J Clin Pharmacol 1979; 7:397–400.
19. Legler U, Frey FJ, Benet LZ. Prednisolone clearance at steady state in humans. J Clin Endocrinol Metab 1982; 55:762–767.
20. Pickp ME, Lowe JR, Leertham PA, Rhina VM, Downie WW. Dose dependent pharmacokinetics of prednisolone. Eur J Clin Pharmacol 1977; 12:213–219.
21. Schalm SW, Summershill WHJ, Go VLW. Prednisone for chronic active liver disease: pharmacokinetics, including conversion to prednisolone. Gastroenterology 1977; 72:910–913.
22. Renner E, Horber FF, Jost G, Frey BM, Frey FJ. Effect of liver functions on the metabolism of prednisone and prednisolone in humans. Gastroenterology 1986; 90:819–828.
23. Madsbad S, Bjerregaard B, Henriksen JH, Juhl E, Kehlet H. Impaired conversion of prednisone to prednisolone in patients with liver cirrhosis. Gut 1980; 21:52–56.
24. Frey FJ, Frey BM. Altered prednisolone kinetics in patients with the nephrotic syndrome. Nephron 1982; 32:45–48.
25. Jacqz E, Hall SD, Branch RA. Genetically determined polymorphism in drug oxidation. Hepatology 1986; 6:1020–1032.
26. Weiersmuller A, Colombo JP, Bircher J. The influence of prednisolone in hepatic function in normal subjects. Effects on galactose elimination capacity, sulfobromophthalein transport maximum and storage capacity, and D-glucaric acid output. Dig Dis 1977; 22:424–428.
27. Petereit LB, Meikle AW. Effectiveness of prednisolone during phenytoin therapy. Clin Pharmacol Ther 1978; 22:912–916.
28. Brooks SM, Werk EE, Ackerman SJ, Sullivan I, Thrasher K. Adverse effects of phenobarbital on corticosteroid metabolism in patients with bronchial asthma. N Engl J Med 1972; 286:1125–1128.
29. Buffington GA, Dominguez JH, Piering WF, Hebert LA, Kauffman HM, Lemann J Jr. Interaction of rifampicin and glucocorticoids. JAMA 1976; 236:1958–1960.
30. Baxter JD, Forsham PH. Tissue effects of glucocorticoids. Am J Med 1972; 53:573–589.
31. Swartz SL, Dluhy RG. Corticosteroids: clinical pharmacology and therapeutic use. Drugs 1978; 16:238–255.
32. Tanner AR, Powell LW. Corticosteroids in liver disease: possible mechanisms of action, pharmacology, and rational use. Gut 1979; 20:1109–1124.
33. Atkinson JP, Frank MM. Effect of cortisone therapy in serum complement components. J Immunol 1973; 111:1061–1066.
34. Nouri-Aria KT, Hegarty JE, Alexander GHM, Eddleston ALWF, Williams R. Effect of corticosteroids in suppressor-cell activity in "autoimmune" and viral chronic active hepatitis. N Engl J Med 1982; 307:1301–1304.
35. Ikeda T, Nikihara M, Daiguji Y, Hasumura Y, Takeuchi J. Immunological mechanisms of corticosteroid therapy in chronic active hepatitis: analysis of peripheral blood suppressor T-cell and interleukin 2 activities. Clin Immunol Immunopathol 1988; 48:371–379.
36. Foote KD, Broncklebank JT, Meadow SR. Height attainment in children with steroid-responsive nephrotic syndrome. Lancet 1985; ii:917–919.
37. Clark JH, Fitzgerald JF. Effect of exogenous corticosteroid therapy on growth in children with HBsAg-negative chronic aggressive hepatitis. J Pediatr Gastroenterol Nutr 1984; 3:72–76.
38. Klein RG, Arnand SB, Gallagher JC. Intestinal calcium absorption in exogenous hypercortisolism. J Clin Invest 1977; 60:253–259.
39. Cutroneo KR, Counts DF. Anti-inflammatory steroids and collagen metabolism, glucocorticoid-mediated alterations of prolyl hydroxylase activity and collagen synthesis. Mol Pharmacol 1975; 11:632–639.
40. Ballardini G, Faccani A, Bianchi FB, Fallarri M, Patrono D, Capelli M, Pisi E. Steroid treatment lowers hepatic fibroplasia, as explored by serum aminoterminal procollagen III peptide, in chronic liver disease. Liver 1984; 4:348–352.
41. Messer J, Reitman D, Sacks HS, Smith H Jr, Chalmers TC. Association of adrenocorticosteroid therapy and peptic-ulcer disease. N Engl J Med 1983; 309:21–24.
42. Van Scoik KG, Johnson CA, Porter WR. The pharmacology and metabolism of the thiopurine drugs 6-mercaptopurine and azathioprine. Drug Metab Rev 1985; 16:157–174.
43. Lennard L, Brown CB, Fox M. Maddocks JL. Azathioprine metabolism in kidney transplant recipients. Br J Clin Pharmacol 1984; 18:693.
44. Elion GB. Significance of azathioprine metabolites. Proc R Soc Med 1976; 65:257–260.
45. Bach J, Dardenne M. Serum immunosuppressive activity of azathioprine in normal subjects and patients with liver disease. Proc R Soc Med 1972; 65:260–263.
46. Al-Safi SA, Maddocks JL. Effects of azathioprine in the mixed lymphocyte reaction. Br J Clin Pharmacol 1983; 15:203–209.
47. Al-Safi SA, Maddocks JL. Azathioprine and 6-mercaptopurine suppress the human mixed lymphocyte reaction by different mechanisms. Br J Clin Pharmacol 1984; 17:417–422.
48. DePinho RA, Goldberg CS, Lefkowitch JH. Azathioprine and the liver. Evidence favoring idiosyncratic, mixed cholestatic-hepatocellular injury in humans. Gastroenterology 1984; 86:162–165.
49. Lennard L, Rees CA, Lilleyman JS, Maddocks JL. Childhood leukemia: a relationship between intracellular 6-mercaptopurine metabolites and neutropenia. Br J Clin Pharmacol 1983; 16:359–363.
50. Weinshilboum R. Pharmacogenetics of methyl conjugation and thiopurine drug toxicity. Bioessays 1987; 7:78–82.
51. Davis M, Eddleston ALWF, Williams R. Hypersensitivity and jaundice due to azathioprine. Postgrad Med J 1980; 56:274–275.
52. Tage-Jensen U, Schlicting P, Thomsen HF, Hoybye G, Thomsen AAC, Copenhagen Study Group for Liver Disease. Malignancies following long-term azathioprine treatment in chronic liver disease. Liver 1987; 7:81–83.
53. Dubois RS, Silverman A. Treatment of chronic active hepatitis in children. Postgrad Med J 1974; 50:386–391.
54. Arasu TS, Wyllie R, Hatch TF, Fitzgerald JF. Management of chronic aggressive hepatitis in children and adolescents. J Pediatr 1979; 95:514.
55. Maggiore G, Bernard O, Hadchouel M, Hadchouel P, Odievre M, Alagille D. Treatment of autoimmune chronic active hepatitis in childhood. J Pediatr 1984; 104:839–844.
56. Hegarty JE, Aria KTN, Portmann B, Eddleston ALWF, Williams R. Relapse following treatment withdrawal in patients with autoimmune chronic active hepatitis. Hepatology 1983; 3:685–689.
57. Summerskill WHJ, Korman MG, Ammon HV, Baggenstoss AH. Prednisone for chronic active liver disease: dose titration, standard dose, and combination with azathioprine compared. Gut 1975; 16:876–883.
58. Stellon AJ, Keating JJ, Johnson PJ, McFarlane IG, Williams R. Maintenance of remission in autoimmune chronic active hepatitis with azathioprine after corticosteroid withdrawal. Hepatology 1988; 8:781–784.
59. Lange J, Schumacher K, Witscher HP. Die Behandkung der chronisch-aggresiven Hepatitis mit D-penicillamin. Dtsh Med Wochenschr 1971; 96:139–145.
60. Stern RB, Wilkinson SP, Horvath PJ, Williams R. Controlled trial of synthetic D-penicillamine and prednisone in maintenance therapy for active chronic hepatitis. Gut 1977; 18:19–22.
61. LaRusso NF, Wiesner RH, Ludwig J, McCarty RL, Beaver SJ, Zinsmeister AR. Prospective trial of penicillamine in primary sclerosing cholangitis. Gastroenterology 1988; 95:1036–1042.

62. El-Shabrawi M, Wilkinson ML, Portmann B, Mieli-Vergani G, Chong SKF, Williams R, Mowat AP. Primary sclerosing cholangitis in childhood. Gastroenterology 1987; 92:1226–1235.
63. Sternlieb I, van den Hamer CJA, Morell AG, Alpert S, Gregoriadis G, Scheinberg IH. Lysosomal defect of copper excretion in Wilson's disease. Gastroenterology 1973;64:99–105.
64. Frommer DJ. Defective biliary excretion of copper in Wilson's disease. Gut 1974; 15:125–129.
65. Epstein O, Sherlock S. Is Wilson's disease caused by a controller gene mutation resulting in perpetuation of the fetal mode of copper metabolism into childhood? Lancet 1981; i:303–305.
66. Walshe JM. Wilson's disease. New oral therapy. Lancet 1956; i:25–26.
67. Walshe JM. The discovery of the therapeutic use of D-penicillamine. J Rheumatol 1981; 8(Suppl 7):3–8.
68. Perratt D. The metabolism and pharmacology of D-penicillamine in man. J Rheumatol 1981; 8(Suppl 7):41–50.
69. Wiesner RH, Dickson ER, Carlson GL, McPhaul LW, Go VLW. The pharmacokinetics of D-penicillamine in man. J Rheumatol 1981; 8(Suppl 7):51–55.
70. Bergstrom RF, Kay DR, Harkcom TM, Wagner JG. Penicillamine kinetics in normal subjects. Clin Pharmacol Ther 1981; 30:404–413.
71. Schuna A, Osman MA, Patel RB, Welling PG, Sundstrom WR. Influence of food in the bioavailability of penicillamine. J Rheumatol 1983; 10:95–97.
72. Kukovetz WR, Beubler E, Kreuzig F, Moritz AJ, Nirnberger G, Werner-Breitenecker L. Bioavailability and pharmacokinetics of D-penicillamine. J Rheumatol 1983; 10:90–94.
73. Wei P, Sass-Kortsak A. Urinary excretion and renal clearance of d-penicillamine in humans and the dog. Gastroenterology 1970; 58:288.
74. Walshe JM. Filterable and non-filterable serum copper. (1) The action of penicillamine. Clin Sci 1963; 25:405–411.
75. Goering PL, Tandon SK, Klaassen CD. Induction of hepatic metallothionein in mouse liver following adminstration of chelating agents. Toxicol Appl Pharmacol 1985; 80:467–472.
76. Heilmeier HE, Viang JL, Greim H, Schramel P, Summer KH. D-Penicillamine induces rat hepatic metallothionein. Toxicology 1986; 43:23–31.
77. Scheinberg IH, Sternlieb I, Schilsky M, Stockert RJ. Penicillamine may detoxify copper in Wilson's disease. Lancet 1987; ii:95.
78. Evans JM, Zerpa H, Nuttall L, Boss M, Sherlock S. Copper chelation therapy in intrahepatic cholestasis of childhood. Gut 1983; 24:42–48.
79. Tanner MS, Bhave SA, Pradham AM, Pandit AN. Clinical trials of penicillamine in Indian childhood cirrhosis. Arch Dis Child 1987; 62:1118–1124.
80. Siegel RC. Collagen cross-linking effect of D-penicillamine on cross-linking in vitro. J Biol Chem 1977; 252:254–259.
81. Merryman P, Jaffe IA. Effect of penicillamine on the proliferative response of human lymphocytes. Proc Soc Exp Biol Med 1978; 157:155–158.
82. Lipsky PE, Ziff M. The effect of D-penicillamine on mitogen-induced human lymphocyte proliferation: synergistic inhibition by D-penicillamine and copper salts. J Immunol 1978; 120:1006–1013.
83. Deiss A, Lynch RE, Lee GR, Cartwright GE. Long-term therapy of Wilson's disease. Ann Intern Med 1971: 75:57–65.
84. Grand RJ, Vawter GF. Juvenile Wilson disease: histologic and functional studies during penicillamine therapy. J Pediatr 1975; 87:1161–1170.
85. Sass-Kortsak A. Wilson's disease. A treatable liver disease in childhood. Pediatr Clin North Am 1975; 22:963–984.
86. Vielhauer W, Eckhardt V, Holtermüller KH, Lüth JB, Schulte B, Prellwitz W, Sonntag W. D-Penicillamine in Wilson's disease presenting as acute liver failure with hemolysis. Dig Dis Sci 1982; 27:1126–1129.
87. Sokol RJ, Francis FD, Gold SH, Ford DM, Lum GM, Ambrusco DR. Othotopic liver transplantation for acute fulminant Wilson's disease. J Pediatr 1985; 107:549–552.
88. Walshe JM, Dixon AK. Dangers of non-compliance in Wilson's disease. Lancet 1986; 1:845–847.
89. Scheinberg IH, Sternlieb I. Major problems in internal medicine. XXIII, Wilson's disease. Philadelphia: WB Saunders, 1984.
90. Polson RJ, Rolles K, Calne RY, Williams R, Marsden D. Reversal of severe neurological manifestations of Wilson's disease following orthotopic liver transplantation. Q J Med 1987; 64:685–691.
91. Neuberger J, Christensen E, Portmann B, Caballeria J, Rodes J, Ranek L, Tygstrup N, Williams R. Double blind controlled trial of d-penicillamine in patients with primary biliary cirrhosis. Gut 1985; 26:114–119.
92. Greer KE, Askew FC, Richardson DR. Skin lesions induced by penicillamine. Arch Dermatol 1976; 112:1267–1269.
93. Harpey JP, Caille B, Moulias R, Goust JM. Lupus-like syndrome induced by D-penicillamine in Wilson's disease. Lancet 1971; i:292.
94. Mjomarod OK, Rasmussen K, Dommerud SA, Gjeruldsen ST. Congenital connective-tissue defect probably due to D-penicillamine treatment in pregnancy. Lancet 1971; i:673–675.
95. Strickland GT. Febrile penicillamine eruption. Arch Neurol 1972; 26:474.
96. Walshe JM. Treatment of Wilson's disease with trientine (triethylene tetramine) dihydrochloride. Lancet 1982; i:643–647.
97. Scheinberg IH, Jaffe ME, Sternlieb I. The use of trientine in preventing the effects of interrupting penicillamine therapy in Wilson's disease. N Engl J Med 1987; 317:209–213.
98. Walshe JM. The management of pregnancy in Wilson's disease treated with trientine. Q J Med 1986; 58:81–87.
99. Borthwick TR, Bensen GD, Schugar HJ. 2,3,2-tetramine—A potent cupruretic agent. Proc Soc Exp Biol Med 1979; 162:227.
100. Borthwick TR, Benson GD, Schugar HJ. Copper chelating agents. A comparison of cupruretic responses to various tetramines and D-penicillamine. J Lab Clin Med 1980; 95:575–580.
101. Epstein O, Sherlock S. Triethylene tetramine dihydrochloride toxicity in primary biliary cirrhosis. Gastroenterology 1980; 78:1442–1445.
102. Walshe JM. Copper chelation in patients with Wilson's disease. A comparison of penicillamine and triethylene tetramine dihydrochloride. Q J Med 1973; 42:441–452.
103. Sarkar B, Sass-Kortsak A, Clarke R, Laurie SH, Wei P. A comparative study of *in vitro* and *in vivo* interaction of D-penicillamine and triethylene-tetramine with copper. Proc R Soc Med 1977; 70(suppl 3):13–18.
104. Walshe JM. The management of Wilson's disease with triethylene tetramine 2HCI (Trien HCI). In: Papadatos J, Bartsocas CS, eds. The management of genetic disorders: proceedings (Progress in Clinical and Biological Research, Vol 34). New York: Alan R Liss, 1979: 271.
105. Hoogenraad TU, Van Haltum J, Van der Hamer CJA. Management of Wilson's disease with zinc sulphate. Experience in a series of 27 patients. J Neurol Sci 1987; 77:137–146.
106. Prasad AS, Brewer GJ, Shoomaker EB, Rabbini P. Hypocupremia induced by zinc therapy in adults. JAMA 1978; 240:2166–2168.
107. Brewer GJ, Hill GM, Prasad AS, Cossack ZT, Rabbani P. Oral zinc therapy for Wilson's disease. Ann Intern Med 1983; 99:314–320.
108. Hill GM, Brewer GJ, Prasad AS, Hydrich CR, Hartmann DE. Treatment of Wilson's disease with zinc. I. Oral zinc therapy regimens. Hepatology 1987; 7:522–528.
109. Brewer GJ, Hill G, Prasad A, Dick R. Treatment of Wilson's disease with zinc. IV. Efficacy monitoring using urine and plasma copper. Proc Soc Exp Biol Med 1987; 184:446–455.
110. Hill GM, Brewer GJ, Juni JE, Prasad AS, Dick RD. Treatment of Wilson's disease with zinc. II. Validation of oral ^{64}copper with copper balance. Am J Med Sci 1986; 29:344–349.
111. Menard MP, McCormick CC, Cousins RJ. Regulation of intestinal metallothionein biosynthesis in rats by dietary zinc. J Nutr 1981; 111:1353–1361.
112. Brewer GJ, Hill GM, Dick RD, Nostrant TT, Sarns JS, Wells JJ, Prasad AS. Treatment of Wilson's disease with zinc. III. Prevention of reaccumulation of hepatic copper. J Lab Clin Med 1987; 109:526–531.
113. Pecoud A, Dozel F, Schelling JL. The effect of foodstuffs on the absorption of zinc sulfate. Clin Pharmacol Ther 1975; 17:469.
114. Chandra RK. Excessive intake of zinc impairs immune responses. JAMA 1984; 252:1443–1446.
115. Yamaguchi M, Takahashi K, Okada S. Zinc-induced hypocalcemia and bone resorption in rats. Toxicol Appl Pharmacol 1983; 67:224–228.
116. Alexiou D, Hatzis T, Kontselinis A. Traitement d'entretien de la maladie de Wilson par le zinc *per os*. Arch Fr Pediatr 1985; 42:447–449.
117. Van Caille-Bertrand M, Degenhaut HJ, Visser HKA, Sinaasappel M, Bouquet J. Oral zinc sulphate for Wilson's disease. Arch Dis Child 1985; 60:656–659.
118. Lipsky MA, Gollan JL. Treatment of Wilson's disease: in D-penicillamine we trust—what about zinc? Hepatology 1987; 7:593–595.
119. Walshe JM. Tetrathiomolybdate (MoS_4) as an anti-copper agent in man. In: Scheinberg I, Walshe JM, eds. Orphan diseases and orphan drugs. Manchester: Manchester University Press, 1986: 76.
120. Walshe JM. Unithiol in Wilson's disease. Br Med J 1985; 290:673–674.
121. Ikeda T, Lever AML, Thomas HC. Evidence for a deficiency of IFN

production in patients with chronic HBV infection acquired in adult life. Hepatology 1986; 6:962–965.
122. Thomas HC, Scully L. Antiviral therapy in hepatitis B infection. Br Med Bull 1985; 41:374–380.
123. Thomas HC, Scully L. Immunomodulators and antiviral drugs for the treatment of viral hepatitis. In: Testa B, Perrisoud D, eds. Liver drugs: from experimental pharmacology to therapeutic application. Baton Rouge: CRC Press, 1988: 175.
124. Stevens CE, Toy PT, Tong MJ, Taylor PE, Vyas GN, Nair PV, Gudavalli M, Krugman S. Perinatal hepatitis B virus transmission in the United States. Prevention by passive-active immunization. JAMA 1985; 253:1740–1745.
125. Yeoh EK, Chang WK, Ip P, Chan KH, Chan E, Fung C. Efficacy and safety of recombinant hepatitis B vaccine in infants born to HBsAg-positive mothers. J Infect Dis 1986; 13(Suppl A): 15–18.
126. Lee GCY, Hwang LY, Beasley RP, Chen SH, Lee TY. Immunogenicity of hepatitis B vaccine in healthy Chinese neonates. J Infect Dis 1983; 148:526–529.
127. Sherlock S. The natural history of hepatitis B. Postgrad Med J 1987; 63(suppl 2):7–11.
128. Sherlock S, Thomas HC. Treatment of chronic hepatitis due to hepatitis B virus. Lancet 1985; ii:1343–1346.
129. Lok ASF, Wilson LA, Thomas HC. Neurotoxicity associated with adenione arabinoside monophosphate in the treatment of chronic hepatitis B infection. J Antimicrob Chemother 1984; 14:93–99.
130. Preiksaitis JK, Lank B, Ng PK, Brox L, LePage GA, Tyrrell DLJ. Effect of liver disease on pharmacokinetics and toxicity of 9-beta-D-arabinofuranosyladenine-5′phosphate. J Infect Dis 1981; 144:358–364.
131. Sacks SL, Scullard GH, Pollard RB, Gregory PB, Robinson WS, Merigan TC. Antiviral treatment of chronic hepatitis B virus infection: pharmacokinetics and side-effects of interferon and adenine arabinoside alone and in combination. Antimicrob Agents Chemother 1982; 21:93–100.
132. Buchanan RA, Kinkel AW, Alford CA, Whitley RJ. Plasma levels and urinary excretion of vidarabine after repeated dosing. Clin Pharmacol Ther 1980; 27:690–696.
133. Whitley RJ, Tucker BC, Kinkel AW, Barton NH, Pass RF, Whelcher JD, Cobbs CG, Diethelm AG, Buchanan RA. Pharmacology, tolerance and antiviral activity of vidarabine monophosphate in humans. Antimicrob Agents Chemother 1980; 18:709.
134. Bassendine MF, Chadwick RG, Salmeron J, Shipton U, Thomas HC, Sherlock S. Adenine arabinoside therapy for HBsAg-positive chronic liver disease: a controlled study. Gastroenterology 1981; 80:1016–1022.
135. Weller IVD, Lok ASF, Mindel A, Karayiannis P, Galpin S, Monjardine J, Sherlock S, Thomas HC. A randomized controlled trial of adenine arabinoside 5-monophosphate (ARA-AMP) in chronic hepatitis B virus infection. Gut 1985; 26:745–751.
136. Hoofnagle JH, Hanson RG, Minuk GY, Pappas SC, Schafer DF, Duskeiko GM, Strauss SE, Popper H, Jones EA. Randomized controlled trial of adenosine arabinoside monophosphate for chronic type B hepatitis. Gastroenterology 1984; 86:150–157.
137. Burke DC. The interferons. Br Med Bull 1985; 41:333–338.
138. Mannering GJ, Deloria LB. The pharmacology and toxicology of the interferons: an overview. Ann Rev Pharmacol Toxicol 1986; 26:455–515.
139. Goldstein D, Laszlo J. Interferon therapy in cancer: from imaginon to interferon. Cancer Res 1986; 46:4315–4329.
140. Peters M, Davis GL, Dooley JS, Hoofnagle JH. The interferon system in acute and chronic viral hepatitis. In: Popper H, Schaffner F, eds. Progress in liver diseases. Vol VIII. New York: Grune and Stratton, 1986: 453.
141. Omata M, Imazeki F, Yokosuka O, Ito Y, Uchiumi K, Mori J, Okuda O. Recombinant leukocyte A interferon treatment in patients with chronic hepatitis B virus infection: pharmacokinetics, tolerance and biologic effects. Gastroenterology 1985; 88:870–880.
142. Lai CL, Lok ASF, Lin HJ, Wu PC, Yeoh EK, Yeung CY. Placebo-controlled trial of recombinant alpha$_2$-interferon in Chinese HBsAg-carrier children. Lancet 1987; ii:877–880.
143. Chang KC, Lauer BD, Beu TD, Chai H. Altered theophylline pharmacokinetics during acute respiratory viral illness. Lancet 1978; 1:1132–1133.
144. Kraemer MJ, Furukawa CT, Koup JR, Shapiro GG, Pierson WE, Fierman CW. Altered theophylline clearance during an influenza B outbreak. Pediatrics 1982; 69:476–480.
145. Renton KW, Mannering GJ. Depression of hepatic cytochrome P-450 dependent monooxygenase system with administered interferon inducing agents. Biochem Biophys Res Commun 1976; 73:343–348.
146. Williams SJ, Craig PI, Cantrill E, Farrell GC. Interferon mediated impairment of hepatic oxidative drug metabolism in rats. Gut 1988; 29:A1460–A1461.
147. Williams SJ, Farrell GC. Inhibition of antipyrine metabolism by interferon. Br J Clin Pharmacol 1986; 22:610–612.
148. Williams SJ, Baird-Lambert JA, Farrell GC. Inhibition of theophylline metabolism by interferon. Lancet 1987; ii:939–941.
149. Dusheiko GM, DiBisceglie A, Bowyer S, Sach SE, Ritchie M, Schoub B, Kew M. Recombinant leukocyte interferon treatment of chronic hepatitis B. Hepatology 1985; 5:556–560.
150. Alexander GJM, Brahm J, Fagan EA, Smith HM, Daniels HM, Edleston ALWF, Williams R. Loss of HBsAg with interferon therapy in chronic hepatitis B infection. Lancet 1987; i:66–68.
151. Hoofnagle JH, Peters M, Mullen KD, Jones DB, Rustgi V, DiBisceglie A, Hallahan C, Park Y, Meshievitz C, Jones EA. Randomized, controlled trial of recombinant human alpha-interferon in patients with chronic hepatitis B. Gastroenterology 1988; 95:1318–1325.
152. Hashida T, Sawada T, Esumi N, Kinugara A, Kusunoki T, Kishida T. Therapeutic effects of human leukocyte interferon on chronic active hepatitis B in children. J Pediatr Gastroenterol Nutr 1985; 4:20–25.
153. LaBanda F, Moreno MR, Carreno V, Bartolome J, Gutiez J, Ramon Y Cajal S, Moreno A, Mora I, Porres JC. Recombinant alpha$_2$-interferon treatment in children with chronic hepatitis B. Lancet 1988; i:250.
154. Lok ASF, Lai CL, Wu PC, Leung EKY. Long-term follow-up in a randomized controlled trial of recombinant alpha$_2$-interferon in Chinese patients with chronic hepatitis B infection. Lancet 1988; ii:298–302.
155. Mizushima N, Kanai K, Matsuda H, Matsumoto M, Tamakoshi K, Ishii H, Nakajima T, Yoshimi T, Kimura M, Nagase M. Improvement of proteinuria in a case of hepatitis B-associated glomerulonephritis after treatment with interferon. Gastroenterology 1987; 92:524–526.
156. v d Heijden AD, de Man RA, ten Cate FW, Schalm SW, Wolff ED. Improvement of hepatitis B associated glomerulonephritis after treatment with antiviral combination therapy. Pediatr Nephrol 1988; 2:C145.
157. Thomson BJ, Doran M, Lever AML, Webster ADB. Alpha-interferon therapy for non-A, non-B hepatitis transmitted by gammaglobulin replacement therapy. Lancet 1987; i:539–541.
158. Hoofnagle JH, Mullen KD, Jones DB, Rustgi V, DiBisceglie A, Peters M, Waggoner JC, Park Y, Jones EA. Treatment of chronic non-A, non-B hepatitis with recombinant human alpha interferon. N Engl J Med 1986; 315:1575–1578.
159. Weller IVD, Carreno V, Fowler MJF, et al. Acyclovir in hepatitis B antigen-positive chronic liver disease: inhibition of viral replication and transient renal impairment with iv bolus administration. J Antimicrob Chemother 1983; 11:223–231.
160. Schalm SW, Heytink RA, Van Buuren HR, de Man RA. Acyclovir enhances the antiviral effect of interferon in chronic hepatitis B. Lancet 1985; 2:358–360.
161. Conn HO, Maddrey WC, Soloway RD. The detrimental effects of adrenocorticoid therapy in HBsAg-positive chronic active hepatitis: fact or artifact? Hepatology 1982; 2:885–887.
162. Van Thiel DH, Dindzans V. Are steroids contraindicated in HBsAg-positive individuals with liver disease? J Pediatr Gastroenterol Nutr 1988; 7:3–6.
163. Schalm SW, Summerskill WHJ, Gitnick GL, Elvebach LR. Contrasting features and responses to treatment of severe chronic active liver disease with and without HBsAg. Gut 1976; 17:781–786.
164. Sagnelli E, Piccinino F, Manzillo G, Felaco FM, Filippini P, Maio G, Pasquale G, Izzo CM. Effect of immunosuppressive therapy in HBsAg-positive chronic active hepatitis in relation to presence or absence of HBeAg and antiHBe. Hepatology 1983; 3:690–695.
165. Lam KC, Lai CL, Ng RP, Trepo C, Wu PC. Deleterious effect of prednisolone in HBsAg positive chronic active hepatitis. N Engl J Med 1981; 304:380–386.
166. Vajro P, Orso G, D'Antonia A, Greco L, Fontanella A, Loffredo G, Oggero V, Buffolano W. Inefficacy of immunosuppressive treatment in HBsAg-positive, delta-negative, moderate chronic active hepatitis in children. J Pediatr Gastroenterol Nutr 1985; 4:26–31.
167. Giusti G, Piccinino F, Sagnelli E, Ruggiero G, Galanti B, Gallo C. Immunosuppressive therapy of HBsAg-Positive chronic active hepatitis in childhood: a multicentric retrospective study in 139 patients. J Pediatr Gastroenterol Nutr 1988; 7:17–21.
168. Maggiore G, DaGiacomo C, Balli F, Barbera C, Guarascio P, Nebbia

G, Palumbo M, Vajro P, Vegnente A. Which treatment for children with hepatitis B surface antigen-positive chronic active hepatitis? J Pediatr Gastroenterol Nutr 1988; 7:788.

169. Giusti G, Piccinino F, Sagnelli E, Ruggiero G, Galanti B, Gallo C. Which treatment for children with hepatitis B surface antigen-positive chronic active hepatitis?—authors' reply. J Pediatr Gastroenterol Nutr 1988; 7:789.
170. Gallo DG, Bailey KR, Scheffner AL. The interaction between cholestyramine and drugs. Proc Soc Exp Biol Med 1965; 120:60–65.
171. Thompson WG. Cholestyramine. Can Med Assoc J 1971; 104:305–309.
172. Datta DV, Sherlock S. Treatment of pruritus of obstructive jaundice with cholestyramine. Br Med J 1963; 1:216–219.
173. Sharp HL. Cholestyramine therapy in patients with a paucity of intrahepatic bile ducts. J Pediatr 1967; 71:723–736.
174. Thompson WG, Thompson GR. Effect of cholestyramine on the absorption of vitamin D_3 and calcium. Gut 1969; 10:717–722.
175. West RJ, Lloyd JK. The effect of cholestyramine on intestinal absorption. Gut 1975; 16:93–98.
176. Primack WA, Gartner LM, McGurk HE, Spitzer A. Hypernatremia associated with cholestyramine therapy. J Pediatr 1977; 90:1024–1025.
177. Bernsten B, Zoger S. Hyperchloremic metabolic acidosis with cholestyramine therapy for biliary cholestasis. Am J Dis Child 1978; 132:1220.
178. Lloyd-Still JD. Cholestyramine therapy and intestinal obstruction in infants. Pediatrics 1977; 89:626–627.
179. Ghent CN, Carruthers G. Treatment of pruritus in primary biliary cirrhosis with rifampin. Gastroenterology 1988; 94:488–493.
180. Banks L, Pares A, Elena M, Piera C, Rodes J. Comparison of rifampicin with phenobarbitone for treatment of pruritus in biliary cirrhosis. Lancet 1989; i:574–576.
181. Hoensch HP, Balzer K, Dylewizi P, Kirch W, Goebell H, Ohnhaus EE. Effect of rifampicin treatment on hepatic drug metabolism and serum bile acids in patients with primary biliary cirrhosis. Eur J Clin Pharmacol 1985; 28:475–477.
182. Toppet M, Vainsel M, Vertrongen F, Fuss M, Cantraine F. Evolution sequentielle des metabolites de la vitamine D sous isoniazide et rifampicine. Arch Fr Pediatr 1988; 45:145–148.
183. Bieri JG, Corash L, Hubbard VS. Medical uses of vitamin E. N Engl J Med 1983; 308:1063–1071.
184. Sokol RJ, Heubi JE, Iannaccone S, Bove KE, Balistreri WF. Mechanism causing vitamin E deficiency during chronic childhood cholestasis. Gastroenterology 1983; 85:1172–1182.
185. Sokol RJ, Farrell MK, Heubi JE, Tsang RC, Balistreri WF. Comparison of vitamin E and 25-hydroxyvitamin D absorption during chronic cholestasis. J Pediatr 1983; 103:712–717.
186. Sokol RJ. The coming of age of vitamin E. Hepatology 1989; 9:649–653.
187. Alvarez F, Landrieu P, Laget P, Lemonnier F, Odievre M, Alagille D. Nervous and ocular disorders in children with cholestasis and vitamin A and E deficiencies. Hepatology 1983; 3:410–414.
188. Muller DPR. Vitamin E—its role in neurological function. Postgrad Med J 1986; 62:107–112.
189. Sung JH, Park SH, Martin AR, Warwick WJ. Axonal dystrophy in the gracile nucleus in congenital biliary atresia and cystic fibrosis (mucoviscidosis): beneficial effect of vitamin E therapy. J Neuropathol Exp Neurol 1980; 39:584–597.
190. Guggenheim MA, Ringel SP, Silverman A, Grabert BE. Progressive neuromuscular disease in children with chronic cholestasis and vitamin E deficiency: diagnosis and treatment with alpha tocopherol. J Pediatr 1982; 100:51–58.
191. Sokol RJ, Guggenheim MA, Iannocccone ST, Barkhaus PE, Miller C, Silverman A, Balistreri WF, Heubi JE. Improved neurologic function after long-term correction of vitamin E deficiency in children with chronic cholestasis. N Engl J Med 1985; 313:1580–1586.
192. Knight ME, Roberts RJ. Disposition of intravenously administered pharmacologic doses of vitamin E in newborn rabbits. J Pediatr 1986; 108:145–150.
193. Gross S, Melhorn DK. Vitamin E-dependent anemia in the premature infant. III. Comparative hemoglobin, vitamin E, and erythrocyte phospholipid responses following absorption of either water-soluble or fat-soluble d-alpha tocopheryl. J Pediatr 1974; 85:753–759.
194. Sokol RJ, Heubi JE, Butler-Simon N, McClung HJ, Lilly JR, Silverman A. Treatment of vitamin E deficiency during chronic childhood cholestasis with oral *d*-alpha-tocopheryl polyethylene glycol-1000 succinate. Gastroenterology 1987; 93:975–985.
195. Sokol RJ, Butler-Simon NA, Bettis D, Smith DJ, Silverman A. Tocopheryl polyethylene glycol 1000 succinate therapy for vitamin E deficiency during chronic childhood cholestasis: neurologic outcome. J Pediatr 1987; 111:830–836.
196. Alagille D. Management of paucity of interlobular bile ducts. J Hepatol 1985; 1:561–565.
197. Perlmutter DH, Gross P, Jones HR, Fulton A, Grand RJ. Intramuscular vitamin E repletion in children with chronic cholestasis. Am J Dis Child 1987; 141:170–174.
198. Bove KE, Kosmetatos N, Wedig KE, Frank DJ, Whitlatch S, Saldivar V, Haas J, Bodenstein C, Balistreri WF. Vasculopathic hepatotoxicity associated with E-Ferol syndrome in low-birth-weight infants. JAMA 1985; 254:2422–2430.
199. Alade SL, Brown RE, Paquet A Jr. Polysorbate 80 and E-ferol toxicity. Pediatrics 1986; 77:593–597.
200. Compston JE. Hepatic osteodystrophy: vitamin D metabolism in patients with liver disease. Gut 1986; 27:1073–1090.
201. Kobayashi A, Kawai S, Ohkubo M, Ohbe Y. Serum 25-hydroxy-vitamin D in hepatobiliary disease in infancy. Arch Dis Child 1979; 54:367–370.
202. Heubi JE, Hollis BW, Specker B, Tsang RC. Bone disease in chronic childhood cholestasis. I. Vitamin D absorption and metabolism. Hepatology 1989; 9:258–264.
203. Kooh SW, Jones G, Reilly BJ, Fraser D. Pathogenesis of rickets in chronic hepatobiliary disease in children. J Pediatr 1979; 94:870–874.
204. Kooh SW, Roberts EA, Theodossiou M, Reilly BJ, Weber JL. Impact of chronic liver disease on bone mineral metabolism in children. J Bone Min Res 1987; 2(suppl 1):95A.
205. Kimura S, Seino Y, Harada T, Nose O, Yamaoka K, Shimizu K, Tanaka H, Yabuuchi H, Fukui Y, Yamata S, Okada A. Vitamin D metabolism in biliary atresia: intestinal absorptions of 25-hydroxyvitamin D_3 and 1,25-dihydroxyvitamin D_3. J Pediatr Gastroenterol Nutr 1988; 7:341–346.
206. Kooh SW, Roberts EA, Fraser D, Curtis J, Jones G, Weber JL, Reilly BJ. Ultraviolet light irradiation therapy for chronic hepatobiliary rickets. Arch Dis Child 1989; 64:617–619.
207. Guarascio P, Portmann B, Visco G, Williams R. Liver damage with reversible portal hypertension from vitamin A intoxication: demonstration of Ito cells. J Clin Pathol 1983; 36:769–771.
208. Price PA, Parthemore JG, Deftos LJ. New biochemical marker for bone metabolism. Measurement by radioimmunoassay of bone Gla-protein in the plasma or normal subjects and patients with bone disease. J Clin Invest 1980; 66:878–893.
209. Cole DEC, Carpenter TO, Gundberg CM. Serum osteocalcin concentrations in children with metabolic bone disease. J Pediatr 1985; 106:770–776.
210. Suttie JW. Recent advances in hepatic vitamin K metabolism and function. Hepatology 1987; 7:367–376.
211. Sundaram KS, Lev M. Warfarin administration reduces synthesis of sulfatides and other sphingolipids in mouse brain. J Lipid Res 1988; 29:1475–1479.
212. Diamond TH, Stiel D, Lunzer M, McDowall D, Eckstein RP, Posen S. Hepatic osteodystrophy. Static and dynamic bone histomorphometry and serum bone Gla-protein in 80 patients with chronic liver disease. Gastroenterology 1989; 96:213–221.
213. Stewart SM, Uauy R, Waller DA, Kennard BD, Andrews WS. Mental and motor development correlates in patients with end-stage biliary atresia awaiting liver transplantation. Pediatrics 1987; 79:882–888.
214. Last PM, Sherlock S. Systemic absorption of orally administered neomycin in liver disease. N Engl J Med 1960; 262:385–389.
215. Lindenbaum J, Manlitz RM, Butler VP Jr. Inhibition of digoxin absorption by neomycin. Gastroenterology 1976; 71:399–404.
216. Avery GS, Davies EF, Brogden RN. Lactulose: a review of its therapeutic and pharmacological properties with particular reference to ammonia metabolism and its mode of action in portal systemic encephalopathy. Drugs 1972; 4:7–48.
217. Dahlqvist A, Gryboski JD. Inability of the human small intestinal lactase to hydrolyze lactulose. Biochim Biophys Acta 1965; 110:635–636.
218. Weber FL Jr. The effect of lactulose on urea metabolism and nitrogen excretion in cirrhotic patients. Gastroenterology 1979; 77:518–523.
219. Weber FL Jr, Fresnard KM. Comparative effects of lactulose and magnesium sulfate on urea metabolism and nitrogen excretion in cirrhotic subjects. Gastroenterology 1981; 80:994–998.
220. Weber FL Jr, Fresnard KM, Lally BR. Effects of lactulose and neomycin on urea metabolism in cirrhotic subjects. Gastroenterology 1982; 83:213–217.

221. Brusilow SW, Danney M, Waber LJ, Batshaw M, Burton B, Levitsky L, Roth K, McKeethren C, Ward J. Treatment of episodic hyperammonemia in children with inborn errors of urea synthesis. N Engl J Med 1984; 310:1630–1634.
222. Mendenhall CL, Ronster S, Marshall L, Weesner R. A new therapy for portal systemic encephalopathy. Am J Gastroenterol 1986; 81:540–543.
223. Uribe M, Bosques F, Poo J, Valdovinos F, Melendez N, de la Mora G, Gil S. A double blind randomized trial of sodium benzoate versus lactulose in patients with chronic portal systemic encephalopathy. Hepatology 1988; 8:1449.
224. Redeker AG, Schweitzer IL, Yamahiro HS. Randomization of corticosteroid therapy in fulminant hepatitis. N Engl J Med 1976; 294:728–729.
225. Gregory PB, Knauer CM, Kempson RL, Miller R. Steroid therapy in severe viral hepatitis. A double-blind, randomized trial of methylprednisolone versus placebo. N Engl J Med 1976; 294:681–687.
226. Ware AJ, Cuthbert JA, Shorey J, Gurian LE, Eigenbrodt EH, Comber B. A prospective trial of steroid therapy in severe viral hepatitis. The prognostic significance of bridging necrosis. Gastroenterology 1981; 80:219–224.
227. Psacharopoulos HT, Mowat AP, Davies M, Portmann B, Silk DBA, Williams R. Fulminant hepatic failure in children. An analysis of 31 cases. Arch Dis Child 1980; 55:252–258.
228. Levin S, Hahn T. Interferon system in acute viral hepatitis. Lancet 1982; i:592–594.

PART 5

Pharmacologic Treatment of Exocrine Pancreatic Insufficiency

Geoffrey J. Cleghorn, M.B.B.S., F.R.A.C.P.

The exocrine pancreas is involved in both the digestion and absorption of orally ingested nutrients. Pancreatic fluid has two major components: a fluid consisting primarily of a solution of sodium bicarbonate and an enzyme component consisting of about 20 digestive enzymes and co-factors. The alkaline fluid serves to neutralize gastric acid entering the duodenum and helps to provide an adequate intraluminal pH for the optimal function of the pancreatic digestive enzymes. These enzymes provide the major route for intraluminal digestion of dietary proteins, triglycerides, and carbohydrates and are also involved in the cleavage of certain vitamins such as A and B_{12}. Therefore, failure of the exocrine pancreas to secrete adequately its enzyme- and electrolyte-rich fluid can lead to major nutritional disturbances manifest clinically as steatorrhea and azotorrhea with resultant growth failure.[1] In addition to the obvious lack of intraluminal digestive activity as a result of the enzyme deficiencies, the failure of bicarbonate secretion also has major effects on both intraluminal pH and enzyme activity. An abnormally low pH can be seen in the late postprandial period, which reduces lipid digestion by inactivating pancreatic lipase and also by precipitating bile salts.

Not all diseases involving the exocrine pancreas have equal effects upon both the enzyme component and the electrolyte component of the gland's secretion. In general, patients with cystic fibrosis have major deficits in both enzyme and electrolyte secretion, although there is a wide range of abnormalities, whereas patients with Shwachman's syndrome have normal fluid and electrolyte secretion with marked disturbances in enzyme output.

Cystic fibrosis (CF) is the most common cause of exocrine pancreatic insufficiency in childhood. Therefore, it is patients with CF who most commonly require oral pancreatic replacement therapy with pancreatic enzymes. Irrespective of the etiology of pancreatic failure, current replacement therapy with oral pancreatic enzymes, although far from ideal in many patients, remains the most important method of correcting the nutritional effects of maldigestion. Despite considerable improvements in the efficacy of pancreatic replacement therapy, it remains difficult to correct malabsorption completely in all patients owing to the many factors adversely affecting the function of exogenously administered enzymes (Table 1).

Since the major clinical manifestation of pancreatic failure is steatorrhea with large, bulky, malodorous stools, early management protocols of patients with pancreatic insufficiency relied heavily upon severe restriction of dietary fat. A low-fat diet did indeed produce socially more acceptable stools but also severely restricted calories and essential fatty acids,

TABLE 1
Factors Adversely Affecting the Efficiency of Pancreatic Enzyme Replacement Therapy

Inadequate enzyme content
Inadequate concentration
Inappropriate type, e.g., tablets
Inappropriate oral administration
Abnormal gastric phase
Inactivation by gastric acid
Insufficient mixing with chyme
Delay in gastric emptying
Abnormal intestinal phase
Prolonged acidic intraluminal pH
Bile acid precipitation
Abnormal intestinal motility preventing complete liberation of available enzymes

which contributed significantly to clinical malnutrition and disease morbidity. Use of a low-fat diet in the management of pancreatic failure is no longer considered acceptable; in fact, some centers have advocated the use of a high-fat diet, in conjunction with optimal pancreatic enzyme replacement therapy, in order to maximize total energy absorption.

PANCREATIC ENZYME REPLACEMENT

Extracts of pancreatic enzymes from animal sources have been available for over 80 years and have been used clinically for a variety of conditions. When crude pancreatic extracts were given to children with pancreatic insufficiency, stool bulk was reduced. Theoretically, these preparations provided enough pancreatic enzyme to prevent the maldigestion associated with exocrine pancreatic insufficiency. Although simple in concept, the normalization of nutrient digestion and absorption has proved more difficult. The earliest pancreatic extracts contained low concentrations of active enzymes. Furthermore, only minimal amounts of these were available for intestinal digestion because of gastric inactivation with acid and pepsin, with degradation of lipase and trypsin occurring below pH 4.5 and 3.5, respectively. Even more active preparations in current use are rapidly degraded in the stomach when unprotected; up to 90 percent of ingested lipase and 80 percent of ingested trypsin have been found to be degraded prior to entering the ligament of Treitz.[2]

The quantity of enzyme required depends upon the amount of active ingredient in the particular commercial preparation and also upon the type and quantity of the meal to be consumed. To abolish malabsorption, the amount and concentration of enzyme present in the duodenum must be 5 to 10 percent of the quantities of endogenously secreted enzymes usually present in normal individuals after postprandial stimulation of the pancreas.[2] In an adult, assuming no inactivation of enzymes in the stomach and duodenum, approximately 30,000 international units of lipase must be taken with an average meal.[3] The amount of lipase varies considerably from preparation to preparation, the average being between 5,000 and 8,000 units per capsule. Theoretically, six to eight capsules are required per meal to abolish steatorrhea. In reality, the quantity of enzymes required becomes much higher, if one considers the degree of gastric inactivation and the consumption of a high-energy diet.

Broadly speaking, research has focused on three avenues of approach in improving nutrient absorption in patients with pancreatic insufficiency (Table 2). As the older enzyme preparations were highly variable in enzyme content, the more modern approach has been to provide increased concentration of enzyme (up to 20,000 lipase units) in a single capsule or tablet. Secondly, methods of protecting enzymes from gastric inactivation have been refined. Intensive research has also been aimed at manipulating the acid-alkaline imbalance in both the gastric and intestinal phases of enzyme activity, and attempts have been made at improving bile salt function.

TABLE 2
Various Methods to Improve the Efficacy of Enzyme Replacement Therapy

Inadequate enzyme content
Increasing enzyme concentration per capsule
Abnormal gastric phase
Enteric coating/microspheres
Acid-resistant enzymes
Lingual lipase
Fungal lipase
Abnormal intestinal phase
Antacids, bicarbonate
H_2-receptor antagonists
Prostaglandin analogues
Modified bile acids (taurine)

Acid-Resistant Preparation

Protective barriers were first used to make the enzyme preparations more resistant to acid inactivation. Initially, this was attempted by coating enzyme tablets with an acid-resistant material, but it was soon discovered that these preparations were no better than conventional preparations, and in some cases the steatorrhea was worse. This was thought to be due to both inefficient mixing of the tablet with the ingested chyme in the stomach and failure of liberation of the active enzyme in the duodenum secondary to slow release of the active ingredients. In fact, these tablets were not infrequently seen intact in the stools of patients taking them.[4]

In order to improve delivery of enzymes to the small intestine, a number of commercial pharmaceutical companies developed techniques capable of coating small "microspheres" with an acid-resistant coating.[5-11] The microspheres in turn were packaged in a gelatin capsule. The rationale behind this preparation is that the acid-resistant layer around the small spheres prevents acid-peptic degradation within the stomach, but their small size permits passage with chyme into the duodenum. When exposed to duodenal contents with a pH in excess of 5.5, the acid-resistant coating breaks down, releasing active pancreatic enzymes. Use of these enteric-coated microspheres has resulted in considerable improvement in fat absorption over that with conventional enzyme therapy.[6] Studies have shown that CF patients with refractory malabsorption on conventional enzyme therapy derive significant benefit with decreased steatorrhea and creatorrhea using fewer capsules.[6] Other studies have found improved compliance as well as improved absorption with these preparations, except in a minority of patients, who appear to have acidic small intestinal contents, thereby preventing dissolution of the acid-resistant coating. Thus, there are few current uses for noncoated enzyme replacement therapy, although even with these modern preparations some patients still have significant malabsorption.

More recently, supplementation with enzymes of nonpancreatic origin has been suggested as a method of achieving improved digestion. Several nonpancreatic lipases have been examined for their acid-resistant properties. Acid-resistant lingual lipase has been proposed as an enzyme worthy of further consideration and investigation. In a preliminary study in animals lingual lipase was found to be stable in the stomach under both fasting and fed conditions but to be less stable

TABLE 3
Suggested Daily Requirements of Pancreatic Enzyme Replacement Therapy

Age	Approximate Daily Fat Intake (g)	Daily Enzyme Dosage*
3 months	50	8–12
9 months	60	12–15
18 months	75	15–20
3 years	100	20–25
5 years	120	25–30
8 years	150	30–35
Teens	170	35–40

*Enzyme = enteric-coated microsphere containing 5,000 to 8,000 lipase units per capsule.

in the duodenum.[12] These experimental studies may be forerunners of in vivo human work examining pancreatic enzyme supplementation containing "foreign" or nonpancreatic enzymes. Human studies have been performed using acid lipase prepared from *Aspergillus niger.*[23] This has been shown to retain enzymatic activity within the stomach of CF patients, but clinical efficacy is currently in doubt. Preliminary studies have shown no improvement in fat absorption over a no-treatment control period in CF patients.[13]

Irrespective of the enzyme preparation used and the amount given, it is imperative that the enzymes be delivered in sufficient amounts to the small intestine to facilitate digestion. It is insufficient simply to take a handful of enzymes at the beginning or end of a meal and hope that this will result in optimal pancreatic replacement (Table 3). For optimal efficacy, it has been suggested that enzymes be distributed throughout the meal and taken in several small aliquots. This, in theory, allows for adequate dispersal within the stomach throughout the meal and therefore allows for maximum exposure of that particular meal to the ingested enzymes. Also, enzyme therapy is not without potential problems in that, being concentrated proteolytic packages, they have the potential for causing quite marked oral excoriation if chewed or held within the mouth too long. This is a particular problem in small infants, in whom gum or mouth injury not infrequently occurs; with rapid transit through the intestinal tract, anal excoriation has also been observed.

Monitoring the effectiveness of pancreatic enzyme replacement is quite imprecise. From a clinical standpoint the patients report less frequent and firmer, less bulky stools. In general, it is not very difficult to ascertain by history alone if a patient's enzyme dosage is insufficient. It is much more difficult to gauge on the basis of history whether a dosage is in fact excessive. The laboratory investigations in this regard are somewhat cumbersome. Quantitative fecal fat estimation is the only reliable method but there are practical limitations. More recently a modification of the standard bentiromide test using para-aminosalicylic acid in addition to the bentiromide has been proposed as useful in monitoring enzyme dosage[14]; further studies are required to confirm the validity of this approach.

Adjunctive Therapy to Acid-Base Equilibrium

The alternative method of improving the efficiency of the ingested pancreatic enzymes has been to modify the acid-base balance within the gastrointestinal (GI) tract. H_2-receptor antagonists such as cimetidine or ranitidine have been used to diminish the secretion of gastric acid, thereby successfully decreasing the gastric inactivation of the ingested enzymes with resultant improvement in nutrient absorption.[3,6,15–19]

As enteric-coated microspheres are pH-dependent and rely upon a luminal pH of greater than 5.5 for dissolution of the acid-resistant coating, it is possible that jejunal hyperacidity may further hinder their activity. It has been shown that postprandial jejunal "hyperacidity" does occur in patients with CF, with 40 percent of a test meal entering the jejunum at a pH below 5.[15] At this pH, bile acids precipitate out of the aqueous solution, leading to a reduction in the aqueous phase bile acid concentration. In addition, lipase activity, which is extremely pH sensitive, is considerably reduced.

A recent study suggested that cimetidine may increase jejunal pH, thus increasing aqueous phase bile acid concentration.[17] In this study of adult CF patients receiving noncoated enzymes, 60 percent of the test meal entered the jejunum at a pH less than 5, compared with only 17 percent in healthy subjects. There was a significant decrease in lipase activity and a decrease in aqueous phase lipid concentration, but the decrease in bile acid precipitation did not reach statistical significance. With the introduction of cimetidine, however, there was significantly less bile acid precipitation, and this resulted in improved lipid solubilization. These workers concluded that the efficacy of pancreatic enzyme therapy is limited both by exogenous enzyme inactivation in the stomach and by the pH-dependent environment within the proximal small intestine and that these effects were both improved by the addition of cimetidine. Data from our unit suggest that patients who had significant steatorrhea while taking enteric-coated microspheres also had improved nutrient absorption with the addition of cimetidine.[18] This improvement could result both from the prevention of gastric inactivation and the reduction in small bowel hyperacidity levels, thus affecting the solubilization of bile salts.

However, the use of cimetidine in improving pancreatic enzyme therapy is still not universally accepted. Boyle et al,[16] who evaluated eight CF patients given 300 mg of cimetidine before each meal in addition to oral pancreatic enzyme therapy, showed a decrease in stool weight and fat, but correction of fat absorption was incomplete. They found that the enzyme replacement therapy increased postprandial serum bile acids and that this increase was abolished with the use of oral cimetidine. As the major effect of the addition of cimetidine appears to be improvement of the small intestinal alkalinity, it is not unreasonable to presume that the addition of antacids or bicarbonate therapy may have some merit. Graham[15] found that the concurrent administration of enzymes with either sodium bicarbonate or aluminum hydroxide yields a greater reduction in steatorrhea than to enzymes alone. Durie et al[19] reported 21 patients with CF in whom sodium bicarbonate (15 g per square meter per 24 hours) was an effective adjunct to enzyme therapy. These workers found that sodium bicarbonate or cimetidine (20 mg per kilogram per day) had equivalent beneficial effects as adjuvant therapy; when both drugs were given simultaneously there was no further improvement in nutrient absorption. Graham did, however, point out that the choice of antacid is critical.[15] The use of magnesium/aluminum hydroxide compounds or calcium carbonate in fact tended to enhance steatorrhoea rather than improve it, and bicarbonate may actually increase gastric acidity. The mechanism through which calcium or magnesium enhances steatorrhea is thought to be due to the formation of calcium soaps and intraluminal precipitation of glycine conjugates of bile salts.

More recently, we have adopted a different approach to adjuvant therapy with the use of prostaglandin agents. In a study of 11 children with CF we evaluated the use of misoprostol, a synthetic methylated prostaglandin E_1 analogue that decreases the secretion of gastric acid and increases duodenal bicarbonate secretion.[20] Prostaglandins of the E and I series inhibit basal and stimulated gastric acid secretion both in vivo and in vitro. In the dog, either PGE_2 or PGI_2 inhibit gastric acid secretion stimulated by food, histamine, pentagastrin, or reserpine. The mechanism by which natural prostaglandins and their analogues inhibit gastric acid secretion is still unknown, but one possibility is that there is direct inhibition of parietal cells by prostaglandins acting from the gastric lumen.[21]

Another mechanism through which prostaglandins might affect gastric secretion is suppression of gastrin release. It has been shown that methylated prostaglandin E_2 analogues given orally in dogs and humans cause a marked suppression of gastrin response to a meal.[22] An important addition to the effect on gastric acid secretion is the effect of prostaglandins, particularly the methylated analogues, in stimulating mucus and bicarbonate secretion. This may account for the reduction in luminal acidity observed with the administration of these prostaglandins.

We found a significant reduction in fat output in the study group as a whole and a significant reduction in the steatorrhea level as a percentage of fat intake in all of the patients who initially had abnormal baseline collections (Fig. 1). Prostaglandin therapy may have some inherent advantages over certain H_2-receptor antagonists as adjuvant therapy in CF patients. Cimetidine may interfere with the metabolism of certain drugs by inhibiting cytochrome P-450 oxygenase in the liver.[23] In CF patients these potential drug interactions may assume some clinical importance by inhibiting metabolism of certain bronchodilators, notably theophylline. As it has no human interactions with cytochromes P-450, misoprostol may be superior as long-term adjuvant therapy in CF.

Bile Acid Dysfunction

In addition to manipulating the acid-alkaline balance in the upper small intestine, other workers have also explored the possibility of improving nutrient absorption with the addition of exogenous taurine.[24–28] As a result of large fecal losses of bile acids, patients with CF develop an increased ratio of glycine to taurine in conjugated bile acids. It has recently been proposed that correction of this elevated ratio by oral taurine supplements may improve absorption and ultimately nutrition by potentiating bile salt micelle formation. Taurine, which is more soluble in an acidic environment, has been administered to patients with CF in doses of 30 mg per kilogram per day, and there has been significant improvement in fat absorption in CF patients on enzyme supplementation.[25] Supplementation with taurine significantly reduced the glycine-to-taurine ratio and bile acid losses in the stools.[25,28] A further disadvantage of preponderant glycine bile salt conjugates is that they are partly and passively absorbed in the proximal portion of the small intestine. Since taurine conjugates are predominantly absorbed in the ileum and are more resistant to bacterial degradation, they are more available to form mixed micelles with fat that may have escaped intestinal absorption more proximally.

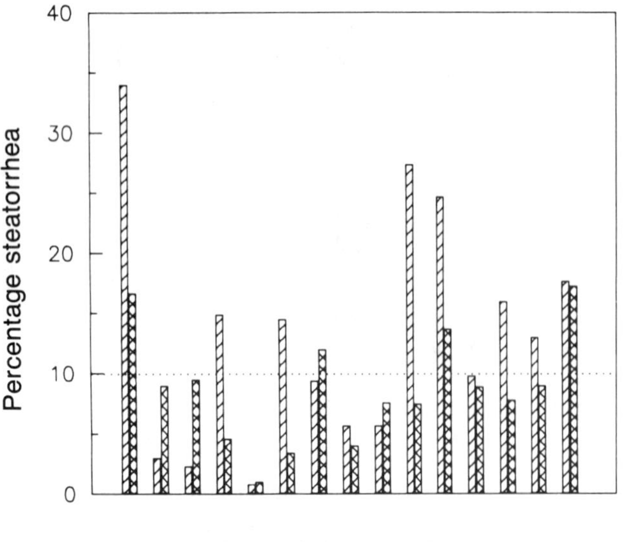

FIGURE 1 Effect of prostaglandin E_1 (misoprostol) upon fecal fat absorption in 15 cystic fibrosis patients who had previously taken enteric-coated microsphere pancreatic enzymes.

REFERENCES

1. DiMagno EP, Go VLW, Summerskill WHJ. Relations between pancreatic enzyme outputs and malabsorption in severe pancreatic insufficiency. N Engl J Med 1973; 288:813–815.
2. DiMagno EP, Malagelada JR, Go VLW, Moertel CG. Fate of orally ingested enzymes in pancreatic insufficiency: comparison of two dosage schedules. N Engl J Med 1977; 296:1318–1322.
3. DiMagno EP. Controversies in the treatment of exocrine pancreatic insufficiency. Dig Dis Sci 1982; 27:481–484.
4. Graham DY. Enzyme replacement therapy of exocrine pancreatic insufficiency in man: relation between in vitro enzyme activities and in vivo potency in commercial pancreatic extracts. N Engl J Med 1977; 296:1314–1318.
5. Salen G, Prakash A. Evaluation of enteric coated microspheres for enzyme replacement therapy in adults with pancreatic insufficiency. Curr Therap Res 1979; 25:650–656.
6. Gow R, Francis P, Bradbear R, Shepherd R. Comparative study of varying regimes to improve steatorrhoea and creatorrhoea in cystic fibrosis: effectiveness of an enteric coated preparation with and without antacids and cimetidine. Lancet 1981; ii:1071–1074.
7. Mischler EH, Farrell S, Farrell P, Odell GB. Comparison of effectiveness of pancreatic enzyme preparations in cystic fibrosis. Am J Dis Child 1982; 136:1060–1063.
8. Sinaasappel M, Bouquet J, Nijens HJ. Problems in the treatment of malabsorption in CF. Acta Pediatr Scand (Suppl) 1985; 317:22–27.
9. Petersen W, Heilmann C, Garne S. Pancreatic enzyme supplementation as acid resistant microspheres versus enteric coated granules in cystic fibrosis. Acta Pediatr Scand (Suppl) 1987; 76:66–69.
10. Beverley DW, Kelleher J, MacDonald A, Littlewood JM, Robinson T, Walters MP. Comparison of four pancreatic extracts in cystic fibrosis. Arch Dis Child 1987; 62:564–568.
11. Stead RJ, Skypala I, Hodson ME, Batten JC. Enteric coated microspheres with pancreatin in the treatment of cystic fibrosis: comparison with a standard enteric coated preparation. Thorax 1987; 42:533–537.
12. Roberts IM, Hanel SI. In vivo studies of co-ordinated lingual lipase (LL), enzyme stability in the stomach and duodenum. (Abstract) 10th International Cystic Fibrosis Congress, Sydney, Australia, 5–10 March, 1988.
13. Assoufi BA, Zentler-Munro P, Cornell S, Northfield TC, Hodson ME. Efficacy of acid resistant fungal lipase in the treatment of steatorrhea due to adult cystic fibrosis. Pediatr Pulmonol 1988; Suppl 2, 134.
14. Smith HL, Berg JD, Booth IW. Small bowel delivery of pancreatic enzyme supplements (PES) as measured by the one-stage bentiromide test in cystic fibrosis patients. Presented at First Pan Pacific Congress of Paediatric Gastroenterology and Nutrition, Queensland, Australia, March 1988.
15. Graham DY. Pancreatic enzyme replacement: the effects of antacids or cimetidine. Dig Dis Sci 1982; 27:485–490.
16. Boyle J, Long WP, Balistreri WF, Widzer SJ, Huang N. Effect of cimetidine in pancreatic enzymes on serum and faecal bile acid and fat absorption in cystic fibrosis. Gastroenterology 1980; 78:950–953.
17. Zentler-Munro PL, Fine DR, Batten JC, Northfield PC. Effect of cimetidine on enzyme inactivation, bile acid precipitation, and lipid solubilization in pancreatic steatorrhoea due to cystic fibrosis. Gut 1985; 26:892–901.
18. Shepherd RW, McGuffie C, Bradbear R. Cimetidine kinetics in CF. Aust Paediatr J 1981; 17:234.
19. Durie PR, Bell L, Linton W, Corey ML, Forstner GG. Effect of cimetidine and sodium bicarbonate on pancreatic replacement therapy in cystic fibrosis. Gut 1980; 21:778–786.
20. Cleghorn GJ, Shepherd RW, Holt TL. The use of a synthetic prostaglandin E_1 analogue (Misoprostal) as an adjunct to pancreatic enzyme replacement in cystic fibrosis. Scand J Gastroenterol 1988; 23(Suppl 143):142–147.
21. Robert A. Prostaglandins in a gastro intestinal tract. In: Johnson LR, ed. Physiology of the gastrointestinal tract. New York: Raven Press, 1981: 1407.
22. Konturek SJ, Tasler J, Kwiecien N, et al. Mechanisms of the inhibitory action of prostaglandins on meal induced gastric secretions. Digestion 1978; 17:281–290.
23. Powell JR, Donn KH. Pharmacokinetic basis for H_2-antagonists drug interactions: concepts and implications. J Clin Gastroenterol 1983; 5(Suppl 1):95–113.
24. Robb TA, Davidson GP, Kirubakaran C. Conjugated bile acids in serum and secretions in response to cholecystokinin/secretin stimulation in children with cystic fibrosis. Gut 1985; 26:1246–1256.
25. Darling PB, Lepage G, Leroy C, Masson P, Roy CC. Effect of taurine supplements on fat absorption in cystic fibrosis. Pediatr Res 1985; 19:578–582.
26. Harries JT, Muller DPR, McCollum JPK, et al. Intestinal bile salts in cystic fibrosis. Arch Dis Child 1979; 54:19–24.
27. Roy CC, Weber AM, Morin CL, et al. Abnormal biliary lipid composition in cystic fibrosis: effect of pancreatic enzymes. N Engl J Med 1977; 297:1301–1305.
28. Thompson GN. Excessive fecal taurine loss predisposes to taurine deficiency in cystic fibrosis. J Pediatr Gastroenterol Nutr 1988; 7:214–219.

PART 6

Pharmacologic Treatment of Gastrointestinal Motility

Michael Spino, B.Sc. Phm., Pharm.D.

The gastrointestinal (GI) tract is richly innervated by several different nervous systems, including the sympathetic, parasympathetic, and enteric nervous systems. It is also influenced by afferent innervation from the gut to the central nervous system (CNS), which integrates input from each of these systems and can modulate motility of the gut itself. It is not surprising, therefore, that many drugs affect GI motility, either directly or indirectly. However, because most agents are nonspecific in action, only a few are suitable for the treatment of GI motility disorders.

In general, the parasympathetic nervous system can be considered to be a stimulant of GI activity, including both motility and secretions. If a nonspecific cholinergic stimulant such as bethanechol is given to increase GI motility, all the

TABLE 1
Partial List of Drugs Affecting Gastrointestinal Motility

Drug	Action
Through the cholinergic nervous system	
Atropine	Blocks effects of acetylcholine at muscarinic receptors
Bethanechol	Direct action on muscarinic receptors
Carbachol	Releases acetylcholine
Dicyclomine	Muscarinic antagonist and a nonspecific smooth muscle relaxant. No CNS activity
Domperidone	Dopamine antagonist, cholinergic agonist, but does not cross blood-brain barrier, therefore little central effect
Hemicholinium	Inhibits acetylcholine synthesis
Metoclopramide	Dopamine antagonist, cholinergic agonist, membrane stabilization, direct smooth muscle contraction
Neostigmine	Acetylcholine esterase inhibitor
Oxyphenonium	Muscarinic and ganglionic blocker
Propantheline	Muscarinic and ganglionic blocker
Through the adrenergic nervous system	
Amphetamine	Enhances norepinephrine release
Cocaine	Enhances norepinephrine release
Epinephrine	Stimulates $alpha_{1\ \&\ 2}$ and $beta_1$ receptors, causing decreased tone and motility and also contracts sphincters. $Alpha_1$ effects may be caused by increased K^+ conductance, causing hyperpolarization, whereas $alpha_2$ effects may be induced on cholinergic PS neurons in the myenteric plexus, which causes decreased acetylcholine release.
Guanethidine	Inhibits norepinephrine release
Methyldopa	Inhibits norepinephrine release
Reserpine	Inhibits norepinephrine release
Tricyclics	Inhibits norepinephrine uptake
Tyramine	Enhances norepinephrine release
Through the modification of intracellular events	
Calcium Antagonists (verapamil, nifedipine)	Antagonize secretions and contractions by inhibiting calcium movement
Miscellaneous	
Narcotics (e.g., morphine)	Decrease propulsive activity and induce stasis in the stomach and small and large intestines and act on epithelial mucosa to decrease net fluid accumulation. They induce increased tone in the stomach and duodenum, which can greatly delay transit of stomach contents. They increase the nonpropulsive type of rhythmic contractions in the small intestine but markedly decrease the propulsive contractions. Similarly, tone is greatly increased in the colon and anal sphincter. Morphine may cause these effects by its action on nerve plexuses within the bowel wall, inhibiting the release of acetylcholine from axon terminals.
Prostaglandins	Inhibit the secretion of gastric acid and decrease the volume of secretions as well as pepsin content. In the small intestine, secretion of pancreatic enzymes and mucus is increased. Because they induce movement of water and electrolytes into the intestinal lumen they cause diarrhea, probably by stimulation of mucosal cyclic AMP.

effects associated with increased parasympathetic stimulation, both in the gut and elsewhere (e.g., bladder, salivary glands, eye), may also be affected. Table 1 lists many of the drugs known to alter GI motility and separates them according to their general mechanism of action.

In practice, only three drugs are extensively used for enhancing GI motility: metoclopramide, domperidone, and cisapride. Cisapride is available only as an investigational drug (phase III) in the United States but is now marketed in Canada and in various European countries. Several studies have already been conducted in pediatric populations. Domperidone, at the time of writing, still has investigational status in the United States but has been on the market in Canada for about 3 years.

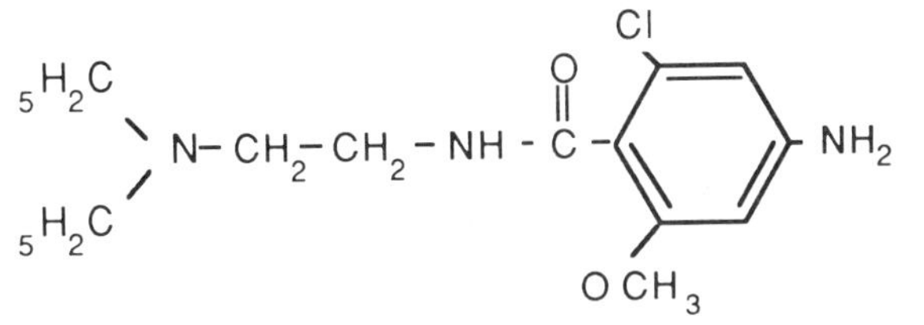

FIGURE 1 Chemical structure of metoclopramide.

METOCLOPRAMIDE

Metoclopramide is a benzamide derivative that differs structurally from procainamide only by the addition of 5-chloro and 2-methoxy aryl substituents (Fig. 1). However, this slight structural modification results in considerable differences in pharmacologic effects. It is photosensitive and degrades when exposed to light. When stored in light-resistant containers, both the tablets and solution are stable for at least 3 years. When mixed with other drugs in an intravenous bag or bottle, it exhibits many incompatibilities.

Metoclopramide is a cholingeric stimulant and a dopamine receptor antagonist with activity in both the GI tract and the brain. In addition, it has some direct smooth muscle stimulant effects. Consequently, the mechanism of action of metoclopramide is complex and may involve several different mechanisms working together for any given effect. The effects do not require an intact vagal nerve, but they are reduced or abolished by anticholingeric drugs such as atropine and potentiated by cholinergic drugs such as carbachol. However, metoclopramide does require neuronal storage sites of acetylcholine.[1-3] A recent study has demonstrated that metoclopramide also exhibits plasma cholinesterase activity at concentrations achieved after a single 10-mg dose.[4]

Metoclopramide accelerates gastric emptying and intestinal transit from the duodenum to the ileocecal valve, and, unlike nonspecific cholinergic-like stimulants, it co-ordinates the gastric, pyloric, and duodenal motor activity. It increases the amplitude and duration of esophageal contractions, the resting tone of the lower esophageal sphincter, and the amplitude and tone of antral contractions while relaxing the pyloric sphincter and the duodenal bulb and increasing peristalsis of the duodenum and jejunum. In most studies, there appears to be little or variable effect on the motility of the colon and gallbladder. These effects are accomplished without stimulation of gastric or pancreatic secretions in normal doses.[1-3]

Metoclopramide readily crosses the blood-brain barrier and is a potent dopamine receptor antagonist in the brain. (Its inhibition of central dopamine receptors is probably responsible for its extrapyramidal effects and worsening of parkinsonism observed in some patients.) Experimentally, it inhibits the emetic effects of apomorphine, Hydergine, and levodopa, probably by blocking dopamine receptors in the chemoreceptor trigger zone (CTZ) of the lateral reticular formation. Enhanced gastric emptying may be an added peripheral component to this antiemetic action.

Stimulation of prolactin secretion from the anterior pituitary is probably a result of inhibiting dopamine receptors in the pituitary and hypothalamus. This action persists during chronic therapy and may induce galactorrhea, amenorrhea, gynecomastia, and impotence. Normally, metoclopramide does not alter the secretion of growth hormone, corticotropin, luteinizing hormone, or follicle-stimulating hormone to a clinically significant degree, although occasionally anecdotal reports of these effects do appear.[1,2,5] However, Massara et al[6] have demonstrated that a 0.17 mg per kilogram *intravenous* bolus dose in children 8 to 17 years old stimulates growth hormone secretion.

Metoclopramide produces a transient increase in plasma aldosterone concentrations as a result of a direct effect on adrenal tissue, which does not appear to be related to its effect on prolactin release. However, it does not alter plasma renin activity or plasma potassium or cortisol concentrations. Unlike prolactin, aldosterone levels appear to return to pretreatment levels on chronic therapy.[1,7]

Metoclopramide is well absorbed after an oral dose (80 to 85 percent) but is extensively metabolized before reaching the systemic circulation (''first-pass effect''). Therefore, intravenous and intramuscular doses achieve higher blood concentrations than oral doses. Variability in the fraction of drug reaching the systemic circulation (bioavailability), ranging from 32 to 97 percent following a 10-mg tablet, was also attributed to the first-pass effect. Increased bioavailability appears to occur in patients with cirrhosis.[8] Peak concentrations are achieved about 1 hour after an oral dose.[9] Although absorption is more variable, rectal administration can be used if the patient is vomiting.[10]

Metoclopramide is minimally bound to plasma proteins, mainly alpha$_1$-acid glycoprotein,[11] and it does not appear to significantly displace bilirubin from albumin-binding sites in infants, at least in concentrations up to 200 ng per milliliter.[11,12] Following an intravenous dose, a two-compartment open model adequately describes the disposition of metoclopramide. This lipid-soluble drug has a large apparent volume of distribution of about 2 to 4 L per kilogram.[13]

Metoclopramide is a high clearance drug with a total body clearance (TBC) in the range of 7 ml per minute per kilogram following a 10-mg dose, mostly due to hepatic metabolism. In human urine, three metabolites of metoclopramide have been identified: the *N*-4 sulfate, accounting for 40 percent or more of an oral dose, the *N*-4 glucuronide, and a side-chain metabolite 4-amino-5-chloro-2-methoxybenzamido-acetic acid, both of which are minor.[9] Earlier reports indicated that there may be some degree of dose-dependent metabolism between a 10- and 20-mg oral dose as evidenced by an increased half-life ($t_{1/2}$) from 3.28 to 5.29 hours.[9] However, within the high-dose group itself, dose-dependent metabolism was not evident.[13] Furthermore, a recent study, using newer, more sensitive assay methods and a longer blood sampling period, has revealed linear kinetics over the 5- to 20-mg dose range in healthy adults.[14] This study draws into question the earlier reports of nonlinearity of metoclopramide metabolism in low doses.

Infants are known to exhibit decreased metabolism of many drugs during the first 1 to 12 months, particularly those drugs dependent on cytochromes P-450. Only one report has appeared on the disposition of metoclopramide (0.15 mg per kilogram orally) in infants ($n = 6$) with gastroesophageal reflux (GER). The mean $t_{1/2}$ (5 hours) and the TBC (uncorrected for absorption, 0.66 L per kilogram per hour) did not appear to differ from those reported for adults.[15]

Approximately 80 percent of an oral dose is excreted in the urine, but only 20 percent of the dose appears as unchanged metoclopramide. The *N*-4 sulfate metabolite accounts for about 40 percent of the dose.[9] With this dispositional profile, one would normally expect that impaired renal function would have a negligible effect on the clearance of metaclopramide from the body. It is surprising, therefore, that both in anephric patients and those with severe renal failure, the terminal $t_{1/2}$ was about 14 hours, double that seen in patients with normal renal function, and the TBC was proportionally decreased. Since this could not be due to decreased elimination of the parent drug, these findings suggest that impaired renal function somehow affects other aspects of metoclopramide elimination, possibly metabolism or enterohepatic recycling.[9] Recently these studies have been confirmed, and it was also demonstrated that hemodialysis is ineffective in removing metoclopramide from the blood.[16]

Metoclopramide is excreted in milk with concentrations rising above those seen in maternal plasma. However, the total amount delivered to the nursing baby is far below therapeutic doses, resulting in estimated "doses" of 24 μg per kilogram per day or less, compared to therapeutic doses of 500 μg per kilogram per day recommended in children.[17] Nevertheless, in a review of dystonic reactions in children, Boulloche et al note that a neonate is reported to have developed a dystonic reaction after breast-feeding from its mother, who was receiving metoclopramide.[18]

Metoclopramide should not be used in patients with pheochromocytoma, GI hemorrhage, GI obstruction (mechanical), or GI perforation. In addition, because it may release catecholamines, it should probably be avoided in hypertensive patients and those receiving monoamine oxidase inhibitors, tricyclic antidepressants, or sympathomimetic amines.[19] Caution should also be exercised in patients undergoing surgery and receiving succinylcholine or ester-type local anesthetics because of the plasma cholinesterase activity exhibited with metoclopramide.[4]

A number of adverse effects are associated with metoclopramide. Transitory, mild hypotension may occur in patients receiving intravenous metoclopramide, but severe hypotension may occur if it is rapidly administered during anesthesia.[20] Drowsiness, fatigue, and lassitude occur in about 10 percent of patients, and insomnia, headache, or dizziness occurs in about 5 percent.[21] Occasionally depression has been reported in patients receiving metoclopramide, but usually improvement is seen with dose reduction.[22] Extrapyramidal effects are caused by metoclopramide, probably as a result of its dopamine-blocking activity in the CNS. Akathisia, or motor restlessness, is the most common extrapyramidal reaction associated with its use. Generally, it occurs shortly after initiation of therapy but is usually reversible upon cessation of metoclopramide. Dystonias, including trismus, torticollis, facial spasms, opisthotonos, and oculogyric crisis, occur most frequently in young patients, although less frequently than akathisia. Occurring shortly after initiation of therapy, they are usually responsive to antihistamines or anticholinergic drugs.[1] Recently some cases of tardive dyskinesia have been reported with long-term use of metoclopramide.[23]

Children receiving high doses of metoclopramide seem to be particularly susceptible to extrapyramidal effects of metoclopramide, leading to the suggestion of a maximum of 0.5 mg per kilogram per day in at least three divided doses.[24] Terrin et al have indicated that dystonic reactions are to be expected in children receiving doses of 0.5 mg per kilogram or more. They also note that intravenous diphenhydramine can reverse these effects within minutes and that, used prophylactically, it can prevent them.[25]

Boulloche et al published their experience of 18 pediatric patients experiencing dystonic reactions on metoclopramide and reviewed 383 cases published from 1968 to 1986. Generally, dystonia occurs shortly after drug administration, and almost always within 72 hours. For girls 11 to 19 years of age, they have suggested that the incidence of dystonic reactions may be 1 per 500 prescriptions, compared to an overall incidence for 1 per 30,000 in the general population.[18]

Metoclopramide increases serum prolactin levels as a result of blockade of dopamine-mediated inhibition of prolactin secretion. Increased serum prolactin concentrations occur in healthy adults, children, pregnant women, and patients with endocrine disorders and occur within 5 minutes of an intravenous dose, lasting 2 to 4 hours. After an oral dose, an effect usually begins within 15 minutes and persists for about 9 hours. Clinically, breast enlargement and increased lactation are observed in women as a result of this effect.[1]

Other endocrine effects of metoclopramide are either transient or inconsistent. Increased aldosterone release from the adrenals is transient, and the effect of metoclopramide on growth hormone is controversial, with some investigators reporting increased and others no response for adolescents and children, respectively, with short stature. It has been suggested that this effect may depend in part on sex hormone status in the individual. Decreased adrenocorticotropic hormone (ACTH)-stimulated growth hormone secretion by metoclopramide has also been reported.[1]

Individual case reports have been published for a variety of adverse events apparently caused by metoclopramide, and some would even seem to have a pharmacologic basis. However, in many cases, insufficient data are available at this time to determine the extent of the problem or validate their occurrence. These include altered taste or smell, urinary incontinence, impotence, agranulocytosis, arrhythmias, hypertensive crisis, depression, mania, asthma, skin rash, and muscle spasms. It appears that metoclopramide does not cause teratogenesis, based on studies published to date.[7]

Children are particularly susceptible to the toxic effects of metoclopramide, which may manifest as agitation, irritability, neck pain and rigidity, and extrapyramidal symptoms. Hypertonia may be misdiagnosed for tetanus, meningitis, or encephalitis.[7] As noted above, a maximum dose of 0.5 mg per kilogram has been recommended for children because of these effects. One study examined the relationship of dose to extrapyramidal effects of 45 pediatric oncology patients (7 to 22 years) who were receiving diphenhydramine prophylactically. They were unable to detect a correlation between increasing dose (0.2 to 3.0 mg per kilogram) and the occurrence of extrapyramidal side effects in these children receiving metoclopramide to prevent chemotherapy-induced vomiting.[26] A recent paper reported that metoclopramide caused methemoglobinemia in a 3-week-old infant due to an accidental 10-fold overdose (1 mg per kilogram every 6 hours).[27]

A number of drug interactions have been reported with metoclopramide, and many of them are related to drug absorption. Since metoclopramide increases gastric emptying, and alters GI motility, one would predict that the rate and possibly the extent of absorption of several drugs would be affected. Indeed, for analgesics, metoclopramide increases the rate of absorption of acetaminophen, acetylsalicylic acid, and tolfenamic acid, but the extent of absorption is not generally affected.[1,28] On the other hand, the mean absorption of a 400-mg dose of cimetidine was reduced by 22 percent in eight healthy control subjects following an oral metoclopramide solution. However, two 7-mg doses were given, one 10 minutes before and one 30 minutes after cimetidine.[29] Since this is not the usual method of metoclopramide administration, the relevance to actual practice is unclear. This is in contrast to cyclosporine; metoclopramide in renal transplant patients increased the mean oral cyclosporine absorption by 29 percent.[30] For the benzodiazepines, the picture is mixed, since metoclopramide induced higher peak serum concentrations and a shorter time to peak for diazepam[31] but had no effect on lorazepam.[1] Interactions with digoxin are unclear. Metoclopramide, 10 mg, three times daily, decreased the mean peak digoxin concentration from 1.5 to 1.1 ng per milliliter in six healthy volunteers (brand of digoxin not stated).[32] Others have reported similar findings with "slowly absorbed" digoxin preparations, but Johnson et al have reported that this difference does not occur with the more rapidly absorbed micronized tablets (Lanoxin) or capsules (Lanoxicaps).[33] Nevertheless, it would be prudent to monitor patients on digoxin if metoclopramide is added to the regimen.

Studies of metoclopramide administered to patients receiving sustained-release preparations of different drugs have been reported, including *quinidine* (Quinidex), *theophylline* (Theo-Dur), and *propranolol*. A mean decrease in absorption of only 10 percent for quinidine[34] and 2 percent for theophylline[35] and a 15 percent increase for propranolol (not significant)[36] were observed when metoclopramide was administered. These studies reveal little, if any, effect of metoclopramide on the absorption of these sustained-release preparations. However, extrapolation to other sustained-release drugs, or even different brands of the same drugs, may be inappropriate.

Metoclopramide, primarily a GI motility drug, is widely used for many indications, not all of which have been approved by governmental regulatory agencies. However, we will limit discussion primarily to its use in disorders of GI motility and related conditions. The use of metoclopramide in migraine, vertigo, neurogenic bladder, peptic ulcer disease, inadequate lactation, parkinsonism-induced orthostatic hypotension, tardive dyskinesia, and arthritis will not be discussed.[1]

Gastroparesis is often a complication of diabetes mellitus or vagotomy and gastric resection, but it may also occur with gastric ulcer or anorexia nervosa, or following infection. Theoretically metoclopramide, by increasing the gastric emptying rate, should relieve symptoms such as early satiety, nausea, vomiting, bloating, weight loss, and anorexia. However, gastroparesis from all causes is not equally sensitive to the effects of metoclopramide.[1]

The use of metoclopramide in *diabetic gastroparesis* has been studied by many investigators with variable results. In some studies, symptoms improved in many patients even if no significant improvement in gastric emptying occurred.[1] One study has provided evidence that chronic administration (1 month) of metoclopramide in diabetic patients may result in a loss of gastrokinetic properties of the drug, although symptomatic relief apparently still occurred.[37] It has been suggested that both a central and peripheral effect combine to relieve symptoms of gastroparesis in diabetic patients.[38] Surgical patients with gastroparesis seem to respond to metoclopramide better than diabetic patients.[39] Metoclopramide may also be a useful adjunct in treating the symptoms of anorexia nervosa.[1]

The actions of metoclopramide to increase lower esophageal sphincter pressure and increase gastric emptying would be expected to relieve symptoms of GER. However, studies have produced inconsistent results. In some cases symptoms were relieved, without significant effect on lower esophageal sphincter pressure. Much of this variability may be related to a dose-response effect of metoclopramide on lower esophageal sphincter pressure.[1]

A combination of metoclopramide and cimetidine, in severe reflux esophagitis, induced improvement in 9 of 12 patients, compared to 3 of 12 patients receiving cimetidine plus a placebo. However, side effects were common with the combination, primarily fatigue, restlessness, drowsiness, confusion, disorientation, and anxiety,[40] suggesting that this combination may not have a net therapeutic advantage.

In general, a favorable response for GER in infants and children is seen. The major adverse effects seem to be drowsiness and irritability.[41–45] However, some studies found it no more effective than placebo in decreasing the frequency or duration of GER.[46]

Metoclopramide has had variable success in the treatment of vomiting, depending, in part, upon the cause and dose employed. In preventing postoperative vomiting, effectiveness may be related to the anesthetic used and the timing of metoclopramide administration, as well as the doses employed. It appears that administration of metoclopramide immediately prior to induction of anesthesia is more likely to be successful.[1]

Some success has also been demonstrated with metoclopramide in nausea and vomiting from a wide range of causes in adults, such as recurrent gastritis, gastroenteritis, gastric carcinoma, hepatic and biliary disorders, chronic renal failure, and cardiac disease.[7] Drug-induced nausea and vomiting are usually treated by termination of the offending agent, but in some cases, the condition might preclude such an action. Thus, it is noteworthy that some studies have demonstrated success of metoclopramide in nausea and vomiting associated with digoxin, tuberculosis therapy, and some antibiotics. Success has also been demonstrated in radiation-induced nausea and vomiting in a double-blind crossover study in which metoclopramide was as effective as prochlorperazine. However, it is not effective as an antiemetic following iodipamide in intravenous cholangiography.[7]

Although early, uncontrolled reports indicated that metoclopramide was effective in preventing vomiting associated with cancer chemotherapy, controlled clinical trials revealed an inadequate protective response. One study found that metoclopramide 20 mg was superior to prochlorperazine 10 mg, but neither treatment was adequate, as the incidence of vomiting exceeded 70 percent in both groups.[47] High-dose metoclopramide, however, has proven very successful in chemotherapy-induced vomiting in adults, even when cisplatin is the agent, but some patients may require more than 2 mg per kilogram intravenously for complete control.[48] Current monographs for the use of metoclopramide in treating chemotherapy-induced vomiting provide details on dilution and suitable intravenous solutions for administration.[21,49] Meyer et al noted that, using the approved protocol, complete protection was achieved in 78 percent of adult patients when concentrations were greater than 850 ng per milliliter immediately prior to the third dose. Concentrations of less than 850 ng per milliliter did not produce complete control of vomiting in any patient.[50] Thus patients not attaining complete protection from vomiting may benefit by increasing the dose up to 3 mg per kilogram.

High-dose metoclopramide has been studied in children, but as noted earlier, large doses may be a problem of increased toxicity, particularly dystonic reactions. In pediatric oncology patients receiving 2 mg per kilogram per dose intravenously prior to and at 1.5, 3.5, 5.5, and 8.5 hours after chemotherapy, 7 of 11 patients reported subjective benefit in terms of severity, duration, and amount of vomiting experienced and degree of discomfort. However, five patients developed dystonic reactions that limited their willingness to continue on metoclopramide, even though diphenhydramine successfully reversed the reactions.[51] In another study, metoclopramide, 0.5 mg per kilogram intravenously 30 minutes before and every 3 hours for five doses, was less effective in preventing chemotherapy-induced vomiting in children than chlorpromazine, and it also resulted in more extrapyramidal effects.[52]

Metoclopramide intravenously facilitates the passage of barium through the GI tract and reduces the time required for examination as well as the time patients are exposed to radiation. However, there is some controversy about whether or not it actually improves the quality of visualization in patients undergoing double-contrast examination of the small bowel.[1,53] A placebo-controlled study of metoclopramide syrup in 18 pediatric patients (19 days to 12 years) revealed a significant decrease in procedure time and fluoroscopy time. Patients fasted for 4 hours or more and were also sedated with promethazine and chlorpromazine. No adverse reactions were reported.[54] In patients undergoing intubation and intestinal biopsy, pretreatment with metoclopramide intravenously facilitates the procedure and decreases time required. In addition, patients with a history of pylorospasm during previous endoscopy may experience pyloric relaxation.[1]

In postoperative adynamic ileus, metoclopramide was reported to have a negative effect in that the condition took significantly longer to resolve than in patients given placebo.[55] The usefulness of metoclopramide in various functional GI disorders such as irritable bowel syndrome, functional vomiting and diarrhea, or spastic constipation is unknown owing to lack of convincing data from well-controlled studies.[1] Some investigators have explored the use of metoclopramide in nursing mothers when other means of stimulating milk production are ineffective.[56,57] Metoclopramide by continuous subcutaneous infusion may also be useful in narcotic bowel syndrome.[58]

DOMPERIDONE

Currently, domperidone is still an investigational drug in the United States, although it has been available in Canada and several other countries for a few years. It does not appear to be more efficacious than metoclopramide for any GI indication, and perhaps not as good for some. However, it exhibits far fewer and generally less serious side effects, which is consistent with its apparent mechanism of action and dispositional characteristics. The intravenous dosage form was withdrawn from the market after reports of sudden death, cardiac arrest, and clinically significant arrhythmias in patients receiving large bolus doses.[59,60] These effects have not occurred after oral administration.

Domperidone is structurally related to the butyrophenone compounds such as haloperidol (Fig. 2). However, it is not used as a neuroleptic because it does not cross the blood-brain barrier well. Domperidone is mainly a peripheral dopamine receptor antagonist and exhibits many of the pharmacologic effects of metoclopramide on the GI tract. In vitro, it has high affinity for dopamine receptors but low affinity for serotonergic and muscarinic sites. Because of its relative inability to cross the blood-brain barrier, it exhibits many fewer CNS adverse effects and extrapyramidal symptoms.[61]

The effect of domperidone on lower esophageal sphincter pressure is inconsistent among studies, with some demonstrating an increased pressure[62] and others not.[63] A study in patients with endoscopically confirmed esophagitis demonstrated no difference between domperidone and placebo on lower esophageal sphincter pressure and a 15-hour pH probe study found no difference in reflux episodes or in the time the esophageal pH was less than 5.[64] It is noteworthy that Di Lorenzo et al found no difference in gastric emptying in children under 3 years, regardless of the presence or absence of GER. By contrast, in children over 6 years, gastric emp-

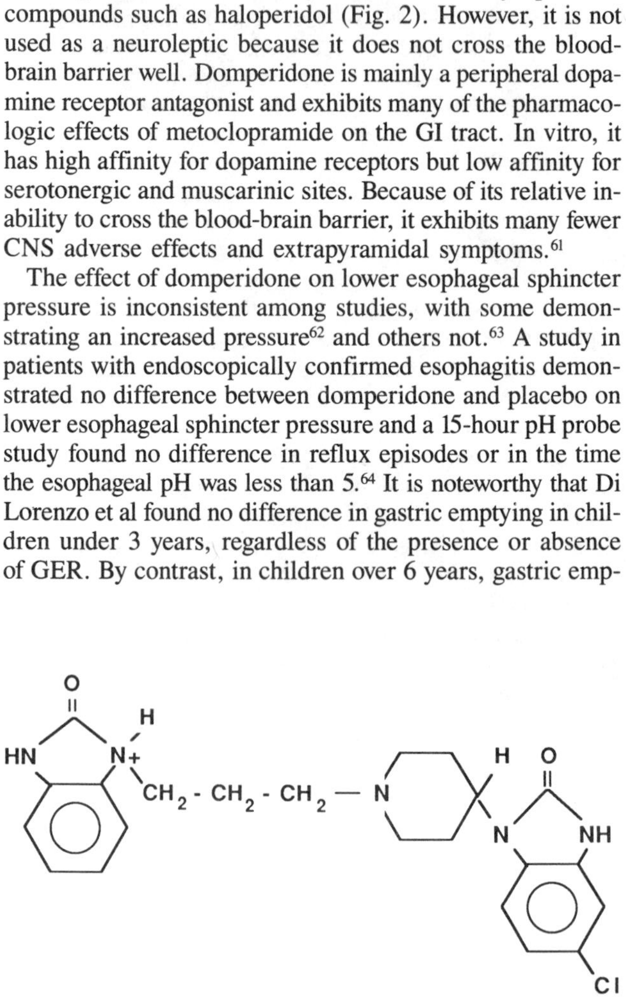

FIGURE 2 Chemical structure of domperidone.

tying was significantly delayed in the presence of reflux.[65] Although the previous studies[62,63] were in adults, Di Lorenzo's study indicates that there probably is not a simple relationship between reflux and gastric emptying, and this may explain some of the variable results with domperidone or other agents.

Increased rate of gastric emptying, comparable to that with metoclopramide, is seen with intravenous domperidone.[66,67] Orally, however, the effect is dose-dependent, with 50-mg and 20-mg doses increasing antral peristalsis, but not a 10-mg dose.[68] Like metoclopramide, domperidone does not affect gastric acid secretion, secretory volume, pH, or serum gastrin levels.[62] It interferes with the inhibitory effects of secretion on the stomach, and it stimulates phasic activity in the gastroduodenal area as well as improves gastroduodenal coordination. Domperidone increases serum prolactin, but not aldosterone.[66]

In animals, domperidone inhibits vomiting of agents that stimulate the CTZ, such as apomorphine, Hydergine, morphine, and levodopa, but not centrally mediated vomiting, such as with copper sulfate.[69] This is consistent with domperidone's strong antidopaminergic effects and CTZ's location outside the blood-brain barrier.

Peak serum concentrations are achieved about 1 hour after an oral dose and tend to be around 20 ng per milliliter after a single 10-mg dose. However, only about 15 percent of an oral dose reaches the systemic circulation, probably as a result of a large first-pass effect. Co-administration with a meal increases absorption to about 23 percent, supporting the concept of low bioavailability due to a large first-pass effect.[70] Unlike metoclopramide, domperidone is highly bound to plasma proteins, in the range of 91 to 93 percent. The apparent volume of distribution is about 5 to 6 L per kilogram, which is of the same order of magnitude as metoclopramide.[70]

The main metabolic pathways are hydroxylation and oxidative *N*-dealkylation, resulting in inactive metabolites. The metabolites are excreted in both the urine and feces.[71] Domperidone is a high-clearance drug, reported to be 700 ml per minute[70] with no evidence of dose-dependent kinetics.[72] The $t_{1/2}$ averages between 7 and 12 hours.[70,72]

Less than 5 percent of domperidone is excreted in the urine unchanged, although about 30 percent of the dose can be collected as glucuronide conjugates of the two main metabolites. Most of the metabolites are excreted in the feces.[70,71] Brogden reported that data on file with the manufacturer (Janssen Pharmaceutica Inc, Piscataway, NJ) indicates that there is a significant prolongation of $t_{1/2}$ to 21 hours in patients with severe renal impairment.[66] Based on the extremely low fraction of drug excreted in the urine unchanged, this is unexpected, although a similar phenomenon was observed for metoclopramide.[9]

Relatively few precautions are required with domperidone. However, like metoclopramide, it should not be used in patients with GI hemorrhage, obstruction (mechanical), or perforation. One concern is that patients should not also receive anticholinergics, since these may antagonize the effects of domperidone, even though little if any of its activity is due to direct cholinergic stimulation of the GI tract.

The overall apparent incidence of adverse effects associated with domperidone use, based upon drug company records in clinical trials, is 7 percent.[73] Most can be attributed to its dopamine receptor antagonism activity, and they disappear upon stopping the drug. Most endocrinologic abnormalities occur as a result of blockade of the inhibition of prolactin release, with the overall incidence of adverse endocrine effects being 1.3 percent.[73] The resultant higher levels of serum prolactin may cause gynecomastia, galactorrhea, and possibly menstrual irregularities.[74,75] Unlike metoclopramide, it does not stimulate growth hormone release.[6] There appears to be no effect on thyroid-stimulating hormone.[76]

In a 4-month-old infant, domperidone induced extrapyramidal effects within 2 hours after the second dose. Upon hospital admission, he continued to experience dystonic movements of both arms. Domperidone was discontinued and no further episodes were observed.[77] A 3-year-old boy also experienced dystonic reactions with domperidone.[78] However, extrapyramidal symptoms occur much less frequently than with metoclopramide.[7,66]

There is little information on drug interactions with domperidone. Because of its effect on GI motility, domperidone has the potential to alter drug absorption. However, the lack of reports suggests that this may not be a problem in practice. Van der Merwe et al demonstrated that although domperidone had no effect on the absorption of acetaminophen, it significantly reduced the saliva-to-plasma ratio of the drug in a dose-dependent manner for unexplained reasons.[79] Whether this is a unique finding for acetaminophen and/or transport into saliva or whether it has a more general application remains to be seen.

Most, but not all, of the indications for domperidone are for disorders of GI motility and related conditions. Domperidone's success in treating reflux esophagitis is equivocal. In an 8-week controlled study, domperidone was compared to a placebo in 23 patients with endoscopically documented esophagitis. While domperidone was significantly better than placebo in relieving regurgitation, it did not improve heartburn or endoscopic healing.[64] A double-blind study found domperidone comparable to ranitidine in 45 patients with reflux esophagitis, but the combination of the two drugs was not significantly superior to either drug alone.[80] A study of GER in infants provided some evidence of improved symptoms related to increased upper GI tract motility.[81] In a multicenter trial, domperidone 0.3 mg per kilogram three times daily for 2 weeks, followed by 0.6 mg per kilogram three times daily for 2 weeks, was superior to placebo in relieving retching, regurgitation, and vomiting.[82]

Dyspepsia is a symptom complex that may be associated with a variety of diseases or may occur in the absence of any known pathology. Domperidone provides symptomatic relief in adult patients, and the large majority of double-blind studies in over 800 such patients suggest that this may be the most responsive indication for the use of domperidone.[61]

In a double-blind, crossover, placebo-controlled study in 12 diabetic gastroparesis patients, domperidone significantly improved gastric emptying rates. When subjects were placed on chronic therapy, their symptoms improved significantly and the gastric emptying rates for the liquid meal remained significantly faster than for placebo, but the solid-phase emptying rates did not.[83] It has also exhibited satisfactory response in postvagotomy gastroparesis patients.[84]

Two studies in patients with irritable bowel syndrome revealed no benefit from domperidone.[61] This is consistent with pharmacologic studies that show little or no activity of domperidone in the colon.

Some studies have found domperidone successful in controlling vomiting in pediatric patients.[66] In one study, increasing the dose of domperidone from 0.5 to 0.7 mg per kilogram in children with cancer chemotherapy increased efficacy from 70 to 89 percent.[85] However, another study in children under 18 years old found domperidone less effective than nabilone in preventing cancer chemotherapy–induced vomiting, although it also produced fewer side effects.[86]

CISAPRIDE

Although cisapride is structurally and mechanistically distinct from metoclopramide and domperidone, it exhibits many of the same therapeutic advantages while expressing distinct activity of its own. It exhibits more specificity for the GI tract. It appears to have fewer and less severe adverse effects. Its place in therapeutics is still being defined, but if studies continue to confirm its efficacy and lack of toxicity, this drug may become the major one of its class.

Structurally, cisapride is a distant relative to metoclopramide: Both are benzamide derivatives, but cisapride is a considerably larger molecule with three cyclic rings (Fig. 3). It is a novel prokinetic drug because it is virtually devoid of antidopaminergic and direct cholinergic effects. It appears to work primarily by causing a release of acetylcholine at the myenteric plexus through an indirect mechanism, without exerting similar effects on secretory glands. Cisapride increases lower esophageal sphincter pressure in both normal subjects and those with abnormally low pressure. It stimulates GI motility from the stomach to the colon, enhances gastric emptying of liquid, solid, and semisolid meals, but does not stimulate gastric secretion. It improves the coordination between antral and duodenal contractions and accelerates gastric emptying. Its actions are not limited to the upper GI tract but include the jejunum, where it increases phase II–type activity and is characterized by a higher number and amplitude of contractions. Unlike domperidone, it exhibits enhanced propulsive contractility in the large intestine. It also appears to enhance the rate of gallbladder refilling.[87–92]

The pharmacokinetics of cisapride have been studied in control volunteers and some patient groups, but no studies in children have been published to date. Approximately 40 to 50 percent of an oral dose of cisapride reaches the systemic circulation, probably as a result of a high first-pass effect. Oral doses of 5 to 20 mg in volunteer subjects demonstrate linear kinetics with maximal plasma concentrations

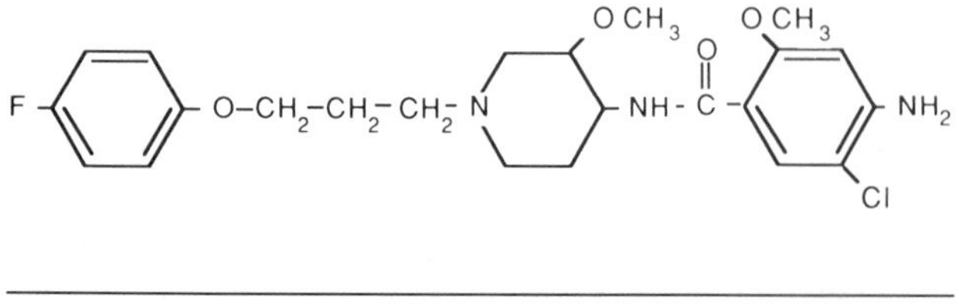

FIGURE 3 Chemical structure of cisapride.

(C_{max}) of about 50 ng per milliliter 1 to 2 hours following a 10-mg tablet when taken 15 minutes before a meal. Food enhances absorption, resulting in about a 20 percent increase in the C_{max} following a 10-mg dose. However, reducing stomach acidity with sodium bicarbonate or cimetidine results in markedly decreased absorption with peak concentrations less than half of those observed in the normal fasting state. In normal volunteers on 10 mg three times daily for several days, there may be some accumulation as evidenced by an increase in the C_{max} of approximately 50 percent.[93,94]

Cisapride is highly bound to plasma proteins (96 to 98 percent). Like metoclopramide and domperidone, it has a large apparent volume of distribution (2.4 L per kilogram). Cisapride concentrates (in rats) in the liver, walls of the stomach and small intestine, lungs, kidneys, cartilage, glandular and lymphatic tissues (in decreasing order), with the liver exhibiting 35 times plasma concentrations and the lymphatics two to six times. Brain concentrations were shown to be two to three times less than plasma concentrations.[93–96]

In humans cisapride is extensively metabolized in the liver, resulting in several identifiable metabolites, the major one being norcisapride (by oxidative *N*-dealkylation). The metabolites, which exhibit negligible activity, are excreted in both urine and feces. In normal volunteers, an intravenous dose exhibits triexponential kinetics, with the $t_{1/2}$ of the terminal phase being 12 to 15 hours. Following an oral dose, the third phase may be more difficult to detect and the drug may appear to have a $t_{1/2}$ of about 7 to 10 hours. The longer $t_{1/2}$ is probably more correct, as it is consistent with a rising C_{max} of about 50 percent over several days.[93] The clearance of cisapride may be decreased in patients with hepatic dysfunction.[93–96] Patients with cystic fibrosis have plasma cisapride concentrations and clearance similar to healthy control subjects.[97]

Normally, less than 1 percent of an oral dose of cisapride is excreted unchanged in the urine, but norcisapride accounts for about 40 percent of the recovered dose. Following an oral dose, 44 percent was excreted as cisapride, norcisapride, and other metabolites in the 0 to 24–hour urine and 37 percent in the 0 to 35–hour feces.[96] Impaired renal function does not appear to have much effect on cisapride disposition, consistent with the small fraction excreted into the urine unchanged.[94] Excretion into breast milk is minimal. Steady-state concentrations in the milk of 20 puerperal women on 20 mg every 8 hours was 6.2 ng per milliliter about 5 percent of the plasma concentrations. Based on these data, nursing infants are unlikely to receive a pharmacologic dose.[98]

The very low affinity of cisapride for dopamine receptors in animal studies[99] would suggest that extrapyramidal effects with cisapride are unlikely. However, this remains to be proved with wider use of the compound. Indeed, 15 cases of abnormal movements have been reported to date in clinical trials, but their relationship to cisapride administration is unknown at this time (Janssen: personal communication January, 1989). Compared with metoclopramide, the incidence of CNS effects such as somnolence was negligible (1.6 versus 15.2 percent, $P < 0.02$).

Based upon data on file with Janssen for over 500 adult subjects treated for 0.5 to 5.6 years, the incidence of adverse reactions was no greater than seen with short-term therapy.[94] Unlike metoclopramide and domperidone, cisapride does not appear to increase prolactin secretion, and thus endocrine problems such as gynecomastia, increased lactation, and menstrual irregularities have not been attributed to the drug.[100,101] Studies have also demonstrated no change in serum glucose, insulin, or gastrin. Interestingly, increased plasma concentrations of pancreatic polypeptide and cholecystokinin were detected after an intravenous dose, and this increase was abolished by 1 mg atropine. However, this effect was not seen with chronic oral administration.[102]

A randomized placebo-controlled, double-blind study in 12 healthy volunteers demonstrated that cisapride did not impair psychomotor function using both objective and subjective criteria, and this is consistent with the low concentrations of the drug found in the brain.[103]

A few cases of hypotension have occurred following intravenous bolus doses of cisapride, causing the company to suspend plans for the marketing of the intravenous form (Janssen: personal communication, January, 1989). As cisapride is released onto the market, it will be given to a much larger population, including patients with more complex and varied diseases. Additional adverse effects may be revealed at that time, including more rarely occurring, idiosyncratic reactions that are too infrequent to detect with certainty in premarketing studies of a few thousand patients. However, to date the drug appears to exhibit fewer adverse effects than either metoclopramide or domperidone, and these are essentially limited to the GI tract.

Based upon its apparent mechanism of action and the relative effects outside the GI tract, it is difficult to specify any precautions in the use of cisapride at this time except for allergies to the drug. However, like metoclopramide, it probably should not be used in patients with GI hemorrhage, obstruction (mechanical), or perforation. Cisapride's few adverse effects can be attributed mainly to its pharmacologic effect on the GI tract, including transient abdominal cramping, borborygmi, and diarrhea. A recent review of 1,576 patients treated for up to 4 weeks revealed an overall incidence of adverse effects of 13.7 percent, compared to 11.2 percent for placebo. However, about 2.5 percent of patients on cisapride discontinued therapy because of diarrhea, compared to 1.3 percent on placebo.[100]

Cisapride, like other drugs that enhance GI motility, may alter absorption of many drugs. Kirch et al compared the effects of metoclopramide and cisapride on digoxin absorption (brand not stated) in six healthy volunteers after 2 weeks of digoxin, 0.25 mg twice daily. C_{max} was reduced by cisapride from 1.5 to 1.3 ng per milliliter (not significant) and to 1.1 ng per milliliter by metoclopramide ($P < 0.05$). Similarly, the 12-hour area under the curve (AUC) was reduced 12 percent by cisapride (not significant), but 19 percent by metoclopramide ($P = 0.06$).[32] These data suggest that while the risk of decreased absorption may be greater for metoclopramide, caution should be exercised with cisapride as well. Whether such a reaction is likely to occur using the Lanoxin preparation is unknown. Nor is it known whether this effect is likely to occur in pediatric patients receiving liquid formulations of digoxin. It appears that cisapride may increase the rate or extent of absorption of diazepam,[31] acenocoumarol, cimetidine, and ranitidine, although the details for the latter three drugs are not available.[94] Serum concentrations of cisapride increased when co-administered with cimetidine, a drug known to inhibit hepatic oxidative metabolism. Ethanol seems to increase the absorption of cisapride.[94]

All of the clinical studies on cisapride published to date are for GI indications. Cisapride's actions of enhanced gastric emptying and increased lower esophageal sphincter pressure suggest that it should be useful in treating GER. Several well-controlled, double-blind randomized trials of cisapride in adults with GER and endoscopically proven mucosal damage demonstrate that cisapride is significantly better than a placebo in terms of objective and subjective criteria.[94,104,105] Compared with other drugs, cisapride was as effective as cimetidine,[106] ranitidine,[107] and metoclopramide.[108] Galmiche has recently reported that the combination of cisapride and cimetidine provided a higher rate of endoscopic healing (70 percent) in severe reflux esophagitis than cimetidine alone (46 percent).[109]

In pediatric patients, open and comparative studies with both placebo and other drugs have demonstrated comparable or superior effectiveness with cisapride.[94] In an acute study, cisapride was comparable to metoclopramide in reducing the number of reflux episodes and the percent of time esophageal pH was less than 4 in 18 infants. It was significantly better than metoclopramide in reducing the number of refluxes longer than 5 minutes as well as esophageal clearance time.[110] A randomized, double-blind, placebo-controlled study of cisapride syrup in 20 children (75 days to 47 months) demonstrated significant improvement of symptoms and histologic damage, but in these patients with "moderate" disease, there was no increase in lower esophageal sphincter pressure detected with cisapride.[111] These and other studies[94] suggest that cisapride may be a useful drug in treating GER in pediatric patients who do not respond to the usual nondrug treatments.

A number of controlled studies have demonstrated the efficacy of cisapride in nonulcer dyspepsia. Evaluation of efficacy is based primarily on subjective criteria such as relief of belching, bloating, abdominal distention, postprandial nausea, vomiting, and heartburn, and cisapride has proved to be more effective than a placebo for such symptomatic relief[94] and comparable to metoclopramide[112] and domperidone.[113]

Several studies in diabetic and nondiabetic patients with gastroparesis have demonstrated symptomatic efficacy of cisapride with faster transit of both solid and liquid meals. The effect appears to occur both after a single dose and during chronic (2 weeks) therapy.[114-116] Placebo-controlled studies of 4 weeks' duration have also demonstrated the effectiveness of cisapride in diabetic gastroparesis.[94,117] Both symptomatic improvement and gastric emptying of solids and liquids were significantly faster than with placebo.[117] At present, there does not appear to be a more effective treatment for diabetic gastroparesis than cisapride, but additional well-controlled studies are needed to confirm this impression.[94]

In three studies of postoperative GI atony, intramuscular cisapride improved GI recovery as judged by time to first flatus and defecation.[94] Cisapride 10 mg, but not 4 mg, was successful in preventing morphine-induced delayed gastric emptying when used as premedication for surgery in 40 adult patients.[118] Manometry and the effectiveness of cisapride were studied in pediatric patients with intestinal obstruction in the absence of a mechanical lesion. Cisapride given intravenously immediately before beginning the meal or orally, 30 minutes before the meal, stimulated proximal duodenal contractions in 9 of 10 patients (8 months to 10 years) with intestinal pseudo-obstruction.[119] Cohen found that cisapride worked for idiopathic intestinal pseudo-obstruction after failure of metoclopramide in an 11-year-old boy.[120] This supports the work of Camilleri et al, which provided objective evidence that, in adults, cisapride improved intestinal motility and transit.[121]

The possibility that cisapride may help cystic fibrosis patients with distal intestinal obstruction syndrome (DIOS) was raised when Hyman successfully treated a 19-month-old boy with cisapride for symptoms associated with absent postprandial duodenal motility.[122] In a double-blind crossover study in 17 patients (12.9 to 34.9 years) with DIOS, Koletzko et al found that cisapride daily for 6 months decreased some of the symptoms, but it did not prevent acute episodes of DIOS at the dose used. On cisapride, 12 patients felt better and three felt worse.[123]

In four studies of patients with chronic constipation from nonorganic conditions, cisapride for 8 to 12 weeks increased stool frequency and quality.[94] One study compared the effectiveness of cisapride with placebo in two groups of chronic constipation patients, one of whom used laxatives. Both groups had significantly greater improvement on cisapride, and this effect was maintained in a 4-week washout period in the laxative users. Intractable constipation in paraplegic patients may also benefit from use of cisapride.[124]

REFERENCES

1. Harrington RA, Hamilton CW, Brogden RN, Linkewich JA, Romankiewicz JA, Heel RC. Metoclopramide: an update review of its pharmacological properties and clinical use. Drugs 1983; 25:451–494.
2. McCallum RW. Review of current status of prokinetic agents in gastroenterology. Am J Gastroenterol 1985; 80:1008–1016.
3. Schulze-Delrieu K. Metoclopramide. Gastroenterology 1979; 77: 768–779.
4. Kambam JR, Parris WCV, Franks JJ, Sastry BVR, Naukam R, Smith BE. The inhibitory effect of metoclopramide on plasma cholinesterase activity. Can J Anaesth 1988; 35:476–478.
5. Cannon JB. Chemistry of dopaminergic agonists. Adv Neurol 1975; 9:177–183.
6. Massara F, Tangolo D, Godano A. Effect of metoclopramide, domperidone and apomorphine on GH secretion in children and adolescents. Acta Endocrinol 1985; 108:451–455.
7. Pinder RM, Brogden RN, Sawyer PR, Speight TM, Avery GS. Metoclopramide: a review of its pharmacological properties and clinical use. Drugs 1976; 12:81–131.
8. Hellstern A, Hellenbrecht D, Saller R, Gatzen M, Manus B, Achert G, Brockmann P, Hausleiter HJ, Leuschner U. Absolute bioavailability of metoclopramide given orally or by enema in patients with normal liver function or with cirrhosis of the liver. Arzneimittelforschung 1987; 37:733–736.
9. Bateman DN. Clinical pharmacokinetics of metoclopramide. Clin Pharmacokinet 1983; 8:523–529.
10. Burgess CD, Chen CT, Siebers RWL, Maling TJB. The bioavailability of rectally administered metoclopramide. Curr Ther Res 1987; 42:1185–1188.
11. Webb D, Buss DC, Fitfield R, Bateman DN, Routledge PA. The plasma protein binding of metoclopramide in health and renal disease. Br J Clin Pharmacol 1986; 21:334–336.
12. Goorley RG, Mogilevsky W, Odell GB. Protein binding of metoclopramide. J Pediatr 1982; 101:631–632.
13. McGovern EM, Grevel J, Bryson SM. Pharmacokinetics of high-dose metoclopramide in cancer patients. Clin Pharmacokinet 1986; 11: 415–424.
14. Wright MR, Axelson JE, Rurak DW, McErlane B, McMorland GH, Ongley RC, Tam YK, Price JDE. Linearity of metoclopramide kinetics at doses of 5-20 mg. Br J Clin Pharmacol 1988; 26:469–473.
15. Kearns GL, Butler HL, Carchman SH, Lane JK, Wright GJ. Metoclopramide pharmacokinetics in infants. Clin Pharmacol Ther 1987; 41:219.
16. Wright MR, Axelson JE, Rurak DW, McErlane B, McMorland GH, Ongley RC, Tam YK, Price JDE. Effect of haemodialysis on metoclopramide kinetics in patients with severe renal failure. Br J Clin Pharmac 1988; 26;474–477.
17. Kauppila A, Arvela P, Koivisto M, Kivinen M, Ylikorkala O, Pelkonen O. Metoclopramide and breast feeding: transfer into milk and the newborn. Eur J Clin Pharmacol 1983; 25:819–823.
18. Boulloche J, Mallet E, Mouterde O, Tron P. Dystonic reactions with metoclopramide: is there a risk population? Helv Paediatr Acta 1988; 42:425–432.
19. Kuchel O, Buu NT, Hamlet P, Larochelle P. Effect of metoclopramide on plasma catecholamine release in essential hypertension. Clin Pharmacol Ther 1985; 37:372–375.
20. Park GR. Hypotension following the intravenous injection of metoclopramide. Anaesthesia 1981; 36:75–76.
21. Maxeran monograph. In: Krogh CME, ed. Compendium of pharmaceuticals and specialties. 23rd ed. Ottawa: Canadian Pharmaceutical Association, 1988: 522.
22. Bottner RK, Tullio CJ. Metoclopramide and depression. Ann Intern Med 1985; 103:482.
23. Patel M, Louis S. Long-term neurologic complications of metoclopramide. NY State J Med 1986; 86:210.
24. Ayers JL, Dawson KP. Acute dystonic reactions in childhood to drugs. NZ Med J 1980; 92:464–465.
25. Terrin BN, McWilliams NB, Maurer HM. Side effects of metoclopramide as an antiemetic in childhood cancer chemotherapy. J Pediatr 1984; 104:138–140.
26. Allen JC, Gralla R, Reilly L, Kellick M, Young C. Metoclopramide: dose-related toxicity and preliminary antiemetic studies in children receiving cancer chemotherapy. J Clin Oncol 1985; 3:1136–1141.
27. Kearns GL, Fiser DH. Metoclopramide-induced methemoglobinemia. Pediatrics 1988; 82:364–366.
28. Tokola RA, Neuvonen PJ. Effects of migraine attack and metoclopramide on the absorption of tolfenamic acid. Br J Clin Pharmacol 1984; 17:67–75.
29. Gugler R, Brand M, Somogyi A. Impaired cimetidine absorption due to antacids and metoclopramide. Eur J Clin Pharmacol 1981; 20:225–228.
30. Wadhwa NK, Scroeder TJ, O'Flaherty E, Pesce AJ, Myre SA, First MR. The effect of oral metoclopramide on the absorption of cyclosporine. Transplantation 1987; 43:211–213.
31. Bateman DN. The action of cisapride on gastric emptying and the pharmacodynamics and pharmacokinetics of oral diazepam. Eur J Clin Pharmacol 1986; 30:205–208.
32. Kirch W, Janisch HD, Santos SR, Duhrsen U, Dylewicz P, Ohnhaus EE. Effect of cisapride and metoclopramide on digoxin bioavailability. Eur J Drug Metab Pharmacokinet 1986; 11:249–250.
33. Johnson BF, Bustrack JA, Urback DR, Hall JH, Marwaha R. Effect of digoxin absorption from tablets and capsules. Clin Pharmacol Ther 1984; 36:724–730.
34. Yuen GJ, Hansten PD, Collins J. Effect of metoclopramide on the absorption of an oral sustained-release quinidine product. Clin Pharm 1987; 6:722–725.
35. Steeves RA, Robinson JD, McKenzie MW, Justus PG. Effects of metoclopramide on the pharmacokinetics of a slow-release theophylline product. Clin Pharm 1982; 1:356–360.
36. Charles BG, Renshaw JJ, Kay JJ, Ravenscroft PJ. Effect of metoclopramide on the bioavailability of long-acting propranolol. Br J Clin Pharmac 1981; 11:517–518.
37. Schade RR, Dugas MC, Lhotsky DM, Gavalers JS, Van Thiel DH. Effect of metoclopramide on gastric liquid emptying in patients with diabetic gastroparesis. Dig Dis Sci 1985; 30:10–15.
38. Snape WJ, Battle WM, Schwartz SS. Metoclopramide to treat gastroparesis due to diabetes mellitus: double-blind controlled trial. Ann Intern Med 1982; 96:444–446.
39. Malagelada JR, Rees WD, Mazzotta LJ, Go VL. Gastric motor abnormalities in diabetic and postvagotomy gastroparesis: effect of

metoclopramide and bethanecol. Gastroenterology 1980; 78:286–293.
40. Lieberman DA, Keefe EB. Treatment of severe reflux esophagitis with cimetidine and metoclopramide. Ann Intern Med 1986; 104:21–26.
41. Hitch DC, Vanhoutte JJ, Torres-Pinedo RB. Enhanced gastroduodenal motility in children. AM J Dis Child 1982; 136:299–302.
42. Hyman PE, Abrams C, Dubois A. Effect of metoclopramide and bethanechol on gastric emptying in infants. Pediatr Res 1985; 19:1029–1032.
43. Leung AKC, Lai PCW. Use of metoclopramide for the treatment of gastroesophageal reflux in infants and children. Curr Ther Res 1984; 36:911–915.
44. Ponte CD. Metoclopramide in the treatment of an infant with gastroesophageal hypomotility. Drug Intell Clin Pharm 1982; 16:965–966.
45. Sankaran K, Yeboah E, Bingham WT. Use of metoclopramide in preterm infants. Dev Pharmacol Ther 1982; 5:114–119.
46. Forbes D, Hodgson M, Hill R. The effects of Gaviscon and metoclopramide in gastroesophageal reflux in children. J Pediatr Gastroenterol Nutr 1986; 5:556–559.
47. Frytak S, Moertel CG. Management of nausea and vomiting in the cancer patient. JAMA 1981; 245:393–396.
48. Gralla RJ, Itri LM, Pisko SE, Squillante AE, Kelsen DP, Braun DWJR, Bordin LA, Braun TJ, Young CW. Antiemetic efficacy of high-dose metoclopramide: randomized trials with placebo and prochlorperazine in patients with chemotherapy-induced nausea and vomiting. N Engl J Med 1981; 305:906–909.
49. Maxeran monograph (USA).
50. Meyer RB, Lewin M, Drayer DE, Pasmantier M, Lonski L, Reidenberg MM. Optimizing metoclopramide control of cisplatin-induced emesis. Ann Intern Med 1984; 100:393–395.
51. Howrie DL, Felix C, Wollman M, Juhl RP, Blatt J. Metoclopramide as an antiemetic agent in pediatric oncology patients. Drug Intel Clin Pharm 1986; 20:122–124.
52. Graham-Pole J, Weare J, Engel S, Gardner R, Mehta P, Gross S. Antiemetics in children receiving cancer chemotherapy: a double-blind prospective randomized study comparing metoclopramide with chlorpromazine. J Clin Oncol 1986; 4:1110–1113.
53. Gopichandran TD, Ring NJ, Beckly DE. Metoclopramide in double contrast barium meals. Clin Radiol 1980; 31:485–488.
54. Grunow JE, Howard S. A randomized study of oral metoclopramide in small bowel biopsy of infants and children. J Pediatr Gastroenterol Nutr 1988; 7:64–67.
55. Jepsen S, Klaerke A, Nielson PH, Simosen O. Negative effect of metoclopramide in postoperative adynamic ileus: a prospective, randomized double-blind study. Br J Surg 1986; 73:290–291.
56. Kauppila A, Anunti P, Kivinen S, Koivisto M, Ruokonen A. Metoclopramide and breast feeding: efficacy and anterior pituitary responses. Eur J Obstet Gynecol Reprod Biol 1985; 19:19–22.
57. Habbick BF, Gerrard JW. Failure to thrive in the contented breast-fed baby. Can Med Assoc J 1984; 131:765–768.
58. Bruera E, Brenneis C, Michaud M, et al. Continuous SC infusion of metoclopramide for treatment of narcotic bowel syndrome. Cancer Treat Rep 1987; 71:1121–1122.
59. Roussak JB, Carey P. Cardiac arrest after treatment with intravenous domperidone. Br Med J 1984; 289:1579.
60. Osborne RJ, Slevin ML, Hunter RW, Hamer J. Cardiotoxicity of intravenous domperidone. Lancet 1985; ii:385.
61. Champion MC. Domperidone. Gen Pharmac 1988; 19:499–505.
62. Brock-Utne JG, Downing JW, Dimopoulos GE, Rubin J, Moshal G. Effect of domperidone on lower esophageal sphincter tone in late pregnancy. Anesthesiology 1980; 52:321–323.
63. Valenzuela JE. Effects of domperidone on the symptoms of reflux esophagitis. R Soc Med Int Cong Symp Series 1981; 36:51–56.
64. Blackwell JN, Heading RC, Fettes MR. Effects of domperidone on lower esophageal sphincter pressure and gastroesophageal reflux in patients with peptic esophagitis. R Soc Med Int Cong Symp Series 1981; 36:57–65.
65. Di Lorenzo C, Peipsz A, Ham H, Cadranel S. Gastric emptying with gastro-oesophageal reflux. Arch Dis Child 1987; 62:449–453.
66. Brogden RN, Carmine AA, Heel RC, Speight JM, Avery GS. Domperidone. A review of its pharmacological activity, pharmacokinetics and therapeutic efficacy in the symptomatic treatment of chronic dyspepsia and as an antiemetic. Drugs 1982; 24:360–400.
67. Baeyens R, Reyntijens A, Van de Velde E. Effects of domperidone (R33,812) on the motor function of the stomach and small intestine. Arzneimittelforschung 1978; 28:682–686.
68. De Schepper A, Wollaert F, Reyntjens A. Effects of oral domperidone on gastric emptying and motility. Arzneimittelforschung 1978; 28:1196–1199.
69. Niemegeers CJE, Schellekens KHL, Janssen PAJ. The antiemetic effects of domperidone a novel potent gastrokinetic. Arch Int Pharmacodyn 1980; 244:130–140.
70. Heykants J, Hendriks R, Meuldermans W, Michiels M, Scheygrond H, Reyntjens H. On the pharmacokinetics of domperidone in animals and man. IV. The pharmacokinetics of intravenous domperidone and its bioavailability in man following intramuscular, oral and rectal administration. Eur J Drug Metab Pharmacokinet 1981; 6:61–70.
71. Meuldermans W, Hurkmans R, Swysen E, Hendrickx J, Michiels M, Lauwers W, Heykants J. On the pharmacokinetics of domperidone in animals and man. III. Comparative study on the secretion and metabolism of domperidone in rats, dogs and man. Eur J Drug Metab Pharmacokinet 1981; 6:49–60.
72. Huang Y-C, Colaizzi JL, Bierman RH, Woestenborghs R, Heykants J. Pharmacokinetics and dose proportionality of domperidone in healthy volunteers. J Clin Pharmacol 1986; 26:628–632.
73. Motilium monograph. In: Krogh CME, ed. Compendium of pharmaceuticals and specialties. 23rd ed. Ottawa: Canadian Pharmaceutical Association, 1988: 569.
74. Maddern GJ. Galactorhoea due to domperidone. Med J Aust 1983; 2:539–540.
75. Cann PA, Read NW, Holdsworth CD. Galactorrhoea as side effect of domperidone. Br Med J 1983; 286:1395–1396.
76. Custro N, Scafidi V, Constanza G, Inglese R, Calanni S. Effect of long-term treatment with therapeutic doses of domperidone on circulating thyroid-stimulating hormone levels in euthyroid patients. Curr Ther Res 1988; 44:287–291.
77. Sol P, Pelet B, Guignard JP. Extrapyramidal reactions due to domperidone. Lancet 1980; ii:802.
78. Franckx J, Noel P. Acute extrapyramidal dysfunction after domperidone administration. Helv Paediat Acta 1984; 39:285–288.
79. Van der Merwe JHD, Van Rooyen JM, Taljaard BPU, Offermeier J. Domperidone reduces the accumulation of paracetamol in saliva. Suid-Afrikaanse Tydskrif Wetenskap 1988; 84:431.
80. Masci E, Testoni PA, Passaretti S, Guslandi M, Thiobello A. Comparison of ranitidine, domperidone maleate and ranitidine +domperidone maleate in the short-term treatment of reflux esophagitis. Drugs Exp Clin Res 1985; 10:1–6.
81. Grill B, Hillemeier AC, Semeraro LA, McCallum RW, Gryboski JD. Effects of domperidone therapy on symptoms and upper gastrointestinal motility in infants with gastroesophageal reflux. J Pediatr 1985; 106:311–316.
82. Clara R. Chronic regurgitation and vomiting treated with domperidone (R33812), a multicenter evaluation. Acta Paediatr Belg 1979; 32:203–207.
83. Horowitz M, Harding PE, Chatterton BE, Collins PJ, Shearman DJ. Acute and chronic effects of domperidone on gastric emptying in diabetic autonomic neuropathy. Dig Dis Sci 1985; 30:1–9.
84. Molino D, Mosca S, Angrisani G, Magliacano V. Symptomatic effects of domperidone in post-vagotomy gastric stasis. Curr Ther Res 1987; 41:13–16.
85. O'Meara A, Mott MG, Domperidone as an antiemetic in paediatric oncology. Cancer Chemother Pharmacol 1981; 6:147–149.
86. Dalzell AM, Bartlett H, Lilleyman JS. Nabilone: an alternative antiemetic for cancer chemotherapy. Arch Dis Child 1986; 61:502–505.
87. Schuurkes JAJ, Akkermans LMA, Van Nueten JM. Stimulating effects of cisapride on antroduodenal motility in the conscious dog. Gastroenterology 1984; 86:1240–1245.
88. Schuurkes JAJ, Van Nueten JM, Van Daele PGH, Reyntjens AJ, Janssen PAJ. Motor-stimulating properties of cisapride on isolated gastrointestinal preparations of the guinea pig. J Pharmacol Exp Ther 1985; 234:775–783.
89. Ceccatelli P, Janssens J, Vantrappen G, Cucchiara S. Cisapride restores the decreased lower oesophageal sphincter pressure in reflux patients. Gut 1988; 29:631–635.
90. Stacher G, Steinringer H, Schneider C, Winklehner S, Mittlebach G, Gaupmann G. Effects of cisapride on jejunal motor activity in fasting healthy humans. Gastroenterology 1986; 90:1210–1216.
91. Krevsky B, Malmud LS, Maurer AH, Somers MG, Siegel JA, Fisher RS. The effect of oral cisapride on colonic transfer. Aliment Pharmacol Ther 1987; 1:293–304.
92. Marzio L, DiGiammarco AM, Capone F, Neri M, Mezzetti A, Capozzi

C, Cuccurullo F. Effect of cisapride on human fasting gallbladder volume: a real-time ultrasonographic study. Eur J Clin Pharmacol 1986; 29:631–633.

93. Van Peer A, Verlinden M, Woestenborghs R, Meuldermans W, Heykants J, Reyntjens A. Clinical pharmacokinetics of cisapride. In: Johnson AG, Lux G, eds. Progress in the treatment of gastrointestinal motility disorders: the role of cisapride. Amsterdam: Excerpta Medica, 1988: 23.

94. McCallum RW, Prakash C, Campoli-Richards DM, Goa KL. Cisapride: a preliminary review of its pharmacodynamic and pharmacokinetic properties, and therapeutic use as a prokinetic agent in gastrointestinal motility disorders. Drugs 1988; 36:652–681.

95. Michiels M, Monbaliu J, Hendriks R, Geerts R, Woestenboroghs R, Heyknats J. Pharmacokinetics and tissue distribution of the new gastrokinetic agent cisapride in rat, rabbit and dog. Arzneimittelforschung 1987; 37:1159–1167.

96. Meuldermans W, Van Peer A, Hendrickx J, Lauwers W, Swysen E, Bockx M, Woestenborghs R, Heykants J. Excretion and biotransformation of cisapride in dogs and humans after oral adminstration. Drugs Metab Dispos 1988; 16:403–409.

97. Spino M, Henderson K, MacLeod SM, Correia J, Koletzko S, Durie P. Cisapride disposition in cystic fibrosis patients and healthy volunteers. Clin Invest Med 1988; 11:17.

98. Hofmeyr GJ, Sonnendecker EWW. Secretion of the gastrokinetic agent cisapride in human milk. Eur J Clin Pharmacol 1986; 30:735–736.

99. Schuurkes JAJ, Megens AA, Niemegeers CJ, Leysen JE, Van Nueten JM. A comparative study of the cholinergic vs the anti-dopaminergic properties of benzamides with gastrointestinal prokinetic activity. In: Szurszewski, ed. Cellular physiology and clinical studies of gastrointestinal smooth muscle. Elsevier Science, 1987: 231.

100. Verlinden M, Reyntjens A, Schuermans V. Safety profile of cisapride. In: Johnson AG, Lux G, eds. Progress in the treatment of gastrointestinal motility disorders: the role of cisapride. Amsterdam: Excerpta Medica, 1988: 30–36.

101. Reyntjens A. Rationale for a new type of gastrointestinal prokinetic. In: Johnson AG, Lux G, eds. Progress in the treatment of gastrointestinal motility disorders: the role of cisapride. Amsterdam: Excerpta Medica, 1988: 5

102. Koop H, Monnikes H, Koop I, Dionysius J, Schwarz C, Arnold R. Effect of the prokinetic drug cisapride on gastrointestinal hormone release. Scand J Gastroenterol 1986; 21:907–913.

103. Stacher G, Gaupmann G, Mittelbach G, Schneider C, Steinringer H, Langer B. Effects of oral cisapride on interdigestive jejunal motor activity, psychomotor function, and side-effect profile in healthy man. Dig Dis Sci 1987; 32:1223–1230.

104. Baldi F, Porro GB, Dobrilla G, Iascone C, Lobello R, Marzio L, Sabbatini F, Tittobello A, Verme G. Cisapride versus placebo in reflux esophagitis. A multicenter double-blind trial. J Clin Gastroenterol 1988; 10:614–618.

105. Lepoutre L, Bollen J, Vandewalle N, Laukens P, Cabooter M, Vanderlinden I. Therapeutic effects of cisapride in reflux esophagitis: a double-blind, placebo-controlled study. In: Johnson AG, Lux G, eds. Progress in the treatment of gastrointestinal motility disorders: the role of cisapride. Amsterdam: Excerpta Medica, 1988: 63.

106. Evreux M, Fournet J, Galmiche JP, Soule J, Vitaux P. Endoscopic and clinical evaluation of cisapride and cimetidine in reflux oesophagitis. Gastroenterology 1988; 94 (Part 2):A120.

107. Janisch HD, Huttermann W, Bouzo MH. Cisapride versus ranitidine in the treatment of reflux esophagitis. Hepatogastroenterology 1988; 35:125–127.

108. Manousos ON, Mandidis A, Michailidis D. Treatment of reflux symptoms in esophagitis patients: comparative trial of cisapride and metoclopramide. Curr Ther Res 1987; 42:807–813.

109. Galmiche JP, Brandstatter G, Evreux M, Hentschel E, Kerstan E, Kratochvil P, Reichel W, Schutze K, Soule JC, Vitaux J. Combined therapy with cisapride and cimetidine in severe reflux oesophagitis: a double blind controlled trial. Gut 1988; 29:675–681.

110. Rode H, Stunden RJ, Miller AJW, Cywes S. Esophageal pH assessment of gastroesophageal reflux in 18 patients and the effect of two prokinetic agents: cisapride and metoclopramide. J Pediatr Surg 1987; 22:931–934.

111. Cucchiara S, Staiano A, Capozzi C, Di Lorenzo C, Boccieri A, Auricchio S. Cisapride for gastro-oesophageal reflux and peptic oesophagitis. Arch Dis Child 1987; 62:454–457.

112. Corinaldesi R, Raiti C, Stanghellini V. Monetti N, Rea E. Salgemini R, Paparo GF, Barbara L. Comparative effects of oral cisapride and metoclopramide on gastric emptying of solids and symptoms in patients with functional dyspepsia and gastroparesis. Curr Ther Res 1987; 42:428–435.

113. Verhaegen H, De Cree J, Leempoels J. Treatment of chronic dyspepsia with cisapride and domperidone. Acta Therapeut 1987; 13:385–394.

114. Testoni PA, Bagnolo F, Fanti L, Passaretti S, Tittobello A. Effect of long-term oral therapy with cisapride on the interdigestive antroduodenal motility pattern in dyspeptic subjects. Curr Ther Res 1988; 43:1118–1126.

115. Urbain J-LC, Siegel JA, Debie NC, Pauwels SP. Effect of cisapride on gastric emptying in dyspeptic patients. Dig Dis Sci 1988; 33:779–783.

116. Horowitz M, Maddern GJ, Maddox A, Wishart J, Chatterton BE, Shearman DJ. Effects of cisapride on gastric and esophageal emptying in progressive systemic sclerosis. J Gastroenterol 1987; 93:311–315.

117. Horowitz M, Maddox A, Harding PE, Maddern GJ, Chatterton BE, Wishart J, Shearman DJ. Effects of cisapride on gastric and esophageal emptying in insulin-dependent diabetes mellitus. Gastroenterology 1987; 93:1899–1907.

118. Rowbotham DJ, Nimmo WS. Effect of cisapride on morphine-induced delay in gastric emptying. Br J Anaesth 1987; 59:536–539.

119. Hyman PE, McDiarmid SV, Napolitano J, Abrams CE, Tomomasa T. Antroduodenal motility in children with chronic intestinal pseudo-obstruction. J Pediatr 1988; 112:899–905.

120. Cohen NP, Booth IW, Parashar K, Corkery JJ. Successful management of idiopathic intestinal pseudo-obstruction with cisapride. J Pediatr Surg 1988; 23:229–230.

121. Camilleri M, Brown ML, Malagelada JR. Impaired transit of chyme in chronic intestinal pseudo-obstruction: correction by cisapride. Gastroenterology 1986; 91:619–626.

122. Hyman PE. Absent postprandial duodenal motility in a child with cystic fibrosis. Correction of the symptoms and manometric abnormality with cisapride. Gastroenterology 1986; 90; 1274–1279.

123. Koletzko S, Corey M, Ellis L, Spino M, Durie P. Effects of cisapride-therapy in patients with cystic fibrosis (CF) and chronic recurrent distal intestinal obstruction syndrome (DIOS). European Society of Pediatric Gastroenterology and Nutrition, Annual Meeting, June 1989.

124. Binnie NR, Creasy G, Edmond P, Smith AN. Action of cisapride on the chronic constipation of paraplegics. Gut 1986; 27:A1241.

CHAPTER 43

Biopsychosocial Care

Beatrice Wood, Ph.D.

Eppur si muove.
Galileo

It has long been appreciated that there is a close association between emotion and gastrointestinal (GI) functioning. The first empirical data for such a link was Beaumont's[1] classic case of a patient whose gastric fistula was covered by a glass plate, permitting the observation of gastric change accompanying anger and fear. These early observations eventually led to psychosomatic theories of GI diseases such as ulcers, Crohn's disease, ulcerative colitis, and irritable bowel syndrome. However, despite repeated empirical demonstration of association between emotional disorder and GI disease, none of the etiologic theories have held up under close scrutiny. Interpretation has thus shifted from emotional disorder as the cause of the disease, to disease as the cause of emotional disorder.[2,3] Yet the latter interpretation also does not satisfy empirical and clinical observation.[4,5] Thus, these linear causal models must give way to more sophisticated models of mutual effect.[6,7]

This chapter presents a systemic biopsychosocial model that assumes interactions among biologic, psychological, and social levels of functioning. The fact of interaction itself is neutral with respect to function and dysfunction, but some types of interaction promote healthy function, whereas others induce dysfunction. The task of the investigator is to identify and distinguish between these two types of interactions. The task of the practitioner is to understand the mutual effect of biologic, psychological, and social levels of functioning in treating disease and to plan treatment accordingly. As research discovers specific patterns of influence among these three levels, fine-tuning of intervention to achieve maximum efficacy can be achieved.

This chapter presents a specific biopsychosocial model for the study and treatment of pediatric GI disease. The origins of the model are outlined, followed by a summary of the biopsychosocial research that both informs such a model and indicates the need for joint psychosocial-medical clinical intervention. The next section presents psychosocial and family factors in pediatric GI illness. Following this, we discuss a controversy regarding how to best deliver psychosocial services to patients and their families. The rest of the chapter describes the structure and evolution of our psychosocial-medical liaison partnership, including the process of developing that partnership, the psychosocial assessment and treatment approach, treatment protocols specific to disease type, shortcomings of the liaison, suggestions for improvement, and directions for the future. The chapter concludes by proposing key features of successful psychosocial-medical liaison partnership.

PHILADELPHIA CHILD GUIDANCE CLINIC PEDIATRIC LIAISON MODEL

Philadelphia Child Guidance Clinic (PCGC) has a long tradition of multidisciplinary clinical-research pediatric liaison projects.[8,9] The PCGC model is an open systems model of biopsychosocial functioning that recognizes the interaction of family, psychological factors, and disease factors in the physical and psychosocial health of a child. The PCGC liaison program emphasizes the value of joint research and clinical endeavors unified under the same biopsychosocial model. Thus, research and clinical intervention build upon one another synergistically to optimize discovery. In addition, joint research and clinical collaboration serve to develop and sustain the liaison partnership between the psychosocial specialist and the physician.

In 1981 a psychologist (author) and a child psychiatrist (Jose Nogueira, M.D.) from PCGC joined the pediatricians at the Division of Gastroenterology and Nutrition at Children's Hospital of Philadelphia. The goal was to develop a liaison partnership for the study and treatment of children with GI disease.

AN EMPIRICAL STUDY OF BIOPSYCHOSOCIAL INTERACTIONS IN CROHN'S DISEASE AND ULCERATIVE COLITIS

Implications for biopsychosocial mechanisms in inflammatory bowel disease (IBD) were explored in a study of Crohn's disease (CD) and ulcerative colitis (UC). Children, aged 6 to 17 years, with CD (n = 51) and UC (n = 37), together with their closest-aged siblings (n = 41 and n = 24, respectively), were evaluated as outpatients. The aim was to analyze multilevel relations among family, psychological factors, and disease factors in IBD.

Disease activity was measured by a modification of the Crohn's disease activity index used in the National Cooperative Study.[10] Psychological variables were psychological status, i.e., degree of psychological health versus disorder, measured by the Child Behavior Check List[11]; explanatory style, i.e., characteristic styles of causal attribution that have been associated with health and disease, measured by the Children's Attribution Style Questionnaire[12]; and psychological style (an empirically derived measure of behavioral tendencies, computed from the Child Behavior Check List). Patients and families answered the questionnaires as part of their outpatient visits. Laboratory values (hematocrit, erythrocyte sedimentation rate, platelet count, and albumin) were obtained through routine clinical assessment.

In addition, 40 families of children with CD, UC, and functional recurrent abdominal pain (RAP) were studied during standard family interaction tasks, lunch, and interview. Videotapes of the families were rated by two independent observers, blind as to diagnosis, according to a previously established system for evaluation of family patterns of interaction.[13] Families were evaluated for characteristics previously associated with uncontrollable disease activity in childhood chronic illness: *enmeshment* (undifferentiated and extreme involvement of family members with one another); *overprotection; rigidity; poor conflict resolution;* and *triangulation* of patient in family conflict. Marital distress and divorce rates were also assessed. These patterns, occurring together, have been interpreted by Minuchin et al as contributing to (as well as being produced by) an unusually severe course of illness for diabetes, asthma, and anorexia nervosa.[8]

Both CD and UC patients were found to have significant and comparable degrees of psychological disorder that was not related to disease activity. Disease activity was, however, related to "internalizing" psychological styles, described as behaviors that reflect anxiety, depression, social withdrawal and somatizing.[5]

CD and UC differed as to the relations among disease activity and psychological and family factors. First, in CD, a tendency toward depression was related to maladaptive explanatory styles (i.e., pessimism), whereas in UC the tendency toward depression appeared to be secondary to disease activity.[14] Second, siblings of CD patients were as dysfunctional as their sick brothers and sisters and had more "internalizing" styles, whereas siblings of UC patients were within the normal range for psychological functioning and had "externalizing" psychological styles.[15] Third, families of children with CD displayed a stronger family pattern of enmeshment, rigidity, poor conflict resolution, triangulation of patient in conflict, and marital distress as compared with families of children with UC and families of children with functional abdominal pain.[16] Accordant with this pattern of family functioning, we found the divorce rate of CD families to be lower than the norm, despite greater observed marital distress. The divorce rates for UC and the functional pain families were comparable to those for the normative populations.[17] The lower divorce rate in CD families is understandable in terms of the particular family patterns found to be more extreme in these families.

These findings indicate different patterns of biopsychosocial interaction for CD families in contrast to UC families. These differences held up even when severity of disease process was taken into account.[16] Specifically, they lead to the speculation that CD may be characterized by a particularly dysfunctional interlocking of family, psychological, and disease mechanisms: Maladaptive family patterns may affect (and be affected by) internalizing psychological style, maladaptive explanatory style, and psychological disorder (in patient and sibling), which in turn affect (and are affected by) disease activity (Fig. 1). UC appears *not* to be characterized by this type of multilevel relationship among family patterns, psychological style, and disease activity (Fig. 2). This may be because the features that organize a maladaptive biopsychosocial relationship in CD (e.g., the chronicity, severity, and/or belief system surrounding the illness) are not present or as extreme in UC. Alternatively, one might speculate that CD may involve a more readily accessible psychophysiologic pathway by which psychological factors may influence physical functioning. New work identifying psychoneuroimmunologic mechanisms in disease offers intriguing possibilities for such pathways.[18-20]

The clinical implications of these findings are clear. Because patients with CD and UC (and CD siblings) are at risk for psychological disorder, they should be assessed and assisted as necessary. Furthermore, since there are multiple relations observed among family, psychological, and disease

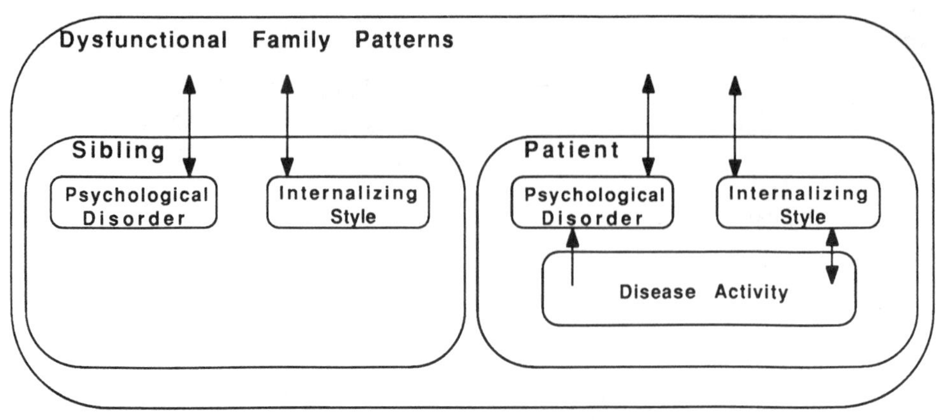

FIGURE 1 Maladaptive biopsychosocial configuration.

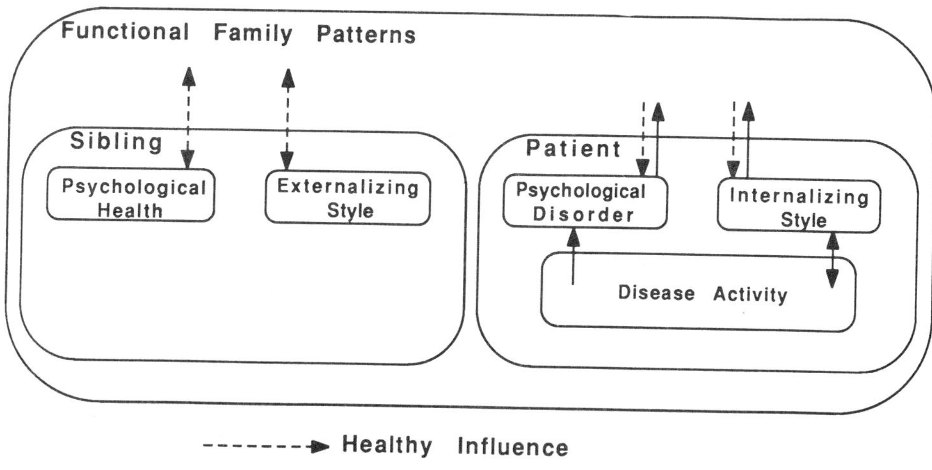

FIGURE 2 Adaptive biopsychosocial configuration.

factors, it would be advisable to evaluate families of CD and UC patients as a whole and to incorporate a family component into the course of treatment.

CLINICAL OBSERVATIONS OF PSYCHOSOCIAL AND FAMILY FACTORS IN PEDIATRIC GASTROINTESTINAL DISEASE

The types of disease most frequently requiring psychosocial/medical collaboration are RAP syndrome,[21,22] encopresis, CD, and UC. Occasionally consultation is requested for nonorganic failure to thrive and liver failure. Anxiety, depression, and somatization are the most common symptoms in children with CD, UC, and RAP.[5] RAP patients also frequently have school and/or peer problems, and school avoidance is not uncommon. Encopresis is often accompanied by conduct disorder and marital conflict. Overt family and marital dysfunction is most common in the families of children with RAP, whereas in families of patients with failure to thrive, CD, and UC, family and marital dysfunction is more covert and easily missed, yet just as serious. In our population of patients, infants with failure to thrive come almost exclusively from highly involved and anxious families. Marital stress and ambivalent parent-child relations are frequent complicating factors, as is dysfunctional involvement of grandparents.

The most seriously emotionally disturbed patients are the adolescents presenting with RAP or children with long histories of encopresis. Conversion symptoms and schizophrenia occasionally accompany these medical syndromes. In particular, the long-term encopretics tend to come from families in which psychosis and other severe psychiatric disorders are present in the nuclear or extended family.

Differential diagnosis of Crohn's disease versus anorexia nervosa sometimes presents a difficulty for primary care physicians. Occasionally we discover that primary physicians, psychologists, and psychiatrists have misdiagnosed a patient with Crohn's disease as having anorexia nervosa. On the other hand, some patients referred to the Division of Gastroenterology for evaluation of what was considered organically caused weight loss, turn out to be suffering from anorexia nervosa or (less often) bulimia. We find a dual diagnosis of primary eating disorder in conjunction with CD or UC to be extremely rare, although one might expect a natural collusion of these two syndromes. However, in contrast to patients with primary eating disorders, CD and UC patients want to gain weight and do not have distorted body images, nor do they have the typically associated psychosocial symptoms of social insecurity and difficulty with intimacy. Sometimes CD and UC patients and their families become locked in a battle over food, because the parents are trying to persuade them to eat more in order to gain weight, which elicits opposition or even refusal to eat. This problem should *not* be diagnosed or treated as a primary eating disorder syndrome. Nonetheless, immediate family and individual therapeutic intervention is required to prevent medical deterioration.

Compliance with medication and diet is not as great a problem in CD and UC as in some other diseases. However, consistency with nutritional supplement and tube feeding can be difficult for these patients, particularly for adolescents, because it constrains the normal mobility of this age group. Compromises need to be made in order to balance the needs of their emotional-social growth and health with their physical growth and health. This is especially important to ensure their ongoing commitment to collaborative efforts in managing their disease.

Sometimes a patient whose disease is nonresponsive to corticosteroids appears to be lying about compliance in order to avoid the cushingoid side effects of the medication. This is discussed with the patient and family, and if necessary the family is assisted in developing a monitoring program. This situation is rare. Usually, once the patients experience how ill they can become, they make a full commitment to their health. Exceptions to this are patients who have become extremely depressed and despondent about their chronic illness. They sometimes stop or want to stop taking their medicine as they express profound hopelessness and, at times, suicidal ideation. If the emotional well-being of patients is being rigorously monitored and managed during follow-up visits, this complication occurs only in cases of unremittingly severe disease activity. In these cases family therapy and individual therapy are intensified, and antidepressant medication is considered as an adjunct therapy.

In the past 5 years, only one IBD patient from our division required psychiatric hospitalization. RAP patients and encopretics more frequently required psychiatric hospitalization because they had become completely nonfunctional psychosocially.

Effects of Chronic Illness on the Family

Chronic illness can severely compromise family functioning. Parents and siblings often become overprotective of the sick child. They become watchful of every move the child makes and do things for the child that a healthy child would be required to do for himself or herself. Parents often feel guilty about having a sick child and may become overly indulgent, failing to set and enforce normal limits for age-appropriate behavior. This encourages dependency and curtails the development of autonomy. Sometimes siblings are unintentionally or unavoidably neglected, causing sibling conflict and sibling psychosocial disorder.[15] Sometimes the child and the disease become the primary focus of the family, thus constraining every decision and plan. Not infrequently, one parent, usually the mother, becomes intensely overinvolved and protective of the sick child, sheltering him or her from appropriate discipline coming from the other parent. This can cause serious marital discord, which stresses the rest of the family, including the sick child. If the family believes that stress can affect the sick child's illness (most families do), they will adopt a strategy of conflict avoidance, thus failing to resolve normal and illness-caused conflicts in the family. This, in particular, is detrimental to marital and sibling relationships. Occasionally, the sick child and his or her illness become a detour around family or marital conflict. This exacerbates the above-described dysfunction, which in turn may increase disease activity.[9,16,17]

Once in a while families are so threatened by the chronic illness or are so preoccupied by other severe physical or psychiatric illnesses or by overwhelming life events or situations that they have difficulty acknowledging and managing the illness. The patient's medical and psychosocial well-being may then be neglected through missed appointments, failure to monitor the child's symptoms or growth, and failure to see that the child adheres to proper diet and medication. The extremely anxious and conscientious families described in the above paragraph sometimes oscillate through periods of burnout and become behaviorally similar to these latter families. Whenever families operate in this manner, they require intensive and consistent psychosocial outreach and intervention.

These clinical observations and the research findings described above strongly indicate the need for a biopsychosocial intervention protocol for children with GI disease. The question is how best to provide such treatment.

BEHAVIORAL PEDIATRICS VERSUS PSYCHOSOCIAL LIAISON: A CONTROVERSY

The prototype for liaison psychiatry has been for the primary physician to determine when and if a patient (or, more recently, a patient's family) needs psychosocial intervention and to refer them to a mental health professional for evaluation and treatment. Medical and psychosocial intervention operates somewhat in parallel. The problem with this intervention model is that often the right hand does not know what the left one is doing. If one accepts that the biopsychosocial levels of an individual's functioning are inter-related, then one can easily appreciate the risk of ineffective treatment and even iatrogenic effects from failure of collaboration. Recognition of this problem has led to more co-ordinated psychosocial-medical intervention.

There are two approaches to this co-ordination. One is the behavioral pediatric approach. The other is a multidisciplinary psychosocial-medical team comprising the appropriate specialists.[23]

Behavioral pediatrics emphasizes training in psychosocial evaluation and treatment as integrated with medical treatment.[24] Both aspects of treatment are provided by the same person, the physician. While this approach seems conceptually ideal, there are practical limitations to implementation. The first limitation is on the amount of time (i.e., money) physicians have to spend with each patient and family, and psychosocial treatment requires a significant time commitment. More important, unless physicians complete a full course of psychiatric or psychological training (about 4 to 6 years), it is unrealistic to expect them to be as expert as they would need to be in assessing and treating the full range of psychosocial, psychiatric, or family dysfunction that can be present along with medical illness. One would not expect a psychiatrist or psychologist to be proficient in treating all types of GI disease after 1 year or so of extra training. On the other hand, it is highly desirable for physicians to become as proficient as possible in understanding and assessing the biopsychosocial levels of the illness they are treating. This improves the efficacy of medical treatment and assists them in making psychosocial interventions as needed and in recognizing when a patient's emotional, psychological, and/or family dysfunction is complex or severe enough to warrant intervention from psychosocial and family specialists. It also enhances collaboration with psychosocial specialists when necessary.

MULTIDISCIPLINARY LIAISON TEAM APPROACH

The liaison described in this chapter is a multidisciplinary one. Our team included pediatric gastroenterologists, nutrition specialists, a nurse clinician, a psychologist, and a child psychiatrist (both of the latter were specialists in family therapy). The nucleus around which the team is organized is the partnership between the psychosocial specialists (psychologist and psychiatrist) and the physician.[23,25]

Psychologist Versus Psychiatrist as Psychosocial Specialist

Mrazek[23] suggests that the child psychiatrist, by virtue of pediatric as well as psychiatric training, has a unique advantage in pediatric liaison activities. Drotar,[26] on the other hand, proposes that child psychologists offer the advantage of developmental and environmental conceptual models in contrast to the disease-oriented and nosologic conceptual models that psychiatry inherits from the medical paradigm. He suggests that psychologists are better suited to intervention in the context of pediatric liaison activity. Certainly, these two professions emphasize different areas in training. For example, psychologists typically receive much more training in research, whereas psychiatrists become more highly proficient in diagnosis and are exposed to more severe psychiatric disorders. Many other important differences exist.[27] It is not possible to make a general recommendation regarding which discipline is more appropriate for liaison work. Ideally a liaison team includes both, since they complement each other so well. In addition, special training in family assessment and therapy is practically indispensable in pediatric liaison intervention. Because the *relationship* between the psychosocial and medical professionals is the nucleus around which the successful liaison develops, a critical factor in selecting a partner is personal compatibility. This may be even more important than type of professional training.

EVOLUTION OF THE LIAISON PARTNERSHIP AT THE DIVISION OF GASTROENTEROLOGY AND NUTRITION, CHILDREN'S HOSPITAL OF PHILADELPHIA

Psychosocial consultation and treatment occurred during two outpatient clinics per week. Inpatient psychosocial consultation and treatment occurred as requested, and joint psychosocial-medical rounds were conducted once a week. Outpatient cases were presented at weekly medical case conferences.

Training

Training of staff and fellows in psychosocial and family issues was provided during rounds, case conferences, and ongoing collaboration on specific cases. *Videotaping* of family assessment and therapy sessions, with both the psychosocial and medical specialists participating, provided a powerfully efficient training and continuing education tool. Tapes of families participating in the IBD/RAP research project also provided additional insight into patterns of family function and dysfunction. Taping occurred with full family knowledge and consent. Most families found this to be acceptable and even desirable, as they understood that it enhanced the quality of their treatment.

Outpatient Consultation

At the very beginning of the liaison relationship, we (the psychologist and the psychiatrist) sat in on cases with a wide variety of diagnoses and complications. The physicians and fellows taught us and provided readings about the various diseases. In return, we introduced conceptual and practical tools with which to recognize, intervene, and/or refer patients for psychosocial consultation and intervention. Through this process we developed a common language and knowledge base. We also studied the belief systems each physician held regarding the interaction of biologic, psychological, and social levels of functioning in chronic illness. Finally, we observed and learned the styles of collaboration with which each physician was most comfortable, and we learned their style of interaction with patients and their families.

Soon we began conjoint treatment of patients. Physicians or the nurse-clinician selected patients for whom they wished psychosocial consultation and collaboration. We sat in on the medical examination and the report to the patient and family. Next we conducted a psychosocial and family interview and assessment with the physician present. Gradually, some physicians joined in the questioning. We would then excuse ourselves so that we could discuss the psychosocial findings and recommendations. Finally, we returned to the family and made our joint recommendations.

We discovered that many patients and families seemed "allergic" to certain words and phrases, such as "therapy," "emotional disturbance," and "psychiatric disorder." "Psychogenic" was frequently translated as "in their head" by parents and patients, which made it difficult, if not impossible, to arrange helpful intervention. We learned to avoid most psychological, psychiatric, and therapy terminology. Families were better able to understand and respond to explanations involving "treatment for the stress-related aspects of this disease." We proposed to them that they come for a few weeks as a family to "help their child manage these aspects of the disease," and/or for "help in dealing with the toll this disease has taken on the family." Sometimes we proposed that the psychosocial specialist have "time alone with the patient to assist him or her in managing the stresses related to their disease." If severe psychiatric disorder was present we found a way to tactfully inform the family and make appropriate recommendations. Usually we continued to follow these cases in our division.

Soon it became redundant for both the physician and psychosocial specialist to be present for all office visits, and in response to the boundless time demands of clinic, we modified the routine. Currently, patients have their initial medical work-up with the physician only, who decides whether psychosocial collaboration would be desirable. If the physician requests psychosocial collaboration and time coordination permits, we try to meet the patient and family in the presence of their physician before they leave the clinic. This is especially important if we think the family might be reluctant to have psychosocial participation in the treatment or if the medical findings are serious. Usually, however, the physician requests psychosocial evaluation for the next follow-up visit. We try, with varying degrees of success, to have the physician persuade the entire family to be available for this evaluation.

After the assessment, we meet with the physician and enlist support, if needed, in presenting the psychosocial findings and recommendations to the family. Families are much better able to accept painful or difficult assessment results and recommendations if the physician demonstrates his or her agreement and is present during feedback to the family. In addition, it is crucial for the physician to actively support and encourage the family to follow through consistently with the psychosocial treatment component.

Occasionally people absolutely refuse psychosocial evaluation. These are among our most disturbed patients and families. In this event we support the physician as best we can by ongoing collaboration and "backseat driving." Frequently they have to provide significant individual or family psychosocial intervention.

Case Report. One 16-year-old boy with functional abdominal pain and his parents were extremely anxious and mistrustful of the diagnosis of organic health. They believed some disease was being missed. Any attempt to involve the psychosocial specialist directly was met with exacerbation of anxiety and reluctance. Finally they agreed to a one-session meeting with both the doctor and the psychologist. Evaluation revealed that this young man was schizophrenic, although not actively psychotic. The family would not allow any more psychosocial intervention, so we coached the physician on a weekly basis. He learned how to gradually educate the family and patient as to the patient's schizophrenia and arrange for appropriate special schooling, while helping the family manage his pain episodes. The pain subsided as the family came to terms with the real limitations this youngster was experiencing in trying to live a normal adolescence.

It is not unheard of for a physician to tell a resistant and dysfunctional family that he or she cannot continue to treat them medically without the psychosocial component. Sometimes this strong commitment on the part of the physician convinces the family to permit psychosocial intervention.

Once in a while we need to intervene with an angry patient or family on behalf of their physician. Frustration can be caused by a delay in test results or in hospitalization, confusion from hearing several conflicting opinions or recommendations, or concern about the way in which their child overheard doctors talking about him on rounds. The anger interferes with treatment and threatens rupture of the doctor-patient-family relationship. Sometimes there is merely a misunderstanding to be clarified. Other times a genuine blunder has occurred and the physician must address this straightforwardly with the patient and family. The presence and support of the psychosocial specialist can assist in the resolution of this difficult situation.

Case Report. One very large, intimidating father was furious because the doctor did not perform a mentioned sigmoidoscopy on his daughter, who had functional abdominal pain. He was a mechanic and simply could not understand how there could be pain in the absence of disease. After all, when his trucks malfunctioned he could always find the mechanical cause and fix it. He also was very frightened, which interfered with his being able to understand what the doctors were saying. It took a 2-hour session to address and modulate his anxiety. It was necessary to listen very carefully to what he had to say in order to understand where his world view (about how things operate) departed from the doctor's. It was then possible to use his own concepts to translate how a human body can malfunction in ways that are not mechanical. It also was necessary to describe RAP to him in great detail, including how it can be treated successfully. After this session he and the doctor were able to resume a collaborative stance vis-à-vis his daughter's treatment.

Inpatient Consultation

Inpatient consultations occur on an as-needed basis. Requests are made for assessment of psychosocial or family factors contributing either to the illness or to difficulty managing the illness. Frequently we are asked to give an opinion as to whether the patient's symptoms could be due to psychogenic factors. (See section on RAP protocol for problems with this kind of request.) Occasionally requests for consultation are made because staff observe behavior in the patient, parents, or family which suggests psychosocial or psychiatric disorder. This request is properly made even if the behavior is not directly interfering with medical management of the illness.

We discuss with the physician and staff the reason for the consultation and also ask what has been said to the patient and family about the reason for the consultation. This is absolutely critical. Before we realized the importance of this detail, we often got off to a confusing and dysfunctional start with families. Subsequently, we coached the physicians on how to prepare patients and families for psychosocial consultations in the least threatening, least constraining, and least labeling way. Simply telling the family a psychiatric consultation has been ordered is disruptive; patients and families become at best anxious and self-conscious and at worst furious or completely closed and defensive. We find that the best approach is for the physician to explain that he or she believes the patient and/or family "could benefit from meeting with the psychosocial member of the team because childhood illness can be so difficult for patients and families to manage." If more persuasion is necessary, he or she can state that "it is in the best interests of the child that the family support the psychosocial component of the treatment." A key point seems to be that families recognize the psychosocial specialist as a regular member of the medical team and not as a "shrink" called in from the outside. It is also extremely important for the family to observe the physician's strong commitment to and trust in psychosocial intervention.

Usually we evaluate the patient alone, first, at bedside. We also ask the doctors to arrange for the entire family to come in for a meeting. We evaluate the family in the physician's absence so that they are free to express any concerns about their care. This is not unusual, given that hospitalization is a frightening and confusing event. We then present our psychosocial opinions and recommendations to the patient and family. If we expect that they will not be receptive, we enlist the support of their physician in providing feedback.

Therapy usually proceeds on a daily or every-other-day basis, as needed and possible. Individual therapy and family therapy are co-ordinated. If necessary, at the end of hospitalization, we have a joint medical-psychosocial session, including the physicians and nurse/clinician, to summarize findings and present a follow-up plan for outpatient psychosocial-medical treatment. Occasionally we recommend transfer to the inpatient psychiatric unit.

BIOPSYCHOSOCIAL ASSESSMENT AND TREATMENT MODEL

The biopsychosocial treatment model we use is partially derived from PCGC's Structural Family Therapy Model.[9,28] This is a systems model, which assumes that family patterns of interaction organize and are organized by individual patterns of functioning. Research has demonstrated that particular family patterns of functioning are associated with and appear to induce psychosocial dysfunction in children. Specifically, weak generational hierarchy (i.e., weak parental authority or poor parental collaboration), cross-generational coalitions, triangulation of the child in family or marital conflict, and extreme patterns of overinvolvement and emotional resonance all have been associated with child psychopathology. In addition, particular dysfunctional patterns of family functioning have been associated with unremitting chronic illness in children.[9] The treatment of choice is considered to be family therapy. Family therapy is to be understood as a model for organizing therapeutic assessment and intervention. It calls for an understanding of family and individual levels of psychosocial functioning and how they interrelate. In order to accomplish this for a given case, it is desirable to have at least one session with the whole family. However, subsequent intervention as organized by the model may involve combinations of treatment of individuals, parents, or the entire family, depending on the areas of dysfunction in the family or family members. We rely heavily on intervention with both the entire family and the individual patient. One major goal is to intervene so as to change maladaptive family patterns into adaptive ones (Figs. 1 and 2).

Individual assessment focuses on evaluation of the patient's psychosocial functioning in the context of his or her family, school, and social life. We assess for symptoms of psychological or emotional disorder and determine whether the psychosocial functioning is developmentally age-appropriate. We look for discrepancies in levels of functioning in the three contexts. For example, it is not unusual for chronically ill children to function more maturely at school or with peers than within the family. We also screen parents and the siblings for psychosocial status. The individual assessment takes place in the context of interviews with the family and with the patient alone.

In our *family assessment* we evaluate the degree to which the family operates in ways (described in the above section) that stress the patient, interfere with management of the child's illness, or undermine his or her age-appropriate functioning. We also assess the level of anxiety and depression present in the family.

We assume that illness organizes most families to be highly involved, protective, and conflict-avoiding. Some degree of these patterns of interaction is no doubt adaptive for the patient and his or her family.[16,17] However, extremes of these patterns, especially when marital distress or patient or sibling emotional disorder is present, suggest possible family dysfunction. In particular we are watchful for a cross-generational coalition between one parent and one child (usually the patient), which isolates and/or undermines the authority of the other parent. We are observant for signs of marital distress, i.e., emotional disengagement and/or overt or covert conflict. Any of these findings indicate that family-level intervention is indicated. *It is very easy to miss the dysfunction in these families during regular medical visits because they present themselves as loving, close, and well-organized families with no conflict. They also tend to deny having any problems or concerns, and they are extremely co-operative with and appreciative of their doctors.*

Families who are neglectful of the patient, chaotic, or conflictual are easier to diagnose and likewise require vigorous intervention.

If indicated, a course of family and/or individual psychosocial intervention is co-ordinated with the medical follow-up visits (or with the inpatient medical treatment) of patients.

DISEASE-SPECIFIC PSYCHOSOCIAL PROTOCOLS

Over the past 8 years we have developed psychosocial-medical protocols that meet the specific needs of the different disease populations. These are not rigidly structured protocols and there are many variations on a theme, depending on the particular physician's approach and on time and scheduling constraints. *Nonetheless, the goals of each of these medical-psychosocial protocols are the same: (1) to minimize the impact of the disease on both physical and psychosocial growth, development, and functioning and (2) to optimize efficacy of medical treatment.*

Recurrent Abdominal Pain Syndrome Protocol

Initially, consistent with the biopsychosocial model, we attempted to conduct a joint psychosocial-medical evaluation for all patients whom we suspected had RAP. Families were extremely disturbed about this because they believed an organic problem was causing their child's pain. They were understandably fearful that we might miss a medical cause if we found evidence of stress or emotional disorder in the patient or family. The psychosocial specialists also observed that early identification of these factors sometimes tended to cause physicians to be biased in favor of psychogenic diagnosis. It is easy to forget that psychogenic diagnosis does not preclude collateral organic disease. Furthermore, if the family perceives any doubt in their physician's mind about the diagnosis of medical health, they become more anxious and request more medical tests, thus postponing the necessary psychosocial work. For these reasons, we adopted a protocol in which the full medical work-up is completed before the psychosocial assessment. If the physician is not fully confident of the RAP diagnosis, we encourage him or her to extend the medical work-up until he or she is certain.

Frequently, by this time the physicians have some psychosocial observations to offer. Based on these, we plan how to present the psychosocial component to the family. The most effective approach is for the physician to report to the entire family that all medical tests are negative and that he or she is convinced that absolutely no disease or organic disorder is present. He or she then explains to the family that an extremely common syndrome, called recurrent abdominal pain syndrome, sometimes seems to be related to stress. He or she describes the syndrome and proposes introducing the psychosocial specialist to assist the family in exploring stress factors and in helping the patient and family manage the pain until it subsides. We then join the session and the physician reviews in detail all the tests done to rule out organic disease. It is extremely useful for the family to hear this again, and the psychosocial specialist assists the family in asking any questions they might need to reassure themselves as to the absence of organic disease. When the family is ready, the physician leaves and we begin the psychosocial evaluation and intervention. It is important to the families that the physician remain interested in their progress. From time to time during the course of therapy, it is necessary for the physician to reappear to reassure the family about his confidence in the diagnosis of organic health.

The physicians we work with do not distinguish RAP from IBS in recommending psychosocial intervention. They believe that these factors are important in both diagnoses. However, for IBS, they sometimes prescribe a bulking agent and/or antispasmodic medication. In addition, all patients with potential RAP diagnoses are given lactose breath tests to screen for milk intolerance.[29] If the test is positive, a nondairy diet is prescribed. Although these treatments may be ameliorative, they usually also undermine a family's already weak (or nonexistent) motivation to pursue psychosocial intervention. However, this is not a significant problem because if psychosocial factors are operative these medical treatments will be ineffective, thus supporting the necessity of psychosocial intervention.

It should be noted that we do not always find psychosocial or family dysfunction in conjunction with RAP. Often, in these cases, the child and family are anxious about illness in general, and a close or distant family member has been ill or has died with similar symptoms. It appears that the child's anxiety and focus on his or her body tends to translate the experience of minor abdominal discomfort into pain. If this seems to be the case, we explain this to families and intervention consists of helping the child and the family to disattend to the child's bodily discomfort. Self-hypnosis and relaxation techniques are taught to the entire family to refocus attention away from the discomfort. These cases usually resolve quickly.

Informal telephone follow-up of this protocol revealed that almost all families reported significant improvement or resolution of the pain. Confidence in the thoroughness of the medical work-up was a key factor in reassuring them and in convincing them to consider psychosocial consultation. Interventions that assisted the family and child in managing the discomfort were highly useful. A few families pursued medical work-up elsewhere because they still believed organic disease was present.

Encopresis Protocol

If a child's encopresis is not secondary to chronic impaction and loss of bowel tone or any other organic factors, the family is followed for psychosocial intervention, combining behavioral contingency (behavior modification) approaches with family therapy. Usually the child has other symptoms of behavioral dyscontrol, which also need addressing. Marital conflict is extremely common in these families, partly because of the stressful nature of this problem and the extreme frustration of being unable to agree on how to manage the child's problem. Mothers are resentful because usually they bear the primary responsibility for dealing with this problem. Fathers often respond well and effectively to becoming involved partners in solving the problem. Once parents devise a joint plan, with shared (but not necessarily equal) responsibility, improvement usually follows.

Frequently, and unfortunately, the encopresis appears to be secondary to chaos in the family, including but not always limited to marital dysfunction. These families are difficult to treat. They require intensive long-term psychosocial-medical intervention. If this is not viable in the context of the medical clinic, they need referral.

If the encopresis is secondary to impaction and loss of bowel tone and normal sphincter reflexes, medical intervention will be made to clean the bowel. The family is informed that it takes months for the child's body to relearn the normal reflexes, and the child must participate actively in this process through regular toilet-sitting and by taking a stool-bulking agent. Frequent follow-up visits are arranged to make sure the bowel stays clean and to track progress. If the physician notices psychosocial or family distress or dysfunction, or if the family is unable to follow the protocol, joint medical-psychosocial visits are arranged.

Early Intervention Protocol for Inflammatory Bowel Disease

IBD patients and their families are uncomfortable with referrals for psychosocial assessment or intervention. Many feel blamed and guilty, wondering whether they are being accused of aggravating the disease. Additionally, the semi-informed lay public still silently holds the belief, or fear, that IBD is caused by emotional or family problems or stress. If some friend or family member communicates this belief to the family of an IBD patient, it can make them nervous about psychosocial evaluation and intervention. Perhaps, in part, as a reaction to this view, some of the informed IBD lay public are vociferously adamant that emotions have noting to do with the disease, except as a response to having it. They reason that psychosocial intervention is thus not indicated or would be ineffective, whereas control of the disease would solve all problems. For these reasons, we decided that IBD patients and their families would be best served by an alternative psychosocial protocol.

The protocol is a multidisciplinary evaluation and education process, which requires several sessions with the family over the course of days. Once the diagnosis of IBD is confirmed, the patient and family are educated by their physician and the nurse/clinician regarding the medical aspects of the disease. Several popular myths are dispelled, including the notion that the etiology is psychosocial or emotional. The nutrition specialist provides an assessment and informs the family as to the nutritional aspects and treatment component for the disease. The physician then introduces the psychosocial specialist to the entire family, describing this person as an integral member of the team who participates in the treatment of all IBD patients and their families. The family is informed that the reason for this is that the stresses of IBD can take a toll on the psychosocial well-being of the child and the family and that many problems can be prevented by early intervention.

The psychosocial specialist then assesses the patient's and family's strengths and weaknesses, while discussing some of the emotional, psychological, and family pitfalls associated with IBD. If the patient and/or family shows signs of dysfunction, beyond the usual stress reaction to the diagnosis of chronic illness, the family is informed that the patient and family will meet with both the psychosocial specialist and their physician for the next few follow-up visits. The follow-up visits are spaced according to the joint medical-psychosocial needs. If patient or family dysfunction is serious, they will be scheduled for an immediate joint follow-up, even if the medical condition is good.

If the patient and family seem functional, they are not followed with ongoing psychosocial intervention. The physician is so informed, and he or she periodically discusses with the psychosocial specialist the progress of the patient and family. Patients or families with minor or marginal dysfunction are reassessed in a few months.

Medical hospitalization for flares calls for psychosocial and family re-evaluation and ongoing intervention, if indicated. For outpatient cases, depression and/or anxiety (in patient or other family member) that interferes with either medical management or normal psychosocial functioning, or is of long duration (more than a few weeks) calls for intervention. So does marital or parent-child relational distress. Sometimes patients begin to withdraw socially or have school problems in the absence of overt emotional or psychological symptoms. The physician must follow these areas of psychosocial functioning, because frequently the family makes allowances too readily on account of the disease. Psychosocial disorder in parents and siblings also can be readily missed. The physician should track their well-being as well.

Treating Patients with Divorced Parents

In evaluating and treating patients whose parents are divorced or remarried, it is important to make sure that the noncustodial parent is appropriately informed and involved in treatment, if indicated. (This does not require joint meetings with the former spouse.) This is especially important in the treatment of the more severe illnesses such as IBD or liver disease. It is not wise to rely on the custodial parent's opinion about whether the other parent should be or wants to be informed. The physician should routinely inform the custodial parent that he or she would like to inform the noncustodial parent as to the child's illness and progress. If consent is not easily forthcoming, a psychosocial consultation may be valuable to assist the family and physician to come to a decision in this regard. This protocol is increasingly important as joint custody becomes more prevalent.

If conflict between the divorced parents is impacting on the patient, the physician and psychosocial specialist must intervene vigorously and probably repeatedly, with both parents and the child, to minimize the effect on the child. We have found this situation to be among the most destructive for our patients. The physician's collaboration in this effort is important, since parents are more willing to suspend their battles in the face of physical injury to the child.

Case Report. One 13-year-old young man with Crohn's disease was followed at the clinic with his mother, who was divorced. The physician noted depression and anxiety in the patient, with somatic complaints that were not explained by laboratory indexes of disease activity. The psychosocial specialist discovered that mother and father were not speaking and that this child was responsible for reporting to his father details regarding his disease, ongoing medical condition, and treatment. He was unable to do so in a way that met father's need for clarity and the father became very anxious, which in turn made the patient worry about himself. Calls to the physician were not sufficient to inform and reassure father, because the physician was reluctant to reveal too much to the noncustodial parent without the mother's permission. The psychosocial specialist arranged that father and mother would alternate in bringing the patient to the clinic, so they both could be fully informed. The psychosocial specialist also intervened to change other divorce-related dysfunctional family patterns and met with the patient individually to help him manage this difficult family situation. This intervention required 2 years of regularly scheduled joint psychosocial-medical visits, including individual treatment for mother, father, and patient.

SUCCESS AND SHORTCOMINGS OF THE LIAISON PROGRAM

We believe that the psychosocial-medical liaison partnership is crucial to successful clinical treatment of both medical and psychosocial aspects of childhood GI disease. Our program has been very successful and cost-effective. Nonetheless there are still many "bugs in the system."

The most serious shortcoming of this liaison program was the difficulty in maintaining ongoing medical-psychosocial co-ordination of treatment for each patient and family for whom there was consultation. Families would sometimes drop out of the psychosocial component of the treatment, with or without informing the physician and psychosocial specialist. In general, this occurred because of a failure of communication between the physician and psychosocial specialist. Much ongoing communication about cases appears to happen naturally through the continual contact among medical staff who share departmental space. In this liaison, the psychosocial specialists were located in the adjacent psychiatry building and were thus isolated from this important avenue of information exchange.

Other significant shortcomings in following our most effective protocols stemmed from the frustrating difficulty of co-ordinating joint sessions and meetings because of the tight schedules of the team members. This problem was again exacerbated by the dual responsibility of the psychosocial specialists to both the Psychiatry Division and the Division of Gastroenterology.

Other problems involved failure in the partnership, usually when the physician made medical decisions involving important psychosocial implications without collaborating with the psychosocial specialist. For example, elective surgery might be scheduled without significant knowledge about the patient's and family's current psychosocial functioning. It is impossible to determine whether this was a failure of judgment on the part of the physician or whether it was another case of "out of sight, out of mind" with regard to psychosocial issues. It appeared that mere presence of a psychosocial specialist made a difference as to whether physicians took into account psychosocial, factors in treatment planning.

Other failures in partnership occurred when the psychosocial specialists were not timely in providing inpatient consultations that were necessary before medical treatment planning could take place.

The most severe failures occurred when the psychosocial specialists were unable to facilitate transfer of a patient from medical hospitalization to the psychiatric unit when needed. This was an unusual event, since psychiatric hospitalization was rarely indicated, yet the frustration in trying to make such transfers probably led to underuse of psychiatric hospitalization. One reason for the difficulty was lack of bed availability. More important, the current psychiatric unit is unequipped to manage a patient needing adjunct medical treatment such as hyperalimentation, intravenous medication, or tube feeding.

Building a Better Liaison

Psychosocial specialists need to have their offices in the same space as the medical staff. Also, they need to be full-time staff. Finally, there should be an inpatient Biopsychosocial Unit, housed in the medical hospital, staffed by the same psychosocial specialists as well as by appropriately trained medical staff. (See reference 25 for a highly successful Psychophysiological Unit.)

FUTURE DIRECTIONS FOR BIOPSYCHOSOCIAL RESEARCH

The exact nature of the processes underlying the biopsychosocial interactions in chronic GI disease must be discovered through further investigations. One approach is to test the direction of effect of the associations observed between family patterns of functioning, psychological style, psychological disorder, and disease activity. Multifactor, multilevel analyses of biopsychosocial function and dysfunction are necessary to elucidate both direction of effect and mechanism underlying the effects. One intriguing avenue for research is to explore whether psychophysiologic mechanisms in CD and/or UC are mediated by interconnections among the behavioral and immune (or other psychophysiologic) systems.

FUTURE DIRECTIONS FOR TREATMENT PROTOCOLS

Families of failure-to-thrive infants require co-ordinated psychosocial-medical treatment, regardless of whether the cause is organic. We have found this to be one of the most stressful medical conditions for families to manage. Ironically, these families are among the most reluctant to accept psychosocial intervention. This appears to be due to the intense focus they understandably have on the medical management of these potentially life-threatening and debilitating illnesses. Nonetheless, involving a psychosocial specialist at the beginning of medical treatment might assist the families in accepting joint psychosocial-medical treatment.

Children with liver disease awaiting (and recovering from) liver transplantation and their families present some of the most challenging and tragic problems for physicians and psychosocial specialists. One problem is how to help the family manage the excruciating wait for a liver, knowing that their child will die without it and that some other child must die to provide it. The guilt and conflicted feelings are virtually insurmountable and do not go away, even after a liver is found. The unremittingly dramatic and draining focus of attention that this situation demands can shred the family. The financial and emotional drain is awesome. The marriage is at risk, and siblings can suffer emotional and psychological neglect and subsequent disorder. The outcome of this procedure with regard to the long-term effects on the patient and the family is unknown. One can only hope that the medical profession will behave responsibly in conducting appropriate studies and in objectively evaluating the cost-to-benefit ratio with regard to the detrimental effects on the patient and family. This must be done for successful as well as unsuccessful transplantation. The possibility must be considered that one may "lose the family" in the process of saving the patient. Finally, any responsible transplant program, if it is to be ethically sound, must include a full complement of psychosocial specialists: social workers, psychologists, and psychiatrists, some of whom have special training in family therapy. Furthermore, there must be a fully functional psychosocial-medical program in place before transplants begin to take place. Anything less that this would constitute, I believe, a violation of the Hippocratic Oath.

KEY ASPECTS OF A SUCCESSFUL PSYCHOSOCIAL-MEDICAL LIAISON

Building a partnership between psychosocial specialists (psychiatrist and/or psychologist) and physicians is a frustrating, rewarding, and endless challenge.[24,26,30] The first step is *developing a common language*. It is necessary to introduce psychosocial concepts and constructs to medical staff using language that is free of jargon. In turn, physicians must define medical terms so that the psychosocial specialist understands the medical issues at hand. The goal is to develop common terminology, concepts, and models that will serve as the foundation upon which a working body of knowledge can evolve. It is also necessary for the psychosocial specialist to learn to present psychosocial aspects of a case succinctly and precisely.

Building trust in each other's special expertise is essential in developing a partnership; otherwise, it is tempting to try to tell the other how to carry out his or her responsibility for the patient's treatment. This can easily deteriorate into a power struggle. A psychosocial specialist best earns trust by demonstrating successful intervention with a few patients. Similarly, the psychosocial specialist must have the opportunity to directly observe successful medical interventions of the physicians with whom he or she will work.

It is intolerable for a professional to work in a setting where *mutual respect* is lacking. It is incumbent upon the psychosocial specialist to find something to respect about each staff member and trainee with whom he or she must work. Earning respect is equally important, but not always easy to obtain, for nonmedical professionals. This author noted a qualitative difference in level of respect after writing a successful grant, carrying out a research project, and presenting papers at "their" conferences. Apparently this was what was called for in a high-caliber university-based hospital. The "coin of the realm" may be different in other settings. One might assume that physicians are automatically accorded respect by virtue of their status as doctors. This is not the case. They also must earn the respect of the psychosocial specialists by demonstrating a scholarly open-mindedness regarding psychological information, constructs, and models.

Loyalty is a critical aspect of a liaison partnership. The psychosocial specialist needs to know that the physicians will make extra efforts to respond when they are needed to reinforce a psychosocial intervention. Sometimes this involves participating jointly in a family or individual therapy session or supporting the advice or directives given to patients and their families. This is crucial because patients and their families see themselves as being treated primarily for a physical disease, and thus the ultimate authority is the medical doctor. (Curiously, this is true even when the intervention is purely psychosocial and out of medical expertise, e.g., recommendation for change of school setting.) This reliance on the doctor is due partly to the fact that he or she has brought the patient and family through multiple medical crises, and thus a strong bond of trust has developed. This trust should be an asset to the psychosocial specialist, to the extent that the physician supports the former's interventions. It should never be challenged by the psychosocial specialist.

Physicians also need the loyalty of the psychosocial specialist so that they can depend on this person to respond promptly to psychiatric, emotional, or family crises, even if it is inconvenient. They also need to be able to count on the psychosocial specialist to support their medical recommendations when the patient or family is reluctant and to facilitate resolution of differences between the family and doctor. Without mutual loyalty between psychosocial and medical specialists the pitfalls in the treatment of complex cases are endless. Nothing builds mutual trust and loyalty better than working together on a difficult and troubling case and following it through to a resolution.

It is crucial that the physician and psychosocial specialist have some *shared model* with respect to the relations among biologic, psychological, and social levels of functioning. (The lack of a shared model may be one reason why so many liaisons falter and fail.) At minimum, the physician must appreciate that disease has some psychological effect and family impact. It is not necessary that the physician hold the view that psychological or family factors influence disease activity in order for there to be effective collaboration. Even the claim that stress is irrelevant to disease activity does not preclude psychosocial intervention, because psychological or family dysfunction can be understood as being secondary to the impact of the disease. Certainly, however, families or patients who avoid psychosocial intervention, despite a clear need, will respond more readily if they and their doctor believe that stress could or does affect the disease process itself.

The psychosocial specialist must understand the psychosocial-disease model held by each physician with whom he or she collaborates. Models become apparent through what doctors say to patients and their families. The psychosocial specialist should use the same model and language as the physician in working with their patients. If he or she cannot work within the physician's model, it would be preferable not to collaborate.

The physician must value and understand the rationale underlying the model of intervention used by the psychosocial specialist. Otherwise, it will be difficult to support the psychosocial intervention. The physician thus may be reluctant to refer patients and unable to encourage them to remain in treatment. If the physician is skeptical of the psychosocial treatment model, the best course of action is for the psychosocial specialist to demonstrate its efficacy with the physician's patients and to explain how the intervention model and strategy contributed to the success.

It helps to have a *sense of humor*. It is invaluable to both the physician and the psychosocial specialist when, despite good intentions, they find themselves at cross-purposes.

Finally, the liaison must have the full and consistent support of the chief of the Division of Pediatric Gastroenterology in order to be successful.

CONCLUSION

A liaison partnership is not a structure that can be quickly orchestrated and implemented. Rather, it is an evolving organic process that requires frequent realignment and new adaptation to changing requirements. It is the people and their relationships that "make or break" a liaison.

Acknowledgments

The author gratefully acknowledges Christine Kodman-Jones, Ph.D., Bruce D. Miller, M.D., Jonathan Schull, Ph.D., and John B. Watkins, M.D., for their helpful comments and criticisms of this chapter.

REFERENCES

1. Beaumont W. Experiments and observations on the gastric juice and the physiology of digestion. Plattsburgh: FP Allen, 1933.

2. Cassileth BR, Lusk EJ, Strouse TB, et al. Psychosocial status in chronic illness. N Engl J Med 1984; 311:506–510.
3. Helzer JE, Stillings WA, Chammas S, et al. A controlled study of the association between ulcerative colitis and psychiatric diagnosis. Dig Dis Sci 1982; 27:513–518.
4. Reinhart JB. Disorders of the gastrointestinal tract in children: consultation-liaison experience. Pediatr Clin North Am 1982; 5:387–397.
5. Wood B, Watkins JB, Boyle JT, Nogueira J, Zimand E, Carroll L. Psychological functioning in children with Crohn's disease and ulcerative colitis: implications for models of psychobiological interaction. J Am Acad Child Adol Psychiatry 1987; 26:744–781.
6. Engel GL. The clinical application of the biopsychosocial model. Am J Psychiatry 1980; 137:535–543.
7. Weiner HM. Psychobiology and human disease. New York: Elsevier North-Holland, 1977.
8. Minuchin S, Rosman B, Baker L, et al. A conceptual model of psychosomatic illness in children: family organization and family therapy. Arch Gen Psychiatry 1975; 32:1031–1038.
9. Minuchin S, Rosman B, Baker L, et al. Psychosomatic families: anorexia nervosa in context. Cambridge: Harvard University Press, 1978.
10. Best WR, Becktel JM, Singleton JW, et al. Development of a Crohn's disease activity index. Gastroenterology 1976; 70:443–444.
11. Achenback TM, Edelbrock C. Manual for the child behavior check list and revised child behavior profile. Burlington: Queen City Printers, 1983.
12. Seligman MEP, Peterson C, Kaslow NJ, et al. Explanatory style and depressive symptoms among children. J Abnorm Psychol 1984; 93:235–238.
13. Wood B. Proximity and hierarchy: orthogonal dimensions of family interconnectedness. Family Process 1985; 4:487–507.
14. Carroll L, Wood B. Learned helplessness in episodic chronic illness: role of explanatory style and disease activity; unpublished manuscript.
15. Wood B, Boyle JT, Watkins JB, Nogueira J, Zimand E, Carroll L. Sibling psychological status and style as related to the disease of their chronically ill brothers and sisters: implications for models of biopsychosocial interaction. J Dev Behav Pediatr 1988; 9:66–72.
16. Wood B, Watkins JB, Nogueira J, Zimand E, Carroll L. The "psychosomatic family": a theoretical and empirical analysis. Fam Proc 1989; 28:399–417.
17. Zimand E, Wood B. Implications of different patterns of divorce in families of children with gastrointestinal disorders. Fam Sys Med 1986; 4:385–397.
18. Glaser R, Rice J, Sheridan J, Fertel R, Stout J, Speicher CE, Pinsky D, Kotur M, Post A, Beck M, Kiecolt-Glaser JK. Stress-related immune suppression: health implications. Brain Behav Immun 1987; 1:7–20
19. Kiecolt-Glaser JK, Glaser R. Methodological issues in behavioral immunology research with humans. Brain Behav Immun 1988; 2:67–78.
20. Locke A, Ader R, Besedovsky H, Hall N, Solomon G, Strom T. Foundations of psychoneuroimmunology. New York: Aldine Publishing, 1985.
21. Apley J. The child with abdominal pain. London: Blackwell Scientific, 1975.
22. Boyle JT. Functional abdominal pain. In: Cohen S, ed. Contemporary issues in gastroenterology. New York: Churchill Livingston.
23. Mrazek D. Child psychiatric consultation and liaison to paediatrics. In: Rutter M, Hersov L, eds. Child and adolescent psychiatry. 2nd ed. Oxford: Blackwell Scientific, 1985: 888.
24. Anders JF, Niehans MN. Promoting the alliance between pediatrics and child psychiatry. Pediatr Clin North Am 1982; 5:241–258.
25. Miller BD. Treatment of the refractory asthmatic child. Am J Asthma Allergy Pediatr 1988; 1:241–247.
26. Drotar D. Transacting with physicians: fact and fiction. J Pediatr Psychol 1983; 8:117–127.
27. Kingsbury SJ. Cognitive differences between clincial psychologists and psychiatrists. Am Psychol 1987; 42:152–156.
28. Minuchin S. Families and family therapy. Cambridge: Harvard University Press, 1974.
29. Barr RG, Watkins JB, Levine MD. Recurrent abdominal pain in childhood due to lactose intolerance: a prospective study. N Engl J Med 1979; 300:1449–1452.
30. Jellinick MS. The present status of child psychiatry in pediatrics. N Engl J Med 1982; 306:1227–1230.

CHAPTER 44

Surgical Treatment

PART 1

General Principles

Sigmund H. Ein, M.D.C.M., FRCSC, F.A.C.S., F.A.A.P.

Some health problems affecting the pediatric population require an operation. Acceptance of this fact of life requires adjustment of our thinking and actions to make the operation as easy as possible for the small patient and his or her family. It is impossible to answer the question "Why?" for the scared, saddened, worried child and parents. Upon reviewing the preoperative and postoperative care of the pediatric patient, much thought, effort, and time are spent to convert the deformed, injured, or sick infant or child into a healed, healthy, happy human being.

This discussion focuses on the general surgical aspects of gastrointestinal (GI) diseases, which affect the intestinal tract (from mouth to anus), liver, biliary tree, and pancreas. It does not list every possible factor involved in the preparation and aftercare of the pediatric surgical patient. General thoughts, trends, and philosophies regarding the perioperative preparation and treatment are presented for physicians whose primary interests focus on pediatric GI diseases. Their aim should be to involve the pediatric surgeon in the investigation of the illness as soon as the question of an operation arises. Once the possibility of surgery becomes a reality, the pediatric patient must be approached with the understanding that, although the GI disease requiring an operation may be "typical" or attributable to a standard illness, its manifestations can be variable. We must not try to fit small patients into specific surgical "slots," thereby making them accommodate a standard operation. The pediatric surgical aim must be to make the small patient as close to perfect as is possible with as much care, compassion, gentleness, and speed as is humanly possible. To paraphrase the words of Willis J. Potts, the pioneer pediatric surgeon from Chicago, we want to help

> the [child] who has the great misfortune of [needing an operation]. All life is before him [or her], and what is done during [the operation] may decide whether life will be a joy or a burden. If this child [could] speak, it would beg imploringly of the surgeon, "Please exercise the greatest gentleness with my miniature tissues and correct the [problem] at the first operation. Give me blood [only if I need it] and the proper amount of fluid and electrolytes; add plenty of oxygen to the anesthesia, and I will show you that I can tolerate a terrific amount of surgery. You will be surprised at the speed of my recovery, and I shall always be grateful to you". . . . [and so will my mom and dad!][1]

PREOPERATIVE EVALUATION AND PREPARATION

Elective Surgery

Before discussing surgery, one must obtain a diagnosis. The urgency with which one proceeds in making the diagnosis of course depends upon the symptoms and signs. The more acute the problem, the more quickly the investigation proceeds with fewer diagnostic tests; the more rapidly the diagnosis is made, the sooner the patient is taken to the operating room. There are only a handful of GI problems affecting the pediatric patient for which surgery is deemed likely: congenital (e.g., obstruction), inflammatory (e.g., appendicitis, inflammatory bowel disease), acquired (e.g., bleeding, obstruction, perforation), and tumor-related (e.g., bowel, liver).

The key to the preoperative evaluation of all potential surgical problems is the history. If the questioning doctor has no idea what the problem is after the history has been taken, then either the history was incomplete (most likely) or the person providing the history (usually the mother) relayed it incorrectly (least likely). Nothing is more worrisome than hearing a mother say something is wrong with her child but she does not know what it is, and the doctor cannot find it.

Pain is a common presenting complaint in the pediatric patient with a GI problem, and of course the younger the patient the less history we have from the actual patient and the more we rely on the mother. Moreover, pain in the younger patient is much more likely to be organic in origin. Teenagers act more like adults within the spectrum of medical diseases, even at presentation, and at this age psychosomatic complaints begin to appear. Any pain that is disabling and lasts more than a short while needs urgent assessment before pain medication is provided, especially if there is a surgical scar on the abdomen. In about one-third of patients with abdominal pain seen in a pediatric emergency department, the pain has a pathologic cause; in another third nothing specific is found and the patient is discharged; in the remaining third, the patients are admitted, observed, and usually go home well within 1 or 2 days. The family history may provide some clues to the correct diagnosis (e.g., cystic fibrosis, pyloric stenosis, appendicitis, Crohn's disease, Peutz-Jeghers syndrome).

Vomiting is a highly common and important symptom and suggests an abnormality within the peritoneal cavity in general and a GI illness specifically. It frequently suggests cessation of GI function from inside (e.g., obstruction due to intussusception) or outside (e.g., peritonitis from appendicitis) the intestinal tract. Bile-stained vomiting must always be considered a symptom of intestinal obstruction due to congenital or acquired causes and must be aggressively investigated and treated.[2]

Blood per rectum is a common symptom in the pediatric patient and must be viewed with concern and urgency if there is more blood than stool; a change in bowel habits usually suggests something abnormal within the GI tract.

When ready to proceed with the physical examination, the examiner should have an idea of the cause of the problem; at this stage it requires confirmation. The abdomen looks, feels, or sounds abnormal, and orifices leading to and exiting from it must also be checked, but not excessively so. The most difficult aspects of the examination should be saved for the end, and the patients and their parents should be told what is being examined and why.

Laboratory and other tests must supplement rather than precede or eliminate the history and physical examination and should be minimized for the sake of the patient and the health care system, without limiting their effectiveness in helping with the diagnosis and plan of treatment. Routine blood work (hemoglobin, white cell count) and urinalysis are important standard tests. Screening for other unforeseen problems that may complicate intraoperative and postoperative care (sickle cell disease, sepsis, electrolyte imbalance) is necessary. Radiologic examinations should be done to identify problems; the two most commonly used screening procedures are abdominal radiography (flat plate and upright) and ultrasonography. If more information is required to localize the GI problem, which is usually intra-abdominal, then contrast and dye studies, along with computed tomography (CT) and magnetic resonance imaging (MRI), should be requested. Endoscopic procedures in pediatric practice may require general anesthesia and therefore, if considered to be of value preoperatively, may be done in the operating room; they may or may not be followed by a laparotomy.

Present-day surgeons seldom practice alone. They should and indeed must make use of their colleagues' experience in evaluating and treating the preoperative pediatric patient. Full use of appropriate tests and opinions of others should be sought to avoid a laparotomy for diagnostic purposes; the surgeon should have an informed idea about what he or she is operating for and where it is located. Once the preoperative diagnosis is made and an elective procedure is planned, preoperative evaluation should lead into the preoperative preparation. To be forewarned is to be forearmed. The chronicity and severity of the illness usually dictate the speed and amount of preparation. A number of areas must be explored and an equal number of questions asked in the surgical preparation of a pediatric patient. The general health of the neonate, infant, and child must be considered; fortunately, most are fit and well. If the problem is congenital, other associated anomalies must be sought, since frequently an adjoining system may have a congenital problem (e.g., esophageal atresia and congenital cardiac defect).[3]

If the chest (lungs) has been secondarily involved, for example, from aspiration due to pharyngoesophageal dyskinesia and/or gastroesophageal reflux (GER), the underlying process must be stopped and the lungs cleared by antibiotics and physiotherapy. The asthmatic child requires bronchodilator therapy preoperatively even though most anesthetic gases are bronchodilators.

When there is a bowel obstruction, the patient's intestinal tract must be decompressed with a nasogastric tube and the frequently occurring electrolyte imbalance and dehydration corrected. Most GI causes of obstruction in pediatrics affect the small bowel and, with the exception of pyloric stenosis and duodenal atresia, produce a metabolic acidosis. With rare exceptions, when an obstruction is present, the emergency is over once the diagnosis is made.

For an inflammatory process, one must determine when it is acute (e.g., appendicitis) or chronic (e.g., Crohn's disease) and whether steroids are being given to the child. Antibiotics are essential, especially those that give anaerobic coverage for organisms living in the lower GI tract.

The nutritional state of the infant or child must be assessed. The severity of malnutrition usually correlates with the length of illness. If the sickness has been longstanding, once the fluid and electrolyte imbalance has been corrected, intravenous alimentation (total parenteral nutrition [TPN]) is worth considering. One can usually estimate the length of time postoperatively before the pediatric patient will be on a regular diet and then correctly determine the need for TPN. A newborn cannot be starved for more than 1 week before negative nitrogen balance becomes obvious; the infant takes 2 or more weeks for this to happen, and the growing child takes about 1 month. In general, no unanimity exists among pediatric surgeons regarding the indications for and timing of TPN, particularly short-term intravenous alimentation. However, little harm can come from an early start with TPN. Although good nutrition can improve wound healing, postoperative morbidity and mortality do not seem to be adversely affected by boosting nutrition.[4]

Is the child immunologically compromised or altered by the illness or previous therapy or both? Severely ill patients are never good surgical candidates at the best of times and need maximum attention and support. The three most common preoperative concerns about these patients are bleeding disorders, immunologic dysfunction, and inability to heal. All attempts should be made to correct any abnormal indices prior to the operation; the more time one has, the easier the task and the more successful the outcome.

The anesthetist almost certainly sees the patient preoperatively to ensure against intraoperative surprises and/or anesthetic problems (e.g., pseudocholinesterase, malignant hyperthermia). In most instances, the anesthetist talks with the patient (if feasible) and the parents.

During the immediate preoperative period, other preparations are required. Because almost all pediatric surgical procedures require a general anesthetic, an appropriate period of fasting must be observed to ensure a clear airway. The length of fast varies according to the pediatric anesthetist's experience and the age and size of the child. If there is a bowel obstruction, a nasogastric tube is of major importance. If a nasogastric tube in needed only postoperatively, it can be passed in the operating room along with other catheters (e.g., urinary) and lines. When a nasogastric tube is used or the child needs fluid replacement, blood transfusion, and/or medications, an intravenous line is essential preoperatively. Most GI surgery is not clean, and preoperative antibiotics may be required for prophylaxis against wound infections (enteric gram-negative bacilli and gram-positive cocci for high-risk gastroduodenal operations; enteric gram-negative bacilli, group D streptococci and clostridia for high-risk biliary tract surgery; and enteric gram-negative bacilli and anaerobes for colorectal operations) and must be given intravenously no earlier than 1 hour before the incision is made.[5] The intestinal tract should be cleansed if a bowel resection is contemplated, and this is best accomplished by warm lactated Ringer's solution infused through a nasogastric tube[6]; enemas and oral antibiotics are now seldom used. Most medications can be given intravenously with few exceptions (e.g., codeine), since intramuscular injections are usually undesirable in pediatric practice. Few pediatric anesthetists sedate the smallest patients before an operation; the older children (especially the ones who are unfortunate enough to need multiple operations) occasionally receive an oral sedative if they are extremely anxious.

Emergency Surgery

Elective surgery becomes emergency surgery when the disease process cannot wait for more than a few hours (e.g., malrotation, ruptured appendix, compromised bowel, or acute bleeding). This places a major strain on both the pediatric patient and his or her parents and doctors because timing is crucial; intervention may be too early (and unprepared) or too late; both situations may create complications. There is really no emergency GI surgical problem in pediatrics that requires an immediate operation without some kind of brief evaluation, preparation, resuscitation, or treatment before the actual operation begins.

When a true emergency of the GI system presents, the history and physical examination, although still important, are often hurriedly intertwined with the investigation and treatment. Only vital investigations should be done, as time is often limited. Resuscitation must be aggressive without compromising the patient's stability. Sometimes the clearing of a pneumonia takes too long and postoperative ventilatory support may be required. Ideally, in patients with bowel obstruction, electrolytes and acid-base balance should be corrected before the obstruction is surgically relieved, but if signs of peritoneal irritation indicate gangrenous bowel or a perforation, correction of the abnormal electrolytes will have to be less than perfect, since attempts to correct imbalances too quickly create rapid electrolyte shifts, especially in potassium, into and out of the cells, resulting in dangerous complications of intraoperative general anesthesia and cardiac instability. Fluid resuscitation is best initiated with lactated Ringer's solution in boluses of 20 ml per kilogram. Although some forms of inflammation are effectively treated with antibiotics, optimal management of any collection of pus requires a scalpel blade, and early intervention is advisable, especially if the patient is septic. Antibiotics may not be totally effective until the pus is evacuated. Aggressive nutritional care is not an immediate concern in the preparation of a patient requiring emergency surgery. The child with hematologic abnormalities may need red cells, white cells, platelets, and/or other blood factors as quickly as possible, sometimes as the operation is beginning; in some cases the underlying pathology is the cause of the hematologic problem, for example, necrotizing enterocolitis (NEC) giving rise to low platelet counts. Sedation should not be given until the diagnosis is made, but if it has been decided what the problem is and when it will be repaired, then some sedation is worthwhile and kind. Successful emergency surgery depends on correct timing; correct timing comes from experience, and experience comes from bad timing.

An emergency operation—for example, acute appendectomy—must proceed whether the child is properly fasted or not, but in many cases the patient has vomited. Even if vomiting has not occurred, once the emergency has declared itself gastric emptying stops, so a full stomach must be considered and watched for during induction of anesthesia. It may be worthwhile in such emergencies to pass a nasogastric tube preoperatively to empty the stomach. Nonetheless, the anesthetic induction is carried out in a "rapid induction sequence" technique with cricoid pressure or in the small baby following awake intubation. Drugs like metoclopramide do not guarantee gastric emptying in such situations. Other monitoring lines and catheters are placed as needed during resuscitation and prior to the operation.

POSTOPERATIVE CARE

Routine Management

The famous New York pediatrician Bela Schick[7] once said: "Children are not simply micro-adults, but have their own specific problems," and indeed they do, especially after an operation.

Postanesthetic Room and Intensive Care Unit

"As the last stitch is tied, postoperative care begins." Most operations for pediatric GI disease are major laparotomies; some are thoracotomies. Sick newborns should be left intubated and taken back to the neonatal intensive care unit (ICU). Small babies less than 4 kg in weight should be closely monitored in a postanesthetic room (PAR); these small patients should be kept in an incubator on a cardiac and apnea monitor and remain in the PAR for at least 4 hours. Depending upon circumstances of surgery and expected complications, older infants and children stay from 1 hour (e.g., hernia repair, appendectomy) to overnight (e.g., pull-through procedure) in a well-staffed PAR. The infant or child requiring ventilation, or one who is very sick, often requires several days in the ICU, where observation and monitoring are closer and more critical.

Regardless of the setting, the immediate postoperative period is for monitoring of all vital signs and to ensure that when the patient arrives on the surgical floor he or she is fully awake and alert enough not to need close attention. All lines and catheters must be watched to make sure they are functioning properly and to make use of the valuable information they deliver; care must always be taken to not focus all the attention on the monitors alone. Some lines, such as arterial lines, may be removed before transfer to a regular surgical floor.

Following arrival in the recovery area (PAR or ICU), the immediate areas of attention upon awakening from a general anesthetic are identical to the ABC's of trauma—airway, breathing, and cardiac. Most infants and children receive mask oxygen upon arrival and are placed on their side until fully awake to prevent aspiration. Close monitoring of respiration and temperature is essential; fevers must be recognized and their etiology diagnosed and treated vigorously (e.g., sepsis, malignant hyperthermia). Since all operations have some blood loss, the second most important area to check is the cardiac status, which includes monitoring of blood pressure, pulse, and records of losses from wounds and drains. These procedures relay information that the cardiovascular system and bleeding and clotting mechanisms are all stable and under control.

As soon as the pediatric patient begins to awaken and appreciate the pain from the operation, the first of several doses of pain medication (morphine, meperidine, or codeine) is given, usually parenterally. This must be co-ordinated with any narcotics or regional local anesthetic blocks given during the operation by the anesthetist and/or surgeon.[8] The ventilated pediatric patient is usually kept sedated with intravenous medication such as morphine.

Intravenous fluids (colloids and crystalloids) are always given in recovery: Colloids may have been initiated intraoperatively or commenced, if indicated, postoperatively once the appropriate blood tests (hemoglobin, hematocrit) were obtained. Most anesthetists use lactated Ringer's solution intravenously in the operating room at a rate of 5 to 10 ml per kilogram per hour; this is often continued at the usual maintenance rate during the few hours of observation in PAR. The alternative is to switch to a maintenance fluid of choice (one-third saline, two-thirds 5 percent dextrose and water). Unless an episode of preoperative or intraoperative shock has compromised renal function, potassium can and should be given immediately postoperatively; often if it is omitted initially it may be forgotten, and unexplained ileus occurs several days later. There is no need to start parenteral nutrition in PAR.

Most wounds are initially covered with a dry sterile dressing; some serosanguinous drainage is to be expected, and the dressings should be reinforced. Drains are meant to drain, but excessive losses from either the wound or drain should be a cause for concern. Drainage from any tube must be checked regularly for quantity and quality. Lack of drainage or unexpected excess losses should not be taken for granted. Drainage tubes should be stable before returning the pediatric patient to the surgical ward. Fluid losses from wounds or drainage tubes must be replaced when appropriate. Regardless of age, the most important drainage tube following GI surgery is the nasogastric (Levin) tube; it is usually placed on low intermittent (Gomco) suction to prevent vomiting from the ever-present gastric ileus. Vomiting should not be accepted when a nasogastric tube is in place. To ensure adequate drainage, it should be irrigated every few hours; antiemetics should not be given.

Commonly ordered and important blood tests include hemoglobin and hematocrit, electrolytes, blood sugar, and blood gases; specific tests are required depending upon the nature of the operation and the postoperative appearance of the patient. If any respiratory or chest problems are anticipated or do occur, chest radiography is mandatory. Parents can and should visit their children in recovery if the stay is longer than a few hours.

Once the patient is awake and stable enough to be transferred to the surgical floor, recovery begins. This process is much shorter in a child. Infants and children who have had a major laparotomy constantly amaze those around them with the rapidity of the healing process; they are very different from adults in their quality of recovery. After a major operation, most adults lie still and stiff, do not move their legs, and do not take big breaths to expand their lungs. Teenagers act much like adults in their postoperative behavior. Infants and young children do exactly the opposite. They move around, yell, and scream; in so doing they aerate their lungs and swallow considerable air. This makes a big difference to their postoperative management and in the resultant complications, which will be discussed under Complications.

Respiration

Postoperative chest problems are relatively uncommon, especially in infants and small children. The older the child the more he or she resembles an adult in the frequency of postoperative complications. Upper abdominal incisions increase postoperative respiratory restriction; vital capacity decreases after major intra-abdominal surgery but returns to normal more quickly in the smaller patient. Functional residual capacity is also affected by shallow breathing without periodic sighs or maximal inflation which normally occurs every hour or less. If periodic sighs or big breaths do not occur (owing to anesthesia, pain, or sedation), alveolar collapse and atelectasis may result.[9] To prevent this, the patient needs to inspire deeply; crying and yelling accomplish this in the younger ones; chest physiotherapy and incentive spirometry accomplish the same in older children and teenagers. The asthmatic child should be given bronchodilator medication as needed.

Fever

On the first or second postoperative day, a slight elevation in the patient's temperature is probably due to the body's normal physiologic reaction to the trauma of the operation, but in general, fever is usually an indication of an infection somewhere in the body. The infection may be a local problem or generalized sepsis. In the younger pediatric patient the fever is likely to be higher, but on occasion hypothermia is indicative of generalized sepsis. In the neonate, sepsis is common, even without surgery, so a pediatric consultation should be sought and a complete septic work-up performed, including lumbar puncture. After 3 or 4 days postoperatively, fever usually points to a chest problem, whereas toward the end of the first week a wound or intra-abdominal infection should be suspected. Steroids and antibiotics mask fevers and should be discontinued as soon as medically feasible. There is no evidence that antibiotics given beyond the perioperative period prevent wound sepsis. The primary method of preventing infection in any operation still remains the operative technique. If an operative infection (wound or otherwise) is not the source of the fever, then a systematic search is necessary to rule out other sources such as intravenous lines. Once the likely site and cause have been identified, the correct antibiotic(s) should be started. When culture results are obtained within 24 to 48 hours, appropriate adjustments of antimicrobial therapy can be made. Antipyretics (acetaminophen) should be used, since fevers increase the metabolic workload of the patient, particularly because the body is expending greater amounts of energy dealing with the metabolic effects of the operation.

Bleeding

If no bleeding has occurred from the operation by the time the infant or child leaves for the surgical ward, the chances are small that bleeding will occur. However, if it occurs, it will be a major hemorrhage requiring immediate attention.

Pain

Pain is difficult to assess in the very young patient. In fact, a newborn may not be able to adequately demonstrate his or her discomfort.[10] It is easier to understand their hunger than their pain. Pain is believed by some to be part of the defense mechanism but also may occur with fear, anxiety, apprehension, and suffering. The presence of pain may cause secondary physiologic alterations in several body systems (pulmonary, GI, circulatory, skeletal muscle), and these in turn may contribute to potential postoperative problems.[9] The location of the incision, its size, and the type of surgery determine the quantity and quality of the pain. Once pain is felt by the patient, the challenge is to find a narcotic dose that is large enough to be effective in relieving the pain and yet small enough to prevent respiratory depression.

The three most common pain drugs currently used in pediatric surgical practice are morphine, meperidine, and codeine. The first is usually used intravenously, frequently intraoperatively, and in the ICU when a patient is being ventilated; it is not usually used during routine recovery in PAR. While giving excellent pain relief, it has the added benefit of providing some sedation at the same time; older children and teenagers tend to get "spaced-out" by it. Meperidine provides adequate pain relief but little sedation. Meperidine causes vomiting more frequently than codeine; vomiting is mediated by stimulation of the central chemoreceptor trigger zone. Most pain medication given on a surgical ward is initially administered intramuscularly every 3 to 4 hours; after a few days, when pain and vomiting have subsided, the dose should be decreased and an attempt made to give it orally. By this time most young pediatric patients seldom need anything for pain, whereas older patients need occasional pain relief; acetaminophen administered orally is often quite sufficient. Although acetylsalicylic acid is an excellent pain medication, it is seldom used because of the risk of bleeding and its ulcerogenic potential. If narcotic pain medication is automatically tapered commencing from the second postoperative day, it is virtually impossible for any infant, young child, or teenager to become addicted. Although regional anesthesia has been tried periodically by some anesthetists, there has not been much demand, interest, or use of this approach for pain control in the surgical patient.

Intravenous Therapy

Most GI pediatric operations require intravenous therapy for up to 1 week postoperatively; maintenance therapy is required with additional replacement of tube, drain, and stoma losses. Consideration must also be given to replacing further losses from fever, hyperventilation, and accumulation of third-space fluid. Many formulas have been developed for calculating replacement requirements and are invariably based on the patient's weight (e.g., doubling the weight in kilograms and adding 10 equals the amount of intravenous fluid required for maintenance in milliliters per hour). If the intravenous fluids are given according to a physiologic formula, routine blood work to check the serum electrolytes need not be done on a daily basis. If, however, a prolonged intravenous course is anticipated, consideration should be given to switching to parenteral nutrition using peripheral veins initially.

Wound Care

The approach to wound care has many variations according to each surgeon's preferences, but all revolve around a few basic principles. Many pediatric wounds are transverse and are closed in layers, and most are sutured with absorbable material. These three factors usually give a neat, strong, trouble-free wound with few postoperative problems. Most wounds are primarily closed, no matter how contaminated they are, because secondary wound closure or wound packing is impractical in pediatric practice; when the latter is done, the dressing may have to be changed with sedation or general anesthesia.

Several factors adversely affect proper wound healing, but none of these is peculiar to the pediatric patient. Infection is probably the biggest concern in preventing early wound healing. The risk of wound infection is definitely reduced if preoperative (or intraoperative) antibiotics are given; whether they need to be continued postoperatively remains a matter of considerable debate.[5] Chemotherapeutic drugs and steroids also prevent wounds from healing quickly; these agents decrease the inflammatory response, fibroblast formation, and protein synthesis.[9] Patients who are malnourished and chronically ill, for example, those with malignant disease, infection, or severe hepatic disease, are usually in negative nitrogen balance and tend to have poor wound healing; whatever is done to their wounds must be delayed from several days up to a week because wound strength and scar formation are both abnormally slow in developing. Supplemental vitamins and minerals should be given postoperatively if and when deficiencies are present, but wound healing cannot be speeded up beyond the normal rate.[9] In pediatric practice, wounds are often closed with absorbable subcuticular sutures and are either not covered at all or covered with collodion glue. Wounds without drains need not have any dressings on them after 24 hours; those with drains require changing when saturated or dirty. Wounds and stomas have to be observed for any unusual discoloration, swelling, or leakage of fluid. It is almost impossible to restrict postoperative activity in all but teenagers, but activity does not seem to affect the eventual wound strength or its healing. Skin stitches are now being replaced with staples because of the relative ease of wound care and "stitch" removal for all concerned. Stitches or staples can be kept clean with warm, soapy washes and an antibiotic ointment. Sutures or staples should be removed after 1 week; the wound may then be taped with small adhesive strips that are waterproof and come off spontaneously.

Drains

The use of drains in pediatric GI surgery is disappearing. There is some evidence that drains do not prevent collections of fluid,[11] and their routine use is seldom necessary other than with a pancreatic fistula. When used, there is rarely a need to bring such drains through the wound, as they increase the risk of infection and weaken the closure. Drains are best used to prevent the collection of any kind of fluid (blood, serum, bile, or pus) within any cavity, for example, the subhepatic space, or under skin flaps; to drain accumulating fluid (e.g., pancreatic); or to drain fluid when it is found at operation (e.g., abscess). Drains can be soft rubber, open sump suction, or closed Silastic suction. The latter minimize influx of outside contaminants, but no matter how sterile one is in drain care, there is always a risk that infection will enter around the drain site; in practice, this is seldom of clinical significance. Drain dressings should be kept clean with an antiseptic gauze soaked in Dakin's solution. The sump suctions usually collect the fluid they drain. Stiff drains or tubes within the abdomen should not be used because of the potential damage they can cause. When drains have served their purpose, they can be removed at one time or can be shortened daily. Most drains are shortened toward the end of a week and are generally removed a few days later; if any fluid collects after removal, the drain tract that has been established will usually reopen to drain further collections of fluid. Many radiologists have become quite proficient at percutaneous radiologically guided needle aspiration of collections of fluid from numerous sites, with placement of closed suction catheters at the source, if necessary.[12]

Gastrointestinal Function

After any laparotomy, GI function or peristalsis comes to a temporary halt, producing gaseous distention, nausea, and vomiting. This occurs for several reasons: handling and surgery of the GI tract or adjoining organs, pain, and drugs (anesthesia, narcotics). Time is required before full peristaltic function returns, which necessitates decompression, bowel rest, and supportive therapy from several days to 1 week (average 5 days). In this regard, there has been considerable discussion pertaining to the use of nasogastric (Levin) tube suction, especially after a laparotomy. Most pediatric surgeons believe that pediatricians use nasogastric suction too infrequently, and conversely many pediatricians believe that their counterparts use it too often. Nevertheless, following abdominal surgery, gastric peristalsis takes a few days to return, the small bowel takes 24 hours, and colonic motility resumes after 48 to 72 hours. For this reason alone, nasogastric decompression is usually used for at least the first few postoperative days to prevent gastric dilatation and vomiting. The pediatric patient swallows considerable air, which prolongs postoperative ileus due to gaseous distention. Recently there has been a trend toward not using a nasogastric tube on a routine basis,[13] or earlier removal. However, routine use will likely continue for a longer period in the pediatric patient than in the adult. Maximum benefit from a nasogastric tube is derived in surgery on the proximal GI tract, postoperative vomiting, ileus, and obstruction and in the unconscious child to prevent aspiration. The tube is usually connected to low, intermittent (Gomco) suction, unless a constant sump nasogastric tube is used, with irrigation every few hours to maintain patency. Vomiting is an unacceptable postoperative symptom. Once GI function returns to normal (bowel sounds, flatus and stool, volume of nasogastric drainage decreases and its color changes from bile to clear), the tube can be clamped or the suction discontinued for a test day and then removed. Radiologists claim that an indwelling nasogastric tube increases GER, but this does not seem to be of major clinical significance. When gastrostomy and jejunostomy tubes are present, they can be connected to suction or to a bedside bag, depending upon the type of tube and the clinical situation.

Once the newborn infant, small child, or teenager returns to the surgical floor, the parents should actively participate in postoperative care; this greatly enhances the time available for the surgical nurses to care for the sicker patients and those patients whose parents are unable to visit. Moreover, it gives the parents the opportunity to help in their child's recovery, and this makes the small patient as happy as possible during an uncomfortable time.

Complications

Virtually all complications occur within the first postoperative week and can develop from the operation, the disease causing the operation, or other unrelated causes. Whatever the cause, the pediatric surgeon must be aware of them, recognize them, and correct them as they arise. It is often difficult for any surgeon to accept that a complication might arise from his or her surgery. As long as the surgeon remembers that postoperative problems are frequently directly related to what was done in the operating room, there will never be a problem in recognizing the complication.

Respiration

Although not nearly as common as in adults, pulmonary complications (e.g., atelectasis, pneumonia) do occur and usually present within the first few days. Pulmonary symptoms are manifested by fever and an increase in the respiratory rate. In the smaller pediatric patient it may be impossible to detect the lung problem by examination alone, and chest radiography is recommended in any patient with a postoperative fever of unknown cause. If a chest complication is found, the patient may require airway suctioning, antibiotics, incentive spirometry (if old enough), and physiotherapy. Overall, morbidity and mortality from chest complications are low, unless there is an underlying pulmonary disease (e.g., cystic fibrosis). Aspiration pneumonia may occur when the pediatric patient has a swallowing disorder, and aggressive tracheobronchial toilet is required as soon as the patient is in recovery. Moreover, the common problem of GER can be aggravated by a nasogastric tube and may contribute to chest contamination. Steroids have not been proven to be of any value in aspiration pneumonia, but antibiotics may be helpful. If an intrathoracic bowel anastomosis is performed, complications frequently occur between 3 and 5 days after surgery, when clinical or radiologic evidence of pyopneumothorax may indicate a leak. Antibiotics, a chest tube, and intubation with ventilation may be needed. If subclavian central lines are inserted, the possibility of a pneumothorax during placement of the line must not be forgotten.

Fever

The presence of fever toward the end of the first week after laparotomy strongly suggests a wound infection. A deep infection may not be clinically evident for several more days. If the wound is not the culprit, then a source of intra-abdominal sepsis must be sought, particularly in the form of an abscess that will "break through" antibiotic therapy and cause a spiking fever. In order of occurrence, intra-abdominal collections of pus are found in the pelvis, between loops of bowel, and in the subphrenic space. When examination (including a rectal examination) fails to reveal an abscess, ultrasonography and/or computed tomography is probably helpful. If percutaneous aspiration and drainage are unsuccessful or technically unfeasible, operative drainage should be done. Any septic focus inside or outside the abdominal cavity causes an ileus in the small patient, which may necessitate discontinuance of feeding and nasogastric tube suction. The ileus continues until the infection is adequately treated.

Phlebitis from angiocatheters is a common complication in the pediatric patient, and the presence of fever requires a check of the intravenous site (or a central line culture) as part of the examination and laboratory assessment. *Staphylococcus epidermidis*, the most common organism cultured from intravenous lines, must be covered by antibiotic therapy until culture results are obtained. The offending angiocatheter or intravenous line must be removed, but a central line infection may be reversed with the appropriate antibiotic coverage except in the case of a fungal infection.

Bleeding

Aside from bleeding into wounds, which is uncommon, intra-abdominal bleeding following GI surgery is indeed rare, especially after the immediate recovery period. Bowel anastomoses do not bleed. Similarly, acquired cardiovascular complications are virtually unknown in pediatric practice. Congenital cardiac lesions require perioperative antibiotic prophylaxis against subacute bacterial endocarditis. Hypertension in postoperative infants and children usually indicates pain. However, hypertensive encephalopathy in children who have surgery for inflammatory bowel disease may result in seizures and coma if not recognized early enough.[14] Apparently prolonged steroid administration alters cerebral electrical activity, diminishes the threshold for seizure activity, and increases the risk of electroencephalographic (EEG) abnormalities. Postoperatively, inappropriate antidiuretic hormone response and the mineralocorticoid effect of the steroids act jointly following the stress of major surgery to cause fluid retention and hypertension. These factors presumably provide sufficient stimuli to trigger convulsive activity in the susceptible patient, as is evident from the commencement of seizure activity at the hypertensive peak. These effects are transitory and reversible upon cessation of the steroid therapy. Preoperative blood pressure and EEG readings as well as evidence of hypertension during the operation may provide a clue to this postoperative occurrence. Once the high blood pressure is recorded, antihypertensive medication should be immediately instituted. The hypertension slowly reverts to normal within the first weeks to months after the operation.

Pain

Complications from pain and pain medication in the pediatric patient are very unusual. Local needle granulomas from intramuscular injections in the anterior thighs are occasionally seen but seldom amount to anything serious. Vomiting from some narcotics is fairly common, and this complication may be confused with postanesthetic vomiting, which occurs in 20 percent of pediatric patients undergoing general anesthesia. Narcotic addiction in the pediatric patient is almost unheard of. Even after the correct dose of a narcotic, respiratory arrest occasionally occurs and is a real concern; it most frequently occurs in small babies under 6 kg in weight. Judicious use of postoperative narcotics in the pediatric patient virtually eliminates these possible complications.

Fluid and Electrolytes

Very few problems arise postoperatively from intravenous fluids and electrolytes. Because the pediatric patient usually has excellent renal function, fluid overload from intravenous therapy is seldom a problem. Technical problems from the intravenous catheters (peripheral and central) occur more frequently than do problems with the fluids they deliver.

Wounds

It is hard to pinpoint the reason for the low incidence of wound complications after the pediatric laparotomy: Stronger tissues; a more nutritionally healthy patient; the frequent use of transverse incisions; better, stronger, longer-lasting synthetic (e.g., polyglycolic acid) suture materials; and possibly closer staff supervision may all play a role. Moreover, wound hematomas and seromas are uncommon, probably because anticoagulant therapy is rarely used in the small patient. Similarly, oral acetylsalicylic acid has fallen into disuse in most children's hospitals.

Spreading cellulitis around a laparotomy wound is an uncommon early development of a wound infection, which may not show itself for several days when it causes a swinging abscess-like fever. Generally speaking, when a wound infection is pointing, it can be drained by removing a skin stitch or two. There is seldom any reason to probe pediatric wounds or to lay them open. These maneuvers are dangerous and add unnecessary morbidity to the child's postoperative recovery. It is also asking for trouble to bring stomas, tubes, or drains through a major laparotomy incision; this practice increases the risk of infection and weakens the wound, even if it is not infected.

Wound dehiscence, which occurs occasionally, often results in an evisceration but tends to occur much less often with the stronger transverse incision. Most frequently it arises due to a local infection or for technical reasons and is always heralded by serosanguinous wound discharge. The incidence of infection in most wounds can be kept to a minimum (less than 5 percent) with a combination of good surgical technique and appropriate antibiotic prophylaxis. Moreover, the newer synthetic dissolvable suture material (polyglycolic acid) has superior tensile strength and resistance to infection and wound stress. A ventral hernia (a wound dehiscence in which the skin sutures are taken out late) is seldom seen in pediatric patients.

There is always a significant risk for poor wound healing in a chronically ill, poorly nourished, infected, or immunosuppressed child who, in spite of attempts to overcome these problems, does not heal in an optimal fashion. Such a child is usually receiving long-term parenteral nutrition and is at risk of developing cholestatic jaundice leading to biliary cirrhosis. On the other hand, it is rare to operate on any pediatric patient for complications of inflammatory bowel disease who is not on steroids, yet in the author's experience wound problems hardly ever occur in these patients.

Leaks and Fistulas

If and when an anastomosis leaks, the intestinal fluid either enters the peritoneal cavity, creating an acute surgical emergency, or makes its way out through the drain site or the wound, forming a fistula. The fistula's contents should be captured like an ostomy (albeit a flush ostomy) and the GI tract put to rest. The fistula heals if there is no distal obstruction, no foreign body in the fistula tract, and no mucosa in the wound indicating the formation of a stoma. Other complications arising from or affecting the GI tract after laparotomy or any surgery of the GI tract will not be discussed in this section. The reader should refer to specific diseases in other chapters of this text. However, some generalized complications that arise from any laparotomy do require further discussion.

The finding of free air on postoperative abdominal radiographs has always been a source of confusion, since it raises the question of a postoperative bowel perforation or leaking anastomosis. Moreover, there is no unanimous opinion regarding the "correct" time for the disappearance of postoperative free air.[15] Generally speaking, all newborns and small infants should have no free air on upright radiographs by the second postoperative day. In older infants and children operated on through small abdominal incisions (e.g., McBurney) free air is usually gone by the third postoperative day, with the longest time being 8 days. Half of the infants and children who have longer operations through larger incisions have no free air by 2 or 3 days, while in the other half, free air disappears slowly over a 3-week period. In the latter cases, there is usually a period of prolonged ileus. There seems to be a correlation between the persistence of free air on one hand and age, thin habitus, size of incision, length of operation, and adynamic ileus on the other hand.

Gastrointestinal Function

Postoperative ileus, which usually resolves after the fifth day in the pediatric patient, may be prolonged if the patient is hypokalemic, hypomagnesemic, or septic (locally or generally). Occasionally, a postoperative ileus blends imperceptibly into a postoperative obstruction, requiring prolonged nasogastric tube decompression. If the bowel obstruction is adhesive in nature, time will usually release the fibrinous adhesion(s). However, one must always strongly consider a forgotten cause of bowel obstruction—intussusception.[16] Obstruction due to intussusception almost always follows 1 to 2 weeks after a major laparotomy and usually involves only the small bowel. There is seldom rectal bleeding or a palpable mass, and contrast studies are usually of no help in the diagnosis or treatment. Surgery is required.

Any time the abdomen is opened there remains forever a 5 percent risk of adhesive bowel obstruction.[17] In a pediatric patient this is manifested by cramps, bilious vomiting, abdominal distention, cessation of bowel function, and radiographs showing air-fluid levels. Over 80 percent of adhesive small bowel obstructions develop within 2 years of the initial operation. Adhesive obstruction is the most common cause of recurrent intestinal obstruction in neonates and is responsible for 7 percent of all cases of intestinal obstruction in the pediatric age range. More than 50 percent of adhesive obstructions occur following laparotomy for inflammatory or neoplastic disease.[17] The relative risk is greatest after subtotal colectomy and ileostomy. Nasogastric decompression is usually successful in correcting the obstruction in the majority of cases, but the obstruction usually recurs in 5 percent of infants and children within 2 years of the previous obstruction. Persistent metabolic acidosis and localized tenderness are the only consistent findings with gangrenous intestine. In addition to adhesive bowel obstruction, localized intra-abdominal obstruction around any stoma must be considered, such as volvulus or internal hernia.

Constipation after laparotomy is common in pediatric practice and can lead to fecal impaction. It is the most common cause of abdominal pain after pediatric laparotomy. If proper attention to stooling is followed, beginning with a suppository on the third postoperative day and a mild laxative if necessary after the GI tract is functioning, this common and annoying problem should be virtually eliminated.

REFERENCES

1. Potts WJ. The surgeon and the child. Philadelphia: WB Saunders, 1959.
2. Millar AJW, Rode H, Brown RA, Cywes S. The deadly vomit: malrotation and midgut volvulus. A review of 137 cases. Pediatr Surg Int 1987; 2:172–176.

3. Ein SH, Shandling B, Wesson D, Filler RM. Esophageal atresia with distal tracheoesophageal fistula: associated anomalies and prognosis in the eighties. J Pediatr Surg 1989; 10:1055–1059.
4. Demling RH. Preoperative care. In: Way LW, ed. Current surgical diagnosis and treatment. Los Altos: Lange, 1985.
5. Antimicrobial prophylaxis in surgery. Med Letter 1987; 29:91–94.
6. Postuma R. Whole bowel irrigation in pediatric patients. J Pediatr Surg 1982; 17:350–352.
7. Singleton EB, Wagner ML, Dutton RV. Radiology of the alimentary tract in infants and children. Philadelphia: WB Saunders, 1977.
8. Langer JC, Shandling B, Rosenberg M. Intraoperative bupivacaine during outpatient hernia repair in children: a randomized double blind trial. J Pediatr Surg 1987; 22:267–270.
9. Pellegrini CA. Postoperative care. In: Way LW, ed. Current surgical diagnosis and treatment. Los Altos: Lange, 1985.
10. Dilworth NM. Children in pain: an underpriviledged group. J Pediatr Surg 1983; 23:103–104.
11. David IB, Buck JR, Filler RM. Rational use of antibiotics for perforated appendicitis in childhood. J Pediatr Surg 1982; 17:494–500.
12. Liu P, Daneman A, Stringer DA, Ein SH. Percutaneous aspiration, drainage and biopsy in children. J Pediatr Surg 1989; 9:865–866.
13. Reasbeck PG, Rice ML, Herbison GP. Nasogastric intubation after intestinal resection. Surg Gynecol Obstet 1984; 158:354–358.
14. Levine AM, Pickett LK, Touloukian RJ. Steroids, hypertension, and fluid retention in the genesis of postoperative seizures with inflammatory bowel disease in childhood. J Pediatr Surg 1974; 9:715–724.
15. Ein SH, Stephens CA, Reilly BJ. The disappearance of free air after pediatric laparotomy. J Pediatr Surg 1985; 20:422–424.
16. Ein SH, Ferguson JM. Intussusception—the forgotten postoperative obstruction. Arch Dis Child 1982; 57:788–790.
17. Janik JS, Ein SH, Filler RM, Shandling B, Simpson JS, Stephens CA. An assessment of the surgical treatment of adhesive small bowel obstruction in infants and children. J Pediatr Surg 1981; 16:225–229.

PART 2

The Pediatric Ostomy

Sigmund H. Ein, M.D.C.M., FRCSC, F.A.C.S., F.A.A.P.

Ostomies have been a boon to infants and children with severe congenital and acquired gastrointestinal (GI) disease, as well as to the doctors, nurses, and parents taking care of their problems. For the purposes of this discussion, pediatric ostomies include tube ostomies and stomas. Fortunately for the pediatric patient, ostomies are almost always temporary and are relatively easy to care for. As they have been developed and subsequently accepted for use in pediatric practice, the treatment of GI diseases has greatly improved. Certainly, the physical and psychological complications from an ostomy in a child must be measured against the morbidity and mortality that may ensue if it is not done.

Although some forms of large bowel stomas were made in adults before 1710, Littre observed a dead 6-day-old baby with an imperforate anus and suggested that a colostomy might have been life-saving. In 1793 Duret created a colostomy in a 3-day-old patient with an imperforate anus, and this individual lived 45 years. This historical fact probably makes this French surgeon the "father of the colostomy," since his observations preceded those of other surgeons by almost 100 years. Over the next 75 years, Dubois, Duret, and Freer made colostomies for babies with an imperforate anus. By the mid-1800s, there were more than 30 case reports of colostomies for imperforate anus. In 1861 Post, in New York City, performed the first infant colostomy in North America.[1] Considerable progress has been made since 1859, when S.D. Gross of Philadelphia wrote,

> We are struck with astonishment that anyone possessed of the proper feeling of humanity should seriously advocate a procedure so fraught with danger and followed, if successful, by such disgusting consequences. I cannot, I must confess, appreciate the benevolence which prompts a surgeon to form an artificial outlet for the discharge of the feces, in a case of imperforate anus. . . .[2]

A planned gastrostomy was first mentioned in the 1830s, but it was not until the 1870s that Verneuil et al performed the first successful pediatric gastrostomies.[3] Almost 100 years later, pediatric gastrostomies were being made without a laparotomy.

Ileostomies were the last type of stoma chronologically to come upon the scene[1,4-7]; it was not until the early 1900s that this stoma began its development. It was soon appreciated that any small bowel stoma could create fluid, electrolyte, and metabolic disturbances.

TYPES OF OSTOMY

Tube Ostomies

Most pediatric GI ostomies are temporary. There are three kinds of tube ostomies: gastrostomy,[3,8,9] jejunostomy,[5,9] and cecostomy[10,11]; the first is commonly used and the latter two much less so. Gastrostomies are generally planned and are always made in the operating room, usually under general anesthesia. They are indicated if the infant or child cannot swallow (esophageal atresia, stricture) or should not swallow (aspiration, esophageal dyskinesia). Gastrostomy tubes can be placed in the stomach either through the endoscopic percutaneous "incisionless" route (usually requiring only sedation), with a small upper abdominal incision, or accompanying a large upper GI operation (antireflux). Increasing numbers of neurologically impaired pediatric patients are now receiving feeding gastrostomies for nutritional benefit, ease of nursing, and prevention of aspiration. However, up to 40 percent of these patients require a subsequent antireflux procedure, since in some cases the gastrostomy seems to interfere with the functioning intact angle of His and the gastroesophageal junction.[13,14] This may refocus attention on placing the gastrostomy tube along the lesser curvature of the stomach and sewing this area to the anterior abdominal wall, a procedure resembling the Boerema gastropexy.[15,16] If the esophagus is patent and functioning normally, oral feeds are started and the gastrostomy tube can be removed if unused for 3 months. Jejunostomy feedings may be delivered either by passing a small feeding tube beside the gastrostomy tube and into the proximal jejunum, by making a tube jejunostomy, or via the percutaneous intraoperative route.[9] The latter two methods are not frequently used in pediatric practice. Similarly a tube cecostomy can be placed electively to decompress left colon surgery, or it is rarely employed as an emergency for a cecal perforation.[10] It decompresses the bowel of gas and some liquid stool, but unlike a stoma it does not completely divert the fecal stream.

Stomas

In general, it is best not to fashion stomas flush with the skin; this renders them similar to fistulas, and their discharge is difficult to capture without irritating the skin. The sutures most commonly used in their construction are absorbable. Unlike the usual practice in adults, the stomas are opened up in the operating room. Some stomas are made as part of a large operation and are brought out a separate opening. In others, stomas are created as the only goal of surgery, and these usually are brought out through the same small incision used to enter the abdomen. As a general rule, a bowel stoma should not be brought out through a large laparotomy wound because of the risk of wound infection, dehiscence, and/or evisceration.

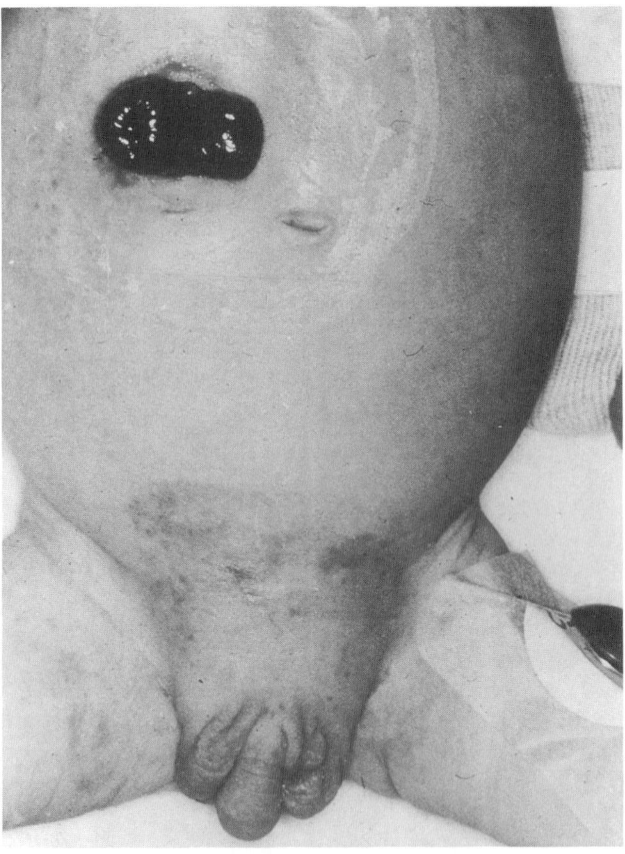

FIGURE 2 Loop colostomy.

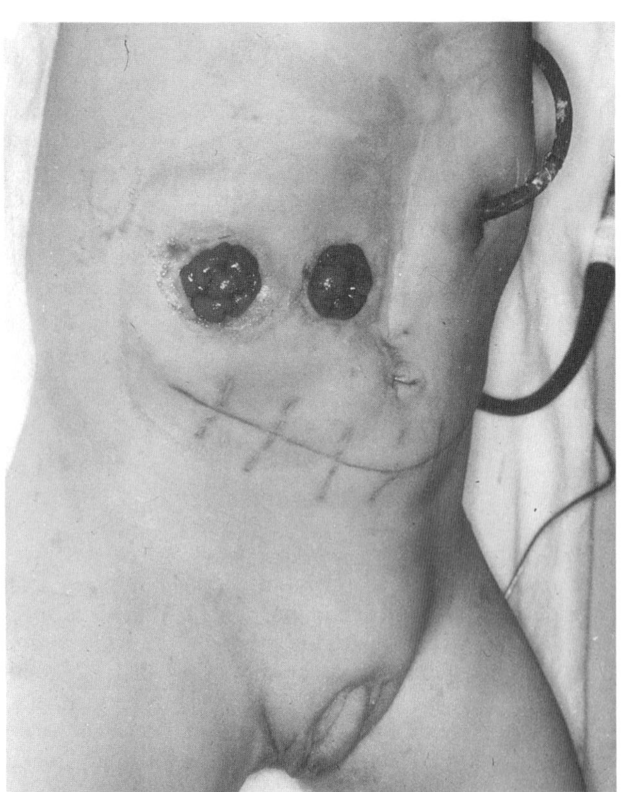

FIGURE 1 End colostomy on left; mucous fistula on right.

Stomas in the pediatric patient are made either as end stomas (Fig. 1) or as loop stomas (Fig. 2).[1,8,17] In the former, the bowel is divided and the proximal stoma is brought through a separate opening and the distal nonfunctioning stoma (called a mucous fistula) is either brought out through another opening or, as in the case with a Hartmann procedure, is closed and dropped back into the peritoneal cavity. When a loop stoma is constructed, the bowel is usually not divided but brought out as a loop over a bridge of some sort (rod, catheter, skin), and both proximal and distal openings adjoin each other. To avoid the very common problem of prolapse, the loop stoma can be divided and the distal limb tunneled subcutaneously and brought out a nearby skin opening.[18,19]

Neck stomas are either from the esophagus or from another piece of bowel (gastric tube or colon) which will eventually join the esophagostomy to form a new swallowing tube (Fig.

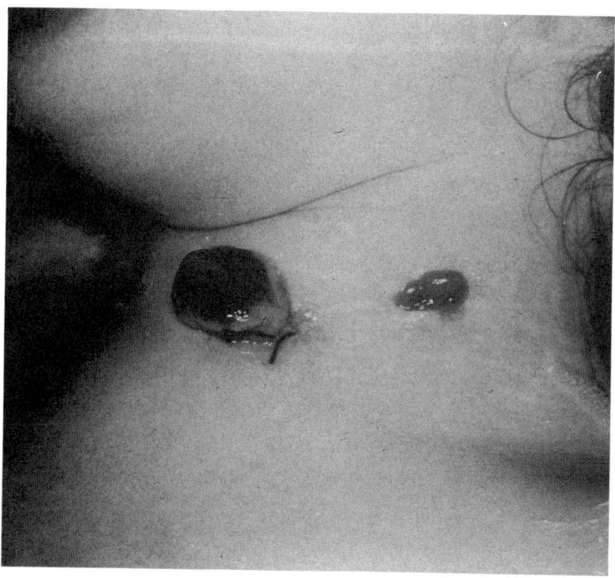

FIGURE 3 Neck stomas (gastric tube on left, esphagostomy on right).

3).[20,21] This form of surgery is necessitated either by the congenital absence of part of the esophagus (in which the proximal and distal halves cannot be joined) or by a severely damaged and strictured esophagus, usually following ingestion of acidic or alkaline agents. Acquired strictures requiring esophagostomy are those that cannot be dilated by mechanical means to a reasonable functioning lumen again. Most neck stomas are made on the left because the esophagus is closer to the neck surface on that side.

Abdominal ostomies can usually be placed anywhere. Gastrostomies or jejunostomies are usually located in the upper abdomen, especially in the left upper quadrant. Jejunostomies are most often needed following perforation in necrotizing enterocolitis (NEC), and occasionally when small bowel atresia cannot be repaired, requiring a temporary ostomy (Fig. 4). In Figure 5, a right upper quadrant jejunostomy is shown from the Roux-en-Y isoperistaltic loop constructed as part of a portoenterostomy procedure to correct biliary atresia.[22] It can be used to measure the bile output from the portoenterostomy anastomotic area draining the liver and is useful to indicate the degree of success of the operation and/or severity of liver damage. The stoma also prevents the common problem of ascending cholangitis that plagues these operations. Most right transverse colostomies are found in newborns or infants with either a high imperforate anus or Hirschsprung's disease and are made in the right upper quadrant; some surgeons prefer to do left transverse colostomies, which are placed in the left upper quadrant. Other surgeons make sigmoid colostomies in the left lower quadrant for these indications and for other rectosigmoid problems. Severe perineal damage following trauma (Fig. 6) or burn (Fig. 7) may require a temporary colostomy until the perineum heals. The most common pediatric stoma in the right lower quadrant is an ileostomy (usually distal ileum), which is frequently performed for NEC or ulcerative colitis (Fig. 8). Rarely a loop cecostomy is required for a cecal perforation from a distal colonic obstruction, NEC, or trauma; initially loop cecostomies are large, edematous, and ugly, but they do shrink in size. In spite of its position in the intestine, it acts like a colostomy, proving how important the ileocecal sphincter is to proper intestinal function.[23]

Urinary stomas are now infrequently used in pediatric patients. These intestinal stomas use ileum and colon as bladder conduits for major congenital anomalies of the lower urinary tract and are always placed in the lower abdomen.[24] The disconnected loop of bowel collects urine from anastomosed ureters and drains into an appliance. However, stomal stenosis (incidence of 80 percent), bacteriuria, stones, high unobstructed intestinal conduit pressures, free ureteroin-

FIGURE 4 Ileostomy for atresia in a baby with gastroschisis and a silon pouch.

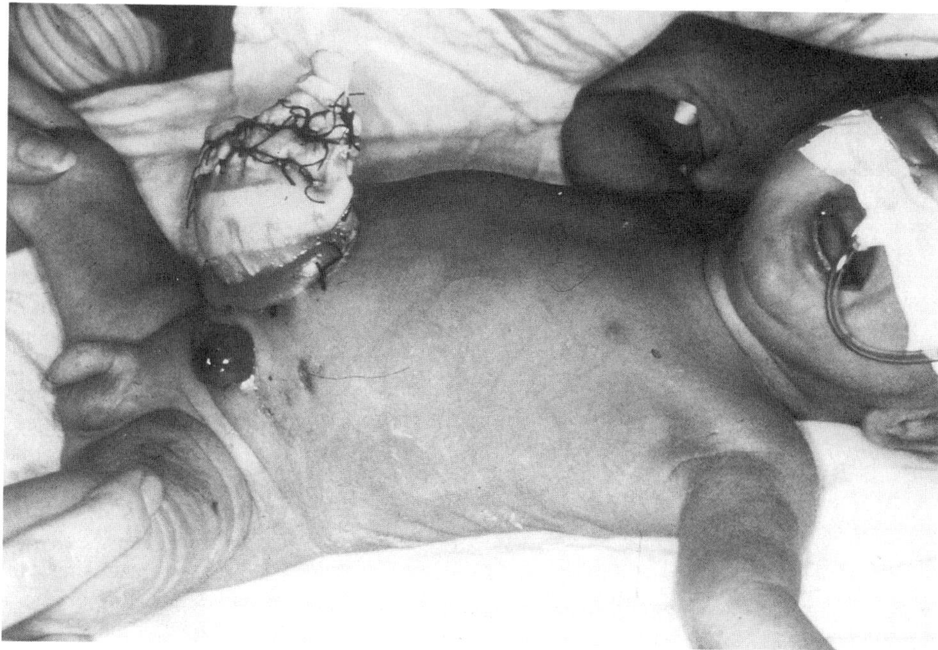

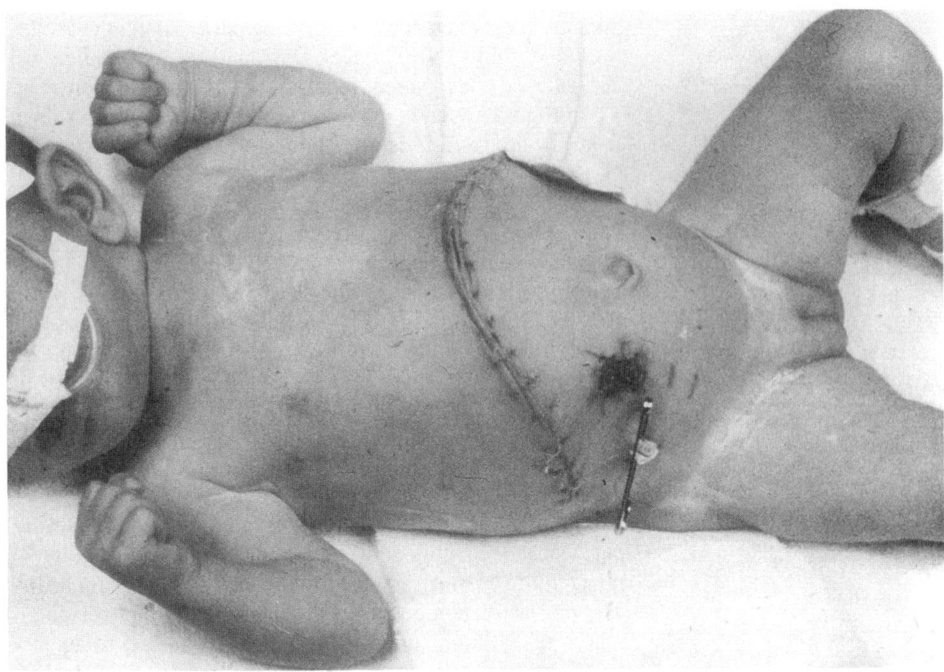

FIGURE 5 Roux-en-Y jejunostomy in a patient with a postoperative portoenterostomy.

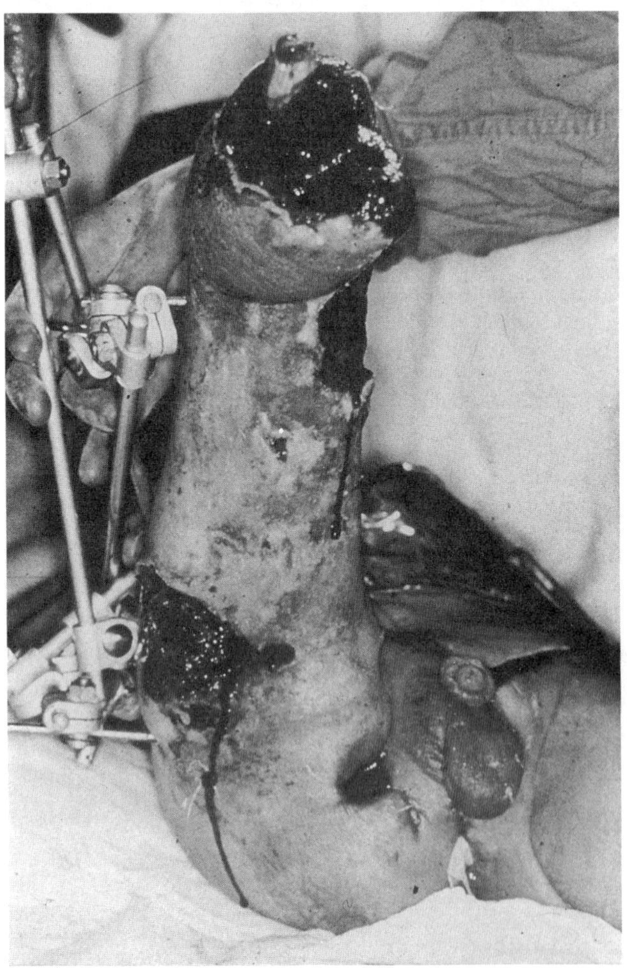

FIGURE 6 Severe perineal trauma required temporary colostomy.

testinal reflux, and renal deterioration over a prolonged period of follow-up have led to their re-evaluation in the pediatric population.[25] Prevention of reflux from the bowel conduit seems easier to achieve using colon, and some studies show that this prevents upper tract destruction. This has led to an interest in the continent Kock pouch, internal diversion, or reconstruction of the lower urinary tract to avoid using an appliance.[24,25]

Rarely, some surgeons have deliberately placed a stoma in the umbilicus, but this is seldom needed and requires preoperative discussion with the patient and/or the family owing to the emotional implications of siting a stoma in the umbilicus.[26]

Fistulas are never planned and usually are difficult to take care of because they produce similar or worse difficulties than flush stomas (Fig. 9).[27] They are commonly seen around stomas and in wounds and are seldom in convenient areas for their care (neck, chest, abdomen, and perineum). Fluid draining from fistulas is difficult to capture, making skin irritation a problem that is both uncomfortable and hard to manage. The two most common causes of fistulas are a leaking bowel anastomosis (technical, distal obstruction) or inflammatory bowel disease (particularly Crohn's disease). A fistula should close spontaneously unless it is lined with mucosa or there is a distal bowel obstruction or a "foreign body" of some kind within the fistula. Apart from several rare exceptions, if one sees "mucosal lips" in the fistula, it almost certainly means that a stoma has developed, and this acts like a flush stoma and requires similar treatment. In Crohn's disease the fistulas do not close until the disease is under control surgically or medically. Treatment usually requires bowel rest using parenteral nutrition, elemental feeds, proximal bowel diversion, bowel resection, or any combination of these methods.

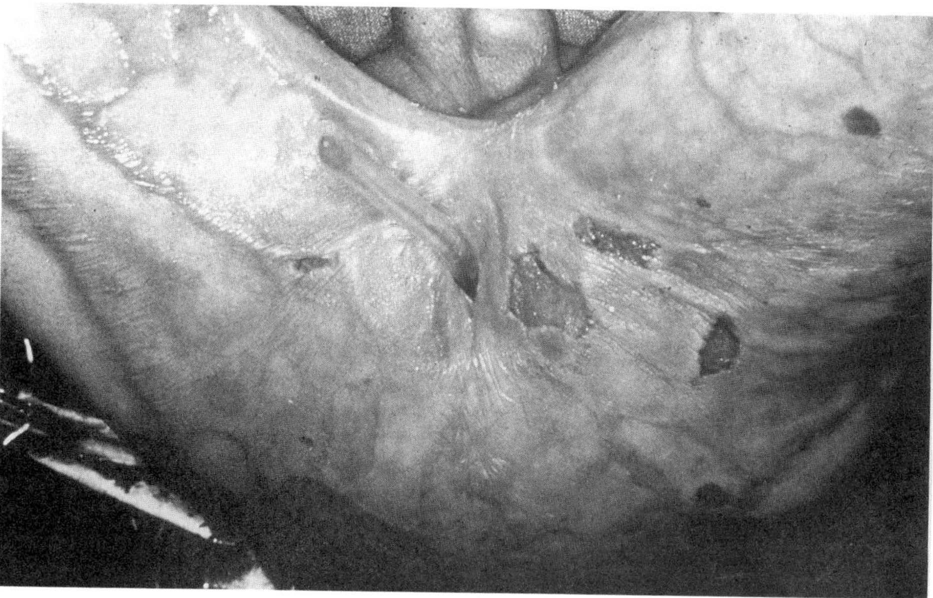

FIGURE 7 Bad perineal burn required colostomy until healing occurred.

PATHOPHYSIOLOGY AND MEDICAL COMPLICATIONS

Aside from the technical considerations of GI stomas, the major concerns of their physiologic care revolve around the stomal output from the GI tract. If it is excessive, acute fluid and electrolyte imbalance may occur. The chance of this complication increases if the patient is young, the stoma is new, and it is created proximally.

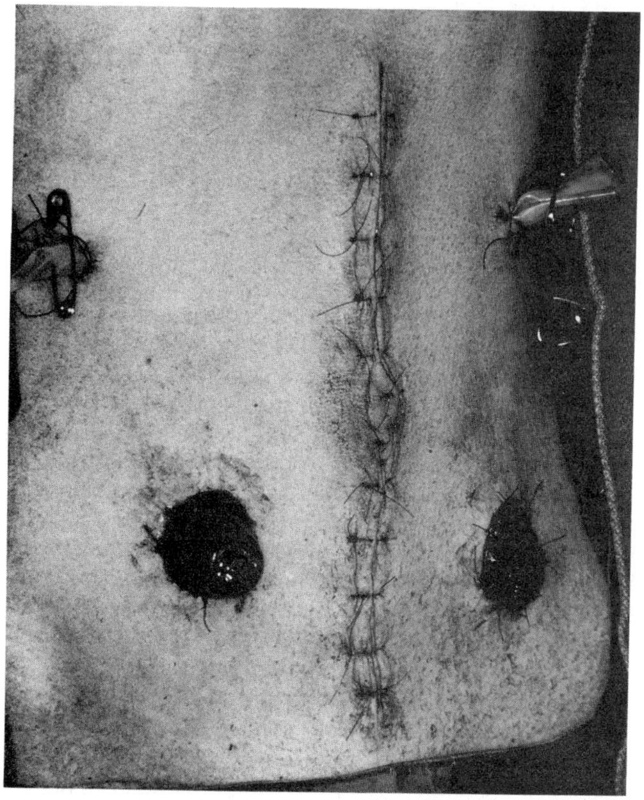

FIGURE 8 Right lower quadrant ileostomy in a teenager with ulcerative colitis. Note left lower quadrant flush sigmoid mucous fistula.

Neck Stoma

The neck esophagostomy or so-called spit fistula produces considerable salt loss, and unless appropriate amounts of sodium, chloride, and potassium are replaced, the serum electrolyte values slowly reach subnormal values. The losses from the neck stoma following a staged gastric tube replace-

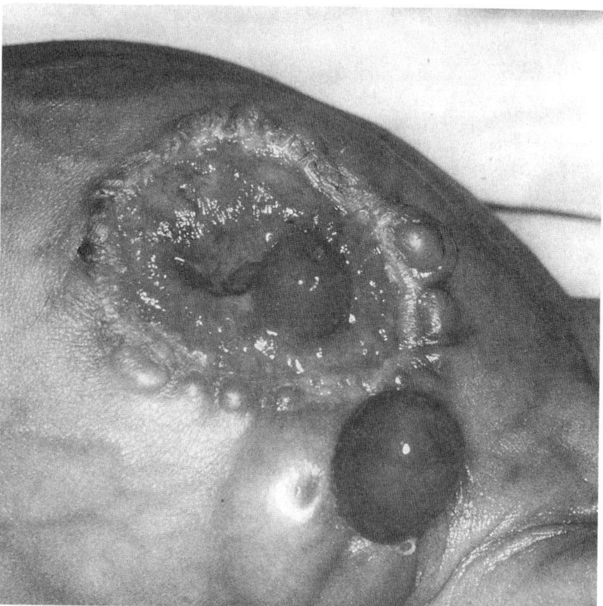

FIGURE 9 Fistulas commonly found around stomas and in wounds are difficult to treat, as shown in this baby with necrotizing enterocolitis.

ment of the esophagus may be considerable owing to reflux of secreted gastric fluids out the neck stoma.[20,21] In contrast, drainage from a neck colostomy does not produce large fluid and electrolyte losses.

Gastrostomy

Gastric fluid and electrolyte losses produce a metabolic alkalosis, but if losses of GI fluid and electrolytes occur beyond the duodenum a metabolic acidosis results. Since gastric losses of saline are generally between half and fully isotonic, and potassium and bicarbonate losses are approximately 20 mmol per liter (Table 1), gastrostomy losses must be replaced with an appropriate intravenous electrolyte solution.

The vast majority of gastrostomies are tube feeding gastrostomies, and since they are clamped when not in use, stomach losses of fluid and electrolytes are minimal. However, when a tube gastrostomy opening becomes too big, the problems of a true gastric fistula are present, as with Dr. William Beaumont and his patient Alexis St. Martin.[3] This problem, which is occasionally seen in pediatric practice, necessitates bagging of the gastric fistula and creates considerable difficulties, since the acidic nature of captured gastric fluid plays havoc with the skin. A gastric fistula acts as a flush stoma and requires surgical closure. Tube gastrostomies almost always close spontaneously following removal of the tube, unless there is distal obstruction, if the tract is lined with mucosa or if it contains a foreign body.

The more proximal the small bowel stoma, the greater are the losses of fluid and electrolytes. Duodenal stomas are almost impossible to create because of the difficulty in bringing the duodenum to the anterior abdominal wall. However, duodenal fistulas occur, most often after traumatic injury, and on occasion following elective surgery. Those high-output fistulas are difficult to bag and cause significant perifistula breakdown of the skin. If some form of constant (sump) suction can be arranged, these problems are somewhat easier to manage.

Jejunostomy

Fluid and electrolyte losses from a proximal jejunostomy virtually equal those of a duodenal fistula except for the concentration of sodium, which is lower; there are additional losses of fluid and electrolytes from both the biliary and pancreatic ducts. Replacement of electrolyte losses requires isotonic saline, 20 mmol of potassium chloride, and 30 mmol of bicarbonate per liter (Table 1). The volume of losses increases greatly when attempting to feed infants and children by mouth. Attempts to replace the proximal stomal drainage into a distal stoma (or mucous fistula) with a tube, constant drip, bolus infusion, or pump have usually met with more frustration than success. Jejunostomy stomas draining a portoenterostomy lose bile, which if possible should be replaced into the distal opening of the stoma several times a day. Tube jejunostomies are usually used for feeding and seldom cause fluid or electrolyte losses.

TABLE 1
Concentration of Electrolytes Within the Intestinal Tract (mmol/liter)

	Na	K	Cl	HCO_3
Gastric juice	60	20	100	20
Bile	140	10	100	40
Pancreatic	140	15	70	90
Jejunostomy	100	20	100	30
New ileostomy	130	20	120	20
Old ileostomy	45	5	30	—
Diarrhea	130	30	90	—

Ileostomy

With more distal small bowel stomas the body is capable of adapting to fluid and electrolyte losses, and the faster this happens, the easier it is to feed the patient. For example, in a new distal ileostomy initial losses of electrolytes are isotonic for sodium and chloride and contain 20 mmol of potassium and bicarbonate per liter, but eventually adaptation of the small bowel facilitates considerable prestomal absorption. Eventually the losses of electrolytes and intestinal water become approximately one-third of that normally passing into the ascending colon (Table 1). Owing to the potential for metabolic disorders, there has been much physiologic investigation of the ileostomy.[28–32] It has been shown, for example, that when the exposed serosa of the ileostomy "matures," fluid and electrolyte losses become markedly reduced.[1,4–7,28] Excessive losses occur only following a partial stomal obstruction, intra-abdominal sepsis, and/or resection of the distal ileum. Daily ileostomy output is closely related to body size and averages about 10 ml per kilogram per day; if the output doubles it should be considered abnormal.[1] A normally functioning ileostomy excretes two to three times the normal amount of salt and water daily, and as a result there may be a marked reduction in both urine volume and renal sodium losses. Occasionally, losses result in dizziness, nausea, and muscle cramps. If excessive, dehydration and metabolic acidosis ensue; the latter situation requires replacement with intravenous saline and potassium. Potassium losses occur only as a result of sodium depletion. Regulatory mechanisms for water absorption are not present in small bowel. Renal regulation of water absorption, on the other hand, is under the influence of antidiuretic hormone (ADH), and renal fluid absorption is usually increased in ileostomy patients, because ADH secretion increases in a state of relative dehydration. Since these patients are constantly thirsty owing to chronic dehydration, urine excretion is decreased and specific gravity is increased. Since patients with longstanding ileostomies have contracted blood and fluid volumes, should they require an operation that takes many hours (e.g., Kock pouch), either preoperative intravenous therapy or up to 10 times their normal intravenous fluids during surgery is recommended to maintain adequate urinary output. Some adaptation of ileal water absorption does occur over weeks or months, but the younger the pediatric patient, the longer this adaptive process takes.[29,31] This adaptive process takes a neonate or young infant at least three times longer than the older child and teenager; who responds as an adult patient. Adaptation enables them to maintain adequate fluid and electrolyte balance without the additional support of an intravenous fluid. Mucosal biopsies of the terminal ileum confirm morphologic adaptation; the villi increase in quantity and length. In infants, sodium losses from ileostomies average 90 mmol per kilogram stool; bicarbonate losses may also be excessive.[29,31] To offset these obligate losses, there is renal conservation of sodium by aldosterone. Nonetheless, renal conservation cannot overcome ileostomy losses, particularly if low-sodium formulas are used, and babies fail to thrive, closely mimicking cystic fibrosis patients. This problem is further exaggerated in the premature baby with an ileostomy. The process may be reversed with salt supplements to twice the normal requirements of 3 mmol per kilogram per day. Babies often suffer from chronic metabolic acidosis because, owing to excessive ileostomy losses of sodium, the kidney cannot secrete an acid urine. In this situation, a low serum sodium stimulates aldosterone to absorb even more renal sodium, but there is inadequate sodium available to exchange with hydrogen ions in the kidney tubules. Metabolic deficits of infancy can be overcome by sodium chloride and bicarbonate supplements when the urine sodium is less than 10 mmol per liter, serum bicarbonate is less than 20 mmol per liter, and serum chlorides is less than 108 mmol per liter. Replacement of stomal losses without salt invariably leads to water intoxication. Early ileostomy closure corrects the problem.

Trace Elements and Vitamins

Excessive losses of other trace elements and vitamins can occur. Losses of magnesium can induce hypomagnesemia leading to hypocalcemic tetany, but this usually manifests only when ileostomy losses are large.[4,5,29] Vitamin B_{12} absorption is reduced in 25 percent of ileostomates after 1 year, and if considerable distal ileum is resected more vitamin B_{12} is malabsorbed. Folic acid malabsorption occurs and may be due to altered intestinal bacterial flora and decreased transit time. Within 5 years of surgery urinary stones (uric acid and calcium) occur in up to 20 percent of patients, compared with a normal incidence of 4 percent.[4,28] Treatment must be directed at decreasing intestinal fluid losses pharmacologically by increasing the fluid intake and urinary output and by alkalinizing the urine. Ileal resection has a damaging effect (decreased absorption) on the enterohepatic circulation of bile acids which predisposes to gallstone formation. Eight percent of the general population have gallstones, but in those with ileostomies, the risk is increased threefold, predominantly involving cholesterol stones.[4,28] The incidence increases to 50 percent in patients who have had an ileostomy longer than 15 years. The major hematologic disorder in these children is an iron deficiency anemia that occurs for unknown reasons. Fat absorption is also influenced by an ileostomy, and daily fat losses are doubled.

Colostomy

Fortunately, with the most common pediatric stoma, a colostomy, difficulties from fluid and electrolyte disorders are minimal. The right-sided (ascending, transverse) colostomy, which is still referred to as a "wet" colostomy, can occasionally cause fluid and electrolyte imbalance in cases of rapid intestinal transit and when fluid and electrolyte losses are excessive, for example, in gastroenteritis. The left-sided (transverse, descending, sigmoid) colostomy, which is referred to as a "dry" colostomy, does not give rise to a fluid and electrolyte problem any more frequently than in the child with an intact intestinal tract (Table 1). However, postassium losses tend to increase as the fluid and electrolyte losses move distally in the pediatric colon.

Pouches

Although pelvic pouches (J and S)[33,34] do not lie proximal to a stoma as does the distal ileal continent ileostomy (Kock pouch),[33,35-39] they provide a good example of colon-like adaptation of the distal ileum due to colonization with bacteria as a result of stasis of intestinal contents. The normally functioning Kock pouch discharges 90 percent of its contents as water; within the pouch there is active absorption of sodium and chloride ions, secretion of bicarbonate ions, and active absorption of vitamin B_{12}.[35-39] Therefore, quantitative similarities exist between absorption of electrolytes from the Kock pouch and the normal ileum. However, a small group of these patients experience high fluid output from the pouch and similarly have greater losses of electrolytes, nitrogen, and fat in the feces. In addition, there may be lesser uptakes of vitamin B_{12}, a lower urinary pH, reduced urinary excretion of sodium and chloride, and a metabolic acidosis. In general, these patients act as if they have had an ileal resection proximal to the pouch, and there may be subclinical dehydration and sodium depletion due to chronic excessive salt and water losses. This type of ileostomy reservoir contains a bacterial ecology somewhere between normal feces and a conventional ileostomy. Coliforms and lactobacilli are the most common aerobes, and *Bacteroides* is the most common anaerobe. The full significance of pouch colonization by bacteria is not completely understood, but the fact that patients with Kock pouches have continued to live without problems for over 10 years seems to indicate that, if severe blind loop stasis exists in the afferent limb, it hardly ever produces clinical effects. Whether or not chronic intermittent stasis in the distal ileal pouch or the underlying disease (or both) contributes to the 10 to 20 percent incidence of pouchitis remains unknown.

Effluent Consistency

In general, the thicker the effluent, the less likely fluid and electrolyte imbalance will occur; this is especially true in the smaller pediatric patient. Jejunostomy drainage always remains liquid, but ileostomy and proximal colostomy (right-sided) drainage can be made pasty; consequently, severe fluid and electrolyte imbalance becomes virtually nonexistent. The dictum "if it is too thick to measure, it doesn't have to be measured; if it is loose enough to be measured, it should be" is a wise one. Attempts to slow the GI transit time and to thicken the stomal drainage with constipating foods (apples, rice, cheese, bananas, peanut butter) and drugs such as kaolin-pectin compound (Kaopectate) or loperamide (Imodium) are relatively safe and may be worthwhile.

SURGICAL COMPLICATIONS

There are two types of problems in pediatric ostomies: metabolic (medical) and mechanical (surgical).[40] The former have been covered under Pathophysiology and Medical Complications; mechanical complications are discussed in this section.

Tube Ostomy

Almost all complications of the tube ostomy are related to the tube itself. By far the most common tube ostomy we deal with is the gastrostomy.[3,9] If the tube becomes dislodged within the first few weeks after the ostomy was created, it must be carefully replaced using a smaller-sized Foley balloon catheter to avoid pushing the newly fixed stomach away from the anterior abdominal wall. Once the catheter has been replaced into the stomach and the balloon inflated, a radiopaque water-soluble dye study must be done to make certain the tube is indeed in the stomach and there is no leakage from the stomach. If leakage is apparent, immediate operative repair is essential. Furthermore, no manipulations, for example esophageal dilatation, should be embarked upon through a new gastrostomy until approximately 1 month postoperatively, when the site is well fixed to the anterior abdominal wall. Rubber tubes (dePezzer, Mallecot) are more difficult to replace but do not dislodge very easily. When a gastrostomy tube is replaced, care must be taken not to damage the posterior stomach wall. Balloon (Foley) catheters are safe and easy to replace, but the balloons often deflate. Newer models (MIC silicon balloon, Bard silicon button) are now frequently being used instead; their advantages include less tissue reactivity and longevity.

A significant problem may occur if a gastrostomy tube is not replaced within hours of coming out; the hole may narrow down rapidly, necessitating dilation to reaccept a regular-sized tube. Occasionally the closed gastrostomy site may have to be reopened in the operating room rather than forcing in another tube in an uncertain direction. All gastrostomy tubes must be fixed to the abdominal wall to prevent the intragastric component from entering the duodenum, thereby causing gastric outlet obstruction. Any patient with a gastrostomy who vomits must have the position of his or her gastrostomy tube checked; frequently pulling the tube back snug up against the abdominal wall solves the problem. If gastric outlet obstruction fails to explain the cause of vomiting, it must be remembered that creating the gastrostomy itself often induces gastroesophageal reflux (GER), which reportedly occurs in 44 percent of patients.[12,13] Most gastrostomies are used for feeding purposes, and eventually nutrients can be delivered by bolus. In the presence of GER, the tube feeds may have to be delivered by constant drip, or alternatively a gastrojejunostomy tube may be inserted with radiologic guidance beside the gastrostomy tube to bypass the stomach.[21] Jejunostomy feeds must, however, be delivered by slow constant drip, using an isotonic formula to avoid dumping.[5,21]

The open type of gastrostomy requires a general anesthetic, but the tube can be placed in the stomach in the desired position. Less GER results if the angle of His is maintained by placing the tube along the lesser curvature of the stomach and then suturing the stomach to the anterior abdominal wall.[14-16] The main disadvantage of the open method is the need for laparotomy. On the other hand, the incisionless gastrostomy,[3] which can be done without anesthesia, is a blind procedure, and fixation of the stomach to the anterior abdominal wall is not as secure. Bleeding and local infection may occur after any gastrostomy operation. The gastrostomy hole may enlarge and leak gastric contents and feeds onto the abdominal wall. Optimal treatment for a leaking gastrostomy requires removal of the gastrostomy tube, use of a barrier agent to protect the skin, the services of an enterostomal therapist, discontinuation of feeds, and time to allow the hole to narrow down, before replacing it with a tube of similar size. Replacing a leaking gastrostomy with a larger tube usually fails to solve the problem. Almost every gastrostomy tube develops some granulation tissue around it, particularly shortly after it has been made. Cauterization provides no permanent solution, but warm soapy washes and antibiotic ointment provide the easiest, cheapest, and most practical way of keeping the area as clean as possible.

Gaseous distention or gastric dilatation from too rapid and too large feeds may lead to considerable discomfort and/or vomiting if the esophagus is patent. However, the gastrostomy may be the only release mechanism for gas when an intact or patent esophagus is not present. These problems can easily be avoided by not pumping large volumes of feed directly into the stomach without an air vent in the system; in addition, the tube should be left open and elevated for 1 hour after each feed to allow the gas to escape and the stomach to empty.

Stomas

Skin Irritation

The most common complication of any pediatric stoma is peristomal skin irritation, the most common culprit being the incontinent flush stoma. Most intestinal stomal discharges are irritating to the skin (proximal more than distal), and if the stoma does not protrude above the skin to permit easy capture of drainage by an appliance, in time the skin invariably breaks down. Rarely a flush stoma is not a problem when there is no discharge from it, as for example in the case of a mucous fistula or the continent ileostomy (Kock pouch) (Fig. 10). Saliva from a neck esophagostomy can be irritating to the skin, but eventually the skin seems to develop a local resistance. Similar observations are made with oral sham feeds. Neck stomas from staged gastric tubes and colon replacements frequently develop peristomal irritation, either from reflux of gastric acid or from gastrostomy feeds. These problems can be eliminated by substituting gastric feedings with gastrojejunostomy tube feedings. Small bowel drainage is very irritating to the skin, especially if the stoma is proximal, and frequently the problem is aggravated by increased stomal output following feeds. Colostomies tend not to cause many skin problems, especially those on the left side of the colon, since the stool in the distal colon is firm. A common skin irritation around pediatric bowel stomas, "thrush rash," is caused by the fungus *Candida albicans* (Fig. 11). It produces a violaceous confluent raised rash that resists all forms of therapy except specific antifungal creams and ointments, which should be given in conjunction with oral antifungal agents to eradicate the intraoral source of this infection.

Prolapse

The next most common stomal complication is retrograde intussusception of the distal limb of the popular loop colostomy, or the so-called prolapsed colostomy (Fig. 12).[5,6] This complication can occur occasionally with the proximal end stoma. Inevitably this complication occurs with virtually every loop colostomy, and the length of the prolapse can vary from inches to a foot or more. Since the colostomy is the most common pediatric stoma, and since the most common colostomy made is the loop, this problems seems frequently to involve the pediatric loop colostomy.[8] Once prolapse develops, permanent reduction is hardly ever achieved.

The prolapsed colostomy has always been the most annoying and difficult mechanical problem to solve. A number of early attempts were made to remedy this problem. In 1841, Schinzinger divided the colonic loop colostomy, closed the distal end, and dropped it back into the abdomen. Subsequently other surgeons, including Madelung, Martini, Billroth, Dittel, Maydl, and Gussenbauer also adopted this maneuver.[6,18] In the 1960s the pediatric surgical literature contained a number of papers dealing with the pediatric colostomy,[18,41] and the authors seemed to take for granted Turnbull and Weakley's statement that "although prolapse of the distal limb of the loop cannot yet be prevented,. . .the complication of prolapse of the distal limb of the colostomy has been corrected only by external conversion of the loop to an end colostomy."[3] Other theories and methods of treatment have been attempted over the last 20 years. Krasna[42] thought that the colostomy prolapse occurred because the colon is very dilated before the colostomy is made, which necessitates the creation of a stomal opening appropriate for the bowel size.

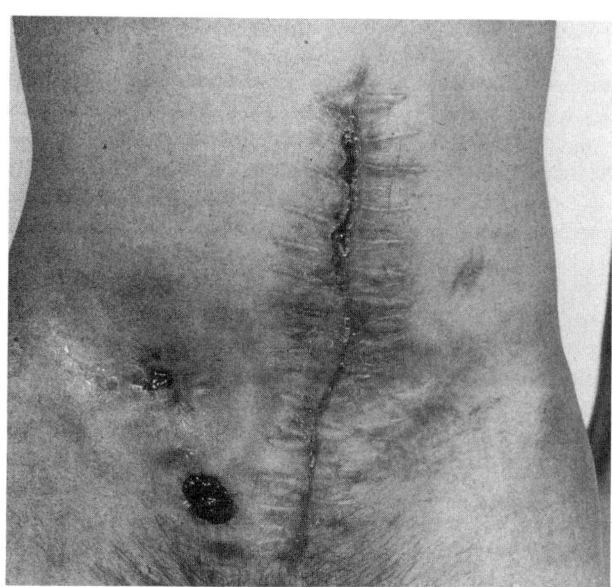

FIGURE 10 Flush Kock pouch ileostomy which is continent.

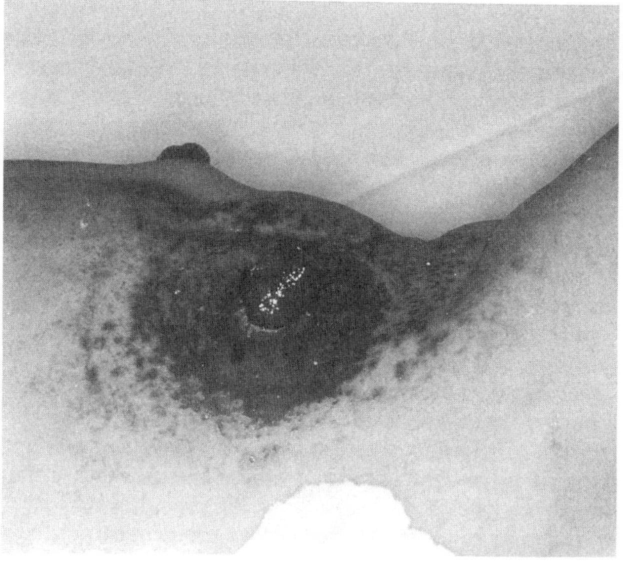

FIGURE 11 Violaceous "thrush rash" due to *Candida albicans*.

After the bowel narrows, the stomal opening becomes too large, permitting the prolapse. He addressed the problem by placing a purse-string suture subcutaneously around the stoma. It appears, therefore, that the smaller the abdominal incision for the loop stoma, the smaller the chance that it will eventually prolapse. However, no author has ventured an explanation for the consistent prolapse of only the nonfunctioning distal limb, which by definition is a retrograde intussusception. One would expect an isoperistaltic intussusception of the more actively functioning proximal colostomy limb to be the major problem.

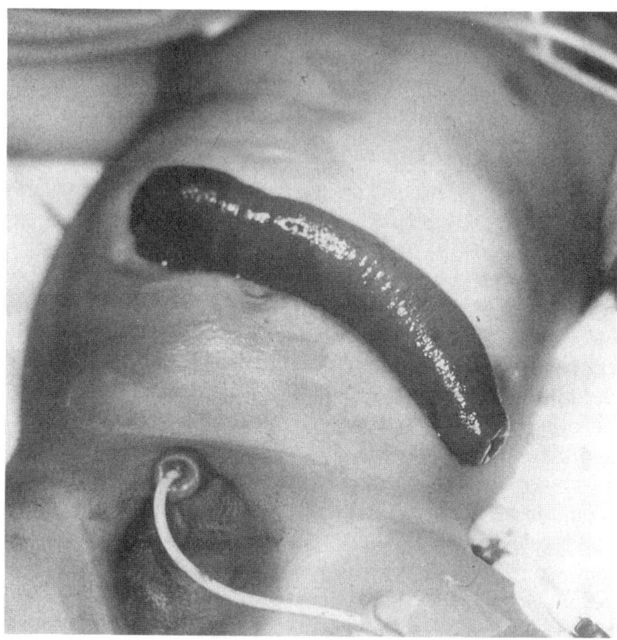

FIGURE 12 Prolapsed colostomy. Note retrograde intussusception of distal limb.

Dividing a loop colostomy and sewing the two loops together before they are matured reduces the incidence of prolapse by 50 percent (Fig. 13). Similarly, Nixon[8] reduced the incidence of colostomy prolapse by using a skin bridge between both limbs of the loop colostomy without actually dividing the loop of colon. These methods greatly reduce but do not eliminate the problem. A virtual guarantee of preventing loop stoma prolapse requires bringing the loop of bowel through the small abdominal wound, dividing the loop, then tunneling and maturing the distal limb to be adequately separated from the proximal one; left open; irrigated if needed prior to further surgery; and excluded from the appliance (see Fig. 1).[18]

Once a stoma prolapses, it is very difficult to reduce, even under general anesthesia. Even if it is successfully reduced, prolapse usually recurs, creating great inconvenience to the pediatric patient and to the care-givers. As a result, further surgery may be required to correct the prolapse, or it may be necessary to repair the distal bowel problem earlier than desired. Occasionally the unknowing or inexperienced general surgeon may excise the prolapsed bowel, making future operative repair of the distal bowel problem difficult if not impossible. Few prolapsed stomas ever become severely discolored and usually appear a bit dusky at the tip of the prolapse; occasionally there is mild blood loss or oozing from mucosal irritation. If possible, a stomal prolapse is best left alone unless it causes major problems to the patient and/or the parents.

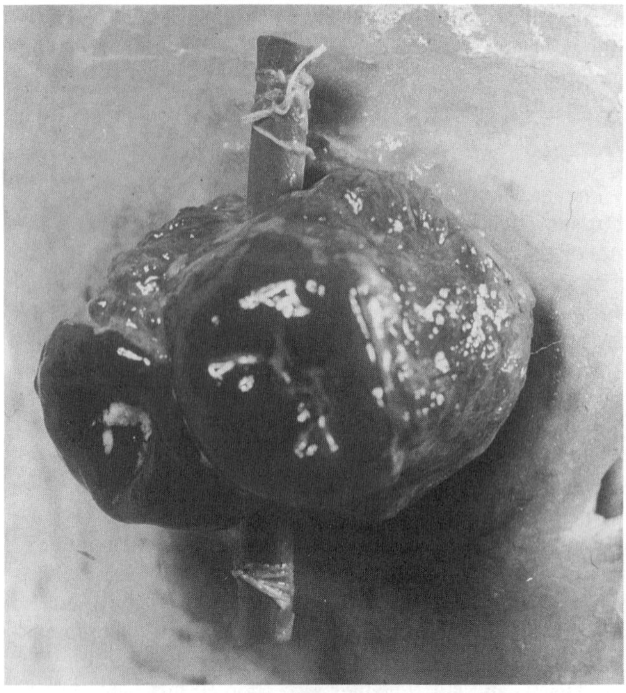

FIGURE 13 Dividing a loop colostomy, but not separating the two stomas, reduces the risk of prolapse but does not prevent it.

Retraction

Retraction of a stoma occasionally occurs, and this usually indicates that the opening of the abdominal fascial wall through which the stoma passes is too wide. Parents often assume that the bowel will disappear into the abdomen. Once a stoma retracts, it will reprotrude spontaneously and for the reasons given above will probably then prolapse. The major problem with a retracted stoma is that it becomes a flush stoma and, unless it is a continent stoma as in a Kock pouch, collection of fecal matter becomes difficult. Treatment should be temporizing, especially if the stoma is not permanent.

Obstruction

Stoma obstruction is quite common and may involve the stoma alone or may be related to the laparotomy. Stomal stricture is relatively infrequent but does occur in a few specific circumstances. A "strictured" stoma may occur only because the newborn or infant grows in size and seems to outgrow his or her stoma; it then begins to act as a partial obstruction and may require revision. Although authorities believe that strictures occur at the fascial level, the site of obstruction seems to be inconsequential—whether it is at the skin, fascial level, or both. Tight stomas need revision, especially if they are required long term. Partial stomal obstruction or "ileostomy dysfunction" causes an excessive outpouring of small bowel contents, which usually requires aggressive intravenous fluid and salt replacement together with radiologic investigations of the cause. Mechanical (abdominal wall, volvulus) or peritoneal (stomal spasm) causes should be considered.

Stomal stricture may be seen in the Kock pouch (continent ileostomy), which requires intubation (and in essence dilatation) by the patient at least three or four times a day (Fig. 14).[37] In spite of daily intubations, one of the most common complications is a mucocutaneous stricture. Regardless of suture material used or how the bowel is sewn to the skin, strictures still occasionally occur and may require revision. Kock himself puzzled over this common problem, which he said affects a proportion of all flush stomas.[1] A devascularized stoma may develop a stricture, and in infancy the most common etiology is NEC. If the stoma is functioning, it may require revision, especially if it begins to retract and obstruct the flow of feces.

Intrinsic stomal obstruction occurs occasionally, particularly in the ileostomy when a bolus of indigested food (celery, corn, fruit rinds) plugs the prestomal lumen. The obstruction can usually be unplugged digitally or with irrigations. Left-sided (dry) colostomies may become obstructed with stool, which will respond to a similar form of treatment.

Any time the abdomen is opened there remains a longstanding risk of adhesive obstruction.[43] In the pediatric patient this is manifested by bilious vomiting, abdominal distention, cramps, cessation of stomal function, and radiologic evidence of obstruction with air-fluid levels. In 80 percent of cases with adhesive small bowel obstruction, symptoms develop within 2 years of the operation. It is the most common cause of recurrent intestinal obstruction in neonates and is responsible for 7 percent of all intestinal obstructions seen in the pediatric age range. More than 50 percent of adhesive obstructions occur following laparotomy for inflammatory or neoplastic disease.[43] The risk of this type of obstruction is greatest af-

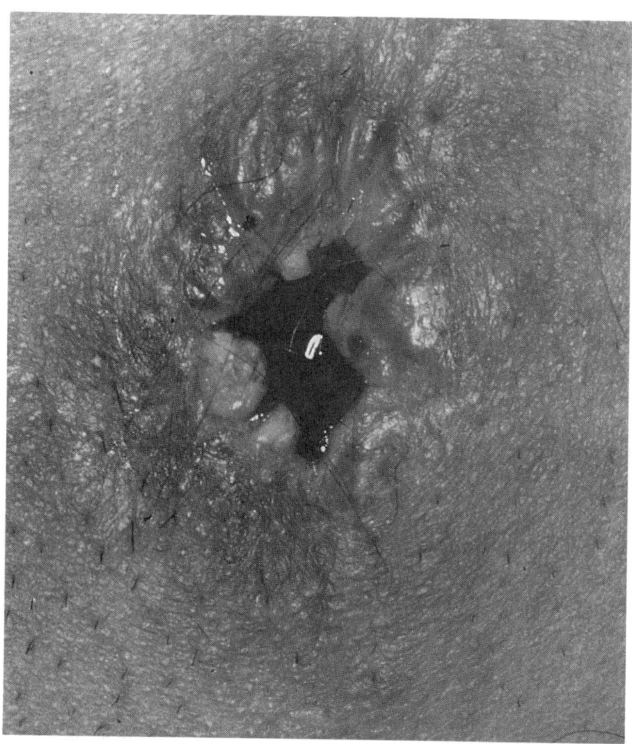

FIGURE 14 Stomal stricture in a Kock pouch flush ileostomy.

ter subtotal colectomy and ileostomy. Nasogastric decompression is usually successful in correcting the obstruction in the majority of cases, but the obstruction usually recurs in 5 percent of infants and children within 2 years. Persistent localized tenderness is the only consistent finding if the intestine becomes gangrenous. Other causes of intra-abdominal obstruction around any stoma, such as internal hernia or volvulus, must always be considered.

Infection, Hernia, and Fistula

The risk of localized infection, such as abscess or cellulitis, exists following the creation of any stoma. If creation of the stoma is planned electively, some benefit is derived from decompressing the intestinal tract with fasting and/or whole bowel irrigations,[44] in combination with perioperative prophylactic antibiotics to cover anaerobic organisms.[45] If the stoma is made during an emergency operation, proper technique combined with antibiotic prophylaxis reduces the risk of infection. If a localized infection does occur, stomal dysfunction persists until the infection is adequately treated medically and/or surgically. Stomal necrosis that occurs within the first 24 hours of surgery is a technical problem that requires immediate revision. Parastomal hernias and parastomal eviscerations are very rare. Hernias may not need revision if asymptomatic, but evisceration is a surgical emergency. Stomal and parastomal fistulas seldom occur, but once present they usually need stomal revision. They occur either from one of the sutures used to fix the stoma to the fascia or from recurrent Crohn's disease proximal to the ileostomy.

Trauma

Amazingly, trauma to the pediatric stoma, either from the unaware infant or toddler or the active child, is a rare event. Stomas are seldom damaged enough to require transfusion, suturing, and/or revision. Bleeding to hemorrhagic proportions from internal portosystemic collaterals around the jejunostomy stoma after portoenterostomy procedure for biliary atresia is a late complication. The solution to this problem is stomal closure.[22] Inflammatory polyps are often seen on pediatric stomas and probably occur from chronic mucosal irritation.[10] They seldom bleed and if troublesome can be removed with cautery. Perforations of stomas require immediate attention. They are usually externally caused, frequently being tube-related, either iatrogenically or patient induced. In incontinent stomas, perforation may occur with irrigations, and in continent stomas (Kock pouch), this complication occurs with attempts to intubate a slipped nipple valve.[3,36,38] Warning signs include immediate local pain followed by increasing peritoneal irritation. Immediate surgical repair or revision with antibiotic coverage is necessary. Needless to say, Kock pouches should be given only to mature teenagers to avoid the potential for such problems.[37,38] In general terms, an end stoma requiring revision may be repaired locally or it may require major repair by placement in a different part of the abdomen. If the stoma is the more common loop, revision may well require division and separation of the two stomas.

Patient Acceptance

Acceptance of an ostomy (especially a stoma) becomes more difficult as the child gets older. If the patient is very ill and the stoma is made on an emergency basis, it will be necessary for the health-care givers to help the child accept the stoma after the fact. On the other hand, if the stoma is a planned event, particularly when it is a permanent or long-term ileostomy for inflammatory bowel disease, it is best to allow time for the older child or teenager to accept it. The patient and his or her parents must first realize that there is no other choice. A sense of body image is crucial to the maturing child, but surprisingly, patients are often more upset by the ravaging effects of the steroids than by an ileostomy, particularly when they realize that surgical remedies may free them of their disease and the need for steroids. Early involvement of the pediatric enterostomal therapist and other specialized care-givers in the planning process is both beneficial and essential (see Part 3 of this chapter).

Ostomy Closure

Ostomy closure[46] usually brings joy to the child who is able to appreciate it and happiness to those around him or her who have struggled to treat the GI problem that required the ostomy to begin with. Stomal closure is a common procedure and is tantamount to a bowel resection. Before closure, a radiopaque contrast study must show a patent GI tract distal to the stoma. Usually preoperative preparation for a bowel resection is required along with perioperative antibiotic prophylaxis. Blood transfusion is seldom necessary. Postoperatively the GI tract is kept decompressed until the bowel distal to the stomal closure begins to function. Wound infection, anastomotic disruption, and fecal fistula are problems that occasionally arise; the most serious of these requires reestablishment of the same stoma.

REFERENCES

1. Kock NG, Darle N, Hulten L, Kewenter J, Myrvold H, Philipson B. Ileostomy. In: Ravitch MM, ed. Current problems in surgery. Chicago: Year Book, 1977: 6.
2. Gross SD. A system of surgery. Philadelphia: Blanchard and Lea, 1866.
3. Gauderer MWL, Stellato TA. Gastrostomies: evolution, techniques, indications, and complications. In: Ravitch MM, ed. Current problems in surgery. Chicago: Year Book, 1986: 659.
4. Hill GL. Ileostomy: surgery, physiology and management. New York: Grune & Stratton, 1976.
5. Kretschmer KP. The intestinal stoma. In: Ebert PA, ed. Major problems in clinical surgery. Philadelphia: WB Saunders, 1978: 1.
6. Turnbull RB Jr, Weakley FL. Atlas of intestinal stomas. St. Louis: CV Mosby, 1967.
7. Brooke BM. Conventional ileostomy. Historical prospectives. In: Dozois RR, ed. Alternatives to conventional ileostomy. Chicago: Year Book, 1985: 19.
8. Nixon HH. Paediatric problems associated with stomas. Intestinal surgical procedures. In: Brooke BN, Jeter KF, Todd IP, eds. Stomas. Clinics in gastroenterology. London: WB Saunders, 1982: 351.
9. Gasson JE. Feeding stomas: gastrostomy and jejunostomy. Surgical procedures and complications. In: Brooke BN, Jeter KF, Todd IP, eds. Stomas. Clinics in gastroenterology. London: WB Saunders, 1982: 337.
10. Thomson JPS. Caecostomy and colostomy. Surgical procedures and complications. In: Brooke BN, Jeter KF, Todd IP, eds. Stomas. Clinics in gastroenterology. London: WB Saunders, 1982: 285.
11. Shaw A. Letter to editor. J Pediatr Surg 1982; 17:685.
12. Langer JC, Wesson DE, Ein SH, Filler RM, Shandling B, Superina RA, Papa M. Feeding gastrostomy in neurologically impaired children: is an antireflux procedure necessary? J Pediatr Gastroenterol Nutr 1988; 7:837–841.
13. Jolley SG, Tunell WP, Hoelzer DJ, Thomas S, Smith EI. Lower esophageal pressure changes with tube gastrostomy: A causative factor of gastroesophageal reflux in children? J Pediatr Surg 1986; 21:624–627.
14. Bardaji C, Boix-Ochoa J. Contribution of the His angle to the gastroesophageal antireflux mechanism. Pediatr Surg Int 1986; 1:172–176.
15. Boerema I. Hiatus hernia: repair by right-sided, subhepatic anterior gastropexy. Surgery 1969; 65:884–893.
16. Heij HA, Vos A. Long-term results of anterior gastropexy for gastroesophageal reflux in children. Pediatr Surg Int 1988; 4:256–259.
17. Irving M. The Brooke ileostomy and loop and split ileostomies. In: Brooke BN, Jeter KF, Todd IP, eds. Stomas. Clinics in gastroenterology. London: WB Saunders, 1982: 237.
18. Ein SH. Divided loop colostomy that does not prolapse. Am J Surg 1984; 147:250–252.
19. DeVries PA. Complications of surgery for congenital anomalies of the anorectum. In: DeVries PA, Shapiro SR, eds. Complications of pediatric surgery. New York: John Wiley, 1982: 233.
20. Ein SH, Shandling B, Simpson JS, Stephens CA. A further look at the gastric tube as an esophageal replacement in infants and children. J Pediatr Surg 1973; 8:859–868.
21. Ein SH, Shandling B, Simpson JS, Stephens CA, Vizas D. Fourteen years of gastric tubes. J Pediatr Surg 1978; 13:638–642.
22. Weber TR, Grosfeld JL. Contemporary management of biliary atresia. Surg Clin North Am 1981; 61:1079–1088.
23. Wilmore DW. Factors correlating with a successful outcome following extensive intestinal resection in newborn infants. J Pediatr 1972; 80: 88–95.
24. Hendry WF. Urinary stomas. Surgical procedures and complications. In: Brooke BN, Jeter KF, Todd IP, eds. Stomas. Clinics in gastroenterology. London: WB Saunders, 1982: 303.
25. Mitchell ME, Rink RC. In: Sheldon CA, Churchill MB, eds. Management principles in pediatric urology. Pediatric clinics of North America. Philadelphia: WB Saunders, 1987: 1319.
26. Cameron GS, Lau GYP. The umbilicus as a site for temporary colostomy in infants. J Pediatr Surg 1982; 17:362–364.
27. Irving M, Beadle C. External intestinal fistulas: nursing care and surgical procedures. In: Brooke BN, Jeter KF, Todd IP, eds. Stomas. Clinics in gastroenterology. London: WB Saunders, 1982: 327.
28. Hill GL. Metabolic complications of ileostomy. In: Brooke BN, Jeter KF, Todd IP, eds. Stomas. Clinics in gastroenterology. London: WB Saunders, 1982: 260.
29. Bower TR, Pringle KC, Soper RT. Sodium deficit causing decreased weight gain and metabolic acidosis in infants with ileostomy. J Pediatr Surg 1988; 23:567–572.
30. Kennedy HJ, Callender ST, Truelove SC, Warner GT. Haematological aspects of life with an ileostomy. Br J Haematol 1982; 52:445–454.
31. Rothstein FC, Halpin TC Jr, Klegman RJ, Izant RJ Jr. Importance of early ileostomy closure to prevent chronic salt and water losses after necrotizing enterocolitis. Pediatrics 1982; 70:249–253.
32. Hill GL. Physiology of conventional ileostomy. In: Dozois RR, ed. Alternatives to conventional ileostomy. Chicago: Year Book, 1985: 29.
33. Goligher JC. The quest for continence in the surgical treatment of ulcerative colitis. In: Jordan GL Jr, ed. Advances in surgery. Chicago: Year Book, 1980: 53.
34. Rothenberger DA, Wong WD, Buls JG, Goldberg SM. The S ileal pouch-anal anastomosis. In: Dozois RR, ed. Alternatives to conventional ileostomy. Chicago: Year Book, 1985: 345.
35. Kock NG. Continent ileostomy. Historical perspective. In: Dozois RR, ed. Alternatives to conventional ileostomy. Chicago: Year Book, 1985: 133.
36. Kock NG, Myrvold HE, Nilsson LO, Philipson BM. Continent ileostomy: The Swedish experience. In: Dozois RR, ed. Alternatives to conventional ileostomy. Chicago: Year Book, 1985: 163.
37. Ein SH. Five years of the pediatric Kock pouch. J Pediatr Surg 1982; 17:644–652.
38. Ein SH. A ten-year experience with the pediatric Kock pouch. J Pediatr Surg 1987; 22:764–766.
39. Phillips SF. Continent ileostomy. Altered physiology. In: Dozois RR, ed. Alternatives to conventional ileostomy. Chicago: Year Book, 1985: 146.
40. Todd IP. Mechanical complications of ileostomy. In: Brooke BN, Jeter KF, Todd IP, eds. Stomas. Clinics in gastroenterology. London: WB Saunders, 1982: 268.
41. Cain WS, Kiesewetter WB. Infant colostomy. Arch Surg 1965; 91: 314–320.
42. Krasna IH. A simple purse string suture technique for treatment of colostomy prolapse and intussusception. J Pediatr Surg 1979; 14:801–802.
43. Janik JS, Ein SH, Filler RM, Shandling B, Simpson JS, Stephens CA. An assessment of the surgical treatment of adhesive small bowel obstruction in infants and children. J Pediatr Surg 1981; 16:225–229.
44. Postuma R. Whole bowel irrigation in pediatric patients. J Pediatr Surg 1982; 17:350–352.
45. Sandusky WR. Use of prophylactic antibiotics in surgical patients. Surg Clin North Am 1980; 60:83–92.
46. Kiely EM, Sparnon AL. Stoma closure in infants and children. Pediatr Surg Int 1987; 2:95–97.

PART 3

Ostomy Care

Patricia Fyvie, R.N., E.T.

The realization that children are not just small adults is nowhere so apparent as in the pediatric medical setting, and all aspects of care should be focused on the child's special needs. Caring for children with ostomies and supporting their concerned families requires some particular skills. This care is best provided by a health care team consisting of many members. Each team member has a specific role to play to achieve a common goal—to provide the very best medical care and emotional support, the end result being a child that returns to a state of good health and independence. A key team member is the enterostomal therapist, who brings to this role the skills of a nurse with special training in the care of persons undergoing ostomy surgery. The enterostomal therapist provides preoperative counseling, postoperative management, and rehabilitative care.[1] The physical and psychological changes that occur as children pass through the normal stages of growth and development must be carefully considered when caring for children with ostomies. The implications of ostomy surgery for infants, young children, and adolescents vary according to the patient's age and present particular challenges to the nurse working in the pediatric setting. Similarly, the role that the parents play in the care and rehabilitation of their special child must be recognized.

PREOPERATIVE COUNSELING

Nothing contributes more to a successful outcome than early preparation for ostomy surgery. The earlier the involvement of the enterostomal therapist in the care of the child being prepared for ostomy surgery, the better the results in terms of the child's adjustment following surgery.[2] To help the parents and children with the educational process, a variety of useful printed resource material is available from several manufacturers (Table 1).

Infants

In newborn infants, ostomy surgery is most often performed as one of a number of corrective steps in the treatment of a congenital anomaly.[3,4] For example, imperforate anus or Hirschsprung's disease frequently requires emergency surgery. In these circumstances, the infant is often taken from the mother's side and transferred to another center where his or her special needs can be met. Nothing prepares the family to deal with this unexpected crisis. The bonding process the mother has been developing with her child during pregnancy comes to an abrupt halt. Early intervention by the enterostomal therapist helps to alleviate parental fears regarding the care of the ostomy and their special child. Frequently, initial contact is made with another member of the family, usually with the father. The enterostomal therapist must provide a clear, simple explanation of the nature of the surgery and his or her role in the care of the infant, because it is this information that is transmitted to the mother and upon which she bases her immediate understanding of their infant's special needs.

Whatever the circumstances surrounding the birth of the infant requiring an ostomy (young single mother or parents

TABLE 1
Printed Resource Material for Children Undergoing Ostomy Surgery and Their Families

Title	Publisher	Comments
Ostomy and Your Child—A Parent's Guide	Convatec-Division of Squibb, Inc	Accurate facts about ostomies. Addresses parents' concerns.
Living with an Ostomy—The Teenage Years	Convatec-Division of Squibb, Inc	Accurate facts about ostomies. Addresses concerns teenagers have regarding ostomy surgery.
All About Jimmy by Carol Norris, Ph.D.	United Ostomy Association	Coloring book that illustrates types of ostomies. Appropriate for school-age children.
The Sneetches and Other Stories by Dr. Seuss	Random House (1961) Toronto, Ontario	Excellent story line for younger children with ostomies. Stimulates discussion.
These Special Children by Katherine Jeter	Bull Publishing Co. (1982) Palo Alto, CA	Resource information for children and parents. Informs, counsels, and comforts. Good for teachers and health-care professionals.

of different cultural beliefs), well-timed, early intervention by the enterostomal therapist can assist the family in coping with this crisis.[5]

Young Children

In the past 5 to 10 years, changing trends in surgical management of various urologic conditions have resulted in a significant decrease in the use of urinary diversions, but the number of young children requiring fecal diversions has increased.[6] For example, it has been recognized that ileostomy surgery in children with severe chronic ulcerative colitis may, on occasion, be preferable to chronic steroid medication, with its attendant side effects.[7,8] Nevertheless, uncertainty regarding the effects of ostomy surgery can have a devastating effect on a young child's family. The child and his family must be approached in a confident, reassuring manner, because often attitudes toward ostomies and ostomy surgery are based upon concepts developed during the initial contact. The child should be directly involved in any discussion about the surgery and an explanation provided at the child's level of understanding. The use of a teaching doll or line drawings is recommended.[8] Often, it is the child's favorite stuffed animal that becomes the model for a demonstration of a pouch application. During the explanation, the experienced enterostomal therapist recognizes the child's needs for maintaining control and independence while still allowing for a parent-child relationship to exist.

Teenagers

It is difficult to convince a teenager who is about to have major abdominal surgery with the creation of an ostomy that this procedure is going to dramatically improve his or her health. However, those who have suffered from the chronic effects of inflammatory bowel disease usually develop a very positive attitude toward surgery once they understand that they will feel better, look better, and regain lost independence.[7]

Once the physician and the family have discussed the need for surgery and the teenager has been informed of this possibility, the enterostomal therapist should be directly involved in the patient's preoperative assessment and care. All pertinent medical, psychological, and social data should be collected prior to visiting the patient's bedside. The enterostomal therapist's first and immediate role is to alleviate any misconceptions that the child and family may have regarding the effects of the surgery. In the author's experience, if time permits, making a series of short visits over a period of days preoperatively is more effective than one long visit on the day immediately prior to surgery.

The fact that the ostomy will be created from the child's own healthy bowel often comes as a surprise. Most children suffering from the effects of inflammatory bowel disease are frequently on limited or restricted diets, and they are surprised to learn that very few dietary restrictions will be imposed upon them postoperatively. In addition, it is hard for them to believe that they will be able to take part in normal activities following surgery. Swimming certainly seems to be out of the question. One must constantly reassure the child and his family that the planned surgery will invariably result in a healthier, more independent life-style.

Determination of preconceived notions is best achieved by asking the patient a simple question "Could you tell me what the doctor told you about your operation?" The use of simple diagrams to describe the nature of the surgery and/or the portion of the bowel that will be removed is extremely helpful, but their use obviously depends upon the age of the child. Other immediate questions the teenager might have include: "What will the stoma look like?" "How much pain will I have after the operation?" and "What is a pouch?" They need to be made aware that the stoma is red in appearance and that it will bleed slightly. In addition, it is important to emphasize that there are no sensory nerves in the stoma capable of causing pain.

Teenagers are particularly interested in the actual appearance of the pouch and where it will be positioned on the abdomen. Stoma models that are available from ostomy product manufacturers (for example, United Surgical Ltd., a division of Smith & Nephew, Inc., and Convatec, a division of Squibb, Inc.) are useful aids in the explanation of the appearance of the stoma and in the application of the appliance. The pouch itself is always of interest, and a demonstration sample should be available at the time of the preoperative visit.

The opportunity to meet another teenager who has undergone ostomy surgery is strongly encouraged for emotional support. However, the patient must be selected with great care in order to match age, sex, ethnic background, and personalities of the particular child. Even in large centers where many children undergo ostomy surgery, it is not always possible to arrange a visit, because frequently when the children have returned to a state of good health and emotional adjustment following ostomy surgery, they are too preoccupied with their daily living to visit at a moment's notice. In certain cases, however, this opportunity should be aggressively pursued, since it often proves invaluable.

STOMA SITE SELECTION

Preoperative preparation of a child for ostomy surgery is not complete without one final step—the selection of the stoma site. This presents a special challenge, as there is no room for error on a small abdomen. The assessment necessary to determine the appropriate stoma site cannot be done in the operating room, so it is important that there be good communication between the surgeon and the enterostomal therapist prior to surgery. This step should be carried out well before surgery, in a relaxed, nonthreatening manner. Several excellent resources are available to assist in the understanding of stoma site selection.[9,10]

A few guidelines should be followed no matter what the age of the patient. The stoma is usually located below the belt line, in the right or left lower quadrant, away from bony prominences, scars, and skin folds. Because creases and wrinkles are often not apparent when the child is recumbent, the site is best selected after the abdomen has been examined with the child in other positions—sitting, standing and bending. If body creases are seen to come across the selected site, then the stoma site must be relocated. The site must be positioned where the child can see it to facilitate self-care when it is appropriate to the child's age. In infants, stoma sites are often constructed above the umbilicus in the upper right or left quadrant.

The use of braces or other devices worn across the stoma site must be accounted for, and in some cases this requires relocating the site or adjusting the device. The selected site is carefully marked using a waterproof permanent marker pen. A well-constructed and appropriately placed stoma permits the appliance to adhere well and maintain healthy peristomal skin. This results in a comfortable, confident child.

POSTOPERATIVE CARE

No matter how well prepared the patient and family are, the first sight of the stoma is frequently a frightening experience. Not uncommonly, a teenager refuses to look at the stoma for a few days and expresses feelings of disgust about its appearance and the pouch contents at the first peek. The first postoperative pouch application (in the operating room or on the ward) may or may not resemble the one that will be selected for long-term management. It will be transparent, odor-proof and drainable. This allows direct inspection of the stoma as well as the drainage, without the need for removing it during the first 24 to 72 hours. Once recovery from the early effects of surgery has occurred, the patient and/or the parents should be encouraged to become directly involved with the care of the ostomy.

Although each child has unique characteristics, he or she shares traits of growth and development with other children of similar age. Obviously, the teaching approach and postoperative care of each child will be determined by age, physical and psychological growth and development, and the family's acceptance of his condition.[6,11,12] Although each age group's characteristics must be considered, some common, basic principles must be adhered to in order to (1) minimize obstacles to mastering ostomy care; (2) encourage participation by the child and the family; (3) provide support and guidance; and (4) maximize the child's self-esteem and body image appropriate to age.[11] The needs and concerns of the family must be considered as well. It has been demonstrated that children adjust better and feel less isolated when all family members are included in the teaching process. However, the parents of a newborn who has undergone ostomy surgery must have the opportunity to reach some level of acceptance before they are introduced to the technical aspects of ostomy care. The more the child and his family know about the anatomy and function of the ostomy, the more confident they will become. At first, following creation of a new stoma, the patient and his family will find ostomy care to be a considerable challenge, but once the basic techniques are mastered, the mechanics of changing the pouch should become a simple routine.

TABLE 2
Some Commonly Used Pediatric Ostomy Appliances

Appliance*	Features
Bongort Pouch (Smith & Nephew—United)	Adhesive backing; skin barrier can be added No precut stoma opening; allows opening to be placed off-center to avoid suture lines or drainage tubes Available in several sizes; drainable and urostomy pouches Appropriate for infants Small pediatric pouch for premature infants
Pediatric Pouch (Hollister, Inc)	Same as Bongort pouch; not available as urostomy pouch One size only Appropriate for infants
Sur-Fit System (Convatec-Division of Squibb, Inc)	Available in two-piece system (flange and pouch) Skin barrier attached Pouch may be changed without removing flange from skin Closed, drainable, or urostomy pouch Appropriate for older children
"Little Ones"	Smaller version appropriate for infants and young children
Sur-Fit System "Active Life" (Convatec-Division of Squibb, Inc)	Available in one-piece system Pre-cut stomal opening Same features as Sur-Fit System, but pouch size/style cannot be changed without removing appliance from skin
"Little Ones"	A smaller version available for infants and young children
Drainage Pouch (Dansac, Denmark)	One-piece system with adhesive flange Skin barrier can be added Available in several pouch sizes/styles
Mini-pouch (Nu-Hope Labs, Inc)	One-piece system with adhesive foam pad Used with or without additional skin barrier Available in drainable or urostomy pouch

*Disposable appliances are preferred; reusable appliances with convex face plates are available for children with ostomies whose construction or location makes it difficult to obtain a secure seal.

TABLE 3
Accessory Ostomy Products

Product	Use	Examples
Skin sealants (wipes, sprays gels, liquids)	Protective film over skin surrounding ostomy Aids adherence of pouch and tape to skin	Skin Prep (United Surgical) Skin Gel (Hollister, Inc) Sween Prep (Sween, Inc)
Skin barriers (wafers, powders, pastes)	Provides protective barrier over skin Increases adhesion Paste fills uneven areas or acts as caulking around base of ostomy	Stomahesive paste (Convatec) Stomahesive wafer (Convatec) Stomahesive powder (Convatec) Premium wafer (Hollister, Inc) Premium paste (Hollister, Inc) Colly-Seel (Mason Labs) Comfeel (Smith & Nephew)
Adhesives (sprays, liquids, and double-sided discs)	Adds adherent strength to appliances Adds adhesive surface to reusable flanges	Medical Spray Adhesive (Hollister, Inc) Skin Bond Cement (United Surgical) Double-faced disc (Marlen, United Surgical)
Convex Inserts (different sizes)	Adds convexity to appliance by applying pressure on skin around base of stoma	Numerous companies
Belts	Adds support (infrequently used on children)	Numerous companies
Tapes	Adds support; waterproofing	Numerous companies

Adapted from Role of the enterostomal nurse. In: Bayless TM, ed. Current management of inflammatory bowel disease. Toronto: BC Decker, 1989.

In the immediate postoperative period, initial stoma assessment and selection of the appropriate appliance should be carried out by the enterostomal therapist. The normal characteristics of the stoma, which were discussed preoperatively, should be reviewed with the child and his family. The selected appliance must protect the surgical incision from stomal drainage. It must adhere securely to the abdomen in order to protect the peristomal skin and to provide protection against odor. It must fit comfortably and be inconspicuously concealed under clothing. The appliance should require a minimal amount of time to apply and be as simple to apply as possible. The appliance and all necessary accessories must be readily available from a supplier in the community. Commonly used appliances and accessory products are itemized in Tables 2 and 3.

Infants

Until recently, very few appropriately sized appliances were available for infants. In recent years, however, with the introduction of new pediatric appliances, the technical aspects of changing pouches have been greatly simplified. The optimal appliance must be capable of protecting the fragile skin from the effects of drainage from the ostomy and must be easily emptied between changes. A well-fitting appliance should remain secure for 24 to 48 hours. Several manufacturers produce pouches of appropriate dimensions to fit an infant or young child's abdomen and offer skin barriers that are flexible enough to contour nicely to the child's body (Tables 2 and 3).

Until recently no appropriately sized appliances were available for tiny premature infants. Certain creativity is helpful when devising appliances in these special situations. Condom catheters as pouches and convex inserts as faceplates have been utilized, but with limited success in achieving a secure seal for any length of time.[7,11] A small pouch is manufactured by Smith & Nephew—United which is appropriate for the very small, premature infant (Table 2).

Although meticulous care of the ostomy is absolutely imperative in the immediate postoperative period, adequate attention must also be given to the needs and care of the baby and his family. Frequently, the needs of the parents of an ill newborn infant are complicated by various social and medical factors. Some parents readily accept the special circumstances of their baby's condition, whereas others first undergo a process of total rejection. The vast majority of parents need constant reassurance and time to work through their feelings.[11] Thus, the enterostomal therapist must support the family as they learn new skills, which invariably previous experience has not provided. Once the basic techniques have been mastered, they will be surprised to discover how easy the technical aspects of stomal care can become. Management of the ostomy must be individualized according to the infant's special needs, and the overall objectives should enhance a positive effect on the child's well-being and his relationship with his parents.

Young Children

A young child presents some unique problems to those caring for his or her ostomy.[7] Nothing can or should prevent an active child from crawling, climbing, and falling. The young child's parents need constant reassurance that the stoma will not be injured during normal activity. The appliance must adhere extremely well to the child's abdomen and be of appropriate size so that it can be easily concealed under clothing. Busy fingers frequently encounter little difficulty in finding the pouch under clothing, so in this age group it is best to keep it well covered.

Obviously, it is important to encourage an environment that affords a feeling of security and trust for the young child. During a pouch change, it is best to establish a regular routine and to prepare the appliance for application before directly involving the child. Appropriate toys should be provided to divert the child's attention. Once an appropriate routine is established in hospital, the same routine should be followed at home. Toddlers should be allowed the opportunity to participate in their care, if only in a minor way. Changing a pouch on their favorite doll might provide them with emotional support, allow them an opportunity to express their feelings about the ostomy, and help them to better understand their circumstances. It is essential that the appliance remain secure during normal activity, since a leaking appliance can lead to ridicule by their playmates.

When the child reaches school age, having an ostomy assumes even greater significance.[6] Teachers and peers may have difficulty in accepting the child as a healthy, normal individual. It is essential for a member of the school staff to be informed of the child's circumstances and to provide assistance if the need arises. However, it is not necessary to inform everyone. The need for privacy when changing a leaking appliance must be considered. The older child should be permitted to decide who to tell about the ostomy and should be encouraged to provide the information if and when the need arises.

Ostomy supplies should be kept at school in case an emergency situation arises. Despite the child's special needs, every other aspect of his educational, emotional, and social development should be regarded as no different from those of his classmates. Inevitably, the size of the appliance will have to be altered to accommodate growth; regular assessment is best carried out by the enterostomal therapist, who in turn will determine the necessary adjustments. By 6 years of age, a young child should be expected to perform most of the routine care of the ostomy and by 10 years of age, care should be completely independent.

Teenagers

When selecting the appropriate appliance for a teenager, one must consider his or her activities carefully. Most commonly used appliances are the same as those selected for adults (Table 2). However, a smaller pouch size may be more appropriate if the teenager is involved in a sport in which the appliance must be concealed under a gymnastic outfit or a bathing suit. Alternatively, a smaller nondrainable pouch may be used during a specific activity. Heavy contact sports such as football or hockey require careful consideration. Adapting an abdominal support to protect the stoma site during contact sports is recommended to provide additional protection. If preparation for discharge from hospital has achieved its objectives, the teenager leaves the hospital feeling confident in the technical aspects of his or her new responsibility.

Except for the first 2 years of life, there is no other time when growth and development move so rapidly as in the early teenage years. Developmental changes are often typically baffling to the adolescent and also to the parents.[12] During this time of onset and development of puberty, dramatic physical, physiologic, and behavioral changes occur that transform a child into a young adult. Even under the best of circumstances, one may expect the adolescent to be paradoxical, inconsistent, rebellious, and unpredictable. He or she is no longer willing to take adult viewpoints on faith. Thus, it is not surprising that the difficulties facing the young adolescent can be quite overwhelming if the need for an ostomy arises. Adolescents are developing strong peer relationships and are often becoming emancipated from their immediate family. Most adolescents who cannot form close relationships or fit into a group feel lonely, unhappy, and isolated. Frequently, following ostomy surgery, a sequence of rejection, adjustment, and acceptance occurs.[12] However, if the individual patient had a poor self-image and low self-esteem before the need for an ostomy occurred, it may be necessary to involve specially trained members of the health care team to assist in making appropriate adjustments.

Any physical change in a teenager's appearance can have a devastating effect on body image and the adolescent's ability to form peer relationships.[13] Children who have been taking steroids chronically for inflammatory bowel disease are often already dealing with the adverse visual and physical effects of these drugs. Frequently, the adolescent with an illness that has made surgery necessary is suffering from impaired growth, delayed pubertal development, and symptoms of fatigue, abdominal cramps, diarrhea, and other discomforts. These symptoms usually resolve following surgery, and the adjustment to the ostomy is made easier by a relative feeling of well-being. Once a general feeling of health has been restored and the technical aspects of ostomy care have been mastered, most teenagers find that their daily activities and interests are not impinged upon by the presence of an ostomy.

Surprisingly, family members are often slower to adjust to their child's new circumstances. They are usually overprotective, but once they are able to see their child gain confidence in the technical aspects of ostomy care and learn more about ostomies themselves, their concerns are alleviated. To what extent the presence of an ostomy affects peer relationships varies considerably with the individual. Whether or not close friends should be told about the ostomy remains an individual choice. A prolonged period of time may be necessary for the young adolescent to accept the changes in body image; friends cannot be expected to adjust any sooner. Newer appliances can be easily concealed under the fashionable and trendy clothes most teenagers like to wear, and there should be no fear that the child's appearance will isolate him or her from friends. Constant encouragement to participate in normal activities of daily living, without undue restrictions, is of vital importance in helping the teenager to adjust and move toward developing meaningful peer relationships. Solid peer relationships in turn reflect how well the individual patient has adjusted with respect to a new body image.

REHABILITATION AND FOLLOW-UP CARE

The supportive relationship between the enterostomal therapist, the child, and his family must be maintained following the child's discharge from hospital. Stoma problems may

TABLE 4
Common Peristomal Problems*

Problem	Cause	Solution
Chemical	Exposure to effluent (stool, urine)	Protect skin from effluent with skin barrier of appropriate opening size (1/16"–1/8" larger than stoma).
	Adhesives, solvents, cleansing agents	Change brand of adhesive, solvent, or cleansing agent. Follow instructions for application closely.
Mechanical	Pressure	Appropriate use of belt (should not slip or be too tight).
	Friction	Select a well-adhering appliance.
	Stripping of barriers, adhesives, and tapes from skin	Reinforce methods of removing barriers, adhesives, and tapes. Do not change more than every 3 to 5 days.
Allergic	Sensitive to parts of appliance, skin barriers, or sealants	Patch test if no obvious visual cause. Substitute with product patient tolerates.
Infectious	Fungal (*Candida* common in children)	Identify source (check mouth, urine, or stool).
	Bacterial (rare)	Mycostatin powder (dust and rub well into affected areas). Severity of infection determines frequency of application.
Leakage	Incorrect size of pouch opening	Opening size of pouch 1/16"–1/8" larger than stoma size.
	Retracted stoma	Use barrier, paste, convex insert.
	Scars or creases near stoma	May require stoma relocation.
	Poor application techniques	Review proper technique.
	Appliance worn too long	Reduce appliance wearing time.
	Excessive perspiration	Use skin sealant.
Itching	Allergy	Identify cause (patch test).
	Leakage	Cleanse skin; remove all soap residue; dry well.
	Inadequate skin cleansing	Expose skin to air. Apply recommended skin creams.

*Adapted from Role of the enterostomal nurse. In: Bayless TM, ed. Current management of inflammatory bowel disease. Toronto: BC Decker, 1989.

occur. Frequently, these problems can be prevented, or early solutions provided, when regular follow-up care is available. Problems like stoma retraction or prolapse most often require a referral to the surgeon, whereas problems related to peristomal skin irritation can be managed by early intervention with the enterostomal therapist (Table 4).

Infants

Since most infants require temporary ostomies, appropriately sized appliances are fitted for the entire time required. Frequently, this period is no more than 6 to 8 months. If corrective surgery is delayed, it may be necessary to change the appliance in order to accommodate growth and increased activity. This ensures a secure system with a larger capacity. The relationship between the enterostomal therapist and the family must be such that the family feels comfortable enough to seek assistance in the selection of appropriate appliances to meet the child's changing needs.

Young Children

As is the case in infancy, young children's needs change as they continue to grow. For example, when considering an appliance change in a 6-year-old, one must consider the fact that the time has arrived for the child to become directly involved in ostomy care. In order to accommodate increasing independence, the selected appliance must be simple to apply and easy to empty. Because the parents have previously been caring for the ostomy themselves, they are often reluctant to relinquish direct responsibility to their "baby." Nevertheless, if it is anticipated that the child in question will continue to have an ostomy during his or her formative years, when body image and self-esteem play such a vital role in growth and development, it is essential to encourage the family to pass on increasing responsibility for certain aspects of ostomy care to the child. In this author's experience, the positive effect of increasing responsibilities on the child's body image and self-esteem is immeasurable.

Teenagers

Although most teenagers are confident in the technical aspects of ostomy care at discharge from hospital, some psychosocial issues may remain unresolved. Once they leave the secure environment of the hospital, the greatest fear they have is rejection by their family and friends.[11-13] However, they usually discover that this fear is unfounded. In most cases, when they do share knowledge of the ostomy with a close friend, they discover considerable support. The role of the enterostomal therapist becomes less significant as the teenager gains self-confidence and develops a positive body image and increased self-esteem in the months following surgery.

SUMMARY

Regardless of the child's age or reasons for an ostomy, the goals of therapy are the same—to provide the very best in preoperative counseling, postoperative management, and rehabilitative care to the child and family. To see an ill child returned to a state of good health and to support the entire family while they master new skills and coping mechanisms is the enterostomal therapist's greatest reward.

REFERENCES

1. Jackson BS, Broadwell DC. Role of the enterostomal therapy practitioner. In: Broadwell DC, Jackson BS, eds. Principles of ostomy care. St Louis: CV Mosby, 1982: 8.
2. Boarini JH. Preoperative considerations. In: Broadwell DC, Jackson BS, eds. Principles of ostomy care. St Louis: CV Mosby, 1982: 321.
3. Goode PS. Nursing management of disorders of the gastrointestinal system. In: Broadwell DC, Jackson BS, eds. Principles of ostomy care. St Louis: CV Mosby, 1982: 257.
4. King AW. Nursing management of stomas of the genitourinary tract. In: Broadwell DC, Jackson BS, eds. Principles of ostomy care. St. Louis: CV Mosby, 1982: 290.
5. Levitt MB. Families at risk: primary prevention in nursing practice. Boston: Little, Brown, 1982.
6. Smith AM. Genitourinary pathophysiology. In: Broadwell DC, Jackson BS, eds. Principles of ostomy care. St. Louis: CV Mosby, 1982: 206.
7. Motta GJ. Life span changes: implications for ostomy care. Nursing Clin North Am June 1987; 22:333–339.
8. Jeter KF. The children. In: These special children. Palo Alto: Bull, 1982: 46.
9. Turnbull RP, Weakley FL. Colectomy and ileostomy for ulcerative colitis. In: Atlas of intestinal stomas. St. Louis: CV Mosby, 1967: 7.
10. Watt RC. Stoma placement. In: Broadwell DC, Jackson BS, eds. Principles of ostomy care. St. Louis: CV Mosby, 1982: 329.
11. Jeter KF. The paediatric patient: ostomy surgery in growing children. In: Broadwell DC, Jackson BS, eds. Principles of ostomy care. St. Louis: CV Mosby, 1982: 489.
12. Bolinger BL. The adolescent patient. In: Broadwell DC, Jackson BS, eds. Principles of ostomy care. St. Louis: CV Mosby, 1982: 534.
13. Yards PS, Howe J. Response to illness and disability. In: Howe J, ed. Nursing care of adolescents. New York: McGraw-Hill, 1980: 86.

Index

Note: Page numbers followed by "f" refer to figures; those followed by "t" refer to tables.